TABLE OF CONTENTS

Visit thePoint http://thepoint.lww.com/QL2011 for exclusive access to:

- Apothecary/Metric Conversions
- Pounds/Kilograms Conversion
- Temperature Conversion
- Pharmaceutical Manufacturers and Distributors
- Multivitamin Products

Refer to the inside front cover of this book for your online access code.

ABOUT THE AUTHORS

Leonard L. Lance, RPh, BSPharm

Leonard L. (Bud) Lance has been directly involved in the pharmaceutical industry since receiving his bachelor's degree in pharmacy from Ohio Northern University in 1970. Upon graduation from ONU, Mr Lance spent four years as a Navy pharmacist in various military assignments and was instrumental in the development and operation of the first whole hospital I.V. admixture program in a military (Portsmouth Naval Hospital) facility.

After completing his military service, he entered the retail pharmacy field and has managed both an independent and a home I.V. franchise pharmacy operation. Since the late 1970s, Mr Lance has focused much of his interest on using computers to improve pharmacy service. The independent pharmacy he worked for was one of the first retail pharmacies in the State of Ohio to computerize (1977).

His love for computers and pharmacy led him to Lexi-Comp, Inc. in 1988. He was the first pharmacist at Lexi-Comp and helped develop Lexi-Comp's first drug database in 1989 and was involved in the editing and publishing of Lexi-Comp's first *Drug Information Handbook* in 1990.

As a result of his strong publishing interest, he serves in the capacity of pharmacy editor and technical advisor. Mr Lance has assisted over 300 major hospitals in producing their own formulary (pharmacy) publications through Lexi-Comp's custom publishing service. Presently, Mr Lance works as a Database Specialist in the Dosage Forms Database in the Medical Sciences Division at Lexi-Comp.

Mr Lance served as president (1984) of the Summit Pharmaceutical Association (SPA). He is a member of the Ohio Pharmacists Association (OPA), the American Pharmaceutical Association (APhA), and the American Society of Health-System Pharmacists (ASHP).

Charles F. Lacy, RPh, MS, PharmD, FCSHP

Dr Lacy is the co-founder and the current Vice President of Executive Affairs at the University of Southern Nevada. In this capacity, Dr Lacy fosters, develops, and maintains new opportunities for the university in the areas of business partnerships, foundational development, external programs development, international affiliations, and outreach project design and coordination. Dr Lacy is Professor of Pharmacy Practice in the Nevada College of Pharmacy and Guest Professor in the MBA program and the College of Nursing.

Prior to his promotion to Executive Affairs, Dr Lacy was Vice President for Information Technologies at the University and the Facilitative Officer for Clinical Programs where he managed the clinical curriculum, clinical faculty activities, student experiential programs, pharmacy residency programs, and the college continuing education programs.

Additionally, he spent 20 years at Cedars-Sinai Medical Center, where he was the Department of Pharmacy's Clinical Coordinator. With over 20 years of clinical experience at one of the nation's largest teaching hospitals, he developed a reputation as an acknowledged expert in drug information, pharmacotherapy, and critical care drug interventions.

Dr Lacy received his doctorate from the University of Southern California School of Pharmacy. Presently, Dr Lacy holds teaching affiliations with the Nevada College of Pharmacy, the University of Southern Nevada, Showa University in Tokyo, Japan, the University of Alberta at Edmonton School of Pharmacy and Health Sciences, KLE University in Bangalore, India, and the Hokkaido College of Pharmacy in Sapporo, Japan. He also received his master's degree from Phillips Graduate Institute in Psychology with an emphasis in Marriage and Family Therapy.

Dr Lacy is an active member of numerous professional associations including the American Society of Health-System Pharmacists (ASHP), the American College of Clinical Pharmacy (ACCP), the American Association of Colleges of Pharmacy (AACP), the American Society of Consultant Pharmacists (ASCP), the American Association of Colleges of Pharmacy (AACP), American Pharmaceutical Association (APhA), the Federation of International Pharmacy (FIP), the Japanese Pharmaceutical Association (JPA), the Nevada Pharmacy Alliance (NPA), and the California Society of Hospital Pharmacists (CSHP), through which he has chaired many committees and subcommittees. He is also an active member of the California Association of Marriage and Family Therapists (CAMFT), American Association of Marriage and Family Therapists (AAMFT), the North American Congress of Clinical Toxicology (NACCT) and the European Congress of Clinical Toxicology (ECCT).

Morton P. Goldman, RPh, PharmD, BCPS, FCCP

Dr Goldman received his bachelor's degree in pharmacy from the University of Pittsburgh, College of Pharmacy and his Doctor of Pharmacy degree from the University of Cincinnati, Division of Graduate Studies and Research. He completed his concurrent 2-year hospital pharmacy residency at the VA Medical Center in Cincinnati. Dr Goldman is presently the Director of Pharmacotherapy Services for the Department of Pharmacy at the Cleveland Clinic Foundation (CCF) after having spent over 4 years at CCF as an Infectious Disease pharmacist and 10 years as Clinical Manager/Assistant Director. He holds faculty appointments from The University of Toledo and Ohio Northern University, Colleges of Pharmacy and Case Western Reserve University, College of Medicine and is the Pharmacology Curriculum Director for the Cleveland Clinic Lerner College of Medicine. Dr Goldman is a Board-Certified Pharmacotherapy Specialist (BCPS) with added qualifications in infectious diseases.

In his capacity as Director of Pharmacotherapy Services at CCF, Dr Goldman remains actively involved in patient care and clinical research with the Department of Infectious Disease, as well as the continuing education of the medical and pharmacy staff. He is an editor of CCF's *Guidelines for Antibiotic Use* and participates in their annual Antimicrobial Review retreat. He is a member of the Pharmacy and Therapeutics Committee and many of its subcommittees. Dr Goldman has authored numerous journal articles and lectures locally and nationally on infectious diseases topics and current drug therapies.

Dr Goldman is an active member of the Ohio College of Clinical Pharmacy, the Society of Infectious Disease Pharmacists, the American College of Clinical Pharmacy (and is a Fellow of the College), and the American Society of Health-Systems Pharmacists.

Lora L. Armstrong, RPh, PharmD, BCPS

Dr Armstrong received her bachelor's degree in pharmacy from Ferris State University and her Doctor of Pharmacy degree from Midwestern University. Dr Armstrong is a Board-Certified Pharmacotherapy Specialist (BCPS).

In her current position, Dr Armstrong serves as Vice President of Clinical Affairs with responsibility for the National Pharmacy & Therapeutics Committee process, Clinical Program Oversight process, and Pharmaceutical Pipeline Services at CVS Caremark. Prior to joining Caremark, Inc, Dr Armstrong served as the Director of Drug Information Services at the University of Chicago Hospitals. She obtained experience in a variety of clinical settings including critical care, hematology, oncology, infectious diseases, and clinical pharmacokinetics. Dr Armstrong played an active role in the education and training of medical, pharmacy, and nursing staff. She coordinated the Drug Information Center, the medical center's Adverse Drug Reaction Monitoring Program, and the continuing Education Program for pharmacists. She also maintained the hospital's strict formulary program and was the editor of the University of Chicago Hospitals' *Formulary of Accepted Drugs* and the drug information center's monthly newsletter *Topics in Drug Therapy*.

Dr Armstrong is an active member of the Academy of Managed Care Pharmacy (AMCP), the American Society of Health-Systems Pharmacists (ASHP), the American Pharmaceutical Association (APhA), the American College of Clinical Pharmacy (ACCP), and the Pharmacy & Therapeutics Society (P & T Society). Dr Armstrong wrote the chapter entitled "Drugs and Hormones Used in Endocrinology" in the 4th edition of the textbook *Endocrinology*. She is an Adjunct Clinical Instructor of Pharmacy Practice at Midwestern University. Dr Armstrong currently serves on the Drug Information Advisory Board for the American Pharmaceutical Association Scientific Review Panel for Evaluations of Drug Interactions (EDI).

EDITORIAL ADVISORY PANEL

Eve Echt, MD
Medical Staff
Department of Radiology
Akron General Medical Center
Akron, Ohio

Michael S. Edwards, PharmD, MBA, BCOP
Chief, Oncology Pharmacy
Director, Oncology Pharmacy Residency Program
Walter Reed Army Medical Center
Washington, DC

Vicki L. Ellingrod, PharmD, BCPP
Associate Professor
University of Iowa
Iowa City, Iowa

Kelley K. Engle, BSPharm
Medical Science Pharmacist
Lexi-Comp, Inc
Hudson, Ohio

Erin Fabian, PharmD, RPh
Pharmacotherapy Specialist
Lexi-Comp, Inc
Hudson, Ohio

Elizabeth Farrington, PharmD, FCCP, FCCM, BCPS
Clinical Specialist, Pediatrics
Department of Pharmacy
University of North Carolina Hospitals and Clinics
Chapel Hill, North Carolina

Margaret A. Fitzgerald, MS, APRN, BC, NP-C, FAANP
President
Fitzgerald Health Education Associates, Inc.
North Andover, Massachusetts
Family Nurse Practitioner
Greater Lawrence Family Health Center
Lawrence, Massachusetts

Lawrence A. Frazee, PharmD, BCPS
Pharmacotherapy Specialist in Internal Medicine
Akron General Medical Center
Akron, Ohio

Matthew A. Fuller, PharmD, BCPS, BCPP, FASHP
Clinical Pharmacy Specialist, Psychiatry
Cleveland Department of
Veterans Affairs Medical Center
Brecksville, Ohio
Associate Clinical Professor of Psychiatry
Clinical Instructor of Psychology
Case Western Reserve University
Cleveland, Ohio
Adjunct Associate Professor of Clinical Pharmacy
University of Toledo
Toledo, Ohio

Jennifer L. Gardner, PharmD
Neonatal Clinical Pharmacy Specialist
Texas Children's Hospital
Houston, Texas

Meredith D. Girard, MD, FACP
Medical Staff
Department of Internal Medicine
Summa Health Systems
Akron, Ohio
Assistant Professor Internal Medicine
Northeast Ohio Universities
College of Medicine (NEOUCOM)
Rootstown, Ohio

Morton P. Goldman, RPh, PharmD, BCPS, FCCP
Director of Pharmacotherapy Services
The Cleveland Clinic Foundation
Cleveland, Ohio

Julie A. Golembiewski, PharmD
Clinical Associate Professor
Colleges of Pharmacy and Medicine
Clinical Pharmacist, Anesthesia/Pain
University of Illinois
Chicago, Illinois

Jeffrey P. Gonzales, PharmD, BCPS
Critical Care Clinical Pharmacy Specialist
University of Maryland Medical Center
Baltimore, Maryland

Roland Grad, MDCM, MSc, CCFP, FCFP
Department of Family Medicine
McGill University
Montreal, Quebec, Canada

Larry D. Gray, PhD, ABMM
Director, Clinical Microbiology
TriHealth Laboratories
Bethesda and Good Samaritan Hospitals
Cincinnati, Ohio

Tracy Hagemann, PharmD
Associate Professor
College of Pharmacy
The University of Oklahoma
Oklahoma City, Oklahoma

Martin D. Higbee, PharmD
Associate Professor
Department of Pharmacy Practice and Science
The University of Arizona
Tucson, Arizona

Jane Hurlburt Hodding, PharmD
Executive Director, Inpatient Pharmacy Services and Clinical Nutrition Services
Long Beach Memorial Medical Center
and Miller Children's Hospital
Long Beach, California

Mark T. Holdsworth, PharmD, BCOP
Associate Professor of Pharmacy & Pediatrics
Pharmacy Practice Area Head
College of Pharmacy
The University of New Mexico
Albuquerque, New Mexico

Edward Horn, PharmD, BCPS
Clinical Specialist, Transplant Surgery
Allegheny General Hospital
Pittsburgh, Pennsylvania

Geralyn M. Meny, MD
Medical Director
American Red Cross, Penn-Jersey Region
Philadelphia, Pennsylvania

Julie Miller, PharmD
Pharmacy Clinical Specialist, Cardiology
Columbus Children's Hospital
Columbus, Ohio

Leah Millstein, MD
Assistant Professor
Division of General Internal Medicine
University of Maryland School of Medicine
Baltimore, Maryland

Kevin M. Mulieri, BS, PharmD
Pediatric Hematology/Oncology Clinical Specialist
Penn State Milton S. Hershey Medical Center
Instructor of Pharmacology
Penn State College of Medicine
Hershey, Pennsylvania

Tom Palma, MS, RPh
Medical Science Pharmacist
Lexi-Comp, Inc
Hudson, Ohio

Susie H. Park, PharmD, BCPP
Assistant Professor of Clinical Pharmacy
University of Southern Califormia
Los Angeles, California

Alpa Patel, PharmD
Antimicrobial Clinical Pharmacist
University of Louisville Hospital
Louisville, Kentucky

Gayle Pearson, BSPharm, MSA
Drug Information Pharmacist
Peter Lougheed Centre,
Alberta Health Services
Calgary, Alberta, Canada

James A. Ponto, MS, RPh, BCNP
Chief Nuclear Pharmacist
Department of Radiology
University of Iowa, Hospitals and Clinics
Professor of Clinical Pharmacy
Department of Pharmacy Practice and Science
University of Iowa College of Pharmacy
Iowa City, Iowa

James Reissig, PharmD
Assistant Director, Clinical Services
Akron General Medical Center
Akron, Ohio

A.J. (Fred) Remillard, PharmD
Assistant Dean, Research and Graduate Affairs
College of Pharmacy and Nutrition
University of Saskatchewan
Saskatoon, Saskatchewan, Canada

Curtis M. Rimmermann, MD, MBA, FACC
Gus P. Karos Chair,
Clinical Cardiovascular Medicine
Department of Cardiovascular Medicine
Cleveland Clinic Foundation
Cleveland, Ohio

P. David Rogers, PharmD, PhD, FCCP
Professor and Associate Dean
for Translational Research
University of Tennessee College of Pharmacy
Memphis, Tennessee

Martha Sajatovic, MD
Professor of Psychiatry
Case Western Reserve University
Cleveland, Ohio
Department of Psychiatry
University Hospitals of Cleveland
Cleveland, Ohio

Jennifer K. Sekeres, PharmD, BCPS
Infectious Diseases Clinical Specialist
The Cleveland Clinic Foundation
Cleveland, Ohio

Todd P. Semla, MS, PharmD, BCPS, FCCP, AGSF
Clinical Pharmacy Specialist
Department of Veterans Affairs
Pharmacy Benefits Management Services
Associate Professor, Clinical
Department of Medicine and
Psychiatry and Behavioral Health
Feinberg School of Medicine
Northwestern University
Chicago, Illinois

Joseph Snoke, RPh, BCPS
Manager
Core Pharmacology Group
Lexi-Comp, Inc
Hudson, Ohio

Joni Lombardi Stahura, BS, PharmD, RPh
Pharmacotherapy Specialist
Lexi-Comp, Inc
Hudson, Ohio

Stephen Marc Stout, PharmD, MS, BCPS
Pharmacotherapy Specialist
Lexi-Comp, Inc
Hudson, Ohio

Dan Streetman, PharmD, RPh
Pharmacotherapy Specialist
Lexi-Comp, Inc
Hudson, Ohio

Darcie-Ann Streetman, PharmD, RPh
Clinical Pharmacist
University of Michigan Health System
Ann Arbor, Michigan

Carol K. Taketomo, PharmD
Director of Pharmacy and Nutrition Services
Children's Hospital Los Angeles
Los Angeles, California

Mary Temple-Cooper, PharmD
Pediatric Clinical Research Specialist
Hillcrest Hospital
Mayfield Heights, Ohio

Elizabeth A. Tomsik, PharmD, BCPS
Manager
Adverse Drug Reactions Group
Lexi-Comp, Inc
Hudson, Ohio

PREFACE

Working with clinical pharmacists, hospital pharmacy and therapeutics committees, and hospital drug information centers, the editors of this handbook have directly assisted in the development and production of hospital-specific formulary documentation for several hundred major U.S. and International medical institutions. The resultant documentation provides relevant detail concerning use of medications within the hospital and other clinical settings. Current information on medications has been extracted from pertinent sources, reviewed, coalesced, and cross-referenced by the editors to create this *Quick Look Drug Book*.

Designed to meet the unique needs of medical transcription, this handbook gives the user quick access to data on over 1800 medications with cross-referencing to 7457 U.S. and Canadian brand or trade names. Selection of the included medications was based on the analysis of those medications offered in a wide range of hospital formularies. The concise standardized format for data used in this handbook was developed to ensure a consistent presentation of information for all medications.

All generic drug names and synonyms appear in lower case, whereas brand or trade names appear in upper/lower case with the proper trademark information. These three items appear as individual entries in the alphabetical listing of drugs and, thus, there is no requirement for an alphabetical index of drugs names.

Chemotherapy regimens along with an index are provided in the section directly following the alphabetical listing of drugs. The mailing and web site addresses for pharmaceutical manufacturers and drug distributors can be accessed online using the code located on the inside front cover of this book.

The Indication/Therapeutic Category Index is an expedient mechanism for locating the medication of choice along with its classification. This index will help the user, with knowledge of the disease state, to identify medications which are most commonly used in treatment. All disease states are cross-referenced to a varying number of medications with the most frequently used medication(s) noted.

— L.L. Lance

USE OF THE HANDBOOK

The *Quick Look Drug Book* is organized into a drug information section, an appendix, and an indication/therapeutic category index.

The drug information section of the handbook, wherein all drugs are listed alphabetically, details information pertinent to each drug. Extensive cross-referencing is provided by brand name and synonyms.

Drug information is presented in a consistent format and for quick reference will provide the following:

Generic Name	U.S. Adopted Name (USAN) or International Nonproprietary Name (INN) If a drug product is only available in Canada, a ***(Canada only)*** will be attached to that product and will appear with every occurrence of that drug throughout the book
Pronunciation Guide	Subjective aid for pronouncing drug names
Sound-Alike/Look-Alike Issues	Lists drugs with similar sounding names or names that look alike
Synonyms	Official names and some slang
Tall-Man	"Tall-Man" lettering revisions recommended by the FDA
U.S./Canadian Brand Names	Common trade names used in the United States and Canada
Therapeutic Category	Lexi-Comp's own system of logical medication classification
Controlled Substance	Drug Enforcement Agency (DEA) classification for federally scheduled controlled substances
Use	Information pertaining to appropriate use of the drug
Dosage Summary	The range of dosing typically used during therapy in children and adults based upon route of administration. The information included is useful for confirming the dose is within the range but should not be used for prescribing purposes. Medications with a variety of indication specific doses that cannot be encompassed by a range will not have a dose.
Product Availability	Provides availability information on products that have been approved by the FDA, but not yet available for use. Estimates for when a product may be available are included, when this information is known. May also provide any unique or critical drug availability issues.
Dosage Forms	Information with regard to form, strength, and availability of the drug in the United States.
Dosage Forms - Canada	Information with regard to form, strength, and availability of products that are uniquely available in Canada, but currently not available in the United States.

Appendix

The appendix offers a compilation of tables, guidelines, and conversion information that can often be helpful when considering patient care.

Indication/Therapeutic Category Index

This index provides a listing of accepted drugs for various disease states thus focusing attention on selection of medications most frequently prescribed in relation to a clinical diagnosis. Diseases may have other nonofficial drugs for their treatment and this indication/therapeutic category index should not be used by itself to determine the appropriateness of a particular therapy. The listed indications may encompass varying degrees of severity and, since certain medications may not be appropriate for a given degree of severity, it should not be assumed that the agents listed for specific indications are interchangeable. Also included as a valuable reference is each medication's therapeutic category.

FDA NAME DIFFERENTIATION PROJECT: THE USE OF TALL-MAN LETTERS

Confusion between similar drug names is an important cause of medication errors. For years, The Institute For Safe Medication Practices (ISMP), has urged generic manufacturers to use a combination of large and small letters as well as bolding (ie, chlorpro**MAZINE** and chlorpro**PAMIDE**) to help distinguish drugs with look-alike names, especially when they share similar strengths. Recently the FDA's Division of Generic Drugs began to issue recommendation letters to manufacturers suggesting this novel way to label their products to help reduce this drug name confusion. Although this project has had marginal success, the method has successfully eliminated problems with products such as diphenhydr**AMINE** and dimenhy**DRINATE**. Hospitals should also follow suit by making similar changes in their own labels, preprinted order forms, computer screens and printouts, and drug storage location labels.

In the *Quick Look Drug Book*, the "Tall-Man" lettering revisions for the drugs suggested by the FDA or recommended by ISMP will be listed in a field called **Tall-Man**.

The following is a list of generic product names and recommended revisions.

Drug Product	Recommended Revision
acetazolamide	aceta**ZOLAMIDE**
acetohexamide	aceto**HEXAMIDE**
alprazolam	**ALPRAZ**olam
amiloride	a**MIL**oride
amlodipine	am**LODIP**ine
azacitidine	aza**CITID**ine
azathioprine	aza**THIO**prine
bupropion	bu**PROP**ion
buspirone	bus**PIR**one
carbamazepine	car**BAM**azepine
carboplatin	**CARBO**platin
cefazolin	ce**FAZ**olin
ceftriaxone	cef**TRIAX**one
chlordiazepoxide	chlordiaze**POXIDE**
chlorpromazine	chlorpro**MAZINE**
chlorpropamide	chlorpro**PAMIDE**
cisplatin	**CIS**platin
clomiphene	clomi**PHENE**
clomipramine	clomi**PRAMINE**
clonazepam	clonaze**PAM**
clonidine	clo**NID**ine
cycloserine	cyclo**SERINE**
cyclosporine	cyclo**SPORINE**
dactinomycin	**DACTIN**omycin
daptomycin	**DAPTO**mycin
daunorubicin	**DAUNO**rubicin
dimenhydrinate	dimenhy**DRINATE**
diphenhydramine	diphenhydr**AMINE**
dobutamine	**DOBUT**amine
dopamine	**DOP**amine
doxorubicin	**DOXO**rubicin
duloxetine	**DUL**oxetine
ephedrine	e**PHED**rine
epinephrine	**EPINEPH**rine
fentanyl	fenta**NYL**

Drug Product	Recommended Revision
fluoxetine	**FLU**oxetine
glipizide	glipi**ZIDE**
glyburide	gly**BURIDE**
guaifenesin	guai**FEN**esin
guanfacine	guan**FACINE**
hydralazine	hydr**ALAZINE**
hydrocodone	**HYDRO**codone
hydromorphone	**HYDRO**morphone
hydroxyzine	hydr**OXY**zine
idarubicin	**IDA**rubicin
infliximab	in**FLIX**imab
lamivudine	lami**VUD**ine
lamotrigine	lamo**TRI**gine
lorazepam	**LOR**azepam
medroxyprogesterone	medroxy**PROGESTER**one
metformin	met**FORMIN**
methylprednisolone	methyl**PREDNIS**olone
methyltestosterone	methyl**TESTOSTER**one
metronidazole	metro**NIDAZOLE**
nicardipine	ni**CAR**dipine
nifedipine	**NIFE**dipine
nimodipine	ni**MOD**ipine
olanzapine	**OLANZ**apine
oxcarbazepine	**OX**carbazepine
oxycodone	oxy**CODONE**
paroxetine	**PAR**oxetine
pentobarbital	**PENT**obarbital
phenobarbital	**PHEN**obarbital
prednisolone	predniso**LONE**
prednisone	predni**SONE**
quetiapine	**QUE**tiapine
quinidine	qui**NID**ine
quinine	qui**NINE**
rituximab	ri**TUX**imab
sitagliptin	sita**GLIP**tin
sufentanil	**SUF**entanil
sulfadiazine	sulf**ADIAZINE**
sulfisoxazole	sulfi**SOXAZOLE**
sumatriptan	**SUMA**triptan
tiagabine	tia**GAB**ine
tizanidine	ti**ZAN**idine
tolazamide	**TOLAZ**amide
tolbutamide	**TOLBUT**amide
tramadol	tra**MAD**ol
trazodone	tra**ZOD**one
valacyclovir	val**ACY**clovir
valganciclovir	val**GANCI**clovir

Drug Product	Recommended Revision
vinblastine	vin**BLAS**tine
vincristine	vin**CRIS**tine

Institute for Safe Medication Practices. "New Tall-Man Lettering Will Reduce Mix-Ups Due to Generic Drug Name Confusion," *ISMP Medication Safety Alert*, September 19, 2001. Available at: http://www.ismp.org.

Institute for Safe Medication Practices. "Prescription Mapping, Can Improve Efficiency While Minimizing Errors With Look-Alike Products," *ISMP Medication Safety Alert*, October 6, 1999. Available at: http://www.ismp.org.

Institute for Safe Medication Practices. "Use of Tall-Man Letters Is Gaining Wide Acceptance," *ISMP Medication Safety Alert*, July 31, 2008. Available at: http://www.ismp.org.

U.S. Pharmacopeia, "USP Quality Review: Use Caution-Avoid Confusion," March 2001, No. 76. Available at: http://www.usp.org.

PREVENTING PRESCRIBING ERRORS

Prescribing errors account for the majority of reported medication errors and have prompted healthcare professionals to focus on the development of steps to make the prescribing process safer. Prescription legibility has been attributed to a portion of these errors and legislation has been enacted in several states to address prescription legibility. However, eliminating handwritten prescriptions and ordering medications through the use of technology [eg, computerized prescriber order entry (CPOE)] has been the primary recommendation. Whether a prescription is electronic, typed, or hand-printed, additional safe practices should be considered for implementation to maximize the safety of the prescribing process. Listed below are suggestions for safer prescribing:

- Ensure correct patient by using at least 2 patient identifiers on the prescription (eg, full name, birth date, or address). Review prescription with the patient or patient's caregiver.
- If pediatric patient, document patient's birth date or age and most recent weight. If geriatric patient, document patient's birth date or age.
- Prevent drug name confusion:
  - Use TALLman lettering (eg, buPROPion, busPIRone, predniSONE, prednisoLONE). For more information see: http://www.fda.gov/Drugs/DrugSafety/MedicationErrors/ucm164587.htm.
  - Avoid abbreviated drug names (eg, MSO_4, $MgSO_4$, MS, HCT, 6MP, MTX), as they may be misinterpreted and cause error.
  - Avoid investigational names for drugs with FDA approval (eg, FK-506, CBDCA).
  - Avoid chemical names such as 6-mercaptopurine or 6-thioguanine, as sixfold overdoses have been given when these were not recognized as chemical names. The proper names of these drugs are mercaptopurine or thioguanine.
  - Use care when prescribing drugs that look or sound similar (eg, look- alike, sound-alike drugs). Common examples include: Celebrex® vs Celexa®, hydroxyzine vs hydralazine, Zyprexa® vs Zyrtec®.
- Avoid dangerous, error-prone abbreviations (eg, regardless of letter-case: U, IU, QD, QOD, µg, cc, @). Do not use apothecary system or symbols. Additionally, text messaging abbreviations (eg, "2Day") should never be used.
  - For more information see: http://www.ismp.org/Tools/errorproneabbreviations.pdf
- Always use a leading zero for numbers less than 1 (0.5 mg is correct and .5 mg is **incorrect**) and never use a trailing zero for whole numbers (2 mg is correct and 2.0 mg is **incorrect**).
- Always use a space between a number and its units as it is easier to read. There should be no periods after the abbreviations mg or mL (10 mg is correct and 10mg is **incorrect**).
- For doses that are greater than 1,000 dosing units, use properly placed commas to prevent 10-fold errors (100,000 units is correct and 100000 units is **incorrect**).
- Do not prescribe drug dosage by the type of container in which the drug is available (eg, do not prescribe "1 amp", "2 vials", etc).
- Do not write vague or ambiguous orders which have the potential for misinterpretation by other healthcare providers. Examples of vague orders to avoid: "resume pre-op medications," "give drug per protocol," or "continue home medications."
- Review each prescription with patient (or patient's caregiver) including the medication name, indication, and directions for use.
- Take extra precautions when prescribing *high alert drugs* (drugs that can cause significant patient harm when prescribed in error). Common examples of these drugs include: Anticoagulants, chemotherapy, insulins, opiates, and sedatives.
  - For more information see: http://www.ismp.org/Tools/highalertmedications.pdf

To Err is Human: Building a Safer Health System, Kohn LT, Corrigan JM, and Donaldson MS, eds, Washington, D.C.: National Academy Press, 2000.

A Complete Outpatient Prescription[1]

A complete outpatient prescription can prevent the prescriber, the pharmacist, and/or the patient from making a mistake and can eliminate the need for further clarification. The complete outpatient prescription should contain:

- Patient's full name
- Medication indication
- Allergies
- Prescriber name and telephone or pager number
- For pediatric patients: Their birth date or age and current weight
- For geriatric patients: Their birth date or age
- Drug name, dosage form and strength
- For pediatric patients: Intended daily weight-based dose so that calculations can be checked by the pharmacist (ie, mg/kg/day or units/kg/day)
- Number or amount to be dispensed
- Complete instructions for the patient or caregiver, including the purpose of the medication, directions for use (including dose), dosing frequency, route of administration, duration of therapy, and number of refills.
- Dose should be expressed in convenient units of measure.
- When there are recognized contraindications for a prescribed drug, the prescriber should indicate knowledge of this fact to the pharmacist (ie, when prescribing a potassium salt for a patient receiving an ACE inhibitor, the prescriber should write "K serum leveling being monitored").

Upon dispensing of the final product, the pharmacist should ensure that the patient or caregiver can effectively demonstrate the appropriate administration technique. An appropriate measuring device should be provided or recommended. Household teaspoons and tablespoons should not be used to measure liquid medications due to their variability and inaccuracies in measurement; oral medication syringes are recommended.

For additional information see: http://www.ppag.org/attachments/files/111/Guidelines_Peds.pdf

[1]Levine SR, Cohen MR, Blanchard NR, et al, "Guidelines for Preventing Medication Errors in Pediatrics," *J Pediatr Pharmacol Ther*, 2001, 6:426-42.

ALPHABETICAL LISTING OF DRUGS

A_1-PI *see* alpha$_1$-proteinase inhibitor *on page 54*
α_1-PI *see* alpha$_1$-proteinase inhibitor *on page 54*
A-25 [US-OTC] *see* vitamin A *on page 987*
A200® Lice [US-OTC] *see* permethrin *on page 744*
A-200® Lice Treatment Kit [US-OTC] *see* pyrethrins and piperonyl butoxide *on page 816*
A-200® Maximum Strength [US-OTC] *see* pyrethrins and piperonyl butoxide *on page 816*
A and D® Original [US-OTC] *see* vitamin A and vitamin D *on page 988*

abacavir (a BAK a veer)

Synonyms abacavir sulfate; ABC

U.S./Canadian Brand Names Ziagen® [US/Can]

Therapeutic Category Antiretroviral Agent, Nucleoside Reverse Transcriptase Inhibitor (NRTI)

Use Treatment of HIV infections in combination with other antiretroviral agents

Dosage Summary

Oral:

Children <3 months: Dosage not established

Children 3 months to 16 years: 8 mg/kg twice daily in combination with other antiretroviral agents (maximum: 300 mg twice daily)

Adults: 600 mg/day in 1-2 divided doses in combination with other antiretroviral agents (maximum: 600 mg/day)

Dosage Forms

Solution, oral:

Ziagen®: 20 mg/mL (240 mL)

Tablet, oral:

Ziagen®: 300 mg

abacavir and lamivudine (a BAK a veer & la MI vyoo deen)

Synonyms abacavir sulfate and lamivudine; lamivudine and abacavir

U.S./Canadian Brand Names Epzicom® [US]; Kivexa™ [Can]

Therapeutic Category Antiretroviral Agent, Nucleoside Reverse Transcriptase Inhibitor (NRTI)

Use Treatment of HIV infections in combination with other antiretroviral agents

Dosage Summary

Oral:

Children: Dosage not established

Adults: One tablet (abacavir 600 mg and lamivudine 300 mg) once daily

Dosage Forms

Tablet:

Epzicom®: Abacavir 600 mg and lamivudine 300 mg

abacavir, lamivudine, and zidovudine
(a BAK a veer, la MI vyoo deen, & zye DOE vyoo deen)

Synonyms 3TC, abacavir, and zidovudine; azidothymidine, abacavir, and lamivudine; AZT, abacavir, and lamivudine; compound S, abacavir, and lamivudine; lamivudine, abacavir, and zidovudine; ZDV, abacavir, and lamivudine; zidovudine, abacavir, and lamivudine

U.S./Canadian Brand Names Trizivir® [US/Can]

Therapeutic Category Antiretroviral Agent, Nucleoside Reverse Transcriptase Inhibitor (NRTI)

Use Treatment of HIV infection (either alone or in combination with other antiretroviral agents) in patients whose regimen would otherwise contain the components of Trizivir®

Dosage Summary Note: Not recommended for patients <40 kg

Oral:

Children: Dosage not established

Adolescents ≥40 kg: 1 tablet twice daily

Adults: 1 tablet twice daily

Dosage Forms

Tablet:

Trizivir®: Abacavir 300 mg, lamivudine 150 mg, and zidovudine 300 mg

abacavir sulfate *see* abacavir *on page 18*
abacavir sulfate and lamivudine *see* abacavir and lamivudine *on page 18*

abarelix *(Discontinued)*

abatacept (ab a TA sept)

Sound-Alike/Look-Alike Issues
Orencia® may be confused with Oracea™

Synonyms BMS-188667; CTLA-4Ig

U.S./Canadian Brand Names Orencia® [US/Can]

Therapeutic Category Antirheumatic, Disease Modifying

Use

Treatment of moderately- to severely-active adult rheumatoid arthritis (RA); may be used as monotherapy or in combination with other DMARDs

Treatment of moderately- to severely-active juvenile idiopathic arthritis (JIA); may be used as monotherapy or in combination with methotrexate

Note: Abatacept should **not** be used in combination with anakinra or TNF-blocking agents

Dosage Summary

I.V.:

Children <6 years: Dosage not established

Children ≥6 years and <75 kg: 10 mg/kg, repeat dose at 2 and 4 weeks after initial infusion, and every 4 weeks thereafter

Children ≥6 years and >75 kg: **Note:** Dosage is according to body weight. Repeat dose at 2 weeks and 4 weeks after initial dose and every 4 weeks thereafter:
75-100 kg: 750 mg
>100 kg: 1000 mg

Adults: **Note:** Dosage is according to body weight. Repeat dose at 2 weeks and 4 weeks after initial dose and every 4 weeks thereafter:
<60 kg: 500 mg
60-100 kg: 750 mg
>100 kg: 1000 mg

Elderly: Use caution

Dosage Forms

Injection, powder for reconstitution [preservative free]:
Orencia®: 250 mg

Abbokinase® *(Discontinued)*

abbott-43818 *see* leuprolide *on page 554*

ABC *see* abacavir *on page 18*

ABCD *see* amphotericin B cholesteryl sulfate complex *on page 74*

abciximab (ab SIK si mab)

Synonyms 7E3; C7E3

U.S./Canadian Brand Names Reopro® [US/Can]

Therapeutic Category Platelet Aggregation Inhibitor

Use Prevention of cardiac ischemic complications in patients undergoing percutaneous coronary intervention (PCI); prevention of cardiac ischemic complications in patients with unstable angina not responding to conventional therapy when PCI is scheduled within 24 hours

Note: Intended for use with aspirin and heparin, at a minimum.

Dosage Summary

I.V.:

Children: Dosage not established

Adults: Bolus: 0.25 mg/kg; Infusion: 0.125 mcg/kg/minute for 12 hours (maximum: 10 mcg/minute)

Dosage Forms

Injection, solution [preservative free]:
Reopro®: 2 mg/mL (5 mL)

Abelcet® [US/Can] *see* amphotericin B lipid complex *on page 75*

Abenol® [Can] *see* acetaminophen *on page 21*

ABI-007 *see* paclitaxel (protein bound) *on page 720*

Abilify® [US/Can] *see* aripiprazole *on page 94*

Abilify Discmelt® [US] *see* aripiprazole *on page 94*

Ablavar™ [US] *see* gadofosveset *on page 434*
ABLC *see* amphotericin B lipid complex *on page 75*

abobotulinumtoxinA (aye bo BOT yoo lin num TOKS in aye)

Synonyms botulinum toxin type A
U.S./Canadian Brand Names Dysport™ [US]
Therapeutic Category Neuromuscular Blocker Agent, Toxin
Use Treatment of cervical dystonia in both toxin-naive and previously treated patients; temporary improvement in the appearance of moderate-severe glabellar lines associated with procerus and corrugator muscle activity
Dosage Summary
I.M.:
Cervical dystonia:
Children: Dosage not established
Adults: Initial: 500 units divided among the affected muscles; subsequent doses: May increase or decrease by 250 units (dosage range: 250-1000 units)
Reduction of glabellar lines:
Children: Dosage not established
Adults <65 years: 10 units (0.05 mL or 0.08 mL) injected into each of 5 sites: 2 in each corrugator muscle and 1 in the procerus muscle (total dose: 50 units)
Adults ≥65 years: Use not indicated
Dosage Forms
Injection, powder for reconstitution:
Dysport™: 500 units

A/B Otic [US] *see* antipyrine and benzocaine *on page 83*
Abraxane® [US] *see* paclitaxel (protein bound) *on page 720*
Abraxane® For Injectable Suspension [Can] *see* paclitaxel *on page 719*
Abreva® [US-OTC] *see* docosanol *on page 321*
absorbable cotton *see* cellulose, oxidized regenerated *on page 195*
absorbable gelatin sponge *see* gelatin (absorbable) *on page 439*
Absorbine® Antifungal *(Discontinued)* *see* tolnaftate *on page 940*
Absorbine® Jock Itch *(Discontinued)* *see* tolnaftate *on page 940*
ABT-335 *see* fenofibric acid *on page 394*
ABX-EGF *see* panitumumab *on page 724*
AC 2993 *see* exenatide *on page 387*
ACAM2000™ [US] *see* smallpox vaccine *on page 880*

acamprosate (a kam PROE sate)

Synonyms acamprosate calcium; calcium acetylhomotaurinate
U.S./Canadian Brand Names Campral® [US/Can]
Therapeutic Category GABA Agonist/Glutamate Antagonist
Use Maintenance of alcohol abstinence
Dosage Summary Note: Treatment should be initiated as soon as possible following the period of alcohol withdrawal, when the patient has achieved abstinence.
Oral:
Children: Dosage not established
Adults: 666 mg 3 times/day (maximum: 1998 mg/day)
Dosage Forms
Tablet, delayed release, enteric coated, oral:
Campral®: 333 mg

acamprosate calcium *see* acamprosate *on page 20*
Acanya™ [US] *see* clindamycin and benzoyl peroxide *on page 233*

acarbose (AY car bose)

Sound-Alike/Look-Alike Issues
Precose® may be confused with PreCare®
U.S./Canadian Brand Names Glucobay™ [Can]; Precose® [US]

Therapeutic Category Antidiabetic Agent, Oral

Use Adjunct to diet and exercise to lower blood glucose in patients with type 2 diabetes mellitus (noninsulin-dependent, NIDDM)

Dosage Summary

Oral:

Children: Dosage not established

Adults: Initial: 25 mg 1-3 times/day with meals; Maintenance: 75-300 mg/day in 3 divided doses with meals (maximum: ≤60 kg: 150 mg/day; >60 kg: 300 mg/day); **Note:** Titration is recommended

Dosage Forms

Tablet, oral: 25 mg, 50 mg, 100 mg

Precose®: 25 mg, 50 mg, 100 mg

A-Caro-25 [US-OTC] *see* beta-carotene *on page 132*

Accel-Amlodipine [Can] *see* amlodipine *on page 68*

Accolate® [US/Can] *see* zafirlukast *on page 996*

AccuHist® Pediatric *(Discontinued)* *see* brompheniramine and pseudoephedrine *on page 148*

AccuNeb® [US] *see* albuterol *on page 43*

Accupril® [US/Can] *see* quinapril *on page 822*

Accuretic® [US/Can] *see* quinapril and hydrochlorothiazide *on page 822*

Accutane® [Can] *see* isotretinoin *on page 530*

Accutane® *(Discontinued)* *see* isotretinoin *on page 530*

Accuzyme® *(Discontinued)*

Accuzyme® SE *(Discontinued)*

ACE *see* captopril *on page 176*

acebutolol (a se BYOO toe lole)

Sound-Alike/Look-Alike Issues

Sectral® may be confused with Factrel®, Seconal®, Septra®

Synonyms acebutolol hydrochloride

U.S./Canadian Brand Names Apo-Acebutolol® [Can]; Mylan-Acebutolol [Can]; Novo-Acebutolol [Can]; Nu-Acebutolol [Can]; Rhotral [Can]; Sandoz-Acebutolol [Can]; Sectral® [US/Can]

Therapeutic Category Antiarrhythmic Agent, Class II; Beta-Adrenergic Blocker

Use Treatment of hypertension; management of ventricular arrhythmias

Dosage Summary

Oral:

Children: Dosage not established

Adults: 200-1200 mg/day in 2 divided doses (maximum: 1200 mg/day)

Elderly: 200-800 mg/day in 2 divided doses (maximum: 800 mg/day)

Dosage Forms

Capsule, oral: 200 mg, 400 mg

Sectral®: 200 mg, 400 mg

acebutolol hydrochloride *see* acebutolol *on page 21*

Aceon® [US] *see* perindopril erbumine *on page 744*

Acephen™ [US-OTC] *see* acetaminophen *on page 21*

Acerola [US-OTC] *see* ascorbic acid *on page 98*

Acetadote® [US] *see* acetylcysteine *on page 34*

Aceta-Gesic [US-OTC] *see* acetaminophen and phenyltoloxamine *on page 26*

acetaminophen (a seet a MIN oh fen)

Sound-Alike/Look-Alike Issues

Acephen™ may be confused with AcipHex®

FeverAll® may be confused with Fiberall®

Tylenol® may be confused with atenolol, timolol, Tuinal®, Tylox®

Synonyms APAP; n-acetyl-p-aminophenol; paracetamol

U.S./Canadian Brand Names Abenol® [Can]; Acephen™ [US-OTC]; APAP 500 [US-OTC]; Apo-Acetaminophen® [Can]; Aspirin Free Anacin® Extra Strength [US-OTC]; Atasol® [Can]; Cetafen® Extra [US-OTC]; Cetafen® [US-OTC]; Excedrin® Tension Headache [US-OTC]; FeverAll® [US-OTC]; Infantaire [US-OTC]; Little Fevers™ [US-OTC]; Mapap® Arthritis Pain [US-OTC]; Mapap® Children's [US-OTC]; Mapap® Extra Strength [US-OTC]; Mapap® Infant's [US-OTC]; Mapap® Junior Rapid Tabs [US-OTC]; Nortemp Children's [US-OTC]; Novo-Gesic [Can]; Pain Eze [US-OTC]; Pediatrix [Can]; Silapap Children's [US-OTC]; Silapap Infant's [US-OTC]; Tempra® [Can]; Tylenol® Jr. Meltaways [US-OTC]; Tylenol® 8 Hour [US-OTC]; Tylenol® Arthritis Pain Extended Relief [US-OTC]; Tylenol® Children's Meltaways [US-OTC]; Tylenol® Children's [US-OTC]; Tylenol® Extra Strength [US-OTC]; Tylenol® Infant's Concentrated [US-OTC]; Tylenol® [US-OTC/Can]; Valorin Extra [US-OTC]; Valorin [US-OTC]

Therapeutic Category Analgesic, Nonnarcotic; Antipyretic

Use Treatment of mild-to-moderate pain and fever (analgesic/antipyretic); does not have antirheumatic or antiinflammatory effects

Dosage Summary

Oral:

Children 0-3 months: 10-15 mg/kg/dose **or** 40 mg/dose every 4-6 hours as needed (maximum: 2.6 g/day)

Children 4-11 months: 10-15 mg/kg/dose **or** 80 mg/dose every 4-6 hours as needed (maximum: 2.6 g/day)

Children 1-2 years: 10-15 mg/kg/dose **or** 120 mg/dose every 4-6 hours as needed (maximum: 2.6 g/day)

Children 2-3 years: 10-15 mg/kg/dose **or** 160 mg/dose every 4-6 hours as needed (maximum: 2.6 g/day)

Children 4-5 years: 10-15 mg/kg/dose **or** 240 mg/dose every 4-6 hours as needed (maximum: 2.6 g/day)

Children 6-8 years: 10-15 mg/kg/dose **or** 320 mg/dose every 4-6 hours as needed (maximum: 2.6 g/day)

Children 9-10 years: 10-15 mg/kg/dose **or** 400 mg/dose every 4-6 hours as needed (maximum: 2.6 g/day)

Children 11 years: 10-15 mg/kg/dose **or** 480 mg/dose every 4-6 hours as needed (maximum: 2.6 g/day)

Adults: 325-650 mg every 4-6 hours as needed **or** 1000 mg 3-4 times/day as needed (maximum: 4 g/day)

Rectal:

Children 0-3 months: 10-15 mg/kg/dose **or** 40 mg every 4-6 hours as needed (maximum: 2.6 g/day)

Children 4-11 months: 10-15 mg/kg/dose **or** 80 mg/dose every 4-6 hours as needed (maximum: 2.6 g/day)

Children 1-2 years: 10-15 mg/kg/dose **or** 120 mg/dose every 4-6 hours as needed (maximum: 2.6 g/day)

Children 2-3 years: 10-15 mg/kg/dose **or** 160 mg/dose every 4-6 hours as needed (maximum: 2.6 g/day)

Children 4-5 years: 10-15 mg/kg/dose **or** 240 mg/dose every 4-6 hours as needed (maximum: 2.6 g/day)

Children 6-8 years: 10-15 mg/kg/dose **or** 320 mg/dose every 4-6 hours as needed (maximum: 2.6 g/day)

Children 9-10 years: 10-15 mg/kg/dose **or** 400 mg/dose every 4-6 hours as needed (maximum: 2.6 g/day)

Children 11 years: 10-15 mg/kg/dose **or** 480 mg/dose every 4-6 hours as needed (maximum: 2.6 g/day)

Adults: 325-650 mg every 4-6 hours as needed **or** 1000 mg 3-4 times/day as needed (maximum: 4 g/day)

Dosage Forms

Caplet, oral: 500 mg

Cetafen® Extra [OTC]: 500 mg

Mapap® Extra Strength [OTC]: 500 mg

Pain Eze [OTC]: 650 mg

Tylenol® [OTC]: 325 mg

Tylenol® Extra Strength [OTC]: 500 mg

Caplet, extended release, oral:

Mapap® Arthritis Pain [OTC]: 650 mg

Tylenol® 8 Hour [OTC]: 650 mg

Tylenol® Arthritis Pain Extended Relief [OTC]: 650 mg

Captab, oral: 500 mg
Elixir, oral:
Mapap® Children's [OTC]: 160 mg/5 mL (118 mL, 480 mL)
Gelcap, oral:
Mapap® [OTC]: 500 mg
Gelcap, rapid release, oral:
Tylenol® Extra Strength [OTC]: 500 mg
Geltab, oral:
Excedrin® Tension Headache [OTC]: 500 mg
Liquid, oral:
APAP 500 [OTC]: 500 mg/5 mL (237 mL)
Silapap Children's [OTC]: 160 mg/5 mL (118 mL, 237 mL, 473 mL)
Tylenol® Extra Strength [OTC]: 500 mg/15 mL (240 mL)
Solution, oral: 160 mg/5 mL (5 mL, 10 mL, 15 mL, 20 mL, 118 mL, 473 mL); 80 mg/0.8 mL (15 mL)
Infantaire [OTC]: 80 mg/0.8 mL (15 mL, 30 mL)
Little Fevers™ [OTC]: 80 mg/mL (30 mL)
Mapap® [OTC]: 80 mg/0.8 mL (15 mL)
Silapap Infant's [OTC]: 80 mg/0.8 mL (15 mL, 30 mL)
Suppository, rectal: 120 mg (12s, 50s, 100s); 325 mg (12s); 650 mg (12s, 50s, 100s)
Acephen™ [OTC]: 120 mg (12s, 50s, 100s); 325 mg (6s, 12s, 50s, 100s); 650 mg (12s, 50s, 100s, 500s)
Feverall® [OTC]: 80 mg (6s, 50s); 120 mg (6s, 50s); 325 mg (6s, 50s); 650 mg (50s)
Suspension, oral: 160 mg/5 mL (5 mL, 10 mL, 10.15 mL, 20 mL, 20.3 mL)
Mapap® Children's [OTC]: 160 mg/5 mL (118 mL)
Mapap® Infant's [OTC]: 80 mg/0.8 mL (15 mL, 30 mL)
Nortemp Children's [OTC]: 160 mg/5 mL (118 mL)
Tylenol® Children's [OTC]: 160 mg/5 mL (60 mL, 120 mL)
Tylenol® Infant's Concentrated [OTC]: 80 mg/0.8 mL (15 mL, 30 mL)
Syrup, oral:
Triaminic™ Children's Fever Reducer Pain Reliever [OTC]: 160 mg/5 mL (118 mL)
Tablet, oral: 325 mg, 500 mg
Aspirin Free Anacin® Extra Strength [OTC]: 500 mg
Cetafen® [OTC]: 325 mg
Mapap® [OTC]: 325 mg
Tylenol® [OTC]: 325 mg
Valorin [OTC]: 325 mg
Valorin Extra [OTC]: 500 mg
Tablet, chewable, oral: 80 mg
Mapap® Children's [OTC]: 80 mg
Tablet, orally disintegrating, oral:
Mapap® Children's [OTC]: 80 mg
Mapap® Junior Rapid Tabs [OTC]: 160 mg
Tylenol® Children's Meltaways [OTC]: 80 mg
Tylenol® Jr. Meltaways [OTC]: 160 mg

acetaminophen and butalbital *see* butalbital and acetaminophen *on page* 159
acetaminophen and chlorpheniramine *see* chlorpheniramine and acetaminophen *on page* 208

acetaminophen and codeine (a seet a MIN oh fen & KOE deen)

Sound-Alike/Look-Alike Issues
Capital® may be confused with Capitrol®
Tylenol® may be confused with atenolol, timolol, Tuinal®, Tylox®

T3 is an error-prone abbreviation (mistaken as liothyronine)

Synonyms codeine and acetaminophen

U.S./Canadian Brand Names Capital® and Codeine [US]; ratio-Emtec [Can]; ratio-Lenoltec [Can]; Triatec-30 [Can]; Triatec-8 Strong [Can]; Triatec-8 [Can]; Tylenol® Elixir with Codeine [Can]; Tylenol® No. 1 Forte [Can]; Tylenol® No. 1 [Can]; Tylenol® No. 2 with Codeine [Can]; Tylenol® No. 3 with Codeine [Can]; Tylenol® No. 4 with Codeine [Can]; Tylenol® with Codeine No. 3 [US]; Tylenol® with Codeine No. 4 [US]

Therapeutic Category Analgesic, Narcotic

Controlled Substance C-III; C-V

Use Relief of mild-to-moderate pain

Dosage Summary

Oral:

Acetaminophen:

Children ≤12 years: 10-15 mg/kg/dose every 4-6 hours as needed (maximum: 2.6 g/day)
Children >12 years: 325-650 mg every 4-6 hours as needed (maximum: 4 g/day)
Adults: 325-650 mg every 4-6 hours as needed (maximum: 4 g/day)

Codeine:

Children: 0.5-1 mg/kg/dose every 4-6 hours (maximum: 60 mg/dose)
Adults: 15-60 mg/dose every 4-6 hours (maximum: 360 mg/day)

Dosage Forms

Solution, oral [C-V]: Acetaminophen 120 mg and codeine 12 mg per 5 mL

Suspension, oral [C-V]: Acetaminophen 120 mg and codeine 12 mg per 5 mL

Capital® and Codeine [C-V]: Acetaminophen 120 mg and codeine 12 mg per 5 mL

Tablet [C-III]: Acetaminophen 300 mg and codeine 15 mg; acetaminophen 300 mg and codeine 30 mg; acetaminophen 300 mg and codeine 60 mg

Tylenol® with Codeine No. 3: Acetaminophen 300 mg and codeine 30 mg
Tylenol® with Codeine No. 4: Acetaminophen 300 mg and codeine 60 mg

Dosage Forms - Canada

Caplet:

ratio-Lenoltec No. 1, Tylenol No. 1: Acetaminophen 300 mg, codeine 8 mg, and caffeine 15 mg
Tylenol No. 1 Forte: Acetaminophen 500 mg, codeine 8 mg, and caffeine 15 mg

Solution, oral:

Tylenol Elixir with Codeine: Acetaminophen 160 mg and codeine 8 mg per 5 mL

Tablet:

ratio-Emtec, Triatec-30: Acetaminophen 300 mg and codeine 30 mg
ratio-Lenoltec No. 1: Acetaminophen 300 mg, codeine 8 mg, and caffeine 15 mg
ratio-Lenoltec No. 2, Tylenol No. 2 with Codeine: Acetaminophen 300 mg, codeine 15 mg, and caffeine 15 mg
ratio-Lenoltec No. 3, Tylenol No. 3 with Codeine: Acetaminophen 300 mg, codeine 30 mg, and caffeine 15 mg
ratio-Lenoltec No. 4, Tylenol No. 4 with Codeine: Acetaminophen 300 mg and codeine 60 mg
Triatec-8: Acetaminophen 325 mg, codeine 8 mg, and caffeine 30 mg
Triatec-8 Strong: Acetaminophen 500 mg, codeine 8 mg, and caffeine 30 mg

acetaminophen and diphenhydramine (a seet a MIN oh fen & dye fen HYE dra meen)

Sound-Alike/Look-Alike Issues

Excedrin® may be confused with Dexatrim®, Dexedrine®
Percogesic® may be confused with paregoric, Percodan®
Tylenol® may be confused with atenolol, timolol, Tuinal®, Tylox®
Tylenol® PM may be confused with Tylenol®

Synonyms diphenhydramine and acetaminophen

U.S./Canadian Brand Names Excedrin PM® [US-OTC]; Goody's PM® [US-OTC]; Legatrin PM® [US-OTC]; Mapap PM [US-OTC]; Percogesic® Extra Strength [US-OTC]; Tylenol® PM [US-OTC]; Tylenol® Severe Allergy [US-OTC]

Therapeutic Category Analgesic, Nonnarcotic

Use Aid in the relief of insomnia accompanied by minor pain

Dosage Summary

Oral:

Children <12 years: Dosage not established
Children ≥12 years: 50 mg of diphenhydramine HCl (76 mg diphenhydramine citrate) at bedtime (maximum: Do not exceed recommended dosage)
Adults: 50 mg of diphenhydramine HCl (76 mg diphenhydramine citrate) at bedtime (maximum: Do not exceed recommended dosage)

Dosage Forms

Caplet, oral: Acetaminophen 500 mg and diphenhydramine 25 mg

Excedrin PM® [OTC]: Acetaminophen 500 mg and diphenhydramine 38 mg
Legatrin PM® [OTC]: Acetaminophen 500 mg and diphenhydramine 50 mg
Mapap PM [OTC], Tylenol® PM [OTC]: Acetaminophen 500 mg and diphenhydramine 25 mg
Percogesic® Extra Strength [OTC]: Acetaminophen 500 mg and diphenhydramine 12.5 mg

Tylenol® Severe Allergy [OTC]: Acetaminophen 500 mg and diphenhydramine 12.5 mg

Gelcap, rapid release, oral:

Tylenol® PM [OTC]: Acetaminophen 500 mg and diphenhydramine 25 mg

Geltab, oral: Acetaminophen 500 mg and diphenhydramine 25 mg

Excedrin® PM [OTC]: Acetaminophen 500 mg and diphenhydramine 38 mg

Tylenol® PM [OTC]: Acetaminophen 500 mg and diphenhydramine 25 mg

Liquid, oral:

Tylenol® PM [OTC]: Acetaminophen 500 mg and diphenhydramine 25 mg per 15 mL

Powder for solution, oral:

Goody's PM® [OTC]: Acetaminophen 500 mg and diphenhydramine 38 mg

Tablet, oral: Acetaminophen 500 mg and diphenhydramine 25 mg

Excedrin® PM [OTC]: Acetaminophen 500 mg and diphenhydramine 38 mg

acetaminophen and hydrocodone *see* hydrocodone and acetaminophen *on page 479*

acetaminophen and oxycodone *see* oxycodone and acetaminophen *on page 715*

acetaminophen and pamabrom (a seet a MIN oh fen & PAM a brom)

Synonyms pamabrom and acetaminophen

U.S./Canadian Brand Names Cramp Tabs [US-OTC]; Midol® Teen Formula [US-OTC]; Tylenol® Women's Menstrual Relief [US-OTC]

Therapeutic Category Analgesic, Miscellaneous; Diuretic, Combination

Use Temporary relief of symptoms associated with premenstrual and menstrual symptoms (eg, cramps, bloating, water-weight gain, headache, backache, muscle aches)

Dosage Summary

Oral:

Children <12 years: Dosage not established

Children ≥12 years: Acetaminophen 650-1000 mg and pamabrom 50 mg every 4-6 hours as needed (maximum: 8 caplets/tablets/24 hours)

Adults: Acetaminophen 650-1000 mg and pamabrom 50 mg every 4-6 hours as needed (maximum: 8 caplets/tablets/24 hours)

Dosage Forms

Caplet:

Midol® Teen Formula: Acetaminophen 500 mg and pamabrom 25 mg

Tylenol® Women's Menstrual Relief: Acetaminophen 500 mg and pamabrom 25 mg

Tablet:

Cramp Tabs: Acetaminophen 325 mg and pamabrom 25 mg

acetaminophen and pentazocine *see* pentazocine and acetaminophen *on page 740*

acetaminophen and phenylephrine (a seet a MIN oh fen & fen il EF rin)

Synonyms phenylephrine hydrochloride and acetaminophen

U.S./Canadian Brand Names Alka-Seltzer Plus® Sinus Formula [US-OTC]; Cetafen Cold® [US-OTC]; Contac® Cold + Flu Maximum Strength Non-Drowsy [US-OTC]; Excedrin® Sinus Headache [US-OTC]; Mapap® Sinus Congestion and Pain Daytime [US-OTC]; Sinus Pain & Pressure [US-OTC]; Sinutab® Sinus [US-OTC]; Sudafed PE® Pressure + Pain [US-OTC]; Tylenol® Sinus Congestion & Pain Daytime [US-OTC]; Vicks® DayQuil® Sinus [US-OTC]

Therapeutic Category Analgesic, Miscellaneous; Decongestant

Use Temporary relief of sinus/nasal congestion and pressure, headache, and minor aches and pains

Dosage Summary

Oral:

Children <12 years: Dosage not established

Children ≥12 years: Acetaminophen 325 mg and phenylephrine 5 mg/caplet: Take 2 caplets every 4 hours as needed; maximum: 12 caplets/24 hours; maximum acetaminophen: 4 g/day

Adults: Acetaminophen 325 mg and phenylephrine 5 mg/caplet: Take 2 caplets every 4 hours as needed; maximum: 12 caplets/24 hours; maximum acetaminophen: 4 g/day

Dosage Forms

Caplet, oral:

Contac® Cold + Flu Maximum Strength Non Drowsy [OTC]: Acetaminophen 500 mg and phenylephrine 5 mg

Excedrin® Sinus Headache [OTC], Mapap® Sinus Congestion and Pain Daytime [OTC], Sinutab® Sinus [OTC], Sudafed PE® Pressure + Pain [OTC]: Acetaminophen 325 mg and phenylephrine 5 mg

Tylenol® Sinus Congestion & Pain Daytime [OTC]: Acetaminophen 325 mg and phenylephrine 5 mg [Cool Burst™ flavor]

Capsule, liquicap, oral:

Vicks® DayQuil® Sinus [OTC]: Acetaminophen 325 mg and phenylephrine 5 mg

Gelcap, oral:

Tylenol® Sinus Congestion & Pain Daytime [OTC]: Acetaminophen 325 mg and phenylephrine 5 mg

Gelcap, rapid release, oral:

Tylenol® Sinus Congestion & Pain Daytime [OTC]: Acetaminophen 325 mg and phenylephrine 5 mg

Tablet for solution, oral [effervescent]:

Alka-Seltzer Plus® Sinus Formula [OTC]: Acetaminophen 250 mg and phenylephrine 5 mg

Tablet, oral:

Cetafen Cold® [OTC], Sinus Pain & Pressure [OTC]: Acetaminophen 500 mg and phenylephrine 5 mg

acetaminophen and phenyltoloxamine (a seet a MIN oh fen & fen il to LOKS a meen)

Sound-Alike/Look-Alike Issues

Percogesic® may be confused with paregoric, Percodan®

Synonyms phenyltoloxamine citrate and acetaminophen

U.S./Canadian Brand Names Aceta-Gesic [US-OTC]; BeFlex [US]; BP Poly 650 [US]; Dologesic® [US]; Flextra-650 [US]; Flextra-DS [US]; Lagesic™ [US]; Phenagesic [US-OTC]; RhinoFlex™ [US]; RhinoFlex™-650 [US]; Staflex [US]; Zgesic [US]

Therapeutic Category Analgesic, Nonnarcotic

Use Relief of mild-to-moderate pain

Dosage Summary

Oral: Based on acetaminophen component:

Children <12 years: 10-15 mg/kg/dose every 4-6 hours as needed (maximum: 2.6 g/day)

Children ≥12 years: 325-650 mg every 4-6 hours as needed (maximum: 4 g/day)

Adults: 325-650 mg every 4-6 hours as needed (maximum: 4 g/day)

Dosage Forms

Caplet:

BeFlex, Staflex: Acetaminophen 500 mg and phenyltoloxamine 55 mg

Dologesic®: Acetaminophen 500 mg and phenyltoloxamine 30 mg

Caplet, extended release [scored]:

Lagesic™: Acetaminophen 600 mg and phenyltoloxamine 66 mg

Capsule:

Dologesic®: Acetaminophen 500 mg and phenyltoloxamine 30 mg

Liquid:

Dologesic®: Acetaminophen 500 mg and phenyltoloxamine 30 mg per 15 mg

Tablet: Acetaminophen 325 mg and phenyltoloxamine 30 mg

Aceta-Gesic [OTC], Phenagesic [OTC]: Acetaminophen 325 mg and phenyltoloxamine 30 mg

BP Poly 650: Acetaminophen 650 mg and phenyltoloxamine 60 mg

RhinoFlex™: Acetaminophen 500 mg and phenyltoloxamine 50 mg

RhinoFlex™-650: Acetaminophen 650 mg and phenyltoloxamine 50 mg

Tablet, prolonged release, oral:

Zgesic: Acetaminophen 600 mg and phenyltoloxamine 66 mg

acetaminophen and propoxyphene *see* propoxyphene and acetaminophen *on page* 805

acetaminophen and pseudoephedrine (a seet a MIN oh fen & soo doe e FED rin)

Sound-Alike/Look-Alike Issues

Ornex® may be confused with Orexin®, Orinase®

Sudafed® may be confused with Sufenta®

Tylenol® may be confused with atenolol, timolol, Tuinal®, Tylox®

Synonyms pseudoephedrine and acetaminophen; pseudoephedrine hydrochloride and acetaminophen

U.S./Canadian Brand Names Contac® Cold and Sore Throat, Non Drowsy, Extra Strength [Can]; Dristan® N.D. [Can]; Dristan® N.D., Extra Strength [Can]; Ornex® Maximum Strength [US-OTC]; Ornex® [US-OTC]; Sinutab® Non Drowsy [Can]; Sudafed® Head Cold and Sinus Extra Strength [Can]; Tylenol® Decongestant [Can]; Tylenol® Sinus [Can]

Therapeutic Category Decongestant/Analgesic

Use Temporary relief of nasal congestion, and minor aches and pains associated with colds, flu, sinusitis, or allergies

Dosage Summary

Oral:

Children <6 years: Dosage not established

Children 6-11 years: Acetaminophen 325 mg/pseudoephedrine 30 mg every 4-6 hours (maximum: 120 mg/day pseudoephedrine)

Children ≥12 years: Acetaminophen 625-1000 mg/pseudoephedrine 60 mg every 4-6 hours (maximum: 240 mg/day pseudoephedrine)

Adults: Acetaminophen 625-1000 mg/pseudoephedrine 60 mg every 4-6 hours (maximum: 240 mg/day pseudoephedrine)

Dosage Forms

Caplet:

Ornex® [OTC]: Acetaminophen 325 mg and pseudoephedrine 30 mg

Ornex® Maximum Strength [OTC]: Acetaminophen 500 mg and pseudoephedrine 30 mg

acetaminophen and tramadol (a seet a MIN oh fen & TRA ma dole)

Sound-Alike/Look-Alike Issues

Ultracet® may be confused with Ultane®, Ultram®

Synonyms APAP and tramadol; tramadol hydrochloride and acetaminophen

U.S./Canadian Brand Names Apo-Tramadol/Acet® [Can]; Tramacet [Can]; Ultracet® [US]

Therapeutic Category Analgesic, Miscellaneous; Analgesic, Nonnarcotic

Use Short-term (≤5 days) management of acute pain

Dosage Summary

Oral:

Children: Dosage not established

Adults: Two tablets every 4-6 hours as needed (maximum: 8 tablets/day)

Dosage Forms

Tablet: Acetaminophen 325 mg and tramadol 37.5 mg

Ultracet®: Acetaminophen 325 mg and tramadol 37.5 mg

acetaminophen, aspirin, and caffeine (a seet a MIN oh fen, AS pir in, & KAF een)

Sound-Alike/Look-Alike Issues

Excedrin® may be confused with Dexatrim®, Dexedrine®

Synonyms aspirin, acetaminophen, and caffeine; aspirin, caffeine, and acetaminophen; caffeine, acetaminophen, and aspirin; caffeine, aspirin, and acetaminophen

U.S./Canadian Brand Names Anacin® Advanced Headache Formula [US-OTC]; Excedrin® Extra Strength [US-OTC]; Excedrin® Migraine [US-OTC]; Fem-Prin® [US-OTC]; Goody's® Extra Strength Headache Powder [US-OTC]; Goody's® Extra Strength Pain Relief [US-OTC]; Pain-Off [US-OTC]; Vanquish® Extra Strength Pain Reliever [US-OTC]

Therapeutic Category Analgesic, Nonnarcotic

Use Relief of mild-to-moderate pain; mild-to-moderate pain associated with migraine headache

Dosage Summary

Oral:

Children ≤12 years: Dosage not established

Children >12 years: 1-2 doses every 4-6 hours as needed (maximum: 4 g/day [based on acetaminophen and aspirin component])

Adults: 1-2 doses every 4-6 hours as needed (maximum: 4 g/day [based on acetaminophen and aspirin component])

Dosage Forms

Caplet: Acetaminophen 250 mg, aspirin 250 mg, and caffeine 65 mg; acetaminophen 194 mg, aspirin 227 mg, and caffeine 33 mg

Excedrin® Extra Strength [OTC], Excedrin® Migraine [OTC]: Acetaminophen 250 mg, aspirin 250 mg, and caffeine 65 mg

Vanquish® Extra Strength Pain Reliever [OTC]: Acetaminophen 194 mg, aspirin 227 mg, and caffeine 33 mg

Geltab: Acetaminophen 250 mg, aspirin 250 mg, and caffeine 65 mg

Excedrin® Extra Strength [OTC], Excedrin® Migraine [OTC]: Acetaminophen 250 mg, aspirin 250 mg, and caffeine 65 mg

Powder: Acetaminophen 260 mg, aspirin 520 mg, and caffeine 32.5 mg

Goody's® Extra Strength Headache Powder [OTC]: Acetaminophen 260 mg, aspirin 520 mg, and caffeine 32.5 mg

Tablet:
Anacin® Advanced Headache Formula [OTC], Excedrin® Extra Strength [OTC], Excedrin® Migraine [OTC], Pain-Off [OTC]: Acetaminophen 250 mg, aspirin 250 mg, and caffeine 65 mg
Fem-Prin® [OTC]: Acetaminophen 194.4 mg, aspirin 226.8 mg, and caffeine 32.4 mg
Goody's® Extra Strength Pain Relief [OTC]: Acetaminophen 130 mg, aspirin 260 mg, and caffeine 16.25 mg

acetaminophen, butalbital, and caffeine *see* butalbital, acetaminophen, and caffeine *on page 159*

acetaminophen, caffeine, and dihydrocodeine

(a seet a MIN oh fen, KAF een, & dye hye droe KOE deen)

Sound-Alike/Look-Alike Issues
Panlor® DC may be confused with Pamelor®

Synonyms caffeine, dihydrocodeine, and acetaminophen; dihydrocodeine bitartrate, acetaminophen, and caffeine

U.S./Canadian Brand Names Panlor® SS [US]; Trezix® [US]; ZerLor™ [US]

Therapeutic Category Analgesic Combination (Opioid)

Controlled Substance C-III

Use Relief of moderate- to moderately-severe pain

Dosage Summary

Oral:
Children: Dosage not established
Adults: 1 tablet or 2 capsules every 4 hours as needed (maximum: 10 capsules/day or 5 tablets/day)

Dosage Forms

Capsule:
Trezix®: Acetaminophen 356.4 mg, caffeine 30 mg, and dihydrocodeine 16 mg

Tablet:
Panlor® SS, ZerLor™: Acetaminophen 712.8 mg, caffeine 60 mg, and dihydrocodeine 32 mg

acetaminophen, caffeine, codeine, and butalbital *see* butalbital, acetaminophen, caffeine, and codeine *on page 159*

acetaminophen, chlorpheniramine, and pseudoephedrine

(a seet a MIN oh fen, klor fen IR a meen, & soo doe e FED rin)

Synonyms acetaminophen, chlorpheniramine maleate, and pseudoephedrine hydrochloride; acetaminophen, pseudoephedrine, and chlorpheniramine; chlorpheniramine, acetaminophen, and pseudoephedrine; chlorpheniramine, pseudoephedrine, and acetaminophen; pseudoephedrine, acetaminophen, and chlorpheniramine; pseudoephedrine, chlorpheniramine, and acetaminophen

U.S./Canadian Brand Names Drinex [US-OTC]; Relief-SF® [US]

Therapeutic Category Antihistamine/Decongestant/Analgesic

Use Temporary relief of cold, allergy, or sinus symptoms

Dosage Summary

Oral:
Children <12 years: Dosage not established
Children ≥12 years: Drinex: 1 tablet 3-4 times/day (maximum: 4 tablets/24 hours); Relief-SF®: 1-2 caplets every 6 hours (maximum: 8 caplets/24 hours)
Adults: Drinex: 1 tablet 3-4 times/day (maximum: 4 tablets/24 hours); Relief-SF®: 1-2 caplets every 6 hours (maximum: 8 caplets/24 hours)

Dosage Forms

Caplet: Acetaminophen 325 mg, chlorpheniramine 2 mg, and pseudoephedrine 30 mg
Relief-SF®: Acetaminophen 500 mg, chlorpheniramine 2 mg, and pseudoephedrine 30 mg

Tablet:
Drinex [OTC]: Acetaminophen 650 mg, chlorpheniramine 4 mg, and pseudoephedrine 60 mg

acetaminophen, chlorpheniramine maleate, and pseudoephedrine hydrochloride *see* acetaminophen, chlorpheniramine, and pseudoephedrine *on page 28*

acetaminophen, codeine, and doxylamine *(Canada only)*

(a seet a MIN oh fen, KOE deen, & dox IL a meen)

Synonyms codeine, doxylamine, and acetaminophen; doxylamine succinate, codeine phosphate, and acetaminophen

U.S./Canadian Brand Names Mersyndol® With Codeine [Can]

Therapeutic Category Analgesic, Opioid; Antihistamine

Controlled Substance CDSA-1

Use Relief of headache, cold symptoms, neuralgia, and muscular aches/pain

Dosage Summary

Oral:

Children ≤12 years: Dosage not established

Children >12 years: 1-2 tablets every 4 hours as needed (maximum: 12 tablets/day)

Adults: 1-2 tablets every 4 hours as needed (maximum: 12 tablets/day)

Dosage Forms - Canada

Tablet:

Mersyndol® With Codeine: Acetaminophen 325 mg, codeine 8 mg, and doxylamine 5 mg

acetaminophen, dextromethorphan, and doxylamine

(a seet a MIN oh fen, deks troe meth OR fan, & dox IL a meen)

Synonyms dextromethorphan hydrobromide, acetaminophen, and doxylamine succinate; doxylamine, acetaminophen, and dextromethorphan

U.S./Canadian Brand Names All-Nite [US-OTC]; Tylenol® Cough & Sore Throat Nighttime [US-OTC]; Vicks® NyQuil® Cold & Flu Multi-Symptom [US-OTC]

Therapeutic Category Analgesic, Miscellaneous; Antitussive; Histamine H_1 Antagonist; Histamine H_1 Antagonist, First Generation

Use Temporary relief of common cold and flu symptoms (eg, minor aches and pain, fever, cough, runny nose, sneezing, sore throat)

Dosage Summary

Oral:

Children <12 years: Dosage not established

Children ≥12 years: Two capsules/caplets **or** 30 mL every 6 hours (maximum: 8 capsules **or** 240 mL/24 hours)

Adults: Two capsules/caplets **or** 30 mL every 6 hours (maximum: 8 capsules **or** 240 mL/24 hours)

Dosage Forms

Caplet:

Vicks® NyQuil® Cold & Flu Multi-Symptom [OTC]: Acetaminophen 325 mg dextromethorphan 15 mg, and doxylamine 6.25 mg

Capsule, liquicap:

Vicks® NyQuil® Cold & Flu Multi-Symptom [OTC]: Acetaminophen 325 mg, dextromethorphan 15 mg, and doxylamine 6.25 mg

Liquid:

All-Nite [OTC]: Acetaminophen 500 mg, dextromethorphan 15 mg, and doxylamine 6.25 mg per 15 mL

Tylenol® Cough & Sore Throat Nighttime [OTC]: Acetaminophen 500 mg, dextromethorphan 15 mg, and doxylamine 6.25 mg per 15 mL

Vicks® NyQuil® Cold & Flu Multi-Symptom [OTC]: Acetaminophen 500 mg, dextromethorphan hydrobromide 15 mg, and doxylamine succinate 6.25 mg per 15 mL

acetaminophen, dextromethorphan, and phenylephrine

(a seet a MIN oh fen, deks troe meth OR fan, & fen il EF rin)

Synonyms dextromethorphan hydrobromide, acetaminophen, and phenylephrine hydrochloride; phenylephrine, acetaminophen, and dextromethorphan; phenylephrine, dextromethorphan, and acetaminophen

U.S./Canadian Brand Names Alka-Seltzer Plus® Day Cold [US-OTC]; Comtrex® Maximum Strength, Non-Drowsy Cold & Cough Relief [US-OTC]; Mapap® Multi-Symptom Cold [US-OTC]; Theraflu® Daytime Severe Cold & Cough [US-OTC]; Theraflu® Warming Relief Daytime Severe Cold & Cough [US-OTC]; Tylenol® Cold Head Congestion Daytime [US-OTC]; Tylenol® Cold Multi-Symptom Daytime [US-OTC]; Vicks® DayQuil® Cold/Flu Multi-Symptom Relief [US-OTC]

Therapeutic Category Analgesic, Miscellaneous; Antitussive; Decongestant

Use Temporary relief of common cold and flu symptoms (eg, pain, fever, cough, congestion)

Dosage Summary Note: Dosage may vary considerably by product; ranges listed are representative. Consult specific product labeling.

Oral:

Vicks® DayQuil® Cold/Flu Multi-Symptom Relief:

Children <6 years: Dosage not established

Children 6-11 years: 15 mL every 4 hours, up to 5 doses per day (maximum: 75 mL/24 hours)

Children ≥12 years: 2 doses every 4 hours or 30 mL every 4 hours (maximum: 6 doses/24 hours)

Adults: 2 doses every 4 hours or 30 mL every 4 hours (maximum: 6 doses/24 hours)

Dosage Forms

Caplet:

Comtrex® Maximum Strength, Non-Drowsy Cold & Cough Relief [OTC], Mapap® Multi-Symptom Cold [OTC], Theraflu® Daytime Severe Cold & Cough [OTC], Tylenol® Cold Head Congestion Daytime [OTC], Tylenol® Cold Multi-Symptom Daytime [OTC]: Acetaminophen 325 mg, dextromethorphan 10 mg, and phenylephrine 5 mg

Capsule, liquid gel:

Alka-Seltzer Plus® Day Cold [OTC]: Acetaminophen 325 mg, dextromethorphan 10 mg, and phenylephrine 5 mg

Capsule, liquicap:

Vicks® DayQuil® Cold/Flu Multi-Symptom Relief [OTC]: Acetaminophen 325 mg, dextromethorphan 10 mg, and phenylephrine 5 mg

Gelcap:

Tylenol® Cold Multi-Symptom Daytime [OTC]: Acetaminophen 325 mg, dextromethorphan 10 mg, and phenylephrine 5 mg

Liquid:

Alka-Seltzer Plus® Day Cold [OTC]: Acetaminophen 162.5 mg, dextromethorphan 5 mg, and phenylephrine 2.5 mg per 5 mL

Tylenol® Cold Multi-Symptom Daytime [OTC], Vicks® DayQuil® Cold/Flu Multi-Symptom Relief [OTC]: Acetaminophen 325 mg, dextromethorphan 10 mg, and phenylephrine 5 mg per 15 mL

Powder for solution:

Theraflu® Daytime Severe Cold & Cough [OTC]: Acetaminophen 650 mg, dextromethorphan 20 mg, and phenylephrine 10 mg/packet (6s)

Syrup:

Theraflu® Warming Relief Daytime Severe Cold & Cough [OTC]: Acetaminophen 325 mg, dextromethorphan 10 mg, and phenylephrine 5 mg per 15 mL

acetaminophen, dextromethorphan, and pseudoephedrine *(Discontinued)*

acetaminophen, dextromethorphan, doxylamine, and pseudoephedrine

(a seet a MIN oh fen, deks troe meth OR fan, dox IL a meen & soo doe e FED rin)

Synonyms dextromethorphan hydrobromide, acetaminophen, doxylamine succinate, and pseudoephedrine hydrochloride; doxylamine, acetaminophen, dextromethorphan, and pseudoephedrine; pseudoephedrine, dextromethorphan, doxylamine, and acetaminophen

U.S./Canadian Brand Names All-Nite Multi-Symptom Cold/Flu [US-OTC]; Vicks® NyQuil® D Cold & Flu Multi-Symptom [US-OTC]

Therapeutic Category Analgesic, Miscellaneous; Antitussive; Decongestant; Histamine H_1 Antagonist; Histamine H_1 Antagonist, First Generation

Use Temporary relief of common cold and flu symptoms (eg, minor aches and pain, fever, cough, congestion, runny nose, sneezing, sore throat)

Dosage Summary

Oral:

Children <12 years: Dosage not established

Children ≥12 years: 30 mL every 6 hours (maximum: 120 mL/24 hours)

Adults: 30 mL every 6 hours (maximum: 120 mL/24 hours)

Dosage Forms

Liquid:

All-Nite Multi-Symptom Cold/Flu [OTC]: Acetaminophen 500 mg, dextromethorphan hydrobromide 15 mg, doxylamine succinate 6.25 mg and pseudoephedrine hydrochloride 30 mg per 15 mL

Vicks® NyQuil® D Cold & Flu Multi-Symptom [OTC]: Acetaminophen 500 mg, dextromethorphan hydrobromide 15 mg, doxylamine succinate 6.25 mg and pseudoephedrine hydrochloride 30 mg per 15 mL

acetaminophen, dichloralphenazone, and isometheptene *see* acetaminophen, isometheptene, and dichloralphenazone *on page 31*

acetaminophen, diphenhydramine, and phenylephrine

(a seet a MIN oh fen, dye fen HYE dra meen, & fen il EF rin)

Synonyms acetaminophen, phenylephrine, and diphenhydramine; diphenhydramine, phenylephrine hydrochloride, and acetaminophen; phenylephrine hydrochloride, acetaminophen, and diphenhydramine

U.S./Canadian Brand Names Benadryl® Allergy and Cold [US-OTC]; Benadryl® Allergy and Sinus Headache [US-OTC]; Benadry® Maximum Strength Severe Allergy and Sinus Headache [US-OTC]; Cold Control PE [US-OTC]; One Tab™ Allergy & Sinus [US-OTC]; One Tab™ Cold & Flu [US-OTC]; Sudafed PE® Nighttime Cold [US-OTC]; Sudafed PE® Severe Cold [US-OTC]; Theraflu® Nighttime Severe Cold & Cough [US-OTC]; Theraflu® Sugar-Free Nighttime Severe Cold & Cough [US-OTC]; Theraflu® Warming Relief ™ Flu & Sore Throat [US-OTC]; Theraflu® Warming Relief™ Nighttime Severe Cold & Cough [US-OTC]; Tylenol® Allergy Multi-Symptom Nighttime [US-OTC]; Tylenol® Children's Plus Cold and Allergy [US-OTC]

Therapeutic Category Analgesic, Miscellaneous; Decongestant; Histamine H_1 Antagonist

Use Temporary relief of symptoms of hay fever and the common cold, including sinus/nasal congestion and pain/pressure, headache, sneezing, runny nose, itchy/watery eyes, sore throat, fever, cough, and minor aches and pains

Dosage Summary

Oral:

Caplet:

Children <6 years: Dosage not established
Children 6-11 years: One caplet every 4 hours as needed (maximum: 5 doses/caplets)
Children ≥12 years: Two caplets every 4 hours as needed (maximum: 12 caplets/24 hours)
Adults: Two caplets every 4 hours as needed (maximum: 12 caplets/24 hours)

Liquid:

Children <6 years and <48 lbs: Dosage not established
Children 6-11 years and 48-95 lbs: 10 mL every 4 hours as needed (maximum: 5 doses/24 hours)
Children ≥12 years and >95 lbs: Use alternative dosage form
Adults: Use alternative dosage form

Powder for solution:

Children <12 years: Dosage not established
Children ≥12 years: One packet every 4 hours as needed (maximum: 6 doses/24 hours)
Adults: One packet every 4 hours as needed (maximum: 6 doses/24 hours)

Syrup:

Children <12 years: Dosage not established
Children ≥12 years: 30 mL every 4 hours as needed (maximum: 6 doses/24 hours)
Adults: 30 mL every 4 hours as needed (maximum: 6 doses/24 hours)

Dosage Forms

Caplet, oral:

Benadryl® Allergy and Cold [OTC], Benadryl® Allergy and Sinus Headache [OTC], Sudafed PE® Severe Cold [OTC]: Acetaminophen 325 mg, diphenhydramine 12.5 mg, and phenylephrine 5 mg

Benadry® Maximum Strength Severe Allergy and Sinus Headache [OTC], Sudafed PE® Nighttime Cold [OTC], Tylenol® Allergy Multi-Symptom Nighttime [OTC]: Acetaminophen 325 mg, diphenhydramine 25 mg, and phenylephrine 5 mg

Cold Control PE [OTC]: Acetaminophen 650 mg, diphenhydramine 25 mg, and phenylephrine 10 mg

One Tab™ Allergy & Sinus, One Tab™ Cold and Flu: Acetaminophen 650 mg, diphenhydramine 25 mg, and phenylephrine 10 mg

Liquid, oral:

Tylenol® Children's Plus Cold and Allergy [OTC]: Acetaminophen 160 mg, diphenhydramine 12.5 mg, and phenylephrine 2.5 mg per 5 mL

Powder for solution, oral:

Theraflu® Nighttime Severe Cold & Cough [OTC], Theraflu® Sugar-Free Nighttime Severe Cold & Cough [OTC]: Acetaminophen 650 mg, diphenhydramine 25 mg, and phenylephrine 10 mg per packet (6s)

Syrup, oral:

Theraflu® Warming Relief™ Flu & Sore Throat [OTC], Theraflu® Warming Relief™ Nighttime Severe Cold & Cough [OTC]: Acetaminophen 325 mg, diphenhydramine 12.5 mg, and phenylephrine 5 mg per 15 mL (245.5 mL)

acetaminophen, isometheptene, and dichloralphenazone

(a seet a MIN oh fen, eye soe me THEP teen, & dye KLOR al FEN a zone)

Sound-Alike/Look-Alike Issues

Midrin® may be confused with midodrine, Mydfrin®

Synonyms acetaminophen, dichloralphenazone, and isometheptene; dichloralphenazone, acetaminophen, and isometheptene; dichloralphenazone, isometheptene, and acetaminophen; isometheptene, acetaminophen, and dichloralphenazone; isometheptene, dichloralphenazone, and acetaminophen

U.S./Canadian Brand Names Epidrin [US]; Midrin® [US]; Migratine [US]
Therapeutic Category Analgesic, Nonnarcotic
Controlled Substance C-IV
Use Relief of migraine and tension headache
Dosage Summary
Oral:
Children: Dosage not established
Adults: 2 capsules initially, then 1 capsule every hour until relief; alternatively, 1-2 capsules every 4 hours (maximum: 5 capsules/12 hours or 8 capsules/day)
Dosage Forms
Capsule:
Epidrin, Midrin®: Acetaminophen 325 mg, isometheptene 65 mg, and dichloralphenazone 100 mg

acetaminophen, phenylephrine, and diphenhydramine *see* acetaminophen, diphenhydramine, and phenylephrine *on page 30*

acetaminophen, pseudoephedrine, and chlorpheniramine *see* acetaminophen, chlorpheniramine, and pseudoephedrine *on page 28*

Acetasol® HC [US] *see* acetic acid, propylene glycol diacetate, and hydrocortisone *on page 33*

acetazolamide (a set a ZOLE a mide)

Sound-Alike/Look-Alike Issues
acetaZOLAMIDE may be confused with acetoHEXAMIDE
Diamox® Sequels® may be confused with Diabinese®, Dobutrex®, Trimox®
Tall-Man aceta**ZOLAMIDE**
U.S./Canadian Brand Names Apo-Acetazolamide® [Can]; Diamox® Sequels® [US]; Diamox® [Can]
Therapeutic Category Anticonvulsant; Carbonic Anhydrase Inhibitor
Use Treatment of glaucoma (chronic simple open-angle, secondary glaucoma, preoperatively in acute angle-closure); drug-induced edema or edema due to congestive heart failure (adjunctive therapy); centrencephalic epilepsies (immediate release dosage form); prevention or amelioration of symptoms associated with acute mountain sickness
Dosage Summary
I.V.:
Children: 20-40 mg/kg/day divided every 6 hours **or** 5 mg/kg (150 mg/m^2) once daily (maximum: 1 g/day)
Adults: 250-500 mg/day (may repeat in 2-4 hours for glaucoma) (maximum: 1 g/day)
Oral:
Immediate release:
Children: 5-30 mg/kg/day (150-900 mg/m^2/day) divided in 1-4 doses (maximum: 1 g/day)
Adults: 250-1000 mg/day in 1-4 divided doses (maximum: 1 g/day)
Elderly: Initial: 250 mg once or twice daily; use lowest effective dose possible.
Extended release:
Children: Dosage not established
Adults: 500 mg every 12-24 hours (maximum: 1 g/day); **Note:** Extended release capsule not recommended for epilepsy.
Dosage Forms
Capsule, extended release, oral: 500 mg
Capsule, sustained release, oral:
Diamox® Sequels®: 500 mg
Injection, powder for reconstitution: 500 mg
Tablet, oral: 125 mg, 250 mg

acetic acid (a SEE tik AS id)

Sound-Alike/Look-Alike Issues
acetic acid for irrigation may be confused with glacial acetic acid
VoSoL® may be confused with Vexol®,VoSol® HC
Synonyms ethanoic acid
U.S./Canadian Brand Names VoSoL® [US]
Therapeutic Category Antibacterial, Otic; Antibacterial, Topical
Use Irrigation of the bladder; periodic irrigation of indwelling catheters; treatment of superficial bacterial infections of the external auditory canal

Dosage Summary

Irrigation: Note: Dosage of an irrigating solution depends on the capacity or surface area of the structure being irrigated

Children: Dosage not established

Adults: Continuous: 0.25% at a rate approximate to urine flow; usually 500-1500 mL/day; Periodic: 50 mL of 0.25%

Otic:

Children <3 years: Dosage not established

Children ≥3 years: Instill 3-5 drops 3-4 times/day

Adults: Instill 5 drops 3-4 times/day

Dosage Forms

Solution, for irrigation: 0.25% (1000 mL)

Solution, for irrigation [preservative free]: 0.25% (250 mL, 500 mL, 1000 mL)

Solution, otic: 2% (15 mL)

VoSoL®: 2% (15 mL)

acetic acid, hydrocortisone, and propylene glycol diacetate *see* acetic acid, propylene glycol diacetate, and hydrocortisone *on page 33*

acetic acid, propylene glycol diacetate, and hydrocortisone

(a SEE tik AS id, PRO pa leen GLY kole dye AS e tate, & hye droe KOR ti sone)

Sound-Alike/Look-Alike Issues

VoSol® may be confused with Vexol®

Synonyms acetic acid, hydrocortisone, and propylene glycol diacetate; hydrocortisone, acetic acid, and propylene glycol diacetate; propylene glycol diacetate, acetic acid, and hydrocortisone

U.S./Canadian Brand Names Acetasol® HC [US]; VoSol® HC [US]

Therapeutic Category Antibiotic/Corticosteroid, Otic

Use Treatment of superficial infections of the external auditory canal caused by organisms susceptible to the action of the antimicrobial, complicated by swelling

Dosage Summary

Otic:

Children ≥3 years: Instill 3-5 drops in ear(s) every 4-6 hours

Adults: Instill 3-5 drops in ear(s) every 4-6 hours

Dosage Forms

Solution, otic [drops]: Acetic acid 2%, propylene glycol diacetate 3%, and hydrocortisone 1% (10 mL)

Acetasol® HC, VoSol® HC: Acetic acid 2%, propylene glycol diacetate 3%, and hydrocortisone 1% (10 mL)

acetohydroxamic acid (a SEE toe hye droks am ik AS id)

Sound-Alike/Look-Alike Issues

Lithostat® may be confused with Lithobid®

Synonyms AHA

U.S./Canadian Brand Names Lithostat® [US/Can]

Therapeutic Category Urinary Tract Product

Use Adjunctive therapy in chronic urea-splitting urinary infection

Dosage Summary

Oral:

Children: Initial: 10 mg/kg/day

Adults: 250 mg 3-4 times/day (maximum: 10-15 mg/kg/day)

Dosage Forms

Tablet, oral:

Lithostat®: 250 mg

Acetoxyl® [Can] *see* benzoyl peroxide *on page 128*

acetoxymethylprogesterone *see* medroxyprogesterone *on page 597*

acetylcholine (a se teel KOE leen)

Sound-Alike/Look-Alike Issues

acetylcholine may be confused with acetylcysteine

Synonyms acetylcholine chloride

U.S./Canadian Brand Names Miochol®-E [US/Can]

Therapeutic Category Cholinergic Agent

Use Produces complete miosis in cataract surgery, keratoplasty, iridectomy, and other anterior segment surgery where rapid miosis is required

Dosage Summary

Intraocular:

Children: Dosage not established

Adults: Instill 0.5-2 mL of 1% injection (5-20 mg) before or after securing sutures

Dosage Forms

Powder for solution, intraocular:

Miochol®-E: 20 mg (2 mL)

acetylcholine chloride *see* acetylcholine *on page* 33

acetylcysteine (a se teel SIS teen)

Sound-Alike/Look-Alike Issues

acetylcysteine may be confused with acetylcholine

Mucomyst® may be confused with Mucinex®

Synonyms *N*-acetyl-L-cysteine; *N*-acetylcysteine; acetylcysteine sodium; mercapturic acid; NAC

U.S./Canadian Brand Names Acetadote® [US]; Acetylcysteine Solution [Can]; Mucomyst® [Can]; Parvolex® [Can]

Therapeutic Category Mucolytic Agent

Use Antidote for acute acetaminophen (APAP) poisoning; repeated supratherapeutic ingestion (RSTI) of APAP; adjunctive mucolytic therapy in patients with abnormal or viscid mucous secretions in acute and chronic bronchopulmonary diseases; pulmonary complications of surgery and cystic fibrosis; diagnostic bronchial studies

Dosage Summary

Inhalation: Note: Patients should receive bronchodilator 10-15 minutes prior to dose

Nebulization:

Infants: 1-2 mL of 20% solution or 2-4 mL 10% solution 3-4 times/day

Children: 1-10 mL of 20% solution or 2-20 mL of 10% solution every 2-6 hours

Adults: 1-10 mL of 20% solution or 2-20 mL of 10% solution every 2-6 hours

Direct instillation:

Children: Dosage not established

Adults: 1-2 mL of 10% or 20% solution every 1-4 hours via tracheostomy **or** 1-2 mL of 20% or 2-4 mL of 10% solution every 1-4 hours via percutaneous intratracheal catheter

I.V.: Acetadote®:

Children: 21-hour regimen: Consists of 3 doses; total dose delivered: 300 mg/kg

Loading dose: 150 mg/kg (maximum: 15 g) infused over 60 minutes

Second dose: 50 mg/kg (maximum: 5 g) infused over 4 hours

Third dose: 100 mg/kg (maximum: 10 g) infused over 16 hours

Adults: 21-hour regimen: Consists of 3 doses; total dose delivered: 300 mg/kg

Loading dose: 150 mg/kg (maximum: 15 g) infused over 60 minutes

Second dose: 50 mg/kg (maximum: 5 g) infused over 4 hours

Third dose: 100 mg/kg (maximum: 10 g) infused over 16 hours

Oral:

Children: Acetaminophen poisoning: 72-hour regimen: Consists of 18 doses; total dose delivered: 1330 mg/kg

Loading dose: 140 mg/kg

Maintenance dose: 70 mg/kg every 4 hours; repeat dose if emesis occurs within 1 hour of administration

Adults:

Acetaminophen poisoning: 72-hour regimen: Consists of 18 doses; total dose delivered: 1330 mg/kg

Loading dose: 140 mg/kg

Maintenance dose: 70 mg/kg every 4 hours; repeat dose if emesis occurs within 1 hour of administration

Renal protectant for radiocontrast: 600-1200 mg twice daily for 2 days

Dosage Forms

Injection, solution:

Acetadote®: 20% [200 mg/mL] (30 mL)

Solution, for inhalation/oral: 10% [100 mg/mL] (10 mL, 30 mL); 20% [200 mg/mL] (10 mL, 30 mL)
Solution, for inhalation/oral [preservative free]: 10% [100 mg/mL] (4 mL, 10 mL); 20% [200 mg/mL] (4 mL, 10 mL, 30 mL)

acetylcysteine, methylcobalamin, and methylfolate *see* methylfolate, methylcobalamin, and acetylcysteine *on page 620*

acetylcysteine, methylfolate, and methylcobalamin *see* methylfolate, methylcobalamin, and acetylcysteine *on page 620*

acetylcysteine sodium *see* acetylcysteine *on page 34*

Acetylcysteine Solution [Can] *see* acetylcysteine *on page 34*

acetylsalicylic acid *see* aspirin *on page 100*

Aches-N-Pain® ***(Discontinued)*** *see* ibuprofen *on page 494*

achromycin *see* tetracycline *on page 922*

aciclovir *see* acyclovir (systemic) *on page 36*

aciclovir *see* acyclovir (topical) *on page 37*

Acid Control [Can] *see* famotidine *on page 390*

Acid Gone [US-OTC] *see* aluminum hydroxide and magnesium carbonate *on page 58*

Acid Gone Extra Strength [US-OTC] *see* aluminum hydroxide and magnesium carbonate *on page 58*

Acid Reducer [Can] *see* ranitidine *on page 828*

Acid Reducer Maximum Strength Non Prescription [Can] *see* ranitidine *on page 828*

acidulated phosphate fluoride *see* fluoride *on page 413*

Aci-jel® ***(Discontinued)*** *see* acetic acid *on page 32*

Acilac [Can] *see* lactulose *on page 544*

AcipHex® [US] *see* rabeprazole *on page 824*

acitretin (a si TRE tin)

Sound-Alike/Look-Alike Issues
Soriatane® may be confused with Loxitane®, sertraline, Sonata®

U.S./Canadian Brand Names Soriatane® [Can]

Therapeutic Category Retinoid-like Compound

Use Treatment of severe psoriasis

Dosage Summary

Oral:
Children: Dosage not established
Adults: 25-50 mg/day as a single dose with the main meal

Aclaro PD™ [US] *see* hydroquinone *on page 487*

Aclasta® [Can] *see* zoledronic acid *on page 1003*

Aclovate® [US] *see* alclometasone *on page 45*

Acne Clear Maximum Strength [US-OTC] *see* benzoyl peroxide *on page 128*

acrivastine and pseudoephedrine (AK ri vas teen & soo doe e FED rin)

Synonyms pseudoephedrine hydrochloride and acrivastine

U.S./Canadian Brand Names Semprex®-D [US]

Therapeutic Category Antihistamine/Decongestant Combination

Use Temporary relief of nasal congestion, decongest sinus openings, running nose, itching of nose or throat, and itchy, watery eyes due to hay fever or other upper respiratory allergies

Dosage Summary

Oral:
Children: Dosage not established
Adults: 1 capsule 3-4 times/day

Dosage Forms

Capsule:
Semprex®-D: Acrivastine 8 mg and pseudoephedrine 60 mg

Act® [US-OTC] *see* fluoride *on page 413*

ACT-D *see* dactinomycin *on page 266*

Actagen® Syrup *(Discontinued)* *see* triprolidine and pseudoephedrine *on page 961*
Actagen® Tablet *(Discontinued)* *see* triprolidine and pseudoephedrine *on page 961*
Act-A-Med® *(Discontinued)* *see* triprolidine and pseudoephedrine *on page 961*
Actemra® [US] *see* tocilizumab *on page 939*
Act® for Kids [US-OTC] *see* fluoride *on page 413*
ACTH *see* corticotropin *on page 251*
ActHIB® [US/Can] *see Haemophilus* B conjugate vaccine *on page 463*
Acthrel® [US] *see* corticorelin *on page 251*
Acticin® [US] *see* permethrin *on page 744*
Actidose®-Aqua [US-OTC] *see* charcoal *on page 200*
Actidose® with Sorbitol [US-OTC] *see* charcoal *on page 200*
Actifed® [Can] *see* triprolidine and pseudoephedrine *on page 961*
Actifed® Allergy Tablet (Night) *(Discontinued)*
Actifed® Cold & Allergy [US-OTC] *[reformulation]* *see* chlorpheniramine and phenylephrine *on page 208*
Actifed® Cold and Allergy *(Discontinued)* *see* triprolidine and pseudoephedrine *on page 961*
Actigall® [US] *see* ursodiol *on page 972*
Actimmune® [US/Can] *see* interferon gamma-1b *on page 516*
actinomycin *see* dactinomycin *on page 266*
actinomycin D *see* dactinomycin *on page 266*
actinomycin CI *see* dactinomycin *on page 266*
Actiq® [US/Can] *see* fentanyl *on page 395*
Activase® [US] *see* alteplase *on page 56*
Activase® rt-PA [Can] *see* alteplase *on page 56*
activated carbon *see* charcoal *on page 200*
activated charcoal *see* charcoal *on page 200*
activated dimethicone *see* simethicone *on page 875*
activated ergosterol *see* ergocalciferol *on page 358*
activated methylpolysiloxane *see* simethicone *on page 875*
activated protein C, human, recombinant *see* drotrecogin alfa *on page 334*
Activella® [US] *see* estradiol and norethindrone *on page 368*
Actonel® [US/Can] *see* risedronate *on page 844*
Actonel® and Calcium [US] *see* risedronate and calcium *on page 845*
Actonel Plus Calcium [Can] *see* risedronate and calcium *on page 845*
Actoplus Met® [US] *see* pioglitazone and metformin *on page 763*
Actoplus Met® XR [US] *see* pioglitazone and metformin *on page 763*
Actos® [US/Can] *see* pioglitazone *on page 762*
Act® x2™ [US-OTC] *see* fluoride *on page 413*
Acular® [US/Can] *see* ketorolac (ophthalmic) *on page 538*
Acular LS® [US/Can] *see* ketorolac (ophthalmic) *on page 538*
Acular® PF *(Discontinued)* *see* ketorolac (ophthalmic) *on page 538*
Acuvail™ [US] *see* ketorolac (ophthalmic) *on page 538*
ACV *see* acyclovir (systemic) *on page 36*
ACV *see* acyclovir (topical) *on page 37*
acycloguanosine *see* acyclovir (systemic) *on page 36*
acycloguanosine *see* acyclovir (topical) *on page 37*

acyclovir (systemic) (ay SYE kloe veer)

Sound-Alike/Look-Alike Issues
acyclovir may be confused with ganciclovir, Retrovir®, valacyclovir
Zovirax® may be confused with Valtrex®, Zithromax®, Zostrix®, Zyloprim®, Zyvox®

Synonyms aciclovir; ACV; acycloguanosine

U.S./Canadian Brand Names Apo-Acyclovir® [Can]; Gen-Acyclovir [Can]; Mylan-Acyclovir [Can]; Novo-Acyclovir [Can]; Nu-Acyclovir [Can]; ratio-Acyclovir [Can]; Zovirax® [US/Can]

Therapeutic Category Antiviral Agent

Use Treatment of genital herpes simplex virus (HSV) and HSV encephalitis

Dosage Summary Note: Obese patients should be dosed using ideal body weight

I.V.:

Neonates: Birth to 3 months: 10-20 mg/kg/dose every 8 hours (maximum: 60 mg/kg/day)
Children <12 years: 10-20 mg/kg/dose every 8 hours (maximum: 60 mg/kg/day)
Children ≥12 years: 5-10 mg/kg/dose **or** 500 mg/m^2/dose every 8 hours (maximum: 45 mg/kg/day)
Adults: 5-10 mg/kg/dose **or** 500 mg/m^2/dose every 8 hours (maximum: 45 mg/kg/day)

Oral:

Children <2 years: Dosage not established
Children ≥2 years and ≤40 kg: 20 mg/kg/dose 4 times/day (maximum: 800 mg/dose)
Children >40 kg: 800 mg/dose 4 times a day
Adults: 200-800 mg/dose 3-5 times/day

Dosage Forms

Capsule, oral: 200 mg
Zovirax®: 200 mg
Injection, powder for reconstitution: 500 mg, 1000 mg
Injection, solution [preservative free]: 50 mg/mL (10 mL, 20 mL)
Suspension, oral: 200 mg/5 mL (473 mL)
Zovirax®: 200 mg/5 mL (473 mL)
Tablet, oral: 400 mg, 800 mg
Zovirax®: 400 mg, 800 mg

acyclovir (topical) (ay SYE kloe veer)

Sound-Alike/Look-Alike Issues

acyclovir may be confused with ganciclovir, Retrovir®, valacyclovir
Zovirax® may be confused with Valtrex®, Zithromax®, Zostrix®, Zyloprim®, Zyvox®

Synonyms aciclovir; ACV; acycloguanosine

U.S./Canadian Brand Names Zovirax® [US/Can]

Therapeutic Category Antiviral Agent, Topical

Use Treatment of herpes labialis (cold sores), mucocutaneous HSV in immunocompromised patients

Dosage Summary

Topical:

Children <12 years: Dosage not established
Children ≥12 years: Cream: Apply 5 times/day
Adults: Cream: Apply 5 times/day; Ointment: 1/2" ribbon of ointment for a 4" square surface area 6 times/day

Dosage Forms

Cream, topical:
Zovirax®: 5% (2 g, 5 g)
Ointment, topical:
Zovirax®: 5% (15 g)

ACZ885 *see* canakinumab *on page* 173
Aczone® [US] *see* dapsone (topical) *on page* 268
AD32 *see* valrubicin *on page* 975
Adacel® [US/Can] *see* diphtheria, tetanus toxoids, and acellular pertussis vaccine *on page* 316
Adagen® [US/Can] *see* pegademase (bovine) *on page* 731
Adalat® XL® [Can] *see* nifedipine *on page* 675
Adalat® CC [US] *see* nifedipine *on page* 675
Adalat® *(Discontinued)* *see* nifedipine *on page* 675

adalimumab (a da LIM yoo mab)

Sound-Alike/Look-Alike Issues

Humira® may be confused with Humulin®, Humalog®
Humira® Pen may be confused with HumaPen® Memoir®

Synonyms antitumor necrosis factor apha (human); D2E7; human antitumor necrosis factor alpha

U.S./Canadian Brand Names Humira® [US/Can]

Therapeutic Category Antirheumatic, Disease Modifying; Monoclonal Antibody

Use

Treatment of active rheumatoid arthritis (moderate-to-severe) and active psoriatic arthritis; may be used alone or in combination with disease-modifying antirheumatic drugs (DMARDs); treatment of ankylosing spondylitis

Treatment of moderately- to severely-active Crohn disease in patients with inadequate response to conventional treatment, or patients who have lost response to or are intolerant of infliximab

Treatment of moderate-to-severe plaque psoriasis

Treatment of moderately- to severely-active juvenile idiopathic arthritis

Dosage Summary

SubQ:

Children <4 years or <15 kg: Dosage not established

Children ≥4 years: 15 kg to <30 kg: 20 mg every other week; ≥30 kg: 40 mg every other week

Adults: 40 mg every other week (maximum: 40 mg every week if not taking methotrexate in rheumatoid arthritis) **or** 160 mg (initially) given as 4 injections on day 1 or over 2 days, then 80 mg 2 weeks later (day 15); Maintenance: 40 mg every 2 weeks beginning day 29 **or** 80 mg (initially) as a single dose, followed by 40 mg every other week, beginning 1 week after initial dose

Dosage Forms

Injection, solution [preservative free]:

Humira®: 20 mg/0.4 mL (0.4 mL); 40 mg/0.8 mL (0.8 mL)

adamantanamine hydrochloride *see* amantadine *on page 61*

adapalene (a DAP a leen)

U.S./Canadian Brand Names Differin® XP [Can]; Differin® [US/Can]

Therapeutic Category Acne Products

Use Treatment of acne vulgaris

Dosage Summary

Topical:

Children ≤12 years: Dosage not established

Children >12 years: Apply once daily at bedtime

Adults: Apply once daily at bedtime

Dosage Forms

Cream, topical:

Differin®: 0.1% (45 g)

Gel, topical: 0.1% (45 g)

Differin®: 0.1% (45 g); 0.3% (45 g)

adapalene and benzoyl peroxide (a DAP a leen & BEN zoe il peer OKS ide)

Synonyms benzoyl peroxide and adapalene

U.S./Canadian Brand Names Epiduo™ [US]

Therapeutic Category Acne Products; Topical Skin Product; Topical Skin Product, Acne

Use Topical treatment of acne vulgaris

Dosage Summary

Topical:

Children ≥12 years: Apply once daily

Adults: Apply once daily

Dosage Forms

Gel, topical:

Epiduo™: Adapalene 0.1% and benzoyl peroxide 2.5% (45 g)

Adcirca™ [US/Can] *see* tadalafil *on page 908*

ADD 234037 *see* lacosamide *on page 541*

Addaprin [US-OTC] *see* ibuprofen *on page 494*

Adderall® [US] *see* dextroamphetamine and amphetamine *on page 286*

Adderall XR® [US/Can] *see* dextroamphetamine and amphetamine *on page 286*

adefovir (a DEF o veer)

Synonyms adefovir dipivoxil; bis-POM PMEA

U.S./Canadian Brand Names Hepsera® [US/Can]

Therapeutic Category Antiretroviral Agent, Nonnucleoside Reverse Transcriptase Inhibitor (NNRTI)

Use Treatment of chronic hepatitis B with evidence of active viral replication (based on persistent elevation of ALT/AST or histologic evidence), including patients with lamivudine-resistant hepatitis B

Dosage Summary

Oral:

Children <12 years: Dosage not established
Children ≥12 years: 10 mg once daily
Adults: 10 mg once daily

Dosage Forms

Tablet, oral:

Hepsera®: 10 mg

adefovir dipivoxil *see* adefovir *on page 38*
ADEKs® [US-OTC] *see* vitamins (multiple/pediatric) *on page 990*
Adenocard® [Can] *see* adenosine *on page 39*
Adenocard® IV [US] *see* adenosine *on page 39*
Adenoscan® [US/Can] *see* adenosine *on page 39*

adenosine (a DEN oh seen)

Synonyms 9-beta-d-ribofuranosyladenine

U.S./Canadian Brand Names Adenocard® IV [US]; Adenocard® [Can]; Adenoscan® [US/Can]; Adenosine Injection, USP [Can]

Therapeutic Category Antiarrhythmic Agent, Class IV; Diagnostic Agent

Use

Adenocard®: Treatment of paroxysmal supraventricular tachycardia (PSVT) including that associated with accessory bypass tracts (Wolff-Parkinson-White syndrome); when clinically advisable, appropriate vagal maneuvers should be attempted prior to adenosine administration; **not effective for conversion of atrial fibrillation, atrial flutter, or ventricular tachycardia**

Adenoscan®: Pharmacologic stress agent used in myocardial perfusion thallium-201 scintigraphy

Dosage Summary

I.V.:

Children <50 kg: Initial: 0.05-0.1 mg/kg/dose (maximum initial dose: 6 mg); repeat: 0.05-0.3 mg/kg/dose (maximum: 0.3 mg/kg/dose or 12 mg/dose)

Children ≥50 kg: Initial: 6 mg; if not effective, 12 mg may be given; may repeat 12 mg if needed (maximum: 12 mg/dose)

Adults: Initial: 6 mg, if not effective, 12 mg may be given; may repeat 12 mg if needed (maximum: 12 mg/dose)

Dosage Forms

Injection, solution [preservative free]: 3 mg/mL (2 mL, 4 mL)
Adenocard® IV: 3 mg/mL (2 mL, 4 mL)
Adenoscan®: 3 mg/mL (20 mL, 30 mL)

Adenosine Injection, USP [Can] *see* adenosine *on page 39*
ADH *see* vasopressin *on page 980*
Adipex-P® [US] *see* phentermine *on page 750*
ADL-2698 *see* alvimopan *on page 60*
Adlone® Injection *(Discontinued)* *see* methylprednisolone *on page 622*
Adoxa® [US] *see* doxycycline *on page 331*
Adoxa® Pak™ 1/75 [US] *see* doxycycline *on page 331*
Adoxa® Pak™ 1/150 [US] *see* doxycycline *on page 331*
Adrenaclick™ [US] *see* epinephrine (systemic, oral inhalation) *on page 352*
Adrenalin® [US/Can] *see* epinephrine (nasal) *on page 354*
Adrenalin® [US/Can] *see* epinephrine (systemic, oral inhalation) *on page 352*
adrenaline *see* epinephrine (nasal) *on page 354*
adrenaline *see* epinephrine (systemic, oral inhalation) *on page 352*
adrenocorticotropic hormone *see* corticotropin *on page 251*
AdreView™ [US] *see* iobenguane I 123 *on page 517*
adria *see* doxorubicin *on page 330*
Adriamycin® [US/Can] *see* doxorubicin *on page 330*

Adrucil® [US] *see* fluorouracil (systemic) *on page* 415
adsorbent charcoal *see* charcoal *on page* 200
Adsorbocarpine® Ophthalmic *(Discontinued)* *see* pilocarpine (ophthalmic) *on page* 760
Adsorbonac® *(Discontinued)* *see* sodium chloride *on page* 882
Adsorbotear® Ophthalmic Solution *(Discontinued)* *see* artificial tears *on page* 97
Advagraf™ [Can] *see* tacrolimus (systemic) *on page* 907
Advair® [Can] *see* fluticasone and salmeterol *on page* 420
Advair Diskus® [US/Can] *see* fluticasone and salmeterol *on page* 420
Advair® HFA [US] *see* fluticasone and salmeterol *on page* 420
Advanced Formula Oxy® Sensitive Gel *(Discontinued)* *see* benzoyl peroxide *on page* 128
Advanced NatalCare® *(Discontinued)* *see* vitamins (multiple/prenatal) *on page* 991
Advanced-RF NatalCare® *(Discontinued)* *see* vitamins (multiple/prenatal) *on page* 991
Advate [US/Can] *see* antihemophilic factor (recombinant) *on page* 81
Advicor® [US/Can] *see* niacin and lovastatin *on page* 672
Advil® [US-OTC/Can] *see* ibuprofen *on page* 494
Advil® Allergy Sinus [US] *see* ibuprofen, pseudoephedrine, and chlorpheniramine *on page* 496
Advil® Children's [US-OTC] *see* ibuprofen *on page* 494
Advil® Cold and Sinus Plus [Can] *see* ibuprofen, pseudoephedrine, and chlorpheniramine *on page* 496
Advil® Cold, Children's *(Discontinued)* *see* pseudoephedrine and ibuprofen *on page* 812
Advil® Cold & Sinus [US-OTC/Can] *see* pseudoephedrine and ibuprofen *on page* 812
Advil® Infants' [US-OTC] *see* ibuprofen *on page* 494
Advil® Junior *(Discontinued)* *see* ibuprofen *on page* 494
Advil® Migraine [US-OTC] *see* ibuprofen *on page* 494
Advil® Multi-Symptom Cold [US] *see* ibuprofen, pseudoephedrine, and chlorpheniramine *on page* 496
Aerius® [Can] *see* desloratadine *on page* 277
Aeroaid® *(Discontinued)*
AeroBid® [US] *see* flunisolide (oral inhalation) *on page* 409
AeroBid®-M [US] *see* flunisolide (oral inhalation) *on page* 409
Aerodine® *(Discontinued)* *see* povidone-iodine (topical) *on page* 784
aerohist plus™ [US] *see* chlorpheniramine, phenylephrine, and methscopolamine *on page* 212
aeroKid™ [US] *see* chlorpheniramine, phenylephrine, and methscopolamine *on page* 212
Afeditab® CR [US] *see* nifedipine *on page* 675
Afinitor® [US] *see* everolimus *on page* 385
Afluria® [US] *see* influenza virus vaccine (inactivated) *on page* 507
A-Free Prenatal [US] *see* vitamins (multiple/prenatal) *on page* 991
Afrin® Children's Nose Drops *(Discontinued)* *see* oxymetazoline (nasal) *on page* 716
Afrin® Extra Moisturizing [US-OTC] *see* oxymetazoline (nasal) *on page* 716
Afrinol® *(Discontinued)* *see* pseudoephedrine *on page* 810
Afrin® Original [US-OTC] *see* oxymetazoline (nasal) *on page* 716
Afrin® Saline Mist *(Discontinued)* *see* sodium chloride *on page* 882
Afrin® Severe Congestion [US-OTC] *see* oxymetazoline (nasal) *on page* 716
Afrin® Sinus [US-OTC] *see* oxymetazoline (nasal) *on page* 716
Aftate® Antifungal *(Discontinued)* *see* tolnaftate *on page* 940

agalsidase alfa *(Canada only)* (aye GAL si days AL fa)

Sound-Alike/Look-Alike Issues
agalsidase alfa may be confused with agalsidase beta, alglucerase, alglucosidase alfa

Synonyms agalsidase alpha; alpha-galactosidase-A (gene-activated)

U.S./Canadian Brand Names Replagal™ [Can]

Therapeutic Category Enzyme

Use Replacement therapy for Fabry disease

Dosage Summary

I.V.:

Children: 0.2 mg/kg every 2 weeks
Adults: 0.2 mg/kg every 2 weeks

Dosage Forms - Canada

Injection, solution [preservative free]:
Replagal™: 1 mg/1mL (3.5 mL)

agalsidase alpha *see* agalsidase alfa *(Canada only) on page 40*

agalsidase beta (aye GAL si days BAY ta)

Sound-Alike/Look-Alike Issues

agalsidase beta may be confused with agalsidase alfa, alglucerase, alglucosidase alfa

Synonyms alpha-galactosidase-A (recombinant); r-h α-GAL

U.S./Canadian Brand Names Fabrazyme® [US/Can]

Therapeutic Category Enzyme

Use Replacement therapy for Fabry disease

Dosage Summary

I.V.:

Children <8 years of age: Dosage not established
Children ≥8 years of age: 1 mg/kg every 2 weeks
Adults: 1 mg/kg every 2 weeks

Dosage Forms

Injection, powder for reconstitution:
Fabrazyme®: 5 mg, 35 mg

Agenerase® ***(Discontinued)***
Aggrastat® [US/Can] *see* tirofiban *on page 936*
Aggrenox® [US/Can] *see* aspirin and dipyridamole *on page 101*
AGN 1135 *see* rasagiline *on page 830*
AgNO$_3$ *see* silver nitrate *on page 875*
Agriflu® [US] *see* influenza virus vaccine (inactivated) *on page 507*
Agrylin® [US/Can] *see* anagrelide *on page 77*
AHA *see* acetohydroxamic acid *on page 33*
AH-Chew® [US] *see* chlorpheniramine, phenylephrine, and methscopolamine *on page 212*
AH-Chew™ Ultra [US] *see* chlorpheniramine, phenylephrine, and methscopolamine *on page 212*
AHF (human) *see* antihemophilic factor (human) *on page 81*
AHF (human) *see* antihemophilic factor/von Willebrand factor complex (human) *on page 82*
AHF (recombinant) *see* antihemophilic factor (recombinant) *on page 81*
Ahist™ [US] *see* chlorpheniramine *on page 207*
A-Hydrocort® [US] *see* hydrocortisone (systemic) *on page 482*
A-hydroCort *see* hydrocortisone (systemic) *on page 482*
A-hydroCort *see* hydrocortisone (topical) *on page 483*
AICC *see* antiinhibitor coagulant complex *on page 83*
Airet® ***(Discontinued)*** *see* albuterol *on page 43*
Airomir [Can] *see* albuterol *on page 43*
AKBeta® ***(Discontinued)*** *see* levobunolol *on page 556*
Ak-Chlor® Ophthalmic ***(Discontinued)*** *see* chloramphenicol *on page 203*
AK Cide Oph [Can] *see* sulfacetamide and prednisolone *on page 900*
AK-Con™ [US] *see* naphazoline (ophthalmic) *on page 658*
AK-Dilate™ [US] *see* phenylephrine (ophthalmic) *on page 752*
AK-Fluor® [US] *see* fluorescein *on page 412*
Ak-Homatropine® Ophthalmic ***(Discontinued)*** *see* homatropine *on page 473*
Akineton® ***(Discontinued)***
AK-Nefrin ***(Discontinued)*** *see* phenylephrine (systemic) *on page 751*
Akne-mycin® [US] *see* erythromycin (topical) *on page 362*
AK-Pentolate™ [US] *see* cyclopentolate *on page 258*

AK-Poly-Bac™ [US] *see* bacitracin and polymyxin B *on page* *113*

AK-Spore® H.C. Ophthalmic ***(Discontinued)*** *see* bacitracin, neomycin, polymyxin B, and hydrocortisone *on page* *114*

AK-Spore® H.C. Otic ***(Discontinued)*** *see* neomycin, polymyxin B, and hydrocortisone *on page* *667*

AK-Spore® Ophthalmic Ointment ***(Discontinued)*** *see* bacitracin, neomycin, and polymyxin B *on page* *114*

AK Sulf Liq [Can] *see* sulfacetamide (ophthalmic) *on page* *899*

AK-Taine® ***(Discontinued)*** *see* proparacaine *on page* *803*

Akten™ [US] *see* lidocaine (ophthalmic) *on page* *562*

AK-Tob™ [US] *see* tobramycin (ophthalmic) *on page* *938*

AK-Tracin® ***(Discontinued)*** *see* bacitracin *on page* *113*

AK-Trol® Ophthalmic Ointment ***(Discontinued)*** *see* neomycin, polymyxin B, and dexamethasone *on page* *666*

AK-Trol® Ophthalmic Suspension ***(Discontinued)*** *see* neomycin, polymyxin B, and dexamethasone *on page* *666*

Akurza ***(Discontinued)*** *see* salicylic acid *on page* *858*

Akwa Tears® [US-OTC] *see* artificial tears *on page* *97*

ALA *see* aminolevulinic acid *on page* *65*

5-ALA *see* aminolevulinic acid *on page* *65*

Alagesic [US] *see* butalbital, acetaminophen, and caffeine *on page* *159*

Alagesic LQ [US] *see* butalbital, acetaminophen, and caffeine *on page* *159*

Alamag [US-OTC] *see* aluminum hydroxide and magnesium hydroxide *on page* *59*

Alamag Plus [US-OTC] *see* aluminum hydroxide, magnesium hydroxide, and simethicone *on page* *59*

Alamast® [US/Can] *see* pemirolast *on page* *736*

Alavert® Allergy 24 Hour [US-OTC] *see* loratadine *on page* *575*

Alavert™ Allergy and Sinus [US-OTC] *see* loratadine and pseudoephedrine *on page* *576*

Alavert® Children's Allergy [US-OTC] *see* loratadine *on page* *575*

Alaway™ [US-OTC] *see* ketotifen *on page* *538*

Alazide® ***(Discontinued)*** *see* hydrochlorothiazide and spironolactone *on page* *478*

Albalon-A® Ophthalmic ***(Discontinued)***

Albalon® ***(Discontinued)*** *see* naphazoline (ophthalmic) *on page* *658*

albendazole (al BEN da zole)

Sound-Alike/Look-Alike Issues

Albenza® may be confused with Aplenzin™, Relenza®

U.S./Canadian Brand Names Albenza® [US]

Therapeutic Category Anthelmintic

Use Treatment of parenchymal neurocysticercosis caused by *Taenia solium* and cystic hydatid disease of the liver, lung, and peritoneum caused by *Echinococcus granulosus*

Dosage Summary

Oral:

Children <60 kg: 15 mg/kg/day in 2 divided doses (maximum: 800 mg/day; exceptions occur [indication specific])

Children ≥60 kg: 800 mg/day in 2 divided doses (maximum: 800 mg/day; exceptions occur [indication specific])

Adults <60 kg: 15 mg/kg/day in 2 divided doses (maximum: 800 mg/day; exceptions occur [indication specific])

Adults ≥60 kg: 800 mg/day in 2 divided doses (maximum: 800 mg/day; exceptions occur [indication specific])

Dosage Forms

Tablet, oral:

Albenza®: 200 mg

Albenza® [US] *see* albendazole *on page* *42*

Albert® Pentoxifylline [Can] *see* pentoxifylline *on page* *742*

albumin (al BYOO min)

Sound-Alike/Look-Alike Issues

Albutein® may be confused with albuterol
Buminate® may be confused with bumetanide

Synonyms albumin (human); normal human serum albumin; normal serum albumin (human); salt-poor albumin; SPA

U.S./Canadian Brand Names Albuminar®-25 [US]; Albuminar®-5 [US]; AlbuRx® 25 [US]; AlbuRx® 5 [US]; Albutein® [US]; Buminate [US]; Flexbumin 25% [US]; Human Albumin Grifols® 25% [US]; Plasbumin®-25 [US/Can]; Plasbumin®-5 [US/Can]

Therapeutic Category Blood Product Derivative

Use Plasma volume expansion and maintenance of cardiac output in the treatment of certain types of shock or impending shock; may be useful for burn patients, ARDS, and cardiopulmonary bypass; other uses considered by some investigators (but not proven) are retroperitoneal surgery, peritonitis, and ascites; unless the condition responsible for hypoproteinemia can be corrected, albumin can provide only symptomatic relief or supportive treatment

Dosage Summary **Note:** Use **5%** solution in intravascularly-depleted patients. Use **25%** solution in hypovolemic patients.

I.V.:

Children: 0.5-1 g/kg/dose (10-20 mL/kg/dose) as needed

Adults: 0.5-1 g/kg/dose as needed **or** 25 g/dose may repeat in 15-30 minutes if response inadequate (maximum: 250 g/48 hours)

Dosage Forms

Injection, solution [preservative free]: 5% [50 mg/mL] (250 mL, 500 mL); 20% [200 mg/mL] (50 mL, 100 mL); 25% [250 mg/mL] (50 mL, 100 mL)
Albuminar®-5: 5% [50 mg/mL] (250 mL, 500 mL)
Albuminar®-25: 25% [250 mg/mL] (50 mL, 100 mL)
AlbuRx® 5: 5% [50 mg/mL] (250 mL, 500 mL)
AlbuRx® 25: 25% [250 mg/mL] (50 mL, 100 mL)
Albutein®: 5% [50 mg/mL] (250 mL, 500 mL); 25% [250 mg/mL] (50 mL, 100 mL)
Buminate: 5% [50 mg/mL] (250 mL, 500 mL); 25% [250 mg/mL] (20 mL)
Flexbumin 25%: 25% [250 mg/mL] (50 mL, 100 mL)
Human Albumin Grifols® 25%: 25% [250 mg/mL] (50 mL, 100 mL)
Plasbumin®-5: 5% [50 mg/mL] (50 mL, 250 mL)
Plasbumin®-25: 25% [250 mg/mL] (20 mL, 50 mL, 100 mL)

Albuminar®-5 [US] *see* albumin *on page 43*
Albuminar®-25 [US] *see* albumin *on page 43*
albumin-bound paclitaxel *see* paclitaxel (protein bound) *on page 720*
albumin (human) *see* albumin *on page 43*
albumin-stabilized nanoparticle paclitaxel *see* paclitaxel (protein bound) *on page 720*
Albumisol® *(Discontinued)* *see* albumin *on page 43*
Albunex® *(Discontinued)* *see* albumin *on page 43*
AlbuRx® 5 [US] *see* albumin *on page 43*
AlbuRx® 25 [US] *see* albumin *on page 43*
Albutein® [US] *see* albumin *on page 43*

albuterol (al BYOO ter ole)

Sound-Alike/Look-Alike Issues

albuterol may be confused with Albutein®, atenolol
Proventil® may be confused with Bentyl®, Prilosec® Prinivil®
salbutamol may be confused with salmeterol
Ventolin® may be confused with phentolamine, Benylin®, Vantin®

Synonyms albuterol sulfate; salbutamol; salbutamol sulphate

U.S./Canadian Brand Names AccuNeb® [US]; Airomir [Can]; Apo-Salvent® CFC Free [Can]; Apo-Salvent® Sterules [Can]; Apo-Salvent® [Can]; Dom-Salbutamol [Can]; Med-Salbutamol [Can]; Mylan-Salbutamol Respirator Solution [Can]; Mylan-Salbutamol Sterinebs P.F. [Can]; Novo-Salbutamol [Can]; Nu-Salbutamol [Can]; PHL-Salbutamol [Can]; PMS-Salbutamol [Can]; ProAir® HFA [US]; Proventil® HFA [US]; ratio-Inspra-Sal [Can]; ratio-Salbutamol [Can]; Sandoz-Salbutamol [Can]; Ventolin® Diskus [Can];

Ventolin® HFA [US/Can]; Ventolin® I.V. Infusion [Can]; Ventolin® Nebules P.F. [Can]; Ventolin® [Can]; VoSpire ER® [US]

Therapeutic Category Adrenergic Agonist Agent

Use Treatment or prevention of bronchospasm in patients with reversible obstructive airway disease; prevention of exercise-induced bronchospasm

Dosage Summary

Inhalation via metered-dose inhaler (90 mcg/puff):

Children ≤4 years: 2 puffs every 4-6 hours as needed [quick relief] **or** 1-2 puffs 5 minutes prior to exercise [prevention] **or** 4-8 puffs 20 minutes for 3 doses then every 1-4 hours as needed [acute, severe exacerbation]

Children >4 years and <12 years: 2 puffs every 4-6 hours as needed (maximum: 12 puffs/day) [bronchospasm, quick-relief] **or** 2 puffs 5-30 minutes prior to exercise [prevention] **or** 4-8 puffs every 20 minutes for 3 doses then every 1-4 hours as needed [acute, severe exacerbation]

Children ≥12 years: 2 puffs every 4-6 hours as needed (maximum: 12 puffs/day) [bronchospasm, quick-relief] **or** 2 puffs 5-30 minutes prior to exercise [prevention] **or** 4-8 puffs every 20 minutes for up to 4 hours then every 1-4 hours as needed [acute, severe exacerbation]

Adults: 2 puffs every 4-6 hours as needed (maximum: 12 puffs/day) [bronchospasm, quick-relief] **or** 2 puffs 5-30 minutes prior to exercise [prevention] **or** 4-8 puffs every 20 minutes for up to 4 hours then every 1-4 hours as needed [acute, severe exacerbation]

Nebulization:

Children ≤12 years: 0.63-2.5 mg/dose every 4-6 hours as needed [bronchospasm, quick-relief] **or** 0.15 mg/kg (minimum: 2.5 mg) every 20 minutes for 3 doses then 0.15-0.3 mg/kg/dose every 1-4 hours as needed [acute, severe exacerbation] **or** continuous nebulization: 0.5 mg/kg/hour [acute, severe exacerbation]

Children >12 years: 1.25-5 mg/dose every 4-8 hours as needed [bronchospasm, quick-relief] **or** 2.5-5 mg every 20 minutes for 3 doses then 2.5-10 mg every 1-4 hours as needed [acute, severe exacerbation] **or** continuous nebulization: 10-15 mg/hour [acute, severe exacerbation]

Adults: 1.25-5 mg/dose every 4-8 hours as needed [bronchospasm, quick-relief] **or** 2.5-5 mg every 20 minutes for 3 doses then 2.5-10 mg every 1-4 hours as needed [acute, severe exacerbation] **or** continuous nebulization: 10-15 mg/hour [acute, severe exacerbation]

Oral:

Regular release:

Children <2 years: Dosage not established
Children 2-6 years: 0.1-0.2 mg/kg/dose 3 times/day (maximum: 12 mg/day)
Children 6-12 years: 2 mg/dose 3-4 times/day (maximum: 24 mg/day)
Children >12 years: 2-4 mg/dose 3-4 times/day (maximum: 32 mg/day)
Adults: 2-4 mg/dose 3-4 times/day (maximum: 32 mg/day)

Extended release:

Children <6 years: Dosage not established
Children 6-12 years: 4 mg every 12 hours (maximum: 24 mg/day)
Children >12 years: 8 mg every 12 hours (maximum: 32 mg/day)
Adults: 8 mg every 12 hours (maximum: 32 mg/day)

Dosage Forms

Aerosol, for oral inhalation:

ProAir® HFA: 90 mcg/inhalation (8.5 g)
Proventil® HFA: 90 mcg/inhalation (6.7 g)
Ventolin® HFA: 90 mcg/inhalation (8 g, 18 g)

Solution, for nebulization: 0.083% [2.5 mg/3 mL] (25s, 30s, 60s); 0.5% [100 mg/20 mL] (1s)

Solution, for nebulization [preservative free]: 0.021% [0.63 mg/3 mL] (25s); 0.042% [1.25 mg/3 mL] (25s, 30s); 0.083% [2.5 mg/3 mL] (10s, 24s, 25s, 30s, 60s); 0.5% [2.5 mg/0.5 mL] (10s, 30s)

AccuNeb®: 0.021% [0.63 mg/3 mL] (25s); 0.042% [1.25 mg/3 mL] (25s)

Syrup, oral: 2 mg/5 mL (473 mL, 480 mL)

Tablet, oral: 2 mg, 4 mg

Tablet, extended release, oral: 4 mg, 8 mg

VoSpire ER®: 4 mg, 8 mg

Dosage Forms - Canada

Injection, solution:

Ventolin® I.V.: 1 mg/1mL (5 mL)

albuterol and ipratropium *see* ipratropium and albuterol *on page 524*

albuterol sulfate *see* albuterol *on page 43*

alcaftadine (al KAF ta deen)

U.S./Canadian Brand Names Lastacaft™ [US]

Therapeutic Category Histamine H_1 Antagonist; Mast Cell Stabilizer

Use Prevention of itching associated with allergic conjunctivitis

Product Availability Lastacaft™: FDA approved July 2010; expected availability is currently undetermined; consult prescribing information for additional information

Alcaine® [US/Can] *see* proparacaine *on page 803*

Alcalak [US-OTC] *see* calcium carbonate *on page 167*

alclometasone (al kloe MET a sone)

Sound-Alike/Look-Alike Issues

Aclovate® may be confused with Accolate®

Synonyms alclometasone dipropionate

U.S./Canadian Brand Names Aclovate® [US]

Therapeutic Category Corticosteroid, Topical

Use Treatment of inflammation of corticosteroid-responsive dermatosis (low to medium potency topical corticosteroid)

Dosage Summary

Topical:

Children <1 year: Dosage not established

Children ≥1 year: Apply a thin film to the affected area 2-3 times/day. Do not use for >3 weeks.

Adults: Apply a thin film to the affected area 2-3 times/day

Dosage Forms

Cream, topical: 0.05% (15 g, 45 g, 60 g)

Aclovate®: 0.05% (15 g, 60 g)

Ointment, topical: 0.05% (15 g, 45 g, 60 g)

Aclovate®: 0.05% (15 g, 45 g, 60 g)

alclometasone dipropionate *see* alclometasone *on page 45*

alcohol, absolute *see* alcohol (ethyl) *on page 45*

alcohol, dehydrated *see* alcohol (ethyl) *on page 45*

alcohol (ethyl) (AL koe hol, ETH il)

Sound-Alike/Look-Alike Issues

ethanol may be confused with Ethyol®, Ethamolin®

Synonyms alcohol, absolute; alcohol, dehydrated; ethanol; ethyl alcohol; EtOH

U.S./Canadian Brand Names Biobase-G™ [Can]; Biobase™ [Can]; Epi-Clenz™ [US-OTC]; Gel-Stat™ [US-OTC]; GelRite™ [US-OTC]; Isagel® [US-OTC]; Lavacol® [US-OTC]; Prevacare® [US-OTC]; Protection Plus® [US-OTC], Purell® 2 in 1 [US-OTC]; Purell® Lasting Care [US-OTC]; Purell® Moisture Therapy [US-OTC]; Purell® with Aloe [US-OTC]; Purell® [US-OTC]

Therapeutic Category Intravenous Nutritional Therapy; Pharmaceutical Aid

Use Topical antiinfective; pharmaceutical aid; therapeutic neurolysis (nerve or ganglion block); replenishment of carbohydrate calories

Dosage Summary

I.V.:

Infusion:

Children: Dosage not established

Adults: 1-2 L/day of alcohol 5% and dextrose 5%

Intraneural:

Children: Dosage not established

Adults: 0.05-1 mL as a single injection per interspace

Topical:

Children: Apply 1-3 times/day as needed

Adults: Apply 1-3 times/day as needed

Dosage Forms

Aerosol, topical:

Epi-Clenz™ [OTC]: 70% (240 mL)

Gel, topical:
Epi-Clenz™ [OTC]: 70% (45 mL, 120 mL, 480 mL)
Gel-Stat™ [OTC]: 62% (120 mL, 480 mL)
GelRite™ [OTC]: 67% (120 mL, 480 mL, 800 mL)
Isagel® [OTC]: 60% (59 mL, 118 mL, 621 mL, 800 mL)
Prevacare® [OTC]: 60% (120 mL, 240 mL, 960 mL, 1200 mL, 1500 mL)
Purell® [OTC]: 62% (15 mL, 30 mL, 59 mL, 60 mL, 120 mL, 236 mL, 240 mL, 250 mL, 360 mL, 500 mL, 800 mL, 1000 mL, 2000 mL)
Purell® Lasting Care [OTC]: 62% (120 mL, 240 mL, 1000 mL)
Purell® Moisture Therapy [OTC]: 62% (75 mL)
Purell® with Aloe [OTC]: 62% (15 mL, 59 mL, 60 mL, 120 mL, 236 mL, 354 mL, 800 mL, 1000 mL, 2000 mL)
Injection, solution [preservative free]: ≥ 98% (1 mL, 5 mL)
Liquid, topical: 70% (480 mL, 3840 mL)
Lavacol® [OTC]: 70% (473 mL)
Lotion, topical:
Purell® 2 in 1 [OTC]: 62% (60 mL, 360 mL, 1000 mL)
Pad, topical:
Isagel® [OTC]: 60% (50s, 300s)
Purell® [OTC]: 62% (24s, 35s, 175s)
Solution, topical:
Protection Plus® [OTC]: 62% (800 mL)

Alconefrin® Nasal Solution *(Discontinued)* *see* phenylephrine (nasal) *on page* 751
Alcortin™ [US] *see* iodoquinol and hydrocortisone *on page* 519
Aldactazide® [US] *see* hydrochlorothiazide and spironolactone *on page* 478
Aldactazide 25® [Can] *see* hydrochlorothiazide and spironolactone *on page* 478
Aldactazide 50® [Can] *see* hydrochlorothiazide and spironolactone *on page* 478
Aldactone® [US/Can] *see* spironolactone *on page* 894
Aldara® [US/Can] *see* imiquimod *on page* 501

aldesleukin (al des LOO kin)

Sound-Alike/Look-Alike Issues
aldesleukin may be confused with oprelvekin
Proleukin® may be confused with oprelvekin

Synonyms IL-2; interleukin 2; interleukin-2; lymphocyte mitogenic factor; recombinant human interleukin-2; T-cell growth factor; TCGF; thymocyte stimulating factor

U.S./Canadian Brand Names Proleukin® [US/Can]

Therapeutic Category Biological Response Modulator

Use Treatment of metastatic renal cell cancer, metastatic melanoma

Dosage Summary
I.V.:
Children: Dosage not established
Adults: 600,000 int. units/kg every 8 hours (maximum: 14 doses); may repeat after 9 days for a total of 28 doses/course

Dosage Forms
Injection, powder for reconstitution:
Proleukin®: 22 x 10^6 int. units

Aldex™ [US] *see* guaifenesin and phenylephrine *on page* 456
Aldex® AN [US] *see* doxylamine *on page* 332
Aldex® CT [US] *see* diphenhydramine and phenylephrine *on page* 312
Aldex®D [US] *see* phenylephrine and pyrilamine *on page* 753
Aldex® DM [US] *see* phenylephrine, pyrilamine, and dextromethorphan *on page* 755
Aldomet® *(Discontinued)* *see* methyldopa *on page* 618
Aldoril® D50 *(Discontinued)* *see* methyldopa and hydrochlorothiazide *on page* 619
Aldoril® *(Discontinued)* *see* methyldopa and hydrochlorothiazide *on page* 619
Aldroxicon I [US-OTC] *see* aluminum hydroxide, magnesium hydroxide, and simethicone *on page* 59
Aldroxicon II [US-OTC] *see* aluminum hydroxide, magnesium hydroxide, and simethicone *on page* 59
Aldurazyme® [US/Can] *see* laronidase *on page* 550

alefacept (a LE fa sept)

Synonyms B 9273; BG 9273; human LFA-3/IgG(1) fusion protein; LFA-3/IgG(1) fusion protein, human

U.S./Canadian Brand Names Amevive® [US/Can]

Therapeutic Category Monoclonal Antibody

Use Treatment of moderate-to-severe chronic plaque psoriasis in adults who are candidates for systemic therapy or phototherapy

Dosage Summary

I.M.:

Children: Dosage not established

Adults: 15 mg once weekly for 12 weeks

Dosage Forms

Injection, powder for reconstitution:

Amevive®: 15 mg

alemtuzumab (ay lem TU zoo mab)

Synonyms anti-CD52 monoclonal antibody; campath-1H; humanized IgG1 anti-CD52 monoclonal antibody; MoAb CD52; monoclonal antibody campath-1H; monoclonal antibody CD52

U.S./Canadian Brand Names Campath® [US]; MabCampath® [Can]

Therapeutic Category Antineoplastic Agent, Monoclonal Antibody

Use Treatment of B-cell chronic lymphocytic leukemia (B-CLL)

Dosage Summary Note: Dose escalation is required

I.V. (infusion):

Children: Dosage not established

Adults: Initial: 3 mg/day, then 10 mg/day; Maintenance: 30 mg/day 3 times/week on alternate days; Maximum dose: 30 mg/day; 90 mg/week (cumulative)

Dosage Forms

Injection, solution [preservative free]:

Campath®: 30 mg/mL (1 mL)

alendronate (a LEN droe nate)

Sound-Alike/Look-Alike Issues

alendronate may be confused with risedronate

Fosamax® may be confused with Flomax®, Fosamax Plus D®, fosinopril, Zithromax®

Synonyms alendronate sodium; alendronic acid monosodium salt trihydrate; MK-217

U.S./Canadian Brand Names Alendronate-FC [Can]; Apo-Alendronate® [Can]; CO Alendronate [Can]; Dom-Alendronate [Can]; Fosamax® [US/Can]; Mylan-Alendronate [Can]; Novo-Alendronate [Can]; PHL-Alendronate [Can]; PMS-Alendronate [Can]; PMS-Alendronate-FC [Can]; ratio-Alendronate [Can]; Riva-Alendronate [Can]; Sandoz Alendronate [Can]; Teva-Alendronate [Can]

Therapeutic Category Bisphosphonate Derivative

Use Treatment and prevention of osteoporosis in postmenopausal females; treatment of osteoporosis in males; Paget disease of the bone in patients who are symptomatic, at risk for future complications, or with alkaline phosphatase ≥2 times the upper limit of normal; treatment of glucocorticoid-induced osteoporosis in males and females with low bone mineral density who are receiving a daily dosage ≥7.5 mg of prednisone (or equivalent)

Dosage Summary

Oral:

Children: Dosage not established

Adults: 5-10 mg/day **or** 35-70 mg once weekly (maximum: 70 mg/week; exceptions occur [indication specific])

Dosage Forms

Solution, oral:

Fosamax®: 70 mg/75 mL (75 mL)

Tablet, oral: 5 mg, 10 mg, 35 mg, 40 mg, 70 mg

Fosamax®: 5 mg, 10 mg, 35 mg, 40 mg, 70 mg

alendronate and cholecalciferol (a LEN droe nate & kole e kal SI fer ole)

Sound-Alike/Look-Alike Issues

Fosamax Plus D® may be confused with Fosamax®

Synonyms alendronate sodium and cholecalciferol; cholecalciferol and alendronate; vitamin D_3 and alendronate

U.S./Canadian Brand Names Fosamax Plus D® [US]; Fosavance [Can]

Therapeutic Category Bisphosphonate Derivative; Vitamin D Analog

Use Treatment of osteoporosis in postmenopausal females; increase bone mass in males with osteoporosis

Dosage Summary

Oral:

Children: Dosage not established

Adults: One tablet once weekly

Dosage Forms

Tablet:

Fosamax Plus D® 70/2800: Alendronate 70 mg and cholecalciferol 2800 int. units

Fosamax Plus D® 70/5600: Alendronate 70 mg and cholecalciferol 5600 int. units

Alendronate-FC [Can] *see* alendronate *on page* 47

alendronate sodium *see* alendronate *on page* 47

alendronate sodium and cholecalciferol *see* alendronate and cholecalciferol *on page* 47

alendronic acid monosodium salt trihydrate *see* alendronate *on page* 47

Alenic Alka *(Discontinued)* *see* aluminum hydroxide and magnesium carbonate *on page* 58

Alenic Alka Tablet [US-OTC] *see* aluminum hydroxide and magnesium trisilicate *on page* 59

Aler-Cap [US-OTC] *see* diphenhydramine (systemic) *on page* 310

Aler-Dryl [US-OTC] *see* diphenhydramine (systemic) *on page* 310

Aler-Tab [US-OTC] *see* diphenhydramine (systemic) *on page* 310

Alertec® [Can] *see* modafinil *on page* 639

Alesse® [US/Can] *see* ethinyl estradiol and levonorgestrel *on page* 376

Aleve® [US-OTC] *see* naproxen *on page* 659

Aleve®-D Sinus & Cold [US-OTC] *see* naproxen and pseudoephedrine *on page* 661

Aleve®-D Sinus & Headache [US-OTC] *see* naproxen and pseudoephedrine *on page* 661

Aleve® Cold & Sinus *(Discontinued)* *see* naproxen and pseudoephedrine *on page* 661

Alfenta® [US/Can] *see* alfentanil *on page* 48

alfentanil (al FEN ta nil)

Sound-Alike/Look-Alike Issues

alfentanil may be confused with Anafranil®, fentanyl, remifentanil, sufentanil

Alfenta® may be confused with Sufenta®

Synonyms alfentanil hydrochloride

U.S./Canadian Brand Names Alfentanil Injection, USP [Can]; Alfenta® [US/Can]

Therapeutic Category Analgesic, Narcotic; General Anesthetic

Controlled Substance C-II

Use Analgesic adjunct for the induction and maintenance of general anesthesia; analgesic component for monitored anesthesia care (MAC)

Dosage Summary Note: Dosage should be based on ideal body weight

I.V.:

Anesthetic Induction:

Children <12 years: Dosage not established

Children ≥12 years: Initial: 130-245 mcg/kg; Maintenance: 0.5-1.5 mcg/kg/minute

Adults: Initial: 130-245 mcg/kg; Maintenance: 0.5-1.5 mcg/kg/minute

Continuous infusion:

Children <12 years: Dosage not established

Children ≥12 years: Initial: 50-75 mcg/kg; Maintenance: 0.5-3 mcg/kg/minute

Adults: Initial: 50-75 mcg/kg; Maintenance: 0.5-3 mcg/kg/minute

Incremental injection:
Children <12 years: Dosage not established
Children ≥12 years:
≤30 minutes anesthesia: Initial: 8-20 mcg/kg; Maintenance: 3-5 mcg/kg **or** 0.5-1 mcg/kg/minute (maximum: 40 mcg/kg total dose)
≥30 minutes anesthesia: Initial: 20-50 mcg/kg; Maintenance: 5-15 mcg/kg (maximum: 75 mcg/kg total dose)
Adults:
≤30 minutes anesthesia: Initial: 8-20 mcg/kg; Maintenance: 3-5 mcg/kg **or** 0.5-1 mcg/kg/minute (maximum: 40 mcg/kg total dose)
≥30 minutes anesthesia: Initial: 20-50 mcg/kg; Maintenance: 5-15 mcg/kg (maximum: 75 mcg/kg total dose)

Dosage Forms
Injection, solution [preservative free]: 500 mcg/mL (2 mL, 5 mL, 10 mL, 20 mL)
Alfenta®: 500 mcg/mL (2 mL, 5 mL)

alfentanil hydrochloride *see* alfentanil *on page 48*
Alfentanil Injection, USP [Can] *see* alfentanil *on page 48*
Alferon® N [US/Can] *see* interferon alfa-n3 *on page 515*

alfuzosin (al FYOO zoe sin)

Synonyms alfuzosin hydrochloride
U.S./Canadian Brand Names Apo-Alfuzosin® [Can]; Sandoz-Alfuzosin [Can]; Uroxatral® [US]; Xatral [Can]
Therapeutic Category Alpha-Adrenergic Blocking Agent
Use Treatment of the functional symptoms of benign prostatic hyperplasia (BPH)
Dosage Summary
Oral:
Children: Dosage not established
Adults: 10 mg once daily
Dosage Forms
Tablet, extended release, oral:
Uroxatral®: 10 mg

alfuzosin hydrochloride *see* alfuzosin *on page 49*

alglucerase (al GLOO ser ase)

Sound-Alike/Look-Alike Issues
alglucerase may be confused with agalsidase alfa, agalsidase beta, alglucosidase alfa
Ceredase® may be confused with Cerezyme®
Synonyms glucocerebrosidase
U.S./Canadian Brand Names Ceredase® [US]
Therapeutic Category Enzyme
Use Replacement therapy for Gaucher disease (type 1)
Dosage Summary Note: Dosage is individualized based on disease severity
I.V.:
Children: Initial: 30-60 units/kg every 2 weeks; Maintenance (range): 2.5 units/kg 3 times/week to 60 units/kg 1-4 times/week
Adults: Initial: 30-60 units/kg every 2 weeks; Maintenance (range): 2.5 units/kg 3 times/week to 60 units/kg once weekly to every 4 weeks
Dosage Forms
Injection, solution [preservative free]:
Ceredase®: 80 units/mL (5 mL)

alglucosidase *see* alglucosidase alfa *on page 49*

alglucosidase alfa (al gloo KOSE i dase AL fa)

Sound-Alike/Look-Alike Issues
alglucosidase alfa may be confused with agalsidase alfa, agalsidase beta, alglucerase
Synonyms alglucosidase; GAA; rhGAA
U.S./Canadian Brand Names Lumizyme™ [US]; Myozyme® [US/Can]

Therapeutic Category Enzyme

Use

Lumizyme™: Replacement therapy for late-onset (noninfantile) Pompe disease without evidence of cardiac hypertrophy in patients 8 years and older

Myozyme®: Replacement therapy for infantile-onset Pompe disease

Dosage Summary

I.V.:

Myozyme®:

Children <1 month: Dosage not established

Children 1 month to 3.5 years (at first infusion): 20 mg/kg over ~4 hours every 2 weeks

Children >3.5 years: Dosage not established

Adults: Dosage not established

Lumizyme™:

Children <8 years: Not recommended

Children ≥8 years: 20 mg/kg over ~4 hours every 2 weeks

Adults: 20 mg/kg over ~4 hours every 2 weeks

Dosage Forms

Injection, powder for reconstitution:

Lumizyme™: 50 mg

Myozyme®: 50 mg

Aliclen™ [US] *see* salicylic acid *on page 858*

Alimta® [US/Can] *see* pemetrexed *on page 735*

Alinia® [US] *see* nitazoxanide *on page 677*

aliskiren (a lis KYE ren)

Sound-Alike/Look-Alike Issues

Tekturna® may be confused with Valturna®

Synonyms aliskiren hemifumarate; SPP100

U.S./Canadian Brand Names Rasilez® [Can]; Tekturna® [US]

Therapeutic Category Renin Inhibitor

Use Treatment of hypertension, alone or in combination with other antihypertensive agents

Dosage Summary

Oral:

Children <18 years: Dosage not established

Adults: 150-300 mg once daily (maximum: 300 mg/day)

Dosage Forms

Tablet, oral:

Tekturna®: 150 mg, 300 mg

aliskiren and hydrochlorothiazide (a lis KYE ren & hye droe klor oh THYE a zide)

Synonyms aliskiren hemifumarate and hydrochlorothiazide; hydrochlorothiazide and aliskiren

U.S./Canadian Brand Names Tekturna HCT® [US]

Therapeutic Category Antihypertensive Agent, Combination; Diuretic, Thiazide; Renin Inhibitor

Use Treatment of hypertension, including use as initial therapy in patients likely to need multiple antihypertensives for adequate control

Dosage Summary

Oral:

Children: Dosage not established

Adults: Aliskiren 150-300 mg and hydrochlorothiazide 12.5-25 mg once daily (maximum: 300 mg/day [aliskiren]; 25 mg/day [hydrochlorothiazide])

Dosage Forms

Tablet:

Tekturna HCT®: 150/12.5: Aliskiren 150 mg and hydrochlorothiazide 12.5 mg; 150/25: Aliskiren 150 mg and hydrochlorothiazide 25 mg; 300/12.5: Aliskiren 300 mg and hydrochlorothiazide 12.5 mg; 300/25: Aliskiren 300 mg and hydrochlorothiazide 25 mg

aliskiren and valsartan (a lis KYE ren & val SAR tan)

Sound-Alike/Look-Alike Issues

Valturna® may be confused with Tekturna®, valsartan

Synonyms aliskiren hemifumarate and valsartan; valsartan and aliskiren

U.S./Canadian Brand Names Valturna® [US]

Therapeutic Category Angiotensin II Receptor Blocker; Renin Inhibitor

Use Treatment of hypertension, including use as initial therapy in patients likely to need multiple antihypertensives for adequate control

Dosage Summary

Oral:

Children: Dosage not established

Adults: Aliskiren 150-300 mg and valsartan 160-320 mg once daily (maximum: 300 mg/day [aliskiren]; 320 mg/day [valsartan])

Dosage Forms

Tablet:

Valturna®: 150/160: Aliskiren 150 mg and valsartan 160 mg; 300/320: Aliskiren 300 mg and valsartan 320 mg

aliskiren hemifumarate *see* aliskiren *on page* 50

aliskiren hemifumarate and hydrochlorothiazide *see* aliskiren and hydrochlorothiazide *on page* 50

aliskiren hemifumarate and valsartan *see* aliskiren and valsartan *on page* 51

alitretinoin (a li TRET i noyn)

Sound-Alike/Look-Alike Issues

Panretin® may be confused with pancreatin

U.S./Canadian Brand Names Panretin® [US/Can]

Therapeutic Category Antineoplastic Agent; Retinoic Acid Derivative

Use Orphan drug: Topical treatment of cutaneous lesions in AIDS-related Kaposi sarcoma

Dosage Summary

Topical:

Children: Dosage not established

Adults: Apply twice daily to cutaneous lesions

Dosage Forms

Gel, topical:

Panretin®: 0.1% (60 g)

Alka-Mints® [US-OTC] *see* calcium carbonate *on page* 167

Alka-Seltzer Plus® Day Cold [US-OTC] *see* acetaminophen, dextromethorphan, and phenylephrine *on page* 29

Alka-Seltzer Plus® Sinus Formula [US-OTC] *see* acetaminophen and phenylephrine *on page* 25

Alka-Seltzer® P.M. [US-OTC] *see* aspirin and diphenhydramine *on page* 101

Alkeran® [US/Can] *see* melphalan *on page* 599

Allanderm-T™ *(Discontinued)* *see* trypsin, balsam Peru, and castor oil *on page* 964

AllanEnzyme *(Discontinued)*

Allanfil 405 *(Discontinued)*

Allanfil Spray *(Discontinued)*

AllanFol RX *(Discontinued)* *see* folic acid, cyanocobalamin, and pyridoxine *on page* 423

AllanHist PDX *(Discontinued)* *see* brompheniramine, pseudoephedrine, and dextromethorphan *on page* 149

AllanTan Pediatric *(Discontinued)* *see* chlorpheniramine and phenylephrine *on page* 208

AllanVan-S *(Discontinued)* *see* phenylephrine and pyrilamine *on page* 753

All Day Allergy [US-OTC] *see* cetirizine *on page* 198

Allegra® [US/Can] *see* fexofenadine *on page* 400

Allegra® 60 mg Capsule *(Discontinued)* *see* fexofenadine *on page* 400

Allegra-D® [Can] *see* fexofenadine and pseudoephedrine *on page* 400

Allegra-D® 12 Hour [US] *see* fexofenadine and pseudoephedrine *on page* 400

Allegra-D® 24 Hour [US] *see* fexofenadine and pseudoephedrine *on page 400*
Allegra® ODT [US] *see* fexofenadine *on page 400*
Aller-Chlor® [US-OTC] *see* chlorpheniramine *on page 207*
Allercon® Tablet *(Discontinued)* *see* triprolidine and pseudoephedrine *on page 961*
Allerdryl® [Can] *see* diphenhydramine (systemic) *on page 310*
AllerDur™ *(Discontinued)* *see* dexchlorpheniramine and pseudoephedrine *on page 283*
Allerest® 12 Hour Nasal Solution *(Discontinued)* *see* oxymetazoline (nasal) *on page 716*
Allerest® Eye Drops *(Discontinued)* *see* naphazoline (ophthalmic) *on page 658*
Allerest® Maximum Strength Allergy and Hay Fever [US-OTC] *see* chlorpheniramine and pseudoephedrine *on page 209*
Allerfrim [US-OTC] *see* triprolidine and pseudoephedrine *on page 961*
Allerfrin® Syrup *(Discontinued)* *see* triprolidine and pseudoephedrine *on page 961*
Allerfrin® Tablet *(Discontinued)* *see* triprolidine and pseudoephedrine *on page 961*
Allerfrin® with Codeine *(Discontinued)* *see* triprolidine, pseudoephedrine, and codeine *(Canada only) on page 961*
Allergen® [US] *see* antipyrine and benzocaine *on page 83*
AllerMax® [US-OTC] *see* diphenhydramine (systemic) *on page 310*
Allernix [Can] *see* diphenhydramine (systemic) *on page 310*
AllerTan™ *(Discontinued)* *see* chlorpheniramine, pyrilamine, and phenylephrine *on page 215*
AlleRx™-D [US] *see* pseudoephedrine and methscopolamine *on page 813*
AlleRx™ Dose Pack *(Discontinued)* *see* chlorpheniramine, pseudoephedrine, and methscopolamine *on page 215*
AlleRx™ Suspension *(Discontinued)* *see* chlorpheniramine and phenylephrine *on page 208*
Allfen [US-OTC] *see* guaifenesin *on page 454*
Allfen DM [US-OTC] *see* guaifenesin and dextromethorphan *on page 455*
Alli™ [US-OTC] *see* orlistat *on page 707*
All-Nite [US-OTC] *see* acetaminophen, dextromethorphan, and doxylamine *on page 29*
All-Nite Multi-Symptom Cold/Flu [US-OTC] *see* acetaminophen, dextromethorphan, doxylamine, and pseudoephedrine *on page 30*
Alloprin® [Can] *see* allopurinol *on page 52*

allopurinol (al oh PURE i nole)

Sound-Alike/Look-Alike Issues

allopurinol may be confused with Apresoline

Zyloprim® may be confused with Xylo-Pfan®, ZORprin®, Zovirax®

Synonyms allopurinol sodium

U.S./Canadian Brand Names Alloprin® [Can]; Aloprim® [US]; Apo-Allopurinol® [Can]; Novo-Purol [Can]; Zyloprim® [US/Can]

Therapeutic Category Xanthine Oxidase Inhibitor

Use

Oral: Prevention of attack of gouty arthritis and nephropathy; treatment of secondary hyperuricemia which may occur during treatment of tumors or leukemia; prevention of recurrent calcium oxalate calculi

I.V.: Treatment of elevated serum and urinary uric acid levels when oral therapy is not tolerated in patients with leukemia, lymphoma, and solid tumor malignancies who are receiving cancer chemotherapy

Dosage Summary

I.V.:

Children ≤10 years: Initial: 200 mg/m^2/day as a single infusion or in equally divided doses at 6-, 8-, or 12-hour intervals

Children >10 years: 200-400 mg/m^2/day as a single infusion or in equally divided doses at 6-, 8-, or 12-hour intervals (maximum: 600 mg/day)

Adults: 200-400 mg/m^2/day as a single infusion or in equally divided doses at 6-, 8-, or 12-hour intervals (maximum: 600 mg/day)

Oral:

Children <6 years: 150 mg/day in 3 divided doses **or** 10 mg/kg/day in 2-3 divided doses **or** 200-300 mg/m^2/day in 2-4 divided doses (maximum: 800 mg/day)

Children 6-10 years: 300 mg/day in 2-3 divided doses **or** 10 mg/kg/day in 2-3 divided doses **or** 200-300 mg/m^2/day in 2-4 divided doses (maximum: 800 mg/day)

Children >10 years: 100-800 mg/day in 1-3 divided doses (maximum: 800 mg/day)
Adults: 100-800 mg/day in 1-3 divided doses (maximum: 800 mg/day)
Elderly: Initial: 100 mg/day; increase until desired uric acid level is obtained

Dosage Forms

Injection, powder for reconstitution: 500 mg (base)
Aloprim®: 500 mg (base)
Tablet, oral: 100 mg, 300 mg
Zyloprim®: 100 mg, 300 mg

allopurinol sodium *see* allopurinol *on page 52*
all-*trans* retinoic acid *see* tretinoin (systemic) *on page 951*
all-*trans* vitamin A acid *see* tretinoin (systemic) *on page 951*
Almacone® [US-OTC] *see* aluminum hydroxide, magnesium hydroxide, and simethicone *on page 59*
Almacone Double Strength® [US-OTC] *see* aluminum hydroxide, magnesium hydroxide, and simethicone *on page 59*

almotriptan (al moh TRIP tan)

Sound-Alike/Look-Alike Issues

Axert® may be confused with Antivert®

Synonyms almotriptan malate

U.S./Canadian Brand Names Axert® [US/Can]

Therapeutic Category Serotonin 5-HT_{1D} Receptor Agonist

Use Acute treatment of migraine with or without aura in adults (with a history of migraine) and adolescents (with a history of migraine lasting ≥4 hours when left untreated)

Dosage Summary

Oral:
Children <12 years: Dosage not established
Children ≥12 years: 6.25-12.5 mg in a single dose; may repeat after 2 hours (maximum daily dose: 25 mg)
Adults: 6.25-12.5 mg in a single dose; may repeat after 2 hours (maximum daily dose: 25 mg)

Dosage Forms

Tablet, oral:
Axert®: 6.25 mg, 12.5 mg

almotriptan malate *see* almotriptan *on page 53*
Alocril® [US/Can] *see* nedocromil *on page 664*
Alodox™ [US] *see* doxycycline *on page 331*
Aloe Vesta® Antifungal [US-OTC] *see* miconazole (topical) *on page 630*
Alomide® [US/Can] *see* lodoxamide *on page 572*
Alophen® [US-OTC] *see* bisacodyl *on page 138*
Aloprim® [US] *see* allopurinol *on page 52*
Alor® 5/500 *(Discontinued)*
Alora® [US] *see* estradiol (systemic) *on page 366*

alosetron (a LOE se tron)

Sound-Alike/Look-Alike Issues

Lotronex® may be confused with Lovenox®, Protonix®

U.S./Canadian Brand Names Lotronex® [US]

Therapeutic Category 5-HT_3 Receptor Antagonist

Use Treatment of women with severe diarrhea-predominant irritable bowel syndrome (IBS) who have failed to respond to conventional therapy

Dosage Summary

Oral:
Children: Dosage not established
Adults: Initial: 0.5 mg twice daily; after 4 weeks of therapy may increase to 1 mg twice daily if needed (maximum: 2 mg/day).

Dosage Forms

Tablet, oral:
Lotronex®: 0.5 mg, 1 mg

Aloxi® [US] *see* palonosetron *on page* 721

Alpain ***(Discontinued)*** *see* acetaminophen and phenyltoloxamine *on page* 26

alpha$_1$-antiprotease *see* alpha$_1$-proteinase inhibitor *on page* 54

alpha$_1$-antitrypsin *see* alpha$_1$-proteinase inhibitor *on page* 54

alpha$_1$-PI *see* alpha$_1$-proteinase inhibitor *on page* 54

alpha$_1$-proteinase inhibitor, human *see* alpha$_1$-proteinase inhibitor *on page* 54

alpha$_1$-proteinase inhibitor (al fa won PRO tee in ase in HI bi tor)

Synonyms A$_1$-PI; alpha$_1$-antiprotease; alpha$_1$-antitrypsin; alpha$_1$-PI; alpha$_1$-proteinase inhibitor, human; α_1-PI

U.S./Canadian Brand Names Aralast NP [US]; Aralast [US]; Prolastin® [Can]; Prolastin®-C [US/Can]; Zemaira® [US]

Therapeutic Category Antitrypsin Deficiency Agent

Use Replacement therapy in congenital alpha$_1$-proteinase inhibitor (alpha$_1$-antitrypsin) deficiency with clinical emphysema

Dosage Summary

I.V.:

Children: Dosage not established

Adults: 60 mg/kg once weekly

Dosage Forms

Injection, powder for reconstitution [preservative free]:

Aralast: ~500 mg, ~1000 mg

Aralast NP: ~500 mg, ~1000 mg

Prolastin®-C: ~1000 mg

Zemaira®: ~1000 mg

alpha-galactosidase (AL fa ga lak TOE si days)

Sound-Alike/Look-Alike Issues

beano® may be confused with B&O (belladonna and opium)

Synonyms *Aspergillus niger*

U.S./Canadian Brand Names beano® [US-OTC]

Therapeutic Category Enzyme

Use Prevention of flatulence and bloating attributed to a variety of grains, cereals, nuts, and vegetables containing the sugars raffinose, stachyose, and/or verbascose

Dosage Summary

Oral:

Children <12 years: Dosage not established

Children ≥12 years:

Drops: 5 drops per serving; 10-15 drops/meal

Tablet: 1 tablet per serving; 2-3 tablets/meal

Adults:

Drops: 5 drops per serving; 10-15 drops/meal

Tablet: 1 tablet per serving; 2-3 tablets/meal

Dosage Forms

Liquid, oral:

beano® [OTC]: 150 Galactosidase units/5 drops (15 mL)

Tablet, oral:

beano® [OTC]: 150 Galactosidase units

alpha-galactosidase-A (gene-activated) *see* agalsidase alfa *(Canada only) on page* 40

alpha-galactosidase-A (recombinant) *see* agalsidase beta *on page* 41

1α-hydroxyergocalciferol *see* doxercalciferol *on page* 329

Alphagan® [Can] *see* brimonidine *on page* 144

Alphagan® ***(Discontinued)*** *see* brimonidine *on page* 144

Alphagan® P [US] *see* brimonidine *on page* 144

Alphamul® ***(Discontinued)*** *see* castor oil *on page* 187

Alphanate® ***[new formulation]*** **[US]** *see* antihemophilic factor/von Willebrand factor complex (human) *on page* 82

AlphaNine® SD [US] *see* factor IX *on page* 389
Alphaquin HP® [US] *see* hydroquinone *on page* 487
Alph-E [US-OTC] *see* vitamin E *on page* 988
Alph-E-Mixed [US-OTC] *see* vitamin E *on page* 988

alprazolam (al PRAY zoe lam)

Sound-Alike/Look-Alike Issues
ALPRAZolam may be confused with alprostadil, LORazepam, triazolam
Xanax® may be confused with Lanoxin®, Tenex®, Tylox®, Xopenex®, Zantac®, Zyrtec®

Tall-Man **ALPRAZ**olam

U.S./Canadian Brand Names Alprazolam Intensol™ [US]; Alti-Alprazolam [Can]; Apo-Alpraz® TS [Can]; Apo-Alpraz® [Can]; Mylan-Alprazolam [Can]; Niravam™ [US]; Novo-Alprazol [Can]; Nu-Alpraz [Can]; Xanax TS™ [Can]; Xanax XR® [US]; Xanax® [US/Can]

Therapeutic Category Benzodiazepine

Controlled Substance C-IV

Use Treatment of anxiety disorder (GAD); panic disorder, with or without agoraphobia; anxiety associated with depression

Dosage Summary

Oral:

Immediate release:

Adults: 0.5-6 mg/day in divided doses (maximum: 10 mg/day); **Note:** Titration is recommended
Elderly: Initial: 0.125-0.25 mg 2-3 times/day; Maintenance: Increase by 0.125 mg/day as needed; smallest effective dose should be used

Extended release:

Children: Dosage not established
Adults: 0.5-6 mg/day as a single dose (maximum: 6 mg/day); **Note:** Titration is recommended
Elderly: Initial: 0.5 mg/day

Dosage Forms

Solution, oral:
Alprazolam Intensol™: 1 mg/mL (30 mL)

Tablet, oral: 0.25 mg, 0.5 mg, 1 mg, 2 mg
Xanax®: 0.25 mg, 0.5 mg, 1 mg, 2 mg

Tablet, extended release, oral: 0.5 mg, 1 mg, 2 mg, 3 mg
Xanax XR®: 0.5 mg, 1 mg, 2 mg, 3 mg

Tablet, orally disintegrating, oral: 0.25 mg, 0.5 mg, 1 mg, 2 mg
Niravam™: 0.25 mg, 0.5 mg, 1 mg, 2 mg

Alprazolam Intensol™ [US] *see* alprazolam *on page* 55

alprostadil (al PROS ta dill)

Sound-Alike/Look-Alike Issues
alprostadil may be confused with ALPRAZolam

Synonyms PGE_1; prostaglandin E_1

U.S./Canadian Brand Names Caverject Impulse® [US]; Caverject® [US/Can]; Edex® [US]; Muse® Pellet [Can]; Muse® [US]; Prostin VR Pediatric® [US]; Prostin® VR [Can]

Therapeutic Category Prostaglandin

Use

Prostin VR Pediatric®: Temporary maintenance of patency of ductus arteriosus in neonates with ductal-dependent congenital heart disease until surgery can be performed. These defects include cyanotic (eg, pulmonary atresia, pulmonary stenosis, tricuspid atresia, Fallot tetralogy, transposition of the great vessels) and acyanotic (eg, interruption of aortic arch, coarctation of aorta, hypoplastic left ventricle) heart disease.

Caverject®: Treatment of erectile dysfunction of vasculogenic, psychogenic, or neurogenic etiology; adjunct in the diagnosis of erectile dysfunction

Edex®, Muse®: Treatment of erectile dysfunction of vasculogenic, psychogenic, or neurogenic etiology

Dosage Summary

I.V.:

Neonates: Initial: 0.05-0.1 mcg/kg/minute; Maintenance: 0.01-0.4 mcg/kg/minute
Children: Dosage not established
Adults: Dosage not established

Intracavernous:

Children: Dosage not established

Adults: Initial: 1.25-2.5 mcg; increase by 2.5 mcg to 5 mcg then in increments of 5-10 mcg until suitable response; Maintenance: Effective dose no more than 3 times/week with at least 24 hours between doses (maximum: 40 mcg/dose [Edex®]; 60 mcg/dose [Caverject®])

Intraurethral:

Children: Dosage not established

Adults: Initial: 125-250 mcg; Maintenance: As needed (maximum: 2 doses/day)

Dosage Forms

Injection, powder for reconstitution:

Caverject Impulse®: 10 mcg, 20 mcg

Caverject®: 20 mcg, 40 mcg

Edex®: 10 mcg, 20 mcg, 40 mcg

Injection, solution: 500 mcg/mL (1 mL)

Prostin VR Pediatric®: 500 mcg/mL (1 mL)

Pellet, urethral:

Muse®: 250 mcg (6s); 500 mcg (6s); 1000 mcg (6s)

Alrex® [US/Can] *see* loteprednol *on page* 578

AL-Rr® Oral *(Discontinued)* *see* chlorpheniramine *on page* 207

Altabax™ [US] *see* retapamulin *on page* 836

Altace® [US/Can] *see* ramipril *on page* 826

Altace® HCT [Can] *see* ramipril and hydrochlorothiazide *(Canada only) on page* 827

Altace® Plus Felodipine [Can] *see* ramipril and felodipine *(Canada only) on page* 827

Altachlore [US-OTC] *see* sodium chloride *on page* 882

Altafrin [US] *see* phenylephrine (ophthalmic) *on page* 752

Altamist [US-OTC] *see* sodium chloride *on page* 882

Altaryl [US-OTC] *see* diphenhydramine (systemic) *on page* 310

alteplase (AL te plase)

Sound-Alike/Look-Alike Issues

alteplase may be confused with Altace®

Activase® may be confused with Cathflo® Activase®, TNKase®

"tPA" abbreviation should not be used when writing orders for this medication; has been misread as TNKase (tenecteplase)

Synonyms alteplase, recombinant; alteplase, tissue plasminogen activator, recombinant; tPA

U.S./Canadian Brand Names Activase® rt-PA [Can]; Activase® [US]; Cathflo® Activase® [US/Can]

Therapeutic Category Fibrinolytic Agent

Use Management of ST-elevation myocardial infarction (STEMI) for the lysis of thrombi in coronary arteries; management of acute ischemic stroke (AIS); management of acute pulmonary embolism

Recommended criteria for treatment:

STEMI: Chest pain ≥20 minutes duration, onset of chest pain within 12 hours of treatment (or within prior 12-24 hours in patients with continuing ischemic symptoms), and ST-segment elevation >0.1 mV in at least two contiguous precordial leads or two adjacent limb leads on ECG or new or presumably new left bundle branch block (LBBB)

AIS: Onset of stroke symptoms within 3 hours of treatment

Acute pulmonary embolism: Age ≤75 years: Documented massive pulmonary embolism by pulmonary angiography or echocardiography or high probability lung scan with clinical shock

Cathflo® Activase®: Restoration of central venous catheter function

Dosage Summary

Intracatheter:

Children <30 kg: 110% of the internal lumen volume of the catheter; retain in catheter for 0.5-2 hours; may repeat once (maximum: 2 mg/2 mL/dose)

Children ≥30 kg: 2 mg (2 mL) retain in catheter for 0.5-2 hours; may repeat once

Adults: 2 mg (2 mL) retain in catheter for 0.5-2 hours; may repeat once

I.V. Infusion:

Children: Dosage not established

Adults:

ST-segment elevation myocardial infarction (STEMI):

Patients >67 kg: Total dose: 100 mg over 1.5 hours; infuse 15 mg over 1-2 minutes. Infuse 50 mg over 30 minutes. Infuse remaining 35 mg of alteplase over the next hour.

Patients ≤67 kg: Bolus: 15 mg over 1-2 minutes; Infusion: 0.75 mg/kg (maximum: 50 mg) over next 30 minutes, followed by 0.5 mg/kg (maximum: 35 mg) over next 60 minutes

Acute ischemic stroke: Bolus: 0.09 mg/kg (10% of the 0.9 mg/kg/dose) over 1 minute; Infusion: 0.81 mg/kg (90% of the 0.9 mg/kg/dose) over 60 minutes (maximum total dose: 90 mg)

Patients ≤100 kg: Load with 0.09 mg/kg (10% of 0.9 mg/kg dose) as an I.V. bolus over 1 minute, followed by 0.81 mg/kg (90% of 0.9 mg/kg dose) as a continuous infusion over 60 minutes.

Patients >100 kg: Load with 9 mg (10% of 90 mg) as an I.V. bolus over 1 minute, followed by 81 mg (90% of 90 mg) as a continuous infusion over 60 minutes.

Acute pulmonary embolism: 100 mg over 2 hours

Dosage Forms

Injection, powder for reconstitution:

Activase®: 50 mg, 100 mg

Cathflo® Activase®: 2 mg

alteplase, recombinant *see* alteplase *on page 56*

alteplase, tissue plasminogen activator, recombinant *see* alteplase *on page 56*

ALternaGel® [US-OTC] *see* aluminum hydroxide *on page 58*

Alti-Alprazolam [Can] *see* alprazolam *on page 55*

Alti-Captopril [Can] *see* captopril *on page 176*

Alti-Clindamycin [Can] *see* clindamycin (systemic) *on page 232*

Alti-Clonazepam [Can] *see* clonazepam *on page 237*

Alti-Desipramine [Can] *see* desipramine *on page 277*

Alti-Doxazosin [Can] *see* doxazosin *on page 328*

Alti-Flunisolide [Can] *see* flunisolide (oral inhalation) *on page 409*

Alti-Flurbiprofen [Can] *see* flurbiprofen (systemic) *on page 418*

Alti-Fluvoxamine [Can] *see* fluvoxamine *on page 422*

Alti-Ipratropium [Can] *see* ipratropium (nasal) *on page 523*

Alti-MPA [Can] *see* medroxyprogesterone *on page 597*

Alti-Nadolol [Can] *see* nadolol *on page 654*

Alti-Nortriptyline [Can] *see* nortriptyline *on page 684*

Alti-Sulfasalazine [Can] *see* sulfasalazine *on page 902*

Alti-Ticlopidine [Can] *see* ticlopidine *on page 932*

Altocor™ ***(Discontinued)*** *see* lovastatin *on page 579*

Altoprev® [US] *see* lovastatin *on page 579*

altretamine (al TRET a meen)

Synonyms hexamethylmelamine; HEXM; HMM; HXM; NSC-13875

U.S./Canadian Brand Names Hexalen® [US/Can]

Therapeutic Category Antineoplastic Agent

Use Palliative treatment of persistent or recurrent ovarian cancer

Dosage Summary

Oral:

Children: Dosage not established

Adults: 260 mg/m^2/day in 4 divided doses for 14 or 21 days of a 28-day cycle

Dosage Forms

Gelcap, oral:

Hexalen®: 50 mg

Alu-Cap® ***(Discontinued)*** *see* aluminum hydroxide *on page 58*

Aludrox® ***(Discontinued)*** *see* aluminum hydroxide and magnesium hydroxide *on page 59*

aluminum chloride hexahydrate (a LOO mi num KLOR ide heks a HYE drate)

Sound-Alike/Look-Alike Issues

Drysol™ may be confused with Drisdol®

U.S./Canadian Brand Names Certain Dri® [US-OTC]; Drysol™ [US]; Hypercare™ [US]; Xerac AC™ [US]

Therapeutic Category Topical Skin Product

Use Astringent in the management of hyperhidrosis

Dosage Summary

Topical:

Children: Dosage not established

Adults: Apply once daily at bedtime

Dosage Forms

Solution, topical:

Certain Dri® [OTC]: 12% (36 mL)

Drysol™: 20% (35 mL, 37.5 mL, 60 mL)

Hypercare™: 20% (35 mL, 37.5 mL, 60 mL)

Xerac AC™: 6.25% (35 mL, 60 mL)

aluminum hydroxide (a LOO mi num hye DROKS ide)

U.S./Canadian Brand Names ALternaGel® [US-OTC]; Amphojel® [Can]; Basaljel® [Can]; Dermagran® [US-OTC]

Therapeutic Category Antacid

Use Treatment of hyperacidity; hyperphosphatemia; temporary protection of minor cuts, scrapes, and burns

Dosage Summary

Oral:

Children: 50-150 mg/kg/day in divided doses every 4-6 hours

Adults: 300-1200 mg 3-4 times/day with meals

Topical:

Children: Apply to affected area as needed; reapply at least every 12 hours

Adults: Apply to affected area as needed; reapply at least every 12 hours

Dosage Forms

Ointment, topical:

Dermagran® [OTC]: 0.275% (113 g)

Suspension, oral: 320 mg/5 mL (30 mL, 355 mL, 473 mL); 600 mg/5 mL (355 mL)

ALternaGel® [OTC]: 600 mg/5 mL (360 mL)

aluminum hydroxide and magnesium carbonate

(a LOO mi num hye DROKS ide & mag NEE zhum KAR bun nate)

Synonyms magnesium carbonate and aluminum hydroxide

U.S./Canadian Brand Names Acid Gone Extra Strength [US-OTC]; Acid Gone [US-OTC]; Gaviscon® Extra Strength [US-OTC]; Gaviscon® Liquid [US-OTC]; Genaton™ [US-OTC]

Therapeutic Category Antacid

Use Temporary relief of symptoms associated with gastric acidity

Dosage Summary

Oral:

Children: Dosage not established

Adults: 15-30 mL **or** 2-4 tablets 4 times/day after meals and at bedtime

Dosage Forms

Liquid: Aluminum hydroxide 31.7 mg and magnesium carbonate 119.3 mg per 5 mL; aluminum hydroxide 84.6 mg and magnesium carbonate 79.1 mg per 5 mL

Acid Gone [OTC], Gaviscon® [OTC], Genaton™ [OTC]: Aluminum hydroxide 31.7 mg and magnesium carbonate 119.3 mg per 5 mL

Gaviscon® Extra Strength [OTC]: Aluminum hydroxide 84.6 mg and magnesium carbonate 79.1 mg per 5 mL

Tablet, chewable: Aluminum hydroxide 160 mg and magnesium carbonate 105 mg

Acid Gone Extra Strength [OTC], Gaviscon® Extra Strength [OTC]: Aluminum hydroxide 160 mg and magnesium carbonate 105 mg

aluminum hydroxide and magnesium hydroxide

(a LOO mi num hye DROKS ide & mag NEE zhum hye DROK side)

Synonyms magnesium hydroxide and aluminum hydroxide

U.S./Canadian Brand Names Alamag [US-OTC]; Diovol® Ex [Can]; Diovol® [Can]; Gelusil® Extra Strength [Can]; Mag-Al Ultimate [US-OTC]; Mag-Al [US-OTC]; Mylanta™ [Can]

Therapeutic Category Antacid

Use Antacid for symptoms related to hyperacidity associated with heartburn, hiatal hernia, upset stomach, peptic ulcer, peptic esophagitis, or gastritis

Dosage Summary

Oral:

Children <12 years: Dosage not established

Children ≥12 years: 10-20 mL 4 times/day (or after meals and at bedtime). (Maximum: Magnesium hydroxide 4500 mg/day; aluminum hydroxide 4500 mg/day) **or** 1-2 tablets as needed (maximum: 16 tablets)

Adults: 10-20 mL 4 times/day (or after meals and at bedtime). (Maximum: Magnesium hydroxide 4500 mg/day; aluminum hydroxide 4500 mg/day) **or** 1-2 tablets as needed (maximum: 16 tablets)

Dosage Forms

Liquid, oral:

Mag-Al [OTC]: Aluminum hydroxide 200 mg and magnesium hydroxide 200 mg per 5 mL

Suspension, oral: Aluminum hydroxide 225 mg and magnesium hydroxide 200 mg per 5 mL

Alamag [OTC]: Aluminum hydroxide 225 mg and magnesium hydroxide 200 mg per 5 mL

Mag-Al Ultimate [OTC]: Aluminum hydroxide 500 mg and magnesium hydroxide 500 mg per 5 mL

Tablet, chewable:

Alamag [OTC]: Aluminum hydroxide 300 mg and magnesium hydroxide 150 mg

aluminum hydroxide and magnesium trisilicate

(a LOO mi num hye DROKS ide & mag NEE zhum trye SIL i kate)

Synonyms magnesium trisilicate and aluminum hydroxide

U.S./Canadian Brand Names Alenic Alka Tablet [US-OTC]; Gaviscon® Tablet [US-OTC]

Therapeutic Category Antacid

Use Temporary relief of hyperacidity

Dosage Summary

Oral:

Children: Dosage not established

Adults: 2-4 tablets 4 times/day

Dosage Forms

Tablet, chewable: Aluminum hydroxide 80 mg and magnesium trisilicate 20 mg

Gaviscon® [OTC]: Aluminum hydroxide 80 mg and magnesium trisilicate 20 mg

aluminum hydroxide, magnesium hydroxide, and simethicone

(a LOO mi num hye DROKS ide, mag NEE zhum hye DROKS ide, & sye METH i kone)

Sound-Alike/Look-Alike Issues

Maalox® may be confused with Maox®, Monodox®

Mylanta® may be confused with Mynatal®

Synonyms magnesium hydroxide, aluminum hydroxide, and simethicone; simethicone, aluminum hydroxide, and magnesium hydroxide

U.S./Canadian Brand Names Alamag Plus [US-OTC]; Aldroxicon I [US-OTC]; Aldroxicon II [US-OTC]; Almacone Double Strength® [US-OTC]; Almacone® [US-OTC]; Diovol Plus® [Can]; Gelusil® [US-OTC/Can]; Maalox® Advanced Maximum Strength Liquid [US-OTC]; Maalox® Advanced Regular Strength [US-OTC]; Mi-Acid [US-OTC]; Mintox Extra Strength [US-OTC]; Mintox Plus [US-OTC]; Mylanta® Double Strength [Can]; Mylanta® Extra Strength [Can]; Mylanta® Liquid [US-OTC]; Mylanta® Maximum Strength Liquid [US-OTC]; Mylanta® Regular Strength [Can]; Rulox [US-OTC]

Therapeutic Category Antacid; Antiflatulent

Use Temporary relief of hyperacidity associated with gas; may also be used for indications associated with other antacids

Dosage Summary

Oral:

Children: Dosage not established

Adults: 10-20 mL or 2-4 tablets 4-6 times/day between meals and at bedtime; **Note:** May be administered every hour for severe symptoms

Dosage Forms

Liquid: Aluminum hydroxide 200 mg, magnesium hydroxide 200 mg, and simethicone 20 mg per 5 mL; aluminum hydroxide 400 mg, magnesium hydroxide 400 mg, and simethicone 40 mg per 5 mL

Aldroxicon I [OTC], Almacone® [OTC], Maalox® Advanced Regular Strength [OTC], Mi-Acid [OTC], Mylanta® Classic Regular Strength [OTC]: Aluminum hydroxide 200 mg, magnesium hydroxide 200 mg, and simethicone 20 mg per 5 mL

Aldroxicon II [OTC], Almacone Double Strength [OTC], Maalox® Advanced Maximum Strength [OTC], Mi-Acid Maximum Strength [OTC], Mylanta® Classic Maximum Strength [OTC]: Aluminum hydroxide 400 mg, magnesium hydroxide 400 mg, and simethicone 40 mg per 5 mL

Suspension: Aluminum hydroxide 225 mg, magnesium hydroxide 200 mg, and simethicone 25 mg per 5 mL

Rulox [OTC]: Aluminum hydroxide 200 mg, magnesium hydroxide 200 mg, and simethicone 25 mg per 5 mL

Tablet, chewable: Aluminum hydroxide 200 mg, magnesium hydroxide 200 mg, and simethicone 25 mg

Alamag Plus [OTC], Gelusil® [OTC], Mintox Plus [OTC]: Aluminum hydroxide 200 mg, magnesium hydroxide 200 mg, and simethicone 25 mg

Almacone® [OTC]: Aluminum hydroxide 200 mg, magnesium hydroxide 200 mg, and simethicone 20 mg

aluminum sucrose sulfate, basic *see* sucralfate *on page 897*

aluminum sulfate and calcium acetate (a LOO mi num SUL fate & KAL see um AS e tate)

Synonyms calcium acetate and aluminum sulfate

U.S./Canadian Brand Names Domeboro® [US-OTC]; Gordon Boro-Packs [US-OTC]; Pedi-Boro® [US-OTC]

Therapeutic Category Topical Skin Product

Use Astringent wet dressing for relief of inflammatory conditions of the skin; reduce weeping that may occur in dermatitis

Dosage Summary

Topical:

Children: Dosage not established

Adults: Soak affected area or wet dressing in the solution 2-4 times/day for 15-30 minutes

Dosage Forms

Powder, for topical solution:

Domeboro® [OTC]: Aluminum sulfate 1191 mg and calcium acetate 839 mg per packet (12s, 100s)

Gordon Boro-Packs: Aluminum sulfate 49% and calcium acetate 51% per packet (100s)

Pedi-Boro® [OTC]: Aluminum sulfate 1191 mg and calcium acetate 839 mg per packet (12s, 100s)

Alupent® *(Discontinued)* *see* metaproterenol *on page 609*

Alupent® Inhalation Solution *(Discontinued)* *see* metaproterenol *on page 609*

Alu-Tab® *(Discontinued)* *see* aluminum hydroxide *on page 58*

Alvesco® [US/Can] *see* ciclesonide (oral inhalation) *on page 220*

alvimopan (al VI moe pan)

Sound-Alike/Look-Alike Issues

alvimopan may be confused with almotriptan

Synonyms ADL-2698; LY246736

U.S./Canadian Brand Names Entereg® [US]

Therapeutic Category Gastrointestinal Agent, Miscellaneous; Opioid Antagonist, Peripherally-Acting

Use Accelerate the time to upper and lower GI recovery following partial large or small bowel resection surgery with primary anastomosis

Dosage Summary

Oral:

Children: Dosage not established

Adults: Initial: 12 mg prior to surgery; Maintenance: 12 mg twice daily (maximum total treatment: 15 doses)

Dosage Forms

Capsule, oral:

Entereg®: 12 mg

amantadine (a MAN ta deen)

Sound-Alike/Look-Alike Issues

amantadine may be confused with ranitidine, rimantadine

Symmetrel® may be confused with Synthroid®

Synonyms adamantanamine hydrochloride; amantadine hydrochloride

U.S./Canadian Brand Names Endantadine® [Can]; Mylan-Amantadine [Can]; PMS-Amantadine [Can]; Symmetrel® [US/Can]

Therapeutic Category Anti-Parkinson Agent (Dopamine Agonist); Antiviral Agent

Use Prophylaxis and treatment of influenza A viral infection (per manufacturer labeling; also refer to current ACIP guidelines for recommendations during current flu season); treatment of parkinsonism; treatment of drug-induced extrapyramidal symptoms

Note: In certain circumstances, the ACIP recommends use of amantadine in combination with oseltamivir for the treatment or prophylaxis of influenza A infection when resistance to oseltamivir is suspected.

Dosage Summary

Oral:

Children <1 year: Dosage not established

Children 1-9 years: 4.4-8.8 mg/kg/day in 2 divided doses (maximum: 150 mg/day)

Children ≥10 years and <40 kg: 5 mg/kg/day in 2 divided doses

Children ≥10 years and ≥40 kg: 100 mg twice daily (maximum: 200 mg/day)

Adults: 200-400 mg/day in 2 divided doses (maximum: 400 mg/day)

Elderly: 100-400 mg/day in 2 divided doses (maximum: 400 mg/day)

Dosage Forms

Capsule, oral: 100 mg

Capsule, softgel, oral: 100 mg

Solution, oral: 50 mg/5 mL (473 mL)

Syrup, oral: 50 mg/5 mL (10 mL, 473 mL, 480 mL)

Tablet, oral: 100 mg

Symmetrel®: 100 mg

amantadine hydrochloride *see* amantadine *on page 61*

Amaphen® ***(Discontinued)***

Amaryl® [US/Can] *see* glimepiride *on page 446*

Amatine® [Can] *see* midodrine *on page 633*

ambenonium (am be NOE nee um)

Synonyms ambenonium chloride

U.S./Canadian Brand Names Mytelase® [US/Can]

Therapeutic Category Cholinergic Agent

Use Treatment of myasthenia gravis

Dosage Summary

Oral:

Children: Dosage not established

Adults: 5-25 mg 3-4 times/day

Dosage Forms

Caplet, oral:

Mytelase®: 10 mg

ambenonium chloride *see* ambenonium *on page 61*

Ambi 10® ***(Discontinued)*** *see* benzoyl peroxide *on page 128*

Ambien® [US] *see* zolpidem *on page 1004*

Ambien CR® [US] *see* zolpidem *on page 1004*

Ambifed [US-OTC] *see* guaifenesin and pseudoephedrine *on page 457*

Ambifed-G [US-OTC] *see* guaifenesin and pseudoephedrine *on page 457*

Ambifed-G DM [US] *see* guaifenesin, pseudoephedrine, and dextromethorphan *on page 460*

Ambi® Skin Tone ***(Discontinued)*** *see* hydroquinone *on page 487*

AmBisome® [US/Can] *see* amphotericin B liposomal *on page 75*

ambrisentan (am bri SEN tan)

Synonyms BSF208075

U.S./Canadian Brand Names Letairis® [US]; Volibris® [Can]

Therapeutic Category Endothelin Antagonist

Use Treatment of pulmonary artery hypertension (PAH) World Health Organization (WHO) Group I in patients with WHO Class II or III symptoms to improve exercise capacity and decrease the rate of clinical deterioration

Dosage Summary

Oral:

Children: Dosage not established

Adults: Initial: 5 mg once daily; if tolerated, may increase to maximum of 10 mg once daily

Dosage Forms

Tablet, oral:

Letairis®: 5 mg, 10 mg

amcinonide (am SIN oh nide)

U.S./Canadian Brand Names Amcort® [Can]; Cyclocort® [Can]; ratio-Amcinonide [Can]; Taro-Amcinonide [Can]

Therapeutic Category Corticosteroid, Topical

Use Relief of the inflammatory and pruritic manifestations of corticosteroid-responsive dermatoses (high potency corticosteroid)

Dosage Summary

Topical:

Children: Dosage not established

Adults: Apply in a thin film 2-3 times/day

Dosage Forms

Cream, topical: 0.1% (15 g, 30 g, 60 g)

Lotion, topical: 0.1% (60 mL)

Ointment, topical: 0.1% (15 g, 30 g, 60 g)

Amcort® [Can] *see* amcinonide *on page 62*

Amcort® Injection *(Discontinued)*

AMD3100 *see* plerixafor *on page 766*

Amdry-C [US] *see* chlorpheniramine, pseudoephedrine, and methscopolamine *on page 215*

Amdry-D *(Discontinued)* *see* pseudoephedrine and methscopolamine *on page 813*

Amerge® [US/Can] *see* naratriptan *on page 661*

Americaine® Anesthetic Lubricant *(Discontinued)* *see* benzocaine *on page 124*

Americaine® Hemorrhoidal [US-OTC] *see* benzocaine *on page 124*

A-Methapred® [US] *see* methylprednisolone *on page 622*

amethocaine hydrochloride *see* tetracaine (ophthalmic) *on page 922*

amethocaine hydrochloride *see* tetracaine (systemic) *on page 921*

amethocaine hydrochloride *see* tetracaine (topical) *on page 922*

amethopterin *see* methotrexate *on page 614*

Ametop™ [Can] *see* tetracaine (topical) *on page 922*

Amevive® [US/Can] *see* alefacept *on page 47*

amfepramone *see* diethylpropion *on page 300*

AMG 073 *see* cinacalcet *on page 223*

AMG-162 *see* denosumab *on page 275*

AMG 531 *see* romiplostim *on page 851*

Amibid DM *(Discontinued)* *see* guaifenesin and dextromethorphan *on page 455*

Amibid LA *(Discontinued)* *see* guaifenesin *on page 454*

Amicar® [US] *see* aminocaproic acid *on page 65*

Amidal *(Discontinued)* *see* guaifenesin and phenylephrine *on page 456*

Amidate® [US/Can] *see* etomidate *on page 384*

Amidrine *(Discontinued)* *see* acetaminophen, isometheptene, and dichloralphenazone *on page 31*

amifostine (am i FOS teen)

Sound-Alike/Look-Alike Issues

Ethyol® may be confused with ethanol

Synonyms ethiofos; gammaphos; WR-2721; YM-08310

U.S./Canadian Brand Names Ethyol® [US/Can]

Therapeutic Category Antidote

Use Reduce the incidence of moderate-to-severe xerostomia in patients undergoing postoperative radiation treatment for head and neck cancer, where the radiation port includes a substantial portion of the parotid glands; reduce the cumulative renal toxicity associated with repeated administration of cisplatin

Dosage Summary **Note:** Antiemetic medication, including dexamethasone 20 mg I.V. and a serotonin 5-HT_3 receptor antagonist, is recommended prior to and in conjunction with amifostine.

I.V.:

Children: Dosage not established

Adults: 910 mg/m^2 once daily over 15 minutes 30 minutes prior to cytotoxic therapy **or** 200 mg/m^2/day over 3 minutes 15-30 minutes prior to radiation therapy

Dosage Forms

Injection, powder for reconstitution: 500 mg

Ethyol®: 500 mg

Amigesic® [Can] *see* salsalate *on page* 862

Amigesic® *(Discontinued)* *see* salsalate *on page* 862

amikacin (am i KAY sin)

Sound-Alike/Look-Alike Issues

amikacin may be confused with Amicar®, anakinra

Amikin® may be confused with Amicar®, Kineret®

Synonyms amikacin sulfate

U.S./Canadian Brand Names Amikacin Sulfate Injection, USP [Can]; Amikin® [Can]

Therapeutic Category Aminoglycoside (Antibiotic)

Use Treatment of serious infections (bone infections, respiratory tract infections, endocarditis, and septicemia) due to organisms resistant to gentamicin and tobramycin, including *Pseudomonas*, *Proteus*, *Serratia*, and other gram-negative bacilli; documented infection of mycobacterial organisms susceptible to amikacin

Dosage Summary **Note:** Use of ideal body weight (IBW) for determining the mg/kg/dose appears to be more accurate than dosing on the basis of total body weight (TBW); **Note:** Individualization of the dose is critical because of the low therapeutic index

I.M.:

Infants: 5-7.5 mg/kg/dose every 8 hours (maximum: 20 mg/kg/day)

Children: 5-7.5 mg/kg/dose every 8 hours (maximum: 20 mg/kg/day)

Adults: 5-7.5 mg/kg/dose every 8 hours (maximum: 20 mg/kg/day)

I.V.:

Infants: 5-7.5 mg/kg/dose every 8 hours (maximum: 20 mg/kg/day)

Children: 5-7.5 mg/kg/dose every 8 hours (maximum: 20 mg/kg/day)

Adults: 5-7.5 mg/kg/dose every 8 hours **or** 15-20 mg/kg as a single daily dose (maximum: 20 mg/kg/day)

Dosage Forms

Injection, solution: 50 mg/mL (2 mL); 250 mg/mL (2 mL, 4 mL)

amikacin sulfate *see* amikacin *on page* 63

Amikacin Sulfate Injection, USP [Can] *see* amikacin *on page* 63

Amikin® [Can] *see* amikacin *on page* 63

amiloride (a MIL oh ride)

Sound-Alike/Look-Alike Issues

aMILoride may be confused with amiodarone, amLODIPine, amrinone

Synonyms amiloride hydrochloride

Tall-Man a**MIL**oride

U.S./Canadian Brand Names Apo-Amiloride® [Can]; Mylan-Amilazide [Can]

Therapeutic Category Diuretic, Potassium Sparing

Use Counteracts potassium loss induced by other diuretics in the treatment of hypertension or edematous conditions including CHF, hepatic cirrhosis, and hypoaldosteronism; usually used in conjunction with more potent diuretics such as thiazides or loop diuretics

Dosage Summary

Oral:

Children: Dosage not established

Adults: 5-10 mg/day in 1-2 divided doses (maximum: 20 mg/day)

Elderly: Initial: 5 mg once daily or every other day; Maintenance: 5-10 mg/day in 1-2 divided doses (maximum: 20 mg/day)

Dosage Forms

Tablet, oral: 5 mg

amiloride and hydrochlorothiazide (a MIL oh ride & hye droe klor oh THYE a zide)

Synonyms hydrochlorothiazide and amiloride

U.S./Canadian Brand Names Apo-Amilzide® [Can]; Gen-Amilazide [Can]; Moduret [Can]; Novamilor [Can]; Nu-Amilzide [Can]

Therapeutic Category Diuretic, Combination

Use Potassium-sparing diuretic; antihypertensive

Dosage Summary

Oral:

Children: Dosage not established

Adults: 1-2 tablets/day as a single dose (maximum: 2 tablets/day)

Elderly: Initial: 1/2 to 1 tablet/day (maximum: 2 tablets/day)

Dosage Forms

Tablet: 5/50: Amiloride 5 mg and hydrochlorothiazide 50 mg

amiloride hydrochloride *see* amiloride *on page 63*

2-amino-6-mercaptopurine *see* thioguanine *on page 927*

2-amino-6-methoxypurine arabinoside *see* nelarabine *on page 664*

2-amino-6-trifluoromethoxy-benzothiazole *see* riluzole *on page 843*

amino acid injection (a MEE noe AS id in JEK shun)

Sound-Alike/Look-Alike Issues

TrophAmine® may be confused with tromethamine

U.S./Canadian Brand Names Aminosyn® II [US]; Aminosyn® [US/Can]; Aminosyn®-HBC [US]; Aminosyn®-PF [US/Can]; Aminosyn®-RF [US/Can]; BranchAmin® [US]; Clinisol® [US]; FreAmine® HBC [US]; FreAmine® III [US]; HepatAmine® [US]; Hepatasol® [US]; NephrAmine® [US]; Premasol™ [US]; Primene® [Can]; Prosol [US]; RenAmin® [US]; Travasol® [US]; TrophAmine® [US]

Therapeutic Category Intravenous Nutritional Therapy

Use As part of parenteral nutrition to prevent nitrogen loss or treat negative nitrogen balance when alimentary tract cannot be used (eg, GI absorption is impaired, bowel rest is needed). Specialty amino acid formulas may be considered only in certain instances.

Dosage Summary

I.V.:

Children: 1-3.85 g/kg/day

Adults: 0.8-2 g/kg/day

Dosage Forms

Injection, solution:

Aminosyn®: 8.5% (500 mL); 10% (500 mL, 1000 mL)

Aminosyn® II: 8.5% (500 mL); 10% (500 mL, 1000 mL, 2000 mL); 15% (2000 mL)

Aminosyn®-HBC: 7% (500 mL)

Aminosyn®-PF: 7% (500 mL); 10% (1000 mL)

Aminosyn®-RF: 5.2% (500 mL)

BranchAmin®: 4% (500 mL)

Clinisol®: 15% (500 mL, 2000 mL)

FreAmine® HBC: 6.9% (750 mL)

FreAmine® III: 8.5% (500 mL); 10% (500 mL, 1000 mL)

HepatAmine®: 8% (500 mL)

Hepatasol®: 8% (500 mL)

NephrAmine®: 5.4% (250 mL)
PremaSol™: 6% (500 mL); 10% (500 mL, 1000 mL, 2000 mL)
Prosol: 20% (2000 mL)
RenAmin®: 6.5% (500 mL)
Travasol®: 10% (500 mL, 1000 mL, 2000 mL)
TrophAmine®: 6% (500 mL); 10% (500 mL)

aminobenzylpenicillin *see* ampicillin *on page 75*

aminocaproic acid (a mee noe ka PROE ik AS id)

Sound-Alike/Look-Alike Issues
Amicar® may be confused with amikacin, Amikin®, Omacor®

Synonyms EACA; epsilon aminocaproic acid

U.S./Canadian Brand Names Amicar® [US]

Therapeutic Category Hemostatic Agent

Use To enhance hemostasis when fibrinolysis contributes to bleeding (causes may include cardiac surgery, hematologic disorders, neoplastic disorders, abruption placentae, hepatic cirrhosis, and urinary fibrinolysis)

Dosage Summary
I.V.:
Adults: Initial: Loading dose: 4-5 g for first hour; Maintenance: 1 g/hour for 8 hours or until bleeding controlled (maximum: 30 g/day) **or** 10 g prior to skin incision, followed by 1-2.5 g/hour (usual dose: 2 g/hour) until the end of operation **or** 10 g prior to skin incision, followed by 10 g after heparin administration then 10 g at discontinuation of cardiopulmonary bypass prior to protamine reversal of heparin
Oral:
Adults: Initial: Loading dose: 4-5 g for first hour; Maintenance: 1 g/hour (or 1.25 g/hour using oral solution) for 8 hours or until bleeding controlled (maximum: 30 g/day)

Dosage Forms
Injection, solution: 250 mg/mL (20 mL)
Solution, oral: 1.25 g/5 mL (237 mL, 473 mL)
Syrup, oral:
Amicar®: 1.25 g/5 mL (473 mL)
Tablet, oral: 500 mg
Amicar®: 500 mg, 1000 mg

aminoglutethimide ***(Discontinued)***

aminolevulinic acid (a MEE noh lev yoo lin ik AS id)

Sound-Alike/Look-Alike Issues
aminolevulinic acid may be confused with methyl aminolevulinate

Synonyms 5-ALA; 5-aminolevulinic acid; ALA; amino levulinic acid; aminolevulinic acid hydrochloride

U.S./Canadian Brand Names Levulan® Kerastick® [US/Can]

Therapeutic Category Photosensitizing Agent, Topical; Porphyrin Agent, Topical

Use Treatment of minimally to moderately thick actinic keratoses (grade 1 or 2) of the face or scalp; to be used in conjunction with blue light illumination

Dosage Summary
Topical:
Children: Dosage not established
Adults: Apply to actinic keratoses followed 14-18 hours later by blue light illumination; may repeat at a treatment site (once) after 8 weeks

Dosage Forms
Powder for solution, topical:
Levulan® Kerastick®: 20% (6s)

amino levulinic acid *see* aminolevulinic acid *on page 65*
5-aminolevulinic acid *see* aminolevulinic acid *on page 65*
aminolevulinic acid hydrochloride *see* aminolevulinic acid *on page 65*

aminophylline (am in OFF i lin)

Sound-Alike/Look-Alike Issues

aminophylline may be confused with amitriptyline, ampicillin

Synonyms theophylline ethylenediamine

U.S./Canadian Brand Names Phyllocontin® [Can]; Phyllocontin®-350 [Can]

Therapeutic Category Theophylline Derivative

Use Bronchodilator in reversible airway obstruction due to asthma or COPD; increase diaphragmatic contractility

Dosage Summary

I.V.:

Children <6 weeks: Dosage not established

Children 6 weeks to 6 months: Loading dose: 6 mg/kg over 20-30 minutes; Maintenance: 0.5 mg/kg/hour as a continuous infusion

Children 6 months to 1 year: Loading dose: 6 mg/kg over 20-30 minutes; Maintenance: 0.6-0.7 mg/kg/hour as a continuous infusion

Children 1-9 years: Loading dose: 6 mg/kg over 20-30 minutes; Maintenance: 1 mg/kg/hour as a continuous infusion

Children 9-16 years: Loading dose: 6 mg/kg over 20-30 minutes; Maintenance: 0.8 mg/kg/hour as a continuous infusion

Adults: Loading dose: 6 mg/kg over 20-30 minutes; Maintenance: 0.1-0.8 mg/kg/hour as a continuous infusion; **Note:** Dose dependent on age, smoker status, and heart/lung status.

Oral:

Children <45 kg: Dosage not established

Children ≥45 kg: Initial: 380 mg/day divided every 6-8 hours; Maintenance: 380-928 mg/day divided every 6-8 hours (maximum: 928 mg/day); **Note:** Titration is recommended

Adults: Initial: 380 mg/day divided every 6-8 hours; Maintenance: 380-928 mg/day divided every 6-8 hours (maximum: 928 mg/day); **Note:** Titration is recommended

Dosage Forms

Injection, solution: 25 mg/mL (10 mL, 20 mL)

Injection, solution [preservative free]: 25 mg/mL (10 mL, 20 mL)

Tablet, oral: 100 mg, 200 mg

4-aminopyridine *see* dalfampridine *on page 266*

aminosalicylate sodium *see* aminosalicylic acid *on page 66*

aminosalicylic acid (a mee noe sal i SIL ik AS id)

Synonyms 4-aminosalicylic acid; aminosalicylate sodium; para-aminosalicylate sodium; PAS; sodium PAS

U.S./Canadian Brand Names Paser® [US]

Therapeutic Category Nonsteroidal Antiinflammatory Drug (NSAID)

Use Adjunctive treatment of tuberculosis used in combination with other antitubercular agents

Dosage Summary

Oral:

Children: 200-300 mg/kg/day in 3-4 equally divided doses

Adults: 150 mg/kg/day in 2-3 equally divided doses

Dosage Forms

Granules, delayed release, oral:

Paser®: 4 g/packet (30s)

4-aminosalicylic acid *see* aminosalicylic acid *on page 66*

5-aminosalicylic acid *see* mesalamine *on page 607*

Aminosyn® [US/Can] *see* amino acid injection *on page 64*

Aminosyn® II [US] *see* amino acid injection *on page 64*

Aminosyn®-HBC [US] *see* amino acid injection *on page 64*

Aminosyn®-HF *(Discontinued)* *see* amino acid injection *on page 64*

Aminosyn®-PF [US/Can] *see* amino acid injection *on page 64*

Aminosyn®-RF [US/Can] *see* amino acid injection *on page 64*

Aminoxin® [US-OTC] *see* pyridoxine *on page 818*

amiodarone (a MEE oh da rone)

Sound-Alike/Look-Alike Issues

amiodarone may be confused with aMILoride, amrinone

Cordarone® may be confused with Cardura®, Cordran®

Synonyms amiodarone hydrochloride

U.S./Canadian Brand Names Apo-Amiodarone® [Can]; Cordarone® [US/Can]; Dom-Amiodarone [Can]; Mylan-Amiodarone [Can]; Novo-Amiodarone [Can]; Pacerone® [US]; PHL-Amiodarone [Can]; PMS-Amiodarone [Can]; PRO-Amiodarone [Can]; ratio-Amiodarone I.V. [Can]; ratio-Amiodarone [Can]; Riva-Amiodarone [Can]; Sandoz-Amiodarone [Can]; Teva-Amiodarone [Can]

Therapeutic Category Antiarrhythmic Agent, Class III

Use Management of life-threatening recurrent ventricular fibrillation (VF) or hemodynamically-unstable ventricular tachycardia (VT) refractory to other antiarrhythmic agents or in patients intolerant of other agents used for these conditions

Dosage Summary

I.O.:

Children (PALS dosing): 5 mg/kg (maximum: 300 mg/day) rapid bolus or over 20-60 minutes; may repeat up to maximum dose of 15 mg/kg/day

Adults: Dosage not established

I.V.:

Children (PALS dosing): 5 mg/kg (maximum: 300 mg/day) rapid bolus or over 20-60 minutes; may repeat up to maximum dose of 15 mg/kg/day

Adults: Initial: 150-300 mg bolus **or** 5-7 mg/kg over 30-60 minutes; Maintenance: 1200-1800 mg/day continuous infusion until 10 g total **or** 1 mg/minute infusion for 6 hours, then 0.5 mg/minute infusion for 18 hours (maximum: 2.1 g/day)

Oral:

Adults: Initial: 800-1600 mg/day in 1-2 doses for 1-3 weeks, then 600-800 mg/day in 1-2 doses for 1 month or 1200-1800 mg/day in divided doses until 10 g total; Maintenance: 100-400 mg/day

Dosage Forms

Injection, solution: 50 mg/mL (3 mL, 9 mL, 18 mL)

Tablet, oral: 200 mg, 400 mg

Cordarone®: 200 mg

Pacerone®: 100 mg, 200 mg, 400 mg

amiodarone hydrochloride *see* amiodarone *on page 67*

Ami-Tex LA *(Discontinued)* *see* guaifenesin and phenylephrine *on page 456*

Amitiza® [US] *see* lubiprostone *on page 580*

Amitone® *(Discontinued)* *see* calcium carbonate *on page 167*

amitriptyline (a mee TRIP ti leen)

Sound-Alike/Look-Alike Issues

amitriptyline may be confused with aminophylline, imipramine, nortriptyline

Elavil® may be confused with Aldoril®, Eldepryl®, enalapril, Equanil®, Mellaril®, Plavix®

Synonyms amitriptyline hydrochloride

U.S./Canadian Brand Names Apo-Amitriptyline® [Can]; Bio-Amitriptyline [Can]; Dom-Amitriptyline [Can]; Levate® [Can]; Novo-Triptyn [Can]; PMS-Amitriptyline [Can]

Therapeutic Category Antidepressant, Tricyclic (Tertiary Amine)

Use Relief of symptoms of depression

Dosage Summary

Oral:

Adolescents: Initial: 25-50 mg/day in divided doses; Maintenance: 25-100 mg/day in divided doses (maximum: 100 mg/day); **Note:** Titration is recommended

Adults: 50-300 mg/day as a single dose at bedtime or in divided doses (maximum: 300 mg/day); **Note:** Titration is recommended

Elderly: Initial: 10-25 mg at bedtime; Maintenance: 25-150 mg/day at bedtime (maximum: 150 mg/day); **Note:** Titration is recommended

Dosage Forms

Tablet, oral: 10 mg, 25 mg, 50 mg, 75 mg, 100 mg, 150 mg

amitriptyline and chlordiazepoxide (a mee TRIP ti leen & klor dye az e POKS ide)

Synonyms chlordiazepoxide and amitriptyline hydrochloride

U.S./Canadian Brand Names Limbitrol® [Can]

Therapeutic Category Antidepressant, Tricyclic (Tertiary Amine)

Controlled Substance C-IV

Use Treatment of moderate-to-severe anxiety and/or agitation and depression

Dosage Summary

Oral:

Children: Dosage not established

Adults: 2-6 tablets/day (maximum: 6 tablets/day); **Note:** Titration is recommended

Dosage Forms

Tablet: 12.5/5: Amitriptyline 12.5 mg and chlordiazepoxide 5 mg; 25/10: Amitriptyline 25 mg and chlordiazepoxide 10 mg

amitriptyline and perphenazine (a mee TRIP ti leen & per FEN a zeen)

Synonyms perphenazine and amitriptyline hydrochloride

U.S./Canadian Brand Names Etrafon® [Can]

Therapeutic Category Antidepressant/Phenothiazine

Use Treatment of patients with moderate-to-severe anxiety and depression

Dosage Summary

Oral:

Children: Dosage not established

Adults: 1 tablet 2-4 times/day

Dosage Forms

Tablet: 2-10: Amitriptyline 10 mg and perphenazine 2 mg; 2-25: Amitriptyline 25 mg and perphenazine 2 mg; 4-10: Amitriptyline 10 mg and perphenazine 4 mg; 4-25: Amitriptyline 25 mg and perphenazine 4 mg; 4-50: Amitriptyline 50 mg and perphenazine 4 mg

amitriptyline hydrochloride *see* amitriptyline *on page* 67

AMJ 9701 *see* palifermin *on page* 720

AmLactin® [US-OTC] *see* lactic acid and ammonium hydroxide *on page* 542

amlexanox (am LEKS an oks)

U.S./Canadian Brand Names Aphthasol® [US]

Therapeutic Category Antiinflammatory Agent, Locally Applied

Use Treatment of aphthous ulcers (ie, canker sores)

Dosage Summary

Topical:

Children: Dosage not established

Adults: Administer ~1/4 inch (0.5 cm) directly on ulcers 4 times/day

Dosage Forms

Paste, oral:

Aphthasol®: 5% (3 g)

amlodipine (am LOE di peen)

Sound-Alike/Look-Alike Issues

amLODIPine may be confused with aMILoride

Norvasc® may be confused with Navane®, Norvir®, Vascor®

Synonyms amlodipine besylate

Tall-Man am**LODIP**ine

U.S./Canadian Brand Names Accel-Amlodipine [Can]; Apo-Amlodipine® [Can]; CO Amlodipine [Can]; Dom-Amlodipine [Can]; GD-Amlodipine [Can]; JAMP-Amlodipine [Can]; Mylan-Amlodipine [Can]; Norvasc® [US/Can]; Novo-Amlodipine [Can]; PHL-Amlodipine [Can]; PMS-Amlodipine [Can]; RAN™-Amlodipine [Can]; ratio-Amlodipine [Can]; Riva-Amlodipine [Can]; Sandoz Amlodipine [Can]; Teva-Amlodipine [Can]; ZYM-Amlodipine [Can]

Therapeutic Category Calcium Channel Blocker

Use Treatment of hypertension; treatment of symptomatic chronic stable angina, vasospastic (Prinzmetal) angina (confirmed or suspected); prevention of hospitalization due to angina with documented CAD (limited to patients without heart failure or ejection fraction <40%)

Dosage Summary

Oral:

Children <6 years: Dosage not established

Children 6-17 years: 2.5-5 mg once daily

Adults: Initial: 5 mg once daily; Maintenance: 2.5-10 mg once daily (maximum: 10 mg/day); **Note:** Titration is recommended

Elderly: 2.5-5 mg once daily

Dosage Forms

Tablet, oral: 2.5 mg, 5 mg, 10 mg

Norvasc®: 2.5 mg, 5 mg, 10 mg

amlodipine and atorvastatin (am LOW di peen & a TORE va sta tin)

Synonyms atorvastatin and amlodipine; atorvastatin calcium and amlodipine besylate

U.S./Canadian Brand Names Caduet® [US/Can]

Therapeutic Category Antilipemic Agent, HMG-CoA Reductase Inhibitor; Calcium Channel Blocker

Use For use when treatment with both amlodipine and atorvastatin is appropriate:

Amlodipine: Treatment of hypertension; treatment of chronic stable angina, vasospastic (Prinzmetal) angina (confirmed or suspected); prevention of hospitalization or to decrease coronary revascularization procedure due to angina with documented CAD (limited to patients without heart failure or ejection fraction <40%)

Atorvastatin: Treatment of dyslipidemias or primary prevention of cardiovascular disease (atherosclerotic) as detailed here:

Primary prevention of cardiovascular disease (high-risk for CVD): To reduce the risk of MI or stroke in patients without evidence of coronary heart disease who have multiple CVD risk factors or type 2 diabetes; also reduces the risk for angina or revascularization procedures in patients with multiple CVD risk factors without evidence of coronary heart disease

Secondary prevention of cardiovascular disease: To reduce the risk of MI, stroke, revascularization procedures, angina, and hospitalization for heart failure

Treatment of dyslipidemias: To reduce elevations in total cholesterol, LDL-C, apolipoprotein B, and triglycerides in patients with elevations of one or more components, and/or to increase low HDL-C as present in heterozygous familial/nonfamilial hypercholesterolemia and mixed dyslipidemia (Fredrickson type IIa and IIb hyperlipidemias); treatment of primary dysbetalipoproteinemia (Fredrickson type III), elevated serum TG levels (Fredrickson type IV), and homozygous familial hypercholesterolemia

Treatment of heterozygous familial hypercholesterolemia (HeFH) in adolescent patients (10-17 years of age, females >1 year postmenarche) having LDL-C ≥190 mg/dL or LDL-C ≥160 mg/dL with positive family history of premature cardiovascular disease (CVD) or with two or more CVD risk factors.

Dosage Summary

Oral:

Children <10 years: Dosage not established

Children 10-17 years (females >1 year postmenarche): 2.5-5 mg (amlodipine) and 10-20 mg (atorvastatin) once daily (maximum: amlodipine 5 mg/day; atorvastatin 20 mg/day)

Adults: 2.5-10 mg (amlodipine) and 10-80 mg (atorvastatin) once daily (maximum: amlodipine 10 mg/day; atorvastatin 80 mg/day)

Dosage Forms

Tablet:

Caduet®:

2.5/10: Amlodipine 2.5 mg and atorvastatin 10 mg; 2.5/20: Amlodipine 2.5 mg and atorvastatin 20 mg; 2.5/40: Amlodipine 2.5 mg and atorvastatin 40 mg

5/10: Amlodipine 5 mg and atorvastatin 10 mg; 5/20: Amlodipine 5 mg and atorvastatin 20 mg; 5/40: Amlodipine 5 mg and atorvastatin 40 mg; 5/80: Amlodipine 5 mg and atorvastatin 80 mg

10/10: Amlodipine 10 mg and atorvastatin 10 mg; 10/20: Amlodipine 10 mg and atorvastatin 20 mg; 10/40: Amlodipine 10 mg and atorvastatin 40 mg; 10/80: Amlodipine 10 mg and atorvastatin 80 mg

amlodipine and benazepril (am LOE di peen & ben AY ze pril)

Synonyms benazepril hydrochloride and amlodipine besylate

U.S./Canadian Brand Names Lotrel® [US]

Therapeutic Category Antihypertensive Agent, Combination

Use Treatment of hypertension

Dosage Summary

Oral:

Children: Dosage not established

Adults: 2.5-10 mg (amlodipine) and 10-40 mg (benazepril) once daily (maximum: amlodipine 10 mg/day; benazepril 80 mg/day)

Elderly: Initial: 2.5 mg/day (based on amlodipine component)

Dosage Forms

Capsule: 2.5/10: Amlodipine 2.5 mg and benazepril 10 mg; 5/10: Amlodipine 5 mg and benazepril 10 mg; 5/20: Amlodipine 5 mg and benazepril 20 mg; 10/20: Amlodipine 10 mg and benazepril 20 mg

Lotrel®: 2.5/10: Amlodipine 2.5 and benazepril 10 mg; 5/10: Amlodipine 5 mg and benazepril 10 mg; 5/20: Amlodipine 5 mg and benazepril 20 mg; 5/40: Amlodipine 5 mg and benazepril 40 mg; 10/20: Amlodipine 10 mg and benazepril 20 mg; 10/40: Amlodipine 10 mg and benazepril 40 mg

amlodipine and olmesartan (am LOE di peen & olme SAR tan)

Synonyms amlodipine besylate and olmesartan medoxomil; olmesartan and amlodipine

U.S./Canadian Brand Names Azor™ [US]

Therapeutic Category Angiotensin II Receptor Blocker Combination; Antihypertensive Agent, Combination; Calcium Channel Blocker

Use Treatment of hypertension, including initial treatment in patients who will require multiple antihypertensives for adequate control

Dosage Summary

Oral:

Children: Dosage not established

Adults: Amlodipine 5-10 mg and olmesartan 20-40 mg once daily (maximum: 10 mg/day [amlodipine]; 40 mg/day [olmesartan]); **Note:** Titration is recommended

Dosage Forms

Tablet:

Azor™: 5/20: Amlodipine 5 mg and olmesartan medoxomil 20 mg; 5/40: Amlodipine 5 mg and olmesartan medoxomil 40 mg; 10/20: Amlodipine 10 mg and olmesartan medoxomil 20 mg; 10/40: Amlodipine 10 mg and olmesartan medoxomil 40 mg

amlodipine and telmisartan *see* telmisartan and amlodipine *on page 913*

amlodipine and valsartan (am LOE di peen & val SAR tan)

Synonyms amlodipine besylate and valsartan; valsartan and amlodipine

U.S./Canadian Brand Names Exforge® [US]

Therapeutic Category Angiotensin II Receptor Blocker Combination; Antihypertensive Agent, Combination; Calcium Channel Blocker

Use Treatment of hypertension

Dosage Summary

Oral:

Children: Dosage not established

Adults: Amlodipine 5-10 mg and valsartan 160-320 mg once daily (maximum: 10 mg/day [amlodipine]; 320 mg/day [valsartan]; **Note:** Titration is recommended

Dosage Forms

Tablet:

Exforge®: 5/160: Amlodipine 5 mg and valsartan 160 mg; 5/320 mg: Amlodipine 5 mg and valsartan 320 mg; 10/160: Amlodipine 10 mg and valsartan 160 mg; 10/320: Amlodipine 10 mg and valsartan 320 mg

amlodipine besylate *see* amlodipine *on page 68*

amlodipine besylate and olmesartan medoxomil *see* amlodipine and olmesartan *on page 70*

amlodipine besylate and telmisartan *see* telmisartan and amlodipine *on page 913*

amlodipine besylate and valsartan *see* amlodipine and valsartan *on page 70*

amlodipine besylate, olmesartan medoxomil, and hydrochlorothiazide *see* olmesartan, amlodipine, and hydrochlorothiazide *on page 698*

amlodipine besylate, valsartan, and hydrochlorothiazide *see* amlodipine, valsartan, and hydrochlorothiazide *on page 71*

amlodipine, hydrochlorothiazide, and olmesartan *see* olmesartan, amlodipine, and hydrochlorothiazide *on page 698*

amlodipine, hydrochlorothiazide, and valsartan *see* amlodipine, valsartan, and hydrochlorothiazide *on page 71*

amlodipine, valsartan, and hydrochlorothiazide

(am LOE di peen, val SAR tan, & hye droe klor oh THYE a zide)

Synonyms amlodipine besylate, valsartan, and hydrochlorothiazide; amlodipine, hydrochlorothiazide, and valsartan; hydrochlorothiazide, amlodipine, and valsartan; valsartan, hydrochlorothiazide, and amlodipine

U.S./Canadian Brand Names Exforge HCT® [US]

Therapeutic Category Angiotensin II Receptor Blocker; Calcium Channel Blocker; Diuretic, Thiazide

Use Treatment of hypertension (not for initial therapy)

Dosage Summary

Oral:

Children: Dosage not established

Adults: Amlodipine 5-10 mg and valsartan 160-320 mg and hydrochlorothiazide 12.5-25 mg once daily (maximum: 10 mg/day [amlodipine]; 25 mg/day [hydrochlorothiazide]; 320 mg/day [valsartan]); **Note:** Titration is recommended

Dosage Forms

Tablet, oral:

Exforge HCT®: Amlodipine 5 mg, valsartan 160 mg, and hydrochlorothiazide 12.5 mg; Amlodipine 5 mg, valsartan 160 mg, and hydrochlorothiazide 25 mg; Amlodipine 10 mg, valsartan 160 mg, and hydrochlorothiazide 12.5 mg; Amlodipine 10 mg, valsartan 160 mg, and hydrochlorothiazide 25 mg; Amlodipine 10 mg, valsartan 320 mg, and hydrochlorothiazide 25 mg

Ammens® Medicated Deodorant *(Discontinued)* *see* aspirin *on page 100*

Ammens® Original Medicated [US-OTC] *see* zinc oxide *on page 1001*

Ammens® Shower Fresh [US-OTC] *see* zinc oxide *on page 1001*

ammonapse *see* sodium phenylbutyrate *on page 886*

ammonia spirit (aromatic) (a MOE nee ah SPEAR it, air oh MAT ik)

Synonyms smelling salts

Therapeutic Category Respiratory Stimulant

Use Respiratory and circulatory stimulant; treatment of fainting

Dosage Summary

Inhalation:

Children: Dosage not established

Adults: Used as "smelling salts" to treat or prevent fainting

Dosage Forms

Solution, for inhalation: 1.7% to 2.1% (0.33 mL, 60 mL)

ammonium chloride (a MOE nee um KLOR ide)

Therapeutic Category Electrolyte Supplement, Oral

Use Treatment of hypochloremic states or metabolic alkalosis

Dosage Summary Note: Calculations may yield different requirements of ammomium chloride.

I.V.:

Children: Dose of mEq NH_4Cl = [0.2 L/kg x body weight (kg)] x [103 - observed serum chloride]; administer 50% of dose over 12 hours, then reevaluate. **Note:** 0.2 L/kg is the estimated chloride volume of distribution and 103 is the average normal serum chloride concentration (mEq/L) **or** Dose of NH_4Cl = [0.5 L/kg x body weight (kg)] x (observed serum HCO_3^- - 24); administer 50% of dose over 12 hours, then reevaluate. **Note:** 0.5 L/kg is the estimated bicarbonate volume of distribution and 24 is the average normal serum bicarbonate concentration (mEq/L)

Adults: Dose of mEq NH_4Cl = [0.2 L/kg x body weight (kg)] x [103 - observed serum chloride]; administer 50% of dose over 12 hours, then reevaluate. **Note:** 0.2 L/kg is the estimated chloride volume of distribution and 103 is the average normal serum chloride concentration (mEq/L) **or** Dose of NH_4Cl = [0.5 L/kg x body weight (kg)] x (observed serum HCO_3^- - 24); administer 50% of dose over 12 hours, then reevaluate. **Note:** 0.5 L/kg is the estimated bicarbonate volume of distribution and 24 is the average normal serum bicarbonate concentration (mEq/L)

Dosage Forms

Injection, solution: Ammonium 5 mEq/mL and chloride 5 mEq/mL (20 mL)

ammonium hydroxide and lactic acid *see* lactic acid and ammonium hydroxide *on page 542*
ammonium lactate *see* lactic acid and ammonium hydroxide *on page 542*
Ammonul® [US] *see* sodium phenylacetate and sodium benzoate *on page 886*
AMN107 *see* nilotinib *on page 676*
Amnesteem® [US] *see* isotretinoin *on page 530*

amobarbital (am oh BAR bi tal)

Synonyms amobarbital sodium; amylobarbitone
U.S./Canadian Brand Names Amytal® [US/Can]
Therapeutic Category Barbiturate
Controlled Substance C-II
Use Hypnotic in short-term treatment of insomnia; reduce anxiety and provide sedation preoperatively
Dosage Summary
I.M.:
Children <6 years: Dosage not established
Children 6-12 years: Sedative: 65-500 mg/dose
Adults:
Hypnotic: 65-200 mg at bedtime (maximum single dose: 1000 mg)
Sedative: 30-50 mg 2-3 times/day (maximum single dose: 1000 mg)
I.V.:
Children <6 years: Dosage not established
Children 6-12 years: Sedative: 65-500 mg/dose
Adults:
Hypnotic: 65-200 mg at bedtime (maximum single dose: 1000 mg)
Sedative: 30-50 mg 2-3 times/day (maximum single dose: 1000 mg)
Dosage Forms
Injection, powder for reconstitution:
Amytal®: 0.5 g

amobarbital sodium *see* amobarbital *on page 72*
Amoclan [US] *see* amoxicillin and clavulanate potassium *on page 73*
AMO Vitrax® ***(Discontinued)*** *see* hyaluronate and derivatives *on page 475*

amoxapine (a MOKS a peen)

Sound-Alike/Look-Alike Issues
amoxapine may be confused with amoxicillin, Amoxil®
Asendin may be confused with aspirin
Therapeutic Category Antidepressant, Tricyclic (Secondary Amine)
Use Treatment of depression, psychotic depression, depression accompanied by anxiety or agitation
Dosage Summary
Oral:
Children <16 years: Dosage not established
Adolescents: Initial: 25-50 mg/day as a single dose or in divided doses; Maintenance: 25-100 mg/day as a single dose at bedtime or in divided doses (maximum: 100 mg/day); **Note:** Titration is recommended
Adults: Initial: 50-75 mg/day in 2-3 divided doses; Maintenance 50-300 mg/day in 2-3 divided doses (maximum: 600 mg/day [inpatient]; 400 mg/day [outpatient]); **Note:** Titration is recommended
Dosage Forms
Tablet, oral: 25 mg, 50 mg, 100 mg, 150 mg

amoxicillin (a moks i SIL in)

Sound-Alike/Look-Alike Issues
amoxicillin may be confused with amoxapine, Amoxil®, Atarax®
Amoxil® may be confused with amoxapine, amoxicillin
Synonyms *p*-hydroxyampicillin; amoxicillin trihydrate; amoxycillin
U.S./Canadian Brand Names Apo-Amoxi® [Can]; Gen-Amoxicillin [Can]; Lin-Amox [Can]; Moxatag™ [US]; Mylan-Amoxicillin [Can]; Novamoxin® [Can]; Nu-Amoxi [Can]; PHL-Amoxicillin [Can]; PMS-Amoxicillin [Can]
Therapeutic Category Penicillin

Use Treatment of otitis media, sinusitis, and infections caused by susceptible organisms involving the upper and lower respiratory tract, skin, and urinary tract; prophylaxis of infective endocarditis in patients undergoing surgical or dental procedures; as part of a multidrug regimen for *H. pylori* eradication

Dosage Summary

Oral:

Infants ≤3 months: 20-30 mg/kg/day divided every 12 hours

Children >3 months and <40 kg: 20-90 mg/kg/day divided every 8-12 hours

Children ≥4 months: 20-100 mg/kg/day divided every 8 hours

Children ≥12 years: Extended-release tablet: 775 mg once daily

Adults: 250-500 mg every 8 hours **or** 500-875 mg twice daily (maximum: 875 mg/dose) **or** extended-release tablet 775 mg once daily

Dosage Forms

Capsule, oral: 250 mg, 500 mg

Powder for suspension, oral: 125 mg/5 mL (80 mL, 100 mL, 150 mL); 200 mg/5 mL (50 mL, 75 mL, 100 mL); 250 mg/5 mL (80 mL, 100 mL, 150 mL); 400 mg/5 mL (50 mL, 75 mL, 100 mL)

Tablet, oral: 500 mg, 875 mg

Tablet, chewable, oral: 125 mg, 200 mg, 250 mg, 400 mg

Tablet, extended release, oral:

Moxatag™: 775 mg

amoxicillin and clavulanate potassium

(a moks i SIL in & klav yoo LAN ate poe TASS ee um)

Sound-Alike/Look-Alike Issues

Augmentin® may be confused with amoxicillin, Azulfidine®

Synonyms amoxicillin and clavulanic acid; clavulanic acid and amoxicillin

U.S./Canadian Brand Names Amoclan [US]; Amoxi-Clav [Can]; Apo-Amoxi-Clav® [Can]; Augmentin ES-600® [US]; Augmentin XR® [US]; Augmentin® [US/Can]; Clavulin® [Can]; Novo-Clavamoxin [Can]; ratio-Aclavulanate [Can]

Therapeutic Category Penicillin

Use Treatment of otitis media, sinusitis, and infections caused by susceptible organisms involving the lower respiratory tract, skin and skin structure, and urinary tract; spectrum same as amoxicillin with additional coverage of beta-lactamase producing *B. catarrhalis*, *H. influenzae*, *N. gonorrhoeae*, and *S. aureus* (not MRSA). The expanded coverage of this combination makes it a useful alternative when amoxicillin resistance is present and patients cannot tolerate alternative treatments.

Dosage Summary Note: Dose in based on the amoxicillin component

Oral:

Immediate release:

Infants <3 months: 30 mg/kg/day divided every 12 hours

Children ≥3 months and <40 kg: 25-90 mg/kg/day divided every 12 hours **or** 20-40 mg/kg/day divided every 8 hours

Children >40 kg: 250-500 mg every 8 hours **or** 875 mg every 12 hours

Adults: 250-500 mg every 8 hours or 875 mg every 12 hours (maximum: 875 mg/dose)

Extended release:

Children <16 years: Dosage not established

Children ≥16 years: Two 1000 mg tablets every 12 hours (maximum: 2000 mg/dose)

Adults: Two 1000 mg tablets every 12 hours (maximum: 2000 mg/dose)

Dosage Forms

Powder for oral suspension: 200: Amoxicillin 200 mg and clavulanate potassium 28.5 mg per 5 mL; 400: Amoxicillin 400 mg and clavulanate potassium 57 mg per 5 mL; 600: Amoxicillin 600 mg and clavulanate potassium 42.9 mg per 5 mL

Amoclan:

200: Amoxicillin 200 mg and clavulanate potassium 28.5 mg per 5 mL

400: Amoxicillin 400 mg and clavulanate potassium 57 mg per 5 mL

600: Amoxicillin 600 mg and clavulanate potassium 42.9 mg per 5 mL

Augmentin®:

125: Amoxicillin 125 mg and clavulanate potassium 31.25 mg per 5 mL

250: Amoxicillin 250 mg and clavulanate potassium 62.5 mg per 5 mL

Augmentin ES-600®: Amoxicillin 600 mg and clavulanate potassium 42.9 mg per 5 mL

Tablet: 500: Amoxicillin 500 mg and clavulanate potassium 125 mg; 875: Amoxicillin 875 mg and clavulanate potassium 125 mg
Augmentin®:
250: Amoxicillin 250 mg and clavulanate potassium 125 mg
500: Amoxicillin 500 mg and clavulanate potassium 125 mg
875: Amoxicillin 875 mg and clavulanate potassium 125 mg
Tablet, chewable: 200: Amoxicillin 200 mg and clavulanate potassium 28.5 mg; 400: Amoxicillin 400 mg and clavulanate potassium 57 mg
Tablet, extended release: Amoxicillin 1000 mg and clavulanate acid 62.5 mg
Augmentin XR®: 1000: Amoxicillin 1000 mg and clavulanate acid 62.5 mg

amoxicillin and clavulanic acid *see* amoxicillin and clavulanate potassium *on page 73*

amoxicillin, clarithromycin, and lansoprazole *see* lansoprazole, amoxicillin, and clarithromycin *on page 549*

amoxicillin trihydrate *see* amoxicillin *on page 72*

Amoxi-Clav [Can] *see* amoxicillin and clavulanate potassium *on page 73*

Amoxil® *(Discontinued)* *see* amoxicillin *on page 72*

amoxycillin *see* amoxicillin *on page 72*

Amphadase™ [US] *see* hyaluronidase *on page 476*

amphetamine and dextroamphetamine *see* dextroamphetamine and amphetamine *on page 286*

Amphocin® *(Discontinued)* *see* amphotericin B (conventional) *on page 74*

Amphojel® [Can] *see* aluminum hydroxide *on page 58*

Amphojel® *(Discontinued)* *see* aluminum hydroxide *on page 58*

Amphotec® [US/Can] *see* amphotericin B cholesteryl sulfate complex *on page 74*

amphotericin B cholesteryl sulfate complex

(am foe TER i sin bee kole LES te ril SUL fate KOM plecks)

Synonyms ABCD; amphotericin B colloidal dispersion

U.S./Canadian Brand Names Amphotec® [US/Can]

Therapeutic Category Antifungal Agent

Use Treatment of invasive aspergillosis in patients who have failed amphotericin B deoxycholate treatment, or who have renal impairment or experience unacceptable toxicity which precludes treatment with amphotericin B deoxycholate in effective doses.

Dosage Summary

I.V.:
Children: 3-4 mg/kg/day (maximum: 7.5 mg/kg/day)
Adults: 3-4 mg/kg/day (maximum: 7.5 mg/kg/day)

Dosage Forms

Injection, powder for reconstitution:
Amphotec®: 50 mg, 100 mg

amphotericin B colloidal dispersion *see* amphotericin B cholesteryl sulfate complex *on page 74*

amphotericin B (conventional) (am foe TER i sin bee con VEN sha nal)

Synonyms amphotericin B desoxycholate

U.S./Canadian Brand Names Fungizone® [Can]

Therapeutic Category Antifungal Agent

Use Treatment of severe systemic and central nervous system infections caused by susceptible fungi such as *Candida* species, *Histoplasma capsulatum*, *Cryptococcus neoformans*, *Aspergillus* species, *Blastomyces dermatitidis*, *Torulopsis glabrata*, and *Coccidioides immitis*; fungal peritonitis; irrigant for bladder fungal infections; used in fungal infection in patients with bone marrow transplantation, amebic meningoencephalitis, ocular aspergillosis (intraocular injection), candidal cystitis (bladder irrigation), chemoprophylaxis (low-dose I.V.), immunocompromised patients at risk of aspergillosis (intranasal/nebulized), refractory meningitis (intrathecal), coccidioidal arthritis (intraarticular/I.M.).

Low-dose amphotericin B has been administered after bone marrow transplantation to reduce the risk of invasive fungal disease.

Dosage Summary

I.V.:

Infants: Test dose: 0.1 mg/kg/dose (maximum: 1 mg); Maintenance: 0.25-1 mg/kg/day given once daily; 1-1.5 mg/kg over 4-6 hours every other day may be given once therapy is established (maximum: 1.5-4 g cumulative dose)

Children: Test dose: 0.1 mg/kg/dose (maximum: 1 mg) infused over 30-60 minutes; Maintenance: 0.25-1 mg/kg/day given once daily; 1-1.5 mg/kg over 4-6 hours every other day may be given once therapy is established (maximum: 1.5-4 g cumulative dose)

Adults: Test dose: 1 mg infused over 20-30 minutes; Maintenance: 0.05-1.5 mg/kg/day given once daily; 1-1.5 mg/kg over 4-6 hours every other day may be given once therapy is established (maximum: 1.5 mg/kg/day)

Dosage Forms

Injection, powder for reconstitution: 50 mg

amphotericin B desoxycholate *see* amphotericin B (conventional) *on page 74*

amphotericin B lipid complex (am foe TER i sin bee LIP id KOM pleks)

Synonyms ABLC

U.S./Canadian Brand Names Abelcet® [US/Can]

Therapeutic Category Antifungal Agent

Use Treatment of aspergillosis or any type of progressive fungal infection in patients who are refractory to or intolerant of conventional amphotericin B therapy

Dosage Summary

I.V.:

Children: 2.5-5 mg/kg/day as a single daily dose (maximum: 5 mg/kg/day)

Adults: 2.5-5 mg/kg/day as a single daily dose (maximum: 5 mg/kg/day)

Dosage Forms

Injection, suspension [preservative free]:

Abelcet®: 5 mg/mL (20 mL)

amphotericin B liposomal (am foe TER i sin bee lye po SO mal)

Synonyms L-AmB

U.S./Canadian Brand Names AmBisome® [US/Can]

Therapeutic Category Antifungal Agent, Systemic

Use Empirical therapy for presumed fungal infection in febrile, neutropenic patients; treatment of patients with *Aspergillus* species, *Candida* species, and/or *Cryptococcus* species infections refractory to amphotericin B desoxycholate (conventional amphotericin), or in patients where renal impairment or unacceptable toxicity precludes the use of amphotericin B desoxycholate; treatment of cryptococcal meningitis in HIV-infected patients; treatment of visceral leishmaniasis

Dosage Summary

I.V.:

Children: 3-6 mg/kg/day as a single daily dose (maximum: 6 mg/kg/day)

Adults: 3-6 mg/kg/day as a single daily dose (maximum: 6 mg/kg/day)

Dosage Forms

Injection, powder for reconstitution:

AmBisome®: 50 mg

ampicillin (am pi SIL in)

Sound-Alike/Look-Alike Issues

ampicillin may be confused with aminophylline

Synonyms aminobenzylpenicillin; ampicillin sodium; ampicillin trihydrate

U.S./Canadian Brand Names Apo-Ampi® [Can]; Novo-Ampicillin [Can]; Nu-Ampi [Can]

Therapeutic Category Penicillin

Use Treatment of susceptible bacterial infections (nonbeta-lactamase-producing organisms); treatment or prophylaxis of infective endocarditis; susceptible bacterial infections caused by streptococci, pneumococci, nonpenicillinase-producing staphylococci, *Listeria*, meningococci; some strains of *H. influenzae*, *Salmonella*, *Shigella*, *E. coli*, *Enterobacter*, and *Klebsiella*

Dosage Summary

I.M.:

Infants: 100-400 mg/kg/day divided every 6 hours (maximum: 12 g/day)
Children: 100-400 mg/kg/day divided every 6 hours (maximum: 12 g/day)
Adults: 250-500 mg every 6 hours or up to 150-250 mg/kg/day divided every 3-4 hours (maximum: 12 g/day)

I.V.:

Infants: 100-400 mg/kg/day divided every 6 hours (maximum: 12 g/day)
Children: 100-400 mg/kg/day divided every 6 hours (maximum: 12 g/day)
Adults: 250-500 mg every 6 hours or up to 150-250 mg/kg/day divided every 3-4 hours (maximum: 12 g/day)

Oral:

Infants: 50-100 mg/kg/day divided every 6 hours (maximum: 4 g/day)
Children: 50-100 mg/kg/day divided every 6 hours (maximum: 4 g/day)
Adults: 250-500 mg every 6 hours

Dosage Forms

Capsule, oral: 250 mg, 500 mg
Injection, powder for reconstitution: 125 mg, 250 mg, 500 mg, 1 g, 2 g, 10 g
Powder for suspension, oral: 125 mg/5 mL (100 mL, 200 mL); 250 mg/5 mL (100 mL, 200 mL)

ampicillin and sulbactam (am pi SIL in & SUL bak tam)

Synonyms sulbactam and ampicillin

U.S./Canadian Brand Names Unasyn® [US/Can]

Therapeutic Category Penicillin

Use Treatment of susceptible bacterial infections involved with skin and skin structure, intraabdominal infections, gynecological infections; spectrum is that of ampicillin plus organisms producing beta-lactamases such as *S. aureus*, *H. influenzae*, *E. coli*, *Klebsiella*, *Acinetobacter*, *Enterobacter*, and anaerobes

Dosage Summary Note: Dosage recommendations based on the ampicillin component

I.M.:

Children: Dosage not established
Adults: 1-2 g (1.5-3 g Unasyn®) ampicillin every 6 hours (maximum: 8 g ampicillin/day)

I.V.:

Children <1 year: Dosage not established
Children ≥1 year: 100-400 mg ampicillin/kg/day divided every 6 hours (maximum: 8 g ampicillin/day)
Adults: 1-2 g (1.5-3 g Unasyn®) ampicillin every 6 hours (maximum: 8 g ampicillin/day)

Dosage Forms

Injection, powder for reconstitution: 1.5 g [ampicillin 1 g and sulbactam 0.5 g]; 3 g [ampicillin 2 g and sulbactam 1 g]; 15 g [ampicillin 10 g and sulbactam 5 g]

Unasyn®: 1.5 g [ampicillin 1 g and sulbactam 0.5 g]; 3 g [ampicillin 2 g and sulbactam 1 g]; 15 g [ampicillin 10 g and sulbactam 5 g]; 15 g [ampicillin 10 g and sulbactam 5 g

ampicillin sodium *see* ampicillin *on page* *75*

ampicillin trihydrate *see* ampicillin *on page* *75*

amprenavir *(Discontinued)*

AMPT *see* metyrosine *on page* *628*

Ampyra™ [US] *see* dalfampridine *on page* *266*

amrinone lactate *see* inamrinone *on page* *504*

Amrix® [US] *see* cyclobenzaprine *on page* *258*

Amvisc® *(Discontinued)* *see* hyaluronate and derivatives *on page* *475*

Amvisc® Plus *(Discontinued)* *see* hyaluronate and derivatives *on page* *475*

amylase, lipase, and protease *see* pancrelipase *on page* *723*

amyl nitrite (AM il NYE trite)

Synonyms isoamyl nitrite

Therapeutic Category Vasodilator

Use Coronary vasodilator in angina pectoris; adjunct in treatment of cyanide poisoning; produce changes in the intensity of heart murmurs

Dosage Summary

Nasal Inhalation:

Children: Dosage not established

Adults: 1-6 inhalations from 1 crushed ampul; may repeat in 3-5 minutes

Dosage Forms

Liquid, for inhalation: USP: 85% to 103% (0.3 mL)

amyl nitrite, sodium nitrite, and sodium thiosulfate *see* sodium nitrite, sodium thiosulfate, and amyl nitrite *on page 885*

amylobarbitone *see* amobarbital *on page 72*

Amytal® [US/Can] *see* amobarbital *on page 72*

AN100226 *see* natalizumab *on page 662*

Anabolin® ***(Discontinued)*** *see* nandrolone *(Canada only) on page 658*

Anacin® Advanced Headache Formula [US-OTC] *see* acetaminophen, aspirin, and caffeine *on page 27*

Anacin® PM Aspirin Free ***(Discontinued)*** *see* acetaminophen and diphenhydramine *on page 24*

Anadrol®-50 [US] *see* oxymetholone *on page 718*

Anafranil® [US/Can] *see* clomipramine *on page 237*

anagrelide (an AG gre lide)

Sound-Alike/Look-Alike Issues

anagrelide may be confused with anastrozole

Synonyms anagrelide hydrochloride; BL4162A; NSC-724577

U.S./Canadian Brand Names Agrylin® [US/Can]; Dom-Anagrelide [Can]; Mylan-Anagrelide [Can]; PMS-Anagrelide [Can]; Sandoz-Anagrelide [Can]

Therapeutic Category Platelet Reducing Agent

Use Treatment of thrombocythemia associated with myeloproliferative disorders (eg, chronic myelogenous leukemia, essential thrombocythemia, polycythemia vera, myeloid metaplasia with myelofibrosis, or other myeloproliferative disorder)

Dosage Summary Note: Maintain initial dose for ≥1 week, then adjust to the lowest effective dose to reduce and maintain platelet count <600,000/µL ideally to the normal range; the dose must not be increased by >0.5 mg/day in any 1 week

Oral:

Children: Initial: 0.5 mg/day; Maintenance: 0.5 mg 1-4 times/day (maximum: 10 mg/day; 2.5 mg/dose)

Adults: Initial: 0.5 mg 4 times/day **or** 1 mg twice daily (maximum: 10 mg/day; 2.5 mg/dose)

Dosage Forms

Capsule, oral: 0.5 mg, 1 mg

Agrylin®: 0.5 mg

anagrelide hydrochloride *see* anagrelide *on page 77*

anakinra (an a KIN ra)

Sound-Alike/Look-Alike Issues

anakinra may be confused with amikacin, Ampyra™

Kineret® may be confused with Amikin®

Synonyms IL-1Ra; interleukin-1 receptor antagonist

U.S./Canadian Brand Names Kineret® [US/Can]

Therapeutic Category Antirheumatic, Disease Modifying

Use Treatment of moderately- to severely-active rheumatoid arthritis in adult patients who have failed one or more disease-modifying antirheumatic drugs (DMARDs); may be used alone or in combination with DMARDs (other than tumor necrosis factor-blocking agents)

Dosage Summary

SubQ:

Children: Dosage not established

Adults: 100 mg once daily

Dosage Forms

Injection, solution [preservative free]:

Kineret®: 100 mg/0.67 mL (0.67 mL)

Ana-Kit® [US] *see* epinephrine and chlorpheniramine *on page 354*

Analpram E™ [US] *see* pramoxine and hydrocortisone *on page 787*
Analpram-HC® [US] *see* pramoxine and hydrocortisone *on page 787*
AnaMantle HC® Cream [US] *see* lidocaine and hydrocortisone *on page 564*
AnaMantle HC® Forte [US] *see* lidocaine and hydrocortisone *on page 564*
AnaMantle HC® Gel [US] *see* lidocaine and hydrocortisone *on page 564*
Anamine® Syrup *(Discontinued)* *see* chlorpheniramine and pseudoephedrine *on page 209*
Anandron® [Can] *see* nilutamide *on page 676*
Anaplex® DM [US] *see* brompheniramine, pseudoephedrine, and dextromethorphan *on page 149*
Anaplex® DMX *(Discontinued)* *see* brompheniramine, pseudoephedrine, and dextromethorphan *on page 149*
Anaplex® Liquid *(Discontinued)* *see* chlorpheniramine and pseudoephedrine *on page 209*
Anaprox® [US/Can] *see* naproxen *on page 659*
Anaprox® DS [US/Can] *see* naproxen *on page 659*
Anaspaz® [US] *see* hyoscyamine *on page 491*

anastrozole (an AS troe zole)

Sound-Alike/Look-Alike Issues
anastrozole may be confused with anagrelide, letrozole
Arimidex® may be confused with Aromasin®

Synonyms ICI-D1033; ZD1033

U.S./Canadian Brand Names Arimidex® [US/Can]

Therapeutic Category Antineoplastic Agent

Use Treatment of locally-advanced or metastatic breast cancer (hormone receptor-positive or unknown) in postmenopausal women; treatment of advanced breast cancer in postmenopausal women with disease progression following tamoxifen therapy; adjuvant treatment of early hormone receptor-positive breast cancer in postmenopausal women

Dosage Summary
Oral:
Children: Dosage not established
Adults: 1 mg once daily

Dosage Forms
Tablet, oral: 1 mg
Arimidex®: 1 mg

Anatrast *(Discontinued)* *see* barium *on page 117*
A-Natural [US-OTC] *see* vitamin A *on page 987*
A-Natural-25 [US-OTC] *see* vitamin A *on page 987*
Anbesol® [US-OTC] *see* benzocaine *on page 124*
Anbesol® Baby [US-OTC/Can] *see* benzocaine *on page 124*
Anbesol® Cold Sore Therapy [US-OTC] *see* benzocaine *on page 124*
Anbesol® Jr. [US-OTC] *see* benzocaine *on page 124*
Anbesol® Maximum Strength [US-OTC] *see* benzocaine *on page 124*
ancef *see* cefazolin *on page 189*
Ancobon® [US/Can] *see* flucytosine *on page 408*
Andehist DM NR *(Discontinued)* *see* brompheniramine, pseudoephedrine, and dextromethorphan *on page 149*
Andehist DM NR Drops *(Discontinued)*
Andehist NR Drops *(Discontinued)*
Andehist NR Syrup *(Discontinued)* *see* brompheniramine and pseudoephedrine *on page 148*
Andriol® [Can] *see* testosterone *on page 919*
Androcur® [Can] *see* cyproterone *(Canada only) on page 262*
Androcur® Depot [Can] *see* cyproterone *(Canada only) on page 262*
Androderm® [US/Can] *see* testosterone *on page 919*
AndroGel® [US/Can] *see* testosterone *on page 919*
Android® [US] *see* methyltestosterone *on page 624*
Andro-L.A.® Injection *(Discontinued)* *see* testosterone *on page 919*

Androlone®-D *(Discontinued)* *see* nandrolone *(Canada only) on page 658*
Androlone® *(Discontinued)* *see* nandrolone *(Canada only) on page 658*
Andropository [Can] *see* testosterone *on page 919*
Andropository® Injection *(Discontinued)* *see* testosterone *on page 919*
Androvite® [US-OTC] *see* vitamins (multiple/oral) *on page 990*
Androxy™ [US] *see* fluoxymesterone *on page 416*
Anectine® [US] *see* succinylcholine *on page 897*
Anestacon® *(Discontinued)* *see* lidocaine (topical) *on page 562*
Anestafoam™ [US-OTC] *see* lidocaine (topical) *on page 562*
aneurine hydrochloride *see* thiamine *on page 927*
Anexate® [Can] *see* flumazenil *on page 409*
Angeliq® [US/Can] *see* drospirenone and estradiol *on page 334*
Angiofluor™ [US] *see* fluorescein *on page 412*
Angiofluor™ Lite [US] *see* fluorescein *on page 412*
Angiomax® [US/Can] *see* bivalirudin *on page 141*
anhydrous glucose *see* dextrose *on page 290*

anidulafungin (ay nid yoo la FUN jin)

Synonyms LY303366

U.S./Canadian Brand Names Eraxis™ [US/Can]

Therapeutic Category Antifungal Agent, Parenteral; Echinocandin

Use Treatment of candidemia and other forms of *Candida* infections (including those of intraabdominal, peritoneal, and esophageal locus)

Dosage Summary

I.V.:

Children: Dosage not established
Adults: Loading dose: 100-200 mg as a single dose; Maintenance: 50-100 mg daily

Dosage Forms

Injection, powder for reconstitution:
Eraxis™: 50 mg, 100 mg

Anodynos-DHC® *(Discontinued)* *see* hydrocodone and acetaminophen *on page 479*
Anolor 300 [US] *see* butalbital, acetaminophen, and caffeine *on page 159*
Anoquan® *(Discontinued)*
Ansaid® [Can] *see* flurbiprofen (systemic) *on page 418*
Ansaid® *(Discontinued)* *see* flurbiprofen (systemic) *on page 418*
ansamycin *see* rifabutin *on page 841*
Antabuse® [US] *see* disulfiram *on page 319*
antagon *see* ganirelix *on page 437*
Antara® [US] *see* fenofibrate *on page 393*
Antazoline-V® Ophthalmic *(Discontinued)*
Anthra-Derm® *(Discontinued)* *see* anthralin *on page 79*
Anthraforte® [Can] *see* anthralin *on page 79*

anthralin (AN thra lin)

Synonyms dithranol

U.S./Canadian Brand Names Anthraforte® [Can]; Anthranol® [Can]; Anthrascalp® [Can]; Dritho-Scalp® [US]; Micanol® [Can]

Therapeutic Category Keratolytic Agent

Use Treatment of psoriasis (quiescent or chronic psoriasis)

Dosage Summary

Topical:

Adults: Generally, apply once a day or as directed.

Dosage Forms

Cream, topical:
Dritho-Scalp®: 0.5% (50 g)

Anthranol® [Can] *see* anthralin *on page 79*

Anthrascalp® [Can] *see* anthralin *on page 79*

anthrax vaccine, adsorbed (AN thraks vak SEEN ad SORBED)

Synonyms AVA

U.S./Canadian Brand Names BioThrax® [US]

Therapeutic Category Vaccine

Use Immunization against *Bacillus anthracis* in persons at high risk for exposure.

The Advisory Committee on Immunization Practices (ACIP) recommends routine vaccination (pre-exposure vaccination) for the following:

- Persons who work directly with the organism in the laboratory
- Persons who handle animals or animal products only when
  - potentially infected in research settings;
  - in areas of high incidence of enzootic anthrax; or
  - where standards and restrictions are not sufficient to prevent exposure
- Military personnel deployed to areas with high risk of exposure as recommended by the Department of Defense (DoD)
- Persons engaged in environmental investigations or remediation efforts

Routine immunization for the general population is not recommended. Routine vaccination may be offered to emergency and other responders (police and fire departments, the National Guard, etc) on a voluntary basis under the direction of a comprehensive occupational health and safety program.

The ACIP recommends postexposure prophylaxis for the following (in the absence of completing a pre-exposure, routine vaccination schedule):

- The general public, including pregnant and breast-feeding women
- Medical professionals
- Children ages 0-18 years as determined on an event-by-event basis
- Persons engaged in handling certain animals or animal products
- Persons who work directly with the organism in the laboratory (postexposure vaccination dependant upon pre-event vaccination status)
- Military personnel as recommended by the DoD
- Persons engaged in environmental investigations or remediation efforts (postexposure vaccination dependant upon pre-event vaccination status)
- Emergency and other responders (police and fire departments, the National Guard, etc)
- Persons working in postal facilities

Dosage Summary

I.M.:

Children <18 years: Dosage not established.

Adults ≤65 years: Five injections of 0.5 mL each given at day 0, week 4, then 6-, 12-, and 18 months; booster injections of 0.5 mL at 1-year intervals are recommended for immunity to be maintained in persons who remain at risk

Elderly >65 years: Dosage not established

SubQ:

Children <18 years: Dosage not established. Use in children is recommended by the ACIP as determined on an event-by-event basis.

Adults: Postexposure prophylaxis: Three injections of 0.5 mL each given at day 0, week 2, and week 4. Administer with a 60-day course of antibiotics. (Refer to guidelines)

Dosage Forms

Injection, suspension:

BioThrax®: *Bacillus anthracis* proteins (5 mL)

anti-4 alpha integrin *see* natalizumab *on page 662*

131 I anti-B1 antibody *see* tositumomab and iodine I 131 tositumomab *on page 944*

131 I-anti-B1 monoclonal antibody *see* tositumomab and iodine I 131 tositumomab *on page 944*

Antiben® ***(Discontinued)*** *see* antipyrine and benzocaine *on page 83*

anti-CD20 monoclonal antibody *see* rituximab *on page 846*

anti-CD20-murine monoclonal antibody I-131 *see* tositumomab and iodine I 131 tositumomab *on page 944*

anti-CD52 monoclonal antibody *see* alemtuzumab *on page 47*

anti-c-erB-2 *see* trastuzumab *on page 948*

Anti-Diarrheal [US-OTC] *see* loperamide *on page 573*

antidigoxin fab fragments, ovine *see* digoxin immune Fab *on page 303*

antidiuretic hormone *see* vasopressin *on page 980*

anti-ERB-2 *see* trastuzumab *on page 948*

Anti-Fungal™ [US-OTC] *see* clotrimazole (topical) *on page 240*

antihemophilic factor (human) (an tee hee moe FIL ik FAK tor HYU man)

Synonyms AHF (human); factor VIII (human)

U.S./Canadian Brand Names Hemofil M [US/Can]; Koāte®-DVI [US]; Monarc-M™ [US]; Monoclate-P® [US]

Therapeutic Category Blood Product Derivative

Use Prevention and treatment of hemorrhagic episodes in patients with hemophilia A (classic hemophilia); perioperative management of hemophilia A; can be of significant therapeutic value in patients with acquired factor VIII inhibitors not exceeding 10 Bethesda units/mL

Dosage Summary Note: Individualize dosage based on coagulation studies performed prior to treatment and at regular intervals during treatment. In general, administration of factor VIII 1 int. unit/kg will increase circulating factor VIII levels by ~2 int. units/dL (consult individual product labeling for specific dosing recommendations). Dose should bring factor VIII levels to 20% to 100% of normal depending on type of hemorrhage.

I.V.:

Children: Desired factor VIII increase (%): Body weight (kg) x 0.5 int. units/kg x desired factor VIII increase (%) = int. units factor VIII required; Expected factor VIII increase (%): (# int. units administered x 2%/int. units/kg) divided by body weight (kg) = expected % factor VIII increase

Adults: Desired factor VIII increase (%): Body weight (kg) x 0.5 int. units/kg x desired factor VIII increase (%) = int. units factor VIII required; Expected factor VIII increase (%): (# int. units administered x 2%/int. units/kg) divided by body weight (kg) = expected % factor VIII increase

Dosage Forms

Injection, powder for reconstitution:

Hemofil M: Vial labeled with international units

Koāte®-DVI: ~250 int. units, ~500 int. units, ~1000 int. units

Monarc-M™: Vial labeled with international units

Monoclate-P®: ~250 int. units, ~500 int. units, ~1000 int. units, ~1500 int. units

antihemophilic factor (recombinant) (an tee hee moe FIL ik FAK tor ree KOM be nant)

Synonyms AHF (recombinant); factor VIII (recombinant); rAHF

U.S./Canadian Brand Names Advate [US/Can]; Helixate® FS [US/Can]; Kogenate® FS [US/Can]; Kogenate® [Can]; Recombinate [US/Can]; ReFacto® [Can]; Xyntha™ [US]

Therapeutic Category Blood Product Derivative

Use Prevention and treatment of hemorrhagic episodes in patients with hemophilia A (classic hemophilia or congenital factor VIII deficiency); perioperative management of hemophilia A; prophylaxis of joint bleeding and to reduce risk of joint damage in children with hemophilia A with no preexisting joint damage; can be of significant therapeutic value in patients with acquired factor VIII inhibitors ≤10 Bethesda units/mL

Dosage Summary Note: Individualize dosage based on coagulation studies performed prior to treatment and at regular intervals during treatment. In general, administration of factor VIII 1 int. unit/kg will increase circulating factor VIII levels by ~2 int. units/dL (consult individual product labeling for specific dosing recommendations). Dose should bring factor VIII levels to 20% to 100% of normal depending on type of hemorrhage.

I.V.:

Children: Desired factor VIII increase (%): [Body weight (kg) x desired factor VIII increase (%)] divided by 2%/int. units/kg = int. units factor VIII required; Expected factor VIII increase (%): (# int. units administered x 2%/int. units/kg) divided by body weight (kg) = expected % factor VIII increase; 25 int. units/kg every other day

Adults: Desired factor VIII increase (%): [Body weight (kg) x desired factor VIII increase (%)] divided by 2%/int. units/kg = int. units factor VIII required; Expected factor VIII increase (%): (# int. units administered x 2%/int. units/kg) divided by body weight (kg) = expected % factor VIII increase

Dosage Forms

Injection, powder for reconstitution [preservative free]:

Advate: 250 int. units, 500 int. units, 1000 int. units, 1500 int. units, 2000 int. units, 3000 int. units
Helixate® FS: 250 int. units, 500 int. units, 1000 int. units, 2000 int. units, 3000 int. units
Kogenate® FS: 250 int. units, 500 int. units, 1000 int. units, 2000 int. units, 3000 int. units
Recombinate: 250 int. units, 500 int. units, 1000 int. units
Xyntha™: 250 int. units, 500 int. units, 1000 int. units, 2000 int. units

antihemophilic factor/von Willebrand factor complex (human)

(an tee hee moe FIL ik FAK tor von WILL le brand FAK tor KOM plex HYU man)

Synonyms AHF (human); factor VIII (human); FVIII/vWF; vWF:RCof

U.S./Canadian Brand Names Alphanate® *[new formulation]* [US]; Humate-P® [US/Can]

Therapeutic Category Antihemophilic Agent; Blood Product Derivative

Use

Prevention and treatment of hemorrhagic episodes in patients with hemophilia A (classical hemophilia) (Alphanate®, Humate-P®) or acquired factor VIII deficiency (Alphanate®)

Prophylaxis with surgical and/or invasive procedures in patients with von Willebrand disease (vWD) when desmopressin is either ineffective or contraindicated (Alphanate®)

Treatment of spontaneous or trauma-induced bleeding, as well as prevention of excessive bleeding during and after surgery, in patients with vWD (mild, moderate, or severe) where use of desmopressin is known or suspected to be inadequate (Humate-P®)

Dosage Summary Note: Dosing is individualized based on coagulation studies.

I.V.:

Children:

Hemophilia A: In general, administration of factor VIII 1 int. unit/kg will increase circulating factor VIII levels by ~2 int. units/dL. Dose should maintain FVIII:C levels at 30% to 50% of normal based on type of hemorrhage.

von Willebrand disease (vWD):

Treatment (Humate-P®): In general, administration of factor VIII 1 int. unit/kg would be expected to raise circulating vWF:RCof approximately 3.5-4 int. units/dL. Usual range: vWF:RCof 40-80 int. units/kg (equivalent to factor VIII 17-33 units in Humate-P®); repeat dose based on clinical and laboratory measures. Dose should maintain vWF:RCof nadir >50%

Surgery/procedure prophylaxis (Alphanate®): Preoperative dose: vWF:RCof 75 int. units /kg; maintenance dose: vWF:RCof 50-75 int. units/kg every 8-12 hours as clinically needed.

Adults:

Hemophilia A: In general, administration of factor VIII 1 int. unit/kg will increase circulating factor VIII levels by ~2 int. units/dL. Dose should maintain FVIII:C levels at 30% to 50% of normal based on type of hemorrhage.

von Willebrand disease (VWD):

Treatment (Humate-P®): In general, administration of factor VIII 1 int. unit/kg would be expected to raise circulating vWF:RCof ~5 int. units/dL. Usual range: vWF:RCof 40-80 int. units/kg (equivalent to factor VIII 17-33 units in Humate-P®); repeat dose based on clinical and laboratory measures. Dose should maintain vWF:RCof nadir >50%

Surgery/procedure prophylaxis (Alphanate®): Preoperative dose: vWF:RCof 60 int. units/kg; maintenance dose: vWF:RCof 40-60 int. units/kg every 8-12 hours as clinically needed.

Dosage Forms

Injection, powder for reconstitution [human derived]:

Alphanate®:

250 int. units [Factor VIII and vWF:RCof ratio varies by lot]
500 int. units [Factor VIII and vWF:RCof ratio varies by lot]
1000 int. units [Factor VIII and vWF:RCof ratio varies by lot]
1500 int. units [Factor VIII and vWF:RCof ratio varies by lot]

Humate-P®:

FVIII 250 int. units and vWF:RCof 600 int. units
FVIII 500 int. units and vWF:RCof 1200 int. units
FVIII 1000 int. units and vWF:RCof 2400 int. units

Anti-Hist [US-OTC] *see* diphenhydramine (systemic) *on page 310*

Antihist-1® *(Discontinued)* *see* clemastine *on page 231*

antiinhibitor coagulant complex (an TEE in HI bi tor coe AG yoo lant KOM pleks)

Synonyms AICC; coagulant complex inhibitor

U.S./Canadian Brand Names Feiba NF [US/Can]; Feiba VH Immuno [Can]; Feiba VH [US]

Therapeutic Category Hemophilic Agent

Use Hemophilia A & B patients with inhibitors who are to undergo surgery or those who are bleeding

Dosage Summary

I.V.:

Children: 50-100 units/kg every 6-12 hours (maximum: 200 units/kg/day)
Adults: 50-100 units/kg every 6-12 hours (maximum: 200 units/kg/day)

Dosage Forms

Injection, powder for reconstitution:

Feiba NF, Feiba VH: ~500 units, ~1000 units, ~2500 units

Antilirium® *(Discontinued)* *see* physostigmine *on page 759*

Antiminth® *(Discontinued)* *see* pyrantel pamoate *on page 816*

Antiphlogistine Rub A-535 No Odour [Can] *see* trolamine *on page 963*

antipyrine and benzocaine (an tee PYE reen & BEN zoe kane)

Synonyms benzocaine and antipyrine

U.S./Canadian Brand Names A/B Otic [US]; Allergen® [US]; Auralgan® [Can]

Therapeutic Category Otic Agent, Analgesic; Otic Agent, Ceruminolytic

Use Temporary relief of pain and reduction of swelling associated with acute congestive and serous otitis media, swimmer's ear, otitis externa; facilitates ear wax removal

Dosage Summary

Otic:

Children: Instill drops 3-4 times/day (ear wax removal) or fill ear canal every 1-2 hours (otitis media)
Adults: Instill drops 3-4 times/day (ear wax removal) or fill ear canal every 1-2 hours (otitis media)

Dosage Forms

Solution, otic [drops]: Antipyrine 5.4% and benzocaine 1.4% (10 mL)

Antispas® Injection *(Discontinued)* *see* dicyclomine *on page 299*

anti-tac monoclonal antibody *see* daclizumab *on page 265*

antithrombin III *see* antithrombin III *on page 83*

antithrombin alfa *see* antithrombin III *on page 83*

antithrombin III (an tee THROM bin)

Synonyms antithrombin alfa; antithrombin III; AT; AT-III; hpAT; rhAT; rhATIII

U.S./Canadian Brand Names Atryn® [US]; Thrombate III® [US/Can]

Therapeutic Category Blood Product Derivative

Use Prophylaxis (ATryn®, Thrombate III®) of thromboembolic events in patients with hereditary antithrombin (AT or AT-III) deficiency undergoing surgical or obstetrical procedures (eg, childbirth); treatment (Thrombate III®) of thromboembolism in patients with hereditary AT deficiency

Dosage Summary Note: Dosing is individualized based on pretherapy antithrombin AT levels.

I.V.:

Human plasma derived (Thrombate III®):

Children: Dosage not established

Adults: Initial dose: Should raise AT levels to 120% and may be calculated based on the following formula: [(desired AT level % - baseline AT level %) x body weight (kg)] **divided** by 1.4 = int. units of antithrombin required; Maintenance dose: Should be targeted to keep levels between 80% to 120% which may be achieved by administering 60% of the initial loading dose every 24 hours. Adjustments may be made by adjusting dose or interval.

Recombinant derived (ATryn®):

Children: Dosage not established

Adults: Dosing should be individualized to raise and maintain AT activity levels to 80-120% of normal and may be calculated based on the following formula:

Surgical patients (nonpregnant): Loading dose: [(100 - baseline AT activity level) **divided** by 2.3] x body weight (kg) = int. units of antithrombin required; Maintenance infusion: [(100 - baseline AT level) **divided** by 10.2] x body weight (kg) = int. units of antithrombin required/hour

Pregnant patients: Loading dose: [(100 - baseline AT activity level) **divided** by 1.3] x body weight (kg) = int. units of antithrombin required; Maintenance infusion: [(100 - baseline AT level) **divided** by 5.4] x body weight (kg) = int. units of antithrombin required/hour

Dosage Forms

Injection, powder for reconstitution [preservative free]:

Atryn®: ~1750 int. units

Thrombate III®: ~500 int. units, ~1000 int. units

antithymocyte globulin (equine) (an te THY moe site GLOB yu lin, E kwine)

Sound-Alike/Look-Alike Issues

antithymocyte globulin equine (Atgam®) may be confused with antithymocyte globulin rabbit (Thymoglobulin®)

Atgam® may be confused with Ativan®

Synonyms antithymocyte immunoglobulin; ATG; horse antihuman thymocyte gamma globulin; lymphocyte immune globulin

U.S./Canadian Brand Names Atgam® [US/Can]

Therapeutic Category Immunosuppressant Agent

Use Prevention and treatment of acute renal allograft rejection; treatment of moderate-to-severe aplastic anemia in patients not considered suitable candidates for bone marrow transplantation

Dosage Summary **Note:** An intradermal skin test is recommended prior to administration of the initial dose of ATG; use 0.1 mL of a fresh 1:1000 dilution of ATG in normal saline. **Note:** Premedication with diphenhydramine, hydrocortisone, and acetaminophen is recommended prior to first dose.

I.V.:

Children: Initial: 5-25 mg/kg/day administered daily for 8-14 days; may be followed by administration every other day (maximum: 21 doses in 28 days).

Adults: Initial: 10-20 mg/kg/day administered daily; may be followed by administration every other day (maximum: 21 doses in 28 days).

Dosage Forms

Injection, solution:

Atgam®: 50 mg/mL (5 mL)

antithymocyte globulin (rabbit) (an te THY moe site GLOB yu lin RAB bit)

Sound-Alike/Look-Alike Issues

antithymocyte globulin rabbit (Thymoglobulin®) may be confused with antithymocyte globulin equine (Atgam®)

Synonyms antithymocyte immunoglobulin; rATG

U.S./Canadian Brand Names Thymoglobulin® [US]

Therapeutic Category Immunosuppressant Agent

Use Treatment of acute rejection of renal transplant; used in conjunction with concomitant immunosuppression

Dosage Summary

I.V.:

Children: 1.5 mg/kg/day as a single daily dose

Adults: 1.5 mg/kg/day as a single daily dose

Dosage Forms

Injection, powder for reconstitution:

Thymoglobulin®: 25 mg

antithymocyte immunoglobulin *see* antithymocyte globulin (equine) *on page 84*

antithymocyte immunoglobulin *see* antithymocyte globulin (rabbit) *on page 84*

antitumor necrosis factor apha (human) *see* adalimumab *on page 37*

Anti-Tuss® Expectorant *(Discontinued)* *see* guaifenesin *on page 454*

anti-VEGF monoclonal antibody *see* bevacizumab *on page 136*

anti-VEGF rhuMAb *see* bevacizumab *on page 136*

antivenin (crotalidae) polyvalent, FAB (ovine) *see* crotalidae polyvalent immune FAB (ovine) *on page 255*

antivenin *(Latrodectus mactans)* (an tee VEN in lak tro DUK tus MAK tans)

Synonyms *Latrodectus mactans* antivenin; *Latrodectus* antivenin; black widow spider species antivenin

U.S./Canadian Brand Names Antivenin (Latrodectus mactans) [US]

Therapeutic Category Antivenin

Use Treatment of patients with moderate-to-severe symptoms (eg, cramping, intractable pain, hypertension) due to black widow spider bites

Dosage Summary

I.M.:

Children <12 years: Dosage not established

Children ≥12 years: 1-2 vials (2.5-5 mL)

I.V.:

Children: 1-2 vials (2.5-5 mL)

Adults: 1-2 vials (2.5-5 mL)

Dosage Forms

Injection, powder for reconstitution:

Antivenin (Latrodectus mactans): 6000 Antivenin units

Antivenin (Latrodectus mactans) [US] *see* antivenin *(Latrodectus mactans) on page 85*

antivenin *(Micrurus fulvius)* (an tee VEN in mye KRU rus FUL vee us)

Synonyms *Micrurus fulvius* antivenin; North American coral snake antivenin

Therapeutic Category Antivenin

Use Neutralization of venoms of Eastern coral snake and Texas coral snake

Dosage Summary

I.V.:

Children: 3-5 vials; some patients may need more than 10 vials

Adults: 3-5 vials; some patients may need more than 10 vials

Note: Each vial of antivenom neutralizes ~2 mg of venom.

Antivert® [US] *see* meclizine *on page 595*

Antizol® [US] *see* fomepizole *on page 425*

Antrizine® *(Discontinued)* *see* meclizine *on page 595*

Anturane® *(Discontinued)*

Anucort-HC™ [US] *see* hydrocortisone (topical) *on page 483*

Anu-Med [US-OTC] *see* phenylephrine (topical) *on page 752*

Anu-med HC [US] *see* hydrocortisone (topical) *on page 483*

Anusol-HC® [US] *see* hydrocortisone (topical) *on page 483*

Anusol HC-1® [US-OTC] *see* hydrocortisone (topical) *on page 483*

Anuzinc [Can] *see* zinc sulfate *on page 1002*

Anxanil® Oral *(Discontinued)* *see* hydroxyzine *on page 490*

Anzemet® [US/Can] *see* dolasetron *on page 323*

4-AP *see* dalfampridine *on page 266*

Apacet® *(Discontinued)* *see* acetaminophen *on page 21*

APAP *see* acetaminophen *on page 21*

APAP 500 [US-OTC] *see* acetaminophen *on page 21*

APAP and tramadol *see* acetaminophen and tramadol *on page 27*

Apaphen® *(Discontinued)* *see* acetaminophen and phenyltoloxamine *on page 26*

APC8015 *see* sipuleucel-T *on page 878*

ApexiCon™ [US] *see* diflorasone *on page 301*

ApexiCon™ E [US] *see* diflorasone *on page 301*

Aphrodyne® *(Discontinued)* *see* yohimbine *on page 996*

Aphthasol® [US] *see* amlexanox *on page 68*

Apidra® [US/Can] *see* insulin glulisine *on page 511*

A.P.L.® *(Discontinued)* *see* chorionic gonadotropin (human) *on page 219*

Aplenzin™ [US] *see* bupropion *on page 156*

Aplisol® [US] *see* tuberculin tests *on page 965*

Aplitest® *(Discontinued)* *see* tuberculin tests *on page 965*

aplonidine *see* apraclonidine *on page* *91*
Apo-Acebutolol® [Can] *see* acebutolol *on page* *21*
Apo-Acetaminophen® [Can] *see* acetaminophen *on page* *21*
Apo-Acetazolamide® [Can] *see* acetazolamide *on page* *32*
Apo-Acyclovir® [Can] *see* acyclovir (systemic) *on page* *36*
Apo-Alendronate® [Can] *see* alendronate *on page* *47*
Apo-Alfuzosin® [Can] *see* alfuzosin *on page* *49*
Apo-Allopurinol® [Can] *see* allopurinol *on page* *52*
Apo-Alpraz® [Can] *see* alprazolam *on page* *55*
Apo-Alpraz® TS [Can] *see* alprazolam *on page* *55*
Apo-Amiloride® [Can] *see* amiloride *on page* *63*
Apo-Amilzide® [Can] *see* amiloride and hydrochlorothiazide *on page* *64*
Apo-Amiodarone® [Can] *see* amiodarone *on page* *67*
Apo-Amitriptyline® [Can] *see* amitriptyline *on page* *67*
Apo-Amlodipine® [Can] *see* amlodipine *on page* *68*
Apo-Amoxi® [Can] *see* amoxicillin *on page* *72*
Apo-Amoxi-Clav® [Can] *see* amoxicillin and clavulanate potassium *on page* *73*
Apo-Ampi® [Can] *see* ampicillin *on page* *75*
Apo-Atenidone® [Can] *see* atenolol and chlorthalidone *on page* *103*
Apo-Atenol® [Can] *see* atenolol *on page* *102*
Apo-Atorvastatin® [Can] *see* atorvastatin *on page* *104*
Apo-Azathioprine® [Can] *see* azathioprine *on page* *109*
Apo-Azithromycin® [Can] *see* azithromycin (systemic) *on page* *111*
Apo-Baclofen® [Can] *see* baclofen *on page* *115*
Apo-Beclomethasone® [Can] *see* beclomethasone (nasal) *on page* *120*
Apo-Benazepril® [Can] *see* benazepril *on page* *122*
Apo-Benztropine® [Can] *see* benztropine *on page* *130*
Apo-Benzydamine® [Can] *see* benzydamine *(Canada only)* *on page* *130*
Apo-Bicalutamide® [Can] *see* bicalutamide *on page* *137*
Apo-Bisacodyl® [Can] *see* bisacodyl *on page* *138*
Apo-Bisoprolol® [Can] *see* bisoprolol *on page* *141*
Apo-Brimonidine® [Can] *see* brimonidine *on page* *144*
Apo-Brimonidine P® [Can] *see* brimonidine *on page* *144*
Apo-Bromazepam® [Can] *see* bromazepam *(Canada only)* *on page* *146*
Apo-Bromocriptine® [Can] *see* bromocriptine *on page* *146*
Apo-Buspirone® [Can] *see* buspirone *on page* *157*
Apo-Butorphanol® [Can] *see* butorphanol *on page* *161*
Apo-Cal® [Can] *see* calcium carbonate *on page* *167*
Apo-Calcitonin® [Can] *see* calcitonin *on page* *165*
Apo-Capto® [Can] *see* captopril *on page* *176*
Apo-Carbamazepine® [Can] *see* carbamazepine *on page* *177*
Apo-Carvedilol® [Can] *see* carvedilol *on page* *186*
Apo-Cefaclor® [Can] *see* cefaclor *on page* *188*
Apo-Cefadroxil® [Can] *see* cefadroxil *on page* *189*
Apo-Cefoxitin® [Can] *see* cefoxitin *on page* *191*
Apo-Cefprozil® [Can] *see* cefprozil *on page* *192*
Apo-Cefuroxime® [Can] *see* cefuroxime *on page* *194*
Apo-Cephalex® [Can] *see* cephalexin *on page* *197*
Apo-Cetirizine® [Can] *see* cetirizine *on page* *198*
Apo-Chlorax® [Can] *see* clidinium and chlordiazepoxide *on page* *231*
Apo-Chlordiazepoxide® [Can] *see* chlordiazepoxide *on page* *203*
Apo-Chlorpropamide® [Can] *see* chlorpropamide *on page* *217*
Apo-Chlorthalidone® [Can] *see* chlorthalidone *on page* *217*

Apo-Levobunolol® [Can] *see* levobunolol *on page 556*
Apo-Levocarb® [Can] *see* carbidopa and levodopa *on page 182*
Apo-Levocarb® CR [Can] *see* carbidopa and levodopa *on page 182*
Apo-Lisinopril® [Can] *see* lisinopril *on page 570*
Apo-Lisinopril®/Hctz [Can] *see* lisinopril and hydrochlorothiazide *on page 570*
Apo-Lithium® Carbonate [Can] *see* lithium *on page 571*
Apo-Lithium® Carbonate SR [Can] *see* lithium *on page 571*
Apo-Loperamide® [Can] *see* loperamide *on page 573*
Apo-Loratadine® [Can] *see* loratadine *on page 575*
Apo-Lorazepam® [Can] *see* lorazepam *on page 576*
Apo-Lovastatin® [Can] *see* lovastatin *on page 579*
Apo-Loxapine® [Can] *see* loxapine *on page 580*
Apo-Medroxy® [Can] *see* medroxyprogesterone *on page 597*
Apo-Mefenamic® [Can] *see* mefenamic acid *on page 597*
Apo-Mefloquine® [Can] *see* mefloquine *on page 598*
Apo-Megestrol® [Can] *see* megestrol *on page 598*
Apo-Meloxicam® [Can] *see* meloxicam *on page 598*
Apo-Metformin® [Can] *see* metformin *on page 609*
Apo-Methazide® [Can] *see* methyldopa and hydrochlorothiazide *on page 619*
Apo-Methazolamide® [Can] *see* methazolamide *on page 612*
Apo-Methoprazine® [Can] *see* methotrimeprazine *(Canada only) on page 615*
Apo-Methotrexate® [Can] *see* methotrexate *on page 614*
Apo-Methyldopa® [Can] *see* methyldopa *on page 618*
Apo-Methylphenidate® [Can] *see* methylphenidate *on page 621*
Apo-Methylphenidate® SR [Can] *see* methylphenidate *on page 621*
Apo-Metoclop® [Can] *see* metoclopramide *on page 624*
Apo-Metoprolol® [Can] *see* metoprolol *on page 625*
Apo-Metoprolol SR® [Can] *see* metoprolol *on page 625*
Apo-Metronidazole® [Can] *see* metronidazole (systemic) *on page 627*
Apo-Midazolam® [Can] *see* midazolam *on page 632*
Apo-Midodrine® [Can] *see* midodrine *on page 633*
Apo-Minocycline® [Can] *see* minocycline *on page 635*
Apo-Mirtazapine [Can] *see* mirtazapine *on page 637*
Apo-Misoprostol® [Can] *see* misoprostol *on page 637*
Apo-Moclobemide® [Can] *see* moclobemide *(Canada only) on page 639*
Apo-Modafinil [Can] *see* modafinil *on page 639*

apomorphine (a poe MOR feen)

Synonyms apomorphine hydrochloride; apomorphine hydrochloride hemihydrate
U.S./Canadian Brand Names Apokyn® [US]
Therapeutic Category Anti-Parkinson Agent (Dopamine Agonist)
Use Treatment of hypomobility, "off" episodes with Parkinson disease
Dosage Summary
SubQ:
Children: Dosage not established
Adults: Initial test dose: 2 mg; Starting dose: 2-3 mg/dose at time of "off" episode; Maintenance dose: 2-6 mg/dose at time of "off episode" (maximum: 20 mg/day; 6 mg/dose; 5 doses/day); **Note:** Titration may be recommended.
Dosage Forms
Injection, solution:
Apokyn®: 10 mg/mL (2 mL, 3 mL)

apomorphine hydrochloride *see* apomorphine *on page 89*
apomorphine hydrochloride hemihydrate *see* apomorphine *on page 89*
Apo-Nabumetone® [Can] *see* nabumetone *on page 654*

Apo-Sertraline® [Can] *see* sertraline *on page* *872*
Apo-Sibutramine® [Can] *see* sibutramine *on page* *873*
Apo-Simvastatin® [Can] *see* simvastatin *on page* *877*
Apo-Sotalol® [Can] *see* sotalol *on page* *892*
Apo-Sulfatrim® [Can] *see* sulfamethoxazole and trimethoprim *on page* *901*
Apo-Sulfatrim® DS [Can] *see* sulfamethoxazole and trimethoprim *on page* *901*
Apo-Sulfatrim® Pediatric [Can] *see* sulfamethoxazole and trimethoprim *on page* *901*
Apo-Sulin® [Can] *see* sulindac *on page* *904*
Apo-Sumatriptan® [Can] *see* sumatriptan *on page* *904*
Apo-Tamox® [Can] *see* tamoxifen *on page* *909*
Apo-Temazepam® [Can] *see* temazepam *on page* *914*
Apo-Terazosin® [Can] *see* terazosin *on page* *917*
Apo-Terbinafine® [Can] *see* terbinafine (systemic) *on page* *917*
Apo-Tetra® [Can] *see* tetracycline *on page* *922*
Apo-Theo LA® [Can] *see* theophylline *on page* *925*
Apo-Tiaprofenic® [Can] *see* tiaprofenic acid *(Canada only) on page* *931*
Apo-Ticlopidine® [Can] *see* ticlopidine *on page* *932*
Apo-Timol® [Can] *see* timolol (systemic) *on page* *933*
Apo-Timop® [Can] *see* timolol (ophthalmic) *on page* *933*
Apo-Tizanidine® [Can] *see* tizanidine *on page* *937*
Apo-Tolbutamide® [Can] *see* tolbutamide *on page* *939*
Apo-Topiramate® [Can] *see* topiramate *on page* *942*
Apo-Tramadol/Acet® [Can] *see* acetaminophen and tramadol *on page* *27*
Apo-Trazodone® [Can] *see* trazodone *on page* *950*
Apo-Trazodone D® [Can] *see* trazodone *on page* *950*
Apo-Triazide® [Can] *see* hydrochlorothiazide and triamterene *on page* *479*
Apo-Triazo® [Can] *see* triazolam *on page* *956*
Apo-Trifluoperazine® [Can] *see* trifluoperazine *on page* *957*
Apo-Trimebutine® [Can] *see* trimebutine *(Canada only) on page* *959*
Apo-Trimethoprim® [Can] *see* trimethoprim *on page* *959*
Apo-Trimip® [Can] *see* trimipramine *on page* *960*
Apo-Valacyclovir® [Can] *see* valacyclovir *on page* *973*
Apo-Valproic® [Can] *see* valproic acid *on page* *974*
Apo-Verap® [Can] *see* verapamil *on page* *981*
Apo-Verap® SR [Can] *see* verapamil *on page* *981*
Apo-Warfarin® [Can] *see* warfarin *on page* *993*
Apo-Zidovudine® [Can] *see* zidovudine *on page* *999*
Apo-Zopiclone® [Can] *see* zopiclone *(Canada only) on page* *1005*
APPG *see* penicillin G procaine *on page* *738*

apraclonidine (a pra KLOE ni deen)

Sound-Alike/Look-Alike Issues
Iopidine® may be confused with indapamide, iodine, Lodine®

Synonyms aplonidine; apraclonidine hydrochloride; p-aminoclonidine

U.S./Canadian Brand Names Iopidine® [US/Can]

Therapeutic Category Alpha$_2$ Agonist, Ophthalmic

Use Prevention and treatment of postsurgical intraocular pressure (IOP) elevation; short-term, adjunctive therapy in patients who require additional reduction of IOP

Dosage Summary

Ophthalmic:

Children: Dosage not established

Adults: 0.5%: Instill 1-2 drops in the affected eye(s) 3 times/day; 1%: Instill 1 drop in operative eye 1 hour prior to and upon completion of surgery

Dosage Forms

Solution, ophthalmic: 0.5% (5 mL, 10 mL)

Iopidine®: 0.5% (5 mL, 10 mL); 1% (0.1 mL)

apraclonidine hydrochloride *see* apraclonidine *on page* 91

Apra *(Discontinued)* *see* acetaminophen *on page* 21

aprepitant (ap RE pi tant)

Sound-Alike/Look-Alike Issues

aprepitant may be confused with fosaprepitant

Emend® (aprepitant) oral capsule formulation may be confused with Emend® for injection (fosaprepitant).

Synonyms L 754030; MK 869

U.S./Canadian Brand Names Emend® [US/Can]

Therapeutic Category Antiemetic

Use Prevention of acute and delayed nausea and vomiting associated with moderately- and highly-emetogenic chemotherapy (in combination with other antiemetics); prevention of postoperative nausea and vomiting (PONV)

Dosage Summary

Oral:

Children: Dosage not established

Adults: 125 mg on day 1, followed by 80 mg on days 2 and 3 **or** 40 mg within 3 hours prior to induction with anesthesia

Dosage Forms

Capsule, oral:

Emend®: 40 mg, 80 mg, 125 mg

Combination package, oral:

Emend®: Capsule: 80 mg (2s) and Capsule: 125 mg (1s)

aprepitant injection *see* fosaprepitant *on page* 427

Apresazide *(Discontinued)* *see* hydralazine and hydrochlorothiazide *on page* 477

Apresoline® [Can] *see* hydralazine *on page* 477

Apresoline® *(Discontinued)* *see* hydralazine *on page* 477

Apri® [US] *see* ethinyl estradiol and desogestrel *on page* 374

Apriso™ [US] *see* mesalamine *on page* 607

Aprodine [US-OTC] *see* triprolidine and pseudoephedrine *on page* 961

aprotinin (a proe TYE nin)

U.S./Canadian Brand Names Trasylol® [Can]

Therapeutic Category Hemostatic Agent

Use Prevention of perioperative blood loss in patients who are at increased risk for blood loss and blood transfusions in association with cardiopulmonary bypass in coronary artery bypass graft surgery

Dosage Summary

I.V.:

Children: Dosage not established

Adults: Test dose: 1 mL (1.4 mg) 10 minutes prior to loading dose; Loading dose: 1-2 million KIU (140-280 mg; 100-200 mL); Pump prime volume: 1-2 million KIU (140-280 mg, 100-200 mL); Infusion: 250,000-500,000 KIU/hour (35-70 mg/hour; 25-50 mL/hour)

Dosage Forms

Injection, solution:

Trasylol®: 1.4 mg/mL [10,000 KIU/mL] (100 mL, 200 mL)

Aptivus® [US/Can] *see* tipranavir *on page* 936

Aqua-Ban® Maximum Strength [US-OTC] *see* pamabrom *on page* 722

Aqua Care® [US-OTC] *see* urea *on page* 970

Aquachloral® Supprettes® *(Discontinued)* *see* chloral hydrate *on page* 202

Aquacort® [Can] *see* hydrocortisone (topical) *on page* 483

AquADEKs™ [US-OTC] *see* vitamins (multiple/pediatric) *on page* 990

Aqua Gem-E™ [US-OTC] *see* vitamin E *on page* 988

AquaLase™ [US] *see* balanced salt solution *on page 116*
AquaMEPHYTON® [Can] *see* phytonadione *on page 759*
AquaMEPHYTON® ***(Discontinued)*** *see* phytonadione *on page 759*
Aquanil HC® [US-OTC] *see* hydrocortisone (topical) *on page 483*
Aquaphilic® with Carbamide [US-OTC] *see* urea *on page 970*
Aquaphyllin® ***(Discontinued)*** *see* theophylline *on page 925*
Aquasol A® [US] *see* vitamin A *on page 987*
Aquasol E® [US-OTC] *see* vitamin E *on page 988*
Aquatab® C ***(Discontinued)*** *see* guaifenesin, pseudoephedrine, and dextromethorphan *on page 460*
Aquatab® D ***(Discontinued)*** *see* guaifenesin and pseudoephedrine *on page 457*
Aquatab® DM ***(Discontinued)*** *see* guaifenesin and dextromethorphan *on page 455*
AquaTar® ***(Discontinued)*** *see* coal tar *on page 242*
aquavan *see* fospropofol *on page 429*
Aquavit-E ***(Discontinued)*** *see* vitamin E *on page 988*
aqueous procaine penicillin G *see* penicillin G procaine *on page 738*
Aquoral™ [US] *see* saliva substitute *on page 861*
ara-C *see* cytarabine *on page 263*
arabinosylcytosine *see* cytarabine *on page 263*
Aralast [US] *see* alpha$_1$-proteinase inhibitor *on page 54*
Aralast NP [US] *see* alpha$_1$-proteinase inhibitor *on page 54*
Aralen® [US/Can] *see* chloroquine *on page 206*
Aranelle™ [US] *see* ethinyl estradiol and norethindrone *on page 378*
Aranesp® [US/Can] *see* darbepoetin alfa *on page 269*
Arava® [US/Can] *see* leflunomide *on page 552*
Arcalyst™ [US] *see* rilonacept *on page 843*
Arduan® ***(Discontinued)***
Aredia® [US/Can] *see* pamidronate *on page 722*
Arestin Microspheres [Can] *see* minocycline *on page 635*

arformoterol (ar for MOE ter ol)

Synonyms (R,R)-formoterol L-tartrate; arformoterol tartrate

U.S./Canadian Brand Names Brovana® [US]

Therapeutic Category Beta$_2$-Adrenergic Agonist

Use Long-term maintenance treatment of bronchoconstriction in chronic obstructive pulmonary disease (COPD), including chronic bronchitis and emphysema

Dosage Summary

Nebulization:

Children <18 years: Dosage not established

Adults: 5 mcg twice daily (maximum: 30 mcg/day)

Dosage Forms

Solution, for nebulization:

Brovana®: 15 mcg/2 mL (30s, 60s)

arformoterol tartrate *see* arformoterol *on page 93*

argatroban (ar GA troh ban)

Sound-Alike/Look-Alike Issues

argatroban may be confused with Aggrastat®, Orgaran®

Therapeutic Category Anticoagulant, Thrombin Inhibitor

Use Prophylaxis or treatment of thrombosis in patients with heparin-induced thrombocytopenia (HIT); adjunct to percutaneous coronary intervention (PCI) in patients who have or are at risk of thrombosis associated with HIT

Dosage Summary

I.V.:

Children: Initial dose: 0.75 mcg/kg/minute; dosage may be adjusted in increments of 0.1-0.25 mcg/kg/minute

Adults: Bolus dose: 150-350 mcg/kg during procedure; Infusion: Initial: 2 mcg/kg/minute **or** 25 mcg/kg/minute during procedure; Maintenance: 0.5-10 mcg/kg/minute (maximum: 10 mcg/kg/minute) **or** 25-40 mcg/kg/minute during procedure

Adults (critically-ill): Initial: 0.2 mcg/kg/minute; Maintenance: 0.5-1.3 mcg/kg/minute

Dosage Forms

Injection, solution: 100 mg/mL (2.5 mL)

arginine (AR ji neen)

Synonyms arginine HCl; arginine hydrochloride; L-arginine; L-arginine hydrochloride

U.S./Canadian Brand Names R-Gene® 10 [US]

Therapeutic Category Diagnostic Agent

Use Pituitary function test (growth hormone)

Dosage Summary

I.V.:

Children: 0.5 g/kg/dose administered over 30 minutes

Adults: 30 g (300 mL) administered over 30 minutes

Dosage Forms

Injection, solution:

R-Gene® 10: 10% [100 mg/mL] (300 mL)

arginine HCl *see* arginine *on page* *94*

arginine hydrochloride *see* arginine *on page* *94*

8-arginine vasopressin *see* vasopressin *on page* *980*

Aricept® [US/Can] *see* donepezil *on page* *326*

Aricept® ODT [US] *see* donepezil *on page* *326*

Aricept® RDT [Can] *see* donepezil *on page* *326*

Arimidex® [US/Can] *see* anastrozole *on page* *78*

aripiprazole (ay ri PIP ray zole)

Sound-Alike/Look-Alike Issues

aripiprazole may be confused with proton pump inhibitors (dexlansoprazole, esomeprazole, lansoprazole, omeprazole, pantoprazole, rabeprazole)

Abilify® may be confused with Ambien®

Synonyms BMS-337039; OPC-14597

U.S./Canadian Brand Names Abilify Discmelt® [US]; Abilify® [US/Can]

Therapeutic Category Antipsychotic Agent, Quinolone

Use

Oral: Acute and maintenance treatment of schizophrenia; stabilization, maintenance, and adjunctive therapy (to lithium or valproate) of bipolar disorder (with acute manic or mixed episodes); adjunctive treatment of major depressive disorder; treatment of irritability associated with autistic disorder

Injection: Agitation associated with schizophrenia or bipolar mania

Dosage Summary Note: Oral solution may be substituted for the oral tablet on a mg-per-mg basis, up to 25 mg. Patients receiving 30 mg tablets should be given 25 mg oral solution. Orally disintegrating tablets (Abilify Discmelt®) are bioequivalent to the immediate release tablets (Abilify®).

Oral:

Children <6 years: Dosage not established

Children 6-9 years: 5-15 mg once daily (maximum: 15 mg/day); **Note:** Titration is recommended

Children ≥10 years: 5-30 mg once daily (maximum: 30 mg/day); **Note:** Titration is recommended

Adults: 10-30 mg once daily (maximum: 30 mg/day); **Note:** Titration is recommended

I.M.:

Children: Dosage not established

Adults: 9.75 mg as a single dose (maximum: 30 mg/day)

Dosage Forms

Injection, solution:

Abilify®: 7.5 mg/mL (1.3 mL)

Solution, oral:
Abilify®: 1 mg/mL (150 mL)
Tablet, oral:
Abilify®: 2 mg, 5 mg, 10 mg, 15 mg, 20 mg, 30 mg
Tablet, orally disintegrating, oral:
Abilify Discmelt®: 10 mg, 15 mg

Aristospan® [US/Can] *see* triamcinolone (systemic, oral inhalation) *on page 952*
Arixtra® [US/Can] *see* fondaparinux *on page 425*
Arm-a-Med® Isoproterenol *(Discontinued)* *see* isoproterenol *on page 528*
Arm-a-Med® Metaproterenol *(Discontinued)*

armodafinil (ar moe DAF i nil)

Synonyms R-modafinil
U.S./Canadian Brand Names Nuvigil™ [US]
Therapeutic Category Stimulant
Controlled Substance C-IV
Use Improve wakefulness in patients with excessive daytime sleepiness associated with narcolepsy and shift work sleep disorder (SWSD); adjunctive therapy for obstructive sleep apnea/hypopnea syndrome (OSAHS)
Dosage Summary
Oral:
Children: Dosage not established
Adults: 150-250 mg once daily
Elderly: Consider lower initial dosage; concentrations were almost doubled in clinical trials (based on modafinil)
Dosage Forms
Tablet, oral:
Nuvigil™: 50 mg, 150 mg, 250 mg

Armour® Thyroid [US] *see* thyroid, desiccated *on page 930*
Aromasin® [US/Can] *see* exemestane *on page 386*
Arranon® [US] *see* nelarabine *on page 664*
Arrestin® *(Discontinued)* *see* trimethobenzamide *on page 959*

arsenic trioxide (AR se nik tri OKS id)

Synonyms As_2O_3; NSC-706363
U.S./Canadian Brand Names Trisenox® [US]
Therapeutic Category Antineoplastic Agent, Miscellaneous
Use Remission induction and consolidation in patients with relapsed or refractory acute promyelocytic leukemia (APL) characterized by t(15;17) translocation or PML/RAR-alpha gene expression
Dosage Summary
I.V.:
Children <4 years: Dosage not established
Children ≥4 years: Induction: 0.15 mg/kg/day (maximum: 60 doses); Consolidation: 0.15 mg/kg/day (maximum: 25 doses over 5 weeks)
Adults: Induction: 0.15 mg/kg/day (maximum: 60 doses); Consolidation: 0.15 mg/kg/day (maximum: 25 doses over 5 weeks)
Dosage Forms
Injection, solution [preservative free]:
Trisenox®: 1 mg/mL (10 mL)

Artane® *(Discontinued)* *see* trihexyphenidyl *on page 958*
artemether and benflumetol *see* artemether and lumefantrine *on page 95*

artemether and lumefantrine (ar TEM e ther & loo me FAN treen)

Synonyms artemether and benflumetol; benflumetol and artemether; lumefantrine and artemether
U.S./Canadian Brand Names Coartem® [US]
Therapeutic Category Antimalarial Agent

Use Treatment of acute, uncomplicated malaria infections due to *Plasmodium falciparum*, including geographical regions where chloroquine resistance has been reported

Dosage Summary

Oral:

Children <2 months: Dosage not established

Children 2 months to ≤16 years:

<5 kg: Dosage not established

5 to <15 kg: Artemether 20 mg/lumefantrine 120 mg twice daily (maximum: 6 tablets per treatment course)

15 to <25 kg: Artemether 40 mg/lumefantrine 240 mg twice daily (maximum: 12 tablets per treatment course)

25 to <35 kg: Artemether 60 mg/lumefantrine 360 mg twice daily (maximum: 18 tablets per treatment course)

≥35 kg: Artemether 80 mg/lumefantrine 480 mg twice daily (maximum: 24 tablets per treatment course)

Children >16 years:

25 to <35 kg: Artemether 60 mg/lumefantrine 360 mg twice daily (maximum: 18 tablets per treatment course)

≥35 kg: Artemether 80 mg/lumefantrine 480 mg twice daily (maximum: 24 tablets per treatment course)

Adults:

25 to <35 kg: Artemether 60 mg/lumefantrine 360 mg twice daily (maximum: 18 tablets per treatment course)

≥35 kg: Artemether 80 mg/lumefantrine 480 mg twice daily (maximum: 24 tablets per treatment course)

Dosage Forms

Tablet:

Coartem®: Artemether 20 mg and lumefantrine 120 mg

Artha-G® ***(Discontinued)*** *see* salsalate *on page* 862

ArthriCare® for Women Extra Moisturizing ***(Discontinued)*** *see* capsaicin *on page* 175

ArthriCare® for Women Multi-Action ***(Discontinued)*** *see* capsaicin *on page* 175

ArthriCare® for Women Silky Dry ***(Discontinued)*** *see* capsaicin *on page* 175

ArthriCare® for Women Ultra Strength ***(Discontinued)*** *see* capsaicin *on page* 175

Arthropan® ***(Discontinued)***

Arthrotec® [US/Can] *see* diclofenac and misoprostol *on page* 298

articaine and epinephrine (AR ti kane & ep i NEF rin)

Synonyms epinephrine and articaine hydrochloride

U.S./Canadian Brand Names Astracaine® with epinephrine 1:200,000 [Can]; Astracaine® with epinephrine forte 1:100,000 [Can]; Septanest® N [Can]; Septanest® SP [Can]; Septocaine® with epinephrine 1:100,000 [US]; Septocaine® with epinephrine 1:200,000 [US]; Ultracaine® DS Forte [Can]; Ultracaine® DS [Can]; Zorcaine™ [US/Can]

Therapeutic Category Local Anesthetic

Use Local, infiltrative, or conductive anesthesia in both simple and complex dental and periodontal procedures

Dosage Summary

Local injection:

Children <4 years: Dosage not established

Children 4-16 years: Maximum: 7 mg/kg (0.175 mL/kg)

Complex procedures: 0.37-7.48 mg/kg (0.7-3.9 mL)

Simple procedures: 0.76-5.65 mg/kg (0.9-5.1 mL)

Adults: Maximum: 7 mg/kg (0.175 mL/kg)

Infiltration: 0.5-2.5 mL of 4% solution; Total dose: 20-100 mg

Nerve block: 0.5-3.4 mL of 4% solution; Total dose: 20-136 mg

Oral surgery: 1-5.1 mL of 4% solution; Total dose: 40-204 mg

Elderly 65-75 years:

Complex procedures: 1.05-4.27 mg/kg (1.3-6.8 mL)

Simple procedures: 0.43-4.76 mg/kg (0.9-11.9 mL)

Elderly ≥75 years:
Complex procedures: 1.12-2.17 mg/kg (1.3-5.1 mL)
Simple procedures: 0.78-4.76 mg/kg (1.3-11.9 mL)

Dosage Forms

Injection, solution [for dental use]:
Septocaine® with epinephrine 1:100,000: Articaine 4% and epinephrine 1:100,000 (1.7 mL)
Septocaine® with epinephrine 1:200,000: Articaine 4% and epinephrine 1:200,000 (1.7 mL)
Zorcaine™: Articaine 4% and epinephrine 1:100,000 (1.7 mL) [contains sodium metabisulfite]

Dosage Forms - Canada

Injection, solution [for dental use]:
Astracaine® with epinephrine 1:200,000: Articaine 4% and epinephrine 1:200,000 (1.8 mL)
Astracaine® Forte with epinephrine forte 1:100,000: Articaine 4% and epinephrine 1:100,000 (1.8 mL)
Septanest® N: Articaine 4% and epinephrine 1:200,000 (1.7 mL)
Septanest® SP: Articaine 4% and epinephrine 1:100,000 (1.7 mL)
Ultracaine® DS: Articaine 4% and epinephrine 1:200,000 (1.7 mL)
Ultracaine® DS Forte: Articaine 4% and epinephrine 1:100,000 (1.7 mL)

artificial saliva *see* saliva substitute *on page 861*

artificial tears (ar ti FISH il tears)

Sound-Alike/Look-Alike Issues
Murocel® may be confused with Murocoll-2®

Synonyms hydroxyethylcellulose; polyvinyl alcohol

U.S./Canadian Brand Names Akwa Tears® [US-OTC]; Bion® Tears [US-OTC]; HypoTears PF [US-OTC]; HypoTears [US-OTC]; Liquifilm® Tears [US-OTC]; Moisture® Eyes PM [US-OTC]; Moisture® Eyes [US-OTC]; Murine® Tears [US-OTC]; Murocel® [US-OTC]; Nature's Tears® [US-OTC]; Nu-Tears® II [US-OTC]; Nu-Tears® [US-OTC]; Refresh Plus® [US-OTC]; Refresh Tears® [US-OTC]; Refresh® [US-OTC]; Soothe® [US-OTC]; Systane® Free [US-OTC]; Systane® [US-OTC]; Teardrops® [Can]; Teargen® II [US-OTC]; Teargen® [US-OTC]; Tearisol® [US-OTC]; Tears Again® [US-OTC]; Tears Naturale® Free [US-OTC]; Tears Naturale® II [US-OTC]; Tears Naturale® [US-OTC]; Tears Plus® [US-OTC]; Tears Renewed® [US-OTC]; Ultra Tears® [US-OTC]; Viva-Drops® [US-OTC]

Therapeutic Category Ophthalmic Agent, Miscellaneous

Use Ophthalmic lubricant; for relief of dry eyes and eye irritation

Dosage Summary

Ophthalmic:
Children: 1-2 drops into eye(s) 3-4 times/day as needed
Adults: 1-2 drops into eye(s) 3-4 times/day as needed

Dosage Forms

Solution, ophthalmic: 15 mL and 30 mL dropper bottles

Artiss™ [US] *see* fibrin sealant *on page 401*
Arzerra™ [US] *see* ofatumumab *on page 695*
As_2O_3 *see* arsenic trioxide *on page 95*
ASA *see* aspirin *on page 100*
5-ASA *see* mesalamine *on page 607*
ASA and diphenhydramine *see* aspirin and diphenhydramine *on page 101*
Asacol® [US/Can] *see* mesalamine *on page 607*
Asacol® 800 [Can] *see* mesalamine *on page 607*
Asacol® HD [US] *see* mesalamine *on page 607*
A.S.A.® *(Discontinued)* *see* aspirin *on page 100*
Asaphen [Can] *see* aspirin *on page 100*
Asaphen E.C. [Can] *see* aspirin *on page 100*
Asclera™ [US] *see* polidocanol *on page 773*
Asco-Caps-500 [US-OTC] *see* ascorbic acid *on page 98*
Asco-Caps-1000 [US-OTC] *see* ascorbic acid *on page 98*
Ascocid® [US-OTC] *see* ascorbic acid *on page 98*
Ascocid®-500 [US-OTC] *see* ascorbic acid *on page 98*
Ascomp® with Codeine [US] *see* butalbital, aspirin, caffeine, and codeine *on page 160*
Ascor L 500® [US] *see* ascorbic acid *on page 98*

Ascor L NC® [US] *see* ascorbic acid *on page 98*

ascorbic acid (a SKOR bik AS id)

Synonyms vitamin C

U.S./Canadian Brand Names Acerola [US-OTC]; Asco-Caps-1000 [US-OTC]; Asco-Caps-500 [US-OTC]; Asco-Tabs-1000 [US-OTC]; Ascocid® [US-OTC]; Ascocid®-500 [US-OTC]; Ascor L 500® [US]; Ascor L NC® [US]; C-Gel [US-OTC]; C-Gram [US-OTC]; C-Time [US-OTC]; Cemill 1000 [US-OTC]; Cemill 500 [US-OTC]; Chew-C [US-OTC]; Dull-C® [US-OTC]; Mild-C® [US-OTC]; One Gram C [US-OTC]; Proflavanol C™ [Can]; Revitalose C-1000® [Can]; Time-C [US-OTC]; Vicks® Vitamin C [US-OTC]; Vita-C® [US-OTC]

Therapeutic Category Vitamin, Water Soluble

Use Prevention and treatment of scurvy; acidify the urine

Dosage Summary

I.M.:

Children: 100-300 mg/day in divided doses
Adults: 100-250 mg 1-2 times/day

I.V.:

Children: 100-300 mg/day in divided doses (up to 500 mg every 6-8 hours for selected indications)
Adults: 100-250 mg 1-2 times/day (up to 4-12 g/day in 3-4 divided doses for selected indications)

Oral:

Children: 100-300 mg/day in divided doses (up to 500 mg every 6-8 hours for selected indications)
Adults: 100-250 mg 1-2 times/day (up to 4-12 g/day in 3-4 divided doses for selected indications)

SubQ:

Children: 100-300 mg/day in divided doses
Adults: 100-250 mg 1-2 times/day

Dosage Forms

Caplet, oral: 1000 mg

Caplet, timed release, oral: 500 mg, 1000 mg

Capsule, oral:
Mild-C® [OTC]: 500 mg

Capsule, softgel, oral:
C-Gel [OTC]: 1000 mg

Capsule, sustained release, oral:
C-Time [OTC]: 500 mg

Capsule, timed release, oral: 500 mg
Asco-Caps-500 [OTC]: 500 mg
Asco-Caps-1000 [OTC]: 1000 mg
Time-C® [OTC]: 500 mg

Crystals for solution, oral: 4000 mg/teaspoon (170 g, 1000 g)
Mild-C® [OTC]: 3600 mg/teaspoon (170 g, 1000 g)
Vita-C® [OTC]: 4000 mg/teaspoon (113 g, 454 g)

Injection, solution: 500 mg/mL (50 mL)
Ascor L 500®: 500 mg/mL (50 mL)

Injection, solution [preservative free]: 500 mg/mL (50 mL)
Ascor L NC®: 500 mg/mL (50 mL)

Liquid, oral: 500 mg/5 mL (118 mL, 120 mL, 473 mL, 480 mL)

Lozenge, oral:
Vicks® Vitamin C [OTC]: 25 mg (20s)

Powder for solution, oral:
Ascocid® [OTC]: 4000 mg/teaspoon (227 g); 4300 mg/teaspoon (227 g, 454 g); 5000 mg/teaspoon (227 g, 454 g)
Dull-C® [OTC]: 4240 mg/teaspoon (113 g, 454 g)

Tablet, oral: 100 mg, 250 mg, 500 mg, 1000 mg
Asco-Tabs-1000 [OTC]: 1000 mg
Ascocid®-500 [OTC]: 500 mg
C-Gram [OTC]: 1000 mg
One Gram C [OTC]: 1000 mg

Tablet, chewable, oral: 250 mg, 500 mg
Acerola [OTC]: 500 mg
Chew-C [OTC]: 500 mg
Mild-C® [OTC]: 250 mg

Tablet, timed release, oral: 500 mg, 1000 mg
Cemill 500 [OTC]: 500 mg
Cemill 1000 [OTC]: 1000 mg
Mild-C® [OTC]: 1000 mg

ascorbic acid and ferrous sulfate *see* ferrous sulfate and ascorbic acid *on page* 399

Ascorbicap® ***(Discontinued)*** *see* ascorbic acid *on page* 98

Asco-Tabs-1000 [US-OTC] *see* ascorbic acid *on page* 98

Ascriptin® Maximum Strength [US-OTC] *see* aspirin *on page* 100

Ascriptin® Regular Strength [US-OTC] *see* aspirin *on page* 100

asenapine (a SEN a peen)

Sound-Alike/Look-Alike Issues
asenapine may be confused with Inapsine®

U.S./Canadian Brand Names Saphris® [US]

Therapeutic Category Antimanic Agent; Antipsychotic Agent, Atypical

Use Acute treatment of schizophrenia; treatment of acute mania or mixed episodes associated with bipolar I disorder

Dosage Summary

Oral:
Children: Dosage not established
Adults: 5-10 mg twice daily; safety of doses >20 mg/day has not been evaluated

Dosage Forms

Tablet, sublingual:
Saphris®: 5 mg, 10 mg

Asendin® ***(Discontinued)*** *see* amoxapine *on page* 72

Asmalix® ***(Discontinued)*** *see* theophylline *on page* 925

Asmanex® Twisthaler® [US] *see* mometasone (oral inhalation) *on page* 641

asparaginase (a SPEAR a ji nase)

Sound-Alike/Look-Alike Issues
asparaginase may be confused with pegaspargase
Elspar® may be confused with Elaprase™, Oncaspar®

Synonyms *E. coli* asparaginase; *Erwinia* asparaginase; L-asparaginase; NSC-106977 (*Erwinia*); NSC-109229 (*E. coli*)

U.S./Canadian Brand Names Elspar® [US]; Kidrolase® [Can]

Therapeutic Category Antineoplastic Agent

Use Treatment of acute lymphocytic leukemia (ALL)

Dosage Summary Note: Refer to individual protocols

I.M.:
Children: 6000 units/m^2/dose 3 times/week **or** 6000 units/m^2 every ~3 days for ~6-9 doses
Adults: 6000 units/m^2/dose 3 times/week for ~6-9 doses **or** 6000 units/m^2 every ~3 days for ~6-9 doses

I.V.:
Children: 6000 units/m^2/dose 3 times/week for ~6-9 doses **or** 6000 units/m^2 every ~3 days for ~6-9 doses **or** 1000 units/kg/day for 10 days
Adults: 6000 units/m^2/dose 3 times/week for ~6-9 doses **or** 6000 units/m^2 every ~3 days for ~6-9 doses **or** 1000 units/kg/day for 10 days **or** 200 units/kg/day (single agent therapy) for 28 days

Intradermal:
Children: Test dose: 0.1-0.2 mL of a 20-250 units/mL concentration
Adults: Test dose: 0.1-0.2 mL of a 20-250 units/mL concentration

Dosage Forms

Injection, powder for reconstitution:
Elspar®: 10,000 int. units

aspart insulin *see* insulin aspart *on page* 509

A-Spas® ***(Discontinued)*** *see* hyoscyamine *on page* 491

Aspercin [US-OTC] *see* aspirin *on page* 100

Aspercreme® [US-OTC] *see* trolamine *on page* 963

Aspergillus niger *see* alpha-galactosidase *on page* 54

Aspergum® [US-OTC] *see* aspirin *on page 100*

aspirin (AS pir in)

Sound-Alike/Look-Alike Issues

aspirin may be confused with Afrin®, Asendin®
Ascriptin® may be confused with Aricept®
Ecotrin® may be confused with Akineton®, Edecrin®, Epogen®
Halfprin® may be confused with Halfan®, Haltran®
ZORprin® may be confused with Zyloprim®

Synonyms acetylsalicylic acid; ASA; baby aspirin

U.S./Canadian Brand Names Asaphen E.C. [Can]; Asaphen [Can]; Ascriptin® Maximum Strength [US-OTC]; Ascriptin® Regular Strength [US-OTC]; Aspercin [US-OTC]; Aspergum® [US-OTC]; Aspir-low [US-OTC]; Aspirtab [US-OTC]; Bayer® Aspirin Extra Strength [US-OTC]; Bayer® Aspirin Regimen Adult Low Strength [US-OTC]; Bayer® Aspirin Regimen Children's [US-OTC]; Bayer® Aspirin Regimen Regular Strength [US-OTC]; Bayer® Genuine Aspirin [US-OTC]; Bayer® Plus Extra Strength [US-OTC]; Bayer® Women's Low Dose Aspirin [US-OTC]; Buffasal [US-OTC]; Bufferin® Extra Strength [US-OTC]; Bufferin® [US-OTC]; Buffinol [US-OTC]; Easprin® [US]; Ecotrin® Arthritis Strength [US-OTC]; Ecotrin® Low Strength [US-OTC]; Ecotrin® [US-OTC]; Entrophen® [Can]; Halfprin® [US-OTC]; Novasen [Can]; Praxis ASA EC 81 Mg Daily Dose [Can]; St. Joseph® Adult Aspirin [US-OTC]; Tri-Buffered Aspirin [US-OTC]

Therapeutic Category Analgesic, Nonnarcotic; Antiplatelet Agent; Antipyretic; Nonsteroidal Antiinflammatory Drug (NSAID)

Use Treatment of mild-to-moderate pain, inflammation, and fever; prevention and treatment of myocardial infarction (MI), acute ischemic stroke, and transient ischemic episodes; management of rheumatoid arthritis, rheumatic fever, osteoarthritis, and gout (high dose); adjunctive therapy in revascularization procedures (coronary artery bypass graft [CABG], percutaneous transluminal coronary angioplasty [PTCA], carotid endarterectomy), stent implantation

Dosage Summary

Oral:

Children: 10-15 mg/kg/dose every 4-6 hours (maximum: 4 g/day) **or** 60-100 mg/kg/day divided every 4-8 hours **or** 1-20 mg/kg/day as a single dose

Adults: 325-650 mg every 4-6 hours (maximum: 4 g/day) **or** 2.4-5.4 g/day in divided doses **or** 40-325 mg/day as a single dose

Rectal:

Children: 10-15 mg/kg/dose every 4-6 hours (maximum: 4 g/day)

Adults: 300-600 mg every 4-6 hours (maximum: 4 g/day)

Dosage Forms

Caplet, oral:
Ascriptin® Maximum Strength [OTC]: 500 mg
Bayer® Aspirin Extra Strength [OTC]: 500 mg
Bayer® Genuine Aspirin [OTC]: 325 mg
Bayer® Plus Extra Strength [OTC]: 500 mg
Bayer® Women's Low Dose Aspirin [OTC]: 81 mg

Caplet, enteric coated, oral:
Bayer® Aspirin Regimen Regular Strength [OTC]: 325 mg

Gum, chewing, oral:
Aspergum® [OTC]: 227 mg (12s)

Suppository, rectal: 300 mg (12s); 600 mg (12s)

Tablet, oral: 325 mg
Ascriptin® Regular Strength [OTC]: 325 mg
Aspercin [OTC]: 325 mg
Aspirtab [OTC]: 325 mg
Bayer® Genuine Aspirin [OTC]: 325 mg
Buffasal [OTC]: 325 mg
Bufferin® [OTC]: 325 mg
Bufferin® Extra Strength [OTC]: 500 mg
Buffinol [OTC]: 324 mg
Tri-Buffered Aspirin [OTC]: 325 mg

Tablet, chewable, oral: 81 mg
Bayer® Aspirin Regimen Children's [OTC]: 81 mg
St Joseph® Adult Aspirin [OTC]: 81 mg

Tablet, delayed release, enteric coated, oral:
Easprin®: 975 mg
Tablet, enteric coated, oral: 81 mg, 325 mg, 650 mg
Aspir-low [OTC]: 81 mg
Bayer® Aspirin Regimen Adult Low Strength [OTC]: 81 mg
Ecotrin® [OTC]: 325 mg
Ecotrin® Arthritis Strength [OTC]: 500 mg
Ecotrin® Low Strength [OTC]: 81 mg
Halfprin® [OTC]: 81 mg, 162 mg
St Joseph® Adult Aspirin [OTC]: 81 mg

aspirin, acetaminophen, and caffeine *see* acetaminophen, aspirin, and caffeine *on page* 27
aspirin and carisoprodol *see* carisoprodol and aspirin *on page* 185

aspirin and diphenhydramine (AS pir in & dye fen HYE dra meen)

Synonyms ASA and diphenhydramine; aspirin and diphenhydramine citrate; diphenhydramine and ASA; diphenhydramine and aspirin; diphenhydramine citrate and aspirin
U.S./Canadian Brand Names Alka-Seltzer® P.M. [US-OTC]; Bayer® PM [US-OTC]
Therapeutic Category Analgesic, Miscellaneous
Use Aid in the relief of insomnia accompanied by minor pain or headache
Dosage Summary
Oral:
Children <12 years: Dosage not established
Children ≥12 years: Two tablets (650 mg aspirin/76 mg diphenhydramine citrate) **or** 2 caplets (1000 mg aspirin/76 mg diphenhydramine citrate) at bedtime (maximum: Do not exceed recommended dosage)
Adults: Two tablets (650 mg aspirin/76 mg diphenhydramine citrate) **or** 2 caplets (1000 mg aspirin/76 mg diphenhydramine citrate) at bedtime (maximum: Do not exceed recommended dosage)
Dosage Forms
Caplet:
Bayer® PM [OTC]: Aspirin 500 mg and diphenhydramine 38.3 mg
Tablet, effervescent:
Alka-Seltzer® P.M. [OTC]: Aspirin 325 mg and diphenhydramine 38 mg

aspirin and diphenhydramine citrate *see* aspirin and diphenhydramine *on page* 101

aspirin and dipyridamole (AS pir in & dye peer ID a mole)

Sound-Alike/Look-Alike Issues
Aggrenox® may be confused with Aggrastat®
Synonyms aspirin and extended-release dipyridamole; dipyridamole and aspirin
U.S./Canadian Brand Names Aggrenox® [US/Can]
Therapeutic Category Antiplatelet Agent
Use Reduction in the risk of stroke in patients who have had transient ischemia of the brain or ischemic stroke due to thrombosis
Dosage Summary
Oral:
Children: Dosage not established
Adults: 1 capsule (200 mg dipyridamole, 25 mg aspirin) twice daily
Dosage Forms
Capsule:
Aggrenox®: Aspirin 25 mg (immediate release) and dipyridamole 200 mg (extended release)

aspirin and extended-release dipyridamole *see* aspirin and dipyridamole *on page* 101
aspirin and meprobamate *see* meprobamate and aspirin *on page* 606
aspirin and oxycodone *see* oxycodone and aspirin *on page* 716
aspirin, caffeine, and acetaminophen *see* acetaminophen, aspirin, and caffeine *on page* 27
aspirin, caffeine, and butalbital *see* butalbital, aspirin, and caffeine *on page* 160
aspirin, caffeine, and orphenadrine *see* orphenadrine, aspirin, and caffeine *on page* 708
aspirin, caffeine, codeine, and butalbital *see* butalbital, aspirin, caffeine, and codeine *on page* 160
aspirin, carisoprodol, and codeine *see* carisoprodol, aspirin, and codeine *on page* 185
Aspirin Free Anacin® ***(Discontinued)*** *see* acetaminophen *on page* 21

Aspirin Free Anacin® Extra Strength [US-OTC] *see* acetaminophen *on page 21*
aspirin, orphenadrine, and caffeine *see* orphenadrine, aspirin, and caffeine *on page 708*
Aspir-low [US-OTC] *see* aspirin *on page 100*
Aspirtab [US-OTC] *see* aspirin *on page 100*
Astelin® [US/Can] *see* azelastine (nasal) *on page 110*
Astepro® [US] *see* azelastine (nasal) *on page 110*
AsthmaHaler® Mist *(Discontinued)* *see* epinephrine (systemic, oral inhalation) *on page 352*
AsthmaNefrin® *(Discontinued)* *see* epinephrine (systemic, oral inhalation) *on page 352*
Astracaine® with epinephrine 1:200,000 [Can] *see* articaine and epinephrine *on page 96*
Astracaine® with epinephrine forte 1:100,000 [Can] *see* articaine and epinephrine *on page 96*
Astramorph/PF™ [US] *see* morphine (systemic) *on page 644*
AT *see* antithrombin III *on page 83*
AT-III *see* antithrombin III *on page 83*
Atacand® [US/Can] *see* candesartan *on page 173*
Atacand HCT® [US] *see* candesartan and hydrochlorothiazide *on page 174*
Atacand® Plus [Can] *see* candesartan and hydrochlorothiazide *on page 174*
Atapryl® *(Discontinued)*
Atarax® [Can] *see* hydroxyzine *on page 490*
Atarax® *(Discontinued)* *see* hydroxyzine *on page 490*
Atasol® [Can] *see* acetaminophen *on page 21*

atazanavir (at a za NA veer)

Synonyms atazanavir sulfate; BMS-232632

U.S./Canadian Brand Names Reyataz® [US/Can]

Therapeutic Category Antiretroviral Agent, Protease Inhibitor

Use Treatment of HIV-1 infections in combination with at least two other antiretroviral agents

Dosage Summary Note: Ritonavir unboosted regimen: Atazanavir without ritonavir is not recommended in antiretroviral-experienced patients with prior virologic failure.

Oral:

Children <6 years: Dosage not established

Children 6-17 years: Antiretroviral-naive patients:

15-24 kg: Atazanavir 150 mg once daily **plus** ritonavir 80 mg once daily
25-31 kg: Atazanavir 200 mg once daily **plus** ritonavir 100 mg once daily
32-38 kg: Atazanavir 250 mg once daily **plus** ritonavir 100 mg once daily
≥39 kg: Atazanavir 300 mg once daily **plus** 100 mg ritonavir once daily. **Note:** Treatment-naive patients ≥39 kg and ≥13 years of age who are unable to tolerate ritonavir, refer to adult dosing.

or

15-19 kg: Atazanavir 8.5 mg/kg/dose once daily (rounded to available capsule strengths) **plus** ritonavir 4 mg/kg/dose once daily
≥20 kg: Atazanavir 7 mg/kg/dose once daily (round to available capsule strengths) (maximum: 300 mg) **plus** ritonavir 4 mg/kg/dose once daily

Children ≥13 years (≥39 kg): 400 mg once daily (antiretroviral-naive) **or** atazanavir 300 mg once daily **plus** ritonavir 100 mg once daily (antiretroviral-experienced)

Children 6-17 years: Antiretroviral-experienced patients:

25-31 kg: Atazanavir 200 mg once daily **plus** ritonavir 100 mg once daily
32-38 kg: Atazanavir 250 mg once daily **plus** ritonavir 100 mg once daily
≥39 kg: Atazanavir 300 mg once daily **plus** 100 mg ritonavir once daily

Adults: Atazanavir 300 mg once daily **plus** ritonavir 100 mg once daily **or** atazanavir 400 mg once daily (antiretroviral-naive unable to tolerate ritonavir)

Dosage Forms

Capsule, oral:

Reyataz®: 100 mg, 150 mg, 200 mg, 300 mg

atazanavir sulfate *see* atazanavir *on page 102*

atenolol (a TEN oh lole)

Sound-Alike/Look-Alike Issues

atenolol may be confused with albuterol, Altenol®, timolol, Tylenol®
Tenormin® may be confused with Imuran®, Norpramin®, thiamine, Trovan®

U.S./Canadian Brand Names Apo-Atenol® [Can]; CO Atenolol [Can]; Dom-Atenolol [Can]; Med-Atenolol [Can]; Mylan-Atenolol [Can]; Nu-Atenol [Can]; PHL-Atenolol [Can]; PMS-Atenolol [Can]; RAN™-Atenolol [Can]; ratio-Atenolol [Can]; Riva-Atenolol [Can]; Sandoz-Atenolol [Can]; Tenormin® [US/Can]; Teva-Atenolol [Can]

Therapeutic Category Beta-Adrenergic Blocker

Use Treatment of hypertension, alone or in combination with other agents; management of angina pectoris; secondary prevention postmyocardial infarction

Dosage Summary

Oral:

Children: 0.5-1 mg/kg/dose given daily; range of 0.5-1.5 mg/kg/day (maximum dose: 2 mg/kg/day up to 100 mg/day)

Adults: 25-100 mg/day as a single daily dose (maximum dose: 100 mg/day)

Dosage Forms

Tablet, oral: 25 mg, 50 mg, 100 mg

Tenormin®: 25 mg, 50 mg, 100 mg

atenolol and chlorthalidone (a TEN oh lole & klor THAL i done)

Synonyms chlorthalidone and atenolol

U.S./Canadian Brand Names Apo-Atenidone® [Can]; Novo-Atenolthalidone [Can]; Tenoretic® [US/Can]

Therapeutic Category Antihypertensive Agent, Combination

Use Treatment of hypertension with a cardioselective beta-blocker and a diuretic

Dosage Summary

Oral:

Children: Dosage not established

Adults: Initial: 50 mg (atenolol) and 25 mg (chlorthalidone) once daily; Maintenance: 50-100 mg (atenolol) and 25 mg (chlorthalidone) once daily (maximum: Atenolol 100 mg/day; chlorthalidone 25 mg/day)

Dosage Forms

Tablet:

50: Atenolol 50 mg and chlorthalidone 25 mg

100: Atenolol 100 mg and chlorthalidone 25 mg

Tenoretic®:

50: Atenolol 50 mg and chlorthalidone 25 mg

100: Atenolol 100 mg and chlorthalidone 25 mg

ATG *see* antithymocyte globulin (equine) *on page* 84

Atgam® [US/Can] *see* antithymocyte globulin (equine) *on page* 84

Ativan® [US/Can] *see* lorazepam *on page* 576

atlizumab *see* tocilizumab *on page* 939

ATNAA [US] *see* atropine and pralidoxime *on page* 107

Atolone® Oral *(Discontinued)*

atomoxetine (AT oh mox e teen)

Sound-Alike/Look-Alike Issues

atomoxetine may be confused with atorvastatin

Synonyms atomoxetine hydrochloride; LY139603; methylphenoxy-benzene propanamine; tomoxetine

U.S./Canadian Brand Names Strattera® [US/Can]

Therapeutic Category Norepinephrine Reuptake Inhibitor, Selective

Use Treatment of attention-deficit/hyperactivity disorder (ADHD)

Dosage Summary

Oral:

Children <6 years: Dosage not established

Children ≥6 years and ≤70 kg: Initial: 0.5 mg/kg/day in 1-2 divided doses; Maintenance: 0.5-1.4 mg/kg/day as a single daily dose or 2 evenly divided doses (maximum: 1.4 mg/kg/day **or** 100 mg/day whichever is less); **Note:** Titration is recommended

Children ≥6 years and >70 kg: Initial: 40 mg/day in 1-2 divided doses; Maintenance: 40-100 mg/day in 1-2 divided doses (maximum: 100 mg/day); **Note:** Titration is recommended

Adults: Initial: 40 mg/day in 1-2 divided doses; Maintenance: 40-100 mg/day in 1-2 divided doses (maximum: 100 mg/day); **Note:** Titration is recommended

Elderly: Dosage not established

Dosage Forms

Capsule, oral:

Strattera®: 10 mg, 18 mg, 25 mg, 40 mg, 60 mg, 80 mg, 100 mg

atomoxetine hydrochloride *see* atomoxetine *on page 103*

atorvastatin (a TORE va sta tin)

Sound-Alike/Look-Alike Issues

atorvastatin may be confused with atomoxetine, lovastatin, nystatin, pitavastatin, pravastatin, rosuvastatin, simvastatin

Lipitor® may be confused with labetalol, Levatol®, lisinopril, Loniten®, Lopid®, Mevacor®, Zocor®, Zyrtec®

Synonyms atorvastatin calcium

U.S./Canadian Brand Names Apo-Atorvastatin® [Can]; CO Atorvastatin [Can]; GD-Atorvastatin [Can]; Lipitor® [US/Can]; Novo-Atorvastatin [Can]; PMS-Atorvastatin [Can]; RAN™-Atorvastatin [Can]; Sandoz-Atorvastatin [Can]

Therapeutic Category HMG-CoA Reductase Inhibitor

Use Treatment of dyslipidemias or primary prevention of cardiovascular disease (atherosclerotic) as detailed below:

Primary prevention of cardiovascular disease (high-risk for CVD): To reduce the risk of MI or stroke in patients without evidence of heart disease who have multiple CVD risk factors or type 2 diabetes. Treatment reduces the risk for angina or revascularization procedures in patients with multiple risk factors.

Secondary prevention of cardiovascular disease: To reduce the risk of nonfatal MI, nonfatal stroke, revascularization procedures, hospitalization for heart failure, and angina in patients with evidence of coronary heart disease.

Treatment of dyslipidemias: To reduce elevations in total cholesterol (C), LDL-C, apolipoprotein B, and triglycerides in patients with elevations of one or more components, and/or to increase low HDL-C as present in Fredrickson type IIa, IIb, III, and IV hyperlipidemias, heterozygous familial and nonfamilial hypercholesterolemia, and homozygous familial hypercholesterolemia

Treatment of heterozygous familial hypercholesterolemia (HeFH) in adolescent patients (10-17 years of age, females >1 year postmenarche) having LDL-C ≥190 mg/dL or LDL-C ≥160 mg/dL with positive family history of premature cardiovascular disease (CVD) or with two or more CVD risk factors.

Dosage Summary Note: Doses should be individualized according to the baseline LDL-cholesterol concentrations, the recommended goal of therapy, and patient response; adjustments should be made at intervals of 2-4 weeks

Oral:

Children <10 years: Dosage not established

Children 10-17 years (females >1 year postmenarche): 10-20 mg/day (maximum: 20 mg/day)

Adults: Initial: 10-20 mg once daily **or** 10-80 mg once daily; Maintenance: 10-80 mg once daily (maximum: 80 mg/day)

Dosage Forms

Tablet, oral:

Lipitor®: 10 mg, 20 mg, 40 mg, 80 mg

atorvastatin and amlodipine *see* amlodipine and atorvastatin *on page 69*

atorvastatin calcium *see* atorvastatin *on page 104*

atorvastatin calcium and amlodipine besylate *see* amlodipine and atorvastatin *on page 69*

atovaquone (a TOE va kwone)

U.S./Canadian Brand Names Mepron® [US/Can]

Therapeutic Category Antiprotozoal

Use Acute oral treatment of mild-to-moderate *Pneumocystis jirovecii* pneumonia (PCP) in patients who are intolerant to co-trimoxazole; prophylaxis of PCP in patients who are intolerant to co-trimoxazole

Dosage Summary

Oral:

Children <1 month: Dosage not established

Children 13-16 years: 1500 mg/day in 1-2 divided doses

Adults: 1500 mg/day in 1-2 divided doses

Dosage Forms

Suspension, oral:

Mepron®: 750 mg/5 mL (5 mL, 210 mL)

atovaquone and proguanil (a TOE va kwone & pro GWA nil)

Synonyms atovaquone and proguanil hydrochloride; proguanil and atovaquone; proguanil hydrochloride and atovaquone

U.S./Canadian Brand Names Malarone® Pediatric [Can]; Malarone® [US/Can]

Therapeutic Category Antimalarial Agent

Use Prevention or treatment of acute, uncomplicated *P. falciparum* malaria

Dosage Summary

Oral:

Children <5 kg: Dosage not established

Children 5-8 kg: Treatment: 125 mg/50 mg as a single daily dose

Children 9-10 kg: Treatment: 187.5 mg/75 mg as a single daily dose

Children 11-20 kg: Prophylaxis: 62.5 mg/25 mg; Treatment: 250 mg/100 mg as a single daily dose

Children 21-30 kg: Prophylaxis: 125 mg/50 mg; Treatment: 500 mg/200 mg as a single daily dose

Children 31-40 kg: Prophylaxis: 187.5 mg/75 mg; Treatment: 750 mg/300 mg as a single daily dose

Children >40 kg: Prophylaxis: 250 mg/100 mg; Treatment: 1 g/400 mg as a single daily dose

Adults: Prophylaxis: 250 mg/100 mg; Treatment: 1 g/400 mg as a single daily dose

Dosage Forms

Tablet:

Malarone®: Atovaquone 250 mg and proguanil 100 mg

Tablet [pediatric]:

Malarone®: Atovaquone 62.5 mg and proguanil 25 mg

atovaquone and proguanil hydrochloride *see* atovaquone and proguanil *on page 105*

Atozine® Oral *(Discontinued)* *see* hydroxyzine *on page 490*

ATRA *see* tretinoin (systemic) *on page 951*

atracurium (a tra KYOO ree um)

Synonyms atracurium besylate

U.S./Canadian Brand Names Atracurium Besylate Injection [Can]

Therapeutic Category Skeletal Muscle Relaxant

Use Adjunct to general anesthesia to facilitate endotracheal intubation and to relax skeletal muscles during surgery; to facilitate mechanical ventilation in ICU patients; does not relieve pain or produce sedation

Dosage Summary

I.V.:

Children <1 month: Dosage not established

Children 1 month to 2 years: Initial: 0.3-0.4 mg/kg; Maintenance: Doses as needed to maintain neuromuscular blockade; Infusion: 10-20 mcg/kg/min

Children >2 years: Initial: 0.4-0.5 mg/kg; Maintenance: 0.08-1 mg/kg at 15- to 25- minute intervals to maintain neuromuscular blockade; Infusion: 5-13 mcg/kg/minute

Adults: Initial: 0.4-0.5 mg/kg; Maintenance: 0.08-1 mg/kg at 15- to 25- minute intervals to maintain neuromuscular blockade; Infusion: 5-13 mcg/kg/minute

Dosage Forms

Injection, solution: 10 mg/mL (10 mL)

Injection, solution [preservative free]: 10 mg/mL (5 mL)

atracurium besylate *see* atracurium *on page 105*

Atracurium Besylate Injection [Can] *see* atracurium *on page 105*

Atralin™ [US] *see* tretinoin (topical) *on page 951*

Atriance™ [Can] *see* nelarabine *on page 664*

Atripla® [US/Can] *see* efavirenz, emtricitabine, and tenofovir *on page 343*

Atropair® *(Discontinued)* *see* atropine *on page 105*

AtroPen® [US] *see* atropine *on page 105*

atropine (A troe peen)

Synonyms atropine sulfate

U.S./Canadian Brand Names AtroPen® [US]; Atropine Care™ [US]; Dioptic's Atropine Solution [Can]; Isopto® Atropine [US/Can]; Sal-Tropine™ [US]

ATROPINE

Therapeutic Category Anticholinergic Agent

Use

Injection: Preoperative medication to inhibit salivation and secretions; treatment of symptomatic sinus bradycardia, AV block (nodal level); antidote for acetylcholinesterase inhibitor poisoning (carbamate insecticides, nerve agents, organophosphate insecticides); adjuvant use with anticholinesterases (eg, edrophonium, neostigmine) to decrease their side effects during reversal of neuromuscular blockade

Ophthalmic: Produce mydriasis and cycloplegia for examination of the retina and optic disc and accurate measurement of refractive errors; uveitis

Oral: Inhibit salivation and secretions

Dosage Summary Note: Doses <0.1 mg (children) and <0.5 mg (adults) have been associated with paradoxical bradycardia

I.M.:

Children ≤5 kg: 0.02 mg/kg/dose every 4-6 hours as needed

Children >5 kg: 0.01-0.2 mg/kg/dose every 4-6 hours as needed (maximum: 0.4 mg/dose; minimum: 0.1 mg/dose)

Adults: 0.4-0.6 mg every 4-6 hours as needed

AtroPen®:

Children <6.8 kg: Dosage not established

Children 6.8-18 kg: 0.5 mg/dose (maximum: 3 doses)

Children >41 kg: 2 mg/dose (maximum: 3 doses)

Adults: 2 mg/dose (maximum: 3 doses)

I.V.:

Children ≤5 kg: 0.02 mg/kg/dose every 4-6 hours as needed **or** 0.02 mg/kg repeated in 5-minute intervals to a maximum total dose of 1 mg (maximum: 0.5 mg/dose; 1 mg total dose) **or** 0.03-0.05 mg/kg every 10-20 minutes until atropine effect, then every 1-4 hours

Children >5 kg: 0.01-0.2 mg/kg/dose every 4-6 hours as needed (maximum: 0.4 mg/dose) **or** 0.02 mg/kg repeated in 5-minute intervals to a maximum total dose of 1 mg (maximum: 0.5 mg/dose; 1 mg total dose) **or** 0.03-0.05 mg/kg every 10-20 minutes until atropine effect, then every 1-4 hours

Adolescents: 0.01-0.2 mg/kg/dose every 4-6 hours as needed (maximum: 0.4 mg/dose) **or** 0.02 mg/kg repeated in 5-minute intervals to a maximum total dose of 1 mg (maximum: 0.5 mg/dose; 2 mg total dose) **or** 0.03-0.05 mg/kg every 10-20 minutes until atropine effect, then every 1-4 hours

Adults: 0.4-0.6 mg every 4-6 hours as needed **or** 0.5-1 mg every 3-5 minutes (maximum: 0.04 mg/kg total dose) **or** 2 mg every 15 minutes until adequate atropinization (maximum: 6 mg) **or** 10% to 20% of loading dose/hour

Intratracheal:

Children: 0.02 mg/kg repeated in 5-minute intervals to a maximum total dose of 1 mg (maximum: 0.5 mg/dose; 1 mg total dose)

Adolescents: 0.02 mg/kg repeated in 5-minute intervals to a maximum total dose of 1 mg (maximum: 0.5 mg/dose; 2 mg total dose)

Adults: Administer 2-2.5 times the recommended I.V. dose

Ophthalmic:

Children: Dosage not established

Adults: Ointment: Apply a small amount in the conjunctival sac up to 3 times/day; Solution (1%): Instill 1-2 drops 4 times/day

Oral:

Children ≤5 kg: 0.02 mg/kg/dose every 4-6 hours as needed

Children >5 kg: 0.01-0.2 mg/kg/dose every 4-6 hours as needed (maximum: 0.4 mg/dose)

Adults: 0.4 mg every 4-6 hours

SubQ:

Children ≤5 kg: 0.02 mg/kg/dose every 4-6 hours as needed

Children >5 kg: 0.01-0.2 mg/kg/dose every 4-6 hours as needed (maximum: 0.4 mg/dose)

Adults: 0.4-0.6 mg every 4-6 hours as needed

Dosage Forms

Injection, solution: 0.05 mg/mL (5 mL); 0.1 mg/mL (5 mL, 10 mL); 0.4 mg/mL (1 mL, 20 mL); 1 mg/mL (1 mL)

AtroPen®: 0.25 mg/0.3 mL (0.3 mL); 0.5 mg/0.7 mL (0.7 mL); 1 mg/0.7 mL (0.7 mL); 2 mg/0.7 mL (0.7 mL)

Injection, solution [preservative free]: 0.4 mg/0.5 mL (0.5 mL); 0.4 mg/mL (1 mL); 1 mg/mL (1 mL)

Ointment, ophthalmic: 1% (3.5 g)
Solution, ophthalmic: 1% (2 mL, 5 mL, 15 mL)
Atropine Care™: 1% (2 mL)
Isopto® Atropine: 1% (5 mL, 15 mL)
Tablet, oral:
Sal-Tropine™: 0.4 mg

atropine and difenoxin *see* difenoxin and atropine *on page 300*

atropine and diphenoxylate *see* diphenoxylate and atropine *on page 313*

atropine and pralidoxime (A troe peen & pra li DOKS eem)

Synonyms atropine and pralidoxime chloride; Mark 1™; NAAK; nerve agent antidote kit; pralidoxime and atropine

U.S./Canadian Brand Names ATNAA [US]; Duodote™ [US]

Therapeutic Category Anticholinergic Agent; Antidote

Use
ATNAA: Treatment of poisoning by susceptible organophosphorous nerve agents having acetylcholinesterase-inhibiting activity for self- or buddy-administration by military personnel
Duodote™: Treatment of poisoning by organophosphorous nerve agents (eg, tabun, sarin, soman) or organophosphorous insecticide for use by trained emergency medical services personnel

Dosage Summary
I.M.:
Children <18 years: Dosage not established
Adults: 1-3 injections (maximum: 3 injections)

Dosage Forms
Injection, solution:
ATNAA, Duodote™: Atropine 2.1 mg/0.7 mL and pralidoxime chloride 600 mg/2 mL [contains benzyl alcohol; prefilled auto-injector]

atropine and pralidoxime chloride *see* atropine and pralidoxime *on page 107*

Atropine Care™ [US] *see* atropine *on page 105*

atropine, hyoscyamine, phenobarbital, and scopolamine *see* hyoscyamine, atropine, scopolamine, and phenobarbital *on page 492*

atropine soluble tablet *(Discontinued)*

atropine sulfate *see* atropine *on page 105*

atropine sulfate and edrophonium chloride *see* edrophonium and atropine *on page 343*

Atropisol® *(Discontinued)* *see* atropine *on page 105*

Atrovent® [US/Can] *see* ipratropium (nasal) *on page 523*

Atrovent® HFA [US/Can] *see* ipratropium (oral inhalation) *on page 523*

Atryn® [US] *see* antithrombin III *on page 83*

Attenuvax® *(Discontinued)* *see* measles virus vaccine (live) *on page 593*

Atuss® HD *(Discontinued)*

Atuss® HX *(Discontinued)*

Augmentin® [US/Can] *see* amoxicillin and clavulanate potassium *on page 73*

Augmentin ES-600® [US] *see* amoxicillin and clavulanate potassium *on page 73*

Augmentin XR® [US] *see* amoxicillin and clavulanate potassium *on page 73*

Auralgan® [Can] *see* antipyrine and benzocaine *on page 83*

auranofin (au RANE oh fin)

Sound-Alike/Look-Alike Issues
Ridaura® may be confused with Cardura®

U.S./Canadian Brand Names Ridaura® [US/Can]

Therapeutic Category Gold Compound

Use Management of active stage of classic or definite rheumatoid arthritis in patients who do not respond to or tolerate other agents; psoriatic arthritis; adjunctive or alternative therapy for pemphigus

Dosage Summary

Oral:

Children: Initial: 0.1 mg/kg/day; Maintenance: 0.15-0.2 mg/kg/day in 1-2 divided doses (maximum: 0.2 mg/kg/day)

Adults: Initial: 6 mg/day; Maintenance: 6-9 mg/day (maximum: 9 mg/day); **Note:** Titration may be recommended

Dosage Forms

Capsule, oral:

Ridaura®: 3 mg

Auraphene B® [US-OTC] *see* carbamide peroxide *on page 178*
Auro® [US-OTC] *see* carbamide peroxide *on page 178*
Aurodex *(Discontinued)* *see* antipyrine and benzocaine *on page 83*
Autoplex® T *(Discontinued)* *see* antiinhibitor coagulant complex *on page 83*
AVA *see* anthrax vaccine, adsorbed *on page 80*
Avagard™ [US-OTC] *see* chlorhexidine gluconate *on page 204*
Avage™ [US] *see* tazarotene *on page 911*
avakine *see* infliximab *on page 506*
Avalide® [US/Can] *see* irbesartan and hydrochlorothiazide *on page 525*
Avamys® [Can] *see* fluticasone (nasal) *on page 419*
Avandamet® [US/Can] *see* rosiglitazone and metformin *on page 853*
Avandaryl® [US] *see* rosiglitazone and glimepiride *on page 853*
Avandia® [US/Can] *see* rosiglitazone *on page 852*
Avapro® [US/Can] *see* irbesartan *on page 525*
Avapro® HCT *see* irbesartan and hydrochlorothiazide *on page 525*
AVAR™ [US] *see* sulfur and sulfacetamide *on page 903*
AVAR™-e [US] *see* sulfur and sulfacetamide *on page 903*
AVAR™-e Green [US] *see* sulfur and sulfacetamide *on page 903*
AVAR™-e LS [US] *see* sulfur and sulfacetamide *on page 903*
AVAR™ LS [US] *see* sulfur and sulfacetamide *on page 903*
Avastin® [US/Can] *see* bevacizumab *on page 136*
Avaxim® [Can] *see* hepatitis A vaccine *on page 468*
Avaxim®-Pediatric [Can] *see* hepatitis A vaccine *on page 468*
AVC™ [US] *see* sulfanilamide *on page 902*
Avelox® [US/Can] *see* moxifloxacin (systemic) *on page 647*
Avelox® ABC Pack [US] *see* moxifloxacin (systemic) *on page 647*
Avelox® I.V. [US/Can] *see* moxifloxacin (systemic) *on page 647*
Aventyl® [Can] *see* nortriptyline *on page 684*
Aventyl® HCl *(Discontinued)* *see* nortriptyline *on page 684*
Aviane™ [US/Can] *see* ethinyl estradiol and levonorgestrel *on page 376*
avian influenza virus vaccine *see* influenza virus vaccine (H5N1) *on page 507*
Avinza® [US] *see* morphine (systemic) *on page 644*
Avita® [US] *see* tretinoin (topical) *on page 951*
Avitene® [US] *see* collagen hemostat *on page 248*
Avitene® Flour [US] *see* collagen hemostat *on page 248*
Avitene® Ultrafoam™ [US] *see* collagen hemostat *on page 248*
Avlosulfon® *(Discontinued)* *see* dapsone (systemic) *on page 268*
Avodart® [US/Can] *see* dutasteride *on page 337*
Avonex® [US/Can] *see* interferon beta-1a *on page 515*
AVP *see* vasopressin *on page 980*
Axert® [US/Can] *see* almotriptan *on page 53*
Axid® [US/Can] *see* nizatidine *on page 681*
Axid® AR [US-OTC] *see* nizatidine *on page 681*
AY-25650 *see* triptorelin *on page 962*
Aygestin® [US] *see* norethindrone *on page 682*

Ayr® Allergy Sinus [US-OTC] *see* sodium chloride *on page* *882*
Ayr® Baby Saline [US-OTC] *see* sodium chloride *on page* *882*
Ayr® Saline [US-OTC] *see* sodium chloride *on page* *882*
Ayr® Saline No-Drip [US-OTC] *see* sodium chloride *on page* *882*
5-Aza-2'-deoxycytidine *see* decitabine *on page* *272*

azacitidine (ay za SYE ti deen)

Sound-Alike/Look-Alike Issues
azaCITIDine may be confused with azaTHIOprine

Synonyms 5-azacytidine; 5-AZC; AZA-CR; azacytidine; ladakamycin

Tall-Man aza**CITID**ine

U.S./Canadian Brand Names Vidaza® [US]

Therapeutic Category Antineoplastic Agent, Antimetabolite (Pyrimidine)

Use Treatment of myelodysplastic syndrome (MDS)

Dosage Summary

I.V.:
Children: Dosage not established
Adults: 75-100 mg/m^2/day for 7 days/28-day treatment cycle

SubQ:
Children: Dosage not established
Adults: 75-100 mg/m^2/day for 7 days/28-day treatment cycle

Dosage Forms

Injection, powder for suspension:
Vidaza®: 100 mg

AZA-CR *see* azacitidine *on page* *109*
Azactam® [US/Can] *see* aztreonam *on page* *112*
azacytidine *see* azacitidine *on page* *109*
5-azacytidine *see* azacitidine *on page* *109*
5-Aza-dCyd *see* decitabine *on page* *272*
azaepothilone B *see* ixabepilone *on page* *532*
Azarga™ [Can] *see* brinzolamide and timolol *(Canada only) on page* *145*
Azasan® [US] *see* azathioprine *on page* *109*
AzaSite® [US] *see* azithromycin (ophthalmic) *on page* *111*

azathioprine (ay za THYE oh preen)

Sound-Alike/Look-Alike Issues
azaTHIOprine may be confused with azaCITIDine, azatadine, azidothymidine, azithromycin, Azulfidine®
Imuran® may be confused with Elmiron®, Enduron®, Imdur®, Inderal®, Tenormin®

Synonyms azathioprine sodium

Tall-Man aza**THIO**prine

U.S./Canadian Brand Names Apo-Azathioprine® [Can]; Azasan® [US]; Imuran® [US/Can]; Mylan-Azathioprine [Can]; Teva-Azathioprine [Can]

Therapeutic Category Immunosuppressant Agent

Use Adjunctive therapy in prevention of rejection of kidney transplants; management of active rheumatoid arthritis (RA)

Dosage Summary

I.V.:
Adults: Transplant immunosuppression: Initial: 3-5 mg/kg/day as a single daily dose; Maintenance: 1-3 mg/kg/day as a single daily dose

Oral:
Adults:
Transplant immunosuppression: Initial: 3-5 mg/kg/day in 1-2 divided doses; Maintenance: 1-3 mg/kg/day in 1-2 divided doses
Rheumatoid arthritis: Initial: 1 mg/kg/day in 1-2 divided doses; Maintenance: 0.5-2.5 mg/kg/day in 1-2 divided doses

Dosage Forms

Injection, powder for reconstitution: 100 mg

Tablet, oral: 50 mg

Azasan®: 75 mg, 100 mg

Imuran®: 50 mg

azathioprine sodium *see* azathioprine *on page 109*

5-AZC *see* azacitidine *on page 109*

Azdone® ***(Discontinued)***

azelaic acid (a zeh LAY ik AS id)

U.S./Canadian Brand Names Azelex® [US]; Finacea® Plus™ [US]; Finacea® [US/Can]

Therapeutic Category Topical Skin Product

Use Topical treatment of inflammatory papules and pustules of mild-to-moderate rosacea; mild-to-moderate inflammatory acne vulgaris

Finacea®: Not FDA-approved for the treatment of acne

Dosage Summary

Topical:

Children <12 years: Dosage not established

Children ≥12 years: Massage gently into affected areas twice daily

Adults: Massage gently into affected areas twice daily

Dosage Forms

Cream, topical:

Azelex®: 20% (30 g, 50 g)

Gel, topical:

Finacea®: 15% (50 g)

Finacea® Plus™: 15% (50 g)

azelastine (nasal) (a ZEL as teen)

Sound-Alike/Look-Alike Issues

Astelin® may be confused with Astepro®

Synonyms azelastine hydrochloride

U.S./Canadian Brand Names Astelin® [US/Can]; Astepro® [US]

Therapeutic Category Histamine H_1 Antagonist; Histamine H_1 Antagonist, Second Generation

Use Treatment of the symptoms of seasonal allergic rhinitis such as rhinorrhea, sneezing, and nasal pruritus; treatment of the symptoms of vasomotor rhinitis

Dosage Summary

Intranasal:

Children <5 years: Dosage not established

Children 5-11 years: 1 spray in each nostril twice daily

Children ≥12 years: 1-2 sprays in each nostril twice daily

Adults: 1-2 sprays in each nostril twice daily

Dosage Forms

Solution, intranasal: 0.1% [137 mcg/spray] (30 mL)

Astelin®: 0.1% [137 mcg/spray] (30 mL)

Astepro®: 0.1% [137 mcg/spray] (30 mL); 0.15% [205.5 mcg/spray] (30 mL)

azelastine (ophthalmic) (a ZEL as teen)

Sound-Alike/Look-Alike Issues

Optivar® may be confused with Optiray®, Optive™

Synonyms azelastine hydrochloride

U.S./Canadian Brand Names Optivar® [US]

Therapeutic Category Histamine H_1 Antagonist; Histamine H_1 Antagonist, Second Generation

Use Treatment of itching of the eye associated with seasonal allergic conjunctivitis

Dosage Summary

Ophthalmic:

Children <3 years: Dosage not established

Children ≥3 years: Instill 1 drop into affected eye(s) twice daily

Adults: Instill 1 drop into affected eye(s) twice daily

Dosage Forms

Solution, ophthalmic: 0.05% (6 mL)

Optivar®: 0.05% (6 mL)

azelastine hydrochloride *see* azelastine (nasal) *on page 110*

azelastine hydrochloride *see* azelastine (ophthalmic) *on page 110*

Azelex® [US] *see* azelaic acid *on page 110*

azidothymidine *see* zidovudine *on page 999*

azidothymidine, abacavir, and lamivudine *see* abacavir, lamivudine, and zidovudine *on page 18*

Azilect® [US] *see* rasagiline *on page 830*

azithromycin (systemic) (az ith roe MYE sin)

Sound-Alike/Look-Alike Issues

azithromycin may be confused with azathioprine, erythromycin

Zithromax® may be confused with Fosamax®, Zinacef®, Zovirax®

Synonyms azithromycin dihydrate; azithromycin hydrogencitrate; azithromycin monohydrate; Z-Pak; Zithromax TRI-PAK™; Zithromax Z-PAK®

U.S./Canadian Brand Names Apo-Azithromycin® [Can]; CO Azithromycin [Can]; Dom-Azithromycin [Can]; Mylan-Azithromycin [Can]; Novo-Azithromycin [Can]; PHL-Azithromycin [Can]; PMS-Azithromycin [Can]; PRO-Azithromycin [Can]; ratio-Azithromycin [Can]; Riva-Azithromycin [Can]; Sandoz-Azithromycin [Can]; Zithromax® [US/Can]; Zmax® [US]

Therapeutic Category Antibiotic, Macrolide

Use Oral, I.V.: Treatment of acute otitis media due to *H. influenzae*, *M. catarrhalis*, or *S. pneumoniae*; pharyngitis/tonsillitis due to *S. pyogenes*; treatment of mild-to-moderate upper and lower respiratory tract infections, infections of the skin and skin structure, community-acquired pneumonia, pelvic inflammatory disease (PID), sexually-transmitted diseases (urethritis/cervicitis), pharyngitis/tonsillitis (alternative to first-line therapy), and genital ulcer disease (chancroid) due to susceptible strains of *Chlamydophila pneumoniae, C. trachomatis*, *M. catarrhalis*, *H. influenzae*, *S. aureus*, *S. pneumoniae*, *Mycoplasma pneumoniae*, and *C. psittaci*; acute bacterial exacerbations of chronic obstructive pulmonary disease (COPD) due to *H. influenzae*, *M. catarrhalis,* or *S. pneumoniae*; acute bacterial sinusitis

Dosage Summary

I.V.:

Children: Dosage not established

Adults: 500 mg as a single daily dose

Oral:

Children <6 months: 10 mg/kg/day

Children ≥6 months: Extended release suspension (Zmax®): 60 mg/kg as a single dose (pediatric patients ≥75 lbs [34 kg] should receive the adult dose).

Children ≥6 months to 2 years: 5-10 mg/kg as a single daily dose (maximum: 500 mg/dose) **or** 30 mg/kg as a single dose (maximum: 1500 mg/dose)

Children ≥2 years: 5-12 mg/kg as single daily dose (maximum: 500 mg/dose) **or** 30 mg/kg as a single dose (maximum: 1500 mg/dose)

Adults: 250-500 mg as a single daily dose **or** 1-2 g as a single dose; Extended release suspension (Zmax®): 2 g as a single dose

Dosage Forms

Injection, powder for reconstitution: 500 mg, 2.5 g

Zithromax®: 500 mg

Microspheres for suspension, extended release, oral:

Zmax®: 2 g/bottle (60 mL)

Powder for suspension, oral: 100 mg/5 mL (15 mL); 200 mg/5 mL (15 mL, 22.5 mL, 30 mL); 1 g/packet (3s, 10s)

Zithromax®: 100 mg/5 mL (15 mL); 200 mg/5 mL (15 mL, 22.5 mL, 30 mL); 1 g/packet (3s, 10s)

Tablet, oral: 250 mg, 500 mg, 600 mg

Zithromax®: 250 mg, 500 mg, 600 mg

Zithromax® TRI-PAK™: 500 mg

Zithromax® Z-PAK®: 250 mg

azithromycin (ophthalmic) (az ith roe MYE sin)

Sound-Alike/Look-Alike Issues

azithromycin may be confused with azathioprine, erythromycin

U.S./Canadian Brand Names AzaSite® [US]

Therapeutic Category Antibiotic, Macrolide; Antibiotic, Ophthalmic

Use Bacterial conjunctivitis

Dosage Summary

Ophthalmic:

Children <1 year: Dosage not established

Children ≥1 year: Days 1 and 2: 1 drop into affected eye(s) twice daily; Days 3-7: 1 drop into affected eye(s) once daily

Adults: Days 1 and 2: 1 drop into affected eye(s) twice daily; Days 3-7: 1 drop into affected eye(s) once daily

Dosage Forms

Solution, ophthalmic:

AzaSite®: 1% (2.5 mL)

azithromycin dihydrate *see* azithromycin (systemic) *on page* 111

azithromycin hydrogencitrate *see* azithromycin (systemic) *on page* 111

azithromycin monohydrate *see* azithromycin (systemic) *on page* 111

Azmacort® *(Discontinued)* *see* triamcinolone (systemic, oral inhalation) *on page* 952

Azo-Gesic™ [US-OTC] *see* phenazopyridine *on page* 746

Azopt® [US/Can] *see* brinzolamide *on page* 145

Azor™ [US] *see* amlodipine and olmesartan *on page* 70

AZO Standard® [US-OTC] *see* phenazopyridine *on page* 746

AZO Standard® Maximum Strength [US-OTC] *see* phenazopyridine *on page* 746

AZT™ [Can] *see* zidovudine *on page* 999

AZT, abacavir, and lamivudine *see* abacavir, lamivudine, and zidovudine *on page* 18

azthreonam *see* aztreonam *on page* 112

aztreonam (AZ tree oh nam)

Sound-Alike/Look-Alike Issues

aztreonam may be confused with azidothymidine

Synonyms azthreonam

U.S./Canadian Brand Names Azactam® [US/Can]; Cayston® [US]

Therapeutic Category Antibiotic, Miscellaneous

Use

Injection: Treatment of patients with urinary tract infections, lower respiratory tract infections, septicemia, skin/skin structure infections, intraabdominal infections, and gynecological infections caused by susceptible gram-negative bacilli

Inhalation: Improve respiratory symptoms in cystic fibrosis (CF) patients with *Pseudomonas aeruginosa*

Dosage Summary

I.M.:

Children ≤1 month: Dosage not established

Children >1 month: 30-50 mg/kg/dose every 6-8 hours (maximum: 8 g/day)

Adults: 500 mg to 1 g every 8-12 hours

I.V.:

Children ≤1 month: Dosage not established

Children >1 month: 30-50 mg/kg/dose every 6-8 hours (maximum: 8 g/day)

Adults: 1-2 g every 6-12 hours (maximum: 8 g/day)

Oral inhalation:

Children <7 years: Dosage not established

Children ≥7 years: 75 mg 3 times daily

Adults: 75 mg 3 times daily

Dosage Forms

Infusion, premixed iso-osmotic solution:

Azactam®: 1 g (50 mL); 2 g (50 mL)

Powder for reconstitution, for oral inhalation [preservative free]:

Cayston®: 75 mg

Azulfidine® [US] *see* sulfasalazine *on page* 902

Azulfidine EN-tabs® [US] *see* sulfasalazine *on page* 902

Azurette® [US] *see* ethinyl estradiol and desogestrel *on page 374*
B6 *see* pyridoxine *on page 818*
B2036-PEG *see* pegvisomant *on page 735*
B 9273 *see* alefacept *on page 47*
baby aspirin *see* aspirin *on page 100*
BabyBIG® [US] *see* botulism immune globulin (intravenous-human) *on page 143*
BAC *see* benzalkonium chloride *on page 124*
Bacid® [US-OTC/Can] *see* Lactobacillus *on page 543*
Baciguent® [US-OTC/Can] *see* bacitracin *on page 113*
BACiiM™ [US] *see* bacitracin *on page 113*
Baciject® [Can] *see* bacitracin *on page 113*
bacillus calmette-Guérin (BCG) live *see* BCG *on page 118*
Baci-Rx [US] *see* bacitracin *on page 113*

bacitracin (bas i TRAY sin)

Sound-Alike/Look-Alike Issues

bacitracin may be confused with Bactrim®, Bactroban®

U.S./Canadian Brand Names Baci-Rx [US]; Baciguent® [US-OTC/Can]; BACiiM™ [US]; Baciject® [Can]

Therapeutic Category Antibiotic, Miscellaneous; Antibiotic, Ophthalmic; Antibiotic, Topical

Use Treatment of susceptible bacterial infections mainly; has activity against gram-positive bacilli; due to toxicity risks, systemic and irrigant uses of bacitracin should be limited to situations where less toxic alternatives would not be effective

Dosage Summary

I.M.:

Infants ≤2.5 kg: 900 units/kg/day in 2-3 divided doses
Infants >2.5 kg: 1000 units/kg/day in 2-3 divided doses
Children: 800-1200 units/kg/day divided every 8 hours
Adults: Dosage not established

Irrigation:

Children: 50-100 units/mL in solution for irrigation, apply 1-5 times/day or as needed during surgical procedures
Adults: 50-100 units/mL in solution for irrigation, apply 1-5 times/day or as needed during surgical procedures

Ophthalmic:

Children: Instill 1/4" to 1/2" ribbon every 3-4 hours (acute infections) or 2-3 times/day (mild-to-moderate infections)
Adults: Instill 1/4" to 1/2" ribbon every 3-4 hours (acute infections) or 2-3 times/day (mild-to-moderate infections)

Oral:

Children: Dosage not established
Adults: 25,000 units 4 times/day

Topical:

Children: Apply 1-5 times/day
Adults: Apply 1-5 times/day

Dosage Forms

Injection, powder for reconstitution: 50,000 units
BACiiM™: 50,000 units
Ointment, ophthalmic: 500 units/g (3.5 g)
Ointment, topical: 500 units/g (0.9 g, 15 g, 28 g, 28.35 g, 30 g, 120 g, 454 g)
Baciguent® [OTC]: 500 units/g (30 g)
Powder, for prescription compounding:
Baci-Rx: 5 million units

bacitracin and polymyxin B (bas i TRAY sin & pol i MIKS in bee)

Synonyms polymyxin B and bacitracin

U.S./Canadian Brand Names AK-Poly-Bac™ [US]; LID-Pack® [Can]; Optimyxin® [Can]; Polysporin® [US-OTC]

Therapeutic Category Antibiotic, Ophthalmic; Antibiotic, Topical

Use Treatment of superficial infections caused by susceptible organisms

Dosage Summary

Ophthalmic:

Children: Instill 1/2" ribbon in the affected eye(s) every 3-4 hours (acute infections) **or** 2-3 times/day (mild-to-moderate infections)

Adults: Instill 1/2" ribbon in the affected eye(s) every 3-4 hours (acute infections) **or** 2-3 times/day (mild-to-moderate infections)

Topical:

Children: Apply to affected area 1-4 times/day

Adults: Apply to affected area 1-4 times/day

Dosage Forms

Ointment, ophthalmic: Bacitracin 500 units and polymyxin B 10,000 units per g (3.5 g)

AK-Poly-Bac™: Bacitracin 500 units and polymyxin B 10,000 units per g (3.5 g)

Ointment, topical: Bacitracin 500 units and polymyxin B 10,000 units per g in white petrolatum (15 g, 30 g)

Polysporin®: Bacitracin 500 units and polymyxin B 10,000 units per g (0.9 g, 15 g, 30 g)

Powder, topical:

Polysporin®: Bacitracin 500 units and polymyxin B 10,000 units per g (10 g)

bacitracin, neomycin, and polymyxin B

(bas i TRAY sin, nee oh MYE sin, & pol i MIKS in bee)

Synonyms neomycin, bacitracin, and polymyxin B; polymyxin B, bacitracin, and neomycin; triple antibiotic

U.S./Canadian Brand Names Neosporin® Neo To Go® [US-OTC]; Neosporin® Topical [US-OTC]

Therapeutic Category Antibiotic, Ophthalmic; Antibiotic, Topical

Use Helps prevent infection in minor cuts, scrapes, and burns; short-term treatment of superficial external ocular infections caused by susceptible organisms

Dosage Summary

Ophthalmic:

Children: Instill 1/2" every 3-4 hours

Adults: Instill 1/2" every 3-4 hours

Topical:

Children: Apply 1-3 times/day

Adults: Apply 1-3 times/day

Dosage Forms

Ointment, ophthalmic: Bacitracin 400 units, neomycin 3.5 mg, and polymyxin B 10,000 units per g (3.5 g)

Ointment, topical: Bacitracin 400 units, neomycin 3.5 mg, and polymyxin B 5000 units per g (0.9 g, 15 g, 30 g, 454 g)

Neosporin® [OTC]: Bacitracin 400 units, neomycin 3.5 mg, and polymyxin B 5000 units per g (15 g, 30 g)

Neosporin® Neo To Go® [OTC]: Bacitracin 400 units, neomycin 3.5 mg, and polymyxin B 5000 units per g (0.9 g)

bacitracin, neomycin, polymyxin B, and hydrocortisone

(bas i TRAY sin, nee oh MYE sin, pol i MIKS in bee, & hye droe KOR ti sone)

Synonyms hydrocortisone, bacitracin, neomycin, and polymyxin B; neomycin, bacitracin, polymyxin B, and hydrocortisone; polymyxin B, bacitracin, neomycin, and hydrocortisone

U.S./Canadian Brand Names Cortisporin® Ointment [US]; Cortisporin® Topical Ointment [Can]

Therapeutic Category Antibiotic/Corticosteroid, Ophthalmic; Antibiotic/Corticosteroid, Topical

Use Prevention and treatment of susceptible inflammatory conditions where bacterial infection (or risk of infection) is present

Dosage Summary

Ophthalmic:

Children: Instill 1/2 inch ribbon to inside of lower lid every 3-4 hours

Adults: Instill 1/2 inch ribbon to inside of lower lid every 3-4 hours

Topical:

Children: Apply sparingly 2-4 times/day

Adults: Apply sparingly 2-4 times/day

Dosage Forms

Ointment, ophthalmic: Bacitracin 400 units, neomycin sulfate 3.5 mg, polymyxin B 10,000 units, and hydrocortisone 10 mg per g (3.5 g)

Ointment, topical:

Cortisporin®: Bacitracin 400 units, neomycin 3.5 mg, polymyxin B 5000 units, and hydrocortisone 10 mg per g (15 g)

bacitracin, neomycin, polymyxin B, and pramoxine

(bas i TRAY sin, nee oh MYE sin, pol i MIKS in bee, & pra MOKS een)

Synonyms neomycin, bacitracin, polymyxin B, and pramoxine; polymyxin B, neomycin, bacitracin, and pramoxine; pramoxine, neomycin, bacitracin, and polymyxin B

U.S./Canadian Brand Names Neosporin® + Pain Relief Ointment [US-OTC]; Tri Biozene [US-OTC]

Therapeutic Category Antibiotic, Topical

Use Prevention and treatment of susceptible superficial topical infections and provide temporary relief of pain or discomfort

Dosage Summary

Topical:

Children <2 years: Dosage not established

Children ≥2 years: Apply 1-3 times/day to infected areas

Adults: Apply 1-3 times/day to infected areas

Dosage Forms

Ointment, topical: Bacitracin 500 units, neomycin 3.5 mg, polymyxin B 10,000 units, and pramoxine 10 mg (15 g, 30 g)

Neosporin® + Pain Relief Ointment [OTC]: Bacitracin 500 units, neomycin 3.5 mg, polymyxin B 10,000 units, and pramoxine 10 mg (15 g, 30 g)

Tri Biozene [OTC]: Bacitracin 500 units, neomycin 3.5 mg, polymyxin B 10,000 units, and pramoxine 10 mg (15 g)

baclofen (BAK loe fen)

Sound-Alike/Look-Alike Issues

baclofen may be confused with Bactroban®

Lioresal® may be confused with lisinopril, Lotensin®

U.S./Canadian Brand Names Apo-Baclofen® [Can]; Dom-Baclofen [Can]; Lioresal® [US/Can]; Liotec [Can]; Med-Baclofen [Can]; Mylan-Baclofen [Can]; Novo-Baclofen [Can]; Nu-Baclo [Can]; PHL-Baclofen [Can]; PMS-Baclofen [Can]; ratio-Baclofen [Can]; Riva-Baclofen [Can]

Therapeutic Category Skeletal Muscle Relaxant

Use Treatment of reversible spasticity associated with multiple sclerosis or spinal cord lesions

Orphan drug: Intrathecal: Treatment of intractable spasticity caused by spinal cord injury, multiple sclerosis, and other spinal disease (spinal ischemia or tumor, transverse myelitis, cervical spondylosis, degenerative myelopathy)

Dosage Summary

Intrathecal:

Children: Test dose: 25-100 mcg; Initial infusion: Infuse at a 24-hourly rate dosed at twice the test dose

Adults: Test dose: 50-100 mcg; Initial infusion: Infuse at a 24-hourly rate dosed at twice the test dose

Oral:

Adults: Initial: 5 mg 3 times/day; Maintenance: Up to 80 mg/day in 2-3 divided doses; **Note:** Titration is recommended

Elderly: Initial: 5 mg 2-3 times/day, increasing gradually as needed

Dosage Forms

Injection, solution, intrathecal [preservative free]:

Lioresal®: 50 mcg/mL (1 mL); 500 mcg/mL (20 mL); 2000 mcg/mL (5 mL, 20 mL)

Tablet, oral: 10 mg, 20 mg

BactoShield® CHG [US-OTC] *see* chlorhexidine gluconate *on page* 204

BactoShield® *(Discontinued)* *see* chlorhexidine gluconate *on page* 204

Bactrim™ [US] *see* sulfamethoxazole and trimethoprim *on page* 901

Bactrim™ DS [US] *see* sulfamethoxazole and trimethoprim *on page* 901

Bactrim™ I.V. Infusion *(Discontinued)* *see* sulfamethoxazole and trimethoprim *on page* 901

Bactroban® [US/Can] *see* mupirocin *on page* 649

Bactroban Cream® [US] *see* mupirocin *on page* 649

Bactroban Nasal® [US] *see* mupirocin *on page 649*
baking soda *see* sodium bicarbonate *on page 882*
BAL *see* dimercaprol *on page 307*
BAL5788 *see* ceftobiprole *(Canada only) on page 193*
BAL9141 *see* ceftobiprole *(Canada only) on page 193*
Balacet 325™ [US] *see* propoxyphene and acetaminophen *on page 805*

balanced salt solution (BAL anced salt soe LOO shun)

U.S./Canadian Brand Names AquaLase™ [US]; BSS Plus® [US/Can]; BSS® [US/Can]; Eye-Stream® [Can]; Navstel® [US]

Therapeutic Category Ophthalmic Agent, Miscellaneous

Use

Irrigation solution for ophthalmic surgery:

AquaLase™, BSS®: Intraocular or extraocular irrigating solution

BSS Plus®, Navstel®: Intraocular irrigating solution

Irrigation solution for eyes, ears, nose, or throat

Dosage Summary

Irrigation:

Children: Based on standard for each surgical procedure

Adults: Based on standard for each surgical procedure

Dosage Forms

Solution, irrigation [preservative free]: Sodium chloride 0.64%, potassium chloride 0.075%, calcium chloride 0.048%, magnesium chloride 0.03%, sodium acetate 0.39%, sodium citrate 0.17% (500 mL)

Solution, ophthalmic [irrigation; preservative free]: Sodium chloride 0.64%, potassium chloride 0.075%, calcium chloride 0.048%, magnesium chloride 0.03%, sodium acetate 0.39%, sodium citrate 0.17% (18 mL, 500 mL)

AquaLase™: Sodium chloride 0.64%, potassium chloride 0.075%, calcium chloride 0.048%, magnesium chloride 0.03%, sodium acetate 0.39%, sodium citrate 0.17% (90 mL)

BSS®: Sodium chloride 0.64%, potassium chloride 0.075%, calcium chloride 0.048%, magnesium chloride 0.03%, sodium acetate 0.39%, sodium citrate 0.17% (15 mL, 30 mL, 250 mL, 500 mL)

BSS Plus®: Sodium chloride 0.71%, potassium chloride 0.038%, calcium chloride 0.015%, magnesium chloride 0.02%, sodium phosphate 0.042%, sodium bicarbonate 0.21%, dextrose 0.092%, glutathione 0.018% (250 mL, 500 mL)

Navstel®: Sodium chloride 0.71%, potassium chloride 0.038%, calcium chloride 0.015%, magnesium chloride 0.02%, sodium phosphate 0.042%, sodium bicarbonate 0.21%, dextrose 0.092%, glutathione 0.018%, hypromellose 0.125% to 0.173% (250 mL, 500 mL)

Baldex® ***(Discontinued)***
BAL in Oil® [US] *see* dimercaprol *on page 307*
Balmex® [US-OTC] *see* zinc oxide *on page 1001*
Balminil Decongestant [Can] *see* pseudoephedrine *on page 810*
Balminil DM D [Can] *see* pseudoephedrine and dextromethorphan *on page 812*
Balminil DM + Decongestant + Expectorant [Can] *see* guaifenesin, pseudoephedrine, and dextromethorphan *on page 460*
Balminil DM E [Can] *see* guaifenesin and dextromethorphan *on page 455*
Balminil Expectorant [Can] *see* guaifenesin *on page 454*
Balnetar® [US-OTC/Can] *see* coal tar *on page 242*

balsalazide (bal SAL a zide)

Sound-Alike/Look-Alike Issues

Colazal® may be confused with Clozaril®

Synonyms balsalazide disodium

U.S./Canadian Brand Names Colazal® [US]

Therapeutic Category 5-Aminosalicylic Acid Derivative; Antiinflammatory Agent

Use Treatment of mild-to-moderate active ulcerative colitis

Dosage Summary

Oral:

Children <5 years: Dosage not established

Children ≥5 years: 750 mg 3 times/day for up to 8 weeks **or** 2.25 g 3 times/day for 8 weeks

Adults: 2.25 g 3 times/day for 8-12 weeks

Dosage Forms

Capsule, oral: 750 mg

Colazal®: 750 mg

balsalazide disodium *see* balsalazide *on page 116*
balsam Peru, castor oil, and trypsin *see* trypsin, balsam Peru, and castor oil *on page 964*
Baltussin *(Discontinued)* *see* dihydrocodeine, chlorpheniramine, and phenylephrine *on page 304*
Balziva™ [US] *see* ethinyl estradiol and norethindrone *on page 378*
Band-Aid® Hurt-Free™ Antiseptic Wash [US-OTC] *see* lidocaine (topical) *on page 562*
Banophen™ [US-OTC] *see* diphenhydramine (systemic) *on page 310*
Banophen™ Anti-Itch [US-OTC] *see* diphenhydramine (topical) *on page 311*
Banophen® Decongestant Capsule *(Discontinued)*
Banzel™ [US] *see* rufinamide *on page 856*
Baraclude® [US/Can] *see* entecavir *on page 351*
Barbidonna® *(Discontinued)* *see* hyoscyamine, atropine, scopolamine, and phenobarbital *on page 492*
Barbita® *(Discontinued)* *see* phenobarbital *on page 747*
Barc™ Liquid *(Discontinued)*
Baricon™ *(Discontinued)* *see* barium *on page 117*
Baridium [US-OTC] *see* phenazopyridine *on page 746*

barium (BA ree um)

Synonyms barium sulfate

U.S./Canadian Brand Names Bar-Test™ [US]; Cat-Pak™ [US]; E-Z-Cat® Dry [US]; E-Z-Cat® [US]; E-Z-Disk™ [US]; Entero VU™ 24% [US]; Esopho-Cat® [US]; Liquid Polibar Plus® [US]; Liquid Polibar® [US]; Readi-Cat® 2 [US]; Readi-Cat® [US]; Varibar® Honey [US]; Varibar® Nectar [US]; Varibar® Pudding [US]; Varibar® Thin Honey [US]; VoLumen® [US]

Therapeutic Category Radiopaque Agents

Use Diagnostic aid for computed tomography or x-ray examinations of the GI tract

Dosage Forms

Cream, oral:
Esopho-Cat®: 3% w/w (30 g)

Paste, oral:
Varibar® Pudding: 40% w/v (230 mL)

Powder for suspension, oral:
E-Z Cat® Dry: 2% w/w (23 g)

Suspension, oral:
E-Z-Cat®: 4.9% w/v (255 mL)
Entero VU™ 24%: 24% w/v (600 mL)
Readi-Cat® 2: 2.1% w/v (250 mL, 450 mL)
Varibar® Honey: 40% w/v (250 mL)
Varibar® Nectar: 40% w/v (240 mL)
Varibar® Thin Honey: 40% w/v (250 mL)
VoLumen®: 0.1% w/v (450 mL)

Suspension, oral/rectal:
Liquid Polibar Plus®: 105% w/v (1900 mL)
Liquid Polibar®: 100% w/v (1900 mL)
Readi-Cat®: 1.3% w/v (450 mL, 900 mL, 1900 mL)
Readi-Cat® 2: 2.1% w/v (450 mL, 900 mL, 1900 mL)

Suspension, rectal:
Cat-Pak™: 1.3% w/v (400 mL)

Tablet, oral:
Bar-Test™: 648 mg
E-Z-Disk™: 648 mg

barium sulfate *see* barium *on page 117*
Barobag® *(Discontinued)* *see* barium *on page 117*
Baro-Cat® *(Discontinued)* *see* barium *on page 117*
Barosperse® *(Discontinued)* *see* barium *on page 117*

Bar-Test™ [US] *see* barium *on page 117*
Basaljel® [Can] *see* aluminum hydroxide *on page 58*
base ointment *see* zinc oxide *on page 1001*

basiliximab (ba si LIK si mab)

U.S./Canadian Brand Names Simulect® [US/Can]

Therapeutic Category Immunosuppressant Agent

Use Prophylaxis of acute organ rejection in renal transplantation (in combination with cyclosporine and corticosteroids)

Dosage Summary

I.V.:

Children <35 kg: 10 mg within 2 hours prior to transplant surgery, followed by a second 10 mg dose 4 days after transplantation

Children ≥35 kg: 20 mg within 2 hours prior to transplant surgery, followed by a second 20 mg dose 4 days after transplantation

Adults: 20 mg within 2 hours prior to transplant surgery, followed by a second 20 mg dose 4 days after transplantation

Dosage Forms

Injection, powder for reconstitution [preservative free]:
Simulect®: 10 mg, 20 mg

BAY 43-9006 *see* sorafenib *on page 892*
BAY 59-7939 *see* rivaroxaban *(Canada only) on page 848*
Baycadron™ [US] *see* dexamethasone (systemic) *on page 281*
Bayer® Aspirin Extra Strength [US-OTC] *see* aspirin *on page 100*
Bayer® Aspirin Regimen Adult Low Strength [US-OTC] *see* aspirin *on page 100*
Bayer® Aspirin Regimen Children's [US-OTC] *see* aspirin *on page 100*
Bayer® Aspirin Regimen Regular Strength [US-OTC] *see* aspirin *on page 100*
Bayer® Genuine Aspirin [US-OTC] *see* aspirin *on page 100*
Bayer® Plus Extra Strength [US-OTC] *see* aspirin *on page 100*
Bayer® PM [US-OTC] *see* aspirin and diphenhydramine *on page 101*
Bayer® with Heart Advantage *(Discontinued)* *see* aspirin *on page 100*
Bayer® Women's Aspirin Plus Calcium *(Discontinued)* *see* aspirin *on page 100*
Bayer® Women's Low Dose Aspirin [US-OTC] *see* aspirin *on page 100*
BayGam® [Can] *see* immune globulin (intramuscular) *on page 501*
BayGam® *(Discontinued)* *see* immune globulin (intramuscular) *on page 501*
BayHepB® *(Discontinued)* *see* hepatitis B immune globulin (human) *on page 469*
BayRab® *(Discontinued)* *see* rabies immune globulin (human) *on page 824*
BayRho-D® Full Dose *(Discontinued)* *see* Rh_o(D) immune globulin *on page 838*
BayRho-D® Mini Dose *(Discontinued)* *see* Rh_o(D) immune globulin *on page 838*
BayTet™ *(Discontinued)* *see* tetanus immune globulin (human) *on page 920*
Baza® Antifungal [US-OTC] *see* miconazole (topical) *on page 630*
Baza® Clear [US-OTC] *see* vitamin A and vitamin D *on page 988*
B-Caro-T™ [US-OTC] *see* beta-carotene *on page 132*

BCG (bee see jee)

Sound-Alike/Look-Alike Issues

BCG (intravesical) may be confused with BCG for immunization

Synonyms bacillus calmette-Guérin (BCG) live; BCG vaccine U.S.P. *(percutaneous use product)*; BCG, live

U.S./Canadian Brand Names BCG Vaccine [US]; ImmuCyst® [Can]; Oncotice™ [Can]; Pacis™ [Can]; TheraCys® [US]; TICE® BCG [US]

Therapeutic Category Biological Response Modulator

Use

BCG intravesical: Treatment and prophylaxis of carcinoma *in situ* of the bladder; prophylaxis of primary or recurrent superficial papillary tumors following transurethral resection

BCG vaccine: Immunization against *Mycobacterium tuberculosis* in persons not previously infected and who are at high risk for exposure

BCG vaccine is not routinely administered for the prevention of *M. tuberculosis* in the United States. The Advisory Committee on Immunization Practices (ACIP) recommends vaccination be considered for the following:

- Children with a negative tuberculin skin test who are continually exposed to (and cannot be separated from) adults who are untreated or ineffectively treated for TB disease when the child cannot be given long-term treatment for infection **or** if the adult has TB caused by strains resistant to isoniazid and rifampin.
- Healthcare workers with a high percentage of patients with *M. tuberculosis* strains resistant to both isoniazid and rifampin, if there is ongoing transmission of the resistant strains and subsequent infection is likely, or if comprehensive infection-control precautions have not been successful. In addition, healthcare workers should be counseled on the risks and benefits of vaccination and treatment of latent TB infection

Dosage Summary

Percutaneous: Note: Initial lesion usually appears after 10-14 days consisting of small, red papule at injection site and reaches maximum diameter of 3 mm in 4-6 weeks.

Children <1 month: 0.2-0.3 mL (half-strength dilution); administer tuberculin test (5 TU) after 2-3 months; repeat vaccination after 1 year of age for negative tuberculin test if indications persist

Children >1 month: 0.2-0.3 mL (full strength dilution); conduct postvaccinal tuberculin test (5 TU of PPD) in 2-3 months; if test is negative, repeat vaccination

Adults: 0.2-0.3 mL (full strength dilution); conduct postvaccinal tuberculin test (5 TU of PPD) in 2-3 months; if test is negative, repeat vaccination

Intravesicular:

Children: Dosage not established

Adults:

TheraCys®: One dose instilled into bladder (for 2 hours) once weekly for 6 weeks followed by 1 treatment at 3, 6, 12, 18, and 24 months after initial treatment

TICE® BCG: One dose instilled into the bladder (for 2 hours) once weekly for 6 weeks (may repeat cycle 1 time), followed by once monthly for 6-12 months

Dosage Forms

Injection, powder for reconstitution, intravesical [preservative free]:

TheraCys®: 81 mg

TICE® BCG: 50 mg

Injection, powder for reconstitution, percutaneous [preservative free]:

BCG Vaccine: 50 mg

BCG, live *see* BCG *on page 118*

BCG Vaccine [US] *see* BCG *on page 118*

BCG vaccine U.S.P. *(percutaneous use product)* *see* BCG *on page 118*

BCNU *see* carmustine *on page 186*

B complex combinations *see* vitamin B complex combinations *on page 988*

BCX-1812 *see* peramivir *on page 743*

BD™ Glucose [US-OTC] *see* dextrose *on page 290*

beano® [US-OTC] *see* alpha-galactosidase *on page 54*

Bebulin® VH [US] *see* factor IX complex (human) *on page 389*

becaplermin (be KAP ler min)

Sound-Alike/Look-Alike Issues

Regranex® may be confused with Granulex®, Repronex®

Synonyms recombinant human platelet-derived growth factor B; rPDGF-BB

U.S./Canadian Brand Names Regranex® [US/Can]

Therapeutic Category Topical Skin Product

Use Adjunctive treatment of diabetic neuropathic ulcers occurring on the lower limbs and feet that extend into subcutaneous tissue (or beyond) and have adequate blood supply

Dosage Summary

Topical:

Children: Dosage not established

Adults: Apply once daily; to determine the length of gel to apply to the ulcer, measure the greatest length of the ulcer by the greatest width of the ulcer. Tube size and unit of measure will determine the formula used in the calculation. Recalculate amount of gel needed every 1-2 weeks, depending on the rate of change in ulcer area.

Centimeters: 15 g tube: [ulcer length (cm) x width (cm)] divided by 4 = length of gel (cm); 2 g tube: [ulcer length (cm) x width (cm)] divided by 2 = length of gel (cm)

Inches: 15 g tube: [length (in) x width (in)] x 0.6 = length of gel (in); 2 g tube: [length (in) x width (in)] x 1.3 = length of gel (in)

Dosage Forms

Gel, topical:

Regranex®: 0.01% (2 g, 15 g)

beclomethasone (oral inhalation) (be kloe METH a sone)

Sound-Alike/Look-Alike Issues

Vanceril® may be confused with Vancenase®

Synonyms Vancenase

U.S./Canadian Brand Names QVAR® [US/Can]; Vanceril® AEM [Can]

Therapeutic Category Corticosteroid, Inhalant (Oral)

Use Oral inhalation: Maintenance and prophylactic treatment of asthma; includes those who require corticosteroids and those who may benefit from a dose reduction/elimination of systemically-administered corticosteroids. Not for relief of acute bronchospasm.

Dosage Summary

Inhalation:

Children <5 years: Dosage not established

Children 5-11 years: Initial: 40 mcg twice daily; Low dose: 80-160 mcg/day in 2 divided doses; Medium dose: >160-320 mcg/day in 2 divided doses; High dose: >320 mcg/day in 2 divided doses

Children ≥12 years: Initial: 40-160 mcg twice daily; Low dose: 80-240 mcg/day in 2 divided doses; Medium dose: >240-480 mcg/day in 2 divided doses; High dose: >480 mcg/day in 2 divided doses

Adults: Initial: 40-160 mcg twice daily; Low dose: 80-240 mcg/day in 2 divided doses; Medium dose: >240-480 mcg/day in 2 divided doses; High dose: >480 mcg/day in 2 divided doses

Dosage Forms

Aerosol, for oral inhalation:

QVAR®: 40 mcg/inhalation (7.3 g); 80 mcg/inhalation (7.3 g)

beclomethasone (nasal) (be kloe METH a sone)

Synonyms beclomethasone dipropionate

U.S./Canadian Brand Names Apo-Beclomethasone® [Can]; Beconase AQ® [US]; Gen-Beclo [Can]; Nu-Beclomethasone [Can]; Rivanase AQ [Can]

Therapeutic Category Corticosteroid, Nasal

Use Symptomatic treatment of seasonal or perennial rhinitis; prevent recurrence of nasal polyps following surgery.

Dosage Summary

Intranasal:

Children <6 years: Dosage not established

Children ≥6 years: 1-2 inhalations each nostril twice daily (maximum: 336 mcg/day)

Adults: 1-2 inhalations each nostril twice daily (maximum: 336 mcg/day)

Dosage Forms

Suspension, intranasal:

Beconase AQ®: 42 mcg/inhalation (25 g)

beclomethasone dipropionate *see* beclomethasone (nasal) *on page* 120

Beclovent® ***(Discontinued)*** *see* beclomethasone (oral inhalation) *on page* 120

Beconase AQ® [US] *see* beclomethasone (nasal) *on page* 120

Beconase® ***(Discontinued)*** *see* beclomethasone (nasal) *on page* 120

Becotin® Pulvules® ***(Discontinued)***

Beepen-VK® ***(Discontinued)*** *see* penicillin V potassium *on page* 739

BeFlex [US] *see* acetaminophen and phenyltoloxamine *on page* 26
behenyl alcohol *see* docosanol *on page* 321
Belix® Oral *(Discontinued)* *see* diphenhydramine (systemic) *on page* 310
belladonna alkaloids with phenobarbital *see* hyoscyamine, atropine, scopolamine, and phenobarbital *on page* 492

belladonna and opium (bel a DON a & OH pee um)

Sound-Alike/Look-Alike Issues
B&O may be confused with beano®

Synonyms opium and belladonna

Therapeutic Category Analgesic, Narcotic

Controlled Substance C-II

Use Relief of moderate-to-severe pain associated with ureteral spasms not responsive to nonopioid analgesics and to space intervals between injections of opiates

Dosage Summary

Rectal:

Children >12 years: 1 suppository 1-2 times/day (maximum: 4 doses/day)
Adults: 1 suppository 1-2 times/day (maximum: 4 doses/day)

Dosage Forms

Suppository: Belladonna extract 16.2 mg and opium 30 mg; belladonna extract 16.2 mg and opium 60 mg

belladonna, phenobarbital, and ergotamine *(Discontinued)*
Bellamine S *(Discontinued)*
Bellatal® *(Discontinued)* *see* hyoscyamine, atropine, scopolamine, and phenobarbital *on page* 492
Bellergal-S® *(Discontinued)*
Bel-Tabs *(Discontinued)*
Benadryl® [Can] *see* diphenhydramine (systemic) *on page* 310
Benadryl-D® Allergy & Sinus [US-OTC] *see* diphenhydramine and phenylephrine *on page* 312
Benadryl-D® Children's Allergy & Sinus [US-OTC] *see* diphenhydramine and phenylephrine *on page* 312
Benadryl® Allergy [US-OTC] *see* diphenhydramine (systemic) *on page* 310
Benadryl® Allergy and Cold [US-OTC] *see* acetaminophen, diphenhydramine, and phenylephrine *on page* 30
Benadryl® Allergy and Sinus Headache [US-OTC] *see* acetaminophen, diphenhydramine, and phenylephrine *on page* 30
Benadryl® Allergy Quick Dissolve [US-OTC] *see* diphenhydramine (systemic) *on page* 310
Benadryl® Children's Allergy [US-OTC] *see* diphenhydramine (systemic) *on page* 310
Benadryl® Children's Allergy Fastmelt® [US-OTC] *see* diphenhydramine (systemic) *on page* 310
Benadryl® Children's Allergy Perfect Measure™ [US-OTC] *see* diphenhydramine (systemic) *on page* 310
Benadryl® Children's Allergy Quick Dissolve *(Discontinued)* *see* diphenhydramine (systemic) *on page* 310
Benadryl® Children's Dye Free Allergy [US-OTC] *see* diphenhydramine (systemic) *on page* 310
Benadryl® Cream [Can] *see* diphenhydramine (topical) *on page* 311
Benadryl® Dye-Free Allergy [US-OTC] *see* diphenhydramine (systemic) *on page* 310
Benadryl® Extra Strength Itch Stopping [US-OTC] *see* diphenhydramine (topical) *on page* 311
Benadryl® Itch Relief Extra Strength [US-OTC] *see* diphenhydramine (topical) *on page* 311
Benadryl® Itch Relief Stick [Can] *see* diphenhydramine (topical) *on page* 311
Benadryl® Itch Stopping [US-OTC] *see* diphenhydramine (topical) *on page* 311
Benadryl® Itch Stopping Extra Strength [US-OTC] *see* diphenhydramine (topical) *on page* 311
Benadryl® Spray [Can] *see* diphenhydramine (topical) *on page* 311
Benadry® Maximum Strength Severe Allergy and Sinus Headache [US-OTC] *see* acetaminophen, diphenhydramine, and phenylephrine *on page* 30
Ben-Allergin-50® Injection *(Discontinued)* *see* diphenhydramine (systemic) *on page* 310
Ben-Aqua® *(Discontinued)* *see* benzoyl peroxide *on page* 128

benazepril (ben AY ze pril)

Sound-Alike/Look-Alike Issues

benazepril may be confused with Benadryl®

Lotensin® may be confused with Lioresal®, lovastatin

Synonyms benazepril hydrochloride

U.S./Canadian Brand Names Apo-Benazepril® [Can]; Lotensin® [US/Can]

Therapeutic Category Angiotensin-Converting Enzyme (ACE) Inhibitor

Use Treatment of hypertension, either alone or in combination with other antihypertensive agents

Dosage Summary

Oral:

Children <6 years: Dosage not established

Children ≥6 years: Initial: 0.2 mg/kg/day (up to 10 mg/day); Maintenance: 0.1-0.6 mg/kg/day (maximum: 40 mg/day)

Adults: Initial: 5-10 mg/day; Maintenance: 20-80 mg/day in 1-2 divided doses

Dosage Forms

Tablet, oral: 5 mg, 10 mg, 20 mg, 40 mg

Lotensin®: 5 mg, 10 mg, 20 mg, 40 mg

benazepril and hydrochlorothiazide (ben AY ze pril & hye droe klor oh THYE a zide)

Synonyms benazepril hydrochloride and hydrochlorothiazide; hydrochlorothiazide and benazepril

U.S./Canadian Brand Names Lotensin HCT® [US]

Therapeutic Category Antihypertensive Agent, Combination

Use Treatment of hypertension

Dosage Summary

Oral:

Children: Dosage not established

Adults: Benazepril 5-20 mg and hydrochlorothiazide 6.25-25 mg daily

Dosage Forms

Tablet:

Generics:

5/6.25: Benazepril 5 mg and hydrochlorothiazide 6.25 mg

10/12.5: Benazepril 10 mg and hydrochlorothiazide 12.5 mg

20/12.5: Benazepril 20 mg and hydrochlorothiazide 12.5 mg

20/25: Benazepril 20 mg and hydrochlorothiazide 25 mg

Brands:

Lotensin HCT® 5/6.25: Benazepril 5 mg and hydrochlorothiazide 6.25 mg

Lotensin HCT® 10/12.5: Benazepril 10 mg and hydrochlorothiazide 12.5 mg

Lotensin HCT® 20/12.5: Benazepril 20 mg and hydrochlorothiazide 12.5 mg

Lotensin HCT® 20/25: Benazepril 20 mg and hydrochlorothiazide 25 mg

benazepril hydrochloride *see* benazepril *on page 122*

benazepril hydrochloride and amlodipine besylate *see* amlodipine and benazepril *on page 69*

benazepril hydrochloride and hydrochlorothiazide *see* benazepril and hydrochlorothiazide *on page 122*

bendamustine (ben da MUS teen)

Sound-Alike/Look-Alike Issues

bendamustine may be confused with carmustine, lomustine

Synonyms bendamustine hydrochloride; cytostasan; SDX-105

U.S./Canadian Brand Names Treanda® [US]

Therapeutic Category Antineoplastic Agent, Alkylating Agent

Use Treatment of chronic lymphocytic leukemia (CLL); treatment of progressed indolent B-cell non-Hodgkin lymphoma (NHL)

Dosage Summary

I.V.:

Children: Dosage not established

Adults: 100 mg/m^2 on days 1 and 2 of a 28-day treatment cycle for up to 6 cycles **or** 120 mg/m^2 on days 1 and 2 of a 21-day treatment cycle for up to 8 cycles

Dosage Forms

Injection, powder for reconstitution:

Treanda®: 25 mg, 100 mg

bendamustine hydrochloride *see* bendamustine *on page 122*

bendroflumethiazide and nadolol *see* nadolol and bendroflumethiazide *on page 654*

BeneFix® [US/Can] *see* factor IX *on page 389*

Benemid® *(Discontinued)* *see* probenecid *on page 795*

benflumetol and artemether *see* artemether and lumefantrine *on page 95*

BenGay® [US-OTC] *see* methyl salicylate and menthol *on page 623*

Benicar® [US] *see* olmesartan *on page 698*

Benicar HCT® [US] *see* olmesartan and hydrochlorothiazide *on page 698*

Benoquin® *(Discontinued)* *see* monobenzone *on page 643*

Benoxyl® [Can] *see* benzoyl peroxide *on page 128*

benserazide and levodopa *(Canada only)* (ben SER a zide & lee voe DOE pa)

Synonyms levodopa and benserazide

U.S./Canadian Brand Names Prolopa® [Can]

Therapeutic Category Anti-Parkinson Agent (Dopamine Agonist)

Use Treatment of Parkinson disease (except drug-induced parkinsonism)

Dosage Summary

Oral:

Children: Dosage not established

Adults: Initial: Levodopa 100 mg/benserazide 25 mg 1-2 times/day; Maintenance: Levodopa 400-800 mg/benserazide 100-200 mg daily in 4-6 divided doses (maximum: Levodopa/benserazide 1200/300 mg/day); **Note:** Titration is recommended

Dosage Forms - Canada

Capsule:

Prolopa®: 50-12.5: Levodopa 50 mg and benserazide 12.5 mg; 100-25: Levodopa 100 mg and benserazide 25 mg; 200-50: Levodopa 200 mg and benserazide 50 mg

Ben-Tann *(Discontinued)* *see* diphenhydramine (systemic) *on page 310*

bentoquatam (BEN toe kwa tam)

Synonyms quaternium-18 bentonite

U.S./Canadian Brand Names Ivy Block® [US-OTC]

Therapeutic Category Protectant, Topical

Use Skin protectant for the prevention of allergic contact dermatitis to poison oak, ivy, and sumac

Dosage Summary

Topical:

Children ≤6 years: Dosage not established

Children >6 years: Apply to skin 15 minutes prior to potential exposure to poison ivy, poison oak, or poison sumac, and reapply every 4 hours

Adults: Apply to skin 15 minutes prior to potential exposure to poison ivy, poison oak, or poison sumac, and reapply every 4 hours

Dosage Forms

Lotion, topical:

Ivy Block® [OTC]: 5% (120 mL)

Bentyl® [US] *see* dicyclomine *on page 299*

Bentyl® Injection *(Discontinued)* *see* dicyclomine *on page 299*

Bentylol® [Can] *see* dicyclomine *on page 299*

Benuryl™ [Can] *see* probenecid *on page 795*

Benylin® 3.3 mg-D-E [Can] *see* guaifenesin, pseudoephedrine, and codeine *on page 459*

Benylin® D for Infants [Can] *see* pseudoephedrine *on page 810*

Benylin® Adult *(Discontinued)* *see* dextromethorphan *on page 287*

Benylin® Cough Syrup *(Discontinued)* *see* diphenhydramine (systemic) *on page 310*

Benylin® DM-D [Can] *see* pseudoephedrine and dextromethorphan *on page 812*

Benylin® DM-D-E [Can] *see* guaifenesin, pseudoephedrine, and dextromethorphan *on page 460*

Benylin® DM ***(Discontinued)*** *see* dextromethorphan *on page 287*
Benylin® DM-E [Can] *see* guaifenesin and dextromethorphan *on page 455*
Benylin® E Extra Strength [Can] *see* guaifenesin *on page 454*
Benylin® Expectorant ***(Discontinued)*** *see* guaifenesin and dextromethorphan *on page 455*
Benylin® Pediatric ***(Discontinued)*** *see* dextromethorphan *on page 287*
Benzac® AC [US/Can] *see* benzoyl peroxide *on page 128*
Benzac® AC Gel ***(Discontinued)*** *see* benzoyl peroxide *on page 128*
BenzaClin® [US/Can] *see* clindamycin and benzoyl peroxide *on page 233*
Benzac® W [US] *see* benzoyl peroxide *on page 128*
Benzac W® Gel [Can] *see* benzoyl peroxide *on page 128*
Benzac W® Wash [Can] *see* benzoyl peroxide *on page 128*
5 Benzagel® [US] *see* benzoyl peroxide *on page 128*
10 Benzagel® [US] *see* benzoyl peroxide *on page 128*
Benzagel® Wash ***(Discontinued)*** *see* benzoyl peroxide *on page 128*

benzalkonium chloride (benz al KOE nee um KLOR ide)

Synonyms BAC

U.S./Canadian Brand Names HandClens® [US-OTC]; Pedi-Pro® [US]; Pronto® Plus Lice Egg Remover Kit [US-OTC]

Therapeutic Category Antibacterial, Topical

Use Antiseptic of skin, mucous membranes, and wounds; surface antiseptic; germicidal preservative

Dosage Summary

Topical antiseptic:

Skin, mucous membranes, or wounds: Apply topically; may require dilution based on standard solution concentration recommendations depending on usage and application site

Dosage Forms

Lotion, topical [foam]:
HandClens® [OTC]: 0.13% (50 mL, 240 mL, 1800 mL)
Lotion, topical [spray]:
HandClens® [OTC]: 0.13% (15 mL)
Powder, topical:
Pedi-Pro®: 1% (60 g)
Solution, topical:
Pronto® Plus Lice Egg Remover Kit [OTC]: 0.1% (60 mL)

Benzamycin® [US] *see* erythromycin and benzoyl peroxide *on page 363*
Benzamycin® Pak [US] *see* erythromycin and benzoyl peroxide *on page 363*
BenzaShave® [US] *see* benzoyl peroxide *on page 128*
benzathine benzylpenicillin *see* penicillin G benzathine *on page 737*
benzathine penicillin G *see* penicillin G benzathine *on page 737*
Benzedrex® [US-OTC] *see* propylhexedrine *on page 807*
BenzEFoam™ [US] *see* benzoyl peroxide *on page 128*
benzene hexachloride *see* lindane *on page 567*
benzhexol hydrochloride *see* trihexyphenidyl *on page 958*
Benziq™ [US] *see* benzoyl peroxide *on page 128*
Benziq™ LS [US] *see* benzoyl peroxide *on page 128*
benzmethyzin *see* procarbazine *on page 797*

benzocaine (BEN zoe kane)

Sound-Alike/Look-Alike Issues

Orabase® may be confused with Orinase®

Synonyms ethyl aminobenzoate

U.S./Canadian Brand Names Americaine® Hemorrhoidal [US-OTC]; Anbesol® Baby [US-OTC/Can]; Anbesol® Cold Sore Therapy [US-OTC]; Anbesol® Jr. [US-OTC]; Anbesol® Maximum Strength [US-OTC]; Anbesol® [US-OTC]; Benzodent® [US-OTC]; Bi-Zets [US-OTC]; Boil-Ease® Pain Relieving [US-OTC]; Cepacol® Fizzlers™ [US-OTC]; Cepacol® Sore Throat Pain Relief [US-OTC]; Cepacol® Sore Throat Plus Coating Relief [US-OTC]; Chiggerex® Plus [US-OTC]; ChiggerTox® [US-OTC]; Dent's Extra

Strength Toothache Gum [US-OTC]; Dentapaine [US-OTC]; Dermoplast® Antibacterial [US-OTC]; Dermoplast® Pain Relieving [US-OTC]; Detane® [US-OTC]; Foille® [US-OTC]; HDA® Toothache [US-OTC]; Hurricaine® [US-OTC]; Ivy-Rid® [US-OTC]; Kank-A® Soft Brush [US-OTC]; Lanacane® Maximum Strength [US-OTC]; Lanacane® [US-OTC]; Little Teethers® [US-OTC]; Medicone® Hemorrhoidal [US-OTC]; Mycinettes® [US-OTC]; Orabase® with Benzocaine [US-OTC]; Orajel® Baby Daytime and Nighttime [US-OTC]; Orajel® Baby Teething Nighttime [US-OTC]; Orajel® Baby Teething [US-OTC]; Orajel® Cold Sore [US-OTC]; Orajel® Denture Plus [US-OTC]; Orajel® Maximum Strength [US-OTC]; Orajel® Medicated Mouth Sore [US-OTC]; Orajel® Medicated Toothache [US-OTC]; Orajel® Mouth Sore [US-OTC]; Orajel® Multi-Action Cold Sore [US-OTC]; Orajel® PM Maximum Strength [US-OTC]; Orajel® Ultra Mouth Sore [US-OTC]; Outgro® [US-OTC]; Red Cross™ Canker Sore [US-OTC]; Rid-A-Pain Dental [US-OTC]; Sepasoothe® [US-OTC]; Skeeter Stik® [US-OTC]; Sore Throat Relief [US-OTC]; Sting-Kill® [US-OTC]; Tanac® [US-OTC]; Thorets [US-OTC]; Trocaine® [US-OTC]; Zilactin Baby® [Can]; Zilactin® Tooth & Gum Pain [US-OTC]; Zilactin®-B [US-OTC/Can]

Therapeutic Category Local Anesthetic

Use Temporary relief of pain associated with pruritic dermatosis, pruritus, minor burns, acute congestive, bee stings, and insect bites; mouth and gum irritations (toothache, minor sore throat pain, canker sores, dentures, orthodontia, teething, mucositis, stomatitis); sunburn; hemorrhoids; anesthetic lubricant for passage of catheters and endoscopic tubes

Dosage Summary

Oral:

Children <5 years: Dosage not established

Children ≥5 years: Allow 1 lozenge (10-15 mg) to dissolve slowly in mouth; may repeat every 2 hours as needed

Adults: Allow 1 lozenge (10-15 mg) to dissolve slowly in mouth; may repeat every 2 hours as needed

Rectal:

Children <12 years: Dosage not established

Children ≥12 years: Apply externally to affected area up to 6 times daily

Adults: Apply externally to affected area up to 6 times daily

Topical:

Children <2 years: Dosage not established

Children ≥2 years: Apply to affected area 3-4 times a day as needed

Adults: Apply to affected area 3-4 times a day as needed

Topical (oral):

Children <4 months: Dosage not established

Children ≥4 months: Apply to affected gum area up to 4 times daily

Adults: Apply thin layer to affected area up to 4 times daily

Dosage Forms

Aerosol, oral:

Hurricaine® [OTC]: 20% (60 mL)

Aerosol, topical: 20% (59.7 g)

Dermoplast® Antibacterial [OTC]: 20% (82.5 mL)

Dermoplast® Pain Relieving [OTC]: 20% (60 mL, 82.5 mL)

Ivy-Rid® [OTC]: 2% (85 g)

Lanacane® Maximum Strength [OTC]: 20% (120 mL)

Combination package, oral:

Orajel® Baby Daytime and Nighttime [OTC]: gel, oral (Daytime Regular formula): benzocaine 7.5% (5.3 g) [1 tube] and gel, oral (Nighttime formula): benzocaine 10% (5.3 g) [1 tube]

Cream, oral:

Benzodent® [OTC]: 20% (7.5 g, 30 g)

Orajel® PM Maximum Strength [OTC]: 20% (5.3 g, 7 g)

Cream, topical:

Lanacane® [OTC]: 6% (28 g, 60 g)

Lanacane® Maximum Strength [OTC]: 20% (28 g)

Gel, oral: 20% (15 g)

Anbesol® [OTC]: 10% (7.1 g)

Anbesol® Baby [OTC]: 7.5% (7.1 g)

Anbesol® Jr. [OTC]: 10% (7.1 g)

Anbesol® Maximum Strength [OTC]: 20% (7.1 g, 10 g)

Dentapaine [OTC]: 20% (11 g)

HDA® Toothache [OTC]: 6.5% (15 mL)

Hurricaine® [OTC]: 20% (30 g); 20% (5.25 g, 30 g)

Kank-A® Soft Brush [OTC]: 20% (2 g)

Little Teethers® [OTC]: 7.5% (9.4 g)
Orabase® with Benzocaine [OTC]: 20% (7 g)
Orajel® [OTC]: 10% (5.3 g, 7 g, 9.4 g)
Orajel® Baby Teething [OTC]: 7.5% (11.9 g); 7.5% (9.4 g)
Orajel® Baby Teething Nighttime [OTC]: 10% (5.3 g)
Orajel® Denture Plus [OTC]: 15% (9 g)
Orajel® Maximum Strength [OTC]: 20% (5.4 g, 7 g, 9.4 g, 11.9 g)
Orajel® Mouth Sore [OTC]: 20% (5.3 g, 9.4 g, 11.9 g)
Orajel® Multi-Action Cold Sore [OTC]: 20% (9.4 g)
Orajel® Ultra Mouth Sore [OTC]: 15% (9.4 g)
Zilactin®-B [OTC]: 10% (7.5 g)

Gel, topical:
Detane® [OTC]: 7.5% (15 g)

Liquid, oral: 20% (15 mL)
Anbesol® [OTC]: 10% (9.3 mL)
Anbesol® Maximum Strength [OTC]: 20% (9.3 mL)
Hurricaine® [OTC]: 20% (30 mL)
Orajel® Baby Teething [OTC]: 7.5% (13.3 mL)
Orajel® Maximum Strength [OTC]: 20% (13.5 mL)
Rid-A-Pain Dental [OTC]: 6.3% (30 mL)
Tanac® [OTC]: 10% (13 mL)

Liquid, topical:
ChiggerTox® [OTC]: 2% (30 mL)
Outgro® [OTC]: 20% (9.3 mL)
Skeeter Stik® [OTC]: 5% (14 mL)

Lozenge, oral: 6 mg (18s)
Bi-Zets [OTC]: 15 mg (10s)
Cepacol® Sore Throat Pain Relief [OTC]: 15 mg (16s, 18s)
Cepacol® Sore Throat Plus Coating Relief [OTC]: 15 mg (18s)
Mycinettes® [OTC]: 15 mg (12s)
Sepasoothe® [OTC]: 10 mg (6s, 24s, 100s, 250s, 500s)
Sore Throat Relief [OTC]: 10 mg (100s, 250s, 500s)
Thorets [OTC]: 18 mg (300s)
Trocaine® [OTC]: 10 mg (50s, 300s)

Ointment, oral:
Anbesol® Cold Sore Therapy [OTC]: 20% (7.1 g)
Red Cross™ Canker Sore [OTC]: 20% (7.5 g)

Ointment, rectal:
Americaine® Hemorrhoidal [OTC]: 20% (30 g)
Medicone® Hemorrhoidal [OTC]: 20% (28.4 g)

Ointment, topical:
Boil-Ease® Pain Relieving [OTC]: 20% (30 g)
Chiggerex® Plus [OTC]: 6% (50 g)
Foille® [OTC]: 5% (3.5 g, 14 g, 28 g)

Pad, topical:
Sting-Kill® [OTC]: 20% (8s)

Paste, oral:
Orabase® with Benzocaine [OTC]: 20% (6 g)

Solution, oral:
Hurricaine® [OTC]: 20% (30 mL)

Swab, oral:
Hurricaine® [OTC]: 20% (8s, 72s)
Orajel® Baby Teething [OTC]: 7.5% (12s)
Orajel® Cold Sore [OTC]: 20% (12s)
Orajel® Medicated Mouth Sore [OTC]: 20% (8s, 12s)
Orajel® Medicated Toothache [OTC]: 20% (8s, 12s)
Zilactin® Tooth & Gum Pain [OTC]: 20% (8s)

Swab, topical:
Boil-Ease® Pain Relieving [OTC]: 20% (12s)
Sting-Kill® [OTC]: 20% (5s)

Tablet, orally dissolving, oral:
Cepacol® Fizzlers™ [OTC]: 6 mg (12s)
Wax, oral:
Dent's Extra Strength Toothache Gum [OTC]: 20% (1 g)

benzocaine and antipyrine *see* antipyrine and benzocaine *on page 83*

benzocaine, butamben, and tetracaine (BEN zoe kane, byoo TAM ben, & TET ra kane)

Synonyms benzocaine, butamben, and tetracaine hydrochloride; benzocaine, butyl aminobenzoate, and tetracaine; butamben, tetracaine, and benzocaine; tetracaine, benzocaine, and butamben

U.S./Canadian Brand Names Cetacaine® [US]; Exactacain™ [US]

Therapeutic Category Local Anesthetic

Use Topical anesthetic to control pain in surgical or endoscopic procedures; anesthetic for accessible mucous membranes except for the eyes

Dosage Summary

Topical:
Children: Dosage not established; dose reduction suggested
Adults:
Cetacaine®:
Aerosol: Apply for ≤1 second; use of sprays >2 seconds is contraindicated
Gel: Apply ~1/2 inch (13 mm) x 3/16 inch (5 mm); application of >1 inch (26 cm) x 3/16 inch (5 mm) is contraindicated
Liquid: Apply 6-7 drops (0.2 mL); application of >12-14 drops (0.4 mL) is contraindicated
Exactacain™: 3 metered sprays (use of >6 metered sprays is contraindicated)
Elderly: Dose reduction is suggested

Dosage Forms

Aerosol, topical [spray]:
Cetacaine®: Benzocaine 14%, butamben 2%, and tetracaine 2% (56 g)
Exactacain™: Benzocaine 14%, butamben 2%, and tetracaine 2% (60 g)
Gel, topical:
Cetacaine®: Benzocaine 14%, butamben 2%, and tetracaine 2% (29 g)
Liquid, topical:
Cetacaine®: Benzocaine 14%, butamben 2%, and tetracaine 2% (56 g)

benzocaine, butamben, and tetracaine hydrochloride *see* benzocaine, butamben, and tetracaine *on page 127*

benzocaine, butyl aminobenzoate, and tetracaine *see* benzocaine, butamben, and tetracaine *on page 127*

Benzocol® *(Discontinued)* *see* benzocaine *on page 124*

Benzodent® [US-OTC] *see* benzocaine *on page 124*

benzoic acid, hyoscyamine, methenamine, methylene blue, and phenyl salicylate *see* methenamine, phenyl salicylate, methylene blue, benzoic acid, and hyoscyamine *on page 613*

benzoic acid, methenamine, methylene blue, phenyl salicylate, and hyoscyamine *see* methenamine, phenyl salicylate, methylene blue, benzoic acid, and hyoscyamine *on page 613*

benzoin (BEN zoin)

Synonyms gum benjamin

U.S./Canadian Brand Names Benz-Protect Swabs™ [US-OTC]; Sprayzoin™ [US-OTC]

Therapeutic Category Pharmaceutical Aid; Protectant, Topical

Use Protective application for irritations of the skin; sometimes used in boiling water as steam inhalants for its expectorant and soothing action

Dosage Summary

Topical:
Children: Apply 1-2 times/day
Adults: Apply 1-2 times/day

Dosage Forms

Tincture, topical: Benzoin Compound USP: Benzoin 10% (30 mL, 59 mL, 60 mL, 120 mL, 473 mL); Benzoin NFXI (59 mL)
Benz-Protect Swabs™: Benzoin Compound USP: Benzoin 10% (3 mL)
Tincture, topical [spray]:
Sprayzoin™: Benzoin Compound USP: Benzoin 10% (120 mL)

benzonatate (ben ZOE na tate)

Synonyms tessalon perles

U.S./Canadian Brand Names Tessalon® [US/Can]; Zonatuss™ [US]

Therapeutic Category Antitussive

Use Symptomatic relief of nonproductive cough

Dosage Summary

Oral:

Children ≤10 years: Dosage not established

Children >10 years: 100 mg 3 times/day **or** every 4 hours (maximum: 600 mg/day)

Adults: 100 mg 3 times/day **or** every 4 hours (maximum: 600 mg/day)

Dosage Forms

Capsule, oral:

Zonatuss™: 150 mg

Capsule, softgel, oral: 100 mg, 200 mg

Tessalon®: 100 mg, 200 mg

benzoyl peroxide (BEN zoe il peer OKS ide)

Sound-Alike/Look-Alike Issues

benzoyl peroxide may be confused with benzyl alcohol

Benoxyl® may be confused with Brevoxyl®, Peroxyl®

Benzac® may be confused with Benza®

Brevoxyl® may be confused with Benoxyl®

U.S./Canadian Brand Names 10 Benzagel® [US]; 5 Benzagel® [US]; Acetoxyl® [Can]; Acne Clear Maximum Strength [US-OTC]; Benoxyl® [Can]; Benzac W® Wash [Can]; Benzac W® Gel [Can]; Benzac® AC [US/Can]; Benzac® W [US]; BenzaShave® [US]; BenzEFoam™ [US]; Benziq™ LS [US]; Benziq™ [US]; BPO; Brevoxyl®-4 [US]; Brevoxyl®-8 [US]; Clearskin [US-OTC]; Clinac® BPO [US]; Desquam-X® 10 [US-OTC]; Desquam-X® 5 [US-OTC]; Desquam-X® [Can]; Inova™ [US]; Levoclen® Acne Wash Kit [US]; Levoclen™-4 [US]; Levoclen™-8 [US]; Neutrogena® Clear Pore™ [US-OTC]; Neutrogena® On The Spot® Acne Treatment [US-OTC]; Oxyderm™ [Can]; OXY® Chill Factor® [US-OTC]; OXY® [US-OTC]; Pacnex™ [US]; Palmer's® Skin Success Invisible Acne [US-OTC]; PanOxyl® Aqua Gel [US-OTC]; PanOxyl® Bar [US-OTC]; PanOxyl® [Can]; Solugel® [Can]; Triaz® [US]; Zapzyt® [US-OTC]; Zoderm® Hydrating Wash™ [US]; Zoderm® Redi-Pads™ [US]; Zoderm® [US]

Therapeutic Category Acne Products

Use Treatment of mild-to-moderate acne vulgaris and acne rosacea

Dosage Summary

Topical:

Children: Dosage not established

Adolescents: Cleanser: Wash once or twice daily; Topical formulations: Apply sparingly once daily; gradually increase to 2-3 times/day if needed

Adults: Cleanser: Wash once or twice daily; Topical formulations: Apply sparingly once daily; gradually increase to 2-3 times/day if needed

Dosage Forms

Aerosol, topical:

BenzEFoam™: 5.3% (60 g)

Bar, topical:

PanOxyl® Bar [OTC]: 5% (113 g); 10% (113 g)

Zapzyt® [OTC]: 10% (113 g)

Cloth, topical:

Triaz®: 3% (60s); 6% (60s)

Cream, topical:

BenzaShave®: 5% (113.4 g); 10% (113.4 g)

Clearskin [OTC]: 10% (28 g)

Neutrogena® Clear Pore™ [OTC]: 3.5% (125 mL)

Neutrogena® On The Spot® Acne Treatment [OTC]: 2.5% (22.5 g)

ZoDerm®: 4.5% (125 mL); 6.5% (125 mL); 8.5% (125 mL)

Gel, topical: 2.5% (60 g); 3% (170 g, 340 g); 5% (45 g, 60 g, 90 g, 150 g, 240 g); 6% (170 g, 340 g); 9% (170 g, 340 g); 10% (45 g, 60 g, 90 g, 150 g, 240 g)

5 Benzagel®: 5% (45 g)

10 Benzagel®: 10% (45 g)

Acne Clear Maximum Strength [OTC]: 10% (42.5 g)

Benzac® AC: 5% (60 g); 10% (60 g)
Benziq™: 5.25% (50 g)
BPO: 4% (42.5 g); 8% (42.5 g)
Brevoxyl®-4: 4% (42.5 g)
Brevoxyl®-8: 8% (42.5 g)
Clinac® BPO: 7% (45 g)
PanOxyl® Aqua Gel [OTC]: 10% (42.5 g)
Triaz®: 3% (170 g, 340 g); 6% (170 g, 340 g); 9% (170 g, 340 g)
Zapzyt® [OTC]: 10% (30 g)
ZoDerm®: 4.5% (125 mL); 6.5% (125 mL); 8.5% (125 mL)

Liquid, topical: 2.5% (240 mL); 5% (120 mL, 150 mL, 240 mL)
Benzac® AC: 5% (240 mL); 10% (240 mL)
Benzac® W: 5% (240 mL); 10% (240 mL)
Benziq™: 5.25% (175 g)
Desquam-X® 5 [OTC]: 5% (140 mL)
Desquam-X® 10 [OTC]: 10% (150 mL)
OXY® [OTC]: 10% (177 mL)
OXY® Chill Factor® [OTC]: 10% (177 mL)
ZoDerm® Hydrating Wash™: 5.75% (473 mL)

Lotion, topical: 5% (30 mL); 10% (30 mL); 4% (170 g); 5% (227 g); 8% (170 g); 10% (227 g)
OXY® [OTC]: 5% (28 g); 10% (28 g)
Pacnex™: 7% (480 mL)
Palmer's® Skin Success Invisible Acne [OTC]: 10% (30 mL)

Pad, topical: 3% (30s); 4.5% (30s); 6% (30s); 6.5% (30s); 8.5% (30s); 9% (30s)
Inova™: 4% (30s); 8% (30s)
Triaz®: 3% (30s, 60s); 6% (30s, 60s); 9% (30s, 60s)
ZoDerm® Redi-Pads™: 4.5% (30s); 6.5% (30s); 8.5% (30s)

Soap, topical: 4.5% (400 mL); 6.5% (400 mL); 8.5% (400 mL)
ZoDerm®: 4.5% (400 mL); 6.5% (400 mL); 8.5% (400 mL)

Wash, topical: 2.5% (227 g); 5% (113 g, 142 g, 227 g); 10% (142 g, 227 g)
Levoclen® Acne Wash Kit: 4% (1s); 8% (1s)
Levoclen™-4: 4% (170 g)
Levoclen™-8: 8% (170 g)

benzoyl peroxide and adapalene *see* adapalene and benzoyl peroxide *on page* 38
benzoyl peroxide and clindamycin *see* clindamycin and benzoyl peroxide *on page* 233
benzoyl peroxide and erythromycin *see* erythromycin and benzoyl peroxide *on page* 363

benzoyl peroxide and hydrocortisone (BEN zoe il peer OKS ide & hye droe KOR ti sone)

Synonyms hydrocortisone and benzoyl peroxide
U.S./Canadian Brand Names Vanoxide-HC® [US/Can]
Therapeutic Category Acne Products
Use Treatment of acne vulgaris and oily skin
Dosage Summary
Topical:
Children: Dosage not established
Adolescents: Apply thin film 1-3 times/day
Adults: Apply thin film 1-3 times/day
Dosage Forms
Lotion:
Vanoxide-HC®: Benzoyl peroxide 5% and hydrocortisone 0.5% (25 mL)

benzphetamine (benz FET a meen)

Synonyms benzphetamine hydrochloride
U.S./Canadian Brand Names Didrex® [US]
Therapeutic Category Anorexiant
Controlled Substance C-III
Use Short-term (few weeks) adjunct to caloric restriction in exogenous obesity

Dosage Summary

Oral:

Children <12 years: Dosage not established

Children ≥12 years: Initial: 25-50 mg once daily; Maintenance: 25-50 mg 1-3 times/day (maximum: 150 mg/day)

Adults: Initial: 25-50 mg once daily; Maintenance: 25-50 mg 1-3 times/day (maximum: 150 mg/day)

Dosage Forms

Tablet, oral: 50 mg

Didrex®: 50 mg

benzphetamine hydrochloride *see* benzphetamine *on page 129*

Benz-Protect Swabs™ [US-OTC] *see* benzoin *on page 127*

benztropine (BENZ troe peen)

Sound-Alike/Look-Alike Issues

benztropine may be confused with bromocriptine

Synonyms benztropine mesylate

U.S./Canadian Brand Names Apo-Benztropine® [Can]; Cogentin® [US]

Therapeutic Category Anti-Parkinson Agent; Anticholinergic Agent

Use Adjunctive treatment of Parkinson disease; treatment of drug-induced extrapyramidal symptoms (except tardive dyskinesia)

Dosage Summary

I.M.:

Children ≤3 years: Dosage not established.

Children >3 years: 0.02-0.05 mg/kg 1-2 times/day

Adults: 1-4 mg/dose 1-2 times/day

I.V.:

Children ≤3 years: Dosage not established.

Children >3 years: 0.02-0.05 mg/kg 1-2 times/day

Adults: 1-4 mg/dose 1-2 times/day

Oral:

Children ≤3 years: Dosage not established.

Children >3 years: 0.02-0.05 mg/kg 1-2 times/day

Adults: 0.5-8 mg/day in 1-2 divided doses; **Note:** Titration is recommended

Elderly: Initial: 0.5 mg 1-2 times/day (maximum: 4 mg/day); **Note:** Titration is recommended

Dosage Forms

Injection, solution: 1 mg/mL (2 mL)

Cogentin®: 1 mg/mL (2 mL)

Tablet, oral: 0.5 mg, 1 mg, 2 mg

benztropine mesylate *see* benztropine *on page 130*

benzydamine *(Canada only)* (ben ZID a meen)

Synonyms benzydamine hydrochloride

U.S./Canadian Brand Names Apo-Benzydamine® [Can]; Dom-Benzydamine [Can]; Novo-Benzydamine [Can]; PMS-Benzydamine [Can]; ratio-Benzydamine [Can]; Sun-Benz® [Can]; Tantum® [Can]

Therapeutic Category Analgesic, Topical

Use Symptomatic treatment of pain associated with acute pharyngitis; treatment of pain associated with radiation-induced oropharyngeal mucositis

Dosage Summary

Oral rinse:

Children: Dosage not established

Adults: Gargle with 15 mL of undiluted solution every 1 1/2-3 hours until symptoms resolve **or** 3-4 times/day

Dosage Forms

Oral rinse: 0.15% (100 mL, 250 mL) [not available in the U.S.]

benzydamine hydrochloride *see* benzydamine *(Canada only) on page 130*

benzyl alcohol (BEN zill AL koe hol)

Sound-Alike/Look-Alike Issues

benzyl alcohol may be confused with benzoyl peroxide

U.S./Canadian Brand Names Ulesfia™ [US]; Zilactin®-L [US-OTC]

Therapeutic Category Antiparasitic Agent, Topical; Pediculocide

Use

Liquid (Zilactin®-L): Temporary relief of pain from cold sores/fever blisters

Lotion (Ulesfia™): Treatment of head lice infestation

Dosage Summary

Topical:

Liquid:

Children <2 years: Dosage not established

Children ≥2 years: Apply to affected area up to 4 times/day

Adults: Apply to affected area up to 4 times/day

Lotion:

Children <6 months: Dosage not established

Children ≥6 months: 4-48 ounces per application; repeat in 7 days

Adults: 4-48 ounces per application; repeat in 7 days

Dosage Forms

Liquid, topical:

Zilactin®-L [OTC]: 10% (5.9 mL)

Lotion, topical:

Ulesfia™: 5% (240 mL)

benzylpenicillin benzathine *see* penicillin G benzathine *on page 737*

benzylpenicillin potassium *see* penicillin G (parenteral/aqueous) *on page 738*

benzylpenicillin sodium *see* penicillin G (parenteral/aqueous) *on page 738*

benzylpenicilloyl-polylysine *(Discontinued)*

bepotastine (be poe TAS teen)

Synonyms bepotastine besilate

U.S./Canadian Brand Names Bepreve™ [US]

Therapeutic Category Histamine H_1 Antagonist; Histamine H_1 Antagonist, Second Generation; Mast Cell Stabilizer

Use Treatment of itching associated with allergic conjunctivitis

Dosage Summary

Ophthalmic:

Children <2 years: Dosage not established

Children ≥2 years: Instill 1 drop into the affected eye(s) twice daily

Adults: Instill 1 drop into the affected eye(s) twice daily

Dosage Forms

Solution, ophthalmic:

Bepreve™: 1.5% (10 mL)

bepotastine besilate *see* bepotastine *on page 131*

Bepreve™ [US] *see* bepotastine *on page 131*

beractant (ber AKT ant)

Sound-Alike/Look-Alike Issues

Survanta® may be confused with Sufenta®

Synonyms bovine lung surfactant; natural lung surfactant

U.S./Canadian Brand Names Survanta® [US/Can]

Therapeutic Category Lung Surfactant

Use Prevention and treatment of respiratory distress syndrome (RDS) in premature infants

Prophylactic therapy: Body weight <1250 g in infants at risk for developing, or with evidence of, surfactant deficiency (administer within 15 minutes of birth)

Rescue therapy: Treatment of infants with RDS confirmed by x-ray and requiring mechanical ventilation (administer as soon as possible - within 8 hours of age)

Dosage Summary

Intratracheal:

Premature infants: Administer 100 mg phospholipids (4 mL/kg), may repeat if needed, no more frequently than every 6 hours to a maximum of 4 doses

Children: Dosage not established

Adults: Dosage not established

Dosage Forms

Suspension, intratracheal [preservative free]:

Survanta®: Phospholipids 25 mg/mL (4 mL, 8 mL)

Berinert® [US] *see* C1 inhibitor (human) *on page 162*

Berocca® ***(Discontinued)***

Berocca® Plus ***(Discontinued)***

Berubigen® ***(Discontinued)*** *see* cyanocobalamin *on page 257*

besifloxacin (be si FLOX a sin)

Synonyms besifloxacin hydrochloride; BOL-303224-A; SS734

U.S./Canadian Brand Names Besivance™ [US]

Therapeutic Category Antibiotic, Ophthalmic; Antibiotic, Quinolone

Use Treatment of bacterial conjunctivitis

Dosage Summary

Ophthalmic:

Children <1 year: Dosage not established

Children ≥1 year: One drop into affected eye(s) 3 times/day (4-12 hours apart)

Adults: One drop into affected eye(s) 3 times/day (4-12 hours apart)

Dosage Forms

Suspension, ophthalmic:

Besivance™: 0.6% (5 mL)

besifloxacin hydrochloride *see* besifloxacin *on page 132*

Besivance™ [US] *see* besifloxacin *on page 132*

β,β-dimethylcysteine *see* penicillamine *on page 737*

Betacaine® [Can] *see* lidocaine (topical) *on page 562*

beta-carotene (BAY ta KARE oh teen)

U.S./Canadian Brand Names A-Caro-25 [US-OTC]; B-Caro-T™ [US-OTC]; Lumitene™ [US-OTC]

Therapeutic Category Vitamin, Fat Soluble

Dosage Summary

Oral:

Children <14 years: 30-150 mg/day

Adults: 30-300 mg/day

Dosage Forms

Capsule, oral:

Lumitene™ [OTC]: 50,000 int. units

Capsule, softgel, oral: 10,000 int. units, 25,000 int. units

A-Caro-25 [OTC]: 25,000 int. units

B-Caro-T™ [OTC]: 25,000 int. units

Tablet, oral: 10,000 int. units

Betachron® ***(Discontinued)*** *see* propranolol *on page 806*

Betaderm [Can] *see* betamethasone *on page 133*

Betadine® [US] *see* povidone-iodine (ophthalmic) *on page 784*

Betadine® [US-OTC/Can] *see* povidone-iodine (topical) *on page 784*

Betadine® First Aid Antibiotics + Moisturizer ***(Discontinued)*** *see* bacitracin and polymyxin B *on page 113*

Betadine® Swab Aids [US-OTC] *see* povidone-iodine (topical) *on page 784*

9-beta-d-ribofuranosyladenine *see* adenosine *on page 39*

Betagan® [US/Can] *see* levobunolol *on page 556*

Beta-HC® [US-OTC] *see* hydrocortisone (topical) *on page 483*

betahistine *(Canada only)* (bay ta HISS teen)

Synonyms betahistine dihydrochloride

U.S./Canadian Brand Names Novo-Betahistine [Can]; Serc® [Can]

Therapeutic Category Antihistamine

Use Treatment of Ménière disease (to decrease episodes of vertigo)

Dosage Summary

Oral:

Children: Dosage not established

Adults: 8-16 mg 3 times/day

Dosage Forms - Canada

Tablet:

Serc®: 16 mg, 24 mg

betahistine dihydrochloride *see* betahistine *(Canada only) on page 133*

betaine (BAY ta een)

Sound-Alike/Look-Alike Issues

betaine may be confused with Betadine®

Cystadane® may be confused with cysteamine, cysteine

Synonyms betaine anhydrous

U.S./Canadian Brand Names Cystadane® [US/Can]

Therapeutic Category Homocystinuria Agent

Use Treatment of homocystinuria (eg, deficiencies or defects in cystathionine beta-synthase [CBS], 5,10-methylene tetrahydrofolate reductase [MTHFR], and cobalamin cofactor metabolism [CBL])

Dosage Summary

Oral:

Children <3 years: Initial: 100 mg/kg/day, then increase weekly by 50 mg/kg increments, as needed

Children ≥3 years: 3 g twice daily; maximum of up to 20 g/day has been necessary to control homocysteine levels in some patients

Adults: 3 g twice daily; maximum of up to 20 g/day has been necessary to control homocysteine levels in some patients

Note: Titration is recommended in all patients, increased gradually until plasma total homocysteine is undetectable or present only in small amounts.

Product Availability Orphan drug; may only be obtained by contacting Accredo Health Group, Inc at 1-888-454-8860.

Dosage Forms

Powder for solution, oral:

Cystadane®: 1 g/scoop (180 g)

betaine anhydrous *see* betaine *on page 133*

Betaject™ [Can] *see* betamethasone *on page 133*

Betalin® S *(Discontinued)* *see* thiamine *on page 927*

Betaloc® [Can] *see* metoprolol *on page 625*

BetaMed™ [US-OTC] *see* pyrithione zinc *on page 819*

betamethasone (bay ta METH a sone)

Sound-Alike/Look-Alike Issues

Luxiq® may be confused with Lasix®

Synonyms betamethasone dipropionate; betamethasone dipropionate, augmented; betamethasone sodium phosphate; betamethasone valerate; flubenisolone

U.S./Canadian Brand Names Beta-Val® [US]; Betaderm [Can]; Betaject™ [Can]; Betnesol® [Can]; Betnovate® [Can]; Celestone® Soluspan® [US/Can]; Celestone® [US]; Diprolene® AF [US]; Diprolene® Glycol [Can]; Diprolene® [US]; Diprosone® [Can]; Ectosone [Can]; Luxíq® [US]; Prevex® B [Can]; Taro-Sone [Can]; Topilene® [Can]; Topisone® [Can]; Valisone® Scalp Lotion [Can]

Therapeutic Category Adrenal Corticosteroid; Corticosteroid, Topical

Use Inflammatory dermatoses such as seborrheic or atopic dermatitis, neurodermatitis, anogenital pruritus, psoriasis, inflammatory phase of xerosis

Dosage Summary

I.M.:

Children ≤12 years: 0.0175-0.125 mg base/kg/day **or** 0.5-7.5 mg base/m^2/day divided every 6-12 hours
Children ≥13 years: 0.6-9 mg/day (generally, 1/3 to 1/2 of oral dose) divided every 12-24 hours
Adults: 0.6-9 mg/day (generally, 1/3 to 1/2 of oral dose) divided every 12-24 hours

Intrabursal, intraarticular, intradermal:

Children: Dosage not established
Adults: 0.25-2 mL

Intralesional:

Children: Dosage not established
Adults: Very large joints: 1-2 mL; Large joints: 1 mL; Medium joints: 0.5-1 mL; Small joints: 0.25-0.5 mL

Oral:

Children ≤12 years: 0.0175-0.25 mg/kg/day **or** 0.5-7.5 mg/m^2/day divided every 6-8 hours
Children ≥13 years: 0.6-7.2 mg/day in 2-4 divided doses
Adults: 0.6-7.2 mg/day in 2-4 divided doses

Topical:

Children ≤12 years: Dosage not established
Children ≥13 years: Apply once or twice daily (maximum: 45-50 g/week; 50 mL/week; 2 weeks total therapy)
Adults: Apply once or twice daily (maximum: 45-50 g/week; 50 mL/week; 2 weeks total therapy)

Dosage Forms

Aerosol, topical:
Luxíq®: 0.12% (50 g, 100 g)

Cream, topical: 0.05% (15 g, 45 g, 50 g); 0.1% (15 g, 45 g)
Beta-Val®: 0.1% (15 g, 45 g)
Diprolene® AF: 0.05% (15 g, 50 g)

Gel, topical: 0.05% (15 g, 50 g)

Injection, suspension: Betamethasone sodium phosphate 3 mg and betamethasone acetate 3 mg per 1 mL (5 mL)
Celestone® Soluspan®: Betamethasone sodium phosphate 3 mg and betamethasone acetate 3 mg per 1 mL (5 mL)

Lotion, topical: 0.05% (30 mL, 60 mL); 0.1% (60 mL)
Beta-Val®: 0.1% (60 mL)
Diprolene®: 0.05% (30 mL, 60 mL)

Ointment, topical: 0.05% (15 g, 45 g, 50 g); 0.1% (15 g, 45 g)
Diprolene®: 0.05% (15 g, 50 g)

Solution, oral:
Celestone®: 0.6 mg/5 mL (118 mL)

betamethasone and clotrimazole (bay ta METH a sone & kloe TRIM a zole)

Sound-Alike/Look-Alike Issues
clotrimazole may be confused with co-trimoxazole
Lotrisone® may be confused with Lotrimin®

Synonyms clotrimazole and betamethasone

U.S./Canadian Brand Names Lotriderm® [Can]; Lotrisone® [US]

Therapeutic Category Antifungal/Corticosteroid

Use Topical treatment of various dermal fungal infections (including tinea pedis, cruris, and corpora in patients ≥17 years of age)

Dosage Summary

Topical:

Children <17 years: Dosage not established.
Adults: Apply to affected area twice daily (maximum: 45 g cream/week; 45 mL lotion/week)

Dosage Forms

Cream: Betamethasone 0.05% and clotrimazole 1% (15 g, 45 g)
Lotrisone®: Betamethasone 0.05% and clotrimazole 1% (15 g, 45 g)

Lotion: Betamethasone 0.05% and clotrimazole 1% (30 mL)
Lotrisone®: Betamethasone 0.05% and clotrimazole 1% (30 mL)

betamethasone dipropionate *see* betamethasone *on page 133*

betamethasone dipropionate and calcipotriene hydrate *see* calcipotriene and betamethasone *on page 164*

betamethasone dipropionate, augmented *see* betamethasone *on page* 133
betamethasone sodium phosphate *see* betamethasone *on page* 133
betamethasone valerate *see* betamethasone *on page* 133
Betapace® [US] *see* sotalol *on page* 892
Betapace AF® [US] *see* sotalol *on page* 892
Beta Sal® [US-OTC] *see* salicylic acid *on page* 858
Betasept® [US-OTC] *see* chlorhexidine gluconate *on page* 204
Betaseron® [US/Can] *see* interferon beta-1b *on page* 516
Betatar® Gel [US-OTC] *see* coal tar *on page* 242
Beta-Val® [US] *see* betamethasone *on page* 133
Betaxin® [Can] *see* thiamine *on page* 927

betaxolol (systemic) (be TAKS oh lol)

Sound-Alike/Look-Alike Issues
betaxolol may be confused with bethanechol, labetalol

Synonyms betaxolol hydrochloride

U.S./Canadian Brand Names Kerlone® [US]; Sandoz-Betaxolol [Can]

Therapeutic Category Beta Blocker, Beta-1 Selective

Use Management of hypertension

Dosage Summary

Oral:
Children: Dosage not established
Adults: 5-20 mg/day
Elderly: Initial dose: 5 mg/day; Range: 5-20 mg/day

Dosage Forms

Tablet, oral: 10 mg, 20 mg
Kerlone®: 10 mg, 20 mg

betaxolol (ophthalmic) (be TAKS oh lol)

Sound-Alike/Look-Alike Issues
Betoptic® S may be confused with Betagan®, Timoptic®

Synonyms betaxolol hydrochloride

U.S./Canadian Brand Names Betoptic S® [US/Can]

Therapeutic Category Ophthalmic Agent, Antiglaucoma

Use Treatment of chronic open-angle glaucoma or ocular hypertension

Dosage Summary

Ophthalmic:
Children:
Solution: Dosage not established
Suspension: Instill 1 drop twice daily
Adults:
Solution: Instill 1-2 drops twice daily
Suspension: Instill 1 drop twice daily

Dosage Forms

Solution, ophthalmic: 0.5% (5 mL, 10 mL, 15 mL)
Suspension, ophthalmic:
Betoptic S®: 0.25% (10 mL, 15 mL)

betaxolol hydrochloride *see* betaxolol (ophthalmic) *on page* 135
betaxolol hydrochloride *see* betaxolol (systemic) *on page* 135

bethanechol (be THAN e kole)

Sound-Alike/Look-Alike Issues
bethanechol may be confused with betaxolol

Synonyms bethanechol chloride

U.S./Canadian Brand Names Duvoid® [Can]; PMS-Bethanechol [Can]; Urecholine® [US]

Therapeutic Category Cholinergic Agent

Use Treatment of acute postoperative and postpartum nonobstructive (functional) urinary retention; treatment of neurogenic atony of the urinary bladder with retention

Dosage Summary

Oral:

Adults: 10-100 mg 2-4 times/day; **Note:** Titration is recommended

Dosage Forms

Tablet, oral: 5 mg, 10 mg, 25 mg, 50 mg

Urecholine®: 5 mg, 10 mg, 25 mg, 50 mg

Dosage Forms - Canada

Tablet:

Duvoid®: 10 mg, 25 mg, 50 mg

bethanechol chloride *see* bethanechol *on page* 135

Betimol® [US] *see* timolol (ophthalmic) *on page* 933

Betnesol® [Can] *see* betamethasone *on page* 133

Betnovate® [Can] *see* betamethasone *on page* 133

Betoptic S® [US/Can] *see* betaxolol (ophthalmic) *on page* 135

bevacizumab (be vuh SIZ uh mab)

Sound-Alike/Look-Alike Issues

bevacizumab may be confused with cetuximab, riTUXimab

Avastin® may be confused with Astelin®

Synonyms anti-VEGF monoclonal antibody; anti-VEGF rhuMAb; rhuMAb-VEGF

U.S./Canadian Brand Names Avastin® [US/Can]

Therapeutic Category Antineoplastic Agent, Monoclonal Antibody; Vaccine, Recombinant

Use Treatment of metastatic colorectal cancer; treatment of advanced nonsquamous, nonsmall cell lung cancer; treatment of metastatic HER-2 negative breast cancer (who have not received chemotherapy for metastatic disease); treatment of progressive glioblastoma; treatment of metastatic renal cell cancer (not an approved use in Canada)

Dosage Summary

I.V.:

Children: Dosage not established

Adults: 5 or 10 mg/kg every 2 weeks **or** 15 mg/kg every 3 weeks

Dosage Forms

Injection, solution [preservative free]:

Avastin®: 25 mg/mL (4 mL, 16 mL)

bexarotene (systemic) (beks AIR oh teen)

U.S./Canadian Brand Names Targretin® [US/Can]

Therapeutic Category Antineoplastic Agent, Miscellaneous

Use Treatment of cutaneous manifestations of cutaneous T-cell lymphoma in patients who are refractory to at least one prior systemic therapy

Dosage Summary

Oral:

Children: Dosage not established

Adults: 300-400 mg/m^2 once daily

Dosage Forms

Capsule, oral:

Targretin®: 75 mg

bexarotene (topical) (beks AIR oh teen)

U.S./Canadian Brand Names Targretin® [US/Can]

Therapeutic Category Antineoplastic Agent, Miscellaneous

Use Treatment of cutaneous lesions in patients with refractory cutaneous T-cell lymphoma (stage 1A and 1B) or who have not tolerated other therapies

Dosage Summary

Topical:

Children: Dosage not established

Adults: Apply once every other day for first week, then increase on a weekly basis to once daily, 2 times/day, 3 times/day, and finally 4 times/day, according to tolerance

Dosage Forms

Gel, topical:

Targretin®: 1% (60 g)

Bextra® ***(Discontinued)***

Bexxar® [US] *see* tositumomab and iodine I 131 tositumomab *on page 944*

bezafibrate *(Canada only)* (be za FYE brate)

U.S./Canadian Brand Names Bezalip® SR [Can]; PMS-Bezafibrate [Can]

Therapeutic Category Antihyperlipidemic Agent, Miscellaneous

Use Adjunct to diet and other therapeutic measures for treatment of type IIa and IIb mixed hyperlipidemia, to regulate lipid and apoprotein levels (reduce serum TG, LDL-cholesterol, and apolipoprotein B, increase HDL-cholesterol and apolipoprotein A); treatment of adult patients with high to very high triglyceride levels (Fredrickson classification type IV and V hyperlipidemias) who are at high risk of sequelae and complications from their dyslipidemia

Dosage Summary

Oral:

Immediate release:

Children: Dosage not established

Adults: 200 mg 2-3 times/day

Sustained release:

Children: Dosage not established

Adults: 400 mg once daily

Dosage Forms - Canada

Tablet, immediate release: 200 mg

PMA-Bezafibrate: 200 mg

Tablet, sustained release:

Bezalip® SR: 400 mg

Bezalip® SR [Can] *see* bezafibrate *(Canada only) on page 137*

BG 9273 *see* alefacept *on page 47*

Biavax® II ***(Discontinued)***

Biaxin® [US/Can] *see* clarithromycin *on page 229*

Biaxin® XL [US/Can] *see* clarithromycin *on page 229*

bicalutamide (bye ka LOO ta mide)

Sound-Alike/Look-Alike Issues

Casodex® may be confused with Kapidex™

Synonyms CDX; ICI-176334

U.S./Canadian Brand Names Apo-Bicalutamide® [Can]; Casodex® [US/Can]; CO Bicalutamide [Can]; Dom-Bicalutamide [Can]; Mylan-Bicalutamide [Can]; Novo-Bicalutamide [Can]; PHL-Bicalutamide [Can]; PMS-Bicalutamide [Can]; PRO-Bicalutamide [Can]; ratio-Bicalutamide [Can]; Sandoz-Bicalutamide [Can]; ZYM-Bicalutamide [Can]

Therapeutic Category Androgen

Use Treatment of metastatic prostate cancer (in combination with an LHRH agonist)

Dosage Summary

Oral:

Children: Dosage not established

Adults: 50 mg once daily

Dosage Forms

Tablet, oral: 50 mg

Casodex®: 50 mg

Bicillin® L-A [US/Can] *see* penicillin G benzathine *on page 737*

Bicillin® C-R [US] *see* penicillin G benzathine and penicillin G procaine *on page 737*

Bicillin® C-R 900/300 [US] *see* penicillin G benzathine and penicillin G procaine *on page 737*
BiCNU® [US/Can] *see* carmustine *on page 186*
Bidhist *(Discontinued)* *see* brompheniramine *on page 147*
BiDil® [US] *see* isosorbide dinitrate and hydralazine *on page 529*
BIG-IV *see* botulism immune globulin (intravenous-human) *on page 143*
Biltricide® [US/Can] *see* praziquantel *on page 789*

bimatoprost (bi MAT oh prost)

U.S./Canadian Brand Names Latisse™ [US]; Lumigan® RC [Can]; Lumigan® [US/Can]

Therapeutic Category Ophthalmic Agent, Miscellaneous

Use Reduction of intraocular pressure (IOP) in patients with open-angle glaucoma or ocular hypertension; hypotrichosis treatment of the eyelashes

Dosage Summary

Ophthalmic:

Children: Dosage not established

Adults: Instill 1 drop into affected eye(s) once daily in the evening

Ophthalmic, topical:

Children: Dosage not established

Adults: Place 1 drop on applicator and apply evenly along the skin of the upper eyelid at base of eyelashes once daily at bedtime; repeat procedure for second eye

Dosage Forms

Solution, ophthalmic:

Latisse™: 0.03% (3 mL)

Lumigan®: 0.03% (2.5 mL, 5 mL, 7.5 mL)

Bio-D-Mulsion® [US-OTC] *see* cholecalciferol *on page 218*
Bio-D-Mulsion Forte® [US-OTC] *see* cholecalciferol *on page 218*
Bio-Amitriptyline [Can] *see* amitriptyline *on page 67*
Biobase™ [Can] *see* alcohol (ethyl) *on page 45*
Biobase-G™ [Can] *see* alcohol (ethyl) *on page 45*
Bio-Carbamazepine [Can] *see* carbamazepine *on page 177*
Bioclate® *(Discontinued)* *see* antihemophilic factor (recombinant) *on page 81*
Biodine® *(Discontinued)* *see* povidone-iodine (topical) *on page 784*
Bio-Hydrochlorothiazide [Can] *see* hydrochlorothiazide *on page 478*
Biolon™ *(Discontinued)* *see* hyaluronate and derivatives *on page 475*
Bionect® [US] *see* hyaluronate and derivatives *on page 475*
Bioniche Promethazine [Can] *see* promethazine *on page 800*
Bion® Tears [US-OTC] *see* artificial tears *on page 97*
Bio-Oxazepam [Can] *see* oxazepam *on page 712*
Biopatch® *(Discontinued)* *see* chlorhexidine gluconate *on page 204*
BioQuin® Durules™ [Can] *see* quinidine *on page 822*
BioThrax® [US] *see* anthrax vaccine, adsorbed *on page 80*
Biozyme-C® *(Discontinued)* *see* collagenase (topical) *on page 247*
biperiden *(Discontinued)*
Biphentin® [Can] *see* methylphenidate *on page 621*
bird flu vaccine *see* influenza virus vaccine (H5N1) *on page 507*
Bisac-Evac™ [US-OTC] *see* bisacodyl *on page 138*

bisacodyl (bis a KOE dil)

Sound-Alike/Look-Alike Issues

Doxidan® may be confused with doxepin

Dulcolax® (bisacodyl) may be confused with Dulcolax® (docusate)

U.S./Canadian Brand Names Alophen® [US-OTC]; Apo-Bisacodyl® [Can]; Bisac-Evac™ [US-OTC]; Biscolax™ [US-OTC]; Carter's Little Pills® [Can]; Correctol® Tablets [US-OTC]; Dacodyl™ [US-OTC]; Doxidan® [US-OTC]; Dulcolax® (bisacodyl) [US-OTC/Can]; ex-lax® Ultra [US-OTC]; Femilax™ [US-OTC]; Fleet® Bisacodyl [US-OTC]; Fleet® Stimulant Laxative [US-OTC]; Gentlax® [Can]; Veracolate® [US-OTC]

Therapeutic Category Laxative

Use Treatment of constipation; colonic evacuation prior to procedures or examination

Dosage Summary

Oral:

Children ≤6 years: Dosage not established
Children >6 years: 5-10 mg (0.3 mg/kg) once daily
Adults: 5-15 mg as a single dose (maximum: 30 mg)

Rectal:

Children <2 years: 5 mg as a single dose
Children ≥2 years: 10 mg as a single dose
Adults: 10 mg as a single dose

Dosage Forms

Solution, rectal:
Fleet® Bisacodyl [OTC]: 10 mg/30 mL (37 mL)

Suppository, rectal: 10 mg (12s, 50s, 100s, 500s)
Bisac-Evac™ [OTC]: 10 mg (8s, 12s, 50s, 100s, 500s, 1000s)
Biscolax™ [OTC]: 10 mg (12s, 100s)
Dulcolax® [OTC]: 10 mg (4s, 8s, 16s, 28s, 50s)

Tablet, delayed release, oral: 5 mg
Doxidan® [OTC]: 5 mg
Fleet® Stimulant Laxative [OTC]: 5 mg

Tablet, enteric coated, oral: 5 mg
Alophen® [OTC]: 5 mg
Bisac-Evac™ [OTC]: 5 mg
Correctol® Tablets [OTC]: 5 mg
Dacodyl™ [OTC]: 5 mg
Dulcolax® [OTC]: 5 mg
ex-lax® Ultra [OTC]: 5 mg
Femilax™ [OTC]: 5 mg
Veracolate® [OTC]: 5 mg

Bisacodyl Uniserts® *(Discontinued)* *see* bisacodyl *on page* 138

bis-chloronitrosourea *see* carmustine *on page* 186

Biscolax™ [US-OTC] *see* bisacodyl *on page* 138

Bismatrol [US-OTC] *see* bismuth *on page* 139

Bismatrol Maximum Strength [US-OTC] *see* bismuth *on page* 139

bismuth (BIZ muth)

Sound-Alike/Look-Alike Issues

Kaopectate® may be confused with Kayexalate®

Synonyms bismuth subsalicylate; pink bismuth

U.S./Canadian Brand Names Bismatrol Maximum Strength [US-OTC]; Bismatrol [US-OTC]; Diotame [US-OTC]; Kao-Tin [US-OTC]; Kaopectate® Extra Strength [US-OTC]; Kaopectate® [US-OTC]; Maalox® Total Relief® [US-OTC]; Peptic Relief [US-OTC]; Pepto Relief [US-OTC]; Pepto-Bismol® Maximum Strength [US-OTC]; Pepto-Bismol® [US-OTC]

Therapeutic Category Antidiarrheal

Use Subsalicylate formulation: Symptomatic treatment of mild, nonspecific diarrhea; control of traveler's diarrhea (enterotoxigenic *Escherichia coli*); as part of a multidrug regimen for *H. pylori* eradication to reduce the risk of duodenal ulcer recurrence

Dosage Summary

Oral:

Subsalicylate based on 262 mg/5 mL liquid or 262 mg tablet (diarrhea):
Children <3 years: Dosage not established
Children 3-6 years: 1/3 tablet **or** 5 mL every 30 minutes to 1 hour as needed (maximum: 8 doses/day)
Children 6-9 years: 2/3 tablet **or** 10 mL every 30 minutes to 1 hour as needed (maximum: 8 doses/day)
Children 9-12 years: 1 tablet **or** 15 mL every 30 minutes to 1 hour as needed (maximum: 8 doses/day)

Subsalicylate based on 262 mg/15 mL liquid or 262 mg tablet:
Children >12 years: Diarrhea: 2 tablets **or** 30 mL every 30 minutes to 1 hour as needed (maximum: 8 doses/day)

Adults:
Diarrhea: 2 tablets **or** 30 mL every 30 minutes to 1 hour as needed (maximum: 8 doses/day)
H. pylori eradication: 524 mg 4 times/day

Dosage Forms

Caplet, oral:
Pepto-Bismol® [OTC]: 262 mg

Liquid, oral: 262 mg/15 mL (237 mL, 240 mL)
Bismatrol [OTC]: 262 mg/15 mL (240 mL)
Bismatrol Maximum Strength [OTC]: 525 mg/15 mL (240 mL)
Diotame [OTC]: 262 mg/15 mL (30 mL)
Kao-Tin [OTC]: 262 mg/15 mL (240 mL, 473 mL)
Kaopectate® [OTC]: 262 mg/15 mL (177 mL, 236 mL, 354 mL)
Kaopectate® Extra Strength [OTC]: 525 mg/15 mL (236 mL)
Maalox® Total Relief® [OTC]: 525 mg/15 mL (360 mL)
Peptic Relief [OTC]: 262 mg/15 mL (237 mL)
Pepto-Bismol® [OTC]: 262 mg/15 mL (120 mL, 240 mL, 360 mL, 480 mL)
Pepto-Bismol® Maximum Strength [OTC]: 525 mg/15 mL (120 mL, 240 mL, 360 mL)

Suspension, oral: 262 mg/15 mL (30 mL)

Tablet, chewable, oral: 262 mg
Bismatrol [OTC]: 262 mg
Diotame [OTC]: 262 mg
Peptic Relief [OTC]: 262 mg
Pepto Relief [OTC]: 262 mg
Pepto-Bismol® [OTC]: 262 mg

bismuth, metronidazole, and tetracycline

(BIZ muth, me troe NI da zole, & tet ra SYE kleen)

Synonyms bismuth subcitrate potassium, tetracycline, and metronidazole; bismuth subsalicylate, tetracycline, and metronidazole; metronidazole, bismuth subcitrate potassium, and tetracycline; metronidazole, bismuth subsalicylate, and tetracycline; tetracycline, metronidazole, and bismuth subcitrate potassium; tetracycline, metronidazole, and bismuth subsalicylate

U.S./Canadian Brand Names Helidac® [US]; Pylera™ [US]

Therapeutic Category Antidiarrheal

Use As part of a multidrug regimen for *H. pylori* eradication to reduce the risk of duodenal ulcer recurrence in combination with an H_2 agonist (Helidac®) or omeprazole (Pylera™)

Dosage Summary

Oral:

Children: Dosage not established

Adults:
Helidac®: Two bismuth subsalicylate 262.4 mg tablets, 1 metronidazole 250 mg tablet, and 1 tetracycline 500 mg capsule 4 times/day at meals and bedtime, plus an H_2 antagonist (at the appropriate dose) for 14 days; follow with 8 oz of water; the H_2 antagonist should be continued for a total of 28 days
Pylera™: Three capsules 4 times/day after meals and at bedtime, plus omeprazole 20 mg twice daily for 10 days; follow each dose with 8 oz of water (each capsule contains bismuth subcitrate potassium 140 mg, metronidazole 125 mg, and tetracycline 125 mg)

Dosage Forms

Capsule:
Pylera™: Bismuth subcitrate potassium 140 mg, metronidazole 125 mg, and tetracycline hydrochloride 125 mg

Combination package:
Helidac® [each package contains 14 blister cards (2-week supply); each card contains the following]:
Capsule: Tetracycline: 500 mg (4)
Tablet, chewable: Bismuth subsalicylate]: 262.4 mg (8)
Tablet: Metronidazole: 250 mg (4)

bismuth subcitrate potassium, tetracycline, and metronidazole *see* bismuth, metronidazole, and tetracycline *on page 140*

bismuth subsalicylate *see* bismuth *on page 139*

bismuth subsalicylate, tetracycline, and metronidazole *see* bismuth, metronidazole, and tetracycline *on page 140*

bisoprolol (bis OH proe lol)

Sound-Alike/Look-Alike Issues

Zebeta® may be confused with DiaBeta®, Zetia®

Synonyms bisoprolol fumarate

U.S./Canadian Brand Names Apo-Bisoprolol® [Can]; Novo-Bisoprolol [Can]; PHL-Bisoprolol [Can]; PMS-Bisoprolol [Can]; PRO-Bisoprolol [Can]; Sandoz-Bisoprolol [Can]; Zebeta® [US]; ZYM-Bisoprolol [Can]

Therapeutic Category Beta-Adrenergic Blocker

Use Treatment of hypertension, alone or in combination with other agents

Dosage Summary

Oral:

Children: Dosage not established

Adults: Initial: 2.5-5 mg once daily; Maintenance: 2.5-20 mg once daily

Elderly: Initial: 2.5 mg/day, increase by 2.5-5 mg/day up to 20 mg/day

Dosage Forms

Tablet, oral: 5 mg, 10 mg

Zebeta®: 5 mg, 10 mg

bisoprolol and hydrochlorothiazide (bis OH proe lol & hye droe klor oh THYE a zide)

Sound-Alike/Look-Alike Issues

Ziac® may be confused with Tiazac®, Zerit®

Synonyms bisoprolol fumarate and hydrochlorothiazide; hydrochlorothiazide and bisoprolol

U.S./Canadian Brand Names Ziac® [US/Can]

Therapeutic Category Antihypertensive Agent, Combination

Use Treatment of hypertension

Dosage Summary

Oral:

Adults: Initial: Bisoprolol 2.5 mg and hydrochlorothiazide 6.25 mg once daily. Titration recommended. Maximum dose (manufacturer recommended): Bisoprolol 20 mg/hydrochlorothiazide 12.5 mg once daily

Add-on/replacement therapy: Bisoprolol 2.5-20 mg and hydrochlorothiazide 6.25-12.5 mg once daily

Dosage Forms

Tablet, oral: 2.5/6.25: Bisoprolol 2.5 mg and hydrochlorothiazide 6.25 mg; 5/6.25: Bisoprolol 5 mg and hydrochlorothiazide 6.25 mg; 10/6.25: Bisoprolol 10 mg and hydrochlorothiazide 6.25 mg

Ziac®: 2.5/6.25: Bisoprolol 2.5 mg and hydrochlorothiazide 6.25 mg; 5/6.25: Bisoprolol 5 mg and hydrochlorothiazide 6.25 mg; 10/6.25: Bisoprolol 10 mg and hydrochlorothiazide 6.25 mg

bisoprolol fumarate *see* bisoprolol *on page 141*

bisoprolol fumarate and hydrochlorothiazide *see* bisoprolol and hydrochlorothiazide *on page 141*

bis-POM PMEA *see* adefovir *on page 38*

bistropamide *see* tropicamide *on page 964*

bivalent human papillomavirus vaccine *see* papillomavirus (types 16, 18) vaccine (human, recombinant) *on page 726*

bivalirudin (bye VAL i roo din)

Synonyms hirulog

U.S./Canadian Brand Names Angiomax® [US/Can]

Therapeutic Category Anticoagulant (Other)

Use Anticoagulant used in conjunction with aspirin for patients with unstable angina undergoing percutaneous transluminal coronary angioplasty (PTCA) or percutaneous coronary intervention (PCI) with provisional glycoprotein IIb/IIIa inhibitor; anticoagulant used in conjunction with aspirin for patients undergoing PCI with (or at risk of) heparin-induced thrombocytopenia (HIT) / thrombosis syndrome (HITTS)

Dosage Summary

I.V.:

Children: Dosage not established

Adults: Bolus: 0.75 mg/kg, may repeat at 0.3 mg/kg if necessary; Infusion: 1.75 mg/kg/hour for duration of procedure and up to 4 hours postprocedure if needed, after 4 hours may continue 0.2 mg/kg/minute for up to 20 hours if needed

Dosage Forms

Injection, powder for reconstitution:

Angiomax®: 250 mg

Bi-Zets [US-OTC] *see* benzocaine *on page 124*

BL4162A *see* anagrelide *on page 77*

Black Draught® [US-OTC] *see* senna *on page 870*

black widow spider species antivenin *see* antivenin *(Latrodectus mactans) on page 85*

BlemErase® Lotion *(Discontinued)* *see* benzoyl peroxide *on page 128*

Blenoxane® [Can] *see* bleomycin *on page 142*

Blenoxane® *(Discontinued)* *see* bleomycin *on page 142*

bleo *see* bleomycin *on page 142*

bleomycin (blee oh MYE sin)

Sound-Alike/Look-Alike Issues

bleomycin may be confused with Cleocin®

Synonyms bleo; bleomycin sulfate; BLM

U.S./Canadian Brand Names Blenoxane® [Can]; Bleomycin Injection, USP [Can]

Therapeutic Category Antineoplastic Agent

Use Treatment of squamous cell carcinomas of the head and neck, penis, cervix, or vulva, testicular carcinoma, Hodgkin lymphoma, and non-Hodgkin lymphoma; sclerosing agent for malignant pleural effusion

Dosage Summary

Intrapleural:

Children: Dosage not established

Adults: 60 units as a single instillation

Dosage Forms

Injection, powder for reconstitution: 15 units, 30 units

Bleomycin Injection, USP [Can] *see* bleomycin *on page 142*

bleomycin sulfate *see* bleomycin *on page 142*

Bleph®-10 [US] *see* sulfacetamide (ophthalmic) *on page 899*

Bleph 10 DPS [Can] *see* sulfacetamide (ophthalmic) *on page 899*

Blephamide® [US/Can] *see* sulfacetamide and prednisolone *on page 900*

BLES [Can] *see* bovine lipid extract surfactant *(Canada only) on page 144*

Blis-To-Sol® [US-OTC] *see* tolnaftate *on page 940*

BLM *see* bleomycin *on page 142*

BMS-188667 *see* abatacept *on page 19*

BMS-232632 *see* atazanavir *on page 102*

BMS-247550 *see* ixabepilone *on page 532*

BMS-337039 *see* aripiprazole *on page 94*

BMS-354825 *see* dasatinib *on page 270*

BMS-477118 *see* saxagliptin *on page 866*

Boil-Ease® Pain Relieving [US-OTC] *see* benzocaine *on page 124*

BOL-303224-A *see* besifloxacin *on page 132*

Bonamine™ [Can] *see* meclizine *on page 595*

Bonefos® [Can] *see* clodronate *(Canada only) on page 236*

Bonine® [US-OTC/Can] *see* meclizine *on page 595*

Boniva® [US] *see* ibandronate *on page 493*

Bontril® [Can] *see* phendimetrazine *on page 747*

Bontril® PDM [US] *see* phendimetrazine *on page 747*

Bontril® Slow-Release [US] *see* phendimetrazine *on page 747*
Boostrix® [US/Can] *see* diphtheria, tetanus toxoids, and acellular pertussis vaccine *on page 316*

bortezomib (bore TEZ oh mib)

Synonyms LDP-341; MLN341; PS-341
U.S./Canadian Brand Names Velcade® [US/Can]
Therapeutic Category Proteasome Inhibitor
Use Treatment of multiple myeloma; treatment of relapsed or refractory mantle cell lymphoma
Dosage Summary
I.V.:
Children: Dosage not established
Adults: 1.3 mg/m^2 days 1, 4, 8, 11, 22, 25, 29, and 32 of a 42-day treatment cycle for 4 cycles, followed by 1.3 mg/m^2 days 1, 8, 22, and 29 of a 42-day treatment cycle for 5 cycles **or** 1.3 mg/m^2 twice weekly for 2 weeks on days 1, 4, 8, and 11 of a 21-day treatment cycle; therapy extending beyond 8 cycles may be given once weekly for 4 weeks (days 1, 8, 15, and 22)
Dosage Forms
Injection, powder for reconstitution:
Velcade®: 3.5 mg

bosentan (boe SEN tan)

Sound-Alike/Look-Alike Issues
Tracleer® may be confused with TriCor©
U.S./Canadian Brand Names Tracleer® [US/Can]
Therapeutic Category Endothelin Antagonist
Use Treatment of pulmonary artery hypertension (PAH) (WHO Group I) in patients with World Health Organization (WHO) Class II, III, or IV symptoms to improve exercise capacity and decrease the rate of clinical deterioration
Dosage Summary
Oral:
Children >12 years and <40 kg: Initial: 62.5 mg twice daily for 4 weeks; Maintenance: 62.5 mg twice daily
Children >12 years and ≥40 kg: Initial: 62.5 mg twice daily for 4 weeks; Maintenance: 125 mg twice daily
Adults <40 kg: Initial: 62.5 mg twice daily for 4 weeks; Maintenance: 62.5 mg twice daily
Adults ≥40 kg: Initial: 62.5 mg twice daily for 4 weeks; Maintenance: 125 mg twice daily
Dosage Forms
Tablet, oral:
Tracleer®: 62.5 mg, 125 mg

B&O Supprettes® ***(Discontinued)*** *see* belladonna and opium *on page 121*
Botox® [US/Can] *see* onabotulinumtoxinA *on page 703*
Botox® Cosmetic [US/Can] *see* onabotulinumtoxinA *on page 703*
botulinum toxin type A *see* abobotulinumtoxinA *on page 20*
botulinum toxin type A *see* incobotulinumtoxinA *on page 504*
botulinum toxin type A *see* onabotulinumtoxinA *on page 703*
botulinum toxin type B *see* rimabotulinumtoxinB *on page 843*

botulism immune globulin (intravenous-human)

(BOT yoo lism i MYUN GLOB you lin, in tra VEE nus, YU man)
Sound-Alike/Look-Alike Issues
BabyBIG® may be confused with HBIG
Synonyms BIG-IV
U.S./Canadian Brand Names BabyBIG® [US]
Therapeutic Category Immune Globulin
Use Treatment of infant botulism caused by toxin type A or B
Dosage Summary
I.V.:
Children <1 year: 100 mg/kg as a single dose
Children ≥1 year: Dosage not established
Adults: Dosage not established

Dosage Forms

Injection, powder for reconstitution [preservative free]:
BabyBIG®: ~100 mg

Boudreaux's® Butt Paste [US-OTC] *see* zinc oxide *on page 1001*

bovine lipid extract surfactant *(Canada only)* (BOH vine LIP id EK strakt ser FAK tunt)

U.S./Canadian Brand Names BLES [Can]

Therapeutic Category Lung Surfactant

Use Treatment of neonatal respiratory distress syndrome (NRDS)

Dosage Summary

Intratracheal:
Infants: 5 mL/kg/dose (equals phospholipids 135 mg/kg/dose); may repeat if needed (maximum: 4 doses)
Children: Dosage not established
Adults: Dosage not established

Dosage Forms - Canada

Suspension, intratracheal [preservative free]:
BLES®: Phospholipids 27 mg/mL (3 mL, 4 mL, 5 mL)

bovine lung surfactant *see* beractant *on page 131*
BP 8 [US] *see* guaifenesin, pseudoephedrine, and dextromethorphan *on page 460*
BP10-1 [US] *see* sulfur and sulfacetamide *on page 903*
BP 50% [US] *see* urea *on page 970*
BP Cleansing Wash [US] *see* sulfur and sulfacetamide *on page 903*
BPM PE [US] *see* brompheniramine and phenylephrine *on page 148*
BPO *see* benzoyl peroxide *on page 128*
BP Poly 650 [US] *see* acetaminophen and phenyltoloxamine *on page 26*
BranchAmin® [US] *see* amino acid injection *on page 64*
Bravelle® [US/Can] *see* urofollitropin *on page 971*
Breathe Free® [US-OTC] *see* sodium chloride *on page 882*
Breezee® Mist Antifungal ***(Discontinued)*** *see* miconazole (topical) *on page 630*
Breonesin® ***(Discontinued)*** *see* guaifenesin *on page 454*
Brethaire® ***(Discontinued)*** *see* terbutaline *on page 918*
brethine *see* terbutaline *on page 918*
Brevibloc® [US/Can] *see* esmolol *on page 364*
Brevicon® [US] *see* ethinyl estradiol and norethindrone *on page 378*
Brevicon® 0.5/35 [Can] *see* ethinyl estradiol and norethindrone *on page 378*
Brevicon® 1/35 [Can] *see* ethinyl estradiol and norethindrone *on page 378*
Brevital® [Can] *see* methohexital *on page 614*
Brevital® Sodium [US] *see* methohexital *on page 614*
Brevoxyl®-4 [US] *see* benzoyl peroxide *on page 128*
Brevoxyl®-8 [US] *see* benzoyl peroxide *on page 128*
Brevoxyl® Acne Wash Kit ***(Discontinued)*** *see* benzoyl peroxide *on page 128*
breze™ ***(Discontinued)*** *see* benzoyl peroxide *on page 128*
Bricanyl® [Can] *see* terbutaline *on page 918*
Bricanyl® ***(Discontinued)*** *see* terbutaline *on page 918*

brimonidine (bri MOE ni deen)

Sound-Alike/Look-Alike Issues
brimonidine may be confused with bromocriptine

Synonyms brimonidine tartrate

U.S./Canadian Brand Names Alphagan® P [US]; Alphagan® [Can]; Apo-Brimonidine P® [Can]; Apo-Brimonidine® [Can]; PMS-Brimonidine Tartrate [Can]; ratio-Brimonidine [Can]; Sandoz-Brimonidine [Can]

Therapeutic Category $Alpha_2$ Agonist, Ophthalmic

Use Lowering of intraocular pressure (IOP) in patients with open-angle glaucoma or ocular hypertension

Dosage Summary

Ophthalmic:

Children <2 years: Dosage not established

Children ≥2 years: Instill 1 drop in affected eye(s) 3 times/day

Adults: Instill 1 drop in affected eye(s) 3 times/day

Dosage Forms

Solution, ophthalmic: 0.15% (5 mL, 10 mL, 15 mL); 0.2% (5 mL, 10 mL, 15 mL)

Alphagan® P: 0.1% (5 mL, 10 mL, 15 mL); 0.15% (5 mL, 10 mL, 15 mL)

brimonidine and timolol (bri MOE ni deen & TIM oh lol)

Synonyms brimonidine tartrate and timolol maleate; timolol and brimonidine

U.S./Canadian Brand Names Combigan® [US/Can]

Therapeutic Category $Alpha_2$ Agonist, Ophthalmic; Beta Blocker, Nonselective; Ophthalmic Agent, Antiglaucoma

Use Reduction of intraocular pressure (IOP) in patients with glaucoma or ocular hypertension

Dosage Summary

Ophthalmic:

Children <2 years: Dosage not established

Children ≥2 years: Instill 1 drop into affected eye(s) twice daily

Adults: Instill 1 drop into affected eye(s) twice daily

Dosage Forms

Solution, ophthalmic [drops]:

Combigan®: Brimonidine 0.2% and timolol 0.5% (5 mL,10 mL)

Dosage Forms - Canada

Solution, ophthalmic [drops]:

Combigan®: Brimonidine 0.2% and timolol 0.5% (2.5 mL, 5 mL,10 mL)

brimonidine tartrate *see* brimonidine *on page 144*

brimonidine tartrate and timolol maleate *see* brimonidine and timolol *on page 145*

brinzolamide (brin ZOH la mide)

U.S./Canadian Brand Names Azopt® [US/Can]

Therapeutic Category Carbonic Anhydrase Inhibitor

Use Lowers intraocular pressure in patients with ocular hypertension or open-angle glaucoma

Dosage Summary

Ophthalmic:

Children: Dosage not established

Adults: Instill 1 drop in affected eye(s) 3 times/day

Dosage Forms

Suspension, ophthalmic:

Azopt®: 1% (10 mL, 15 mL)

brinzolamide and timolol *(Canada only)* (brin ZOH la mide & TIM oh lol)

Synonyms brinzolamide and timolol maleate; timolol maleate and brinzolamide

U.S./Canadian Brand Names Azarga™ [Can]

Therapeutic Category Beta-Adrenergic Blocker, Nonselective; Carbonic Anhydrase Inhibitor; Ophthalmic Agent, Antiglaucoma

Use Treatment of elevated intraocular pressure in patients with ocular hypertension or open-angle glaucoma

Dosage Summary

Ophthalmic:

Children: Dosage not established

Adults: Instill 1 drop twice daily

Dosage Forms - Canada

Solution, ophthalmic [drops]:

Azarga™: Brinzolamide 1% and timolol maleate 0.5% (5 mL)

brinzolamide and timolol maleate *see* brinzolamide and timolol *(Canada only) on page 145*

Brioschi® [US-OTC] *see* sodium bicarbonate *on page 882*

British anti-lewisite *see* dimercaprol *on page 307*

BRL 43694 *see* granisetron *on page 452*

Bromaline® [US-OTC] *see* brompheniramine and pseudoephedrine *on page 148*

Bromaline® DM [US-OTC] *see* brompheniramine, pseudoephedrine, and dextromethorphan *on page 149*

Bromarest® ***(Discontinued)*** *see* brompheniramine *on page 147*

Bromatane DX [US] *see* brompheniramine, pseudoephedrine, and dextromethorphan *on page 149*

Bromaxefed RF ***(Discontinued)*** *see* brompheniramine and pseudoephedrine *on page 148*

bromazepam *(Canada only)* (broe MA ze pam)

U.S./Canadian Brand Names Apo-Bromazepam® [Can]; Gen-Bromazepam [Can]; Lectopam® [Can]; Novo-Bromazepam [Can]; Nu-Bromazepam [Can]; PRO-Doc Limitee Bromazepam [Can]

Therapeutic Category Benzodiazepine; Sedative

Use Short-term, symptomatic treatment of anxiety

Dosage Summary

Oral:

Children: Dosage not established

Adults: Initial: 6-18 mg/day in divided doses; Maintenance: 6-30 mg/day in divided doses

Elderly: Initial: 3 mg/day in divided doses

Dosage Forms - Canada

Tablet: 1.5 mg, 3 mg, 6 mg

Lectopam®: 3 mg, 6 mg

Brombay® ***(Discontinued)*** *see* brompheniramine *on page 147*

Brometane DX ***(Discontinued)*** *see* brompheniramine, pseudoephedrine, and dextromethorphan *on page 149*

Bromfed® [US] *see* brompheniramine and phenylephrine *on page 148*

Bromfed® DM [US] *see* brompheniramine, pseudoephedrine, and dextromethorphan *on page 149*

Bromfed®-PD [US] *see* brompheniramine and phenylephrine *on page 148*

bromfenac (BROME fen ak)

Synonyms bromfenac sodium

U.S./Canadian Brand Names Xibrom™ [US]

Therapeutic Category Analgesic, Nonnarcotic; Nonsteroidal Antiinflammatory Drug (NSAID), Ophthalmic

Use Treatment of postoperative inflammation and reduction in ocular pain following cataract removal

Dosage Summary

Ophthalmic:

Children: Dosage not established

Adults: Instill 1 drop into affected eye(s) twice daily

Dosage Forms

Solution, ophthalmic:

Xibrom™: 0.09% (2.5 mL, 5 mL)

bromfenac sodium *see* bromfenac *on page 146*

Bromfenex® ***(Discontinued)*** *see* brompheniramine and pseudoephedrine *on page 148*

Bromfenex® PD ***(Discontinued)*** *see* brompheniramine and pseudoephedrine *on page 148*

Bromhist DM ***(Discontinued)*** *see* brompheniramine, pseudoephedrine, and dextromethorphan *on page 149*

Bromhist-NR ***(Discontinued)*** *see* brompheniramine and pseudoephedrine *on page 148*

Bromhist PDX ***(Discontinued)*** *see* brompheniramine, pseudoephedrine, and dextromethorphan *on page 149*

Bromhist Pediatric ***(Discontinued)*** *see* brompheniramine and pseudoephedrine *on page 148*

bromocriptine (broe moe KRIP teen)

Sound-Alike/Look-Alike Issues

bromocriptine may be confused with benztropine, brimonidine

Cycloset® may be confused with Glyset®

Parlodel® may be confused with pindolol, Provera®

Synonyms bromocriptine mesylate

U.S./Canadian Brand Names Apo-Bromocriptine® [Can]; Parlodel® SnapTabs® [US]; Parlodel® [US/Can]; PMS-Bromocriptine [Can]

Therapeutic Category Anti-Parkinson Agent (Dopamine Agonist); Ergot Alkaloid and Derivative

Use Treatment of hyperprolactinemia associated with amenorrhea with or without galactorrhea, infertility, or hypogonadism; treatment of prolactin-secreting adenomas; treatment of acromegaly; treatment of Parkinson disease

Dosage Summary

Oral:

Children <11 years: Dosage not established

Children 11-15 years: Initial: 1.25-2.5 mg daily; Maintenance: 2.5-10 mg/day; **Note:** Titration is recommended

Children ≥16 years: Initial: 1.25-2.5 mg daily; Maintenance: 2.5-15 mg/day; **Note:** Titration is recommended

Adults:

Initial: 1.25-2.5 mg/day in 1-2 divided doses

Maintenance: Acromegaly: 20-30 mg/day; Hyperprolactinemia: 2.5-15 mg/day; Parkinsonism: 30-90 mg/day; maximum: 100 mg/day; **Note:** Titration is recommended

Product Availability

Cycloset®: FDA approved May 2009; availability currently undetermined

Cycloset® has been approved for the treatment of type 2 diabetes.

Dosage Forms

Capsule, oral: 5 mg

Parlodel®: 5 mg

Tablet, oral: 2.5 mg

Parlodel® SnapTabs®: 2.5 mg

bromocriptine mesylate *see* bromocriptine *on page 146*

Bromphen® *(Discontinued)* *see* brompheniramine *on page 147*

Bromphenex™ DM [US-OTC] *see* brompheniramine, pseudoephedrine, and dextromethorphan *on page 149*

brompheniramine (brome fen IR a meen)

Synonyms brompheniramine maleate; brompheniramine tannate

U.S./Canadian Brand Names Lodrane® 12 Hour [US]; Lodrane® 24 [US]; Lodrane® XR [US]; LoHist-12 [US]; TanaCof-XR [US]

Therapeutic Category Antihistamine

Use Symptomatic relief of perennial and seasonal allergic rhinitis, vasomotor rhinitis, and other respiratory allergies

Dosage Summary

Oral:

Children 2-6 years: TanaCof-XR: 1.25 mL every 12 hours (maximum: 2.5 mL/day)

Children 6-12 years:

Lodrane® 24: One capsule once daily

LoHist-12: One tablet every 12 hours (maximum: 2 tablets/day)

TanaCof-XR: 2.5 mL every 12 hours (maximum: 5 mL/day)

Children >12 years:

Lodrane® 24: 1-2 capsules once daily

LoHist-12: 1-2 tablets every 12 hours (maximum: 4 tablets/day)

TanaCof-XR: 5 mL every 12 hours (maximum: 10 mL/day)

Adults:

Lodrane® 24: 1-2 capsules once daily

LoHist-12: 1-2 tablets every 12 hours (maximum: 4 tablets/day)

TanaCof-XR: 5 mL every 12 hours (maximum: 10 mL/day)

Dosage Forms

Capsule, extended release, oral:

Lodrane® 24: 12 mg

Suspension, oral: 12 mg/5 mL (118 mL)

TanaCof-XR: 8 mg/5 mL (480 mL)

Tablet, chewable, oral: 12 mg

Tablet, extended release, oral:

LoHist-12: 6 mg

Tablet, timed release, oral: 6 mg

brompheniramine and phenylephrine (brome fen IR a meen & fen il EF rin)

Sound-Alike/Look-Alike Issues

Bromfed® may be confused with Bromphen®

Synonyms brompheniramine maleate and phenylephrine hydrochloride; brompheniramine tannate and phenylephrine tannate; phenylephrine and brompheniramine

U.S./Canadian Brand Names BPM PE [US]; Bromfed® [US]; Bromfed®-PD [US]; C-Tan D Plus [US]; C-Tan D [US]; Dimaphen Cold & Allergy [US-OTC]; Dimetapp® Children's Cold & Allergy [US-OTC]

Therapeutic Category Alpha/Beta Agonist; Histamine H_1 Antagonist; Histamine H_1 Antagonist, First Generation

Use Temporary relief of upper respiratory conditions such as nasal congestion, runny nose, itchy/watery eyes, and sneezing due to the common cold, hay fever, or upper respiratory allergies

Dosage Summary

Oral:

Children <2 years: Dosage not established

Children 6-11 years:

C-Tann D, C-Tann D Plus: 5 mL every 12 hours (maximum: 10 mL/24 hours)

BPM PE: 2.5 mL every 6 hours as needed (maximum: 15 mL/24 hours)

Bromfed®-PD: One capsule every 12 hours

Dimaphen Cold & Allergy: 10 mL every 4-6 hours as needed (maximum: 60 mL/24 hours)

Dimetapp® chewable tablet: Two tablets every 4 hours as needed (maximum: 12 tablets/24 hours)

Dimetapp® syrup: 10 mL every 4 hours as needed (maximum: 60 mL/24 hours)

Children ≥12 years:

C-Tann D, C-Tann D Plus: 5-10 mL every 12 hours (maximum: 20 mL/24 hours)

BPM PE: 5 mL every 6 hours as needed (maximum: 30 mL/24 hours)

Bromfed®: One capsule every 12 hours

Bromfed®-PD: 1-2 capsules every 12 hours

Dimaphen Cold & Allergy: 20 mL every 4-6 hours as needed (maximum: 120 mL/24 hours)

Dimetapp® syrup: 20 mL every 4 hours as needed (maximum: 120 mL/24 hours)

Adults:

C-Tann D, C-Tann D Plus: 5-10 mL every 12 hours (maximum: 20 mL/24 hours)

BPM PE: 5 mL every 6 hours as needed (maximum: 30 mL/24 hours)

Bromfed®: One capsule every 12 hours

Bromfed®-PD: 1-2 capsules every 12 hours

Dimaphen Cold & Allergy: 20 mL every 4-6 hours as needed (maximum: 120 mL/24 hours)

Dimetapp® syrup: 20 mL every 4 hours as needed (maximum: 120 mL/24 hours)

Dosage Forms

Capsule, extended release: Brompheniramine 6 mg and phenylephrine 7.5 mg; Brompheniramine 12 mg and phenylephrine 15 mg

Bromfed®: Brompheniramine 12 mg and phenylephrine 15 mg

Bromfed®-PD: Brompheniramine 6 mg and phenylephrine 7.5 mg

Elixir, oral:

Dimaphen Cold & Allergy [OTC]: Brompheniramine 1 mg and phenylephrine 2. 5 mg per 5 mL

Liquid, oral:

BPM PE: Brompheniramine 4 mg and phenylephrine 7.5 mg per 5 mL

Suspension, oral: Brompheniramine 12 mg and phenylephrine 20 mg per 5 mL

C-Tan D: Brompheniramine 4 mg and phenylephrine 5 mg per 5 mL

C-Tan D Plus: Brompheniramine 5 mg and phenylephrine 5 mg per 5 mL

Syrup:

Dimetapp® Children's Cold & Allergy [OTC]: Brompheniramine 1 mg and phenylephrine 2.5 mg per 5 mL

Tablet, chewable:

Dimetapp® Children's Cold & Allergy [OTC]: Brompheniramine 1 mg and phenylephrine 2.5 mg

brompheniramine and pseudoephedrine (brome fen IR a meen & soo doe e FED rin)

Synonyms brompheniramine maleate and pseudoephedrine hydrochloride; brompheniramine maleate and pseudoephedrine sulfate; pseudoephedrine and brompheniramine

U.S./Canadian Brand Names Bromaline® [US-OTC]; Brotapp [US]; Histex® SR [US]; Lodrane® 12D [US]; Lodrane® 24D [US]; LoHist 12D [US]; LoHist LQ [US]; Respahist® [US]; Sildec Syrup [US]

Therapeutic Category Antihistamine/Decongestant Combination

Use Temporary relief of symptoms of seasonal and perennial allergic rhinitis, and vasomotor rhinitis, including nasal obstruction

Dosage Summary

Oral:

Extended release:

Children <6 years: Dosage not established

Children 6-12 years: 45 mg pseudoephedrine every 12 hours

Children ≥12 years: 45-90 mg every 12 hours

Adults: 45-90 mg every 12 hours

Immediate release:

Children <1 month: Dosage not established

Children 1-3 months: Brompheniramine 0.25 mg/pseudoephedrine 3.75 mg 4 times/daily

Children 3-6 months: Brompheniramine 0.5 mg/pseudoephedrine 7.5 mg 4 times/daily

Children 6-12 months: Brompheniramine 0.5-0.75 mg/pseudoephedrine 7.5-11.25 mg every 6-8 hours (maximum: 4 doses/day)

Children 12-24 months: Brompheniramine 0.75-1 mg/pseudoephedrine 11.25-15 mg every 6-8 hours (maximum: 4 doses/day)

Children 2-6 years: Brompheniramine 1-2 mg/pseudoephedrine 15-22.5 mg every 6-8 hours (maximum: 4 doses/day)

Children 6-12 years: Brompheniramine 2-4 mg/pseudoephedrine 30-45 mg every 6-8 hours (maximum: 4 doses/day)

Children ≥12 years: Brompheniramine 4 mg/pseudoephedrine 45-60 mg every 4-8 hours (maximum: 4 doses/day)

Adults: Brompheniramine 4 mg/pseudoephedrine 45-60 mg every 4-8 hours (maximum: 4 doses/day)

Long acting:

Children <6 years: Dosage not established

Children 6-12 years: 60 mg pseudoephedrine every 12 hours

Children ≥12 years: 60-120 mg pseudoephedrine every 12 hours

Adults: 60-120 mg pseudoephedrine every 12 hours

Dosage Forms

Caplet, extended release:

Histex® SR: Brompheniramine 10 mg and pseudoephedrine 120 mg

Capsule, extended release:

Lodrane® 24D: Brompheniramine 12 mg and pseudoephedrine 90 mg

Liquid: Brompheniramine 4 mg and pseudoephedrine 60 mg per 5 mL (480 mL)

Brotapp: Brompheniramine 1 mg and pseudoephedrine 15 mg per 5 mL

LoHist LQ: Brompheniramine 4 mg and pseudoephedrine 60 mg per 5 mL

Solution:

Bromaline® [OTC]: Brompheniramine 1 mg and pseudoephedrine 15 mg per 5 mL

Syrup:

Sildec: Brompheniramine 4 mg and pseudoephedrine 45 mg per 5 mL

Tablet, extended release:

Lodrane® 12D, LoHist 12D: Brompheniramine 6 mg and pseudoephedrine 45 mg

Tablet, sustained release: Brompheniramine 6 mg and pseudoephedrine 45 mg

brompheniramine maleate *see* brompheniramine *on page 147*

brompheniramine maleate and phenylephrine hydrochloride *see* brompheniramine and phenylephrine *on page 148*

brompheniramine maleate and pseudoephedrine hydrochloride *see* brompheniramine and pseudoephedrine *on page 148*

brompheniramine maleate and pseudoephedrine sulfate *see* brompheniramine and pseudoephedrine *on page 148*

brompheniramine, pseudoephedrine, and dextromethorphan

(brome fen IR a meen, soo doe e FED rin, & deks troe meth OR fan)

Synonyms dextromethorphan hydrobromide, brompheniramine maleate, and pseudoephedrine hydrochloride; pseudoephedrine tannate, dextromethorphan tannate, and brompheniramine tannate

U.S./Canadian Brand Names Anaplex® DM [US]; Bromaline® DM [US-OTC]; Bromatane DX [US]; Bromfed® DM [US]; Bromphenex™ DM [US-OTC]; Bromplex DX [US]; Brotapp-DM [US]; EndaCof-DM [US]; EndaCof-PD [US]; Histacol™ BD [US]; Myphetane DX [US]; PediaHist DM [US]

Therapeutic Category Antihistamine; Cough Preparation; Decongestant

Use Relief of cough and upper respiratory symptoms (including nasal congestion) associated with allergy or the common cold

Dosage Summary

Oral:

Children 1-3 months: EndaCof-PD: 0.25 mL 4 times/day
Children 3-6 months: EndaCof-PD: 0.5 mL 4 times/day
Children 6-12 months: EndaCof-PD: 0.75 mL 4 times/day
Children 12-24 months: EndaCof-PD: 1 mL 4 times/day
Children 2-6 years:
Anaplex® DM, EndaCof-DM: 1.25 mL every 4-6 hours (maximum: 4 doses/day)
Children 6-12 years:
Anaplex® DM, EndaCof-DM: 2.5 mL every 4-6 hours (maximum: 4 doses/day)
Bromaline® DM: 10 mL every 4-6 hours (maximum: 4 doses/day)
Children >12 years:
Anaplex® DM, EndaCof-DM: 5 mL every 4-6 hours (maximum: 4 doses/day)
Bromaline® DM: 20 mL every 4-6 hours (maximum: 4 doses/day)
Adults:
Anaplex® DM, EndaCof-DM: 5 mL every 4-6 hours (maximum: 4 doses/day)
Bromaline® DM: 20 mL every 4-6 hours (maximum: 4 doses/day)

Dosage Forms

Elixir, oral:
Bromaline® DM [OTC]: Brompheniramine 1 mg, pseudoephedrine 15 mg, and dextromethorphan 5 mg per 5 mL

Liquid, oral:
Bromphenex™ DM [OTC], Bromplex DM: Brompheniramine 4 mg, pseudoephedrine 60 mg, and dextromethorphan 30 mg per 5 mL
Brotapp-DM: Brompheniramine 1 mg, pseudoephedrine 15 mg, and dextromethorphan 5 mg per 5 mL

Solution, oral [drops]:
EndaCof-PD, Histacol™ BD: Brompheniramine 1 mg, pseudoephedrine 12.5 mg, and dextromethorphan 3 mg per 1 mL
PediaHist DM: Brompheniramine 1 mg, pseudoephedrine 15 mg, and dextromethorphan 4 mg per 1 mL
Resperal-DM: Brompheniramine 1 mg, pseudoephedrine 12 mg, and dextromethorphan 5 mg per 1 mL

Suspension, oral: Brompheniramine 8 mg, pseudoephedrine 90 mg, and dextromethorphan 60 mg per 5 mL

Syrup, oral:
Anaplex® DM, EndaCof-DM: Brompheniramine 4 mg, pseudoephedrine 60 mg, and dextromethorphan 30 mg per 5 mL
Bromatane DX, Myphetane DX: Brompheniramine 2 mg, pseudoephedrine 30 mg, and dextromethorphan 10 mg per 5 mL

brompheniramine tannate *see* brompheniramine *on page 147*

brompheniramine tannate and phenylephrine tannate *see* brompheniramine and phenylephrine *on page 148*

Brompheril® ***(Discontinued)*** *see* dexbrompheniramine and pseudoephedrine *on page 282*

Bromplex DX [US] *see* brompheniramine, pseudoephedrine, and dextromethorphan *on page 149*

Bronchial® ***(Discontinued)***

Bronchial Mist® ***(Discontinued)*** *see* epinephrine (systemic, oral inhalation) *on page 352*

Broncho Saline® ***(Discontinued)*** *see* sodium chloride *on page 882*

Bronitin® Mist ***(Discontinued)*** *see* epinephrine (systemic, oral inhalation) *on page 352*

Brontex® ***(Discontinued)*** *see* guaifenesin and codeine *on page 455*

Brotane® ***(Discontinued)*** *see* brompheniramine *on page 147*

Brotapp [US] *see* brompheniramine and pseudoephedrine *on page 148*

Brotapp-DM [US] *see* brompheniramine, pseudoephedrine, and dextromethorphan *on page 149*

Brovana® [US] *see* arformoterol *on page 93*

BroveX™ CT ***(Discontinued)*** *see* brompheniramine *on page 147*

BroveX™ ***(Discontinued)*** *see* brompheniramine *on page 147*

Brovex SR ***(Discontinued)*** *see* brompheniramine and pseudoephedrine *on page 148*

BSF208075 *see* ambrisentan *on page 62*

BSS® [US/Can] *see* balanced salt solution *on page 116*

BSS Plus® [US/Can] *see* balanced salt solution *on page* 116
B-Tuss™ [US] *see* phenylephrine, hydrocodone, and chlorpheniramine *on page* 754
BTX-A *see* onabotulinumtoxinA *on page* 703
B-type natriuretic peptide (human) *see* nesiritide *on page* 669
Budeprion XL® [US] *see* bupropion *on page* 156
Budeprion SR® [US] *see* bupropion *on page* 156

budesonide (systemic, oral inhalation) (byoo DES oh nide)

U.S./Canadian Brand Names Entocort® EC [US]; Entocort® [Can]; Pulmicort Flexhaler® [US]; Pulmicort Respules® [US]; Pulmicort® [Can]

Therapeutic Category Corticosteroid, Inhalant (Oral); Corticosteroid, Systemic

Use

Nebulization: Maintenance and prophylactic treatment of asthma

Oral capsule: Treatment of active Crohn disease (mild-to-moderate) involving the ileum and/or ascending colon; maintenance of remission (for up to 3 months) of Crohn disease (mild-to-moderate) involving the ileum and/or ascending colon

Oral inhalation: Maintenance and prophylactic treatment of asthma; includes patients who require oral corticosteroids and those who may benefit from systemic dose reduction/elimination

Dosage Summary

Inhalation:

Children <6 years: Dosage not established

Children ≥6 years: 180-360 mcg twice daily; Low dose: 180-400 mcg/day in 2 divided doses; Medium dose: >400-800 mcg/day in 2 divided doses; High dose: >800 mcg/day in 2 divided doses

Adults: 180-720 mcg twice daily, Low dose: 180-600 mcg/day in 2 divided doses; Medium dose: >600-1200 mcg/day in 2 divided doses; High dose: >1200 mcg/day in 2 divided doses

Nebulization:

Children <12 months: Dosage not established

Children 12 months to 8 years: 0.25-1 mg in 1-2 divided doses

Children >8 years: Dosage not established

Adults: Dosage not established

Oral:

Children: Dosage not established

Adults: Initial: 9 mg once daily; Maintenance: 6 mg once daily

Dosage Forms

Capsule, enteric coated, oral:

Entocort® EC: 3 mg

Powder, for oral inhalation:

Pulmicort Flexhaler®: 90 mcg/inhalation (165 mg); 180 mcg/inhalation (225 mg)

Suspension, for nebulization: 0.25 mg/2 mL (30s); 0.5 mg/2 mL (30s)

Pulmicort Respules®: 0.25 mg/2 mL (30s); 0.5 mg/2 mL (30s); 1 mg/2 mL (30s)

Dosage Forms - Canada

Powder for oral inhalation:

Pulmicort Turbuhaler®: 100 mcg/inhalation, 200 mcg/inhalation, 400 mcg/inhalation

budesonide (nasal) (byoo DES oh nide)

U.S./Canadian Brand Names Gen-Budesonide AQ [Can]; Mylan-Budesonide AQ [Can]; Rhinocort Aqua® [US/Can]; Rhinocort® Turbuhaler® [Can]

Therapeutic Category Corticosteroid, Nasal

Use Management of symptoms of seasonal or perennial rhinitis

Canadian labeling: Additional use (not in U.S. labeling): Prevention and treatment of nasal polyps

Dosage Summary

Intranasal inhalation:

Children <6 years: Dosage not established

Children ≥6 years: 64 mcg/day as a single 32 mcg spray in each nostril (maximum: 129 mcg/day [children <12 years])

Adults: 64 mcg/day as a single 32 mcg spray in each nostril (maximum: 256 mcg/day)

Dosage Forms

Suspension, intranasal:

Rhinocort Aqua®: 32 mcg/inhalation (8.6 g)

Dosage Forms - Canada

Powder for nasal inhalation:

Rhinocort® Turbuhaler®: 100 mcg/inhalation

Suspension, intranasal [spray]:

Rhinocort® Aqua®: 64 mcg/inhalation

budesonide and eformoterol *see* budesonide and formoterol *on page* 152

budesonide and formoterol (byoo DES oh nide & for MOH te rol)

Synonyms budesonide and eformoterol; eformoterol and budesonide; formoterol and budesonide; formoterol fumarate dihydrate and budesonide

U.S./Canadian Brand Names Symbicort® [US/Can]

Therapeutic Category $Beta_2$-Adrenergic Agonist Agent; Corticosteroid, Inhalant (Oral)

Use Treatment of asthma in patients ≥12 years of age where combination therapy is indicated; maintenance treatment of airflow obstruction associated with chronic obstructive pulmonary disease (COPD; including chronic bronchitis and emphysema)

Dosage Summary

Inhalation:

Children <5 years: Dosage not established

Children 5-11 years: (NIH Guidelines): Symbicort® 80/4.5: Two inhalations twice daily. Do not exceed 4 inhalations per day.

Children ≥12 years: Two inhalations once or twice daily (maximum: 4 inhalations/day).

Adults: Two inhalations twice daily (maximum: 4 inhalations/day)

Dosage Forms

Aerosol for oral inhalation:

Symbicort® 80/4.5: Budesonide 80 mcg and formoterol fumarate dihydrate 4.5 mcg per actuation (6.9 g) [60 metered inhalations]; budesonide 80 mcg and formoterol fumarate dihydrate 4.5 mcg per actuation (10.2 g) [120 metered inhalations]

Symbicort® 160/4.5: Budesonide 160 mcg and formoterol fumarate dihydrate 4.5 mcg per actuation (6 g) [60 metered inhalations]; budesonide 160 mcg and formoterol fumarate dihydrate 4.5 mcg per actuation (10.2 g) [120 metered inhalations]

Dosage Forms - Canada

Powder for oral inhalation:

Symbicort® 100 Turbuhaler®: Budesonide 100 mcg and formoterol dihydrate 6 mcg per inhalation (available in 60 or 120 metered doses) [delivers ~80 mcg budesonide and 4.5 mcg formoterol per inhalation]

Symbicort® 200 Turbuhaler®: Budesonide 200 mcg and formoterol dihydrate 6 mcg per inhalation (available in 60 or 120 metered doses) [delivers ~160 mcg budesonide and 4.5 mcg formoterol per inhalation]

Buffasal [US-OTC] *see* aspirin *on page* 100

Bufferin® [US-OTC] *see* aspirin *on page* 100

Bufferin® Extra Strength [US-OTC] *see* aspirin *on page* 100

Buffinol [US-OTC] *see* aspirin *on page* 100

Bulk-K [US-OTC] *see* psyllium *on page* 814

bumetanide (byoo MET a nide)

Sound-Alike/Look-Alike Issues

bumetanide may be confused with Buminate®

Bumex® may be confused with Brevibloc®, Buprenex®, Permax®

U.S./Canadian Brand Names Burinex® [Can]

Therapeutic Category Diuretic, Loop

Use Management of edema secondary to heart failure or hepatic or renal disease (including nephrotic syndrome)

Dosage Summary

I.M.:

Infants and children: 0.015-0.1 mg/kg/dose every 6-24 hours (maximum: 10 mg/day)

Adults: 0.5-1 mg/dose; may repeat in 2-3 hours for up to 2 doses (maximum: 10 mg/day)

I.V.:

Infants and children: 0.015-0.1 mg/kg/dose every 6-24 hours (maximum: 10 mg/day)

Adults: 0.5-1 mg/dose; may repeat in 2-3 hours for up to 2 doses (maximum: 10 mg/day)

Oral:

Infants and children: 0.015-0.1 mg/kg/dose every 6-24 hours (maximum: 10 mg/day)

Adults: 0.5-2 mg 1-2 times/day; may repeat in 4-5 hours for up to 2 doses (maximum: 5 mg/day [HTN]; 10 mg/day [edema])

Dosage Forms

Injection, solution: 0.25 mg/mL (2 mL, 4 mL, 5 mL, 10 mL)

Tablet, oral: 0.5 mg, 1 mg, 2 mg

Bumex® ***(Discontinued)*** *see* bumetanide *on page* 152

Bumex® Injection ***(Discontinued)*** *see* bumetanide *on page* 152

Buminate [US] *see* albumin *on page* 43

Bupap [US] *see* butalbital and acetaminophen *on page* 159

Buphenyl® [US] *see* sodium phenylbutyrate *on page* 886

bupivacaine (byoo PIV a kane)

Sound-Alike/Look-Alike Issues

bupivacaine may be confused with mepivacaine, ropivacaine

Marcaine® may be confused with Narcan®

Synonyms bupivacaine hydrochloride

U.S./Canadian Brand Names Bupivacaine Spinal [US]; Marcaine® Spinal [US]; Marcaine® [US/Can]; Sensorcaine® [US/Can]; Sensorcaine®-MPF Spinal [US]; Sensorcaine®-MPF [US]

Therapeutic Category Local Anesthetic

Use Peripheral nerve block; infiltration; sympathetic block; spinal, caudal, or epidural block; retrobulbar block

Dosage Summary Note: Dose varies with procedure, depth of anesthesia, vascularity of tissues, duration of anesthesia, and condition of patient. Do not use solutions containing preservatives for caudal or epidural block.

Caudal block:

Children ≤12 years: Dosage not established

Children >12 years: 15-30 mL of 0.25% or 0.5%

Adults: 15-30 mL of 0.25% or 0.5%

Epidural block:

Children ≤12 years: Dosage not established

Children >12 years: 10-20 mL of 0.25% or 0.5% in 3-5 mL increments **or** 10-20 mL of 0.75% if high degree of muscle relaxation and prolonged effects needed

Adults: 10-20 mL of 0.25% or 0.5% in 3-5 mL increments **or** 10-20 mL of 0.75% if high degree of muscle relaxation and prolonged effects needed

Infiltration (local):

Children ≤12 years: Dosage not established

Children >12 years: 0.25% (maximum: 175 mg)

Adults: 0.25% (maximum: 175 mg)

Nerve block:

Children ≤12 years: Dosage not established

Children >12 years: Peripheral: 5 mL of 0.25% or 0.5% (maximum: 400 mg/day); Sympathetic: 20-50 mL of 0.25%

Adults: Peripheral: 5 mL of 0.25% or 0.5% (maximum: 400 mg/day); Sympathetic: 20-50 mL of 0.25%

Retrobulbar anesthesia:

Children ≤12 years: Dosage not established

Children >12 years: 2-4 mL of 0.75%

Adults: 2-4 mL of 0.75%

Spinal:

Children: Dosage not established

Adults: Preservative free solution of 0.75% bupivacaine in 8.25% dextrose:

Cesarean section: 1-1.4 mL

Lower abdominal procedures: 1.6 mL

Lower extremity and perineal procedures: 1 mL

Normal vaginal delivery: 0.8 mL (higher doses may be required in some patients)

Dosage Forms

Injection, solution: 0.25% [2.5 mg/mL] (50 mL); 0.5% [5 mg/mL] (50 mL)

Marcaine®: 0.5% [5 mg/mL] (50 mL)

Sensorcaine®: 0.25% [2.5 mg/mL] (50 mL); 0.5% [5 mg/mL] (50 mL)

Injection, solution [preservative free]: 0.25% [2.5 mg/mL] (10 mL, 20 mL, 30 mL, 50 mL); 0.5% [5 mg/mL] (10 mL, 20 mL, 30 mL); 0.75% [7.5 mg/mL] (10 mL, 20 mL, 30 mL)

Marcaine®: 0.25% [2.5 mg/mL] (10 mL, 30 mL, 50 mL); 0.5% [5 mg/mL] (10 mL, 30 mL); 0.75% [7.5 mg/mL] (10 mL, 30 mL)

Sensorcaine®-MPF: 0.25% [2.5 mg/mL] (10 mL, 30 mL); 0.5% [5 mg/mL] (10 mL, 30 mL); 0.75% [7.5 mg/mL] (10 mL, 30 mL)

Injection, solution, premixed in $D_{8.25}W$ [preservative free]:

Bupivacaine Spinal: 0.75% [7.5 mg/mL] (2 mL)

Marcaine® Spinal: 0.75% [7.5 mg/mL] (2 mL)

Sensorcaine®-MPF Spinal: 0.75% [7.5 mg/mL] (2 mL)

bupivacaine and epinephrine (byoo PIV a kane & ep i NEF rin)

Synonyms epinephrine bitartrate and bupivacaine hydrochloride

U.S./Canadian Brand Names Marcaine® with Epinephrine [US]; Sensorcaine® with Epinephrine [US/Can]; Sensorcaine®-MPF with Epinephrine [US]; Vivacaine™ [US]

Therapeutic Category Local Anesthetic

Use Local anesthetic (injectable) for peripheral nerve block, infiltration, sympathetic block, caudal or epidural block, retrobulbar block

Dosage Summary Note: Dose varies with procedure, depth of anesthesia, vascularity of tissues, duration of anesthesia, and condition of patient. Do not use solutions containing preservatives for caudal or epidural block.

Caudal block (preservative free):

Children ≤12 years: Dosage not established

Children >12 years: 15-30 mL of 0.25% or 0.5%

Adults: 15-30 mL of 0.25% or 0.5%

Epidural block (preservative free):

Children ≤12 years: Dosage not established

Children >12 years: 10-20 mL of 0.25% or 0.5% in 3-5 mL increments **or** 10-20 mL of 0.75% if high degree of muscle relaxation or prolonged effects needed

Adults: 10-20 mL of 0.25% or 0.5% in 3-5 mL increments **or** 10-20 mL of 0.75% if high degree of muscle relaxation or prolonged effects needed

Infiltration (local):

Children ≤12 years: Dosage not established

Children >12 years: 0.25% (maximum: 175 mg [bupivacaine])

Adults: 0.25% (maximum: 175 mg [bupivacaine])

Infiltration and nerve block (maxillary; mandibular):

Children ≤12 years: Dosage not established

Children >12 years: 9 mg (1.8 mL) of bupivacaine as a 0.5% solution with epinephrine 1:200,000 per injection site; may repeat after 10 minutes if needed (maximum: 90 mg bupivacaine/appointment)

Adults: 9 mg (1.8 mL) of bupivacaine as a 0.5% solution with epinephrine 1:200,000 per injection site; may repeat after 10 minutes if needed (maximum: 90 mg bupivacaine/appointment)

Nerve block:

Children ≤12 years: Dosage not established

Children >12 years: Peripheral: 5 mL of 0.25 or 0.5% (maximum: 400 mg/day [bupivacaine]); Sympathetic: 20-50 mL of 0.25%

Adults: Peripheral: 5 mL of 0.25 or 0.5% (maximum: 400 mg/day [bupivacaine]); Sympathetic: 20-50 mL of 0.25%

Retrobulbar anesthesia:

Children ≤12 years: Dosage not established

Children >12 years: 2-4 mL of 0.75%

Adults: 2-4 mL of 0.75%

Dosage Forms

Injection, solution [preservative free]: Bupivacaine 0.25% and epinephrine 1:200,000 (10 mL, 30 mL); bupivacaine 0.5% and epinephrine 1:200,000 (10 mL, 30 mL)

Marcaine® with Epinephrine: Bupivacaine 0.25% and epinephrine 1:200,000 (10 mL, 30 mL); bupivacaine 0.5% and epinephrine 1:200,000 (10 mL, 30 mL)

Sensorcaine® MPF with Epinephrine: Bupivacaine 0.25% and epinephrine 1:200,000 (10 mL, 30 mL); bupivacaine 0.5% and epinephrine 1:200,000 (10 mL, 30 mL); bupivacaine 0.75% and epinephrine 1:200,000 (30 mL)

Injection, solution: Bupivacaine 0.25% and epinephrine 1:200,000 (50 mL); bupivacaine 0.5% and epinephrine 1:200,000 (50 mL)

Marcaine® with Epinephrine, Sensorcaine® with Epinephrine: Bupivacaine 0.25% and epinephrine 1:200,000 (50 mL); bupivacaine 0.5% and epinephrine 1:200,000 (50 mL)

Injection, solution [for dental use]:

Marcaine® with Epinephrine, Vivacaine™: Bupivacaine 0.5% and epinephrine 1:200,000 (1.8 mL)

bupivacaine hydrochloride *see* bupivacaine *on page 153*

Bupivacaine Spinal [US] *see* bupivacaine *on page 153*

Buprenex® [US/Can] *see* buprenorphine *on page 155*

buprenorphine (byoo pre NOR feen)

Sound-Alike/Look-Alike Issues

Buprenex® may be confused with Brevibloc®, Bumex®

Synonyms buprenorphine hydrochloride; Butrans™

U.S./Canadian Brand Names Buprenex® [US/Can]; Subutex® [US/Can]

Therapeutic Category Analgesic, Narcotic

Controlled Substance Injection: C-V/C-III; Tablet: C-III

Use

Injection: Management of moderate-to-severe pain

Tablet: Treatment of opioid dependence

Dosage Summary

I.M.:

Children <2 years: Dosage not established

Children 2-12 years: 2-6 mcg/kg every 4-6 hours

Children ≥13 years: Initial: 0.3 mg, may repeat once in 30-60 minutes then every 6-8 hours as needed; Maintenance: 0.15-0.6 mg every 4-8 hours as needed

Adults: Initial: 0.3 mg, may repeat once in 30-60 minutes then every 6-8 hours as needed; Maintenance: 0.15-0.6 mg every 4-8 hours as needed

Elderly: 0.15 mg every 6 hours

I.V.:

Children <2 years: Dosage not established

Children 2-12 years: 2-6 mcg/kg every 4-6 hours

Children ≥13 years: Initial: 0.3 mg, may repeat once in 30-60 minutes then every 6-8 hours as needed

Adults: Initial: 0.3 mg, may repeat once in 30-60 minutes then every 6-8 hours as needed

Elderly: 0.15 mg every 6 hours

Sublingual:

Children <16 years: Dosage not established

Children ≥16 years: Induction: 12-16 mg/day; Maintenance: 4-24 mg/day (target dose: 16 mg/day)

Adults: Induction: 12-16 mg/day; Maintenance: 4-24 mg/day (target dose: 16 mg/day)

Product Availability

Butrans™: FDA approved June 2010; availability expected in early 2011

Butrans™ is a transdermal system indicated for moderate-to-severe chronic pain in patients requiring an around-the-clock opioid analgesic for an extended period of time.

Dosage Forms

Injection, solution: 0.3 mg/mL (1 mL)

Buprenex®: 0.3 mg/mL (1 mL)

Tablet, sublingual: 2 mg, 8 mg

Subutex®: 2 mg, 8 mg

buprenorphine and naloxone (byoo pre NOR feen & nal OKS one)

Synonyms buprenorphine hydrochloride and naloxone hydrochloride dihydrate; naloxone and buprenorphine; naloxone hydrochloride dihydrate and buprenorphine hydrochloride

U.S./Canadian Brand Names Suboxone® [US]

Therapeutic Category Analgesic, Narcotic

Controlled Substance C-III

Use Treatment of opioid dependence

Dosage Summary

Sublingual:

Children <16 years: Dosage not established

Children ≥16 years: Initial: Begin with buprenorphine tablets, combination not recommended; Maintenance: 4-24 mg/day (target dose: 16 mg/day)

Adults: Initial: Begin with buprenorphine tablets, combination not recommended; Maintenance: 4-24 mg/day (target dose: 16 mg/day)

Product Availability

Suboxone® sublingual film: FDA approved August 2010; availability expected in early October 2010

Suboxone® sublingual film was shown to have a faster dissolution rate and improved palatability when compared with Suboxone® sublingual tablets, thereby gaining patient preference

Dosage Forms

Tablet, sublingual:

Suboxone®: Buprenorphine 2 mg and naloxone 0.5 mg; buprenorphine 8 mg and naloxone 2 mg

buprenorphine hydrochloride *see* buprenorphine *on page 155*

buprenorphine hydrochloride and naloxone hydrochloride dihydrate *see* buprenorphine and naloxone *on page 155*

Buproban® [US] *see* bupropion *on page 156*

bupropion (byoo PROE pee on)

Sound-Alike/Look-Alike Issues

buPROPion may be confused with busPIRone

Aplenzin™ may be confused with Albenza®, Relenza®

Wellbutrin SR® may be confused with Wellbutrin XL®

Wellbutrin XL® may be confused with Wellbutrin SR®

Zyban® may be confused with Zagam®, Diovan®

Synonyms bupropion hydrobromide; bupropion hydrochloride

Tall-Man bu**PROP**ion

U.S./Canadian Brand Names Aplenzin™ [US]; Budeprion SR® [US]; Budeprion XL® [US]; Buproban® [US]; Bupropion SR® [Can]; Novo-Bupropion SR [Can]; PMS-Bupropion SR [Can]; ratio-Bupropion SR [Can]; Sandoz-Bupropion SR [Can]; Wellbutrin SR® [US/Can]; Wellbutrin XL® [US/Can]; Wellbutrin® [US]; Zyban® [US/Can]

Therapeutic Category Antidepressant, Aminoketone

Use Treatment of major depressive disorder, including seasonal affective disorder (SAD); adjunct in smoking cessation

Dosage Summary

Oral:

Extended release:

Children: Dosage not established

Adults: Initial: Hydrochloride salt:150 mg once daily; Maintenance: 300 mg once daily (maximum: 450 mg/day); Hydrobromide salt: 174-522 mg/day

Immediate release hydrochloride salt:

Adults: Initial: 100 mg twice daily; Maintenance: 100 mg 3 times/day (maximum: 450 mg/day)

Elderly: Initial: 37.5 mg twice daily, increase by 37.5-100 mg every 3-4 days as tolerated

Sustained release hydrochloride salt:

Children: Dosage not established

Adults: Initial: 150 mg once daily; Maintenance: 150 mg twice daily (maximum: 400 mg/day)

Elderly: Initial: 100 mg/day, increase by 37.5-100 mg every 3-4 days as tolerated

Dosage Forms

Tablet, oral: 75 mg, 100 mg

Wellbutrin®: 75 mg, 100 mg

Tablet, extended release, oral: 100 mg, 150 mg, 200 mg, 300 mg

Aplenzin™: 174 mg, 348 mg, 522 mg

Budeprion SR®: 100 mg, 150 mg

Budeprion XL®: 150 mg, 300 mg

Buproban®: 150 mg

Wellbutrin XL®: 150 mg, 300 mg

Tablet, sustained release, oral:

Wellbutrin SR®: 100 mg, 150 mg, 200 mg

Zyban®: 150 mg

bupropion hydrobromide *see* bupropion *on page 156*
bupropion hydrochloride *see* bupropion *on page 156*
Bupropion SR® [Can] *see* bupropion *on page 156*
Burinex® [Can] *see* bumetanide *on page 152*
Burn Jel® [US-OTC] *see* lidocaine (topical) *on page 562*
Burn Jel Plus [US-OTC] *see* lidocaine (topical) *on page 562*
Buscopan® [Can] *see* scopolamine derivatives (systemic) *on page 866*

buserelin acetate *(Canada only)* (BYOO se rel in AS e tate)

Sound-Alike/Look-Alike Issues
Suprefact® may be confused with Suprane®

U.S./Canadian Brand Names Suprefact® Depot [Can]; Suprefact® [Can]

Therapeutic Category Luteinizing Hormone-Releasing Hormone Analog

Use Palliative treatment in patients with hormone-dependent advanced prostate cancer (stage D); treatment of endometriosis in women who do not require surgical intervention as first-line therapy (length of therapy is usually 6 months, but no longer than 9 months)

Dosage Summary

Intranasal:
Children: Dosage not established
Adults: 400 mcg (200 mcg into each nostril) 3 times/day; **Note:** Treatment is 6-9 months for endometriosis

SubQ:
Children: Dosage not established
Adults:
Implants: 6.3 mg every 8 weeks **or** 9.45 mg every 12 weeks
Injection: Initial: 500 mcg every 8 hours for 7 days; maintenance: 200 mcg once daily

Dosage Forms - Canada

Injection, solution:
Suprefact®: 1 mg/mL (5.5 mL, 10 mL)

Solution, intranasal:
Suprefact®: 1mg/1mL (10 mL)

Implant, subcutaneous:
Suprefact® Depot: 6.3 mg, 9.45 mg

BuSpar® [Can] *see* buspirone *on page 157*
BuSpar® *(Discontinued)* *see* buspirone *on page 157*
Buspirex [Can] *see* buspirone *on page 157*

buspirone (byoo SPYE rone)

Sound-Alike/Look-Alike Issues
busPIRone may be confused with buPROPion

Synonyms buspirone hydrochloride

Tall-Man bus**PIR**one

U.S./Canadian Brand Names Apo-Buspirone® [Can]; BuSpar® [Can]; Buspirex [Can]; Bustab® [Can]; CO Buspirone [Can]; Dom-Buspirone [Can]; Gen-Buspirone [Can]; Lin-Buspirone [Can]; Mylan-Buspirone [Can]; Novo-Buspirone [Can]; Nu-Buspirone [Can]; PMS-Buspirone [Can]; ratio-Buspirone [Can]; Riva-Buspirone [Can]

Therapeutic Category Antianxiety Agent

Use Management of generalized anxiety disorder (GAD)

Dosage Summary

Oral:
Children <6 years: Dosing not established
Children ≥6 years: Initial: 5 mg daily; Maintenance: Up to 60 mg/day in 2-3 divided doses; **Note:** Titration is recommended
Adolescents: Initial: 5 mg daily; Maintenance: Up to 60 mg/day in 2-3 divided doses; **Note:** Titration is recommended
Adults: Initial: 7.5 mg twice daily; Maintenance: Up to 60 mg/day in 2 divided doses (target dose: 10-15 mg twice daily); **Note:** Titration is recommended

Elderly: Initial: 5 mg twice daily; Maintenance: 20-30 mg/day (maximum: 60 mg/day); **Note:** Titration is recommended

Dosage Forms

Tablet, oral: 5 mg, 7.5 mg, 10 mg, 15 mg, 30 mg

buspirone hydrochloride *see* buspirone *on page 157*

Bustab® [Can] *see* buspirone *on page 157*

busulfan (byoo SUL fan)

Sound-Alike/Look-Alike Issues

busulfan may be confused with Butalan®

Myleran® may be confused with Alkeran®, Leukeran®, melphalan, Mylicon®

Synonyms NSC-750

U.S./Canadian Brand Names Busulfex® [US/Can]; Myleran® [US/Can]

Therapeutic Category Antineoplastic Agent

Use

Oral: Chronic myelogenous leukemia (CML); conditioning regimens for bone marrow transplantation

I.V.: Combination therapy with cyclophosphamide as a conditioning regimen prior to allogeneic hematopoietic progenitor cell transplantation for chronic myelogenous leukemia

Dosage Summary

I.V.:

Children ≤12 kg: **BMT:** 1.1 mg/kg (ideal body weight) every 6 hours for 16 doses

Children >12 kg: **BMT:** 0.8 mg/kg (ideal body weight) every 6 hours for 16 doses

Adults: **BMT:** 0.8 mg/kg (ideal body weight or actual body weight, whichever is lower) every 6 hours for 16 doses

Oral:

Children: Induction: 0.06-0.12 mg/kg/day **or** 1.8-4.6 mg/m^2/day; Maintenance: Titrate to maintain leukocyte counts above 40,000/mm^3; **BMT:** 1 mg/kg (ideal body weight) every 6 hours for 16 doses

Adults: Induction: 60 mcg/kg/day or 1.8 mg/m^2/day; usual range: 4-12 mg/day; Maintenance: 1-4 mg/day to 2 mg/week; **BMT:** 1 mg/kg (ideal body weight) every 6 hours for 16 doses

Dosage Forms

Injection, solution:

Busulfex®: 6 mg/mL (10 mL)

Tablet, oral:

Myleran®: 2 mg

Busulfex® [US/Can] *see* busulfan *on page 158*

butabarbital (byoo ta BAR bi tal)

Sound-Alike/Look-Alike Issues

butabarbital may be confused with butalbital

U.S./Canadian Brand Names Butisol Sodium® [US]

Therapeutic Category Barbiturate

Controlled Substance C-III

Use Sedative; hypnotic

Dosage Summary

Oral:

Children: 2-6 mg/kg preoperatively (maximum: 100 mg)

Adults: 15-30 mg 3-4 times/day **or** 50-100 mg prior to bedtime or surgery

Elderly: Use with caution; reduce dose if use is needed

Dosage Forms

Elixir, oral:

Butisol Sodium®: 30 mg/5 mL (480 mL)

Tablet, oral:

Butisol Sodium®: 30 mg, 50 mg

Butalan® ***(Discontinued)***

butalbital, acetaminophen, and caffeine

(byoo TAL bi tal, a seet a MIN oh fen, & KAF een)

Sound-Alike/Look-Alike Issues

Fioricet® may be confused with Fiorinal®, Lorcet®

Repan® may be confused with Riopan®

Synonyms acetaminophen, butalbital, and caffeine

U.S./Canadian Brand Names Alagesic LQ [US]; Alagesic [US]; Anolor 300 [US]; Dolgic® Plus [US]; Esgic-Plus™ [US]; Esgic® [US]; Fioricet® [US]; Margesic [US]; Orbivan™ [US]; Repan® [US]; Zebutal® [US]

Therapeutic Category Barbiturate/Analgesic

Use Relief of the symptomatic complex of tension or muscle contraction headache

Dosage Summary

Oral:

Children: Dosage not established

Adults: 1-2 tablets/capsules or 15-30 mL every 4 hours (maximum: 6 tablets/capsules daily; 180 mL/day)

Elderly: Use not recommended

Dosage Forms

Capsule, oral:

Anolor 300, Esgic®, Margesic: Butalbital 50 mg, acetaminophen 325 mg, and caffeine 40 mg

Esgic-Plus™, Zebutal®: Butalbital 50 mg, acetaminophen 500 mg, and caffeine 40 mg

Orbivan™: Butalbital 50 mg, acetaminophen 300 mg, and caffeine 40 mg

Liquid, oral:

Alagesic LQ: Butalbital 50 mg, acetaminophen 325 mg, and caffeine 40 mg per 15 mL

Tablet, oral: Butalbital 50 mg, acetaminophen 325 mg, and caffeine 40 mg; butalbital 50 mg, acetaminophen 500 mg, and caffeine 40 mg

Dolgic® Plus: Butalbital 50 mg, acetaminophen 750 mg, and caffeine 40 mg

Esgic®, Fioricet®, Repan®: Butalbital 50 mg, acetaminophen 325 mg, and caffeine 40 mg

Esgic-Plus™: Butalbital 50 mg, acetaminophen 500 mg, and caffeine 40 mg

butalbital, acetaminophen, caffeine, and codeine

(byoo TAL bi tal, a seet a MIN oh fen, KAF een, & KOE deen)

Sound-Alike/Look-Alike Issues

Fioricet® may be confused with Fiorinal®, Florinef®, Lorcet®, Percocet®

Phrenilin® may be confused with Phenergan®, Trinalin®

Synonyms acetaminophen, caffeine, codeine, and butalbital; caffeine, acetaminophen, butalbital, and codeine; codeine, acetaminophen, butalbital, and caffeine

U.S./Canadian Brand Names Fioricet® with Codeine [US]

Therapeutic Category Analgesic Combination (Opioid); Barbiturate

Controlled Substance C-III

Use Relief of symptoms of complex tension (muscle contraction) headache

Dosage Summary

Oral:

Children: Dosage not established

Adults: 1-2 capsules every 4 hours (maximum: 6 capsules/day)

Dosage Forms

Capsule: Butalbital 50 mg, acetaminophen 325 mg, caffeine 40 mg, and codeine 30 mg

Fioricet® with Codeine: Butalbital 50 mg, acetaminophen 325 mg, caffeine 40 mg, and codeine 30 mg

butalbital and acetaminophen (byoo TAL bi tal & a seet a MIN oh fen)

Synonyms acetaminophen and butalbital

U.S./Canadian Brand Names Bupap [US]; Cephadyn [US]; Phrenilin® Forte [US]; Phrenilin® [US]; Promacet [US]; Sedapap® [US]

Therapeutic Category Analgesic, Miscellaneous; Barbiturate

Use Relief of the symptomatic complex of tension or muscle contraction headache

Dosage Summary

Oral:

Children: Dosage not established

Adults: One tablet/capsule every 4 hours as needed (maximum: 6 doses/day) **or** Phrenilin®: 1-2 tablets every 4 hours as needed (maximum: 6 tablets/day)

Dosage Forms

Tablet:

Phrenilin®: Butalbital 50 mg and acetaminophen 325 mg

Bupap, Cephadyn, Promacet, Sedapap®: Butalbital 50 mg and acetaminophen 650 mg

Capsule:

Phrenilin® Forte: Butalbital 50 mg and acetaminophen 650 mg

butalbital, aspirin, and caffeine (byoo TAL bi tal, AS pir in, & KAF een)

Sound-Alike/Look-Alike Issues

Fiorinal® may be confused with Fioricet®, Florical®, Florinef®

Synonyms aspirin, caffeine, and butalbital; butalbital compound

U.S./Canadian Brand Names Fiorinal® [US/Can]

Therapeutic Category Barbiturate/Analgesic

Controlled Substance C-III

Use Relief of the symptomatic complex of tension or muscle contraction headache

Dosage Summary

Oral:

Children: Dosage not established

Adults: 1-2 tablets/capsules every 4 hours (maximum: 6 tablets/capsules daily)

Elderly: Use not recommended

Dosage Forms

Capsule: Butalbital 50 mg, aspirin 325 mg, and caffeine 40 mg

Fiorinal®: Butalbital 50 mg, aspirin 325 mg, and caffeine 40 mg

Tablet: Butalbital 50 mg, aspirin 325 mg, and caffeine 40 mg

butalbital, aspirin, caffeine, and codeine

(byoo TAL bi tal, AS pir in, KAF een, & KOE deen)

Sound-Alike/Look-Alike Issues

Fiorinal® may be confused with Fioricet®, Florical®, Florinef®

Synonyms aspirin, caffeine, codeine, and butalbital; butalbital compound and codeine; codeine and butalbital compound; codeine, butalbital, aspirin, and caffeine

U.S./Canadian Brand Names Ascomp® with Codeine [US]; Fiorinal® with Codeine [US]; Fiorinal®-C 1/2 [Can]; Fiorinal®-C 1/4 [Can]; Tecnal C 1/2 [Can]; Tecnal C 1/4 [Can]

Therapeutic Category Analgesic, Narcotic; Barbiturate

Controlled Substance C-III

Use Relief of symptoms of complex tension (muscle contraction) headache

Dosage Summary

Oral:

Children: Dosage not established

Adults: 1-2 capsules every 4 hours as needed (maximum: 6 capsules/day)

Elderly: Use with caution; however, barbiturates (butalbital) are generally not recommended in the elderly.

Dosage Forms

Capsule: Butalbital 50 mg, aspirin 325 mg, caffeine 40 mg, and codeine 30 mg

Ascomp® with Codeine, Fiorinal® with Codeine: Butalbital 50 mg, aspirin 325 mg, caffeine 40 mg, and codeine 30 mg

butalbital compound *see* butalbital, aspirin, and caffeine *on page* 160

butalbital compound and codeine *see* butalbital, aspirin, caffeine, and codeine *on page* 160

butamben, tetracaine, and benzocaine *see* benzocaine, butamben, and tetracaine *on page* 127

butenafine (byoo TEN a feen)

Sound-Alike/Look-Alike Issues

Lotrimin® may be confused with Lotrisone®, Otrivin®

Synonyms butenafine hydrochloride

U.S./Canadian Brand Names Lotrimin® ultra™ [US-OTC]; Mentax® [US]

Therapeutic Category Antifungal Agent

Use Topical treatment of tinea pedis (athlete's foot), tinea cruris (jock itch), tinea corporis (ringworm), and tinea versicolor

Dosage Summary

Topical:

Children ≤12 years: Dosage not established

Children >12 years: Apply to affected area once or twice daily

Adults: Apply to affected area once or twice daily

Dosage Forms

Cream, topical:

Lotrimin® ultra™ [OTC]: 1% (12 g, 24 g)

Mentax®: 1% (15 g, 30 g)

butenafine hydrochloride *see* butenafine *on page 160*

Buticaps® ***(Discontinued)***

Butisol Sodium® [US] *see* butabarbital *on page 158*

butoconazole (byoo toe KOE na zole)

Synonyms butoconazole nitrate

U.S./Canadian Brand Names Femstat® One [Can]; Gynazole-1® [US/Can]

Therapeutic Category Antifungal Agent

Use Local treatment of vulvovaginal candidiasis

Dosage Summary

Intravaginal:

Children: Dosage not established

Adults: Insert 1 applicatorful at bedtime

Dosage Forms

Cream, vaginal:

Gynazole-1®: 2% (5 g)

butoconazole nitrate *see* butoconazole *on page 161*

butorphanol (byoo TOR fa nole)

Sound-Alike/Look-Alike Issues

Stadol® may be confused with Haldol®, sotalol

Synonyms butorphanol tartrate

U.S./Canadian Brand Names Apo-Butorphanol® [Can]; PMS-Butorphanol [Can]

Therapeutic Category Analgesic, Narcotic

Controlled Substance C-IV

Use

Parenteral: Management of moderate-to-severe pain; preoperative medication; supplement to balanced anesthesia; management of pain during labor

Nasal spray: Management of moderate-to-severe pain, including migraine headache pain

Dosage Summary

I.M.:

Children: Dosage not established

Adults: Initial: 2 mg, may repeat every 3-4 hours as needed; Usual range: 1-4 mg every 3-4 hours as needed **or** 2 mg prior to surgery

Elderly: Initial: 1/2 of the recommended dose, repeated dosing generally should be at least 6 hours apart

I.V.:

Children: Dosage not established

Adults: Initial: 1 mg, may repeat every 3-4 hours as needed; Usual range: 0.5-2 mg every 3-4 hours as needed **or** 2 mg and/or an incremental dose of 0.5-1 mg (up to 0.06 mg/kg) as supplement to surgery

Elderly: Initial: 1/2 of the recommended dose, repeated dosing generally should be at least 6 hours apart

Intranasal:

Children: Dosage not established

Adults: Initial: 1 spray (~1 mg) in 1 nostril, may repeat in 60-90 minutes, then repeat initial dose sequence in 3-4 hours after last dose as needed; may use initial dose of 1 spray in each nostril (2 mg) in patients who will remain recumbent

Elderly: Initial: Should not exceed 1 mg, may repeat after 90-120 minutes

Dosage Forms

Injection, solution: 1 mg/mL (1 mL); 2 mg/mL (1 mL, 2 mL, 10 mL)
Injection, solution [preservative free]: 1 mg/mL (1 mL); 2 mg/mL (1 mL, 2 mL)
Solution, intranasal: 10 mg/mL (2.5 mL)

butorphanol tartrate *see* butorphanol *on page 161*
Butrans™ *see* buprenorphine *on page 155*
B-Vex D *(Discontinued)* *see* brompheniramine and phenylephrine *on page 148*
B-Vex *(Discontinued)* *see* brompheniramine *on page 147*
B vitamin combinations *see* vitamin B complex combinations *on page 988*
BW-430C *see* lamotrigine *on page 546*
BW524W91 *see* emtricitabine *on page 347*
Byclomine® Injection *(Discontinued)* *see* dicyclomine *on page 299*
Bydramine® Cough Syrup *(Discontinued)* *see* diphenhydramine (systemic) *on page 310*
Byetta® [US] *see* exenatide *on page 387*
Bystolic® [US] *see* nebivolol *on page 663*
C1 esterase inhibitor *see* C1 inhibitor (human) *on page 162*
C1-INH *see* C1 inhibitor (human) *on page 162*
C1-inhibitor *see* C1 inhibitor (human) *on page 162*
C1INHRP *see* C1 inhibitor (human) *on page 162*
C2B8 monoclonal antibody *see* rituximab *on page 846*
C7E3 *see* abciximab *on page 19*
C8-CCK *see* sincalide *on page 877*
311C90 *see* zolmitriptan *on page 1004*
C225 *see* cetuximab *on page 199*

C1 inhibitor (human) (cee won in HIB i ter HYU man)

Synonyms C1 esterase inhibitor; C1-INH; C1-inhibitor; C1INHRP; human C1 inhibitor

U.S./Canadian Brand Names Berinert® [US]; Cinryze™ [US]

Therapeutic Category Blood Product Derivative

Use

Berinert®: Treatment of acute abdominal or facial attacks of hereditary angioedema (HAE)
Cinryze™: Routine prophylaxis against angioedema attacks in patients with HAE or inherited C1 inhibitor deficiency

Dosage Summary

Oral:
Children: Dosage not established
Adolescents: 1000 units every 3-4 days **or** 20 units/kg
Adults: 1000 units every 3-4 days **or** 20 units/kg

Dosage Forms

Injection, powder for reconstitution:
Berinert®: 500 units
Cinryze™: 500 units

cabazitaxel (ca baz i TAKS el)

Synonyms RPR-116258A; XRP6258

U.S./Canadian Brand Names Jevtana® [US]

Use Treatment of hormone-refractory metastatic prostate cancer (in patients previously treated with a docetaxel-containing regimen)

Dosage Summary

I.V.:
Children: Dosage not established
Adults: 25 mg/m^2 once every 3 weeks

Dosage Forms

Injection, solution:
Jevtana®: 40 mg/mL (1.5 mL)

cabergoline (ca BER goe leen)

U.S./Canadian Brand Names CO Cabergoline [Can]; Dostinex® [Can]

Therapeutic Category Ergot-like Derivative

Use Treatment of hyperprolactinemic disorders, either idiopathic or due to pituitary adenomas

Dosage Summary

Oral:

Children: Dosage not established

Adults: Initial: 0.25 mg twice weekly; Maintenance: Up to 1 mg twice weekly; **Note:** Titration is recommended

Dosage Forms

Tablet, oral: 0.5 mg

Ca-DTPA [US] *see* diethylene triamine penta-acetic acid *on page 300*

Caduet® [US/Can] *see* amlodipine and atorvastatin *on page 69*

CaEDTA *see* edetate CALCIUM disodium *on page 341*

Caelyx® [Can] *see* doxorubicin (liposomal) *on page 330*

Cafatine-PB® ***(Discontinued)*** *see* ergotamine *on page 359*

Cafcit® [US] *see* caffeine *on page 163*

CAFdA *see* clofarabine *on page 236*

Cafergor® [Can] *see* ergotamine and caffeine *on page 359*

Cafergot® [US] *see* ergotamine and caffeine *on page 359*

Cafetrate® ***(Discontinued)*** *see* ergotamine *on page 359*

caffeine (KAF een)

Synonyms caffeine and sodium benzoate; caffeine citrate; sodium benzoate and caffeine

U.S./Canadian Brand Names Cafcit® [US]; Enerjets [US-OTC]; No Doz® Maximum Strength [US-OTC]; Vivarin® [US-OTC]

Therapeutic Category Stimulant

Use

Caffeine citrate: Treatment of idiopathic apnea of prematurity

Caffeine and sodium benzoate: Treatment of acute respiratory depression (not a preferred agent)

Caffeine [OTC labeling]: Restore mental alertness or wakefulness when experiencing fatigue

Dosage Summary

I.M. (caffeine and sodium benzoate):

Children: 8 mg/kg every 4 hours as needed

Adults: 250 mg as a single dose; may repeat as needed (maximum: 500 mg/dose; 2500 mg/day)

I.V.:

Neonates (caffeine citrate): Loading dose: 10-20 mg/kg; Maintenance: 5 mg/kg once daily

Children (caffeine and sodium benzoate): 8 mg/kg every 4 hours as needed

Adults (caffeine and sodium benzoate): 250 mg as a single dose; may repeat as needed (maximum: 500 mg/dose; 2500 mg/day) **or** 300-2000 mg (electroconvulsive therapy)

Oral:

Neonates (caffeine citrate): Loading dose: 10-20 mg/kg; Maintenance: 5 mg/kg once daily

Children <12 years: Dosage not established

Children ≥12 years (caffeine and sodium benzoate): 100-200 mg every 3-4 hours as needed (OTC labeling)

Adults (caffeine and sodium benzoate): 100-200 mg every 3-4 hours as needed (OTC labeling)

SubQ (caffeine and sodium benzoate):

Children: 8 mg/kg every 4 hours as needed

Adults: Dosing with this route not established

Dosage Forms

Caplet:

No Doz® Maximum Strength [OTC], Vivarin® [OTC]: 200 mg

Injection, solution [preservative free]: 20 mg/mL (3 mL)

Cafcit®: 20 mg/mL (3 mL)

Lozenge:

Enerjets® [OTC]: 75 mg

Solution, oral [preservative free]: 20 mg/mL (3 mL)

Cafcit®: 20 mg/mL

Tablet: 200 mg
Vivarin® [OTC]: 200 mg

caffeine, acetaminophen, and aspirin *see* acetaminophen, aspirin, and caffeine *on page* 27

caffeine, acetaminophen, butalbital, and codeine *see* butalbital, acetaminophen, caffeine, and codeine *on page* 159

caffeine and ergotamine *see* ergotamine and caffeine *on page* 359

caffeine and sodium benzoate *see* caffeine *on page* 163

caffeine, aspirin, and acetaminophen *see* acetaminophen, aspirin, and caffeine *on page* 27

caffeine citrate *see* caffeine *on page* 163

caffeine, dihydrocodeine, and acetaminophen *see* acetaminophen, caffeine, and dihydrocodeine *on page* 28

caffeine, orphenadrine, and aspirin *see* orphenadrine, aspirin, and caffeine *on page* 708

Cal-C-Caps [US-OTC] *see* calcium citrate *on page* 169

Caladryl® Clear™ [US-OTC] *see* pramoxine *on page* 787

Calan® [US/Can] *see* verapamil *on page* 981

Calan® SR [US] *see* verapamil *on page* 981

Calcarb 600 [US-OTC] *see* calcium carbonate *on page* 167

Cal-Cee [US-OTC] *see* calcium citrate *on page* 169

Calci-Chew® [US-OTC] *see* calcium carbonate *on page* 167

Calciday-667® *(Discontinued)* *see* calcium carbonate *on page* 167

Calciferol™ [US-OTC] *see* ergocalciferol *on page* 358

Calciferol™ Injection *(Discontinued)* *see* ergocalciferol *on page* 358

CalciFolic-D™ [US] *see* vitamins (multiple/oral) *on page* 990

Calcijex® [US/Can] *see* calcitriol *on page* 165

Calcimar® [Can] *see* calcitonin *on page* 165

Calcimar® *(Discontinued)* *see* calcitonin *on page* 165

Calci-Mix® [US-OTC] *see* calcium carbonate *on page* 167

Calcionate [US-OTC] *see* calcium glubionate *on page* 170

calcipotriene (kal si POE try een)

U.S./Canadian Brand Names Dovonex® [US/Can]

Therapeutic Category Antipsoriatic Agent

Use Treatment of plaque psoriasis; chronic, moderate-to-severe psoriasis of the scalp

Dosage Summary

Topical:

Children: Dosage not established

Adults: Apply (cream, use thin film) to the affected skin or scalp twice daily

Dosage Forms

Cream, topical:

Dovonex®: 0.005% (60 g, 120 g)

Solution, topical: 0.005% (60 mL)

Dovonex®: 0.005% (60 mL)

calcipotriene and betamethasone (kal si POE try een & bay ta METH a sone)

Synonyms betamethasone dipropionate and calcipotriene hydrate; calcipotriol and betamethasone dipropionate

U.S./Canadian Brand Names Dovobet® [Can]; Taclonex Scalp® [US]; Taclonex® [US]; Xamiol® [Can]

Therapeutic Category Corticosteroid, Topical; Vitamin D Analog

Use Treatment of psoriasis vulgaris

Dosage Summary

Topical:

Children: Dosage not established

Adults: Apply to affected area once daily (maximum: 100 g/week)

Dosage Forms

Ointment, topical:

Taclonex®: Calcipotriene 0.005% and betamethasone 0.064% (60 g, 100 g)

Suspension, topical:
Taclonex Scalp®: Calcipotriene 0.005% and betamethasone 0.064% (15 g, 30 g, 60 g, 2 x 60 g)

Dosage Forms - Canada

Gel, topical:
Xamiol®: Calcipotriol 50 mcg/g and betamethasone 0.5 mg/g (30 g, 60 g, 2 x 60 g)

Ointment, topical:
Dovobet®: Calcipotriol 50 mcg/g and betamethasone 0.5 mg/g (30 g, 60 g, 120 g)

calcipotriol and betamethasone dipropionate *see* calcipotriene and betamethasone *on page* 164
Calcite-500 [Can] *see* calcium carbonate *on page* 167

calcitonin (kal si TOE nin)

Sound-Alike/Look-Alike Issues
calcitonin may be confused with calcitriol
Miacalcin® may be confused with Micatin®

Synonyms calcitonin (salmon)

U.S./Canadian Brand Names Apo-Calcitonin® [Can]; Calcimar® [Can]; Caltine® [Can]; Fortical® [US]; Miacalcin® NS [Can]; Miacalcin® [US]; PRO-Calcitonin [Can]; Sandoz-Calcitonin [Can]

Therapeutic Category Polypeptide Hormone

Use Treatment of Paget disease of bone (osteitis deformans); adjunctive therapy for hypercalcemia; treatment of osteoporosis in women >5 years postmenopause

Dosage Summary

I.M.:
Children: Dosage not established
Adults: Paget disease/osteoporosis: 50-100 units every 1-3 days; Hypercalcemia: 4-8 units/kg every 12 hours (maximum: 8 units/kg every 6 hours)

Intranasal:
Children: Dosage not established
Adults: 200 units (1 spray) in one nostril daily

SubQ:
Children: Dosage not established
Adults: Paget disease/osteoporosis: 50-100 units every 1-3 days; Hypercalcemia: 4-8 units/kg every 12 hours (maximum: 8 units/kg every 6 hours)

Dosage Forms

Injection, solution:
Miacalcin®: 200 int. units/mL (2 mL)

Solution, intranasal: 200 int. units/actuation (3.7 mL, 3.8 mL)
Fortical®: 200 int. units/actuation (3.7 mL)
Miacalcin®: 200 int. units/actuation (3.7 mL)

calcitonin (salmon) *see* calcitonin *on page* 165
Calcitrate [US-OTC] *see* calcium citrate *on page* 169
Cal-Citrate™ 225 [US-OTC] *see* calcium citrate *on page* 169

calcitriol (kal si TRYE ole)

Sound-Alike/Look-Alike Issues
calcitriol may be confused with calcifediol, Calciferol®, calcitonin, calcium carbonate, captopril, colestipol, paricalcitol, ropinirole

Synonyms 1,25 dihydroxycholecalciferol

U.S./Canadian Brand Names Calcijex® [US/Can]; Rocaltrol® [US/Can]; Vectical™ [US]

Therapeutic Category Vitamin D Analog

Use
Oral, injection: Management of hypocalcemia in patients on chronic renal dialysis; management of secondary hyperparathyroidism in patients with chronic kidney disease (CKD); management of hypocalcemia in hypoparathyroidism and pseudohypoparathyroidism
Topical: Management of mild-to-moderate plaque psoriasis

Dosage Summary Note: Individualize dosage

I.V.:
Children (K/DOQI guidelines, CKD stage 5): 0.0075-0.025 mcg/kg (maximum range: 0.25 mcg-1 mcg/day) (refer to K/DOQI guidelines for detail)
Adults: 0.5-4 mcg 3 times/week (refer to K/DOQI guidelines for dosing by stage of CKD)

Oral:

Children: 0.25-0.2 mcg/day **or** 0.01-0.015 mcg/kg/day (maximum: 0.5 mcg/day); (refer to K/DOQI guidelines for dosing by stage of CKD, age and weight)

Adults: 0.25 mcg every other day to 2 mcg once daily (refer to K/DOQI guidelines for dosing by stage of CKD)

Topical:

Children: Dosage not established

Adults: Apply to affected areas twice daily (maximum: 200 g/week)

Dosage Forms

Capsule, softgel, oral: 0.25 mcg, 0.5 mcg

Rocaltrol®: 0.25 mcg, 0.5 mcg

Injection, solution: 1 mcg/mL (1 mL, 2 mL)

Calcijex®: 1 mcg/mL (1 mL)

Ointment, topical:

Vectical™: 3 mcg/g (100 g)

Solution, oral: 1 mcg/mL (15 mL)

Rocaltrol®: 1 mcg/mL (15 mL)

calcium acetate (KAL see um AS e tate)

Sound-Alike/Look-Alike Issues

PhosLo® may be confused with Phos-Flur®, ProSom™

U.S./Canadian Brand Names Eliphos™ [US]; PhosLo® [US/Can]

Therapeutic Category Electrolyte Supplement, Oral

Use Control of hyperphosphatemia in end-stage renal failure; does not promote aluminum absorption

Dosage Summary

Oral:

Children 0-6 months: RDA: 210 mg/day

Children 7-12 months: RDA: 270 mg/day

Children 1-3 years: RDA: 500 mg/day

Children 4-8 years: RDA: 800 mg/day

Children 9-18 years: RDA: 1300 mg/day

Adults: Initial: 1334 mg with each meal; Maintenance: 2001-2668 mg with each meal

Dosage Forms

Gelcap, oral: 667 mg

PhosLo®: 667 mg

Tablet, oral:

Eliphos™: 667 mg

calcium acetate and aluminum sulfate *see* aluminum sulfate and calcium acetate *on page 60*

calcium acetylhomotaurinate *see* acamprosate *on page 20*

calcium and risedronate *see* risedronate and calcium *on page 845*

calcium and vitamin D (KAL see um & VYE ta min dee)

Sound-Alike/Look-Alike Issues

Os-Cal® may be confused with Asacol®

Synonyms vitamin D and calcium carbonate

U.S./Canadian Brand Names Cal-CYUM [US-OTC]; Caltrate® 600+ Soy™ [US-OTC]; Caltrate® 600+D [US-OTC]; Caltrate® ColonHealth™ [US-OTC]; Chew-Cal [US-OTC]; Liqua-Cal [US-OTC]; Os-Cal® 500+D [US-OTC]; Oysco 500+D [US-OTC]; Oysco D [US-OTC]; Oyst-Cal-D 500 [US-OTC]; Oyst-Cal-D [US-OTC]

Therapeutic Category Calcium Salt; Electrolyte Supplement, Oral; Vitamin, Fat Soluble

Use Dietary supplement, antacid

Dosage Summary

Oral: Adults: Refer to individual monographs for dietary reference intake.

Dosage Forms

Capsule, softgel: Calcium 500 mg and vitamin D 500 int. units; calcium 600 mg and vitamin D 100 int. units; calcium 600 mg and vitamin D 200 int. units

Liqua-Cal: Calcium 600 mg and vitamin D 200 int. units

Tablet: Calcium 250 mg and vitamin D 125 int. units; calcium 500 mg and vitamin D 125 int. units; calcium 500 mg and vitamin D 200 int. units; calcium 600 mg and vitamin D 125 int. units; calcium 600 mg and vitamin D 200 int. units

Caltrate® 600+D: Calcium 600 mg and vitamin D 200 int. units

Caltrate® 600+Soy™: Calcium 600 mg and vitamin D 200 int. units

Caltrate® ColonHealth™: Calcium 600 mg and vitamin D 200 int. units

Oysco D: Calcium 250 mg and vitamin D 125 int. units

Oysco 500+D: Calcium 500 mg and vitamin D 200 int. units

Oyst-Cal-D: Calcium 250 mg and vitamin D 125 int. units

Oyst-Cal-D 500: Calcium 500 mg and vitamin D 200 int. units

Tablet, chewable: Calcium 500 mg and vitamin D 100 int. units; calcium 600 mg and vitamin D 400 int. units

Os-Cal® 500+D: Calcium 500 mg and vitamin D 400 int. units

Wafer, chewable:

Cal-CYUM: Calcium 519 mg and vitamin D 150 int. units (50s)

Chew-Cal: Calcium 333 mg and vitamin D 40 int. units (100s, 250s)

calcium carbonate (KAL see um KAR bun ate)

Sound-Alike/Look-Alike Issues

calcium carbonate may be confused with calcitriol

Florical® may be confused with Fiorinal®

Mylanta® may be confused with Mynatal®

Nephro-Calci® may be confused with Nephrocaps®

Synonyms oscal

U.S./Canadian Brand Names Alcalak [US-OTC]; Alka-Mints® [US-OTC]; Apo-Cal® [Can]; Cal-Gest [US-OTC]; Cal-Mint [US-OTC]; Calcarb 600 [US-OTC]; Calci-Chew® [US-OTC]; Calci-Mix® [US-OTC]; Calcite-500 [Can]; Caltrate® 600 [US-OTC]; Caltrate® Select [Can]; Caltrate® [Can]; Children's Pepto [US-OTC]; Chooz® [US-OTC]; Florical® [US-OTC]; Maalox® Children's [US-OTC]; Maalox® Regular Strength [US-OTC]; Nephro-Calci® [US-OTC]; Nutralox® [US-OTC]; Os-Cal® [Can]; Oysco 500 [US-OTC]; Oystercal™ 500 [US-OTC]; Rolaids® Extra Strength [US-OTC]; Super Calcium 600 [US-OTC]; Titralac™ [US-OTC]; Tums® E-X [US-OTC]; Tums® Extra Strength Sugar Free [US-OTC]; Tums® Quickpak [US-OTC]; Tums® Smoothies™ [US-OTC]; Tums® Ultra [US-OTC]; Tums® [US-OTC]

Therapeutic Category Antacid; Electrolyte Supplement, Oral

Use As an antacid; treatment and prevention of calcium deficiency or hyperphosphatemia (eg, osteoporosis, osteomalacia, mild/moderate renal insufficiency, hypoparathyroidism, postmenopausal osteoporosis, rickets); has been used to bind phosphate

Dosage Summary

Oral:

Neonates: 50-150 mg/kg/day in 4-6 divided doses (maximum: 1 g/day)

Children <2 years: 45-65 mg/kg/day in 4 divided doses

Children 2-5 years (24-47 lbs): Antacid: 161 mg (elemental calcium) as needed (maximum: 483 mg/day); Hypocalcemia: 45-65 mg/kg/day in 4 divided doses

Children 6-11 years (48-95 lbs): Antacid: 322 mg (elemental calcium) as needed (maximum: 966 mg/day); Hypocalcemia: 45-65 mg/kg/day in 4 divided doses

Children >11 years: 45-65 mg/kg/day in 4 divided doses

Adults ≤51 years: Antacid: 1-2 tablets or 5-10 mL every 2 hours (maximum: 7000 mg/day); Hypocalcemia/dietary: 500-2000 mg/day in 2-4 divided doses

Adults >51 years: Antacid: 1-2 tablets or 5-10 mL every 2 hours (maximum: 7000 mg/day); Hypocalcemia/dietary: 500-2000 mg/day in 2-4 divided doses; Osteoporosis: 1200 mg/day

Dosage Forms

Capsule, oral:

Calci-Mix® [OTC]: 1250 mg

Florical® [OTC]: 364 mg

Gum, chewing, oral:

Chooz® [OTC]: 500 mg (12s)

Powder, oral: 4000 mg/teaspoon (480 g)

Tums® Quickpak [OTC]: 1000 mg/packet (24s)

Suspension, oral: 1250 mg/5 mL (5 mL, 500 mL)

Tablet, oral: 648 mg, 650 mg, 1250 mg, 1500 mg

Calcarb 600 [OTC]: 1500 mg

Caltrate® 600 [OTC]: 1500 mg

Florical® [OTC]: 364 mg
Nephro-Calci® [OTC]: 1500 mg
Oysco 500 [OTC]: 1250 mg
Oystercal™ 500 [OTC]: 1250 mg
Super Calcium 600 [OTC]: 1500 mg

Tablet, chewable, oral: 420 mg, 500 mg, 600 mg, 650 mg, 750 mg, 1250 mg
Alcalak [OTC]: 420 mg
Alka-Mints® [OTC]: 850 mg
Cal-Gest [OTC]: 500 mg
Cal-Mint [OTC]: 650 mg
Calci-Chew® [OTC]: 1250 mg
Children's Pepto [OTC]: 400 mg
Maalox® Children's [OTC]: 400 mg
Maalox® Regular Strength [OTC]: 600 mg
Nutralox® [OTC]: 420 mg
Titralac™ [OTC]: 420 mg
Tums® [OTC]: 500 mg
Tums® E-X [OTC]: 750 mg
Tums® Extra Strength Sugar Free [OTC]: 750 mg
Tums® Smoothies™ [OTC]: 750 mg
Tums® Ultra [OTC]: 1000 mg

Tablet, softchew, oral:
Rolaids® Extra Strength [OTC]: 1177 mg

calcium carbonate and etidronate disodium *see* etidronate and calcium carbonate *(Canada only) on page* 383

calcium carbonate and magnesium hydroxide

(KAL see um KAR bun ate & mag NEE zhum hye DROKS ide)

Sound-Alike/Look-Alike Issues
Mylanta® may be confused with Mynatal®

Synonyms magnesium hydroxide and calcium carbonate

U.S./Canadian Brand Names Mi-Acid™ Double Strength [US-OTC]; Mylanta® Gelcaps® [US-OTC]; Mylanta® Supreme [US-OTC]; Mylanta® Ultra [US-OTC]; Rolaids® Extra Strength [US-OTC]; Rolaids® [US-OTC]

Therapeutic Category Antacid

Use Hyperacidity

Dosage Summary

Oral:
Children: Dosage not established
Adults: 2-4 tablets between meals and at bedtime

Dosage Forms

Gelcap:
Mylanta® Gelcaps® [OTC]: Calcium carbonate 550 mg and magnesium hydroxide 125 mg

Liquid:
Mylanta® Supreme [OTC]: Calcium carbonate 400 mg and magnesium hydroxide 135 mg per 5 mL

Tablet, chewable: Calcium carbonate 550 mg and magnesium hydroxide 110 mg; calcium carbonate 675 mg and magnesium hydroxide 135 mg; calcium carbonate 700 mg and magnesium hydroxide 300 mg
Mi-Acid™ Double Strength [OTC], Mylanta® Ultra [OTC]: Calcium carbonate 700 mg and magnesium hydroxide 300 mg
Rolaids® [OTC]: Calcium carbonate 550 mg and magnesium hydroxide 110 mg
Rolaids® Extra Strength [OTC]: Calcium carbonate 675 mg and magnesium hydroxide 135 mg

calcium carbonate and simethicone (KAL see um KAR bun ate & sye METH i kone)

Synonyms simethicone and calcium carbonate

U.S./Canadian Brand Names Gas Ban™ [US-OTC]; Maalox® Advanced Maximum Strength [US-OTC]; Maalox® Junior Plus Antigas [US-OTC]; Titralac® Plus [US-OTC]

Therapeutic Category Antacid; Antiflatulent

Use Relief of acid indigestion, heartburn, bloating, pressure, and discomfort of gas

Dosage Summary

Oral:

Children <6 years: Dosage not established

Children 6-11 years: Maalox® Junior Plus Antigas: Two tablets as symptoms occur or as directed by healthcare provider (maximum: 6 tablets/24 hours)

Children ≥12 years; Maalox® Advanced Maximum Strength: 1-2 tablets as symptoms occur or as directed by healthcare provider (maximum: 8 tablets/24 hours)

Adults: Maalox® Advanced Maximum Strength: 1-2 tablets as symptoms occur or as directed by healthcare provider (maximum: 8 tablets/24 hours); Titralac® Plus: Two tablets every 2-3 hours as needed (maximum: 19 tablets/24 hours)

Dosage Forms

Tablet, chewable:

Gas Ban™ [OTC]: Calcium carbonate 300 mg and simethicone 40 mg

Maalox® Advanced Maximum Strength [OTC]: Calcium carbonate 1000 mg and simethicone 60 mg

Maalox® Junior Plus Antigas [OTC]: Calcium carbonate 400 mg and simethicone 24 mg

Titralac® Plus [OTC]: Calcium carbonate 420 mg and simethicone 21 mg

calcium carbonate, folic acid, and magnesium carbonate *see* magnesium carbonate, calcium carbonate, and folic acid *on page 583*

calcium carbonate, magnesium hydroxide, and famotidine *see* famotidine, calcium carbonate, and magnesium hydroxide *on page 391*

calcium chloride (KAL see um KLOR ide)

Therapeutic Category Electrolyte Supplement, Oral

Use Treatment of acute symptomatic hypocalcemia; cardiac disturbances of hyperkalemia or hypocalcemia; emergent treatment of hypocalcemic tetany; treatment of severe hypermagnesemia

Dosage Summary **Note:** One gram of calcium chloride is equal to 270 mg of elemental calcium. **Dosages are expressed in terms of the calcium chloride salt based on a solution concentration of 100 mg/mL (10%) containing 1.4 mEq (27.3 mg)/mL elemental calcium.**

I.V.:

Neonates:

Acute, symptomatic ionized hypocalcemia, hyperkalemia, or magnesium toxicity. **Note:** Routine use in cardiac arrest is not recommended due to the lack of improved survival [PALS 2005 Guidelines]: 20 mg/kg; may repeat as necessary

Hypocalcemia secondary to citrated blood transfusion: Give 32 mg (0.45 mEq elemental calcium) for each 100 mL citrated blood infused

Hypocalcemic tetany: 40-60 mg/kg/dose repeated every 6-8 hours

Infants and Children:

Acute, symptomatic ionized hypocalcemia, hyperkalemia, or magnesium toxicity. **Note:** Routine use in cardiac arrest is not recommended due to the lack of improved survival [PALS 2005 Guidelines]: 20 mg/kg, may repeat as necessary

Hypocalcemia secondary to citrated blood transfusion: Give 32 mg (0.45 mEq elemental calcium) for each 100 mL citrated blood infused

Hypocalcemic tetany: 10 mg/kg over 5-10 minutes, may repeat after 6-8 hours or follow with an infusion (maximum: 200 mg/kg/day) **or** 35-50 mg/kg every 6-8 hours

Adults:

Acute, symptomatic ionized hypocalcemia, hyperkalemia, or magnesium toxicity. **Note:** Routine use in cardiac arrest is not recommended due to the lack of improved survival [ACLS 2005 Guidelines]: 500-1000 mg, may repeat as necessary

Hypocalcemia secondary to citrated blood transfusion: 200-500 mg per 500 mL of citrated blood

Hypocalcemic tetany: 1000 mg, may repeat after 6 hours

Dosage Forms

Injection, solution: 10% (10 mL)

Injection, solution [preservative free]: 10% (10 mL)

calcium citrate (KAL see um SIT rate)

Sound-Alike/Look-Alike Issues

Citracal® may be confused with Citrucel®

U.S./Canadian Brand Names Cal-C-Caps [US-OTC]; Cal-Cee [US-OTC]; Cal-Citrate™ 225 [US-OTC]; Calcitrate [US-OTC]; Osteocit® [Can]

Therapeutic Category Electrolyte Supplement, Oral

Use Antacid; treatment and prevention of calcium deficiency or hyperphosphatemia (eg, osteoporosis, osteomalacia, mild/moderate renal insufficiency, hypoparathyroidism, postmenopausal osteoporosis, rickets)

Dosage Summary

Oral:

Children 0-6 months: RDA: 210 mg/day
Children 7-12 months: RDA: 270 mg/day
Children 1-3 years: RDA: 500 mg/day
Children 4-8 years: RDA: 800 mg/day
Children 9-18 years: RDA: 1300 mg/day
Adults: 500-2000 mg divided 2-4 times/day

Dosage Forms

Capsule, oral:

Cal-C-Caps [OTC]: Elemental calcium 180 mg
Cal-Citrate™ 225 [OTC]: Elemental calcium 225 mg

Granules, oral: Elemental calcium 760 mg/teaspoon (480 g)

Tablet, oral: Elemental calcium 250 mg

Cal-Cee [OTC]: Elemental calcium 250 mg
Calcitrate [OTC]: Elemental calcium 200 mg

calcium disodium edetate *see* edetate CALCIUM disodium *on page 341*

Calcium Disodium Versenate® [US] *see* edetate CALCIUM disodium *on page 341*

calcium glubionate (KAL see um gloo BYE oh nate)

Sound-Alike/Look-Alike Issues

calcium glubionate may be confused with calcium gluconate

U.S./Canadian Brand Names Calcionate [US-OTC]

Therapeutic Category Electrolyte Supplement, Oral

Use Dietary supplement

Dosage Summary

Oral:

Children 0-6 months: RDA: 210 mg/day
Children 7-12 months: RDA: 270 mg/day
Children 1-3 years: RDA: 500 mg/day
Children 4-8 years: RDA: 800 mg/day
Children 9-18 years: RDA: 1300 mg/day
Adults 19-50 years: RDA: 1000 mg/day
Adults ≥51 years: RDA: 1200 mg/day

Dosage Forms

Syrup, oral:

Calcionate [OTC]: 1.8 g/5 mL (473 mL)

calcium gluconate (KAL see um GLOO koe nate)

Sound-Alike/Look-Alike Issues

calcium gluconate may be confused with calcium glubionate

U.S./Canadian Brand Names Cal-G [US-OTC]; Cal-GLU™ [US-OTC]

Therapeutic Category Electrolyte Supplement, Oral

Use Treatment and prevention of hypocalcemia; treatment of tetany, cardiac disturbances of hyperkalemia, cardiac resuscitation when epinephrine fails to improve myocardial contractions, hypocalcemia; calcium supplementation; hydrofluoric acid (HF) burns

Dosage Summary **Note:** 1 gram of calcium gluconate is equal to 90 mg of elemental calcium. The following dosages are expressed in terms of the calcium gluconate salt based on a solution concentration of 100 mg/mL (10%) containing 0.465 mEq (9.3 mg)/mL elemental calcium

I.V.:

Neonates:

Hypocalcemia: 200-800 mg/kg/day as a continuous infusion or in 4 divided doses (maximum: 1 g/dose)

Hypocalcemia secondary to citrated blood infusion: Give 98 mg (0.45 mEq elemental calcium) for each 100 mL citrated blood infused

Infants and Children:
Cardiac arrest or magnesium intoxication: 60-100 mg/kg/dose (maximum: 3 g/dose)
Hypocalcemia: 200-500 mg/kg/day as a continuous infusion or in 4 divided doses (maximum: 2-3 g/dose)
Hypocalcemia secondary to citrated blood infusion: Give 98 mg (0.45 mEq elemental calcium) for each 100 mL citrated blood infused
Hypocalcemic tetany: 100-200 mg/kg, may repeat every 6-8 hours or follow with an infusion of 500 mg/kg/day
Adults:
Cardiac arrest or magnesium intoxication: 500-800 mg/dose (maximum: 3 g/dose)
Hypocalcemia: 2-15 g/24 hours as a continuous infusion or in divided doses
Hypocalcemia secondary to citrated blood infusion: 500 mg to 1 g per 500 mL of citrated blood **or** up to 2 g as a single dose
Hypocalcemic tetany: 1-3 g/dose, may repeat until therapeutic response occurs
Maintenance electrolyte requirements for TPN: 1.7-3.4 g/1000 kcal/24 hours
Oral:
Children: Hypocalcemia: 200-500 mg/kg/day divided every 6 hours
Adults: Hypocalcemia: 500 mg to 2 g 2-4 times/day

Dosage Forms
Capsule, oral:
Cal-G [OTC]: 700 mg
Cal-GLU™ [OTC]: 515 mg
Injection, solution [preservative free]: 10% (10 mL, 50 mL, 100 mL, 200 mL)
Powder, oral: 3727 mg/tablespoon (480 g)
Tablet, oral: 500 mg, 648 mg

calcium lactate (KAL see um LAK tate)

Therapeutic Category Electrolyte Supplement, Oral
Use Adjunct in prevention of postmenopausal osteoporosis; treatment and prevention of calcium depletion
Dosage Summary
Oral:
Children 0-6 months: RDA: 210 mg/day
Children 7-12 months: RDA: 270 mg/day
Children 1-3 years: RDA: 500 mg/day
Children 4-8 years: RDA: 800 mg/day
Children 9-18 years: RDA: 1300 mg/day
Adults 19-50 years: RDA: 1000 mg/day
Adults ≥51 years: RDA: 1200 mg/day
Dosage Forms
Tablet, oral: 648 mg, 650 mg

calcium leucovorin *see* leucovorin calcium *on page* 553
calcium levoleucovorin *see* LEVOleucovorin *on page* 558
calcium pantothenate *see* pantothenic acid *on page* 726

calcium phosphate (tribasic) (KAL see um FOS fate tri BAY sik)

Synonyms tricalcium phosphate
U.S./Canadian Brand Names Posture® [US-OTC]
Therapeutic Category Electrolyte Supplement, Oral
Use Dietary supplement
Dosage Summary
Oral:
Children 0-6 months: RDA: 210 mg/day
Children 7-12 months: RDA: 270 mg/day
Children 1-3 years: RDA: 500 mg/day
Children 4-8 years: RDA: 800 mg/day
Children 9-18 years: RDA: 1300 mg/day
Adults: 2 tablets daily
Dosage Forms
Caplet:
Posture® [OTC]: Calcium 600 mg and phosphorus 280 mg

calcium polystyrene sulfonate *(Canada only)* (KAL see um pol i STI reen sul fo NATE)

Sound-Alike/Look-Alike Issues

calcium polystyrene sulfonate may be confused with sodium polystyrene sulfonate

Synonyms calcium polystyrene sulphonate

U.S./Canadian Brand Names Resonium Calcium® [Can]

Therapeutic Category Antidote

Use Treatment of hyperkalemia

Dosage Summary

Oral:

Children: 0.5-1 g/kg/day
Adults: 15 g 3-4 times/day

Rectal:

Children: 0.5-1 g/kg/day
Adults: 30 g once daily

Dosage Forms - Canada

Powder for suspension, oral/rectal:

Resonium Calcium®: 300 g

calcium polystyrene sulphonate *see* calcium polystyrene sulfonate *(Canada only) on page 172*
Cal-CYUM [US-OTC] *see* calcium and vitamin D *on page 166*
Caldecort® [US-OTC] *see* hydrocortisone (topical) *on page 483*
Caldolor™ [US] *see* ibuprofen *on page 494*

calfactant (kaf AKT ant)

U.S./Canadian Brand Names Infasurf® [US]

Therapeutic Category Lung Surfactant

Use Prevention of respiratory distress syndrome (RDS) in premature infants at high risk for RDS and for the treatment ("rescue") of premature infants who develop RDS

Prophylaxis: Therapy at birth with calfactant is indicated for premature infants <29 weeks of gestational age at significant risk for RDS. Should be administered as soon as possible, preferably within 30 minutes after birth.

Treatment: For infants ≤72 hours of age with RDS (confirmed by clinical and radiologic findings) and requiring endotracheal intubation.

Dosage Summary

Intratracheal:

Premature infants: 3 mL/kg (body weight at birth) every 12 hours for a total of 3 doses
Children: Dosage not established
Adults: Dosage not established

Dosage Forms

Suspension, intratracheal [preservative free]:

Infasurf®: 35 mg/mL (3 mL, 6 mL)

Cal-G [US-OTC] *see* calcium gluconate *on page 170*
Cal-Gest [US-OTC] *see* calcium carbonate *on page 167*
Cal-GLU™ [US-OTC] *see* calcium gluconate *on page 170*
Callergy Clear [US-OTC] *see* pramoxine *on page 787*
Calm-X® Oral *(Discontinued)* *see* dimenhydrinate *on page 307*
Cal-Mint [US-OTC] *see* calcium carbonate *on page 167*
Calmoseptine® [US-OTC] *see* menthol and zinc oxide (topical) *on page 603*
Calmylin with Codeine [Can] *see* guaifenesin, pseudoephedrine, and codeine *on page 459*
Calna [US-OTC] *see* vitamins (multiple/prenatal) *on page 991*
Cal-Nate™ *(Discontinued)* *see* vitamins (multiple/prenatal) *on page 991*
CaloMist™ [US] *see* cyanocobalamin *on page 257*
Calphron® *(Discontinued)* *see* calcium acetate *on page 166*
Cal-Plus® *(Discontinued)* *see* calcium carbonate *on page 167*
Caltine® [Can] *see* calcitonin *on page 165*
Caltrate® [Can] *see* calcium carbonate *on page 167*

Caltrate® 600 [US-OTC] *see* calcium carbonate *on page* 167
Caltrate® 600+D [US-OTC] *see* calcium and vitamin D *on page* 166
Caltrate® 600+ Soy™ [US-OTC] *see* calcium and vitamin D *on page* 166
Caltrate® ColonHealth™ [US-OTC] *see* calcium and vitamin D *on page* 166
Caltrate® Jr. *(Discontinued)* *see* calcium carbonate *on page* 167
Caltrate® Select [Can] *see* calcium carbonate *on page* 167
Cambia™ [US] *see* diclofenac (systemic) *on page* 296
Camila® [US] *see* norethindrone *on page* 682
Campath® [US] *see* alemtuzumab *on page* 47
campath-1H *see* alemtuzumab *on page* 47
Campho-Phenique® [US-OTC] *see* camphor and phenol *on page* 173

camphor and phenol (KAM for & FEE nole)

Synonyms phenol and camphor
U.S./Canadian Brand Names Campho-Phenique® [US-OTC]
Therapeutic Category Topical Skin Product
Use Relief of pain and itching associated with minor burns, sunburn, minor cuts, insect bites, minor skin irritation; temporary relief of pain from cold sores
Dosage Summary
Topical:
Children: Dosage not established
Adults: Apply 1-3 times/day
Dosage Forms
Gel, topical:
Campho-Phenique® [OTC]: Camphor 10.8% and phenol 4.7% (7 g, 14 g)
Liquid, topical: Camphor 10.8% and phenol 4.7% (45 mL)
Campho-Phenique® [OTC]: Camphor 10.8% and phenol 4.7% (22.5 mL, 45 mL)

Campral® [US/Can] *see* acamprosate *on page* 20
Camptosar® [US/Can] *see* irinotecan *on page* 525
camptothecin-11 *see* irinotecan *on page* 525

canakinumab (can a KIN ue mab)

Synonyms ACZ885
U.S./Canadian Brand Names Ilaris® [US]
Therapeutic Category Interleukin-1 Beta Inhibitor; Interleukin-1 Inhibitor; Monoclonal Antibody
Use Treatment of cryopyrin-associated periodic syndromes (CAPS), including familial cold autoinflammatory syndrome (FCAS) and Muckle-Wells syndrome (MWS)
Dosage Summary
SubQ:
Children <4 years and <15 kg: Dosage not established
Children ≥4 years and 15-40 kg: 2 mg/kg every 8 weeks; may increase to 3 mg/kg if response inadequate
Children ≥4 years and >40 kg: 150 mg every 8 weeks
Adults >40 kg: 150 mg every 8 weeks
Dosage Forms
Injection, powder for reconstitution:
Ilaris®: 180 mg

Canasa® [US] *see* mesalamine *on page* 607
Cancidas® [US/Can] *see* caspofungin *on page* 187

candesartan (kan de SAR tan)

Sound-Alike/Look-Alike Issues
Atacand® may be confused with antacid
Synonyms candesartan cilexetil
U.S./Canadian Brand Names Atacand® [US/Can]
Therapeutic Category Angiotensin II Receptor Antagonist

Use Alone or in combination with other antihypertensive agents in treating essential hypertension; treatment of heart failure (NYHA class II-IV)

Dosage Summary

Oral:

Children: Dosage not established

Adults: Initial: 4-16 mg once daily; Maintenance: 4-32 mg/day in 1-2 divided doses; CHF target dose: 32 mg/day

Dosage Forms

Tablet, oral:

Atacand®: 4 mg, 8 mg, 16 mg, 32 mg

candesartan and hydrochlorothiazide (kan de SAR tan & hye droe klor oh THYE a zide)

Synonyms candesartan cilexetil and hydrochlorothiazide

U.S./Canadian Brand Names Atacand HCT® [US]; Atacand® Plus [Can]

Therapeutic Category Antihypertensive Agent, Combination

Use Treatment of hypertension; combination product should not be used for initial therapy

Dosage Summary

Oral:

Children: Dosage not established

Adults: Candesartan 16-32 mg/day in 1-2 divided doses and hydrochlorothiazide 12.5-25 mg once daily

Dosage Forms

Tablet:

Atacand HCT®: 16/12.5: Candesartan 16 mg and hydrochlorothiazide 12.5 mg; 32/12.5: Candesartan 32 mg and hydrochlorothiazide 12.5 mg; 32/25: Candesartan 32 mg and hydrochlorothiazide 25 mg

candesartan cilexetil *see* candesartan *on page 173*

candesartan cilexetil and hydrochlorothiazide *see* candesartan and hydrochlorothiazide *on page 174*

Candida albicans (Monilia) (KAN dee da AL bi kans mo NIL ya)

Synonyms *Monilia* skin test

U.S./Canadian Brand Names Candin® [US]

Therapeutic Category Diagnostic Agent

Use Screen for detection of nonresponsiveness to antigens in immunocompromised individuals

Dosage Summary

Intradermal:

Children: 0.1 mL, examine reaction site in 24-48 hours

Adults: 0.1 mL, examine reaction site in 24-48 hours

Dosage Forms

Injection, solution:

Candin®: 0.1 mL/dose (1 mL)

Candin® [US] *see Candida albicans (Monilia) on page 174*

Candistatin® [Can] *see* nystatin (topical) *on page 693*

CanesOral® [Can] *see* fluconazole *on page 407*

Canesten® Topical [Can] *see* clotrimazole (topical) *on page 240*

Canesten® Vaginal [Can] *see* clotrimazole (topical) *on page 240*

Cankaid® [US-OTC] *see* carbamide peroxide *on page 178*

cannabidiol and tetrahydrocannabinol *see* tetrahydrocannabinol and cannabidiol *(Canada only) on page 923*

Cantil® [US/Can] *see* mepenzolate *on page 603*

Capastat® Sulfate [US] *see* capreomycin *on page 175*

CAPE *see* capecitabine *on page 174*

capecitabine (ka pe SITE a been)

Sound-Alike/Look-Alike Issues

Xeloda® may be confused with Xenical®

Synonyms CAPE

U.S./Canadian Brand Names Xeloda® [US/Can]

Therapeutic Category Antineoplastic Agent, Antimetabolite

Use Treatment of metastatic colorectal cancer; adjuvant therapy of Dukes C colon cancer; treatment of metastatic breast cancer

Dosage Summary

Oral:

Children: Dosage not established

Adults: 1250 mg/m^2 twice daily for 2 weeks, every 21 days

Dosage Forms

Tablet, oral:

Xeloda®: 150 mg, 500 mg

Capex® [US/Can] *see* fluocinolone (topical) *on page* *411*

Caphosol® [US] *see* saliva substitute *on page* *861*

Capital® and Codeine [US] *see* acetaminophen and codeine *on page* *23*

Capitrol® *(Discontinued)*

Capoten® [Can] *see* captopril *on page* *176*

Capoten® *(Discontinued)* *see* captopril *on page* *176*

Capozide® [US/Can] *see* captopril and hydrochlorothiazide *on page* *176*

capreomycin (kap ree oh MYE sin)

Sound-Alike/Look-Alike Issues

Capastat® may be confused with Cepastat®

Synonyms capreomycin sulfate

U.S./Canadian Brand Names Capastat® Sulfate [US]

Therapeutic Category Antibiotic, Miscellaneous

Use Treatment of tuberculosis in conjunction with at least one other antituberculosis agent

Dosage Summary

I.M.:

Adults: 1 g/day (maximum: 20 mg/kg/day) for 60-120 days, followed by 1 g 2-3 times/week

I.V.:

Adults: 1 g/day (maximum: 20 mg/kg/day) for 60-120 days, followed by 1 g 2-3 times/week

Dosage Forms

Injection, powder for reconstitution:

Capastat® Sulfate: 1 g

capreomycin sulfate *see* capreomycin *on page* *175*

capsaicin (kap SAY sin)

Sound-Alike/Look-Alike Issues

Zostrix® may be confused with Zestril®, Zovirax®

Synonyms NGX-4010

U.S./Canadian Brand Names Capzasin-HP® [US-OTC]; Capzasin-P® [US-OTC]; DiabetAid® Pain and Tingling Relief [US-OTC]; Qutenza™ [US]; Salonpas® Hot [US-OTC]; Zostrix® Diabetic Foot Pain [US-OTC]; Zostrix® [US-OTC/Can]; Zostrix®-HP [US-OTC/Can]

Therapeutic Category Analgesic, Topical

Use

Topical patch (Qutenza™): Management of postherpetic neuralgia (PHN)

OTC labeling: Temporary treatment of minor pain associated with muscles and joints due to backache, strains, sprains, bruises, cramps or arthritis; temporary relief of pain associated with diabetic neuropathy

Dosage Summary

Topical:

Children ≤11 years: Dosage not established

Children ≥12 years: OTC labeling: Patch (Salonpas®-Hot): Apply patch to affected area up to 3-4 times/day

Adults:

Patch (Qutenza™[capsaicin 8%]): Apply patch to most painful area for 60 minutes (maximum: 4 patches in a single application)

OTC labeling:

Patch (Salonpas®-Hot): Apply patch to affected area up to 3-4 times/day

Topical products (cream, gel, liquid, lotion): Apply to affected area 3-4 times/day

Dosage Forms

Cream, topical: 0.025% (60 g); 0.075% (60 g)
Capzasin-HP® [OTC]: 0.1% (42.5 g)
Capzasin-P® [OTC]: 0.035% (42.5 g)
Zostrix® [OTC]: 0.025% (60 g)
Zostrix® Diabetic Foot Pain [OTC]: 0.075% (60 g)
Zostrix®-HP [OTC]: 0.075% (60 g)

Gel, topical:
Capzasin-P® [OTC]: 0.025% (42.5 g)

Liquid, topical:
Capzasin-P® [OTC]: 0.15% (29.5 mL)

Lotion, topical:
DiabetAid® Pain and Tingling Relief [OTC]: 0.025% (120 mL)

Patch, topical:
Qutenza™: 8% (1s, 2s)
Salonpas® Hot [OTC]: 0.025% (1s)

captopril (KAP toe pril)

Sound-Alike/Look-Alike Issues
captopril may be confused with calcitriol, Capitrol®, carvedilol

Synonyms ACE

U.S./Canadian Brand Names Alti-Captopril [Can]; Apo-Capto® [Can]; Capoten® [Can]; Gen-Captopril [Can]; Mylan-Captopril [Can]; Novo-Captopril [Can]; Nu-Capto [Can]; PMS-Captopril [Can]

Therapeutic Category Angiotensin-Converting Enzyme (ACE) Inhibitor

Use Management of hypertension; treatment of heart failure, left ventricular dysfunction after myocardial infarction, diabetic nephropathy

Dosage Summary

Oral:
Infants: Initial: 0.15-0.3 mg/kg/dose; Maintenance: 2.5-6 mg/kg/day in 1-4 divided doses
Children: Initial: 0.5 mg/kg/dose; Maintenance: Up to 6 mg/kg/day in 2-4 divided doses
Older Children: Initial: 6.25-12.5 mg every 12-24 hours; Maintenance: Up to 6 mg/kg/day
Adolescents: Initial: 12.5-25 mg every 8-12 hours; Maintenance: Up tp 450 mg/day divided every 8-12 hours
Adults: Initial: 6.25-25 mg 2-3 times/day; Maintenance: 25-450 mg/day in 2-3 divided doses; HF target dose: 50 mg 3 times/day; Usual dosage range (JNC 7): 25-100 mg in 2 divided doses

Dosage Forms

Tablet, oral: 12.5 mg, 25 mg, 50 mg, 100 mg

captopril and hydrochlorothiazide (KAP toe pril & hye droe klor oh THYE a zide)

Synonyms hydrochlorothiazide and captopril

U.S./Canadian Brand Names Capozide® [US/Can]

Therapeutic Category Antihypertensive Agent, Combination

Use Management of hypertension

Dosage Summary

Oral:
Children: Dosage not established
Adults: Captopril 25-150 mg and hydrochlorothiazide 15-50 mg once daily

Dosage Forms

Tablet:
Generics:
25/15: Captopril 25 mg and hydrochlorothiazide 15 mg
25/25: Captopril 25 mg and hydrochlorothiazide 25 mg
50/15: Captopril 50 mg and hydrochlorothiazide 15 mg
50/25: Captopril 50 mg and hydrochlorothiazide 25 mg
Brands:
Capozide®:
25/15: Captopril 25 mg and hydrochlorothiazide 15 mg
25/25: Captopril 25 mg and hydrochlorothiazide 25 mg
50/15: Captopril 50 mg and hydrochlorothiazide 15 mg
50/25: Captopril 50 mg and hydrochlorothiazide 25 mg

Capzasin-HP® [US-OTC] *see* capsaicin *on page 175*

Capzasin-P® [US-OTC] *see* capsaicin *on page 175*

Carac® [US] *see* fluorouracil (topical) *on page 415*

Carafate® [US] *see* sucralfate *on page 897*

Carapres® [Can] *see* clonidine *on page 238*

carbachol (KAR ba kole)

Sound-Alike/Look-Alike Issues
Isopto® Carbachol may be confused with Isopto® Carpine

Synonyms carbacholine; carbamylcholine chloride

U.S./Canadian Brand Names Isopto® Carbachol [US/Can]; Miostat® [US/Can]

Therapeutic Category Cholinergic Agent

Use Lowers intraocular pressure in the treatment of glaucoma; cause miosis during surgery

Dosage Summary

Ophthalmic:
Children: Dosage not established
Adults: Instill 1-2 drops up to 3 times/day **or** 0.5 mL instilled during surgery

Dosage Forms

Solution, intraocular:
Miostat®: 0.01% (1.5 mL)

Solution, ophthalmic:
Isopto® Carbachol: 1.5% (15 mL); 3% (15 mL)

carbacholine *see* carbachol *on page 177*

Carbaglu® [US] *see* carglumic acid *on page 184*

carbamazepine (kar ba MAZ e peen)

Sound-Alike/Look-Alike Issues
carBAMazepine may be confused with OXcarbazepine
Carbatrol® may be confused with Cartrol®
Epitol® may be confused with Epinal®
Tegretol®, Tegretol®-XR may be confused with Mebaral®, Toprol-XL®, Toradol®, Trental®

Synonyms CBZ; SPD417

Tall-Man car**BAM**azepine

U.S./Canadian Brand Names Apo-Carbamazepine® [Can]; Bio-Carbamazepine [Can]; Carbamazepine [Can]; Carbatrol® [US]; Dom-Carbamazepine [Can]; Epitol® [US]; Equetro® [US]; Gen-Carbamazepine CR [Can]; Mapezine® [Can]; Mylan-Carbamazepine CR [Can]; Novo-Carbamaz [Can]; Nu-Carbamazepine [Can]; PHL-Carbamazepine [Can]; PMS-Carbamazepine [Can]; Sandoz-Carbamazepine [Can]; Taro-Carbamazepine Chewable [Can]; Tegretol® [US/Can]; Tegretol®-XR [US]

Therapeutic Category Anticonvulsant

Use
Carbatrol®, Tegretol®, Tegretol®-XR: Partial seizures with complex symptomatology (psychomotor, temporal lobe), generalized tonic-clonic seizures (grand mal), mixed seizure patterns, trigeminal neuralgia
Equetro®: Acute manic and mixed episodes associated with bipolar 1 disorder

Dosage Summary

Oral:
Extended release:
Capsules:
Children <12 years: Receiving ≥400 mg/day of carbamazepine may be converted to extended release capsules (Carbatrol®) using the same total daily dosage divided twice daily
Children 12-15 years: Initial: 400 mg/day; Maintenance: 800-1000 mg/day in 2 divided doses (maximum: 1000 mg/day); **Note:** Titration is recommended
Adolescents >15 years: Initial: 400 mg/day; Maintenance: 800-1200 mg/day in 2 divided doses (maximum: 1200 mg/day); **Note:** Titration is recommended

Adults:

Bipolar disorder (Equetro®): Initial: 400 mg/day in 2 divided doses: Maintenance: Adjust by 200 mg daily increments (maximum: 1600 mg/day)

Epilepsy: Initial: 400 mg/day; Maintenance: 800-1200 mg/day in 2 divided doses (maximum: 2400 mg/day); **Note:** Titration is recommended

Tablets:

Children <6 years: Dosage not established

Children 6-12 years: Initial: 200 mg/day; Maintenance: 400-800 mg/day in 2 divided doses (maximum: 1000 mg/day); **Note:** Titration is recommended

Children 12-15 years: Initial: 400 mg/day; Maintenance: 800-1000 mg/day in 2 divided doses (maximum: 1000 mg/day); **Note:** Titration is recommended

Adolescents >15 years: Initial: 400 mg/day; Maintenance: 800-1200 mg/day in 2 divided doses (maximum: 1200 mg/day); **Note:** Titration is recommended

Adults: Epilepsy: Initial: 400 mg/day; Maintenance: 800-1200 mg/day in 2 divided doses (maximum: 2400 mg/day); **Note:** Titration is recommended

Immediate release:

Children <6 years: Initial: 10-20 mg/kg/day in 2-3 divided doses (tablets) **or** 4 divided doses (suspension); Maintenance: Up to 35 mg/kg/day in in 3-4 divided doses; **Note:** Titration is recommended

Children 6-12 years: Initial: 200 mg/day in 2 divided doses (tablets) **or** 4 divided doses (suspension); Maintenance: 400-800 mg/day in 2-4 divided doses (maximum: 1000 mg/day); **Note:** Titration is recommended

Children 12-15 years: Initial: 400 mg/day in 2 divided doses (tablets) **or** 4 divided doses (suspension); Maintenance: 800-1000 mg/day in 3-4 divided doses (maximum: 1000 mg/day); **Note:** Titration is recommended

Adolescents >15 years: Initial: 400 mg/day in 2 divided doses (tablets) **or** 4 divided doses (suspension); Maintenance: 800-1200 mg/day in 3-4 divided doses (maximum: 1200 mg/day); **Note:** Titration is recommended

Adults:

Epilepsy: Initial: 400 mg/day in 2 divided doses (tablets) **or** 4 divided doses (suspension); Maintenance: 800-1200 mg/day in 3-4 divided doses (maximum: 2400 mg/day); **Note:** Titration is recommended

Trigeminal or glossopharyngeal neuralgia: Initial: 200 mg/day in 2 divided doses; Maintenance: 400-800 mg/day in 2 divided doses (maximum: 1200 mg/day); **Note:** Titration is recommended

Dosage Forms

Capsule, extended release, oral:

Carbatrol®: 100 mg, 200 mg, 300 mg

Equetro®: 100 mg, 200 mg, 300 mg

Suspension, oral: 100 mg/5 mL (5 mL, 10 mL, 450 mL)

Tegretol®: 100 mg/5 mL (450 mL)

Tablet, oral: 200 mg

Epitol®: 200 mg

Tegretol®: 200 mg

Tablet, chewable, oral: 100 mg

Tegretol®: 100 mg

Tablet, extended release, oral: 200 mg, 400 mg

Tegretol®-XR: 100 mg, 200 mg, 400 mg

Carbamazepine [Can] *see* carbamazepine *on page 177*

carbamide *see* urea *on page 970*

carbamide peroxide (KAR ba mide per OKS ide)

Synonyms urea peroxide

U.S./Canadian Brand Names Auraphene B® [US-OTC]; Auro® [US-OTC]; Cankaid® [US-OTC]; Debrox® [US-OTC]; E-R-O® [US-OTC]; Gly-Oxide® [US-OTC]; Murine® Ear Wax Removal Kit [US-OTC]; Murine® Ear [US-OTC]; Otix® [US-OTC]

Therapeutic Category Antiinfective Agent, Oral; Otic Agent, Ceruminolytic

Use Relief of minor inflammation of gums, oral mucosal surfaces, and lips including canker sores and dental irritation; emulsify and disperse ear wax

Dosage Summary

Otic:

Children <12 years: Instill 1-5 drops twice daily

Children ≥12 years: Instill 5-10 drops twice daily
Adults: Instill 5-10 drops twice daily
Topical (oral):
Children <2 years: Dosage not established
Children ≥2 years: Apply several drops on affected area, expectorate after 2-3 minutes 4 times/day **or** place 10 drops on tongue, swish for several minutes, expectorate
Adults: Apply several drops on affected area, expectorate after 2-3 minutes 4 times/day **or** place 10 drops on tongue, swish for several minutes, expectorate

Dosage Forms
Liquid, oral: 10% (60 mL)
Cankaid® [OTC]: 10% (15 mL)
Gly-Oxide® [OTC]: 10% (15 mL, 60 mL)
Solution, otic: 6.5% (15 mL)
Auraphene B® [OTC]: 6.5% (15 mL)
Auro® [OTC]: 6.5% (22.2 mL)
Debrox® [OTC]: 6.5% (15 mL, 30 mL)
E-R-O® [OTC]: 6.5% (15 mL)
Murine® Ear [OTC]: 6.5% (15 mL)
Murine® Ear Wax Removal Kit [OTC]: 6.5% (15 mL)
Otix® [OTC]: 6.5% (15 mL)

carbamylcholine chloride *see* carbachol *on page 177*
Carbaphen 12® [US] *see* carbetapentane, phenylephrine, and chlorpheniramine *on page 180*
Carbaphen 12 Ped® [US] *see* carbetapentane, phenylephrine, and chlorpheniramine *on page 180*
Carbastat® *(Discontinued)* *see* carbachol *on page 177*
Carbatrol® [US] *see* carbamazepine *on page 177*
Carbaxefed DM RF *(Discontinued)*
Carbaxefed RF *(Discontinued)*
carbenicillin *(Discontinued)*

carbetapentane and chlorpheniramine (kar bay ta PEN tane & klor fen IR a meen)

Synonyms carbetapentane tannate and chlorpheniramine tannate; chlorpheniramine and carbetapentane

U.S./Canadian Brand Names C-Tanna 12 [US]; Tussi-12 S™ [US]; Tussi-12® [US]; Tussizone-12 RF™ [US]; Tustan 12S™ [US]

Therapeutic Category Antihistamine/Antitussive

Use Symptomatic relief of cough associated with upper respiratory tract conditions, such as the common cold, bronchitis, bronchial asthma

Dosage Summary
Oral:
Children <2 years: Dosage not established
Children 2-6 years: Carbetapentane 15-30 mg and chlorpheniramine 2-4 mg every 12 hours
Children >6 years: Carbetapentane 30-60 mg and chlorpheniramine 4-8 mg every 12 hours
Adults: Carbetapentane 60-120 mg and chlorpheniramine 5-10 mg every 12 hours

Dosage Forms
Suspension:
C-Tanna 12: Carbetapentane 30 mg and chlorpheniramine 4 mg per 5 mL
Tablet:
Tussi-12®, Tussizone-12 RF™: Carbetapentane 60 mg and chlorpheniramine 5 mg

carbetapentane and phenylephrine (kar bay ta PEN tane & fen il EF rin)

Synonyms phenylephrine tannate and carbetapentane tannate

Therapeutic Category Antitussive; Antitussive/Decongestant; Sympathomimetic

Use Symptomatic relief of upper respiratory tract conditions such as the common cold, bronchial asthma, and bronchitis (acute and chronic)

Dosage Summary
Oral:
Children <2 years: Dosage not established
Children 2-6 years: 2.5 mL every 12 hours (maximum: 5 mL/24 hours)
Children 6-12 years: 5 mL every 12 hours (maximum: 10 mL/24 hours)
Children >12 years: 5-10 mL every 12 hours (maximum: 20 mL/24 hours)
Adults: 5-10 mL every 12 hours (maximum: 20 mL/24 hours)

carbetapentane and pseudoephedrine (kar bay ta PEN tane & soo doe e FED rin)

Synonyms carbetapentane tannate and pseudoephedrine tannate; pseudoephedrine and carbetapentane

U.S./Canadian Brand Names Pseudacarb™ [US]

Therapeutic Category Antitussive/Decongestant

Use Relief of cough and congestion due to the common cold, influenza, sinusitis, or bronchitis

Dosage Summary

Oral:

Children <2 years: Dosage not established
Children 2-6 years: 1/2 tablet **or** 2.5 mL every 12 hours (maximum: 4 doses/day)
Children 6-12 years: 1 tablet **or** 5 mL every 12 hours (maximum: 4 doses/day)
Children >12 years: 2 tablets **or** 10 mL every 12 hours (maximum: 4 doses/day)
Adults: 2 tablets **or** 10 mL every 12 hours (maximum: 4 doses/day)

Dosage Forms

Suspension: Carbetapentane 25 mg and pseudoephedrine 75 mg per 5 mL

Tablet, chewable:

Pseudacarb™: Carbetapentane 25 mg and pseudoephedrine 75 mg

carbetapentane, ephedrine, phenylephrine, and chlorpheniramine *see* chlorpheniramine, ephedrine, phenylephrine, and carbetapentane *on page 210*

carbetapentane, guaifenesin, and phenylephrine

(kar bay ta PEN tane, gwye FEN e sin, & fen il EF rin)

Synonyms guaifenesin, carbetapentane citrate, and phenylephrine hydrochloride; phenylephrine hydrochloride, carbetapentane citrate, and guaifenesin

U.S./Canadian Brand Names Carbetaplex [US]; Extendryl® GCP [US]; Gentex LQ [US]; Phencarb GG [US]

Therapeutic Category Antitussive; Expectorant; Expectorant/Decongestant/Antitussive; Sympathomimetic

Use Relief of nonproductive cough accompanying respiratory tract congestion associated with the common cold, influenza, sinusitis, and bronchitis

Dosage Summary

Oral:

Children <2 years: Dosage not established
Children 2-6 years: Gentex LQ: 2.5 mL every 4-6 hours
Children 6-12 years: Gentex LQ: 5 mL every 4-6 hours
Children ≥12 years: Gentex LQ: 5-10 mL every 4-6 hours
Adults: Gentex LQ: 5-10 mL every 4-6 hours

Dosage Forms

Liquid:

Carbetaplex: Carbetapentane 20 mg, guaifenesin 100 mg, and phenylephrine 15 mg per 5 mL
Gentex LQ: Carbetapentane 20 mg, guaifenesin 100 mg, and phenylephrine 10 mg per 5 mL
Phencarb GG: Carbetapentane 20 mg, guaifenesin 100 mg, and phenylephrine 10 mg per 5 mL

Solution, oral:

Extendryl® GCP: Carbetapentane 15 mg, guaifenesin 100 mg, and phenylephrine 5 mg per 5 mL

carbetapentane, phenylephrine, and chlorpheniramine

(kar bay ta PEN tane, fen il EF rin, & klor fen IR a meen)

Synonyms chlorpheniramine, carbetapentane, and phenylephrine; phenylephrine, chlorpheniramine, and carbetapentane

U.S./Canadian Brand Names Carbaphen 12 Ped® [US]; Carbaphen 12® [US]

Therapeutic Category Antihistamine/Decongestant/Antitussive; Antitussive; Sympathomimetic

Use Symptomatic relief of cough, nasal congestion, and discharge associated with the common cold, bronchial asthma, acute and chronic bronchitis, and other respiratory tract conditions

Dosage Summary

Oral:

Children <2 years: Dosage not established
Children 2-6 years: Carbaphen 12 Ped®: 1-2 mL every 12 hours
Children 6-12 years: Carbaphen 12 Ped®: 2-4 mL every 12 hours

Children >12 years: Carbaphen 12®: 5-10 mL every 12 hours
Adults: Carbaphen 12®: 5-10 mL every 12 hours

Dosage Forms

Suspension:

Carbaphen 12®: Carbetapentane 60 mg, phenylephrine 20 mg, and chlorpheniramine 8 mg per 5 mL
Carbaphen 12 Ped®: Carbetapentane 15 mg, phenylephrine 2.5 mg, and chlorpheniramine 2 mg per 1 mL

carbetapentane, phenylephrine, and pyrilamine

(kar bay ta PEN tane, fen il EF rin, & peer II a meen)

Synonyms phenylephrine tannate, carbetapentane tannate, and pyrilamine tannate; pyrilamine, phenylephrine, and carbetapentane

U.S./Canadian Brand Names C-Tanna 12D [US]; Tussi-12® D [US]; Tussi-12® DS [US]

Therapeutic Category Antihistamine; Antihistamine/Decongestant/Antitussive; Antitussive; Decongestant

Use Symptomatic relief of cough associated with respiratory tract conditions such as the common cold, bronchial asthma, acute and chronic bronchitis

Dosage Summary

Oral:

Children <2 years: Dosage not established
Children 2-6 years: Tussi-12® DS: 2.5-5 mL every 12 hours
Children 6-11 years:
Tussi-12® D: 1/2 to 1 tablet every 12 hours
Tussi-12® DS: 5-10 mL every 12 hours
Children ≥12 years: Tussi-12® D: 1-2 tablets every 12 hours
Adults: Tussi-12® D: 1-2 tablets every 12 hours

Dosage Forms

Suspension:

C-Tanna 12D: Carbetapentane 30 mg, pyrilamine 30 mg, and phenylephrine 5 mg per 5 mL
Tussi-12® DS: Carbetapentane 30 mg, pyrilamine 30 mg, and phenylephrine 5 mg per 5 mL

Tablet:

C-Tanna 12D, Tussi-12® D: Carbetapentane 60 mg, pyrilamine 40 mg, and phenylephrine 10 mg

carbetapentane tannate and chlorpheniramine tannate *see* carbetapentane and chlorpheniramine *on page 179*

carbetapentane tannate and pseudoephedrine tannate *see* carbetapentane and pseudoephedrine *on page 180*

Carbetaplex [US] *see* carbetapentane, guaifenesin, and phenylephrine *on page 180*

carbetocin *(Canada only)* (kar BE toe sin)

U.S./Canadian Brand Names Duratocin™ [Can]

Therapeutic Category Oxytocic Agent

Use Prevention of uterine atony and postpartum hemorrhage following elective cesarean section under anesthesia (epidural or spinal)

Dosage Summary

I.V.:

Children: Dosage not established
Adults: 100 mcg (single dose)

Dosage Forms - Canada

Injection, solution:

Duratocin™: 100 mcg/mL (1 mL)

carbidopa (kar bi DOE pa)

U.S./Canadian Brand Names Lodosyn® [US]

Therapeutic Category Anti-Parkinson Agent (Dopamine Agonist)

Use Given with levodopa in the treatment of parkinsonism to enable a lower dosage of levodopa to be used and a more rapid response to be obtained and to decrease side effects; for details of administration and dosage, see Levodopa; has no effect without levodopa

Dosage Summary Note: Must be given with levodopa to have effect
Oral:
Children: Dosage not established
Adults: 70-100 mg/day (maximum: 200 mg/day)
Dosage Forms
Tablet, oral:
Lodosyn®: 25 mg

carbidopa and levodopa (kar bi DOE pa & lee voe DOE pa)

Sound-Alike/Look-Alike Issues
Sinemet® may be confused with Serevent®
Synonyms levodopa and carbidopa
U.S./Canadian Brand Names Apo-Levocarb® CR [Can]; Apo-Levocarb® [Can]; Dom-Levo-Carbidopa [Can]; Endo®-Levodopa/Carbidopa [Can]; Novo-Levocarbidopa [Can]; Nu-Levocarb [Can]; Parcopa® [US]; PRO-Levocarb [Can]; Sinemet® CR [US/Can]; Sinemet® [US/Can]
Therapeutic Category Anti-Parkinson Agent (Dopamine Agonist)
Use Idiopathic Parkinson disease; postencephalitic parkinsonism; symptomatic parkinsonism
Dosage Summary
Oral:
Immediate release:
Children: Dosage not established
Adults: Initial: Carbidopa 25 mg/levodopa 100 mg 3 times/day (maximum: 8 tablets of any strength/day **or** 200 mg of carbidopa and 2000 mg of levodopa); **Note:** Titration is recommended
Elderly: Initial: Carbidopa 25 mg/levodopa 100 mg twice daily, increase as necessary
Sustained release:
Children: Dosage not established
Adults: Initial: Carbidopa 50 mg/levodopa 200 mg 2 times/day, at intervals not <6 hours (maximum: 8 tablets/day); **Note:** Titration is recommended every 3 days
Dosage Forms
Tablet: 10/100: Carbidopa 10 mg and levodopa 100 mg; 25/100: Carbidopa 25 mg and levodopa 100 mg; 25/250: Carbidopa 25 mg and levodopa 250 mg
Sinemet®:
10/100: Carbidopa 10 mg and levodopa 100 mg
25/100: Carbidopa 25 mg and levodopa 100 mg
25/250: Carbidopa 25 mg and levodopa 250 mg
Tablet, extended release: 25/100: Carbidopa 25 mg and levodopa 100 mg; 50/200: Carbidopa 50 mg and levodopa 200 mg
Tablet, orally disintegrating: 10/100: Carbidopa 10 mg and levodopa 100 mg; 25/100: Carbidopa 25 mg and levodopa 100 mg; 25/250: Carbidopa 25 mg and levodopa 250 mg
Parcopa®:
10/100: Carbidopa 10 mg and levodopa 100 mg [contains phenylalanine 3.4 mg/tablet; mint flavor]
25/100: Carbidopa 25 mg and levodopa 100 mg [contains phenylalanine 3.4 mg/tablet; mint flavor]
25/250: Carbidopa 25 mg and levodopa 250 mg [contains phenylalanine 8.4 mg/tablet; mint flavor]
Tablet, sustained release: 25/100: Carbidopa 25 mg and levodopa 100 mg; 50/200: Carbidopa 50 mg and levodopa 200 mg
Sinemet® CR:
25/100: Carbidopa 25 mg and levodopa 100 mg
50/200: Carbidopa 50 mg and levodopa 200 mg

carbidopa, entacapone, and levodopa *see* levodopa, carbidopa, and entacapone *on page 557*
carbidopa, levodopa, and entacapone *see* levodopa, carbidopa, and entacapone *on page 557*
Carbihist *(Discontinued)* *see* carbinoxamine *on page 182*

carbinoxamine (kar bi NOKS a meen)

Synonyms carbinoxamine maleate
U.S./Canadian Brand Names Palgic® [US]
Therapeutic Category Antihistamine
Use Seasonal and perennial allergic rhinitis; vasomotor rhinitis; urticaria; decrease severity of other allergic reactions

Dosage Summary

Oral:

Children ≤3 years: Dosage not established
Children >3-6 years: Palgic®: 2-5 mg 3-4 times/day
Children >6 years: Palgic®: 4-6 mg 3-4 times/day
Adults: Palgic®: 4-8 mg 3-4 times/day

Dosage Forms

Solution, oral:
Palgic®: 4 mg/5 mL (480 mL)

Tablet, oral:
Palgic®: 4 mg

carbinoxamine and pseudoephedrine ***(Discontinued)***

carbinoxamine maleate *see* carbinoxamine *on page* 182

Carbinoxamine PD ***(Discontinued)*** *see* carbinoxamine *on page* 182

carbinoxamine, pseudoephedrine, and dextromethorphan ***(Discontinued)***

Carbiset® Tablet ***(Discontinued)***

Carbiset-TR® Tablet ***(Discontinued)***

Carbocaine® [US/Can] *see* mepivacaine *on page* 604

Carbocaine® 2% with Neo-Cobefrin® [US] *see* mepivacaine and levonordefrin *on page* 605

Carbodec® Syrup ***(Discontinued)***

Carbodec® Tablet ***(Discontinued)***

Carbodec® TR Tablet ***(Discontinued)***

Carbofed DM ***(Discontinued)*** *see* brompheniramine, pseudoephedrine, and dextromethorphan *on page* 149

carbolic acid *see* phenol *on page* 748

Carbolith™ [Can] *see* lithium *on page* 571

carboplatin (KAR boe pla tin)

Sound-Alike/Look-Alike Issues
CARBOplatin may be confused with CISplatin, oxaliplatin
Paraplatin® may be confused with Platinol®

Synonyms CBDCA; NSC-241240

Tall-Man **CARBO**platin

U.S./Canadian Brand Names Paraplatin-AQ [Can]

Therapeutic Category Antineoplastic Agent

Use Treatment of ovarian cancer

Dosage Summary

I.V.:

Adults: 300-360 mg/m^2 every 4 weeks **or** AUC of 4-8 (using Calvert formula)
Elderly: The Calvert formula should be used to calculate dosing for elderly patients.

Dosage Forms

Injection, powder for reconstitution: 50 mg, 150 mg, 450 mg
Injection, solution: 10 mg/mL (5 mL, 15 mL, 45 mL, 60 mL)
Injection, solution [preservative free]: 10 mg/mL (5 mL, 15 mL, 45 mL)

carboprost *see* carboprost tromethamine *on page* 183

carboprost tromethamine (KAR boe prost tro METH a meen)

Synonyms carboprost; prostaglandin F_2

U.S./Canadian Brand Names Hemabate® [US/Can]

Therapeutic Category Prostaglandin

Use Termination of pregnancy; treatment of refractory postpartum uterine bleeding

Dosage Summary

I.M.:

Children: Dosage not established
Adults (females):
Abortion: 250 mcg at 1.5- to 3.5-hour intervals, a 500 mcg dose may be given if uterine response is not adequate after several 250 mcg doses (maximum total dose: 12 mg)

Postpartum bleeding: 250 mcg; if needed, may repeat at 15- to 90-minute intervals (maximum total dose: 2 mg [8 doses])

Dosage Forms

Injection, solution:

Hemabate®: Carboprost 250 mcg and tromethamine 83 mcg per mL (1 mL)

carbose D *see* carboxymethylcellulose *on page 184*

Carboxine ***(Discontinued)*** *see* carbinoxamine *on page 182*

Carboxine-PSE ***(Discontinued)***

carboxymethylcellulose (kar boks ee meth il SEL yoo lose)

Sound-Alike/Look-Alike Issues

Optive™ may be confused with Optivar®

Synonyms carbose D; carboxymethylcellulose sodium

U.S./Canadian Brand Names Celluvisc™ [Can]; Optive™ [US-OTC]; Refresh Liquigel™ [US-OTC]; Refresh Plus® [US-OTC/Can]; Refresh Tears® [US-OTC/Can]; Tears Again® Gel Drops™ [US-OTC]; Tears Again® Night and Day™ [US-OTC]; Theratears® [US]

Therapeutic Category Ophthalmic Agent, Miscellaneous

Use Artificial tear substitute

Dosage Summary

Ophthalmic:

Children: Dosage not established

Adults: Instill 1-2 drops into eye(s) 3-4 times/day

Dosage Forms

Gel, ophthalmic:

Tears Again® Night & Day™ [OTC]: 1.5% (3.5 g)

Liquid, ophthalmic:

Refresh Liquigel™ [OTC]: 1% (15 mL)

Solution, ophthalmic:

Optive™ [OTC]: 0.5% (15 mL, 30 mL)

Refresh Tears® [OTC]: 0.5% (15 mL)

Tears Again® Gel Drops™ [OTC]: 0.7% (15 mL)

Solution, ophthalmic [preservative free]:

Refresh Plus® [OTC]: 0.5% (0.4 mL)

Theratears® [OTC]: 0.25% (0.6 mL, 15 mL)

carboxymethylcellulose sodium *see* carboxymethylcellulose *on page 184*

Cardene® [US] *see* nicardipine *on page 673*

Cardene® I.V. [US] *see* nicardipine *on page 673*

Cardene® SR [US] *see* nicardipine *on page 673*

Cardio-Green® ***(Discontinued)*** *see* indocyanine green *on page 505*

Cardioquin® ***(Discontinued)*** *see* quinidine *on page 822*

Cardizem® [US] *see* diltiazem *on page 306*

Cardizem® CD [US/Can] *see* diltiazem *on page 306*

Cardizem® Injection ***(Discontinued)*** *see* diltiazem *on page 306*

Cardizem® LA [US] *see* diltiazem *on page 306*

Cardizem® SR ***(Discontinued)*** *see* diltiazem *on page 306*

Cardura® [US] *see* doxazosin *on page 328*

Cardura-1™ [Can] *see* doxazosin *on page 328*

Cardura-2™ [Can] *see* doxazosin *on page 328*

Cardura-4™ [Can] *see* doxazosin *on page 328*

Cardura® XL [US] *see* doxazosin *on page 328*

CareNatal™ DHA ***(Discontinued)*** *see* vitamins (multiple/prenatal) *on page 991*

carglumic acid (kar GLU mik AS id)

Synonyms N-carbamoyl-L-glutamic acid; N-carbamylglutamate

U.S./Canadian Brand Names Carbaglu® [US]

Therapeutic Category Antidote; Metabolic Alkalosis Agent; Urea Cycle Disorder (UCD) Treatment Agent

Use Adjunctive treatment of acute hyperammonemia and maintenance therapy of chronic hyperammonemia due to the deficiency of the hepatic enzyme N-acetylglutamate synthase (NAGS)

Product Availability Carbaglu®: FDA approved March 2010; availability expected in third quarter 2010; consult prescribing information for additional information

Carimune™ *(Discontinued)* *see* immune globulin (intravenous) *on page* *502*

Carimune® NF [US] *see* immune globulin (intravenous) *on page* *502*

carisoprodate *see* carisoprodol *on page* *185*

carisoprodol (kar eye soe PROE dole)

Synonyms carisoprodate; isobamate

U.S./Canadian Brand Names Soma® [US]

Therapeutic Category Skeletal Muscle Relaxant

Use Short-term (2-3 weeks) treatment of acute musculoskeletal pain

Dosage Summary Note: Carisoprodol should only be used for short periods (2-3 weeks) due to lack of evidence of effectiveness with prolonged use.

Oral:

Children <16 years: Dosage not established

Children ≥16 years: 250-350 mg 3 times/day and at bedtime

Adults: 250-350 mg 3 times/day and at bedtime

Elderly: Use not recommended

Dosage Forms

Tablet, oral: 350 mg

Soma®: 250 mg, 350 mg

carisoprodol and aspirin (kar eye soe PROE dole & AS pir in)

Synonyms aspirin and carisoprodol

U.S./Canadian Brand Names Soma® Compound [US]

Therapeutic Category Skeletal Muscle Relaxant

Use Relief of discomfort associated with acute, painful skeletal muscle conditions

Dosage Summary

Oral:

Children <16 years: Dosage not established

Children ≥16 years: 1-2 tablets 4 times/day (maximum: 8 tablets/24 hours)

Adults: 1-2 tablets 4 times/day (maximum: 8 tablets/24 hours)

Elderly: Use not recommended

Dosage Forms

Tablet: Carisoprodol 200 mg and aspirin 325 mg

Soma® Compound: Carisoprodol 200 mg and aspirin 325 mg

carisoprodol, aspirin, and codeine (kar eye soe PROE dole, AS pir in, and KOE deen)

Synonyms aspirin, carisoprodol, and codeine; codeine, aspirin, and carisoprodol

Therapeutic Category Skeletal Muscle Relaxant

Controlled Substance C-III

Use Skeletal muscle relaxant

Dosage Summary

Oral:

Children: Dosage not established

Adults: 1-2 tablets 4 times/day (maximum: 8 tablets/day)

Dosage Forms

Tablet: Carisoprodol 200 mg, aspirin 325 mg, and codeine 16 mg

Carmol® 10 [US-OTC] *see* urea *on page* *970*

Carmol® 20 [US-OTC] *see* urea *on page* *970*

Carmol® 40 [US] *see* urea *on page* *970*

Carmol® Deep Cleansing [US-OTC] *see* urea *on page* *970*

Carmol-HC® [US] *see* urea and hydrocortisone *on page* *971*

Carmol® Scalp Treatment [US] *see* sulfacetamide (topical) *on page* *900*

carmustine (kar MUS teen)

Sound-Alike/Look-Alike Issues
carmustine may be confused with bendamustine, lomustine

Synonyms BCNU; bis-chloronitrosourea; carmustinum; WR-139021

U.S./Canadian Brand Names BiCNU® [US/Can]; Gliadel Wafer® [Can]; Gliadel® [US]

Therapeutic Category Antineoplastic Agent

Use

Injection: Treatment of brain tumors (glioblastoma, brainstem glioma, medulloblastoma, astrocytoma, ependymoma, and metastatic brain tumors), multiple myeloma, Hodgkin disease (relapsed or refractory), non-Hodgkin lymphomas (relapsed or refractory),

Wafer (implant): Adjunct to surgery in patients with recurrent glioblastoma multiforme; adjunct to surgery and radiation in patients with high-grade malignant glioma

Dosage Summary

I.V.:
Adults: 150-200 mg/m^2 every 6-8 weeks **or** 75-100 mg/m^2/day for 2 days every 6-8 weeks

Implantation:
Children: Dosage not established
Adults: Up to 8 wafers may be placed in the resection cavity (total dose: 62.6 mg)

Dosage Forms

Injection, powder for reconstitution:
BiCNU®: 100 mg

Wafer, for implantation:
Gliadel®: 7.7 mg (8s)

carmustinum *see* carmustine *on page 186*
Carnation Instant Breakfast® [US-OTC] *see* nutritional formula, enteral/oral *on page 692*
Carnitine-300 [US-OTC] *see* levocarnitine *on page 556*
Carnitor® [US/Can] *see* levocarnitine *on page 556*
Carnitor® SF [US] *see* levocarnitine *on page 556*
Carrington® Antifungal [US-OTC] *see* miconazole (topical) *on page 630*
Carrington® Oral Wound Rinse [US-OTC] *see* maltodextrin *on page 589*

carteolol (ophthalmic) (KAR tee oh lole)

Sound-Alike/Look-Alike Issues
carteolol may be confused with carvedilol

Synonyms carteolol hydrochloride

Therapeutic Category Ophthalmic Agent, Antiglaucoma

Use Treatment of chronic open-angle glaucoma and intraocular hypertension

Dosage Summary

Ophthalmic:
Children: Dosage not established
Adults: Instill 1 drop in affected eye(s) twice daily

Dosage Forms

Solution, ophthalmic: 1% (5 mL, 10 mL, 15 mL)

carteolol hydrochloride *see* carteolol (ophthalmic) *on page 186*
Carter's Little Pills® [Can] *see* bisacodyl *on page 138*
Carter's Little Pills® *(Discontinued)* *see* bisacodyl *on page 138*
Cartia XT® [US] *see* diltiazem *on page 306*

carvedilol (KAR ve dil ole)

Sound-Alike/Look-Alike Issues
carvedilol may be confused with atenolol, captopril, carbidopa, carteolol
Coreg® may be confused with Corgard®, Cortef®, Cozaar®

U.S./Canadian Brand Names Apo-Carvedilol® [Can]; Coreg CR® [US]; Coreg® [US/Can]; Dom-Carvedilol [Can]; Mylan-Carvedilol [Can]; Novo-Carvedilol [Can]; PHL-Carvedilol [Can]; PMS-Carvedilol [Can]; RAN™-Carvedilol [Can]; ratio-Carvedilol [Can]; ZYM-Carvedilol [Can]

Therapeutic Category Beta-Adrenergic Blocker

Use Mild-to-severe heart failure of ischemic or cardiomyopathic origin (usually in addition to standard therapy); left ventricular dysfunction following myocardial infarction (MI) (clinically stable with LVEF ≤40%); management of hypertension

Dosage Summary

Oral:

Children: Dosage not established

Adults:

HF: Immediate release: Initial: 3.125 mg twice daily for 2 weeks; Maintenance: 6.25-50 mg twice daily (maximum: 50 mg/day [<85 kg]; 100 mg/day [>85 kg]). Extended release: Initial: 10 mg once daily; range 10-80 mg once daily. **Note:** Titration is recommended.

HTN: Immediate release: Initial: 6.25 mg twice daily; Maintenance: 12.5-25 mg twice daily (maximum: 50 mg/day). Extended release: Initial: 20 mg; range: 20-80 mg once daily. **Note:** Titration is recommended.

Left ventricular dysfunction following MI: Immediate release: Initial: 3.125-6.25 mg twice daily; Target dose: 25 mg twice daily. Extended release: Initial: 20 mg once daily; range 20-80 mg once daily. **Note:** Titration is recommended.

Dosage Forms

Capsule, extended release, oral:

Coreg CR®: 10 mg, 20 mg, 40 mg, 80 mg

Tablet, oral: 3.125 mg, 6.25 mg, 12.5 mg, 25 mg

Coreg®: 3.125 mg, 6.25 mg, 12.5 mg, 25 mg

Casodex® [US/Can] *see* bicalutamide *on page* 137

caspofungin (kas poe FUN jin)

Synonyms caspofungin acetate

U.S./Canadian Brand Names Cancidas® [US/Can]

Therapeutic Category Antifungal Agent, Systemic

Use Treatment of invasive *Aspergillus* infections in patients who are refractory or intolerant of other therapy; treatment of candidemia and other *Candida* infections (intraabdominal abscesses, esophageal, peritonitis, pleural space); empirical treatment for presumed fungal infections in febrile neutropenic patient

Dosage Summary

I.V.:

Children <3 months: Dosage not established

Children 3 months to 17 years: 70 mg/m^2 on day 1, subsequent dosing: 50 mg/m^2 once daily, if clinical response inadequate, may increase to 70 mg/m^2 once daily if tolerated, but increased efficacy not demonstrated (maximum dose: 70 mg/day)

Adults: Initial: 70 mg on day 1; Subsequent dose: 50 mg once daily; may increase to 70 mg once daily if clinical response inadequate or concomitant use with enzyme inducer

Dosage Forms

Injection, powder for reconstitution:

Cancidas®: 50 mg, 70 mg

caspofungin acetate *see* caspofungin *on page* 187

Castellani Paint Modified [US-OTC] *see* phenol *on page* 748

castor oil (KAS tor oyl)

Synonyms oleum ricini

Therapeutic Category Laxative

Use Preparation for rectal or bowel examination or surgery; rarely used to relieve constipation; also applied to skin as emollient and protectant

Dosage Summary

Oral:

Children <2 years: Dosage not established

Children 2-11 years: 5-15 mL as a single dose

Children ≥12 years: 15-60 mL as a single dose

Adults: 15-60 mL as a single dose

Dosage Forms

Oil, oral: 100% (60 mL, 120 mL, 180 mL, 480 mL, 3840 mL)

cefaclor (SEF a klor)

Sound-Alike/Look-Alike Issues

cefaclor may be confused with cephalexin

U.S./Canadian Brand Names Apo-Cefaclor® [Can]; Ceclor® [Can]; Novo-Cefaclor [Can]; Nu-Cefaclor [Can]; PMS-Cefaclor [Can]; Raniclor™ [US]

Therapeutic Category Cephalosporin (Second Generation)

Use Treatment of susceptible bacterial infections including otitis media, lower respiratory tract infections, acute exacerbations of chronic bronchitis, pharyngitis and tonsillitis, urinary tract infections, skin and skin structure infections

Dosage Summary

Oral:

Children ≤1 month: Dosage not established

Children >1 month: 20-40 mg/kg/day divided every 8-12 hours (maximum: 1 g/day)

Adults: 250-500 mg every 8 hours

Dosage Forms

Capsule, oral: 250 mg, 500 mg

Powder for suspension, oral: 125 mg/5 mL (75 mL, 150 mL); 250 mg/5 mL (75 mL, 150 mL); 375 mg/5 mL (50 mL, 100 mL)

Tablet, chewable, oral:
Raniclor™: 250 mg, 375 mg
Tablet, extended release, oral: 500 mg

cefadroxil (sef a DROKS il)

Synonyms cefadroxil monohydrate

U.S./Canadian Brand Names Apo-Cefadroxil® [Can]; Novo-Cefadroxil [Can]; PRO-Cefadroxil [Can]

Therapeutic Category Cephalosporin (First Generation)

Use Treatment of susceptible bacterial infections, including those caused by group A beta-hemolytic *Streptococcus*

Dosage Summary

Oral:
Children: 30 mg/kg/day in 2 divided doses (maximum: 2 g/day)
Adults: 1-2 g/day in 2 divided doses

Dosage Forms

Capsule, oral: 500 mg
Powder for suspension, oral: 250 mg/5 mL (50 mL, 100 mL); 500 mg/5 mL (75 mL, 100 mL)
Tablet, oral: 1 g

cefadroxil monohydrate *see* cefadroxil *on page* 189
Cefanex® ***(Discontinued)*** *see* cephalexin *on page* 197

cefazolin (sef A zoe lin)

Sound-Alike/Look-Alike Issues
ceFAZolin may be confused with cefprozil, cefTRIAXone, cephalexin, cephalothin
Kefzol® may be confused with Cefzil®

Synonyms ancef; cefazolin sodium

Tall-Man ce**FAZ**olin

Therapeutic Category Cephalosporin (First Generation)

Use Treatment of respiratory tract, skin, genital, urinary tract, biliary tract, bone and joint infections, and septicemia due to susceptible gram-positive cocci (except enterococcus); some gram-negative bacilli including *E. coli*, *Proteus*, and *Klebsiella* may be susceptible; surgical prophylaxis

Dosage Summary

I.M.:
Children ≤1 month: Dosage not established
Children >1 month: 25-100 mg/kg/day divided every 6-8 hours (maximum: 6 g/day)
Adults: 250 mg to 1.5 g every 6-12 hours (maximum: 12 g/day)

I.V.:
Children ≤1 month: Dosage not established
Children >1 month: 25-100 mg/kg/day divided every 6-8 hours (maximum: 6 g/day)
Adults: 250 mg to 1.5 g every 6-12 hours (maximum: 12 g/day)

Dosage Forms

Infusion, premixed iso-osmotic dextrose solution: 1 g (50 mL)
Injection, powder for reconstitution: 500 mg, 1 g, 10 g, 20 g, 100 g, 300 g

cefazolin sodium *see* cefazolin *on page* 189

cefdinir (SEF di ner)

Synonyms CFDN

U.S./Canadian Brand Names Omnicef® [US/Can]

Therapeutic Category Cephalosporin (Third Generation)

Use Treatment of community-acquired pneumonia, acute exacerbations of chronic bronchitis, acute bacterial otitis media, acute maxillary sinusitis, pharyngitis/tonsillitis, and uncomplicated skin and skin structure infections.

Dosage Summary

Oral:
Children <6 months: Dosage not established
Children 6 months to 12 years: 14 mg/kg/day in 1-2 divided doses (maximum: 600 mg/day)
Children >12 years: 600 mg/day in 1-2 divided doses
Adults: 600 mg/day in 1-2 divided doses

Dosage Forms

Capsule, oral: 300 mg

Omnicef®: 300 mg

Powder for suspension, oral: 125 mg/5 mL (60 mL, 100 mL); 250 mg/5 mL (60 mL, 100 mL)

Omnicef®: 125 mg/5 mL (60 mL, 100 mL); 250 mg/5 mL (60 mL, 100 mL)

cefditoren (sef de TOR en)

Synonyms cefditoren pivoxil

U.S./Canadian Brand Names Spectracef® [US]

Therapeutic Category Antibiotic, Cephalosporin

Use Treatment of acute bacterial exacerbation of chronic bronchitis or community-acquired pneumonia (due to susceptible organisms including *Haemophilus influenzae*, *Haemophilus parainfluenzae*, *Streptococcus pneumoniae*-penicillin susceptible only, *Moraxella catarrhalis*); pharyngitis or tonsillitis (*Streptococcus pyogenes*); and uncomplicated skin and skin-structure infections (*Staphylococcus aureus* - not MRSA, *Streptococcus pyogenes*)

Dosage Summary

Oral:

Children <12 years: Dosage not established

Children ≥12 years: 200-400 mg twice daily

Adults: 200-400 mg twice daily

Dosage Forms

Tablet, oral: 200 mg, 400 mg

Spectracef®: 200 mg, 400 mg

cefditoren pivoxil *see* cefditoren *on page 190*

cefepime (SEF e pim)

Sound-Alike/Look-Alike Issues

cefepime may be confused with cefixime, ceftazidime

Synonyms cefepime hydrochloride

U.S./Canadian Brand Names Maxipime® [US/Can]

Therapeutic Category Cephalosporin (Fourth Generation)

Use Treatment of uncomplicated and complicated urinary tract infections, including pyelonephritis caused by *Escherichia coli, Klebsiella pneumoniae*, or *Proteus mirabilis*; monotherapy for febrile neutropenia; uncomplicated skin and skin structure infections caused by *Streptococcus pyogenes* or methicillin-susceptible staphylococci; moderate-to-severe pneumonia caused by *Streptococcus pneumoniae, Pseudomonas aeruginosa, Klebsiella pneumoniae*, or *Enterobacter* species; complicated intraabdominal infections (in combination with metronidazole) caused by *E. coli, P. aeruginosa, K. pneumoniae, Enterobacter* species, or *Bacteroides fragilis* against methicillin-susceptible staphylococci, *Enterobacter* sp, and many other gram-negative bacilli.

Children 2 months to 16 years: Empiric therapy of febrile neutropenia patients, uncomplicated skin/soft tissue infections, pneumonia, and uncomplicated/complicated urinary tract infections, including pyelonephritis.

Dosage Summary

I.M.:

Children <2 months: Dosage not established

Children ≥2 months: 50 mg/kg/dose every 12 hours

Adults: 500-1000 mg every 12 hours

I.V.:

Children <2 months: Dosage not established

Children ≥2 months: 50 mg/kg/dose every 8-12 hours

Adults: 1-2 g every 8-12 hours

Dosage Forms

Infusion, premixed iso-osmotic dextrose solution: 1 g (50 mL); 2 g (100 mL)

Injection, powder for reconstitution: 1 g, 2 g

Maxipime®: 500 mg, 1 g, 2 g

cefepime hydrochloride *see* cefepime *on page 190*

Cefizox® [US/Can] *see* ceftizoxime *on page 193*

Cefotan® ***(Discontinued)***

cefotaxime (sef oh TAKS eem)

Sound-Alike/Look-Alike Issues
cefotaxime may be confused with cefoxitin, ceftizoxime, cefuroxime

Synonyms cefotaxime sodium

U.S./Canadian Brand Names Claforan® [US/Can]

Therapeutic Category Cephalosporin (Third Generation)

Use Treatment of susceptible infection in respiratory tract, skin and skin structure, bone and joint, urinary tract, gynecologic as well as septicemia, and documented or suspected meningitis. Active against most gram-negative bacilli (not *Pseudomonas*) and gram-positive cocci (not enterococcus). Active against many penicillin-resistant pneumococci.

Dosage Summary

I.M.:

Children <1 month: Dosage not established

Children 1 month to 12 years and <50 kg: 50-200 mg/kg/day in divided doses every 6-8 hours (maximum: 12 g/day)

Children >12 years and ≥50 kg: 1-2 g every 8-12 hours **or** as a single dose

Adults: 1-2 g every 8-12 hours **or** as a single dose

I.V.:

Children <1 month: Dosage not established

Children 1 month to 12 years and <50 kg: 50-200 mg/kg/day in divided doses every 6-8 hours (maximum: 12 g/day)

Children >12 years and ≥50 kg: 1-2 g every 4-12 hours

Adults: 1-2 g every 4-12 hours

Dosage Forms

Infusion, premixed iso-osmotic solution:
Claforan®: 1 g (50 mL); 2 g (50 mL)

Injection, powder for reconstitution: 500 mg, 1 g, 2 g, 10 g, 20 g
Claforan®: 500 mg, 1 g, 2 g, 10 g

cefotaxime sodium *see* cefotaxime *on page 191*

cefoxitin (se FOKS i tin)

Sound-Alike/Look-Alike Issues
cefoxitin may be confused with cefotaxime, cefotetan, Cytoxan
Mefoxin® may be confused with Lanoxin®

Synonyms cefoxitin sodium

U.S./Canadian Brand Names Apo-Cefoxitin® [Can]; Mefoxin® [US]

Therapeutic Category Cephalosporin (Second Generation)

Use Less active against staphylococci and streptococci than first generation cephalosporins, but active against anaerobes including *Bacteroides fragilis*; active against gram-negative enteric bacilli including *E. coli*, *Klebsiella*, and *Proteus*; used predominantly for respiratory tract, skin, bone and joint, urinary tract and gynecologic as well as septicemia; surgical prophylaxis; intraabdominal infections and other mixed infections; indicated for bacterial *Eikenella corrodens* infections

Dosage Summary

I.M.:

Children ≤3 months: Dosage not established

Children >3 months: 80-160 mg/kg/day divided every 4-6 hours (maximum: 12 g/day)

Adolescents: 80-160 mg/kg/day divided every 4-6 hours (maximum: 12 g/day) **or** 1-2 g prior to surgery

Adults: 1-2 g every 4-8 hours (maximum: 12 g/day) **or** 1-2 g prior to surgery

I.V.:

Children ≤3 months: Dosage not established

Children >3 months: 80-160 mg/kg/day divided every 4-6 hours (maximum: 12 g/day) **or** 30-40 mg/kg prior to surgery

Adolescents: 80-160 mg/kg/day divided every 4-6 hours (maximum: 12 g/day) **or** 1-2 g prior to surgery

Adults: 1-2 g every 4-8 hours (maximum: 12 g/day) **or** 1-2 g prior to surgery

Dosage Forms

Infusion, premixed iso-osmotic dextrose solution:
Mefoxin®: 1 g (50 mL); 2 g (50 mL)

Injection, powder for reconstitution: 1 g, 2 g, 10 g

Powder, for prescription compounding: 100 g

cefoxitin sodium *see* cefoxitin *on page 191*

cefpodoxime (sef pode OKS eem)

Synonyms cefpodoxime proxetil

Therapeutic Category Cephalosporin (Second Generation)

Use Treatment of susceptible acute, community-acquired pneumonia caused by *S. pneumoniae* or nonbeta-lactamase producing *H. influenzae*; acute uncomplicated gonorrhea caused by *N. gonorrhoeae*; uncomplicated skin and skin structure infections caused by *S. aureus* or *S. pyogenes*; acute otitis media caused by *S. pneumoniae*, *H. influenzae*, or *M. catarrhalis*; pharyngitis or tonsillitis; and uncomplicated urinary tract infections caused by *E. coli*, *Klebsiella*, and *Proteus*

Dosage Summary

Oral:

Children <2 months: Dosage not established

Children 2 months to 12 years: 10 mg/kg/day divided every 12 hours (maximum: 400 mg/day)

Children ≥12 years: 100-400 mg every 12 hours **or** 200 mg as a single dose

Adults: 100-400 mg every 12 hours **or** 200 mg as a single dose

Dosage Forms

Granules for suspension, oral: 50 mg/5 mL (50 mL, 100 mL); 100 mg/5 mL (50 mL, 100 mL)

Tablet, oral: 100 mg, 200 mg

cefpodoxime proxetil *see* cefpodoxime *on page 192*

cefprozil (sef PROE zil)

Sound-Alike/Look-Alike Issues

cefprozil may be confused with ceFAZolin, cefuroxime

Cefzil® may be confused with Cefol®, Ceftin®, Kefzol®

U.S./Canadian Brand Names Apo-Cefprozil® [Can]; Cefzil® [Can]; Mint-Cefprozil [Can]; RAN™-Cefprozil [Can]; Sandoz-Cefprozil [Can]

Therapeutic Category Cephalosporin (Second Generation)

Use Treatment of otitis media and infections involving the respiratory tract and skin and skin structure; active against methicillin-sensitive staphylococci, many streptococci, and various gram-negative bacilli including *E. coli*, some *Klebsiella*, *P. mirabilis*, *H. influenzae*, and *Moraxella*.

Dosage Summary

Oral:

Children ≤6 months: Dosage not established

Children 6 months to 2 years: 7.5-30 mg/kg/day divided every 12 hours

Children 2-12 years: 7.5-30 mg/kg/day divided every 12 hours **or** 20 mg/kg every 24 hours (maximum: 1 g/day)

Adolescents >12 years: 250-500 mg every 12 hours **or** 500 mg every 24 hours

Adults: 250-500 mg every 12 hours **or** 500 mg every 24 hours

Dosage Forms

Powder for suspension, oral: 125 mg/5 mL (50 mL, 75 mL, 100 mL); 250 mg/5 mL (50 mL, 75 mL, 100 mL)

Tablet, oral: 250 mg, 500 mg

ceftazidime (SEF tay zi deem)

Sound-Alike/Look-Alike Issues

ceftazidime may be confused with cefepime, ceftizoxime

Ceptaz® may be confused with Septra®

Tazicef® may be confused with Tazidime®

U.S./Canadian Brand Names Fortaz® [US/Can]; Tazicef® [US]

Therapeutic Category Cephalosporin (Third Generation)

Use Treatment of documented susceptible *Pseudomonas aeruginosa* infection and infections due to other susceptible aerobic gram-negative organisms; empiric therapy of a febrile, granulocytopenic patient

Dosage Summary

I.M.:

Children: Dosage not established

Adults: 500 mg to 2 g every 8-12 hours

Elderly: Do not administer more frequently than every 12 hours

I.V.:

Children <1 month: Dosage not established

Children 1 month to 12 years: 30-50 mg/kg every 8 hours (maximum: 6 g/day)

Children ≥12 years: 500 mg to 2 g every 8-12 hours (maximum: 6 g/day)

Adults: 500 mg to 2 g every 8-12 hours (maximum: 6 g/day)

Elderly: Do not administer more frequently than every 12 hours

Dosage Forms

Infusion, premixed iso-osmotic solution:

Fortaz®: 1 g (50 mL); 2 g (50 mL)

Injection, powder for reconstitution: 1 g, 2 g, 6 g

Fortaz®: 500 mg, 1 g, 2 g, 6 g

Tazicef®: 1 g, 2 g, 6 g

ceftibuten (sef TYE byoo ten)

Sound-Alike/Look-Alike Issues

Cedax® may be confused with Cidex®

U.S./Canadian Brand Names Cedax® [US]

Therapeutic Category Cephalosporin (Third Generation)

Use Treatment of acute exacerbations of chronic bronchitis, acute bacterial otitis media, and pharyngitis/tonsillitis

Dosage Summary

Oral:

Children <6 months: Dosage not established

Children 6 months to <12 years: 9 mg/kg/day (maximum: 400 mg/day)

Children ≥12 years: 400 mg once daily

Adults: 400 mg once daily

Dosage Forms

Capsule, oral:

Cedax®: 400 mg

Powder for suspension, oral:

Cedax®: 90 mg/5 mL (60 mL, 90 mL, 120 mL)

Ceftin® [US/Can] *see* cefuroxime *on page* 194

Ceftin® Tablet 125 mg *(Discontinued)* *see* cefuroxime *on page* 194

ceftizoxime (sef ti ZOKS eem)

Sound-Alike/Look-Alike Issues

ceftizoxime may be confused with cefotaxime, ceftazidime, cefuroxime

Synonyms ceftizoxime sodium

U.S./Canadian Brand Names Cefizox® [US/Can]

Therapeutic Category Cephalosporin (Third Generation)

Use Treatment of susceptible bacterial infections, mainly respiratory tract, skin and skin structure, bone and joint, urinary tract and gynecologic, as well as septicemia; active against many gram-negative bacilli (not *Pseudomonas*), some gram-positive cocci (not *Enterococcus*), and some anaerobes

Dosage Summary

I.M.:

Children <6 months: Dosage not established

Children ≥6 months: 150-200 mg/kg/day divided every 6-8 hours (maximum: 12 g/day)

Adults: 1-2 g every 4-12 hours **or** 4 g every 8 hours (life-threatening infections) **or** 1 g as a single dose

I.V.:

Children <6 months: Dosage not established

Children ≥6 months: 150-200 mg/kg/day divided every 6-8 hours (maximum: 12 g/day)

Adults: 1-2 g every 4 hours **or** 1-4 g every 8-12 hours

Dosage Forms

Infusion, premixed in D_5W [preservative free]:

Cefizox®: 1 g (50 mL); 2 g (50 mL)

ceftizoxime sodium *see* ceftizoxime *on page* 193

ceftobiprole *(Canada only)* (sef toe BYE prole)

Synonyms BAL5788; BAL9141; ceftobiprole medocaril

U.S./Canadian Brand Names Zeftera™ [Can]

Therapeutic Category Antibiotic, Cephalosporin

Use Treatment of complicated skin and skin structure infections, including diabetic foot infections without concurrent osteomyelitis, caused by *Enterobacter cloacae, Escherichia coli, Klebsiella pneumoniae, Proteus mirabilis, Staphylococcus aureus* (including methicillin-resistant staphylococcus aureus [MRSA]) and *Streptococcus pyogenes*

Dosage Summary

I.V.:

Children: Dosage not established
Adults: 500 mg every 8-12 hours

Dosage Forms - Canada

Injection, powder for reconstitution:

Zeftera™: 500 mg

ceftobiprole medocaril *see* ceftobiprole *(Canada only) on page 193*

ceftriaxone (sef trye AKS one)

Sound-Alike/Look-Alike Issues

cefTRIAXone may be confused with CeFAZolin, Cetraxal®
Rocephin® may be confused with Roferon®

Synonyms ceftriaxone sodium

Tall-Man cef**TRIAX**one

U.S./Canadian Brand Names Rocephin® [US/Can]

Therapeutic Category Cephalosporin (Third Generation)

Use Treatment of lower respiratory tract infections, acute bacterial otitis media, skin and skin structure infections, bone and joint infections, intraabdominal and urinary tract infections, pelvic inflammatory disease (PID), uncomplicated gonorrhea, bacterial septicemia, and meningitis; used in surgical prophylaxis

Dosage Summary

I.M.:

Children: 50-100 mg/kg/day divided every 12-24 hours (maximum: 4 g/day) **or** 125 mg or 50 mg/kg as a single dose
Adults: 1-2 g every 12-24 hours **or** 125-250 mg as a single dose

I.V.:

Children: 50-100 mg/kg/day divided every 12-24 hours (maximum: 4 g/day)
Adults: 1-2 g every 12-24 hours

Dosage Forms

Infusion, premixed in D_5W: 1 g (50 mL); 2 g (50 mL)
Injection, powder for reconstitution: 250 mg, 500 mg, 1 g, 2 g, 10 g
Rocephin®: 500 mg, 1 g

ceftriaxone sodium *see* ceftriaxone *on page 194*

cefuroxime (se fyoor OKS eem)

Sound-Alike/Look-Alike Issues

cefuroxime may be confused with cefotaxime, cefprozil, ceftizoxime, deferoxamine
Ceftin® may be confused with Cefzil®, Cipro®
Zinacef® may be confused with Zithromax®

Synonyms cefuroxime axetil; cefuroxime sodium

U.S./Canadian Brand Names Apo-Cefuroxime® [Can]; Ceftin® [US/Can]; Cefuroxime For Injection [Can]; PRO-Cefuroxime [Can]; ratio-Cefuroxime [Can]; Zinacef® [US]

Therapeutic Category Cephalosporin (Second Generation)

Use Treatment of infections caused by staphylococci, group B streptococci, *H. influenzae* (type A and B), *E. coli*, *Enterobacter*, *Salmonella*, and *Klebsiella*; treatment of susceptible infections of the upper and lower respiratory tract, otitis media, urinary tract, uncomplicated skin and soft tissue, bone and joint, sepsis, uncomplicated gonorrhea, and early Lyme disease; surgical prophylaxis

Dosage Summary

I.M.:

Children 3 months to 12 years: 75-150 mg/kg/day divided every 8 hours (maximum: 6 g/day)
Adolescents >12 years: 750 mg to 1.5 g every 6-8 hours (maximum: 6 g/day) **or** 1.5 g as a single dose
Adults: 750 mg to 1.5 g every 6-8 hours (maximum: 6 g/day) **or** 1.5 g as a single dose

I.V.:

Children 3 months to 12 years: 75-150 mg/kg/day divided every 8 hours (maximum: 6 g/day)

Adolescents >12 years: 750 mg to 1.5 g every 6-8 hours (maximum: 6 g/day) **or** 1.5 g prior to surgery

Adults: 750 mg to 1.5 g every 6-8 hours (maximum: 6 g/day) **or** 1.5 g prior to surgery

Oral:

Children <3 months: Dosage not established

Children 3 months to 12 years: 20-30 mg/kg/day in 2 divided doses **or** 125-250 mg every 12 hours (maximum: 1 g/day)

Adolescents >12 years: 125-500 mg every 12 hours **or** 1 g as a single dose

Adults: 125-500 mg every 12 hours **or** 1 g as a single dose

Dosage Forms

Infusion, premixed iso-osmotic solution:

Zinacef®: 750 mg (50 mL); 1.5 g (50 mL)

Injection, powder for reconstitution: 750 mg, 1.5 g, 7.5 g, 75 g, 225 g

Zinacef®: 750 mg, 1.5 g, 7.5 g

Powder for suspension, oral: 125 mg/5 mL (100 mL); 250 mg/5 mL (50 mL, 100 mL)

Ceftin®: 125 mg/5 mL (100 mL); 250 mg/5 mL (50 mL, 100 mL)

Tablet, oral: 250 mg, 500 mg

Ceftin®: 250 mg, 500 mg

cefuroxime axetil *see* cefuroxime *on page 194*

Cefuroxime For Injection [Can] *see* cefuroxime *on page 194*

cefuroxime sodium *see* cefuroxime *on page 194*

Cefzil® [Can] *see* cefprozil *on page 192*

Celebrex® [US/Can] *see* celecoxib *on page 195*

celecoxib (se le KOKS ib)

Sound-Alike/Look-Alike Issues

Celebrex® may be confused with Celexa®, cerebra, Cerebyx®, Cervarix®, Clarinex®

U.S./Canadian Brand Names Celebrex® [US/Can]

Therapeutic Category Nonsteroidal Antiinflammatory Drug (NSAID), COX-2 Selective

Use Relief of the signs and symptoms of osteoarthritis, ankylosing spondylitis, juvenile rheumatoid arthritis (JRA), and rheumatoid arthritis; management of acute pain; treatment of primary dysmenorrhea; to reduce the number of intestinal polyps in familial adenomatous polyposis (FAP)

Dosage Summary

Oral:

Children <2 years or <10 kg: Dosage not established

Children ≥2 years and ≥10 kg to ≤25 kg: 50 mg twice daily

Children ≥2 years and >25 kg: 100 mg twice daily

Adults: 100-400 mg/day in 1-2 divided doses **or** acute pain/dysmenorrhea: Initial: 400 mg followed by 200 mg on day 1 if needed; maintenance: 200 mg twice daily if needed **or** FAP: 400 mg twice daily

Dosage Forms

Capsule, oral:

Celebrex®: 50 mg, 100 mg, 200 mg, 400 mg

Celestone® [US] *see* betamethasone *on page 133*

Celestone® Soluspan® [US/Can] *see* betamethasone *on page 133*

Celexa® [US/Can] *see* citalopram *on page 227*

CellCept® [US/Can] *see* mycophenolate *on page 650*

Cellugel® [US] *see* hydroxypropyl methylcellulose *on page 489*

cellulose, oxidized regenerated (SEL yoo lose, OKS i dyzed re JEN er aye ted)

Sound-Alike/Look-Alike Issues

Surgicel® may be confused with Serentil®

Synonyms absorbable cotton; oxidized regenerated cellulose

U.S./Canadian Brand Names Surgicel® Fibrillar [US]; Surgicel® NuKnit [US]; Surgicel® [US]

Therapeutic Category Hemostatic Agent

Use Hemostatic; temporary packing for the control of capillary, venous, or small arterial hemorrhage

Dosage Summary

Topical:

Children: Dosage not established

Adults: Lay or hold firmly minimal amounts of the fabric strip on the bleeding site

Dosage Forms

Fabric, fibrous:

Surgicel® Fibrillar:

1" x 2" (10s)

2" x 4" (10s)

4" x 4" (10s)

Fabric, knitted:

Surgicel® NuKnit:

1" x 1" (24s)

1" x 3 1/2" (10s)

3" x 4" (24s)

6" x 9" (10s)

Fabric, sheer weave:

Surgicel®:

1/2" x 2" (24s)

2" x 3" (24s)

2" x 14" (24s)

4" x 8" (24s)

Celluvisc™ [Can] *see* carboxymethylcellulose *on page 184*

Celontin® [US/Can] *see* methsuximide *on page 617*

Celsentri™ [Can] *see* maraviroc *on page 591*

Cemill 500 [US-OTC] *see* ascorbic acid *on page 98*

Cemill 1000 [US-OTC] *see* ascorbic acid *on page 98*

Cena-K® *(Discontinued)* *see* potassium chloride *on page 781*

Cenestin® [US/Can] *see* estrogens (conjugated A/synthetic) *on page 369*

Cenolate® *(Discontinued)* *see* ascorbic acid *on page 98*

Centamin [US-OTC] *see* vitamins (multiple/oral) *on page 990*

Centany™ *(Discontinued)* *see* mupirocin *on page 649*

Centrum® [US-OTC] *see* vitamins (multiple/oral) *on page 990*

Centrum Cardio® [US-OTC] *see* vitamins (multiple/oral) *on page 990*

Centrum Kids® Complete Dora the Explorer™ [US-OTC] *see* vitamins (multiple/pediatric) *on page 990*

Centrum Kids® Complete Rugrats™ [US-OTC] *see* vitamins (multiple/pediatric) *on page 990*

Centrum Kids® Complete SpongeBob SquarePants™ [US-OTC] *see* vitamins (multiple/pediatric) *on page 990*

Centrum Performance® [US-OTC] *see* vitamins (multiple/oral) *on page 990*

Centrum® Silver® [US-OTC] *see* vitamins (multiple/oral) *on page 990*

Centrum® Silver® Ultra Men's [US-OTC] *see* vitamins (multiple/oral) *on page 990*

Centrum® Silver® Ultra Women's [US-OTC] *see* vitamins (multiple/oral) *on page 990*

Centrum® Ultra Men's [US-OTC] *see* vitamins (multiple/oral) *on page 990*

Centrum® Ultra Women's [US-OTC] *see* vitamins (multiple/oral) *on page 990*

Cepacol® [US-OTC] *see* cetylpyridinium *on page 199*

Cepacol® Fizzlers™ [US-OTC] *see* benzocaine *on page 124*

Cepacol® Maximum Strength [US-OTC] *see* dyclonine *on page 338*

Cepacol® Sore Throat Pain Relief [US-OTC] *see* benzocaine *on page 124*

Cepacol® Sore Throat Plus Coating Relief [US-OTC] *see* benzocaine *on page 124*

Cepastat® [US-OTC] *see* phenol *on page 748*

Cepastat® Extra Strength [US-OTC] *see* phenol *on page 748*

Cephadyn [US] *see* butalbital and acetaminophen *on page 159*

cephalexin (sef a LEKS in)

Sound-Alike/Look-Alike Issues

cephalexin may be confused with cefaclor, ceFAZolin, cephalothin, ciprofloxacin

Keflex® may be confused with Keppra®, Valtrex®

Synonyms cephalexin monohydrate

U.S./Canadian Brand Names Apo-Cephalex® [Can]; Dom-Cephalexin [Can]; Keflex® [US/Can]; Keftab® [Can]; Novo-Lexin [Can]; Nu-Cephalex [Can]; PMS-Cephalexin [Can]

Therapeutic Category Cephalosporin (First Generation)

Use Treatment of susceptible bacterial infections including respiratory tract infections, otitis media, skin and skin structure infections, bone infections, and genitourinary tract infections, including acute prostatitis; alternative therapy for acute infective endocarditis prophylaxis

Dosage Summary

Oral:

Children ≤1 year: Dosage not established

Children >1-15 years: 25-100 mg/kg/day divided every 6-12 hours (maximum: 4 g/day) **or** 50 mg/kg prior to procedure (maximum: 2 g)

Adolescents >15 years: 25-100 mg/kg/day divided every 6-12 hours (maximum: 4 g/day) **or** 50 mg/kg prior to procedure (maximum: 2 g) **or** 500 mg every 12 hours (uncomplicated cystitis)

Adults: 250-1000 mg every 6 hours **or** 500 mg every 12 hours (maximum: 4 g/day) **or** 2 g prior to procedure

Dosage Forms

Capsule, oral: 250 mg, 500 mg

Keflex®: 250 mg, 500 mg, 750 mg

Powder for suspension, oral: 125 mg/5 mL (100 mL, 200 mL); 250 mg/5 mL (100 mL, 200 mL)

Tablet, oral: 250 mg, 500 mg

cephalexin monohydrate *see* cephalexin *on page 197*

cephalothin *(Discontinued)*

Cephulac® *(Discontinued)* *see* lactulose *on page 544*

Ceprotin [US] *see* protein C concentrate (human) *on page 809*

Ceptaz® *(Discontinued)* *see* ceftazidime *on page 192*

Cerebyx® [US/Can] *see* fosphenytoin *on page 429*

Ceredase® [US] *see* alglucerase *on page 49*

Cerefolin® NAC [US] *see* methylfolate, methylcobalamin, and acetylcysteine *on page 620*

Cerezyme® [US/Can] *see* imiglucerase *on page 500*

Ceron [US] *see* chlorpheniramine and phenylephrine *on page 208*

Ceron-DM [US] *see* chlorpheniramine, phenylephrine, and dextromethorphan *on page 211*

Cerovel™ *(Discontinued)* *see* urea *on page 970*

Certain Dri® [US-OTC] *see* aluminum chloride hexahydrate *on page 58*

certolizumab pegol (cer to LIZ u mab PEG ol)

Synonyms CDP870

U.S./Canadian Brand Names Cimzia® [US/Can]

Therapeutic Category Gastrointestinal Agent, Miscellaneous; Tumor Necrosis Factor (TNF) Blocking Agent

Use Treatment of moderately- to severely-active Crohn disease in patients who have inadequate response to conventional therapy; moderately- to severely-active rheumatoid arthritis (as monotherapy or in combination with nonbiological disease-modifying antirheumatic drugs [DMARDS])

Dosage Summary

SubQ:

Children: Dosage not established

Adults: Initial: 400 mg, repeat dose 2 and 4 weeks after initial dose; Maintenance: 400 mg every 4 weeks **or** 200 mg every other week

Dosage Forms

Injection, powder for reconstitution [preservative free]:

Cimzia®: 200 mg

Injection, solution [preservative free]:

Cimzia®: 200 mg/mL (1 mL)

Certuss-D® [US] *see* guaifenesin, dextromethorphan, and phenylephrine *on page 458*
Cerubidine® [US/Can] *see* daunorubicin hydrochloride *on page 271*
Cerumenex® *(Discontinued)*
Cervarix® [US/Can] *see* papillomavirus (types 16, 18) vaccine (human, recombinant) *on page 726*
Cervidil® [US/Can] *see* dinoprostone *on page 308*
C.E.S.® [Can] *see* estrogens (conjugated/equine, systemic) *on page 370*
C.E.S. *see* estrogens (conjugated/equine, systemic) *on page 370*
C.E.S. *see* estrogens (conjugated/equine, topical) *on page 371*
Cesia™ [US] *see* ethinyl estradiol and desogestrel *on page 374*
Cetacaine® [US] *see* benzocaine, butamben, and tetracaine *on page 127*
Cetacort® *(Discontinued)* *see* hydrocortisone (topical) *on page 483*
Cetafen® [US-OTC] *see* acetaminophen *on page 21*
Cetafen Cold® [US-OTC] *see* acetaminophen and phenylephrine *on page 25*
Cetafen® Extra [US-OTC] *see* acetaminophen *on page 21*
Cetapred® Ophthalmic *(Discontinued)* *see* sulfacetamide and prednisolone *on page 900*

cetirizine (se TI ra zeen)

Sound-Alike/Look-Alike Issues
Zyrtec® may be confused with Lipitor©, Serax®, Xanax®, Zantac®, Zerit®, Zocor®, Zyprexa®, Zyrtec-D®
Zyrtec® (cetirizine) may be confused with Zyrtec® Itchy Eye (ketotifen)

Synonyms cetirizine hydrochloride; P-071; UCB-P071

U.S./Canadian Brand Names All Day Allergy [US-OTC]; Apo-Cetirizine® [Can]; PMS-Cetirizine [Can]; Reactine™ [Can]; Zyrtec® Allergy [US-OTC]; Zyrtec® Children's Allergy [US-OTC]; Zyrtec® Children's Hives Relief [US-OTC]

Therapeutic Category Antihistamine

Use Perennial and seasonal allergic rhinitis and other allergic symptoms including urticaria; chronic idiopathic urticaria

Dosage Summary
Oral:
Children <6 months: Dosage not established
Children 6-12 months: 2.5 mg once daily
Children 12 months to <2 years: 2.5 mg once or twice daily
Children 2-5 years: 2.5-5 mg/day in 1-2 divided doses
Children ≥6 years: 5-10 mg once daily
Adults: 5-10 mg once daily
Elderly: Initial: 5 mg once daily

Dosage Forms
Capsule, liquid gel, oral:
Zyrtec® Allergy [OTC]: 10 mg
Syrup, oral: 5 mg/5 mL (5 mL, 118 mL, 120 mL, 473 mL, 480 mL)
Zyrtec® Children's Allergy [OTC]: 5 mg/5 mL (118 mL)
Zyrtec® Children's Hives Relief [OTC]: 5 mg/5 mL (118 mL)
Tablet, oral: 5 mg, 10 mg
All Day Allergy [OTC]: 10 mg
Zyrtec® Allergy [OTC]: 10 mg
Tablet, chewable, oral: 5 mg, 10 mg
Zyrtec® Children's Allergy [OTC]: 5 mg, 10 mg

cetirizine and pseudoephedrine (se TI ra zeen & soo doe e FED rin)

Sound-Alike/Look-Alike Issues
Zyrtec® may be confused with Lipitor®, Serax®, Xanax®, Zantac®, Zocor®, Zyprexa®, Zyrtec-D®
Zyrtec-D® may be confused with Zyrtec®

Synonyms cetirizine hydrochloride and pseudoephedrine hydrochloride; pseudoephedrine hydrochloride and cetirizine hydrochloride

U.S./Canadian Brand Names Reactine® Allergy and Sinus [Can]; Zytrec-D® Allergy & Congestion [US-OTC]

Therapeutic Category Antihistamine/Decongestant Combination

Use Treatment of symptoms of seasonal or perennial allergic rhinitis

Dosage Summary

Oral:

Children <12 years: Dosage not established

Children ≥12 years: 1 tablet twice daily (maximum: 2 tablets/day)

Adults: 1 tablet twice daily (maximum: 2 tablets/day)

Dosage Forms

Tablet, extended release: Cetirizine hydrochloride 5 mg and pseudoephedrine hydrochloride 120 mg

Zyrtec-D® Allergy & Congestion [OTC]: Cetirizine 5 mg and pseudoephedrine 120 mg

cetirizine hydrochloride *see* cetirizine *on page 198*

cetirizine hydrochloride and pseudoephedrine hydrochloride *see* cetirizine and pseudoephedrine *on page 198*

Cetraxal® [US] *see* ciprofloxacin (otic) *on page 225*

cetrorelix (set roe REL iks)

Synonyms cetrorelix acetate

U.S./Canadian Brand Names Cetrotide® [US/Can]

Therapeutic Category Antigonadotropic Agent

Use Inhibits premature luteinizing hormone (LH) surges in women undergoing controlled ovarian stimulation

Dosage Summary

SubQ:

Children: Dosage not established

Adults (females): 0.25 mg once daily **or** 3 mg as a single dose

Elderly ≥65 years: Dosage not established

Dosage Forms

Injection, powder for reconstitution:

Cetrotide®: 0.25 mg, 3 mg

cetrorelix acetate *see* cetrorelix *on page 199*

Cetrotide® [US/Can] *see* cetrorelix *on page 199*

cetuximab (se TUK see mab)

Sound-Alike/Look-Alike Issues

cetuximab may be confused with bevacizumab

Synonyms C225; IMC-C225; MOAB C225

U.S./Canadian Brand Names Erbitux® [US/Can]

Therapeutic Category Antineoplastic Agent, Monoclonal Antibody; Epidermal Growth Factor Receptor (EGFR) Inhibitor

Use Treatment of metastatic colorectal cancer; treatment of squamous cell cancer of the head and neck

Note: Subset analyses (retrospective) in metastatic colorectal cancer trials have not shown a benefit with EGFR inhibitor treatment in patients whose tumors have codon 12 or 13 *KRAS* mutations; use is not recommended in these patients.

Dosage Summary

I.V.:

Children: Dosage not established

Adults: Loading dose: 400 mg/m^2; Maintenance: 250 mg/m^2 weekly

Dosage Forms

Injection, solution [preservative free]:

Erbitux®: 2 mg/mL (50 mL, 100 mL)

cetyl alcohol, glycerin, lanolin, mineral oil, and petrolatum *see* lanolin, cetyl alcohol, glycerin, petrolatum, and mineral oil *on page 548*

cetylpyridinium (SEE til peer i DI nee um)

Synonyms cetylpyridinium chloride; CPC

U.S./Canadian Brand Names Cepacol® [US-OTC]; DiabetAid Therapeutic Gingivitis Mouth Rinse [US-OTC]

Therapeutic Category Local Anesthetic

Use Antiseptic to aid in the prevention and reduction of plaque and gingivitis, and to freshen breath

Dosage Summary

Oral:

Children <6 years: Dosage not established

Children ≥6 years: Rinse or gargle in mouth

Adults: Rinse or gargle in mouth

Dosage Forms

Liquid, oral:

Cepacol® [OTC]: 0.05% (360 mL, 720 mL)

DiabetAid Therapeutic Gingivitis Mouth Rinse [OTC]: 0.1% (480 mL)

cetylpyridinium chloride *see* cetylpyridinium *on page 199*

Cevalin® ***(Discontinued)*** *see* ascorbic acid *on page 98*

cevimeline (se vi ME leen)

Sound-Alike/Look-Alike Issues

cevimeline may be confused with Savella™

Evoxac® may be confused with Eurax®

Synonyms cevimeline hydrochloride

U.S./Canadian Brand Names Evoxac® [US/Can]

Therapeutic Category Cholinergic Agent

Use Treatment of symptoms of dry mouth in patients with Sjögren syndrome

Dosage Summary

Oral:

Children: Dosage not established

Adults: 30 mg 3 times/day

Dosage Forms

Capsule, oral:

Evoxac®: 30 mg

cevimeline hydrochloride *see* cevimeline *on page 200*

CFDN *see* cefdinir *on page 189*

CG *see* chorionic gonadotropin (human) *on page 219*

CG5503 *see* tapentadol *on page 910*

C-Gel [US-OTC] *see* ascorbic acid *on page 98*

CGP 33101 *see* rufinamide *on page 856*

CGP-39393 *see* desirudin *on page 277*

CGP-42446 *see* zoledronic acid *on page 1003*

CGP-57148B *see* imatinib *on page 499*

C-Gram [US-OTC] *see* ascorbic acid *on page 98*

CGS-20267 *see* letrozole *on page 553*

Champix® [Can] *see* varenicline *on page 978*

Chantix® [US] *see* varenicline *on page 978*

Charcadole® [Can] *see* charcoal *on page 200*

Charcadole®, Aqueous [Can] *see* charcoal *on page 200*

Charcadole® TFS [Can] *see* charcoal *on page 200*

Char-Caps [US-OTC] *see* charcoal *on page 200*

CharcoAid® ***(Discontinued)*** *see* charcoal *on page 200*

charcoal (CHAR kole)

Sound-Alike/Look-Alike Issues

Actidose® may be confused with Actos®

Synonyms activated carbon; activated charcoal; adsorbent charcoal; liquid antidote; medicinal carbon; medicinal charcoal

U.S./Canadian Brand Names Actidose® with Sorbitol [US-OTC]; Actidose®-Aqua [US-OTC]; Char-Caps [US-OTC]; Charcadole® TFS [Can]; Charcadole® [Can]; Charcadole®, Aqueous [Can]; Charcoal Plus® DS [US-OTC]; CharcoCaps® [US-OTC]; EZ-Char® [US-OTC]; Kerr Insta-Char® [US-OTC]; Requa® Activated Charcoal [US-OTC]

Therapeutic Category Antidote

Use Emergency treatment in poisoning by drugs and chemicals; aids the elimination of certain drugs and improves decontamination of excessive ingestions of sustained-release products or in the presence of bezoars; repetitive doses have proven useful to enhance the elimination of certain drugs (eg, carbamazepine, dapsone, phenobarbital, quinine, or theophylline); repetitive doses for gastric dialysis in uremia to adsorb various waste products; dietary supplement (digestive aid)

Dosage Summary **Note:** ~10 g of activated charcoal for each 1 g of toxin is considered adequate

Oral:

Children <1 year: 10-25 g **or** 0.5-1 g/kg as a single dose; additional doses can be given as 0.25 g/kg/hour or equivalent

Children 1-12 years: 25-50 g **or** 0.5-1 g/kg as a single dose; additional doses can be given as 0.25 g/kg/hour or equivalent

Children >12 years: 25-100 g **or** 1 g/kg as a single dose, additional doses can be given as 12.5 g/hour (0.25 g/kg/hour) or equivalent

Adults:

Acute poisoning: 25-100 mg as a single dose, additional doses can be given as 12.5 g/hour or equivalent

Dietary supplement: 500-520 mg after meals, may repeat in 2 hours (maximum: 10 g/day)

Dosage Forms

Capsule, oral:

Char-Caps [OTC]: 260 mg

CharcoCaps® [OTC]: 260 mg

Pellets for suspension, oral:

EZ-Char® [OTC]: 25 g/bottle (1s)

Powder for suspension, oral: USP: 100% (30 g, 240 g)

Suspension, oral:

Actidose® with Sorbitol [OTC]: 25 g (120 mL); 50 g (240 mL)

Actidose®-Aqua [OTC]: 15 g (72 mL); 25 g (120 mL); 50 g (240 mL)

Kerr Insta-Char® [OTC]: 25 g (120 mL); 50 g (240 mL)

Tablet, oral:

Requa® Activated Charcoal [OTC]: 250 mg

Tablet, enteric coated, oral:

Charcoal Plus® DS [OTC]: 250 mg

Charcoal Plus® DS [US-OTC] *see* charcoal *on page 200*

CharcoCaps® [US-OTC] *see* charcoal *on page 200*

Chealamide® ***(Discontinued)*** *see* edetate disodium *on page 342*

CheeTah® ***(Discontinued)*** *see* barium *on page 117*

Chemet® [US/Can] *see* succimer *on page 896*

Chenodal™ [US] *see* chenodiol *on page 201*

chenodeoxycholic acid *see* chenodiol *on page 201*

chenodiol (kee noe DYE ole)

Synonyms CDCA; chenodeoxycholic acid

U.S./Canadian Brand Names Chenodal™ [US]

Therapeutic Category Bile Acid

Use Oral dissolution of radiolucent cholesterol gallstones in selected patients as an alternative to surgery

Dosage Summary

Oral:

Adults: Initial: 250 mg twice daily; maintenance: 13-16 mg/kg/day in 2 divided doses

Dosage Forms

Tablet, oral:

Chenodal™: 250 mg

Cheracol® D [US-OTC] *see* guaifenesin and dextromethorphan *on page 455*

Cheracol® ***(Discontinued)*** *see* guaifenesin and codeine *on page 455*

Cheracol® Plus [US-OTC] *see* guaifenesin and dextromethorphan *on page 455*

Cheracol® Spray [US-OTC] *see* phenol *on page 748*

cheratussin *see* guaifenesin *on page 454*

Chew-C [US-OTC] *see* ascorbic acid *on page 98*

Chew-Cal [US-OTC] *see* calcium and vitamin D *on page 166*
CHG *see* chlorhexidine gluconate *on page 204*
Chibroxin® *(Discontinued)* *see* norfloxacin *on page 684*
chickenpox vaccine *see* varicella virus vaccine *on page 978*
Chiggerex® Plus [US-OTC] *see* benzocaine *on page 124*
ChiggerTox® [US-OTC] *see* benzocaine *on page 124*
Children's Advil® Cold [Can] *see* pseudoephedrine and ibuprofen *on page 812*
Children's Dimetapp® Elixir Cold & Allergy *(Discontinued)* *see* brompheniramine and pseudoephedrine *on page 148*
Children's Hold® *(Discontinued)* *see* dextromethorphan *on page 287*
Children's Kaopectate® *(Discontinued)*
Children's Motion Sickness Liquid [Can] *see* dimenhydrinate *on page 307*
Children's Nasal Decongestant [US-OTC] *see* pseudoephedrine *on page 810*
Children's Pepto [US-OTC] *see* calcium carbonate *on page 167*
children's vitamins *see* vitamins (multiple/pediatric) *on page 990*
ChiRhoStim® [US] *see* secretin *on page 868*
Chirocaine® *(Discontinued)*
Chlo-Amine® Oral *(Discontinued)* *see* chlorpheniramine *on page 207*
chloditan *see* mitotane *on page 638*
chlodithane *see* mitotane *on page 638*
Chlorafed® Liquid *(Discontinued)* *see* chlorpheniramine and pseudoephedrine *on page 209*
chloral *see* chloral hydrate *on page 202*

chloral hydrate (KLOR al HYE drate)

Synonyms chloral; hydrated chloral; trichloroacetaldehyde monohydrate

U.S./Canadian Brand Names PMS-Chloral Hydrate [Can]; Somnote® [US]

Therapeutic Category Hypnotic, Nonbarbiturate

Controlled Substance C-IV

Use Short-term sedative and hypnotic (<2 weeks); sedative/hypnotic for diagnostic procedures; sedative prior to EEG evaluations

Dosage Summary

Oral:

Children:

Conscious sedation: 50-75 mg/kg prior to procedure, may repeat (maximum total: 1 g)
Hypnotic: 20-50 mg/kg (maximum: 1 g/dose or 2 g/day)
Prior to EEG: 20-25 mg/kg, may repeat (maximum total: 2 g)
Sedation/anxiolytic: 5-15 mg/kg every 8 hours (maximum: 500 mg/dose)

Adults: 250 mg 3 times/day **or** 500-1000 mg at bedtime or prior to procedure (maximum: 2 g/day)

Elderly: Hypnotic: Initial: 250 mg at bedtime

Rectal:

Children:

Conscious sedation: 50-75 mg/kg prior to procedure, may repeat (maximum total: 1 g)
Hypnotic: 20-50 mg/kg (maximum: 2 g/day)
Prior to EEG: 20-25 mg/kg, may repeat (maximum total: 2 g)
Sedation/anxiolytic: 5-15 mg/kg every 8 hours (maximum: 500 mg/dose)

Adults: 250 mg 3 times/day **or** 500-1000 mg at bedtime or prior to procedure (maximum: 2 g/day)

Dosage Forms

Capsule, oral:

Somnote®: 500 mg

Suppository, rectal: 500 mg (25s)

Syrup, oral: 500 mg/5 mL (5 mL, 473 mL, 480 mL)

chlorambucil (klor AM byoo sil)

Sound-Alike/Look-Alike Issues

chlorambucil may be confused with Chloromycetin®
Leukeran® may be confused with Alkeran®, leucovorin, Leukine®, Myleran®

Synonyms CB-1348; chlorambucilum; chloraminophene; chlorbutinum; WR-139013

U.S./Canadian Brand Names Leukeran® [US/Can]

Therapeutic Category Antineoplastic Agent

Use Management of chronic lymphocytic leukemia (CLL), Hodgkin lymphoma, non-Hodgkin lymphoma (NHL)

Dosage Summary

Oral:

Adults: 0.1-0.2 mg/kg/day for 3-6 weeks **or** 0.4 mg/kg biweekly or monthly (may increase by 0.1 mg/kg/dose) **or** 0.03-0.1 mg/kg/day

Elderly: Use lowest recommended dose; usual dose: 2-4 mg/day

Dosage Forms

Tablet, oral:

Leukeran®: 2 mg

chlorambucilum *see* chlorambucil *on page 202*

chloraminophene *see* chlorambucil *on page 202*

chloramphenicol (klor am FEN i kole)

Sound-Alike/Look-Alike Issues

Chloromycetin® may be confused with chlorambucil, Chlor-Trimeton®

U.S./Canadian Brand Names Chloromycetin® Succinate [Can]; Chloromycetin® [Can]; Diochloram® [Can]; Pentamycetin® [Can]

Therapeutic Category Antibiotic, Miscellaneous

Use Treatment of serious infections due to organisms resistant to other less toxic antibiotics or when its penetrability into the site of infection is clinically superior to other antibiotics to which the organism is sensitive; useful in infections caused by *Bacteroides*, *H. influenzae*, *Neisseria meningitidis*, *Salmonella*, and *Rickettsia*; active against many vancomycin-resistant enterococci

Dosage Summary

I.V.:

Neonates: Loading dose: 20 mg/kg, followed by maintenance dose based on postnatal age:

≤7 days: 25 mg/kg/day once every 24 hours

>7 days, ≤2000 g: 25 mg/kg/day once every 24 hours

>7 days, >2000 g: 50 mg/kg/day divided every 12 hours

Infants >30 days and Children: 50-100 mg/kg/day divided every 6 hours (maximum: 4 g/day)

Adults: 50-100 mg/kg/day divided every 6 hours (maximum: 4 g/day)

Dosage Forms

Injection, powder for reconstitution: 1 g

ChloraPrep® [US-OTC] *see* chlorhexidine gluconate *on page 204*

ChloraPrep® Frepp® [US-OTC] *see* chlorhexidine gluconate *on page 204*

ChloraPrep® Sepp® [US-OTC] *see* chlorhexidine gluconate *on page 204*

Chlorascrub™ [US-OTC] *see* chlorhexidine gluconate *on page 204*

Chlorascrub™ Maxi [US-OTC] *see* chlorhexidine gluconate *on page 204*

Chloraseptic® Kids Sore Throat Spray [US-OTC] *see* phenol *on page 748*

Chloraseptic® Mouth Pain [US-OTC] *see* phenol *on page 748*

Chloraseptic® Sore Throat Gargle [US-OTC] *see* phenol *on page 748*

Chloraseptic® Sore Throat Spray [US-OTC] *see* phenol *on page 748*

Chlorate® Oral *(Discontinued)* *see* chlorpheniramine *on page 207*

chlorbutinum *see* chlorambucil *on page 202*

Chlordex GP [US] *see* dextromethorphan, chlorpheniramine, phenylephrine, and guaifenesin *on page 290*

chlordiazepoxide (klor dye az e POKS ide)

Sound-Alike/Look-Alike Issues

chlordiazePOXIDE may be confused with chlorproMAZINE

Librium® may be confused with Librax®

Synonyms methaminodiazepoxide hydrochloride

Tall-Man chlordiaze**POXIDE**

U.S./Canadian Brand Names Apo-Chlordiazepoxide® [Can]

Therapeutic Category Benzodiazepine

Controlled Substance C-IV

Use Management of anxiety disorder or for the short-term relief of symptoms of anxiety; withdrawal symptoms of acute alcoholism; preoperative apprehension and anxiety

Dosage Summary

I.M.:

Children ≤6 years: Dosage not established

Children >6 years: 0.5 mg/kg/day divided every 6-8 hours

Adults: Initial: 50-100 mg followed by 25-50 mg 3-4 times/day as needed **or** 50-100 mg prior to surgery (maximum: 300 mg/day)

I.V.:

Children: Dosage not established

Adults: Initial: 50-100 mg followed by 25-50 mg 3-4 times/day as needed **or** 50-100 mg to start, may repeat in 2-4 hours as needed (maximum: 300 mg/day)

Oral:

Children ≤6 years: Dosage not established

Children >6 years: 0.5 mg/kg/day divided every 6-8 hours

Adults: 15-100 mg/day in 3-4 divided doses **or** 50-100 mg to start, may repeat in 2-4 hours as needed (maximum: 300 mg/day)

Elderly: Anxiety: 5 mg 2-4 times/day

Dosage Forms

Capsule, oral: 5 mg, 10 mg, 25 mg

chlordiazepoxide and amitriptyline hydrochloride *see* amitriptyline and chlordiazepoxide *on page 68*

chlordiazepoxide and clidinium *see* clidinium and chlordiazepoxide *on page 231*

chlorethazine *see* mechlorethamine *on page 594*

chlorethazine mustard *see* mechlorethamine *on page 594*

Chlorex-A 12 *(Discontinued)* *see* chlorpheniramine, pyrilamine, and phenylephrine *on page 215*

Chlorex-A *(Discontinued)* *see* chlorpheniramine, phenylephrine, and phenyltoloxamine *on page 213*

chlorhexidine gluconate (klor HEKS i deen GLOO koe nate)

Sound-Alike/Look-Alike Issues

Peridex® may be confused with Precedex™

Synonyms CHG

U.S./Canadian Brand Names Avagard™ [US-OTC]; BactoShield® CHG [US-OTC]; Betasept® [US-OTC]; ChloraPrep® Frepp® [US-OTC]; ChloraPrep® Sepp® [US-OTC]; ChloraPrep® [US-OTC]; Chlorascrub™ Maxi [US-OTC]; Chlorascrub™ [US-OTC]; Dyna-Hex® [US-OTC]; Hibiclens® [US-OTC]; Hibidil® 1:2000 [Can]; Hibistat® [US-OTC]; Operand® Chlorhexidine Gluconate [US-OTC]; ORO-Clense [Can]; Peridex® Oral Rinse [Can]; Peridex® [US]; PerioChip® [US]; PerioGard® [US-OTC]

Therapeutic Category Antibiotic, Oral Rinse; Antibiotic, Topical

Use Skin cleanser for line placement, skin wounds, preoperative skin preparation; germicidal hand rinse; antibacterial dental rinse. Chlorhexidine is active against gram-positive and gram-negative organisms, facultative anaerobes, aerobes, and yeast.

Orphan drug: Peridex®: Oral mucositis with cytoreductive therapy when used for patients undergoing bone marrow transplant

Dosage Summary

Oral:

Periodontal chip:

Children: Dosage not established

Adults: One chip is inserted into a periodontal pocket, repeat every 3 months in pockets with depth ≥5 mm (maximum: 8 chips/visit)

Rinse:

Children: Dosage not established

Adults: Swish 15 mL in mouth, then expectorate twice daily

Topical:

Rinse/wash:

Children: Dosage not established

Adults: Apply for 15 seconds and rinse

Sanitizer:
Children: Dosage not established
Adults: Dispense 1 pumpful in each palm and spread evenly over hands, nails and just above elbow, then dispense additional pumpful in each hand and reapply up to wrist
Scrub:
Children: Dosage not established
Adults: Scrub 3 minutes and rinse, then wash for additional 3 minutes

Dosage Forms

Chip, for periodontal pocket insertion:
PerioChip®: 2.5 mg (20s)
Liquid, oral: 0.12% (473 mL, 475 mL, 480 mL)
Peridex®: 0.12% (118 mL, 473 mL, 1920 mL)
PerioGard® [OTC]: 0.12% (480 mL)
Liquid, topical:
Betasept® [OTC]: 4% (118 mL, 237 mL, 473 mL, 946 mL, 3840 mL)
Dyna-Hex® [OTC]: 2% (120 mL, 480 mL, 960 mL, 3840 mL); 4% (120 mL, 240 mL, 480 mL, 960 mL, 3840 mL)
Hibiclens® [OTC]: 4% (15 mL, 118 mL, 236 mL, 473 mL, 946 mL, 3840 mL)
Operand® Chlorhexidine Gluconate [OTC]: 2% (118 mL); 4% (118 mL, 237 mL, 472 mL, 946 mL, 3785 mL)
Lotion, topical:
Avagard™ [OTC]: 1% (500 mL)
Solution, topical:
Bactoshield® CHG [OTC]: 2% (120 mL, 480 mL, 750 mL, 960 mL, 3840 mL); 4% (120 mL, 473 mL, 960 mL, 3840 mL)
Sponge, topical:
ChloraPrep® [OTC]: 2% (25s); 2% (25s); 2% (25s); 2% (25s); 2% (25s); 2% (25s); 2% (25s); 2% (25s)
ChloraPrep® Frepp® [OTC]: 2% (20s)
ChloraPrep® Sepp® [OTC]: 2% (200s)
Sponge/Brush, topical:
Bactoshield® CHG [OTC]: 4% (300s)
Swab, topical:
Chlorascrub™ [OTC]: 3.15% (100s)
Swabsticks, topical:
ChloraPrep® [OTC]: 2% (48s, 120s)
Chlorascrub™ [OTC]: 3.15% (50s)
Chlorascrub™ Maxi [OTC]: 3.15% (30s)
Wipe, topical:
Hibistat® [OTC]: 0.5% (50s)

Chlor Hist [US-OTC] *see* chlorpheniramine *on page 207*
chlormeprazine *see* prochlorperazine *on page 797*
Chlor-Mes-D [US] *see* chlorpheniramine, phenylephrine, and methscopolamine *on page 212*
Chlor-Mes *(Discontinued)* *see* chlorpheniramine, phenylephrine, and methscopolamine *on page 212*
2-chlorodeoxyadenosine *see* cladribine *on page 229*
chloroethane *see* ethyl chloride *on page 382*
Chloromag® [US] *see* magnesium chloride *on page 583*
Chloromycetin® [Can] *see* chloramphenicol *on page 203*
Chloromycetin® Succinate [Can] *see* chloramphenicol *on page 203*

chlorophyll (KLOR oh fil)

Synonyms chlorophyllin
U.S./Canadian Brand Names Nullo® [US-OTC]
Therapeutic Category Gastrointestinal Agent, Miscellaneous
Use Control fecal odors in colostomy or ileostomy

Dosage Summary

Oral:
Children ≤12 years: Dosage not established
Children >12 years: 100-200 mg/day in divided doses (maximum: 300 mg/day)
Adults: 100-200 mg/day in divided doses (maximum: 300 mg/day)

Ostomy:

Children ≤12 years: Dosage not established

Children >12 years: Place 1-2 tablets in empty pouch each time it is reused or changed

Adults: Place 1-2 tablets in empty pouch each time it is reused or changed

Dosage Forms

Caplet, oral:

Nullo® [OTC]: Chlorophyllin copper complex 100 mg

chlorophyllin *see* chlorophyll *on page 205*

chlorophyllin, papain, and urea *(Discontinued)*

chloroprocaine (klor oh PROE kane)

Sound-Alike/Look-Alike Issues

Nesacaine® may be confused with Neptazane®

Synonyms chloroprocaine hydrochloride

U.S./Canadian Brand Names Nesacaine® [US]; Nesacaine®-CE [Can]; Nesacaine®-MPF [US]

Therapeutic Category Local Anesthetic

Use Infiltration anesthesia, peripheral nerve block, epidural anesthesia

Dosage Summary

Caudal block:

Children: Dosage not established

Adults: Preservative-free: 2% or 3%: 15-25 mL; may repeat at 40-60 minute intervals

Infiltration and peripheral nerve block:

Children ≤3 years: Dosage not established

Children >3 years: Infiltration: Concentrations of 0.5-1% (maximum without epinephrine: 11 mg/kg); Nerve block: Concentrations of 1% to 1.5% (maximum without epinephrine: 11 mg/kg)

Adults: **Note:** Maximum single dose (without epinephrine): 11 mg/kg (800 mg); Maximum single dose (with epinephrine): 14 mg/kg (1000 mg)

Brachial plexus: 2%; 30-40 mL; Total dose 600-800 mg

Digital (without epinephrine): 1%; 3-4 mL; Total dose: 30-40 mg

Infraorbital: 2%: 0.5-1 mL; Total dose 10-20 mg

Mandibular: 2%: 2-3 mL; Total dose 40-60 mg

Paracervical: 1%; 3 mL per each of four sites

Pudendal: 2%; 10 mL each side; Total dose: 400 mg

Lumbar epidural block:

Children: Dosage not established

Adults: Preservative-free: 2% or 3%: 2-2.5 mL per segment; Usual total volume: 15-25 mL, may repeat with doses that are 2-6 mL less than total initial dose every 40-50 minutes

Dosage Forms

Injection, solution: 2% [20 mg/mL] (30 mL); 3% [30 mg/mL] (30 mL)

Nesacaine®: 1% [10 mg/mL] (30 mL); 2% [20 mg/mL] (30 mL)

Injection, solution [preservative free]: 2% [20 mg/mL] (20 mL); 3% [30 mg/mL] (20 mL)

Nesacaine®-MPF: 2% [20 mg/mL] (20 mL); 3% [30 mg/mL] (20 mL)

chloroprocaine hydrochloride *see* chloroprocaine *on page 206*

Chloroptic® Ophthalmic Solution *(Discontinued)* *see* chloramphenicol *on page 203*

Chloroptic® SOP *(Discontinued)* *see* chloramphenicol *on page 203*

chloroquine (KLOR oh kwin)

Synonyms chloroquine phosphate

U.S./Canadian Brand Names Aralen® [US/Can]; Novo-Chloroquine [Can]

Therapeutic Category Aminoquinoline (Antimalarial)

Use Suppression/chemoprophylaxis or treatment of acute malaria due to susceptible *Plasmodium malariae, P. vivax, P. ovale, P. falciparum*; extraintestinal amebiasis

Dosage Summary

Oral:

Children:

Malaria prophylaxis:

No pretreatment: 10 mg/kg (base) in 2 divided doses given 6 hours apart, followed by normal prophylactic regimen

Prior to exposure: 5 mg base/kg/week (maximum: 300 mg base/dose)

Malaria treatment: 10 mg/kg (base) on day 1, followed by 5 mg/kg (base) 6-, 24-, and 36 hours after first dose (or administer the final dose 48 hours after the initial dose [CDC guideline table, 2009])

Adults:

Extraintestinal amebiasis: 1 g/day (600 mg base) for 2 days, then 500 mg/day (300 mg base)

Malaria prophylaxis:

No pretreatment: 1 g (600 mg base) in 2 divided doses given 6 hours apart, followed by normal prophylactic regimen

Prior to exposure: 500 mg/week (300 mg base)

Malaria treatment: 1 g (600 mg base) on day 1, followed by 500 mg (300 mg base) 6 hours later and 500 mg (300 mg base) on days 2 and 3

Dosage Forms

Tablet, oral: 250 mg, 500 mg

Aralen®: 500 mg

chloroquine phosphate *see* chloroquine *on page 206*

chlorothiazide (klor oh THYE a zide)

U.S./Canadian Brand Names Diuril® [US/Can]; Sodium Diuril® [US]

Therapeutic Category Diuretic, Thiazide

Use Management of mild-to-moderate hypertension; adjunctive treatment of edema

Dosage Summary

I.V.:

Adults: 250-1000 mg once or twice daily (maximum: 1000 mg/day)

Oral:

Children <6 months: 10-30 mg/kg/day in 2 divided doses (maximum: 375 mg/day)

Children ≥6 months: 10-20 mg/kg/day in 1-2 divided doses (maximum: 375 mg/day)

Adults: 250-2000 mg/day in 1-2 divided doses (maximum: 1000 mg/day [CHF])

Dosage Forms

Injection, powder for reconstitution: 500 mg

Sodium Diuril®: 0.5 g

Suspension, oral:

Diuril®: 250 mg/5 mL (237 mL)

Tablet, oral: 250 mg, 500 mg

Chlorphed® *(Discontinued)* *see* brompheniramine *on page 147*

Chlorphed®-LA Nasal Solution *(Discontinued)* *see* oxymetazoline (nasal) *on page 716*

Chlorphen [US-OTC] *see* chlorpheniramine *on page 207*

chlorpheniramine (klor fen IR a meen)

Sound-Alike/Look-Alike Issues

Chlor-Trimeton® may be confused with Chloromycetin®

Synonyms chlorpheniramine maleate; CTM

U.S./Canadian Brand Names Ahist™ [US]; Aller-Chlor® [US-OTC]; Chlor Hist [US-OTC]; Chlor-Trimeton® Allergy [US-OTC]; Chlor-Tripolon® [Can]; Chlorphen [US-OTC]; Diabetic Tussin® for Children Allergy Relief [US-OTC]; Ed Chlorped [US]; Ed-Chlortan [US]; Novo-Pheniram [Can]; P-Tann [US]; Teldrin® HBP [US-OTC]

Therapeutic Category Antihistamine

Use Perennial and seasonal allergic rhinitis and other allergic symptoms including urticaria

Dosage Summary

Oral:

Immediate release:

Children <2 years: 0.35 mg/kg/day divided every 4-6 hours

Children 2-6 years: 1 mg every 4-6 hours **or** 0.35 mg/kg/day divided every 4-6 hours (maximum: 6 mg/day)

Children 6-12 years: 2 mg every 4-6 hours or 0.35 mg/kg/day divided every 4-6 hours (maximum: 12 mg/day)

Children >12 years: 4 mg every 4-6 hours (maximum: 24 mg/day)

Adults: 4 mg every 4-6 hours (maximum: 24 mg/day)

Elderly: 4 mg once or twice daily

Sustained release:
Children <6 years: Dosage not established
Children 6-12 years: 8 mg at bedtime
Children >12 years: 8-12 mg every 8-12 hours (maximum: 24 mg/day)
Adults: 8-12 mg every 8-12 hours (maximum: 24 mg/day)
Elderly: 8 mg at bedtime

Dosage Forms

Suspension, oral:
Ed Chlorped: 2 mg/mL (60 mL)
P-Tann: 8 mg/5 mL (473 mL)

Syrup, oral:
Aller-Chlor® [OTC]: 2 mg/5 mL (118 mL)
Diabetic Tussin® for Children Allergy Relief [OTC]: 2 mg/5 mL (118 mL)

Tablet, oral: 4 mg
Aller-Chlor® [OTC]: 4 mg
Chlor Hist [OTC]: 4 mg
Chlor-Trimeton® Allergy [OTC]: 4 mg
Chlorphen [OTC]: 4 mg
Ed-Chlortan: 4 mg
Teldrin® HBP [OTC]: 4 mg

Tablet, extended release, oral:
Chlor-Trimeton® Allergy [OTC]: 12 mg

Tablet, long acting, oral:
Ahist™: 12 mg

chlorpheniramine, acetaminophen, and pseudoephedrine *see* acetaminophen, chlorpheniramine, and pseudoephedrine *on page 28*

chlorpheniramine and acetaminophen (klor fen IR a meen & a seet a MIN oh fen)

Synonyms acetaminophen and chlorpheniramine

U.S./Canadian Brand Names Coricidin HBP® Cold and Flu [US-OTC]

Therapeutic Category Antihistamine/Analgesic

Use Symptomatic relief of congestion, headache, aches and pains of colds and flu

Dosage Summary

Oral:
Children: Dosage not established
Adults: 2 tablets every 4 hours

Dosage Forms

Tablet:
Coricidin HBP® Cold and Flu [OTC]: Chlorpheniramine 2 mg and acetaminophen 325 mg

chlorpheniramine and carbetapentane *see* carbetapentane and chlorpheniramine *on page 179*

chlorpheniramine and dextromethorphan *see* dextromethorphan and chlorpheniramine *on page 288*

chlorpheniramine and phenylephrine (klor fen IR a meen & fen il EF rin)

Sound-Alike/Look-Alike Issues
Rynatan® may be confused with Rynatuss®

Synonyms chlorpheniramine maleate and phenylephrine hydrochloride; chlorpheniramine tannate and phenylephrine tannate; phenylephrine and chlorpheniramine

U.S./Canadian Brand Names Actifed® Cold & Allergy [US-OTC] *[reformulation]*; C-Phen [US]; Ceron [US]; Dallergy Drops [US]; Dallergy®-JR [US]; Dec-Chlorphen [US]; Ed A-Hist™ [US]; Ed ChlorPed D [US]; NoHist [US]; PD-Hist-D [US]; PediaTan™ D [US]; Phenabid® [US]; R-Tanna Pediatric [US]; R-Tanna [US]; Rinate™ Pediatric [US]; Rondec® [US]; Rynatan® Pediatric [US]; Rynatan® [US]; Sudafed PE® Sinus + Allergy [US-OTC]; Tannate Pediatric [US]; Triaminic® Cold and Allergy [US-OTC]

Therapeutic Category Antihistamine/Decongestant Combination

Use Temporary relief of upper respiratory conditions such as nasal congestion, runny nose, and sneezing due to the common cold, hay fever, or allergic or vasomotor rhinitis

Dosage Summary

Oral:

Children <6 months: Dosage not established
Children 6-12 months: Rondec® Drops: 0.75 mL 4 times/day
Children 1-2 years: Rondec® Drops: 1 mL 4 times/day
Children 2-6 years:
Rondec® Syrup: 1.25 mL every 4-6 hours (maximum: 7.5 mL/day)
Rynatan®: Suspension: 2.5-5 mL every 12 hours
Children 6-12 years:
Dallergy® Jr: One capsule every 12 hours (maximum: 2 capsules/day)
Ed A-Hist™: One-half caplet every 12 hours
Rondec®: 2.5 mL every 4-6 hours (maximum: 15 mL/day)
Rynatan®: Suspension: 5-10 mL every 12 hours
Children ≥12 years:
Dallergy® Jr: Two capsules every 12 hours (maximum: 4 capsules/day)
Ed A-Hist™: One caplet every 12 hours
R-Tanna: 1-2 tablets every 12 hours
Rondec®: 5 mL every 4-6 hours (maximum: 30 mL/day)
Rynatan®: Tablet: 1-2 tablets every 12 hours
Adults:
Dallergy® Jr: Two capsules every 12 hours (maximum: 4 capsules/day)
Ed A-Hist™: One caplet every 12 hours
R-Tanna: 1-2 tablets every 12 hours
Rondec®: 5 mL every 4-6 hours (maximum: 30 mL/day)
Rynatan®: Tablet: 1-2 tablets every 12 hours

Dosage Forms

Caplet, prolonged release:
Ed A-Hist™, NoHist: Chlorpheniramine 8 mg and phenylephrine 20 mg
Capsule, extended release:
Dallergy®-JR: Chlorpheniramine 4 mg and phenylephrine 20 mg
Liquid:
Ed A-Hist™: Chlorpheniramine 4 mg and phenylephrine 10 mg per 5 mL
Triaminic® Cold and Allergy [OTC]: Chlorpheniramine 1 mg and phenylephrine 2.5 mg per 5 mL
Liquid, oral [drops]:
Dallergy: Chlorpheniramine 1 mg and phenylephrine 2 mg per 1 mL
Solution, oral [drops]:
C-Phen, Dec-Chlorphen, PD-Hist-D: Chlorpheniramine 1 mg and phenylephrine 3.5 mg per 1 mL
Suspension, oral: Chlorpheniramine 4 mg and phenylephrine 20 mg per 5 mL
Dallergy®-JR: Chlorpheniramine 4 mg and phenylephrine 20 mg per 5 mL
PediaTan™ D: Chlorpheniramine 8 mg and phenylephrine 10 mg per 5 mL
R-Tanna Pediatric, Rinate™ Pediatric, Rynatan® Pediatric: Chlorpheniramine 4.5 mg and phenylephrine 5 mg per 5 mL
Suspension, oral [drops]:
Ed ChlorPed D: Chlorpheniramine 2 mg and phenylephrine 6 mg per 1 mL
Syrup:
Ceron, C-Phen, Dec-Chlorphen, PD-Hist-D, Rondec®: Chlorpheniramine 4 mg and phenylephrine 12.5 mg per 5 mL
Tablet:
Actifed® Cold & Allergy [OTC], Sudafed PE® Sinus + Allergy [OTC]: Chlorpheniramine 4 mg and phenylephrine 10 mg
R-Tanna, Rynatan®: Chlorpheniramine 9 mg and phenylephrine 25 mg
Tablet, chewable:
Rynatan®: Chlorpheniramine 4.5 mg and phenylephrine 5 mg
Tablet, timed release:
Phenabid®: Chlorpheniramine 8 mg and phenylephrine 20 mg

chlorpheniramine and pseudoephedrine (klor fen IR a meen & soo doe e FED rin)

Sound-Alike/Look-Alike Issues

Allerest® may be confused with Sinarest®
Chlor-Trimeton® may be confused with Chloromycetin®
Sudafed® may be confused with Sufenta®

Synonyms chlorpheniramine maleate and pseudoephedrine hydrochloride; chlorpheniramine tannate and pseudoephedrine tannate; pseudoephedrine and chlorpheniramine

U.S./Canadian Brand Names Allerest® Maximum Strength Allergy and Hay Fever [US-OTC]; Dicel™ [US]; LoHist-D [US]; Suclor™ [US]; Sudafed® Sinus & Allergy [US-OTC]; SudaHist® [US]; Sudal® 12 [US]; Triaminic® Cold & Allergy [Can]

Therapeutic Category Antihistamine/Decongestant Combination

Use Relief of nasal congestion associated with the common cold, hay fever, and other allergies, sinusitis, eustachian tube blockage, and vasomotor and allergic rhinitis

Dosage Summary Note: General dosing guidelines; consult specific product labeling

Oral:

Immediate release:

Children <2 years: Dosage not established

Children 2-6 years: Chlorpheniramine maleate 1 mg and pseudoephedrine hydrochloride 15 mg every 4-6 hours **or** chlorpheniramine tannate 4.5 mg and pseudoephedrine tannate 75 mg: 2.5-5 mL every 12 hours (maximum: 10 mL/day)

Children 6-12 years: Chlorpheniramine maleate 2 mg and pseudoephedrine hydrochloride 30 mg every 4-6 hours

Children ≥12 years: Chlorpheniramine maleate 4 mg and pseudoephedrine hydrochloride 60 mg every 4-6 hours **or** chlorpheniramine tannate 4.5 mg and pseudoephedrine tannate 75 mg: 10-20 mL every 12 hours (maximum: 40 mL/day)

Adults: Chlorpheniramine maleate 4 mg and pseudoephedrine hydrochloride 60 mg every 4-6 hours **or** chlorpheniramine tannate 4.5 mg and pseudoephedrine tannate 75 mg: 10-20 mL every 12 hours (maximum: 40 mL/day)

Sustained release:

Children <12 years: Dosage not established

Children ≥12 years: Deconamine® SR: Chlorpheniramine maleate 8 mg and pseudoephedrine hydrochloride 120 mg every 12 hours

Adults: Deconamine® SR: Chlorpheniramine maleate 8 mg and pseudoephedrine hydrochloride 120 mg every 12 hours

Dosage Forms

Capsule, extended release, oral: Chlorpheniramine 8 mg and pseudoephedrine 120 mg; chlorpheniramine 12 mg and pseudoephedrine 100 mg

Suclor™: Chlorpheniramine 8 mg and pseudoephedrine 120 mg

Liquid, oral:

LoHist-D: Chlorpheniramine 2 mg and pseudoephedrine 30 mg per 5 mL

Liquid, oral [drops]:

Neutrahist Pediatric [OTC]: Chlorpheniramine 0.8 mg and pseudoephedrine 9 mg per 1 mL

Suspension, oral:

Dicel®: Chlorpheniramine 5 mg and pseudoephedrine 75 mg per 5 mL

Syrup, oral: Chlorpheniramine 2 mg and pseudoephedrine 30 mg per 5 mL

Tablet, oral: Chlorpheniramine 4 mg and pseudoephedrine 60 mg

Tablet, sustained release:

SudaHist®: Chlorpheniramine 12 mg and pseudoephedrine 120 mg

chlorpheniramine, carbetapentane, and phenylephrine *see* carbetapentane, phenylephrine, and chlorpheniramine *on page 180*

chlorpheniramine, dextromethorphan, phenylephrine, and guaifenesin *see* dextromethorphan, chlorpheniramine, phenylephrine, and guaifenesin *on page 290*

chlorpheniramine, dihydrocodeine, and pseudoephedrine *see* pseudoephedrine, dihydrocodeine, and chlorpheniramine *on page 813*

chlorpheniramine, ephedrine, phenylephrine, and carbetapentane

(klor fen IR a meen, e FED rin, fen il EF rin, & kar bay ta PEN tane)

Sound-Alike/Look-Alike Issues

Rynatuss® may be confused with Rynatan®

Synonyms carbetapentane, ephedrine, phenylephrine, and chlorpheniramine; ephedrine, chlorpheniramine, phenylephrine, and carbetapentane; phenylephrine, ephedrine, chlorpheniramine, and carbetapentane

U.S./Canadian Brand Names Quad Tann® [US]; Rynatuss® [US]; Tetra Tannate Pediatric [US]

Therapeutic Category Antihistamine/Decongestant/Antitussive

Use Symptomatic relief of cough with a decongestant and an antihistamine

Dosage Summary

Oral:

Children <2 years: Titrate dose individually
Children 2-6 years: 2.5-5 mL every 12 hours
Children >6 years: 5-10 mL every 12 hours
Adults: 1-2 tablets every 12 hours

Dosage Forms

Suspension:

Tetra Tannate Pediatric: Chlorpheniramine 4 mg, ephedrine 5 mg, phenylephrine 5 mg, and carbetapentane 30 mg per 5 mL

Tablet:

Rynatuss®: Chlorpheniramine 5 mg, ephedrine 10 mg, phenylephrine 10 mg, and carbetapentane 50 mg

Tablet, long acting:

Quad Tann®: Chlorpheniramine 5 mg, ephedrine 10 mg, phenylephrine 10 mg, and carbetapentane 60 mg

chlorpheniramine, hydrocodone, and phenylephrine *see* phenylephrine, hydrocodone, and chlorpheniramine *on page 754*

chlorpheniramine maleate *see* chlorpheniramine *on page 207*

chlorpheniramine maleate and dextromethorphan hydrobromide *see* dextromethorphan and chlorpheniramine *on page 288*

chlorpheniramine maleate and hydrocodone bitartrate *see* hydrocodone and chlorpheniramine *on page 480*

chlorpheniramine maleate and phenylephrine hydrochloride *see* chlorpheniramine and phenylephrine *on page 208*

chlorpheniramine maleate and pseudoephedrine hydrochloride *see* chlorpheniramine and pseudoephedrine *on page 209*

chlorpheniramine maleate, dihydrocodeine bitartrate, and phenylephrine hydrochloride *see* dihydrocodeine, chlorpheniramine, and phenylephrine *on page 304*

chlorpheniramine maleate, ibuprofen, and pseudoephedrine *see* ibuprofen, pseudoephedrine, and chlorpheniramine *on page 496*

chlorpheniramine maleate, phenylephrine hydrochloride, and guaifenesin *see* chlorpheniramine, phenylephrine, and guaifenesin *on page 212*

chlorpheniramine maleate, pseudoephedrine hydrochloride, and dextromethorphan hydrobromide *see* chlorpheniramine, pseudoephedrine, and dextromethorphan *on page 214*

chlorpheniramine, phenylephrine, and dextromethorphan

(klor fen IR a meen, fen il EF rin, & deks troe meth OR fan)

Synonyms dextromethorphan, chlorpheniramine, and phenylephrine; phenylephrine, chlorpheniramine, and dextromethorphan

U.S./Canadian Brand Names C-Phen DM [US]; Ceron-DM [US]; Corfen DM [US]; De-Chlor DM [US]; De-Chlor DR [US]; Dex PC [US]; Ed A-Hist DM [US]; Father John's® Plus [US-OTC]; Mintuss DR [US]; Neo DM [US]; Norel DM™ [US]; PD-Cof [US]; PE-Hist DM [US]; Phenabid DM® [US]; Poly Tussin DM [US]; Robitussin® Cough and Cold Nighttime [US-OTC]; Robitussin® Pediatric Cough and Cold Nighttime [US-OTC]; Rondec®-DM [US]; Statuss™ DM [US]; Trital DM [US]; Tussplex™ DM [US]

Therapeutic Category Antihistamine/Decongestant/Antitussive

Use Temporary relief of cough and upper respiratory symptoms associated with allergies or the common cold

Dosage Summary

Oral:

Children <6 months: Dosage not established
Children 6-12 months: Rondec®-DM Drops: 0.75 mL 4 times/day
Children 1-2 years: Rondec®-DM Drops: 1 mL 4 times/day
Children 2-6 years: Rondec®-DM Syrup: 1.25 mL every 4-6 hours (maximum: 7.5 mL/day)
Children 6-12 years: Rondec®-DM Syrup: 2.5 mL every 4-6 hours (maximum: 15 mL/day)
Children ≥12 years: Rondec®-DM Syrup: 5 mL every 4-6 hours (maximum: 30 mL/day)
Adults: Rondec®-DM Syrup: 5 mL every 4-6 hours (maximum: 30 mL/day)

Dosage Forms

Liquid:

Corfen DM, Norel DM™, Trital DM: Chlorpheniramine 4 mg, phenylephrine 10 mg, and dextromethorphan 15 mg per 5 mL

De-Chlor DM: Chlorpheniramine 2 mg, phenylephrine 10 mg, and dextromethorphan 15 mg per 5 mL

De-Chlor DR: Chlorpheniramine 2 mg, phenylephrine 6 mg, and dextromethorphan 15 mg per 5 mL

Father John's® Plus [OTC]: Chlorpheniramine 2 mg, phenylephrine 5 mg, and dextromethorphan 5 mg per 15 mL

Liquid, oral [drops]:

C-Phen DM, PD-Cof, Rondec®-DM: Chlorpheniramine 1 mg, phenylephrine 3.5 mg, and dextromethorphan 3 mg per 1 mL

Neo DM: Chlorpheniramine 0.75 mg, phenylephrine 1.75 mg, and dextromethorphan 2.75 mg per 1 mL

Syrup:

Ceron-DM, C-Phen DM, PD-Cof, Rondec®-DM: Chlorpheniramine 4 mg, phenylephrine 12.5 mg, and dextromethorphan 15 mg per 5 mL

Dex PC, Mintuss DR: Chlorpheniramine 2 mg, phenylephrine 6 mg, and dextromethorphan 15 mg per 5 mL

Ed A-Hist DM: Chlorpheniramine 4 mg, phenylephrine 10 mg, and dextromethorphan 15 mg per 5 mL

PE-Hist DM, Tussplex™ DM: Chlorpheniramine 2 mg, phenylephrine 5 mg, and dextromethorphan 15 mg per 5 mL

Robitussin® Cough and Cold Nighttime [OTC], Robitussin® Pediatric Cough and Cold Nighttime [OTC]: Chlorpheniramine 1 mg, phenylephrine 2.5 mg, and dextromethorphan 5 mg per 5 mL

Statuss™ DM: Chlorpheniramine 2 mg, phenylephrine 10 mg, and dextromethorphan 15 mg per 5 mL

Tablet, timed release:

Phenabid DM®: Chlorpheniramine 8 mg, phenylephrine 20 mg, and dextromethorphan 30 mg

chlorpheniramine, phenylephrine, and guaifenesin

(klor fen IR a meen, fen il EF rin, & gwye FEN e sin)

Synonyms chlorpheniramine maleate, phenylephrine hydrochloride, and guaifenesin; chlorpheniramine tannate, phenylephrine tannate, and guaifenesin; guaifenesin, phenylephrine, and chlorpheniramine; phenylephrine, chlorpheniramine, and guaifenesin

U.S./Canadian Brand Names P Chlor GG [US]

Therapeutic Category Cough and Cold Combination

Use Symptomatic relief of upper respiratory symptoms associated with infections such as the common cold or allergies

Dosage Summary

Oral:

Children <3 months: 2-3 2-3 drops per month of age every 4-6 hours as needed (maximum: 4 doses/day)

Children 3-6 months: 0.3-0.6 mL every 4-6 hours as needed (maximum: 4 doses/day)

Children 6 months to 1 year: 0.6-1 mL every 4-6 hours as needed (maximum: 4 doses/day)

Children 1-2 years: 1-2 mL every 4-6 hours as needed (maximum: 4 doses/day)

Dosage Forms

Liquid:

P Chlor GG [drops]: Chlorpheniramine 1 mg, phenylephrine 2 mg, and guaifenesin 20 mg per 1 mL

chlorpheniramine, phenylephrine, and methscopolamine

(klor fen IR a meen, fen il EF rin, & meth skoe POL a meen)

Synonyms methscopolamine nitrate, chlorpheniramine maleate, and phenylephrine hydrochloride; phenylephrine tannate, chlorpheniramine tannate, and methscopolamine nitrate

U.S./Canadian Brand Names aerohist plus™ [US]; aeroKid™ [US]; AH-Chew® [US]; AH-Chew™ Ultra [US]; Chlor-Mes-D [US]; Dallergy® [US]; Dehistine [US]; Duradyl® [US]; Durahist™ PE [US]; Histatab PH [US]; OMNIhist® II L.A. [US]; Phenylephrine CM [US]; Rescon® [US]; Triall™ [US]

Therapeutic Category Antihistamine/Decongestant/Anticholinergic

Use Treatment of upper respiratory symptoms such as respiratory congestion, allergic rhinitis, vasomotor rhinitis, sinusitis, and allergic skin reactions of urticaria and angioedema

Dosage Summary

Oral:

aeroKid™:

Children <6 years: Dosage not established

Children 6-11 years: 2.5-5 mL every 12 hours

Children ≥12 years: 5-10 mL every 12 hours
Adults: 5-10 mL every 12 hours
AH-Chew®:
Children <6 years: Dosage not established
Children 6-11 years: 2.5-5 mL every 4 hours
Children ≥12 years: 5-10 mL every 3-4 hours
Adults: 5-10 mL every 3-4 hours
Dallergy®:
Children <6 years: Dosage not established
Children 6-11 years: One-half caplet every 12 hours
Children ≥12 years: 1 capsule every 12 hours
Adults: 1 capsule every 12 hours

Dosage Forms

Caplet, extended release:
aerohist plus™: Chlorpheniramine 8 mg, phenylephrine 20 mg, and methscopolamine 2.5 mg
Dallergy®: Chlorpheniramine 12 mg, phenylephrine 20 mg, and methscopolamine 2.5 mg

Liquid:
Chlor-Mes-D: Chlorpheniramine 2 mg, phenylephrine 10 mg, and methscopolamine 0.625 mg per 5 mL

Suspension:
AH-Chew®: Chlorpheniramine, phenylephrine, and methscopalamine 1.5 mg per 5 mL

Syrup:
aeroKid™: Chlorpheniramine 4 mg, phenylephrine 1 mg, and methscopolamine 1.25 mg per 5 mL
Dallergy®: Chlorpheniramine 2 mg, phenylephrine 8 mg, and methscopolamine 0.75 mg per 5 mL
Dehistine, Duradryl®: Chlorpheniramine 2 mg, phenylephrine 10 mg, and methscopolamine 1.25 mg per 5 mL
Triall™: Chlorpheniramine 2 mg, phenylephrine 8 mg, and methscopolamine 0.75 mg per 5 mL

Tablet [scored]:
Dallergy®: Chlorpheniramine 4 mg, phenylephrine 10 mg, and methscopolamine 1.25 mg

Tablet, chewable:
AH-Chew™ Ultra: Chlorpheniramine 2 mg, phenylephrine 10 mg, and methscopolamine 1.5 mg

Tablet, extended release: Chlorpheniramine 8 mg, phenylephrine 20 mg, and methscopolamine 1.25 mg
Durahist™ PE: Chlorpheniramine 8 mg, phenylephrine 20 mg, and methscopolamine 1.25 mg [scored]

Tablet, long acting [scored]:
OMNIhist® II L.A.: Chlorpheniramine 8 mg, phenylephrine 25 mg, and methscopolamine 2.5 mg

Tablet, sustained release:
Histatab PH: Chlorpheniramine 8 mg, phenylephrine 20 mg, and methscopolamine 1.25 mg

Tablet, timed release:
Phenylephrine CM: Chlorpheniramine 8 mg, phenylephrine 40 mg, and methscopolamine 2.5 mg

Tablet, variable release:
Rescon®: Chlorpheniramine 12 mg and phenylephrine 40 mg [sustained release] and methscopolamine 2 mg [immediate release] [MaxRelent release]

chlorpheniramine, phenylephrine, and phenyltoloxamine

(klor fen IR a meen, fen il EF rin, & fen il tole LOKS a meen)

Synonyms phenylephrine, chlorpheniramine, and phenyltoloxamine; phenyltoloxamine, chlorpheniramine, and phenylephrine

U.S./Canadian Brand Names Nalex®-A [US]; NoHist-A [US]; Rhinacon A [US]

Therapeutic Category Antihistamine/Decongestant Combination

Use Symptomatic relief of rhinitis and nasal congestion due to colds or allergy

Dosage Summary

Oral:
Children <2 years: Dosage not established
Children 2-6 years: Nalex®-A: 1.25-2.5 mL every 4-6 hours
Children 6-12 years: Nalex®-A: 5 mL every 4-6 hours **or** one-half tablet 2-3 times/day
Children >12 years: Nalex®-A: 10 mL every 4-6 hours **or** 1 tablet 2-3 times/day
Adults: Nalex®-A: 10 mL every 4-6 hours **or** 1 tablet 2-3 times/day

Dosage Forms

Liquid: Chlorpheniramine 2.5 mg, phenylephrine 5 mg, and phenyltoloxamine 7.5 mg per 5 mL
Nalex®-A, NoHist-A, Rhinacon A: Chlorpheniramine 2.5 mg, phenylephrine 5 mg, and phenyltoloxamine 7.5 mg per 5 mL

Tablet, extended release:
Rhinacon A: Chlorpheniramine 4 mg, phenylephrine 20 mg, and phenyltoloxamine 40 mg

Tablet, prolonged release:
Nalex®-A: Chlorpheniramine 4 mg, phenylephrine 20 mg, and phenyltoloxamine 40 mg

chlorpheniramine, phenylephrine, and pyrilamine *see* chlorpheniramine, pyrilamine, and phenylephrine *on page 215*

chlorpheniramine, phenylephrine, codeine, and potassium iodide *(Discontinued)*

chlorpheniramine, pseudoephedrine, and acetaminophen *see* acetaminophen, chlorpheniramine, and pseudoephedrine *on page 28*

chlorpheniramine, pseudoephedrine, and codeine

(klor fen IR a meen, soo doe e FED rin, & KOE deen)

Synonyms codeine, chlorpheniramine, and pseudoephedrine; pseudoephedrine, chlorpheniramine, and codeine

Therapeutic Category Antihistamine/Decongestant/Antitussive

Controlled Substance C-V

Use Temporary relief of cough associated with minor throat or bronchial irritation or nasal congestion due to common cold, allergic rhinitis, or sinusitis

Dosage Summary

Oral:

Children <25 lbs: Dosage not established
Children 25-50 lbs: 1.25-2.5 mL every 4-6 hours (maximum: 4 doses/day)
Children 50-90 lbs: 2.5-5 mL every 4-6 hours (maximum: 4 doses/day)
Adults: 10 mL every 4-6 hours (maximum: 4 doses/day)

chlorpheniramine, pseudoephedrine, and dextromethorphan

(klor fen IR a meen, soo doe e FED rin, & deks troe meth OR fan)

Synonyms chlorpheniramine maleate, pseudoephedrine hydrochloride, and dextromethorphan hydrobromide; chlorpheniramine tannate, pseudoephedrine tannate, and dextromethorphan tannate; dexchlorpheniramine tannate, pseudoephedrine tannate, and dextromethorphan tannate; dextromethorphan, chlorpheniramine, and pseudoephedrine; pseudoephedrine, chlorpheniramine, and dextromethorphan

U.S./Canadian Brand Names Dicel™ DM [US]; DuraTan™ Forte [US]; Entre-S [US]; Kidkare Children's Cough and Cold [US-OTC]; Pedia Relief™ [US-OTC]; Rescon DM [US-OTC]; Tanafed DMX™ [US]; Tannate PD-DM [US]

Therapeutic Category Antihistamine/Decongestant/Antitussive

Use Temporarily relieves nasal congestion, runny nose, cough, and sneezing due to the common cold, hay fever, or allergic rhinitis

Dosage Summary Note: General dosing guidelines; consult specific product labeling.

Oral:

Chlorpheniramine maleate 1 mg, pseudoephedrine 15 mg, and dextromethorphan hydrobromide 7.5 mg per 5 mL:
Children <6 years: Dosage not established
Children 6-12 years: 10 mL every 6 hours
Children >12 years: 20 mL every 6 hours

Chlorpheniramine maleate 1 mg, pseudoephedrine 15 mg, and dextromethorphan hydrobromide 5 mg per tablet or 5 mL:
Children <6 years: Dosage not established
Children 6-12 years: 2 tablets **or** 10 mL every 4-6 hours (maximum: 4 doses/day)

Chlorpheniramine maleate 2 mg, pseudoephedrine 30 mg, and dextromethorphan hydrobromide 10 mg per tablet or 5 mL (Rescon DM):
Children <6 years: Dosage not established
Children 6-12 years: 5 mL every 4-6 hours (maximum: 4 doses/day)
Children >12 years: 10 mL every 4-6 hours (maximum: 4 doses/day)
Adults: 10 mL every 4-6 hours (maximum: 4 doses/day)

Dexchlorpheniramine tannate 2.5 mg, pseudoephedrine tannate 75 mg, and dextromethorphan tannate 25 mg (Tanafed DMX™):
Children <2 years: Dosage not established
Children 2-6 years: 2.5-5 mL every 12 hours (maximum: 10 mL/day)
Children 6-12 years: 5-10 mL every 12 hours (maximum: 20 mL/day)

Children ≥12 years: 10-20 mL every 12 hours (maximum: 40 mL/day)
Adults: 10-20 mL every 12 hours (maximum: 40 mL/day)

Dosage Forms

Liquid, oral: Chlorpheniramine 1 mg, pseudoephedrine 15 mg, and dextromethorphan 5 mg per 5 mL
Kidkare Children's Cough and Cold [OTC], Pedia Relief™ [OTC]: Chlorpheniramine 1 mg, pseudoephedrine 15 mg, and dextromethorphan 5 mg per 5 mL
Rescon DM [OTC]: Chlorpheniramine 2 mg, pseudoephedrine 30 mg, and dextromethorphan 10 mg per 5 mL

Liquid, oral [drops]:
Neutrahist PDX: Chlorpheniramine 0.8 mg, pseudoephedrine 9 mg, and dextromethorphan 3 mg per 1 mL

Suspension, oral:
Dicel™ DM: Chlorpheniramine 5 mg, pseudoephedrine 75 mg, and dextromethorphan 25 mg per 5 mL
Entre-S: Chlorpheniramine maleate 4 mg, pseudoephedrine 30 mg, and dextromethorphan 30 mg per 5 mL
Tanafed DMX™: Dexchlorpheniramine 2.5 mg, pseudoephedrine 75 mg, and dextromethorphan 25 mg per 5 mL

chlorpheniramine, pseudoephedrine, and methscopolamine

(klor fen IR a meen, soo doe e FED rin, & meth skoe POL a meen)

Synonyms methscopolamine, chlorpheniramine, and pseudoephedrine; methscopolamine, pseudoephedrine, and chlorpheniramine; pseudoephedrine hydrochloride, methscopolamine nitrate, and chlorpheniramine maleate; pseudoephedrine, methscopolamine, and chlorpheniramine

U.S./Canadian Brand Names Amdry-C [US]; Coldamine [US]

Therapeutic Category Antihistamine/Decongestant/Anticholinergic

Use Relief of symptoms of allergic rhinitis, vasomotor rhinitis, sinusitis, and the common cold

Dosage Summary

Oral:
Children <6 years: Dosage not established
Children 6-11 years:: One-half tablet every 12 hours (maximum: 1 tablet/day)
Children ≥12 years: : One tablet every 12 hours (maximum: 2 tablets/day)
Adults:: One tablet every 12 hours (maximum: 2 tablets/day)

Dosage Forms

Tablet, extended release:
Coldamine: Chlorpheniramine 8 mg, pseudoephedrine 90 mg, and methscopolamine 2.5 mg

Tablet, sustained release: Chlorpheniramine maleate 8 mg, pseudoephedrine hydrochloride 60 mg, and methscopolamine nitrate 1.25 mg; chlorpheniramine maleate 8 mg, pseudoephedrine hydrochloride 90 mg, and methscopolamine nitrate 2.5 mg
Amdry-C: Chlorpheniramine 8 mg, pseudoephedrine 120 mg, and methscopolamine 2.5 mg [scored]

chlorpheniramine, pyrilamine, and phenylephrine

(klor fen IR a meen, pye RIL a meen, & fen il EF rin)

Synonyms chlorpheniramine, phenylephrine, and pyrilamine; phenylephrine, chlorpheniramine, and pyrilamine; pyrilamine, chlorpheniramine, and phenylephrine

U.S./Canadian Brand Names MyHist-PD [US]; Nalex A 12 [US]; Poly Hist Forte® [US]; Poly Hist PD [US]; Ru-Hist Forte [US]; Triplex™ AD [US]

Therapeutic Category Alpha/Beta Agonist; Histamine H_1 Antagonist; Histamine H_1 Antagonist, First Generation

Use Symptomatic relief of rhinitis and nasal congestion due to colds or allergy

Dosage Summary Oral:

Tablet:
Children <6 years: Dosage not established.
Children 6-12 years: 1/2 tablet 2-3 times/day
Children >12 years: 1 tablet 2-3 times/day
Adults: 1 tablet 2-3 times/day

Liquid (MyHist-PD, Poly Hist PD):
Children <6 years: Dosage not established.
Children 2-6 years: 2.5 mL every 4-6 hours (maximum: 10 mL/day)
Children 6-12 years: 5 mL every 4-6 hours (maximum: 20 mL/day)
Children >12 years: 5-10 mL every 4-6 hours (maximum: 40 mL/day)
Adults: 5-10 mL every 4-6 hours (maximum: 40 mL/day)

Liquid (Triplex™ AD):
Children <6 years: Dosage not established
Children 6-12 years: 5 mL every 4-6 hours (maximum: 20 mL/day)
Children >12: 5-10 mL every 4-6 hours (maximum: 40 mL/day)
Adults: 5-10 mL every 4-6 hours (maximum: 40 mL/day)

Suspension:
Children 2-6 years: 2.5 mL every 12 hours (maximum: 5 mL/day)
Children 6-12 years: 5 mL every 12 hours (maximum: 10 mL/day)
Children >12 years and Adults: 5-10 mL every 12 hours (maximum: 20 mL/day)

Dosage Forms

Liquid, oral:
MyHist-PD, Triplex™ AD: Chlorpheniramine 2 mg, pyrilamine 12.5 mg, and phenylephrine 7.5 mg per 5 mL (473 mL)

Suspension, oral:
Nalex A 12: Chlorpheniramine 2 mg, pyrilamine 12.5 mg, and phenylephrine 5 mg per 5 mL

Tablet, time-released, oral: Chlorpheniramine 4 mg, pyrilamine 25 mg, and phenylephrine 10 mg
Ru-Hist Forte: Chlorpheniramine 4 mg, pyrilamine 25 mg, and phenylephrine 10 mg

chlorpheniramine tannate and phenylephrine tannate *see* chlorpheniramine and phenylephrine *on page 208*

chlorpheniramine tannate and pseudoephedrine tannate *see* chlorpheniramine and pseudoephedrine *on page 209*

chlorpheniramine tannate, phenylephrine tannate, and guaifenesin *see* chlorpheniramine, phenylephrine, and guaifenesin *on page 212*

chlorpheniramine tannate, pseudoephedrine tannate, and dextromethorphan tannate *see* chlorpheniramine, pseudoephedrine, and dextromethorphan *on page 214*

Chlor-Pro® Injection *(Discontinued)* *see* chlorpheniramine *on page 207*

chlorpromazine (klor PROE ma zeen)

Sound-Alike/Look-Alike Issues
chlorproMAZINE may be confused with chlordiazePOXIDE, chlorproPAMIDE, clomiPRAMINE, prochlorperazine, promethazine
Thorazine® may be confused with thiamine, thioridazine

Synonyms chlorpromazine hydrochloride; CPZ

Tall-Man chlorpro**MAZINE**

U.S./Canadian Brand Names Largactil® [Can]; Novo-Chlorpromazine [Can]

Therapeutic Category Phenothiazine Derivative

Use Management of psychotic disorders (control of mania, treatment of schizophrenia); control of nausea and vomiting; relief of restlessness and apprehension before surgery; acute intermittent porphyria; adjunct in the treatment of tetanus; intractable hiccups; combativeness and/or explosive hyperexcitable behavior in children 1-12 years of age and in short-term treatment of hyperactive children

Dosage Summary

I.M.:
Children <6 months: Dosage not established
Children ≥6 months: 0.5-1 mg/kg every 6-8 hours (maximum: <5 years [<22.7 kg]: 40 mg/day; 5-12 years [22.7-45.5 kg]: 75 mg/day)
Adults:
Hiccups/nausea/vomiting: Initial: 25 mg, may repeat (25-50 mg) in 1-4 hours, gradually increase to a maximum of 400 mg every 4-6 hours; Usual dose: 25-50 mg every 4-8 hours
Schizophrenia/psychosis: Initial: 25 mg, may repeat (25-50 mg) in 1-4 hours, gradually increase to a maximum of 400 mg every 4-6 hours; Usual dose: 300-800 mg/day

I.V.:
Children <6 months: Dosage not established
Children ≥6 months: 0.5-1 mg/kg every 6-8 hours (maximum: <5 years [<22.7 kg]: 40 mg/day; 5-12 years [22.7-45.5 kg]: 75 mg/day)
Adults:
Hiccups/nausea/vomiting: Initial: 25 mg, may repeat (25-50 mg) in 1-4 hours, gradually increase to a maximum of 400 mg every 4-6 hours; Usual dose: 25-50 mg every 4-6 hours via slow I.V. infusion
Schizophrenia/psychosis: Initial: 25 mg, may repeat (25-50 mg) in 1-4 hours, gradually increase to a maximum of 400 mg every 4-6 hours; Usual dose: 300-800 mg/day

Oral:
Children <6 months: Dosage not established
Children ≥6 months: 0.5-1 mg/ kg every 4-6 hours as needed
Adults:
Hiccups: 25-50 mg 3-4 times/day
Nausea/vomiting: 10-25 mg every 4-6 hours
Schizophrenia/psychosis: 30-800 mg/day in 1-4 divided doses; some patient may require 1-2 g/day
Elderly (unlabeled use): Dementia: Initial: 10-25 mg 1-2 times/day, titrate up to 800 mg/day

Dosage Forms
Injection, solution: 25 mg/mL (1 mL, 2 mL)
Tablet, oral: 10 mg, 25 mg, 50 mg, 100 mg, 200 mg

chlorpromazine hydrochloride *see* chlorpromazine *on page 216*

chlorpropamide (klor PROE pa mide)

Sound-Alike/Look-Alike Issues
chlorproPAMIDE may be confused with chlorproMAZINE
Diabinese® may be confused with DiaBeta®, Dialume®, Diamox®

Tall-Man chlorpro**PAMIDE**

U.S./Canadian Brand Names Apo-Chlorpropamide® [Can]; Novo-Propamide [Can]

Therapeutic Category Antidiabetic Agent, Oral

Use Management of blood sugar in type 2 diabetes mellitus (noninsulin-dependent, NIDDM)

Dosage Summary
Oral:
Children: Dosage not established
Adults: Initial: 250 mg/day; Maintenance: 100-500 mg/day (maximum: 750 mg/day); **Note:** Titration is recommended
Elderly: Initial: 100-125 mg/day

Dosage Forms
Tablet, oral: 100 mg, 250 mg

Chlor-Tan A 12 ***(Discontinued)*** *see* chlorpheniramine, pyrilamine, and phenylephrine *on page 215*

chlorthalidone (klor THAL i done)

U.S./Canadian Brand Names Apo-Chlorthalidone® [Can]; Thalitone® [US]

Therapeutic Category Diuretic, Miscellaneous

Use Management of mild-to-moderate hypertension when used alone or in combination with other agents; treatment of edema associated with heart failure or nephrotic syndrome. Recent studies have found chlorthalidone effective in the treatment of isolated systolic hypertension in the elderly.

Dosage Summary
Oral:
Adults: 12.5-100 mg/day **or** 100 mg 3 times/week (maximum: 200 mg/day)
Elderly: Initial: 12.5-25 mg/day or every other day

Dosage Forms
Tablet, oral: 25 mg, 50 mg
Thalitone®: 15 mg

chlorthalidone and atenolol *see* atenolol and chlorthalidone *on page 103*
chlorthalidone and clonidine *see* clonidine and chlorthalidone *on page 238*
Chlor-Trimeton® Allergy [US-OTC] *see* chlorpheniramine *on page 207*
Chlor-Trimeton® Allergy D ***(Discontinued)*** *see* chlorpheniramine and pseudoephedrine *on page 209*
Chlor-Trimeton® Syrup ***(Discontinued)*** *see* chlorpheniramine *on page 207*
Chlor-Tripolon® [Can] *see* chlorpheniramine *on page 207*
Chlor-Tripolon ND® [Can] *see* loratadine and pseudoephedrine *on page 576*

chlorzoxazone (klor ZOKS a zone)

Sound-Alike/Look-Alike Issues
Parafon Forte® may be confused with Fam-Pren Forte

U.S./Canadian Brand Names Parafon Forte® DSC [US]; Parafon Forte® [Can]; Strifon Forte® [Can]

Therapeutic Category Skeletal Muscle Relaxant

Use Symptomatic treatment of muscle spasm and pain associated with acute musculoskeletal conditions

Dosage Summary

Oral:

Children: 20 mg/kg/day **or** 600 mg/m^2/day in 3-4 divided doses

Adults: 250-750 mg 3-4 times/day

Elderly: Initial: 250 mg 2-4 times/day, increase up to maximum of 750 mg 3-4 times/day

Dosage Forms

Caplet, oral:

Parafon Forte® DSC: 500 mg

Tablet, oral: 500 mg

cholecalciferol (kole e kal SI fer ole)

Sound-Alike/Look-Alike Issues

cholecalciferol may be confused with ergocalciferol

Synonyms D_3

U.S./Canadian Brand Names Bio-D-Mulsion Forte® [US-OTC]; Bio-D-Mulsion® [US-OTC]; D-3 [US-OTC]; D-Vi-Sol® [Can]; D3-50™ [US-OTC]; D3-5™ [US-OTC]; DDrops® Baby [US-OTC]; DDrops® Kids [US-OTC]; DDrops® [US-OTC]; DDrops® [US]; Delta® D3 [US-OTC]; Enfamil® D-Vi-Sol™ [US-OTC]; Maximum D3® [US-OTC]; Vitamin D3 [US-OTC]

Therapeutic Category Vitamin D Analog

Use Dietary supplement, treatment of vitamin D deficiency, or prophylaxis of deficiency

Dosage Summary

Oral:

Children: Dosage not established

Adults: 200-1000 units/day

Dosage Forms

Capsule, oral:

D-3 [OTC]: 1000 int. units

D3-50™ [OTC]: 50,000 int. units

D3-5™ [OTC]: 5000 int. units

Maximum D3® [OTC]: 10,000 int. units

Capsule, softgel, oral:

D-3 [OTC]: 2000 int. units

Solution, oral:

Bio-D-Mulsion Forte® [OTC]: 2000 int. units/drop (30 mL)

Bio-D-Mulsion® [OTC]: 400 int. units/drop (30 mL)

DDrops® [OTC]: 2000 int. units/drop (10 mL); 1000 units/drop (10 mL)

DDrops® Baby [OTC]: 400 int. units/drop (10 mL)

DDrops® Kids [OTC]: 400 int. units/drop (10 mL)

Enfamil® D-Vi-Sol™ [OTC]: 400 int. units/mL (50 mL)

Tablet, oral: 400 int. units, 1000 units

Delta® D3 [OTC]: 400 int. units

Vitamin D3 [OTC]: 1000 int. units

cholecalciferol and alendronate *see* alendronate and cholecalciferol *on page 47*

cholera and traveler's diarrhea vaccine *see* traveler's diarrhea and cholera vaccine *(Canada only) on page 949*

cholera vaccine *see* traveler's diarrhea and cholera vaccine *(Canada only) on page 949*

cholestyramine resin (koe LES teer a meen REZ in)

U.S./Canadian Brand Names Novo-Cholamine Light [Can]; Novo-Cholamine [Can]; PMS-Cholestyramine [Can]; Prevalite® [US]; Questran® Light Sugar Free [Can]; Questran® Light [US]; Questran® [US/Can]; ZYM-Cholestyramine-Light [Can]; ZYM-Cholestyramine-Regular [Can]

Therapeutic Category Bile Acid Sequestrant

Use Adjunct in the management of primary hypercholesterolemia; pruritus associated with elevated levels of bile acids; diarrhea associated with excess fecal bile acids; binding toxicologic agents; pseudomembraneous colitis

Dosage Summary

Oral:

Children: 240 mg/kg/day in 3 divided doses

Adults: 4-24 g/day in 1-6 divided doses

Dosage Forms

Powder for suspension, oral: Cholestyramine resin 4 g/5 g of powder (210 g); Cholestyramine resin 4 g/5.7 g of powder (239.4 g); Cholestyramine resin 4 g/9 g of powder (378 g); Cholestyramine resin 4 g/5 g packet (60s); Cholestyramine resin 4 g/5.7 g packet (60s); Cholestyramine resin 4 g/9 g packet (60s)

Prevalite®: Cholestyramine resin 4 g/5.5 g of powder (231 g); Cholestyramine resin 4 g/5.5 g packet (42s, 60s)

Questran®: Cholestyramine resin 4 g/9 g of powder (378 g); Cholestyramine resin 4 g/9 g packet (60s)

Questran® Light: Cholestyramine resin 4 g/5 g of powder (210 g); Cholestyramine resin 4 g/5 g packet (60s)

choline fenofibrate *see* fenofibric acid *on page* 394

choline magnesium trisalicylate (KOE leen mag NEE zhum trye sa LIS i late)

Synonyms tricosal

Therapeutic Category Analgesic, Nonnarcotic; Nonsteroidal Antiinflammatory Drug (NSAID)

Use Management of osteoarthritis, rheumatoid arthritis, and other arthritis; acute painful shoulder

Dosage Summary

Oral:

Children <37 kg: 50 mg/kg/day in 2 divided doses

Children ≥37 kg: 2250 mg/day in divided doses

Adults: 500 mg to 1.5 g 2-3 times/day **or** 3 g at bedtime

Elderly: 750 mg 3 times/day

Dosage Forms

Liquid, oral: 500 mg/5 mL (240 mL)

Cholografin® Meglumine [US] *see* iodipamide meglumine *on page* 518

chondroitin sulfate and sodium hyaluronate *see* sodium chondroitin sulfate and sodium hyaluronate *on page* 884

Chooz® [US-OTC] *see* calcium carbonate *on page* 167

choriogonadotropin alfa *see* chorionic gonadotropin (recombinant) *on page* 219

Chorionic Gonadotropin for Injection [Can] *see* chorionic gonadotropin (human) *on page* 219

chorionic gonadotropin (human) (kor ee ON ik goe NAD oh troe pin, HYU man)

Synonyms CG; hCG

U.S./Canadian Brand Names Chorionic Gonadotropin for Injection [Can]; Novarel® [US]; Pregnyl® [US/Can]

Therapeutic Category Gonadotropin

Use Induces ovulation and pregnancy in anovulatory, infertile females; treatment of hypogonadotropic hypogonadism, prepubertal cryptorchidism; spermatogenesis induction with follitropin alfa

Dosage Summary

I.M.:

Children: 4000 units 3 times/week for 3 weeks **or** 5000 units every second day for 4 injections **or** 500 units 3 times/week for 4-6 weeks **or** 15 injections of 500-1000 units given over 6 weeks

Children (males): Hypogonadism: 500-1000 units 3 times/week for 3 weeks, followed by the same dose twice weekly for 3 weeks **or** 4000 units 3 times/week for 6-9 months, then reduce dosage to 2000 units 3 times/week for additional 3 months

Adults (females): 5000-10,000 units 1 day following last dose of menotropins

Adults (males): 1000-2000 units 2-3 times/week

Dosage Forms

Injection, powder for reconstitution: 10,000 units

Novarel®: 10,000 units

Pregnyl®: 10,000 units

chorionic gonadotropin (recombinant)

(kor ee ON ik goe NAD oh troe pin ree KOM be nant)

Synonyms choriogonadotropin alfa; r-hCG

U.S./Canadian Brand Names Ovidrel® [US/Can]

Therapeutic Category Gonadotropin; Ovulation Stimulator

Use As part of an assisted reproductive technology (ART) program, induces ovulation in infertile females who have been pretreated with follicle-stimulating hormones (FSH); induces ovulation and pregnancy in infertile females when the cause of infertility is functional

Dosage Summary

SubQ:

Children: Dosage not established

Adults (female): 250 mcg given 1 day following last dose of follicle stimulating agent

Dosage Forms

Injection, solution:

Ovidrel®: 257.5 mcg/0.515 mL (0.515 mL)

Choron® ***(Discontinued)*** *see* chorionic gonadotropin (human) *on page 219*

chromic phosphate P 32 (KROME ik FOS fate pe THUR tee too)

Synonyms P32; phosphorus p32

U.S./Canadian Brand Names Phosphocol® P 32 [US]

Therapeutic Category Radiopharmaceutical

Use Treatment of peritoneal or pleural effusions caused by metastatic disease by intracavitary instillation; may be injected interstitially for the treatment of cancer

Dosage Summary

Intraperitoneal instillation:

Children: Dosage not established

Adults: 370-740 megabecquerels (10-20 millicuries)

Intrapleural instillation:

Children: Dosage not established

Adults: 222-444 megabecquerels (6-12 millicuries)

Interstitial instillation:

Children: Dosage not established

Adults: ~3.7-18.5 megabecquerels/g of tumor weight (0.1-0.5 millicuries/g)

Dosage Forms

Injection, suspension:

Phosphocol® P 32: 185 MBq (5mCi) per mL

chromium *see* trace metals *on page 945*

Chronovera® [Can] *see* verapamil *on page 981*

Chronulac® ***(Discontinued)*** *see* lactulose *on page 544*

CI-1008 *see* pregabalin *on page 792*

Cialis® [US/Can] *see* tadalafil *on page 908*

Cibacalcin® ***(Discontinued)*** *see* calcitonin *on page 165*

ciclesonide (oral inhalation) (sye KLES oh nide)

U.S./Canadian Brand Names Alvesco® [US/Can]

Therapeutic Category Corticosteroid, Inhalant (Oral)

Use Prophylactic management of bronchial asthma

Dosage Summary

Oral inhalation:

Children <12 years: Dosage not established

Children ≥12 years: 100-800 mcg/day (1-2 puffs once or twice daily) (maximum: 640 mcg/day)

Adults: 100-800 mcg/day (1-2 puffs once or twice daily) (maximum 640 mcg/day)

Dosage Forms

Aerosol, for oral inhalation:

Alvesco®: 80 mcg/inhalation (6.1 g); 160 mcg/inhalation (6.1 g)

Dosage Forms - Canada

Aerosol for oral inhalation:

Alvesco®: 50 mcg/inhalation; 100 mcg/inhalation; 200 mcg/inhalation

ciclesonide (nasal) (sye KLES oh nide)

U.S./Canadian Brand Names Omnaris™ [US/Can]

Therapeutic Category Corticosteroid, Nasal

Use Management of seasonal and perennial allergic rhinitis

Dosage Summary

Intranasal:

Children <6 years: Dosage not established

Children ≥6 years: 2 sprays (50 mcg/spray) per nostril once daily (maximum: 200 mcg/day)

Adults: 2 sprays (50 mcg/spray) per nostril once daily (maximum: 200 mcg/day)

Dosage Forms

Suspension, intranasal:

Omnaris™: 50 mcg/inhalation (12.5 g)

ciclopirox (sye kloe PEER oks)

Sound-Alike/Look-Alike Issues

Loprox® may be confused with Lonox®

Synonyms ciclopirox olamine

U.S./Canadian Brand Names Loprox® [US/Can]; Penlac® [US/Can]; Stieprox® [Can]

Therapeutic Category Antifungal Agent

Use

Cream/suspension: Treatment of tinea pedis (athlete's foot), tinea cruris (jock itch), tinea corporis (ringworm), cutaneous candidiasis, and tinea versicolor (pityriasis)

Gel: Treatment of tinea pedis (athlete's foot), tinea corporis (ringworm); seborrheic dermatitis of the scalp

Lacquer (solution): Topical treatment of mild-to-moderate onychomycosis of the fingernails and toenails due to *Trichophyton rubrum* (not involving the lunula) and the immediately-adjacent skin

Shampoo: Treatment of seborrheic dermatitis of the scalp

Dosage Summary

Topical:

Cream/suspension:

Children ≤10 years: Dosage not established

Children >10 years: Apply twice daily

Adults: Apply twice daily

Gel:

Children ≤16 years: Dosage not established

Children >16 years: Apply twice daily

Adults: Apply twice daily

Lacquer:

Children <12 years: Dosage not established

Children ≥12 years: Apply to adjacent skin and affected nails daily; remove with alcohol every 7 days

Adults: Apply to adjacent skin and affected nails daily; remove with alcohol every 7 days

Shampoo:

Children ≤16 years: Dosage not established

Children >16 years: Apply 5-10 mL to wet hair, lather, and leave in place ~3 minutes, rinse; repeat twice weekly (allow minimum of 3 days between applications)

Adults: Apply 5-10 mL to wet hair, lather, and leave in place ~3 minutes, rinse; repeat twice weekly (allow minimum of 3 days between applications)

Dosage Forms

Cream, topical: 0.77% (15 g, 30 g, 90 g)

Gel, topical: 0.77% (30 g, 45 g, 100 g)

Loprox®: 0.77% (30 g, 45 g, 100 g)

Shampoo, topical: 1% (120 mL)

Loprox®: 1% (120 mL)

Solution, topical: 8% (6.6 mL)

Penlac®: 8% (6.6 mL)

Suspension, topical: 0.77% (30 mL, 60 mL); 0.77% (30 mL, 60 mL)

ciclopirox olamine *see* ciclopirox *on page* *221*

cidecin *see* daptomycin *on page* *269*

cidofovir (si DOF o veer)

U.S./Canadian Brand Names Vistide® [US]

Therapeutic Category Antiviral Agent

Use Treatment of cytomegalovirus (CMV) retinitis in patients with acquired immunodeficiency syndrome (AIDS). **Note:** Should be administered with probenecid.

Dosage Summary Note: Probenecid must be administered orally with each dose of cidofovir

I.V.:

Children: Dosage not established

Adults: Induction: 5 mg/kg once weekly for 2 consecutive weeks; Maintenance: 5 mg/kg once every 2 weeks

Dosage Forms

Injection, solution [preservative free]:

Vistide®: 75 mg/mL (5 mL)

cilazapril and hydrochlorothiazide *(Canada only)*

(sye LAY za pril & hye droe klor oh THYE a zide)

Synonyms cilazapril monohydrate and hydrochlorothiazide; hydrochlorothiazide and cilazapril

U.S./Canadian Brand Names Apo-Cilazapril®/Hctz [Can]; Inhibace® Plus [Can]; Novo-Cilazapril/HCTZ [Can]

Therapeutic Category Angiotensin-Converting Enzyme (ACE) Inhibitor

Use Treatment of mild-to-moderate hypertension in patients who have been stabilized on the individual agents given in the same proportions; not indicated for initial treatment of hypertension

Dosage Summary

Oral:

Children: Dosage not established

Adults: One tablet administered once daily; dose is individualized

Dosage Forms - Canada

Tablet: 5/12.5: Cilazapril 5 mg and hydrochlorothiazide 12.5 mg

Inhibace® Plus 5/12.5: Cilazapril 5 mg and hydrochlorothiazide 12.5 mg

cilazapril *(Canada only)* (sye LAY za pril)

Synonyms cilazapril monohydrate

U.S./Canadian Brand Names Apo-Cilazapril® [Can]; CO Cilazapril [Can]; Inhibace® [Can]; Mylan-Cilazapril [Can]; Novo-Cilazapril [Can]; PHL-Cilazapril [Can]; PMS-Cilazapril [Can]

Therapeutic Category Angiotensin-Converting Enzyme (ACE) Inhibitor

Use Management of hypertension; treatment of heart failure

Dosage Summary

Oral:

Children: Dosage not established

Adults: Initial: 0.5-5 mg once daily (maximum: 2.5 mg/day [CHF]; 10 mg/day [HTN])

Elderly: Initial: 1.25 mg once daily

Dosage Forms - Canada

Tablet:

Inhibace®, Novo-Cilazapril: 1 mg, 2.5 mg, 5 mg

cilazapril monohydrate *see* cilazapril *(Canada only) on page 222*

cilazapril monohydrate and hydrochlorothiazide *see* cilazapril and hydrochlorothiazide *(Canada only) on page 222*

cilostazol (sil OH sta zol)

Sound-Alike/Look-Alike Issues

Pletal® may be confused with Plendil®

Synonyms OPC-13013

U.S./Canadian Brand Names Pletal® [US/Can]

Therapeutic Category Platelet Aggregation Inhibitor

Use Symptomatic management of peripheral vascular disease, primarily intermittent claudication

Dosage Summary

Oral:

Children: Dosage not established

Adults: 100 mg twice daily; reduce to 50 mg twice daily during concurrent therapy with inhibitors of CYP3A4 or CYP2C19

Dosage Forms

Tablet, oral: 50 mg, 100 mg

Pletal®: 50 mg, 100 mg

Ciloxan® [US/Can] *see* ciprofloxacin (ophthalmic) *on page 224*

cimetidine (sye MET i deen)

Sound-Alike/Look-Alike Issues

cimetidine may be confused with simethicone

U.S./Canadian Brand Names Apo-Cimetidine® [Can]; Dom-Cimetidine [Can]; Mylan-Cimetidine [Can]; Novo-Cimetidine [Can]; Nu-Cimet [Can]; PMS-Cimetidine [Can]; Tagamet HB 200® [US-OTC]; Tagamet® HB [Can]

Therapeutic Category Histamine H_2 Antagonist

Use Short-term treatment of active duodenal ulcers and benign gastric ulcers; maintenance therapy of duodenal ulcer; treatment of gastric hypersecretory states; treatment of gastroesophageal reflux disease (GERD); prevention of upper GI bleeding in critically-ill patients

OTC labeling: Prevention or relief of heartburn, acid indigestion, or sour stomach

Dosage Summary

I.M.:

Children: 20-40 mg/kg/day divided every 6 hours

Adults: 300-600 mg every 6 hours

I.V.:

Children: 20-40 mg/kg/day divided every 6 hours

Adults: 300-600 mg every 6 hours **or** 37.5-50 mg/hour continuous infusion

Oral:

Children <12 years: 20-40 mg/kg/day divided every 6 hours

Children ≥12 years: 20-40 mg/kg/day divided every 6 hours **or** 200 mg 1-2 times/day [OTC]

Adults: 300-600 mg 4 times/day **or** 400-800 mg 1-2 times/day **or** 200 mg 1-2 times/day [OTC]

Dosage Forms

Solution, oral: 300 mg/5 mL (237 mL, 240 mL, 250 mL, 473 mL, 480 mL)

Tablet, oral: 200 mg, 300 mg, 400 mg, 800 mg

Tagamet HB 200® [OTC]: 200 mg

Cimzia® [US/Can] *see* certolizumab pegol *on page 197*

cinacalcet (sin a KAL cet)

Synonyms AMG 073; cinacalcet hydrochloride

U.S./Canadian Brand Names Sensipar® [US/Can]

Therapeutic Category Calcimimetic

Use Treatment of secondary hyperparathyroidism in patients with chronic kidney disease (CKD) on dialysis; treatment of hypercalcemia in patients with parathyroid carcinoma

Canadian labeling (additional use; not in U.S. labeling): Reduction of significant hypercalcemia in patients with primary hyperparathyroidism and who are not candidates for parathyroidectomy

Dosage Summary

Oral:

Children: Dosage not established

Adults:

Parathyroid carcinoma: Initial: 30 mg twice daily; Maintenance: Increase dose incrementally every 2-4 weeks to normalize calcium levels (maximum: 360 mg/day)

Secondary hyperparathyroidism: Initial: 30 mg once daily; Maintenance: Increase dose incrementally every 2-4 weeks to maintain iPTH level (maximum: 180 mg/day)

Dosage Forms

Tablet, oral:

Sensipar®: 30 mg, 60 mg, 90 mg

cinacalcet hydrochloride *see* cinacalcet *on page 223*

Cinryze™ [US] *see* C1 inhibitor (human) *on page* 162
Cipralex® [Can] *see* escitalopram *on page* 363
Cipro® [US/Can] *see* ciprofloxacin (systemic) *on page* 224
Cipro® XL [Can] *see* ciprofloxacin (systemic) *on page* 224
Ciprodex® [US/Can] *see* ciprofloxacin and dexamethasone *on page* 225

ciprofloxacin (systemic) (sip roe FLOKS a sin)

Sound-Alike/Look-Alike Issues

ciprofloxacin may be confused with cephalexin
Cipro® may be confused with Ceftin®

Synonyms ciprofloxacin hydrochloride

U.S./Canadian Brand Names Apo-Ciproflox® [Can]; Cipro® I.V. [US]; Cipro® XL [Can]; Cipro® XR [US]; Cipro® [US/Can]; CO Ciprofloxacin [Can]; Dom-Ciprofloxacin [Can]; Mint-Ciprofloxacin [Can]; Mylan-Ciprofloxacin [Can]; Novo-Ciprofloxacin [Can]; PHL-Ciprofloxacin [Can]; PMS-Ciprofloxacin [Can]; PRO-Ciprofloxacin [Can]; Proquin® XR [US]; RAN™-Ciprofloxacin [Can]; ratio-Ciprofloxacin [Can]; Riva-Ciprofloxacin [Can]; Sandoz-Ciprofloxacin [Can]; Taro-Ciprofloxacin [Can]

Therapeutic Category Antibiotic, Quinolone

Use

Children: Complicated urinary tract infections and pyelonephritis due to *E. coli*. **Note:** Although effective, ciprofloxacin is not the drug of first choice in children.

Children and Adults: To reduce incidence or progression of disease following exposure to aerolized *Bacillus anthracis*.

Adults: Treatment of the following infections when caused by susceptible bacteria: Urinary tract infections; acute uncomplicated cystitis in females; chronic bacterial prostatitis; lower respiratory tract infections (including acute exacerbations of chronic bronchitis); acute sinusitis; skin and skin structure infections; bone and joint infections; complicated intraabdominal infections (in combination with metronidazole); infectious diarrhea; typhoid fever due to *Salmonella typhi* (eradication of chronic typhoid carrier state has not been proven); uncomplicated cervical and urethra gonorrhea (due to *N. gonorrhoeae*); nosocomial pneumonia; empirical therapy for febrile neutropenic patients (in combination with piperacillin)

Note: As of April 2007, the CDC no longer recommends the use of fluoroquinolones for the treatment of gonococcal disease.

Dosage Summary

I.V.:

Children: 20-30 mg/kg/day divided every 12 hours (maximum: 800 mg/day)
Adults: 200-400 mg every 8-12 hours

Oral:

Extended release:
Children: Dosage not established
Adults: 500-1000 mg every 24 hours

Immediate release:
Children: 20-30 mg/kg/day in 2 divided doses; (maximum: 1.5 g/day)
Adults: 250-750 mg every 12 hours or 250 mg to 1 g as a single dose

Dosage Forms

Infusion, premixed in D_5W: 200 mg (100 mL); 400 mg (200 mL)
Cipro® I.V.: 200 mg (100 mL); 400 mg (200 mL)
Infusion, premixed in D_5W [preservative free]: 200 mg (100 mL); 400 mg (200 mL)
Injection, solution: 10 mg/mL (20 mL, 40 mL, 120 mL)
Injection, solution [preservative free]: 10 mg/mL (20 mL)
Microcapsules for suspension, oral:
Cipro®: 250 mg/5 mL (100 mL); 500 mg/5 mL (100 mL)
Tablet, oral: 100 mg, 250 mg, 500 mg, 750 mg
Cipro®: 250 mg, 500 mg
Tablet, extended release, oral: 500 mg, 1000 mg
Cipro® XR: 500 mg, 1000 mg
Proquin® XR: 500 mg

ciprofloxacin (ophthalmic) (sip roe FLOKS a sin)

Sound-Alike/Look-Alike Issues

ciprofloxacin may be confused with cephalexin
Ciloxan® may be confused with cinoxacin, Cytoxan

Synonyms ciprofloxacin hydrochloride

U.S./Canadian Brand Names Ciloxan® [US/Can]

Therapeutic Category Antibiotic, Ophthalmic; Antibiotic, Quinolone

Use Treatment of superficial ocular infections (corneal ulcers, conjunctivitis) due to susceptible strains

Dosage Summary

Ophthalmic:

Ointment:

Children ≤2 years: Dosage not established

Children >2 years: Apply a 1/2" ribbon into the conjunctival sac 3 times/day for the first 2 days, followed by a 1/2" ribbon applied twice daily

Adults: Apply a 1/2" ribbon into the conjunctival sac 3 times/day for the first 2 days, followed by a 1/2" ribbon applied twice daily

Solution:

Children ≤1 year: Dosage not established

Children >1 year:

Conjunctivitis: Instill 1-2 drops in eye(s) every 2 hours while awake for 2 days, then 1-2 drops every 4 hours while awake

Corneal ulcer: Instill 2 drops into affected eye every 15 minutes for the first 6 hours, then 2 drops every 30 minutes for the remainder of the first day, on day 2 instill 2 drops into the affected eye hourly, on days 3-14 instill 2 drops every 4 hours

Adults:

Conjunctivitis: Instill 1-2 drops in eye(s) every 2 hours while awake for 2 days, then 1-2 drops every 4 hours while awake

Corneal ulcer: Instill 2 drops into affected eye every 15 minutes for the first 6 hours, then 2 drops every 30 minutes for the remainder of the first day, on day 2 instill 2 drops into the affected eye hourly, on days 3-14 instill 2 drops every 4 hours

Dosage Forms

Ointment, ophthalmic:

Ciloxan®: 3.33 mg/g (3.5 g)

Solution, ophthalmic: 3.5 mg/mL (2.5 mL, 5 mL, 10 mL); 0.3% (2.5 mL, 5 mL)

Ciloxan®: 3.5 mg/mL (5 mL)

ciprofloxacin (otic) (sip roe FLOKS a sin)

Sound-Alike/Look-Alike Issues

ciprofloxacin may be confused with cephalexin

Cetraxal® may be confused with cefTRIAXone

Synonyms ciprofloxacin hydrochloride

U.S./Canadian Brand Names Cetraxal® [US]

Therapeutic Category Antibiotic, Otic; Antibiotic, Quinolone

Use Treatment of acute otitis externa due to susceptible strains of *Pseudomonas aeruginosa* or *Staphylococcus aureus*

Dosage Summary

Otic:

Children <1 year: Dosage not established

Children ≥1 year: 0.5 mg (0.25 mL) every 12 hours

Adults: 0.5 mg (0.25 mL) every 12 hours

Dosage Forms

Solution, otic [preservative free]:

Cetraxal®: 0.5 mg/0.25 mL (14s)

ciprofloxacin and dexamethasone (sip roe FLOKS a sin & deks a METH a sone)

Synonyms ciprofloxacin hydrochloride and dexamethasone; dexamethasone and ciprofloxacin

U.S./Canadian Brand Names Ciprodex® [US/Can]

Therapeutic Category Antibiotic/Corticosteroid, Otic

Use Treatment of acute otitis media in pediatric patients with tympanostomy tubes or acute otitis externa in children and adults

Dosage Summary

Otic:

Children: Instill 4 drops into affected ear(s) twice daily
Adults: Instill 4 drops into affected ear(s) twice daily

Dosage Forms

Suspension, otic:

Ciprodex®: Ciprofloxacin 0.3% and dexamethasone 0.1% (7.5 mL)

ciprofloxacin and hydrocortisone (sip roe FLOKS a sin & hye droe KOR ti sone)

Synonyms ciprofloxacin hydrochloride and hydrocortisone; hydrocortisone and ciprofloxacin

U.S./Canadian Brand Names Cipro® HC [US/Can]

Therapeutic Category Antibiotic/Corticosteroid, Otic

Use Treatment of acute otitis externa, sometimes known as "swimmer's ear"

Dosage Summary

Otic:

Children ≤1 year: Dosage not established
Children >1 year: Three drops into affected ear(s) twice daily
Adults: Three drops into affected ear(s) twice daily

Dosage Forms

Suspension, otic:

Cipro® HC: Ciprofloxacin 0.2% and hydrocortisone 1% (10 mL)

ciprofloxacin hydrochloride *see* ciprofloxacin (ophthalmic) *on page 224*
ciprofloxacin hydrochloride *see* ciprofloxacin (otic) *on page 225*
ciprofloxacin hydrochloride *see* ciprofloxacin (systemic) *on page 224*
ciprofloxacin hydrochloride and dexamethasone *see* ciprofloxacin and dexamethasone *on page 225*
ciprofloxacin hydrochloride and hydrocortisone *see* ciprofloxacin and hydrocortisone *on page 226*
Cipro® HC [US/Can] *see* ciprofloxacin and hydrocortisone *on page 226*
Cipro® I.V. [US] *see* ciprofloxacin (systemic) *on page 224*
Cipro® XR [US] *see* ciprofloxacin (systemic) *on page 224*

cisapride (SIS a pride)

Sound-Alike/Look-Alike Issues

Propulsid® may be confused with propranolol

U.S./Canadian Brand Names Propulsid® [US]

Therapeutic Category Gastrointestinal Agent, Prokinetic

Use Treatment of nocturnal symptoms of gastroesophageal reflux disease (GERD); has demonstrated effectiveness for gastroparesis, refractory constipation, and nonulcer dyspepsia

Dosage Summary

Oral:

Children: 0.15-0.3 mg/kg 3-4 times/day (maximum: 10 mg/dose)
Adults: Initial: 5-10 mg 4 times/day, may increase to 20 mg 4 times/day if needed

cisatracurium (sis a tra KYOO ree um)

Sound-Alike/Look-Alike Issues

Nimbex® may be confused with Revex®

Synonyms cisatracurium besylate

U.S./Canadian Brand Names Nimbex® [US/Can]

Therapeutic Category Skeletal Muscle Relaxant

Use Adjunct to general anesthesia to facilitate endotracheal intubation and to relax skeletal muscles during surgery; to facilitate mechanical ventilation in ICU patients; does not relieve pain or produce sedation

Dosage Summary

I.V.:

Children <1month: Dosage not established
Children 1-23 months: Intubating dose: 0.15 mg/kg
Children 2-12 years: Intubating dose: 0.1-0.15 mg/kg over 5-15 seconds; Infusion: Initial: 3 mcg/kg/minute; Maintenance: 1-2 mcg/kg/minute (surgery) **or** 0.5-10 mcg/kg/minute (ICU)

Children >12 years: Infusion: Initial: 3 mcg/kg/minute; Maintenance: 1-2 mcg/kg/minute (surgery) **or** 0.5-10 mcg/kg/minute (ICU)

Adults: Intubating dose: 0.1-0.2 mg/kg; Infusion: Initial: 3 mcg/kg/minute; Maintenance: 1-2 mcg/kg/minute (surgery) **or** 0.5-10 mcg/kg/minute (ICU)

Dosage Forms

Injection, solution:

Nimbex®: 2 mg/mL (5 mL, 10 mL); 10 mg/mL (20 mL)

cisatracurium besylate *see* cisatracurium *on page 226*

cisplatin (SIS pla tin)

Sound-Alike/Look-Alike Issues

CISplatin may be confused with CARBOplatin, oxaliplatin

Synonyms CDDP

Tall-Man CISplatin

Therapeutic Category Antineoplastic Agent

Use Treatment of advanced bladder cancer, metastatic testicular cancer, and metastatic ovarian cancer

Dosage Summary

I.V.:

Adults: 50-70 mg/m^2 every 3-4 weeks **or** 75-100 mg/m^2/day every 4 weeks **or** 20 mg/m^2/day for 5 days every 3 weeks

Dosage Forms

Injection, solution [preservative free]: 1 mg/mL (50 mL, 100 mL, 200 mL)

13-*cis*-retinoic acid *see* isotretinoin *on page 530*

citalopram (sye TAL oh pram)

Sound-Alike/Look-Alike Issues

Celexa® may be confused with Celebrex®, Cerebra®, Cerebyx®, Ranexa™, Zyprexa®

Synonyms citalopram hydrobromide; nitalapram

U.S./Canadian Brand Names Apo-Citalopram® [Can]; Celexa® [US/Can]; Citalopram-Odan [Can]; CO Citalopram [Can]; CTP 30 [Can]; Dom-Citalopram [Can]; JAMP-Citalopram [Can]; Mint-Citalopram [Can]; Mylan-Citalopram [Can]; NG-Citalopram [Can]; Novo-Citalopram [Can]; PHL-Citalopram [Can]; PMS-Citalopram [Can]; RAN™-Citalopram [Can]; ratio-Citalopram [Can]; Riva-Citalopram [Can]; Sandoz-Citalopram [Can]

Therapeutic Category Antidepressant

Use Treatment of depression

Dosage Summary

Oral:

Adults: Initial: 20 mg/day; Maintenance: 20-60 mg/day

Elderly: Initial: 20 mg once daily; may increase to 40 mg/day in nonresponsive patients

Dosage Forms

Solution, oral: 10 mg/5 mL (240 mL)

Tablet, oral: 10 mg, 20 mg, 40 mg

Celexa®: 10 mg, 20 mg, 40 mg

citalopram hydrobromide *see* citalopram *on page 227*

Citalopram-Odan [Can] *see* citalopram *on page 227*

Citanest® Plain [Can] *see* prilocaine *on page 794*

Citanest® Plain Dental [US] *see* prilocaine *on page 794*

Citracal® Kosher *(Discontinued)* *see* calcium citrate *on page 169*

Citracal® Prenatal 90+ DHA *(Discontinued)* *see* vitamins (multiple/prenatal) *on page 991*

Citracal® Prenatal + DHA *(Discontinued)* *see* vitamins (multiple/prenatal) *on page 991*

CitraNatal™ 90 DHA [US] *see* vitamins (multiple/prenatal) *on page 991*

CitraNatal™ DHA [US] *see* vitamins (multiple/prenatal) *on page 991*

CitraNatal™ Rx [US] *see* vitamins (multiple/prenatal) *on page 991*

citrate of magnesia *see* magnesium citrate *on page 584*

citric acid and D-gluconic acid irrigant *see* citric acid, magnesium carbonate, and glucono-delta-lactone *on page 228*

citric acid and potassium citrate *see* potassium citrate and citric acid *on page* 782
citric acid bladder mixture *see* citric acid, magnesium carbonate, and glucono-delta-lactone *on page* 228

citric acid, magnesium carbonate, and glucono-delta-lactone

(SI trik AS id, mag NEE see um KAR bo nate, and GLOO kon o DEL ta LAK tone)

Sound-Alike/Look-Alike Issues

Renacidin® may be confused with Remicade®

Synonyms citric acid and D-gluconic acid irrigant; citric acid bladder mixture; citric acid, magnesium hydroxycarbonate, D-gluconic acid, magnesium acid citrate, and calcium carbonate; hemiacidrin

U.S./Canadian Brand Names Renacidin® [US]

Therapeutic Category Irrigating Solution

Use Prevention of formation of calcifications of indwelling urinary tract catheters; treatment of renal and bladder calculi of the apatite or struvite type

Dosage Summary

Irrigation:

Children: Dosage not established

Adults: 30-60 mL into catheter 2-3 times/day **or** 30 mL into bladder, retained for 30-60 minutes then drained 4-6 times **or** 60-120 mL/hour

Dosage Forms

Solution, irrigation:

Renacidin®: Citric acid 6.602 g, magnesium carbonate 3.177 g, glucono-delta-lactone 0.198 g per 100 mL (500 mL)

citric acid, magnesium hydroxycarbonate, D-gluconic acid, magnesium acid citrate, and calcium carbonate *see* citric acid, magnesium carbonate, and glucono-delta-lactone *on page* 228

citric acid, sodium citrate, and potassium citrate

(SIT rik AS id, SOW dee um SIT rate, & poe TASS ee um SIT rate)

Sound-Alike/Look-Alike Issues

polycitra may be confused with Bicitra®

Synonyms polycitra; potassium citrate, citric acid, and sodium citrate; sodium citrate, citric acid, and potassium citrate

U.S./Canadian Brand Names Cytra-3 [US]; Tricitrates [US]

Therapeutic Category Alkalinizing Agent

Use Conditions where long-term maintenance of an alkaline urine is desirable as in control and dissolution of uric acid and cystine calculi of the urinary tract

Dosage Summary

Oral:

Children: 5-15 mL diluted in water after meals and at bedtime

Adults: 15-30 mL diluted in water after meals and at bedtime

Dosage Forms

Solution, oral:

Cytra-3, Tricitrates: Citric acid 334 mg, sodium citrate 500 mg, and potassium citrate 550 mg per 5 mL

Citroma® [US-OTC] *see* magnesium citrate *on page* 584
Citro-Mag® [Can] *see* magnesium citrate *on page* 584
Citrotein® [US-OTC] *see* nutritional formula, enteral/oral *on page* 692
citrovorum factor *see* leucovorin calcium *on page* 553
Citrucel® [US-OTC] *see* methylcellulose *on page* 618
Citrucel® Fiber Shake *(Discontinued)* *see* methylcellulose *on page* 618
Citrucel® Fiber Smoothie *(Discontinued)* *see* methylcellulose *on page* 618
CL-118,532 *see* triptorelin *on page* 962
Cl-719 *see* gemfibrozil *on page* 440
CL-184116 *see* porfimer *on page* 779
CL-232315 *see* mitoxantrone *on page* 638

cladribine (KLA dri been)

Sound-Alike/Look-Alike Issues

cladribine may be confused with clevidipine, clofarabine, fludarabine
Leustatin® may be confused with lovastatin

Synonyms 2-CdA; 2-chlorodeoxyadenosine; NSC-105014

U.S./Canadian Brand Names Leustatin® [US/Can]

Therapeutic Category Antineoplastic Agent

Use Treatment of hairy cell leukemia

Dosage Summary

I.V.:

Adults: Continuous infusion: 0.09 mg/kg/day days 1-7 every 28-35 days

Dosage Forms

Injection, solution [preservative free]: 1 mg/mL (10 mL)
Leustatin®: 1 mg/mL (10 mL)

Claforan® [US/Can] *see* cefotaxime *on page* 191
Claravis™ [US] *see* isotretinoin *on page* 530
Clarifoam™ EF [US] *see* sulfur and sulfacetamide *on page* 903
Clarinex® [US] *see* desloratadine *on page* 277
Clarinex-D® 12 Hour [US] *see* desloratadine and pseudoephedrine *on page* 278
Clarinex-D® 24 Hour [US] *see* desloratadine and pseudoephedrine *on page* 278
Claripel™ *(Discontinued)* *see* hydroquinone *on page* 487

clarithromycin (kla RITH roe mye sin)

Sound-Alike/Look-Alike Issues

clarithromycin may be confused with Claritin®, clindamycin, erythromycin

U.S./Canadian Brand Names Apo-Clarithromycin® [Can]; Biaxin® XL [US/Can]; Biaxin® [US/Can]; Mylan-Clarithromycin [Can]; PMS-Clarithromycin [Can]; ratio-Clarithromycin [Can]; Riva-Clarithromycin [Can]; Sandoz-Clarithromycin [Can]

Therapeutic Category Macrolide (Antibiotic)

Use

Children:

- Acute otitis media (*H. influenzae*, *M. catarrhalis*, or *S. pneumoniae*)
- Community-acquired pneumonia due to susceptible *Mycoplasma pneumoniae*, *S. pneumoniae*, or *Chlamydia pneumoniae* (TWAR)
- Pharyngitis/tonsillitis due to susceptible *S. pyogenes*, acute maxillary sinusitis due to susceptible *H. influenzae, S. pneumoniae,* or *Moraxella catarrhalis*, uncomplicated skin/skin structure infections due to susceptible *S. aureus, S. pyogenes,* and mycobacterial infections
- Prevention of disseminated mycobacterial infections due to MAC disease in patients with advanced HIV infection

Adults:

- Pharyngitis/tonsillitis due to susceptible *S. pyogenes*
- Acute maxillary sinusitis due to susceptible *H. influenzae, M. catarrhalis,* or *S. pneumoniae*
- Acute exacerbation of chronic bronchitis due to susceptible *H. influenzae*, *H. parainfluenzae*, *M. catarrhalis*, or *S. pneumoniae*
- Community-acquired pneumonia due to susceptible *H. influenzae, H. parainfluenzae, Mycoplasma pneumoniae, S. pneumoniae,* or *Chlamydia pneumoniae* (TWAR), *Moraxella catarrhalis*
- Uncomplicated skin/skin structure infections due to susceptible *S. aureus*, *S. pyogenes*
- Disseminated mycobacterial infections due to *M. avium* or *M. intracellulare*
- Prevention of disseminated mycobacterial infections due to *M. avium* complex (MAC) disease (eg, patients with advanced HIV infection)
- Duodenal ulcer disease due to *H. pylori* in regimens with other drugs including amoxicillin and lansoprazole or omeprazole, ranitidine bismuth citrate, bismuth subsalicylate, tetracycline, and/or an H_2 antagonist

Dosage Summary

Oral:

Extended release:

Children: Dosage not established
Adults: 1000 mg once daily

Immediate release:

Children: 15 mg/kg/day divided every 12 hours (maximum: 1 g/day) **or** 15 mg/kg prior to procedure (maximum: 500 mg)

Adults: 250-500 mg every 8-12 hours **or** 500 mg prior to procedure

Dosage Forms

Granules for suspension, oral: 125 mg/5 mL (50 mL, 100 mL); 250 mg/5 mL (50 mL, 100 mL)

Biaxin®: 125 mg/5 mL (50 mL, 100 mL); 250 mg/5 mL (50 mL, 100 mL)

Tablet, oral: 250 mg, 500 mg

Biaxin®: 250 mg, 500 mg

Tablet, extended release, oral: 500 mg

Biaxin® XL: 500 mg

clarithromycin, lansoprazole, and amoxicillin *see* lansoprazole, amoxicillin, and clarithromycin *on page 549*

Claritin® [Can] *see* loratadine *on page 575*

Claritin® 24 Hour Allergy [US-OTC] *see* loratadine *on page 575*

Claritin-D® 12 Hour Allergy & Congestion [US-OTC] *see* loratadine and pseudoephedrine *on page 576*

Claritin-D® 24 Hour Allergy & Congestion [US-OTC] *see* loratadine and pseudoephedrine *on page 576*

Claritin® Allergic Decongestant [Can] *see* oxymetazoline (nasal) *on page 716*

Claritin® Children's Allergy [US-OTC] *see* loratadine *on page 575*

Claritin® *(Discontinued)* *see* loratadine *on page 575*

Claritin® Extra [Can] *see* loratadine and pseudoephedrine *on page 576*

Claritin™ Eye [US-OTC] *see* ketotifen *on page 538*

Claritin® Hives Relief *(Discontinued)* *see* loratadine *on page 575*

Claritin® Kids [Can] *see* loratadine *on page 575*

Claritin® Liberator [Can] *see* loratadine and pseudoephedrine *on page 576*

Claritin® Liqui-Gels® 24 Hour Allergy [US-OTC] *see* loratadine *on page 575*

Claritin® RediTabs® 24 Hour Allergy [US-OTC] *see* loratadine *on page 575*

Claritin® Reditabs *(Discontinued)* *see* loratadine *on page 575*

Clarus™ [Can] *see* isotretinoin *on page 530*

Clasteon® [Can] *see* clodronate *(Canada only) on page 236*

clavulanic acid and amoxicillin *see* amoxicillin and clavulanate potassium *on page 73*

Clavulin® [Can] *see* amoxicillin and clavulanate potassium *on page 73*

Clean & Clear® Advantage® Acne Cleanser [US-OTC] *see* salicylic acid *on page 858*

Clean & Clear® Advantage® Acne Spot Treatment [US-OTC] *see* salicylic acid *on page 858*

Clean & Clear® Advantage® Invisible Acne Patch [US-OTC] *see* salicylic acid *on page 858*

Clean & Clear® Advantage® Oil-Free Acne [US-OTC] *see* salicylic acid *on page 858*

Clean & Clear® Blackhead Clearing Daily Cleansing [US-OTC] *see* salicylic acid *on page 858*

Clean & Clear® Blackhead Clearing Scrub [US-OTC] *see* salicylic acid *on page 858*

Clean & Clear® Continuous Control® Acne Wash [US-OTC] *see* salicylic acid *on page 858*

Clean & Clear® Deep Cleaning [US-OTC] *see* salicylic acid *on page 858*

Clean & Clear® Dual Action Moisturizer [US-OTC] *see* salicylic acid *on page 858*

Clean & Clear® Invisible Blemish Treatment [US-OTC] *see* salicylic acid *on page 858*

Clear Away® Disc *(Discontinued)* *see* salicylic acid *on page 858*

Clear By Design® Gel *(Discontinued)* *see* benzoyl peroxide *on page 128*

Clear eyes® for Dry Eyes Plus ACR Relief [US-OTC] *see* naphazoline (ophthalmic) *on page 658*

Clear eyes® for Dry Eyes plus Redness Relief [US-OTC] *see* naphazoline (ophthalmic) *on page 658*

Clear eyes® Redness Relief [US-OTC] *see* naphazoline (ophthalmic) *on page 658*

Clear eyes® Seasonal Relief [US-OTC] *see* naphazoline (ophthalmic) *on page 658*

Clearsil® Maximum Strength *(Discontinued)* *see* benzoyl peroxide *on page 128*

Clearskin [US-OTC] *see* benzoyl peroxide *on page 128*

Clear Tussin® 30 *(Discontinued)* *see* guaifenesin and dextromethorphan *on page 455*

clemastine (KLEM as teen)

Synonyms clemastine fumarate

U.S./Canadian Brand Names Tavist® Allergy [US-OTC]

Therapeutic Category Antihistamine

Use Perennial and seasonal allergic rhinitis and other allergic symptoms including urticaria

Dosage Summary

Oral:

Children <6 years: 0.05 mg/kg/day (base) **or** 0.335-0.67 mg/day (fumarate) in 2-3 divided doses (maximum: 1.34 mg/day [fumarate] or 1 mg/day [base])

Children 6-12 years: 0.67-1.34 mg fumarate (0.5-1 mg base) twice daily (maximum: 4.02 mg/day [3 mg base])

Children ≥12 years: 1.34-2.68 mg fumarate (1-2 mg base) 2-3 times/day (maximum: 8.04 mg/day [6 mg base])

Adults: 1.34-2.68 mg fumarate (1-2 mg base) 2-3 times/day (maximum: 8.04 mg/day [6 mg base])

Dosage Forms

Syrup, oral: 0.67 mg/5 mL (120 mL, 473 mL)

Tablet, oral: 1.34 mg, 2.68 mg

Tavist® Allergy [OTC]: 1.34 mg

clemastine fumarate *see* clemastine *on page* *231*

Clenia™ [US] *see* sulfur and sulfacetamide *on page* *903*

Cleocin® [US] *see* clindamycin (topical) *on page* *232*

Cleocin HCl® [US] *see* clindamycin (systemic) *on page* *232*

Cleocin Pediatric® [US] *see* clindamycin (systemic) *on page* *232*

Cleocin Phosphate® [US] *see* clindamycin (systemic) *on page* *232*

Cleocin T® [US] *see* clindamycin (topical) *on page* *232*

Cleocin® Vaginal Ovule [US] *see* clindamycin (topical) *on page* *232*

clevidipine (klev ID i peen)

Sound-Alike/Look-Alike Issues

clevidipine may be confused with cladribine, clofarabine, clomiPRAMINE

Cleviprex™ may be confused with Claravis™

Synonyms clevidipine butyrate

U.S./Canadian Brand Names Cleviprex™ [US]

Therapeutic Category Calcium Channel Blocker

Use Management of hypertension when oral treatment is not feasible or not desirable

Dosage Summary

I.V.:

Children: Dosage not established

Adults: Initial: 1-2 mg/hour; usual maintenance: 4-6 mg/hour; maximum: 21 mg/hour (1000 mL/24 hours)

Elderly: Refer to adult dosing

Dosage Forms

Injection, emulsion:

Cleviprex™: 0.5 mg/mL (50 mL, 100 mL)

clevidipine butyrate *see* clevidipine *on page* *231*

Cleviprex™ [US] *see* clevidipine *on page* *231*

clidinium and chlordiazepoxide (kli DI nee um & klor dye az e POKS ide)

Sound-Alike/Look-Alike Issues

Librax® may be confused with Librium®

Synonyms chlordiazepoxide and clidinium

U.S./Canadian Brand Names Apo-Chlorax® [Can]; Librax® *[original formulation]* [US/Can]

Therapeutic Category Anticholinergic Agent

Use Adjunct treatment of peptic ulcer; treatment of irritable bowel syndrome

Dosage Summary

Oral:

Children: Dosage not established

Adults: 1-2 capsules 3-4 times/day

Dosage Forms

Capsule: Clidinium 2.5 mg and chlordiazepoxide 5 mg

Librax® [original formulation]: Clidinium 2.5 mg and chlordiazepoxide 5 mg

Climara® [US/Can] *see* estradiol (systemic) *on page* 366

ClimaraPro® [US] *see* estradiol and levonorgestrel *on page* 368

Clinac® BPO [US] *see* benzoyl peroxide *on page* 128

Clindagel® [US] *see* clindamycin (topical) *on page* 232

ClindaMax® [US] *see* clindamycin (topical) *on page* 232

clindamycin (systemic) (klin da MYE sin)

Sound-Alike/Look-Alike Issues

clindamycin may be confused with clarithromycin, Claritin®, vancomycin

Cleocin® may be confused with bleomycin, Clinoril®, Cubicin®, Lincocin®

Synonyms clindamycin hydrochloride; clindamycin palmitate

U.S./Canadian Brand Names Alti-Clindamycin [Can]; Apo-Clindamycin® [Can]; Cleocin HCl® [US]; Cleocin Pediatric® [US]; Cleocin Phosphate® [US]; Clindamycin Injection, USP [Can]; Clindamycine [Can]; Gen-Clindamycin [Can]; Novo-Clindamycin [Can]; PMS-Clindamycin [Can]; ratio-Clindamycin [Can]; Riva-Clindamycin [Can]

Therapeutic Category Antibiotic, Lincosamide

Use Treatment of susceptible bacterial infections, mainly those caused by anaerobes, streptococci, pneumococci, and staphylococci; pelvic inflammatory disease (I.V.)

Dosage Summary

I.M.:

Children <1 month: 15-20 mg/kg/day in 3-4 divided doses

Children >1 month: 20-40 mg/kg/day in 3-4 divided doses

Adults: 1.2-2.7 g/day in 2-4 divided doses (maximum: 4.8 g/day)

I.V.:

Children <1 month: 15-20 mg/kg/day in 3-4 divided doses

Children >1 month: 20-40 mg/kg/day in 3-4 divided doses

Adults: 1.2-2.7 g/day in 2-4 divided doses (maximum: 4.8 g/day)

Oral:

Children: 8-20 mg/kg/day as hydrochloride or 8-25 mg/kg/day as palmitate in 3-4 divided doses (minimum dose of palmitate: 37.5 mg 3 times/day)

Adults: 150-450 mg every 6-8 hours (maximum: 1.8 g/day)

Dosage Forms

Capsule, oral: 75 mg, 150 mg, 300 mg

Cleocin HCl®: 75 mg, 150 mg, 300 mg

Granules for solution, oral: 75 mg/5 mL (100 mL)

Cleocin Pediatric®: 75 mg/5 mL (100 mL)

Infusion, premixed in D_5W:

Cleocin Phosphate®: 300 mg (50 mL); 600 mg (50 mL); 900 mg (50 mL)

Injection, solution: 150 mg/mL (2 mL, 4 mL, 6 mL, 60 mL)

Cleocin Phosphate®: 150 mg/mL (2 mL, 4 mL, 6 mL, 60 mL)

clindamycin (topical) (klin da MYE sin)

Sound-Alike/Look-Alike Issues

clindamycin may be confused with clarithromycin, Claritin®, vancomycin

Cleocin® may be confused with bleomycin, Clinoril®, Cubicin®, Lincocin®

Synonyms clindamycin phosphate

U.S./Canadian Brand Names Cleocin T® [US]; Cleocin® Vaginal Ovule [US]; Cleocin® [US]; Clinda-T [Can]; Clindagel® [US]; ClindaMax® [US]; ClindaReach® [US]; Clindasol™ [Can]; Clindesse® [US]; Clindets [Can]; Dalacin® C [Can]; Dalacin® T [Can]; Dalacin® Vaginal [Can]; Evoclin® [US]; Taro-Clindamycin [Can]

Therapeutic Category Antibiotic, Lincosamide; Topical Skin Product, Acne

Use Treatment of susceptible bacterial infections, mainly those caused by anaerobes, streptococci, pneumococci, and staphylococci; bacterial vaginosis (vaginal cream, vaginal suppository); topically in treatment of severe acne; vaginally for *Gardnerella vaginalis*

Dosage Summary

Intravaginal:

Children: Dosage not established

Adults: Insert one ovule or applicatorful once daily or one applicatorful as a single dose (Clindesse®)

Topical:

Children <12 years: Dosage not established

Children ≥12 years: Apply once or twice daily

Adults: Apply once or twice daily

Dosage Forms

Aerosol, topical:

Evoclin®: 1% (50 g, 100 g)

Cream, vaginal: 2% (40 g)

Cleocin®: 2% (40 g)

Clindesse®: 2% (5 g)

Gel, topical: 1% (30 g, 60 g)

Cleocin T®: 1% (30 g, 60 g)

Clindagel®: 1% (40 mL, 75 mL)

ClindaMax®: 1% (30 g, 60 g)

Lotion, topical: 1% (60 mL)

Cleocin T®: 1% (60 mL)

ClindaMax®: 1% (60 mL)

Pledget, topical: 1% (60s, 69s)

Cleocin T®: 1% (60s)

ClindaReach®: 1% (120s)

Solution, topical: 1% (30 mL, 60 mL)

Cleocin T®: 1% (30 mL, 60 mL)

Suppository, vaginal:

Cleocin® Vaginal Ovule: 100 mg (3s)

clindamycin and benzoyl peroxide (klin da MYE sin & BEN zoe il peer OKS ide)

Synonyms benzoyl peroxide and clindamycin; clindamycin phosphate and benzoyl peroxide

U.S./Canadian Brand Names Acanya™ [US]; BenzaClin® [US/Can]; Clindoxyl [Can]; Duac® CS [US]

Therapeutic Category Topical Skin Product; Topical Skin Product, Acne

Use Topical treatment of acne vulgaris

Dosage Summary

Topical:

Children <12 years: Dosage not established

Children ≥12 years: Apply once daily (Acanya®, Duac® CS) **or** twice daily (BenzaClin®) to affected areas

Adults: Apply once daily (Acanya®, Duac® CS) **or** twice daily (BenzaClin®) to affected areas

Dosage Forms

Gel, topical: Clindamycin 1% and benzoyl peroxide 5% (50 g)

Acanya®: Clindamycin 1.2% and benzoyl peroxide 2.5% (50 g)

BenzaClin®: Clindamycin 1% and benzoyl peroxide 5% (25 g, 35 g, 50 g)

Duac® CS: Clindamycin 1% and benzoyl peroxide 5% (45 g)

clindamycin and tretinoin (klin da MYE sin & TRET i noyn)

Synonyms clindamycin phosphate and tretinoin; tretinoin and clindamycin; Veltin™

U.S./Canadian Brand Names Ziana™ [US]

Therapeutic Category Acne Products; Retinoic Acid Derivative; Topical Skin Product; Topical Skin Product, Acne

Use Treatment of acne vulgaris

Dosage Summary

Topical:

Children <12 years: Dosage not established

Children ≥12 years: Apply pea-size amount to entire face once daily at bedtime

Adults: Apply pea-size amount to entire face once daily at bedtime

Product Availability
Veltin™: FDA approved July 2010; anticipated availability is undetermined
Veltin™ gel is indicated for the topical treatment of acne vulgaris

Dosage Forms

Gel, topical:
Ziana™: Clindamycin phosphate 1.2% and tretinoin 0.025% (30 g, 60 g)

Clindamycine [Can] *see* clindamycin (systemic) *on page* *232*
clindamycin hydrochloride *see* clindamycin (systemic) *on page* *232*
Clindamycin Injection, USP [Can] *see* clindamycin (systemic) *on page* *232*
clindamycin palmitate *see* clindamycin (systemic) *on page* *232*
clindamycin phosphate *see* clindamycin (topical) *on page* *232*
clindamycin phosphate and benzoyl peroxide *see* clindamycin and benzoyl peroxide *on page* *233*
clindamycin phosphate and tretinoin *see* clindamycin and tretinoin *on page* *233*
ClindaReach® [US] *see* clindamycin (topical) *on page* *232*
Clindasol™ [Can] *see* clindamycin (topical) *on page* *232*
Clinda-T [Can] *see* clindamycin (topical) *on page* *232*
Clindesse® [US] *see* clindamycin (topical) *on page* *232*
Clindets [Can] *see* clindamycin (topical) *on page* *232*
Clindets® *(Discontinued)* *see* clindamycin (topical) *on page* *232*
Clindex® *(Discontinued)* *see* clidinium and chlordiazepoxide *on page* *231*
Clindoxyl [Can] *see* clindamycin and benzoyl peroxide *on page* *233*
Clinisol® [US] *see* amino acid injection *on page* *64*
Clinoril® [US] *see* sulindac *on page* *904*

clioquinol and flumethasone *(Canada only)* (klye ok KWIN ole & floo METH a sone)

Synonyms flumethasone and clioquinol; iodochlorhydroxyquin and flumethasone

U.S./Canadian Brand Names Locacorten® Vioform® [Can]

Therapeutic Category Antibiotic, Topical; Corticosteroid, Topical

Use Treatment of corticosteroid-responsive dermatoses complicated by infection with bacterial and/or fungal agents

Dosage Summary

Otic:
Children ≤2 years: Dosage not established
Children >2 years: Instill 2-3 drops into affected ear(s) 2 times/day
Adults: Instill 2-3 drops into affected ear(s) 2 times/day

Topical:
Children ≤2 years: Dosage not established
Children >2 years: Apply a thin layer to affected area 2-3 times/day
Adults: Apply a thin layer to affected area 2-3 times/day

Dosage Forms - Canada

Cream, topical:
Locacorten® Vioform®: Clioquinol 3% and flumethasone 0.02% (15 g, 50 g)

Solution, otic:
Locacorten® Vioform®: Clioquinol 1% and flumethasone 0.02% (10 mL)

Clobazam-10 [Can] *see* clobazam *(Canada only)* *on page* *234*

clobazam *(Canada only)* (KLOE ba zam)

U.S./Canadian Brand Names Apo-Clobazam® [Can]; Clobazam-10 [Can]; Dom-Clobazam [Can]; Frisium® [Can]; Novo-Clobazam [Can]; PMS-Clobazam [Can]; ratio-Clobazam [Can]

Therapeutic Category Anticonvulsant; Antidepressant

Use Adjunctive treatment of epilepsy

Dosage Summary Note: Daily doses of up to 30 mg may be taken as a single dose at bedtime; higher doses should be divided

Oral:
Children <2 years: 0.5-1 mg/kg/day
Children 2-16 years: Initial: 5 mg/day; Maintenance: Up to 40 mg/day; **Note:** Titration is recommended
Adults: Initial: 5-15 mg/day; Maintenance: Up to 80 mg/day; **Note:** Titration is recommended

Dosage Forms - Canada

Tablet:

Alti-Clobazam, Apo-Clobazam®, Clobazam-10, Dom-Clobazam, Frisium®, Novo-Clobazam, PMS-Clobazam, ratio-Clobazam: 10 mg

clobetasol (kloe BAY ta sol)

Synonyms clobetasol propionate

U.S./Canadian Brand Names Clobex® [US/Can]; Cormax® [US]; Dermovate® [Can]; Gen-Clobetasol [Can]; Mylan-Clobetasol Cream [Can]; Mylan-Clobetasol Ointment [Can]; Mylan-Clobetasol Scalp Application [Can]; Novo-Clobetasol [Can]; Olux-E™ [US]; Olux® [US]; Olux®/Olux-E™ CP [US]; PMS-Clobetasol [Can]; ratio-Clobetasol [Can]; Taro-Clobetasol [Can]; Temovate E® [US]; Temovate® [US]

Therapeutic Category Corticosteroid, Topical

Use Short-term relief of inflammation of moderate-to-severe corticosteroid-responsive dermatoses (very high potency topical corticosteroid)

Dosage Summary

Topical:

Children <12 years: Dosage not established

Children ≥12 years: Apply to affected area twice daily (maximum: 50 g/week; 50 mL/week)

Adults: Apply to affected area twice daily **or** apply shampoo to dry scalp once daily (maximum: 50 g/week; 50 mL/week)

Dosage Forms

Aerosol, topical: 0.05% (50 g, 100 g)

Olux-E™: 0.05% (50 g, 100 g)

Olux®: 0.05% (50 g, 100 g)

Olux®/Olux-E™ CP: Olux-E™: 0.05% (50 g) and Olux® 0.05% (50 g) [contains ethanol 60%] (1s); Olux-E™: 0.05% (10 g) and Olux® 0.05% (100 g) [contains ethanol 60%] (1s)

Cream, topical: 0.05% (15 g, 30 g, 45 g, 60 g, 60s)

Temovate E®: 0.05% (60 g)

Temovate®: 0.05% (30 g, 60 g)

Gel, topical: 0.05% (15 g, 30 g, 60 g)

Temovate®: 0.05% (60 g)

Lotion, topical:

Clobex®: 0.05% (30 mL, 59 mL, 118 mL)

Ointment, topical: 0.05% (15 g, 30 g, 45 g, 60 g)

Cormax®: 0.05% (15 g, 45 g)

Temovate®: 0.05% (15 g, 30 g)

Shampoo, topical:

Clobex®: 0.05% (118 mL)

Solution, topical: 0.05% (25 mL, 50 mL)

Clobex®: 0.05% (59 mL, 125 mL)

Cormax®: 0.05% (25 mL, 50 mL)

Temovate®: 0.05% (50 mL)

clobetasol propionate *see* clobetasol *on page 235*

Clobevate® *(Discontinued)* *see* clobetasol *on page 235*

Clobex® [US/Can] *see* clobetasol *on page 235*

clocortolone (kloe KOR toe lone)

Sound-Alike/Look-Alike Issues

Cloderm® may be confused with Clocort®

Synonyms clocortolone pivalate

U.S./Canadian Brand Names Cloderm® [US/Can]

Therapeutic Category Corticosteroid, Topical

Use Inflammation of corticosteroid-responsive dermatoses (intermediate-potency topical corticosteroid)

Dosage Summary

Topical:

Children: Dosage not established

Adults: Apply sparingly to affected area 1-4 times/day until control is achieved

Dosage Forms
Cream, topical:
Cloderm®: 0.1% (30 g, 45 g, 90 g)

clocortolone pivalate *see* clocortolone *on page 235*
Cloderm® [US/Can] *see* clocortolone *on page 235*

clodronate *(Canada only)* (KLOE droh nate)

Synonyms clodronate disodium
U.S./Canadian Brand Names Bonefos® [Can]; Clasteon® [Can]
Therapeutic Category Bisphosphonate Derivative
Use Management of hypercalcemia of malignancy; management of osteolysis due to bone metastases of malignancy
Dosage Summary
I.V.:
Children: Dosage not established
Adults: 1500 mg as single dose (Clasteon®) **or** 300 mg/day (Clasteon®, Bonefos®); maximum therapy: 10 days (Clasteon®); 7 days (Bonefos®)
Oral:
Children: Dosage not established
Adults: 1600-2400 mg/day in 1-2 divided doses (maximum: 3200 mg/day); **Note:** I.V. therapy should be used first
Dosage Forms - Canada
Injection:
Bonefos®: 60 mg/mL (5 mL)
Clasteon®; 30 mg/mL (10 mL)
Capsule:
Bonefos®, Clasteon®: 400 mg

clodronate disodium *see* clodronate *(Canada only) on page 236*

clofarabine (klo FARE a been)

Sound-Alike/Look-Alike Issues
clofarabine may be confused with cladribine, clevidipine
Synonyms CAFdA; clofarex; NSC606869
U.S./Canadian Brand Names Clolar® [US]
Therapeutic Category Antineoplastic Agent, Antimetabolite (Purine Antagonist)
Use Treatment of relapsed or refractory acute lymphoblastic leukemia (ALL)
Dosage Summary
I.V.:
Children <1 years: Dosage not established
Children >1 year: 52 mg/m^2/day days 1 through 5; repeat every 2-6 weeks
Adults ≤21 years: 52 mg/m^2/day days 1 through 5; repeat every 2-6 weeks
Adults >21 years: Dosage not established
Dosage Forms
Injection, solution [preservative free]:
Clolar®: 1 mg/mL (20 mL)

clofarex *see* clofarabine *on page 236*
Clolar® [US] *see* clofarabine *on page 236*
Clomid® [US/Can] *see* clomiphene *on page 236*

clomiphene (KLOE mi feen)

Sound-Alike/Look-Alike Issues
clomiPHENE may be confused with clomiPRAMINE, clonidine
Clomid® may be confused with clonidine
Serophene® may be confused with Sarafem®
Synonyms clomiphene citrate
Tall-Man clomi**PHENE**
U.S./Canadian Brand Names Clomid® [US/Can]; Milophene® [Can]; Serophene® [US/Can]

Therapeutic Category Ovulation Stimulator

Use Treatment of ovulatory failure in patients desiring pregnancy

Dosage Summary

Oral:

Children: Dosage not established

Adults (females): First course: 50 mg/day for 5 days; Second course (if needed): 100 mg/day for 5 days; **Note:** If ovulation does not occur after 3 courses, or if 3 ovulatory responses occur but pregnancy is not achieved, further treatment is not recommended.

Dosage Forms

Tablet, oral: 50 mg

Clomid®: 50 mg

Serophene®: 50 mg

clomiphene citrate *see* clomiphene *on page* 236

clomipramine (kloe MI pra meen)

Sound-Alike/Look-Alike Issues

clomiPRAMINE may be confused with chlorproMAZINE, clevidipine, clomiPHENE, desipramine, Norpramin®

Anafranil® may be confused with alfentanil, enalapril, nafarelin

Synonyms clomipramine hydrochloride

Tall-Man clomi**PRAMINE**

U.S./Canadian Brand Names Anafranil® [US/Can]; Apo-Clomipramine® [Can]; CO Clomipramine [Can]; Gen-Clomipramine [Can]

Therapeutic Category Antidepressant, Tricyclic (Tertiary Amine)

Use Treatment of obsessive-compulsive disorder (OCD)

Dosage Summary

Oral:

Children <10 years: Dosage not established

Children ≥10 years: Initial: 25 mg/day; Maintenance: Up to 3 mg/kg/day (maximum: 200 mg/day); **Note:** Titration is recommended

Adults: Initial: 25 mg/day; Maintenance: Up to 250 mg/day; **Note:** Titration is recommended

Dosage Forms

Capsule, oral: 25 mg, 50 mg, 75 mg

Anafranil®: 25 mg, 50 mg, 75 mg

clomipramine hydrochloride *see* clomipramine *on page* 237

Clonapam [Can] *see* clonazepam *on page* 237

clonazepam (kloe NA ze pam)

Sound-Alike/Look-Alike Issues

clonazePAM may be confused with clofazimine, cloNIDine, clorazepate, clozapine, LORazepam

Klonopin® may be confused with clofazimine, clonNIDine, clorazepate, clozapine, LORazepam

Tall-Man clonaze**PAM**

U.S./Canadian Brand Names Alti-Clonazepam [Can]; Apo-Clonazepam® [Can]; Clonapam [Can]; CO Clonazepam [Can]; Gen-Clonazepam [Can]; Klonopin® [US/Can]; Mylan-Clonazepam [Can]; Novo-Clonazepam [Can]; Nu-Clonazepam [Can]; PMS-Clonazepam [Can]; PRO-Clonazepam [Can]; Rho®-Clonazepam [Can]; Rivotril® [Can]; Sandoz-Clonazepam [Can]; ZYM-Clonazepam [Can]

Therapeutic Category Benzodiazepine

Controlled Substance C-IV

Use Alone or as an adjunct in the treatment of petit mal variant (Lennox-Gastaut), akinetic, and myoclonic seizures; petit mal (absence) seizures unresponsive to succimides; panic disorder with or without agoraphobia

Dosage Summary

Oral:

Children <10 years or <30 kg: Initial: 0.01-0.03 mg/kg/day in 2-3 divided doses (maximum: 0.05 mg/kg/day); Maintenance: 0.1-0.2 mg/kg/day in 3 divided doses (maximum: 0.2 mg/kg/day); **Note:** Titration is recommended

Children ≥10 years or ≥30 kg:
Panic disorders: Initial: 0.25 mg twice daily; Maintenance: 1-4 mg/day in 2 divided doses; **Note:** Titration is recommended
Seizure disorders: Initial: Up to 1.5 mg/day in 3 divided doses; Maintenance: 0.05-2 mg/kg/day (maximum: 20 mg/day); **Note:** Titration is recommended
Adults:
Panic disorders: Initial: 0.25 mg twice daily; Maintenance: 1-4 mg/day in 2 divided doses; **Note:** Titration is recommended
Seizure disorders: Initial: Up to 1.5 mg/day in 3 divided doses; Maintenance: 0.05-2 mg/kg/day (maximum: 20 mg/day); **Note:** Titration is recommended

Dosage Forms
Tablet, oral: 0.5 mg, 1 mg, 2 mg
Klonopin®: 0.5 mg, 1 mg, 2 mg
Tablet, orally disintegrating, oral: 0.125 mg, 0.25 mg, 0.5 mg, 1 mg, 2 mg

clonidine (KLON i deen)

Sound-Alike/Look-Alike Issues
cloNIDine may be confused with Clomid®, clomiPHENE, clonazePAM, clozapine, Klonopin®, quiNIDine
Catapres® may be confused with Cataflam®, Cetapred®, Combipres®
Synonyms clonidine hydrochloride
Tall-Man clo**NID**ine
U.S./Canadian Brand Names Apo-Clonidine® [Can]; Carapres® [Can]; Catapres-TTS®-1 [US]; Catapres-TTS®-2 [US]; Catapres-TTS®-3 [US]; Catapres® [US]; Dixarit® [Can]; DOM-Clonidine [Can]; Duraclon® [US]; Novo-Clonidine [Can]; Nu-Clonidine [Can]
Therapeutic Category Alpha-Adrenergic Agonist
Use Management of mild-to-moderate hypertension; either used alone or in combination with other antihypertensives
Orphan drug: Duraclon®: For continuous epidural administration as adjunctive therapy with intraspinal opioids for treatment of cancer pain in patients tolerant to or unresponsive to intraspinal opioids

Dosage Summary
Epidural:
Children: Initial: 0.5 mcg/kg/**hour**; adjust with caution, based on clinical effect
Adults: Initial: 30 mcg/hour, titrate as required (maximum: 40 mcg/hour)
Oral:
Children: Children ≥12 years: Initial: 0.2 mg/day in 2 divided doses; increase gradually at 5- to 7-day intervals (maximum: 2.4 mg/day) **or** 0.15 mg/m^2 or 4 mcg/kg as single dose (tolerance test)
Adults: Initial: 0.1 mg twice daily; Maintenance: 0.1-0.8 mg/day in 2 divided doses (maximum: 2.4 mg/day) **or** 0.1-0.2 mg, followed by 0.1 mg every hour (up to 0.6 mg) if needed (HTN urgency)
Elderly: Initial: 0.1 mg once daily at bedtime, increase gradually as needed
Transdermal:
Children: Dosage not established
Adults: Initial: 0.1 mg once weekly; Maintenance: 0.1-0.3 mg once weekly (maximum: 0.6 mg); **Note:** Titration is recommended

Dosage Forms
Injection, solution [preservative free]: 100 mcg/mL (10 mL); 500 mcg/mL (10 mL)
Duraclon®: 100 mcg/mL (10 mL); 500 mcg/mL (10 mL)
Patch, transdermal: 0.1 mg/24 hours (4s); 0.2 mg/24 hours (4s); 0.3 mg/24 hours (4s)
Catapres-TTS®-1: 0.1 mg/24 hours (4s)
Catapres-TTS®-2: 0.2 mg/24 hours (4s)
Catapres-TTS®-3: 0.3 mg/24 hours (4s)
Tablet, oral: 0.1 mg, 0.2 mg, 0.3 mg
Catapres®: 0.1 mg, 0.2 mg, 0.3 mg

clonidine and chlorthalidone (KLON i deen & klor THAL i done)

Sound-Alike/Look-Alike Issues
Combipres® may be confused with Catapres®
Synonyms chlorthalidone and clonidine
U.S./Canadian Brand Names Clorpres® [US]
Therapeutic Category Antihypertensive Agent, Combination
Use Management of mild-to-moderate hypertension

Dosage Summary

Oral:

Children: Dosage not established

Adults: 1 tablet 1-2 times/day (maximum: clonidine 0.6 mg; chlorthalidone 30 mg)

Dosage Forms

Tablet:

Clorpres®: 0.1: Clonidine 0.1 mg and chlorthalidone 15 mg; 0.2: Clonidine 0.2 mg and chlorthalidone 15 mg; 0.3: Clonidine 0.3 mg and chlorthalidone 15 mg

clonidine hydrochloride *see* clonidine *on page 238*

clopidogrel (kloh PID oh grel)

Sound-Alike/Look-Alike Issues

Plavix® may be confused with Elavil®, Paxil®

Synonyms clopidogrel bisulfate

U.S./Canadian Brand Names Plavix® [US/Can]

Therapeutic Category Antiplatelet Agent

Use Reduces rate of atherothrombotic events (myocardial infarction, stroke, vascular deaths) in patients with recent MI or stroke, or established peripheral arterial disease; reduces rate of atherothrombotic events in patients with unstable angina (UA) or non-ST-segment elevation MI (NSTEMI) managed medically or with percutaneous coronary intervention (PCI) (with or without stent) or CABG; reduces rate of death and atherothrombotic events in patients with ST-segment elevation MI (STEMI) managed medically

Dosage Summary

Oral:

Children: Dosage not established

Adults: Loading dose: 300 mg (maximum: 600 mg); Maintenance: 75 mg once daily

Dosage Forms

Tablet, oral:

Plavix®: 75 mg, 300 mg

clopidogrel bisulfate *see* clopidogrel *on page 239*

Clopixol® [Can] *see* zuclopenthixol *(Canada only) on page 1006*

Clopixol-Acuphase® [Can] *see* zuclopenthixol *(Canada only) on page 1006*

Clopixol® Depot [Can] *see* zuclopenthixol *(Canada only) on page 1006*

clorazepate (klor AZ e pate)

Sound-Alike/Look-Alike Issues

clorazepate may be confused with clofibrate, clonazepam

Synonyms clorazepate dipotassium

U.S./Canadian Brand Names Apo-Clorazepate® [Can]; Novo-Clopate [Can]; Tranxene® T-Tab® [US]

Therapeutic Category Anticonvulsant; Benzodiazepine

Controlled Substance C-IV

Use Treatment of generalized anxiety disorder; management of ethanol withdrawal; adjunct anticonvulsant in management of partial seizures

Dosage Summary

Oral:

Children <9 years: Dosage not established

Children 9-12 years: Initial: 3.75-7.5 mg twice daily; Maintenance: Up to 60 mg/day in 2-3 divided doses; **Note:** Titration is recommended

Children >12 years: Initial: Up to 7.5 mg 2-3 times/day; Maintenance: Up to 90 mg/day; **Note:** Titration is recommended

Adults:

Anxiety: 7.5-15 mg 2-4 times/day

Ethanol withdrawal: Initial: 30 mg, then 15 mg 2-4 times/day on first day (maximum: 90 mg/day); Maintenance: Gradually decrease dose over subsequent days

Seizures: Initial: Up to 7.5 mg 2-3 times/day; Maintenance: Up to 90 mg/day; **Note:** Titration is recommended

Elderly: Use not recommended; Anxiety: 7.5 mg 1-2 times/day

Dosage Forms

Tablet, oral: 3.75 mg, 7.5 mg, 15 mg

Tranxene® T-Tab®: 3.75 mg, 7.5 mg, 15 mg

clorazepate dipotassium *see* clorazepate *on page 239*

Clorpactin® WCS-90 [US-OTC] *see* oxychlorosene *on page 714*

Clorpres® [US] *see* clonidine and chlorthalidone *on page 238*

Clotrimaderm [Can] *see* clotrimazole (topical) *on page 240*

clotrimazole (oral) (kloe TRIM a zole)

Sound-Alike/Look-Alike Issues

clotrimazole may be confused with co-trimoxazole

Mycelex® may be confused with Myoflex®

Synonyms Mycelex

U.S./Canadian Brand Names Mycelex® [US]

Therapeutic Category Antifungal Agent, Oral Nonabsorbed

Use Treatment of susceptible fungal infections, including oropharyngeal candidiasis; limited data suggest that clotrimazole troches may be effective for prophylaxis against oropharyngeal candidiasis in neutropenic patients

Dosage Summary

Oral:

Children ≤3 years: Dosage not established

Children >3 years: Prophylaxis: 10 mg 3 times/day; Treatment: 10 mg 5 times/day

Adults: Prophylaxis: 10 mg 3 times/day; Treatment: 10 mg 5 times/day

Dosage Forms

Troche, oral: 10 mg

clotrimazole (topical) (kloe TRIM a zole)

Sound-Alike/Look-Alike Issues

clotrimazole may be confused with co-trimoxazole

Lotrimin® may be confused with Lotrisone®, Otrivin®

U.S./Canadian Brand Names Anti-Fungal™ [US-OTC]; Canesten® Topical [Can]; Canesten® Vaginal [Can]; Clotrimaderm [Can]; Cruex® [US-OTC]; Gyne-Lotrimin® 3 [US-OTC]; Gyne-Lotrimin® 7 [US-OTC]; Lotrimin® AF Athlete's Foot [US-OTC]; Lotrimin® AF for Her [US-OTC]; Lotrimin® AF Jock Itch [US-OTC]; Trivagizole-3® [Can]

Therapeutic Category Antifungal Agent, Topical; Antifungal Agent, Vaginal

Use Treatment of susceptible fungal infections, including dermatophytoses, superficial mycoses, and cutaneous candidiasis, as well as vulvovaginal candidiasis

Dosage Summary

Intravaginal:

Children ≤12 years: Dosage not established

Children >12 years: Cream: Insert 1 applicatorful once daily; Tablet: Insert 100 mg/day **or** 500 mg as a single dose

Adults: Cream: Insert 1 applicatorful once daily; Tablet: Insert 100 mg/day **or** 500 mg as a single dose

Topical:

Children ≤3 years: Dosage not established

Children >3 years: Apply twice daily

Adults: Apply twice daily

Dosage Forms

Cream, topical: 1% (15 g, 30 g, 45 g)

Anti-Fungal™ [OTC]: 1% (113 g)

Cruex® [OTC]: 1% (15 g)

Lotrimin® AF Athlete's Foot [OTC]: 1% (12 g)

Lotrimin® AF for Her [OTC]: 1% (24 g)

Lotrimin® AF Jock Itch [OTC]: 1% (12 g)

Cream, vaginal: 1% (45 g); 2% (21 g)

Gyne-Lotrimin® 7 [OTC]: 1% (45 g)

Gyne-Lotrimin® 3 [OTC]: 2% (21 g)

Solution, topical: 1% (10 mL, 30 mL)

clotrimazole and betamethasone *see* betamethasone and clotrimazole *on page 134*

Cloxacillin [Can] *see* cloxacillin *(Canada only) on page 241*

cloxacillin *(Canada only)* (kloks a SIL in)

Synonyms cloxacillin sodium

U.S./Canadian Brand Names Apo-Cloxi® [Can]; Cloxacillin [Can]; Novo-Cloxin [Can]; Nu-Cloxi [Can]

Therapeutic Category Penicillin

Use Treatment of susceptible bacterial infections, including beta-hemolytic streptococci, pneumococci, and penicillinase-producing staphylococci causing respiratory tract, skin and skin structure, bone and joint, urinary tract infections

Dosage Summary

I.M.:

Children ≤20 kg: 25-50 mg/kg/day in divided doses every 6 hours; exceptions occur [indication specific]

Children >20 kg: 250-500 mg every 6 hours; exceptions occur [indication specific]

Adults: 250-500 mg every 6 hours (manufacturer recommended maximum dose: 6 g/day); exceptions occur [indication specific]

I.V.:

Children ≤20 kg: 25-50 mg/kg/day in divided doses every 6 hours; exceptions occur [indication specific]

Children >20 kg: 250-500 mg every 6 hours; exceptions occur [indication specific]

Adults: 250-500 mg every 6 hours (manufacturer recommended maximum dose: 6 g/day); exceptions occur [indication specific]

Oral:

Children ≤20 kg: 25-50 mg/kg/day in divided doses every 6 hours

Children >20 kg: 250-500 mg every 6 hours

Adults: 250-500 mg every 6 hours (manufacturer recommended maximum dose: 6 g/day); exceptions occur [indication specific]

Dosage Forms - Canada

Capsule: 250 mg, 500 mg

Injection, powder for reconstitution: 250 mg, 500 mg, 1000 mg, 2000 mg

Powder for suspension, oral: 125 mg/5 mL

cloxacillin sodium *see* cloxacillin *(Canada only) on page 241*

Cloxapen® ***(Discontinued)*** *see* cloxacillin *(Canada only) on page 241*

clozapine (KLOE za peen)

Sound-Alike/Look-Alike Issues

clozapine may be confused with clofazimine, clonidine, Klonopin®

Clozaril® may be confused with Clinoril®, Colazal®

U.S./Canadian Brand Names Apo-Clozapine® [Can]; Clozaril® [US/Can]; FazaClo® [US]; Gen-Clozapine [Can]; PMS-Clozapine [Can]

Therapeutic Category Antipsychotic Agent, Dibenzodiazepine

Use Treatment-refractory schizophrenia; to reduce risk of recurrent suicidal behavior in schizophrenia or schizoaffective disorder

Dosage Summary

Oral:

Adults: Initial: 12.5 mg once or twice daily; Maintenance: 12.5-900 mg/day (maximum: 900 mg/day); **Note:** Titration is recommended

Elderly: Initial: 12.5-25 mg/day, increase by 25 mg/day as tolerated; **Note:** Titrate cautiously as daily increases may not be tolerated

Dosage Forms

Tablet, oral: 25 mg, 50 mg, 100 mg, 200 mg

Clozaril®: 25 mg, 100 mg

Tablet, orally disintegrating, oral:

FazaClo®: 12.5 mg, 25 mg, 100 mg

Clozaril® [US/Can] *see* clozapine *on page 241*

Clysodrast® ***(Discontinued)*** *see* bisacodyl *on page 138*

CMA-676 *see* gemtuzumab ozogamicin *on page 441*

CMV-IGIV *see* cytomegalovirus immune globulin (intravenous-human) *on page 264*

CNJ-016® [US] *see* vaccinia immune globulin (intravenous) *on page 973*

CNTO-148 *see* golimumab *on page 451*

CNTO 1275 *see* ustekinumab *on page 972*
CoActifed® [Can] *see* triprolidine, pseudoephedrine, and codeine *(Canada only) on page 961*
coagulant complex inhibitor *see* antiinhibitor coagulant complex *on page 83*
coagulation factor I *see* fibrinogen concentrate (human) *on page 401*
coagulation factor VIIa *see* factor VIIa (recombinant) *on page 388*
CO Alendronate [Can] *see* alendronate *on page 47*

coal tar (KOLE tar)

Synonyms crude coal tar; LCD; pix carbonis

U.S./Canadian Brand Names Balnetar® [US-OTC/Can]; Betatar® Gel [US-OTC]; Cutar® [US-OTC]; Denorex® Therapeutic Protection 2-in-1 Shampoo + Conditioner [US-OTC]; Denorex® Therapeutic Protection [US-OTC]; DHS® Tar [US-OTC]; DHS™ Tar Gel [US-OTC]; Doak® Tar Distillate [US]; Doak® Tar Oil [US-OTC]; Doak® Tar [US-OTC]; Estar® [Can]; Exorex® Penetrating Emulsion #2 [US-OTC]; Exorex® Penetrating Emulsion [US-OTC]; ionil-T® Plus [US-OTC]; ionil-T® [US-OTC]; MG217® Medicated Tar Extra Strength [US-OTC]; MG217® Medicated Tar Intensive Strength [US-OTC]; MG217® Medicated Tar [US-OTC]; Neutrogena® T/Gel® Extra Strength [US-OTC]; Neutrogena® T/Gel® Stubborn Itch Control [US-OTC]; Neutrogena® T/Gel® [US-OTC]; Oxipor® VHC [US-OTC]; Pentrax® [US-OTC]; Scytera™ [US-OTC]; Targel® [Can]; Tera-Gel™ [US-OTC]; Thera-Gel [US-OTC]; Zetar® [US-OTC]

Therapeutic Category Antipsoriatic Agent; Antiseborrheic Agent, Topical

Use Topically for controlling dandruff, seborrheic dermatitis, or psoriasis

Dosage Summary

Topical:

Children: Dosage not established

Adults:

Bath: Add 60-90 mL (5-20%) or 15-25 mL (30%) to bath water, soak 5-20 minutes, use once daily to every 3 days

Scalp: Apply to lesions 3-12 hours before each shampoo

Shampoo: Rub into wet hair, rinse, repeat leaving on 5 minutes; apply twice weekly for 2 weeks then once weekly

Skin: Apply to affected areas 1-4 times/day, decrease to 2-3 times/week once condition controlled

Soap: Use on affected areas instead of regular soap

Dosage Forms

Aerosol, topical:

Scytera™ [OTC]: Coal tar solution 10% (100 g)

Emulsion, topical:

Cutar® [OTC]: Coal tar solution 7.5% (180 mL, 3840 mL)
Exorex® Penetrating Emulsion [OTC]: Coal tar 1% (100 mL, 250 mL)
Exorex® Penetrating Emulsion #2 [OTC]: Coal tar 2% (100 mL, 250 mL)

Gel, topical:

DHS™ Tar Gel [OTC]: Solubilized coal tar extract 2.9% (240 mL)
Thera-Gel [OTC]: 0.5% (255 mL)

Liquid, topical:

Doak® Tar Distillate: Coal tar 40% (59 mL)

Lotion, topical:

MG217® Medicated Tar [OTC]: Coal tar solution 5% (120 mL)
Oxipor® VHC [OTC]: Coal tar solution 25% (56 mL, 120 mL)

Oil, topical:

Balnetar® [OTC]: Coal tar 2.5% (221 mL)
Doak® Tar Oil [OTC]: Coal tar distillate 2% (237 mL)

Ointment, topical:

MG217® Medicated Tar Intensive Strength [OTC]: Coal tar solution 10% (107 g)

Shampoo, topical:

Betatar Gel® [OTC]: Coal tar solution 12.5% (480 mL)
Denorex® Therapeutic Protection [OTC]: Coal tar solution 12.5% (118 mL, 240 mL, 300 mL)
DHS® Tar [OTC]: Solubilized coal tar extract 2.9% (120 mL, 240 mL, 480 mL)
Doak® Tar [OTC]: Coal tar distillate 3% (237 mL)
ionil-T® [OTC]: Coal tar 1% (240 mL, 480 mL, 960 mL)
ionil-T® Plus [OTC]: Coal tar 2% (240 mL)
MG217® Medicated Tar Extra Strength [OTC]: Coal tar solution 15% (120 mL, 240 mL)

Neutrogena® T/Gel® [OTC]: Solubilized coal tar extract 2% (130 mL, 255 mL, 480 mL)
Neutrogena® T/Gel® Extra Strength [OTC]: Solubilized coal tar extract 4% (177 mL)
Neutrogena® T/Gel® Stubborn Itch Control [OTC]: Coal tar extract 2% (130 mL)
Pentrax® [OTC]: Coal tar 5% (236 mL)
Tera-Gel™ [OTC]: Solubilized coal tar extract 2% (120 mL, 255 mL)
Zetar® [OTC]: Coal tar 1% (177 mL)

Shampoo/Conditioner, topical:
Denorex® Therapeutic Protection 2-in-1 Shampoo + Conditioner [OTC]: Coal tar solution 12.5% (120 mL, 240 mL, 300 mL)

Solution, topical: 20% (473 mL)

coal tar and salicylic acid (KOLE tar & sal i SIL ik AS id)

Synonyms salicylic acid and coal tar

U.S./Canadian Brand Names Sebcur/T® [Can]; Tarsum® [US-OTC]; X-Seb T® Pearl [US-OTC]; X-Seb T® Plus [US-OTC]

Therapeutic Category Antipsoriatic Agent; Antiseborrheic Agent, Topical

Use Seborrheal dermatitis, dandruff, psoriasis

Dosage Summary

Topical:
Gel:
Children: Dosage not established
Adults: Apply to plaques, leave on up to 1 hour then rinse
Shampoo:
Children: Dosage not established
Adults: Apply to wet hair, massage into scalp then rinse

Dosage Forms

Gel [shampoo]: Coal tar solution 10% [equivalent to coal tar 2%] and salicylic acid (120 mL, 240 mL)
Tarsum® [OTC]: Coal tar solution 10% [equivalent to coal tar 2%] and salicylic acid (120 mL, 240 mL)

Shampoo, topical: Coal tar solution 10% [equivalent to coal tar 2%] and salicylic acid (120 mL, 240 mL)
X-Seb T® Pearl [OTC], X-Seb T® Plus [OTC]: Coal tar solution 10% [equivalent to coal tar 2%] and salicylic acid (120 mL, 240 mL)

CO Amlodipine [Can] *see* amlodipine *on page 68*
Coartem® [US] *see* artemether and lumefantrine *on page 95*
CO Atenolol [Can] *see* atenolol *on page 102*
CO Atorvastatin [Can] *see* atorvastatin *on page 104*
CO Azithromycin [Can] *see* azithromycin (systemic) *on page 111*
Cobex® *(Discontinued)* *see* cyanocobalamin *on page 257*
CO Bicalutamide [Can] *see* bicalutamide *on page 137*
CO Buspirone [Can] *see* buspirone *on page 157*
CO Cabergoline [Can] *see* cabergoline *on page 163*

cocaine (koe KANE)

Synonyms cocaine hydrochloride

Therapeutic Category Local Anesthetic

Controlled Substance C-II

Use Topical anesthesia for mucous membranes

Dosage Summary

Topical:
Children: Use reduced dosages
Adults: Do not exceed 1 mg/kg (1% to 10% concentration); **Note:** Dosage depends on the area to be anesthetized, tissue vascularity, technique of anesthesia, and individual patient tolerance
Elderly: Use reduced dosages

Dosage Forms

Powder, for prescription compounding: USP: 100% (1 g, 5 g, 25 g)
Solution, topical: 4% (4 mL, 10 mL); 10% (4 mL, 10 mL)

cocaine hydrochloride *see* cocaine *on page 243*
CO Cilazapril [Can] *see* cilazapril *(Canada only) on page 222*
CO Ciprofloxacin [Can] *see* ciprofloxacin (systemic) *on page 224*

CO Citalopram [Can] *see* citalopram *on page 227*
CO Clomipramine [Can] *see* clomipramine *on page 237*
CO Clonazepam [Can] *see* clonazepam *on page 237*
Codal-DM [US-OTC] *see* phenylephrine, pyrilamine, and dextromethorphan *on page 755*
Codamine® *(Discontinued)*
Codamine® Pediatric *(Discontinued)*
Codehist® DH *(Discontinued)* *see* chlorpheniramine, pseudoephedrine, and codeine *on page 214*

codeine (KOE deen)

Sound-Alike/Look-Alike Issues
codeine may be confused with Cardene®, Cophene®, Cordran®, iodine, Lodine®

Synonyms codeine phosphate; codeine sulfate; methylmorphine

U.S./Canadian Brand Names Codeine Contin® [Can]

Therapeutic Category Analgesic, Narcotic; Antitussive

Controlled Substance C-II

Use Treatment of mild-to-moderate pain; antitussive in lower doses

Dosage Summary

I.M.:

Children: 0.5-1 mg/kg every 4-6 hours as needed (maximum: 60 mg/dose; 1.5 mg/kg/dose)

Adults: Initial: 30 mg every 4-6 hours; Usual range: 15-120 mg every 4-6 hours as needed (maximum: 1.5 mg/kg/dose)

Oral:

Children:

Analgesic: 0.5-1 mg/kg every 4-6 hours as needed (maximum: 60 mg/dose; 1.5 mg/kg/dose)

Antitussive: 1-1.5 mg/kg/day divided every 4-6 hours as needed (maximum: 30 mg/day [2-6 years]; 60 mg/day [6-12 years])

Adults:

Analgesic: Initial: 30 mg every 4-6 hours as needed; Usual range: 15-120 mg every 4-6 hours as needed (maximum: 1.5 mg/kg/dose)

Antitussive: 10-20 mg every 4-6 hours as needed (maximum: 120 mg/day)

SubQ:

Children: 0.5-1 mg/kg every 4-6 hours as needed (maximum: 60 mg/dose; 1.5 mg/kg/dose)

Adults: Initial: 30 mg every 4-6 hours; Usual range: 15-120 mg every 4-6 hours as needed (maximum: 1.5 mg/kg/dose)

Dosage Forms

Powder, for prescription compounding: USP: 100% (10 g, 25 g)

Tablet, oral: 15 mg, 30 mg, 60 mg

Dosage Forms - Canada

Tablet, controlled release:

Codeine Contin®: 50 mg, 100 mg, 150 mg, 200 mg

codeine, acetaminophen, butalbital, and caffeine *see* butalbital, acetaminophen, caffeine, and codeine *on page 159*
codeine and acetaminophen *see* acetaminophen and codeine *on page 23*
codeine and butalbital compound *see* butalbital, aspirin, caffeine, and codeine *on page 160*
codeine and guaifenesin *see* guaifenesin and codeine *on page 455*
codeine and promethazine *see* promethazine and codeine *on page 801*
codeine and pseudoephedrine *see* pseudoephedrine and codeine *on page 811*
codeine, aspirin, and carisoprodol *see* carisoprodol, aspirin, and codeine *on page 185*
codeine, butalbital, aspirin, and caffeine *see* butalbital, aspirin, caffeine, and codeine *on page 160*
codeine, chlorpheniramine, and pseudoephedrine *see* chlorpheniramine, pseudoephedrine, and codeine *on page 214*
Codeine Contin® [Can] *see* codeine *on page 244*
codeine, doxylamine, and acetaminophen *see* acetaminophen, codeine, and doxylamine *(Canada only) on page 28*
codeine, guaifenesin, and pseudoephedrine *see* guaifenesin, pseudoephedrine, and codeine *on page 459*

codeine, phenylephrine, and promethazine *see* promethazine, phenylephrine, and codeine *on page 802*
codeine phosphate *see* codeine *on page 244*
codeine phosphate and pseudoephedrine hydrochloride *see* pseudoephedrine and codeine *on page 811*
codeine, pseudoephedrine, and triprolidine *see* triprolidine, pseudoephedrine, and codeine *(Canada only) on page 961*
codeine sulfate *see* codeine *on page 244*
codeine, triprolidine, and pseudoephedrine *see* triprolidine, pseudoephedrine, and codeine *(Canada only) on page 961*
Codiclear® DH *(Discontinued)*
codimal® DM *(Discontinued)* *see* phenylephrine, pyrilamine, and dextromethorphan *on page 755*
cod liver oil *see* vitamin A and vitamin D *on page 988*
CO Enalapril [Can] *see* enalapril *on page 348*
CO-Etidrocal [Can] *see* etidronate and calcium carbonate *(Canada only) on page 383*
Co-Etidronate [Can] *see* etidronate *on page 383*
CO Famciclovir [Can] *see* famciclovir *on page 390*
CO Fluconazole [Can] *see* fluconazole *on page 407*
CO Fluoxetine [Can] *see* fluoxetine *on page 415*
CO Gabapentin [Can] *see* gabapentin *on page 433*
Cogentin® [US] *see* benztropine *on page 130*
Co-Gesic® *(Discontinued)* *see* hydrocodone and acetaminophen *on page 479*
CO Glimepiride [Can] *see* glimepiride *on page 446*
Cognex® *(Discontinued)*
CO Ipra-Sal [Can] *see* ipratropium and albuterol *on page 524*
Colace® [US-OTC/Can] *see* docusate *on page 321*
Colace® Glycerin Suppositories*(Discontinued)* *see* glycerin *on page 449*
Colax-C® [Can] *see* docusate *on page 321*
Colazal® [US] *see* balsalazide *on page 116*
ColBenemid® *(Discontinued)* *see* colchicine and probenecid *on page 245*

colchicine (KOL chi seen)

Sound-Alike/Look-Alike Issues
colchicine may be confused with Cortrosyn®

U.S./Canadian Brand Names Colcrys® [US]

Therapeutic Category Antigout Agent

Use Prevention and treatment of acute gout flares; treatment of familial Mediterranean fever (FMF)

Dosage Summary

Oral:

Children <4 years: Dosage not established.
Children 4-6 years: 0.3-1.8 mg/day in 1-2 divided doses
Children 6-12 years: 0.9-1.8 mg/day in 1-2 divided doses
Children 12-16 years: 1.2-2.4 mg/day in 1-2 divided doses
Children >16 years: FMF: 1.2-2.4 mg/day in 1-2 divided doses; Gout prophylaxis: 0.6 mg once or twice daily; Gout treatment: Initial: 1.2 mg; repeat with 0.6 mg in 1 hour (maximum total therapy: 1.8 mg)
Adults: FMF: 1.2-2.4 mg/day in 1-2 divided doses; Gout prophylaxis: 0.6 mg once or twice daily; Gout treatment: Initial: 1.2 mg; repeat with 0.6 mg in 1 hour (maximum total therapy: 1.8 mg)

Dosage Forms

Tablet, oral: 0.6 mg
Colcrys®: 0.6 mg

colchicine and probenecid (KOL chi seen & proe BEN e sid)

Synonyms probenecid and colchicine

Therapeutic Category Antigout Agent

Use Treatment of chronic gouty arthritis when complicated by frequent, recurrent acute attacks of gout

Dosage Summary

Oral:

Children: Dosage not established

Adults: Initial: 1 tablet daily for 1 week; Maintenance: 1 tablet twice daily

Dosage Forms

Tablet: Colchicine 0.5 mg and probenecid 0.5 g

Colcrys® [US] *see* colchicine *on page 245*

Coldamine [US] *see* chlorpheniramine, pseudoephedrine, and methscopolamine *on page 215*

Cold Control PE [US-OTC] *see* acetaminophen, diphenhydramine, and phenylephrine *on page 30*

Coldcough [US] *see* pseudoephedrine, dihydrocodeine, and chlorpheniramine *on page 813*

Coldcough HC *(Discontinued)*

Coldcough PD [US] *see* dihydrocodeine, chlorpheniramine, and phenylephrine *on page 304*

Coldlac-LA® *(Discontinued)*

Coldloc® *(Discontinued)*

Coldmist DM *(Discontinued)* *see* guaifenesin, pseudoephedrine, and dextromethorphan *on page 460*

Coldtuss DR *(Discontinued)* *see* chlorpheniramine, phenylephrine, and dextromethorphan *on page 211*

colesevelam (koh le SEV a lam)

U.S./Canadian Brand Names Welchol® [US/Can]

Therapeutic Category Antihyperlipidemic Agent, Miscellaneous; Bile Acid Sequestrant

Use Management of elevated LDL in primary hypercholesterolemia (Fredrickson type IIa) when used alone or in combination with an HMG-CoA reductase inhibitor; management of heterozygous familial hypercholesterolemia (heFH) in adolescent patients (males and postmenarchal females 10-17 years of age) when used alone or in combination with an HMG-CoA reductase inhibitor, in patients who after an adequate trial of dietary therapy have LDL-C ≥190 mg/dL or LDL-C ≥160 mg/dL with positive family history of premature cardiovascular disease (CVD) or with two or more CVD risk factors; improve glycemic control in type 2 diabetes mellitus (noninsulin-dependent, NIDDM) in conjunction with diet, exercise, and insulin or oral antidiabetic agents

Dosage Summary

Oral:

Children <10 years: Dosage not established

Children 10-17 years (males and postmenarchal females): 3.75 g/day in 1-2 divided doses

Adults: 3.75 g/day in 1-2 divided doses

Dosage Forms

Granules for suspension, oral:

Welchol®: 3.75 g/packet (30s)

Tablet, oral:

Welchol®: 625 mg

Colestid® [US/Can] *see* colestipol *on page 246*

Colestid® Flavored [US] *see* colestipol *on page 246*

colestipol (koe LES ti pole)

Sound-Alike/Look-Alike Issues

colestipol may be confused with calcitriol

Synonyms colestipol hydrochloride

U.S./Canadian Brand Names Colestid® Flavored [US]; Colestid® [US/Can]

Therapeutic Category Antihyperlipidemic Agent, Miscellaneous

Use Adjunct in management of primary hypercholesterolemia; regression of arteriolosclerosis; relief of pruritus associated with elevated levels of bile acids; possibly used to decrease plasma half-life of digoxin in toxicity

Dosage Summary

Oral:

Children: Dosage not established

Adults:

Granules: Initial: 5 g 1-2 times/day; Maintenance: 5-30 g/day in 1-4 divided doses; **Note:** Titration is recommended

Tablets: Initial: 2 g 1-2 times/day; Maintenance: 2-16 g/day; **Note:** Titration is recommended

Dosage Forms

Granules for suspension, oral: 5 g/scoop (500 g); 5 g/packet (30s, 90s)

Colestid®: 5 g/teaspoon (300 g, 500 g); 5 g/packet (30s, 90s)

Colestid® Flavored: 5 g/scoop (450 g); 5 g/packet (60s)

Tablet, oral: 1 g

Colestid®: 1 g

colestipol hydrochloride *see* colestipol *on page 246*

CO Levetiracetam [Can] *see* levetiracetam *on page 555*

CO Lisinopril [Can] *see* lisinopril *on page 570*

colistimethate (koe lis ti METH ate)

Synonyms colistimethate sodium; colistin methanesulfonate; colistin sulfomethate; pentasodium colistin methanesulfonate

U.S./Canadian Brand Names Coly-Mycin® M [US/Can]

Therapeutic Category Antibiotic, Miscellaneous

Use Treatment of infections due to sensitive strains of certain gram-negative bacilli which are resistant to other antibacterials or in patients allergic to other antibacterials

Dosage Summary

I.M.:

Children: 2.5-5 mg/kg/day in 2-4 divided doses

Adults: 2.5-5 mg/kg/day in 2-4 divided doses

I.V.:

Children: 2.5-5 mg/kg/day in 2-4 divided doses

Adults: 2.5-5 mg/kg/day in 2-4 divided doses

Inhalation, nebulization (unlabeled):

Children: 50-75 mg in NS (3-4 mL total) 2-3 times/day

Adults: 50-75 mg in NS (3-4 mL total) 2-3 times/day

Dosage Forms

Injection, powder for reconstitution: 150 mg

Coly-Mycin® M: 150 mg

colistimethate sodium *see* colistimethate *on page 247*

colistin, hydrocortisone, neomycin, and thonzonium *see* neomycin, colistin, hydrocortisone, and thonzonium *on page 666*

colistin methanesulfonate *see* colistimethate *on page 247*

colistin sulfomethate *see* colistimethate *on page 247*

collagen *see* collagen hemostat *on page 248*

collagen absorbable hemostat *see* collagen hemostat *on page 248*

collagenase (systemic) (KOL la je nase)

Sound-Alike/Look-Alike Issues

collagenase clostridium histolyticum (Xiaflex™) may be confused with topical collagenase formulation (ie, Santyl™)

Xiaflex™ may be confused with Zanaflex®

Synonyms collagenase clostridium histolyticum

U.S./Canadian Brand Names Xiaflex™ [US]

Therapeutic Category Enzyme

Use Treatment of Dupuytren contracture with a palpable cord

Dosage Summary

Intralesional:

Children: Dosage not established

Adults: 0.58 mg per cord

Dosage Forms

Injection, powder for reconstitution:

Xiaflex™: 0.9 mg

collagenase (topical) (KOL la je nase)

Sound-Alike/Look-Alike Issues

Topical collagenase formulation (Santyl®) may be confused with the injectable collagenase clostridium histolyticum (Xiaflex™)

U.S./Canadian Brand Names Santyl® [US]
Therapeutic Category Enzyme
Use Promotes debridement of necrotic tissue in dermal ulcers and severe burns
Dosage Summary
Topical:
Children: Apply once daily
Adults: Apply once daily
Dosage Forms
Ointment, topical:
Santyl®: 250 units/g (15 g, 30 g)

collagenase clostridium histolyticum *see* collagenase (systemic) *on page* 247

collagen hemostat (KOL la jen HEE moe stat)

Sound-Alike/Look-Alike Issues
Avitene® may be confused with Ativan®
Synonyms collagen; collagen absorbable hemostat; MCH; microfibrillar collagen hemostat
U.S./Canadian Brand Names Avitene® Flour [US]; Avitene® Ultrafoam™ [US]; Avitene® [US]; EndoAvitene® [US]; Helistat® [US]; Helitene® [US]; Instat™ MCH [US]; Instat™ [US]; SyringeAvitene™ [US]
Therapeutic Category Hemostatic Agent
Use Adjunct to hemostasis when control of bleeding by ligature is ineffective or impractical
Dosage Summary
Topical:
Children: Dosage not established
Adults: Apply dry directly to source of bleeding; remove excess material after ~10-15 minutes
Dosage Forms
Powder, topical:
Avitene® Flour: (0.5 g, 1 g, 5 g)
Helitene®: (0.5 g, 1 g)
Instat™ MCH: (0.5 g, 1 g)
SyringeAvitene™: (1 g)
Sheet, topical:
Avitene®: (1s, 6s)
EndoAvitene®: (6s)
Sponge:
Avitene® Ultrafoam™: (6s)
Sponge, topical:
Helistat®: (10s, 18s)

Colocort® [US] *see* hydrocortisone (topical) *on page* 483
CO Lovastatin [Can] *see* lovastatin *on page* 579
Coly-Mycin® M [US/Can] *see* colistimethate *on page* 247
Coly-Mycin® S [US] *see* neomycin, colistin, hydrocortisone, and thonzonium *on page* 666
Colyte® [US/Can] *see* polyethylene glycol-electrolyte solution *on page* 775
Combantrin™ [Can] *see* pyrantel pamoate *on page* 816
ComBgen™ *(Discontinued)* *see* folic acid, cyanocobalamin, and pyridoxine *on page* 423
Combigan® [US/Can] *see* brimonidine and timolol *on page* 145
CombiPatch® [US] *see* estradiol and norethindrone *on page* 368
Combipres® *(Discontinued)* *see* clonidine and chlorthalidone *on page* 238
ComBi Rx™ *(Discontinued)* *see* vitamins (multiple/prenatal) *on page* 991
Combivent® [US] *see* ipratropium and albuterol *on page* 524
Combivent UDV [Can] *see* ipratropium and albuterol *on page* 524
Combivir® [US/Can] *see* zidovudine and lamivudine *on page* 1000
Combunox™ *(Discontinued)* *see* oxycodone and ibuprofen *on page* 716
CO Meloxicam [Can] *see* meloxicam *on page* 598
CO Memantine [Can] *see* memantine *on page* 599
CO Metformin [Can] *see* metformin *on page* 609

Comfort® Ophthalmic ***(Discontinued)*** *see* naphazoline (ophthalmic) *on page 658*
Comfort® Tears Solution ***(Discontinued)*** *see* artificial tears *on page 97*
Comhist® ***(Discontinued)*** *see* chlorpheniramine, phenylephrine, and phenyltoloxamine *on page 213*
CO Mirtazapine [Can] *see* mirtazapine *on page 637*
Commit® [US-OTC] *see* nicotine *on page 674*
Compazine® ***(Discontinued)*** *see* prochlorperazine *on page 797*
Compound 347™ [US] *see* enflurane *on page 349*
compound E *see* cortisone acetate *on page 252*
compound F *see* hydrocortisone (systemic) *on page 482*
compound F *see* hydrocortisone (topical) *on page 483*
compound S *see* zidovudine *on page 999*
compound S, abacavir, and lamivudine *see* abacavir, lamivudine, and zidovudine *on page 18*
Compound W® [US-OTC] *see* salicylic acid *on page 858*
Compound W® One Step Invisible Strip [US-OTC] *see* salicylic acid *on page 858*
Compound W® One Step Wart Remover [US-OTC] *see* salicylic acid *on page 858*
Compound W® One Step Wart Remover for Feet [US-OTC] *see* salicylic acid *on page 858*
Compound W® One Step Wart Remover for Kids [US-OTC] *see* salicylic acid *on page 858*
Compoz® [US-OTC] *see* diphenhydramine (systemic) *on page 310*
Compro® [US] *see* prochlorperazine *on page 797*
Comtan® [US/Can] *see* entacapone *on page 350*
Comtrex® Maximum Strength, Non-Drowsy Cold & Cough Relief [US-OTC] *see* acetaminophen, dextromethorphan, and phenylephrine *on page 29*
Comtrex® Maximum Strength Sinus and Nasal Decongestant ***(Discontinued)*** *see* acetaminophen, chlorpheniramine, and pseudoephedrine *on page 28*
Comtrex® Non-Drowsy Cold and Cough Relief ***(Discontinued)***
Comvax® [US] *see Haemophilus* B conjugate and hepatitis B vaccine *on page 463*
Conal ***(Discontinued)*** *see* chlorpheniramine, pyrilamine, and phenylephrine *on page 215*
Conceptrol® [US-OTC] *see* nonoxynol 9 *on page 681*
Concerta® [US/Can] *see* methylphenidate *on page 621*
Condyline™ [Can] *see* podofilox *on page 773*
Condylox® [US] *see* podofilox *on page 773*
Conex® ***(Discontinued)***
Congess® Jr ***(Discontinued)*** *see* guaifenesin and pseudoephedrine *on page 457*
Congess® Sr ***(Discontinued)*** *see* guaifenesin and pseudoephedrine *on page 457*
Congestac® [US-OTC] *see* guaifenesin and pseudoephedrine *on page 457*

conivaptan (koe NYE vap tan)

Synonyms conivaptan hydrochloride; YM087

U.S./Canadian Brand Names Vaprisol® [US]

Therapeutic Category Vasopressin Antagonist

Use Treatment of euvolemic and hypervolemic hyponatremia in hospitalized patients

Dosage Summary

I.V.:

Children: Dosage not established

Adults: Loading dose: 20 mg bolus, followed by 20 mg as continuous infusion over 24 hours; Maintenance: 20-40 mg/day as a continuous infusion over 24 hours (maximum therapy: 4 days)

Dosage Forms

Infusion, premixed in D_5W:

Vaprisol®: 20 mg (100 mL)

conivaptan hydrochloride *see* conivaptan *on page 249*
conjugated estrogen *see* estrogens (conjugated/equine, systemic) *on page 370*
conjugated estrogen *see* estrogens (conjugated/equine, topical) *on page 371*
conjugated estrogen and methyltestosterone *see* estrogens (esterified) and methyltestosterone *on page 372*
CO Norfloxacin [Can] *see* norfloxacin *on page 684*

Conray® [US] *see* iothalamate meglumine *on page* 521
Conray® 30 [US] *see* iothalamate meglumine *on page* 521
Conray® 43 [US] *see* iothalamate meglumine *on page* 521
Conray® 400 ***(Discontinued)***
Constulose [US] *see* lactulose *on page* 544
Contac® Cold 12 Hour Relief Non Drowsy [Can] *see* pseudoephedrine *on page* 810
Contac® Cold 12 Hour Relief Non Drowsy ***(Discontinued)*** *see* pseudoephedrine *on page* 810
Contac® Cold and Sore Throat, Non Drowsy, Extra Strength [Can] *see* acetaminophen and pseudoephedrine *on page* 26
Contac® Cold-Chest Congestion, Non Drowsy, Regular Strength [Can] *see* guaifenesin and pseudoephedrine *on page* 457
Contac® Cold ***(Discontinued)*** *see* pseudoephedrine *on page* 810
Contac® Cold + Flu Maximum Strength Non-Drowsy [US-OTC] *see* acetaminophen and phenylephrine *on page* 25
Contac® Cough Formula Liquid ***(Discontinued)*** *see* guaifenesin and dextromethorphan *on page* 455
continuous renal replacement therapy *see* electrolyte solution, renal replacement *on page* 345
ControlRx® [US] *see* fluoride *on page* 413
Contuss® ***(Discontinued)***
Contuss® XT ***(Discontinued)***
CO Olanzapine [Can] *see* olanzapine *on page* 696
CO Olanzapine ODT [Can] *see* olanzapine *on page* 696
CO Ondansetron [Can] *see* ondansetron *on page* 704
CO Pantoprazole [Can] *see* pantoprazole *on page* 725
CO Paroxetine [Can] *see* paroxetine *on page* 729
Copaxone® [US/Can] *see* glatiramer acetate *on page* 445
COPD [US] *see* dyphylline and guaifenesin *on page* 339
Copegus® [US] *see* ribavirin *on page* 839
Cophene-B® ***(Discontinued)*** *see* brompheniramine *on page* 147
Cophene XP® ***(Discontinued)***
CO Pioglitazone [Can] *see* pioglitazone *on page* 762
copolymer-1 *see* glatiramer acetate *on page* 445

copper (KOP er)

Synonyms cupric chloride; cupric chloride dihydrate

Therapeutic Category Trace Element, Parenteral

Use Supplement to intravenous solutions given for total parenteral nutrition (TPN) to maintain copper serum levels and to prevent depletion of endogenous stores and subsequent deficiency symptoms

Dosage Summary

I.V. (as a parenteral nutrition component):
Infants: 20 mcg/kg/day
Children: 20 mcg/kg/day
Adults: 0.3-1.5 mg/day

Dosage Forms

Injection, solution [preservative free]: 0.4 mg/mL (10 mL)

copper *see* trace metals *on page* 945
CO Pramipexole [Can] *see* pramipexole *on page* 786
CO Pravastatin [Can] *see* pravastatin *on page* 789
Co-Pyronil® 2 Pulvules® ***(Discontinued)*** *see* chlorpheniramine and pseudoephedrine *on page* 209
CO Quetiapine [Can] *see* quetiapine *on page* 821
CO Ramipril [Can] *see* ramipril *on page* 826
CO Ranitidine [Can] *see* ranitidine *on page* 828
Cordarone® [US/Can] *see* amiodarone *on page* 67
Cordran® [US/Can] *see* flurandrenolide *on page* 417
Cordran® SP [US] *see* flurandrenolide *on page* 417

Cordron-D NR ***(Discontinued)***

Cordron-DM NR ***(Discontinued)***

Cordron-HC ***(Discontinued)***

Cordron-HC NR ***(Discontinued)***

Coreg® [US/Can] *see* carvedilol *on page 186*

Coreg CR® [US] *see* carvedilol *on page 186*

Corfen DM [US] *see* chlorpheniramine, phenylephrine, and dextromethorphan *on page 211*

Corgard® [US/Can] *see* nadolol *on page 654*

Coricidin HBP® Chest Congestion and Cough [US-OTC] *see* guaifenesin and dextromethorphan *on page 455*

Coricidin HBP® Cold and Flu [US-OTC] *see* chlorpheniramine and acetaminophen *on page 208*

Coricidin® HBP Cough & Cold [US-OTC] *see* dextromethorphan and chlorpheniramine *on page 288*

CO Risperidone [Can] *see* risperidone *on page 845*

Corlopam® [US/Can] *see* fenoldopam *on page 394*

Cormax® [US] *see* clobetasol *on page 235*

CO Ropinirole [Can] *see* ropinirole *on page 851*

Correctol® [US-OTC] *see* docusate *on page 321*

Correctol® Tablets [US-OTC] *see* bisacodyl *on page 138*

Cortaid® Intensive Therapy [US-OTC] *see* hydrocortisone (topical) *on page 483*

Cortaid® Maximum Strength [US-OTC] *see* hydrocortisone (topical) *on page 483*

Cortamed® [Can] *see* hydrocortisone (topical) *on page 483*

Cortatrigen® Otic ***(Discontinued)*** *see* neomycin, polymyxin B, and hydrocortisone *on page 667*

Cortef® [US/Can] *see* hydrocortisone (systemic) *on page 482*

Cortenema® [US/Can] *see* hydrocortisone (topical) *on page 483*

CortiCool® [US-OTC] *see* hydrocortisone (topical) *on page 483*

corticorelin (kor ti koe REL in)

Sound-Alike/Look-Alike Issues

corticorelin may be confused with corticotropin

Acthrel® may be confused with Acthar®

Synonyms corticorelin ovine triflutate; human corticotrophin-releasing hormone, analogue; ovine corticotrophin-releasing hormone

U.S./Canadian Brand Names Acthrel® [US]

Therapeutic Category Diagnostic Agent, ACTH-Dependent Hypercortisolism

Use Diagnostic test used in adrenocorticotropic hormone (ACTH)-dependent Cushing syndrome to differentiate between pituitary and ectopic production of ACTH

Dosage Summary

I.V.:

Children: Dosage not established

Adults: 1 mcg/kg; dosages >100 mcg have been associated with an increase in adverse effects

Dosage Forms

Injection, powder for reconstitution:

Acthrel®: 100 mcg

corticorelin ovine triflutate *see* corticorelin *on page 251*

corticotropin (kor ti koe TROE pin)

Sound-Alike/Look-Alike Issues

corticotropin may be confused with corticorelin

Synonyms ACTH; adrenocorticotropic hormone; corticotropin, repository

U.S./Canadian Brand Names H.P. Acthar® [US]

Therapeutic Category Adrenal Corticosteroid

Use Acute exacerbations of multiple sclerosis; diagnostic aid in adrenocortical insufficiency, severe muscle weakness in myasthenia gravis

Cosyntropin is preferred over corticotropin for diagnostic test of adrenocortical insufficiency (cosyntropin is less allergenic and test is shorter in duration)

Dosage Summary

I.M.:

Children:

Antiinflammatory/immunosuppressant: 0.8 units/kg/day or 25 units/m^2/day divided every 12-24 hours

Infantile spasms: Initial: 20 units/day for 2 weeks, if no response increase to 30 units/day for 4 weeks; Usual range: 5-160 units/day

Adults: 80-120 units/day for 2-3 weeks **or** 40-80 units every 24-72 hours

SubQ:

Children: Dosage not established

Adults: 40-80 units every 24-72 hours

Dosage Forms

Injection, gelatin:

H.P. Acthar®: 80 units/mL (5 mL)

corticotropin, repository *see* corticotropin *on page 251*

Cortifoam® [US/Can] *see* hydrocortisone (topical) *on page 483*

Cortimyxin® [Can] *see* neomycin, polymyxin B, and hydrocortisone *on page 667*

cortisol *see* hydrocortisone (systemic) *on page 482*

cortisol *see* hydrocortisone (topical) *on page 483*

cortisone acetate (KOR ti sone AS e tate)

Sound-Alike/Look-Alike Issues

cortisone may be confused with Cardizem®, Cortizone®

Synonyms compound E

Therapeutic Category Adrenal Corticosteroid

Use Management of adrenocortical insufficiency

Dosage Summary

Oral:

Children: 0.5-10 mg/kg/day **or** 20-300 mg/m^2/day divided every 6-8 hours

Adults: 25-300 mg /day divided every 12-24 hours

Dosage Forms

Tablet, oral: 25 mg

Cortisporin® Cream [US] *see* neomycin, polymyxin B, and hydrocortisone *on page 667*

Cortisporin® Ointment [US] *see* bacitracin, neomycin, polymyxin B, and hydrocortisone *on page 114*

Cortisporin® Ophthalmic *(Discontinued)* *see* neomycin, polymyxin B, and hydrocortisone *on page 667*

Cortisporin® Otic [US/Can] *see* neomycin, polymyxin B, and hydrocortisone *on page 667*

Cortisporin®-TC [US] *see* neomycin, colistin, hydrocortisone, and thonzonium *on page 666*

Cortisporin® Topical Cream *(Discontinued)* *see* neomycin, polymyxin B, and hydrocortisone *on page 667*

Cortisporin® Topical Ointment [Can] *see* bacitracin, neomycin, polymyxin B, and hydrocortisone *on page 114*

Cortizone-10® Maximum Strength [US-OTC] *see* hydrocortisone (topical) *on page 483*

Cortizone-10® Maximum Strength Cooling Relief [US-OTC] *see* hydrocortisone (topical) *on page 483*

Cortizone-10® Maximum Strength Easy Relief [US-OTC] *see* hydrocortisone (topical) *on page 483*

Cortizone-10® Maximum Strength Intensive Healing Formula [US-OTC] *see* hydrocortisone (topical) *on page 483*

Cortizone-10® Plus Maximum Strength [US-OTC] *see* hydrocortisone (topical) *on page 483*

Cortizone-10® Quick Shot *(Discontinued)* *see* hydrocortisone (topical) *on page 483*

Cortone® *(Discontinued)*

Cortrosyn® [US/Can] *see* cosyntropin *on page 253*

Corvert® [US] *see* ibutilide *on page 496*

Corzide® [US] *see* nadolol and bendroflumethiazide *on page 654*

CO Sertraline [Can] *see* sertraline *on page 872*

CO Simvastatin [Can] *see* simvastatin *on page* 877
Cosmegen® [US/Can] *see* dactinomycin *on page* 266
Cosopt® [US/Can] *see* dorzolamide and timolol *on page* 327
CO Sotalol [Can] *see* sotalol *on page* 892
CO Sumatriptan [Can] *see* sumatriptan *on page* 904

cosyntropin (koe sin TROE pin)

Sound-Alike/Look-Alike Issues
Cortrosyn® may be confused with colchicine, Cotazym®

Synonyms synacthen; tetracosactide

U.S./Canadian Brand Names Cortrosyn® [US/Can]

Therapeutic Category Diagnostic Agent

Use Diagnostic test to differentiate primary adrenal from secondary (pituitary) adrenocortical insufficiency

Dosage Summary

I.M.:
Children <2 years: 0.125 mg
Children ≥2 years: 0.25-0.75 mg
Adults: 0.25-0.75 mg

I.V.:
Children <2 years: 0.125 mg
Children ≥2 years: 0.25-0.75 mg; **Note:** An infusion of 0.04 mg/hour over 6 hours (0.25 mg total) may be used when greater cortisol stimulation needed
Adults: 0.25-0.75 mg; **Note:** An infusion of 0.04 mg/hour over 6 hours (0.25 mg total) may be used when greater cortisol stimulation needed

Dosage Forms

Injection, powder for reconstitution: 0.25 mg
Cortrosyn®: 0.25 mg
Injection, solution [preservative free]: 0.25 mg/mL (1 mL)

Cotazym® [Can] *see* pancrelipase *on page* 723
Cotazym® *(Discontinued)* *see* pancrelipase *on page* 723
Cotazym-S® *(Discontinued)* *see* pancrelipase *on page* 723
CO Temazepam [Can] *see* temazepam *on page* 914
CO Terbinafine [Can] *see* terbinafine (systemic) *on page* 917
CO Topiramate [Can] *see* topiramate *on page* 942
co-trimoxazole *see* sulfamethoxazole and trimethoprim *on page* 901
Coughcold HCM *(Discontinued)*
Coughtuss [US] *see* phenylephrine, hydrocodone, and chlorpheniramine *on page* 754
Coumadin® [US/Can] *see* warfarin *on page* 993
CoVan® [Can] *see* triprolidine, pseudoephedrine, and codeine *(Canada only) on page* 961
Covaryx® [US] *see* estrogens (esterified) and methyltestosterone *on page* 372
Covaryx® H.S. [US] *see* estrogens (esterified) and methyltestosterone *on page* 372
CO Venlafaxine XR [Can] *see* venlafaxine *on page* 981
Covera® [Can] *see* verapamil *on page* 981
Covera-HS® [US/Can] *see* verapamil *on page* 981
Coversyl® [Can] *see* perindopril erbumine *on page* 744
Coversyl® Plus [Can] *see* perindopril erbumine and indapamide *(Canada only) on page* 744
co-vidarabine *see* pentostatin *on page* 742
coviracil *see* emtricitabine *on page* 347
Cozaar® [US/Can] *see* losartan *on page* 577
CO Zopiclone [Can] *see* zopiclone *(Canada only) on page* 1005
CP358774 *see* erlotinib *on page* 360
CPC *see* cetylpyridinium *on page* 199
C-Phen [US] *see* chlorpheniramine and phenylephrine *on page* 208
C-Phen DM [US] *see* chlorpheniramine, phenylephrine, and dextromethorphan *on page* 211
CPM *see* cyclophosphamide *on page* 259

CPM-12 *(Discontinued)* *see* chlorpheniramine *on page 207*
CPT-11 *see* irinotecan *on page 525*
CPZ *see* chlorpromazine *on page 216*
Cramp Tabs [US-OTC] *see* acetaminophen and pamabrom *on page 25*
Crantex HC *(Discontinued)*
Crantex LA [US] *see* guaifenesin and phenylephrine *on page 456*
Creomulsion® Adult Formula [US-OTC] *see* dextromethorphan *on page 287*
Creomulsion® for Children [US-OTC] *see* dextromethorphan *on page 287*
Creon® [US/Can] *see* pancrelipase *on page 723*
Creo-Terpin® [US-OTC] *see* dextromethorphan *on page 287*
Crestor® [US/Can] *see* rosuvastatin *on page 853*
Cresylate® [US] *see* m-cresyl acetate *on page 592*
Crinone® [US/Can] *see* progesterone *on page 799*
Critic-Aid® Clear AF [US-OTC] *see* miconazole (topical) *on page 630*
Critic-Aid Skin Care® [US-OTC] *see* zinc oxide *on page 1001*
Criticare HN® [US-OTC] *see* nutritional formula, enteral/oral *on page 692*
Crixivan® [US/Can] *see* indinavir *on page 505*
CroFab® [US] *see* crotalidae polyvalent immune FAB (ovine) *on page 255*
Crolom® [US] *see* cromolyn (ophthalmic) *on page 255*
cromoglycic acid *see* cromolyn (nasal) *on page 255*
cromoglycic acid *see* cromolyn (ophthalmic) *on page 255*
cromoglycic acid *see* cromolyn (systemic, oral inhalation) *on page 254*

cromolyn (systemic, oral inhalation) (KROE moe lin)

Sound-Alike/Look-Alike Issues

Intal® may be confused with Endal®

Synonyms cromoglycic acid; cromolyn sodium; disodium cromoglycate; DSCG

U.S./Canadian Brand Names Gastrocrom® [US]; Intal® [Can]; Nalcrom® [Can]; Nu-Cromolyn [Can]; PMS-Sodium Cromoglycate [Can]

Therapeutic Category Mast Cell Stabilizer

Use

Inhalation: May be used as an adjunct in the prophylaxis of allergic disorders, including asthma; prevention of exercise-induced bronchospasm

Oral: Systemic mastocytosis

Dosage Summary

Inhalation:

Metered spray:

Children <5 years: Dosage not established

Children 5-12 years: Initial: 2 inhalations 4 times/day; Maintenance: 1-2 inhalations 3-4 times/day **or** 2 inhalations prior to exercise or allergen exposure

Children >12 years: Initial: 2 inhalations 4 times/day; Maintenance: 2-4 inhalations 3-4 times/day **or** 2 inhalations prior to exercise or allergen exposure

Adults: Initial: 2 inhalations 4 times/day; Maintenance: 2-4 inhalations 3-4 times/day **or** 2 inhalations prior to exercise or allergen exposure

Nebulization:

Children <2 years: Dosage not established

Children ≥2 years: Initial: 20 mg 4 times/day; Maintenance: 20 mg 3-4 times/day **or** 20 mg prior to exercise or allergen exposure

Adults: Initial: 20 mg 4 times/day; Maintenance: 20 mg 3-4 times/day **or** 20 mg prior to exercise or allergen exposure

Oral:

Children <2 years: Dosage not established

Children 2-12 years: 100 mg 4 times/day (maximum: 40 mg/kg/day)

Children >12 years: 200 mg 4 times/day (maximum: 40 mg/kg/day)

Adults: 200 mg 4 times/day (maximum: 40 mg/kg/day)

Dosage Forms

Solution, for nebulization: 20 mg/2 mL (60s, 120s)

Solution, oral:

Gastrocrom®: 100 mg/5 mL (96s)

cromolyn (nasal) (KROE moe lin)

Sound-Alike/Look-Alike Issues

NasalCrom® may be confused with Nasacort®, Nasalide®

Synonyms cromoglycic acid; cromolyn sodium; disodium cromoglycate; DSCG

U.S./Canadian Brand Names NasalCrom® [US-OTC]; Rhinaris-CS Anti-Allergic Nasal Mist [Can]

Therapeutic Category Mast Cell Stabilizer

Use Prevention and treatment of seasonal and perennial allergic rhinitis

Dosage Summary

Intranasal:

Children <2 years: Dosage not established

Children ≥2 years: Instill 1 spray in each nostril 3-4 times/day

Adults: Instill 1 spray in each nostril 3-4 times/day

Dosage Forms

Solution, intranasal: 40 mg/mL (13 mL, 26 mL)

NasalCrom® [OTC]: 40 mg/mL (13 mL, 26 mL)

cromolyn (ophthalmic) (KROE moe lin)

Synonyms cromoglycic acid; cromolyn sodium; disodium cromoglycate; DSCG

U.S./Canadian Brand Names Crolom® [US]; Opticrom® [Can]

Therapeutic Category Mast Cell Stabilizer

Use Treatment of vernal keratoconjunctivitis, vernal conjunctivitis, and vernal keratitis

Dosage Summary

Ophthalmic:

Children: Dosage not established

Adults: 1-2 drops in each eye 4-6 times/day

Dosage Forms

Solution, ophthalmic: 4% (10 mL)

Crolom®: 4% (10 mL)

cromolyn sodium *see* cromolyn (nasal) *on page 255*

cromolyn sodium *see* cromolyn (ophthalmic) *on page 255*

cromolyn sodium *see* cromolyn (systemic, oral inhalation) *on page 254*

Crosseal™ [US] *see* fibrin sealant *on page 401*

crotalidae polyvalent immune FAB (ovine)

(kroe TAL ih die pol i VAY lent i MYUN fab (oh vine))

Synonyms antivenin (crotalidae) polyvalent, FAB (ovine); crotaline antivenin, polyvalent, FAB (ovine); FabAV, FAB (ovine); North American antisnake-bite serum, FAB (ovine); snake antivenin, FAB (ovine)

U.S./Canadian Brand Names CroFab® [US]

Therapeutic Category Antivenin

Use Neutralization of venoms of North American crotalids: Rattlesnakes (*Crotalus*, *Sistrurus*); copperhead and cottonmouth moccasins (*Agkistrodon*)

Dosage Summary

I.V.:

Children: Initial dose: 4-6 vials, may repeat with 4-6 vials; Maintenance dose: Administer 2 vials every 6 hours for up to 18 hours

Adults: Initial dose: 4-6 vials, may repeat with 4-6 vials; Maintenance dose: Administer 2 vials every 6 hours for up to 18 hours

Dosage Forms

Injection, powder for reconstitution:

CroFab®: Derived from *Crotalus adamanteus, C. atrox, C. scutulatus*, and *Agkistrodon piscivorus* snake venoms

crotaline antivenin, polyvalent, FAB (ovine) *see* crotalidae polyvalent immune FAB (ovine) *on page 255*

crotamiton (kroe TAM i tonn)

Sound-Alike/Look-Alike Issues

Eurax® may be confused with Efudex®, Eulexin®, Evoxac™, Serax®, Urex®

U.S./Canadian Brand Names Eurax® [US]

Therapeutic Category Scabicides/Pediculicides

Use Treatment of scabies (*Sarcoptes scabiei*) and symptomatic treatment of pruritus

Dosage Summary

Topical:

Children:

Pruritus: Massage into affected areas, repeat as needed

Scabies: Apply a thin layer from the neck to the toes, repeat in 24 hours; take a cleansing bath 48 hours after final application, may repeat after 7-10 days

Adults:

Pruritus: Massage into affected areas, repeat as needed

Scabies: Apply a thin layer from the neck to the toes, repeat in 24 hours; take a cleansing bath 48 hours after final application, may repeat after 7-10 days

Dosage Forms

Cream, topical:

Eurax®: 10% (60 g)

Lotion, topical:

Eurax®: 10% (60 mL, 480 mL)

CRRT *see* electrolyte solution, renal replacement *on page* 345

crude coal tar *see* coal tar *on page* 242

Cruex® [US-OTC] *see* clotrimazole (topical) *on page* 240

Cryselle® 28 [US] *see* ethinyl estradiol and norgestrel *on page* 380

crystalline penicillin *see* penicillin G (parenteral/aqueous) *on page* 738

Crystamine® *(Discontinued)* *see* cyanocobalamin *on page* 257

Crystapen® [Can] *see* penicillin G (parenteral/aqueous) *on page* 738

Crysti 1000® *(Discontinued)* *see* cyanocobalamin *on page* 257

CS-747 *see* prasugrel *on page* 788

CsA *see* cyclosporine (ophthalmic) *on page* 260

CsA *see* cyclosporine (systemic) *on page* 260

C-Tan D [US] *see* brompheniramine and phenylephrine *on page* 148

C-Tan D Plus [US] *see* brompheniramine and phenylephrine *on page* 148

C-Tanna 12 [US] *see* carbetapentane and chlorpheniramine *on page* 179

C-Tanna 12D [US] *see* carbetapentane, phenylephrine, and pyrilamine *on page* 181

C-Time [US-OTC] *see* ascorbic acid *on page* 98

CTLA-4Ig *see* abatacept *on page* 19

CTM *see* chlorpheniramine *on page* 207

CTP 30 [Can] *see* citalopram *on page* 227

CTX *see* cyclophosphamide *on page* 259

Cubicin® [US/Can] *see* daptomycin *on page* 269

Culturelle® [US-OTC] *see* Lactobacillus *on page* 543

cupric chloride *see* copper *on page* 250

cupric chloride dihydrate *see* copper *on page* 250

Cuprimine® [US/Can] *see* penicillamine *on page* 737

Curad® Mediplast® [US-OTC] *see* salicylic acid *on page* 858

Curasore® [US-OTC] *see* pramoxine *on page* 787

Curosurf® [US/Can] *see* poractant alfa *on page* 778

Cutar® [US-OTC] *see* coal tar *on page* 242

Cutivate® [US/Can] *see* fluticasone (topical) *on page* 420

Cuvposa™ *see* glycopyrrolate *on page* 450

CVT-3146 *see* regadenoson *on page* 833

CyA *see* cyclosporine (ophthalmic) *on page* 260

CyA *see* cyclosporine (systemic) *on page* 260

cyanide antidote kit *see* sodium nitrite, sodium thiosulfate, and amyl nitrite *on page 885*
Cyanide Antidote Package [US] *see* sodium nitrite, sodium thiosulfate, and amyl nitrite *on page 885*

cyanocobalamin (sye an oh koe BAL a min)

Synonyms vitamin B_{12}

U.S./Canadian Brand Names CaloMist™ [US]; Ener-B® [US-OTC]; Nascobal® [US]; Twelve Resin-K [US-OTC]

Therapeutic Category Vitamin, Water Soluble

Use Treatment of pernicious anemia; vitamin B_{12} deficiency due to dietary deficiencies or malabsorption diseases, inadequate secretion of intrinsic factor, and inadequate utilization of B_{12} (eg, during neoplastic treatment); increased B_{12} requirements due to pregnancy, thyrotoxicosis, hemorrhage, malignancy, liver or kidney disease

CaloMist™: Maintenance of vitamin B_{12} concentrations after initial correction in patients with B_{12} deficiency without CNS involvement

Dosage Summary

I.M.:

Children:

B_{12} deficiency (dosage not well established): 0.2 mcg/kg for 2 days, followed by 1000 mcg/day for 2-7 days, followed by 100 mcg/week for one month, then 100 mcg monthly **or** 100 mcg/day for 10-15 days, then once or twice weekly for several months

Pernicious anemia: Initial: 30-50 mcg/day for 2 or more weeks (total dose: 1000-5000 mcg); Maintenance: 100 mcg/month

Adults:

B_{12} deficiency: Initial: 30 mcg/day for 5-10 days; Maintenance: 100-200 mcg/month

Pernicious anemia: Initial: 100 mcg/day for 6-7 days; if improvement, administer same dose on alternate days for 7 doses, then every 3-4 days for 2-3 weeks; Maintenance: 100-1000 mcg/month **or** 1000 mcg/day for 5 days, followed by 500-1000 mcg/month

Intranasal:

Children: Dosage not established

Adults: Nascobal®: 500 mcg in one nostril once weekly; CaloMist™: Maintenance therapy (following correction of vitamin B_{12} deficiency): 50-100 mcg/day

Oral:

Children: B_{12} deficiency: Dosage not established

Adults:

B_{12} deficiency: 250 mcg/day

Pernicious anemia: 1000-2000 mcg/day

SubQ:

Children:

B_{12} deficiency (dosage not well established): 0.2 mcg/kg for 2 days, followed by 1000 mcg/day for 2-7 days, followed by 100 mcg/week for one month, then 100 mcg monthly **or** 100 mcg/day for 10-15 days, then once or twice weekly for several months

Pernicious anemia: Initial: 30-50 mcg/day for 2 or more weeks (total dose: 1000-5000 mcg); Maintenance: 100 mcg/month

Adults:

B_{12} deficiency: Initial: 30 mcg/day for 5-10 days; Maintenance: 100-200 mcg/month

Pernicious anemia: Initial: 100 mcg/day for 6-7 days; if improvement, administer same dose on alternate days for 7 doses, then every 3-4 days for 2-3 weeks; Maintenance: 100-1000 mcg/month **or** 1000 mcg/day for 5 days, followed by 500-1000 mcg/month

Dosage Forms

Injection, solution: 1000 mcg/mL (1 mL, 10 mL, 30 mL)

Lozenge, oral: 50 mcg (100s); 100 mcg (100s); 250 mcg (100s, 250s); 500 mcg (100s, 250s)

Lozenge, sublingual: 500 mcg (100s)

Solution, intranasal:

CaloMist™: 25 mcg/spray (10.7 mL)

Nascobal®: 500 mcg/spray (2.3 mL)

Tablet, for buccal application/oral/sublingual:

Twelve Resin-K [OTC]: 1000 mcg

Tablet, oral: 50 mcg, 100 mcg, 250 mcg, 500 mcg, 1000 mcg

Ener-B® [OTC]: 100 mcg, 500 mcg, 1000 mcg

Tablet, sublingual: 1000 mcg, 2500 mcg, 5000 mcg

Tablet, timed release, oral: 1000 mcg

Ener-B® [OTC]: 1500 mcg

cyanocobalamin, folic acid, and pyridoxine *see* folic acid, cyanocobalamin, and pyridoxine *on page* 423

Cyanoject® *(Discontinued)* *see* cyanocobalamin *on page* 257

Cyclen® [Can] *see* ethinyl estradiol and norgestimate *on page* 380

Cyclessa® [US/Can] *see* ethinyl estradiol and desogestrel *on page* 374

cyclobenzaprine (sye kloe BEN za preen)

Sound-Alike/Look-Alike Issues

cyclobenzaprine may be confused with cycloSERINE, cyproheptadine

Flexeril® may be confused with Floxin®

Synonyms cyclobenzaprine hydrochloride

U.S./Canadian Brand Names Amrix® [US]; Apo-Cyclobenzaprine® [Can]; Dom-Cyclobenzaprine [Can]; Fexmid® [US]; Flexeril® [US/Can]; Flexitec [Can]; Gen-Cyclobenzaprine [Can]; Mylan-Cyclobenzaprine [Can]; Novo-Cycloprine [Can]; Nu-Cyclobenzaprine [Can]; PHL-Cyclobenzaprine [Can]; PMS-Cyclobenzaprine [Can]; ratio-Cyclobenzaprine [Can]; Riva-Cycloprine [Can]

Therapeutic Category Skeletal Muscle Relaxant

Use Treatment of muscle spasm associated with acute, painful musculoskeletal conditions

Dosage Summary

Oral capsule, extended release:

Children <18 years: Dosage not established

Adults: Usual: 15 mg once daily (maximum: 30 mg once daily; maximum duration: 3 weeks)

Elderly: Dosage not established

Oral tablet, immediate release:

Children <15 years: Dosage not established

Children ≥15 years: Initial: 5 mg 3 times/day; Maintenance: 5-10 mg 3 times/day (maximum duration: 3 weeks)

Adults: Initial: 5 mg 3 times/day; Maintenance: 5-10 mg 3 times/day (maximum duration: 3 weeks)

Elderly: Initial: 5 mg; titrate slowly and consider less frequent dosing

Dosage Forms

Capsule, extended release, oral:

Amrix®: 15 mg, 30 mg

Tablet, oral: 5 mg, 10 mg

Fexmid®: 7.5 mg

Flexeril®: 5 mg, 10 mg

cyclobenzaprine hydrochloride *see* cyclobenzaprine *on page* 258

Cyclocort® [Can] *see* amcinonide *on page* 62

Cyclocort® *(Discontinued)* *see* amcinonide *on page* 62

Cyclogyl® [US/Can] *see* cyclopentolate *on page* 258

Cyclomen® [Can] *see* danazol *on page* 267

Cyclomydril® [US] *see* cyclopentolate and phenylephrine *on page* 259

cyclopentolate (sye kloe PEN toe late)

Synonyms cyclopentolate hydrochloride

U.S./Canadian Brand Names AK-Pentolate™ [US]; Cyclogyl® [US/Can]; Cylate™ [US]; Diopentolate® [Can]

Therapeutic Category Anticholinergic Agent

Use Diagnostic procedures requiring mydriasis and cycloplegia

Dosage Summary

Ophthalmic:

Neonates: Cyclopentolate and phenylephrine combination formulation is the preferred agent

Children: Instill 1 drop of 0.5%, 1%, or 2% in eye followed by 1 drop of 0.5% or 1% in 5 minutes, if necessary

Adults: Instill 1 drop of 1% followed by another drop in 5 minutes; 2% solution in heavily pigmented iris

Dosage Forms

Solution, ophthalmic: 1% (2 mL, 5 mL, 15 mL)

AK-Pentolate™: 1% (2 mL, 15 mL)

Cyclogyl®: 0.5% (15 mL); 1% (2 mL, 5 mL, 15 mL); 2% (2 mL, 5 mL, 15 mL)

Cylate™: 1% (2 mL, 15 mL)

cyclopentolate and phenylephrine (sye kloe PEN toe late & fen il EF rin)

Synonyms phenylephrine and cyclopentolate

U.S./Canadian Brand Names Cyclomydril® [US]

Therapeutic Category Anticholinergic/Adrenergic Agonist

Use Induce mydriasis greater than that produced with cyclopentolate HCl alone

Dosage Summary

Ophthalmic:

Neonates: Instill 1 drop into eyes every 5-10 minutes, for up to 3 doses

Children: Instill 1 drop into eyes every 5-10 minutes, for up to 3 doses

Adults: Instill 1 drop into eyes every 5-10 minutes, for up to 3 doses

Dosage Forms

Solution, ophthalmic:

Cyclomydril®: Cyclopentolate 0.2% and phenylephrine 1% (2 mL, 5 mL)

cyclopentolate hydrochloride *see* cyclopentolate *on page* 258

cyclophosphamide (sye kloe FOS fa mide)

Sound-Alike/Look-Alike Issues

cyclophosphamide may be confused with cycloSPORINE, ifosfamide

Cytoxan® may be confused with cefoxitin, Centoxin®, Ciloxan®, cytarabine, CytoGam®, Cytosar®, Cytosar-U®, Cytotec®

Synonyms CPM; CTX; CYT; neosar

U.S./Canadian Brand Names Procytox® [Can]

Therapeutic Category Antineoplastic Agent

Use

Oncology-related uses: Treatment of Hodgkin lymphoma, non-Hodgkin lymphoma (including Burkitt lymphoma), chronic lymphocytic leukemia (CLL), chronic myelocytic leukemia (CML), acute myelocytic leukemia (AML), acute lymphocytic leukemia (ALL), mycosis fungoides, multiple myeloma, neuroblastoma, retinoblastoma; breast cancer; ovarian adenocarcinoma

Nononcology uses: Treatment of refractory nephrotic syndrome in children

Dosage Summary

Oral:

Children: 1-5 mg/kg/day

Adults: 1-5 mg/kg/day

Dosage Forms

Injection, powder for reconstitution: 500 mg, 1 g, 2 g

Tablet, oral: 25 mg, 50 mg

cycloserine (sye kloe SER een)

Sound-Alike/Look-Alike Issues

cycloSERINE may be confused with cyclobenzaprine, cycloSPORINE

Tall-Man cyclo**SERINE**

U.S./Canadian Brand Names Seromycin® [US]

Therapeutic Category Antibiotic, Miscellaneous

Use Adjunctive treatment in pulmonary or extrapulmonary tuberculosis

Dosage Summary

Oral:

Children: 10-20 mg/kg/day in 2 divided doses (maximum: 1000 mg/day)

Adults: Initial: 250 mg every 12 hours for 14 days; Maintenance: 500-1000 mg/day in 2 divided doses

Dosage Forms

Capsule, oral:

Seromycin®: 250 mg

cyclosporin A *see* cyclosporine (ophthalmic) *on page* 260

cyclosporin A *see* cyclosporine (systemic) *on page* 260

cyclosporine (systemic) (SYE kloe spor een)

Sound-Alike/Look-Alike Issues

cycloSPORINE may be confused with cyclophosphamide, Cyklokapron®, cycloSERINE

cycloSPORINE modified (Neoral®, Gengraf®) may be confused with cycloSPORINE nonmodified (Sandimmne®)

Gengraf® may be confused with Prograf®

Neoral® may be confused with Neurontin®, Nizoral®

Sandimmune® may be confused with Sandostatin®

Synonyms CsA; CyA; cyclosporin A

Tall-Man cyclo**SPORINE**

U.S./Canadian Brand Names Apo-Cyclosporine® [Can]; Gengraf® [US]; Neoral® [US/Can]; Rhoxal-cyclosporine [Can]; Sandimmune® I.V. [Can]; Sandimmune® [US]; Sandoz-Cyclosporine [Can]

Therapeutic Category Immunosuppressant Agent

Use Prophylaxis of organ rejection in kidney, liver, and heart transplants, has been used with azathioprine and/or corticosteroids; severe, active rheumatoid arthritis (RA) not responsive to methotrexate alone; severe, recalcitrant plaque psoriasis in nonimmunocompromised adults unresponsive to or unable to tolerate other systemic therapy

Dosage Summary Note: Modified (Neoral®/Genraf®) and non-modified (Sandimmune®) cyclosporine products are not bioequivalent and cannot be used interchangeably.

I.V. (non-modified):

Children: Initial dose: 5-6 mg/kg/day or one-third of the oral dose as a single dose; Maintenance: 3-7.5 mg/kg/day; **Note:** May divided into 2-3 doses for day or give as continuous infusion over 24 hours

Adults: Initial dose: 5-6 mg/kg/day or one-third of the oral dose as a single dose; Maintenance: 3-7.5 mg/kg/day; **Note:** May divided into 2-3 doses for day or give as continuous infusion over 24 hours

Oral:

Modified:

Children: Transplant: Heart: 7 ± 3 mg/kg/day in 2 divided doses; Liver: 8 ± 4 mg/kg/day in 2 divided doses; Renal: 9 ± 3 mg/kg/day in 2 divided doses

Adults:

Psoriasis: Initial: 2.5 mg/kg/day in 2 divided doses; Maintenance: May increase by 0.5 mg/kg/day after 4 weeks, if insufficient response; additional dosage increases may be made every 2 weeks if needed (maximum: 4 mg/kg/day; 1 year).

Rheumatoid arthritis: Initial: 2.5 mg/kg/day in 2 divided doses; Maintenance: May increase by 0.5-0.75 mg/kg/day after 8 weeks, if insufficient response; additional dosage increases may be made again at 12 weeks (maximum: 4 mg/kg/day)

Transplant: Heart: 7 ± 3 mg/kg/day in 2 divided doses; Liver: 8 ± 4 mg/kg/day in 2 divided doses; Renal: 9 ± 3 mg/kg/day in 2 divided doses

Non-modified:

Children: Initial: 10-14 mg/kg/day for 1-2 weeks; Maintenance: Taper by 5% per week to 3-10 mg/kg/day

Adults: Initial: 10-14 mg/kg/day for 1-2 weeks; Maintenance: Taper by 5% per week to 3-10 mg/kg/day

Dosage Forms

Capsule, oral: 25 mg, 100 mg

Gengraf®: 25 mg, 100 mg

Capsule, softgel, oral: 25 mg, 50 mg, 100 mg

Neoral®: 25 mg, 100 mg

Sandimmune®: 25 mg, 100 mg

Injection, solution: 50 mg/mL (5 mL)

Sandimmune®: 50 mg/mL (5 mL)

Injection, solution [preservative free]: 50 mg/mL (5 mL)

Solution, oral: 100 mg/mL (50 mL)

Gengraf®: 100 mg/mL (50 mL)

Neoral®: 100 mg/mL (50 mL)

Sandimmune®: 100 mg/mL (50 mL)

cyclosporine (ophthalmic) (SYE kloe spor een)

Sound-Alike/Look-Alike Issues

cycloSPORINE may be confused with cyclophosphamide, Cyklokapron®, cycloSERINE

Synonyms CsA; CyA; cyclosporin A

Tall-Man cyclo**SPORINE**

U.S./Canadian Brand Names Restasis® [US]

Therapeutic Category Immunosuppressant Agent

Use Increase tear production when suppressed tear production is presumed to be due to keratoconjunctivitis sicca-associated ocular inflammation (in patients not already using topical antiinflammatory drugs or punctal plugs)

Dosage Summary

Ophthalmic (Restasis®):

Children <16 years: Dosage not established

Children ≥16 years: Instill 1 drop in each eye every 12 hours

Adults: Instill 1 drop in each eye every 12 hours

Dosage Forms

Emulsion, ophthalmic [preservative free]:

Restasis®: 0.05% (0.4 mL)

Cycofed® Pediatric *(Discontinued)* *see* guaifenesin, pseudoephedrine, and codeine *on page* 459

Cyestra-35 [Can] *see* cyproterone and ethinyl estradiol *(Canada only) on page* 261

Cyklokapron® [US/Can] *see* tranexamic acid *on page* 947

Cylate™ [US] *see* cyclopentolate *on page* 258

Cylex® *(Discontinued)* *see* benzocaine *on page* 124

Cymbalta® [US/Can] *see* duloxetine *on page* 336

Cyomin® *(Discontinued)* *see* cyanocobalamin *on page* 257

cyproheptadine (si proe HEP ta deen)

Sound-Alike/Look-Alike Issues

cyproheptadine may be confused with cyclobenzaprine

Periactin may be confused with Perative®, Percodan®, Persantine®

Synonyms cyproheptadine hydrochloride

Therapeutic Category Antihistamine

Use Perennial and seasonal allergic rhinitis and other allergic symptoms including urticaria

Dosage Summary

Oral:

Children <12 years: 0.25 mg/kg/day or 8 mg/m^2/day in 2-3 divided doses **or** 2-4 mg 2-3 times/day

Children ≥12 years: 0.25 mg/kg/day or 8 mg/m^2/day in 2-3 divided doses **or** 2-8 mg 2-4 times/day **or** 4 mg at bedtime, increasing by 4 mg every 3-4 days up to 36 mg/day in divided doses (spasticity with spinal cord damage)

Adults: 4-32 mg/day in 3-4 divided doses **or** 4 mg at bedtime, increasing by 4 mg every 3-4 days up to 36 mg/day in divided doses (spasticity with spinal cord damage)

Elderly: Initial: 4 mg twice daily

Dosage Forms

Syrup, oral: 2 mg/5 mL (473 mL)

Tablet, oral: 4 mg

cyproheptadine hydrochloride *see* cyproheptadine *on page* 261

cyproterone acetate *see* cyproterone *(Canada only) on page* 262

cyproterone and ethinyl estradiol *(Canada only)*

(sye PROE ter one & ETH in il es tra DYE ole)

Synonyms ethinyl estradiol and cyproterone acetate

U.S./Canadian Brand Names Cyestra-35 [Can]; Diane-35® [Can]; Novo-Cyproterone/Ethinyl Estradiol [Can]

Therapeutic Category Acne Products; Estrogen and Androgen Combination

Use Treatment of females with severe acne, unresponsive to other therapies, with associated symptoms of androgenization (including mild hirsutism or seborrhea). **Should not be used solely for contraception;** however, will provide reliable contraception if taken as recommended for approved indications.

Dosage Summary

Oral:

Children: Not for use prior to menarche

Adults (female): One tablet daily for 21 days, followed by 7 days off

Dosage Forms - Canada

Tablet:

Diane-35: Cyproterone 2 mg and ethinyl estradiol 0.035 mg (21s)

cyproterone *(Canada only)* (sye PROE ter one)

Synonyms cyproterone acetate

U.S./Canadian Brand Names Androcur® Depot [Can]; Androcur® [Can]; Apo-Cyproterone® [Can]; Gen-Cyproterone [Can]; Mylan-Cyproterone [Can]; Novo-Cyproterone [Can]

Therapeutic Category Antiandrogen; Progestin

Use Palliative treatment of advanced prostate carcinoma

Dosage Summary

I.M.:

Children: Dosage not established

Adults (males): 300 mg (3 mL) once weekly **or** every 2 weeks

Oral:

Children: Dosage not established

Adults (males): 100-300 mg/day in 2-3 divided doses

Dosage Forms - Canada

Injection, solution: 100 mg/mL (3 mL)

Androcur® Depot: 100 mg/mL (3 mL)

Tablet: 50 mg

Androcur®, Apo-Cyproterone®, Gen-Cyproterone: 50 mg

Cystadane® [US/Can] *see* betaine *on page* 133

Cystagon® [US] *see* cysteamine *on page* 262

cysteamine (sis TEE a meen)

Synonyms cysteamine bitartrate

U.S./Canadian Brand Names Cystagon® [US]

Therapeutic Category Urinary Tract Product

Use Treatment of nephropathic cystinosis

Dosage Summary Note: Initial dose should be 1/4 to 1/6 of maintenance dose

Oral:

Children <12 years: Maintenance: 1.3 g/m^2/day **or** 60 mg/kg/day in 4 divided doses (maximum dose: 1.95 g/m^2/day; 90 mg/kg/day)

Children ≥12 years and >110 lbs: Maintenance: 2 g/day in 4 divided doses (maximum: 1.95 g/m^2/day; 90 mg/kg/day)

Adults >110 lbs: Maintenance: 2 g/day in 4 divided doses (maximum: 1.95 g/m^2/day; 90 mg/kg/day)

Dosage Forms

Capsule, oral:

Cystagon®: 50 mg, 150 mg

cysteamine bitartrate *see* cysteamine *on page* 262

cysteine (SIS te een)

Synonyms cysteine hydrochloride

U.S./Canadian Brand Names Cysteine-500 [US]

Therapeutic Category Nutritional Supplement

Use Supplement to crystalline amino acid solutions, in particular the specialized pediatric formulas (eg, Aminosyn® PF, TrophAmine®) to meet the intravenous amino acid nutritional requirements of infants receiving parenteral nutrition (PN)

Dosage Summary

I.V.:

Neonates and infants: Added as a fixed ratio to crystalline amino acid solution: 40 mg cysteine per g of amino acids; dosage will vary with the daily amino acid dosage; individual doses of cysteine of 0.8-1 mmol/kg/day have also been added directly to the daily PN solution

Children >2 years: Dosage not established

Adults: Dosage not established

Dosage Forms

Capsule, oral:

Cysteine-500: 500 mg

Injection, solution: 50 mg/mL (10 mL, 50 mL)

Cysteine-500 [US] *see* cysteine *on page* 262

cysteine hydrochloride *see* cysteine *on page* 262

Cystistat® [Can] *see* hyaluronate and derivatives *on page* 475

Cysto-Conray® II [US] *see* iothalamate meglumine *on page* 521

Cystografin® [US] *see* diatrizoate meglumine *on page* 292

Cystografin® Dilute [US] *see* diatrizoate meglumine *on page* 292

Cystospaz-M® ***(Discontinued)*** *see* hyoscyamine *on page* 491

CYT *see* cyclophosphamide *on page* 259

Cytadren® ***(Discontinued)***

cytarabine (sye TARE a been)

Sound-Alike/Look-Alike Issues

cytarabine may be confused with Cytadren®, Cytosar®, Cytoxan®, vidarabine

cytarabine (conventional) may be confused with cytarabine liposomal

Cytosar-U may be confused with cytarabine, Cytovene®, Cytoxan®, Neosar®

Synonyms ara-C; arabinosylcytosine; cytarabine (conventional); cytarabine hydrochloride; Cytosar-U; cytosine arabinosine hydrochloride

U.S./Canadian Brand Names Cytosar® [Can]

Therapeutic Category Antineoplastic Agent

Use Remission induction in acute myeloid leukemia (AML), treatment of acute lymphocytic leukemia (ALL) and chronic myelocytic leukemia (CML; blast phase); prophylaxis and treatment of meningeal leukemia

Dosage Summary

I.T.:

Children <1 year: 15-20 mg/dose

Children 1-2 years: 16-30 mg/dose

Children 2-3 years: 20-50 mg/dose

Children ≥3 years: 20-70 mg/dose

Adults: 40-100 mg/dose

I.V.:

Children: Induction: 100-200 mg/m^2/day for 7 days

Adults: Induction: 100-200 mg/m^2/day for 7 days

SubQ:

Children: Dosage not established

Adults: Dosage not established

Dosage Forms

Injection, powder for reconstitution: 100 mg, 500 mg, 1 g, 2 g

Injection, solution: 20 mg/mL (25 mL); 100 mg/mL (20 mL)

Injection, solution [preservative free]: 20 mg/mL (5 mL, 50 mL); 100 mg/mL (20 mL)

cytarabine (conventional) *see* cytarabine *on page* 263

cytarabine hydrochloride *see* cytarabine *on page* 263

cytarabine (liposomal) (sye TARE a been lip po SOE mal)

Sound-Alike/Look-Alike Issues

cytarabine may be confused with Cytadren®, Cytosar®, Cytoxan®, vidarabine

cytarabine (liposomal) may be confused with conventional cytarabine

DepoCyt® may be confused with Depoject®

U.S./Canadian Brand Names DepoCyt® [US/Can]

Therapeutic Category Antineoplastic Agent, Antimetabolite (Purine)

Use Treatment of lymphomatous meningitis

Dosage Summary

I.T.:

Children: Dosage not established

Adults: Induction: 50 mg every 14 days for a total of 2 doses (weeks 1 and 3); Consolidation: 50 mg every 14 days for 3 doses (weeks 5, 7, and 9), followed by 50 mg at week 13; Maintenance: 50 mg every 28 days for 4 doses (weeks 17, 21, 25, and 29)

Dosage Forms

Injection, suspension, intrathecal [preservative free]:

DepoCyt®: 10 mg/mL (5 mL)

CytoGam® [US/Can] *see* cytomegalovirus immune globulin (intravenous-human) *on page* 264

cytomegalovirus immune globulin (intravenous-human)

(sye toe meg a low VYE rus i MYUN GLOB yoo lin in tra VEE nus HYU man)

Sound-Alike/Look-Alike Issues

CytoGam® may be confused with Cytoxan®, Gamimune® N

Synonyms CMV-IGIV

U.S./Canadian Brand Names CytoGam® [US/Can]

Therapeutic Category Immune Globulin

Use Prophylaxis of cytomegalovirus (CMV) disease associated with kidney, lung, liver, pancreas, and heart transplants; concomitant use with ganciclovir should be considered in organ transplants (other than kidney) from CMV seropositive donors to CMV seronegative recipients

Dosage Summary

I.V.:

Children: Dosage not established

Adults: Initial: 150 mg/kg with 72 hours of transplant; 2-, 4-, 6- and 8 weeks after transplant: 100 mg/kg (kidney) **or** 150 mg/kg (liver, lung, pancreas, heart); 12 and 16 weeks after transplant: 50 mg/kg (kidney) **or** 100 mg/kg (liver, lung, pancreas, heart)

Dosage Forms

Injection, solution [preservative free]:

CytoGam®: 50 mg ± 10 mg/mL (50 mL)

Cytomel® [US/Can] *see* liothyronine *on page* 568

Cytosar® [Can] *see* cytarabine *on page* 263

Cytosar-U *see* cytarabine *on page* 263

cytosine arabinosine hydrochloride *see* cytarabine *on page* 263

cytostasan *see* bendamustine *on page* 122

Cytotec® [US] *see* misoprostol *on page* 637

Cytovene® [Can] *see* ganciclovir (systemic) *on page* 437

Cytovene®-IV [US] *see* ganciclovir (systemic) *on page* 437

Cytoxan® *(Discontinued)* *see* cyclophosphamide *on page* 259

Cytra-3 [US] *see* citric acid, sodium citrate, and potassium citrate *on page* 228

Cytra-K [US] *see* potassium citrate and citric acid *on page* 782

Cytuss HC [US] *see* phenylephrine, hydrocodone, and chlorpheniramine *on page* 754

D2 *see* ergocalciferol *on page* 358

D2E7 *see* adalimumab *on page* 37

D-3 [US-OTC] *see* cholecalciferol *on page* 218

D_3 *see* cholecalciferol *on page* 218

D3-5™ [US-OTC] *see* cholecalciferol *on page* 218

D3-50™ [US-OTC] *see* cholecalciferol *on page* 218

D-3-mercaptovaline *see* penicillamine *on page* 737

d4T *see* stavudine *on page* 894

D_5W *see* dextrose *on page* 290

$D_{10}W$ *see* dextrose *on page* 290

$D_{25}W$ *see* dextrose *on page* 290

$D_{30}W$ *see* dextrose *on page* 290

$D_{40}W$ *see* dextrose *on page* 290

$D_{50}W$ *see* dextrose *on page* 290

$D_{60}W$ *see* dextrose *on page* 290

$D_{70}W$ *see* dextrose *on page* 290

DAB$_{389}$IL-2 *see* denileukin diftitox *on page 275*
DAB389 interleukin-2 *see* denileukin diftitox *on page 275*

dabigatran etexilate *(Canada only)* (da BIG a tran ett EX ill ate)

Synonyms dabigatran etexilate mesilate
U.S./Canadian Brand Names Pradax™ [Can]
Therapeutic Category Anticoagulant, Thrombin Inhibitor
Use Postoperative thromboprophylaxis in patients who have undergone total hip or knee replacement procedures
Dosage Summary
Oral:
Children: Dosage not established
Adults: Initial: 110-220 mg once; Maintenance: 200 mg/day
Elderly >75 years: 150 mg/day
Dosage Forms - Canada
Capsule:
Pradax™: 75 mg, 110 mg

dabigatran etexilate mesilate *see* dabigatran etexilate *(Canada only) on page 265*
DABIL2 *see* denileukin diftitox *on page 275*

dacarbazine (da KAR ba zeen)

Sound-Alike/Look-Alike Issues
dacarbazine may be confused with Dicarbosil®, procarbazine
Synonyms DIC; dimethyl triazeno imidazole carboxamide; DTIC; DTIC-dome; imidazole carboxamide; imidazole carboxamide dimethyltriazene; WR-139007
U.S./Canadian Brand Names Dacarbazine for Injection [Can]
Therapeutic Category Antineoplastic Agent
Use Treatment of malignant melanoma, Hodgkin disease
Dosage Summary
I.V.:
Children: 375 mg/m^2 on days 1 and 15, repeat every 28 days
Adults: 375 mg/m^2 days 1 and 15 every 4 weeks **or** 250 mg/m^2 days 1-5 every 3 weeks
Dosage Forms
Injection, powder for reconstitution: 100 mg, 200 mg

Dacarbazine for Injection [Can] *see* dacarbazine *on page 265*
Dacex-DM ***(Discontinued)*** *see* guaifenesin, dextromethorphan, and phenylephrine *on page 458*
dacliximab *see* daclizumab *on page 265*

daclizumab (dac KLYE zue mab)

Synonyms anti-tac monoclonal antibody; dacliximab; MOAB anti-tac
U.S./Canadian Brand Names Zenapax® [Can]
Therapeutic Category Immunosuppressant Agent
Use Prophylaxis of acute rejection in renal transplantation (in combination with cyclosporine and corticosteroids)
Dosage Summary
I.V.:
Children: 1 mg/kg within 24 hours before transplantation (day 0), then every 14 days for 4 additional doses
Adults: 1 mg/kg within 24 hours before transplantation (day 0), then every 14 days for 4 additional doses
Product Availability Zenapax®: Due to diminishing market demand, the manufacturer of daclizumab has discontinued production; it is anticipated that available supplies will be depleted in January 2010; all remaining lots will expire in 2011.

Dacodyl™ [US-OTC] *see* bisacodyl *on page 138*
Dacogen™ [US] *see* decitabine *on page 272*
DACT *see* dactinomycin *on page 266*

dactinomycin (dak ti noe MYE sin)

Sound-Alike/Look-Alike Issues

DACTINomycin may be confused with DAPTOmycin, DAUNOrubicin
actinomycin may be confused with achromycin

Synonyms ACT-D; actinomycin; actinomycin Cl; actinomycin D; DACT

Tall-Man **DACTIN**omycin

U.S./Canadian Brand Names Cosmegen® [US/Can]

Therapeutic Category Antineoplastic Agent

Use Treatment of Wilms tumor, childhood rhabdomyosarcoma, Ewing sarcoma, metastatic testicular tumors (nonseminomatous), gestational trophoblastic neoplasm; regional perfusion (palliative or adjunctive) of locally recurrent or locoregional solid tumors (sarcomas, carcinomas, and adenocarcinomas)

Dosage Summary

I.V.:

Children ≤6 months: Dosage not established

Children >6 months: 15 mcg/kg/day for 5 days every 3-6 weeks **or** 400-600 mcg/m^2/day for 5 days every 3-6 weeks

Adults: 12-15 mcg/kg/day for 5 days every 3-6 weeks **or** 400-600 mcg/m^2/day for 5 days every 3-6 weeks **or** 1000 mcg/m^2 on day 1 **or** 500 mcg/dose days 1 and 2

Regional perfusion:

Children: Dosage not established

Adults: Lower extremity or pelvis: 50 mcg/kg; Upper extremity: 35 mcg/kg

Dosage Forms

Injection, powder for reconstitution: 0.5 mg

Cosmegen®: 0.5 mg

Dairyaid® [Can] *see* lactase *on page 542*

Dakin's Solution [US] *see* sodium hypochlorite solution *on page 884*

Dakrina® Ophthalmic Solution *(Discontinued)* *see* artificial tears *on page 97*

Dalacin® C [Can] *see* clindamycin (topical) *on page 232*

Dalacin® T [Can] *see* clindamycin (topical) *on page 232*

Dalacin® Vaginal [Can] *see* clindamycin (topical) *on page 232*

dalfampridine (dal FAM pri deen)

Sound-Alike/Look-Alike Issues

dalfampridine may be confused with delavirdine, desipramine
Ampyra™ may be confused with anakinra

Synonyms 4-aminopyridine; 4-AP; EL-970; fampridine-SR

U.S./Canadian Brand Names Ampyra™ [US]

Therapeutic Category Potassium Channel Blocker

Use Treatment to improve walking in multiple sclerosis (MS) patients

Dosage Summary

Oral: Extended release:

Children: Dosage not established

Adults: 10 mg every 12 hours

Dosage Forms

Tablet, extended release, oral:

Ampyra™: 10 mg

dalfopristin and quinupristin *see* quinupristin and dalfopristin *on page 823*

Dallergy® [US] *see* chlorpheniramine, phenylephrine, and methscopolamine *on page 212*

Dallergy-D® Syrup *(Discontinued)* *see* chlorpheniramine and phenylephrine *on page 208*

Dallergy Drops [US] *see* chlorpheniramine and phenylephrine *on page 208*

Dallergy®-JR [US] *see* chlorpheniramine and phenylephrine *on page 208*

Dalmane® [Can] *see* flurazepam *on page 417*

Dalmane® *(Discontinued)* *see* flurazepam *on page 417*

d-Alpha-Gems™ [US-OTC] *see* vitamin E *on page 988*

***d*-alpha tocopherol** *see* vitamin E *on page 988*

dalteparin (dal TE pa rin)

Synonyms dalteparin sodium; NSC-714371

U.S./Canadian Brand Names Fragmin® [US/Can]

Therapeutic Category Anticoagulant (Other)

Use Prevention of deep vein thrombosis which may lead to pulmonary embolism, in patients requiring abdominal surgery who are at risk for thromboembolism complications (eg, patients >40 years of age, obesity, patients with malignancy, history of deep vein thrombosis or pulmonary embolism, and surgical procedures requiring general anesthesia and lasting >30 minutes); prevention of DVT in patients undergoing hip-replacement surgery; patients immobile during an acute illness; acute treatment of unstable angina or non-Q-wave myocardial infarction; prevention of ischemic complications in patients on concurrent aspirin therapy; in patients with cancer, extended treatment (6 months) of acute symptomatic venous thromboembolism (DVT and/or PE) to reduce the recurrence of venous thromboembolism

Dosage Summary

SubQ:

Children: Dosage not established

Adults: Prophylaxis: 2500-5000 int. units daily; Treatment: 120 int. units/kg every 12 hours (maximum: 10,000 int. units/dose) or 200 int. units/kg (maximum 18,000 int. units/dose) once daily for 30 days, then ~150 int. units/kg once daily.

Dosage Forms

Injection, solution:

Fragmin®: 25,000 anti-Xa int. units/mL (3.8 mL)

Injection, solution [preservative free]:

Fragmin®: 10,000 anti-Xa int. units/mL (1 mL); 2500 anti-Xa int. units/0.2 mL (0.2 mL); 5000 anti-Xa int. units/0.2 mL (0.2 mL); 7500 anti-Xa int. units/0.3 mL (0.3 mL); 12,500 anti-Xa int. units/0.5 mL (0.5 mL); 15,000 anti-Xa int. units/0.6 mL (0.6 mL); 18,000 anti-Xa int. units/0.72 mL (0.72 mL)

dalteparin sodium *see* dalteparin *on page* 267

Damason-P® ***(Discontinued)***

danaparoid *(Canada only)* (da NAP a roid)

Sound-Alike/Look-Alike Issues

Orgaran® may be confused with argatroban

Synonyms danaparoid sodium

U.S./Canadian Brand Names Orgaran® [Can]

Therapeutic Category Anticoagulant (Other)

Use Prevention of postoperative deep vein thrombosis following elective hip replacement surgery

Dosage Summary

SubQ:

Children: Dosage not established

Adults: 750 anti-Xa units every 12 hours

Dosage Forms - Canada

Injection, solution:

Orgaran®: 750 anti-Xa units/0.6 mL (0.6 mL)

danaparoid sodium *see* danaparoid *(Canada only) on page* 267

danazol (DA na zole)

Sound-Alike/Look-Alike Issues

danazol may be confused with Dantrium®

Danocrine® may be confused with Dacriose®

U.S./Canadian Brand Names Cyclomen® [Can]

Therapeutic Category Androgen

Use Treatment of endometriosis, fibrocystic breast disease, and hereditary angioedema

Dosage Summary

Oral:

Children: Dosage not established

Adults (females): 100-800 mg/day in 2 divided doses

Adults (females/males): Hereditary angioedema: Initial: 200 mg 2-3 times/day, after favorable response decrease dosage by 50% or less at intervals of 1-3 months

Dosage Forms
Capsule, oral: 50 mg, 100 mg, 200 mg

Dandrex [US] *see* selenium sulfide *on page 869*
Danocrine® *(Discontinued)* *see* danazol *on page 267*
Dantrium® [US/Can] *see* dantrolene *on page 268*

dantrolene (DAN troe leen)

Sound-Alike/Look-Alike Issues
Dantrium® may be confused with danazol, Daraprim®
Synonyms dantrolene sodium
U.S./Canadian Brand Names Dantrium® [US/Can]; Revonto™ [US]
Therapeutic Category Skeletal Muscle Relaxant
Use Treatment of spasticity associated with upper motor neuron disorders (eg, spinal cord injury, stroke, cerebral palsy, or multiple sclerosis); management of malignant hyperthermia; prevention of malignant hyperthermia in susceptible individuals (preoperative/postoperative administration)
Dosage Summary
I.V.:
Children: Malignant hyperthermia: 1-2.5 mg/kg, may repeat up to cumulative dose of 10 mg/kg **or** 2.5 mg/kg prior to surgery
Adults: Malignant hyperthermia: 1-2.5 mg/kg, may repeat up to cumulative dose of 10 mg/kg **or** 2.5 mg/kg prior to surgery
Oral:
Children:
Malignant hyperthermia: 4-8 mg/kg/day in 4 divided doses
Spasticity: 0.5-2 mg/kg/dose 1-3 times/day (maximum: 400 mg/day)
Adults:
Malignant hyperthermia: 4-8 mg/kg/day in 4 divided doses
Spasticity: 25-100 mg 1-3 times/day (maximum: 400 mg/day)
Dosage Forms
Capsule, oral: 25 mg, 50 mg, 100 mg
Dantrium®: 25 mg, 50 mg, 100 mg
Injection, powder for reconstitution:
Dantrium®: 20 mg
Revonto™: 20 mg

dantrolene sodium *see* dantrolene *on page 268*
dapcin *see* daptomycin *on page 269*
dapiprazole *(Discontinued)*

dapsone (systemic) (DAP sone)

Sound-Alike/Look-Alike Issues
dapsone may be confused with Diprosone®
Synonyms diaminodiphenylsulfone
Therapeutic Category Antibiotic, Miscellaneous
Use Treatment of leprosy and dermatitis herpetiformis (infections caused by *Mycobacterium leprae*)
Dosage Summary
Oral:
Children: 1-2 mg/kg once daily (maximum: 100 mg/day)
Adults: 50-300 mg once daily
Dosage Forms
Tablet, oral: 25 mg, 100 mg

dapsone (topical) (DAP sone)

Sound-Alike/Look-Alike Issues
dapsone may be confused with Diprosone®
Synonyms diaminodiphenylsulfone
U.S./Canadian Brand Names Aczone® [US]
Therapeutic Category Topical Skin Product, Acne

Use Topical treatment of acne vulgaris

Dosage Summary

Topical:

Children <12 years: Dosage not established

Children ≥12 years: Apply pea-sized amount (approximately) in thin layer to affected areas twice daily

Adults: Apply pea-sized amount (approximately) in thin layer to affected areas twice daily

Dosage Forms

Gel, topical:

Aczone®: 5% (30 g, 60 g)

Daptacel® [US] *see* diphtheria, tetanus toxoids, and acellular pertussis vaccine *on page 316*

daptomycin (DAP toe mye sin)

Sound-Alike/Look-Alike Issues

DAPTOmycin may be confused with DACTINomycin

Cubicin® may be confused with Cleocin®

Synonyms cidecin; dapcin; LY146032

Tall-Man DAPTOmycin

U.S./Canadian Brand Names Cubicin® [US/Can]

Therapeutic Category Antibiotic, Cyclic Lipopeptide

Use Treatment of complicated skin and skin structure infections caused by susceptible aerobic gram-positive organisms; *Staphylococcus aureus* bacteremia, including right-sided infective endocarditis caused by MSSA or MRSA

Dosage Summary

I.V.:

Children: Dosage not established

Adults: 4-6 mg/kg once daily

Dosage Forms

Injection, powder for reconstitution:

Cubicin®: 500 mg

Daranide® ***(Discontinued)***

Daraprim® [US/Can] *see* pyrimethamine *on page 818*

darbepoetin alfa (dar be POE e tin AL fa)

Sound-Alike/Look-Alike Issues

darbepoetin alfa may be confused with dalteparin, epoetin alfa, epoetin beta

Aranesp® may be confused with Aralast, Aricept®

Synonyms erythropoiesis-stimulating agent (ESA); erythropoiesis-stimulating protein; NESP; novel erythropoiesis-stimulating protein

U.S./Canadian Brand Names Aranesp® [US/Can]

Therapeutic Category Colony-Stimulating Factor; Growth Factor; Recombinant Human Erythropoietin

Use Treatment of anemia (elevate or maintain red blood cell level and decrease the need for transfusions) associated with chronic renal failure (including patients on dialysis and not on dialysis); treatment of anemia due to concurrent chemotherapy in patients with metastatic cancer (nonmyeloid malignancies)

Note: Darbepoetin is **not** indicated for use in cancer patients under the following conditions:

- receiving hormonal therapy, therapeutic biologic products, or radiation therapy unless also receiving concurrent myelosuppressive chemotherapy
- receiving myelosuppressive therapy when the expected outcome is curative

Dosage Summary

I.V.:

Children <1 year: Dosage not established

Children 1-18 years: 6.25-200 mcg/week

Adults: 0.45 mcg/kg once weekly **or** 0.75 mcg/kg once every 2 weeks (alternate dose for nondialysis patients); titrate to hemoglobin response

SubQ:

Children <1 year: Dosage not established

Children 1-18 years: 6.25-200 mcg/week

Adults: 0.45-4.5 mcg/kg/week **or** 0.75 mcg/kg once every 2 weeks (alternate dose for nondialysis patients) or 500 mcg once every 3 weeks; titrate to hemoglobin response

Dosage Forms

Injection, solution [preservative free]:

Aranesp®: 25 mcg/mL (1 mL); 40 mcg/mL (1 mL); 25 mcg/0.42 mL (0.42 mL); 60 mcg/mL (1 mL); 40 mcg/0.4 mL (0.4 mL); 100 mcg/mL (1 mL); 60 mcg/0.3 mL (0.3 mL); 100 mcg/0.5 mL (0.5 mL); 150 mcg/0.75 mL (0.75 mL); 200 mcg/mL (1 mL); 300 mcg/mL (1 mL); 150 mcg/0.3 mL (0.3 mL); 200 mcg/0.4 mL (0.4 mL); 300 mcg/0.6 mL (0.6 mL); 500 mcg/mL (1 mL)

darifenacin (dar i FEN a sin)

Synonyms darifenacin hydrobromide; UK-88,525

U.S./Canadian Brand Names Enablex® [US/Can]

Therapeutic Category Anticholinergic Agent

Use Management of symptoms of bladder overactivity (urge incontinence, urgency, and frequency)

Dosage Summary

Oral:

Children: Dosage not established

Adults: Initial: 7.5 mg once daily, may increase to 15 mg once daily if response not adequate after 2 weeks

Note: Dosage should not exceed 7.5 mg/day with concurrent CYP3A4 inhibitors

Dosage Forms

Tablet, extended release, oral:

Enablex®: 7.5 mg, 15 mg

darifenacin hydrobromide *see* darifenacin *on page* 270

darunavir (dar OO na veer)

Synonyms darunavir ethanolate; TMC-114

U.S./Canadian Brand Names Prezista® [US/Can]

Therapeutic Category Antiretroviral Agent, Protease Inhibitor

Use Treatment of HIV-1 infections in combination with ritonavir and other antiretroviral agents

Dosage Summary

Oral:

Children <6 years: Dosage not established

Children ≥6 years: 375-600 mg twice daily; **Note:** Coadministration with ritonavir (50-100 mg twice daily) is required

Adults: 600 mg twice daily **or** 800 mg twice daily; **Note:** Coadministration with ritonavir (100 mg once or twice daily) is required

Dosage Forms

Tablet, oral:

Prezista®: 75 mg, 150 mg, 400 mg, 600 mg

Dosage Forms - Canada

Tablet:

Prezista®: 300 mg, 400 mg, 600 mg

darunavir ethanolate *see* darunavir *on page* 270

Darvocet A500® [US] *see* propoxyphene and acetaminophen *on page* 805

Darvocet-N® 50 [US/Can] *see* propoxyphene and acetaminophen *on page* 805

Darvocet-N® 100 [US/Can] *see* propoxyphene and acetaminophen *on page* 805

Darvon® [US] *see* propoxyphene *on page* 805

Darvon® Compound *(Discontinued)*

Darvon-N® [US/Can] *see* propoxyphene *on page* 805

dasatinib (da SA ti nib)

Sound-Alike/Look-Alike Issues

dasatinib may be confused with imatinib, nilotinib

Synonyms BMS-354825

U.S./Canadian Brand Names Sprycel® [US/Can]

Therapeutic Category Antineoplastic Agent, Tyrosine Kinase Inhibitor

Use Treatment of chronic myelogenous leukemia (CML) in chronic, accelerated or blast (myeloid or lymphoid) phase resistant or intolerant to prior therapy (including imatinib); treatment of Philadelphia chromosome-positive (Ph+) acute lymphoblastic leukemia (ALL) resistant or intolerant to prior therapy

Dosage Summary

Oral:

Children: Dosage not established

Adults: 100 mg or 140 mg once daily

Dosage Forms

Tablet, oral:

Sprycel®: 20 mg, 50 mg, 70 mg, 100 mg

daunomycin *see* daunorubicin hydrochloride *on page 271*

daunorubicin citrate (liposomal) (daw noe ROO bi sin SI trate lip po SOE mal)

Sound-Alike/Look-Alike Issues

DAUNOrubicin liposomal may be confused with DACTINomycin, DOXOrubicin, DOXOrubicin liposomal, epirubicin, IDArubicin, valrubicin

Liposomal formulation (DaunoXome®) may be confused with the conventional formulation (Cerubidine®, Rubex®)

Synonyms DAUNOrubicin liposomal; liposomal DAUNOrubicin; NSC-697732

Tall-Man DAUNOrubicin citrate (liposomal)

U.S./Canadian Brand Names DaunoXome® [US]

Therapeutic Category Antineoplastic Agent

Use First-line treatment of advanced HIV-associated Kaposi sarcoma (KS)

Dosage Summary

I.V.:

Children: Dosage not established

Adults: 40 mg/m^2 every 2 weeks

Dosage Forms

Injection, solution [preservative free]:

DaunoXome®: 2 mg/mL (25 mL)

daunorubicin hydrochloride (daw noe ROO bi sin hye droe KLOR ide)

Sound-Alike/Look-Alike Issues

DAUNOrubicin may be confused with DACTINomycin, DOXOrubicin, DOXOrubicin liposomal, epirubicin, IDArubicin, valrubicin

Conventional formulation (Cerubidine®, DAUNOrubicin hydrochloride) may be confused with the liposomal formulation (DaunoXome®)

Synonyms daunomycin; rubidomycin hydrochloride

Tall-Man DAUNOrubicin hydrochloride

U.S./Canadian Brand Names Cerubidine® [US/Can]

Therapeutic Category Antineoplastic Agent

Use Treatment of acute lymphocytic leukemia (ALL) and acute myeloid leukemia (AML)

Dosage Summary

I.V.:

Children <2 years or BSA <0.5 m^2: Dose should be based on weight, 1 mg/kg/dose per protocol with frequency dependent on regimen employed (maximum cumulative dose: 10 mg/kg)

Children ≥2 years and BSA ≥0.5 m^2: on day 1 every week for 4 cycles **or** 30-60 mg/m^2/day for 3 days (maximum cumulative dose: 300 mg/m^2)

Adults <60 years: 30-60 mg/m^2/day for 2-3 days (maximum cumulative dose: 550 mg/m^2; 400 mg/m^2 with chest irradiation)

Adults ≥60 years: 30 mg/m^2/day for 2-3 days (maximum cumulative dose: 550 mg/m^2; 400 mg/m^2 with chest irradiation)

Dosage Forms

Injection, powder for reconstitution: 20 mg

Cerubidine®: 20 mg

Injection, solution [preservative free]: 5 mg/mL (4 mL, 10 mL)

DAUNOrubicin liposomal *see* daunorubicin citrate (liposomal) *on page 271*

DaunoXome® [US] *see* daunorubicin citrate (liposomal) *on page 271*

1-Day™ [US-OTC] *see* tioconazole *on page* 935
Dayhist® Allergy ***(Discontinued)*** *see* clemastine *on page* 231
Daypro® [US/Can] *see* oxaprozin *on page* 711
Dayto Himbin® ***(Discontinued)*** *see* yohimbine *on page* 996
Daytrana™ [US] *see* methylphenidate *on page* 621
DC 240® Softgel® ***(Discontinued)*** *see* docusate *on page* 321
dCF *see* pentostatin *on page* 742
DDAVP® [US/Can] *see* desmopressin acetate *on page* 278
DDAVP® Melt [Can] *see* desmopressin acetate *on page* 278
ddI *see* didanosine *on page* 299
DDrops® [US-OTC] *see* cholecalciferol *on page* 218
DDrops® Baby [US-OTC] *see* cholecalciferol *on page* 218
DDrops® Kids [US-OTC] *see* cholecalciferol *on page* 218
1-deamino-8-D-arginine vasopressin *see* desmopressin acetate *on page* 278
Debrox® [US-OTC] *see* carbamide peroxide *on page* 178
Decadron® Phosphate ***(Discontinued)*** *see* dexamethasone (systemic) *on page* 281
Deca-Durabolin® [Can] *see* nandrolone *(Canada only) on page* 658
Deca-Durabolin® ***(Discontinued)*** *see* nandrolone *(Canada only) on page* 658
Decahist-DM ***(Discontinued)***
Decavac® [US] *see* diphtheria and tetanus toxoid *on page* 313
Dec-Chlorphen [US] *see* chlorpheniramine and phenylephrine *on page* 208
Dec-Chlorphen DM ***(Discontinued)*** *see* chlorpheniramine, phenylephrine, and dextromethorphan *on page* 211
De-Chlor DM [US] *see* chlorpheniramine, phenylephrine, and dextromethorphan *on page* 211
De-Chlor DR [US] *see* chlorpheniramine, phenylephrine, and dextromethorphan *on page* 211
De-Chlor G ***(Discontinued)***
De-Chlor HC [US] *see* phenylephrine, hydrocodone, and chlorpheniramine *on page* 754

decitabine (de SYE ta been)

Synonyms 5-Aza-2'-deoxycytidine; 5-Aza-dCyd; deoxyazacytidine; dezocitidine
U.S./Canadian Brand Names Dacogen™ [US]
Therapeutic Category Antineoplastic Agent, Antimetabolite (Pyrimidine)
Use Treatment of myelodysplastic syndrome (MDS)
Dosage Summary
I.V.:
Children: Dosage not established
Adults: MDS: 15 mg/m^2 over 3 hours every 8 hours for 3 days every 6 weeks **or** 20 mg/m^2 over 1 hour daily for 5 days every 28 days
Dosage Forms
Injection, powder for reconstitution:
Dacogen™: 50 mg

Declomycin® [Can] *see* demeclocycline *on page* 274
Declomycin® ***(Discontinued)*** *see* demeclocycline *on page* 274
Deconamine® SR ***(Discontinued)*** *see* chlorpheniramine and pseudoephedrine *on page* 209
Deconsal® II [US] *see* guaifenesin and phenylephrine *on page* 456
Deconsal® CT ***(Discontinued)*** *see* phenylephrine and pyrilamine *on page* 753
Deconsal® DM ***(Discontinued)*** *see* phenylephrine, pyrilamine, and dextromethorphan *on page* 755
Deep Sea [US-OTC] *see* sodium chloride *on page* 882
Defen-LA® ***(Discontinued)*** *see* guaifenesin and pseudoephedrine *on page* 457

deferasirox (de FER a sir ox)

Sound-Alike/Look-Alike Issues
deferasirox may be confused with deferoxamine
Synonyms ICL670
U.S./Canadian Brand Names Exjade® [US/Can]

Therapeutic Category Antidote; Chelating Agent

Use Treatment of chronic iron overload due to blood transfusions (transfusional hemosiderosis)

Dosage Summary

Oral:

Children <2 years: Dosage not established

Children ≥2 years: Initial: 20 mg/kg once daily; Maintenance: 20-30 mg/kg once daily; **Note:** Titration is recommended. Maximum dose: 40 mg/kg/day.

Adults: Initial: 20 mg/kg once daily; Maintenance: 20-30 mg/kg once daily; **Note:** Titration is recommended. Maximum dose: 40 mg/kg/day.

Dosage Forms

Tablet for suspension, oral:

Exjade®: 125 mg, 250 mg, 500 mg

deferoxamine (de fer OKS a meen)

Sound-Alike/Look-Alike Issues

deferoxamine may be confused with cefuroxime, deferasirox

Desferal® may be confused with desflurane, Dexferrum®, Disophrol®

Synonyms deferoxamine mesylate; desferrioxamine; NSC-644468

U.S./Canadian Brand Names Desferal® [US/Can]; PMS-Deferoxamine [Can]

Therapeutic Category Antidote

Use Acute iron intoxication or when clinical signs of significant iron toxicity exist; chronic iron overload secondary to multiple transfusions

Dosage Summary

I.M.:

Children <3 years: Dosage not established

Children ≥3 years: 90 mg/kg/dose every 8 hours (maximum: 6 g/24 hours)

Adults: Initial: 1000 mg, followed by 500 mg every 4 hours for up to 2 doses; Maintenance: 500 mg every 4-12 hours or 500-1000 mg once daily (maximum: 6 g/day)

I.V.:

Children <3 years: Dosage not established

Children ≥3 years: 15 mg/kg/hour (maximum: 6-12 g/24 hours)

Adults: Initial: 1000 mg, followed by 500 mg every 4 hours for up to 2 doses; Maintenance: 500 mg every 4-12 hours or 2000 mg with each unit of blood (maximum: 1-6 g/day)

SubQ:

Children <3 years: Dosage not established

Children ≥3 years: 20-40 mg/kg/day over 8-12 hours (maximum: 2000 mg/day)

Adults: 1-2 g once daily over 8-24 hours

Dosage Forms

Injection, powder for reconstitution: 500 mg, 2 g

Desferal®: 500 mg, 2 g

deferoxamine mesylate *see* deferoxamine *on page* 273

Deficol® ***(Discontinued)*** *see* bisacodyl *on page* 138

Definity® [US/Can] *see* perflutren lipid microspheres *on page* 743

degarelix (deg a REL ix)

Sound-Alike/Look-Alike Issues

degarelix may be confused with cetrorelix, ganirelix

Synonyms degarelix acetate; FE200486

U.S./Canadian Brand Names Firmagon® [US/Can]

Therapeutic Category Antineoplastic Agent, Gonadotropin-Releasing Hormone Antagonist; Gonadotropin Releasing Hormone Antagonist

Use Treatment of advanced prostate cancer

Dosage Summary

SubQ:

Children: Dosage not established

Adults: Loading dose: 240 mg; Maintenance dose: 80 mg every 28 days

Dosage Forms

Injection, powder for reconstitution:

Firmagon®: 80 mg, 120 mg

degarelix acetate *see* degarelix *on page 273*

Degest® 2 Ophthalmic *(Discontinued)* *see* naphazoline (ophthalmic) *on page 658*

Dehistine [US] *see* chlorpheniramine, phenylephrine, and methscopolamine *on page 212*

Dehydral® [Can] *see* methenamine *on page 612*

dehydrobenzperidol *see* droperidol *on page 334*

Delacort [US-OTC] *see* hydrocortisone (topical) *on page 483*

Delatest® Injection *(Discontinued)* *see* testosterone *on page 919*

Delatestryl® [US/Can] *see* testosterone *on page 919*

delavirdine (de la VIR deen)

Sound-Alike/Look-Alike Issues

delavirdine may be confused with dalfampridine

Synonyms U-90152S

U.S./Canadian Brand Names Rescriptor® [US/Can]

Therapeutic Category Antiviral Agent

Use Treatment of HIV-1 infection in combination with at least two additional antiretroviral agents

Dosage Summary

Oral:

Children <16 years: Dosage not established

Children ≥16 years: 400 mg 3 times/day

Adults: 400 mg 3 times/day

Dosage Forms

Tablet, oral:

Rescriptor®: 100 mg, 200 mg

Delestrogen® [US] *see* estradiol (systemic) *on page 366*

Delfen® [US-OTC] *see* nonoxynol 9 *on page 681*

Delsym® [US-OTC] *see* dextromethorphan *on page 287*

delta-9-tetrahydro-cannabinol *see* dronabinol *on page 333*

delta-9-tetrahydrocannabinol and cannabinol *see* tetrahydrocannabinol and cannabidiol *(Canada only) on page 923*

delta-9 THC *see* dronabinol *on page 333*

deltacortisone *see* prednisone *on page 792*

Delta® D3 [US-OTC] *see* cholecalciferol *on page 218*

deltadehydrocortisone *see* prednisone *on page 792*

Del-Vi-A® *(Discontinued)* *see* vitamin A *on page 987*

Demadex® [US] *see* torsemide *on page 943*

demeclocycline (dem e kloe SYE kleen)

Synonyms demeclocycline hydrochloride; demethylchlortetracycline

U.S./Canadian Brand Names Declomycin® [Can]

Therapeutic Category Tetracycline Derivative

Use Treatment of susceptible bacterial infections (acne, gonorrhea, pertussis, and urinary tract infections) caused by both gram-negative and gram-positive organisms

Dosage Summary

Oral:

Children <8 years: Dosage not established

Children ≥8 years: 8-12 mg/kg/day divided every 6-12 hours

Adults: 600 mg/day in 2 or 4 divided doses

Dosage Forms

Tablet, oral: 150 mg, 300 mg

demeclocycline hydrochloride *see* demeclocycline *on page 274*

Demerol® [US/Can] *see* meperidine *on page 603*

4-demethoxydaunorubicin *see* idarubicin *on page 497*
demethylchlortetracycline *see* demeclocycline *on page 274*
Demser® [US/Can] *see* metyrosine *on page 628*
Demulen® 30 [Can] *see* ethinyl estradiol and ethynodiol diacetate *on page 376*
Demulen® *(Discontinued)* *see* ethinyl estradiol and ethynodiol diacetate *on page 376*
Denavir® [US] *see* penciclovir *on page 736*

denileukin diftitox (de ni LOO kin DIF ti toks)

Synonyms DAB389 interleukin-2; DAB_{389}IL-2; DABIL2
U.S./Canadian Brand Names ONTAK® [US]
Therapeutic Category Antineoplastic Agent, Miscellaneous
Use Treatment of persistent or recurrent cutaneous T-cell lymphoma (CTCL) whose malignant cells express the CD25 component of the IL-2 receptor
Dosage Summary
I.V.:
Children: Dosage not established
Adults: 9 or 18 mcg/kg/day days 1-5 every 21 days
Dosage Forms
Injection, solution:
ONTAK®: 150 mcg/mL (2 mL)

Denorex® Extra Strength Protection [US-OTC] *see* salicylic acid *on page 858*
Denorex® Extra Strength Protection 2-in-1 [US-OTC] *see* salicylic acid *on page 858*
Denorex® Therapeutic Protection [US-OTC] *see* coal tar *on page 242*
Denorex® Therapeutic Protection 2-in-1 Shampoo + Conditioner [US-OTC] *see* coal tar *on page 242*

denosumab (den OH sue mab)

Synonyms AMG-162
U.S./Canadian Brand Names Prolia™ [US]
Therapeutic Category Monoclonal Antibody
Use Treatment of osteoporosis in postmenopausal women at high risk for fracture
Dosage Summary
SubQ:
Children: Dosage not established
Adults, male: Dosage not established
Adults, female, postmenopausal: 60 mg every 6 months
Dosage Forms
Injection, solution [preservative free]:
Prolia™: 60 mg/mL (1 mL)

Denta 5000 Plus [US] *see* fluoride *on page 413*
DentaGel [US] *see* fluoride *on page 413*
Dentapaine [US-OTC] *see* benzocaine *on page 124*
Dent's Ear Wax *(Discontinued)* *see* carbamide peroxide *on page 178*
Dent's Extra Strength Toothache Gum [US-OTC] *see* benzocaine *on page 124*
deoxyazacytidine *see* decitabine *on page 272*
2′-deoxycoformycin *see* pentostatin *on page 742*
deoxycoformycin *see* pentostatin *on page 742*
Depacon® [US] *see* valproic acid *on page 974*
Depade® [US] *see* naltrexone *on page 657*
Depakene® [US/Can] *see* valproic acid *on page 974*
Depakote® [US] *see* divalproex *on page 319*
Depakote® ER [US] *see* divalproex *on page 319*
Depakote® Sprinkle [US] *see* divalproex *on page 319*
depAndro® Injection *(Discontinued)* *see* testosterone *on page 919*
Depen® [US/Can] *see* penicillamine *on page 737*

depGynogen® Injection *(Discontinued)* *see* estradiol (systemic) *on page 366*
Deplin™ [US] *see* methylfolate *on page 620*
depMedalone® Injection *(Discontinued)* *see* methylprednisolone *on page 622*
DepoCyt® [US/Can] *see* cytarabine (liposomal) *on page 263*
DepoDur® [US] *see* morphine (liposomal) *on page 645*
Depo®-Estradiol [US/Can] *see* estradiol (systemic) *on page 366*
Depoject® Injection *(Discontinued)* *see* methylprednisolone *on page 622*
Depo-Medrol® [US/Can] *see* methylprednisolone *on page 622*
Deponit® Patch *(Discontinued)* *see* nitroglycerin *on page 679*
Depo-Prevera® [Can] *see* medroxyprogesterone *on page 597*
Depo-Provera® [US/Can] *see* medroxyprogesterone *on page 597*
Depo-Provera® Contraceptive [US] *see* medroxyprogesterone *on page 597*
depo-subQ provera 104™ [US] *see* medroxyprogesterone *on page 597*
Depotest® 100 [Can] *see* testosterone *on page 919*
Depotest® Injection *(Discontinued)* *see* testosterone *on page 919*
Depo®-Testosterone [US] *see* testosterone *on page 919*
deprenyl *see* selegiline *on page 869*
depsipeptide *see* romidepsin *on page 850*
Dermaflex® Gel *(Discontinued)* *see* lidocaine (topical) *on page 562*
DermaFungal [US-OTC] *see* miconazole (topical) *on page 630*
Dermagran® [US-OTC] *see* aluminum hydroxide *on page 58*
Dermagran® AF [US-OTC] *see* miconazole (topical) *on page 630*
Dermamycin® [US-OTC] *see* diphenhydramine (topical) *on page 311*
Dermarest® Psoriasis Medicated Lotion [US-OTC] *see* hydrocortisone (topical) *on page 483*
Dermarest® Psoriasis Medicated Moisturizer [US-OTC] *see* salicylic acid *on page 858*
Dermarest® Psoriasis Medicated Scalp Treatment [US-OTC] *see* salicylic acid *on page 858*
Dermarest® Psoriasis Medicated Shampoo/Conditioner [US-OTC] *see* salicylic acid *on page 858*
Dermarest® Psoriasis Medicated Skin Treatment [US-OTC] *see* salicylic acid *on page 858*
Dermarest® Psoriasis Overnight Treatment [US-OTC] *see* salicylic acid *on page 858*
Dermarest® Psoriasis Scalp Treatment Mousse *(Discontinued)* *see* salicylic acid *on page 858*
Dermarest® Skin Correcting Cream Plus [US-OTC] *see* hydroquinone *on page 487*
Derma-Smoothe/FS® [US/Can] *see* fluocinolone (topical) *on page 411*
Dermatop® [US/Can] *see* prednicarbate *on page 790*
Dermatophytin-O *(Discontinued)*
Dermazene® [US] *see* iodoquinol and hydrocortisone *on page 519*
DermaZinc™ [US-OTC] *see* pyrithione zinc *on page 819*
Dermazole [Can] *see* miconazole (topical) *on page 630*
Dermoplast® Antibacterial [US-OTC] *see* benzocaine *on page 124*
Dermoplast® Pain Relieving [US-OTC] *see* benzocaine *on page 124*
DermOtic® [US] *see* fluocinolone (otic) *on page 410*
Dermovate® [Can] *see* clobetasol *on page 235*
Dermtex® HC [US-OTC] *see* hydrocortisone (topical) *on page 483*
Desferal® [US/Can] *see* deferoxamine *on page 273*
desferrioxamine *see* deferoxamine *on page 273*

desflurane (DES flure ane)

Sound-Alike/Look-Alike Issues
desflurane may be confused with Desferal®

U.S./Canadian Brand Names Suprane® [US/Can]

Therapeutic Category General Anesthetic

Use Induction and/or maintenance of general anesthesia in adults; maintenance of anesthesia in intubated children; **Note:** Use of desflurane for induction of general anesthesia is not recommended due to its irritant properties and unpleasant odor which causes coughing, breath holding, laryngospasm, oxygen desaturation, increased secretions, hypertension, and tachycardia.

Dosage Summary

Inhalation:

Children (intubated): 5.2% to 10% to maintain surgical levels of anesthesia

Adults: 2.5% to 8.5% to maintain surgical levels of anesthesia

Dosage Forms

Liquid, for inhalation:

Suprane®: 100% (240 mL)

desiccated thyroid *see* thyroid, desiccated *on page* 930

desipramine (des IP ra meen)

Sound-Alike/Look-Alike Issues

desipramine may be confused with clomiPRAMINE, dalfampridine, deserpidine, diphenhydrAMINE, disopyramide, imipramine, nortriptyline

Norpramin® may be confused with clomiPRAMINE, imipramine, Normodyne®, Norpace®, nortriptyline, Tenormin®

Synonyms desipramine hydrochloride; desmethylimipramine hydrochloride

U.S./Canadian Brand Names Alti-Desipramine [Can]; Apo-Desipramine® [Can]; Norpramin® [US/Can]; Nu-Desipramine [Can]; PMS-Desipramine [Can]

Therapeutic Category Antidepressant, Tricyclic (Secondary Amine)

Use Treatment of depression

Dosage Summary

Oral:

Children <6 years: Dosage not established

Adolescents: Initial: 25-50 mg once daily; Maintenance: 25-100 mg/day in single or divided doses (maximum: 150 mg/day); **Note:** Increase gradually

Adults: Initial: 75 mg/day in divided doses; Maintenance: 75-200 mg/day in single or divided doses (maximum: 300 mg/day); **Note:** Increase gradually

Elderly: Initial: 10-25 mg/day; Maintenance: 75-150 mg/day; **Note:** Titration is recommended

Dosage Forms

Tablet, oral: 10 mg, 25 mg, 50 mg, 75 mg, 100 mg, 150 mg

Norpramin®: 10 mg, 25 mg, 50 mg, 75 mg, 100 mg, 150 mg

desipramine hydrochloride *see* desipramine *on page* 277

desirudin (des i ROO din)

Synonyms CGP-39393; desulfato-hirudin; desulfatohirudin; desulphatohirudin; r-hirudin; recombinant desulfatohirudin; recombinant hirudin

U.S./Canadian Brand Names Iprivask® [US]

Therapeutic Category Anticoagulant, Thrombin Inhibitor

Use Prophylaxis of deep vein thrombosis (DVT) in patients undergoing surgery for hip replacement

Dosage Summary

SubQ:

Children: Dosage not established

Adults: 15 mg every 12 hours

Dosage Forms

Injection, powder for reconstitution [preservative free]:

Iprivask®: 15 mg

Desitin® [US-OTC] *see* zinc oxide *on page* 1001

Desitin® Creamy [US-OTC] *see* zinc oxide *on page* 1001

desloratadine (des lor AT a deen)

Sound-Alike/Look-Alike Issues

Clarinex® may be confused with Celebrex®

U.S./Canadian Brand Names Aerius® [Can]; Clarinex® [US]

Therapeutic Category Antihistamine, Nonsedating

Use Relief of nasal and non-nasal symptoms of seasonal allergic rhinitis (SAR) and perennial allergic rhinitis (PAR); treatment of chronic idiopathic urticaria (CIU)

Dosage Summary

Oral:

Children <6 months: Dosage not established
Children 6-11 months: 1 mg once daily
Children 1-5 years: 1.25 mg once daily
Children 6-11 years: 2.5 mg once daily
Children ≥12 years: 5 mg once daily
Adults: 5 mg once daily

Dosage Forms

Syrup, oral:
Clarinex®: 0.5 mg/mL (480 mL)

Tablet, oral:
Clarinex®: 5 mg

Tablet, orally disintegrating, oral:
Clarinex®: 2.5 mg, 5 mg

desloratadine and pseudoephedrine (des lor AT a deen & soo doe e FED rin)

Synonyms pseudoephedrine and desloratadine

U.S./Canadian Brand Names Clarinex-D® 12 Hour [US]; Clarinex-D® 24 Hour [US]

Therapeutic Category Antihistamine/Decongestant Combination, Nonsedating

Use Relief of symptoms of seasonal allergic rhinitis, in children ≥12 years of age and adults

Dosage Summary

Oral:

Children <12 years: Dosage not established
Children ≥12 years: 12 hour: 1 tablet twice daily; 24 hour: 1 tablet once daily
Adults: 12 hour: 1 tablet twice daily; 24 hour: 1 tablet once daily

Dosage Forms

Tablet, variable release:

Clarinex-D® 12 Hour: Desloratadine 2.5 mg [immediate release] and pseudoephedrine 120 mg [extended release]

Clarinex-D® 24 Hour: Desloratadine 5 mg [immediate release] and pseudoephedrine 240 mg [extended release]

desmethylimipramine hydrochloride *see* desipramine *on page* 277

desmopressin acetate (des moe PRES in AS e tate)

Synonyms 1-deamino-8-D-arginine vasopressin

U.S./Canadian Brand Names Apo-Desmopressin® [Can]; DDAVP® Melt [Can]; DDAVP® [US/Can]; Minirin® [Can]; Nove-Desmopressin [Can]; Octostim® [Can]; PMS-Desmopressin [Can]; Stimate® [US]

Therapeutic Category Vasopressin Analog, Synthetic

Use

Injection: Treatment of diabetes insipidus; maintenance of hemostasis and control of bleeding in hemophilia A with factor VIII coagulant activity levels >5% and mild-to-moderate classic von Willebrand disease (type 1) with factor VIII coagulant activity levels >5%

Nasal solutions (DDAVP® Nasal Spray and DDAVP® Rhinal Tube): Treatment of central diabetes insipidus

Nasal spray (Stimate®): Maintenance of hemostasis and control of bleeding in hemophilia A with factor VIII coagulant activity levels >5% and mild-to-moderate classic von Willebrand disease (type 1) with factor VIII coagulant activity levels >5%

Tablet: Treatment of central diabetes insipidus, temporary polyuria and polydipsia following pituitary surgery or head trauma, primary nocturnal enuresis

Dosage Summary

I.V.:

Children <3 months: Dosage not established
Children ≥3 months: 0.3 mcg/kg 30 minutes prior to procedure, may repeat dose if needed
Adults: 2-4 mcg/day in 2 divided doses **or** 1/10 of the intranasal maintenance dose **or** 0.3 mcg/kg 30 minutes prior to procedure

Intranasal:

Children <3 months: Dosage not established
Children 3-11 months: Initial: 5 mcg/day (0.05 mL/day) in 1-2 divided doses; Maintenance: 5-30 mcg/day (0.05-0.3 mL/day) in 1-2 divided doses

Children 12 months to 12 years: Initial: 5 mcg/day (0.05 mL/day) in 1-2 divided doses; Maintenance: 5-30 mcg/day (0.05-0.3 mL/day) in 1-2 divided doses **or** 150 mcg (1 spray of high concentration) 2 hours prior to surgery

Children >12 years and <50 kg: 10-40 mcg/day (0.1-0.4 mL) in 1-3 divided doses **or** 150 mcg (1 spray of high concentration spray) 2 hours prior to surgery

Children >12 years and ≥50 kg: 10-40 mcg/day in 1-3 divided doses **or** 300 mcg (1 spray each nostril of high concentration spray) 2 hours prior to surgery

Adults <50 kg: 10-40 mcg/day in 1-3 divided doses **or** 150 mcg (1 spray of high concentration spray) 2 hours prior to surgery

Adults ≥50 kg: 10-40 mcg/day in 1-3 divided doses **or** 300 mcg (1 spray each nostril of high concentration spray) 2 hours prior to surgery

Oral:

Children <4 years: Dosage not established

Children 4-5 years: Initial: 0.05 mg twice daily; Maintenance: 0.1-1.2 mg/day in 2-3 divided doses

Children ≥6 years: Initial: 0.05 mg twice daily **or** 0.2 mg at bedtime; Maintenance: 0.1-1.2 mg/day in 2-3 divided doses **or** 0.2-0.6 mg at bedtime

Adults: 0.2-0.6 mg at bedtime **or** 0.1-1.2 mg/day in 2-3 divided doses

SubQ:

Children: Dosage not established

Adults: 2-4 mcg/day in 2 divided doses **or** 1/10 of the intranasal maintenance dose

Dosage Forms

Injection, solution: 4 mcg/mL (1 mL, 10 mL)

DDAVP®: 4 mcg/mL (1 mL, 10 mL)

Solution, intranasal: 0.1 mg/mL (2.5 mL, 5 mL)

DDAVP®: 0.1 mg/mL (2.5 mL, 5 mL)

Stimate®: 1.5 mg/mL (2.5 mL)

Tablet, oral: 0.1 mg, 0.2 mg

DDAVP®: 0.1 mg, 0.2 mg

Dosage Forms - Canada

Tablet, sublingual:

DDAVP® Melt: 60 mcg, 120 mcg, 240 mcg

Desocort® [Can] *see* desonide *on page* 279

Desogen® [US] *see* ethinyl estradiol and desogestrel *on page* 374

desogestrel and ethinyl estradiol *see* ethinyl estradiol and desogestrel *on page* 374

Desonate® [US] *see* desonide *on page* 279

desonide (DES oh nide)

U.S./Canadian Brand Names Desocort® [Can]; Desonate® [US]; DesOwen® [US]; LoKara™ [US]; PMS-Desonide [Can]; Verdeso™ [US]

Therapeutic Category Corticosteroid, Topical

Use Treatment of inflammatory and pruritic manifestations of corticosteroid responsive dermatosis (low-to-medium potency corticosteroid); mild-to-moderate atopic dermatitis

Dosage Summary

Topical:

Children <3 months: Dosage not established.

Children ≥3 months: Aerosol, gel: Apply 2 times/day sparingly

Adults: Apply 2-3 times/day sparingly

Dosage Forms

Aerosol, topical:

Verdeso™: 0.05% (50 g, 100 g)

Cream, topical: 0.05% (15 g, 60 g)

DesOwen®: 0.05% (60 g)

Gel, topical:

Desonate®: 0.05% (60 g)

Lotion, topical: 0.05% (59 mL, 60 mL, 118 mL)

DesOwen®: 0.05% (60 mL, 120 mL)

LoKara™: 0.05% (59 mL, 118 mL)

Ointment, topical: 0.05% (15 g, 60 g)

DesOwen®: 0.05% (60 g)

DesOwen® [US] *see* desonide *on page* 279

desoximetasone (des oks i MET a sone)

Sound-Alike/Look-Alike Issues

desoximetasone may be confused with dexamethasone
Topicort® may be confused with Topic®

U.S./Canadian Brand Names Taro-Desoximetasone [Can]; Topicort® [US/Can]; Topicort®-LP [US]

Therapeutic Category Corticosteroid, Topical

Use Relieves inflammation and pruritic symptoms of corticosteroid-responsive dermatosis (intermediate- to high-potency topical corticosteroid)

Dosage Summary

Topical:

Cream, gel:
Children: Apply a thin film to affected area twice daily
Adults: Apply a thin film to affected area twice daily

Ointment:
Children <10 years: Apply a thin film to affected area twice daily
Children ≥10 years: Apply a thin film to affected area twice daily
Adults: Apply a thin film to affected area twice daily

Dosage Forms

Cream, topical: 0.05% (15 g, 60 g); 0.25% (15 g, 60 g)
Topicort®: 0.25% (15 g, 60 g)
Topicort®-LP: 0.05% (15 g, 60 g)

Gel, topical: 0.05% (15 g, 60 g)
Topicort®: 0.05% (15 g, 60 g)

Ointment, topical: 0.25% (15 g, 60 g)
Topicort®: 0.25% (15 g, 60 g)

desoxyephedrine hydrochloride *see* methamphetamine *on page 611*
Desoxyn® [US/Can] *see* methamphetamine *on page 611*
desoxyphenobarbital *see* primidone *on page 795*
Desquam-X® [Can] *see* benzoyl peroxide *on page 128*
Desquam-X® 5 [US-OTC] *see* benzoyl peroxide *on page 128*
Desquam-X® 10 [US-OTC] *see* benzoyl peroxide *on page 128*
Desquam-X® Wash *(Discontinued)* *see* benzoyl peroxide *on page 128*
Desquam-E™ *(Discontinued)* *see* benzoyl peroxide *on page 128*
desulfato-hirudin *see* desirudin *on page 277*
desulphatohirudin *see* desirudin *on page 277*

desvenlafaxine (des ven la FAX een)

Synonyms O-desmethylvenlafaxine; ODV

U.S./Canadian Brand Names Pristiq® [US/Can]

Therapeutic Category Antidepressant, Serotonin/Norepinephrine Reuptake Inhibitor

Use Treatment of major depressive disorder

Dosage Summary

Oral:

Children: Dosage not established.
Adults: Initial: 50 mg once daily

Dosage Forms

Tablet, extended release, oral:
Pristiq®: 50 mg, 100 mg

Desyrel® *(Discontinued)* *see* trazodone *on page 950*
Detane® [US-OTC] *see* benzocaine *on page 124*
detemir insulin *see* insulin detemir *on page 510*
Detrol® [US/Can] *see* tolterodine *on page 941*
Detrol® LA [US/Can] *see* tolterodine *on page 941*
detryptoreline *see* triptorelin *on page 962*
Detuss *(Discontinued)*
Detussin® Expectorant *(Discontinued)*

Dex4® [US-OTC] *see* dextrose *on page* 290
Dexacidin® ***(Discontinued)*** *see* neomycin, polymyxin B, and dexamethasone *on page* 666
Dexacine™ ***(Discontinued)*** *see* neomycin, polymyxin B, and dexamethasone *on page* 666

dexamethasone (systemic) (deks a METH a sone)

Sound-Alike/Look-Alike Issues
dexamethasone may be confused with desoximetasone, dextroamphetamine
Decadron® may be confused with Percodan®

Synonyms dexamethasone sodium phosphate

U.S./Canadian Brand Names Apo-Dexamethasone® [Can]; Baycadron™ [US]; Dexamethasone Intensol™ [US]; Dexasone® [Can]; DexPak® 10 Day TaperPak® [US]; DexPak® 13 Day TaperPak® [US]; DexPak® 6 Day TaperPak® [US]

Therapeutic Category Antiemetic; Antiinflammatory Agent; Corticosteroid, Systemic

Use Primarily as an antiinflammatory or immunosuppressant agent in the treatment of a variety of diseases including those of allergic, dermatologic, endocrine, hematologic, inflammatory, neoplastic, nervous system, renal, respiratory, rheumatic, and autoimmune origin; may be used in management of cerebral edema, chronic swelling, as a diagnostic agent, diagnosis of Cushing syndrome, antiemetic

Dosage Summary Note: Dosage varies considerably by indication; ranges listed are representative

I.M.:
Children: 0.03-2 mg/kg/day **or** 0.6-10 mg/m²/day divided every 6-12 hours
Adults: 0.75-9 mg/day **or** 0.03-2 mg/kg/day **or** 0.6-0.75 mg/m²/day in divided doses every 6-12 hours **or** 4 mg every 4-6 hours

I.V.:
Children: 0.03-2 mg/kg/day **or** 0.6-10 mg/m²/day divided every 6-12 hours **or** 5-20 mg prior to chemotherapy
Adults: 0.75-9 mg/day **or** 0.03-2 mg/kg/day **or** 0.6-0.75 mg/m²/day in divided doses every 6-12 hours **or** 4 mg every 4-6 hours **or** 10-20 mg prior to chemotherapy **or** 10 mg every 12 hours **or** 40 mg **or** 1-6 mg/kg every 2-6 hours (shock)

Intra-articular, intralesional, or soft tissue:
Children: Dosage not established
Adults: 0.4-6 mg/day

Oral:
Children: 0.03-2 mg/kg/day **or** 0.6-10 mg/m²/day divided every 6-12 hours
Adults: 0.75-9 mg/day **or** 0.03-2 mg/kg/day **or** 0.6-0.75 mg/m²/day in divided doses every 6-12 hours **or** 10-20 mg prior to chemotherapy **or** 4-10 mg 1-2 times/day **or** 4 mg every 4-6 hours **or** 30 mg /day for 1 week, then 4-12 mg/day (MS) **or** 40 mg once daily (Multiple myeloma)

Dosage Forms
Elixir, oral: 0.5 mg/5 mL (237 mL)
Baycadron™: 0.5 mg/5 mL (237 mL)
Injection, solution: 4 mg/mL (1 mL, 5 mL, 30 mL); 10 mg/mL (1 mL, 10 mL)
Injection, solution [preservative free]: 10 mg/mL (1 mL)
Solution, oral: 0.5 mg/5 mL (240 mL, 500 mL)
Dexamethasone Intensol™: 1 mg/mL (30 mL)
Tablet, oral: 0.5 mg, 0.75 mg, 1 mg, 1.5 mg, 2 mg, 4 mg, 6 mg
DexPak® 6 Day TaperPak®: 1.5 mg
DexPak® 10 Day TaperPak®: 1.5 mg
DexPak® 13 Day TaperPak®: 1.5 mg

dexamethasone (ophthalmic) (deks a METH a sone)

Sound-Alike/Look-Alike Issues
dexamethasone may be confused with desoximetasone, dextroamphetamine
Maxidex® may be confused with Maxzide®

Synonyms dexamethasone sodium phosphate

U.S./Canadian Brand Names Diodex® [Can]; Maxidex® [US/Can]; Ozurdex™ [US]

Therapeutic Category Antiinflammatory Agent, Ophthalmic; Corticosteroid, Ophthalmic

Use Management of steroid responsive inflammatory conditions such as allergic conjunctivitis, iritis, or cyclitis; symptomatic treatment of corneal injury from chemical, radiation, or thermal burns, or penetration of foreign bodies

Ophthalmic intravitreal implant (Ozurdex™): Treatment of macular edema following branch retinal vein occlusion (BRVO) or central retinal vein occlusion (CRVO)

Dosage Summary

Intravitreal:

Children: Dosage not established

Adults: 0.7 mg implant in affected eye

Ophthalmic:

Solution:

Children: Dosage not established

Adults: Instill 1-2 drops into conjunctival sac every hour during the day and every other hour during the night; gradually reduce dose to every 3-4 hours, then to 3-4 times/day

Suspension:

Children: Dosage not established

Adults: Instill 1-2 drops up to 4-6 times/day or hourly in severe cases

Dosage Forms

Implant, intravitreal:

Ozurdex™: 0.7 mg (1s)

Solution, ophthalmic: 0.1% (5 mL)

Suspension, ophthalmic:

Maxidex®: 0.1% (5 mL)

dexamethasone and ciprofloxacin *see* ciprofloxacin and dexamethasone *on page* 225

dexamethasone and tobramycin *see* tobramycin and dexamethasone *on page* 938

Dexamethasone Intensol™ [US] *see* dexamethasone (systemic) *on page* 281

dexamethasone, neomycin, and polymyxin B *see* neomycin, polymyxin B, and dexamethasone *on page* 666

dexamethasone sodium phosphate *see* dexamethasone (ophthalmic) *on page* 281

dexamethasone sodium phosphate *see* dexamethasone (systemic) *on page* 281

Dexasone® [Can] *see* dexamethasone (systemic) *on page* 281

dexbrompheniramine and pseudoephedrine

(deks brom fen EER a meen & soo doe e FED rin)

Synonyms pseudoephedrine and dexbrompheniramine

U.S./Canadian Brand Names Drixoral® [Can]

Therapeutic Category Antihistamine/Decongestant Combination

Use Relief of symptoms of upper respiratory mucosal congestion in seasonal and perennial nasal allergies, acute rhinitis, rhinosinusitis, and eustachian tube blockage

Dosage Summary

Oral:

Children ≤12 years: Dosage not established

Children >12 years: 1 tablet every 8-12 hours

Adults: 1 tablet every 8-12 hours

Dosage Forms

Tablet, sustained action: Dexbrompheniramine 6 mg and pseudoephedrine 120 mg

Dexchlor® ***(Discontinued)*** *see* dexchlorpheniramine *on page* 282

dexchlorpheniramine (deks klor fen EER a meen)

Synonyms dexchlorpheniramine maleate

Therapeutic Category Antihistamine

Use Perennial and seasonal allergic rhinitis and other allergic symptoms including urticaria

Dosage Summary

Oral:

Regular release:

Children <2 years: Dosage not established

Children 2-5 years: 0.5 mg every 4-6 hours

Children 6-11 years: 1 mg every 4-6 hours

Adults: 2 mg every 4-6 hours

Timed release:

Children <5 years: Dosage not established

Children 6-11 years: 4 mg at bedtime

Adults: 4-6 mg at bedtime **or** every 8-10 hours

Dosage Forms

Syrup, oral: 2 mg/5 mL (473 mL, 3840 mL)

dexchlorpheniramine and pseudoephedrine

(deks klor fen EER a meen & soo doe e FED rin)

Synonyms pseudoephedrine tannate and dexchlorpheniramine tannate

Therapeutic Category Alpha/Beta Agonist; Antihistamine

Use Relief of nasal congestion associated with the common cold, hay fever, and other allergies, sinusitis, and vasomotor and allergic rhinitis

Dosage Summary

Oral:

Children <2 years: Dosage not established

Children 2-6 years: AllerDur™ or DuoTan PD: 2.5-5 mL every 12 hours (maximum: 10 mL/day)

Children 6-12 years: AllerDur™ 5-7.5 mL every 12 hours (maximum: 15 mL/24 hours) or DuoTan PD 5-10 mL every 12 hours (maximum: 20 mL/day)

Children ≥12 years: AllerDur™ 15 mL every 12 hours (maximum: 30 mL/24 hours) or DuoTan PD 10-20 mL every 12 hours (maximum: 40 mL/day)

Adults: AllerDur™ 15 mL every 12 hours (maximum: 30 mL/24 hours) or DuoTan PD 10-20 mL every 12 hours (maximum: 40 mL/day)

dexchlorpheniramine maleate *see* dexchlorpheniramine *on page* 282

dexchlorpheniramine tannate, pseudoephedrine tannate, and dextromethorphan tannate *see* chlorpheniramine, pseudoephedrine, and dextromethorphan *on page* 214

Dexcon-DM *(Discontinued)* *see* guaifenesin, dextromethorphan, and phenylephrine *on page* 458

Dexcon-PE *(Discontinued)* *see* guaifenesin, dextromethorphan, and phenylephrine *on page* 458

Dexedrine® [Can] *see* dextroamphetamine *on page* 285

Dexedrine® Spansule® [US] *see* dextroamphetamine *on page* 285

Dexferrum® [US] *see* iron dextran complex *on page* 525

Dexilant™ [US/Can] *see* dexlansoprazole *on page* 283

Dexiron™ [Can] *see* iron dextran complex *on page* 525

dexlansoprazole (deks lan SOE pra zole)

Sound-Alike/Look-Alike Issues

dexlansoprazole may be confused with aripiprazole, lansoprazole

Synonyms TAK-390MR

U.S./Canadian Brand Names Dexilant™ [US/Can]

Therapeutic Category Proton Pump Inhibitor; Substituted Benzimidazole

Use Short-term (4 weeks) treatment of heartburn associated with nonerosive GERD; short-term (up to 8 weeks) treatment of all grades of erosive esophagitis; to maintain healing of erosive esophagitis for up to 6 months

Dosage Summary

Oral:

Children: Dosage not established.

Adults: 30-60 mg once daily

Dosage Forms

Capsule, delayed release, oral:

Dexilant™: 30 mg, 60 mg

dexmedetomidine (deks MED e toe mi deen)

Sound-Alike/Look-Alike Issues

Precedex® may be confused with Peridex®

Synonyms dexmedetomidine hydrochloride

U.S./Canadian Brand Names Precedex® [US/Can]

Therapeutic Category Alpha-Adrenergic Agonist - Central-Acting (Alpha$_2$-Agonists); Sedative

Use Sedation of initially intubated and mechanically ventilated patients during treatment in an intensive care setting; sedation prior to and/or during surgical or other procedures of nonintubated patients

Dosage Summary **Note:** Errors have occurred due to misinterpretation of dosing information. Maintenance dose expressed as mcg/kg/**hour**.

I.V.:
Children: Dosage not established
Adults: Loading infusion: 0.5-1 mcg/kg; Maintenance infusion: 0.2-1 mcg/kg/**hour**

Dosage Forms
Injection, solution [preservative free]:
Precedex®: 100 mcg/mL (2 mL)

dexmedetomidine hydrochloride *see* dexmedetomidine *on page 283*

dexmethylphenidate (dex meth il FEN i date)

Sound-Alike/Look-Alike Issues
dexmethylphenidate may be confused with methadone
Focalin® may be confused with Folotyn™

Synonyms dexmethylphenidate hydrochloride

U.S./Canadian Brand Names Focalin® XR [US]; Focalin® [US]

Therapeutic Category Central Nervous System Stimulant, Nonamphetamine

Controlled Substance C-II

Use Treatment of attention-deficit/hyperactivity disorder (ADHD)

Dosage Summary
Oral:
Extended release:
Children <6 years: Dosage not established
Children ≥6 years: Initial: 5 mg once daily; Maintenance: Up to 30 mg/day; **Note:** Titration is recommended
Adults: Initial: 10 mg once daily; Maintenance: Up to 40 mg/day; **Note:** Titration is recommended
Immediate release:
Children <6 years: Dosage not established
Children ≥6 years: Initial: 2.5 mg twice daily; Maintenance: Up to 20 mg/day in 2 divided doses (at least 4 hours apart); **Note:** Titration is recommended
Adults: Initial: 2.5 mg twice daily; Maintenance: Up to 20 mg/day in 2 divided doses (at least 4 hours apart); **Note:** Titration is recommended

Dosage Forms
Capsule, extended release, oral:
Focalin® XR: 5 mg, 10 mg, 15 mg, 20 mg, 30 mg
Tablet, oral: 2.5 mg, 5 mg, 10 mg
Focalin®: 2.5 mg, 5 mg, 10 mg

dexmethylphenidate hydrochloride *see* dexmethylphenidate *on page 284*
DexPak® 6 Day TaperPak® [US] *see* dexamethasone (systemic) *on page 281*
DexPak® 10 Day TaperPak® [US] *see* dexamethasone (systemic) *on page 281*
DexPak® 13 Day TaperPak® [US] *see* dexamethasone (systemic) *on page 281*
DexPak® TaperPak® *(Discontinued)* *see* dexamethasone (systemic) *on page 281*

dexpanthenol (deks PAN the nole)

Synonyms pantothenyl alcohol

Therapeutic Category Gastrointestinal Agent, Stimulant

Use Prophylactic use to minimize paralytic ileus; treatment of postoperative distention; topical to relieve itching and to aid healing of minor dermatoses

Dosage Summary
I.M.:
Children: Dosage not established
Adults: Initial: 250-500 mg; repeat in 2 hours, followed by doses every 6 hours if needed

Dosage Forms
Injection, solution [preservative free]: 250 mg/mL (2 mL)

Dex PC [US] *see* chlorpheniramine, phenylephrine, and dextromethorphan *on page 211*

dexrazoxane (deks ray ZOKS ane)

Sound-Alike/Look-Alike Issues
Zinecard® may be confused with Gemzar®

Synonyms ICRF-187

U.S./Canadian Brand Names Totect® [US]; Zinecard® [US/Can]

Therapeutic Category Cardiovascular Agent, Other

Use

Zinecard®: Reduction of the incidence and severity of cardiomyopathy associated with doxorubicin administration in women with metastatic breast cancer who have received a cumulative doxorubicin dose of 300 mg/m^2 and who would benefit from continuing therapy with doxorubicin. (Not recommended for use with initial doxorubicin therapy.)

Totect®: Treatment of anthracycline-induced extravasation.

Dosage Summary

I.V.:

Children: Dosage not established

Adults:

Prevention of cardiomyopathy: A 10:1 ratio of dexrazoxane:doxorubicin (500 mg/m^2 dexrazoxane: 50 mg/m^2 doxorubicin)

Anthracycline-induced extravasation: 1000 mg/m^2 on days 1 and 2 (maximum dose: 2000 mg), followed by 500 mg/m^2 on day 3 (maximum dose: 1000 mg)

Dosage Forms

Injection, powder for reconstitution: 250 mg, 500 mg

Totect®: 500 mg

Zinecard®: 250 mg, 500 mg

dextran (DEKS tran)

Sound-Alike/Look-Alike Issues

dextran may be confused with Dexatrim®, Dexedrine®

Synonyms dextran 40; dextran 70; dextran, high molecular weight; dextran, low molecular weight

U.S./Canadian Brand Names LMD® [US]

Therapeutic Category Plasma Volume Expander

Use Blood volume expander used in treatment of shock or impending shock when blood or blood products are not available; dextran 40 is also used as a priming fluid in cardiopulmonary bypass and for prophylaxis of venous thrombosis and pulmonary embolism in surgical procedures associated with a high risk of thromboembolic complications

Dosage Summary

I.V.:

Dextran 40:

Children: Total dose should not exceed 20 mL/kg during first 24 hours

Adults: 500-1000 mL at a rate of 20-40 mL/minute (maximum: 20 mL/kg/day for first 24 hours); 10 mL/kg/day thereafter (5 days total therapy) **or** 50-100 g on the day of surgery, then 50 g (4 mL/minute) every 2-3 days during the period of risk

Dextran 70:

Children: Total dose should not exceed 20 mL/kg during first 24 hours

Adults: 500-1000 mL at a rate of 20-40 mL/minute (maximum: 20 mL/kg/day for first 24 hours)

Dosage Forms

Infusion, premixed in D$_5$W:

LMD®: 10% Dextran 40 (500 mL)

Infusion, premixed in NS:

LMD®: 10% Dextran 40 (500 mL)

dextran 1 ***(Discontinued)***

dextran 40 *see* dextran *on page 285*

dextran 70 *see* dextran *on page 285*

dextran, high molecular weight *see* dextran *on page 285*

dextran, low molecular weight *see* dextran *on page 285*

dextroamphetamine (deks troe am FET a meen)

Sound-Alike/Look-Alike Issues

dextroamphetamine may be confused with dexamethasone

Dexedrine® may be confused with dextran, Excedrin®

Synonyms dextroamphetamine sulfate

U.S./Canadian Brand Names Dexedrine® Spansule® [US]; Dexedrine® [Can]; DextroStat® [US]
Therapeutic Category Amphetamine
Controlled Substance C-II
Use Narcolepsy; attention-deficit/hyperactivity disorder (ADHD)
Dosage Summary
Oral:
Children <3 years: Dosage not established
Children 3-5 years: ADHD: Initial: 2.5 mg once daily; Maintenance: 0.1-0.5 mg/kg once daily (maximum: 40 mg/day); **Note:** Titration is recommended
Children 6-12 years: Initial: 5 mg once or twice daily; Maintenance: 5-20 mg (0.1-0.5 mg/kg) once daily (maximum: 40 mg [ADHD]: 60 mg [narcolepsy]); **Note:** Titration is recommended
Children >12 years: Initial: 5-10 mg/day in 1-2 divided doses; Maintenance: Up to 40 mg/day [ADHD] or 60 mg/day [narcolepsy]; **Note:** Titration is recommended
Adults: Initial: 10 mg once daily; Maintenance: Up to 60 mg/day; **Note:** Titration is recommended
Dosage Forms
Capsule, extended release, oral: 5 mg, 10 mg, 15 mg
Capsule, sustained release, oral:
Dexedrine® Spansule®: 5 mg, 10 mg, 15 mg
Tablet, oral: 5 mg, 10 mg
DextroStat®: 5 mg, 10 mg

dextroamphetamine and amphetamine (deks troe am FET a meen & am FET a meen)

Sound-Alike/Look-Alike Issues
Adderall® may be confused with Inderal®
Synonyms amphetamine and dextroamphetamine
U.S./Canadian Brand Names Adderall XR® [US/Can]; Adderall® [US]
Therapeutic Category Amphetamine
Controlled Substance C-II
Use Attention-deficit/hyperactivity disorder (ADHD); narcolepsy
Dosage Summary
Oral:
Extended release:
Children <5 years: Dosage not established
Children 6-12 years: ADHD: Initial: 5-10 mg once daily; Maintenance: Up to 30 mg/day; **Note:** Titration is recommended
Adolescents 13-17 years: ADHD: Initial: 10 mg once daily; Maintenance: 10-20 mg once daily; **Note:** Doses up to 60 mg/day have been used, but no evidence of additional benefit
Adults: ADHD: 20 mg once daily; **Note:** Doses up to 60 mg/day have been used, but no evidence of additional benefit
Immediate release:
Children <3 years: Dosage not established
Children 3-5 years: ADHD: Initial: 2.5 mg once daily; Maintenance: Up to 40 mg/day in 1-3 divided doses; **Note:** Titration is recommended
Children 6-12 years: Initial: 5 mg once or twice daily; Maintenance: Up to 40 mg/day [ADHD] or 60 mg/day [narcolepsy] in 1-3 divided doses; **Note:** Titration is recommended
Children >12 years: Initial: 5-10 mg in 1-2 divided doses; Maintenance: Up to 40 mg/day [ADHD] or 60 mg/day [narcolepsy] in 1-3 divided doses; **Note:** Titration is recommended
Adults: Initial: 5-10 mg in 1-2 divided doses; Maintenance: Up to 40 mg/day [ADHD] or 60 mg/day [narcolepsy] in 1-3 divided doses; **Note:** Titration is recommended
Dosage Forms
Capsule, extended release:
5 mg [dextroamphetamine sulfate 1.25 mg, dextroamphetamine saccharate 1.25 mg, amphetamine aspartate monohydrate 1.25 mg, amphetamine sulfate 1.25 mg]
10 mg [dextroamphetamine sulfate 2.5 mg, dextroamphetamine saccharate 2.5 mg, amphetamine aspartate monohydrate 2.5 mg, amphetamine sulfate 2.5 mg]
15 mg [dextroamphetamine sulfate 3.75 mg, dextroamphetamine saccharate 3.75 mg, amphetamine aspartate monohydrate 3.75 mg, amphetamine sulfate 3.75 mg]
20 mg [dextroamphetamine sulfate 5 mg, dextroamphetamine saccharate 5 mg, amphetamine aspartate monohydrate 5 mg, amphetamine sulfate 5 mg]

25 mg [dextroamphetamine sulfate 6.25 mg, dextroamphetamine saccharate 6.25 mg, amphetamine aspartate monohydrate 6.25 mg, amphetamine sulfate 6.25 mg]
30 mg [dextroamphetamine sulfate 7.5 mg, dextroamphetamine saccharate 7.5 mg, amphetamine aspartate monohydrate 7.5 mg, amphetamine sulfate 7.5 mg]
Adderall XR®:
5 mg [dextroamphetamine 1.25 mg, dextroamphetamine saccharate 1.25 mg, amphetamine aspartate monohydrate 1.25 mg, amphetamine sulfate 1.25 mg]
10 mg [dextroamphetamine sulfate 2.5 mg, dextroamphetamine saccharate 2.5 mg, amphetamine aspartate monohydrate 2.5 mg, amphetamine sulfate 2.5 mg]
15 mg [dextroamphetamine sulfate 3.75 mg, dextroamphetamine saccharate 3.75 mg, amphetamine aspartate monohydrate 3.75 mg, amphetamine sulfate 3.75 mg]
20 mg [dextroamphetamine sulfate 5 mg, dextroamphetamine saccharate 5 mg, amphetamine aspartate monohydrate 5 mg, amphetamine sulfate 5 mg]
25 mg [dextroamphetamine sulfate 6.25 mg, dextroamphetamine saccharate 6.25 mg, amphetamine aspartate monohydrate 6.25 mg, amphetamine sulfate 6.25 mg]
30 mg [dextroamphetamine sulfate 7.5 mg, dextroamphetamine saccharate 7.5 mg, amphetamine aspartate monohydrate 7.5 mg, amphetamine sulfate 7.5 mg]

Tablet: 5 mg, 7.5 mg, 10 mg, 12.5 mg, 15 mg, 20 mg, 30 mg
5 mg [dextroamphetamine sulfate 1.25 mg, dextroamphetamine saccharate 1.25 mg, amphetamine aspartate monohydrate 1.25 mg, amphetamine sulfate 1.25 mg]
7.5 mg [dextroamphetamine sulfate 1.875 mg, dextroamphetamine saccharate 1.875 mg, amphetamine aspartate monohydrate 1.875 mg, amphetamine sulfate 1.875 mg]
10 mg [dextroamphetamine sulfate 2.5 mg, dextroamphetamine saccharate 2.5 mg, amphetamine aspartate monohydrate 2.5 mg, amphetamine sulfate 2.5 mg]
12.5 mg [dextroamphetamine sulfate 3.125 mg, dextroamphetamine saccharate 3.125 mg, amphetamine aspartate monohydrate 3.125 mg, amphetamine sulfate 3.125 mg]
15 mg [dextroamphetamine sulfate 3.75 mg, dextroamphetamine saccharate 3.75 mg, amphetamine aspartate monohydrate 3.75 mg, amphetamine sulfate 3.75 mg]
20 mg [dextroamphetamine sulfate 5 mg, dextroamphetamine saccharate 5 mg, amphetamine aspartate monohydrate 5 mg, amphetamine sulfate 5 mg]
30 mg [dextroamphetamine sulfate 7.5 mg, dextroamphetamine saccharate 7.5 mg, amphetamine aspartate monohydrate 7.5 mg, amphetamine sulfate 7.5 mg]
Adderall®:
5 mg [dextroamphetamine sulfate 1.25 mg, dextroamphetamine saccharate 1.25 mg, amphetamine aspartate monohydrate 1.25 mg, amphetamine sulfate 1.25 mg]
7.5 mg [dextroamphetamine 1.875 mg, dextroamphetamine saccharate 1.875 mg, amphetamine aspartate monohydrate 1.875 mg, amphetamine sulfate 1.875 mg]
10 mg [dextroamphetamine sulfate 2.5 mg, dextroamphetamine saccharate 2.5 mg, amphetamine aspartate monohydrate 2.5 mg, amphetamine sulfate 2.5 mg]
12.5 mg [dextroamphetamine sulfate 3.125 mg, dextroamphetamine saccharate 3.125 mg, amphetamine aspartate monohydrate 3.125 mg, amphetamine sulfate 3.125 mg]
15 mg [dextroamphetamine sulfate 3.75 mg, dextroamphetamine saccharate 3.75 mg, amphetamine aspartate monohydrate 3.75 mg, amphetamine sulfate 3.75 mg]
20 mg [dextroamphetamine sulfate 5 mg, dextroamphetamine saccharate 5 mg, amphetamine aspartate monohydrate 5 mg, amphetamine sulfate 5 mg]
30 mg [dextroamphetamine sulfate 7.5 mg, dextroamphetamine saccharate 7.5 mg, amphetamine aspartate monohydrate 7.5 mg, amphetamine sulfate 7.5 mg]

dextroamphetamine sulfate *see* dextroamphetamine *on page 285*

dextromethorphan (deks troe meth OR fan)

Sound-Alike/Look-Alike Issues
Benylin® may be confused with Benadryl®, Ventolin®
Delsym® may be confused with Delfen®, Desyrel®

U.S./Canadian Brand Names Creo-Terpin® [US-OTC]; Creomulsion® Adult Formula [US-OTC]; Creomulsion® for Children [US-OTC]; Delsym® [US-OTC]; Father John's® [US-OTC]; Hold® DM [US-OTC]; Nycoff [US-OTC]; PediaCare® Children's Long-Acting Cough [US-OTC]; Robafen Cough [US-OTC]; Robitussin® Children's Cough Long Acting [US-OTC]; Robitussin® Cough Long-Acting [US-OTC]; Robitussin® CoughGels™ Long-Acting [US-OTC]; Scot-Tussin® Diabetes [US-OTC]; Silphen DM® [US-OTC]; Triaminic® Children's Cough Long Acting [US-OTC]; Triaminic® Thin Strips® Children's Long Acting Cough [US-OTC]; Trocal® [US-OTC]; Vicks® 44® Cough Relief [US-OTC]; Vicks® DayQuil® Cough [US-OTC]

Therapeutic Category Antitussive

Use Symptomatic relief of coughs caused by the common cold or inhaled irritants

Dosage Summary

Oral:

Extended release:

Children <4 years: Not for OTC use

Children 4-6 years: 15 mg twice daily (maximum: 30 mg/day)

Children 6-12 years: 30 mg twice daily (maximum: 60 mg/day)

Children >12 years: 60 mg twice daily (maximum: 120 mg/day)

Adults: 60 mg twice daily (maximum: 120 mg/day)

Immediate release:

Children <4 years: Not for OTC use

Children 4-6 years: 2.5-7.5 mg every 4-8 hours (maximum: 30 mg/day)

Children 6-12 years: 5-10 mg every 4 hours **or** 15 mg every 6-8 hours (maximum: 60 mg/day)

Children >12 years: 10-20 mg every 4 hours **or** 30 mg every 6-8 hours (maximum: 120 mg/day)

Adults: 10-20 mg every 4 hours **or** 30 mg every 6-8 hours (maximum: 120 mg/day)

Dosage Forms

Capsule, liquid filled, oral:

Robafen Cough [OTC]: 15 mg

Robitussin® CoughGels™ Long-Acting [OTC]: 15 mg

Liquid, oral: 15 mg/5 mL (120 mL)

Creo-Terpin® [OTC]: 10 mg/15 mL (120 mL)

Scot-Tussin® Diabetes [OTC]: 10 mg/5 mL (118 mL)

Vicks® 44® Cough Relief [OTC]: 10 mg/5 mL (120 mL)

Lozenge, oral:

Hold® DM [OTC]: 5 mg (10s)

Trocal® [OTC]: 7.5 mg (50s, 300s)

Solution, oral:

PediaCare® Children's Long-Acting Cough [OTC]: 7.5 mg/5 mL (118 mL)

Vicks® DayQuil® Cough [OTC]: 15 mg/15 mL (177 mL, 295 mL)

Strip, orally disintegrating, oral:

Triaminic Thin Strips® Children's Long Acting Cough [OTC]: 7.5 mg (14s, 16s)

Suspension, extended release, oral:

Delsym® [OTC]: Dextromethorphan polistirex [equivalent to dextromethorphan hydrobromide] 30 mg/5 mL (89 mL, 148 mL)

Syrup, oral:

Creomulsion® Adult Formula [OTC]: 20 mg/15 mL (120 mL)

Creomulsion® for Children [OTC]: 5 mg/5 mL (120 mL)

Father John's® [OTC]: 10 mg/5 mL (118 mL, 236 mL)

Robitussin® Children's Cough Long-Acting [OTC]: 7.5 mg/5 mL (118 mL)

Robitussin® Cough Long Acting [OTC]: 15 mg/5 mL (240 mL)

Silphen-DM [OTC]: 10 mg/5 mL (120 mL)

Triaminic® Children's Cough Long Acting [OTC]: 7.5 mg/5 mL (118 mL)

Tablet, oral:

Nycoff [OTC]: 15 mg

dextromethorphan and chlorpheniramine (deks troe meth OR fan & klor fen IR a meen)

Synonyms chlorpheniramine and dextromethorphan; chlorpheniramine maleate and dextromethorphan hydrobromide; dextromethorphan hydrobromide and chlorpheniramine maleate

U.S./Canadian Brand Names Coricidin® HBP Cough & Cold [US-OTC]; Dimetapp® Children's Long Acting Cough Plus Cold [US-OTC]; Robitussin® Children's Cough & Cold Long-Acting [US-OTC]; Robitussin® Cough & Cold Long-Acting [US-OTC]; Scot-Tussin® DM Maximum Strength [US-OTC]; Triaminic® Children's Softchews® Cough & Runny Nose [US-OTC]

Therapeutic Category Antitussive; Histamine H_1 Antagonist; Histamine H_1 Antagonist, First Generation

Use Symptomatic relief of runny nose, sneezing, itchy/watery eyes, cough, and other upper respiratory symptoms associated with hay fever, common cold, or upper respiratory allergies

Dosage Summary

Oral:

Children <6 years: Dosage not established

Children 6-11 years: Dextromethorphan 10-15 mg and chlorpheniramine 2 mg every 4-6 hours as needed (maximum: 60 mg dextromethorphan and 10 mg chlorpheniramine/24 hours)

Children ≥12 years: Dextromethorphan 30 mg and chlorpheniramine 4 mg every 6 hours as needed (maximum: 120 mg dextromethorphan and 16 mg chlorpheniramine/24 hours)

Adults: Dextromethorphan 30 mg and chlorpheniramine 4 mg every 6 hours as needed (maximum: 120 mg dextromethorphan and 16 mg chlorpheniramine/24 hours)

Dosage Forms

Syrup:

Dimetapp® Children's Long Acting Cough Plus Cold [OTC]: Dextromethorphan 7.5 mg and chlorpheniramine 1 mg per 5 mL (118 mL)

Robitussin® Children's Cough and Cold Long-Acting [OTC]: Dextromethorphan 15 mg and chlorpheniramine 2 mg per 5 mL (118 mL)

Robitussin® Cough and Cold Long-Acting [OTC]: Dextromethorphan 15 mg and chlorpheniramine 2 mg per 5 mL (118 mL)

Scot-Tussin® DM Maximum Strength [OTC]: Dextromethorphan 15 mg and chlorpheniramine 2 mg per 5 mL (118 mL)

Tablet:

Coricidin® HBP Cough and Cold [OTC]: Dextromethorphan 30 mg and chlorpheniramine 4 mg

Tablet, softchew:

Triaminic® Children's Softchews® Cough & Runny Nose [OTC]: Dextromethorphan 5 mg and chlorpheniramine 1 mg

dextromethorphan and guaifenesin *see* guaifenesin and dextromethorphan *on page* 455

dextromethorphan and phenylephrine (deks troe meth OR fan & fen il EF rin)

Synonyms dextromethorphan hydrobromide and phenylephrine hydrochloride; phenylephrine and dextromethorphan

U.S./Canadian Brand Names PediaCare® Children's Multi-Symptom Cold [US-OTC]; Safetussin® CD [US-OTC]; Sudafed PE® Children's Cold & Cough [US-OTC]; Triaminic Thin Strips® Children's Day Time Cold & Cough [US-OTC]; Triaminic® Day Time Cold & Cough [US-OTC]

Therapeutic Category Antitussive; Decongestant

Use Temporary relief of symptoms of hay fever, the common cold, and upper respiratory allergies including sinus/nasal congestion, minor bronchial/throat irritation, and cough

Dosage Summary

Oral:

Children <4 years: Dosage not established

Children 4-6 years: PediaCare® Children's Multi-Symptom Cold, Sudafed PE® Children's Cold & Cough, Triaminic® Day Time Cold & Cough: 5 mL every 4 hours as needed (maximum: 30 mL/24 hours); Triaminic Thin Strips® Children's Day Time Cold & Cough: Allow 1 strip to dissolve on tongue every 4 hours as needed (maximum: 6 strips/24 hours)

Children 6-12 years: PediaCare® Children's Multi-Symptom Cold, Sudafed PE® Children's Cold & Cough, Triaminic® Day Time Cold & Cough: 10 mL every 4 hours as needed (maximum: 60 mL/24 hours); Safetussin® CD: 5 mL every 6 hours as needed (maximum: 20 mL/24 hours); Triaminic Thin Strips® Children's Day Time Cold & Cough: Allow 2 strips to dissolve on tongue every 4 hours as needed (maximum: 12 strips/24 hours)

Children ≥12 years: Safetussin® CD: 10 mL every 6 hours as needed (maximum: 40 mL/24 hours)

Adults: Safetussin® CD: 10 mL every 6 hours as needed (maximum: 40 mL/24 hours)

Dosage Forms

Liquid, oral:

Sudafed PE® Children's Cold + Cough [OTC]: Dextromethorphan 5 mg and phenylephrine 2.5 mg per 5 mL (118 mL)

Strip, orally disintegrating:

Triaminic Thin Strips® Children's Day Time Cold & Cough [OTC]: Dextromethorphan bromide 5 mg and phenylephrine 2.5 mg (14s, 16s, 48s)

Syrup:

PediaCare® Children's Multi-Symptom Cold [OTC], Triaminic® Day Time Cold & Cough [OTC]: Dextromethorphan 5 mg and phenylephrine 2.5 mg per 5 mL

Safetussin® CD [OTC]: Dextromethorphan 15 mg and phenylephrine 2.5 mg per 5 mL

dextromethorphan and promethazine *see* promethazine and dextromethorphan *on page* 801

dextromethorphan and pseudoephedrine *see* pseudoephedrine and dextromethorphan *on page* 812

dextromethorphan, chlorpheniramine, and phenylephrine *see* chlorpheniramine, phenylephrine, and dextromethorphan *on page* 211

dextromethorphan, chlorpheniramine, and pseudoephedrine *see* chlorpheniramine, pseudoephedrine, and dextromethorphan *on page 214*

dextromethorphan, chlorpheniramine, phenylephrine, and guaifenesin

(deks troe meth OR fan, klor fen IR a meen, fen il EF rin, & gwye FEN e sin)

Synonyms chlorpheniramine, dextromethorphan, phenylephrine, and guaifenesin; guaifenesin, chlorpheniramine, phenylephrine, and dextromethorphan; phenylephrine hydrochloride, chlorpheniramine maleate, dextromethorphan hydrobromide, and guaifenesin

U.S./Canadian Brand Names Chlordex GP [US]; Donatussin [US]; Quartuss™ [US]

Therapeutic Category Antihistamine/Decongestant/Antitussive/Expectorant

Use Symptomatic relief of dry, nonproductive cough and upper respiratory symptoms associated with infections such as the common cold, bronchitis, or sinusitis

Dosage Summary

Oral:

Children <2 year: Dosage not established
Children 2-6 years: 2.5 mL every 6 hours as needed (maximum: 10 mL/24 hours)
Children 6-12 years: 5 mL every 6 hours as needed (maximum: 20 mL/24 hours)
Children ≥12 years: 10 mL every 6 hours as needed (maximum: 40 mL/24 hours)
Adults: 10 mL every 6 hours as needed (maximum: 40 mL/24 hours)

Dosage Forms

Syrup:

Chlordex GP: Dextromethorphan 7.5 mg, chlorpheniramine 2 mg, phenylephrine 10 mg, and guaifenesin 100 mg per 5 mL (480 mL)

Donatussin, Quartuss™: Dextromethorphan 15 mg, chlorpheniramine 2 mg, phenylephrine 10 mg, and guaifenesin 100 mg per 5 mL (480 mL)

dextromethorphan, guaifenesin, and pseudoephedrine *see* guaifenesin, pseudoephedrine, and dextromethorphan *on page 460*

dextromethorphan hydrobromide, acetaminophen, and doxylamine succinate *see* acetaminophen, dextromethorphan, and doxylamine *on page 29*

dextromethorphan hydrobromide, acetaminophen, and phenylephrine hydrochloride *see* acetaminophen, dextromethorphan, and phenylephrine *on page 29*

dextromethorphan hydrobromide, acetaminophen, doxylamine succinate, and pseudoephedrine hydrochloride *see* acetaminophen, dextromethorphan, doxylamine, and pseudoephedrine *on page 30*

dextromethorphan hydrobromide and chlorpheniramine maleate *see* dextromethorphan and chlorpheniramine *on page 288*

dextromethorphan hydrobromide and phenylephrine hydrochloride *see* dextromethorphan and phenylephrine *on page 289*

dextromethorphan hydrobromide, brompheniramine maleate, and pseudoephedrine hydrochloride *see* brompheniramine, pseudoephedrine, and dextromethorphan *on page 149*

dextromethorphan hydrobromide, guaifenesin, and phenylephrine hydrochloride *see* guaifenesin, dextromethorphan, and phenylephrine *on page 458*

dextromethorphan tannate, pyrilamine tannate, and phenylephrine tannate *see* phenylephrine, pyrilamine, and dextromethorphan *on page 755*

dextropropoxyphene *see* propoxyphene *on page 805*

dextrose (DEKS trose)

Sound-Alike/Look-Alike Issues

Glutose™ may be confused with Glutofac®

Synonyms anhydrous glucose; $D_{10}W$; $D_{25}W$; $D_{30}W$; $D_{40}W$; $D_{50}W$; D_5W; $D_{60}W$; $D_{70}W$; dextrose monohydrate; glucose; glucose monohydrate; glycosum

U.S./Canadian Brand Names BD™ Glucose [US-OTC]; Dex4® [US-OTC]; Enfamil® Glucose [US-OTC]; GlucoBurst® [US-OTC]; Glutol™ [US-OTC]; Glutose 15™ [US-OTC]; Glutose 45™ [US-OTC]; Insta-Glucose® [US-OTC]; Similac® Glucose [US-OTC]

Therapeutic Category Antidote, Hypoglycemia; Intravenous Nutritional Therapy

Use

Oral: Treatment of hypoglycemia

5% and 10% solutions: Peripheral infusion to provide calories and fluid replacement

25% (hypertonic) solution: Treatment of acute symptomatic episodes of hypoglycemia in infants and children to restore depressed blood glucose levels; adjunctive treatment of hyperkalemia when combined with insulin

50% (hypertonic) solution: Treatment of insulin-induced hypoglycemia (hyperinsulinemia or insulin shock) and adjunctive treatment of hyperkalemia in adolescents and adults

≥10% solutions: Infusion after admixture with amino acids for nutritional support

Dosage Summary

I.V.:

Infants ≤6 months: 0.25-1 g/kg/dose (maximum: 25 g/dose)

Children >6 months to 12 years: 0.5-1 g/kg/dose (maximum: 25 g/dose)

Adolescents: 10-50 g/dose

Adults: 10-50 g/dose

Oral:

Children ≤2 years: Dosage not established

Children >2 years: 10-20 g as a single dose, may repeat if needed

Adults: 10-20 g as a single dose, may repeat if needed

Dosage Forms

Gel, oral:

Dex4® [OTC]: 40% (38 g)

GlucoBurst® [OTC]: 40% (37.5 g)

Glutose 15™ [OTC]: 40% (37.5 g)

Glutose 45™ [OTC]: 40% (112.5 g)

Insta-Glucose® [OTC]: 40% (31 g)

Infusion: 5% (25 mL, 50 mL, 100 mL, 150 mL, 250 mL, 500 mL, 1000 mL); 10% (150 mL, 250 mL, 500 mL, 1000 mL); 20% (500 mL, 1000 mL); 30% (500 mL, 1000 mL); 40% (500 mL, 1000 mL); 50% (50 mL, 500 mL, 1000 mL, 2000 mL, 5000 mL); 60% (500 mL, 1000 mL); 70% (250 mL, 500 mL, 1000 mL, 2000 mL)

Injection, solution: 10% (3 mL, 5 mL); 25% (10 mL); 50% (50 mL)

Liquid, oral:

Dex4® [OTC]: 15 g/60 mL (60 mL)

Solution, oral:

Enfamil® Glucose [OTC]: 5% (89 mL); 10% (89 mL)

Glutol™ [OTC]: 55% (180 mL)

Similac® Glucose [OTC]: 5% (59 mL); 10% (59 mL)

Tablet, chewable, oral:

BD™ Glucose [OTC]: 5 g

Dex4® [OTC]: 4 g

GlucoBurst® [OTC]: 5 g

dextrose, levulose and phosphoric acid *see* fructose, dextrose, and phosphoric acid *on page 430*

dextrose monohydrate *see* dextrose *on page 290*

DextroStat® [US] *see* dextroamphetamine *on page 285*

Dex-Tuss [US] *see* guaifenesin and codeine *on page 455*

Dey-Dose® Isoproterenol *(Discontinued)* *see* isoproterenol *on page 528*

Dey-Dose® Metaproterenol *(Discontinued)*

dezocitidine *see* decitabine *on page 272*

DFMO *see* eflornithine *on page 344*

DHAD *see* mitoxantrone *on page 638*

DHAQ *see* mitoxantrone *on page 638*

DHC® *(Discontinued)* *see* hydrocodone and acetaminophen *on page 479*

DHC Plus® *(Discontinued)*

DHE *see* dihydroergotamine *on page 305*

D.H.E. 45® [US] *see* dihydroergotamine *on page 305*

DHPG sodium *see* ganciclovir (systemic) *on page 437*

DHS™ Sal [US-OTC] *see* salicylic acid *on page 858*

DHS® Tar [US-OTC] *see* coal tar *on page 242*

DHS™ Tar Gel [US-OTC] *see* coal tar *on page 242*

DHS™ Zinc [US-OTC] *see* pyrithione zinc *on page 819*

DHT™ *(Discontinued)*

DHT™ Intensol™ *(Discontinued)*
DiabetAid® Antifungal Foot Bath [US-OTC] *see* miconazole (topical) *on page 630*
DiabetAid® Pain and Tingling Relief [US-OTC] *see* capsaicin *on page 175*
DiabetAid Therapeutic Gingivitis Mouth Rinse [US-OTC] *see* cetylpyridinium *on page 199*
Diabetic Siltussin DAS-Na [US-OTC] *see* guaifenesin *on page 454*
Diabetic Siltussin-DM DAS-Na [US-OTC] *see* guaifenesin and dextromethorphan *on page 455*
Diabetic Siltussin-DM DAS-Na Maximum Strength [US-OTC] *see* guaifenesin and dextromethorphan *on page 455*
Diabetic Tussin® DM [US-OTC] *see* guaifenesin and dextromethorphan *on page 455*
Diabetic Tussin® DM Maximum Strength [US-OTC] *see* guaifenesin and dextromethorphan *on page 455*
Diabetic Tussin® EX [US-OTC] *see* guaifenesin *on page 454*
Diabetic Tussin® for Children Allergy Relief [US-OTC] *see* chlorpheniramine *on page 207*
Diabinese® *(Discontinued)* *see* chlorpropamide *on page 217*
Diaβeta® [US/Can] *see* glyburide *on page 448*
Dialose® Tablet *(Discontinued)* *see* docusate *on page 321*
Dialume® *(Discontinued)* *see* aluminum hydroxide *on page 58*
Diamicron® [Can] *see* gliclazide *(Canada only) on page 445*
Diamicron® MR [Can] *see* gliclazide *(Canada only) on page 445*
Diamine T.D.® *(Discontinued)* *see* brompheniramine *on page 147*
diaminocyclohexane oxalatoplatinum *see* oxaliplatin *on page 711*
diaminodiphenylsulfone *see* dapsone (systemic) *on page 268*
diaminodiphenylsulfone *see* dapsone (topical) *on page 268*
Diamode [US-OTC] *see* loperamide *on page 573*
Diamox® [Can] *see* acetazolamide *on page 32*
Diamox® 250 mg Tablet *(Discontinued)* *see* acetazolamide *on page 32*
Diamox® Sequels® [US] *see* acetazolamide *on page 32*
Diane-35® [Can] *see* cyproterone and ethinyl estradiol *(Canada only) on page 261*
Diar-aid® *(Discontinued)* *see* loperamide *on page 573*
Diarr-Eze [Can] *see* loperamide *on page 573*
Diastat® [US/Can] *see* diazepam *on page 294*
Diastat® AcuDial™ [US] *see* diazepam *on page 294*
Diastat® Rectal Delivery System [Can] *see* diazepam *on page 294*

diatrizoate meglumine (dye a tri ZOE ate MEG loo meen)

U.S./Canadian Brand Names Cystografin® Dilute [US]; Cystografin® [US]

Therapeutic Category Iodinated Contrast Media; Radiological/Contrast Media, Ionic

Use

Solution for instillation: Retrograde cystourethrography; retrograde or ascending pyelography

Solution for injection: Arthrography, cerebral angiography, direct cholangiography, discography, drip infusion pyelography, excretory urography, peripheral arteriography, splenoportography, venography; contrast enhancement of computed tomographic head and body imaging

Dosage Forms

Solution, for instillation:

Cystografin®: 30% (100 mL, 300 mL)

Cystografin® Dilute: 18% (300 mL)

diatrizoate meglumine and diatrizoate sodium

(dye a tri ZOE ate MEG loo meen & dye a tri ZOE ate SOW dee um)

Synonyms diatrizoate sodium and diatrizoate meglumine

U.S./Canadian Brand Names Gastrografin® [US]; MD-76®R [US]; MD-Gastroview® [US]

Therapeutic Category Iodinated Contrast Media; Radiological/Contrast Media, Ionic

Use

Oral/rectal: Examination of GI tract; adjunct to contrast enhancement in computed tomography of the torso

Injection: Angiocardiography, aortography, central venography, cerebral angiography, cholangiography, digital arteriography, excretory urography, nephrotomography, peripheral angiography, peripheral arteriography, renal arteriography, renal venography, splenoportography, visceral arteriography; contrast enhancement of computed tomographic imaging

Dosage Summary

Oral:

Children <5 years: 30 mL, dilute 1:1 (if <10 kg or debilitated, dilute 1:3)
Children 5-10 years: 60 mL, dilute 1:1 (if <10 kg or debilitated, dilute 1:3)
Adults: 30-90 mL **or** 25-77 mL in 1000 mL tap water

Rectal:

Children <5 years: Dilute 1:5 in tap water
Children ≥5 years: Dilute 90 mL in 500 mL tap water
Adults: Dilute 240 mL in 1000 mL tap water

Dosage Forms

Solution, injection:

MD-76®R: Diatrizoate meglumine 660 mg and diatrizoate sodium 100 mg per 1 mL (50 mL, 100 mL, 200 mL)

Solution, oral/rectal:

Gastrografin®: Diatrizoate meglumine 660 mg and diatrizoate sodium 100 mg per 1 mL
MD-Gastroview®: Diatrizoate meglumine 660 mg and diatrizoate sodium 100 mg per 1 mL

diatrizoate meglumine and iodipamide meglumine

(dye a tri ZOE ate MEG loo meen & eye oh DI pa mide MEG loo meen)

Synonyms iodipamide meglumine and diatrizoate meglumine

U.S./Canadian Brand Names Sinografin® [US]

Therapeutic Category Iodinated Contrast Media; Radiological/Contrast Media, Ionic

Use Hysterosalpingography

Dosage Summary

Intrauterine:

Children: Dosage not established
Adults: Usual dose: 3-4 mL; Total dosage range: 1.5-10 mL

Dosage Forms

Injection, solution [for intrauterine instillation]:

Sinografin®: Diatrizoate meglumine 524 mg and iodipamide meglumine 268 mg per mL (10 mL)

diatrizoate sodium (dye a tri ZOE ate SOW dee um)

U.S./Canadian Brand Names Hypaque™ Sodium [US]

Therapeutic Category Iodinated Contrast Media; Radiological/Contrast Media, Ionic

Use Radiographic examination of GI tract

Dosage Summary

Oral:

Infants: 20% to 40% solution: 30-75 mL
Children: 20% to 40% solution: 30-75 mL
Adults: 25% to 40% solution: 90-180 mL

Rectal: Enema:

Infants: 10% to 15% solution: 100-500 mL depending on weight of patient
Children: 10% to 15% solution: 100-500 mL depending on weight of patient
Adults: 15% to 25% solution: 500-1000 mL

Dosage Forms

Powder for solution, oral/rectal:

Hypaque™ Sodium: 100% (250 g)

diatrizoate sodium and diatrizoate meglumine *see* diatrizoate meglumine and diatrizoate sodium *on page* 292

Diatx®Zn [US] *see* vitamins (multiple/oral) *on page* 990

Diazemuls® [Can] *see* diazepam *on page* 294

Diazemuls® Injection *(Discontinued)* *see* diazepam *on page* 294

diazepam (dye AZ e pam)

Sound-Alike/Look-Alike Issues

diazepam may be confused with diazoxide, diltiazem, Ditropan®, LORazepam

Valium® may be confused with Valcyte®

U.S./Canadian Brand Names Apo-Diazepam® [Can]; Diastat® AcuDial™ [US]; Diastat® Rectal Delivery System [Can]; Diastat® [US/Can]; Diazemuls® [Can]; Diazepam Intensol™ [US]; Novo-Dipam [Can]; Valium® [US/Can]

Therapeutic Category Benzodiazepine

Controlled Substance C-IV

Use Management of anxiety disorders, ethanol withdrawal symptoms; skeletal muscle relaxant; treatment of convulsive disorders; preoperative or preprocedural sedation and amnesia

Rectal gel: Management of selected, refractory epilepsy patients on stable regimens of antiepileptic drugs requiring intermittent use of diazepam to control episodes of increased seizure activity

Dosage Summary

I.M.:

Children <30 days: Dosage not established

Children >30 days to <5 years: 1-2 mg every 3-4 hours as needed **or** 0.04-0.3 mg/kg every 2-4 hours (maximum: 0.6 mg/kg/8 hours)

Children ≥5 years: 5-10 mg every 3-4 hours as needed **or** 0.04-0.3 mg/kg every 2-4 hours (maximum: 0.6 mg/kg/8 hours)

Adults: 2-10 mg, may repeat in 3-4 hours if needed

I.V.:

Children <30 days: Dosage not established

Children >30 days to <5 years:

Anxiety/sedation/skeletal muscle relaxant: 0.04-0.3 mg/kg every 2-4 hours (maximum: 0.6 mg/kg/8 hours)

Muscle spasm associated with tetanus: 1-2 mg every 3-4 hours as needed

Status epilepticus: 0.1-0.3 mg/kg given over ≤5 mg/minute; may repeat dose after 5-10 minutes; maximum: 10 mg/dose

Children ≥5 years:

Anxiety/sedation/skeletal muscle relaxant: 0.04-0.3 mg/kg every 2-4 hours (maximum: 0.6 mg/kg/8 hours)

Muscle spasm associated with tetanus: 5-10 mg every 3-4 hours as needed

Status epilepticus: 0.1-0.3 mg/kg given over ≤5 mg/minute; may repeat dose after 5-10 minutes; maximum: 10 mg/dose

Adolescents:

Anxiety/sedation/skeletal muscle relaxant: 0.04-0.3 mg/kg every 2-4 hours (maximum: 0.6 mg/kg/8 hours)

Muscle spasm associated with tetanus: 5-10 mg every 3-4 hours as needed

Procedures: 5 mg may repeat with 2.5 mg if needed prior to procedures

Status epilepticus: 0.1-0.3 mg/kg given over ≤5 mg/minute; may repeat dose after 5-10 minutes; maximum: 10 mg/dose

Adults:

Anxiety/sedation/skeletal muscle relaxant: 2-10 mg, may repeat in 3-4 hours if needed

ICU sedation: 0.03-0.1 mg/kg every 30 minutes to 6 hours

Muscle spasm: Initial: 5-10 mg; then 5-10 mg in 3-4 hours, if necessary; larger doses may be required if associated with tetanus

Status epilepticus: 5-10 mg every 5-10 minutes given over ≤5 mg/minute; maximum dose: 30 mg

Oral:

Children: 0.12-1mg/kg/day divided every 6-8 hours **or** 0.2-0.3 mg/kg (maximum: 10 mg) prior to procedures

Adolescents: 0.12-0.8 mg/kg/day divided every 6-8 hours **or** 10 mg prior to procedures

Adults:

Acute ethanol withdrawal: 10 mg 3-4 times during first 24 hours, then decrease to 5 mg 3-4 times/day as needed

Anxiety (symptoms/disorders): 2-10 mg 2-4 times/day

Skeletal muscle relaxant (adjunct therapy): 2-10 mg 3-4 times/day

Tranquilization of agitated patient: 5-10 mg every 30-60 minutes; average total dose: 20-60 mg

Elderly/debilitated patients: 2-2.5 mg 1-2 times/day initially; increase gradually as needed and tolerated

Rectal:
Gel:
Children <2 years: Dosage not established
Children 2-5 years: Initial: 0.5 mg/kg, may repeat in 4-12 hours if needed
Children 6-11 years: Initial: 0.3 mg/kg, may repeat in 4-12 hours if needed
Children ≥12 years: Initial: 0.2 mg/kg, may repeat in 4-12 hours if needed
Adults: Initial: 0.2 mg/kg, may repeat in 4-12 hours if needed
Elderly: Consider reducing dose
Parenteral formulation prep:
Children: 0.5 mg/kg/dose then 0.25 mg/kg/dose in 10 minutes if needed
Adults: Dosage not established

Dosage Forms
Gel, rectal: 10 mg (2 mL); 20 mg (4 mL); 5 mg/mL (0.5 mL)
Diastat®: 5 mg/mL (0.5 mL)
Diastat® AcuDial™: 10 mg (2 mL); 20 mg (4 mL)
Injection, solution: 5 mg/mL (2 mL, 10 mL)
Solution, oral: 5 mg/5 mL (5 mL, 500 mL)
Diazepam Intensol™: 5 mg/mL (30 mL)
Tablet, oral: 2 mg, 5 mg, 10 mg
Valium®: 2 mg, 5 mg, 10 mg

Diazepam Intensol™ [US] *see* diazepam *on page* *294*

diazoxide (dye az OKS ide)

Sound-Alike/Look-Alike Issues
diazoxide may be confused with diazepam, Dyazide®

U.S./Canadian Brand Names Proglycem® [US/Can]

Therapeutic Category Antihypertensive Agent; Antihypoglycemic Agent

Use Hypoglycemia related to islet cell adenoma, carcinoma, hyperplasia, or adenomatosis; nesidioblastosis; leucine sensitivity; extrapancreatic malignancy

Dosage Summary
Oral:
Infants: 8-15 mg/kg/day in divided doses every 8-12 hours
Children: 3-8 mg/kg/day in divided doses every 8-12 hours
Adults: 3-8 mg/kg/day in divided doses every 8-12 hours

Dosage Forms
Suspension, oral:
Proglycem®: 50 mg/mL (30 mL)

Dosage Forms - Canada
Capsule, oral:
Proglycem®: 50 mg

Dibent® Injection *(Discontinued)* *see* dicyclomine *on page* *299*
Dibenzyline® [US/Can] *see* phenoxybenzamine *on page* *749*

dibucaine (DYE byoo kane)

U.S./Canadian Brand Names Nupercainal® [US-OTC]

Therapeutic Category Local Anesthetic

Use Fast, temporary relief of pain and itching due to hemorrhoids, minor burns

Dosage Summary
Topical:
Children: Apply to affected areas (maximum 7.5 g/24 hour period)
Adults: Apply to affected areas (maximum: 30 g/24 hour period)

Dosage Forms
Ointment, topical: 1% [10 mg/g] (30 g, 454 g)
Nupercainal® [OTC]: 1% [10 mg/g] (30 g, 60 g)

DIC *see* dacarbazine *on page* *265*
Dicarbosil® *(Discontinued)* *see* calcium carbonate *on page* *167*
Dicel™ [US] *see* chlorpheniramine and pseudoephedrine *on page* *209*
Dicel™ DM [US] *see* chlorpheniramine, pseudoephedrine, and dextromethorphan *on page* *214*

Dicetel® [Can] *see* pinaverium *(Canada only) on page 761*

dichloralphenazone, acetaminophen, and isometheptene *see* acetaminophen, isometheptene, and dichloralphenazone *on page 31*

dichloralphenazone, isometheptene, and acetaminophen *see* acetaminophen, isometheptene, and dichloralphenazone *on page 31*

dichlorodifluoromethane and trichloromonofluoromethane

(dye klor oh dye flor oh METH ane & tri klor oh mon oh flor oh METH ane)

Synonyms trichloromonofluoromethane and dichlorodifluoromethane

U.S./Canadian Brand Names Fluori-Methane® [US]

Therapeutic Category Analgesic, Topical

Use Management of pain associated with injections

Dosage Summary

Topical:

Children: Dosage not established

Adults: Invert bottle over treatment area, allow liquid to stream from bottle until entire muscle covered

Dosage Forms

Aerosol, topical:

Fluori-Methane®: Dichlorodifluoromethane 15% and trichloromonofluoromethane 85% (103 mL)

dichlorotetrafluoroethane and ethyl chloride *see* ethyl chloride and dichlorotetrafluoroethane *on page 382*

dichlorphenamide *(Discontinued)*

Dickinson's® Witch Hazel [US-OTC] *see* witch hazel *on page 994*

Dickinson's® Witch Hazel Astringent Cleanser [US-OTC] *see* witch hazel *on page 994*

Dickinson's® Witch Hazel Cleansing Astringent [US-OTC] *see* witch hazel *on page 994*

Diclectin® [Can] *see* doxylamine and pyridoxine *(Canada only) on page 332*

diclofenac (systemic) (dye KLOE fen ak)

Sound-Alike/Look-Alike Issues

diclofenac may be confused with Diflucan®, Duphalac®

Cataflam® may be confused with Catapres®

Voltaren® may be confused with traMADol, Ultram®, Verelan®

Synonyms diclofenac potassium; diclofenac sodium

U.S./Canadian Brand Names Apo-Diclo Rapide® [Can]; Apo-Diclo SR® [Can]; Apo-Diclo® [Can]; Cambia™ [US]; Cataflam® [US/Can]; Diclofenac ECT [Can]; Diclofenac Sodium SR [Can]; Diclofenac Sodium [Can]; Diclofenac SR [Can]; Dom-Diclofenac SR [Can]; Dom-Diclofenac [Can]; Novo-Difenac ECT [Can]; Novo-Difenac K [Can]; Novo-Difenac Suppositories [Can]; Novo-Difenac-SR [Can]; Nu-Diclo [Can]; Nu-Diclo-SR [Can]; Pennsaid® [Can]; PMS-Diclofenac SR [Can]; PMS-Diclofenac [Can]; PMS-Diclofenac-K [Can]; PRO-Diclo-Rapide [Can]; Sandoz-Diclofenac Rapide [Can]; Sandoz-Diclofenac SR [Can]; Sandoz-Diclofenac [Can]; Voltaren Rapide® [Can]; Voltaren SR® [Can]; Voltaren® [Can]; Voltaren®-XR [US]; Zipsor™ [US]

Therapeutic Category Nonsteroidal Antiinflammatory Drug (NSAID)

Use

Capsule: Relief of mild-to-moderate acute pain

Immediate-release tablet: Ankylosing spondylitis; primary dysmenorrhea; acute and chronic treatment of rheumatoid arthritis, osteoarthritis

Delayed-release tablet: Acute and chronic treatment of rheumatoid arthritis, osteoarthritis, ankylosing spondylitis

Extended-release tablet: Chronic treatment of osteoarthritis, rheumatoid arthritis

Oral solution: Treatment of acute migraine with or without aura

Suppository (CAN; not available in U.S.): Symptomatic treatment of rheumatoid arthritis and osteoarthritis (including degenerative joint disease of hip)

Dosage Summary

Oral:

Immediate release capsule:

Children: Dosage not established

Adults: 100 mg/day in 4 divided doses

Immediate release tablet:
Children: Dosage not established
Adults: 100-200 mg/day in 2-5 divided doses
Extended release tablet:
Children: Dosage not established
Adults: 100-200 mg/day
Oral solution:
Children: Dosage not established
Adults: 50 mg once

Dosage Forms

Capsule, liquid filled, oral:
Zipsor™: 25 mg
Powder for solution, oral:
Cambia™: 50 mg/packet (1s)
Tablet, oral: 50 mg
Cataflam®: 50 mg
Tablet, delayed release, enteric coated, oral: 25 mg, 50 mg, 75 mg
Tablet, extended release, oral: 100 mg
Voltaren®-XR: 100 mg

diclofenac (ophthalmic) (dye KLOE fen ak)

Sound-Alike/Look-Alike Issues
diclofenac may be confused with Diflucan®, Duphalac®

Synonyms diclofenac sodium

U.S./Canadian Brand Names Voltaren Ophthalmic® [US]; Voltaren Ophtha® [Can]

Therapeutic Category Nonsteroidal Antiinflammatory Drug (NSAID), Ophthalmic

Use Postoperative inflammation following cataract extraction; temporary relief of pain and photophobia in patients undergoing corneal refractive surgery

Dosage Summary

Ophthalmic:
Children: Dosage not established
Adults: 1-2 drops into affected eye 4 times/day

Dosage Forms

Solution, ophthalmic: 0.1% (2.5 mL, 5 mL)
Voltaren Ophthalmic®: 0.1% (2.5 mL, 5 mL)

diclofenac (topical) (dye KLOE fen ak)

Sound-Alike/Look-Alike Issues
diclofenac may be confused with Diflucan®, Duphalac®
Voltaren® may be confused with traMADol, Ultram®, Verelan®

Synonyms diclofenac diethylamine [CAN]; diclofenac epolamine; diclofenac sodium

U.S./Canadian Brand Names Flector® [US]; Pennsaid® [US]; Solaraze® [US]; Voltaren® Emulgel™ [Can]; Voltaren® Gel [US]

Therapeutic Category Nonsteroidal Antiinflammatory Drug (NSAID), Topical

Use

Topical gel 1%: Relief of osteoarthritis pain in joints amenable to topical therapy (eg, ankle, elbow, foot, hand, knee, wrist)
Canadian labeling (not in U.S. labeling): Relief of pain associated with acute, localized joint/muscle injuries (eg, sports injuries, strains) in patients ≥16 years of age
Topical gel 3%: Actinic keratosis (AK) in conjunction with sun avoidance
Topical patch: Acute pain due to minor strains, sprains, and contusions
Topical solution: Relief of osteoarthritis pain of the knee

Dosage Summary

Topical:
Children: Dosage not established
Adults:
1% gel: Apply 2-4 g to affected joint 4 times daily (maximum: 16 g/day single joint of lower extremity, 8 g/day single joint of upper extremity); Maximum total body dose of 1% gel should not exceed 32 g per day.
3% gel: Apply to lesion area twice daily

Patch: Apply 1 patch twice daily
Solution: Apply 40 drops to each affected knee 4 times daily

Dosage Forms

Gel, topical:
Solaraze®: 3% (100 g)
Voltaren® Gel: 1% (100 g)

Patch, transdermal:
Flector®: 1.3% (30s)

Solution, topical:
Pennsaid®: 1.5% (150 mL)

Dosage Forms - Canada

Gel, topical:
Voltaren® Emulgel™: 1.16% (20 g, 50 g, 100 g)

diclofenac and misoprostol (dye KLOE fen ak & mye soe PROST ole)

Synonyms misoprostol and diclofenac

U.S./Canadian Brand Names Arthrotec® [US/Can]

Therapeutic Category Analgesic, Nonnarcotic; Prostaglandin

Use Treatment of osteoarthritis and rheumatoid arthritis in patients at high risk for NSAID-induced gastric and duodenal ulceration

Dosage Summary

Oral:
Children: Dosage not established
Adults: Arthrotec® 50: One tablet 3-4 times/day; may administer Arthrotec® 50 or Arthrotec® 75 one tablet twice daily if recommended dose is not tolerated

Dosage Forms

Tablet:
Arthrotec® 50: Diclofenac 50 mg and misoprostol 200 mcg
Arthrotec® 75: Diclofenac 75 mg and misoprostol 200 mcg

diclofenac diethylamine [CAN] *see* diclofenac (topical) *on page 297*
Diclofenac ECT [Can] *see* diclofenac (systemic) *on page 296*
diclofenac epolamine *see* diclofenac (topical) *on page 297*
diclofenac potassium *see* diclofenac (systemic) *on page 296*
diclofenac sodium *see* diclofenac (ophthalmic) *on page 297*
Diclofenac Sodium [Can] *see* diclofenac (systemic) *on page 296*
diclofenac sodium *see* diclofenac (systemic) *on page 296*
diclofenac sodium *see* diclofenac (topical) *on page 297*
Diclofenac Sodium SR [Can] *see* diclofenac (systemic) *on page 296*
Diclofenac SR [Can] *see* diclofenac (systemic) *on page 296*

dicloxacillin (dye kloks a SIL in)

Synonyms dicloxacillin sodium

U.S./Canadian Brand Names Dycill® [Can]; Pathocil® [Can]

Therapeutic Category Penicillin

Use Treatment of systemic infections such as pneumonia, skin and soft tissue infections, and osteomyelitis caused by penicillinase-producing staphylococci

Dosage Summary

Oral:
Children <40 kg: 12.5-100 mg mg/kg/day divided every 6 hours
Children >40 kg: 125-250 mg every 6 hours
Adults: 125-1000 mg every 6-8 hours

Dosage Forms

Capsule, oral: 250 mg, 500 mg

dicloxacillin sodium *see* dicloxacillin *on page 298*

dicyclomine (dye SYE kloe meen)

Sound-Alike/Look-Alike Issues

dicyclomine may be confused with diphenhydrAMINE, doxycycline, dyclonine

Bentyl® may be confused with Aventyl®, Benadryl®, Bontril®, Cantil®, Proventil®, Trental®

Synonyms dicyclomine hydrochloride; dicycloverine hydrochloride

U.S./Canadian Brand Names Bentylol® [Can]; Bentyl® [US]; Formulex® [Can]; Lomine [Can]; Riva-Dicyclomine [Can]

Therapeutic Category Anticholinergic Agent

Use Treatment of functional bowel/irritable bowel syndrome

Dosage Summary

I.M.:

Children: Dosage not established

Adults: 80 mg/day in 4 divided doses

Oral:

Children: Dosage not established

Adults: Initial: 20 mg 4 times/day; Maintenance: Up to 160 mg/day in 4 divided doses

Elderly: Initial: 10-20 mg 4 times/day; Maintenance: Up to 160 mg/day in 4 divided doses

Dosage Forms

Capsule, oral: 10 mg

Bentyl®: 10 mg

Injection, solution: 10 mg/mL (2 mL)

Bentyl®: 10 mg/mL (2 mL)

Syrup, oral:

Bentyl®: 10 mg/5 mL (480 mL)

Tablet, oral: 20 mg

Bentyl®: 20 mg

dicyclomine hydrochloride *see* dicyclomine *on page* 299

dicycloverine hydrochloride *see* dicyclomine *on page* 299

Di-Dak-Sol [US] *see* sodium hypochlorite solution *on page* 884

didanosine (dye DAN oh seen)

Sound-Alike/Look-Alike Issues

Videx® may be confused with Lidex®

Synonyms ddI; dideoxyinosine

U.S./Canadian Brand Names Videx® EC [US/Can]; Videx® [US/Can]

Therapeutic Category Antiviral Agent

Use Treatment of HIV infection; always to be used in combination with at least two other antiretroviral agents

Dosage Summary

Oral:

Delayed release:

Children <20 kg: Dosage not established

Children 20 kg to <25 kg: 200 mg once daily

Children 25 kg to <60 kg: 250 mg once daily

Children ≥60 kg: 400 mg once daily

Adults <60 kg: 250 mg once daily

Adults ≥60 kg: 400 mg once daily

Pediatric powder for oral solution (Videx®):

Neonates <2 weeks: Dosage not established

Infants 2 weeks to 8 months: 100 mg/m^2 twice daily

Children >8 months to 12 years: 120 mg/m^2 twice daily

Adolescents <60 kg: 125 mg twice daily **or** 250 mg once daily

Adolescents ≥60 kg: 200 mg twice daily **or** 400 mg once daily

Adults <60 kg: 125 mg twice daily **or** 250 mg once daily

Adults ≥60 kg: 200 mg twice daily **or** 400 mg once daily

Dosage Forms

Capsule, delayed release, enteric coated beadlets, oral: 125 mg, 200 mg, 250 mg, 400 mg

Videx® EC: 125 mg, 200 mg, 250 mg, 400 mg

Capsule, delayed release, enteric coated pellets, oral: 200 mg, 250 mg, 400 mg

Powder for solution, oral:
Videx®: 2 g/bottle, 4 g/bottle

dideoxyinosine *see* didanosine *on page* 299
Didrex® [US] *see* benzphetamine *on page* 129
Didrocal™ [Can] *see* etidronate and calcium carbonate *(Canada only) on page* 383
Didronel® [US/Can] *see* etidronate *on page* 383
dienogest and estradiol *see* estradiol and dienogest *on page* 367
dietary supplements *see* nutritional formula, enteral/oral *on page* 692

diethylene triamine penta-acetic acid

(dye ETH i leen TRYE a meen PEN ta a SEE tik AS id)

Synonyms diethylenetriamine pentaacetic acid; DTPA; pentetate calcium trisodium; pentetate zinc trisodium; trisodium calcium diethylenetriaminepentaacetate (Ca-DTPA); zinc diethylenetriaminepentaacetate (Zn-DTPA)

U.S./Canadian Brand Names Ca-DTPA [US]; Zn-DTPA [US]

Therapeutic Category Antidote

Use Treatment of known or suspected internal contamination with plutonium, americium, or curium

Dosage Summary

I.V.:

Children <12 years: Initial: Ca-DTPA: 14 mg/kg/day (maximum dose: 1 g/day); Maintenance: Zn-DTPA: 14 mg/kg/day (maximum: 1 g/day)

Children ≥12 years: Initial: Ca-DTPA: 1 g/day; Maintenance: Zn-DTPA: 1 g/day

Adults: Initial: Ca-DTPA: 1 g/day; Maintenance: Zn-DTPA: 1 g/day

Pregnant females: Initial: Zn-DTPA: 1 g/day, unless high internal contamination then use Ca-DTPA; Maintenance: Zn-DTPA: 1 g/day

Dosage Forms

Injection, solution:
Ca-DTPA: 200 mg/mL (5 mL)
Zn-DTPA: 200 mg/mL (5 mL)

diethylenetriamine pentaacetic acid *see* diethylene triamine penta-acetic acid *on page* 300

diethylpropion (dye eth il PROE pee on)

Synonyms amfepramone; diethylpropion hydrochloride

U.S./Canadian Brand Names Tenuate® Dospan® [Can]; Tenuate® [Can]

Therapeutic Category Anorexiant

Controlled Substance C-IV

Use Short-term (few weeks) adjunct in the management of exogenous obesity

Dosage Summary

Oral:

Controlled release:

Children ≤16 years: Dosage not established
Children >16 years: 75 mg at midmorning
Adults: 75 mg at midmorning

Immediate release:

Children ≤16 years: Dosage not established
Children >16 years: 25 mg 3 times/day before meals or food
Adults: 25 mg 3 times/day before meals or food

Dosage Forms

Tablet, oral: 25 mg
Tablet, controlled release, oral: 75 mg

diethylpropion hydrochloride *see* diethylpropion *on page* 300

difenoxin and atropine (dye fen OKS in & A troe peen)

Synonyms atropine and difenoxin

U.S./Canadian Brand Names Motofen® [US]

Therapeutic Category Antidiarrheal

Controlled Substance C-IV

Use Treatment of diarrhea

Dosage Summary

Oral:

Children: Dosage not established

Adults: 2 tablets (each tablet contains difenoxin hydrochloride 1 mg and atropine sulfate 0.025 mg) initially, then 1 tablet after each loose stool (maximum: 8 tablets/day)

Dosage Forms

Tablet, oral:

Motofen®: Difenoxin 1 mg and atropine 0.025 mg

Differin® [US/Can] *see* adapalene *on page 38*

Differin® XP [Can] *see* adapalene *on page 38*

Difil-G [US] *see* dyphylline and guaifenesin *on page 339*

Difil®-G Forte [US] *see* dyphylline and guaifenesin *on page 339*

diflorasone (dye FLOR a sone)

Synonyms diflorasone diacetate

U.S./Canadian Brand Names ApexiCon™ E [US]; ApexiCon™ [US]

Therapeutic Category Corticosteroid, Topical

Use Relieves inflammation and pruritic symptoms of corticosteroid-responsive dermatosis (high to very high potency topical corticosteroid)

Dosage Summary

Topical:

Cream:

Children: Dosage not established

Adults: Apply 2-4 times/day

Ointment:

Children: Dosage not established

Adults: Apply 1-3 times/day

Dosage Forms

Cream, topical: 0.05% (15 g, 30 g, 60 g)

ApexiCon™ E: 0.05% (30 g, 60 g)

Ointment, topical: 0.05% (15 g, 30 g, 60 g)

ApexiCon™: 0.05% (30 g, 60 g)

diflorasone diacetate *see* diflorasone *on page 301*

Diflucan® [US/Can] *see* fluconazole *on page 407*

diflunisal (dye FLOO ni sal)

Sound-Alike/Look-Alike Issues

Dolobid® may be confused with Slo-Bid®

U.S./Canadian Brand Names Apo-Diflunisal® [Can]; Novo-Diflunisal [Can]; Nu-Diflunisal [Can]

Therapeutic Category Analgesic, Nonnarcotic; Nonsteroidal Antiinflammatory Drug (NSAID)

Use Management of inflammatory disorders usually including rheumatoid arthritis and osteoarthritis; can be used as an analgesic for treatment of mild-to-moderate pain

Dosage Summary

Oral:

Children: Dosage not established

Adults: 250-500 mg every 8-12 hours (maximum: 1.5 g/day)

Dosage Forms

Tablet, oral: 500 mg

difluprednate (dye floo PRED nate)

Sound-Alike/Look-Alike Issues

Durezol® may be confused with Durasal

U.S./Canadian Brand Names Durezol® [US]

Therapeutic Category Corticosteroid, Ophthalmic

Use Treatment of inflammation and pain following ocular surgery

Dosage Summary

Ophthalmic:

Children: Dosage not established

Adults: Instill 1 drop in affected eye(s) 2-4 times/day

Dosage Forms

Emulsion, ophthalmic:

Durezol®: 0.05% (5 mL)

Digibind® [US/Can] *see* digoxin immune Fab *on page 303*

DigiFab® [US] *see* digoxin immune Fab *on page 303*

digitalis *see* digoxin *on page 302*

digoxin (di JOKS in)

Sound-Alike/Look-Alike Issues

digoxin may be confused with Desoxyn®, doxepin

Lanoxin® may be confused with Lasix®, levothyroxine, Levoxyl®, Levsinex®, Lomotil®, Lonox®, Mefoxin®, naloxone, Xanax®

Synonyms digitalis

U.S./Canadian Brand Names Apo-Digoxin® [Can]; Digoxin CSD [Can]; Lanoxin® [US/Can]; Pediatric Digoxin CSD [Can]; PMS-Digoxin [Can]; Toloxin® [Can]

Therapeutic Category Antiarrhythmic Agent, Miscellaneous; Cardiac Glycoside

Use Treatment of mild-to-moderate (or stage C as recommended by the ACCF/AHA) heart failure (HF); atrial fibrillation (rate-control)

Note: In treatment of atrial fibrillation (AF), use is not considered first-line unless AF coexistent with heart failure or in sedentary patients.

Dosage Summary

I.M. (not preferred due to severe injection site pain):

Preterm infants: Digitalizing dose: 15-25 mcg/kg; Maintenance: 4-6 mcg/kg/day in divided doses every 12 hours

Full-term infants: Digitalizing dose: 20-30 mcg/kg; Maintenance: 5-8 mcg/kg/day in divided doses every 12 hours

Children 1 month to 2 years: Digitalizing dose: 30-50 mcg/kg; Maintenance: 7.5-12 mcg/kg/day in divided doses every 12 hours

Children 2-5 years: Digitalizing dose: 25-35 mcg/kg; Maintenance: 6-9 mcg/kg/day in divided doses every 12 hours

Children 5-10 years: Digitalizing dose: 15-30 mcg/kg; Maintenance: 4-8 mcg/kg/day in divided doses every 12 hours

Children >10 years: Digitalizing dose: 8-12 mcg/kg; Maintenance: 2-3 mcg/kg once daily

Adults: Digitalizing dose: 0.5-1 mg; Maintenance: 0.1-0.4 mg once daily

I.V.:

Preterm infants: Digitalizing dose: 15-25 mcg/kg; Maintenance: 4-6 mcg/kg/day in divided doses every 12 hours

Full-term infants: Digitalizing dose: 20-30 mcg/kg; Maintenance: 5-8 mcg/kg/day in divided doses every 12 hours

Children 1 month to 2 years: Digitalizing dose: 30-50 mcg/kg; Maintenance: 7.5-12 mcg/kg/day in divided doses every 12 hours

Children 2-5 years: Digitalizing dose: 25-35 mcg/kg; Maintenance: 6-9 mcg/kg/day in divided doses every 12 hours

Children 5-10 years: Digitalizing dose: 15-30 mcg/kg; Maintenance: 4-8 mcg/kg/day in divided doses every 12 hours

Children >10 years: Digitalizing dose: 8-12 mcg/kg; Maintenance: 2-3 mcg/kg once daily

Adults: Digitalizing dose: 0.5-1 mg; Maintenance: 0.1-0.4 mg once daily

Oral:

Preterm infants: Digitalizing dose: 20-30 mcg/kg; Maintenance: 5-7.5 mcg/kg/day in divided doses every 12 hours

Full-term infants: Digitalizing dose: 25-35 mcg/kg; Maintenance: 6-10 mcg/kg/day in divided doses every 12 hours

Children 1 month to 2 years: Digitalizing dose: 35-60 mcg/kg; Maintenance: 10-15 mcg/kg/day in divided doses every 12 hours

Children 2-5 years: Digitalizing dose: 30-40 mcg/kg; Maintenance: 7.5-10 mcg/kg/day in divided doses every 12 hours

Children 5-10 years: Digitalizing dose: 20-35 mcg/kg; Maintenance: 5-10 mcg/kg/day in divided doses every 12 hours

Children >10 years: Digitalizing dose: 10-15 mcg/kg; Maintenance: 2.5-5 mcg/kg once daily

Adults: Digitalizing dose: 0.75-1.5 mg; Maintenance: 0.125-0.5 mg once daily

Dosage Forms

Injection, solution: 250 mcg/mL (1 mL, 2 mL)

Lanoxin®: 100 mcg/mL (1 mL); 250 mcg/mL (2 mL)

Solution, oral: 50 mcg/mL (2.5 mL, 5 mL, 60 mL)

Tablet, oral: 125 mcg, 250 mcg

Lanoxin®: 125 mcg, 250 mcg

Dosage Forms - Canada

Tablet, oral:

Apo-Digoxin®: 62.5 mcg, 125 mcg, 250 mcg

Digoxin CSD [Can] *see* digoxin *on page* 302

digoxin immune Fab (di JOKS in i MYUN fab)

Synonyms antidigoxin fab fragments, ovine

U.S./Canadian Brand Names Digibind® [US/Can]; DigiFab® [US]

Therapeutic Category Antidote

Use Treatment of life-threatening or potentially life-threatening digoxin intoxication, including:

- acute digoxin ingestion (ie, >10 mg in adults or >4 mg in children)
- chronic ingestions leading to steady-state digoxin concentrations >6 ng/mL in adults or >4 ng/mL in children
- manifestations of digoxin toxicity due to overdose (life-threatening ventricular arrhythmias, progressive bradycardia, second- or third-degree heart block not responsive to atropine, serum potassium >5 mEq/L in adults or >6 mEq in children)

Dosage Summary

I.V.:

Acute ingestion of known amount: Children and Adults:

Dose (vials) = Total body load (mg) / (0.5 mg digitalis bound/vial)

Based on steady-state digoxin concentration:

Infants and Children ≤20 kg:

Dose (mg) = [(serum digoxin concentration [ng/mL] x weight [kg]) / 10] x (mg/vial)[1]

[1]Digibind® 38 mg/vial or DigiFab™ 40 mg/vial

Adults:

Dose (vials) = [(serum digoxin concentration [ng/mL] x weight [kg]) / 100

Amount ingested and blood level unknown:

Children ≤20 kg: Acute toxicity: 20 vials total in 2 divided doses; Chronic toxicity: 1 vial may be sufficient

Children >20 kg: Acute toxicity: 20 vials total in 2 divided doses; Chronic toxicity: 6 vials

Adults: Acute toxicity: 20 vials total in 2 divided doses; Chronic toxicity: 6 vials

Dosage Forms

Injection, powder for reconstitution:

Digibind®: 38 mg

DigiFab®: 40 mg

dihematoporphyrin ether *see* porfimer *on page* 779

Dihistine® DH *(Discontinued)* *see* chlorpheniramine, pseudoephedrine, and codeine *on page* 214

dihydrocodeine, aspirin, and caffeine (dye hye droe KOE deen, AS pir in, & KAF een)

Sound-Alike/Look-Alike Issues

Synalgos®-DC may be confused with Synagis®

Synonyms dihydrocodeine compound

U.S./Canadian Brand Names Synalgos®-DC [US]

Therapeutic Category Analgesic, Narcotic

Controlled Substance C-III

Use Management of mild-to-moderate pain that requires relaxation

Dosage Summary

Oral:

Children: Dosage not established

Adults: 1-2 capsules every 4-6 hours as needed

Dosage Forms

Capsule, oral:

Synalgos®-DC: Dihydrocodeine 16 mg, aspirin 356.4 mg, and caffeine 30 mg

dihydrocodeine bitartrate, acetaminophen, and caffeine *see* acetaminophen, caffeine, and dihydrocodeine *on page 28*

dihydrocodeine bitartrate, phenylephrine hydrochloride, and chlorpheniramine maleate *see* phenylephrine, hydrocodone, and chlorpheniramine *on page 754*

dihydrocodeine bitartrate, pseudoephedrine hydrochloride, and chlorpheniramine maleate *see* pseudoephedrine, dihydrocodeine, and chlorpheniramine *on page 813*

dihydrocodeine, chlorpheniramine, and phenylephrine

(dye hye droe KOE deen, klor fen IR a meen, & fen il EF rin)

Synonyms chlorpheniramine maleate, dihydrocodeine bitartrate, and phenylephrine hydrochloride; phenylephrine, chlorpheniramine, and dihydrocodeine

U.S./Canadian Brand Names Coldcough PD [US]; Novahistine DH [US]

Therapeutic Category Antihistamine; Antihistamine/Decongestant/Antitussive; Antitussive; Decongestant

Controlled Substance C-III/C-V

Use Symptomatic relief of cough and congestion associated with the upper respiratory tract

Dosage Summary

Oral:

Children <2 years: Dosage not established

Children 2-6 years: Novahistine DH: 1.25-2.5 mL every 4-6 hours as needed (maximum: 10 mL/day)

Children 6-12 years:

Baltussin: 2.5 mL every 4-6 hours as needed

Novahistine DH: 2.5-5 mL every 4-6 hours as needed (maximum: 20 mL/day)

Children >12 years:

Baltussin: 5 mL every 4-6 hours as needed

Novahistine DH: 5-10 mL every 4-6 hours as needed (maximum: 40 mL/day)

Adults:

Baltussin: 5 mL every 4-6 hours as needed

Novahistine DH: 5-10 mL every 4-6 hours as needed (maximum: 40 mL/day)

Dosage Forms

Liquid, oral:

Novahistine DH: Dihydrocodeine 7.5 mg, chlorpheniramine 2 mg and phenylephrine 5 mg per 5 mL

Syrup, oral:

Coldcough PD, DiHydro-PE [OTC]: Dihydrocodeine 3 mg, chlorpheniramine 2 mg, and phenylephrine 7.5 mg per 5 mL

dihydrocodeine compound *see* dihydrocodeine, aspirin, and caffeine *on page 303*

dihydrocodeine, pseudoephedrine, and guaifenesin

(dye hye droe KOE deen, soo doe e FED rin, & gwye FEN e sin)

Synonyms guaifenesin, dihydrocodeine, and pseudoephedrine; pseudoephedrine hydrochloride, guaifenesin, and dihydrocodeine bitartrate

U.S./Canadian Brand Names DiHydro-GP [US]; Pancof®-EXP [US]

Therapeutic Category Antitussive/Decongestant/Expectorant

Use Temporary relief of cough and congestion associated with upper respiratory tract infections and allergies

Dosage Summary

Oral:

Children <2 years: Dosage not established

Children 2-6 years: 1.25-2.5 mL every 4-6 hours as needed

Children 6-12 years: 2.5-5 mL every 4-6 hours as needed

Children ≥12 years: 5-10 mL every 4-6 hours as needed

Adults: 5-10 mL every 4-6 hours as needed

Dosage Forms

Syrup:

DiHydro-GP, Pancof®-EXP: Dihydrocodeine 7.5 mg, pseudoephedrine 15 mg, and guaifenesin 100 mg per 5 mL

DiHydro-CP [US] *see* pseudoephedrine, dihydrocodeine, and chlorpheniramine *on page* 813

dihydroergotamine (dye hye droe er GOT a meen)

Synonyms DHE; dihydroergotamine mesylate

U.S./Canadian Brand Names D.H.E. 45® [US]; Migranal® [US/Can]

Therapeutic Category Ergot Alkaloid and Derivative

Use Treatment of migraine headache with or without aura; injection also indicated for treatment of cluster headaches

Dosage Summary

I.M.:

Children: Dosage not established

Adults: 1 mg initially, may repeat hourly up to 3 mg total (maximum: 6 mg/week)

I.V.:

Children: Dosage not established

Adults: 1 mg initially, may repeat hourly up to 2 mg total (maximum: 6 mg/week)

Intranasal:

Children: Dosage not established

Adults: 1 spray (0.5 mg) in each nostril initially, may repeat after 15 minutes up to 4 sprays total (maximum: 6 sprays/24 hours; 8 sprays/week)

SubQ:

Children: Dosage not established

Adults: 1 mg initially, may repeat hourly up to 3 mg total (maximum: 6 mg/week)

Dosage Forms

Injection, solution: 1 mg/mL (1 mL)

D.H.E. 45®: 1 mg/mL (1 mL)

Solution, intranasal:

Migranal®: 4 mg/mL (1 mL)

dihydroergotamine mesylate *see* dihydroergotamine *on page* 305

dihydroergotoxine *see* ergoloid mesylates *on page* 358

dihydrogenated ergot alkaloids *see* ergoloid mesylates *on page* 358

DiHydro-GP [US] *see* dihydrocodeine, pseudoephedrine, and guaifenesin *on page* 304

dihydrohydroxycodeinone *see* oxycodone *on page* 714

dihydromorphinone *see* hydromorphone *on page* 485

dihydroxyanthracenedione *see* mitoxantrone *on page* 638

dihydroxyanthracenedione dihydrochloride *see* mitoxantrone *on page* 638

1,25 dihydroxycholecalciferol *see* calcitriol *on page* 165

dihydroxydeoxynorvinkaleukoblastine *see* vinorelbine *on page* 986

dihydroxypropyl theophylline *see* dyphylline *on page* 339

Dihyrex® Injection *(Discontinued)* *see* diphenhydramine (systemic) *on page* 310

diiodohydroxyquin *see* iodoquinol *on page* 519

Dilacor XR® [US] *see* diltiazem *on page* 306

Dilantin® [US/Can] *see* phenytoin *on page* 756

Dilantin-125® [US] *see* phenytoin *on page* 756

Dilatrate®-SR [US] *see* isosorbide dinitrate *on page* 529

Dilaudid® [US/Can] *see* hydromorphone *on page* 485

Dilaudid® Cough Syrup *(Discontinued)* *see* hydromorphone *on page* 485

Dilaudid-HP® [US/Can] *see* hydromorphone *on page* 485

Dilaudid-HP-Plus® [Can] *see* hydromorphone *on page* 485

Dilaudid® Sterile Powder [Can] *see* hydromorphone *on page* 485

Dilaudid-XP® [Can] *see* hydromorphone *on page* 485

Dilex-G [US] *see* dyphylline and guaifenesin *on page* 339

Dilocaine® Injection *(Discontinued)* *see* lidocaine (systemic) *on page* 561

Dilomine® Injection *(Discontinued)* *see* dicyclomine *on page 299*

Dilor® [Can] *see* dyphylline *on page 339*

Dilt-CD [US] *see* diltiazem *on page 306*

Diltia XT® [US] *see* diltiazem *on page 306*

diltiazem (dil TYE a zem)

Sound-Alike/Look-Alike Issues

diltiazem may be confused with Calan®, diazepam, Dilantin®

Cardizem® may be confused with Cardene®, Cardene SR®, Cardizem CD®, Cardizem SR®, cardiem, cortisone

Cartia XT® may be confused with Procardia XL®

Tiazac® may be confused with Tigan®, Tiazac® XC [CAN], Ziac®

Synonyms diltiazem hydrochloride

U.S./Canadian Brand Names Apo-Diltiaz CD® [Can]; Apo-Diltiaz SR® [Can]; Apo-Diltiaz TZ® [Can]; Apo-Diltiaz® Injectable [Can]; Apo-Diltiaz® [Can]; Cardizem® CD [US/Can]; Cardizem® LA [US]; Cardizem® [US]; Cartia XT® [US]; Dilacor XR® [US]; Dilt-CD [US]; Dilt-XR [US]; Diltia XT® [US]; Diltiazem HCl ER® [Can]; Diltiazem Hydrochloride Injection [Can]; Diltiazem TZ [Can]; Diltzac [US]; Med-Diltiazem [Can]; Novo-Diltazem [Can]; Novo-Diltazem-CD [Can]; Novo-Diltiazem HCl ER [Can]; Nu-Diltiaz [Can]; Nu-Diltiaz-CD [Can]; ratio-Diltiazem CD [Can]; Sandoz-Diltiazem CD [Can]; Sandoz-Diltiazem T [Can]; Taztia XT® [US]; Tiazac® XC [Can]; Tiazac® [US/Can]

Therapeutic Category Calcium Channel Blocker

Use

Oral: Essential hypertension; chronic stable angina or angina from coronary artery spasm

Injection: Atrial fibrillation or atrial flutter; paroxysmal supraventricular tachycardia (PSVT)

Dosage Summary

I.V.:

Children: Dosage not established

Adults: Bolus: 0.25 mg/kg, may repeat 0.35 mg/kg after 15 minutes; Infusion: 5-15 mg/hour

Oral:

Extended release:

Children: Dosage not established

Adults: Initial: 120-240 mg once daily **or** 60-120 mg twice daily; Maintenance: 120-540 mg once daily **or** 240-360 mg/day in 2 divided doses

Immediate release:

Children (unlabeled use): Initial: 1.5-2 mg/kg/day in 3 divided doses (maximum: 6 mg/kg/day, up to 360 mg/day)

Adults: Initial: 30 mg 4 times/day; Maintenance: 120-320 mg/day in divided doses

Dosage Forms

Capsule, extended release, oral: 60 mg, 90 mg, 120 mg, 180 mg, 240 mg, 300 mg, 360 mg, 420 mg

Cardizem® CD: 120 mg, 180 mg, 240 mg, 300 mg, 360 mg

Cartia XT®: 120 mg, 180 mg, 240 mg, 300 mg

Dilacor XR®: 240 mg

Dilt-CD: 120 mg, 180 mg, 240 mg, 300 mg

Dilt-XR: 120 mg, 180 mg, 240 mg

Diltia XT®: 120 mg, 180 mg, 240 mg

Diltzac: 120 mg, 180 mg, 240 mg, 300 mg, 360 mg

Taztia XT®: 120 mg, 180 mg, 240 mg, 300 mg, 360 mg

Tiazac®: 120 mg, 180 mg, 240 mg, 300 mg, 360 mg, 420 mg

Injection, powder for reconstitution: 100 mg

Injection, solution: 5 mg/mL (5 mL, 10 mL, 25 mL)

Tablet, oral: 30 mg, 60 mg, 90 mg, 120 mg

Cardizem®: 30 mg, 60 mg, 90 mg, 120 mg

Tablet, extended release, oral: 180 mg, 240 mg, 300 mg, 360 mg, 420 mg

Cardizem® LA: 120 mg, 180 mg, 240 mg, 300 mg, 360 mg, 420 mg

Dosage Forms - Canada

Tablet, extended release:

Tiazac® XC: 120 mg, 180 mg, 240 mg, 300 mg, 360 mg

Diltiazem HCl ER® [Can] *see* diltiazem *on page 306*

diltiazem hydrochloride *see* diltiazem *on page 306*

Diltiazem Hydrochloride Injection [Can] *see* diltiazem *on page 306*

Diltiazem TZ [Can] *see* diltiazem *on page 306*

Dilt-XR [US] *see* diltiazem *on page 306*

Diltzac [US] *see* diltiazem *on page 306*

Dimaphen Cold & Allergy [US-OTC] *see* brompheniramine and phenylephrine *on page 148*

Dimaphen DM *(Discontinued)* *see* brompheniramine, pseudoephedrine, and dextromethorphan *on page 149*

dimenhydrinate (dye men HYE dri nate)

Sound-Alike/Look-Alike Issues

dimenhyDRINATE may be confused with diphenhydrAMINE

Tall-Man dimenhy**DRINATE**

U.S./Canadian Brand Names Apo-Dimenhydrinate® [Can]; Children's Motion Sickness Liquid [Can]; Dimenhydrinate Injection [Can]; Dinate® [Can]; Dramamine® [US-OTC]; Driminate [US-OTC]; Gravol® [Can]; Nauseatol [Can]; Novo-Dimenate [Can]; PMS-Dimenhydrinate [Can]; Sandoz-Dimenhydrinate [Can]; TripTone® [US-OTC]

Therapeutic Category Antihistamine

Use Treatment and prevention of nausea, vertigo, and vomiting associated with motion sickness

Dosage Summary

Oral:

Children <2 years: Dosage not established

Children 2-5 years: 12.5-25 mg every 6-8 hours (maximum: 75 mg/day)

Children 6-12 years: 25-50 mg every 6-8 hours (maximum: 150 mg/day)

I.M.:

Children: 1.25 mg/kg **or** 37.5 mg/m^2 4 times/day; maximum: 300 mg/day

Adults: 50-100 mg every 4 hours

I.V.:

Children: Dosage not established

Adults: 50-100 mg every 4 hours

Dosage Forms

Injection, solution: 50 mg/mL (1 mL)

Tablet, oral:

Dramamine® [OTC]: 50 mg

Driminate [OTC]: 50 mg

TripTone® [OTC]: 50 mg

Tablet, chewable, oral:

Dramamine® [OTC]: 50 mg

Dimenhydrinate Injection [Can] *see* dimenhydrinate *on page 307*

dimercaprol (dye mer KAP role)

Synonyms BAL; British anti-lewisite; dithioglycerol

U.S./Canadian Brand Names BAL in Oil® [US]

Therapeutic Category Chelating Agent

Use Antidote to gold, arsenic (except arsine), or acute mercury poisoning (except nonalkyl mercury); adjunct to edetate CALCIUM disodium in lead poisoning

Dosage Summary

I.M.:

Children:

Arsenic or gold poisoning (mild): 2.5 mg/kg every 6 hours for 2 days, then every 12 hours for 1 day, followed by once daily for 10 days

Arsenic or gold poisoning (severe): 3 mg/kg every 4 hours for 2 days, then every 6 hours for 1 day, followed by every 12 hours for 10 days

Lead encephalopathy: 4 mg/kg (75 mg/m^2) loading dose, followed by 4 mg/kg (75 mg/m^2) every 4 hours for 2-7 days

Symptomatic lead poisoning or blood lead levels ≥70 mcg/dL: 4 mg/kg/dose (75 mg/m^2) loading dose, followed by 3 mg/kg/dose (50 mg/m^2) every 4 hours for 2-7 days

Mercury poisoning: 5 mg/kg initially, followed by 2.5 mg/kg 1-2 times/day for 10 days

Adults:

Arsenic or gold poisoning (mild): 2.5 mg/kg every 6 hours for 2 days, then every 12 hours for 1 day, followed by once daily for 10 days

Arsenic or gold poisoning (severe): 3 mg/kg every 4 hours for 2 days, then every 6 hours for 1 day, followed by every 12 hours for 10 days

Lead encephalopathy: 4 mg/kg (75 mg/m^2) loading dose, followed by 4 mg/kg (75 mg/m^2) every 4 hours for 2-7 days

Symptomatic lead poisoning or blood lead levels ≥70 mcg/dL: 4 mg/kg/dose (75 mg/m^2) loading dose, followed by 3 mg/kg/dose (50 mg/m^2) every 4 hours for 2-7 days

Mercury poisoning: 5 mg/kg initially, followed by 2.5 mg/kg 1-2 times/day for 10 days

Dosage Forms

Injection, oil:

BAL in Oil®: 100 mg/mL (3 mL)

Dimetabs® Oral *(Discontinued)* *see* dimenhydrinate *on page 307*

Dimetapp® 12-Hour Non-Drowsy Extentabs® *(Discontinued)* *see* pseudoephedrine *on page 810*

Dimetapp® Children's ND *(Discontinued)* *see* loratadine *on page 575*

Dimetapp® Children's Cold & Allergy [US-OTC] *see* brompheniramine and phenylephrine *on page 148*

Dimetapp® Children's Long Acting Cough Plus Cold [US-OTC] *see* dextromethorphan and chlorpheniramine *on page 288*

Dimetapp® Children's Nighttime Cold & Congestion [US-OTC] *see* diphenhydramine and phenylephrine *on page 312*

Dimetapp® Decongestant Infant *(Discontinued)* *see* pseudoephedrine *on page 810*

Dimetapp® DM Children's Cold and Cough *(Discontinued)* *see* brompheniramine, pseudoephedrine, and dextromethorphan *on page 149*

Dimetapp® Infant Decongestant Plus Cough *(Discontinued)* *see* pseudoephedrine and dextromethorphan *on page 812*

Dimetapp® ND Children's *(Discontinued)* *see* loratadine *on page 575*

Dimetapp® Sinus Caplets *(Discontinued)* *see* pseudoephedrine and ibuprofen *on page 812*

dimethyl sulfoxide (dye meth il sul FOKS ide)

Synonyms DMSO

U.S./Canadian Brand Names Dimethyl Sulfoxide Irrigation, USP [Can]; Kemsol® [Can]; Rimso-50® [US/Can]

Therapeutic Category Urinary Tract Product

Use Symptomatic relief of interstitial cystitis

Dosage Summary

Bladder instillation:

Children: Dosage not established

Adults: Instill 50 mL and allow to remain for 15 minutes, may repeat every 1-2 weeks

Dosage Forms

Solution, intravesical:

Rimso-50®: 50% (50 mL)

Dimethyl Sulfoxide Irrigation, USP [Can] *see* dimethyl sulfoxide *on page 308*

dimethyl triazeno imidazole carboxamide *see* dacarbazine *on page 265*

Dinate® [Can] *see* dimenhydrinate *on page 307*

Dinate® Injection *(Discontinued)* *see* dimenhydrinate *on page 307*

dinoprostone (dye noe PROST one)

Sound-Alike/Look-Alike Issues

Prepidil® may be confused with Bepridil®

Synonyms PGE_2; prostaglandin E_2

U.S./Canadian Brand Names Cervidil® [US/Can]; Prepidil® [US/Can]; Prostin E2® [US/Can]

Therapeutic Category Prostaglandin

Use

Endocervical gel: Promote cervical ripening in patients at or near term in whom there is a medical or obstetrical indication for the induction of labor

Suppositories: Terminate pregnancy from 12th through 20th week of gestation; evacuate uterus in cases of missed abortion or intrauterine fetal death up to 28 weeks of gestation; manage benign hydatidiform mole (nonmetastatic gestational trophoblastic disease)

Vaginal insert: Initiation and/or continuation of cervical ripening in patients at or near term in whom there is a medical or obstetrical indication for the induction of labor

Dosage Summary

Endocervical:

Children: Females of reproductive age: 0.5 mg; may repeat every 6 hours if needed. Maximum cumulative dose: 1.5 mg/24 hours

Adults (females): 0.5 mg; may repeat every 6 hours if needed. Maximum cumulative dose: 1.5 mg/24 hours

Intravaginal:

Children: Females of reproductive age: Insert: 10 mg; remove at onset of active labor or after 12 hours; Suppository: 20 mg every 3-5 hours until abortion occurs

Adults (females): Insert: 10 mg remove at onset of active labor or after 12 hours; Suppository: 20 mg every 3-5 hours until abortion occurs

Dosage Forms

Gel, endocervical:

Prepidil®: 0.5 mg/3 g (3 g)

Insert, vaginal:

Cervidil®: 10 mg (1s)

Suppository, vaginal:

Prostin E2®: 20 mg (5s)

Diocaine® [Can] *see* proparacaine *on page* *803*

Diocarpine [Can] *see* pilocarpine (ophthalmic) *on page* *760*

Diochloram® [Can] *see* chloramphenicol *on page* *203*

Diocto [US-OTC] *see* docusate *on page* *321*

Diocto C® ***(Discontinued)***

Diocto-K® ***(Discontinued)*** *see* docusate *on page* *321*

Diocto-K Plus® ***(Discontinued)*** *see* docusate *on page* *321*

dioctyl calcium sulfosuccinate *see* docusate *on page* *321*

dioctyl sodium sulfosuccinate *see* docusate *on page* *321*

Diodex® [Can] *see* dexamethasone (ophthalmic) *on page* *281*

Diodoquin® [Can] *see* iodoquinol *on page* *519*

Diogent® [Can] *see* gentamicin (ophthalmic) *on page* *443*

Diomycin® [Can] *see* erythromycin (ophthalmic) *on page* *362*

Dionephrine® [Can] *see* phenylephrine (ophthalmic) *on page* *752*

Diopentolate® [Can] *see* cyclopentolate *on page* *258*

Diopred® [Can] *see* prednisolone (ophthalmic) *on page* *791*

Dioptic's Atropine Solution [Can] *see* atropine *on page* *105*

Dioptimyd® [Can] *see* sulfacetamide and prednisolone *on page* *900*

Dioptrol® [Can] *see* neomycin, polymyxin B, and dexamethasone *on page* *666*

Diosulf™ [Can] *see* sulfacetamide (ophthalmic) *on page* *899*

Diotame [US-OTC] *see* bismuth *on page* *139*

Diotrope® [Can] *see* tropicamide *on page* *964*

Dioval® Injection ***(Discontinued)*** *see* estradiol (systemic) *on page* *366*

Diovan® [US/Can] *see* valsartan *on page* *976*

Diovan HCT® [US/Can] *see* valsartan and hydrochlorothiazide *on page* *976*

Diovol® [Can] *see* aluminum hydroxide and magnesium hydroxide *on page* *59*

Diovol® Ex [Can] *see* aluminum hydroxide and magnesium hydroxide *on page* *59*

Diovol Plus® [Can] *see* aluminum hydroxide, magnesium hydroxide, and simethicone *on page* *59*

Dipentum® [US/Can] *see* olsalazine *on page* *699*

Diphen [US-OTC] *see* diphenhydramine (systemic) *on page* *310*

Diphenacen 50® Injection ***(Discontinued)*** *see* diphenhydramine (systemic) *on page 310*
Diphenatol® ***(Discontinued)*** *see* diphenoxylate and atropine *on page 313*
Diphenhist® [US-OTC] *see* diphenhydramine (systemic) *on page 310*
Diphenhist® [US-OTC] *see* diphenhydramine (topical) *on page 311*

diphenhydramine (systemic) (dye fen HYE dra meen)

Sound-Alike/Look-Alike Issues

diphenhydrAMINE may be confused with desipramine, dicyclomine, dimenhyDRINATE
Benadryl® may be confused with benazepril, Bentyl®, Benylin®, Caladryl®

Synonyms diphenhydramine citrate; diphenhydramine hydrochloride; diphenhydramine tannate

Tall-Man diphenhydr**AMINE**

U.S./Canadian Brand Names Aler-Cap [US-OTC]; Aler-Dryl [US-OTC]; Aler-Tab [US-OTC]; Allerdryl® [Can]; AllerMax® [US-OTC]; Allernix [Can]; Altaryl [US-OTC]; Anti-Hist [US-OTC]; Banophen™ [US-OTC]; Benadryl® Allergy Quick Dissolve [US-OTC]; Benadryl® Allergy [US-OTC]; Benadryl® Children's Allergy Fastmelt® [US-OTC]; Benadryl® Children's Allergy Perfect Measure™ [US-OTC]; Benadryl® Children's Allergy [US-OTC]; Benadryl® Children's Dye Free Allergy [US-OTC]; Benadryl® Dye-Free Allergy [US-OTC]; Benadryl® [Can]; Compoz® [US-OTC]; Diphen [US-OTC]; Diphenhist® [US-OTC]; Genahist™ [US-OTC]; Histaprin [US-OTC]; Nytol® Extra Strength [Can]; Nytol® Quick Caps [US-OTC]; Nytol® Quick Gels [US-OTC]; Nytol® [Can]; PediaCare® Children's Allergy [US-OTC]; PediaCare® Children's NightTime Cough [US-OTC]; PMS-Diphenhydramine [Can]; Siladryl Allergy [US-OTC]; Silphen [US-OTC]; Simply Sleep® [US-OTC/Can]; Sleep-ettes D [US-OTC]; Sleep-Tabs [US-OTC]; Sleepinal® [US-OTC]; Sominex® Maximum Strength [US-OTC]; Sominex® [US-OTC/Can]; Theraflu® Thin Strips® Multi Symptom [US-OTC]; Triaminic Thin Strips® Children's Cough & Runny Nose [US-OTC]; Twilite® [US-OTC]; Unisom® SleepGels® Maximum Strength [US-OTC]; Unisom® SleepMelts™ [US-OTC]

Therapeutic Category Histamine H_1 Antagonist; Histamine H_1 Antagonist, First Generation

Use Symptomatic relief of allergic symptoms caused by histamine release including nasal allergies and allergic dermatosis; adjunct to epinephrine in the treatment of anaphylaxis; nighttime sleep aid; prevention or treatment of motion sickness; antitussive; management of parkinsonian syndrome including drug-induced extrapyramidal symptoms

Dosage Summary Note: Dosages are expressed as the hydrochloride salt.

I.M.:

Children: 5 mg/kg/day **or** 150 mg/m^2/day in divided every 6-8 hours (maximum: 300 mg/day)
Adults: 10-100 per dose (maximum: 400 mg/day)
Elderly: Initial: 25 mg 2-3 times/day increasing as needed

I.V.:

Children: 5 mg/kg/day **or** 150 mg/m^2/day in divided every 6-8 hours (maximum: 300 mg/day)
Adults: 10-100 mg every 2-4 hours (maximum: 400 mg/day)
Elderly: Initial: 25 mg 2-3 times/day increasing as needed

Oral:

Children: 5 mg/kg/day **or** 150 mg/m^2/day in divided every 6-8 hours (maximum: 300 mg/day)
Children 2 to <6 years: 5 mg/kg/day **or** 150 mg/m^2/day in divided every 6-8 hours (maximum: 300 mg/day) **or** 6.25 mg every 4-6 hours (maximum: 37.5 mg/day)
Children 6 to <12 years: 5 mg/kg/day **or** 150 mg/m^2/day in divided every 6-8 hours (maximum: 300 mg/day) **or** 12.5-25 mg every 4-6 hours (maximum: 150 mg/day)
Children ≥12 years: 5 mg/kg/day **or** 150 mg/m^2/day in divided doses every 6-8 hours **or** 25-50 mg every 4-6 hours (maximum: 300 mg/day) **or** 50 mg at bedtime
Adults: 25-50 mg every 4-6 hours (maximum: 400 mg/day) **or** 50 mg at bedtime
Elderly: Initial: 25 mg 2-3 times/day increasing as needed

Dosage Forms

Caplet, oral:

Aler-Dryl [OTC]: 50 mg
AllerMax® [OTC]: 50 mg
Anti-Hist [OTC]: 25 mg
Compoz® [OTC]: 50 mg
Histaprin [OTC]: 25 mg
Nytol® Quick Caps [OTC]: 25 mg
Simply Sleep® [OTC]: 25 mg
Sleep-ettes D [OTC]: 50 mg
Sominex® Maximum Strength [OTC]: 50 mg
Twilite® [OTC]: 50 mg

Capsule, oral: 25 mg, 50 mg
Aler-Cap [OTC]: 25 mg
Banophen™ [OTC]: 25 mg
Benadryl® Allergy [OTC]: 25 mg
Diphen [OTC]: 25 mg
Diphenhist® [OTC]: 25 mg
Sleepinal® [OTC]: 50 mg
Capsule, softgel, oral:
Benadryl® Dye-Free Allergy [OTC]: 25 mg
Compoz® [OTC]: 50 mg
Nytol® Quick Gels [OTC]: 50 mg
Unisom® SleepGels® Maximum Strength [OTC]: 50 mg
Captab, oral:
Diphenhist® [OTC]: 25 mg
Elixir, oral:
Altaryl [OTC]: 12.5 mg/5 mL (120 mL, 480 mL, 3840 mL)
Banophen™ [OTC]: 12.5 mg/5 mL (120 mL, 480 mL)
Injection, solution: 50 mg/mL (1 mL, 10 mL)
Injection, solution [preservative free]: 50 mg/mL (1 mL)
Liquid, oral:
AllerMax® [OTC]: 12.5 mg/5 mL (120 mL)
Benadryl® Children's Allergy [OTC]: 12.5 mg/5 mL (118 mL, 236 mL)
Benadryl® Children's Allergy Perfect Measure™ [OTC]: 12.5 mg/5 mL (5 mL)
Benadryl® Children's Dye Free Allergy [OTC]: 12.5 mg/5 mL (118 mL)
Siladryl Allergy [OTC]: 12.5 mg/5 mL (118 mL, 237 mL, 473 mL)
Solution, oral: 12.5 mg/5 mL (5 mL, 10 mL, 20 mL)
Diphenhist® [OTC]: 12.5 mg/5 mL (120 mL, 480 mL)
Strip, orally disintegrating, oral:
Benadryl® Allergy Quick Dissolve [OTC]: 25 mg (10s)
Theraflu® Thin Strips® Multi Symptom [OTC]: 25 mg (12s, 24s)
Triaminic Thin Strips® Children's Cough & Runny Nose [OTC]: 12.5 mg (14s)
Syrup, oral:
PediaCare® Children's Allergy [OTC]: 12.5 mg/5 mL (118 mL)
PediaCare® Children's NightTime Cough [OTC]: 12.5 mg/5 mL (118 mL)
Silphen [OTC]: 12.5 mg/5 mL (118 mL, 237 mL, 473 mL)
Tablet, oral: 25 mg, 50 mg
Aler-Tab [OTC]: 25 mg
Banophen™ [OTC]: 25 mg
Benadryl® Allergy [OTC]: 25 mg
Sleep-Tabs [OTC]: 25 mg
Sominex® [OTC]: 25 mg
Tablet, orally dissolving, oral:
Benadryl® Children's Allergy FastMelt® [OTC]: 12.5 mg
Unisom® SleepMelts™ [OTC]: 25 mg

diphenhydramine (topical) (dye fen HYE dra meen)

Sound-Alike/Look-Alike Issues
diphenhydrAMINE may be confused with desipramine, dicyclomine, dimenhyDRINATE
Benadryl® may be confused with benazepril, Bentyl®, Benylin®, Caladryl®

Synonyms diphenhydramine hydrochloride

Tall-Man diphenhydr**AMINE**

U.S./Canadian Brand Names Banophen™ Anti-Itch [US-OTC]; Benadryl® Cream [Can]; Benadryl® Extra Strength Itch Stopping [US-OTC]; Benadryl® Itch Relief Extra Strength [US-OTC]; Benadryl® Itch Relief Stick [Can]; Benadryl® Itch Stopping Extra Strength [US-OTC]; Benadryl® Itch Stopping [US-OTC]; Benadryl® Spray [Can]; Dermamycin® [US-OTC]; Diphenhist® [US-OTC]

Therapeutic Category Histamine H_1 Antagonist; Histamine H_1 Antagonist, First Generation; Topical Skin Product

Use Topically for relief of pain and itching associated with insect bites, minor cuts and burns, or rashes due to poison ivy, poison oak, and poison sumac

Dosage Summary

Topical:

Children ≥2 years: Apply 1% or 2% up to 3-4 times/day

Adults: Apply 1% or 2% up to 3-4 times/day

Dosage Forms

Cream, topical: 2% (30 g)

Banophen™ Anti-Itch [OTC]: 2% (28.4 g)

Benadryl® Itch Stopping [OTC]: 1% (14.2 g, 28.3 g)

Benadryl® Itch Stopping Extra Strength [OTC]: 2% (14.2 g, 28.3 g)

Dermamycin® [OTC]: 2% (28 g)

Diphenhist® [OTC]: 2% (28.4 g)

Gel, topical:

Benadryl® Extra Strength Itch Stopping [OTC]: 2% (120 mL)

Liquid, topical:

Benadryl® Itch Relief Extra Strength [OTC]: 2% (14 mL)

Benadryl® Itch Stopping Extra Strength [OTC]: 2% (59 mL)

Dermamycin® [OTC]: 2% (60 mL)

diphenhydramine and acetaminophen *see* acetaminophen and diphenhydramine *on page 24*

diphenhydramine and ASA *see* aspirin and diphenhydramine *on page 101*

diphenhydramine and aspirin *see* aspirin and diphenhydramine *on page 101*

diphenhydramine and phenylephrine (dye fen HYE dra meen & fen il EF rin)

Synonyms diphenhydramine hydrochloride and phenylephrine hydrochloride; diphenhydramine tannate and phenylephrine tannate; phenylephrine and diphenhydramine; phenylephrine hydrochloride and diphenhydramine hydrochloride; phenylephrine tannate and diphenhydramine tannate

U.S./Canadian Brand Names Aldex® CT [US]; Benadryl-D® Allergy & Sinus [US-OTC]; Benadryl-D® Children's Allergy & Sinus [US-OTC]; Dimetapp® Children's Nighttime Cold & Congestion [US-OTC]; Robitussin® Night Time Cough & Cold [US-OTC]; Triaminic® Children's Night Time Cold & Cough [US-OTC]; Triaminic® Children's Thin Strips® Night Time Cold & Cough [US-OTC]

Therapeutic Category Alpha/Beta Agonist; Histamine H_1 Antagonist; Histamine H_1 Antagonist, First Generation

Use Temporary relief of symptoms of allergic rhinitis, sinusitis, and other upper respiratory conditions, including sinus/nasal congestion, sneezing, stuffy/runny nose, itchy/watery eyes, and cough

Dosage Summary

Oral:

Children <2 years: Dosage not established

Children 2-5 years: D-Tann: 1.25-2.5 mL every 12 hours

Children 6-11 years: Aldex® CT: One-half to 1 tablet every 6 hours; D-Tann: 2.5-5 mL **or** 1/2 to 1 tablet every 12 hours; OTC labeling: 5-10 mL or 1 strip every 4 hours as needed (maximum: 6 doses/24 hours)

Children ≥12 years: Aldex® CT: 1-2 tablets every 6 hours; D-Tann: 5-10 mL **or** 1-2 tablets every 12 hours; OTC labeling: 10-20 mL every 4 hours as needed or 1 tablet every 4 hours as needed (maximum: 6 doses/24 hours)

Adults: Aldex® CT: 1-2 tablets every 6 hours; D-Tann: 5-10 mL **or** 1-2 tablets every 12 hours; OTC labeling: 10-20 mL every 4 hours as needed or 1 tablet every 4 hours as needed (maximum: 6 doses/24 hours)

Dosage Forms

Liquid, oral:

Benadryl-D® Children's Allergy & Sinus [OTC]: Diphenhydramine 12.5 mg and phenylephrine 5 mg per 5 mL (118 mL)

Strip, orally disintegrating:

Triaminic® Children's Thin Strips® Night Time Cold & Cough [OTC]: Diphenhydramine 12.5 mg and phenylephrine 5 mg

Syrup, oral:

Dimetapp® Children's Nighttime Cold and Congestion [OTC]: Diphenhydramine 6.25 mg and phenylephrine 2.5 mg per 5 mL (120 mL)

Robitussin® Night Time Cough & Cold [OTC]: Diphenhydramine 6.25 mg and phenylephrine 2.5 mg per 5 mL (120 mL)

Triaminic® Children's Night Time Cold & Cough [OTC]: Diphenhydramine 6.25 mg and phenylephrine 2.5 mg per 5 mL (118 mL)

Tablet, oral:

Benadryl-D® Allergy & Sinus [OTC]: Diphenhydramine 25 mg and phenylephrine 10 mg

Tablet, chewable, oral:

Aldex® CT: Diphenhydramine 12.5 mg and phenylephrine 5 mg

diphenhydramine and pseudoephedrine *(Discontinued)*

diphenhydramine citrate *see* diphenhydramine (systemic) *on page 310*

diphenhydramine citrate and aspirin *see* aspirin and diphenhydramine *on page 101*

diphenhydramine hydrochloride *see* diphenhydramine (systemic) *on page 310*

diphenhydramine hydrochloride *see* diphenhydramine (topical) *on page 311*

diphenhydramine hydrochloride and phenylephrine hydrochloride *see* diphenhydramine and phenylephrine *on page 312*

diphenhydramine, phenylephrine hydrochloride, and acetaminophen *see* acetaminophen, diphenhydramine, and phenylephrine *on page 30*

diphenhydramine tannate *see* diphenhydramine (systemic) *on page 310*

diphenhydramine tannate and phenylephrine tannate *see* diphenhydramine and phenylephrine *on page 312*

diphenoxylate and atropine (dye fen OKS i late & A troe peen)

Sound-Alike/Look-Alike Issues

Lomotil® may be confused with Lamictal®, Lamisil®, lamoTRIgine, Lanoxin®, Lasix®, ludiomil

Synonyms atropine and diphenoxylate

U.S./Canadian Brand Names Lomotil® [US/Can]

Therapeutic Category Antidiarrheal

Controlled Substance C-V

Use Treatment of diarrhea

Dosage Summary

Oral:

Children <2 years: Dosage not established

Children 2-12 years: Initial: Diphenoxylate 0.3-0.4 mg/kg/day in 4 divided doses (maximum: 10 mg/day); Maintenance: Reduce as needed, may be as low as 25% of the initial daily dose

Adults: Initial: Diphenoxylate 5 mg 4 times/day (maximum: 20 mg/day); Maintenance: Reduce as needed, may be as low as 5 mg/day

Dosage Forms

Solution, oral: Diphenoxylate 2.5 mg and atropine 0.025 mg per 5 mL

Tablet: Diphenoxylate 2.5 mg and atropine 0.025 mg

Diphenylan Sodium® *(Discontinued)* *see* phenytoin *on page 756*

diphenylhydantoin *see* phenytoin *on page 756*

diphtheria and tetanus toxoid (dif THEER ee a & TET a nus TOKS oyds)

Sound-Alike/Look-Alike Issues

diphtheria and Tetanus Toxoids (Td) may be confused with tuberculin purified protein derivative (PPD)

Synonyms DT; Td; tetanus and diphtheria toxoid

U.S./Canadian Brand Names Decavac® [US]; Td Adsorbed [Can]

Therapeutic Category Toxoid

Use

Diphtheria and tetanus toxoids adsorbed for pediatric use (DT): Infants and children through 6 years of age: Active immunization against diphtheria and tetanus when pertussis vaccine is contraindicated

Tetanus and diphtheria toxoids adsorbed for adult use (Td) (Decavac™): Children ≥7 years of age and Adults: Active immunization against diphtheria and tetanus; tetanus prophylaxis in wound management

The Advisory Committee on Immunization Practices (ACIP) recommends routine vaccination for the following:

- Adults and children ≥7 years should receive a booster dose of Td every 10 years; persons <65 years of age may substitute a single Td booster dose with Tdap
- Children 7-10 years, adults, and the elderly (≥65 years) who are wounded in bombings or similar mass casualty events who have penetrating injuries or nonintact skin exposure and who cannot confirm receipt of a tetanus booster within the previous 5 years, may also receive a single dose of Td; children ≥11 years may also receive Td if Tdap is unavailable

Dosage Summary

I.M.:

DT:

Children <6 weeks: Dosage not established

Children 6 weeks to 1 year: Three 0.5 mL doses at least 4 weeks apart, administer a reinforcing dose 6-12 months after the third injection

Children 1-6 years: Two 0.5 mL doses at least 4-8 weeks apart; reinforcing dose 6-12 months after second injection

Children 4-6 years (booster immunization): 0.5 mL, repeat at 10-year intervals with the adult preparation

Td:

Children ≥7 years: Two 0.5 mL doses 4-8 weeks apart, then a third (reinforcing) dose of 0.5 mL 6-12 months later; Booster: 0.5 mL every 10 years

Adults: Two 0.5 mL doses 4-8 weeks apart, then a third (reinforcing) dose of 0.5 mL 6-12 months later; Booster: 0.5 mL every 10 years

Dosage Forms

Injection, suspension [Td, adult; preservative free]: Diphtheria 2 Lf units and tetanus 2 Lf units per 0.5 mL (0.5 mL)

Decavac™: Diphtheria 2 Lf units and tetanus 5 Lf units per 0.5 mL (0.5 mL)

Injection, suspension [DT, pediatric; preservative free]: Diphtheria 6.7 Lf units and tetanus 5 Lf units per 0.5 mL (0.5 mL)

diphtheria and tetanus toxoids, acellular pertussis, and poliovirus vaccine

(dif THEER ee a & TET a nus TOKS oyds, ay CEL yoo lar per TUS sis & POE lee oh VYE rus vak SEEN)

Synonyms diphtheria and tetanus toxoids and acellular pertussis adsorbed, and inactivated poliovirus vaccine combined; diphtheria, tetanus toxoids, acellular pertussis (DTaP); DTaP-IPV; poliovirus, inactivated (IPV)

U.S./Canadian Brand Names Kinrix™ [US]

Therapeutic Category Vaccine, Inactivated

Use Active immunization against diphtheria, tetanus, pertussis, and poliomyelitis, used as the 5th dose in the DTaP series and the 4th dose in the IPV series

The Advisory Committee on Immunization Practices (ACIP) recommends routine vaccination for use as the fifth dose in the DTaP series and the fourth dose in the IPV series in children who received DTaP (Infanrix®) and/or DTaP-Hepatitis B-IPV (Pediarix®) as the first 3 doses and DTaP (Infanrix®) as the fourth dose. Whenever feasible, the same manufacturer should be used to provide the pertussis component; however, vaccination should not be deferred if a specific brand is not known or is not available.

Dosage Summary

I.M.:

Children <4 years: Dosage not established

Children 4-6 years: 0.5 mL

Children ≥7 years: Dosage not established

Adults: Dosage not established

Dosage Forms

Injection, suspension [preservative free]:

Kinrix™: Diphtheria toxoid 25 Lf, tetanus toxoid 10 Lf, acellular pertussis antigens [inactivated pertussis toxin 25 mcg, filamentous hemagglutinin 25 mcg, pertactin 8 mcg], type 1 poliovirus 40 D-antigen units, type 2 poliovirus 8 D-antigen units, and type 3 poliovirus 32 D-antigen units per 0.5 mL (0.5 mL)

diphtheria and tetanus toxoids, acellular pertussis, poliovirus and *Haemophilus* b conjugate vaccine

(dif THEER ee a & TET a nus TOKS oyds ay CEL yoo lar per TUS sis POE lee oh VYE rus & hem OF fi lus in floo EN za bee KON joo gate vak SEEN)

Synonyms *Haemophilus* B conjugate (Hib); *Haemophilus* B polysaccharide; diphtheria toxoid; diphtheria, tetanus toxoids, acellular pertussis (DTaP); DTaP-IPV/Hib; pertussis, acellular (adsorbed); poliovirus, inactivated (IPV); tetanus toxoid

U.S./Canadian Brand Names Pediacel® [Can]; Pentacel® [US/Can]

Therapeutic Category Vaccine, Inactivated

Use Active immunization against diphtheria, tetanus, pertussis, poliomyelitis, and invasive disease caused by *H. influenzae* type b in children 6 weeks through 4 years of age

Advisory Committee on Immunization Practices (ACIP) recommends that Pentacel® (DTaP-IPV/Hib) may be used to provide the recommended DTaP, IPV, and Hib immunization in children <5 years of age. Whenever feasible, the same manufacturer should be used to provide the pertussis component; however, vaccination should not be deferred if a specific brand is not known or is not available. The Hib component in Pentacel® contains a tetanus toxoid conjugate. A Hib vaccine containing the PRP-OMP conjugate (PedvaxHIB®) may provide a more rapid seroconversion following the first dose and may be preferable to use in certain populations (eg, American Indian or Alaska Native children).

Dosage Summary

I.M.:

Children 6 weeks to ≤4 years: 0.5 mL per dose administered at 2, 4, 6, and 15-18 months (total of 4 doses)

Children ≥5 years: Dosage not established

Adults: Dosage not established

Dosage Forms

Injection, suspension:

Pentacel®: Diphtheria toxoid 15 Lf, tetanus toxoid 5 Lf, acellular pertussis antigens, poliovirus, and *Haemophilus* b capsular polysaccharide 10 mcg per 0.5 mL (0.5 mL)

diphtheria and tetanus toxoids and acellular pertussis adsorbed, and inactivated poliovirus vaccine combined *see* diphtheria and tetanus toxoids, acellular pertussis, and poliovirus vaccine *on page 314*

diphtheria and tetanus toxoids and acellular pertussis adsorbed, hepatitis B (recombinant) and inactivated poliovirus vaccine combined *see* diphtheria, tetanus toxoids, acellular pertussis, hepatitis B (recombinant), and poliovirus (inactivated) vaccine *on page 315*

diphtheria antitoxin (dif THEER ee a an tee TOKS in)

Therapeutic Category Antitoxin

Use Treatment of diphtheria (neutralizes unbound toxin, available from CDC)

Dosage Summary

I.M.:

Children: 20,000-120,000 units

Adults: 20,000-120,000 units

I.V.:

Children: Infusion: 20,000-120,000 units

Adults: Infusion: 20,000-120,000 units

diphtheria CRM$_{197}$ protein *see* pneumococcal conjugate vaccine (7-valent) *on page 771*

diphtheria CRM$_{197}$ protein *see* pneumococcal conjugate vaccine (13-valent) *on page 770*

diphtheria, tetanus toxoids, acellular pertussis (DTaP) *see* diphtheria and tetanus toxoids, acellular pertussis, and poliovirus vaccine *on page 314*

diphtheria, tetanus toxoids, acellular pertussis (DTaP) *see* diphtheria and tetanus toxoids, acellular pertussis, poliovirus and *Haemophilus* b conjugate vaccine *on page 314*

diphtheria, tetanus toxoids, acellular pertussis, hepatitis B (recombinant), and poliovirus (inactivated) vaccine

(dif THEER ee a, TET a nus TOKS oyds, ay CEL yoo lar per TUS sis, hep a TYE tis bee ree KOM be nant, & POE lee oh VYE rus vak SEEN)

Synonyms diphtheria and tetanus toxoids and acellular pertussis adsorbed, hepatitis B (recombinant) and inactivated poliovirus vaccine combined; DTap-HepB-IPV

U.S./Canadian Brand Names Pediarix® [US/Can]

Therapeutic Category Vaccine

Use Combination vaccine for the active immunization against diphtheria, tetanus, pertussis, hepatitis B virus (all known subtypes), and poliomyelitis (caused by poliovirus types 1, 2, and 3)

The Advisory Committee on Immunization Practices (ACIP) recommends Pediarix® for the following:

- Primary vaccination for DTaP, Hep B, and IPV in children at 2, 4, and 6 months of age.
- To complete the primary vaccination series in children who have received DTaP (Infanrix®) and who are scheduled to receive the other components of the vaccine. Whenever feasible, the same manufacturer should be used to provide the pertussis component; however, vaccination should not be

deferred if a specific brand is not known or is not available. HepB and IPV from different manufacturers are interchangeable.

Dosage Summary

I.M.:

Children <6 weeks: Dosage not established

Children 6 weeks to <7 years: 0.5 mL every 6-8 weeks for a total of 3 doses

Adults: Dosage not established

Dosage Forms

Injection, suspension [preservative free]:

Pediarix®: Diphtheria toxoid 25 Lf, tetanus toxoid 10 Lf, acellular pertussis antigens per 0.5 mL (0.5 mL)

diphtheria, tetanus toxoids, and acellular pertussis vaccine

(dif THEER ee a & TET a nus TOKS oyds & ay CEL yoo lar per TUS sis vak SEEN)

Sound-Alike/Look-Alike Issues

Adacel® (Tdap) may be confused with Daptacel® (DTap)

Synonyms DTaP; dTpa; Tdap; tetanus toxoid, reduced diphtheria toxoid, and acellular pertussis, adsorbed

U.S./Canadian Brand Names Adacel® [US/Can]; Boostrix® [US/Can]; Daptacel® [US]; Infanrix® [US]; Tripedia® [US]

Therapeutic Category Toxoid

Use

Daptacel®, Infanrix®, Tripedia® (DTaP): Active immunization against diphtheria, tetanus, and pertussis from age 6 weeks through 6 years of age (prior to seventh birthday)

Adacel®, Boostrix® (Tdap): Active booster immunization against diphtheria, tetanus, and pertussis

The Advisory Committee on Immunization Practices (ACIP) recommends routine vaccination for the following:

Children 6 weeks to <7 years (DTaP): For primary immunization against diphtheria, tetanus and pertussis

Adolescents 11-18 years (Tdap):

- A single dose of Tdap as a booster dose in adolescents who have completed the recommended childhood DTaP vaccination series (preferred age of administration is 11-12 years)
- A single dose of Tdap should be given to replace a single dose of Td if the last dose of Td was ≥5 years earlier; lesser intervals may be used if the benefit outweighs the risk (not for multiple administrations; recommendations are for the replacement of a single dose of Td only)
- Persons wounded in bombings or similar mass casualty events and who cannot confirm receipt of a tetanus booster within the previous 5 years and who have penetrating injuries or nonintact skin exposure should receive a single dose of Tdap

Adults 19-64 years: A single dose of Tdap should be given to replace a single dose of Td if the last dose of Td was ≥10 years earlier (not for multiple administrations; recommendations are for the replacement of a single dose of Td only). A shorter interval (<10 years but at least 2 years since last dose of Td) may be considered in the following situations:

- To protect against pertussis
- To protect against pertussis transmission to infants in adults who anticipate close contact with children <12 months of age; Tdap should be administered at least 2 weeks prior to beginning close contact
- Healthcare providers with direct patient contact
- Persons wounded in bombings or similar mass casualty events and who cannot confirm receipt of a tetanus booster within the previous 5 years and who have penetrating injuries or nonintact skin exposure, should receive a single dose of Tdap

Dosage Summary

I.M.:

Children 6 weeks to <7 years: Primary immunization: Daptacel®, Infanrix®, Tripedia®: 0.5 mL per dose, total of 5 doses: Three doses, usually given at 2, 4, and 6 months of age; Fourth dose given at ~15-20 months of age; Fifth dose given at 4-6 years of age

Children ≥10 years: Booster immunization: Boostrix®: 0.5 mL as a single dose

Children ≥11 years: Booster immunization: Adacel®: 0.5 mL as a single dose

Adults ≤64 years: Booster immunization: Adacel®, Boostrix®: 0.5 mL as a single dose

Dosage Forms

Injection, suspension [Tdap, booster formulation]:

Adacel®: Diphtheria 2 Lf units, tetanus 5 Lf units, and acellular pertussis antigens per 0.5 mL (0.5 mL)

Boostrix®: Diphtheria 2.5 Lf units, tetanus 5 Lf units, and acellular pertussis antigens per 0.5 mL (0.5 mL)

Injection, suspension [DTaP, active immunization formulation]:

Daptacel®: Diphtheria 15 Lf units, tetanus 5 Lf units, and acellular pertussis antigens per 0.5 mL (0.5 mL)

Infanrix®: Diphtheria 25 Lf units, tetanus 10 Lf units, and acellular pertussis antigens per 0.5 mL (0.5 mL) [preservative free]

Tripedia®: Diphtheria 6.7 Lf units, tetanus 5 Lf units, and acellular pertussis antigens per 0.5 mL (0.5 mL)

Note: Tripedia® vaccine is also used to reconstitute ActHIB® to prepare TriHIBit® vaccine (diphtheria, tetanus toxoids, and acellular pertussis and *Haemophilus influenzae* b conjugate vaccine combination)

diphtheria, tetanus toxoids, and acellular pertussis vaccine and *Haemophilus influenzae* b conjugate vaccine

(dif THEER ee a & TET a nus TOKS oyds, ay CEL yoo lar per TUS sis & hem OF fi lus in floo EN za bee KON joo gate vak SEEN)

Synonyms *Haemophilus influenzae* b conjugate vaccine and diphtheria, tetanus toxoids, and acellular pertussis vaccine; DTaP/Hib

U.S./Canadian Brand Names TriHIBit® [US]

Therapeutic Category Toxoid; Vaccine, Inactivated Bacteria

Use Active immunization of children 15-18 months of age for prevention of diphtheria, tetanus, pertussis, and invasive disease caused by *H. influenzae* type b

The Advisory Committee on Immunization Practices (ACIP) recommends the use of TriHIBit® for the fourth dose of the diphtheria, tetanus, pertussis, and *Haemophilus* vaccine series. Whenever feasible, the same manufacturer should be used to provide the pertussis component; however, vaccination should not be deferred if a specific brand is not known or is not available.

Dosage Summary

I.M.:

Children <12 months: Dosage not established

Children 12-20 months: 0.5 mL (as part of a general vaccination schedule)

Adults: Dosage not established

Dosage Forms

Injection, suspension [preservative free]:

TriHIBit®: Diphtheria 6.7 Lf units, tetanus 5 Lf units, acellular pertussis antigens [inactivated pertussis toxin 23.4 mcg, filamentous hemagglutinin 23.4 mcg], and *Haemophilus* b capsular polysaccharide 10 mcg [bound to tetanus toxoid 24 mcg] per 0.5 mL (0.5 mL) [Tripedia® vaccine used to reconstitute ActHIB® forms TriHIBit®]

diphtheria toxoid *see* diphtheria and tetanus toxoids, acellular pertussis, poliovirus and *Haemophilus* b conjugate vaccine *on page* 314

diphtheria toxoid conjugate *see Haemophilus* B conjugate vaccine *on page* 463

dipivalyl epinephrine *see* dipivefrin *on page* 317

dipivefrin (dye PI ve frin)

Synonyms dipivalyl epinephrine; dipivefrin hydrochloride; DPE

U.S./Canadian Brand Names Ophtho-Dipivefrin™ [Can]; PMS-Dipivefrin [Can]; Propine® [Can]

Therapeutic Category Adrenergic Agonist Agent

Use Reduces elevated intraocular pressure in chronic open-angle glaucoma; also used to treat ocular hypertension, low tension, and secondary glaucomas

Dosage Summary

Ophthalmic:

Children: Dosage not established

Adults: Instill 1 drop every 12 hours

dipivefrin hydrochloride *see* dipivefrin *on page* 317

Diprivan® [US/Can] *see* propofol *on page* 804

Diprolene® [US] *see* betamethasone *on page* 133

Diprolene® AF [US] *see* betamethasone *on page* 133

Diprolene® Glycol [Can] *see* betamethasone *on page* 133

dipropylacetic acid *see* valproic acid *on page* 974

Diprosone® [Can] *see* betamethasone *on page 133*

dipyridamole (dye peer ID a mole)

Sound-Alike/Look-Alike Issues

dipyridamole may be confused with disopyramide
Persantine® may be confused with Periactin®, Permitil®

U.S./Canadian Brand Names Apo-Dipyridamole FC® [Can]; Dipyridamole For Injection [Can]; Persantine® [US/Can]

Therapeutic Category Antiplatelet Agent; Vasodilator

Use

Oral: Used with warfarin to decrease thrombosis in patients after artificial heart valve replacement
I.V.: Diagnostic agent in CAD

Dosage Summary

I.V.:

Children: Dosage not established
Adults: 0.14 mg/kg/minute for 4 minutes (maximum: 60 mg)

Oral:

Children ≥12 years: 75-100 mg 4 times/day
Adults: 75-100 mg 4 times/day

Dosage Forms

Injection, solution: 5 mg/mL (2 mL, 10 mL)
Tablet, oral: 25 mg, 50 mg, 75 mg
Persantine®: 25 mg, 50 mg, 75 mg

dipyridamole and aspirin *see* aspirin and dipyridamole *on page 101*
Dipyridamole For Injection [Can] *see* dipyridamole *on page 318*
Disalcid® ***(Discontinued)*** *see* salsalate *on page 862*
disalicylic acid *see* salsalate *on page 862*
DisCoVisc® [US] *see* sodium chondroitin sulfate and sodium hyaluronate *on page 884*
Disobrom® ***(Discontinued)*** *see* dexbrompheniramine and pseudoephedrine *on page 282*
disodium cromoglycate *see* cromolyn (nasal) *on page 255*
disodium cromoglycate *see* cromolyn (ophthalmic) *on page 255*
disodium cromoglycate *see* cromolyn (systemic, oral inhalation) *on page 254*
disodium thiosulfate pentahydrate *see* sodium thiosulfate *on page 888*
***d*-isoephedrine hydrochloride** *see* pseudoephedrine *on page 810*
Disonate® ***(Discontinued)*** *see* docusate *on page 321*

disopyramide (dye soe PEER a mide)

Sound-Alike/Look-Alike Issues

disopyramide may be confused with desipramine, dipyridamole
Norpace® may be confused with Norpramin®

Synonyms disopyramide phosphate

U.S./Canadian Brand Names Norpace® CR [US]; Norpace® [US/Can]; Rythmodan® [Can]; Rythmodan®-LA [Can]

Therapeutic Category Antiarrhythmic Agent, Class I-A

Use Suppression and prevention of unifocal and multifocal atrial and premature, ventricular premature complexes, coupled ventricular tachycardia; effective in the conversion of atrial fibrillation, atrial flutter, and paroxysmal atrial tachycardia to normal sinus rhythm and prevention of the recurrence of these arrhythmias after conversion by other methods

Dosage Summary

Oral:

Controlled release:

Children: Dosage not established
Adults <50 kg: 200 mg every 12 hours
Adults ≥50 kg: 300 mg every 12 hours

Immediate release:

Children <1 year: 10-30 mg/kg/day in 4 divided doses
Children 1-4 years: 10-20 mg/kg/day in 4 divided doses
Children 4-12 years: 10-15 mg/kg/day in 4 divided doses

Children 12-18 years: 6-15 mg/kg/day in 4 divided doses
Adults <50 kg: 100 mg every 6 hours
Adults ≥50 kg: Initial: 150 mg every 6 hours; Maintenance: 150-400 mg every 6 hours

Dosage Forms

Capsule, oral: 100 mg, 150 mg
Norpace®: 100 mg, 150 mg
Capsule, controlled release, oral:
Norpace® CR: 100 mg, 150 mg
Capsule, extended release, oral: 150 mg

disopyramide phosphate *see* disopyramide *on page 318*
Disotate® *(Discontinued)* *see* edetate disodium *on page 342*
Di-Spaz® Injection *(Discontinued)* *see* dicyclomine *on page 299*
Di-Spaz® Oral *(Discontinued)* *see* dicyclomine *on page 299*
DisperMox™ *(Discontinued)* *see* amoxicillin *on page 72*

disulfiram (dye SUL fi ram)

Sound-Alike/Look-Alike Issues

disulfiram may be confused with Diflucan®
Antabuse® may be confused with Anturane®

U.S./Canadian Brand Names Antabuse® [US]

Therapeutic Category Aldehyde Dehydrogenase Inhibitor Agent

Use Management of chronic alcoholism

Dosage Summary

Oral:
Children: Dosage not established
Adults: Initial: 500 mg once daily; Maintenance: 125-500 mg once daily (maximum: 500 mg/day)

Dosage Forms

Tablet, oral:
Antabuse®: 250 mg, 500 mg

Dital® *(Discontinued)* *see* phendimetrazine *on page 747*
dithioglycerol *see* dimercaprol *on page 307*
dithranol *see* anthralin *on page 79*
Ditropan® [US/Can] *see* oxybutynin *on page 713*
Ditropan XL® [US/Can] *see* oxybutynin *on page 713*
diurex® [US-OTC] *see* pamabrom *on page 722*
diurex® Aquagels® [US-OTC] *see* pamabrom *on page 722*
diurex® Maximum Relief [US-OTC] *see* pamabrom *on page 722*
Diurigen® *(Discontinued)* *see* chlorothiazide *on page 207*
Diuril® [US/Can] *see* chlorothiazide *on page 207*

divalproex (dye VAL proe ex)

Sound-Alike/Look-Alike Issues

Depakote® may be confused with Depakene®, Depakote® ER, Senokot®
Depakote® ER may be confused with Depakote®, divalproex enteric coated

Synonyms divalproex sodium; valproic acid derivative

U.S./Canadian Brand Names Apo-Divalproex® [Can]; Depakote® ER [US]; Depakote® Sprinkle [US]; Depakote® [US]; Dom-Divalproex [Can]; Epival® [Can]; Mylan-Divalproex [Can]; Novo-Divalproex [Can]; Nu-Divalproex [Can]; PHL-Divalproex [Can]; PMS-Divalproex [Can]

Therapeutic Category Anticonvulsant, Miscellaneous; Antimanic Agent; Histone Deacetylase Inhibitor

Use Monotherapy and adjunctive therapy in the treatment of patients with complex partial seizures; monotherapy and adjunctive therapy of simple and complex absence seizures; adjunctive therapy in patients with multiple seizure types that include absence seizures
Depakote®, Depakote® ER: Mania associated with bipolar disorder; migraine prophylaxis

Dosage Summary

Oral:

Children: Simple and complex absence seizures: Initial: 15 mg/kg/day; increase by 5-10 mg/kg/day at weekly intervals until therapeutic levels are achieved; maximum: 60 mg/kg/day. **Note:** Titration recommended. Administer doses >250 mg/day in divided doses.

Children ≥10 years: Complex partial seizures: Initial: 10-15 mg/kg/day; increase by 5-10 mg/kg/day at weekly intervals until therapeutic levels are achieved; maximum: 60 mg/kg/day. **Note:** Titration recommended. Administer doses >250 mg/day in divided doses.

Children ≥16 years: Migraine prophylaxis: Depakote® ER 500 mg once daily for 7 days, then increase to 1000 mg once daily **or** Depakote® tablets 250 mg twice daily; adjust dose based on patient response, up to 1000 mg/day

Adults:

Seizure disorders: Initial: 10-15 mg/kg/day in 1-3 divided doses; increase by 5-10 mg/kg/day at weekly intervals until therapeutic levels are achieved; maximum: 60 mg/kg/day. **Note:** Titration recommended. Administer doses >250 mg/day in divided doses.

Mania: Depakote® tablet: Initial: 750 mg/day in divided doses; Depakote® ER: Initial: 25 mg/kg/day given once daily; dose should be adjusted as rapidly as possible to desired clinical effect; maximum recommended dose: 60 mg/kg/day

Migraine prophylaxis: Depakote® ER 500 mg once daily for 7 days, then increase to 1000 mg once daily **or** Depakote® tablets 250 mg twice daily; adjust dose based on patient response, up to 1000 mg/day

Dosage Forms

Capsule, sprinkle, oral: 125 mg

Depakote® Sprinkle: 125 mg

Tablet, delayed release, oral: 125 mg, 250 mg, 500 mg

Depakote®: 125 mg, 250 mg, 500 mg

Tablet, extended release, oral: 250 mg, 500 mg

Depakote® ER: 250 mg, 500 mg

divalproex sodium *see* divalproex *on page 319*

Divigel® [US] *see* estradiol (systemic) *on page 366*

Dixarit® [Can] *see* clonidine *on page 238*

Dizac® Injectable Emulsion *(Discontinued)* *see* diazepam *on page 294*

Dizmiss® *(Discontinued)* *see* meclizine *on page 595*

5071-1DL(6) *see* megestrol *on page 598*

***dl*-alpha tocopherol** *see* vitamin E *on page 988*

4-DMDR *see* idarubicin *on page 497*

***D*-mannitol** *see* mannitol *on page 590*

D-Med® Injection *(Discontinued)* *see* methylprednisolone *on page 622*

DMSA *see* succimer *on page 896*

DMSO *see* dimethyl sulfoxide *on page 308*

Doak® Tar [US-OTC] *see* coal tar *on page 242*

Doak® Tar Distillate [US] *see* coal tar *on page 242*

Doak® Tar Oil [US-OTC] *see* coal tar *on page 242*

Doan's® Extra Strength [US-OTC] *see* magnesium salicylate *on page 587*

dobutamine (doe BYOO ta meen)

Sound-Alike/Look-Alike Issues

DOBUTamine may be confused with DOPamine

Synonyms dobutamine hydrochloride

Tall-Man DOBUTamine

U.S./Canadian Brand Names Dobutamine Injection, USP [Can]; Dobutrex® [Can]

Therapeutic Category Adrenergic Agonist Agent

Use Short-term management of patients with cardiac decompensation

Dosage Summary

I.V.:

Children: 2.5-20 mcg/kg/minute (maximum: 40 mcg/kg/minute)

Adults: 2.5-20 mcg/kg/minute (maximum: 40 mcg/kg/minute)

Dosage Forms

Infusion, premixed in D_5W: 1 mg/mL (250 mL, 500 mL); 2 mg/mL (250 mL); 4 mg/mL (250 mL)

Injection, solution: 12.5 mg/mL (20 mL, 40 mL, 100 mL)

dobutamine hydrochloride *see* dobutamine *on page* 320

Dobutamine Injection, USP [Can] *see* dobutamine *on page* 320

Dobutrex® [Can] *see* dobutamine *on page* 320

docetaxel (doe se TAKS el)

Sound-Alike/Look-Alike Issues

Taxotere® may be confused with Taxol®

Synonyms NSC-628503; RP-6976

U.S./Canadian Brand Names Taxotere® [US/Can]

Therapeutic Category Antineoplastic Agent

Use Treatment of breast cancer (locally advanced/metastatic or adjuvant treatment of operable node-positive); locally-advanced or metastatic nonsmall cell lung cancer (NSCLC); hormone refractory, metastatic prostate cancer; advanced gastric adenocarcinoma; locally-advanced squamous cell head and neck cancer

Dosage Summary

I.V.:

Children: Dosage not established

Adults: 60-100 mg/m^2 every 3 weeks

Dosage Forms

Injection, solution:

Taxotere®: 20 mg/0.5 mL (0.5 mL, 2 mL)

docosanol (doe KOE san ole)

Synonyms *n*-docosanol; behenyl alcohol

U.S./Canadian Brand Names Abreva® [US-OTC]

Therapeutic Category Antiviral Agent, Topical

Use Treatment of herpes simplex of the face or lips

Dosage Summary

Topical:

Children <12 years: Dosage not established

Children ≥12 years: Apply 5 times/day to affected area

Adults: Apply 5 times/day to affected area

Dosage Forms

Cream, topical:

Abreva® [OTC]: 10% (2 g)

docusate (DOK yoo sate)

Sound-Alike/Look-Alike Issues

docusate may be confused with Doxinate®

Colace® may be confused with Calan®, Cozaar®

Dulcolax® (docusate) may be confused with Dulcolax® (bisacodyl)

Surfak® may be confused with Surbex®

Synonyms dioctyl calcium sulfosuccinate; dioctyl sodium sulfosuccinate; docusate calcium; docusate potassium; docusate sodium; DOSS

U.S./Canadian Brand Names Apo-Docusate-Sodium® [Can]; Colace® [US-OTC/Can]; Colax-C® [Can]; Correctol® [US-OTC]; Diocto [US-OTC]; Docu-Soft [US-OTC]; DocuSoft S™ [US-OTC]; Dok™ [US-OTC]; DSS® [US-OTC]; Dulcolax® (docusate) [US-OTC]; Dulcolax® Stool Softener [US-OTC]; Enemeez® Plus [US-OTC]; Enemeez® [US-OTC]; Fleet® Pedia-Lax™ Liquid Stool Softener [US-OTC]; Fleet® Sof-lax® [US-OTC]; Kaopectate® Stool Softener [US-OTC]; Novo-Docusate Calcium [Can]; Novo-Docusate Sodium [Can]; Phillips'® Liquid-Gels® [US-OTC]; Phillips'® Stool Softener Laxative [US-OTC]; PMS-Docusate Calcium [Can]; PMS-Docusate Sodium [Can]; Regulex® [Can]; Selax® [Can]; Silace [US-OTC]; Soflax™ [Can]

Therapeutic Category Stool Softener

Use Stool softener in patients who should avoid straining during defecation and constipation associated with hard, dry stools; prophylaxis for straining (Valsalva) following myocardial infarction. A safe agent to be used in elderly; some evidence that doses <200 mg are ineffective; stool softeners are unnecessary if stool is well hydrated or "mushy" and soft; shown to be ineffective used long-term.

Dosage Summary

Oral:

Children <3 years: 10-40 mg/day in 1-4 divided doses
Children 3-6 years: 20-60 mg/day in 1-4 divided doses
Children 6-12 years: 40-150 mg/day in 1-4 divided doses
Adolescents: 50-500 mg/day in 1-4 divided doses
Adults: 50-500 mg/day in 1-4 divided doses

Rectal:

Young children: Dosage not established
Older children: Add 50-100 mg to enema fluid, give as retention or flushing enema
Adults: Add 50-100 mg to enema fluid, give as a retention or flushing enema

Dosage Forms

Capsule, oral:
Colace® [OTC]: 50 mg, 100 mg

Capsule, liquid, oral:
DocuSoft S™ [OTC]: 100 mg

Capsule, softgel, oral: 100 mg, 240 mg, 250 mg
Correctol® [OTC]: 100 mg
Docu-Soft [OTC]: 100 mg
Dok™ [OTC]: 100 mg, 250 mg
DSS® [OTC]: 100 mg, 250 mg
Dulcolax® [OTC]: 100 mg
Dulcolax® Stool Softener [OTC]: 100 mg
Fleet® Sof-lax® [OTC]: 100 mg
Kaopectate® Stool Softener [OTC]: 240 mg
Phillips'® Liquid-Gels® [OTC]: 100 mg
Phillips'® Stool Softener Laxative [OTC]: 100 mg

Liquid, oral: 50 mg/5 mL (10 mL, 25 mL, 473 mL); 150 mg/15 mL (480 mL)
Diocto [OTC]: 150 mg/15 mL (480 mL)
Fleet® Pedia-Lax™ Liquid Stool Softener [OTC]: 50 mg/15 mL (118 mL)
Silace [OTC]: 150 mg/15 mL (473 mL)

Solution, rectal:
Enemeez® [OTC]: 283 mg/5 mL (5 mL)
Enemeez® Plus [OTC]: 283 mg/5 mL (5 mL)

Syrup, oral: 20 mg/5 mL (25 mL, 473 mL)
Colace® [OTC]: 60 mg/15 mL (473 mL)
Diocto [OTC]: 60 mg/15 mL (480 mL)
Silace [OTC]: 60 mg/15 mL (480 mL)

Tablet, oral:
Dok™ [OTC]: 100 mg

docusate and senna (DOK yoo sate & SEN na)

Sound-Alike/Look-Alike Issues
Senokot® may be confused with Depakote®

Synonyms senna and docusate; senna-S

U.S./Canadian Brand Names Dok™ Plus [US-OTC]; Peri-Colace® [US-OTC]; Senokot-S® [US-OTC]; SenoSol™-SS [US-OTC]

Therapeutic Category Laxative, Stimulant; Stool Softener

Use Short-term treatment of constipation

Dosage Summary

Oral:

Children <2 years: Dosage not established
Children 2-6 years: Initial: 4.3 mg sennosides plus 25 mg docusate (1/2 tablet) once daily (maximum: 1 tablet twice daily)
Children 6-12 years: Initial: 8.6 sennosides plus 50 mg docusate (1 tablet) once daily (maximum: 2 tablets twice daily)

Children ≥12 years: Initial: 2 tablets (17.2 mg sennosides plus 100 mg docusate) once daily (maximum: 4 tablets twice daily)

Adults: Initial: 2 tablets (17.2 mg sennosides plus 100 mg docusate) once daily (maximum: 4 tablets twice daily)

Dosage Forms

Tablet: Docusate 50 mg and sennosides 8.6 mg

Dok™ Plus, Peri-Colace® [OTC], Senokot-S® [OTC], SenoSol™-SS: Docusate 50 mg and sennosides 8.6 mg

docusate calcium *see* docusate *on page* 321

docusate potassium *see* docusate *on page* 321

docusate sodium *see* docusate *on page* 321

Docu-Soft [US-OTC] *see* docusate *on page* 321

Docusoft Plus™ *(Discontinued)*

DocuSoft S™ [US-OTC] *see* docusate *on page* 321

dofetilide (doe FET il ide)

U.S./Canadian Brand Names Tikosyn® [US/Can]

Therapeutic Category Antiarrhythmic Agent, Class III

Use Maintenance of normal sinus rhythm in patients with chronic atrial fibrillation/atrial flutter of longer than 1-week duration who have been converted to normal sinus rhythm; conversion of atrial fibrillation and atrial flutter to normal sinus rhythm

Dosage Summary Note: QT_c must be determined prior to first dose. If QT_c >440 msec (>500 msec in patients with ventricular conduction abnormalities), dofetilide is contraindicated

Oral:

Children: Dosage not established

Adults: Initial: 500 mcg twice daily; Maintenance: 125-500 mcg twice daily **or** 125 mcg once daily

Dosage Forms

Capsule, oral:

Tikosyn®: 125 mcg, 250 mcg, 500 mcg

Dofus [US-OTC] *see* Lactobacillus *on page* 543

Dok™ [US-OTC] *see* docusate *on page* 321

Dok™ Plus [US-OTC] *see* docusate and senna *on page* 322

Doktors® Nasal Solution *(Discontinued)* *see* phenylephrine (nasal) *on page* 751

Dolacet® Forte *(Discontinued)* *see* hydrocodone and acetaminophen *on page* 479

dolasetron (dol A se tron)

Sound-Alike/Look-Alike Issues

dolasetron may be confused with granisetron, ondansetron, palonosetron

Anzemet® may be confused with Aldomet®, Antivert®, Avandamet®

Synonyms dolasetron mesylate; MDL 73,147EF

U.S./Canadian Brand Names Anzemet® [US/Can]

Therapeutic Category Selective 5-HT_3 Receptor Antagonist

Use Prevention of nausea and vomiting associated with emetogenic cancer chemotherapy (initial and repeat courses); prevention of postoperative nausea and vomiting; treatment of postoperative nausea and vomiting (injectable form only).

Note: In Canada, dolasetron is not indicated for use in children and adolescents <18 years of age or for the prevention and treatment of postoperative nausea and vomiting (contraindicated for both).

Dosage Summary

I.V.:

Children <2 years: Dosage not established

Children 2-16 years: 1.8 mg/kg before chemotherapy (maximum: 100 mg/dose) **or** 0.35 mg/kg as a single dose before cessation of anesthesia **or** 0.35 mg/kg as soon as nausea or vomiting present (maximum: 12.5 mg)

Adults: 1.8 mg/kg or 100 mg before chemotherapy **or** 12.5 mg before cessation of anesthesia

Oral:

Children <2 years: Dosage not established

Children 2-16 years: 1.8 mg/kg before chemotherapy **or** 1.2 mg/kg before surgery (maximum: 100 mg/dose)

Adults: 100 mg before chemotherapy or surgery

Dosage Forms

Injection, solution:

Anzemet®: 20 mg/mL (0.625 mL, 5 mL, 25 mL)

Tablet, oral:

Anzemet®: 50 mg, 100 mg

Dom-Indapamide [Can] *see* indapamide *on page 504*
Dom-Levetiracetam [Can] *see* levetiracetam *on page 555*
Dom-Levo-Carbidopa [Can] *see* carbidopa and levodopa *on page 182*
Dom-Lisinopril [Can] *see* lisinopril *on page 570*
Dom-Loperamide [Can] *see* loperamide *on page 573*
Dom-Lorazepam [Can] *see* lorazepam *on page 576*
Dom-Lovastatin [Can] *see* lovastatin *on page 579*
Dom-Mefenamic Acid [Can] *see* mefenamic acid *on page 597*
Dom-Meloxicam [Can] *see* meloxicam *on page 598*
Dom-Metformin [Can] *see* metformin *on page 609*
Dom-Methimazole [Can] *see* methimazole *on page 613*
Dom-Metoprolol [Can] *see* metoprolol *on page 625*
Dom-Minocycline [Can] *see* minocycline *on page 635*
Dom-Mirtazapine [Can] *see* mirtazapine *on page 637*
Dom-Moclobemide [Can] *see* moclobemide *(Canada only) on page 639*
Dom-Ondansetron [Can] *see* ondansetron *on page 704*
Dom-Oxybutynin [Can] *see* oxybutynin *on page 713*
Dom-Paroxetine [Can] *see* paroxetine *on page 729*

domperidone *(Canada only)* (dom PE ri done)

Sound-Alike/Look-Alike Issues
domperidone may be confused with iloperidone

Synonyms domperidone maleate

U.S./Canadian Brand Names Apo-Domperidone® [Can]; Dom-Domperidone [Can]; Mylan-Domperidone [Can]; Novo-Domperidone [Can]; Nu-Domperidone [Can]; PHL-Domperidone [Can]; PMS-Domperidone [Can]; RAN™-Domperidone [Can]; ratio-Domperidone [Can]

Therapeutic Category Dopamine Antagonist

Use Symptomatic management of upper GI motility disorders associated with chronic and subacute gastritis and diabetic gastroparesis; prevention of GI symptoms associated with use of dopamine-agonist anti-Parkinson agents

Dosage Forms - Canada
Tablet: 10 mg
Alti-Domperidone, Apo-Domperidone®, Dom-Domperidone, Novo-Domperidone, Nu-Domperidone, PHL-Domperidone, PMS-Domperidone, ratio-Domperidone: 10 mg

domperidone maleate *see* domperidone *(Canada only) on page 325*
Dom-Pioglitazone [Can] *see* pioglitazone *on page 762*
Dom-Piroxicam [Can] *see* piroxicam *on page 764*
Dom-Pravastatin [Can] *see* pravastatin *on page 789*
Dom-Propranolol [Can] *see* propranolol *on page 806*
Dom-Ranitidine [Can] *see* ranitidine *on page 828*
Dom-Risperidone [Can] *see* risperidone *on page 845*
Dom-Salbutamol [Can] *see* albuterol *on page 43*
Dom-Sertraline [Can] *see* sertraline *on page 872*
Dom-Simvastatin [Can] *see* simvastatin *on page 877*
Dom-Sotalol [Can] *see* sotalol *on page 892*
Dom-Sumatriptan [Can] *see* sumatriptan *on page 904*
Dom-Temazepam [Can] *see* temazepam *on page 914*
Dom-Terazosin [Can] *see* terazosin *on page 917*
Dom-Tiaprofenic [Can] *see* tiaprofenic acid *(Canada only) on page 931*
Dom-Timolol [Can] *see* timolol (ophthalmic) *on page 933*
Dom-Topiramate [Can] *see* topiramate *on page 942*
Dom-Trazodone [Can] *see* trazodone *on page 950*
Dom-Ursodiol C [Can] *see* ursodiol *on page 972*
Dom-Verapamil SR [Can] *see* verapamil *on page 981*
Dom-Zopiclone [Can] *see* zopiclone *(Canada only) on page 1005*

Donatussin [US] *see* dextromethorphan, chlorpheniramine, phenylephrine, and guaifenesin *on page 290*

Donatussin DC *(Discontinued)*

Donatussin DM *(Discontinued)* *see* chlorpheniramine, phenylephrine, and dextromethorphan *on page 211*

Donatussin Drops [US] *see* guaifenesin and phenylephrine *on page 456*

donepezil (doh NEP e zil)

Sound-Alike/Look-Alike Issues

Aricept® may be confused with AcipHex®, Ascriptin®, and Azilect®

Synonyms E2020

U.S./Canadian Brand Names Aricept® ODT [US]; Aricept® RDT [Can]; Aricept® [US/Can]

Therapeutic Category Acetylcholinesterase Inhibitor; Cholinergic Agent

Use Treatment of mild, moderate, or severe dementia of the Alzheimer type

Dosage Summary

Oral:

Children: Dosage not established

Adults: 5 mg once daily; Maintenance: 5-23 mg once daily

Dosage Forms

Tablet, oral:

Aricept®: 5 mg, 10 mg, 23 mg

Tablet, orally disintegrating, oral:

Aricept® ODT: 5 mg, 10 mg

Donnamar® *(Discontinued)* *see* hyoscyamine *on page 491*

Donnapine® *(Discontinued)* *see* hyoscyamine, atropine, scopolamine, and phenobarbital *on page 492*

Donnatal® [US] *see* hyoscyamine, atropine, scopolamine, and phenobarbital *on page 492*

Donnatal Extentabs® [US] *see* hyoscyamine, atropine, scopolamine, and phenobarbital *on page 492*

dopamine (DOE pa meen)

Sound-Alike/Look-Alike Issues

DOPamine may be confused with DOBUTamine, Dopram®

Synonyms dopamine hydrochloride

Tall-Man DOPamine

Therapeutic Category Adrenergic Agonist Agent

Use Adjunct in the treatment of shock (eg, MI, open heart surgery, renal failure, cardiac decompensation) which persists after adequate fluid volume replacement

Dosage Summary

I.V.:

Neonates: 1-20 mcg/kg/minute

Children: 1-20 mcg/kg/minute (maximum: 50 mcg/kg/minute)

Adults: 1-50 mcg/kg/minute

Dosage Forms

Infusion, premixed in D_5W: 0.8 mg/mL (250 mL, 500 mL); 1.6 mg/mL (250 mL, 500 mL); 3.2 mg/mL (250 mL)

Injection, solution: 40 mg/mL (5 mL, 10 mL); 80 mg/mL (5 mL, 10 mL); 160 mg/mL (5 mL)

dopamine hydrochloride *see* dopamine *on page 326*

Dopram® [US] *see* doxapram *on page 328*

Doral® [US/Can] *see* quazepam *on page 820*

Doribax™ [Can] *see* doripenem *on page 326*

doripenem (dore i PEN em)

Synonyms S-4661

U.S./Canadian Brand Names Doribax™ [Can]

Therapeutic Category Antibiotic, Carbapenem

Use Treatment of complicated intraabdominal infections and complicated urinary tract infections (including pyelonephritis) due to susceptible gram-positive, gram-negative (including *Pseudomonas aeruginosa*), and anaerobic bacteria

Dosage Summary

I.V.:

Children: Dosage not established
Adults: 500 mg every 8 hours

Dosage Forms

Injection, powder for reconstitution:
Doribax®: 500 mg

Dormarex® 2 Oral ***(Discontinued)*** *see* diphenhydramine (systemic) *on page 310*

dornase alfa (DOOR nase AL fa)

Synonyms recombinant human deoxyribonuclease; rhDNase

U.S./Canadian Brand Names Pulmozyme® [US/Can]

Therapeutic Category Enzyme

Use Management of cystic fibrosis patients to reduce the frequency of respiratory infections that require parenteral antibiotics in patients with FVC ≥40% of predicted; in conjunction with standard therapies, to improve pulmonary function in patients with cystic fibrosis

Dosage Summary

Inhalation:

Children <3 months: Dosage not established
Children ≥3 months: 2.5 mg once daily
Adults: 2.5 mg once daily

Dosage Forms

Solution, for nebulization [preservative free]:
Pulmozyme®: 2.5 mg/2.5 mL (30s)

Doryx® [US] *see* doxycycline *on page 331*

dorzolamide (dor ZOLE a mide)

Synonyms dorzolamide hydrochloride

U.S./Canadian Brand Names Trusopt® [US/Can]

Therapeutic Category Carbonic Anhydrase Inhibitor

Use Treatment of elevated intraocular pressure in patients with ocular hypertension or open-angle glaucoma

Dosage Summary

Ophthalmic:

Children: Instill 1 drop into affected eye(s) 3 times/day
Adults: Instill 1 drop into affected eye(s) 3 times/day

Dosage Forms

Solution, ophthalmic: 2% (10 mL)
Trusopt®: 2% (10 mL)

Dosage Forms - Canada

Solution, ophthalmic [drops; preservative free]:
Trusopt®: 2% (0.2 mL)

dorzolamide and timolol (dor ZOLE a mide & TYE moe lole)

Synonyms timolol and dorzolamide

U.S./Canadian Brand Names Cosopt® [US/Can]

Therapeutic Category Beta-Adrenergic Blocker; Carbonic Anhydrase Inhibitor

Use Treatment of elevated intraocular pressure in patients with ocular hypertension or open-angle glaucoma

Dosage Summary

Ophthalmic:

Children <2 years: Dosage not established
Children ≥2 years: Instill 1 drop into affected eye(s) twice daily
Adults: Instill 1 drop into affected eye(s) twice daily

Dosage Forms

Solution, ophthalmic [drops]: Dorzolamide 2% and timolol 0.5% (10 mL)
Cosopt®: Dorzolamide 2% and timolol 0.5% (10 mL)

Dosage Forms - Canada

Solution, ophthalmic [drops; preservative free]:

Cosopt®: Dorzolamide hydrochloride 2% and timolol maleate 0.5% (0.2 mL)

dorzolamide hydrochloride *see* dorzolamide *on page* 327

DOSS *see* docusate *on page* 321

Dostinex® [Can] *see* cabergoline *on page* 163

Dostinex® *(Discontinued)* *see* cabergoline *on page* 163

Double Tussin DM [US-OTC] *see* guaifenesin and dextromethorphan *on page* 455

Dovobet® [Can] *see* calcipotriene and betamethasone *on page* 164

Dovonex® [US/Can] *see* calcipotriene *on page* 164

doxacurium *(Discontinued)*

doxapram (DOKS a pram)

Sound-Alike/Look-Alike Issues

doxapram may be confused with doxacurium, doxazosin, doxepin, Doxinate®, DOXOrubicin

Dopram® may be confused with DOPamine

Synonyms doxapram hydrochloride

U.S./Canadian Brand Names Dopram® [US]

Therapeutic Category Respiratory Stimulant

Use Respiratory and CNS stimulant for respiratory depression secondary to anesthesia, drug-induced CNS depression; acute hypercapnia secondary to COPD

Dosage Summary

I.V.:

Children: Dosage not established

Adults: 0.5-1 mg/kg every 5 minutes until response (maximum total dose: 2 mg/kg) **or** 1-5 mg/minute until response, should not be continued >2 hours (maximum total dose: 4 mg/kg; 3 g/day)

Dosage Forms

Injection, solution: 20 mg/mL (20 mL)

Dopram®: 20 mg/mL (20 mL)

doxapram hydrochloride *see* doxapram *on page* 328

doxazosin (doks AY zoe sin)

Sound-Alike/Look-Alike Issues

doxazosin may be confused with doxapram, doxepin, DOXOrubicin

Cardura® may be confused with Cardene®, Cordarone®, Cordran®, Coumadin®, K-Dur®, Ridaura®

Synonyms doxazosin mesylate

U.S./Canadian Brand Names Alti-Doxazosin [Can]; Apo-Doxazosin® [Can]; Cardura-1™ [Can]; Cardura-2™ [Can]; Cardura-4™ [Can]; Cardura® XL [US]; Cardura® [US]; Gen-Doxazosin [Can]; Mylan-Doxazosin [Can]; Novo-Doxazosin [Can]

Therapeutic Category Alpha-Adrenergic Blocking Agent

Use

Immediate release formulation: Treatment of hypertension as monotherapy or in conjunction with diuretics, ACE inhibitors, beta-blockers, or calcium antagonists

Immediate release and extended release formulations: Treatment of urinary outflow obstruction and/or obstructive and irritative symptoms associated with benign prostatic hyperplasia (BPH)

Dosage Summary

Oral:

Extended release:

Children: Dosage not established

Adults: Initial: 4 mg once daily; Maintenance: 4-8 mg/day (maximum: 8 mg/day)

Immediate release:

Adults: Initial: 1-4 mg once daily; Maintenance: 4-8 mg/day

BPH: Goal: 4-8 mg/day (maximum: 8 mg/day)

Hypertension: Maximum: 16 mg/day

Elderly: Initial: 0.5 mg once daily

Dosage Forms

Tablet, oral: 1 mg, 2 mg, 4 mg, 8 mg

Cardura®: 1 mg, 2 mg, 4 mg, 8 mg

Tablet, extended release, oral:
Cardura® XL: 4 mg, 8 mg

doxazosin mesylate *see* doxazosin *on page 328*

doxepin (systemic) (DOKS e pin)

Sound-Alike/Look-Alike Issues
doxepin may be confused with digoxin, doxapram, doxazosin, Doxidan®, doxycycline
Sinequan® may be confused with saquinavir, Serentil®, Seroquel®, Singulair®, Zonegran®

Synonyms doxepin hydrochloride

U.S./Canadian Brand Names Apo-Doxepin® [Can]; Doxepine [Can]; Novo-Doxepin [Can]; Sinequan® [Can]

Therapeutic Category Antidepressant, Tricyclic (Tertiary Amine)

Use Depression; treatment of insomnia (with difficulty of sleep maintenance)

Dosage Summary

Oral:
Adolescents: Initial: 25-50 mg/day in single or divided doses; Maintenance: 100 mg/day; titrate gradually
Adults: Initial: 10-150 mg/day in 1-3 divided doses; Maintenance: Up to 300 mg/day in a single (≤150 mg) or divided doses
Elderly: Initial: 10-25 mg at bedtime; Maintenance: Up to 75 mg at bedtime

Dosage Forms

Capsule, oral: 10 mg, 25 mg, 50 mg, 75 mg, 100 mg, 150 mg
Solution, oral: 10 mg/mL (120 mL)
Tablet, oral:
Silenor®: 3 mg, 6 mg

doxepin (topical) (DOKS e pin)

Sound-Alike/Look-Alike Issues
doxepin may be confused with digoxin, doxapram, doxazosin, Doxidan®, doxycycline
Zonalon® may be confused with Zone-A Forte®

Synonyms doxepin hydrochloride

U.S./Canadian Brand Names Prudoxin™ [US]; Zonalon® [US/Can]

Therapeutic Category Topical Skin Product

Use Short-term (<8 days) management of moderate pruritus in adults with atopic dermatitis or lichen simplex chronicus

Dosage Summary

Dental:
Children: Dosage not established
Adults: Apply 3-4 times daily

Topical:
Children: Dosage not established
Adults: Apply a thin film 4 times/day (maximum total therapy: 8 days)

Dosage Forms

Cream, topical:
Prudoxin™: 5% (45 g)
Zonalon®: 5% (30 g, 45 g)

Doxepine [Can] *see* doxepin (systemic) *on page 329*
doxepin hydrochloride *see* doxepin (systemic) *on page 329*
doxepin hydrochloride *see* doxepin (topical) *on page 329*

doxercalciferol (doks er kal si fe FEER ole)

Synonyms 1α-hydroxyergocalciferol

U.S./Canadian Brand Names Hectorol® [US/Can]

Therapeutic Category Vitamin D Analog

Use Treatment of secondary hyperparathyroidism in patients with chronic kidney disease

Dosage Summary

I.V.:
Children: Dosage not established

Adults: Initial: 4 mcg 3 times/week after dialysis; Titration: Dose can be increased by 1-2 mcg at 8-week intervals, as necessary (maximum: 18 mcg/week)

Oral:

Children: Dosage not established

Adults (dialysis patients): Initial: 10 mcg 3 times/week at dialysis; Titration: Dose can be increased by 2.5 mcg at 8-week intervals (maximum: 60 mcg/week)

Adults (predialysis patients): Initial: 1 mcg/day; Titration: Increase dose by 0.5 mcg at 2-week intervals (maximum: 3.5 mcg/day)

Dosage Forms

Capsule, softgel, oral:

Hectorol®: 0.5 mcg, 1 mcg, 2.5 mcg

Injection, solution:

Hectorol®: 2 mcg/mL (2 mL)

Doxidan® [US-OTC] *see* bisacodyl *on page 138*

Doxil® [US] *see* doxorubicin (liposomal) *on page 330*

doxorubicin (doks oh ROO bi sin)

Sound-Alike/Look-Alike Issues

DOXOrubicin may be confused with DACTINomycin, DAUNOrubicin, DAUNOrubicin liposomal, doxacurium, doxapram, doxazosin, DOXOrubicin liposomal, epirubicin, IDArubicin, valrubicin

Adriamycin PFS® may be confused with achromycin, Aredia®, Idamycin®

ADR is an error-prone abbreviation

Conventional formulation (Adriamycin PFS®, Adriamycin RDF®) may be confused with the liposomal formulation (Doxil®)

Synonyms adria; doxorubicin hydrochloride; hydroxydaunomycin hydrochloride; hydroxyldaunorubicin hydrochloride

Tall-Man DOXOrubicin

U.S./Canadian Brand Names Adriamycin® [US/Can]

Therapeutic Category Antineoplastic Agent

Use Treatment of acute lymphocytic leukemia (ALL), acute myeloid leukemia (AML), Hodgkin disease, malignant lymphoma, soft tissue and bone sarcomas, thyroid cancer, small cell lung cancer, breast cancer, gastric cancer, ovarian cancer, bladder cancer, neuroblastoma, and Wilms tumor

Dosage Summary

I.V.:

Children: 35-75 mg/m^2/dose every 21 days **or** 20-30 mg/m^2/dose once weekly **or** 60-90 mg/m^2 infusion over 96 hours every 3-4 weeks

Adults: 60-75 mg/m^2/dose every 21 days **or** 60 mg/m^2/dose every 2 weeks **or** 40-60 mg/m^2/dose every 3-4 weeks **or** 20-30 mg/m^2/day for 2-3 days every 4 weeks **or** 20 mg/m^2/dose once weekly.

Dosage Forms

Injection, powder for reconstitution:

Adriamycin®: 10 mg, 20 mg, 50 mg

Injection, solution [preservative free]: 2 mg/mL (5 mL, 10 mL, 25 mL, 37.5 mL, 75 mL, 100 mL)

Adriamycin®: 2 mg/mL (5 mL, 10 mL, 25 mL, 100 mL)

doxorubicin hydrochloride *see* doxorubicin *on page 330*

DOXOrubicin hydrochloride (liposomal) *see* doxorubicin (liposomal) *on page 330*

DOXOrubicin hydrochloride liposome *see* doxorubicin (liposomal) *on page 330*

doxorubicin (liposomal) (doks oh ROO bi sin lip pah SOW mal)

Sound-Alike/Look-Alike Issues

DOXOrubicin liposomal may be confused with DACTINomycin, DAUNOrubicin, DAUNOrubicin liposomal, doxacurium, doxapram, doxazosin, DOXOrubicin, epirubicin, IDArubicin, valrucibin

DOXOrubicin liposomal may be confused with DAUNOrubicin liposomal

Doxil® may be confused with Doxy®, Paxil®

Liposomal formulation (Doxil®) may be confused with the conventional formulation (Adriamycin PFS®, Adriamycin RDF®)

Synonyms DOXOrubicin hydrochloride (liposomal); DOXOrubicin hydrochloride liposome; liposomal DOXOrubicin; pegylated DOXOrubicin liposomal; pegylated liposomal DOXOrubicin

Tall-Man DOXOrubicin (liposomal)

U.S./Canadian Brand Names Caelyx® [Can]; Doxil® [US]

Therapeutic Category Antineoplastic Agent

Use Treatment of ovarian cancer, multiple myeloma, and AIDS-related Kaposi sarcoma

Dosage Summary

I.V.:

Children: Dosage not established

Adults: 20-30 mg/m^2 every 3 weeks **or** 50 mg/m^2/dose every 4 weeks

Dosage Forms

Injection, solution:

Doxil®: 2 mg/mL (10 mL, 25 mL)

Doxy 100™ [US] *see* doxycycline *on page 331*

Doxycin [Can] *see* doxycycline *on page 331*

doxycycline (doks i SYE kleen)

Sound-Alike/Look-Alike Issues

doxycycline may be confused with dicyclomine, doxepin, doxylamine
Doxy100™ may be confused with Doxil®
Monodox® may be confused with Maalox®
Oracea™ may be confused with Orencia®
Vibramycin® may be confused with vancomycin, Vibativ™

Synonyms doxycycline calcium; doxycycline hyclate; doxycycline monohydrate

U.S./Canadian Brand Names Adoxa® Pak™ 1/150 [US]; Adoxa® Pak™ 1/75 [US]; Adoxa® [US]; Alodox™ [US]; Apo-Doxy Tabs® [Can]; Apo-Doxy® [Can]; Dom-Doxycycline [Can]; Doryx® [US]; Doxy 100™ [US]; Doxycin [Can]; Doxytab [Can]; Monodox® [US]; Novo-Doxylin [Can]; Nu-Doxycycline [Can]; Oracea® [US]; Oraxyl™ [US]; Periostat® [US/Can]; PHL-Doxycycline [Can]; PMS-Doxycycline [Can]; Vibra-Tabs® [Can]; Vibramycin® [US/Can]

Therapeutic Category Tetracycline Derivative

Use Principally in the treatment of infections caused by susceptible *Rickettsia*, *Chlamydia*, and *Mycoplasma*; alternative to mefloquine for malaria prophylaxis; treatment for syphilis, uncomplicated *Neisseria gonorrhoeae*, *Listeria*, *Actinomyces israelii*, and *Clostridium* infections in penicillin-allergic patients; used for community-acquired pneumonia and other common infections due to susceptible organisms; anthrax due to *Bacillus anthracis,* including inhalational anthrax (postexposure); treatment of infections caused by uncommon susceptible gram-negative and gram-positive organisms including *Borrelia recurrentis*, *Ureaplasma urealyticum*, *Haemophilus ducreyi*, *Yersinia pestis*, *Francisella tularensis*, *Vibrio cholerae*, *Campylobacter fetus*, *Brucella* spp, *Bartonella bacilliformis*, and *Calymmatobacterium granulomatis,* Q fever, Lyme disease; treatment of inflammatory lesions associated with rosacea; intestinal amebiasis; severe acne

Dosage Summary

I.V.:

Children ≤8 years: Anthrax, tickborne rickettsial disease: 2.2 mg/kg every 12 hours
Children >8 years and ≤45 kg: 2-5 mg/kg/day in 1-2 divided doses (maximum: 200 mg/day)
Children >8 years and >45 kg: 100-200 mg/day in 1-2 divided doses
Adults: 100-200 mg/day in 1-2 divided doses

Oral:

Children ≤8 years: Anthrax, tickborne rickettsial disease: 2.2 mg/kg every 12 hours
Children >8 years and ≤45 kg: 2-5 mg/kg/day in 1-2 divided doses (maximum: 200 mg/day)
Children >8 years and >45 kg: 100-200 mg/day in 1-2 divided doses
Adults: 100-200 mg/day in 1-2 divided doses **or** 300 mg as a single dose (*Vibrio cholerae*) **or** 40 mg once daily (rosacea; Oracea™) **or** 20 mg twice daily (periodontitis)

Dosage Forms

Capsule, oral: 50 mg, 100 mg

Adoxa®: 150 mg
Monodox®: 50 mg, 75 mg, 100 mg
Oracea®: 40 mg [30 mg (immediate release) and 10 mg (delayed release)]
Oraxyl™: 20 mg
Vibramycin®: 100 mg

Capsule, variable release, oral:

Oracea®: 40 mg [30 mg (immediate release) and 10 mg (delayed release)]

Injection, powder for reconstitution: 100 mg

Doxy 100™: 100 mg

Powder for suspension, oral:
Vibramycin®: 25 mg/5 mL (60 mL)
Syrup, oral:
Vibramycin®: 50 mg/5 mL (473 mL)
Tablet, oral: 20 mg, 50 mg, 75 mg, 100 mg, 150 mg
Adoxa®: 50 mg, 75 mg, 100 mg
Adoxa® Pak™ 1/150: 150 mg
Adoxa® Pak™ 1/75: 75 mg
Alodox™: 20 mg
Periostat®: 20 mg
Tablet, delayed release coated pellets, oral:
Doryx®: 75 mg, 100 mg, 150 mg

doxycycline calcium *see* doxycycline *on page 331*
doxycycline hyclate *see* doxycycline *on page 331*
doxycycline monohydrate *see* doxycycline *on page 331*

doxylamine (dox IL a meen)

Sound-Alike/Look-Alike Issues
doxylamine may be confused with doxycycline
Synonyms doxylamine succinate
U.S./Canadian Brand Names Aldex® AN [US]; Unisom®-2 [Can]
Therapeutic Category Antihistamine
Use Treatment of short-term insomnia
Dosage Summary
Oral:
Children: Dosage not established
Adults: One tablet 30 minutes before bedtime
Dosage Forms
Tablet, chewable, oral:
Aldex® AN: 5 mg

doxylamine, acetaminophen, and dextromethorphan *see* acetaminophen, dextromethorphan, and doxylamine *on page 29*
doxylamine, acetaminophen, dextromethorphan, and pseudoephedrine *see* acetaminophen, dextromethorphan, doxylamine, and pseudoephedrine *on page 30*

doxylamine and pyridoxine *(Canada only)* (dox IL a meen & peer i DOX een)

Sound-Alike/Look-Alike Issues
doxylamine may be confused with doxycycline
Synonyms doxylamine succinate and pyridoxine hydrochloride; pyridoxine and doxylamine
U.S./Canadian Brand Names Diclectin® [Can]
Therapeutic Category Antihistamine; Vitamin
Use Treatment of pregnancy-associated nausea and vomiting
Dosage Summary
Oral:
Children: Dosage not established
Adults: 2 tablets (a total of doxylamine 20 mg and pyridoxine 20 mg) at bedtime, may increase by 1 tablet in the morning and/or afternoon in severe cases
Dosage Forms - Canada
Tablet, delayed release:
Diclectin®: Doxylamine 10 mg and pyridoxine 10 mg

doxylamine succinate *see* doxylamine *on page 332*
doxylamine succinate and pyridoxine hydrochloride *see* doxylamine and pyridoxine *(Canada only) on page 332*
doxylamine succinate, codeine phosphate, and acetaminophen *see* acetaminophen, codeine, and doxylamine *(Canada only) on page 28*
Doxytab [Can] *see* doxycycline *on page 331*
DPA *see* valproic acid *on page 974*

D-Pan® *(Discontinued)* *see* dexpanthenol *on page 284*
DPE *see* dipivefrin *on page 317*
D-penicillamine *see* penicillamine *on page 737*
DPH *see* phenytoin *on page 756*
D-Phen 1000 [US] *see* guaifenesin and phenylephrine *on page 456*
DPM™ [US-OTC] *see* urea *on page 970*
Dramamine® [US-OTC] *see* dimenhydrinate *on page 307*
Dramamine® Less Drowsy Formula [US-OTC] *see* meclizine *on page 595*
Dramilin® Injection *(Discontinued)* *see* dimenhydrinate *on page 307*
Driminate [US-OTC] *see* dimenhydrinate *on page 307*
Drinex [US-OTC] *see* acetaminophen, chlorpheniramine, and pseudoephedrine *on page 28*
Drinkables® Fruits and Vegetables [US-OTC] *see* vitamins (multiple/oral) *on page 990*
Drinkables® MultiVitamins [US-OTC] *see* vitamins (multiple/oral) *on page 990*
Drisdol® [US-OTC] *see* ergocalciferol *on page 358*
Dristan® [US-OTC] *see* oxymetazoline (nasal) *on page 716*
Dristan® Long Lasting Nasal [Can] *see* oxymetazoline (nasal) *on page 716*
Dristan® Long Lasting Nasal Solution *(Discontinued)* *see* oxymetazoline (nasal) *on page 716*
Dristan® N.D. [Can] *see* acetaminophen and pseudoephedrine *on page 26*
Dristan® N.D., Extra Strength [Can] *see* acetaminophen and pseudoephedrine *on page 26*
Dristan® Saline Spray *(Discontinued)* *see* sodium chloride *on page 882*
Drithocreme® HP 1% *(Discontinued)* *see* anthralin *on page 79*
Dritho-Scalp® [US] *see* anthralin *on page 79*
Drixoral® [Can] *see* dexbrompheniramine and pseudoephedrine *on page 282*
Drixoral® Cough & Congestion Liquid Caps *(Discontinued)* *see* pseudoephedrine and dextromethorphan *on page 812*
Drixoral® Cough Liquid Caps *(Discontinued)* *see* dextromethorphan *on page 287*
Drixoral® Nasal [Can] *see* oxymetazoline (nasal) *on page 716*
Drixoral® ND [Can] *see* pseudoephedrine *on page 810*
Drixoral® Non-Drowsy *(Discontinued)* *see* pseudoephedrine *on page 810*
Drize®-R *(Discontinued)* *see* chlorpheniramine, phenylephrine, and methscopolamine *on page 212*

dronabinol (droe NAB i nol)

Sound-Alike/Look-Alike Issues
dronabinol may be confused with droperidol

Synonyms delta-9 THC; delta-9-tetrahydro-cannabinol; tetrahydrocannabinol; THC

U.S./Canadian Brand Names Marinol® [US/Can]

Therapeutic Category Antiemetic

Controlled Substance C-III

Use Chemotherapy-associated nausea and vomiting refractory to other antiemetic(s); AIDS-related anorexia

Dosage Summary

Oral:

Children: Initial: 5 mg/m^2 before chemotherapy, then 5 mg/m^2/dose every 2-4 hours after chemotherapy for a total of 4-6 doses/day; Titration: Increase in increments of 2.5 mg/m^2 (maximum: 15 mg/m^2/dose)

Adults:

Antiemetic: Initial: 5 mg/m^2 before chemotherapy, then 5 mg/m^2/dose every 2-4 hours after chemotherapy for a total of 4-6 doses/day; Titration: Increase in increments of 2.5 mg/m^2 (maximum: 15 mg/m^2/dose)

Appetite stimulant: Initial: 2.5 mg twice daily; Maintenance: Titrate up to 20 mg/day in 2 divided doses

Dosage Forms

Capsule, soft gelatin, oral: 2.5 mg, 5 mg, 10 mg
Marinol®: 2.5 mg, 5 mg, 10 mg

dronedarone (droe NE da rone)

Synonyms dronedarone hydrochloride; SR33589

U.S./Canadian Brand Names Multaq® [US/Can]

Therapeutic Category Antiarrhythmic Agent, Miscellaneous

Use To reduce the risk of hospitalization related to paroxysmal or persistent atrial fibrillation (AF) or atrial flutter (AFl) in patients with a recent episode of AF/AFl and associated cardiovascular risk factors (eg, age >70 years, hypertension, diabetes, prior cerebrovascular accident, left atrial diameter ≥50 mm or left ventricular ejection fraction <40%), who are in normal sinus rhythm or will be cardioverted

Dosage Summary

Oral:

Children: Dosage not established

Adults: 400 mg twice daily with morning and evening meals

Dosage Forms

Tablet, oral:

Multaq®: 400 mg

dronedarone hydrochloride *see* dronedarone *on page* *333*

droperidol (droe PER i dole)

Sound-Alike/Look-Alike Issues

droperidol may be confused with dronabinol

Inapsine® may be confused with asenapine, Nebcin®

Synonyms dehydrobenzperidol

U.S./Canadian Brand Names Droperidol Injection, USP [Can]

Therapeutic Category Antiemetic; Antipsychotic Agent, Butyrophenone

Use Prevention and/or treatment of nausea and vomiting from surgical and diagnostic procedures

Dosage Summary

I.M.:

Children <2 years: Dosage not established

Children 2-12 years: Maximum: 0.1 mg/kg; additional doses may be repeated

Adults: Maximum initial dose: 2.5 mg, additional doses of 1.25 mg may be administered

I.V.:

Children <2 years: Dosage not established

Children 2-12 years: Maximum: 0.1 mg/kg; additional doses may be repeated

Adults: Maximum initial dose: 2.5 mg; additional doses of 1.25 mg may be administered

Dosage Forms

Injection, solution: 2.5 mg/mL (2 mL)

Injection, solution [preservative free]: 2.5 mg/mL (2 mL)

Droperidol Injection, USP [Can] *see* droperidol *on page* *334*

drospirenone and estradiol (droh SPYE re none & es tra DYE ole)

Synonyms E2 and DRSP; estradiol and drospirenone

U.S./Canadian Brand Names Angeliq® [US/Can]

Therapeutic Category Estrogen and Progestin Combination

Use Treatment of moderate-to-severe vasomotor symptoms associated with menopause; treatment of vulvar and vaginal atrophy associated with menopause

Dosage Summary

Oral:

Children: Dosage not established

Adults (females): One tablet daily

Dosage Forms

Tablet:

Angeliq®: Drospirenone 0.5 mg and estradiol 1 mg

drospirenone and ethinyl estradiol *see* ethinyl estradiol and drospirenone *on page* *375*

drotrecogin alfa (dro TRE coe jin AL fa)

Sound-Alike/Look-Alike Issues

Dosing issues:

Use caution when interpreting dosing information. Maintenance dose expressed as mcg/kg/**hour**.

Synonyms activated protein C, human, recombinant; drotrecogin alfa, activated; protein C (activated), human, recombinant; rhAPC

U.S./Canadian Brand Names Xigris® [US/Can]

Therapeutic Category Protein C (Activated)

Use Reduction of mortality from severe sepsis (associated with organ dysfunction) in adults at high risk of death (eg, APACHE II score ≥25)

Dosage Summary

I.V.:

Adults: 24 mcg/kg/**hour** for 96 hours

Dosage Forms

Injection, powder for reconstitution [preservative free]:

Xigris®: 5 mg, 20 mg

D-Trp(6)-LHRH *see* triptorelin *on page* 962
Duac® CS [US] *see* clindamycin and benzoyl peroxide *on page* 233
Duac® *(Discontinued)* *see* clindamycin and benzoyl peroxide *on page* 233
Duet® [US] *see* vitamins (multiple/prenatal) *on page* 991
Duetact™ [US] *see* pioglitazone and glimepiride *on page* 762
Duet® DHA [US] *see* vitamins (multiple/prenatal) *on page* 991
Duet® DHA[ec] [US] *see* vitamins (multiple/prenatal) *on page* 991
Dukoral® [Can] *see* traveler's diarrhea and cholera vaccine *(Canada only) on page* 949
Dulcolax Balance® [US-OTC] *see* polyethylene glycol 3350 *on page* 775
Dulcolax® (bisacodyl) [US-OTC/Can] *see* bisacodyl *on page* 138
Dulcolax® (docusate) [US-OTC] *see* docusate *on page* 321
Dulcolax® Stool Softener [US-OTC] *see* docusate *on page* 321
Dulera® [US] *see* mometasone and formoterol *on page* 642
Dull-C® [US-OTC] *see* ascorbic acid *on page* 98

duloxetine (doo LOX e teen)

Sound-Alike/Look-Alike Issues
DULoxetine may be confused with FLUoxetine
Cymbalta® may be confused with Symbyax®

Synonyms (+)-(*S*)-*N*-methyl-γ-(1-naphthyloxy)-2-thiophenepropylamine hydrochloride; duloxetine hydrochloride; LY248686

Tall-Man DULoxetine

U.S./Canadian Brand Names Cymbalta® [US/Can]

Therapeutic Category Antidepressant, Serotonin/Norepinephrine Reuptake Inhibitor

Use Acute and maintenance treatment of major depressive disorder (MDD); treatment of generalized anxiety disorder (GAD); management of pain associated with diabetic neuropathy; management of fibromyalgia

Dosage Summary

Oral:
Children: Dosage not established
Adults: 30-60 mg/day in 1-2 divided doses (maximum: 120 mg/day)
Elderly: Initial: 20 mg 1-2 times/day; Maintenance: 40-60 mg/day as a single or divided dose

Dosage Forms

Capsule, delayed release, enteric coated pellets, oral:
Cymbalta®: 20 mg, 30 mg, 60 mg

duloxetine hydrochloride *see* duloxetine *on page* 336
Duocaine™ *(Discontinued)*
DuoCet™ *(Discontinued)* *see* hydrocodone and acetaminophen *on page* 479
Duodote™ [US] *see* atropine and pralidoxime *on page* 107
DuoFilm® [US-OTC/Can] *see* salicylic acid *on page* 858
Duoforte® 27 [Can] *see* salicylic acid *on page* 858
Duomax [US] *see* guaifenesin and phenylephrine *on page* 456
DuoNeb® [US] *see* ipratropium and albuterol *on page* 524
DuoPlant® *(Discontinued)* *see* salicylic acid *on page* 858
Duotan PD *(Discontinued)* *see* dexchlorpheniramine and pseudoephedrine *on page* 283
Duo-Trach® Injection *(Discontinued)* *see* lidocaine (systemic) *on page* 561
DuoTrav™ [Can] *see* travoprost and timolol *(Canada only) on page* 950
Duovent® UDV [Can] *see* ipratropium and fenoterol *(Canada only) on page* 524
DuP 753 *see* losartan *on page* 577
Duphalac® *(Discontinued)* *see* lactulose *on page* 544
Duraclon® [US] *see* clonidine *on page* 238
Duradrin® *(Discontinued)* *see* acetaminophen, isometheptene, and dichloralphenazone *on page* 31
Duradyl® [US] *see* chlorpheniramine, phenylephrine, and methscopolamine *on page* 212
Duradyne DHC® *(Discontinued)* *see* hydrocodone and acetaminophen *on page* 479
Duragesic® [US/Can] *see* fentanyl *on page* 395

Duragesic® MAT [Can] *see* fentanyl *on page 395*
Dura-Gest® ***(Discontinued)***
Durahist™ ***(Discontinued)*** *see* chlorpheniramine, pseudoephedrine, and methscopolamine *on page 215*
Durahist™ PE [US] *see* chlorpheniramine, phenylephrine, and methscopolamine *on page 212*
Duralith® [Can] *see* lithium *on page 571*
Duralone® Injection ***(Discontinued)*** *see* methylprednisolone *on page 622*
Duramist Plus [US-OTC] *see* oxymetazoline (nasal) *on page 716*
Duramorph® [US] *see* morphine (systemic) *on page 644*
Duraphen™ II DM [US] *see* guaifenesin, dextromethorphan, and phenylephrine *on page 458*
Duraphen™ DM ***(Discontinued)*** *see* guaifenesin, dextromethorphan, and phenylephrine *on page 458*
Duraphen™ Forte [US] *see* guaifenesin, dextromethorphan, and phenylephrine *on page 458*
Durasal™ [US] *see* salicylic acid *on page 858*
DuraTan™ Forte [US] *see* chlorpheniramine, pseudoephedrine, and dextromethorphan *on page 214*
Duratest® Injection ***(Discontinued)*** *see* testosterone *on page 919*
Durathate® Injection ***(Discontinued)*** *see* testosterone *on page 919*
Duration® ***(Discontinued)*** *see* oxymetazoline (nasal) *on page 716*
Duratocin™ [Can] *see* carbetocin *(Canada only) on page 181*
Duratuss® [US] *see* guaifenesin and phenylephrine *on page 456*
Duratuss® DA ***(Discontinued)*** *see* chlorpheniramine and pseudoephedrine *on page 209*
Duratuss® DM ***(Discontinued)*** *see* guaifenesin and dextromethorphan *on page 455*
Duratuss GP® [US] *see* guaifenesin and phenylephrine *on page 456*
Duratuss® HD ***(Discontinued)***
Dura-Vent®/DA ***(Discontinued)*** *see* chlorpheniramine, phenylephrine, and methscopolamine *on page 212*
Dura-Vent® ***(Discontinued)***
Durezol® [US] *see* difluprednate *on page 301*
Duricef® ***(Discontinued)*** *see* cefadroxil *on page 189*
Duricef® Oral Suspension 125 mg/5 mL ***(Discontinued)*** *see* cefadroxil *on page 189*
Durolane® [Can] *see* hyaluronate and derivatives *on page 475*
Durrax® Oral ***(Discontinued)*** *see* hydroxyzine *on page 490*

dutasteride (doo TAS teer ide)

U.S./Canadian Brand Names Avodart® [US/Can]

Therapeutic Category Antineoplastic Agent, Anthracenedione

Use Treatment of symptomatic benign prostatic hyperplasia (BPH) as monotherapy or combination therapy with tamsulosin

Dosage Summary

Oral:

Children: Dosage not established

Adults (males): 0.5 mg once daily

Dosage Forms

Capsule, softgel, oral:

Avodart®: 0.5 mg

dutasteride and tamsulosin (doo TAS teer ide & tam SOO loe sin)

Synonyms tamsulosin and dutasteride; tamsulosin hydrochloride and dutasteride

U.S./Canadian Brand Names Jalyn™ [US]

Therapeutic Category 5 Alpha-Reductase Inhibitor; Alpha$_1$ Blocker

Use Treatment of symptomatic benign prostatic hyperplasia (BPH)

Dosage Summary

Oral:

Children: Dosage not established

Adults (males): One capsule (0.5 mg dutasteride/0.4 mg tamsulosin) once daily

Dosage Forms

Capsule, oral:

Jalyn™: Dutasteride 0.5 mg and tamsulosin hydrochloride 0.4 mg

Duvoid® [Can] *see* bethanechol *on page* 135

Duvoid® ***(Discontinued)*** *see* bethanechol *on page* 135

D-Vi-Sol® [Can] *see* cholecalciferol *on page* 218

DW286 *see* gemifloxacin *on page* 441

Dwelle® Ophthalmic Solution ***(Discontinued)*** *see* artificial tears *on page* 97

DX-88 *see* ecallantide *on page* 340

Dyazide® [US] *see* hydrochlorothiazide and triamterene *on page* 479

Dycill® [Can] *see* dicloxacillin *on page* 298

Dycill® ***(Discontinued)*** *see* dicloxacillin *on page* 298

Dyclone® ***(Discontinued)*** *see* dyclonine *on page* 338

dyclonine (DYE kloe neen)

Sound-Alike/Look-Alike Issues

dyclonine may be confused with dicyclomine

Synonyms dyclonine hydrochloride

U.S./Canadian Brand Names Cepacol® Maximum Strength [US-OTC]; Orajel® Maximum Strength Overnight Cold Sore [US-OTC]; Sucrets® Children's [US-OTC]; Sucrets® Maximum Strength [US-OTC]; Sucrets® Regular Strength [US-OTC]

Therapeutic Category Local Anesthetic

Use Temporary relief of pain associated with oral mucosa

Dosage Summary

Oral:

Lozenge:

Children <2 years: Dosage not established

Children ≥2 years: One lozenge every 2 hours as needed (maximum: 10 lozenges/day)

Adults: One lozenge every 2 hours as needed (maximum: 10 lozenges/day)

Spray:

Children <3 years: Dosage not established

Children 3-12 years: 1-3 sprays, up to 4 times/day

Children ≥12 years: 1-4 sprays, up to 4 times/day

Adults: 1-4 sprays, up to 4 times/day

Dosage Forms

Lozenge, oral:

Sucrets® Children's [OTC]: 1.2 mg (18s)

Sucrets® Maximum Strength [OTC]: 3 mg (18s)

Sucrets® Regular Strength [OTC]: 2 mg (18s)

Patch, topical:

Orajel® Maximum Strength Overnight Cold Sore [OTC]: 3 mg (8s)

Solution, oral:

Cepacol® Maximum Strength [OTC]: 0.1% (118 mL)

dyclonine hydrochloride *see* dyclonine *on page* 338

Dygase ***(Discontinued)*** *see* pancreatin *on page* 723

Dylix [US] *see* dyphylline *on page* 339

Dymenate® Injection ***(Discontinued)*** *see* dimenhydrinate *on page* 307

Dynabac® ***(Discontinued)***

Dynacin® [US] *see* minocycline *on page* 635

DynaCirc® [Can] *see* isradipine *on page* 531

DynaCirc CR® [US] *see* isradipine *on page* 531

DynaCirc® ***(Discontinued)*** *see* isradipine *on page* 531

Dyna-Hex® [US-OTC] *see* chlorhexidine gluconate *on page* 204

Dynahist-ER Pediatric® ***(Discontinued)*** *see* chlorpheniramine and pseudoephedrine *on page* 209

Dynapen® ***(Discontinued)*** *see* dicloxacillin *on page* 298

Dynatuss-EX ***(Discontinued)*** *see* guaifenesin, dextromethorphan, and phenylephrine *on page* 458

Dynex ***(Discontinued)*** *see* guaifenesin and pseudoephedrine *on page* *457*

dyphylline (DYE fi lin)

Synonyms dihydroxypropyl theophylline

U.S./Canadian Brand Names Dilor® [Can]; Dylix [US]; Lufyllin® [US/Can]

Therapeutic Category Theophylline Derivative

Use Bronchodilator in reversible airway obstruction due to asthma, chronic bronchitis, or emphysema

Dosage Summary

Oral:

Children: Dosage not established

Adults: Up to 15 mg/kg 4 times/day, individualize dosage

Dosage Forms

Elixir, oral:

Dylix: 100 mg/15 mL (473 mL)

Tablet, oral:

Lufyllin®: 200 mg, 400 mg

dyphylline and guaifenesin (DYE fi lin & gwye FEN e sin)

Synonyms guaifenesin and dyphylline

U.S./Canadian Brand Names COPD [US]; Difil-G [US]; Difil®-G Forte [US]; Dilex-G [US]; Lufyllin®-GG [US]

Therapeutic Category Expectorant; Theophylline Derivative

Use Treatment of bronchial asthma and reversible bronchospasm associated with chronic bronchitis and emphysema

Dosage Summary

Oral:

Children <6 years: Dosage not established

Children 6-12 years:

Elixir: Lufyllin®-GG: 15-30 mL 3 or 4 times/day

Syrup: Dilex-G:

18-27 kg: 1.25-1.6 mL 4 times/day

27-36 kg: 2.5-3.3 mL 4 times/day

36.5-45 kg: 3.3-3.7 mL 4 times/day

Tablet: Lufyllin®-GG: 1/2 -1 tablet 3 or 4 times/day

Children >12 years:

Elixir: Lufyllin®-GG: 30 mL 4 times/day

Syrup:

Dilex-G: 5-10 mL 4 times/day

Difil®-G Forte: 5-10 mL 3 or 4 times/day; may double or triple (in severe cases) according to patient response

Tablet: Difil®-G, Dilex-G, Lufyllin®-GG: One tablet 3 or 4 times/day

Adults:

Elixir: Lufyllin®-GG: 30 mL 4 times/day

Syrup:

Dilex-G: 5-10 mL 4 times/day

Difil®-G Forte: 5-10 mL 3 or 4 times/day; may double or triple (in severe cases) according to patient response

Tablet: Difil®-G, Dilex-G, Lufyllin®-GG: One tablet 3 or 4 times/day

Dosage Forms

Elixir: Dyphylline 100 mg and guaifenesin 100 mg per 15 mL

Lufyllin®-GG: Dyphylline 100 mg and guaifenesin 100 mg per 15 mL

Liquid: Dyphylline 100 mg and guaifenesin 100 mg per 5 mL

Difil®-G Forte: Dyphylline 100 mg and guaifenesin 100 mg per 5 mL

Syrup:

Dilex-G: Dyphylline 100 mg and guaifenesin 200 mg per 5 mL

Tablet: Dyphylline 200 mg and guaifenesin 200 mg

COPD, Lufyllin®-GG: Dyphylline 200 mg and guaifenesin 200 mg

Difil-G: Dyphylline 200 mg and guaifenesin 300 mg

Dilex-G: Dyphylline 200 mg and guaifenesin 400 mg

Dyrenium® [US] *see* triamterene *on page* *955*

Dyrexan-OD® *(Discontinued)* *see* phendimetrazine *on page 747*
Dysport™ [US] *see* abobotulinumtoxinA *on page 20*
Dytan™ *(Discontinued)* *see* diphenhydramine (systemic) *on page 310*
E2 and DRSP *see* drospirenone and estradiol *on page 334*
7E3 *see* abciximab *on page 19*
E2020 *see* donepezil *on page 326*
E 2080 *see* rufinamide *on page 856*
EACA *see* aminocaproic acid *on page 65*
Easprin® [US] *see* aspirin *on page 100*
Ebixa® [Can] *see* memantine *on page 599*

ecallantide (e KAL lan tide)

Synonyms DX-88

U.S./Canadian Brand Names Kalbitor® [US]

Therapeutic Category Kallikrein Inhibitor

Use Treatment of acute attacks of hereditary angioedema (HAE)

Dosage Summary

SubQ:

Children <16 years: Dosage not established
Children ≥16 years: 30 mg; may repeat once within 24 hours (maximum: 60 mg/24 hours)
Adults: 30 mg; may repeat once within 24 hours (maximum: 60 mg/24 hours)

Dosage Forms

Injection, solution [preservative free]:
Kalbitor®: 10 mg/mL (1 mL)

echothiophate iodide (ek oh THYE oh fate EYE oh dide)

Synonyms ecostigmine iodide

U.S./Canadian Brand Names Phospholine Iodide® [US]

Therapeutic Category Cholinesterase Inhibitor

Use Used as miotic in treatment of chronic, open-angle glaucoma; may be useful in specific cases of angle-closure glaucoma (postiridectomy or where surgery refused/contraindicated); postcataract surgery-related glaucoma; accommodative esotropia

Dosage Summary

Ophthalmic:

Children: Diagnosis: Instill 1 drop of (0.125%) into both eyes at bedtime for 2-3 weeks; Treatment: Instill 1 drop of 0.06% once daily **or** 0.125% every other day (maximum: 0.125% daily)
Adults: Initial: 1 drop (0.03%) twice daily; Maintenance: 1 dose daily or every other day

Dosage Forms

Powder for reconstitution, ophthalmic:
Phospholine Iodide®: 6.25 mg (5 mL)

EC-Naprosyn® [US] *see* naproxen *on page 659*
***E. coli* asparaginase** *see* asparaginase *on page 99*

econazole (e KONE a zole)

Synonyms econazole nitrate

Therapeutic Category Antifungal Agent

Use Topical treatment of tinea pedis (athlete's foot), tinea cruris (jock itch), tinea corporis (ringworm), tinea versicolor, and cutaneous candidiasis

Dosage Summary

Topical:

Children: Apply sufficient quantity once or twice daily
Adults: Apply sufficient quantity once or twice daily

Dosage Forms

Cream, topical: 1% (15 g, 30 g, 85 g)

econazole nitrate *see* econazole *on page 340*
ecostigmine iodide *see* echothiophate iodide *on page 340*

Ecotrin® [US-OTC] *see* aspirin *on page* 100
Ecotrin® Arthritis Strength [US-OTC] *see* aspirin *on page* 100
Ecotrin® Low Strength [US-OTC] *see* aspirin *on page* 100
Ectosone [Can] *see* betamethasone *on page* 133

eculizumab (e kue LIZ oo mab)

Sound-Alike/Look-Alike Issues

eculizumab may be confused with efalizumab

U.S./Canadian Brand Names Soliris® [US/Can]

Therapeutic Category Monoclonal Antibody; Monoclonal Antibody, Complement Inhibitor

Use Treatment of paroxysmal nocturnal hemoglobinuria (PNH) to reduce hemolysis

Dosage Summary

I.V.:

Children: Dosage not established

Adults: 600 mg once weekly for 4 weeks, followed by 900 mg 1 week later; then maintenance: 900 mg every 2 weeks thereafter

Dosage Forms

Injection, solution [preservative free]:

Soliris®: 10 mg/mL (30 mL)

Ed A-Hist™ [US] *see* chlorpheniramine and phenylephrine *on page* 208
Ed A-Hist DM [US] *see* chlorpheniramine, phenylephrine, and dextromethorphan *on page* 211
edathamil disodium *see* edetate disodium *on page* 342
Ed Chlorped [US] *see* chlorpheniramine *on page* 207
Ed ChlorPed D [US] *see* chlorpheniramine and phenylephrine *on page* 208
Ed-Chlortan [US] *see* chlorpheniramine *on page* 207
Ed-Chlor-Tan*(Discontinued)* *see* chlorpheniramine *on page* 207
Edecrin® [US/Can] *see* ethacrynic acid *on page* 373

edetate CALCIUM disodium (ED e tate KAL see um dye SOW dee um)

Sound-Alike/Look-Alike Issues

edetate CALCIUM disodium (CaEDTA) may be confused with edetate disodium (Na_2EDTA). To avoid potentially serious errors, the abbreviation "EDTA" should **never** be used. CDC recommends that edetate disodium should **never** be used for chelation therapy in children. Fatal hypocalcemia may result if edetate disodium is used for chelation therapy instead of edetate calcium disodium. ISMP recommends confirming the diagnosis to help distinguish between the two drugs prior to dispensing and/or administering either drug.

edetate CALCIUM disodium may be confused with etomidate

Synonyms CaEDTA; calcium disodium edetate; edetate disodium CALCIUM

U.S./Canadian Brand Names Calcium Disodium Versenate® [US]

Therapeutic Category Chelating Agent

Use Treatment of symptomatic acute and chronic lead poisoning or for symptomatic patients with high blood lead levels

Dosage Summary

I.M.:

Children:

Asymptomatic lead poisoning with blood lead level >20 mcg/dL and <70 mcg/dL: 1000 mg/m^2/day (25-50 mg/kg/day) for 5 days

Symptomatic lead poisoning or blood lead levels ≥70 mcg/dL: 1000 mg/m^2/day (25-50 mg/kg/day) for 5 days

Lead encephalopathy: 1500 mg/m^2/day (50-75 mg/kg/day)

Adults:

Asymptomatic lead poisoning with blood lead level >20 mcg/dL and <70 mcg/dL: 1000 mg/m^2/day (25-50 mg/kg/day) for 5 days

Symptomatic lead poisoning or blood lead levels ≥70 mcg/dL: 1000 mg/m^2/day (25-50 mg/kg/day) for 5 days

Lead encephalopathy: 1500 mg/m^2/day (50-75 mg/kg/day)

I.V.:

Children:

Asymptomatic lead poisoning with blood lead level >20 mcg/dL and <70 mcg/dL: 1000 mg/m^2/day (25-50 mg/kg/day) for 5 days

Symptomatic lead poisoning or blood lead levels ≥70 mcg/dL: 1000 mg/m^2/day (25-50 mg/kg/day) for 5 days

Lead encephalopathy: 1500 mg/m^2/day (50-75 mg/kg/day)

Adults:

Asymptomatic lead poisoning with blood lead level >20 mcg/dL and <70 mcg/dL: 1000 mg/m^2/day (25-50 mg/kg/day) for 5 days

Symptomatic lead poisoning or blood lead levels ≥70 mcg/dL: 1000 mg/m^2/day (25-50 mg/kg/day) for 5 days

Lead encephalopathy: 1500 mg/m^2/day (50-75 mg/kg/day)

Dosage Forms

Injection, solution:

Calcium Disodium Versenate®: 200 mg/mL (2.5 mL)

edetate disodium (ED e tate dye SOW dee um)

Sound-Alike/Look-Alike Issues

edetate disodium (Na_2EDTA) may be confused with edetate calcium disodium (CaEDTA). To avoid potentially serious errors, the abbreviation "EDTA" should **never** be used. CDC recommends that edetate disodium should **never** be used for chelation therapy in children. Fatal hypocalcemia may result if edetate disodium is used for chelation therapy instead of edetate calcium disodium. ISMP recommends confirming the diagnosis to help distinguish between the two drugs prior to dispensing and/or administering either drug.

edetate disodium may be confused with etomidate

EDTA (Disodium) (error-prone abbreviation)

Synonyms edathamil disodium; endrate; Na_2EDTA; sodium edetate

Therapeutic Category Chelating Agent

Use Emergency treatment of hypercalcemia in adults

Dosage Summary

I.V.:

Adults: 50 mg/kg/day (maximum: 3 g/day)

Dosage Forms

Injection, solution: 150 mg/mL (20 mL)

edetate disodium CALCIUM *see* edetate CALCIUM disodium *on page 341*

Edex® [US] *see* alprostadil *on page 55*

Edluar™ [US] *see* zolpidem *on page 1004*

edrophonium (ed roe FOE nee um)

Synonyms edrophonium chloride

U.S./Canadian Brand Names Enlon® [US/Can]; Tensilon® [Can]

Therapeutic Category Cholinergic Agent

Use Diagnosis of myasthenia gravis; differentiation of cholinergic crises from myasthenia crises; reversal of nondepolarizing neuromuscular blockers

Dosage Summary

I.M.:

Infants: 0.5-1 mg

Children ≤34 kg: 1 mg

Children >34 kg: 5 mg

Adults: 10 mg, if no cholinergic reactions administer 2 mg 30 minutes later

I.V.: Note: Following doses may be administered I.M. or SubQ if no I.V. access

Infants: 0.1 mg, followed by 0.4 mg if no response (maximum total dose: 0.5 mg)

Children ≤34 kg: 0.04 mg/kg, followed by 0.16 mg/kg if no response **or** 1 mg, followed by 1mg every 30-45 seconds if no response (maximum total dose: 5 mg) **or** 0.04 mg/kg as a single dose 1 hour after oral anticholinesterase therapy

Children >34 kg: 0.04 mg/kg, followed by 0.16 mg/kg if no response **or** 2 mg, followed by 1 mg every 30-45 seconds if no response (maximum total dose: 10 mg) **or** 0.04 mg/kg as a single dose 1 hour after oral anticholinesterase therapy

Adults: 2 mg test dose, followed by 8 mg after 30 minutes if no response **or** 1-2 mg as a single dose 1 hour after oral anticholinesterase therapy **or** 10 mg every 5-10 minutes up to 40 mg **or** 5-10 mg as a single dose **or** 1 mg, may repeat after 1 minute

Dosage Forms

Injection, solution:

Enlon®: 10 mg/mL (15 mL)

edrophonium and atropine (ed roe FOE nee um & A troe peen)

Synonyms atropine sulfate and edrophonium chloride; edrophonium chloride and atropine sulfate

U.S./Canadian Brand Names Enlon-Plus® [US]

Therapeutic Category Anticholinergic Agent; Antidote; Cholinergic Agonist

Use Reversal of nondepolarizing neuromuscular blockers; adjunct treatment of respiratory depression caused by curare overdose

Dosage Summary

I.V.:

Children: Dosage not established

Adults: 0.05-0.1 mL/kg (0.5-1 mg/kg of edrophonium and 0.007-0.014 mg/kg of atropine)

Dosage Forms

Injection, solution:

Enlon-Plus®: Edrophonium 10 mg/mL and atropine 0.14 mg/mL (5 mL, 15 mL)

edrophonium chloride *see* edrophonium *on page 342*

edrophonium chloride and atropine sulfate *see* edrophonium and atropine *on page 343*

ED-SPAZ® *(Discontinued)* *see* hyoscyamine *on page 491*

ED-TLC [US] *see* phenylephrine, hydrocodone, and chlorpheniramine *on page 754*

ED-Tuss HC [US] *see* phenylephrine, hydrocodone, and chlorpheniramine *on page 754*

EEMT™ [US] *see* estrogens (esterified) and methyltestosterone *on page 372*

EEMT™ HS [US] *see* estrogens (esterified) and methyltestosterone *on page 372*

E.E.S.® [US/Can] *see* erythromycin (systemic) *on page 361*

efalizumab *(Discontinued)*

efavirenz (e FAV e renz)

U.S./Canadian Brand Names Sustiva® [US/Can]

Therapeutic Category Antiretroviral Agent, Nonnucleoside Reverse Transcriptase Inhibitor (NNRTI)

Use Treatment of HIV-1 infections in combination with at least two other antiretroviral agents

Dosage Summary

Oral:

Children <3 years: Dosage not established

Children ≥3 years and 10 kg to <15 kg: 200 mg once daily

Children ≥3 years and 15 kg to <20 kg: 250 mg once daily

Children ≥3 years and 20 kg to <25 kg: 300 mg once daily

Children ≥3 years and 25 kg to <32.5 kg: 350 mg once daily

Children ≥3 years and 32.5 kg to <40 kg: 400 mg once daily

Children ≥3 years and ≥40 kg: 600 mg once daily

Adults: 600 mg once daily

Dosage Forms

Capsule, oral:

Sustiva®: 50 mg, 200 mg

Tablet, oral:

Sustiva®: 600 mg

efavirenz, emtricitabine, and tenofovir

(e FAV e renz, em trye SYE ta been, & te NOE fo veer)

Synonyms emtricitabine, efavirenz, and tenofovir; FTC, TDF, and EFV; tenofovir disoproxil fumarate, efavirenz, and emtricitabine

U.S./Canadian Brand Names Atripla® [US/Can]

Therapeutic Category Antiretroviral Agent, Nonnucleoside Reverse Transcriptase Inhibitor (NNRTI); Antiretroviral Agent, Nucleoside Reverse Transcriptase Inhibitor (NRTI); Antiretroviral Agent, Reverse Transcriptase Inhibitor (Nucleotide)

Use Treatment of HIV infection

Dosage Summary

Oral:

Children: Dosage not established

Adults: One tablet once daily

Dosage Forms

Tablet:

Atripla®: Efavirenz 600 mg, emtricitabine 200 mg, and tenofovir disoproxil fumarate 300 mg

Effer-K® [US] *see* potassium bicarbonate and potassium citrate *on page 780*

Effer-Syllium® *(Discontinued)* *see* psyllium *on page 814*

Effexor® [US] *see* venlafaxine *on page 981*

Effexor XR® [US/Can] *see* venlafaxine *on page 981*

Effient™ [US] *see* prasugrel *on page 788*

Eflone® *(Discontinued)* *see* fluorometholone *on page 414*

eflornithine (ee FLOR ni theen)

Sound-Alike/Look-Alike Issues

Vaniqa® may be confused with Viagra®

Synonyms DFMO; eflornithine hydrochloride

U.S./Canadian Brand Names Vaniqa® [US/Can]

Therapeutic Category Antiprotozoal; Topical Skin Product

Use Cream: Females ≥12 years: Reduce unwanted hair from face and adjacent areas under the chin

Orphan status: Injection: Treatment of meningoencephalitic stage of *Trypanosoma brucei gambiense* infection (sleeping sickness)

Dosage Summary

I.V.:

Children: Dosage not established

Adults: 100 mg/kg/dose every 6 hours

Topical:

Children: Apply thin layer to affected areas twice daily (at least 8 hours apart)

Adults: Apply thin layer to affected areas twice daily (at least 8 hours apart)

Dosage Forms

Cream, topical:

Vaniqa®: 13.9% (30 g)

eflornithine hydrochloride *see* eflornithine *on page 344*

Efodine® *(Discontinued)* *see* povidone-iodine (topical) *on page 784*

eformoterol and budesonide *see* budesonide and formoterol *on page 152*

Efudex® [US/Can] *see* fluorouracil (topical) *on page 415*

E-Gem® [US-OTC] *see* vitamin E *on page 988*

E-Gem® Lip Care [US-OTC] *see* vitamin E *on page 988*

E-Gems® [US-OTC] *see* vitamin E *on page 988*

E-Gems® Elite [US-OTC] *see* vitamin E *on page 988*

E-Gems® Plus [US-OTC] *see* vitamin E *on page 988*

EHDP *see* etidronate *on page 383*

EL-970 *see* dalfampridine *on page 266*

Elaprase™ [US/Can] *see* idursulfase *on page 497*

Elavil® *(Discontinued)* *see* amitriptyline *on page 67*

Eldepryl® [US] *see* selegiline *on page 869*

Eldopaque® [US/Can] *see* hydroquinone *on page 487*

Eldopaque Forte® [US] *see* hydroquinone *on page 487*

Eldoquin® [US/Can] *see* hydroquinone *on page 487*

Eldoquin Forte® [US] *see* hydroquinone *on page 487*

electrolyte lavage solution *see* polyethylene glycol-electrolyte solution *on page 775*

electrolyte lavage solution *see* polyethylene glycol-electrolyte solution and bisacodyl *on page 776*

electrolyte solution, renal replacement

(ee LEK trow lite soe LOO shun REE nil ree PLASE ment)

Synonyms continuous renal replacement therapy; CRRT; renal replacement solution

U.S./Canadian Brand Names Normocarb HF™ [US]; PrismaSol [US]

Therapeutic Category Alkalinizing Agent; Electrolyte Supplement

Use Used as a replacement solution to replenish water, correct electrolytes, and adjust acid-base balance depleted by hemofiltration or hemodiafiltration (continuous renal replacement therapy [CRRT])

Dosage Summary

Continuous renal replacement circuit:

Children:

Pre- or post-filter: Volume of solution administered depends upon the patient's fluid balance, target fluid balance, body weight, and amount of fluid removed during hemofiltration process.

Post-filter replacement: Volume infused/hour should not be greater than 1/3 of blood flow rate (eg, blood flow rate 100 mL/minute [6000 mL/hour], post-filter replacement rate ≤2000 mL/hour)

Adults:

Pre- or post-filter: Volume of solution administered depends upon the patient's fluid balance, target fluid balance, body weight, and amount of fluid removed during hemofiltration process.

Post-filter replacement: Volume infused/hour should not be greater than 1/3 of blood flow rate (eg, blood flow rate 100 mL/minute [6000 mL/hour], post-filter replacement rate ≤2000 mL/hour)

Dosage Forms

Injection, solution [concentrate; preservative free]:

Normocarb HF™ 25: Bicarbonate 25 mEq/L, chloride 116.5 mEq/L, magnesium 1.5 mEq/L, sodium 140 mEq/L (240 mL) [strength represents final solution after mixing; when diluted as directed, makes 3240 mL of infusate]

Normocarb HF™ 35: Bicarbonate 35 mEq/L, chloride 106.5 mEq/L, magnesium 1.5 mEq/L, sodium 140 mEq/L (240 mL) [strength represents final solution after mixing; when diluted as directed, makes 3240 mL of infusate]

Injection, solution [preservative free]:

PrimaSol B22GK 2/0: Bicarbonate 22 mEq/L, chloride 118.5 mEq/L, dextrose 100 mg/dL, lactate 3 mEq/L, magnesium 1.5 mEq/L, potassium 2 mEq/L, sodium 140 mEq/L (5000 mL) [strength represents final solution after mixing]

PrismaSol BGK 2/0: Bicarbonate 32 mEq/L, chloride 108 mEq/L, dextrose 100 mg/dL, lactate 3 mEq/L, magnesium 1 mEq/L, potassium 2 mEq/L, sodium 140 mEq/L (5000 mL) [strength represents final solution after mixing]

PrismaSol BGK 2/3.5: Bicarbonate 32 mEq/L, calcium 3.5 mEq/L, chloride 111.5 mEq/L, dextrose 100 mg/dL, lactate 3 mEq/L, magnesium 1 mEq/L, potassium 2 mEq/L, sodium 140 mEq/L (5000 mL) [strength represents final solution after mixing]

PrimaSol BGK 4/0/1.2: Bicarbonate 32 mEq/L, chloride 110.2 mEq/L, dextrose 100 mg/dL, lactate 3 mEq/L, magnesium 1.2 mEq/L, potassium 4 mEq/L, sodium 140 mEq/L (5000 mL) [strength represents final solution after mixing]

PrismaSol BGK 4/2.5: Bicarbonate 32 mEq/L, calcium 2.5 mEq/L, chloride 113 mEq/L, dextrose 100 mg/dL, lactate 3 mEq/L, magnesium 1.5 mEq/L, potassium 4 mEq/L, sodium 140 mEq/L (5000 mL) [strength represents final solution after mixing]

PrimaSol BK 0/0/1.2: Bicarbonate 32 mEq/L, chloride 106.2 mEq/L, lactate 3 mEq/L, magnesium 1.2 mEq/L, sodium 140 mEq/L (5000 mL) [strength represents final solution after mixing]

Elestat™ [US] *see* epinastine *on page* 352

Elestrin™ [US] *see* estradiol (systemic) *on page* 366

eletriptan (el e TRIP tan)

Synonyms eletriptan hydrobromide

U.S./Canadian Brand Names Relpax® [US/Can]

Therapeutic Category Serotonin 5-$HT_{1B,\ 1D}$ Receptor Agonist

Use Acute treatment of migraine, with or without aura

Dosage Summary

Oral:

Children: Dosage not established

Adults: 20-40 mg as a single dose, may repeat after 2 hours (maximum: 80 mg/day)

Dosage Forms

Tablet, oral:

Relpax®: 20 mg, 40 mg

eletriptan hydrobromide *see* eletriptan *on page 345*

Elidel® [US/Can] *see* pimecrolimus *on page 761*

Eligard® [US/Can] *see* leuprolide *on page 554*

Elimite® [US] *see* permethrin *on page 744*

Eliphos™ [US] *see* calcium acetate *on page 166*

Elitek™ [US] *see* rasburicase *on page 830*

Elixomin® *(Discontinued)* *see* theophylline *on page 925*

Elixophyllin® [US] *see* theophylline *on page 925*

Elixophyllin-GG® *(Discontinued)*

ElixSure™ Fever/Pain *(Discontinued)* *see* acetaminophen *on page 21*

ella® [US] *see* ulipristal *on page 968*

Ellence® [US/Can] *see* epirubicin *on page 355*

Elmiron® [US/Can] *see* pentosan polysulfate sodium *on page 741*

Elocom® [Can] *see* mometasone (topical) *on page 641*

Elocon® [US] *see* mometasone (topical) *on page 641*

Eloxatin® [US/Can] *see* oxaliplatin *on page 711*

Elspar® [US] *see* asparaginase *on page 99*

Eltor® [Can] *see* pseudoephedrine *on page 810*

eltrombopag (el TROM boe pag)

Synonyms eltrombopag olamine; Revolade®; SB-497115; SB-497115-GR

U.S./Canadian Brand Names Promacta® [US]

Therapeutic Category Colony Stimulating Factor; Thrombopoietic Agent

Use Treatment of thrombocytopenia in patients with chronic immune (idiopathic) thrombocytopenic purpura (ITP) at risk for bleeding who have had insufficient response to corticosteroids, immune globulin, or splenectomy

Dosage Summary

Oral:

Children: Dosage not established

Adults: 50 mg once daily (maximum dose: 75 mg/day)

Dosage Forms

Tablet, oral:

Promacta®: 25 mg, 50 mg

eltrombopag olamine *see* eltrombopag *on page 346*

Eltroxin® [Can] *see* levothyroxine *on page 560*

Emadine® [US] *see* emedastine *on page 346*

Embeda™ [US] *see* morphine and naltrexone *on page 646*

Embeline™ *(Discontinued)* *see* clobetasol *on page 235*

Embeline™ E *(Discontinued)* *see* clobetasol *on page 235*

Emcyt® [US/Can] *see* estramustine *on page 369*

Emecheck® *(Discontinued)*

emedastine (em e DAS teen)

Synonyms emedastine difumarate

U.S./Canadian Brand Names Emadine® [US]

Therapeutic Category Antihistamine, H_1 Blocker, Ophthalmic

Use Treatment of allergic conjunctivitis

Dosage Summary

Ophthalmic:

Children <3 years: Dosage not established

Children ≥3 years: Instill 1 drop in affected eye up to 4 times/day

Adults: Instill 1 drop in affected eye up to 4 times/day

Dosage Forms

Solution, ophthalmic:

Emadine®: 0.05% (5 mL)

emedastine difumarate *see* emedastine *on page* *346*

Emend® [US/Can] *see* aprepitant *on page* *92*

Emend® for Injection [US] *see* fosaprepitant *on page* *427*

Emetrol® [US-OTC] *see* fructose, dextrose, and phosphoric acid *on page* *430*

Emitrip® *(Discontinued)* *see* amitriptyline *on page* *67*

Emko® *(Discontinued)* *see* nonoxynol 9 *on page* *681*

EMLA® [US/Can] *see* lidocaine and prilocaine *on page* *565*

Emo-Cort® [Can] *see* hydrocortisone (topical) *on page* *483*

Emsam® [US] *see* selegiline *on page* *869*

emtricitabine (em trye SYE ta been)

Synonyms BW524W91; coviracil; FTC

U.S./Canadian Brand Names Emtriva® [US/Can]

Therapeutic Category Antiretroviral Agent, Nucleoside Reverse Transcriptase Inhibitor (NRTI)

Use Treatment of HIV infection in combination with at least two other antiretroviral agents

Dosage Summary

Oral:

Capsule:

Children <3 months: Use solution

Children ≥3 months and ≤33 kg: Use solution

Children 3 months to 17 years and >33 kg: 200 mg once daily

Adults: 200 mg once daily

Solution:

Children <3 months: 3 mg/kg/day

Children 3 months to 17 years: 6 mg/kg once daily (maximum: 240 mg/day)

Adults: 240 mg once daily

Dosage Forms

Capsule, oral:

Emtriva®: 200 mg

Solution, oral:

Emtriva®: 10 mg/mL (170 mL)

emtricitabine and tenofovir (em trye SYE ta been & te NOE fo veer)

Synonyms tenofovir and emtricitabine

U.S./Canadian Brand Names Truvada® [US/Can]

Therapeutic Category Antiretroviral Agent, Nucleoside Reverse Transcriptase Inhibitor (NRTI); Antiretroviral Agent, Reverse Transcriptase Inhibitor (Nucleotide)

Use Treatment of HIV infection in combination with other antiretroviral agents

Dosage Summary

Oral:

Children: Dosage not established

Adults: One tablet (emtricitabine 200 mg and tenofovir 300 mg) once daily

Dosage Forms

Tablet:

Truvada®: Emtricitabine 200 mg and tenofovir 300 mg

emtricitabine, efavirenz, and tenofovir *see* efavirenz, emtricitabine, and tenofovir *on page* *343*

Emtriva® [US/Can] *see* emtricitabine *on page* *347*

Emulsoil® *(Discontinued)* *see* castor oil *on page* *187*

E-Mycin® *(Discontinued)*

E-Mycin-E® *(Discontinued)*

ENA 713 *see* rivastigmine *on page* *848*

Enablex® [US/Can] *see* darifenacin *on page* *270*

enalapril (e NAL a pril)

Sound-Alike/Look-Alike Issues

enalapril may be confused with Anafranil®, Elavil®, Eldepryl®, ramipril

Synonyms enalapril maleate; enalaprilat

U.S./Canadian Brand Names Apo-Enalapril® [Can]; CO Enalapril [Can]; Mylan-Enalapril [Can]; Novo-Enalapril [Can]; PMS-Enalapril [Can]; PRO-Enalapril [Can]; RAN™-Enalapril [Can]; ratio-Enalapril [Can]; Riva-Enalapril [Can]; Sandoz-Enalapril [Can]; Sig-Enalapril [Can]; Taro-Enalapril [Can]; Vasotec® I.V. [Can]; Vasotec® [US/Can]

Therapeutic Category Angiotensin-Converting Enzyme (ACE) Inhibitor

Use Treatment of hypertension; treatment of symptomatic heart failure; treatment of asymptomatic left ventricular dysfunction

Dosage Summary

I.V.:

Children: Dosage not established

Adults: 0.625-5 mg every 6 hours

Oral:

Children <1 month: Dosage not established

Children 1 month to 17 years: Initial: 0.08 mg/kg/day (up to 5 mg) in 1-2 divided doses; Maintenance: Up to 0.58 mg/kg (40 mg)

Adults: Initial: 2.5-5 mg/day in 1-2 divided doses; Maintenance: 2.5-40 mg/day in 1-2 divided doses; Target dose for HF: 10-20 mg twice daily

Dosage Forms

Injection, solution: 1.25 mg/mL (1 mL, 2 mL)

Tablet, oral: 2.5 mg, 5 mg, 10 mg, 20 mg

Vasotec®: 2.5 mg, 5 mg, 10 mg, 20 mg

enalapril and felodipine (e NAL a pril & fe LOE di peen)

Synonyms enalapril maleate and felodipine; felodipine and enalapril

U.S./Canadian Brand Names Lexxel® [Can]

Therapeutic Category Antihypertensive Agent, Combination

Use Treatment of hypertension, however, not indicated for initial treatment of hypertension; replacement therapy in patients receiving separate dosage forms (for patient convenience); when monotherapy with one component fails to achieve desired antihypertensive effect, or when dose-limiting adverse effects limit upward titration of monotherapy

Dosage Summary

Oral:

Children: Dosage not established

Adults: Enalapril 5-20 mg and felodipine 2.5-10 mg once daily

Elderly: Initial dose of felodipine is 2.5 mg daily

enalapril and hydrochlorothiazide (e NAL a pril & hye droe klor oh THYE a zide)

Synonyms enalapril maleate and hydrochlorothiazide; hydrochlorothiazide and enalapril

U.S./Canadian Brand Names Vaseretic® [US/Can]

Therapeutic Category Antihypertensive Agent, Combination

Use Treatment of hypertension

Dosage Summary

Oral:

Children: Dosage not established

Adults: Enalapril 5-10 mg and hydrochlorothiazide 12.5-25 mg once daily (maximum: 40 mg/day [enalapril]; 50 mg/day [hydrochlorothiazide])

Dosage Forms

Tablet: 5/12.5: Enalapril 5 mg and hydrochlorothiazide 12.5 mg; 10/25: Enalapril 10 mg and hydrochlorothiazide 25 mg

Vaseretic®: 10/25: enalapril 10 mg and hydrochlorothiazide 25 mg

enalaprilat *see* enalapril *on page 348*

enalapril maleate *see* enalapril *on page 348*

enalapril maleate and felodipine *see* enalapril and felodipine *on page 348*

enalapril maleate and hydrochlorothiazide *see* enalapril and hydrochlorothiazide *on page 348*

Enbrel® [US/Can] *see* etanercept *on page 373*
Encare® [US-OTC] *see* nonoxynol 9 *on page 681*
Encora® [US] *see* vitamins (multiple/oral) *on page 990*
EndaCof *(Discontinued)*
EndaCof-DM [US] *see* brompheniramine, pseudoephedrine, and dextromethorphan *on page 149*
EndaCof-PD [US] *see* brompheniramine, pseudoephedrine, and dextromethorphan *on page 149*
EndaCof-XP *(Discontinued)*
Endagen™-HD *(Discontinued)* *see* phenylephrine, hydrocodone, and chlorpheniramine *on page 754*
Endantadine® [Can] *see* amantadine *on page 61*
EndoAvitene® [US] *see* collagen hemostat *on page 248*
Endocet® [US/Can] *see* oxycodone and acetaminophen *on page 715*
Endocodone® *(Discontinued)* *see* oxycodone *on page 714*
Endodan® [US/Can] *see* oxycodone and aspirin *on page 716*
Endo®-Levodopa/Carbidopa [Can] *see* carbidopa and levodopa *on page 182*
Endolor® *(Discontinued)*
Endometrin® [US] *see* progesterone *on page 799*
endrate *see* edetate disodium *on page 342*
Enduron® *(Discontinued)* *see* methyclothiazide *on page 617*
Enduronyl® Forte *(Discontinued)*
Enecat™ *(Discontinued)* *see* barium *on page 117*
Enemeez® [US-OTC] *see* docusate *on page 321*
Enemeez® Plus [US-OTC] *see* docusate *on page 321*
Ener-B® [US-OTC] *see* cyanocobalamin *on page 257*
Enerjets [US-OTC] *see* caffeine *on page 163*
Enfamil® D-Vi-Sol™ [US-OTC] *see* cholecalciferol *on page 218*
Enfamil® Glucose [US-OTC] *see* dextrose *on page 290*

enflurane (EN floo rane)

Sound-Alike/Look-Alike Issues
enflurane may be confused with isoflurane

U.S./Canadian Brand Names Compound 347™ [US]

Therapeutic Category General Anesthetic

Use Maintenance of general anesthesia

Note: Use for induction of general anesthesia is an FDA-labeled indication; however, it is not recommended clinically due to its irritant properties and unpleasant odor which causes breath-holding and coughing. In addition, other labeled indications that are not routinely used and/or recommended clinically include use as analgesia during vaginal delivery and use as an adjunct to other general anesthetic agents during Cesarean section delivery.

Dosage Summary

Inhalation:
Children: Dosage not established
Adults: Maintenance: 0.5% to 3% (maximum concentration: 3%)

Dosage Forms

Liquid, for inhalation:
Compound 347™: >99.9% (250 mL)

enfuvirtide (en FYOO vir tide)

Synonyms T-20

U.S./Canadian Brand Names Fuzeon® [US/Can]

Therapeutic Category Antiretroviral Agent, Fusion Protein Inhibitor

Use Treatment of HIV-1 infection in combination with other antiretroviral agents in treatment-experienced patients with evidence of HIV-1 replication despite ongoing antiretroviral therapy

Dosage Summary

SubQ:
Children <6 years: Dosage not established
Children 6-16 years: 2 mg/kg twice daily (maximum: 90 mg/dose)

Adolescents ≥16 years: 90 mg twice daily
Adults: 90 mg twice daily

Dosage Forms

Injection, powder for reconstitution [preservative free]:
Fuzeon®: 108 mg

ENG *see* etonogestrel *on page 384*
Engerix-B® [US/Can] *see* hepatitis B vaccine (recombinant) *on page 470*
Engerix-B® and Havrix® *see* hepatitis A and hepatitis B recombinant vaccine *on page 468*
enhanced-potency inactivated poliovirus vaccine *see* poliovirus vaccine (inactivated) *on page 774*
Enhancer ***(Discontinued)*** *see* barium *on page 117*
Enisyl® ***(Discontinued)*** *see* l-lysine *on page 572*
Enjuvia™ [US] *see* estrogens (conjugated B/synthetic) *on page 370*
Enlon® [US/Can] *see* edrophonium *on page 342*
Enlon-Plus® [US] *see* edrophonium and atropine *on page 343*
Enomine® ***(Discontinued)***
Enovil® ***(Discontinued)*** *see* amitriptyline *on page 67*

enoxaparin (ee noks a PA rin)

Sound-Alike/Look-Alike Issues

Lovenox® may be confused with Lasix®, Levaquin®, Lotronex®, Protonix®

Synonyms enoxaparin sodium

U.S./Canadian Brand Names Enoxaparin Injection [Can]; Lovenox® HP [Can]; Lovenox® [US/Can]

Therapeutic Category Anticoagulant (Other)

Use

Acute coronary syndromes: Unstable angina (UA), non-ST-elevation (NSTEMI), and ST-elevation myocardial infarction (STEMI)

DVT prophylaxis: Following hip or knee replacement surgery, abdominal surgery, or in medical patients with severely-restricted mobility during acute illness who are at risk for thromboembolic complications

DVT treatment (acute): Inpatient treatment (patients with and without pulmonary embolism) and outpatient treatment (patients without pulmonary embolism)

Note: High-risk patients include those with one or more of the following risk factors: >40 years of age, obesity, general anesthesia lasting >30 minutes, malignancy, history of deep vein thrombosis or pulmonary embolism

Dosage Summary

SubQ:

Adults: Prophylaxis: 30 mg every 12 hours **or** 40 mg once daily; Treatment: 1 mg/kg every 12 hours **or** 1.5 mg/kg once daily

STEMI indication only:

<75 years: 30 mg I.V. bolus plus 1 mg/kg SubQ every 12 hours

≥75 years: 0.75 mg/kg SubQ every 12 hours; **Note:** I.V. bolus is omitted

Elderly: Refer to adult dosing.

Dosage Forms

Injection, solution:
Lovenox®: 100 mg/mL (3 mL)

Injection, solution [preservative free]: 30 mg/0.3 mL (0.3 mL); 40 mg/0.4 mL (0.4 mL); 60 mg/0.6 mL (0.6 mL); 80 mg/0.8 mL (0.8 mL); 100 mg/mL (1 mL); 120 mg/0.8 mL (0.8 mL); 150 mg/mL (1 mL)
Lovenox®: 30 mg/0.3 mL (0.3 mL); 40 mg/0.4 mL (0.4 mL); 60 mg/0.6 mL (0.6 mL); 80 mg/0.8 mL (0.8 mL); 100 mg/mL (1 mL); 120 mg/0.8 mL (0.8 mL); 150 mg/mL (1 mL)

Enoxaparin Injection [Can] *see* enoxaparin *on page 350*
enoxaparin sodium *see* enoxaparin *on page 350*
Enpresse™ [US] *see* ethinyl estradiol and levonorgestrel *on page 376*
Ensure® [US-OTC] *see* nutritional formula, enteral/oral *on page 692*
Ensure Plus® [US-OTC] *see* nutritional formula, enteral/oral *on page 692*

entacapone (en TA ka pone)

U.S./Canadian Brand Names Comtan® [US/Can]

Therapeutic Category Anti-Parkinson Agent; Reverse COMT Inhibitor

Use Adjunct to levodopa/carbidopa therapy in patients with idiopathic Parkinson disease who experience "wearing-off" symptoms at the end of a dosing interval

Dosage Summary

Oral:

Children: Dosage not established

Adults: 200 mg with each dose of levodopa/carbidopa (maximum: 1600 mg/day)

Dosage Forms

Tablet, oral:

Comtan®: 200 mg

entacapone, carbidopa, and levodopa *see* levodopa, carbidopa, and entacapone *on page 557*

entecavir (en TE ka veer)

U.S./Canadian Brand Names Baraclude® [US/Can]

Therapeutic Category Antiretroviral Agent, Reverse Transcriptase Inhibitor (Nucleoside)

Use Treatment of chronic hepatitis B infection in adults with evidence of active viral replication and either evidence of persistent transaminase elevations or histologically-active disease

Dosage Summary

Oral:

Children <16 years: Dosage not established

Adolescents ≥16 years: Nucleoside naive: 0.5 mg once daily; Lamivudine- or telbivudine-resistant: 1 mg once daily

Adults: Nucleoside-naive: 0.5 mg once daily; Lamivudine- or telbivudine-resistant: 1 mg once daily

Dosage Forms

Solution, oral:

Baraclude®: 0.05 mg/mL (210 mL)

Tablet, oral:

Baraclude®: 0.5 mg, 1 mg

Entereg® [US] *see* alvimopan *on page 60*
enterotoxigenic *Escherichia coli* and *Vibrio cholera* vaccine *see* traveler's diarrhea and cholera vaccine *(Canada only) on page 949*
Entero VU™ 24% [US] *see* barium *on page 117*
Entertainer's Secret® [US-OTC] *see* saliva substitute *on page 861*
Entex® *(Discontinued)* *see* guaifenesin and phenylephrine *on page 456*
Entex® ER *(Discontinued)* *see* guaifenesin and phenylephrine *on page 456*
Entex® HC *(Discontinued)*
Entex® LA [Can] *see* guaifenesin and pseudoephedrine *on page 457*
Entex® LA *(Discontinued)* *see* guaifenesin and phenylephrine *on page 456*
Entex® PSE *(Discontinued)* *see* guaifenesin and pseudoephedrine *on page 457*
Entocort® [Can] *see* budesonide (systemic, oral inhalation) *on page 151*
Entocort® EC [US] *see* budesonide (systemic, oral inhalation) *on page 151*
Entre-S [US] *see* chlorpheniramine, pseudoephedrine, and dextromethorphan *on page 214*
Entrobar® *(Discontinued)* *see* barium *on page 117*
EntroEase® *(Discontinued)* *see* barium *on page 117*
Entrophen® [Can] *see* aspirin *on page 100*
Entsol® [US-OTC] *see* sodium chloride *on page 882*
Entuss-D® Liquid *(Discontinued)*
Enulose [US] *see* lactulose *on page 544*
Eovist® [US] *see* gadoxetate *on page 435*
Eperbel-S *(Discontinued)*

ephedrine (systemic) (e FED rin)

Sound-Alike/Look-Alike Issues

ePHEDrine may be confused with Epifrin®, EPINEPHrine

Synonyms ephedrine sulfate

Tall-Man ePHEDrine

Therapeutic Category Alpha/Beta Agonist

Use Treatment of nasal congestion, idiopathic orthostatic hypotension, anesthesia-induced hypotension

Dosage Summary

I.V.:

Children: 0.2-0.3 mg/kg/dose every 4-6 hours

Adults: 5-25 mg/dose, repeat after 5-10 minutes as needed, then every 3-4 hours (maximum: 150 mg/day)

Oral:

Children <12 years: Dosage not established

Children ≥12 years: 12.5-50 mg every 4 hours as needed (maximum: 150 mg/day)

Adults: 12.5-50 mg every 4 hours as needed (maximum: 150 mg/day)

Dosage Forms

Capsule, oral: 25 mg

Injection, solution [preservative free]: 50 mg/mL (1 mL)

ephedrine, chlorpheniramine, phenylephrine, and carbetapentane *see* chlorpheniramine, ephedrine, phenylephrine, and carbetapentane *on page 210*

ephedrine sulfate *see* ephedrine (systemic) *on page 351*

Epi-Clenz™ [US-OTC] *see* alcohol (ethyl) *on page 45*

epidoxorubicin *see* epirubicin *on page 355*

Epidrin [US] *see* acetaminophen, isometheptene, and dichloralphenazone *on page 31*

Epiduo™ [US] *see* adapalene and benzoyl peroxide *on page 38*

Epi E-Z Pen® [Can] *see* epinephrine (systemic, oral inhalation) *on page 352*

Epiflur™ [US] *see* fluoride *on page 413*

Epifoam® [US] *see* pramoxine and hydrocortisone *on page 787*

Epifrin® *(Discontinued)* *see* epinephrine (systemic, oral inhalation) *on page 352*

Epiklor™ [US] *see* potassium chloride *on page 781*

Epiklor™/25 [US] *see* potassium chloride *on page 781*

epinastine (ep i NAS teen)

Synonyms epinastine hydrochloride

U.S./Canadian Brand Names Elestat™ [US]

Therapeutic Category Antihistamine, H_1 Blocker, Ophthalmic

Use Treatment of allergic conjunctivitis

Dosage Summary

Ophthalmic:

Children <3 years: Dosage not established

Children ≥3 years: Instill 1 drop into each eye twice daily

Adults: Instill 1 drop into each eye twice daily

Dosage Forms

Solution, ophthalmic:

Elestat™: 0.05% (5 mL)

epinastine hydrochloride *see* epinastine *on page 352*

epinephrine (systemic, oral inhalation) (ep i NEF rin)

Sound-Alike/Look-Alike Issues

EPINEPHrine may be confused with ePHEDrine

Epifrin® may be confused with ephedrine, EpiPen®

EpiPen® may be confused with Epifrin®

Synonyms adrenaline; epinephrine bitartrate; epinephrine hydrochloride; racemic epinephrine; racepinephrine

Tall-Man EPINEPHrine

U.S./Canadian Brand Names Adrenaclick™ [US]; Adrenalin® [US/Can]; Epi E-Z Pen® [Can]; EpiPen 2-Pak® [US]; EpiPen Jr 2-Pak® [US]; EpiPen® Jr [US/Can]; EpiPen® [US/Can]; Primatene® Mist [US-OTC]; S2® [US-OTC]; Twinject® [US/Can]

Therapeutic Category Alpha/Beta Agonist

Use Treatment of bronchospasms, bronchial asthma, viral croup, anaphylactic reactions, cardiac arrest; added to local anesthetics to decrease systemic absorption of intraspinal and local anesthetics and increase duration of action; decrease superficial hemorrhage

Dosage Summary

I.M.:

Children: Consult specific product labeling

Adults: 0.3-0.5 mg (**1:1000** solution) every 15-20 minutes **or** consult specific product labeling

EpiPen® Jr.:

Children <15 kg: Dosage not established

Children 15-29 kg: 0.15 mg; if anaphylactic symptoms persist, dose may be repeated in 5-15 minutes using an additional EpiPen® Jr

EpiPen®:

Children <30 kg: Refer to EpiPen® Jr dosing

Children ≥30 kg: 0.3 mg; if anaphylactic symptoms persist, dose may be repeated in 5-15 minutes using an additional EpiPen®

Adults: 0.3 mg; if anaphylactic symptoms persist, dose may be repeated in 5-15 minutes using an additional EpiPen®

Twinject®:

Children <15 kg: Dosage not established

Children 15-29 kg: 0.15 kg; if anaphylactic symptoms persist, dose may be repeated in 5-15 minutes using the same device after partial disassembly

Children ≥30 kg: 0.3 mg; if anaphylactic symptoms persist, dose may be repeated in 5-15 minutes using the same device after partial disassembly

Adults: 0.3 mg; if anaphylactic symptoms persist, dose may be repeated in 5-15 minutes using the same device after partial disassembly

Inhalation:

Children <4 years: Dosage not established

Children ≥4 years: One inhalation, may repeat once after 1 minute, then do not use again for at least 3 hours

Adults: One inhalation, may repeat once after 1 minute, then do not use again for at least 3 hours

I.O.:

Children: 0.01 mg/kg kg (maximum single dose: 1 mg) every 3-5 minutes as needed

Adults: 1 mg every 3-5 minutes (up to 0.2 mg/kg may be needed for specific problems)

I.V. (1:10,000):

Neonates: 0.01-0.03 mg/kg every 3-5 minutes as needed

Children: 0.01 mg/kg kg (maximum single dose: 1 mg) every 3-5 minutes as needed **or** 0.1-1 mcg/kg/minute as a continuous infusion **or** 0.01 mg/kg every 20 minutes (hypersensitivity reaction)

Adults: 1 mg every 3-5 minutes (up to 0.2 mg/kg may be needed for specific problems) **or** 1-10 mcg/minute as a continuous infusion

Intratracheal:

Neonates: Up to 0.1 mg/kg every 3-5 minutes until I.V. access obtained

Children: 0.1 mg/kg (maximum single dose: 10 mg) every 3-5 minutes until I.V./I.O access established or return of spontaneous circulation

Adults: 2-2.5 mg every 3-5 minutes until I.V./I.O access established or return of spontaneous circulation; dilute in 5-10 mL NS or distilled water

Nebulization (S2® Racepinephrine, OTC):

Children <4 years: Jet nebulizer: 0.05 mL/kg (maximum dose: 0.5 mL) diluted in 3 mL NS up to every 2 hours

Children ≥4 years:

Hand-bulb nebulizer: Add 0.5 mL (~10 drops) to nebulizer; 1-3 inhalations up to every 3 hours if needed

Jet nebulizer: Add 0.5 mL (~10 drops) to nebulizer and dilute with 3 mL of NS. Administer over ~15 minutes every 3-4 hours as needed.

Adults:

Hand-bulb nebulizer: Add 0.5 mL (~10 drops) to nebulizer; 1-3 inhalations up to every 3 hours if needed

Jet nebulizer: Add 0.5 mL (~10 drops) to nebulizer and dilute with 3 mL of NS. Administer over ~15 minutes every 3-4 hours as needed.

SubQ:

Children: 0.01 mg/kg (**1:1000** solution) every 20 minutes for 3 doses or as condition requires (maximum: 0.5 mg/dose) **or** EpiPen®/Twinject® (Consult specific product labeling)

Adults: 0.3-0.5 mg (**1:1000** solution) every 15-20 minutes for 3 doses or as condition requires **or** EpiPen®/Twinject® (Consult specific product labeling)

EpiPen® Jr:

Children <15 kg: Dosage not established

Children 15-29 kg: 0.15 mg; if anaphylactic symptoms persist, dose may be repeated in 5-15 minutes using an additional EpiPen® Jr

EpiPen®:

Children <30 kg: Refer to EpiPen® Jr dosing

Children ≥30 kg: 0.3 mg; if anaphylactic symptoms persist, dose may be repeated in 5-15 minutes using an additional EpiPen®

Adults: 0.3 mg; if anaphylactic symptoms persist, dose may be repeated in 5-15 minutes using an additional EpiPen®

Twinject®:

Children <15 kg: Dosage not established

Children 15-29 kg: 0.15 mg; if anaphylactic symptoms persist, dose may be repeated in 5-15 minutes using the same device after partial disassembly

Children ≥30 kg: 0.3 mg; if anaphylactic symptoms persist, dose may be repeated in 5-15 minutes using the same device after partial disassembly

Adults: 0.3 mg; if anaphylactic symptoms persist, dose may be repeated in 5-15 minutes using the same device after partial disassembly

Dosage Forms

Aerosol, for oral inhalation:

Primatene® Mist [OTC]: 0.22 mg/inhalation (15 mL)

Injection, solution: 0.1 mg/mL, 0.3 mg/3 mL, 0.15 mg/0.15 mL, 1 mg/mL

Adrenaclick™: 0.15 mg/0.15 mL, 0.3 mg/0.3 mL

Adrenalin®: 1 mg/mL

EpiPen 2-Pak®: 0.3 mg/0.3 mL

EpiPen Jr 2-Pak®: 0.15 mg/0.3 mL

EpiPen®: 0.3 mg/0.3 mL

EpiPen® Jr.: 0.15 mg/0.3 mL

Twinject®: 0.15 mg/0.15 mL, 0.3 mg/0.3 mL

Injection, solution [preservative free]: 1 mg/mL

Solution, for oral inhalation [preservative free]:

S2® [OTC]: 2.25% (0.5 mL)

epinephrine (nasal) (ep i NEF rin)

Sound-Alike/Look-Alike Issues

EPINEPHrine may be confused with ePHEDrine

Synonyms adrenaline; epinephrine hydrochloride

Tall-Man EPINEPHrine

U.S./Canadian Brand Names Adrenalin® [US/Can]

Therapeutic Category Alpha/Beta Agonist

Use Treatment of nasal congestion

Dosage Summary

Intranasal:

Children <6 years: Dosage not established

Children ≥6 years: Apply **1:1000** solution locally as drops, spray or with sterile swab

Adults: Apply **1:1000** solution locally as drops, spray or with sterile swab

Dosage Forms

Solution, intranasal:

Adrenalin®: 1 mg/mL (30 mL)

epinephrine and articaine hydrochloride *see* articaine and epinephrine *on page* 96

epinephrine and chlorpheniramine (ep i NEF rin & klor fen IR a meen)

Synonyms insect sting kit

U.S./Canadian Brand Names Ana-Kit® [US]

Therapeutic Category Antidote

Use Anaphylaxis emergency treatment of insect bites or stings by the sensitive patient that may occur within minutes of insect sting or exposure to an allergic substance

Dosage Summary

I.M. or SubQ:

Epinephrine (1:1000):

Children <2 years: 0.05-0.1 mL

Children 2-6 years: 0.15 mL

Children 6-12 years: 0.2 mL

Children >12 years: 0.3 mL

Adults: 0.3 mL

Oral:

Chlorpheniramine (2 mg/tablet):

Children <6 years: 1 tablet

Children 6-12 years: 2 tablets

Children >12 years: 4 tablets

Adults: 4 tablets

Dosage Forms

Kit:

Ana-Kit®: Epinephrine 1:1000 (1 mL), chlorpheniramine chewable tablet 2 mg (4), sterile alcohol pads (2), tourniquet (1)

epinephrine and lidocaine *see* lidocaine and epinephrine *on page 563*

epinephrine bitartrate *see* epinephrine (systemic, oral inhalation) *on page 352*

epinephrine bitartrate and bupivacaine hydrochloride *see* bupivacaine and epinephrine *on page 154*

epinephrine hydrochloride *see* epinephrine (nasal) *on page 354*

epinephrine hydrochloride *see* epinephrine (systemic, oral inhalation) *on page 352*

EpiPen® [US/Can] *see* epinephrine (systemic, oral inhalation) *on page 352*

EpiPen 2-Pak® [US] *see* epinephrine (systemic, oral inhalation) *on page 352*

EpiPen® Jr [US/Can] *see* epinephrine (systemic, oral inhalation) *on page 352*

EpiPen Jr 2-Pak® [US] *see* epinephrine (systemic, oral inhalation) *on page 352*

epipodophyllotoxin *see* etoposide *on page 384*

EpiQuin™ Micro [US] *see* hydroquinone *on page 487*

epirubicin (ep i ROO bi sin)

Sound-Alike/Look-Alike Issues

epirubicin may be confused with DAUNOrubicin, DOXOrubicin, idarubicin

Ellence® may be confused with Elase®

Synonyms epidoxorubicin; epirubicin hydrochloride; pidorubicin; pidorubicin hydrochloride

U.S./Canadian Brand Names Ellence® [US/Can]; Pharmorubicin® [Can]

Therapeutic Category Antineoplastic Agent, Anthracycline; Antineoplastic Agent, Antibiotic

Use Adjuvant therapy for primary breast cancer

Dosage Summary

I.V.:

Children: Dosage not established

Adults: 100 mg/m^2 day 1 every 3 weeks **or** 60 mg/m^2 days 1 and 8 every 4 weeks

Dosage Forms

Injection, powder for reconstitution: 50 mg

Injection, solution [preservative free]: 2 mg/mL (25 mL, 100 mL)

Ellence®: 2 mg/mL (25 mL, 100 mL)

epirubicin hydrochloride *see* epirubicin *on page 355*

Epitol® [US] *see* carbamazepine *on page 177*

Epival® [Can] *see* divalproex *on page 319*

Epival® I.V. [Can] *see* valproic acid *on page 974*

Epivir® [US] *see* lamivudine *on page 545*

Epivir-HBV® [US] *see* lamivudine *on page 545*

eplerenone (e PLER en one)

Sound-Alike/Look-Alike Issues

Inspra™ may be confused with Spiriva®

U.S./Canadian Brand Names Inspra™ [US]

Therapeutic Category Antihypertensive Agent; Selective Aldosterone Blocker

Use Treatment of hypertension (may be used alone or in combination with other antihypertensive agents); treatment of heart failure (HF) following acute MI

Dosage Summary

Oral:

Children: Dosage not established

Adults: Initial: 25-50 mg once daily; Maintenance: 50 mg once or twice daily (maximum: 100 mg/day); **Note:** Dosage may be adjusted according to serum potassium concentrations

Dosage Forms

Tablet, oral: 25 mg, 50 mg

Inspra™: 25 mg, 50 mg

EPO *see* epoetin alfa *on page* *356*

epoetin alfa (e POE e tin AL fa)

Sound-Alike/Look-Alike Issues

epoetin alfa may be confused with darbepoetin alfa, epoetin beta

Epogen® may be confused with Neupogen®

Synonyms *r*HuEPO-α; EPO; erythropoiesis-stimulating agent (ESA); erythropoietin

U.S./Canadian Brand Names Epogen® [US]; Eprex® [Can]; Procrit® [US]

Therapeutic Category Colony-Stimulating Factor

Use Treatment of anemia (elevate or maintain red blood cell level and decrease the need for transfusions) associated with HIV (zidovudine) therapy, chronic renal failure (including patients on dialysis and not on dialysis); reduction of allogeneic blood transfusion for elective, noncardiac, nonvascular surgery; treatment of anemia due to concurrent chemotherapy in patients with metastatic cancer (nonmyeloid malignancies) receiving chemotherapy for a minimum of 2 months

Note: Erythropoietin is **not** indicated for use in cancer patients under the following conditions:

- receiving hormonal therapy, therapeutic biologic products, or radiation therapy unless also receiving concurrent myelosuppressive chemotherapy
- receiving myelosuppressive therapy when the expected outcome is curative
- anemia due to other factors (eg, iron deficiency, folate deficiency, or gastrointestinal bleed)

Not intended for patients who require immediate correction of severe anemia or as a substitute for emergency transfusion.

Dosage Summary

I.V.:

Children: Initial: 50 units/kg 3 times/week; Maintenance: 50-400 units/kg 1-3 times/week **or** 600 units/kg once weekly (maximum: 40,000 units)

Adults: Initial: 50-100 units/kg 3 times/week; Maintenance: 75-150 units/kg/week **or** 100-300 units/kg 3 times/week

SubQ:

Children: Initial: 50 units/kg 3 times/week; Maintenance: 50-400 units/kg 1-3 times/week

Adults: Initial: 50-100 units/kg 3 times/week; Maintenance: 75 units/kg 1-3 times/week **or** 75-150 units/kg/week **or** 100-300 units/kg 3 times/week **or** 10,000 units 3 times/week to 40,000-60,000 units once weekly (cancer patients) **or** 300 units/kg/day for 10 days before surgery, on the day of surgery, and for 4 days after surgery **or** 600 units/kg in once weekly doses (21, 14, and 7 days before surgery) plus a fourth dose on the day of surgery

Dosage Forms

Injection, solution:

Epogen®: 10,000 units/mL (2 mL); 20,000 units/mL (1 mL)

Procrit®: 10,000 units/mL (2 mL); 20,000 units/mL (1 mL)

Injection, solution [preservative free]:

Epogen®: 2000 units/mL (1 mL); 3000 units/mL (1 mL); 4000 units/mL (1 mL); 10,000 units/mL (1 mL)

Procrit®: 2000 units/mL (1 mL); 3000 units/mL (1 mL); 4000 units/mL (1 mL); 10,000 units/mL (1 mL); 40,000 units/mL (1 mL)

Dosage Forms - Canada

Injection, solution [preservative free]:

Eprex®: 1000 units/0.5 mL (0.5 mL), 2000 units/0.5 mL (0.5 mL), 3000 units/0.3 mL (0.3 mL), 4000 units/0.4 mL (0.4 mL), 5000 units/0.5 mL (0.5 mL), 6000 units/0.6 mL (0.6 mL), 8000 units/0.8 mL (0.8 mL), 10,000 units/mL (1 mL), 20,000 units/0.5 mL (0.5 mL), 30,000 units/0.75 mL (0.75 mL), 40,000 units/mL (1 mL) [contains polysorbate 80; prefilled syringe, free of human serum albumin]

Epogen® [US] *see* epoetin alfa *on page 356*

epoprostenol (e poe PROST en ole)

Synonyms epoprostenol sodium; PGI_2; PGX; prostacyclin

U.S./Canadian Brand Names Flolan® [US/Can]

Therapeutic Category Platelet Inhibitor

Use Treatment of idiopathic pulmonary arterial hypertension (IPAH); pulmonary hypertension associated with the scleroderma spectrum of disease (SSD) in NYHA Class III and Class IV patients who do not respond adequately to conventional therapy

Dosage Summary

I.V.:

Adults: Initial: 1-2 ng/kg/minute, increase dose in increments of 1-2 ng/kg/minute every 15 minutes or longer until dose-limiting side effects are noted or response to epoprostenol plateaus

Dosage Forms

Injection, powder for reconstitution: 0.5 mg, 1.5 mg

Flolan®: 0.5 mg, 1.5 mg

epoprostenol sodium *see* epoprostenol *on page 357*

epothilone B lactam *see* ixabepilone *on page 532*

Eprex® [Can] *see* epoetin alfa *on page 356*

eprosartan (ep roe SAR tan)

U.S./Canadian Brand Names Teveten® [US/Can]

Therapeutic Category Angiotensin II Receptor Antagonist

Use Treatment of hypertension; may be used alone or in combination with other antihypertensives

Dosage Summary

Oral:

Children: Dosage not established

Adults: Initial: 400-600 mg once daily; Maintenance: 400-800 mg/day in 1-2 divided doses

Dosage Forms

Tablet, oral:

Teveten®: 400 mg, 600 mg

eprosartan and hydrochlorothiazide (ep roe SAR tan & hye droe klor oh THYE a zide)

Synonyms eprosartan mesylate and hydrochlorothiazide; hydrochlorothiazide and eprosartan

U.S./Canadian Brand Names Teveten® HCT [US/Can]; Teveten® Plus [Can]

Therapeutic Category Angiotensin II Antagonist Combination; Antihypertensive Agent, Combination; Diuretic, Thiazide

Use Treatment of hypertension (not indicated for initial treatment)

Dosage Summary

Oral:

Children: Dosage not established

Adults: Eprosartan 600 mg and hydrochlorothiazide 12.5-25 mg once daily

Dosage Forms

Tablet:

Teveten® HCT: 600 mg/12.5 mg: Eprosartan 600 mg and hydrochlorothiazide 12.5 mg; 600 mg/25 mg: Eprosartan 600 mg and hydrochlorothiazide 25 mg

eprosartan mesylate and hydrochlorothiazide *see* eprosartan and hydrochlorothiazide *on page 357*

epsilon aminocaproic acid *see* aminocaproic acid *on page 65*

epsom salts *see* magnesium sulfate *on page 588*

EPT *see* teniposide *on page 916*

eptacog alfa (activated) *see* factor VIIa (recombinant) *on page 388*

eptifibatide (ep TIF i ba tide)

Synonyms intrifiban

U.S./Canadian Brand Names Integrilin® [US/Can]

Therapeutic Category Antiplatelet Agent

Use Treatment of patients with acute coronary syndrome (unstable angina/non-Q wave myocardial infarction [UA/NQMI]), including patients who are to be managed medically and those undergoing percutaneous coronary intervention (PCI including angioplasty, intracoronary stenting)

Dosage Summary

I.V.:

Children: Dosage not established

Adults: Bolus: 180 mcg/kg (maximum: 22.6 mg), repeat once for PCI; Infusion: 2 mcg/kg/minute (maximum: 15 mg/hour)

Dosage Forms

Injection, solution:

Integrilin®: 0.75 mg/mL (100 mL); 2 mg/mL (10 mL, 100 mL)

Epzicom® [US] *see* abacavir and lamivudine *on page 18*

Equagesic® [US] *see* meprobamate and aspirin *on page 606*

Equalactin® [US-OTC] *see* polycarbophil *on page 774*

Equalizer Gas Relief [US-OTC] *see* simethicone *on page 875*

Equanil® *(Discontinued)* *see* meprobamate *on page 605*

Equetro® [US] *see* carbamazepine *on page 177*

Equilet® *(Discontinued)* *see* calcium carbonate *on page 167*

Eraxis™ [US/Can] *see* anidulafungin *on page 79*

Erbitux® [US/Can] *see* cetuximab *on page 199*

ergocalciferol (er goe kal SIF e role)

Sound-Alike/Look-Alike Issues

ergocalciferol may be confused with cholecalciferol

Calciferol™ may be confused with calcitriol

Drisdol® may be confused with Drysol™

Synonyms activated ergosterol; D2; viosterol; vitamin D2

U.S./Canadian Brand Names Calciferol™ [US-OTC]; Drisdol® [US-OTC]; Drisdol® [US/Can]; Ostoforte® [Can]

Therapeutic Category Vitamin D Analog

Use Treatment of refractory rickets, hypophosphatemia, hypoparathyroidism; dietary supplement

Dosage Summary Note: Dosage varies considerably by indication; ranges listed are representative

Oral:

Children: 5-5000 mcg/day (200-200,000 int. units/day)

Adults 18-50 years: 5-7500 mcg/day (200-300,000 int. units/day)

Adults: 51-70 years: 10-7500 mcg/day (400-300,000 int. units/day)

Elderly >70 years: 15-7500 mcg/day (600-300,000 int. units/day)

Dosage Forms

Capsule, oral:

Drisdol®: 50,000 int. units

Capsule, softgel, oral: 50,000 int. units, 50,000 units

Solution, oral: 8000 int. units/mL (60 mL)

Calciferol™ [OTC]: 8000 int. units/mL (60 mL)

Drisdol® [OTC]: 8000 int. units/mL (60 mL)

Tablet, oral: 400 int. units

ergoloid mesylates (ER goe loid MES i lates)

Synonyms dihydroergotoxine; dihydrogenated ergot alkaloids

U.S./Canadian Brand Names Hydergine® [Can]

Therapeutic Category Ergot Alkaloid and Derivative

Use Treatment of cerebrovascular insufficiency in primary progressive dementia, Alzheimer dementia, and senile onset

Dosage Summary

Oral:

Children: Dosage not established

Adults: Initial: 1 mg 3 times/day; Maintenance: 3-12 mg/day in 3 divided doses

Dosage Forms

Tablet, oral: 1 mg

Ergomar® [US] *see* ergotamine *on page 359*

ergometrine maleate *see* ergonovine *on page 359*

ergonovine (er goe NOE veen)

Synonyms ergometrine maleate; ergonovine maleate

U.S./Canadian Brand Names Ergotrate® [US]

Therapeutic Category Ergot Alkaloid and Derivative

Use Prevention and treatment of postpartum and postabortion hemorrhage caused by uterine atony or subinvolution

Dosage Summary

I.M.:

Children: Dosage not established

Adults: 0.2 mg, may repeat in 2-4 hours if needed

I.V.:

Children: Dosage not established

Adults: 0.2 mg, may repeat in 2-4 hours if needed

Oral:

Children: Dosage not established

Adults: 0.2-0.4 mg every 6-12 hours

SL:

Children: Dosage not established

Adults: 0.2-0.4 mg every 6-12 hours

Dosage Forms

Injection, solution:

Ergotrate®: 0.2 mg/mL (1 mL)

Tablet, oral:

Ergotrate®: 0.2 mg

ergonovine maleate *see* ergonovine *on page 359*

ergotamine (er GOT a meen)

Synonyms ergotamine tartrate

U.S./Canadian Brand Names Ergomar® [US]

Therapeutic Category Ergot Alkaloid and Derivative

Use Abort or prevent vascular headaches, such as migraine, migraine variants, or so-called "histaminic cephalalgia"

Dosage Summary

SL:

Children: Dosage not established

Adults: One tablet initially, then 1 tablet every 30 minutes if needed (maximum: 3 tablets/day; 5 tablets/week)

Dosage Forms

Tablet, sublingual:

Ergomar®: 2 mg

ergotamine and caffeine (er GOT a meen & KAF een)

Sound-Alike/Look-Alike Issues

Cafergot® may be confused with Carafate®

Synonyms caffeine and ergotamine; ergotamine tartrate and caffeine

U.S./Canadian Brand Names Cafergor® [Can]; Cafergot® [US]; Migergot [US]

Therapeutic Category Antimigraine Agent; Ergot Derivative; Stimulant

Use Abort or prevent vascular headaches, such as migraine, migraine variants, or so-called "histaminic cephalalgia"

Dosage Summary

Oral:

Children: Dosage not established

Adults: Two tablets initially, then 1 tablet every 30 minutes as needed (maximum: 6 tablets/attack; 10 tablets/week)

Rectal:

Children: Dosage not established

Adults: One suppository initially, may repeat after 1 hour if needed (maximum: 2 doses/attack; 5 doses/week)

Dosage Forms

Suppository, rectal:

Migergot: Ergotamine tartrate 2 mg and caffeine 100 mg (12s)

Tablet: Ergotamine tartrate 1 mg and caffeine 100 mg

Cafergot®: Ergotamine tartrate 1 mg and caffeine 100 mg

ergotamine tartrate *see* ergotamine *on page* 359

ergotamine tartrate and caffeine *see* ergotamine and caffeine *on page* 359

Ergotamine Tartrate and Caffeine Cafatine® ***(Discontinued)*** *see* ergotamine *on page* 359

Ergotrate® [US] *see* ergonovine *on page* 359

erlotinib (er LOE tye nib)

Sound-Alike/Look-Alike Issues

erlotinib may be confused with gefitinib, imatinib

Synonyms CP358774; erlotinib hydrochloride; OSI-774

U.S./Canadian Brand Names Tarceva® [US/Can]

Therapeutic Category Antineoplastic Agent, Tyrosine Kinase Inhibitor

Use Treatment of locally advanced or metastatic nonsmall cell lung cancer (NSCLC) refractory to at least 1 prior chemotherapy regimen (as monotherapy); maintenance treatment of locally advanced or metastatic NCSLC which has not progressed after 4-6 cycles of first line platinum-based chemotherapy; locally advanced, unresectable or metastatic pancreatic cancer (first-line therapy in combination with gemcitabine)

Dosage Summary

Oral:

Children: Dosage not established

Adults: 150 mg/day **or** 100 mg/day with gemcitabine

Dosage Forms

Tablet, oral:

Tarceva®: 25 mg, 100 mg, 150 mg

erlotinib hydrochloride *see* erlotinib *on page* 360

E-R-O® [US-OTC] *see* carbamide peroxide *on page* 178

Errin® [US] *see* norethindrone *on page* 682

Ertaczo® [US] *see* sertaconazole *on page* 872

ertapenem (er ta PEN em)

Sound-Alike/Look-Alike Issues

ertapenem may be confused with imipenem, meropenem

Invanz® may be confused with Avinza™, I.V. vancomycin

Synonyms ertapenem sodium; L-749,345; MK0826

U.S./Canadian Brand Names Invanz® [US/Can]

Therapeutic Category Antibiotic, Carbapenem

Use Treatment of the following moderate-to-severe infections: Complicated intraabdominal infections, complicated skin and skin structure infections (including diabetic foot infections without osteomyelitis), complicated UTI (including pyelonephritis), acute pelvic infections (including postpartum endomyometritis, septic abortion, postsurgical gynecologic infections), and community-acquired pneumonia. Prophylaxis of surgical site infection following elective colorectal surgery. Antibacterial coverage includes aerobic gram-positive organisms, aerobic gram-negative organisms, anaerobic organisms.

Note: Methicillin-resistant *Staphylococcus*, *Enterococcus* spp, penicillin-resistant strains of *Streptococcus pneumoniae*, beta-lactamase-positive strains of *Haemophilus influenzae* are **resistant** to ertapenem, as are most *Pseudomonas aeruginosa*.

Dosage Summary

I.M.:

Children <3 months: Dosage not established
Children 3 months to 12 years: 15 mg/kg twice daily (maximum: 1 g/day)
Adolescents ≥13 years: 1 g once daily
Adults: 1 g once daily

I.V.:

Children <3 months: Dosage not established
Children 3 months to 12 years: 15 mg/kg twice daily (maximum: 1 g/day)
Adolescents ≥13 years: 1 g once daily
Adults: 1 g once daily **or** 1 g given 1 hour prior to surgery

Dosage Forms

Injection, powder for reconstitution:

Invanz®: 1 g

ertapenem sodium *see* ertapenem *on page* 360
***Erwinia* asparaginase** *see* asparaginase *on page* 99
Ery [US] *see* erythromycin (topical) *on page* 362
Erybid™ [Can] *see* erythromycin (systemic) *on page* 361
Eryc® [Can] *see* erythromycin (systemic) *on page* 361
Eryc® *(Discontinued)* *see* erythromycin (systemic) *on page* 361
Eryderm® *(Discontinued)* *see* erythromycin (topical) *on page* 362
Erygel® *(Discontinued)* *see* erythromycin (topical) *on page* 362
EryPed® [US] *see* erythromycin (systemic) *on page* 361
Ery-Tab® [US] *see* erythromycin (systemic) *on page* 361
Erythrocin® [US] *see* erythromycin (systemic) *on page* 361
Erythrocin® Lactobionate-I.V. [US] *see* erythromycin (systemic) *on page* 361

erythromycin (systemic) (er ith roe MYE sin)

Sound-Alike/Look-Alike Issues

erythromycin may be confused with azithromycin, clarithromycin, Ethmozine®
Akne-Mycin® may be confused with AK-Mycin®
E.E.S.® may be confused with DES®
Eryc® may be confused with Emcyt®, Ery-Tab®
Ery-Tab® may be confused with Eryc®
Erythrocin® may be confused with Ethmozine®

Synonyms erythromycin base; Erythromycin ethylsuccinate; erythromycin lactobionate; erythromycin stearate

U.S./Canadian Brand Names Apo-Erythro Base® [Can]; Apo-Erythro E-C® [Can]; Apo-Erythro-ES® [Can]; Apo-Erythro-S® [Can]; E.E.S.® [US/Can]; Ery-Tab® [US]; Erybid™ [Can]; Eryc® [Can]; EryPed® [US]; Erythro-RX [US]; Erythrocin® Lactobionate-I.V. [US]; Erythrocin® [US]; Novo-Rythro Estolate [Can]; Novo-Rythro Ethylsuccinate [Can]; Nu-Erythromycin-S [Can]; PCE® [US/Can]

Therapeutic Category Antibiotic, Macrolide

Use Treatment of susceptible bacterial infections including *S. pyogenes*, some *S. pneumoniae,* some *S. aureus*, *M. pneumoniae*, *Legionella pneumophila*, diphtheria, pertussis, *Chlamydia*, erythrasma, *N. gonorrhoeae*, *E. histolytica*, syphilis and nongonococcal urethritis, and *Campylobacter* gastroenteritis; used in conjunction with neomycin for decontaminating the bowel

Dosage Summary Note: Due to differences in absorption, 400 mg erythromycin ethylsuccinate produces the same serum levels as 250 mg erythromycin base or stearate).

I.V.:

Children: 15-50 mg/kg/day divided every 6 hours (maximum: 4 g/day)
Adults: 15-20 mg/kg/day divided every 6 hours **or** 500 mg to 1 g every 6 hours or as a continuous infusion over 24 hours (maximum: 4 g/day)

Oral:

Children: 30-50 mg/kg/day in 2-4 divided doses; maximum base or stearate: 2 g/day; maximum ethylsuccinate: 3.2 g/day

Adults: Base: 250-500 mg every 6-12 hours; maximum base or ethylsuccinate: 400-800 mg every 6-12 hours

Dosage Forms

Capsule, delayed release, enteric coated pellets, oral: 250 mg

Granules for suspension, oral:

E.E.S.®: 200 mg/5 mL (100 mL, 200 mL)

Injection, powder for reconstitution:

Erythrocin® Lactobionate-I.V.: 500 mg

Powder, for prescription compounding:

Erythro-RX: USP: 100% (50 g)

Powder for suspension, oral:

EryPed®: 200 mg/5 mL (100 mL); 400 mg/5 mL (100 mL)

Tablet, oral: 250 mg, 400 mg, 500 mg

E.E.S.®: 400 mg

Erythrocin®: 250 mg, 500 mg

Tablet, delayed release, enteric coated, oral:

Ery-Tab®: 250 mg, 333 mg, 500 mg

Tablet, polymer coated particles, oral:

PCE®: 333 mg, 500 mg

erythromycin (ophthalmic) (er ith roe MYE sin)

Sound-Alike/Look-Alike Issues

erythromycin may be confused with azithromycin

Synonyms erythromycin base

U.S./Canadian Brand Names Diomycin® [Can]; PMS-Erythromycin [Can]

Therapeutic Category Antibiotic, Macrolide; Antibiotic, Ophthalmic

Use Treatment of superficial eye infections involving the conjunctiva or cornea; neonatal ophthalmia

Dosage Summary

Ophthalmic:

Neonates: 0.5-1 cm ribbon of ointment should be instilled into each conjunctival sac

Children: Instill 1/2" (1.25 cm) 2-6 times/day depending on the severity of the infection

Adults: Instill 1/2" (1.25 cm) 2-6 times/day depending on the severity of the infection

Dosage Forms

Ointment, ophthalmic: 0.5% (1 g, 3.5 g, 3.75 g)

Ointment, ophthalmic [preservative free]: 0.5% (3.5 g)

erythromycin (topical) (er ith roe MYE sin)

Sound-Alike/Look-Alike Issues

erythromycin may be confused with azithromycin, clarithromycin, Ethmozine®

Akne-Mycin® may be confused with AK-Mycin®

U.S./Canadian Brand Names Akne-mycin® [US]; Ery [US]; Sans Acne® [Can]

Therapeutic Category Acne Products; Antibiotic, Macrolide; Antibiotic, Topical; Topical Skin Product; Topical Skin Product, Acne

Use Treatment of acne vulgaris

Dosage Summary

Topical:

Children: Apply over the affected area twice daily

Adults: Apply over the affected area twice daily

Dosage Forms

Gel, topical: 2% (30 g, 60 g)

Ointment, topical:

Akne-mycin®: 2% (25 g)

Pledget, topical:

Ery: 2% (60s)

Solution, topical: 2% (60 mL)

Dosage Forms - Canada

Solution, topical:

Sans Acne®: 2% (60 mL)

erythromycin and benzoyl peroxide (er ith roe MYE sin & BEN zoe il per OKS ide)

Synonyms benzoyl peroxide and erythromycin

U.S./Canadian Brand Names Benzamycin® Pak [US]; Benzamycin® [US]

Therapeutic Category Acne Products

Use Topical control of acne vulgaris

Dosage Summary

Topical:

Children: Dosage not established
Adolescents ≥12 years: Apply twice daily
Adults: Apply twice daily

Dosage Forms

Gel, topical: Erythromycin 30 mg and benzoyl peroxide 50 mg per g (23 g, 47g)
Benzamycin®: Erythromycin 30 mg and benzoyl peroxide 50 mg per g (47 g)
Benzamycin® Pak: Erythromycin 30 mg and benzoyl peroxide 50 mg per 0.8 g packet (60s)

erythromycin and sulfisoxazole (er ith roe MYE sin & sul fi SOKS a zole)

Sound-Alike/Look-Alike Issues

Pediazole® may be confused with Pediapred®

Synonyms sulfisoxazole and erythromycin

U.S./Canadian Brand Names E.S.P.® [US]; Pediazole® [Can]

Therapeutic Category Macrolide (Antibiotic); Sulfonamide

Use Treatment of susceptible bacterial infections of the upper and lower respiratory tract, otitis media in children caused by susceptible strains of *Haemophilus influenzae*, and many other infections in patients allergic to penicillin

Dosage Summary

Oral:

Children <2 months: Dosage not established
Children ≥2 months: 50 mg/kg/day erythromycin and 150 mg/kg/day sulfisoxazole in divided doses every 6 hours
Adults: 400 mg erythromycin and 1200 mg sulfisoxazole every 6 hours
Elderly: Use not recommended

Dosage Forms

Powder for oral suspension: Erythromycin 200 mg and sulfisoxazole 600 mg per 5 mL
E.S.P.®: Erythromycin 200 mg and sulfisoxazole 600 mg per 5 mL

erythromycin base *see* erythromycin (ophthalmic) *on page 362*
erythromycin base *see* erythromycin (systemic) *on page 361*
Erythromycin ethylsuccinate *see* erythromycin (systemic) *on page 361*
erythromycin lactobionate *see* erythromycin (systemic) *on page 361*
erythromycin stearate *see* erythromycin (systemic) *on page 361*
erythropoiesis-stimulating agent (ESA) *see* darbepoetin alfa *on page 269*
erythropoiesis-stimulating agent (ESA) *see* epoetin alfa *on page 356*
erythropoiesis-stimulating protein *see* darbepoetin alfa *on page 269*
erythropoietin *see* epoetin alfa *on page 356*
Erythro-RX [US] *see* erythromycin (systemic) *on page 361*

escitalopram (es sye TAL oh pram)

Sound-Alike/Look-Alike Issues

Lexapro® may be confused with Loxitane®

Synonyms escitalopram oxalate; Lu-26-054; S-citalopram

U.S./Canadian Brand Names Cipralex® [Can]; Lexapro® [US]

Therapeutic Category Antidepressant, Selective Serotonin Reuptake Inhibitor

Use Treatment of major depressive disorder; generalized anxiety disorders (GAD)

Dosage Summary

Oral:

Children <12 years: Dosage not established
Children ≥12 years: Initial: 10 mg once daily; Maintenance: 10-20 mg once daily
Adults: Initial: 10 mg once daily; Maintenance: 10-20 mg once daily
Elderly: 10 mg once daily

Dosage Forms

Solution, oral:

Lexapro®: 1 mg/mL (240 mL)

Tablet, oral:

Lexapro®: 5 mg, 10 mg, 20 mg

Dosage Forms - Canada

Tablet:

Cipralex®: 10 mg, 20 mg

escitalopram oxalate *see* escitalopram *on page* 363

eserine salicylate *see* physostigmine *on page* 759

Esgic® [US] *see* butalbital, acetaminophen, and caffeine *on page* 159

Esgic-Plus™ [US] *see* butalbital, acetaminophen, and caffeine *on page* 159

Esidrix Tablets *(Discontinued)* *see* hydrochlorothiazide *on page* 478

Eskalith CR® *(Discontinued)* *see* lithium *on page* 571

Eskalith® *(Discontinued)* *see* lithium *on page* 571

esmolol (ES moe lol)

Sound-Alike/Look-Alike Issues

esmolol may be confused with Osmitrol®

Brevibloc® may be confused with Brevital®, Bumex®, Buprenex®

Synonyms esmolol hydrochloride

U.S./Canadian Brand Names Brevibloc® [US/Can]

Therapeutic Category Antiarrhythmic Agent, Class II; Beta-Adrenergic Blocker

Use Treatment of supraventricular tachycardia (SVT) and atrial fibrillation/flutter (control ventricular rate); treatment of intraoperative and postoperative tachycardia and/or hypertension; treatment of non-compensatory sinus tachycardia

Dosage Summary

I.V.:

Children: Dosage not established

Adults: Bolus: 80 mg **or** 500 mcg/kg; Infusion: 50-200 mcg/kg/minute (maximum: 300 mcg/kg/minute)

Dosage Forms

Infusion, premixed in NS [preservative free]:

Brevibloc: 2000 mg (100 mL); 2500 mg (250 mL)

Injection, solution [preservative free]: 10 mg/mL (10 mL)

Brevibloc: 10 mg/mL (10 mL)

esmolol hydrochloride *see* esmolol *on page* 364

E-Solve-2® Topical *(Discontinued)*

esomeprazole (es oh ME pray zol)

Sound-Alike/Look-Alike Issues

esomeprazole may be confused with aripiprazole

Nexium® may be confused with Nexavar®

Synonyms esomeprazole magnesium; esomeprazole sodium

U.S./Canadian Brand Names Nexium® I.V. [US]; Nexium® [US/Can]

Therapeutic Category Proton Pump Inhibitor

Use

Oral: Short-term (4-8 weeks) treatment of erosive esophagitis; maintaining symptom resolution and healing of erosive esophagitis; treatment of symptomatic gastroesophageal reflux disease (GERD); as part of a multidrug regimen for *Helicobacter pylori* eradication in patients with duodenal ulcer disease (active or history of within the past 5 years); prevention of gastric ulcers in patients at risk (age ≥60 years and/or history of gastric ulcer) associated with continuous NSAID therapy; long-term treatment of pathological hypersecretory conditions including Zollinger-Ellison syndrome

Canadian labeling: Additional use (not in U.S. labeling): Oral: Treatment of nonerosive reflux disease (NERD)

I.V.: Short-term (≤10 days) treatment of gastroesophageal reflux disease (GERD) when oral therapy is not possible or appropriate

Dosage Summary

I.V.:

Children: Dosage not established

Adults: 20-40 mg once daily

Oral:

Children 1-11 years <20 kg: 10 mg once daily; ≥20 kg: 10-20 mg once daily

Children 12-17 years: 20-40 mg once daily

Adults: 20-40 mg once daily **or** 80-240 mg/day in divided doses (hypersecretory conditions)

Dosage Forms

Capsule, delayed release, oral:

Nexium®: 20 mg, 40 mg

Granules for suspension, delayed release, oral:

Nexium®: 10 mg/packet (30s); 20 mg/packet (30s); 40 mg/packet (30s)

Injection, powder for reconstitution:

Nexium® I.V.: 20 mg, 40 mg

Dosage Forms - Canada Note: Strength expressed as base.

Granules, for oral suspension, delayed release, as magnesium:

Nexium®: 10 mg/packet (28s)

Tablet, extended release, as magnesium:

Nexium®: 20 mg, 40 mg

esomeprazole and naproxen *see* naproxen and esomeprazole *on page 660*

esomeprazole magnesium *see* esomeprazole *on page 364*

esomeprazole sodium *see* esomeprazole *on page 364*

Esopho-Cat® [US] *see* barium *on page 117*

Esoterica® Daytime [US-OTC] *see* hydroquinone *on page 487*

Esoterica® Nighttime [US-OTC] *see* hydroquinone *on page 487*

E.S.P.® [US] *see* erythromycin and sulfisoxazole *on page 363*

Estalis® [Can] *see* estradiol and norethindrone *on page 368*

Estalis-Sequi® [Can] *see* estradiol and norethindrone *on page 368*

Estar® [Can] *see* coal tar *on page 242*

estazolam (es TA zoe lam)

Sound-Alike/Look-Alike Issues

ProSom® may be confused with PhosLo®, Proscar®, Pro-Sof® Plus, Prozac®, Psorcon®

Therapeutic Category Benzodiazepine

Controlled Substance C-IV

Use Short-term management of insomnia

Dosage Summary

Oral:

Children: Dosage not established

Adults: 0.5-2 mg at bedtime

Elderly: Initial: 0.5 mg at bedtime in small or debilitated patients

Dosage Forms

Tablet, oral: 1 mg, 2 mg

Ester-E™ [US-OTC] *see* vitamin E *on page 988*

esterified estrogen and methyltestosterone *see* estrogens (esterified) and methyltestosterone *on page 372*

esterified estrogens *see* estrogens (esterified) *on page 371*

Estivin® II Ophthalmic *(Discontinued)* *see* naphazoline (ophthalmic) *on page 658*

Estra-L® Injection *(Discontinued)* *see* estradiol (systemic) *on page 366*

Estrace® [US] *see* estradiol (systemic) *on page 366*

Estrace® [US/Can] *see* estradiol (topical) *on page 367*

Estraderm® [US/Can] *see* estradiol (systemic) *on page 366*

estradiol *see* estradiol (systemic) *on page 366*

17β-estradiol *see* estradiol (topical) *on page 367*

estradiol (systemic) (es tra DYE ole)

Sound-Alike/Look-Alike Issues

Alora® may be confused with Aldara®
Elestrin™ may be confused with alosetron
Estraderm® may be confused with Testoderm®

Synonyms estradiol; estradiol acetate; estradiol transdermal; estradiol valerate

U.S./Canadian Brand Names Alora® [US]; Climara® [US/Can]; Delestrogen® [US]; Depo®-Estradiol [US/Can]; Divigel® [US]; Elestrin™ [US]; Estrace® [US]; Estraderm® [US/Can]; Estradot® [Can]; Estrasorb® [US]; EstroGel® [US/Can]; Evamist™ [US]; Femring® [US]; Femtrace® [US]; Menostar® [US/Can]; Oesclim® [Can]; Sandoz-Estradiol Derm 100 [Can]; Sandoz-Estradiol Derm 50 [Can]; Sandoz-Estradiol Derm 75 [Can]; Vivelle-Dot® [US]

Therapeutic Category Estrogen Derivative

Use Treatment of moderate-to-severe vasomotor symptoms associated with menopause; treatment of vulvar and vaginal atrophy; hypoestrogenism (due to hypogonadism, castration, or primary ovarian failure); prostatic cancer (palliation), breast cancer (palliation), advanced prostatic cancer (palliation), metastatic breast cancer (palliation) in men and postmenopausal women, osteoporosis (prophylaxis); abnormal uterine bleeding due to hormonal imbalance; postmenopausal urogenital symptoms of the lower urinary tract (urinary urgency, dysuria)

Dosage Summary

I.M.:

Children: Dosage not established
Cypionate:
Females (hypogonadism): 1.5-2 mg monthly
Adults (females): Menopause: 1-5 mg every 3-4 weeks
Valerate:
Females (hypogonadism): 10-20 mg every 4 weeks
Adults (females): Menopause: 10-20 mg every 4 weeks
Adults (males): Prostate cancer: ≥30 mg or more every 1-2 weeks

Oral:

Children: Dosage not established
Females (hypogonadism): 1-2 mg/day
Adults (females):
Breast cancer: 10 mg 3 times/day
Other indications: 0.5-2 mg/day cyclically (3 weeks on, 1 week off)
Adults (males): Prostate cancer: 1-2 mg 3 times/day; Breast cancer: 10 mg 3 times/day

Topical:

Children: Dosage not established
Adults (females):
Emulsion: 3.48 g applied once daily in the morning
Gel: 1.25 g/day (EstroGel®) or 0.87 g/day (Elestrin™) or 0.25-1 g/day (Divigel®) applied at the same time each day
Spray: One spray (1.53 mg) per day; dosing range: 1-3 sprays/day

Transdermal:

Children: Dosage not established
Adults (females):
Alora®, Estraderm®, Vivelle-Dot®: Apply twice weekly continuously or cyclically (3 weeks on, 1 week off)
Climara®, Menostar®: Apply once weekly continuously or cyclically (3 weeks on, 1 week off)

Dosage Forms

Emulsion, topical:
Estrasorb®: 2.5 mg/g (56s)

Gel, topical:
Divigel®: 0.1% (30s)
Elestrin™: 0.06% (144 g)
EstroGel®: 0.06% (50 g)

Injection, oil: 20 mg/mL (5 mL); 40 mg/mL (5 mL)
Delestrogen®: 10 mg/mL (5 mL); 20 mg/mL (5 mL); 40 mg/mL (5 mL)
Depo®-Estradiol: 5 mg/mL (5 mL)

Patch, transdermal: 0.025 mg/24 hours (4s); 0.0375 mg/24 hours (4s); 0.05 mg/24 hours (4s); 0.06 mg/24 hours (4s); 0.075 mg/24 hours (4s); 0.1 mg/24 hours (4s)
Alora®: 0.025 mg/24 hours (8s); 0.05 mg/24 hours (8s); 0.075 mg/24 hours (8s); 0.1 mg/24 hours (8s)
Climara®: 0.025 mg/24 hours (4s); 0.0375 mg/24 hours (4s); 0.05 mg/24 hours (4s); 0.06 mg/24 hours (4s); 0.075 mg/24 hours (4s); 0.1 mg/24 hours (4s)
Estraderm®: 0.05 mg/24 hours (8s); 0.1 mg/24 hours (8s)
Menostar®: 0.014 mg/24 hours (4s)
Vivelle-Dot®: 0.025 mg/24 hours (24s); 0.0375 mg/24 hours (24s); 0.05 mg/24 hours (24s); 0.075 mg/24 hours (24s); 0.1 mg/24 hours (24s)
Ring, vaginal:
Femring®: 0.05 mg/24 hours (1s); 0.1 mg/24 hours (1s)
Solution, topical:
Evamist™: 1.53 mg/spray (8.1 mL)
Tablet, oral: 0.5 mg, 1 mg, 2 mg
Estrace®: 0.5 mg, 1 mg, 2 mg
Femtrace®: 0.45 mg, 0.9 mg, 1.8 mg

estradiol (topical) (es tra DYE ole)

Synonyms 17β-estradiol

U.S./Canadian Brand Names Estrace® [US/Can]; Estring® [US/Can]; Vagifem® [US/Can]

Therapeutic Category Estrogen Derivative

Use Treatment of vulvar and vaginal atrophy; postmenopausal urogenital symptoms of the lower urinary tract (urinary urgency, dysuria)

Dosage Summary

Intravaginal:
Children: Dosage not established
Adults (females):
Cream: Initial: 2-4 g/day for 2 weeks, then 1/2 the initial dose for 2 weeks; Maintenance: 1 g 1-3 times/week
Ring: Estring®: Insert 2 mg, leave in place for 3 months
Tablet: Initial: Insert 1 tablet once daily for 2 weeks; Maintenance: Insert 1 tablet twice weekly

Dosage Forms

Cream, vaginal:
Estrace®: 0.1 mg/g (42.5 g)
Ring, vaginal:
Estring®: 2 mg (1s)
Tablet, vaginal:
Vagifem®: 10 mcg

estradiol acetate *see* estradiol (systemic) *on page* 366

estradiol and dienogest (es tra DYE ole & dye EN oh jest)

Synonyms dienogest and estradiol; estradiol valerate and dienogest

U.S./Canadian Brand Names Natazia™ [US]

Therapeutic Category Contraceptive; Estrogen and Progestin Combination

Use Prevention of pregnancy

Dosage Summary

Oral:
Children (premenarche): Use not indicated
Children (postmenarche): Take 1 tablet daily
Adults (females): Take 1 tablet daily

Dosage Forms

Tablet, oral [four-phasic formulation]:
Natazia™:
Days 1-2: Estradiol valerate 3 mg [2 dark yellow tablets]
Days 3-7: Estradiol valerate 2 mg and dienogest 2 mg [5 medium red tablets]
Days 8-24: Estradiol valerate 2 mg and dienogest 3 mg [17 light yellow tablets]
Days 25-26: Estradiol valerate 1 mg [2 dark red tablets]
Days 27-28: 2 white inactive tablets (28s)

estradiol and drospirenone *see* drospirenone and estradiol *on page* 334

estradiol and levonorgestrel (es tra DYE ole & LEE voe nor jes trel)

Synonyms levonorgestrel and estradiol

U.S./Canadian Brand Names ClimaraPro® [US]

Therapeutic Category Estrogen and Progestin Combination

Use Women with an intact uterus: Treatment of moderate-to-severe vasomotor symptoms associated with menopause; prevention of postmenopausal osteoporosis

Dosage Summary

Transdermal:

Children: Dosage not established

Adults (females): Apply 1 patch (estradiol 0.045 mg/levonorgestrel 0.015 mg) weekly

Dosage Forms

Patch, transdermal:

ClimaraPro®: Estradiol 0.045 mg/24 hours and levonorgestrel 0.015 mg/24 hours (4s) [once-weekly patch]

estradiol and NGM *see* estradiol and norgestimate *on page 369*

estradiol and norethindrone (es tra DYE ole & nor eth IN drone)

Synonyms norethindrone and estradiol

U.S./Canadian Brand Names Activella® [US]; CombiPatch® [US]; Estalis-Sequi® [Can]; Estalis® [Can]; Mimvey™ [US]

Therapeutic Category Estrogen and Progestin Combination

Use Women with an intact uterus:

Tablet: Treatment of moderate-to-severe vasomotor symptoms associated with menopause; treatment of vulvar and vaginal atrophy; prophylaxis for postmenopausal osteoporosis

Transdermal patch: Treatment of moderate-to-severe vasomotor symptoms associated with menopause; treatment of vulvar and vaginal atrophy; treatment of hypoestrogenism due to hypogonadism, castration, or primary ovarian failure

Dosage Summary

Oral:

Children: Dosage not established

Adults (females): One tablet daily

Transdermal:

Children: Dosage not established

Adults (females): Apply 1 patch twice weekly

Dosage Forms

Patch, transdermal:

CombiPatch®:

0.05/0.14: Estradiol 0.05 mg and norethindrone 0.14 mg per day (8s) [9 sq cm]

0.05/0.25: Estradiol 0.05 mg and norethindrone 0.25 mg per day (8s) [16 sq cm]

Tablet, oral: Estradiol 1 mg and norethindrone acetate 0.5 mg (28s)

Activella® 0.5/0.1: Estradiol 0.5 mg and norethindrone acetate 0.1 mg (28s)

Activella® 1/0.5, Mimvey™: Estradiol 1 mg and norethindrone acetate 0.5 mg (28s)

Dosage Forms - Canada

Combination pack:

Estalis-Sequi® 140/50:

Patch, transdermal (Vivelle®): Estradiol 50 mcg per day (4s) [14.5 sq cm; total estradiol 4.33 mg]

Patch, transdermal (Estalis®): Norethindrone 140 mcg and estradiol 50 mcg per day (4s) [9 sq cm; total norethindrone 2.7 mg, total estradiol 0.62 mg]

Estalis-Sequi® 250/50:

Patch, transdermal (Vivelle®): Estradiol 50 mcg per day (4s) [14.5 sq cm; total estradiol 4.33 mg]

Patch, transdermal (Estalis®): Norethindrone 250 mcg and estradiol 50 mcg per day (4s) [16 sq cm; total norethindrone 4.8 mg, total estradiol 0.51 mg]

Patch, transdermal:

Estalis®:

140/50: Norethindrone 140 mcg and estradiol 50 mcg per day (8s) [9 sq cm; total norethindrone 2.7 mg, total estradiol 0.62 mg]

250/50 Norethindrone 250 mcg and estradiol 50 mcg per day (8s) [16 sq cm; total norethindrone 4.8 mg, total estradiol 0.51 mg]

estradiol and norgestimate (es tra DYE ole & nor JES ti mate)

Synonyms estradiol and NGM; norgestimate and estradiol; ortho prefest

U.S./Canadian Brand Names Prefest™ [US]

Therapeutic Category Estrogen and Progestin Combination

Use Women with an intact uterus: Treatment of moderate-to-severe vasomotor symptoms associated with menopause; treatment of atrophic vaginitis; prevention of osteoporosis

Dosage Summary

Oral:

Children: Dosage not established

Adults (females): One tablet of estradiol 1 mg once daily for 3 days, followed by 1 tablet of estradiol 1 mg and norgestimate 0.09 mg once daily for 3 days; repeat sequence continuously

Dosage Forms

Tablet, oral:

Prefest™: Estradiol 1 mg [15 peach tablets] and estradiol 1 mg and norgestimate 0.09 mg [15 white tablets]

estradiol transdermal *see* estradiol (systemic) *on page 366*

estradiol valerate *see* estradiol (systemic) *on page 366*

estradiol valerate and dienogest *see* estradiol and dienogest *on page 367*

Estradot® [Can] *see* estradiol (systemic) *on page 366*

estramustine (es tra MUS teen)

Sound-Alike/Look-Alike Issues

estramustine may be confused with exemestane

Emcyt® may be confused with Eryc®

Synonyms estramustine phosphate; estramustine phosphate sodium; NSC-89199

U.S./Canadian Brand Names Emcyt® [US/Can]

Therapeutic Category Antineoplastic Agent

Use Palliative treatment of progressive or metastatic prostate cancer

Dosage Summary

Oral:

Children: Dosage not established

Adults (males): 14 mg/kg/day (range: 10-16 mg/kg/day) in 3 or 4 divided doses

Dosage Forms

Capsule, oral:

Emcyt®: 140 mg

estramustine phosphate *see* estramustine *on page 369*

estramustine phosphate sodium *see* estramustine *on page 369*

Estrasorb® [US] *see* estradiol (systemic) *on page 366*

Estratab® [Can] *see* estrogens (esterified) *on page 371*

Estratab® *(Discontinued)* *see* estrogens (esterified) *on page 371*

Estratest® [Can] *see* estrogens (esterified) and methyltestosterone *on page 372*

Estratest® *(Discontinued)* *see* estrogens (esterified) and methyltestosterone *on page 372*

Estratest® H.S. *(Discontinued)* *see* estrogens (esterified) and methyltestosterone *on page 372*

Estring® [US/Can] *see* estradiol (topical) *on page 367*

Estro-Cyp® Injection *(Discontinued)* *see* estradiol (systemic) *on page 366*

EstroGel® [US/Can] *see* estradiol (systemic) *on page 366*

estrogenic substances, conjugated *see* estrogens (conjugated/equine, systemic) *on page 370*

estrogenic substances, conjugated *see* estrogens (conjugated/equine, topical) *on page 371*

estrogens (conjugated A/synthetic) (ES troe jenz, KON joo gate ed, aye, sin THET ik)

Sound-Alike/Look-Alike Issues

Cenestin® may be confused with Senexon®

U.S./Canadian Brand Names Cenestin® [US/Can]

Therapeutic Category Estrogen Derivative

Use Treatment of moderate-to-severe vasomotor symptoms of menopause; treatment of vulvar and vaginal atrophy

Dosage Summary

Oral:

Children: Dosage not established

Adults (females): 0.3-1.25 mg once daily; **Note:** Titration is recommended

Dosage Forms

Tablet, oral:

Cenestin®: 0.3 mg, 0.45 mg, 0.625 mg, 0.9 mg, 1.25 mg

estrogens (conjugated B/synthetic) (ES troe jenz, KON joo gate ed, bee, sin THET ik)

Sound-Alike/Look-Alike Issues

Enjuvia™ may be confused with Januvia™

U.S./Canadian Brand Names Enjuvia™ [US]

Therapeutic Category Estrogen Derivative

Use Treatment of moderate-to-severe vasomotor symptoms of menopause; treatment of vulvar and vaginal atrophy associated with menopause; treatment of moderate-to-severe vaginal dryness and pain with intercourse associated with menopause

Dosage Summary

Oral:

Children: Dosage not established

Adults (females): 0.3-1.25 mg once daily; **Note:** Titration is recommended

Dosage Forms

Tablet, oral:

Enjuvia™: 0.3 mg, 0.45 mg, 0.625 mg, 0.9 mg, 1.25 mg

estrogens (conjugated/equine, systemic) (ES troe jenz KON joo gate ed, EE kwine)

Sound-Alike/Look-Alike Issues

Premarin® may be confused with Primaxin®, Provera®, Remeron®

Synonyms C.E.S.; CE; CEE; conjugated estrogen; estrogenic substances, conjugated

U.S./Canadian Brand Names C.E.S.® [Can]; Premarin® [US/Can]

Therapeutic Category Estrogen Derivative

Use Treatment of moderate-to-severe vasomotor symptoms associated with menopause; treatment of vulvar and vaginal atrophy; hypoestrogenism (due to hypogonadism, castration, or primary ovarian failure); prostatic cancer (palliation); breast cancer (palliation); osteoporosis (prophylaxis, postmenopausal women at significant risk only); abnormal uterine bleeding; moderate-to-severe dyspareunia (pain during intercourse) due to vaginal/vulvar atrophy of menopause

Dosage Summary **Note:** Cyclic administration: Either 3 weeks on, 1 week off **or** 25 days on, 5 days off

I.M.:

Children (premenarche): Dosage not established

Children (postmenarche): Abnormal uterine bleeding: 25 mg, may repeat in 6-12 hours if needed

Adults (females): Abnormal uterine bleeding: 25 mg, may repeat in 6-12 hours if needed

I.V.:

Children (premenarche): Dosage not established

Children (postmenarche): Abnormal uterine bleeding: 25 mg, may repeat in 6-12 hours if needed

Adults (females): Abnormal uterine bleeding: 25 mg, may repeat in 6-12 hours if needed

Oral:

Females (hypogonadism): 0.3-0.625 mg/day given cyclically

Adults (females):

Breast cancer: 10 mg 3 times/day

Other indications: 0.3-1.25 mg daily or cyclically; **Note:** Titration is recommended

Adults (males):

Breast cancer: 10 mg 3 times/day

Prostate cancer: 1.25-2.5 mg 3 times/day

Dosage Forms

Injection, powder for reconstitution:

Premarin®: 25 mg

Tablet, oral:

Premarin®: 0.3 mg, 0.45 mg, 0.625 mg, 0.9 mg, 1.25 mg

estrogens (conjugated/equine, topical) (ES troe jenz KON joo gate ed, EE kwine)

Sound-Alike/Look-Alike Issues

Premarin® may be confused with Primaxin®, Provera®, Remeron®

Synonyms C.E.S.; CE; CEE; conjugated estrogen; estrogenic substances, conjugated

U.S./Canadian Brand Names Premarin® [US/Can]

Therapeutic Category Estrogen Derivative

Use Treatment of vulvar and vaginal atrophy; moderate-to-severe dyspareunia (pain during intercourse) due to vaginal/vulvar atrophy of menopause

Dosage Summary

Intravaginal:

Children: Dosage not established

Adults (females): Vaginal atrophy: 0.5-2 g/day given cyclically; Moderate-to-severe dyspareunia: 0.5 g twice weekly (eg, Monday and Thursday) or once daily cyclically - either 3 weeks on, 1 week off **or** 25 days on, 5 days off

Dosage Forms

Cream, vaginal:

Premarin®: 0.625 mg/g (42.5 g)

estrogens (conjugated/equine) and medroxyprogesterone

(ES troe jenz KON joo gate ed/EE kwine & me DROKS ee proe JES te rone)

Sound-Alike/Look-Alike Issues

Premphase® may be confused with Prempro®

Prempro® may be confused with Premphase®

Synonyms medroxyprogesterone and estrogens (conjugated); MPA and estrogens (conjugated)

U.S./Canadian Brand Names Premphase® [US/Can]; Premplus® [Can]; Prempro® [US/Can]

Therapeutic Category Estrogen and Progestin Combination

Use Women with an intact uterus: Treatment of moderate-to-severe vasomotor symptoms associated with menopause; treatment of moderate-to-severe vulvar and vaginal atrophy due to menopause; postmenopausal osteoporosis (prophylaxis)

Dosage Summary

Oral:

Children: Dosage not established

Adults (females): Prempro®: Conjugated estrogen 0.3-0.625 mg/MPA 1.5-5 mg once daily or Premphase®: One 0.625 mg tablet daily on days 1 through 14 and 1 conjugated estrogen 0.625 mg/MPA 5 mg tablet daily on days 15 through 28

Dosage Forms

Tablet:

Premphase® [therapy pack contains two separate tablet formulations]: Conjugated estrogens 0.625 mg [14 maroon tablets] and conjugated estrogen 0.625 mg/medroxyprogesterone 5 mg [14 light blue tablets] (28s)

Prempro®:

0.3/1.5: Conjugated estrogens 0.3 mg and medroxyprogesterone 1.5 mg (28s)

0.45/1.5: Conjugated estrogens 0.45 mg and medroxyprogesterone 1.5 mg (28s)

0.625/2.5: Conjugated estrogens 0.625 mg and medroxyprogesterone 2.5 mg (28s)

0.625/5: Conjugated estrogens 0.625 mg and medroxyprogesterone 5 mg (28s)

estrogens (esterified) (ES troe jenz, es TER i fied)

Sound-Alike/Look-Alike Issues

Estratab® may be confused with Estratest®, Estratest® H.S.

Synonyms esterified estrogens

U.S./Canadian Brand Names Estratab® [Can]; Menest® [US/Can]

Therapeutic Category Estrogen Derivative

Use Treatment of moderate-to-severe vasomotor symptoms associated with menopause; treatment of vulvar and vaginal atrophy; hypoestrogenism (due to hypogonadism, castration, or primary ovarian failure); prostatic cancer (palliation); breast cancer (palliation); osteoporosis (prophylaxis, in women at significant risk only)

Dosage Summary

Oral:

Females (hypogonadism): 2.5-7.5 mg daily for 20 days followed by a 10-day rest, repeat until response

Adults (females):

Breast cancer: 10 mg 3 times/day

Other indications: 0.3-1.25 mg daily or cyclically (3 weeks on and 1 week off)

Adults (males):

Breast cancer: 10 mg 3 times/day

Prostate cancer: 1.25-2.5 mg 3 times/day

Dosage Forms

Tablet, oral:

Menest®: 0.3 mg, 0.625 mg, 1.25 mg, 2.5 mg

estrogens (esterified) and methyltestosterone

(ES troe jenz es TER i fied & meth il tes TOS te rone)

Sound-Alike/Look-Alike Issues

Estratest® may be confused with Eskalith®, Estratab®, Estratest® H.S.

Estratest® H.S. may be confused with Eskalith®, Estratab®, Estratest®

Synonyms conjugated estrogen and methyltestosterone; esterified estrogen and methyltestosterone

U.S./Canadian Brand Names Covaryx® H.S. [US]; Covaryx® [US]; EEMT™ HS [US]; EEMT™ [US]; Estratest® [Can]

Therapeutic Category Estrogen and Androgen Combination

Use Vasomotor symptoms of menopause

Dosage Summary

Oral:

Children: Dosage not established

Adults (females): Lowest dose that will control symptoms should be chosen, normally given 3 weeks on and 1 week off

Dosage Forms

Tablet: Esterified estrogens 1.25 mg and methyltestosterone 2.5 mg; esterified estrogen 0.625 mg and methyltestosterone 1.25 mg

Covaryx®, EEMT™: Esterified estrogen 1.25 mg and methyltestosterone 2.5 mg

Covaryx® H.S., EEMT™ HS: Esterified estrogen 0.625 mg and methyltestosterone 1.25 mg

estropipate (ES troe pih pate)

Synonyms piperazine estrone sulfate

U.S./Canadian Brand Names Ogen® [Can]

Therapeutic Category Estrogen Derivative

Use Treatment of moderate-to-severe vasomotor symptoms associated with menopause; treatment of vulvar and vaginal atrophy; hypoestrogenism (due to hypogonadism, castration, or primary ovarian failure); osteoporosis (prophylaxis, in women at significant risk only)

Dosage Summary

Oral:

Children: Dosage not established

Adults (females): 0.75-6 mg once daily or cyclically [menopause] **or** 1.5-9 mg for the first 3 weeks, followed by a rest period of 8-10 days [hypoestrogenism] **or** 0.75 mg for 25 days of a 31 day cycle [osteoporosis]

Dosage Forms

Tablet, oral: 0.625 mg, 1.25 mg, 2.5 mg

Estrostep® 21 *(Discontinued)* *see* ethinyl estradiol and norethindrone *on page 378*

Estrostep® Fe [US] *see* ethinyl estradiol and norethindrone *on page 378*

eszopiclone (es zoe PIK lone)

Sound-Alike/Look-Alike Issues

Lunesta® may be confused with Neulasta®

U.S./Canadian Brand Names Lunesta® [US]

Therapeutic Category Hypnotic, Nonbenzodiazepine

Controlled Substance C-IV

Use Treatment of insomnia

Dosage Summary

Oral:

Children: Dosage not established

Adults: Initial: 1-2 mg immediately before bedtime (maximum: 3 mg/day)

Elderly: Initial: 1-2 mg immediately before bedtime (maximum: 2 mg/day)

Dosage Forms

Tablet, oral:

Lunesta®: 1 mg, 2 mg, 3 mg

etanercept (et a NER sept)

Sound-Alike/Look-Alike Issues

Enbrel® may be confused with Levbid®

U.S./Canadian Brand Names Enbrel® [US/Can]

Therapeutic Category Antirheumatic, Disease Modifying

Use Treatment of moderately- to severely-active rheumatoid arthritis (RA); moderately- to severely-active polyarticular juvenile idiopathic arthritis (JIA); psoriatic arthritis; active ankylosing spondylitis (AS); moderate-to-severe chronic plaque psoriasis

Dosage Summary

SubQ:

Children <2 years: Dosage not established

Children 2-17 years: 0.8 mg/kg (maximum: 50 mg) once weekly **or** 0.4 mg/kg (maximum: 25 mg) twice weekly

Adults: 50 mg once weekly **or** 25-50 mg twice weekly

Dosage Forms

Injection, powder for reconstitution:

Enbrel®: 25 mg

Injection, solution [preservative free]:

Enbrel®: 50 mg/mL (0.51 mL, 0.98 mL)

ethacrynate sodium *see* ethacrynic acid *on page* 373

ethacrynic acid (eth a KRIN ik AS id)

Sound-Alike/Look-Alike Issues

Edecrin® may be confused with Eulexin®, Ecotrin®

Synonyms ethacrynate sodium

U.S./Canadian Brand Names Edecrin® [US/Can]; Sodium Edecrin® [US]

Therapeutic Category Diuretic, Loop

Use Management of edema associated with congestive heart failure; hepatic cirrhosis or renal disease; short-term management of ascites due to malignancy, idiopathic edema, and lymphedema

Dosage Summary

I.V.:

Children: Dosage not established

Adults: 0.5-1 mg/kg/dose (maximum: 100 mg/dose); **Note:** Occasionally may need to give second dose

Oral:

Children: 1-3 mg/kg/day

Adults: 50-400 mg/day in 1-2 divided doses

Elderly: Initial: 25-50 mg/day

Dosage Forms

Injection, powder for reconstitution:

Sodium Edecrin®: 50 mg

Tablet, oral:

Edecrin®: 25 mg

ethambutol (e THAM byoo tole)

Sound-Alike/Look-Alike Issues

Myambutol® may be confused with Nembutal®

Synonyms ethambutol hydrochloride

U.S./Canadian Brand Names Etibi® [Can]; Myambutol® [US]

Therapeutic Category Antimycobacterial Agent

Use Treatment of pulmonary tuberculosis in conjunction with other antituberculosis agents

Dosage Summary

Oral:

Children: 15-20 mg/kg/day (maximum: 1 g/day) **or** 50 mg/kg twice weekly (maximum: 2.5 g/dose)

Adults:

Daily therapy: 15-25 mg/kg/day (maximum 1600 mg)

Three times/week DOT: 25-30 mg/kg/dose (maximum: 2.4 g/dose)

Twice weekly DOT: 50 mg/kg/dose (maximum: 4 g/dose)

Dosage Forms

Tablet, oral: 100 mg, 400 mg

Myambutol®: 100 mg, 400 mg

ethambutol hydrochloride *see* ethambutol *on page 373*

Ethamolin® [US] *see* ethanolamine oleate *on page 374*

ethanoic acid *see* acetic acid *on page 32*

ethanol *see* alcohol (ethyl) *on page 45*

ethanolamine oleate (ETH a nol a meen OH lee ate)

Sound-Alike/Look-Alike Issues

Ethamolin® may be confused with ethanol

Synonyms monoethanolamine

U.S./Canadian Brand Names Ethamolin® [US]

Therapeutic Category Sclerosing Agent

Use Orphan drug: Sclerosing agent used for bleeding esophageal varices

Dosage Summary

Injection:

Children: Dosage not established

Adults: 1.5-5 mL per varix (maximum: 20 mL total)

Dosage Forms

Injection, solution:

Ethamolin®: 5% (2 mL)

EtheDent™ ***(Discontinued)*** *see* fluoride *on page 413*

EthexDERM™ BPW-5 ***(Discontinued)*** *see* benzoyl peroxide *on page 128*

EthexDERM™ BPW-10 ***(Discontinued)*** *see* benzoyl peroxide *on page 128*

Ethezyme™ 650 ***(Discontinued)***

Ethezyme™ 830 ***(Discontinued)***

Ethezyme™ ***(Discontinued)***

ethinyl estradiol and cyproterone acetate *see* cyproterone and ethinyl estradiol *(Canada only) on page 261*

ethinyl estradiol and desogestrel (ETH in il es tra DYE ole & des oh JES trel)

Sound-Alike/Look-Alike Issues

Apri® may be confused with Apriso™

Ortho-Cept® may be confused with Ortho-Cyclen®

Synonyms desogestrel and ethinyl estradiol

U.S./Canadian Brand Names Apri® [US]; Azurette® [US]; Cesia™ [US]; Cyclessa® [US/Can]; Desogen® [US]; Kariva™ [US]; Linessa® [Can]; Marvelon® [Can]; Mircette® [US]; Ortho-Cept® [US/Can]; Reclipsen™ [US]; Solia™ [US]; Velivet™ [US]

Therapeutic Category Contraceptive, Oral

Use Prevention of pregnancy

Dosage Summary

Oral:

Children (premenarche): Dosage not established

Children (postmenarche): 21-tablet package: 1 tablet daily for 21 days, followed by 7 days off; 28-tablet package: 1 tablet daily

Adults (females): 21-tablet package: 1 tablet daily for 21 days, followed by 7 days off; 28-tablet package: 1 tablet daily

Dosage Forms

Tablet, low-dose formulations:

Azurette™:

Day 1-21: Ethinyl estradiol 0.02 mg and desogestrel 0.15 mg [21 white tablets]
Day 22-23: 2 inactive green tablets
Day 24-28: Ethinyl estradiol 0.01 mg [5 blue tablets] (28s)

Kariva®:

Day 1-21: Ethinyl estradiol 0.02 mg and desogestrel 0.15 mg [21 white tablets]
Day 22-23: 2 inactive light green tablets
Day 24-28: Ethinyl estradiol 0.01 mg [5 light blue tablets] (28s)

Mircette®:

Day 1-21: Ethinyl estradiol 0.02 mg and desogestrel 0.15 mg [21 white tablets]
Day 22-23: 2 inactive green tablets
Day 24-28: Ethinyl estradiol 0.01 mg [5 yellow tablets] (28s)

Tablet, monophasic formulations:

Apri® 28: Ethinyl estradiol 0.03 mg and desogestrel 0.15 mg (28s) [21 rose tablets and 7 white inactive tablets]

Desogen®, Reclipsen™, Solia®: Ethinyl estradiol 0.03 mg and desogestrel 0.15 mg (28s) [21 white tablets and 7 green inactive tablets]

Ortho-Cept® 28: Ethinyl estradiol 0.03 mg and desogestrel 0.15 mg (28s) [21 light orange tablets and 7 green inactive tablets]

Tablet, triphasic formulations:

Caziant®:

Day 1-7: Ethinyl estradiol 0.025 mg and desogestrel 0.1 mg [7 white tablets]
Day 8-14: Ethinyl estradiol 0.025 mg and desogestrel 0.125 mg [7 light blue tablets]
Day 15-21: Ethinyl estradiol 0.025 mg and desogestrel 0.15 mg [7 blue tablets]
Day 22-28: 7 green inactive tablets (28s)

Cesia®, Cyclessa®:

Day 1-7: Ethinyl estradiol 0.025 mg and desogestrel 0.1 mg [7 light yellow tablets]
Day 8-14: Ethinyl estradiol 0.025 mg and desogestrel 0.125 mg [7 orange tablets]
Day 15-21: Ethinyl estradiol 0.025 mg and desogestrel 0.15 mg [7 red tablets]
Day 22-28: 7 green inactive tablets (28s)

Velivet™:

Day 1-7: Ethinyl estradiol 0.025 mg and desogestrel 0.1 mg [7 beige tablets]
Day 8-14: Ethinyl estradiol 0.025 mg and desogestrel 0.125 mg [7 orange tablets]
Day 15-21: Ethinyl estradiol 0.025 mg and desogestrel 0.15 mg [7 pink tablets]
Day 22-28: 7 white inactive tablets (28s)

ethinyl estradiol and drospirenone (ETH in il es tra DYE ole & droh SPYE re none)

Sound-Alike/Look-Alike Issues

Yasmin® may be confused with Yaz®
Yaz® may be confused with Yasmin®

Synonyms drospirenone and ethinyl estradiol

U.S./Canadian Brand Names Gianvi™ [US]; Ocella™ [US]; Yasmin® [US/Can]; Yaz® [US/Can]

Therapeutic Category Contraceptive, Oral

Use Females: Prevention of pregnancy; treatment of premenstrual dysphoric disorder (PMDD); treatment of acne

Dosage Summary

Oral:

Children (premenarche): Use not indicated
Children (females, postmenarche): One tablet daily
Adults (females): One tablet daily

Dosage Forms

Tablet:

Gianvi™: Ethinyl estradiol 0.03 mg and drospirenone 3 mg (28s) [24 pink active tablets and 4 white inactive tablets]

Ocella™, Yasmin®: Ethinyl estradiol 0.03 mg and drospirenone 3 mg (28s) [21 yellow active tablets and 7 white inactive tablets]

Yaz®: Ethinyl estradiol 0.02 mg and drospirenone 3 mg (28s) [24 light pink active tablets and 4 white inactive tablets]

Zarah™: Ethinyl estradiol 0.03 mg and drospirenone 3 mg (28s) [21 blue active tablets and 7 peach inactive tablets]

ethinyl estradiol and ethynodiol diacetate

(ETH in il es tra DYE ole & e thye noe DYE ole dye AS e tate)

Sound-Alike/Look-Alike Issues

Demulen® may be confused with Dalmane®, Demerol®

Synonyms ethynodiol diacetate and ethinyl estradiol

U.S./Canadian Brand Names Demulen® 30 [Can]; Kelnor™ [US]; Zovia® [US]

Therapeutic Category Contraceptive, Oral

Use Prevention of pregnancy

Dosage Summary

Oral:

Children (premenarche): Dosage not established

Children (postmenarche): 21-tablet package: 1 tablet daily for 21 days, followed by 7 days off; 28-tablet package: 1 tablet daily

Adults (females): 21-tablet package: 1 tablet daily for 21 days, followed by 7 days off; 28-tablet package: 1 tablet daily

Dosage Forms

Tablet, monophasic formulations:

Kelnor™ 1/35: Ethinyl estradiol 0.035 mg and ethynodiol diacetate 1 mg [21 light yellow tablets and 7 white inactive tablets] (28s)

Zovia® 1/35-28: Ethinyl estradiol 0.035 mg and ethynodiol diacetate 1 mg [21 light pink tablets and 7 white inactive tablets] (28s)

Zovia® 1/50-28: Ethinyl estradiol 0.05 mg and ethynodiol diacetate 1 mg [21 pink tablets and 7 white inactive tablets] (28s)

ethinyl estradiol and etonogestrel (ETH in il es tra DYE ole & et oh noe JES trel)

Synonyms etonogestrel and ethinyl estradiol

U.S./Canadian Brand Names NuvaRing® [US/Can]

Therapeutic Category Contraceptive, Oral; Estrogen and Progestin Combination

Use Prevention of pregnancy

Dosage Summary

Vaginal:

Children (females, premenarche): Dosage not established

Children (females, postmenarche): Insert one ring and leave in place for 3 consecutive weeks, then remove for 1 week

Adults (females): Insert one ring and leave in place for 3 consecutive weeks, then remove for 1 week

Dosage Forms

Ring, vaginal:

NuvaRing®: Ethinyl estradiol 0.015 mg/day and etonogestrel 0.12 mg/day (1s) [3-week duration]

ethinyl estradiol and levonorgestrel (ETH in il es tra DYE ole & LEE voe nor jes trel)

Sound-Alike/Look-Alike Issues

Alesse® may be confused with Aleve®

Nordette® may be confused with Nicorette®

Seasonale® may be confused with Seasonique™

Seasonique™ may be confused with Seasonale®

Tri-Levlen® may be confused with Trilafon®

Triphasil® may be confused with Tri-Norinyl®

Synonyms levonorgestrel and ethinyl estradiol

U.S./Canadian Brand Names Alesse® [US/Can]; Aviane™ [US/Can]; Enpresse™ [US]; Jolessa™ [US]; Lessina™ [US]; Levlen® [US]; Levlite™ [US]; Levora® [US]; LoSeasonique™ [US]; Lutera™ [US]; Lybrel® [US]; Min-Ovral® [Can]; Nordette® [US]; Portia™ [US]; Quasense™ [US]; Seasonale® [US/Can]; Seasonique™ [US]; Sronyx™ [US]; Triphasil® [US/Can]; Triquilar® [Can]; Trivora® [US]

Therapeutic Category Contraceptive, Oral

Use Prevention of pregnancy; postcoital contraception

Dosage Summary

Oral:

Children (premenarche): Use not indicated

Children (postmenarche):

Contraception: 21-tablet package: 1 tablet daily for 21 days, followed by 7 days off; 28-tablet package: 1 tablet daily

Emergency contraception: 2 tablets as soon as possible (but within 72 hours of unprotected intercourse), followed by 2 tablets 12 hours later

Adults (females):

Contraception: 21-tablet package: 1 tablet daily for 21 days, followed by 7 days off; 28-tablet package: 1 tablet daily

Emergency contraception: 2 tablets as soon as possible (but within 72 hours of unprotected intercourse), followed by 2 tablets 12 hours later

Dosage Forms

Tablet, oral [low-dose formulation]:

Alesse® 28: Ethinyl estradiol 0.02 mg and levonorgestrel 0.1 mg (28s) [21 pink tablets and 7 light green inactive tablets]

Aviane™ 28: Ethinyl estradiol 0.02 mg and levonorgestrel 0.1 mg (28s) [21 orange tablets and 7 light green inactive tablets]

Lessina™ 28, Levlite™ 28: Ethinyl estradiol 0.02 mg and levonorgestrel 0.1 mg (28s) [21 pink tablets and 7 white inactive tablets]

Lutera™, Sronyx™: Ethinyl estradiol 0.02 mg and levonorgestrel 0.1 mg (28s) [21 white tablets and 7 peach inactive tablets]

Tablet, oral [monophasic formulation]:

Levlen® 28: Ethinyl estradiol 0.03 mg and levonorgestrel 0.15 mg (28s) [21 light orange tablets and 7 pink inactive tablets]

Levora® 28: Ethinyl estradiol 0.03 mg and levonorgestrel 0.15 mg (28s) [21 white tablets and 7 peach inactive tablets]

Nordette® 28: Ethinyl estradiol 0.03 mg and levonorgestrel 0.15 mg (28s) [21 light orange tablets and 7 pink inactive tablets]

Portia™ 28: Ethinyl estradiol 0.03 mg and levonorgestrel 0.15 mg (28s) [21 pink tablets and 7 white inactive tablets]

Tablet, oral [extended cycle regimen]:

Jolessa™, Seasonale®: Ethinyl estradiol 0.03 mg and levonorgestrel 0.15 mg (91s) [84 pink tablets and 7 white inactive tablets]

LoSeasonique™: Ethinyl estradiol 0.02 mg and levonorgestrel 0.1 mg (91s) [84 orange tablets] and ethinyl estradiol 0.01 mg [7 yellow tablets]

Quasense™: Ethinyl estradiol 0.03 mg and levonorgestrel 0.15 mg] (91s) [84 white tablets and 7 peach inactive tablets]

Seasonique™: Ethinyl estradiol 0.03 mg and levonorgestrel 0.15 mg (91s) [84 light blue-green tablets] and ethinyl estradiol 0.01 mg [7 yellow tablets]

Tablet, oral [noncyclic regimen]:

Lybrel®: Ethinyl estradiol 0.02 mg and levonorgestrel 0.09 mg (28s) [28 yellow tablets]

Tablet, oral [triphasic formulation]:

Enpresse™ 28:

Day 1-6: Ethinyl estradiol 0.03 mg and levonorgestrel 0.05 mg [6 pink tablets]
Day 7-11: Ethinyl estradiol 0.04 mg and levonorgestrel 0.075 mg [5 white tablets]
Day 12-21: Ethinyl estradiol 0.03 mg and levonorgestrel 0.125 mg [10 orange tablets]
Day 22-28: 7 light green inactive tablets (28s)

Triphasil® 28:

Day 1-6: Ethinyl estradiol 0.03 mg and levonorgestrel 0.05 mg [6 brown tablets]
Day 7-11: Ethinyl estradiol 0.04 mg and levonorgestrel 0.075 mg [5 white tablets]
Day 12-21: Ethinyl estradiol 0.03 mg and levonorgestrel 0.125 mg [10 light yellow tablets]
Day 22-28: 7 light green inactive tablets (28s)

Trivora® 28:

Day 1-6: Ethinyl estradiol 0.03 mg and levonorgestrel 0.05 mg [6 blue tablets]
Day 7-11: Ethinyl estradiol 0.04 mg and levonorgestrel 0.075 mg [5 white tablets]
Day 12-21: Ethinyl estradiol 0.03 mg and levonorgestrel 0.125 mg [10 pink tablets]
Day 22-28: 7 peach inactive tablets (28s)

ethinyl estradiol and NGM *see* ethinyl estradiol and norgestimate *on page* *380*

ethinyl estradiol and norelgestromin (ETH in il es tra DYE ole & nor el JES troe min)

Synonyms norelgestromin and ethinyl estradiol

U.S./Canadian Brand Names Evra® [Can]; Ortho Evra® [US]

Therapeutic Category Contraceptive, Oral; Estrogen and Progestin Combination

Use Prevention of pregnancy

Dosage Summary

Topical:

Children (premenarche): Dosage not established

Children (postmenarche): Apply one patch weekly for 3 weeks, followed by one week that is patch-free

Adults (females): Apply one patch weekly for 3 weeks, followed by one week that is patch-free

Dosage Forms

Patch, transdermal:

Ortho Evra®: Ethinyl estradiol 0.75 mg and norelgestromin 6 mg [releases ethinyl estradiol 20 mcg and norelgestromin 150 mcg per day] (1s, 3s)

Dosage Forms - Canada

Patch, transdermal:

Evra®: Ethinyl estradiol 0.6 mg and norelgestromin 6 mg (1s, 3s)

ethinyl estradiol and norethindrone (ETH in il es tra DYE ole & nor eth IN drone)

Sound-Alike/Look-Alike Issues

femhrt® may be confused with Femara®

Modicon® may be confused with Mylicon®

Norinyl® may be confused with Nardil®

Tri-Norinyl® may be confused with Triphasil®

Synonyms norethindrone acetate and ethinyl estradiol

U.S./Canadian Brand Names Aranelle™ [US]; Balziva™ [US]; Brevicon® 0.5/35 [Can]; Brevicon® 1/35 [Can]; Brevicon® [US]; Estrostep® Fe [US]; Femcon® Fe [US]; femhrt® [US/Can]; Junel™ Fe [US]; Junel™ [US]; Leena™ [US]; Loestrin® 24 Fe [US]; Loestrin® Fe [US]; Loestrin® [US]; Loestrin™ 1.5/30 [Can]; Microgestin™ Fe [US]; Microgestin™ [US]; Minestrin™ 1/20 [Can]; Modicon® [US]; Necon® 0.5/35 [US]; Necon® 1/35 [US]; Necon® 10/11 [US]; Necon® 7/7/7 [US]; Norinyl® 1+35 [US]; Nortrel™ 7/7/7 [US]; Nortrel™ [US]; Ortho-Novum® 7/7/7 [US]; Ortho-Novum® [US]; Ortho® 0.5/35 [Can]; Ortho® 1/35 [Can]; Ortho® 7/7/7 [Can]; Ovcon® [US]; Select™ 1/35 [Can]; Synphasic® [Can]; Tilia™ Fe [US]; Tri-Legest™ Fe [US]; Tri-Norinyl® [US]; Zenchent™ [US]

Therapeutic Category Contraceptive, Oral

Use Prevention of pregnancy; treatment of acne; moderate-to-severe vasomotor symptoms associated with menopause; prevention of osteoporosis (in women at significant risk only)

Dosage Summary

Oral:

Children (premenarche): Dosage not established

Children (postmenarche): 21-tablet package: 1 tablet daily for 21 days, followed by 7 days off; 28-tablet package: 1 tablet daily

Adults (females): 21-tablet package: 1 tablet daily for 21 days, followed by 7 days off; 28-tablet package: 1 tablet daily

Dosage Forms

Tablet, oral:

femhrt® 1/5: Ethinyl estradiol 0.005 mg and norethindrone acetate 1 mg (28s, 90s) [white tablets]

femhrt® Lo 0.5/2.5: Ethinyl estradiol 0.0025 mg and norethindrone acetate 0.5 mg (28s, 90s) [white tablets]

Tablet, oral, monophasic formulations:

Balziva™: Ethinyl estradiol 0.035 mg and norethindrone 0.4 mg (28s) [21 light peach tablets and 7 white inactive tablets]

Brevicon®: Ethinyl estradiol 0.035 mg and norethindrone 0.5 mg (28s) [21 blue tablets and 7 orange inactive tablets]

Junel® 1/20: Ethinyl estradiol 0.02 mg and norethindrone acetate 1 mg (21s) [yellow tablets]

Junel® 1.5/30, Loestrin® 21 1.5/30: Ethinyl estradiol 0.03 mg and norethindrone acetate 1.5 mg (21s) [pink tablets]

Junel® Fe 1/20: Ethinyl estradiol 0.02 mg and norethindrone acetate 1 mg (28s) [21 yellow tablets] and ferrous fumarate 75 mg [7 brown tablets]

Junel® Fe 1.5/30, Loestrin® Fe 21 1.5/30: Ethinyl estradiol 0.03 mg and norethindrone acetate 1.5 mg (28s) [21 pink tablets] and ferrous fumarate 75 mg [7 brown tablets]
Loestrin® 21 1/20: Ethinyl estradiol 0.02 mg and norethindrone acetate 1 mg (21s) [light yellow tablets]
Loestrin® 24 Fe: Ethinyl estradiol 0.02 mg and norethindrone acetate 1 mg (28s) [24 white tablets] and ferrous fumarate 75 mg [4 brown tablets]
Loestrin® Fe 21 1/20: Ethinyl estradiol 0.02 mg and norethindrone acetate 1 mg (28s) [21 light yellow tablets] and ferrous fumarate 75 mg [7 brown tablets]
Microgestin® 1/20: Ethinyl estradiol 0.02 mg and norethindrone acetate 1 mg (21s) [white tablets]
Microgestin® 1.5/30: Ethinyl estradiol 0.03 mg and norethindrone acetate 1.5 mg (21s) [green tablets]
Microgestin® Fe 1/20: Ethinyl estradiol 0.02 mg and norethindrone acetate 1 mg (28s) [21 white tablets] and ferrous fumarate 75 mg [7 brown tablets]
Microgestin® Fe 1.5/30: Ethinyl estradiol 0.03 mg and norethindrone acetate 1.5 mg (28s) [21 green tablets] and ferrous fumarate 75 mg [7 brown tablets]
Modicon®: Ethinyl estradiol 0.035 mg and norethindrone 0.5 mg (28s) [21 white tablets and 7 green inactive tablets]
Necon® 0.5/35, Nortrel® 0.5/35: Ethinyl estradiol 0.035 mg and norethindrone 0.5 mg (28s) [21 light yellow tablets and 7 white inactive tablets]
Necon® 1/35: Ethinyl estradiol 0.035 mg and norethindrone 1 mg (28s) [21 dark yellow tablets and 7 white inactive tablets]
Norinyl® 1+35: Ethinyl estradiol 0.035 mg and norethindrone 1 mg (28s) [21 yellow-green tablets and 7 orange inactive tablets]
Nortrel® 1/35:
Ethinyl estradiol 0.035 mg and norethindrone 1 mg (21s) [yellow tablets]
Ethinyl estradiol 0.035 mg and norethindrone 1 mg (28s) [21 yellow tablets and 7 white inactive tablets]
Ortho-Novum® 1/35: Ethinyl estradiol 0.035 mg and norethindrone 1 mg (28s) [21 peach tablets and 7 green inactive tablets]
Ovcon® 35: Ethinyl estradiol 0.035 mg and norethindrone 0.4 mg (28s) [21 light peach tablets and 7 green inactive tablets]
Ovcon® 50: Ethinyl estradiol 0.05 mg and norethindrone 1 mg (28s) [21 yellow tablets and 7 green inactive tablets]
Zenchent™: Ethinyl estradiol 0.035 mg and norethindrone 0.4 mg (28s) [21 orange tablets and 7 white inactive tablets]

Tablet, chewable, oral, monophasic formulations:
Femcon® Fe: Ethinyl estradiol 0.035 mg and norethindrone 0.4 mg (28s) [21 white tablets] and ferrous fumarate 75 mg [7 brown tablets] [spearmint flavor]

Tablet, oral, biphasic formulations:
Necon® 10/11:
Day 1-10: Ethinyl estradiol 0.035 mg and norethindrone 0.5 mg [10 light yellow tablets]
Day 11-21: Ethinyl estradiol 0.035 mg and norethindrone 1 mg [11 dark yellow tablets]
Day 22-28: 7 white inactive tablets (28s)

Tablet, oral, triphasic formulations:
Aranelle®:
Day 1-7: Ethinyl estradiol 0.035 mg and norethindrone 0.5 mg [7 light yellow tablets]
Day 8-16: Ethinyl estradiol 0.035 mg and norethindrone 1 mg [9 white tablets]
Day 17-21: Ethinyl estradiol 0.035 mg and norethindrone 0.5 mg [5 light yellow tablets]
Day 22-28: 7 peach inactive tablets (28s)
Estrostep® Fe, Tilia™ Fe::
Day 1-5: Ethinyl estradiol 0.02 mg and norethindrone acetate 1 mg [5 white triangular tablets]
Day 6-12: Ethinyl estradiol 0.03 mg and norethindrone acetate 1 mg [7 white square tablets]
Day 13-21: Ethinyl estradiol 0.035 mg and norethindrone acetate 1 mg [9 white round tablets]
Day 22-28: Ferrous fumarate 75 mg [7 brown tablets] (28s)
Leena®:
Day 1-7: Ethinyl estradiol 0.035 mg and norethindrone 0.5 mg [7 light blue tablets]
Day 8-16: Ethinyl estradiol 0.035 mg and norethindrone 1 mg [9 light yellow-green tablets]
Day 17-21: Ethinyl estradiol 0.035 mg and norethindrone 0.5 mg [5 light blue tablets]
Day 22-28: 7 orange inactive tablets (28s)
Necon® 7/7/7, Ortho-Novum® 7/7/7:
Day 1-7: Ethinyl estradiol 0.035 mg and norethindrone 0.5 mg [7 white tablets]
Day 8-14: Ethinyl estradiol 0.035 mg and norethindrone 0.75 mg [7 light peach tablets]
Day 15-21: Ethinyl estradiol 0.035 mg and norethindrone 1 mg [7 peach tablets]
Day 22-28: 7 green inactive tablets (28s)

Nortrel® 7/7/7:
Day 1-7: Ethinyl estradiol 0.035 mg and norethindrone 0.5 mg [7 light yellow tablets]
Day 8-14: Ethinyl estradiol 0.035 mg and norethindrone 0.75 mg [7 blue tablets]
Day 15-21: Ethinyl estradiol 0.035 mg and norethindrone 1 mg [7 peach tablets]
Day 22-28: 7 white inactive tablets (28s)
Tri-Legest™ Fe:
Day 1-5: Ethinyl estradiol 0.02 mg and norethindrone acetate 1 mg [5 light pink tablets]
Day 6-12: Ethinyl estradiol 0.03 mg and norethindrone acetate 1 mg [7 light yellow tablets]
Day 13-21: Ethinyl estradiol 0.035 mg and norethindrone acetate 1 mg [9 light blue tablets]
Day 22-28: Ferrous fumarate 75 mg [7 brown tablets] (28s)
Tri-Norinyl®:
Day 1-7: Ethinyl estradiol 0.035 mg and norethindrone 0.5 mg [7 blue tablets]
Day 8-16: Ethinyl estradiol 0.035 mg and norethindrone 1 mg [9 yellow-green tablets]
Day 17-21: Ethinyl estradiol 0.035 mg and norethindrone 0.5 mg [5 blue tablets]
Day 22-28: 7 orange inactive tablets (28s)

ethinyl estradiol and norgestimate (ETH in il es tra DYE ole & nor JES ti mate)

Sound-Alike/Look-Alike Issues
Ortho-Cyclen® may be confused with Ortho-Cept®
Ortho Tri-Cyclen® may be confused with Ortho Tri-Cyclen® Lo
Ortho Tri-Cyclen® Lo may be confused with Ortho Tri-Cyclen®

Synonyms ethinyl estradiol and NGM; norgestimate and ethinyl estradiol

U.S./Canadian Brand Names Cyclen® [Can]; MonoNessa® [US]; Ortho Tri-Cyclen® Lo [US]; Ortho Tri-Cyclen® [US]; Ortho-Cyclen® [US]; Sprintec® [US]; Tri-Cyclen® Lo [Can]; Tri-Cyclen® [Can]; Tri-Sprintec® [US]; TriNessa® [US]

Therapeutic Category Contraceptive, Oral

Use Prevention of pregnancy; treatment of acne

Dosage Summary

Oral:
Children (premenarche): Dosage not established
Children (postmenarche): 21-tablet package: 1 tablet daily for 21 days, followed by 7 days off; 28-tablet package: 1 tablet daily
Adults (females): 21-tablet package: 1 tablet daily for 21 days, followed by 7 days off; 28-tablet package: 1 tablet daily

Dosage Forms

Tablet, monophasic formulations:
MonoNessa®, Ortho-Cyclen®: Ethinyl estradiol 0.035 mg and norgestimate 0.25 mg (28s) [21 blue tablets and 7 green inactive tablets]
Sprintec®: Ethinyl estradiol 0.035 mg and norgestimate 0.25 mg (28s) [21 blue tablets and 7 white inactive tablets]

Tablet, triphasic formulations:
Ortho Tri-Cyclen®, TriNessa®:
Day 1-7: Ethinyl estradiol 0.035 mg and norgestimate 0.18 mg [7 white tablets]
Day 8-14: Ethinyl estradiol 0.035 mg and norgestimate 0.215 mg [7 light blue tablets]
Day 15-21: Ethinyl estradiol 0.035 mg and norgestimate 0.25 mg [7 blue tablets]
Day 22-28: 7 green inactive tablets (28s)
Tri-Sprintec®:
Day 1-7: Ethinyl estradiol 0.035 mg and norgestimate 0.18 mg [7 gray tablets]
Day 8-14: Ethinyl estradiol 0.035 mg and norgestimate 0.215 mg [7 light blue tablets]
Day 15-21: Ethinyl estradiol 0.035 mg and norgestimate 0.25 mg [7 blue tablets]
Day 22-28: 7 white inactive tablets (28s)
Ortho Tri-Cyclen® Lo:
Day 1-7: Ethinyl estradiol 0.025 mg and norgestimate 0.18 mg [7 white tablets]
Day 8-14: Ethinyl estradiol 0.025 mg and norgestimate 0.215 mg [7 light blue tablets]
Day 15-21: Ethinyl estradiol 0.025 mg and norgestimate 0.25 mg [7 dark blue tablets]
Day 22-28: 7 green inactive tablets (28s)

ethinyl estradiol and norgestrel (ETH in il es tra DYE ole & nor JES trel)

Synonyms morning after pill; norgestrel and ethinyl estradiol

U.S./Canadian Brand Names Cryselle® 28 [US]; Lo/Ovral®-28 [US]; Low-Ogestrel® [US]; Ogestrel® [US]; Ovral® [Can]

Therapeutic Category Contraceptive, Oral

Use Prevention of pregnancy; postcoital contraceptive or "morning after" pill

Dosage Summary

Oral:

Children (premenarche): Dosage not established

Children (females, postmenarche):

Contraception: 21-tablet package: 1 tablet daily for 21 days, followed by 7 days off; 28-tablet package: 1 tablet daily

Postcoital contraception: Ethinyl estradiol 0.03 mg and norgestrel 0.3 mg formulation: 4 tablets within 72 hours of unprotected intercourse and 4 tablets 12 hours after first dose **or** ethinyl estradiol 0.05 mg and norgestrel 0.5 mg formulation: 2 tablets within 72 hours of unprotected intercourse and 2 tablets 12 hours after first dose

Adults (females):

Contraception: 21-tablet package: 1 tablet daily for 21 days, followed by 7 days off; 28-tablet package: 1 tablet daily

Postcoital contraception: Ethinyl estradiol 0.03 mg and norgestrel 0.3 mg formulation: 4 tablets within 72 hours of unprotected intercourse and 4 tablets 12 hours after first dose **or** ethinyl estradiol 0.05 mg and norgestrel 0.5 mg formulation: 2 tablets within 72 hours of unprotected intercourse and 2 tablets 12 hours after first dose

Dosage Forms

Tablet, monophasic formulations:

Cryselle® 28: Ethinyl estradiol 0.03 mg and norgestrel 0.3 mg [21 white tablets and 7 light green inactive tablets] (28s)

Low-Ogestrel®: Ethinyl estradiol 0.03 mg and norgestrel 0.3 mg [21 white tablets and 7 peach inactive tablets] (28s)

Lo/Ovral®-28: Ethinyl estradiol 0.03 mg and norgestrel 0.3 mg [21 white tablets and 7 pink inactive tablets] (28s)

Ogestrel®: Ethinyl estradiol 0.05 mg and norgestrel 0.5 mg [21 white tablets and 7 peach inactive tablets] (28s)

ethiofos *see* amifostine *on page 63*

ethionamide (e thye on AM ide)

U.S./Canadian Brand Names Trecator® [US/Can]

Therapeutic Category Antimycobacterial Agent

Use Treatment of tuberculosis and other mycobacterial diseases, in conjunction with other antituberculosis agents, when first-line agents have failed or resistance has been demonstrated

Dosage Summary

Oral:

Children: 15-20 mg/kg/day in 2-3 divided doses (maximum: 1 g/day)

Adults: 250-750 mg/day in 1-4 divided doses (maximum: 1 g/day)

Dosage Forms

Tablet, oral:

Trecator®: 250 mg

Ethmozine® ***(Discontinued)***

ethosuximide (eth oh SUKS i mide)

Sound-Alike/Look-Alike Issues

ethosuximide may be confused with methsuximide

Zarontin® may be confused with Neurontin®, Xalatan®, Zantac®, Zaroxolyn®

U.S./Canadian Brand Names Zarontin® [US/Can]

Therapeutic Category Anticonvulsant

Use Management of absence (petit mal) seizures

Dosage Summary

Oral:

Children <3 years: Dosage not established

Children 3-6 years: Initial: 250 mg/day; Maintenance: 20 mg/kg/day (maximum dose: 1.5 g/day in divided doses)

Children ≥6 years: Initial: 500 mg/day; Maintenance: 20 mg/kg/day (maximum dose: 1.5 g/day in divided doses)
Adults: Initial: 500 mg/day (maximum dose: 1.5 g/day in divided doses)

Dosage Forms

Capsule, softgel, oral: 250 mg
Zarontin®: 250 mg
Solution, oral: 250 mg/5 mL (473 mL)
Zarontin®: 250 mg/5 mL (480 mL)
Syrup, oral: 250 mg/5 mL (473 mL)

ethotoin (ETH oh toyn)

Synonyms ethylphenylhydantoin

U.S./Canadian Brand Names Peganone® [US/Can]

Therapeutic Category Hydantoin

Use Generalized tonic-clonic or complex-partial seizures

Dosage Summary

Oral:
Children <1 year: Dosage not established
Children ≥1 year: Maximum initial dose: 750 mg/day; usual maintenance dose: 0.5-1 g/day; maximum dose: 3 g/day
Adults: Initial dose: ≤1 g/day; usual maintenance dose: 2-3 g/day

Dosage Forms

Tablet, oral:
Peganone®: 250 mg

ETH-Oxydose™ *(Discontinued)* *see* oxycodone *on page 714*
ethoxynaphthamido penicillin sodium *see* nafcillin *on page 655*
ethyl alcohol *see* alcohol (ethyl) *on page 45*
ethyl aminobenzoate *see* benzocaine *on page 124*

ethyl chloride (ETH il KLOR ide)

Synonyms chloroethane

U.S./Canadian Brand Names Gebauer's Ethyl Chloride® [US]

Therapeutic Category Local Anesthetic

Use Local anesthetic in minor operative procedures and to relieve pain caused by insect stings and burns, and irritation caused by myofascial and visceral pain syndromes

Dosage Summary

Topical:
Children: Dosage not established
Adults: Dosage varies with use

Dosage Forms

Aerosol, topical:
Gebauer's Ethyl Chloride®: 100% (103.5 mL)

ethyl chloride and dichlorotetrafluoroethane

(ETH il KLOR ide & dye klor oh te tra floo or oh ETH ane)

Synonyms dichlorotetrafluoroethane and ethyl chloride

Therapeutic Category Local Anesthetic

Use Topical refrigerant anesthetic to control pain associated with minor surgical procedures, dermabrasion, injections, contusions, and minor strains

Dosage Summary

Topical:
Children: Dosage not established
Adults: Apply as a fine mist approximately 2" to 4" from site of application

ethyl esters of omega-3 fatty acids *see* omega-3-acid ethyl esters *on page 701*
ethylphenylhydantoin *see* ethotoin *on page 382*
ethynodiol diacetate and ethinyl estradiol *see* ethinyl estradiol and ethynodiol diacetate *on page 376*
Ethyol® [US/Can] *see* amifostine *on page 63*

Etibi® [Can] *see* ethambutol *on page* 373

etidronate (e ti DROE nate)

Sound-Alike/Look-Alike Issues

etidronate may be confused with etidocaine, etomidate, etretinate

Synonyms EHDP; sodium etidronate

U.S./Canadian Brand Names Co-Etidronate [Can]; Didronel® [US/Can]; Mylan-Etidronate [Can]

Therapeutic Category Bisphosphonate Derivative

Use Symptomatic treatment of Paget disease; prevention and treatment of heterotopic ossification due to spinal cord injury or after total hip replacement

Dosage Summary

Oral:

Children: Dosage not established

Adults:

Heterotopic ossification:

Caused by spinal cord injury: 20 mg/kg/day for 2 weeks, then 10 mg/kg/day for 10 weeks (total treatment period: 12 weeks)

Complicating total hip replacement: 20 mg/kg/day for 1 month preoperatively then 20 mg/kg/day for 3 months postoperatively (total treatment period: 4 months)

Paget disease: 5-10 mg/kg/day for up to 6 months or 11-20 mg/kg/day for up to 3 months; may retreat after etidronate-free period ≥90 days

Dosage Forms

Tablet, oral: 200 mg, 400 mg

Didronel®: 400 mg

etidronate and calcium carbonate *(Canada only)*

(e ti DROE nate & KAL see um KAR bun ate)

Synonyms calcium carbonate and etidronate disodium

U.S./Canadian Brand Names CO-Etidrocal [Can]; Didrocal™ [Can]; Mylan-Eti-Cal Carepac [Can]; Novo-Etidronatecal [Can]

Therapeutic Category Bisphosphonate Derivative; Calcium Salt

Use Treatment and prevention of postmenopausal osteoporosis; prevention of corticosteroid-induced osteoporosis

Dosage Summary

Oral:

Children: Dosage not established

Adults: Etidronate disodium 400 mg once daily for 14 days, followed by calcium carbonate 1250 mg (500 mg elemental calcium) once daily for 76 days

Dosage Forms - Canada

Combination package [each package contains 5 blister cards (90-day supply)]:

Didrocal™:

Tablet, etidronate: 400 mg (14s) [first card (white tablets)]

Tablet, calcium: 1250 mg (76s) [remaining cards (blue tablets)]

etodolac (ee toe DOE lak)

Sound-Alike/Look-Alike Issues

Lodine® may be confused with codeine, iodine, Iopidine®, Lopid®

Synonyms etodolic acid

U.S./Canadian Brand Names Apo-Etodolac® [Can]; Utradol™ [Can]

Therapeutic Category Analgesic, Nonnarcotic; Nonsteroidal Antiinflammatory Drug (NSAID)

Use Acute and long-term use in the management of signs and symptoms of osteoarthritis; rheumatoid arthritis and juvenile rheumatoid arthritis; management of acute pain

Dosage Summary

Oral:

Extended release:

Children <6 years: Dosage not established

Children 6-16 years and 20-30 kg: 400 mg once daily

Children 6-16 years and 31-45 kg: 600 mg once daily

Children 6-16 years and 46-60 kg: 800 mg once daily

Children 6-16 years and >60 kg: 1000 mg once daily
Adults: 400-1000 mg once daily
Regular release:
Children: Dosage not established
Adults: 200-400 mg every 6-12 hours as needed **or** 500 mg 2 times/day (maximum: 1 g/day)

Dosage Forms
Capsule, oral: 200 mg, 300 mg
Tablet, oral: 400 mg, 500 mg
Tablet, extended release, oral: 400 mg, 500 mg, 600 mg

etodolic acid *see* etodolac *on page 383*

EtOH *see* alcohol (ethyl) *on page 45*

etomidate (e TOM i date)

Sound-Alike/Look-Alike Issues
etomidate may be confused with etidronate

U.S./Canadian Brand Names Amidate® [US/Can]

Therapeutic Category General Anesthetic

Use Induction and maintenance of general anesthesia

Dosage Summary
I.V.:
Children ≤10 years: Dosage not established
Children >10 years: Induction: 0.2-0.6 mg/kg; Maintenance: 5-20 mcg/kg/minute
Adults: Induction: 0.2-0.6 mg/kg; Maintenance: 5-20 mcg/kg/minute

Dosage Forms
Injection, solution: 2 mg/mL (10 mL, 20 mL)
Amidate®: 2 mg/mL (10 mL, 20 mL)

etonogestrel (e toe noe JES trel)

Synonyms 3-keto-desogestrel; ENG

U.S./Canadian Brand Names Implanon™ [US]

Therapeutic Category Contraceptive; Progestin

Use Prevention of pregnancy; for use in women who request long-acting (up to 3 years) contraception

Dosage Summary
Subdermal:
Children: Not for use prior to menarche
Adults: Implant 1 rod for up to 3 years
Elderly: Not for use after menopause

Dosage Forms
Rod, subdermal:
Implanon™: 68 mg

etonogestrel and ethinyl estradiol *see* ethinyl estradiol and etonogestrel *on page 376*

Etopophos® [US] *see* etoposide phosphate *on page 385*

etoposide (e toe POE side)

Sound-Alike/Look-Alike Issues
etoposide may be confused with teniposide
VePesid® may be confused with Versed

Synonyms epipodophyllotoxin; VP-16; VP-16-213

U.S./Canadian Brand Names Toposar® [US]

Therapeutic Category Antineoplastic Agent

Use Treatment of refractory testicular tumors; treatment of small cell lung cancer

Dosage Summary
I.V.:
Adults: 35 mg/m^2/day for 4 days every 3-4 weeks **or** 50-100 mg/m^2/day for 5 days every 3-4 weeks **or** 60-100 mg/m^2/day for 3 days **or** 500 mg/m^2 over 24 hours every 3 weeks **or** 100 mg/m^2 every other day for 3 doses repeated every 3-4 weeks

Oral:
Children: Dosage not established
Adults: Doses should be twice the I.V. dose (rounded to the nearest 50 mg) given once daily

Dosage Forms
Capsule, softgel, oral: 50 mg
Injection, solution: 20 mg/mL (5 mL, 25 mL, 50 mL, 100 mL)
Toposar®: 20 mg/mL (5 mL, 25 mL, 50 mL)

etoposide phosphate (e toe POE side FOS fate)

Sound-Alike/Look-Alike Issues
etoposide may be confused with teniposide

U.S./Canadian Brand Names Etopophos® [US]

Therapeutic Category Antineoplastic Agent

Use Treatment of refractory testicular tumors; treatment of small cell lung cancer

Dosage Summary Note: Etoposide phosphate is a prodrug of etoposide, doses should be expressed as the desired ETOPOSIDE dose; not as the etoposide phosphate dose.
I.V.:
Children: Dosage not established
Adults: 35 mg/m^2/day for 4 days to 50-100 mg/m^2/day for 5 days every 3-4 weeks **or** 100 mg/m^2/day on days 1, 3, and 5 every 3-4 weeks

Dosage Forms
Injection, powder for reconstitution:
Etopophos®: 100 mg

Etrafon® [Can] *see* amitriptyline and perphenazine *on page 68*

etravirine (et ra VIR een)

Synonyms TMC125

U.S./Canadian Brand Names Intelence™ [US/Can]

Therapeutic Category Antiretroviral Agent, Nonnucleoside Reverse Transcriptase Inhibitor (NNRTI)

Use Treatment of HIV-1 infection in combination with at least two additional antiretroviral agents in treatment-experienced patients exhibiting viral replication with documented nonnucleoside reverse transcriptase inhibitor (NNRTI) resistance

Dosage Summary
Oral:
Children: Dosage not established
Adults: 200 mg twice daily after meals

Dosage Forms
Tablet, oral:
Intelence®: 100 mg

ETS-2% Topical *(Discontinued)*
Euflex® [Can] *see* flutamide *on page 418*
Euflexxa™ [US] *see* hyaluronate and derivatives *on page 475*
Euglucon® [Can] *see* glyburide *on page 448*
Eulexin® [Can] *see* flutamide *on page 418*
Eurax® [US] *see* crotamiton *on page 256*
Euro-Lithium [Can] *see* lithium *on page 571*
Euthyrox [Can] *see* levothyroxine *on page 560*
Evac-Q-Mag® *(Discontinued)* *see* magnesium citrate *on page 584*
Evac-U-Gen® [US-OTC] *see* senna *on page 870*
Evalose® *(Discontinued)* *see* lactulose *on page 544*
Evamist™ [US] *see* estradiol (systemic) *on page 366*

everolimus (e ver OH li mus)

Sound-Alike/Look-Alike Issues
everolimus may be confused with sirolimus, tacrolimus, temsirolimus

Synonyms RAD001

U.S./Canadian Brand Names Afinitor® [US]; Zortress® [US]

Therapeutic Category Antineoplastic Agent, mTOR Kinase Inhibitor; mTOR Kinase Inhibitor

Use Treatment of advanced renal cell cancer (RCC), after sunitinib or sorafenib failure (Afinitor®); prophylaxis of organ rejection in patients at low-moderate immunologic risk receiving renal transplants (Zortress®)

Dosage Summary

Oral:

Children: Dosage not established

Adults: 10 mg once daily **or** Initial: 0.75 mg twice daily; adjust maintenance dose if needed at a 4- to 5-day interval (from prior dose adjustment) based on serum concentrations, tolerability, and response

Dosage Forms

Tablet, oral:

Afinitor®: 2.5 mg, 5 mg, 10 mg

Zortress®: 0.25 mg, 0.5 mg, 0.75 mg

Everone® 200 [Can] *see* testosterone *on page 919*

Everone® Injection *(Discontinued)* *see* testosterone *on page 919*

Evicel™ [US] *see* fibrin sealant *on page 401*

Evista® [US/Can] *see* raloxifene *on page 825*

Evithrom™ [US] *see* thrombin (topical) *on page 929*

Evoclin® [US] *see* clindamycin (topical) *on page 232*

Evoxac® [US/Can] *see* cevimeline *on page 200*

Evra® [Can] *see* ethinyl estradiol and norelgestromin *on page 378*

Exactacain™ [US] *see* benzocaine, butamben, and tetracaine *on page 127*

Exalgo™ [US] *see* hydromorphone *on page 485*

Excedrin® Extra Strength [US-OTC] *see* acetaminophen, aspirin, and caffeine *on page 27*

Excedrin® IB *(Discontinued)* *see* ibuprofen *on page 494*

Excedrin® Migraine [US-OTC] *see* acetaminophen, aspirin, and caffeine *on page 27*

Excedrin PM® [US-OTC] *see* acetaminophen and diphenhydramine *on page 24*

Excedrin® Sinus Headache [US-OTC] *see* acetaminophen and phenylephrine *on page 25*

Excedrin® Tension Headache [US-OTC] *see* acetaminophen *on page 21*

ExeClear-C [US] *see* guaifenesin and codeine *on page 455*

ExeClear *(Discontinued)*

ExeCof [US] *see* guaifenesin, dextromethorphan, and phenylephrine *on page 458*

ExeCof-XP *(Discontinued)*

ExeFen-DMX [US] *see* guaifenesin, pseudoephedrine, and dextromethorphan *on page 460*

ExeFen-IR [US] *see* guaifenesin and pseudoephedrine *on page 457*

ExeFen-PD [US] *see* guaifenesin and phenylephrine *on page 456*

Exelderm® [US/Can] *see* sulconazole *on page 899*

Exelon® [US/Can] *see* rivastigmine *on page 848*

exemestane (ex e MES tane)

Sound-Alike/Look-Alike Issues

exemestane may be confused with estramustine

Aromasin® may be confused with Arimidex®

U.S./Canadian Brand Names Aromasin® [US/Can]

Therapeutic Category Antineoplastic Agent, Miscellaneous

Use Treatment of advanced breast cancer in postmenopausal women whose disease has progressed following tamoxifen therapy; adjuvant treatment of postmenopausal estrogen receptor-positive early breast cancer following 2-3 years of tamoxifen (for a total of 5 years of adjuvant therapy)

Dosage Summary

Oral:

Children: Dosage not established

Adults (postmenopausal females): 25 mg once daily (50 mg once daily with CYP3A4 inducers)

Dosage Forms

Tablet, oral:

Aromasin®: 25 mg

exenatide (ex EN a tide)

Synonyms AC 2993; AC002993; exendin-4; LY2148568

U.S./Canadian Brand Names Byetta® [US]

Therapeutic Category Antidiabetic Agent, Incretin Mimetic

Use Treatment of type 2 diabetes mellitus (noninsulin-dependent, NIDDM) to improve glycemic control

Dosage Summary

SubQ:

Children: Dosage not established

Adults: Initial: 5 mcg twice daily for 1 month; Maintenance: 5-10 mcg twice daily

Dosage Forms

Injection, solution:

Byetta®: 250 mcg/mL (1.2 mL, 2.4 mL)

exendin-4 *see* exenatide *on page 387*

ExeTuss *(Discontinued)* *see* guaifenesin and phenylephrine *on page 456*

ExeTuss-DM [US] *see* guaifenesin, dextromethorphan, and phenylephrine *on page 458*

ExeTuss-GP [US] *see* guaifenesin and phenylephrine *on page 456*

ExeTuss HC *(Discontinued)*

Exforge® [US] *see* amlodipine and valsartan *on page 70*

Exforge HCT® [US] *see* amlodipine, valsartan, and hydrochlorothiazide *on page 71*

Exidine® Scrub *(Discontinued)* *see* chlorhexidine gluconate *on page 204*

Exjade® [US/Can] *see* deferasirox *on page 272*

ex-lax® [US-OTC] *see* senna *on page 870*

ex-lax® Maximum Strength [US-OTC] *see* senna *on page 870*

ex-lax® Ultra [US-OTC] *see* bisacodyl *on page 138*

Exorex® Penetrating Emulsion [US-OTC] *see* coal tar *on page 242*

Exorex® Penetrating Emulsion #2 [US-OTC] *see* coal tar *on page 242*

Exsel® *(Discontinued)* *see* selenium sulfide *on page 869*

Extavia® [US/Can] *see* interferon beta-1b *on page 516*

extended release epidural morphine *see* morphine (liposomal) *on page 645*

Extendryl® *(Discontinued)* *see* chlorpheniramine, phenylephrine, and methscopolamine *on page 212*

Extendryl® GCP [US] *see* carbetapentane, guaifenesin, and phenylephrine *on page 180*

Extendryl® HC *(Discontinued)*

Extendryl® JR *(Discontinued)* *see* chlorpheniramine, phenylephrine, and methscopolamine *on page 212*

Extendryl PSE [US] *see* pseudoephedrine and methscopolamine *on page 813*

Extendryl® SR *(Discontinued)* *see* chlorpheniramine, phenylephrine, and methscopolamine *on page 212*

Extina® [US] *see* ketoconazole (topical) *on page 536*

Extra Action Cough Syrup *(Discontinued)* *see* guaifenesin and dextromethorphan *on page 455*

Extraneal [US] *see* icodextrin *on page 497*

EYE001 *see* pegaptanib *on page 732*

Eye-Lube-A® Solution *(Discontinued)* *see* artificial tears *on page 97*

Eye-Sed® Ophthalmic *(Discontinued)* *see* zinc sulfate *on page 1002*

Eye-Sine™ *(Discontinued)* *see* tetrahydrozoline (ophthalmic) *on page 923*

Eyestil [Can] *see* hyaluronate and derivatives *on page 475*

Eye-Stream® [Can] *see* balanced salt solution *on page 116*

E-Z-Cat® [US] *see* barium *on page 117*

E-Z-Cat® Dry [US] *see* barium *on page 117*

EZ-Char® [US-OTC] *see* charcoal *on page 200*

E-Z-Disk™ [US] *see* barium *on page 117*

ezetimibe (ez ET i mibe)

Sound-Alike/Look-Alike Issues

Zetia® may be confused with Zebeta®, Zestril®

U.S./Canadian Brand Names Ezetrol® [Can]; Zetia® [US]

Therapeutic Category Antilipemic Agent, 2-Azetidinone

Use Use in combination with dietary therapy for the treatment of primary hypercholesterolemia (as monotherapy or in combination with HMG-CoA reductase inhibitors); homozygous sitosterolemia; homozygous familial hypercholesterolemia (in combination with atorvastatin or simvastatin); mixed hyperlipidemia (in combination with fenofibrate)

Dosage Summary

Oral:

Children <10 years: Dosage not established

Children ≥10 years: 10 mg once daily

Adults: 10 mg once daily

Dosage Forms

Tablet, oral:

Zetia®: 10 mg

ezetimibe and simvastatin (ez ET i mibe & SIM va stat in)

Sound-Alike/Look-Alike Issues

Vytorin® may be confused with Vyvanse™

Synonyms simvastatin and ezetimibe

U.S./Canadian Brand Names Vytorin® [US]

Therapeutic Category Antilipemic Agent, 2-Azetidinone

Use Used in combination with dietary modification for the treatment of primary hypercholesterolemia and homozygous familial hypercholesterolemia

Dosage Summary

Oral:

Children: Dosage not established

Adults: Ezetimibe 10 mg and simvastatin 10-80 mg once daily

Dosage Forms

Tablet:

Vytorin®:

10/10: Ezetimibe 10 mg and simvastatin 10 mg

10/20: Ezetimibe 10 mg and simvastatin 20 mg

10/40: Ezetimibe 10 mg and simvastatin 40 mg

10/80: Ezetimibe 10 mg and simvastatin 80 mg

Ezetrol® [Can] *see* ezetimibe *on page 387*

Ezide® *(Discontinued)* *see* hydrochlorothiazide *on page 478*

F_3T *see* trifluridine *on page 958*

FabAV, FAB (ovine) *see* crotalidae polyvalent immune FAB (ovine) *on page 255*

FaBB [US] *see* folic acid, cyanocobalamin, and pyridoxine *on page 423*

Fabrazyme® [US/Can] *see* agalsidase beta *on page 41*

Factive® [US/Can] *see* gemifloxacin *on page 441*

factor VIIa (recombinant) (FAK ter SEV en aye ree KOM be nant)

Sound-Alike/Look-Alike Issues

NovoSeven® RT may be confused with Novacet®

Synonyms coagulation factor VIIa; eptacog alfa (activated); rFVIIa

U.S./Canadian Brand Names Niastase® [Can]; NovoSeven® RT [US]

Therapeutic Category Antihemophilic Agent; Blood Product Derivative

Use Treatment of bleeding episodes and prevention of bleeding in surgical interventions in patients with either hemophilia A or B with inhibitors to factor VIII or factor IX, acquired hemophilia, or congenital factor VII deficiency

Dosage Summary

I.V.:

Children:

Congenital factor VII deficiency: 10-30 mcg/kg every 4-6 hours until hemostasis is achieved

Hemophilia A or B with inhibitors: 90 mcg/kg every 2 hours until hemostasis is achieved **or** immediately before surgery and every 2 hours for 48 hours, then every 2-6 hours until healed (minor surgery) **or** every 2 hours for 5 days, then every 4 hours until healed (major surgery)

Acquired hemophilia: 70-90 mcg/kg every 2-3 hours until hemostasis is achieved

Adults:

Congenital factor VII deficiency: 10-30 mcg/kg every 4-6 hours until hemostasis is achieved

Hemophilia A or B with inhibitors: 90 mcg/kg every 2 hours until hemostasis is achieved **or** immediately before surgery and every 2 hours for 48 hours, then every 2-6 hours until healed (minor surgery) **or** every 2 hours for 5 days, then every 4 hours until healed (major surgery)

Acquired hemophilia: 70-90 mcg/kg every 2-3 hours until hemostasis is achieved

Dosage Forms

Injection, powder for reconstitution [preservative free]:

NovoSeven® RT: 1 mg, 2 mg, 5 mg

factor VIII (human) *see* antihemophilic factor (human) *on page* 81

factor VIII (human) *see* antihemophilic factor/von Willebrand factor complex (human) *on page* 82

factor VIII (recombinant) *see* antihemophilic factor (recombinant) *on page* 81

factor IX (FAK ter nyne)

Synonyms factor IX concentrate

U.S./Canadian Brand Names AlphaNine® SD [US]; BeneFix® [US/Can]; Immunine® VH [Can]; Mononine® [US/Can]

Therapeutic Category Antihemophilic Agent

Use Prevention and control of bleeding in patients with factor IX deficiency (hemophilia B or Christmas disease)

Dosage Summary Note: Dosage is expressed in int. units of factor IX activity and must be individualized

I.V.:

AlphaNine® SD, Mononine®:

Children: Number of factor IX int. units required = body weight (in kg) x desired factor IX level increase (as %) x 1 int. unit/kg every 12-24 hours or every 18-30 hours

Adults: Number of factor IX int. units required = body weight (in kg) x desired factor IX level increase (as %) x 1 int. unit/kg every 12-24 hours or every 18-30 hours

BeneFix®:

Children <15 years: Number of factor IX int. units required = body weight (in kg) x desired factor IX level increase (as %) x 1.4 int. units/kg every 12-24 hours or every 18-30 hours

Children ≥15 years: Number of factor IX int. units required = body weight (in kg) x desired factor IX level increase (as %) x 1.3 int. units/kg every 12-24 hours or every 18-30 hours

Adults: Number of factor IX int. units required = body weight (in kg) x desired factor IX level increase (as %) x 1.3 int. units/kg every 12-24 hours or every 18-30 hours

Dosage Forms

Injection, powder for reconstitution [recombinant]:

BeneFix®: ~250 int. units, ~500 int. units, ~1000 int. units, ~2000 int. units [exact potency labeled on each vial]

Injection, powder for reconstitution [human derived]:

AlphaNine® SD: ~500 int. units, ~1000 int. units, ~1500 int. units [exact potency labeled on each vial]

Mononine®: ~500 int. units, ~1000 int. units [exact potency labeled on each vial]

factor IX complex (human) (FAK ter nyne KOM pleks HYU man)

Synonyms PCC; prothrombin complex concentrate

U.S./Canadian Brand Names Bebulin® VH [US]; Profilnine® SD [US]

Therapeutic Category Antihemophilic Agent

Use Prevention and control of bleeding in patients with factor IX deficiency (hemophilia B or Christmas disease)

Dosage Summary Note: Dosage is expressed in units of factor IX activity and must be individualized

I.V.:

Children:

Bebulin® VH: In general, Factor IX 1 int. unit/kg will increase the plasma factor IX level by 0.8%: Number of Factor IX int. units required = body weight (kg) x desired factor IX increase (% of normal) x 1.2 int. units/kg

Profilnine® SD: In general, Factor IX 1 int. unit/kg will increase the plasma factor IX level by 1%: Number of Factor IX int. units required = bodyweight (kg) x desired factor IX increase (% of normal) x 1 int. unit/kg

Adults:

Bebulin® VH: In general, Factor IX 1 int. unit/kg will increase the plasma factor IX level by 0.8%: Number of Factor IX int. units required = body weight (kg) x desired factor IX increase (% of normal) x 1.2 int. units/kg

Profilnine® SD: In general, Factor IX 1 int. unit/kg will increase the plasma factor IX level by 1%: Number of Factor IX int. units required = bodyweight (kg) x desired factor IX increase (% of normal) x 1 int. unit/kg

Dosage Forms

Injection, powder for reconstitution:

Bebulin® VH: Exact potency labeled on each vial

Profilnine® SD: ~500 int. units, ~1000 int. units, ~1500 int. units [exact potency labeled on each vial]

factor IX concentrate *see* factor IX *on page 389*

Factrel® *(Discontinued)*

famciclovir (fam SYE kloe veer)

Sound-Alike/Look-Alike Issues

Famvir® may be confused with Femara®

U.S./Canadian Brand Names Apo-Famciclovir® [Can]; CO Famciclovir [Can]; Famvir® [US/Can]; PMS-Famciclovir [Can]; Sandoz-Famciclovir [Can]

Therapeutic Category Antiviral Agent

Use Treatment of acute herpes zoster (shingles); treatment and suppression of recurrent episodes of genital herpes in immunocompetent patients; treatment of herpes labialis (cold sores) in immunocompetent patients; treatment of recurrent mucocutaneous/genital herpes simplex in HIV-infected patients

Dosage Summary

Oral:

Children: Dosage not established

Adults: 125-1000 mg twice daily **or** 500 mg every 8 hours **or** 1500 mg once

Dosage Forms

Tablet, oral: 125 mg, 250 mg, 500 mg

Famvir®: 125 mg, 250 mg, 500 mg

famotidine (fa MOE ti deen)

Sound-Alike/Look-Alike Issues

famotidine may be confused with FLUoxetine, furosemide

U.S./Canadian Brand Names Acid Control [Can]; Apo-Famotidine® Injectable [Can]; Apo-Famotidine® [Can]; Famotidine Omega [Can]; Heartburn Relief Maximum Strength [US-OTC]; Heartburn Relief [US-OTC]; Mylan-Famotidine [Can]; Novo-Famotidine [Can]; Nu-Famotidine [Can]; Pepcid® AC Maximum Strength [US-OTC]; Pepcid® AC [US-OTC/Can]; Pepcid® I.V. [Can]; Pepcid® [US/Can]; Ulcidine [Can]

Therapeutic Category Histamine H_2 Antagonist

Use Maintenance therapy and treatment of duodenal ulcer; treatment of gastroesophageal reflux disease (GERD), active benign gastric ulcer; pathological hypersecretory conditions

OTC labeling: Relief of heartburn, acid indigestion, and sour stomach

Dosage Summary

I.V.:

Children <1 year: Dosage not established

Children 1-16 years: 0.25 mg/kg every 12 hours (maximum: 40 mg/day)

Adults: 20 mg every 12 hours

Oral:

Children <3 months: 0.5 mg/kg once daily

Children 3-12 months: 0.5 mg/kg twice daily

Children 1-11 years: 0.5-1 mg/kg/day in 1-2 divided doses (maximum: 80 mg/day; exceptions occur [indication specific])

Children 12-16 years: 0.5-1 mg/kg/day in 1-2 divided doses (maximum: 80 mg/day; exceptions occur [indication specific])

OTC dosing: 10-20 mg every 12 hours (OTC dosing)

Adults: 20-40 mg/day in 1-2 divided doses

OTC dosing: 10-20 mg every 12 hours

Hypersecretory conditions: 20 mg every 6 hours, may increase in increments up to 160 mg every 6 hours

Dosage Forms

Infusion, premixed in NS [preservative free]: 20 mg (50 mL)
Injection, solution: 10 mg/mL (4 mL, 20 mL, 50 mL)
Injection, solution [preservative free]: 10 mg/mL (2 mL)
Powder for suspension, oral: 40 mg/5 mL (50 mL)
Pepcid®: 40 mg/5 mL (50 mL)
Tablet, oral: 10 mg, 20 mg, 40 mg
Heartburn Relief [OTC]: 10 mg
Heartburn Relief Maximum Strength [OTC]: 20 mg
Pepcid®: 20 mg, 40 mg
Pepcid® AC [OTC]: 10 mg
Pepcid® AC Maximum Strength [OTC]: 20 mg
Tablet, chewable, oral:
Pepcid® AC Maximum Strength [OTC]: 20 mg

famotidine, calcium carbonate, and magnesium hydroxide

(fa MOE ti deen, KAL see um KAR bun ate, & mag NEE zhum hye DROKS ide)

Synonyms calcium carbonate, magnesium hydroxide, and famotidine; magnesium hydroxide, famotidine, and calcium carbonate

U.S./Canadian Brand Names Pepcid® Complete® [US-OTC/Can]; Tums® Dual Action [US-OTC]

Therapeutic Category Antacid; Histamine H_2 Antagonist

Use Relief of heartburn due to acid indigestion

Dosage Summary

Oral:
Children <12 years: Dosage not established
Children ≥12 years: 1 tablet as needed (maximum: 2 tablets/day)
Adults: 1 tablet as needed (maximum: 2 tablets/day)

Dosage Forms

Tablet, chewable, oral:
Pepcid® Complete® [OTC], Tums® Dual Action [OTC]: Famotidine 10 mg, calcium carbonate 800 mg, and magnesium hydroxide 165 mg

Famotidine Omega [Can] *see* famotidine *on page 390*
fampridine-SR *see* dalfampridine *on page 266*
Famvir® [US/Can] *see* famciclovir *on page 390*
Fanapt™ [US] *see* iloperidone *on page 498*
Fansidar® ***(Discontinued)*** *see* sulfadoxine and pyrimethamine *on page 901*
2F-ara-AMP *see* fludarabine *on page 408*
Fareston® [US/Can] *see* toremifene *on page 943*
Faslodex® [US] *see* fulvestrant *on page 431*
Fasturtec® [Can] *see* rasburicase *on page 830*

fat emulsion (fat e MUL shun)

Synonyms intravenous fat emulsion

U.S./Canadian Brand Names Intralipid® [US/Can]; Liposyn® II [Can]; Liposyn® III [US]

Therapeutic Category Intravenous Nutritional Therapy

Use Source of calories and essential fatty acids for patients requiring parenteral nutrition of extended duration; prevention and treatment of essential fatty acid deficiency (EFAD)

Dosage Summary Note: Dose should not exceed 60% of the total daily calories

I.V.:
Premature infants: Initial: 0.25-0.5 g/kg/day; Maintenance: Up to 3 g/kg/day (≤1 g/kg/day if on phototherapy); **Note:** Titration is recommended
Infants: Initial: 0.5-1 g/kg/day; Maintenance: Up to 3 g/kg/day; **Note:** Titration is recommended
Children: Initial: 0.5-1 g/kg/day; **Note:** Titration is recommended
Adults: Initial: 1 g/kg/day; Maintenance: Up to 2.5-3 g/kg/day **or** 500 mL twice weekly (prevention of fatty acid deficiency); **Note:** Titration is recommended

Dosage Forms

Injection, emulsion:
Intralipid®: 20% (100 mL, 250 mL, 500 mL, 1000 mL); 30% (500 mL)
Liposyn® III: 10% (500 mL); 20% (500 mL); 30% (500 mL)

Father John's® [US-OTC] *see* dextromethorphan *on page 287*

Father John's® Plus [US-OTC] *see* chlorpheniramine, phenylephrine, and dextromethorphan *on page 211*

FazaClo® [US] *see* clozapine *on page 241*

5-FC *see* flucytosine *on page 408*

FC1157a *see* toremifene *on page 943*

FE200486 *see* degarelix *on page 273*

febuxostat (feb UX oh stat)

Synonyms TEI-6720; TMX-67

U.S./Canadian Brand Names Uloric® [US]

Therapeutic Category Xanthine Oxidase Inhibitor

Use Chronic management of hyperuricemia in patients with gout

Dosage Summary

Oral:

Children: Dosage not established

Adults: 40-80 mg once daily

Dosage Forms

Tablet, oral:

Uloric®: 40 mg, 80 mg

Fedahist® Expectorant *(Discontinued)* *see* guaifenesin and pseudoephedrine *on page 457*

Fedahist® Expectorant Pediatric *(Discontinued)* *see* guaifenesin and pseudoephedrine *on page 457*

Fedahist® Tablet *(Discontinued)* *see* chlorpheniramine and pseudoephedrine *on page 209*

Feen-A-Mint® *(Discontinued)* *see* bisacodyl *on page 138*

Feiba NF [US/Can] *see* antiinhibitor coagulant complex *on page 83*

Feiba VH [US] *see* antiinhibitor coagulant complex *on page 83*

Feiba VH Immuno [Can] *see* antiinhibitor coagulant complex *on page 83*

felbamate (FEL ba mate)

U.S./Canadian Brand Names Felbatol® [US]

Therapeutic Category Anticonvulsant

Use Not as a first-line antiepileptic treatment; only in those patients who respond inadequately to alternative treatments and whose epilepsy is so severe that a substantial risk of aplastic anemia and/or liver failure is deemed acceptable in light of the benefits conferred by its use. Patient must be fully advised of risk and provide signed written informed consent. Felbamate can be used as either monotherapy or adjunctive therapy in the treatment of partial seizures (with and without generalization) and in adults with epilepsy. Used as adjunctive therapy in the treatment of partial and generalized seizures associated with Lennox-Gastaut syndrome in children.

Dosage Summary

Oral:

Adjunctive therapy: **Note:** Dose of concomitant carbamazepine, phenobarbital, phenytoin, or valproic acid should be decreased by 20% to 33% when initiating felbamate therapy. Further dosage reductions may be necessary as dose of felbamate is increased.

Children <2 years: Dosage not established

Children 2-14 years: Initial: 15 mg/kg/day in divided doses 3 or 4 times/day; may increase once per week by 15 mg/kg/day increments up to 45 mg/kg/day in divided doses 3 or 4 times/day (maximum: 3600 mg/day)

Children >14 years: Initial: 1200 mg/day in divided doses 3 or 4 times/day; may increase once per week by 1200 mg/day increments up to 3600 mg/day in divided doses 3 or 4 times/day.

Adults: Initial: 1200 mg/day in divided doses 3 or 4 times/day; may increase once per week by 1200 mg/day increments up to 3600 mg/day in divided doses 3 or 4 times/day.

Monotherapy:

Children ≤14 years: Dosage not established

Children >14 years: Initial: 1200 mg/day in 3-4 divided doses; Maintenance: 2400-3600 mg/day in 3-4 divided doses; **Note:** Titration is recommended

Adults: Initial: 1200 mg/day in 3-4 divided doses; Maintenance: 2400-3600 mg/day in 3-4 divided doses; **Note:** Titration is recommended

Dosage Forms

Suspension, oral:
Felbatol®: 600 mg/5 mL (240 mL, 960 mL)

Tablet, oral:
Felbatol®: 400 mg

Felbatol® [US] *see* felbamate *on page* 392

Feldene® [US] *see* piroxicam *on page* 764

felodipine (fe LOE di peen)

Sound-Alike/Look-Alike Issues
Plendil® may be confused with Isordil®, pindolol, Pletal®, Prilosec®, Prinivil®

U.S./Canadian Brand Names Plendil® [Can]; Renedil® [Can]

Therapeutic Category Calcium Channel Blocker

Use Treatment of hypertension

Dosage Summary

Oral:
Adults: Initial: 2.5-10 mg once daily; Maintenance: 2.5-20 mg once daily (maximum: 20 mg/day)
Elderly: Initial: 2.5 mg/day

Dosage Forms

Tablet, extended release, oral: 2.5 mg, 5 mg, 10 mg

felodipine and enalapril *see* enalapril and felodipine *on page* 348

felodipine and ramipril *see* ramipril and felodipine *(Canada only) on page* 827

Femara® [US/Can] *see* letrozole *on page* 553

Femcet® ***(Discontinued)***

Femcon® Fe [US] *see* ethinyl estradiol and norethindrone *on page* 378

Femguard® ***(Discontinued)*** *see* sulfabenzamide, sulfacetamide, and sulfathiazole *on page* 899

femhrt® [US/Can] *see* ethinyl estradiol and norethindrone *on page* 378

Femilax™ [US-OTC] *see* bisacodyl *on page* 138

Femiron® [US-OTC] *see* ferrous fumarate *on page* 398

Fem-Prin® [US-OTC] *see* acetaminophen, aspirin, and caffeine *on page* 27

Femring® [US] *see* estradiol (systemic) *on page* 366

Femstat® One [Can] *see* butoconazole *on page* 161

Femtrace® [US] *see* estradiol (systemic) *on page* 366

Fenesin DM IR [US] *see* guaifenesin and dextromethorphan *on page* 455

Fenesin IR [US-OTC] *see* guaifenesin *on page* 454

Fenesin PE IR [US] *see* guaifenesin and phenylephrine *on page* 456

fenofibrate (fen oh FYE brate)

Sound-Alike/Look-Alike Issues
TriCor® may be confused with Fibricor®, Tracleer®

Synonyms procetofene; proctofene

U.S./Canadian Brand Names Antara® [US]; Apo-Feno-Micro® [Can]; Apo-Fenofibrate® [Can]; Dom-Fenofibrate Micro [Can]; Feno-Micro-200 [Can]; Fenofibrate Micro [Can]; Fenoglide® [US]; Fenomax [Can]; Lipidil EZ® [Can]; Lipidil Micro® [Can]; Lipidil Supra® [Can]; Lipofen® [US]; Lofibra® [US]; Mylan-Fenofibrate Micro [Can]; Novo-Fenofibrate [Can]; Novo-Fenofibrate-S [Can]; Nu-Fenofibrate [Can]; PHL-Fenofibrate Supra [Can]; PMS-Fenofibrate Micro [Can]; PRO-Feno-Super [Can]; ratio-Fenofibrate MC [Can]; Riva-Fenofibrate Micro [Can]; Sandoz-Fenofibrate S [Can]; TriCor® [US]; Triglide® [US]

Therapeutic Category Antihyperlipidemic Agent, Miscellaneous

Use Adjunct to dietary therapy for the treatment of adults with elevations of serum triglyceride levels (types IV and V hyperlipidemia); adjunct to dietary therapy for the reduction of low density lipoprotein cholesterol (LDL-C), total cholesterol (total-C), triglycerides, and apolipoprotein B (apo B) in adult patients with primary hypercholesterolemia or mixed dyslipidemia (Fredrickson types IIa and IIb)

Dosage Summary

Oral:
Children: Dosage not established

Adults:
Antara® (micronized): 43-130 mg/day (maximum dose: 130 mg/day)
Fenoglide®: 40-120 mg/day (maximum dose: 120 mg/day)
Lipofen®: 50-150 mg/day (maximum dose: 150 mg/day)
Lofibra® (micronized): 67-200 mg/day with meals (maximum dose: 200 mg/day)
Lofibra® (tablets): 54-160 mg/day (maximum dose: 160 mg/day)
TriCor®: 48-145 mg/day (maximum dose: 145 mg/day)
Triglide®: 50-160 mg/day (maximum dose: 160 mg/day)

Elderly:
Antara® (micronized): 43 mg/day
Fenoglide®: Adjust dosage based on creatinine clearance
Lipofen®: 50 mg/day
Lofibra® (micronized): 67 mg/day
Lofibra® (tablets): 54 mg/day
TriCor®: Adjust dosage based on creatinine clearance
Triglide®: 50 mg/day

Dosage Forms

Capsule, oral: 67 mg, 134 mg, 200 mg
Antara®: 43 mg, 130 mg
Lipofen®: 50 mg, 150 mg
Lofibra®: 67 mg, 134 mg, 200 mg

Tablet, oral: 54 mg, 160 mg
Fenoglide®: 40 mg, 120 mg
Lofibra®: 54 mg, 160 mg
TriCor®: 48 mg, 145 mg
Triglide®: 50 mg, 160 mg

Fenofibrate Micro [Can] *see* fenofibrate *on page* 393

fenofibric acid (fen oh FYE brik AS id)

Sound-Alike/Look-Alike Issues
Fibricor™ may be confused with Tricor®
TriLipix® may be confused with Trileptal®, TriLyte®

Synonyms ABT-335; choline fenofibrate

U.S./Canadian Brand Names Fibricor™ [US]; TriLipix® [US]

Therapeutic Category Antilipemic Agent, Fibric Acid

Use Adjunct to dietary therapy for the treatment of severely elevated serum triglyceride levels; adjunct to dietary therapy for the reduction of low density lipoprotein cholesterol (LDL-C), total cholesterol (total-C), triglycerides, and apolipoprotein B (apo B) and to increase high density lipoprotein cholesterol (HDL-C) in patients with primary hypercholesterolemia or mixed dyslipidemia

TriLipix® is also indicated as adjunct to dietary therapy concomitantly with a statin to reduce triglyceride levels and increase HDL-C levels in patients with mixed dyslipidemia and coronary heart disease (CHD) or at risk for CHD

Dosage Summary

Oral:
Children: Dosage not established
Adults: Fibricor™: 35-105 mg once daily (maximum: 105 mg/day); TriLipix™: 45-135 mg once daily (maximum: 135 mg/day)

Dosage Forms

Capsule, delayed release, oral:
TriLipix®: 45 mg, 135 mg

Tablet, oral: 35 mg, 105 mg
Fibricor™: 35 mg, 105 mg

Fenoglide® [US] *see* fenofibrate *on page* 393

fenoldopam (fe NOL doe pam)

Synonyms fenoldopam mesylate

U.S./Canadian Brand Names Corlopam® [US/Can]

Therapeutic Category Antihypertensive Agent

Use Treatment of severe hypertension (up to 48 hours in adults), including in patients with renal compromise; short-term (up to 4 hours) blood pressure reduction in pediatric patients

Dosage Summary

I.V.:

Children: Initial: 0.2 mcg/kg/minute, may increase to 0.3-0.5 mcg/kg/minute every 20-30 minutes (maximum: 0.8 mcg/kg/minute)

Adults: Initial: 0.1-0.3 mcg/kg/minute, may increase in increments of 0.05-0.1 mcg/kg/minute every 15 minutes (maximum: 1.6 mcg/kg/minute)

Dosage Forms

Injection, solution: 10 mg/mL (1 mL, 2 mL)

Corlopam®: 10 mg/mL (1 mL, 2 mL)

fenoldopam mesylate *see* fenoldopam *on page* 394

Fenomax [Can] *see* fenofibrate *on page* 393

Feno-Micro-200 [Can] *see* fenofibrate *on page* 393

fenoprofen (fen oh PROE fen)

Sound-Alike/Look-Alike Issues

fenoprofen may be confused with flurbiprofen

Nalfon® may be confused with Naldecon®

Synonyms fenoprofen calcium

U.S./Canadian Brand Names Nalfon® [US/Can]

Therapeutic Category Analgesic, Nonnarcotic; Nonsteroidal Antiinflammatory Drug (NSAID)

Use Symptomatic treatment of acute and chronic rheumatoid arthritis and osteoarthritis; relief of mild-to-moderate pain

Dosage Summary

Oral:

Children: Dosage not established

Adults: 200 mg every 4-6 hours as needed **or** 300-600 mg 3-4 times/day (maximum: 3.2 g/day)

Dosage Forms

Capsule, oral:

Nalfon®: 200 mg

Tablet, oral: 600 mg

fenoprofen calcium *see* fenoprofen *on page* 395

fenoterol and ipratropium *see* ipratropium and fenoterol *(Canada only) on page* 524

fenoterol hydrobromide and ipratropium bromide *see* ipratropium and fenoterol *(Canada only) on page* 524

fentanyl (FEN ta nil)

Sound-Alike/Look-Alike Issues

fentaNYL may be confused with alfentanil, SUFentanil

Synonyms fentanyl citrate; fentanyl hydrochloride; fentanyl patch; OTFC (oral transmucosal fentanyl citrate)

Tall-Man fenta**NYL**

U.S./Canadian Brand Names Actiq® [US/Can]; Duragesic® MAT [Can]; Duragesic® [US/Can]; Fentanyl Citrate Injection, USP [Can]; Fentora® [US]; Novo-Fentanyl [Can]; Onsolis™ [US]; PMS-Fentanyl MTX [Can]; RAN™-Fentanyl Matrix Patch [Can]; RAN™-Fentanyl Transdermal System [Can]; ratio-Fentanyl [Can]

Therapeutic Category Analgesic, Narcotic; General Anesthetic

Controlled Substance C-II

Use

Injection: Relief of pain, preoperative medication, adjunct to general or regional anesthesia

Iontophoretic transdermal system (Ionsys™): Short-term, in-hospital management of acute postoperative pain

Transdermal patch (eg, Duragesic®): Management of persistent moderate-to-severe chronic pain

Transmucosal lozenge (eg, Actiq®), buccal tablet (Fentora®), buccal film (Onsolis™): Management of breakthrough cancer pain in opioid-tolerant patients

Dosage Summary Note: These are guidelines and do not represent the maximum doses that may be required in all patients. Doses should be titrated to pain relief/prevention.

I.M.:

Children: Dosage not established

Adults: 50-100 mcg/dose every 1-2 hours as needed (unlabeled) **or** 50-100 mcg/dose prior to surgery

I.V.:

Children <2 year: Dosage not established

Transmucosal buccal film (Onsolis™):

Children <18 years: Dosage not established

Adults: Initial: 200 mcg; titration, if needed, may be done in increments of 200 mcg per episode of breakthrough pain; maintenance dose range: 200-1200 mcg; maximum dose: 1200 mcg film; maximum frequency: 4 applications/day; do not exceed 4 simultaneous applications of the 200 mcg films

Transmucosal buccal tablet (Fentora®):

Children <18 years: Dosage not established

Adults: Initial: 100 mcg; a second dose, if needed, may be started 30 minutes after the start of the first dose (maximum: 2 doses per breakthrough pain episode every 4 hours)

Transmucosal lozenge (Actiq®):

Children <16 years: Dosage not established

Children ≥16 years: Initial: 200 mcg; the second dose may be started 15 minutes after completion of the first dose if pain unrelieved (maximum: 2 doses per breakthrough pain episode every 4 hours; maximum daily dose: 4 units/day)

Adults: Initial: 200 mcg; the second dose may be started 15 minutes after completion of the first dose if pain unrelieved (maximum: 2 doses per breakthrough pain episode every 4 hours; maximum daily dose: 4 units/day)

Elderly: In clinical trials, patients who were >65 years of age were titrated to a mean dose that was 200 mcg less than that of younger patients.

Transdermal:

Patch:

Children <2 years: Dosage not established

Children ≥2 years: Initial: Opioid-tolerant: Convert 24-hour analgesic requirements to patch using tables; Fentanyl infusion: Dose at rate equivalent to the I.V. rate; Patches range from 12.5-300 mcg/hour applied every 72 hours; **Note:** Titration is recommended

Adults: Initial: Opioid-tolerant: Convert 24-hour analgesic requirements to patch using tables; Fentanyl infusion: Dose at rate equivalent to the I.V. rate; Patches range from 12.5-300 mcg/hour applied every 72 hours; **Note:** Titration is recommended

Dosage Forms

Film, for buccal application:

Onsolis™: 200 mcg (30s); 400 mcg (30s); 600 mcg (30s); 800 mcg (30s); 1200 mcg (30s)

Injection, solution [preservative free]: 0.05 mg/mL (2 mL, 5 mL, 10 mL, 20 mL, 30 mL, 50 mL)

Lozenge, oral: 200 mcg (30s); 400 mcg (30s); 600 mcg (30s); 800 mcg (30s); 1200 mcg (30s); 1600 mcg (30s)

Actiq®: 200 mcg (30s); 400 mcg (30s); 600 mcg (30s); 800 mcg (30s); 1200 mcg (30s); 1600 mcg (30s)

Patch, transdermal: 12.5 mcg/hr (5s); 25 mcg/hr (5s); 50 mcg/hr (5s); 75 mcg/hr (5s); 100 mcg/hr (5s)

Duragesic®: 12.5 mcg/hr (5s); 25 mcg/hr (5s); 50 mcg/hr (5s); 75 mcg/hr (5s); 100 mcg/hr (5s)

Powder, for prescription compounding: USP: 100% (1 g)

Tablet, for buccal application:

Fentora®: 100 mcg (28s); 200 mcg (28s); 400 mcg (28s); 600 mcg (28s); 800 mcg (28s)

Dosage Forms - Canada

Patch, transdermal, as base: 12 mcg/hr (5s); 25 mcg/hr (5s); 50 mcg/hr (5s); 75 mcg/hr (5s); 100 mcg/hr (5s)

Duragesic® MAT: 12 mcg/hr (5s); 25 mcg/hr (5s); 50 mcg/hr (5s); 75 mcg/hr (5s); 100 mcg/hr (5s)

fentanyl citrate *see* fentanyl *on page 395*

Fentanyl Citrate Injection, USP [Can] *see* fentanyl *on page 395*

fentanyl hydrochloride *see* fentanyl *on page 395*

Fentanyl Oralet® ***(Discontinued)*** *see* fentanyl *on page 395*

fentanyl patch *see* fentanyl *on page 395*

Fentora® [US] *see* fentanyl *on page 395*

Feosol® [US-OTC] *see* ferrous sulfate *on page 398*

Feosol® Elixir ***(Discontinued)*** *see* ferrous sulfate *on page 398*

Feostat® ***(Discontinued)*** *see* ferrous fumarate *on page 398*

Feraheme™ [US] *see* ferumoxytol *on page 399*

Ferancee® *(Discontinued)* *see* ferrous sulfate and ascorbic acid *on page 399*
Feratab® *(Discontinued)* *see* ferrous sulfate *on page 398*
Fer-Gen-Sol *(Discontinued)* *see* ferrous sulfate *on page 398*
Fergon® [US-OTC] *see* ferrous gluconate *on page 398*
Feridex I.V.® *(Discontinued)* *see* ferumoxides *on page 399*
Fer-In-Sol® [US-OTC/Can] *see* ferrous sulfate *on page 398*
Fer-In-Sol® Syrup *(Discontinued)* *see* ferrous sulfate *on page 398*
Fer-iron [US-OTC] *see* ferrous sulfate *on page 398*
Fermalac [Can] *see* Lactobacillus *on page 543*
Ferodan™ [Can] *see* ferrous sulfate *on page 398*
Fero-Grad 500® *(Discontinued)* *see* ferrous sulfate and ascorbic acid *on page 399*
Fero-Gradumet® *(Discontinued)* *see* ferrous sulfate *on page 398*
Ferospace® *(Discontinued)* *see* ferrous sulfate *on page 398*
Ferralet® *(Discontinued)* *see* ferrous gluconate *on page 398*
Ferralyn® Lanacaps® *(Discontinued)* *see* ferrous sulfate *on page 398*
Ferra-TD® *(Discontinued)* *see* ferrous sulfate *on page 398*
Ferretts® [US-OTC] *see* ferrous fumarate *on page 398*
Ferrex™ 150 [US-OTC] *see* polysaccharide-iron complex *on page 777*
Ferrex™ 150 Forte [US] *see* polysaccharide-iron complex, vitamin B12, and folic acid *on page 778*
Ferrex™ 150 Forte Plus [US] *see* polysaccharide-iron complex, vitamin B12, and folic acid *on page 778*
Ferrex™ 150 Plus [US-OTC] *see* polysaccharide-iron complex *on page 777*
ferric (III) hexacyanoferrate (II) *see* ferric hexacyanoferrate *on page 397*

ferric gluconate (FER ik GLOO koe nate)

Sound-Alike/Look-Alike Issues
ferric gluconate may be confused with ferumoxytol
Ferrlecit® may be confused with Ferralet®

Synonyms sodium ferric gluconate

U.S./Canadian Brand Names Ferrlecit® [US/Can]

Therapeutic Category Iron Salt

Use Repletion of total body iron content in patients with iron-deficiency anemia who are undergoing hemodialysis in conjunction with erythropoietin therapy

Dosage Summary

I.V.:
Children <6 years: Dosage not established
Children ≥6 years: 1.5 mg/kg of elemental iron at 8 sequential dialysis sessions (maximum: 125 mg/dose)
Adults: 125 mg of elemental iron at ~8 sequential dialysis treatments to make a cumulative dose of 1 g

Dosage Forms

Injection, solution:
Ferrlecit®: Elemental iron 12.5 mg/mL (5 mL)

ferric hexacyanoferrate (FER ik hex a SYE an oh fer ate)

Synonyms ferric (III) hexacyanoferrate (II); insoluble prussian blue; prussian blue

U.S./Canadian Brand Names Radiogardase® [US]

Therapeutic Category Antidote

Use Treatment of known or suspected internal contamination with radioactive cesium and/or radioactive or nonradioactive thallium

Dosage Summary

Oral:
Children <2 years: Dosage not established
Children 2-12 years: 1 g 3 times/day
Children >12 years: 3 g 3 times/day, may reduce to 1-2 g 3 times/day once internal radioactivity is substantially decreased with cesium exposure
Adults: 3 g 3 times/day, may reduce to 1-2 g 3 times/day once internal radioactivity is substantially decreased with cesium exposure

Dosage Forms

Capsule, oral:

Radiogardase®: 0.5 g

Ferrlecit® [US/Can] *see* ferric gluconate *on page 397*

Ferro-Sequels® [US-OTC] *see* ferrous fumarate *on page 398*

ferrous fumarate (FER us FYOO ma rate)

Synonyms iron fumarate

U.S./Canadian Brand Names Femiron® [US-OTC]; Ferretts® [US-OTC]; Ferro-Sequels® [US-OTC]; Hemocyte® [US-OTC]; Ircon® [US-OTC]; Palafer® [Can]

Therapeutic Category Electrolyte Supplement, Oral

Use Prevention and treatment of iron-deficiency anemias

Dosage Summary Doses expressed in terms of elemental iron.

Oral:

Children: 1-6 mg elemental iron/kg/day in 1-3 divided doses

Adults: 60 mg elemental iron 2-4 times/day

Dosage Forms

Tablet, oral: 324 mg

Femiron® [OTC]: 63 mg

Ferretts® [OTC]: 325 mg

Hemocyte® [OTC]: 324 mg

Ircon® [OTC]: 200 mg

Tablet, timed release, oral:

Ferro-Sequels® [OTC]: 150 mg

ferrous gluconate (FER us GLOO koe nate)

Synonyms iron gluconate

U.S./Canadian Brand Names Apo-Ferrous Gluconate® [Can]; Fergon® [US-OTC]; Novo-Ferrogluc [Can]

Therapeutic Category Electrolyte Supplement, Oral

Use Prevention and treatment of iron-deficiency anemias

Dosage Summary

Oral:

Children: 1-6 mg Fe/kg/day in 1-3 divided doses

Adults: 60 mg 1-4 times/day

Dosage Forms

Tablet, oral: 246 mg, 324 mg, 325 mg

Fergon® [OTC]: 240 mg

ferrous sulfate (FER us SUL fate)

Sound-Alike/Look-Alike Issues

Feosol® may be confused with Fer-In-Sol®

Fer-In-Sol® may be confused with Feosol®

Slow FE® may be confused with Slow-K®

Synonyms $FeSO_4$; iron sulfate

U.S./Canadian Brand Names Apo-Ferrous Sulfate® [Can]; Feosol® [US-OTC]; Fer-In-Sol® [US-OTC/Can]; Fer-iron [US-OTC]; Ferodan™ [Can]; MyKidz Iron 10™ [US-OTC]; Slow FE® [US-OTC]

Therapeutic Category Electrolyte Supplement, Oral

Use Prevention and treatment of iron-deficiency anemias

Dosage Summary

Oral:

Extended release:

Children: Dosage not established

Adults: 250 mg 1-2 times/day

Immediate release:

Children: 1-6 mg Fe/kg/day in 1-3 divided doses (maximum: 15 mg/day [prophylaxis dosing])

Adults: 300 mg 1-4 times/day

Dosage Forms

Elixir, oral: 220 mg/5 mL (473 mL, 480 mL)

Liquid, oral: 300 mg/5 mL (5 mL); 75 mg/mL (50 mL); 75 mg/0.6 mL (50 mL)

Fer-In-Sol® [OTC]: 75 mg/mL (50 mL)

Fer-iron [OTC]: 75 mg/mL (50 mL)

Suspension, oral:

MyKidz Iron 10™ [OTC]: 75 mg/1.5 mL (118 mL)

Tablet, oral: 324 mg, 325 mg

Feosol® [OTC]: 200 mg

Tablet, enteric coated, oral: 324 mg, 325 mg

Tablet, extended release, oral: 160 mg

Tablet, slow release, oral: 160 mg

Tablet, timed release, oral:

Slow FE® [OTC]: 160 mg

ferrous sulfate and ascorbic acid (FER us SUL fate & a SKOR bik AS id)

Synonyms ascorbic acid and ferrous sulfate; iron sulfate and vitamin C

Therapeutic Category Vitamin

Use Treatment of iron deficiency in nonpregnant adults; treatment and prevention of iron deficiency in pregnant adults

Dosage Summary

Oral:

Children: Dosage not established

Adults: 1 tablet daily

Fertinorm® H.P. [Can] *see* urofollitropin *on page* *971*

ferumoxides (fer yoo MOX ides)

Sound-Alike/Look-Alike Issues

Feridex I.V.® may be confused with Fertinex®

Therapeutic Category Radiopaque Agents

Use For I.V. administration as an adjunct to MRI (in adult patients) to enhance the T2 weighted images used in the detection and evaluation of lesions of the liver

Dosage Summary

I.V.:

Children: Dosage not established

Adults: 0.56 mg of iron (0.05 mL Feridex I.V.®)/kg body weight) as a single dose as an adjunct to MRI

ferumoxytol (fer ue MOX i tol)

Sound-Alike/Look-Alike Issues

ferumoxytol may be confused with ferric gluconate, iron dextran complex, iron sucrose

U.S./Canadian Brand Names Feraheme™ [US]

Therapeutic Category Iron Salt

Use Treatment of iron-deficiency anemia in chronic kidney disease

Dosage Summary

I.V.:

Children: Dosage not established

Adults: 510 mg (17 mL) as a single dose, followed by a second 510 mg dose 3-8 days after initial dose

Dosage Forms

Injection, solution:

Feraheme™: Elemental iron 30 mg/mL (17 mL)

FESO *see* fesoterodine *on page* *399*

$FeSO_4$ *see* ferrous sulfate *on page* *398*

fesoterodine (fes oh TER oh deen)

Sound-Alike/Look-Alike Issues

fesoterodine may be confused with fexofenadine, tolterodine

Synonyms FESO; fesoterodine fumarate

U.S./Canadian Brand Names Toviaz™ [US]

Therapeutic Category Anticholinergic Agent

Use Treatment of patients with an overactive bladder with symptoms of urinary frequency, urgency, or urge incontinence.

Dosage Summary

Oral:

Children <18 years: Dosage not established

Adults: 4-8 mg once daily; Adjusted dosage: 4 mg/day

Dosage Forms

Tablet, extended release, oral:

Toviaz™: 4 mg, 8 mg

fesoterodine fumarate *see* fesoterodine *on page* *399*

Fe-Tinic™ 150 ***(Discontinued)*** *see* polysaccharide-iron complex *on page* *777*

FeverAll® [US-OTC] *see* acetaminophen *on page* *21*

Fexmid® [US] *see* cyclobenzaprine *on page* *258*

fexofenadine (feks oh FEN a deen)

Sound-Alike/Look-Alike Issues

fexofenadine may be confused with fesoterodine

Allegra® may be confused with Viagra®

Synonyms fexofenadine hydrochloride

U.S./Canadian Brand Names Allegra® ODT [US]; Allegra® [US/Can]

Therapeutic Category Antihistamine

Use Relief of symptoms associated with seasonal allergic rhinitis; treatment of chronic idiopathic urticaria

Dosage Summary

Oral:

Children 6 months to <2 years: 15 mg twice daily

Children 2-11 years: 30 mg twice daily

Children ≥12 years: 60 mg twice daily **or** 180 mg once daily

Adults: 60 mg twice daily **or** 180 mg once daily

Elderly: Initial: 60 mg once daily

Dosage Forms

Suspension, oral:

Allegra®: 6 mg/mL (300 mL)

Tablet, oral: 30 mg, 60 mg, 180 mg

Allegra®: 60 mg, 180 mg

Tablet, orally disintegrating, oral:

Allegra® ODT: 30 mg

fexofenadine and pseudoephedrine (feks oh FEN a deen & soo doe e FED rin)

Sound-Alike/Look-Alike Issues

Allegra-D® may be confused with Viagra®

Synonyms pseudoephedrine and fexofenadine

U.S./Canadian Brand Names Allegra-D® 12 Hour [US]; Allegra-D® 24 Hour [US]; Allegra-D® [Can]

Therapeutic Category Antihistamine/Decongestant Combination

Use Relief of symptoms associated with seasonal allergic rhinitis in adults and children ≥12 years of age

Dosage Summary

Oral:

Children <12 years: Dosage not established

Children ≥12 years:

Allegra-D® 12 Hour: One tablet twice daily

Allegra-D® 24 Hour: One tablet once daily

Adults:

Allegra-D® 12 Hour: One tablet twice daily

Allegra-D® 24 Hour: One tablet once daily

Dosage Forms

Tablet, extended release: Fexofenadine 60 mg [immediate release] and pseudoephedrine 120 mg [extended release]

Allegra-D® 12 Hour: Fexofenadine 60 mg [immediate release] and pseudoephedrine 120 mg [extended release]

Allegra-D® 24 Hour: Fexofenadine 180 mg [immediate release] and pseudoephedrine 240 mg [extended release]

fexofenadine hydrochloride *see* fexofenadine *on page 400*

Fiberall® [US-OTC] *see* psyllium *on page 814*

FiberCon® [US-OTC] *see* polycarbophil *on page 774*

Fiber-Lax [US-OTC] *see* polycarbophil *on page 774*

Fiber-Tabs™ [US-OTC] *see* polycarbophil *on page 774*

Fibricor™ [US] *see* fenofibric acid *on page 394*

fibrinogen concentrate (human) (fi BRIN o gin KON suhn trate HYU man)

Synonyms coagulation factor I

U.S./Canadian Brand Names RiaSTAP™ [US]

Therapeutic Category Blood Product Derivative

Use Treatment of acute bleeding episodes in patients with congenital fibrinogen deficiency (afibrinogenemia and hypofibrinogenemia)

Dosage Summary

I.V.:

Children:

When baseline fibrinogen level is known: Dose (mg/kg) = [Target level (mg/dL) - measured level (mg/dL)] **divided by** 1.7 (mg/dL per mg/kg body weight)

When baseline fibrinogen level is not known: 70 mg/kg

Adults:

When baseline fibrinogen level is known: Dose (mg/kg) = [Target level (mg/dL) - measured level (mg/dL)] **divided by** 1.7 (mg/dL per mg/kg body weight)

When baseline fibrinogen level is not known: 70 mg/kg

Dosage Forms

Injection, powder for reconstitution:

RiaSTAP™: 900-1300 mg [contains albumin (human); exact potency labeled on vial]

fibrin sealant (FI brin SEEL ent)

Synonyms fibrin sealant (human); FS; FS VH S/D; TachoSil®

U.S./Canadian Brand Names Artiss™ [US]; Crosseal™ [US]; Evicel™ [US]; Tisseel® VH S/D [US]; Tisseel® VH [Can]

Therapeutic Category Hemostatic Agent

Use

Artiss™: Aid in adhering autologous skin grafts in burn patients (not indicated for hemostasis)

Evicel™: Adjunct to hemostasis in surgery when control of bleeding by conventional surgical techniques is ineffective or impractical

Tisseel® VH: Adjunct to hemostasis in cardiopulmonary bypass surgery and splenic injury (due to blunt or penetrating trauma to the abdomen) when the control of bleeding by conventional surgical techniques is ineffective or impractical; adjunctive sealant for closure of colostomies; hemostatic agent in heparinized patients undergoing cardiopulmonary bypass

Dosage Summary

Topical:

Children ≤6 months: Dosage not established

Children >6 months: Evicel™: To cover layer of 1 mm thickness: Apply 1 mL for every 20 cm^2 coverage area needed; may apply second layer if needed

Children ≥1 year: Artiss™: Spray a thin layer; ~1 mL for every 50 cm^2 graft area needed

Adults:

Artiss™: Spray a thin layer; ~1 mL for every 50 cm^2 graft area needed

Evicel™: To cover layer of 1 mm thickness: Apply 1 mL for every 20 cm^2 coverage area needed; may apply second layer if needed

Tisseel® VH: Apply thin layers of ~2 mL for every 8 cm^2 coverage area needed

Product Availability

TachoSil®: FDA approved April 2010; availability expected in the second half of 2010

TachoSil® is an absorbable fibrin sealant patch approved as an adjunct to hemostasis in cardiovascular surgery when control of bleeding by conventional surgical techniques is ineffective or impractical.

Dosage Forms

Kit [each 2 mL kit contains]: Tisseel® VH S/D:
- Powder for solution, topical:
  - Fibrinogen 67-106 mg/mL
  - Thrombin 400-625 int. units/mL
- Solution, topical:
  - Aprotinin 2250-3750 KIU/mL
  - Calcium chloride 36-44 µmol/mL

Kit [each 2 mL kit contains, preservative free]: Evicel™: Solution, topical:
- Fibrinogen 55-85 mg/mL (1 mL)
- Thrombin 800-1200 int. units/mL
- Calcium chloride 5.6-6.2 mg/mL (1 mL)

Kit [each 4 mL kit contains]:
- Artiss™:
  - Powder for solution, topical:
    - Fibrinogen 67-106 mg/mL
    - Thrombin 2.5-6.5 int. units/mL
  - Solution, topical:
    - Aprotinin 2250-3750 KIU/mL
    - Calcium chloride 36-44 µmol/mL
- Tisseel® VH S/D:
  - Powder for solution, topical:
    - Fibrinogen 67-106 mg/mL
    - Thrombin 400-625 int. units/mL
  - Solution, topical:
    - Aprotinin 2250-3750 KIU/mL
    - Calcium chloride 36-44 µmol/mL

Kit [each 4 mL kit contains, preservative free]: Evicel™: Solution, topical:
- Calcium chloride 5.6-6.2 mg/mL (2 mL)
- Fibrinogen 55-85 mg/mL (2 mL)
- Thrombin 800-1200 int. units/mL

Kit [each 10 mL kit contains]:
- Artiss™:
  - Powder, for solution, topical:
    - Fibrinogen 67-106 mg/mL
    - Thrombin 2.5-6.5 int. units/mL
  - Solution, topical:
    - Calcium chloride 36-44 µmol/mL
    - Aprotinin 2250-3750 KIU/mL
- Tisseel® VH S/D:
  - Powder for solution, topical:
    - Fibrinogen 67-106 mg/mL
    - Thrombin 400-625 int. units/mL
  - Solution, topical:
    - Aprotinin 2250-3750 KIU/mL
    - Calcium chloride 36-44 µmol/mL

Kit [each 10 mL kit contains, preservative free]: Evicel™:
- Solution, topical:
  - Fibrinogen 55-85 mg/mL (5 mL)
  - Thrombin 800-1200 int. units/mL
  - Calcium chloride 5.6-6.2 mg/mL (5 mL)

Kit, topical [each kit contains]: Crosseal™:
- Calcium chloride 5.6-6.0 mg/mL
- Fibrinogen 40-60 mg/mL
- Spray application device: Thrombin 800-1200 int. units/mL (1 mL, 2 mL, 5 mL)

Solution, topical [each dual-chamber 2 mL prefilled syringe contains]: Tisseel™ VH S/D:
Sealer protein chamber:
Aprotinin 2250-3750 KIU/mL
Fibrinogen 67-106 mg/mL
Thrombin chamber:
Calcium chloride 36-44 µmol/mL
Thrombin 400-625 int. units/mL

Solution, topical [each dual-chamber 4 mL prefilled syringe contains]: Tisseel™ VH S/D:
Sealer protein chamber:
Aprotinin 2250-3750 KIU/mL
Fibrinogen 67-106 mg/mL
Thrombin chamber:
Calcium chloride 36-44 µmol/mL
Thrombin 400-625 int. units/mL

Solution, topical [each dual-chamber 10 mL prefilled syringe contains]: Tisseel™ VH S/D:
Sealer protein chamber:
Aprotinin 2250-3750 KIU/mL
Fibrinogen 67-106 mg/mL
Thrombin chamber:
Calcium chloride 36-44 µmol/mL
Thrombin 400-625 int. units/mL

fibrin sealant (human) *see* fibrin sealant *on page 401*
Fibro-XL [US-OTC] *see* psyllium *on page 814*
Fibro-Lax [US-OTC] *see* psyllium *on page 814*

filgrastim (fil GRA stim)

Sound-Alike/Look-Alike Issues
Neupogen® may be confused with Epogen®, Neulasta®, Neumega®, Neupro®, Nutramigen®

Synonyms G-CSF; granulocyte colony-stimulating factor; NSC-614629

U.S./Canadian Brand Names Neupogen® [US/Can]

Therapeutic Category Colony-Stimulating Factor

Use Stimulation of granulocyte production in chemotherapy-induced neutropenia (nonmyeloid malignancies, acute myeloid leukemia, and bone marrow transplantation); severe chronic neutropenia (SCN); moblilization of hematopoietic progenitor cells in patients undergoing peripheral blood progenitor cell (PBPC) collection

Dosage Summary **Note:** Dosing should be based on actual body weight (even in morbidly obese patients).
I.V.:
Children: 5-10 mcg/kg/day
Adults: 5-10 mcg/kg/day
SubQ:
Children: 5-10 mcg/kg/day **or** 6 mcg/kg twice daily
Adults: 5-10 mcg/kg/day **or** 6 mcg/kg twice daily

Dosage Forms
Injection, solution [preservative free]:
Neupogen®: 300 mcg/mL (1 mL, 1.6 mL); 600 mcg/mL (0.5 mL, 0.8 mL)

Finacea® [US/Can] *see* azelaic acid *on page 110*
Finacea® Plus™ [US] *see* azelaic acid *on page 110*

finasteride (fi NAS teer ide)

Sound-Alike/Look-Alike Issues
finasteride may be confused with furosemide
Proscar® may be confused with ProSom®, Provera®, Prozac®, Psorcon®

U.S./Canadian Brand Names PMS-Finasteride [Can]; Propecia® [US/Can]; Proscar® [US/Can]; ratio-Finasteride [Can]; Sandoz-Finasteride [Can]

Therapeutic Category Antiandrogen

Use

Propecia®: Treatment of male pattern hair loss in **men only**. Safety and efficacy were demonstrated in men between 18-41 years of age.

Proscar®: Treatment of symptomatic benign prostatic hyperplasia (BPH); can be used in combination with an alpha-blocker, doxazosin

Dosage Summary

Oral:

Children: Dosage not established

Adults:

BPH: 5 mg once daily

Male pattern baldness: 1 mg once daily

Dosage Forms

Tablet, oral: 5 mg

Propecia®: 1 mg

Proscar®: 5 mg

Fiorgen PF® ***(Discontinued)***

Fioricet® [US] *see* butalbital, acetaminophen, and caffeine *on page 159*

Fioricet® with Codeine [US] *see* butalbital, acetaminophen, caffeine, and codeine *on page 159*

Fiorinal® [US/Can] *see* butalbital, aspirin, and caffeine *on page 160*

Fiorinal®-C 1/2 [Can] *see* butalbital, aspirin, caffeine, and codeine *on page 160*

Fiorinal®-C 1/4 [Can] *see* butalbital, aspirin, caffeine, and codeine *on page 160*

Fiorinal® with Codeine [US] *see* butalbital, aspirin, caffeine, and codeine *on page 160*

Firmagon® [US/Can] *see* degarelix *on page 273*

First™-Progesterone VGS 25 [US] *see* progesterone *on page 799*

First™-Progesterone VGS 50 [US] *see* progesterone *on page 799*

First™-Progesterone VGS 100 [US] *see* progesterone *on page 799*

First™-Progesterone VGS 200 [US] *see* progesterone *on page 799*

First™-Progesterone VGS 400 [US] *see* progesterone *on page 799*

First®-Testosterone [US] *see* testosterone *on page 919*

First®-Testosterone MC [US] *see* testosterone *on page 919*

fisalamine *see* mesalamine *on page 607*

fish oil *see* omega-3-acid ethyl esters *on page 701*

FK228 *see* romidepsin *on page 850*

FK506 *see* tacrolimus (systemic) *on page 907*

Flagyl® [US/Can] *see* metronidazole (systemic) *on page 627*

Flagyl® 375 [US] *see* metronidazole (systemic) *on page 627*

Flagyl® ER [US] *see* metronidazole (systemic) *on page 627*

Flagystatin® [Can] *see* metronidazole and nystatin *(Canada only) on page 628*

Flamazine® [Can] *see* silver sulfadiazine *on page 875*

Flarex® [US/Can] *see* fluorometholone *on page 414*

flavan *see* flavocoxid *on page 404*

flavocoxid (fla vo KOKS id)

Synonyms flavan; flavonoid

U.S./Canadian Brand Names Limbrel 250™ [US]; Limbrel 500™ [US]

Therapeutic Category Antiinflammatory Agent

Use Clinical dietary management of the metabolic processes of osteoarthritis

Dosage Summary

Oral:

Children: Dosage not established

Adults: 250-500 mg every 12 hours

Dosage Forms

Capsule, oral:

Limbrel 250™: 250 mg

Limbrel 500™: 500 mg

flavonoid *see* flavocoxid *on page 404*

Flavorcee® ***(Discontinued)*** *see* ascorbic acid *on page 98*

flavoxate (fla VOKS ate)

Sound-Alike/Look-Alike Issues

flavoxate may be confused with fluvoxamine
Urispas® may be confused with Urised®

Synonyms flavoxate hydrochloride

U.S./Canadian Brand Names Apo-Flavoxate® [Can]; Urispas® [US/Can]

Therapeutic Category Antispasmodic Agent, Urinary

Use Antispasmodic to provide symptomatic relief of dysuria, nocturia, suprapubic pain, urgency, and incontinence due to detrusor instability and hyperreflexia in elderly with cystitis, urethritis, urethrocystitis, urethrotrigonitis, and prostatitis

Dosage Summary

Oral:

Children ≤12 years: Dosage not established
Children >12 years: 100-200 mg 3-4 times/day
Adults: 100-200 mg 3-4 times/day

Dosage Forms

Tablet, oral: 100 mg

flavoxate hydrochloride *see* flavoxate *on page 405*
Flebogamma® [US] *see* immune globulin (intravenous) *on page 502*
Flebogamma® DIF [US] *see* immune globulin (intravenous) *on page 502*

flecainide (fle KAY nide)

Sound-Alike/Look-Alike Issues

flecainide may be confused with fluconazole
Tambocor™ may be confused with Pamelor®, Temodar®, tamoxifen, Tamiflu®

Synonyms flecainide acetate

U.S./Canadian Brand Names Apo-Flecainide® [Can]; Tambocor™ [US/Can]

Therapeutic Category Antiarrhythmic Agent, Class I-C

Use Prevention and suppression of documented life-threatening ventricular arrhythmias (eg, sustained ventricular tachycardia); controlling symptomatic, disabling supraventricular tachycardias in patients without structural heart disease in whom other agents fail

Dosage Summary

Oral:

Children: Initial: 3 mg/kg/day **or** 50-100 mg/m^2/day in 3 divided doses; Maintenance: 3-6 mg/kg/day **or** 100-150 mg/m^2/day in 3 divided doses (maximum: 11 mg/kg/day; 200 mg/m^2/day)
Adults: Initial: 50-100 mg every 12 hours; Maintenance: 100-400 mg/day in 2 divided doses (maximum: 400 mg/day; exceptions occur [indication specific]); **Note:** Titration is recommended

Dosage Forms

Tablet, oral: 50 mg, 100 mg, 150 mg
Tambocor™: 50 mg, 100 mg, 150 mg

flecainide acetate *see* flecainide *on page 405*
Flector® [US] *see* diclofenac (topical) *on page 297*
Fleet® Babylax® ***(Discontinued)*** *see* glycerin *on page 449*
Fleet® Bisacodyl [US-OTC] *see* bisacodyl *on page 138*
Fleet® Enema [US-OTC/Can] *see* sodium phosphates *on page 887*
Fleet® Enema Extra® [US-OTC] *see* sodium phosphates *on page 887*
Fleet® Flavored Castor Oil ***(Discontinued)*** *see* castor oil *on page 187*
Fleet® Glycerin Maximum Strength [US-OTC] *see* glycerin *on page 449*
Fleet® Glycerin Suppositories [US-OTC] *see* glycerin *on page 449*
Fleet® Laxative ***(Discontinued)*** *see* bisacodyl *on page 138*
Fleet® Liquid Glycerin [US-OTC] *see* glycerin *on page 449*
Fleet® Pedia-Lax™ Chewable Tablet [US-OTC] *see* magnesium hydroxide *on page 585*
Fleet® Pedia-Lax™ Enema [US-OTC] *see* sodium phosphates *on page 887*
Fleet® Pedia-Lax™ Glycerin Suppositories [US-OTC] *see* glycerin *on page 449*

Fleet® Pedia-Lax™ Liquid Glycerin Suppositories [US-OTC] *see* glycerin *on page* 449
Fleet® Pedia-Lax™ Liquid Stool Softener [US-OTC] *see* docusate *on page* 321
Fleet® Pedia-Lax™ Quick Dissolve [US-OTC] *see* senna *on page* 870
Fleet® Phospho-soda® *(Discontinued)* *see* sodium phosphates *on page* 887
Fleet® Phospho-soda® EZ-Prep™ *(Discontinued)* *see* sodium phosphates *on page* 887
Fleet® Sof-lax® [US-OTC] *see* docusate *on page* 321
Fleet® Stimulant Laxative [US-OTC] *see* bisacodyl *on page* 138
Fletcher's® [US-OTC] *see* senna *on page* 870
Flexaphen® *(Discontinued)* *see* chlorzoxazone *on page* 217
Flexbumin 25% [US] *see* albumin *on page* 43
Flexeril® [US/Can] *see* cyclobenzaprine *on page* 258
Flexitec [Can] *see* cyclobenzaprine *on page* 258
Flex-Power [US-OTC] *see* trolamine *on page* 963
Flextra-650 [US] *see* acetaminophen and phenyltoloxamine *on page* 26
Flextra-DS [US] *see* acetaminophen and phenyltoloxamine *on page* 26
Flintstones™ Complete [US-OTC] *see* vitamins (multiple/pediatric) *on page* 990
Flintstones™ Gummies [US-OTC] *see* vitamins (multiple/pediatric) *on page* 990
Flintstones™ Gummies Vita-Packs [US-OTC] *see* vitamins (multiple/pediatric) *on page* 990
Flintstones™ Plus Bone Building Support [US-OTC] *see* vitamins (multiple/pediatric) *on page* 990
Flintstones™ Plus Immunity Support [US-OTC] *see* vitamins (multiple/pediatric) *on page* 990
Flintstones™ Plus Iron [US-OTC] *see* vitamins (multiple/pediatric) *on page* 990
Flintstones™ Sour Gummies [US-OTC] *see* vitamins (multiple/pediatric) *on page* 990
floctafenina *see* floctafenine *(Canada only) on page* 406

floctafenine *(Canada only)* (flok ta FEN een)

Synonyms floctafenina; floctafeninum

U.S./Canadian Brand Names Apo-Floctafenine® [Can]

Therapeutic Category Nonsteroidal Antiinflammatory Drug (NSAID), Oral

Use Short-term management of acute, mild-to-moderate pain

Dosage Summary

Oral:

Children: Dosage not established

Adults: 200-400 mg every 6-8 hours as needed (maximum: 1200 mg/day)

Dosage Forms - Canada

Tablet:

Apo-Floctafenine®: 200 mg, 400 mg

floctafeninum *see* floctafenine *(Canada only) on page* 406
Flolan® [US/Can] *see* epoprostenol *on page* 357
Flomax® [US] *see* tamsulosin *on page* 909
Flomax® CR [Can] *see* tamsulosin *on page* 909
Flonase® [US/Can] *see* fluticasone (nasal) *on page* 419
Floranex™ [US-OTC] *see* Lactobacillus *on page* 543
Flora-Q™ [US-OTC] *see* Lactobacillus *on page* 543
Florastor® [US-OTC] *see Saccharomyces boulardii on page* 857
Florastor® Kids [US-OTC] *see Saccharomyces boulardii on page* 857
Florazole® ER [Can] *see* metronidazole (systemic) *on page* 627
Florical® [US-OTC] *see* calcium carbonate *on page* 167
Florinef® [Can] *see* fludrocortisone *on page* 408
Florinef® *(Discontinued)* *see* fludrocortisone *on page* 408
Florone E® *(Discontinued)* *see* diflorasone *on page* 301
Flovent® Diskus® [US/Can] *see* fluticasone (oral inhalation) *on page* 419
Flovent® HFA [US/Can] *see* fluticasone (oral inhalation) *on page* 419
Floxin® [Can] *see* ofloxacin (otic) *on page* 696

Floxin® *(Discontinued)* *see* ofloxacin (otic) *on page 696*
floxin otic singles *see* ofloxacin (otic) *on page 696*

floxuridine (floks YOOR i deen)

Sound-Alike/Look-Alike Issues
floxuridine may be confused with Fludara®, fludarabine
FUDR® may be confused with Fludara®

Synonyms fluorodeoxyuridine; FUDR

U.S./Canadian Brand Names FUDR® [Can]

Therapeutic Category Antineoplastic Agent

Use Management of hepatic metastases of colorectal and gastric cancers

Dosage Summary
Intra-arterial:
Children: Dosage not established
Adults: 0.1-0.6 mg/kg/day

Dosage Forms
Injection, powder for reconstitution: 500 mg

Fluanxol® [Can] *see* flupenthixol *(Canada only) on page 416*
Fluarix® [US] *see* influenza virus vaccine (inactivated) *on page 507*
flubenisolone *see* betamethasone *on page 133*
Flucaine® [US] *see* proparacaine and fluorescein *on page 804*

fluconazole (floo KOE na zole)

Sound-Alike/Look-Alike Issues
fluconazole may be confused with flecainide, FLUoxetine, furosemide, itraconazole
Diflucan® may be confused with diclofenac, Diprivan®, disulfiram

U.S./Canadian Brand Names Apo-Fluconazole® [Can]; CanesOral® [Can]; CO Fluconazole [Can]; Diflucan® [US/Can]; Dom-Fluconazole [Can]; Fluconazole Injection [Can]; Fluconazole Omega [Can]; Mylan-Fluconazole [Can]; Novo-Fluconazole [Can]; PHL-Fluconazole [Can]; PMS-Fluconazole [Can]; PRO-Fluconazole [Can]; Riva-Fluconazole [Can]; Taro-Fluconazole [Can]; Zym-Fluconazole [Can]

Therapeutic Category Antifungal Agent

Use Treatment of candidiasis (vaginal, oropharyngeal, esophageal, urinary tract infections, peritonitis, pneumonia, and systemic infections); cryptococcal meningitis; antifungal prophylaxis in allogeneic bone marrow transplant recipients

Dosage Summary
I.V.:
Neonates: Loading dose: 6-12 mg/kg; Maintenance: 3-12 mg/kg every 72 hours
Children: Loading dose: 6-12 mg/kg; Maintenance: 3-12 mg/kg/day
Adults: 100-1000 mg once daily
Oral:
Neonates: Loading dose: 6-12 mg/kg; Maintenance: 3-12 mg/kg every 72 hours
Children: Loading dose: 6-12 mg/kg; Maintenance: 3-12 mg/kg/day
Adults: 100-1000 mg once daily **or** 150 mg as a single dose

Dosage Forms
Infusion, premixed iso-osmotic dextrose solution: 200 mg (100 mL); 400 mg (200 mL)
Diflucan®: 400 mg (200 mL)
Infusion, premixed iso-osmotic sodium chloride solution: 100 mg (50 mL); 200 mg (100 mL); 400 mg (200 mL)
Diflucan®: 200 mg (100 mL); 400 mg (200 mL)
Infusion, premixed iso-osmotic sodium chloride solution [preservative free]: 200 mg (100 mL); 400 mg (200 mL)
Powder for suspension, oral: 10 mg/mL (35 mL); 40 mg/mL (35 mL)
Diflucan®: 10 mg/mL (35 mL); 40 mg/mL (35 mL)
Tablet, oral: 50 mg, 100 mg, 150 mg, 200 mg
Diflucan®: 50 mg, 100 mg, 150 mg, 200 mg

Fluconazole Injection [Can] *see* fluconazole *on page 407*
Fluconazole Omega [Can] *see* fluconazole *on page 407*

flucytosine (floo SYE toe seen)

Sound-Alike/Look-Alike Issues

flucytosine may be confused with fluorouracil

Ancobon® may be confused with Oncovin®

Synonyms 5-FC; 5-fluorocytosine; 5-flurocytosine

U.S./Canadian Brand Names Ancobon® [US/Can]

Therapeutic Category Antifungal Agent

Use Adjunctive treatment of systemic fungal infections (eg, septicemia, endocarditis, UTI, meningitis, or pulmonary) caused by susceptible strains of *Candida* or *Cryptococcus*

Dosage Summary

Oral:

Adults: 50-150 mg/kg/day in divided doses every 6 hours

Dosage Forms

Capsule, oral:

Ancobon®: 250 mg, 500 mg

Fludara® [US/Can] *see* fludarabine *on page 408*

fludarabine (floo DARE a been)

Sound-Alike/Look-Alike Issues

fludarabine may be confused with cladribine, floxuridine, Flumadine®

Fludara® may be confused with FUDR®

Synonyms 2F-ara-AMP; fludarabine phosphate; NSC-312887

U.S./Canadian Brand Names Fludara® [US/Can]; Oforta™ [US]

Therapeutic Category Antineoplastic Agent

Use

U.S. labeling: Treatment of progressive or refractory B-cell chronic lymphocytic leukemia (CLL)

Canadian labeling: Second-line treatment of chronic lymphocytic leukemia (CLL); second-line treatment of low-grade, refractory non-Hodgkin lymphoma (NHL)

Dosage Summary

Oral:

Children: Dosage not established

Adults: 40 mg/m2/day for 5 days every 28 days

I.V.:

Adults: 25 mg/m^2/day for 5 days every 28 days

Dosage Forms

Injection, powder for reconstitution: 50 mg

Fludara®: 50 mg

Injection, solution [preservative free]: 25 mg/mL (2 mL)

Tablet, oral:

Oforta™: 10 mg

Dosage Forms - Canada

Tablet, oral:

Fludara®: 10 mg

fludarabine phosphate *see* fludarabine *on page 408*

fludrocortisone (floo droe KOR ti sone)

Sound-Alike/Look-Alike Issues

Florinef® may be confused with Fioricet®, Fiorinal®

Synonyms 9α-fluorohydrocortisone acetate; fludrocortisone acetate; fluohydrisone acetate; fluohydrocortisone acetate

U.S./Canadian Brand Names Florinef® [Can]

Therapeutic Category Adrenal Corticosteroid (Mineralocorticoid)

Use Partial replacement therapy for primary and secondary adrenocortical insufficiency in Addison disease; treatment of salt-losing adrenogenital syndrome

Dosage Summary

Oral:

Children: 0.05-0.1 mg/day

Adults: 0.05-0.2 mg/day with ranges of 0.1 mg 3 times/week to 0.2 mg/day

Dosage Forms

Tablet, oral: 0.1 mg

fludrocortisone acetate *see* fludrocortisone *on page* *408*

FluLaval® [US] *see* influenza virus vaccine (inactivated) *on page* *507*

Flumadine® [US/Can] *see* rimantadine *on page* *844*

flumazenil (FLOO may ze nil)

Sound-Alike/Look-Alike Issues

flumazenil may be confused with influenza virus vaccine

U.S./Canadian Brand Names Anexate® [Can]; Flumazenil Injection [Can]; Flumazenil Injection, USP [Can]; Romazicon® [US/Can]

Therapeutic Category Antidote

Use Benzodiazepine antagonist; reverses sedative effects of benzodiazepines used in conscious sedation and general anesthesia; treatment of benzodiazepine overdose

Dosage Summary

I.V.:

Children: Initial: 0.01 mg/kg (maximum dose: 0.2 mg), may repeat 0.005-0.01 mg/kg (maximum dose: 0.2 mg) after 45 seconds, and then every minute (maximum cumulative total: 4 doses; 1 mg; 0.05 mg/kg)

Adults:

Benzodiazepine overdose: Initial: 0.2 mg, may repeat with 0.3 mg, then 0.5 mg at 1-minute intervals (maximum total dose: 5 mg)

Reversal of conscious sedation/general anesthesia: Initial: 0.2 mg, may repeat at 1-minute intervals (maximum total dose: 1 mg)

Dosage Forms

Injection, solution: 0.1 mg/mL (5 mL, 10 mL)

Romazicon®: 0.1 mg/mL (5 mL, 10 mL)

Flumazenil Injection [Can] *see* flumazenil *on page* *409*

Flumazenil Injection, USP [Can] *see* flumazenil *on page* *409*

flumethasone and clioquinol *see* clioquinol and flumethasone *(Canada only) on page* *234*

FluMist® [US] *see* influenza virus vaccine (live/attenuated) *on page* *508*

flunarizine *(Canada only)* (floo NAR i zeen)

Synonyms flunarizine hydrochloride

U.S./Canadian Brand Names Apo-Flunarizine® [Can]; Novo-Flunarizine [Can]; Sibelium® [Can]

Therapeutic Category Calcium-Entry Blocker (Selective)

Use Prophylaxis of classic (with aura) or common (without aura) migraine; symptomatic treatment of vestibular vertigo (due to a diagnosed functional disorder of the vestibular system)

Dosage Summary

Oral:

Children: Dosage not established

Adults <65 years: 5-10 mg once daily, usually at bedtime

Elderly ≥65 years: Decrease dosage by 50% and administer at same frequency

Dosage Forms - Canada

Capsule:

Apo-Flunarizine®, Novo-Flunarizine, Sibelium®: 5 mg

flunarizine hydrochloride *see* flunarizine *(Canada only) on page* *409*

flunisolide (oral inhalation) (floo NISS oh lide)

Sound-Alike/Look-Alike Issues

flunisolide may be confused with Flumadine®, fluocinonide

U.S./Canadian Brand Names AeroBid® [US]; AeroBid®-M [US]; Alti-Flunisolide [Can]; Apo-Flunisolide® [Can]; PMS-Flunisolide [Can]

Therapeutic Category Corticosteroid, Inhalant (Oral)

Use Steroid-dependent asthma

Dosage Summary

Oral inhalation:

AeroBid®, AeroBid®-M:

Children <6 years: Dosage not established

Children 6-15 years: 2 inhalations twice daily (maximum: 4 inhalations/day)

Children >15 years: 2 inhalations twice daily (maximum: 8 inhalations/day)

Adults: 2 inhalations twice daily (maximum: 8 inhalations/day)

Dosage Forms

Aerosol, for oral inhalation:

AeroBid®: 250 mcg/actuation (7 g)

AeroBid®-M: 250 mcg/actuation (7 g)

flunisolide (nasal) (floo NISS oh lide)

Sound-Alike/Look-Alike Issues

flunisolide may be confused with Flumadine®, fluocinonide

Nasarel® may be confused with Nizoral®

U.S./Canadian Brand Names Apo-Flunisolide® [Can]; Nasalide® [Can]; Rhinalar® [Can]

Therapeutic Category Corticosteroid, Nasal

Use Seasonal or perennial rhinitis

Dosage Summary

Intranasal:

Children <6 years: Dosage not established

Children 6-14 years: 1-2 sprays 2-3 times daily (maximum: 4 sprays/day in each nostril)

Children ≥15 years: 2 sprays twice daily (maximum: 8 sprays/day in each nostril)

Adults: 2 sprays twice daily (maximum 8 sprays/day in each nostril)

Dosage Forms

Solution, intranasal: 25 mcg/actuation (25 mL); 29 mcg/actuation (25 mL)

fluocinolone (ophthalmic) (floo oh SIN oh lone)

Sound-Alike/Look-Alike Issues

fluocinolone may be confused with fluocinonide

Synonyms fluocinolone acetonide

U.S./Canadian Brand Names Retisert® [US]

Therapeutic Category Corticosteroid, Ophthalmic

Use Treatment of chronic, noninfectious uveitis affecting the posterior segment of the eye

Dosage Summary

Ocular implant:

Children <12 years: Dosage not established

Children ≥12 years: One silicone-encased tablet (0.59 mg) is designed to release 0.6 mcg/day, decreasing over 30 days to a steady-state release rate of 0.3-0.4 mcg/day for 30 months

Adults: One silicone-encased tablet (0.59 mg) is designed to release 0.6 mcg/day, decreasing over 30 days to a steady-state release rate of 0.3-0.4 mcg/day for 30 months

Dosage Forms

Implant, intravitreal:

Retisert®: 0.59 mg (1s)

fluocinolone (otic) (floo oh SIN oh lone)

Sound-Alike/Look-Alike Issues

fluocinolone may be confused with fluocinonide

Synonyms fluocinolone acetonide

U.S./Canadian Brand Names DermOtic® [US]

Therapeutic Category Corticosteroid, Otic

Use Relief of chronic eczematous external otitis

Dosage Summary

Otic:

Children <2 years: Dosage not established

Children ≥2 years: 5 drops into affected ear twice daily
Adults: 5 drops into affected ear twice daily

Dosage Forms

Oil, otic:
DermOtic®: 0.01% (20 mL)

fluocinolone (topical) (floo oh SIN oh lone)

Sound-Alike/Look-Alike Issues
fluocinolone may be confused with fluocinonide

Synonyms fluocinolone acetonide

U.S./Canadian Brand Names Capex® [US/Can]; Derma-Smoothe/FS® [US/Can]; Synalar® [Can]

Therapeutic Category Corticosteroid, Topical

Use Relief of susceptible inflammatory dermatosis [low, medium corticosteroid]; dermatitis or psoriasis of the scalp; atopic dermatitis in adults and children ≥3 months of age

Dosage Summary

Topical:
Children <3 months: Dosage not established
Children ≥3 months: Apply a thin layer to affected area 2-4 times/day; Derma-Smoothe/FS® body oil: Apply thin film to affected area twice daily
Adults: Apply thin layer to affected area 2-4 times/day
Capex®: Apply no more than 1 ounce to scalp once daily; work into lather and allow to remain on scalp for ~5 minutes. Remove from hair and scalp by rinsing thoroughly with water.
Derma-Smoothe/FS® body oil: Apply thin film to affected area 3 times/day
Derma-Smoothe/FS® scalp oil: Massage thoroughly into wet or dampened hair/scalp; cover with shower cap. Leave on overnight (or for at least 4 hours). Remove by washing hair with shampoo and rinsing thoroughly.

Dosage Forms

Cream, topical: 0.01% (15 g, 60 g); 0.025% (15 g, 60 g)
Oil, topical:
Derma-Smoothe/FS®: 0.01% (120 mL)
Ointment, topical: 0.025% (15 g, 60 g)
Shampoo, topical:
Capex®: 0.01% (120 mL)
Solution, topical: 0.01% (60 mL)

fluocinolone acetonide *see* fluocinolone (ophthalmic) *on page* *410*
fluocinolone acetonide *see* fluocinolone (otic) *on page* *410*
fluocinolone acetonide *see* fluocinolone (topical) *on page* *411*

fluocinolone, hydroquinone, and tretinoin

(floo oh SIN oh lone, HYE droe kwin one, & TRET i noyn)

Synonyms hydroquinone, fluocinolone acetonide, and tretinoin; tretinoin, fluocinolone acetonide, and hydroquinone

U.S./Canadian Brand Names Tri-Luma™ [US]

Therapeutic Category Corticosteroid, Topical; Depigmenting Agent; Retinoic Acid Derivative

Use Short-term treatment of moderate-to-severe melasma of the face

Dosage Summary

Topical:
Children: Dosage not established
Adults: Apply a thin film 30 minutes prior to bedtime daily to hyperpigmented areas of melasma (including 1/2 inch of normal-appearing surrounding skin)

Dosage Forms

Cream, topical:
Tri-Luma™: Hydroquinone 4%, tretinoin 0.05%, fluocinolone 0.01% (30 g)

fluocinonide (floo oh SIN oh nide)

Sound-Alike/Look-Alike Issues
fluocinonide may be confused with flunisolide, fluocinolone
Lidex® may be confused with Lasix®, Videx®, Wydase®

U.S./Canadian Brand Names Lidemol® [Can]; Lidex® [Can]; Lyderm® [Can]; Tiamol® [Can]; Topactin [Can]; Topsyn® [Can]; Vanos™ [US]

Therapeutic Category Corticosteroid, Topical

Use Antiinflammatory, antipruritic; treatment of plaque-type psoriasis (up to 10% of body surface area) [high-potency topical corticosteroid]

Dosage Summary

Topical:

Children <12 years: Apply thin layer of 0.05% cream to affected area 2-4 times/day

Children ≥12 years: Apply thin layer of 0.05% cream to affected area 2-4 times/day **or** apply a thin layer of 0.1% cream once or twice daily to affected area

Adults: Apply thin layer of 0.05% cream to affected area 2-4 times/day **or** apply a thin layer of 0.1% cream once or twice daily to affected area

Dosage Forms

Cream, topical:

Vanos™: 0.1% (30 g, 60 g)

Cream, anhydrous, emollient, topical: 0.05% (15 g, 30 g, 60 g, 120 g)

Cream, aqueous, emollient, topical: 0.05% (15 g, 30 g, 60 g)

Gel, topical: 0.05% (15 g, 30 g, 60 g)

Ointment, topical: 0.05% (15 g, 30 g, 60 g)

Solution, topical: 0.05% (20 mL, 60 mL)

fluohydrisone acetate *see* fludrocortisone *on page* *408*

fluohydrocortisone acetate *see* fludrocortisone *on page* *408*

Fluonid® Topical *(Discontinued)* *see* fluocinolone (topical) *on page* *411*

Fluor-I-Strip® *(Discontinued)* *see* fluorescein *on page* *412*

Fluorabon™ [US] *see* fluoride *on page* *413*

Fluoracaine® *(Discontinued)* *see* proparacaine and fluorescein *on page* *804*

Fluor-A-Day [US/Can] *see* fluoride *on page* *413*

FluorCare® Neutral *(Discontinued)* *see* fluoride *on page* *413*

fluorescein (FLURE e seen)

Synonyms fluorescein sodium; sodium fluorescein; soluble fluorescein

U.S./Canadian Brand Names AK-Fluor® [US]; Angiofluor™ Lite [US]; Angiofluor™ [US]; Fluorescite® [US/Can]; Fluorets® [US]; Ful-Glo® [US]

Therapeutic Category Diagnostic Agent

Use

Injection: Diagnostic aid in ophthalmic angiography and angioscopy

Topical: To stain the anterior segment of the eye for procedures (such as fitting contact lenses), disclosing corneal injury, and in applanation tonometry

Dosage Summary

I.V.:

Children: 3.5 mg/lb (7.7 mg/kg) injected rapidly into antecubital vein

Adults: 500-750 mg injected rapidly into antecubital vein

Ophthalmic:

Children: Apply moistened strip until desired amount of staining obtained

Adults: Apply moistened strip until desired amount of staining obtained

Dosage Forms

Injection, solution: 10% (5 mL); 25% (2 mL)

AK-Fluor®: 10% (5 mL)

Angiofluor™: 10% (5 mL); 25% (2 mL)

Angiofluor™ Lite: 10% (5 mL); 25% (2 mL)

Fluorescite®: 10% (5 mL); 25% (2 mL)

Injection, solution [preservative free]:

Fluorescite®: 10% (5 mL)

Strip, ophthalmic:

Fluorets®: 1 mg (100s)

Ful-Glo®: 0.6 mg (300s); 1 mg (100s)

fluorescein and proparacaine *see* proparacaine and fluorescein *on page* *804*

fluorescein sodium *see* fluorescein *on page* *412*

Fluorescite® [US/Can] *see* fluorescein *on page* 412
Fluorets® [US] *see* fluorescein *on page* 412

fluoride (FLOR ide)

Sound-Alike/Look-Alike Issues
EtheDent™ may be confused with Effient™
Luride® may be confused with Lortab®
Phos-Flur® may be confused with PhosLo®
Thera-Flur-N® may be confused with Thera-Flu®

Synonyms acidulated phosphate fluoride; sodium fluoride; stannous fluoride

U.S./Canadian Brand Names Act® for Kids [US-OTC]; Act® x2™ [US-OTC]; Act® [US-OTC]; CaviRinse™ [US]; ControlRx® [US]; Denta 5000 Plus [US]; DentaGel [US]; Epiflur™ [US]; Fluor-A-Day [US/Can]; Fluorabon™ [US]; Fluorigard® [US-OTC]; Fluorinse® [US]; Flura-Drops® [US]; Gel-Kam® Rinse [US]; Gel-Kam® [US-OTC]; Gel-Kam® [US]; Just for Kids™ [US-OTC]; Lozi-Flur™ [US]; NeutraCare® [US-OTC]; NeutraGard® Advanced [US]; NeutraGard® Plus [US]; NeutraGard® [US-OTC]; Omnii Gel™ [US-OTC]; PerioMed™ [US]; Phos-Flur® Rinse [US-OTC]; Phos-Flur® [US]; PreviDent® 5000 Plus® [US]; PreviDent® [US]; StanGard® Perio [US]; StanGard® [US]; Stop® [US]

Therapeutic Category Mineral, Oral

Use Prevention of dental caries

Dosage Summary

Oral:

Cream:
Children <6 years: Dosage not established
Children ≥6 years: Brush on teeth once daily
Adults: Brush on teeth once daily

Fluorinse®, PreviDent® rinse:
Children ≤6 years: Dosage not established
Children >6 years: Once weekly, vigorously swish 5-10 mL (Fluorinse®) or 10 mL (PreviDent®) in mouth for 1 minute, then spit
Adults: Once weekly, vigorously swish 5-10 mL (Fluorinse®) or 10 mL (PreviDent®) in mouth for 1 minute, then spit

Gel or Rinse:
Children <6 years: Dosage not established
Children 6-12 years: 5-10 mL rinse or apply to teeth and spit daily after brushing
Adults: 10 mL rinse or apply to teeth and spit daily after brushing

Lozenge:
Adults: One daily

Lozenge/oral drops/tablets:
Fluoride content of drinking water <0.3 ppm:
Children 0-6 months: None
Children 6 months to 3 years: 0.25 mg/day
Children 3-6 years: 0.5 mg/day
Children 6-16 years: 1 mg/day
Fluoride content of drinking water 0.3-0.6 ppm:
Children 0-3 years: None
Children 3-6 years: 0.25 mg/day
Children 6-16 years: 0.5 mg/day

Dosage Forms

Cream, oral: 1.1% (51 g)
Denta 5000 Plus: 1.1% (51 g)
PreviDent® 5000 Plus®: 1.1% (51 g)

Gel, topical: 1.1% (56 g)
DentaGel: 1.1% (56 g)
Gel-Kam® [OTC]: 0.4% (129 g); 0.4% (129 g)
Just For Kids™ [OTC]: 0.4% (122 g)
NeutraCare® [OTC]: 1.1% (60 g)
NeutraGard® Advanced: 1.1% (60 g)
Omnii Gel™ [OTC]: 0.4% (122 g)
Phos-Flur®: 1.1% (51 g)
PreviDent®: 1.1% (60 g)
StanGard®: 0.4% (122 g)
Stop®: 0.4% (120 g)

Lozenge, oral:
Lozi-Flur™: 2.21 mg (90s)
Paste, oral:
ControlRx®: 1.1% (56 g)
Solution, oral: 1.1 mg/mL (50 mL); 0.2% (473 mL); 0.63% (300 mL)
Act® [OTC]: 0.05% (530 mL)
Act® for Kids [OTC]: 0.05% (530 mL)
Act® x2™ [OTC]: 0.05% (530 mL)
CaviRinse™: 0.2% (240 mL)
Fluor-A-Day: 0.125 mg/drop (30 mL)
Fluorabon™: 0.25 mg/0.6 mL (60 mL)
Fluorigard® [OTC]: 0.05% (473 mL)
Fluorinse®: 0.2% (480 mL)
Flura-Drops®: 0.55 mg/drop (24 mL)
Gel-Kam® Rinse: 0.63% (300 mL)
NeutraGard® [OTC]: 0.05% (480 mL)
NeutraGard® Plus: 0.2% (480 mL)
PerioMed™: 0.63% (284 mL)
Phos-Flur® Rinse [OTC]: 0.044% (500 mL)
PreviDent®: 0.2% (473 mL, 1920 mL)
StanGard® Perio: 0.63% (284 mL)
Tablet, chewable, oral: 0.55 mg, 1.1 mg, 2.2 mg
Epiflur™: 0.55 mg, 1.1 mg, 2.2 mg
Fluor-A-Day: 0.56 mg, 1.1 mg, 2.21 mg

Fluorigard® [US-OTC] *see* fluoride *on page* 413
Fluori-Methane® [US] *see* dichlorodifluoromethane and trichloromonofluoromethane *on page* 296
Fluorinse® [US] *see* fluoride *on page* 413
Fluoritab® *(Discontinued)* *see* fluoride *on page* 413
5-fluorocytosine *see* flucytosine *on page* 408
fluorodeoxyuridine *see* floxuridine *on page* 407
9α-fluorohydrocortisone acetate *see* fludrocortisone *on page* 408

fluorometholone (flure oh METH oh lone)

U.S./Canadian Brand Names Flarex® [US/Can]; FML Forte® [US/Can]; FML® [US/Can]; PMS-Fluorometholone [Can]

Therapeutic Category Adrenal Corticosteroid

Use Treatment of steroid-responsive inflammatory conditions of the eye

Dosage Summary

Ophthalmic:

Ointment:
Children ≤2 years: Dosage not established
Children >2 years: Apply small amount (~1/2 inch ribbon) every 4 hours (initial: 24-48 hours) **or** 1-3 times/day
Adults: Apply small amount (~1/2 inch ribbon) every 4 hours (initial: 24-48 hours) **or** 1-3 times/day

Solution:
Children ≤2 years: Dosage not established
Children >2 years: Instill 1 drop every 4 hours (initial: 24-48 hours) **or** 1 drop 2-4 times/day
Adults: Instill 2 drops (initial: 24-48 hours) **or** 1-2 drops 2-4 times/day

Dosage Forms

Ointment, ophthalmic:
FML®: 0.1% (3.5 g)
Suspension, ophthalmic: 0.1% (5 mL, 10 mL, 15 mL)
Flarex®: 0.1% (5 mL)
FML Forte®: 0.25% (5 mL, 10 mL)
FML®: 0.1% (5 mL, 10 mL, 15 mL)

Fluor-Op® *(Discontinued)* *see* fluorometholone *on page* 414
Fluoroplex® [US/Can] *see* fluorouracil (topical) *on page* 415
5-fluorouracil *see* fluorouracil (systemic) *on page* 415

5-fluorouracil *see* fluorouracil (topical) *on page 415*

fluorouracil (systemic) (flure oh YOOR a sil)

Sound-Alike/Look-Alike Issues

fluorouracil may be confused with flucytosine

Synonyms 5-fluorouracil; 5-FU; FU

U.S./Canadian Brand Names Adrucil® [US]

Therapeutic Category Antineoplastic Agent, Antimetabolite (Pyrimidine Analog)

Use Treatment of carcinomas of the breast, colon, rectum, pancreas, or stomach

Dosage Summary

I.V.:

Bolus:

Children: Dosage not established

Adults: 500-600 mg/m^2 every 3 weeks **or** 500-600 mg/m^2/dose days 1 and 8 every 4 weeks **or** 500 mg/m^2/dose days 1 and 8 every 3 weeks **or** 500 mg/m^2/dose days 1 and 4 every 3 weeks **or** 500 mg/m^2/dose days 1, 8, 15, 22, 29, and 36 of an 8-week treatment cycle **or** 425 mg/m^2 on days 1-5 every 4 weeks

Infusion:

Children: Dosage not established

Adults: 500-750 mg/m^2/day for 5 days every 3 weeks **or** 1000 mg/m^2/day for 4-5 days every 3-4 weeks **or** 2600 mg/m^2 on day 1 every week **or** 1600 mg/m^2/day for 2 days every 2 weeks **or** 400 mg/m^2 bolus followed by 1200 mg/m^2/day for 2 days every 2 weeks

Dosage Forms

Injection, solution: 50 mg/mL (10 mL, 20 mL, 50 mL, 100 mL)

Adrucil®: 50 mg/mL (10 mL, 50 mL, 100 mL)

fluorouracil (topical) (flure oh YOOR a sil)

Sound-Alike/Look-Alike Issues

fluorouracil may be confused with flucytosine

Carac® may be confused with Kuric™

Efudex® may be confused with Efidac (Efidac 24®), Eurax®

Synonyms 5-fluorouracil; 5-FU; FU

U.S./Canadian Brand Names Carac® [US]; Efudex® [US/Can]; Fluoroplex® [US/Can]

Therapeutic Category Antineoplastic Agent, Antimetabolite (Pyrimidine Analog)

Use Management of actinic or solar keratoses and superficial basal cell carcinomas

Dosage Summary

Topical:

Children: Dosage not established

Adults: Apply to lesions once (Carac™) or twice daily (Efudex®; Fluoroplex®)

Dosage Forms

Cream, topical: 5% (40 g)

Carac®: 0.5% (30 g)

Efudex®: 5% (40 g)

Fluoroplex®: 1% (30 g)

Solution, topical: 2% (10 mL); 5% (10 mL)

Efudex®: 5% (10 mL)

Fluorouracil® ***(Discontinued)*** *see* fluorouracil (topical) *on page 415*

Fluothane® ***(Discontinued)***

fluoxetine (floo OKS e teen)

Sound-Alike/Look-Alike Issues

FLUoxetine may be confused with DULoxetine, famotidine, Feldene®, fluconazole, fluvastatin, fluvoxamine, fosinopril, furosemide, PARoxetine, thiothixene

Prozac® may be confused with Paxil®, Prelone®, Prilosec®, Prograf®, Proscar®, ProSom®, ProStep®, Provera®

Sarafem® may be confused with Serophene®

Synonyms fluoxetine hydrochloride

Tall-Man **FLU**oxetine

U.S./Canadian Brand Names Apo-Fluoxetine® [Can]; CO Fluoxetine [Can]; Dom-Fluoxetine [Can]; Fluoxetine [Can]; FXT 40 [Can]; Gen-Fluoxetine [Can]; Mylan-Fluoxetine [Can]; Novo-Fluoxetine [Can]; Nu-Fluoxetine [Can]; PHL-Fluoxetine [Can]; PMS-Fluoxetine [Can]; PRO-Fluoxetine [Can]; Prozac® Weekly™ [US]; Prozac® [US/Can]; ratio-Fluoxetine [Can]; Riva-Fluoxetine [Can]; Sandoz-Fluoxetine [Can]; Sarafem® [US]; Selfemra® [US]; ZYM-Fluoxetine [Can]

Therapeutic Category Antidepressant, Selective Serotonin Reuptake Inhibitor

Use Treatment of major depressive disorder (MDD); treatment of binge-eating and vomiting in patients with moderate-to-severe bulimia nervosa; obsessive-compulsive disorder (OCD); premenstrual dysphoric disorder (PMDD); panic disorder with or without agoraphobia; in combination with olanzapine for treatment-resistant or bipolar I depression

Dosage Summary

Oral:

Children <7 years: Dosage not established

Children 7-18 years: Initial: 10-20 mg once daily; Maintenance: 10-60 mg once daily; **Note:** Titration is recommended

Adults: 10-80 mg once daily **or** 90 mg once weekly; **Note:** Titration is recommended

Elderly: Some patients may require an initial dose of 10 mg/day with dosage increases of 10 mg and 20 mg every several weeks as tolerated

Dosage Forms

Capsule, oral: 10 mg, 20 mg, 40 mg

Prozac®: 10 mg, 20 mg, 40 mg

Selfemra®: 10 mg, 20 mg

Capsule, delayed release, enteric coated pellets, oral: 90 mg

Prozac® Weekly™: 90 mg

Solution, oral: 20 mg/5 mL (5 mL, 120 mL)

Tablet, oral: 10 mg, 20 mg

Sarafem®: 10 mg, 15 mg, 20 mg

Fluoxetine [Can] *see* fluoxetine *on page 415*

fluoxetine and olanzapine *see* olanzapine and fluoxetine *on page 697*

fluoxetine hydrochloride *see* fluoxetine *on page 415*

fluoxymesterone (floo oks i MES te rone)

U.S./Canadian Brand Names Androxy™ [US]

Therapeutic Category Androgen

Controlled Substance C-III

Use Replacement of endogenous testicular hormone; in females, palliative treatment of breast cancer

Dosage Summary

Oral:

Children: Dosage not established

Adults (females): 10-40 mg/day in divided doses

Adults (males): 2.5-20 mg/day

Dosage Forms

Tablet, oral:

Androxy™: 10 mg

flupenthixol *(Canada only)* (floo pen THIKS ol)

Synonyms flupenthixol decanoate; flupenthixol dihydrochloride

U.S./Canadian Brand Names Fluanxol® [Can]

Therapeutic Category Antipsychotic Agent; Thioxanthene Derivative

Use Maintenance therapy of chronic schizophrenic patients whose main manifestations do **not** include excitement, agitation, or hyperactivity

Dosage Summary

I.M. (Depot):

Children: Dosage not established

Adults: Initial test dose: 5-20 mg; Maintenance: 2- to 3-week intervals

Oral:

Children: Dosage not established

Adults: Initial: 1 mg 3 times/day; Maintenance: 3-6 mg/day in divided doses; **Note:** Titration is recommended

Dosage Forms - Canada

Injection, solution [depot]:

Fluanxol®: 20 mg/mL (10 mL); 100 mg/mL (2 mL)

Tablet:

Fluanxol®: 0.5 mg, 3 mg

flupenthixol decanoate *see* flupenthixol *(Canada only) on page 416*

flupenthixol dihydrochloride *see* flupenthixol *(Canada only) on page 416*

fluphenazine (floo FEN a zeen)

Synonyms fluphenazine decanoate

U.S./Canadian Brand Names Apo-Fluphenazine Decanoate® [Can]; Apo-Fluphenazine® [Can]; Modecate® Concentrate [Can]; Modecate® [Can]; PMS-Fluphenazine Decanoate [Can]

Therapeutic Category Phenothiazine Derivative

Use Management of manifestations of psychotic disorders and schizophrenia; depot formulation may offer improved outcome in individuals with psychosis who are nonadherent with oral antipsychotics

Dosage Summary

I.M.:

Children: Dosage not established

Adults: 2.5-10 mg/day in divided doses every 6-8 hours **or** 12.5 mg every 3 weeks (depot)

Oral:

Adults: 0.5-10 mg/day in divided doses every 6-8 hours (maximum: 40 mg/day)

SubQ (Depot):

Children: Dosage not established

Adults: 12.5 mg every 3 weeks

Dosage Forms

Elixir, oral: 2.5 mg/5 mL (60 mL, 473 mL)

Injection, oil: 25 mg/mL (5 mL)

Injection, solution: 2.5 mg/mL (10 mL)

Solution, oral: 5 mg/mL (118 mL)

Tablet, oral: 1 mg, 2.5 mg, 5 mg, 10 mg

fluphenazine decanoate *see* fluphenazine *on page 417*

Flura® *(Discontinued)* *see* fluoride *on page 413*

Flura-Drops® [US] *see* fluoride *on page 413*

flurandrenolide (flure an DREN oh lide)

Sound-Alike/Look-Alike Issues

Cordran® may be confused with Cardura®, codeine, Cordarone®

Synonyms flurandrenolone

U.S./Canadian Brand Names Cordran® SP [US]; Cordran® [US/Can]

Therapeutic Category Corticosteroid, Topical

Use Inflammation of corticosteroid-responsive dermatoses [medium potency topical corticosteroid]

Dosage Summary

Topical:

Children: Apply 1-2 times/day

Adults: Apply 2-3 times/day

Dosage Forms

Cream, topical:

Cordran® SP: 0.05% (15 g, 30 g, 60 g)

Lotion, topical:

Cordran®: 0.05% (15 mL, 60 mL)

Tape, topical:

Cordran®: 4 mcg/cm2 (24 inch, 80 inch)

flurandrenolone *see* flurandrenolide *on page 417*

Flurate® Ophthalmic Solution *(Discontinued)* *see* fluorescein *on page 412*

flurazepam (flure AZ e pam)

Sound-Alike/Look-Alike Issues

flurazepam may be confused with temazepam

Dalmane® may be confused with Demulen®, Dialume®

Synonyms flurazepam hydrochloride

U.S./Canadian Brand Names Apo-Flurazepam® [Can]; Dalmane® [Can]; Som Pam [Can]

Therapeutic Category Benzodiazepine

Controlled Substance C-IV

Use Short-term treatment of insomnia

Dosage Summary

Oral:

Children <15 years: Dosage not established
Children ≥15 years: 15 mg at bedtime
Adults: 15-30 mg at bedtime
Elderly: 15 mg at bedtime

Dosage Forms

Capsule, oral: 15 mg, 30 mg

flurazepam hydrochloride *see* flurazepam *on page 417*

flurbiprofen (systemic) (flure BI proe fen)

Sound-Alike/Look-Alike Issues

flurbiprofen may be confused with fenoprofen
Ansaid® may be confused with Asacol®, Axid®

Synonyms flurbiprofen sodium

U.S./Canadian Brand Names Alti-Flurbiprofen [Can]; Ansaid® [Can]; Apo-Flurbiprofen® [Can]; Froben-SR® [Can]; Froben® [Can]; Novo-Flurprofen [Can]; Nu-Flurprofen [Can]

Therapeutic Category Nonsteroidal Antiinflammatory Drug (NSAID)

Use Treatment of rheumatoid arthritis and osteoarthritis

Dosage Summary

Oral:

Children: Dosage not established
Adults: 200-300 mg/day in 2-4 divided doses (maximum: 100 mg/dose; 300 mg/day)

Dosage Forms

Tablet, oral: 50 mg, 100 mg

flurbiprofen (ophthalmic) (flure BI proe fen)

Sound-Alike/Look-Alike Issues

flurbiprofen may be confused with fenoprofen
Ocufen® may be confused with Ocuflox®, Ocupress®

Synonyms flurbiprofen sodium

U.S./Canadian Brand Names Ocufen® [US/Can]

Therapeutic Category Nonsteroidal Antiinflammatory Drug (NSAID), Ophthalmic

Use Inhibition of intraoperative miosis

Dosage Summary

Ophthalmic:

Children: Dosage not established
Adults: Instill 1 drop to each eye every 30 minutes, beginning 2 hours prior to surgery (maximum: 4 doses)

Dosage Forms

Solution, ophthalmic: 0.03% (2.5 mL)
Ocufen®: 0.03% (2.5 mL)

flurbiprofen sodium *see* flurbiprofen (ophthalmic) *on page 418*
flurbiprofen sodium *see* flurbiprofen (systemic) *on page 418*
5-flurocytosine *see* flucytosine *on page 408*
Fluro-Ethyl® ***(Discontinued)*** *see* ethyl chloride and dichlorotetrafluoroethane *on page 382*
Flurosyn® Topical ***(Discontinued)*** *see* fluocinolone (topical) *on page 411*

flutamide (FLOO ta mide)

Sound-Alike/Look-Alike Issues

flutamide may be confused with Flumadine®, thalidomide

Eulexin® may be confused with Edecrin®, Eurax®

Synonyms 4′-nitro-3′-trifluoromethylisobutyrantide; niftolid; NSC-147834; SCH 13521

U.S./Canadian Brand Names Apo-Flutamide® [Can]; Euflex® [Can]; Eulexin® [Can]; Novo-Flutamide [Can]

Therapeutic Category Antiandrogen

Use Treatment of metastatic prostatic carcinoma in combination therapy with LHRH agonist analogues

Dosage Summary

Oral:

Children: Dosage not established

Adults: 250 mg 3 times/day

Dosage Forms

Capsule, oral: 125 mg

fluticasone (oral inhalation) (floo TIK a sone)

Sound-Alike/Look-Alike Issues

Flovent® may be confused with Flonase®

Synonyms fluticasone propionate

U.S./Canadian Brand Names Flovent® Diskus® [US/Can]; Flovent® HFA [US/Can]

Therapeutic Category Corticosteroid, Inhalant (Oral)

Use Maintenance treatment of asthma as prophylactic therapy; also indicated for patients requiring oral corticosteroid therapy for asthma to assist in total discontinuation or reduction of total oral dose

Dosage Summary

Inhalation:

Flovent® HFA:

Children <4 years: Dosage not established

Children 4-11 years: 88 mcg twice daily; Low dose: 88-176 mcg/day in 2 divided doses; Medium dose: 176->352 mcg/day in 2 divided doses; High dose: >352 mcg/day in 2 divided doses

Children ≥12 years: 88-880 mcg twice daily; Low dose: 88-264 mcg/day in 2 divided doses; Medium dose: >264-440 mcg/day in 2 divided doses; High dose: >440 mcg/day in 2 divided doses

Adults: 88-880 mcg twice daily; Low dose: 88-264 mcg/day in 2 divided doses; Medium dose: >264-440 mcg/day in 2 divided doses; High dose: >440 mcg/day in 2 divided doses

Flovent® Diskus®:

Children <4 years: Dosage not established

Children 4-11 years: 50-100 mcg twice daily

Children >11 years: 100-1000 mcg twice daily

Adults: 100-1000 mcg twice daily

Dosage Forms

Aerosol, for oral inhalation:

Flovent® HFA: 44 mcg/inhalation (10.6 g); 110 mcg/inhalation (12 g); 220 mcg/inhalation (12 g)

Powder, for oral inhalation:

Flovent® Diskus®: 50 mcg (60s); 100 mcg (60s); 250 mcg (60s)

Dosage Forms - Canada

Powder, for oral inhalation [prefilled blister pack]:

Flovent® Diskus®: 50 mcg (28s, 60s); 100 mcg (28s, 60s); 250 mcg (28s, 60s); 500 mcg (28s, 60s)

fluticasone (nasal) (floo TIK a sone)

Sound-Alike/Look-Alike Issues

Flonase® may be confused with Flovent®

Synonyms fluticasone furoate; fluticasone propionate

U.S./Canadian Brand Names Apo-Fluticasone® [Can]; Avamys® [Can]; Flonase® [US/Can]; ratio-Fluticasone [Can]; Veramyst® [US]

Therapeutic Category Corticosteroid, Nasal

Use

Flonase®: Management of seasonal and perennial allergic rhinitis and nonallergic rhinitis

Veramyst®, Avamys® [CAN]: Management of seasonal and perennial allergic rhinitis

Dosage Summary

Intranasal, propionate:

Flonase®:

Children <4 years: Dosage not established

Children ≥4 years: Initial: 1 spray (50 mcg/spray) per nostril once daily; Maintenance: 1-2 sprays (100 mcg) per nostril once daily (maximum: 2 sprays in each nostril [200 mcg]/day)
Adults: Initial: 2 sprays (50 mcg/spray) per nostril once daily; Maintenance: 1-2 sprays per nostril once daily

Intranasal, furoate:
Veramyst®:
Children <2 years: Dosage not established
Children 2-11 years: Initial: 1 spray (27.5 mcg/spray) per nostril once daily; Maintenance 1-2 sprays per nostril once daily (55-110 mcg/day) (maximum: 2 sprays in each nostril [110 mcg]/day)
Children ≥12 years: Initial: 2 sprays (27.5 mcg/spray) per nostril once daily; Maintenance 1-2 sprays per nostril once daily (55-110 mcg/day) (maximum: 2 sprays in each nostril [110 mcg]/day)
Adults: Initial: 2 sprays (27.5 mcg/spray) per nostril once daily; Maintenance 1-2 sprays per nostril once daily (55-110 mcg/day)

Dosage Forms
Suspension, intranasal: 50 mcg/inhalation (16 g)
Flonase®: 50 mcg/inhalation (16 g)
Veramyst®: 27.5 mcg/inhalation (10 g)

Dosage Forms - Canada
Suspension, intranasal, as furoate [spray]:
Avamys®: 27.5 mcg/inhalation (4.5 g, 10 g)

fluticasone (topical) (floo TIK a sone)

Sound-Alike/Look-Alike Issues
Cutivate® may be confused with Ultravate®

Synonyms fluticasone propionate

U.S./Canadian Brand Names Cutivate® [US/Can]

Therapeutic Category Corticosteroid, Topical

Use Relief of inflammation and pruritus associated with corticosteroid-responsive dermatoses; atopic dermatitis

Dosage Summary
Topical:
Cream:
Children <3 months: Dosage not established
Children ≥3 months: Apply sparingly to affected area once or twice daily
Adults: Apply sparingly to affected area once or twice daily
Lotion:
Children <1 year: Dosage not established
Children ≥1 year: Apply sparingly to affected area once daily
Adults: Apply sparingly to affected area once or twice daily

Dosage Forms
Cream, topical: 0.05% (15 g, 30 g, 60 g)
Cutivate®: 0.05% (30 g, 60 g)
Lotion, topical:
Cutivate®: 0.05% (120 mL)
Ointment, topical: 0.005% (15 g, 30 g, 60 g)
Cutivate®: 0.005% (30 g, 60 g)

fluticasone and salmeterol (floo TIK a sone & sal ME te role)

Sound-Alike/Look-Alike Issues
Advair® may be confused with Adcirca™, Advicor®

Synonyms fluticasone propionate and salmeterol xinafoate; salmeterol and fluticasone

U.S./Canadian Brand Names Advair Diskus® [US/Can]; Advair® HFA [US]; Advair® [Can]

Therapeutic Category $Beta_2$-Adrenergic Agonist Agent; Corticosteroid, Inhalant

Use Maintenance treatment of asthma; maintenance treatment of COPD

Dosage Summary
Oral inhalation:
Children <4 years: Advair Diskus®: Dosage not established
Children 4-11 years: Advair Diskus®: Fluticasone 100 mcg/salmeterol 50 mcg/inhalation: One inhalation twice daily (maximum dose)
Children <12 years: Advair® HFA: Dosage not established

Children ≥12 years: Asthma:

Advair Diskus®: Fluticasone 100-500 mcg/salmeterol 50 mcg/inhalation: One inhalation twice daily. Maximum: Fluticasone 500 mcg/salmeterol 50 mcg/inhalation twice daily

Advair® HFA: Fluticasone 45-230 mcg/salmeterol 21 mcg/inhalation: Two inhalations twice daily

Advair® 125 or Advair® 250 [Canadian labeling; not in approved U.S. labeling]: Fluticasone 125-250 mcg/salmeterol 25 mcg/inhalation: Two inhalations twice daily

Adults:

COPD:

Advair Diskus®: Initial, maximum: Fluticasone 250 mcg/salmeterol 50 mcg twice daily

Advair Diskus® [Canadian labeling; not in approved U.S. labeling]: Fluticasone 250-500 mcg/ salmeterol 50 mcg: One inhalation twice daily

Asthma:

Advair Diskus®: Maximum dose: Fluticasone 500 mcg/salmeterol 50 mcg/inhalation: One inhalation twice daily

Advair® HFA: Fluticasone 45-230 mcg/salmeterol 50 mcg/inhalation: Two inhalations twice daily

Advair® 125 or Advair® 250 [Canadian labeling; not in approved U.S. labeling]: Fluticasone 125-250 mcg/salmeterol 25 mcg/inhalation: Two inhalations twice daily

Dosage Forms Excipient information presented when available (limited, particularly for generics); consult specific product labeling. [DSC] = Discontinued product

Aerosol, for oral inhalation:

Advair® HFA:

45/21: Fluticasone propionate 45 mcg and salmeterol 21 mcg (8 g, 12 g) [chlorofluorocarbon free]

115/21: Fluticasone propionate 115 mcg and salmeterol 21 mcg (8 g, 12 g) [chlorofluorocarbon free]

230/21: Fluticasone propionate 230 mcg and salmeterol 21 mcg (8 g, 12 g) [chlorofluorocarbon free]

Powder, for oral inhalation:

Advair Diskus®:

100/50: Fluticasone propionate 100 mcg and salmeterol 50 mcg (14s, 60s)

250/50: Fluticasone propionate 250 mcg and salmeterol 50 mcg (60s)

500/50: Fluticasone propionate 500 mcg and salmeterol 50 mcg (60s)

Dosage Forms - Canada

Aerosol, for oral inhalation:

Advair®: 125/25: Fluticasone propionate 125 mcg and salmeterol 25 mcg (12 g); 250/25: Fluticasone propionate 250 mcg and salmeterol 25 mcg (12 g)

fluticasone furoate *see* fluticasone (nasal) *on page 419*

fluticasone propionate *see* fluticasone (nasal) *on page 419*

fluticasone propionate *see* fluticasone (oral inhalation) *on page 419*

fluticasone propionate *see* fluticasone (topical) *on page 420*

fluticasone propionate and salmeterol xinafoate *see* fluticasone and salmeterol *on page 420*

fluvastatin (FLOO va sta tin)

Sound-Alike/Look-Alike Issues

fluvastatin may be confused with fluoxetine, nystatin, pitavastatin

U.S./Canadian Brand Names Lescol® XL [US/Can]; Lescol® [US/Can]

Therapeutic Category HMG-CoA Reductase Inhibitor

Use To be used as a component of multiple risk factor intervention in patients at risk for atherosclerosis vascular disease due to hypercholesterolemia

Adjunct to dietary therapy to reduce elevated total cholesterol (total-C), LDL-C, triglyceride, and apolipoprotein B (apo-B) levels and to increase HDL-C in primary hypercholesterolemia and mixed dyslipidemia (Fredrickson types IIa and IIb); to slow the progression of coronary atherosclerosis in patients with coronary heart disease; reduce risk of coronary revascularization procedures in patients with coronary heart disease

Dosage Summary

Oral:

Extended release:

Children <10 years: Dosage not established

Children 10-16 years (females 1 year postmenarche): 80 mg once daily

Adults: 80 mg once daily

Immediate release:

Children <10 years: Dosage not established

Adolescents 10-16 years (females 1 year postmenarche): Initial: 20 mg once daily; Maintenance: Up to 80 mg/day in 2 divided doses

Adults: Initial: 20-40 mg once daily; Maintenance: Up to 80 mg/day in 2 divided doses

Dosage Forms

Capsule, oral:

Lescol®: 20 mg, 40 mg

Tablet, extended release, oral:

Lescol® XL: 80 mg

Fluviral S/F® [Can] *see* influenza virus vaccine (inactivated) *on page 507*

Fluvirin® [US] *see* influenza virus vaccine (inactivated) *on page 507*

fluvoxamine (floo VOKS a meen)

Sound-Alike/Look-Alike Issues

fluvoxamine may be confused with flavoxate, fluoxetine

Luvox may be confused with Lasix®, Levoxyl®, Lovenox®

U.S./Canadian Brand Names Alti-Fluvoxamine [Can]; Apo-Fluvoxamine® [Can]; Luvox® CR [US]; Luvox® [Can]; Novo-Fluvoxamine [Can]; Nu-Fluvoxamine [Can]; PMS-Fluvoxamine [Can]; Rhoxal-fluvoxamine [Can]; Riva-Fluvox [Can]; Sandoz-Fluvoxamine [Can]

Therapeutic Category Antidepressant, Selective Serotonin Reuptake Inhibitor

Use Treatment of obsessive-compulsive disorder (OCD); treatment of social anxiety disorder

Dosage Summary

Oral:

Children <8 years: Dosage not established

Children 8-11 years: Initial: 25 mg at bedtime; Maintenance: 50-200 mg/day (maximum: 200 mg/day); **Note:** Titration is recommended

Children 12-17 years: Initial: 25 mg at bedtime; Maintenance: 50-200 mg/day (maximum: 300 mg/day); **Note:** Titration is recommended

Adults: Initial: 50-100 mg at bedtime; Maintenance: 100-300 mg/day in 1-2 divided doses; **Note:** Titration is recommended

Dosage Forms

Capsule, extended release, oral:

Luvox® CR: 100 mg, 150 mg

Tablet, oral: 25 mg, 50 mg, 100 mg

Fluzone® [US] *see* influenza virus vaccine (inactivated) *on page 507*

Fluzone® High-Dose [Can] *see* influenza virus vaccine (inactivated) *on page 507*

FML® [US/Can] *see* fluorometholone *on page 414*

FML Forte® [US/Can] *see* fluorometholone *on page 414*

FML-S® ***(Discontinued)***

Focalin® [US] *see* dexmethylphenidate *on page 284*

Focalin® XR [US] *see* dexmethylphenidate *on page 284*

Foille® [US-OTC] *see* benzocaine *on page 124*

folacin *see* folic acid *on page 423*

Folacin-800 [US-OTC] *see* folic acid *on page 423*

folacin, vitamin B_{12}, and vitamin B_6 *see* folic acid, cyanocobalamin, and pyridoxine *on page 423*

Folamin™ ***(Discontinued)*** *see* folic acid, cyanocobalamin, and pyridoxine *on page 423*

folate *see* folic acid *on page 423*

Folbee [US] *see* folic acid, cyanocobalamin, and pyridoxine *on page 423*

Folbic [US] *see* folic acid, cyanocobalamin, and pyridoxine *on page 423*

Folcaps™ [US] *see* folic acid, cyanocobalamin, and pyridoxine *on page 423*

Folex® PFS™ ***(Discontinued)*** *see* methotrexate *on page 614*

Folgard® [US-OTC] *see* folic acid, cyanocobalamin, and pyridoxine *on page 423*

Folgard RX® [US] *see* folic acid, cyanocobalamin, and pyridoxine *on page 423*

Folgard RX 2.2® ***(Discontinued)*** *see* folic acid, cyanocobalamin, and pyridoxine *on page 423*

folic acid (FOE lik AS id)

Sound-Alike/Look-Alike Issues

folic acid may be confused with folinic acid

Synonyms folacin; folate; pteroylglutamic acid

U.S./Canadian Brand Names Apo-Folic® [Can]; Folacin-800 [US-OTC]

Therapeutic Category Vitamin, Water Soluble

Use Treatment of megaloblastic and macrocytic anemias due to folate deficiency; dietary supplement to prevent neural tube defects

Dosage Summary

I.M.:

Infants: 0.1 mg/day
Children <4 years: Up to 0.3 mg/day
Children ≥4 years: 0.4 mg/day
Adults: 0.4 mg/day
Pregnant and lactating women: 0.8 mg/day

I.V.:

Infants: 0.1 mg/day
Children <4 years: Up to 0.3 mg/day
Children ≥4 years: 0.4 mg/day
Adults: 0.4 mg/day
Pregnant and lactating women: 0.8 mg/day

Oral:

Infants: 0.1 mg/day
Children <4 years: Up to 0.3 mg/day
Children ≥4 years: 0.4 mg/day
Adults: 0.4 mg/day
Pregnant and lactating women: 0.8 mg/day (anemia) **or** 4 mg/day (prevention neural tube defects)
Females of childbearing potential: Prevention of neural tube defects: 0.4-0.8 mg/day

SubQ:

Infants: 0.1 mg/day
Children <4 years: Up to 0.3 mg/day
Children ≥4 years: 0.4 mg/day
Adults: 0.4 mg/day
Pregnant and lactating women: 0.8 mg/day

Dosage Forms

Injection, solution: 5 mg/mL (10 mL)
Tablet, oral: 0.4 mg, 0.8 mg, 1 mg
Folacin-800 [OTC]: 0.8 mg

folic acid, cyanocobalamin, and pyridoxine

(FOE lik AS id, sye an oh koe BAL a min, & peer i DOKS een)

Synonyms cyanocobalamin, folic acid, and pyridoxine; folacin, vitamin B_{12}, and vitamin B_6; pyridoxine, folic acid, and cyanocobalamin

U.S./Canadian Brand Names FaBB [US]; Folbee [US]; Folbic [US]; Folcaps™ [US]; Folgard RX® [US]; Folgard® [US-OTC]; Foltx® [US]; Tricardio B [US]

Therapeutic Category Vitamin

Use Nutritional supplement in end-stage renal failure, dialysis, hyperhomocysteinemia, homocystinuria, malabsorption syndromes, dietary deficiencies

Dosage Summary

Oral:

Children: Dosage not established
Adults: One tablet daily

Dosage Forms

Tablet: Folic acid 0.8 mg, cyanocobalamin 1000 mcg, and pyridoxine 50 mg
FaBB, Folgard RX®: Folic acid 2.2 mg, cyanocobalamin 1000 mcg, and pyridoxine 25 mg
Folbee: Folic acid 2.5 mg, cyanocobalamin 1000 mcg, and pyridoxine 25 mg
Folbic, Foltx®: Folic acid 2.5 mg, cyanocobalamin 2000 mcg, and pyridoxine 25 mg
Folcaps™: Folic acid 2.2 mg, cyanocobalamin 500 mcg, and pyridoxine 25 mg
Folgard® [OTC]: Folic acid 0.8 mg, cyanocobalamin 115 mcg, and pyridoxine 10 mg
Tricardio B: Folic acid 0.4 mg, cyanocobalamin 250 mcg, and pyridoxine 25 mg

folic acid, magnesium carbonate, and calcium carbonate *see* magnesium carbonate, calcium carbonate, and folic acid *on page 583*

follicle-stimulating hormone, human *see* urofollitropin *on page 971*

follicle stimulating hormone, recombinant *see* follitropin alfa *on page 424*

follicle stimulating hormone, recombinant *see* follitropin beta *on page 424*

Follistim® AQ [US] *see* follitropin beta *on page 424*

Follistim® AQ Cartridge [US] *see* follitropin beta *on page 424*

follitropin alfa (foe li TRO pin AL fa)

Synonyms follicle stimulating hormone, recombinant; FSH; rFSH-alpha; rhFSH-alpha

U.S./Canadian Brand Names Gonal-f® Pen [Can]; Gonal-f® RFF [US]; Gonal-f® [US/Can]

Therapeutic Category Ovulation Stimulator

Use

Gonal-f®: Ovulation induction in patients in whom the cause of infertility is functional and not caused by primary ovarian failure; development of multiple follicles with Assisted Reproductive Technology (ART); spermatogenesis induction

Gonal-f® RFF: Ovulation induction in patients in whom the cause of infertility is functional and not caused by primary ovarian failure; development of multiple follicles with ART

Dosage Summary

SubQ:

Gonal-f®:

Children: Dosage not established

Adults (females):

ART: Initial: 150-225 int. units once daily for 5 days; Maintenance: Dose adjustments of ≤75-150 int. units can be made every 3-5 days up to 450 int. units/day

Ovulation induction: Initial: 75 int. units/day for 5-7 days; Maintenance: Dose adjustments of up to 37.5 int. units after 14 days initially, then every 7-14 days up to 300 int. units/day

Adults (males): Initial: 150 int. units 3 times/week; Maintenance: Up to 300 int. units 3 times/week (maximum: 18 months of therapy)

Gonal-f® RFF:

Children: Dosage not established

Adults (females):

ART: Initial: 150-225 int. units once daily for 5 days; Maintenance: Dose adjustments of ≤75-150 int. units can be made every 3-5 days up to 450 int. units/day

Ovulation induction: Initial: 75 int. units/day for 5-7 days; Maintenance: Dose adjustments of up to 37.5 int. units every 7-14 days up to 300 int. units/day

Adults (males): Dosage not established

Dosage Forms

Injection, powder for reconstitution:

Gonal-f®: 450 int. units

Gonal-f® RFF: 75 int. units

Injection, solution:

Gonal-f® RFF: 300 int. units/0.5 mL (0.5 mL); 450 int. units/0.75 mL (0.75 mL); 900 int. units/1.5 mL (1.5 mL)

follitropin beta (foe li TRO pin BAY ta)

Synonyms follicle stimulating hormone, recombinant; FSH; rFSH-beta; rhFSH-beta

U.S./Canadian Brand Names Follistim® AQ Cartridge [US]; Follistim® AQ [US]; Puregon® [Can]

Therapeutic Category Ovulation Stimulator

Use Ovulation induction in patients in whom the cause of infertility is functional and not caused by primary ovarian failure; development of multiple follicles with Assisted Reproductive Technology (ART)

Dosage Summary

I.M., SubQ:

Children: Dosage not established

Adults (females):

ART: Initial: 150-225 int. units for at least the first 4-5 days; Maintenance: Adjust dose based on patient response up to 450-600 int. units/day

Ovulation induction: Initial: 75 int. units/day for up to 7-14 days; Maintenance: Adjust dose based on patient response up to 175-300 int. units/day

Adults (males): Dosage not established

Dosage Forms

Injection, solution:

Follistim® AQ: 75 int. units/0.5 mL (0.5 mL); 150 int. units/0.5 mL (0.5 mL)

Follistim® AQ Cartridge: 175 int. units/0.21 mL (0.21 mL); 350 int. units/0.42 mL (0.42 mL); 650 int. units/0.78 mL (0.78 mL); 975 int. units/1.17 mL (1.17 mL)

Folotyn™ [US] *see* pralatrexate *on page* *785*

Foltrin® [US] *see* vitamins (multiple/oral) *on page* *990*

Foltx® [US] *see* folic acid, cyanocobalamin, and pyridoxine *on page* *423*

Folvite® *(Discontinued)* *see* folic acid *on page* *423*

fomepizole (foe ME pi zole)

Sound-Alike/Look-Alike Issues

fomepizole may be confused with omeprazole

Synonyms 4-methylpyrazole; 4-MP

U.S./Canadian Brand Names Antizol® [US]

Therapeutic Category Antidote

Use Treatment of methanol or ethylene glycol poisoning alone or in combination with hemodialysis

Dosage Summary

I.V.:

Adults: Loading dose of 15 mg/kg, followed by 10 mg/kg every 12 hours for 4 doses, then 15 mg/kg every 12 hours until levels have been reduced <20 mg/dL and patient is asymptomatic

Dosage Forms

Injection, solution [preservative free]: 1 g/mL (1.5 mL)

Antizol®: 1 g/mL (1.5 mL)

fondaparinux (fon da PARE i nuks)

Synonyms fondaparinux sodium

U.S./Canadian Brand Names Arixtra® [US/Can]

Therapeutic Category Factor Xa Inhibitor

Use Prophylaxis of deep vein thrombosis (DVT) in patients undergoing surgery for hip replacement, knee replacement, hip fracture (including extended prophylaxis following hip fracture surgery), or abdominal surgery (in patients at risk for thromboembolic complications); treatment of acute pulmonary embolism (PE); treatment of acute DVT without PE

Note: Additional Canadian approvals (not approved in U.S.): Unstable angina or non-ST segment elevation myocardial infarction (UA/NSTEMI) for the prevention of death and subsequent MI; ST segment elevation MI (STEMI) for the prevention of death and myocardial reinfarction

Dosage Summary

SubQ:

Children: Dosage not established

Adults <50 kg: Treatment: 5 mg once daily

Adults 50-100 kg: Prophylaxis: 2.5 mg once daily; Treatment: 7.5 mg once daily

Adults >100 kg: Prophylaxis: 2.5 mg once daily; Treatment: 10 mg once daily

Dosage Forms

Injection, solution [preservative free]:

Arixtra®: 2.5 mg/0.5 mL (0.5 mL); 5 mg/0.4 mL (0.4 mL); 7.5 mg/0.6 mL (0.6 mL); 10 mg/0.8 mL (0.8 mL)

fondaparinux sodium *see* fondaparinux *on page* *425*

Foradil® [Can] *see* formoterol *on page* *425*

Foradil® Aerolizer® [US] *see* formoterol *on page* *425*

Forane® [US/Can] *see* isoflurane *on page* *527*

formoterol (for MOH te rol)

Sound-Alike/Look-Alike Issues

Foradil® may be confused with Toradol®

Synonyms formoterol fumarate; formoterol fumarate dihydrate

U.S./Canadian Brand Names Foradil® Aerolizer® [US]; Foradil® [Can]; Oxeze® Turbuhaler® [Can]; Perforomist™ [US]

Therapeutic Category $Beta_2$-Adrenergic Agonist Agent

Use Maintenance treatment of asthma and prevention of bronchospasm in patients ≥5 years of age with reversible obstructive airway disease, including patients with symptoms of nocturnal asthma, who require regular treatment with inhaled, short-acting $beta_2$-agonists; maintenance treatment of bronchoconstriction in patients with COPD; prevention of exercise-induced bronchospasm in patients ≥5 years of age

Note:

Oxeze® is also approved in Canada for acute relief of symptoms ("on demand" treatment) in patients ≥6 years of age.

Perforomist™ is only indicated for maintenance treatment of bronchoconstriction in patients with COPD.

Dosage Summary

Inhalation:

Foradil®:

Children <5 years: Dosage not established

Children ≥5 years: 12 mcg capsule inhaled every 12 hours **or** 12 mcg capsule inhaled prior to exercise

Adults: 12 mcg capsule inhaled every 12 hours **or** 12 mcg capsule inhaled prior to exercise

Perforomist™:

Children <18 years: Dosage not established

Adults: 20 mcg twice daily (maximum dose: 40 mcg/day)

Dosage Forms

Powder, for oral inhalation:

Foradil® Aerolizer®: 12 mcg/capsule (12s, 60s)

Solution, for nebulization:

Perforomist™: 20 mcg/2 mL (60s)

Dosage Forms - Canada

Powder for oral inhalation:

Oxeze® Turbuhaler®: 6 mcg/inhalation, 12 mcg/inhalation

formoterol and budesonide *see* budesonide and formoterol *on page 152*

formoterol and mometasone *see* mometasone and formoterol *on page 642*

formoterol and mometasone furoate *see* mometasone and formoterol *on page 642*

formoterol fumarate *see* formoterol *on page 425*

formoterol fumarate dihydrate *see* formoterol *on page 425*

formoterol fumarate dihydrate and budesonide *see* budesonide and formoterol *on page 152*

formoterol fumarate dihydrate and mometasone *see* mometasone and formoterol *on page 642*

Formula EM [US-OTC] *see* fructose, dextrose, and phosphoric acid *on page 430*

Formula Q® *(Discontinued)* *see* quinine *on page 823*

Formulation R™ [US-OTC] *see* phenylephrine (topical) *on page 752*

Formulex® [Can] *see* dicyclomine *on page 299*

5-formyl tetrahydrofolate *see* leucovorin calcium *on page 553*

Fortamet® [US] *see* metformin *on page 609*

Fortaz® [US/Can] *see* ceftazidime *on page 192*

Forteo® [US/Can] *see* teriparatide *on page 919*

Fortical® [US] *see* calcitonin *on page 165*

Fortovase® *(Discontinued)* *see* saquinavir *on page 865*

Fosamax® [US/Can] *see* alendronate *on page 47*

Fosamax Plus D® [US] *see* alendronate and cholecalciferol *on page 47*

fosamprenavir (FOS am pren a veer)

Sound-Alike/Look-Alike Issues

Lexiva® may be confused with Levitra®

Synonyms fosamprenavir calcium; GW433908G

U.S./Canadian Brand Names Lexiva® [US]; Telzir® [Can]

Therapeutic Category Antiretroviral Agent, Protease Inhibitor

Use Treatment of HIV infections in combination with at least two other antiretroviral agents

Dosage Summary Note: The adult regimen of 1400 mg twice daily may be used for pediatric patients who weigh ≥47 kg. When combined with ritonavir, the adult regimen of fosamprenavir 700 mg plus ritonavir 100 mg twice daily can be used in children who weigh ≥39 kg while ritonavir capsules may be used for pediatric patients who weigh ≥33 kg.

Oral:

Children <2 years: Dosage not established

Children 2-5 years: 30 mg/kg/dose twice daily (maximum: 1400 mg twice daily)

Children ≥6 years:

Unboosted regimen: 30 mg/kg/dose twice daily (maximum: 1400 mg twice daily)

Ritonavir-boosted regimen: 18 mg/kg/dose twice daily (maximum: 700 mg twice daily)

Adults:

Unboosted regimen: 1400 mg twice daily

Ritonavir-boosted regimen: 700 mg twice daily **or** 1400 mg once daily

Dosage Forms

Suspension, oral:

Lexiva®: 50 mg/mL (225 mL)

Tablet, oral:

Lexiva®: 700 mg

Dosage Forms - Canada

Tablet:

Telzir®: 700 mg

Suspension, oral:

Telzir®: 50 mg/mL

fosamprenavir calcium *see* fosamprenavir *on page 426*

fosaprepitant (fos a PRE pi tant)

Sound-Alike/Look-Alike Issues

fosaprepitant may be confused with aprepitant, fosamprenavir, fospropofol

Emend® for injection (fosaprepitant) may be confused with Emend® (aprepitant) which is an oral capsule formulation.

Synonyms aprepitant injection; fosaprepitant dimeglumine; L-758,298; MK 0517

U.S./Canadian Brand Names Emend® for Injection [US]

Therapeutic Category Antiemetic; Substance P/Neurokinin 1 Receptor Antagonist

Use Prevention of acute and delayed nausea and vomiting associated with moderately- and highly-emetogenic chemotherapy (in combination with other antiemetics)

Dosage Summary

I.V.:

Children: Dosage not established

Adults: 115 mg 30 minutes prior to chemotherapy on day 1

Dosage Forms

Injection, powder for reconstitution:

Emend® for Injection: 115 mg

fosaprepitant dimeglumine *see* fosaprepitant *on page 427*

Fosavance [Can] *see* alendronate and cholecalciferol *on page 47*

foscarnet (fos KAR net)

Synonyms PFA; phosphonoformate; phosphonoformic acid

U.S./Canadian Brand Names Foscavir® [Can]

Therapeutic Category Antiviral Agent

Use Treatment of acyclovir-resistant mucocutaneous herpes simplex virus (HSV) infections in immunocompromised persons (eg, with advanced AIDS); treatment of CMV retinitis in persons with HIV

Dosage Summary

I.V.:

Children ≤12 years: Dosage not established

Adolescents: Induction: CMV: 60 mg/kg every 8 hours **or** 90 mg/kg every 12 hours for 14-21 day; HSV: 40 mg/kg/dose every 8-12 hours for 14-21 days; Maintenance: CMV: 90-120 mg/kg once daily

Adults: Induction: CMV: 60 mg/kg every 8 hours **or** 90 mg/kg every 12 hours for 14-21 day; HSV: 40 mg/kg/dose every 8-12 hours for 14-21 days; Maintenance: CMV: 90-120 mg/kg once daily

Dosage Forms

Injection, solution [preservative free]: 24 mg/mL (250 mL, 500 mL)

Foscavir® [Can] *see* foscarnet *on page 427*

Foscavir® *(Discontinued)* *see* foscarnet *on page 427*

fosfomycin (fos foe MYE sin)

Sound-Alike/Look-Alike Issues

Monurol® may be confused with Monopril®

Synonyms fosfomycin tromethamine

U.S./Canadian Brand Names Monurol® [US/Can]

Therapeutic Category Antibiotic, Miscellaneous

Use Single oral dose in the treatment of uncomplicated urinary tract infections in women due to susceptible strains of *E. coli* and *Enterococcus faecalis*

Dosage Summary

Oral:

Children: Dosage not established

Adults (females): Single dose of 3 g in 3-4 oz (90-120 mL) of water

Dosage Forms

Powder for solution, oral:

Monurol®: 3 g/sachet (3s)

fosfomycin tromethamine *see* fosfomycin *on page 428*

fosinopril (foe SIN oh pril)

Sound-Alike/Look-Alike Issues

fosinopril may be confused with FLUoxetine, Fosamax®, furosemide, lisinopril

Monopril® may be confused with Accupril®, minoxidil, moexipril, Monoket®, Monurol®, ramipril

Synonyms fosinopril sodium

U.S./Canadian Brand Names Apo-Fosinopril® [Can]; Monopril® [Can]; Mylan-Fosinopril [Can]; PMS-Fosinopril [Can]; RAN™-Fosinopril [Can]; Riva-Fosinopril [Can]; Teva-Fosinopril [Can]

Therapeutic Category Angiotensin-Converting Enzyme (ACE) Inhibitor

Use Treatment of hypertension, either alone or in combination with other antihypertensive agents; treatment of heart failure (HF)

Dosage Summary

Oral:

Children ≤50 kg: Dosage not established

Children ≥6 years and >50 kg: Initial: 5-10 mg once daily (maximum: 40 mg/day)

Adults: Initial: 10 mg once daily; Maintenance: 10-40 mg/day in 1-2 divided doses (maximum: 80 mg/day)

Dosage Forms

Tablet, oral: 10 mg, 20 mg, 40 mg

fosinopril and hydrochlorothiazide (foe SIN oh pril & hye droe klor oh THYE a zide)

Sound-Alike/Look-Alike Issues

Monopril® may be confused with Accupril®, minoxidil, moexipril, Monoket®, Monurol®, ramipril

Synonyms hydrochlorothiazide and fosinopril

U.S./Canadian Brand Names Monopril-HCT® [Can]

Therapeutic Category Angiotensin-Converting Enzyme (ACE) Inhibitor

Use Treatment of hypertension; not indicated for first-line treatment

Dosage Summary

Oral:

Children: Dosage not established

Adults: Fosinopril 10-80 mg and hydrochlorothiazide 12.5-50 mg once daily; **Note:** JNC 7 recommends fosinopril 10-40 mg/day

Dosage Forms

Tablet: 0/12.5: Fosinopril 10 mg and hydrochlorothiazide 12.5 mg; 20/12.5: Fosinopril 20 mg and hydrochlorothiazide 12.5 mg

fosinopril sodium *see* fosinopril *on page 428*

fosphenytoin (FOS fen i toyn)

Sound-Alike/Look-Alike Issues

fosphenytoin may be confused with fospropofol

Cerebyx® may be confused with Celebrex®, Celexa™, Cerezyme®, Cervarix®

Synonyms fosphenytoin sodium

U.S./Canadian Brand Names Cerebyx® [US/Can]

Therapeutic Category Hydantoin

Use Used for the control of generalized convulsive status epilepticus and prevention and treatment of seizures occurring during neurosurgery; indicated for short-term parenteral administration when other means of phenytoin administration are unavailable, inappropriate, or deemed less advantageous (the safety and effectiveness of fosphenytoin use for more than 5 days has not been systematically evaluated)

Dosage Summary Note: The dose, concentration in solutions, and infusion rates for fosphenytoin are expressed as phenytoin sodium equivalents (PE); fosphenytoin should always be prescribed and dispensed in phenytoin sodium equivalents (PE)

I.M.:

Children: Dosage not established

Adults: Loading: 15-20 mg PE/kg; Maintenance: 4-6 mg PE/kg/day

I.V.:

Adults: Loading: 10-20 mg PE/kg; Maintenance: 4-6 mg PE/kg/day

Dosage Forms

Injection, solution: 75 mg/mL (2 mL, 10 mL)

Cerebyx®: 75 mg/mL (2 mL)

fosphenytoin sodium *see* fosphenytoin *on page* 429

fospropofol (fos PROE po fole)

Sound-Alike/Look-Alike Issues

fospropofol may be confused with fosaprepitant, fosphenytoin, propofol

Synonyms aquavan; fospropofol disodium; GPI 15715

U.S./Canadian Brand Names Lusedra™ [US]

Therapeutic Category Sedative

Controlled Substance C-IV

Use Monitored anesthesia care (MAC) sedation in patients undergoing diagnostic or therapeutic procedures

Dosage Summary

I.V.:

Children: Dosage not established

Adults:

Healthy adults <65 years or with mild systemic disease (ASA-PS1 or -PS2): Initial: 6.5 mg/kg (maximum initial dose: 577.5 mg or 16.5 mL); supplemental: 1.6 mg/kg (maximum supplemental dose: 140 mg or 4 mL) no more frequently than every 4 minutes as needed

Elderly patients ≥65 years or patients with severe systemic disease (ASA-PS3 or -PS4): Initial: 4.9 mg/kg (maximum initial dose: 437.5 mg or 12.5 mL); supplemental 1.2 mg/kg (maximum supplemental dose: 105 mg or 3 mL) no more frequently than every 4 minutes as needed

Dosage Forms

Injection, solution [preservative free]:

Lusedra™: 35 mg/mL (30 mL)

fospropofol disodium *see* fospropofol *on page* 429

Fosrenol® [US/Can] *see* lanthanum *on page* 550

Fototar® ***(Discontinued)*** *see* coal tar *on page* 242

FR901228 *see* romidepsin *on page* 850

Fragmin® [US/Can] *see* dalteparin *on page* 267

Fraxiparine™ [Can] *see* nadroparin *(Canada only) on page* 654

Fraxiparine™ Forte [Can] *see* nadroparin *(Canada only) on page* 654

FreAmine® III [US] *see* amino acid injection *on page* 64

FreAmine® HBC [US] *see* amino acid injection *on page* 64

Freedavite [US-OTC] *see* vitamins (multiple/oral) *on page* 990

Freezone® [US-OTC] *see* salicylic acid *on page* 858

Frisium® [Can] *see* clobazam *(Canada only) on page 234*
Froben® [Can] *see* flurbiprofen (systemic) *on page 418*
Froben-SR® [Can] *see* flurbiprofen (systemic) *on page 418*
Frova® [US/Can] *see* frovatriptan *on page 430*

frovatriptan (froe va TRIP tan)

Synonyms frovatriptan succinate
U.S./Canadian Brand Names Frova® [US/Can]
Therapeutic Category Antimigraine Agent; Serotonin 5-$HT_{1B,\ 1D}$ Receptor Agonist
Use Acute treatment of migraine with or without aura
Dosage Summary
Oral:
Children: Dosage not established
Adults: 2.5 mg as a single dose, may repeat after 2 hours (maximum: 7.5 mg/day)
Dosage Forms
Tablet, oral:
Frova®: 2.5 mg

frovatriptan succinate *see* frovatriptan *on page 430*

fructose, dextrose, and phosphoric acid (FRUK tose, DEKS trose, & foss FOR ik AS id)

Sound-Alike/Look-Alike Issues
Emetrol® may be confused with emetine
Synonyms dextrose, levulose and phosphoric acid; levulose, dextrose and phosphoric acid; phosphorated carbohydrate solution; phosphoric acid, levulose and dextrose
U.S./Canadian Brand Names Emetrol® [US-OTC]; Formula EM [US-OTC]; Kalmz [US-OTC]; Nausea Relief [US-OTC]; Nausetrol® [US-OTC]
Therapeutic Category Antiemetic
Use Relief of nausea associated with upset stomach that occurs with intestinal or stomach flu, and food indiscretions
Dosage Summary
Oral:
Children <2 years: Dosage not established
Children ≥2-12 years: 5-10 mL every 15 minutes as needed; do not take for more than 1 hour (5 doses)
Children ≥12 years: 15-30 mL every 15 minutes as needed; do not take for more than 1 hour (5 doses)
Adults: 15-30 mL every 15 minutes as needed; do not take for more than 1 hour (5 doses)
Dosage Forms
Liquid, oral: Fructose 1.87 g, dextrose 1.87 g, and phosphoric acid 21.5 mg per 5 mL
Formula EM [OTC], Kalmz [OTC], Nausea Relief [OTC], Nausetrol® [OTC]: Fructose 1.87 g, dextrose 1.87 g, and phosphoric acid 21.5 mg per 5 mL

frusemide *see* furosemide *on page 431*
FS *see* fibrin sealant *on page 401*
FSH *see* follitropin alfa *on page 424*
FSH *see* follitropin beta *on page 424*
FSH *see* urofollitropin *on page 971*
FS Shampoo® Topical *(Discontinued)* *see* fluocinolone (topical) *on page 411*
FS VH S/D *see* fibrin sealant *on page 401*
FTC *see* emtricitabine *on page 347*
FTC, TDF, and EFV *see* efavirenz, emtricitabine, and tenofovir *on page 343*
FU *see* fluorouracil (systemic) *on page 415*
FU *see* fluorouracil (topical) *on page 415*
5-FU *see* fluorouracil (systemic) *on page 415*
5-FU *see* fluorouracil (topical) *on page 415*
Fucidin® [Can] *see* fusidic acid *(Canada only) on page 432*
Fucithalmic® [Can] *see* fusidic acid *(Canada only) on page 432*
FUDR® [Can] *see* floxuridine *on page 407*
FUDR *see* floxuridine *on page 407*

Ful-Glo® [US] *see* fluorescein *on page 412*

fulvestrant (fool VES trant)

Synonyms ICI-182,780; zeneca 182,780; ZM-182,780

U.S./Canadian Brand Names Faslodex® [US]

Therapeutic Category Antineoplastic Agent, Estrogen Receptor Antagonist

Use Treatment of hormone receptor-positive metastatic breast cancer in postmenopausal women with disease progression following antiestrogen therapy

Dosage Summary

I.M.:

Children: Dosage not established

Adults: 250 mg at 1-month intervals

Dosage Forms

Injection, solution:

Faslodex®: 50 mg/mL (5 mL)

Fumasorb® ***(Discontinued)*** *see* ferrous fumarate *on page 398*

Fumerin® ***(Discontinued)*** *see* ferrous fumarate *on page 398*

Funduscein® Injection ***(Discontinued)*** *see* fluorescein *on page 412*

Fungi-Nail® [US-OTC] *see* undecylenic acid and derivatives *on page 969*

Fungizone® [Can] *see* amphotericin B (conventional) *on page 74*

Fung-O® [US-OTC] *see* salicylic acid *on page 858*

Fungoid® [US-OTC] *see* miconazole (topical) *on page 630*

Furacin® Topical ***(Discontinued)***

Furadantin® [US] *see* nitrofurantoin *on page 678*

Furalan® ***(Discontinued)*** *see* nitrofurantoin *on page 678*

Furan® ***(Discontinued)*** *see* nitrofurantoin *on page 678*

Furanite® ***(Discontinued)*** *see* nitrofurantoin *on page 678*

furazosin *see* prazosin *on page 789*

furosemide (fyoor OH se mide)

Sound-Alike/Look-Alike Issues

furosemide may be confused with famotidine, finasteride, fluconazole, FLUoxetine, fosinopril, loperamide, torsemide

Lasix® may be confused with Esidrix®, Lanoxin®, Lidex®, Lomotil®, Lovenox®, Luvox®, Luxiq®

Synonyms frusemide

U.S./Canadian Brand Names Apo-Furosemide® [Can]; Dom-Furosemide [Can]; Furosemide Injection, USP [Can]; Furosemide Special [Can]; Lasix® Special [Can]; Lasix® [US/Can]; Novo-Semide [Can]; Nu-Furosemide [Can]; PMS-Furosemide [Can]

Therapeutic Category Diuretic, Loop

Use Management of edema associated with heart failure and hepatic or renal disease; acute pulmonary edema; treatment of hypertension (alone or in combination with other antihypertensives)

Dosage Summary

I.M.:

Children: Initial: 1 mg/kg/dose, may increase dose by 1 mg/kg/dose administered not sooner than 2 hours after previous dose until satisfactory response achieved. May administer maintenance dose at intervals of 6-12 hours (maximum: 6 mg/kg/dose).

Adults: Initial: 20-40 mg/dose, may repeat the same dose or increase dose by 20 mg/dose and administer 1-2 hours after previous dose. Usual maintenance dose interval: 6-12 hours (maximum: 200 mg/dose).

Elderly: Initial: 20 mg/day; increase slowly to desired response

I.V.:

Children: Initial: 1 mg/kg/dose, may increase dose by 1 mg/kg/dose administered not sooner than 2 hours after previous dose until satisfactory response achieved. May administer maintenance dose at intervals of 6-12 hours (maximum: 6 mg/kg/dose).

Adults: Initial: 20-40 mg/dose, may repeat the same dose or increase dose by 20 mg/dose and administer 1-2 hours after previous dose; Usual maintenance dose interval: 6-12 hours (maximum: 200 mg/dose) **or** 40 mg, followed by 80 mg within 1 hour or 20-40 mg bolus, followed by continuous I.V. infusion doses of 10-40 mg/hour, doubled as needed up to a maximum 160 mg/hour.

Elderly: Initial: 20 mg/day; increase slowly to desired response

Oral:

Children: Initial: 2 mg/kg/dose, increasing in increments of 1-2 mg/kg/dose with each succeeding dose at intervals of 6-8 hours until a satisfactory response is achieved (maximum: 6 mg/kg/dose).

Adults: Initial: 20-80 mg/dose, may repeat same dose or increase dose in increments of 20-40 mg/dose at intervals of 6-8 hours. Usual maintenance dose interval is once or twice daily (maximum: 600 mg/day).

Elderly: Initial: 20 mg/day; increase slowly to desired response

Dosage Forms

Injection, solution [preservative free]: 10 mg/mL (2 mL, 4 mL, 10 mL)

Solution, oral: 40 mg/5 mL (5 mL, 500 mL); 10 mg/mL (4 mL, 60 mL, 120 mL)

Tablet, oral: 20 mg, 40 mg, 80 mg

Lasix®: 20 mg, 40 mg, 80 mg

Furosemide Injection, USP [Can] *see* furosemide *on page 431*

Furosemide Special [Can] *see* furosemide *on page 431*

fusidic acid *(Canada only)* (fyoo SI dik AS id)

Synonyms sodium fusidate

U.S./Canadian Brand Names Fucidin® [Can]; Fucithalmic® [Can]

Therapeutic Category Antifungal Agent, Systemic

Use

Systemic: Treatment of skin and soft tissue infections, or osteomyelitis, caused by susceptible organisms, including *Staphylococcus aureus* (penicillinase-producing or nonpenicillinase strains); may be used in the treatment of pneumonia, septicemia, endocarditis, burns, and cystic fibrosis caused by susceptible organisms when other antibiotics have failed

Topical: Treatment of primary and secondary skin infections caused by susceptible organisms

Ophthalmic: Treatment of superficial infections of the eye and conjunctiva caused by susceptible organisms

Dosage Summary

I.V.:

Children ≤12 years: 20 mg/kg/day in 3 divided doses

Children >12 years: 500 mg 3 times/day

Adults: 500 mg 3 times/day

Ophthalmic:

Children <2 years: Dosage not established

Children ≥2 years: Instill 1 drop in each eye every 12 hours

Adults: Instill 1 drop in each eye every 12 hours

Oral:

Children: Dosage not established

Adults: 500-1000 mg 3 times/day

Topical:

Children: Apply to affected area 3-4 times/day or 1-2 times/day if gauze dressing used

Adults: Apply to affected area 3-4 times/day or 1-2 times/day if gauze dressing used

Dosage Forms - Canada

Cream:

Fucidin®: 2% (15 g, 30 g)

Injection, powder for reconstitution:

Fucidin®: 500 mg

Ointment, topical:

Fucidin®: 2% (15 g, 30 g)

Suspension, ophthalmic:

Fucithalmic®: 10 mg/g [1%] (0.2 g) [unit-dose, without preservative]; (3 g, 5 g) [multidose, contains benzalkonium chloride]

Tablet:

Fucidin® [CAN]: 250 mg [not available in the U.S.]

Fusilev™ [US] *see* LEVOleucovorin *on page 558*

Fuzeon® [US/Can] *see* enfuvirtide *on page 349*

FVIII/vWF *see* antihemophilic factor/von Willebrand factor complex (human) *on page 82*

FXT 40 [Can] *see* fluoxetine *on page 415*

GAA *see* alglucosidase alfa *on page 49*

gabapentin (GA ba pen tin)

Sound-Alike/Look-Alike Issues
Neurontin® may be confused with Motrin®, Neoral®, nitrofurantoin, Noroxin®, Zarontin®

U.S./Canadian Brand Names Apo-Gabapentin® [Can]; CO Gabapentin [Can]; Dom-Gabapentin [Can]; Mylan-Gabapentin [Can]; Neurontin® [US/Can]; PHL-Gabapentin [Can]; PMS-Gabapentin [Can]; PRO-Gabapentin [Can]; RAN™-Gabapentin [Can]; ratio-Gabapentin [Can]; Riva-Gabapentin [Can]; Teva-Gabapentin [Can]

Therapeutic Category Anticonvulsant

Use Adjunct for treatment of partial seizures with and without secondary generalized seizures in patients >12 years of age with epilepsy; adjunct for treatment of partial seizures in pediatric patients 3-12 years of age; management of postherpetic neuralgia (PHN) in adults

Dosage Summary

Oral:

Children <3 years: Dosage not established

Children 3-4 years: Initial: 10-15 mg/kg/day in 3 divided doses; Maintenance: 40 mg/kg/day in 3 divided doses (maximum: 50 mg/kg/day); **Note:** Titration is recommended

Children 5-12 years: Initial: 10-15 mg/kg/day in 3 divided doses; Maintenance: 25-35 mg/kg/day in 3 divided doses (maximum: 50 mg/kg/day); **Note:** Titration is recommended

Children >12 years: Initial: 300 mg 3 times/day; Maintenance: 900-1800 mg/day in 3 divided doses (maximum: 3600 mg/day [short-term]); **Note:** Titration is recommended

Adults:

Anticonvulsant: Initial: 300 mg 3 times/day; Maintenance: 900-1800 mg/day in 3 divided doses (maximum: 3600 mg/day [short-term]); **Note:** Titration is recommended

Postherpetic neuralgia: Initial: Day 1: 300 mg, Day 2: 300 mg twice daily, Day 3: 300mg 3 times/day; Maintenance: 1800-3600 mg/day; **Note:** Titration is recommended

Dosage Forms

Capsule, oral: 100 mg, 300 mg, 400 mg
Neurontin®: 100 mg, 300 mg, 400 mg

Solution, oral:
Neurontin®: 250 mg/5 mL (470 mL)

Tablet, oral: 600 mg, 800 mg
Neurontin®: 600 mg, 800 mg

Gabitril® [US/Can] *see* tiagabine *on page 931*

gadobenate dimeglumine (gad oh BEN ate dye MEG loo meen)

Synonyms gadolinum-BOPTA; Gd-BOPTA

U.S./Canadian Brand Names Multihance® Multipak™ [US]; Multihance® [US]

Therapeutic Category Diagnostic Agent; Radiological/Contrast Media, Nonionic

Use Contrast medium for magnetic resonance imaging (MRI) to visualize CNS lesions with abnormal vascularity in the brain, spine, and associated tissues

Dosage Summary

I.V.:

Children: Dosage not established

Adults: 0.1 mmol/kg (0.2 mL/kg)

Dosage Forms

Injection, solution [preservative free]:
Multihance®: 529 mg/mL (5 mL, 10 mL, 15 mL, 20 mL)
Multihance® Multipack™: 529 mg/mL (50 mL, 100 mL)

gadobutrol *(Canada only)* (gad oh BYOO trol)

Sound-Alike/Look-Alike Issues
Gadovist® may be confused with Magnevist®, Vasovist™

Synonyms gadovist 1.0

U.S./Canadian Brand Names Gadovist® [Can]

Therapeutic Category Gadolinium-Containing Contrast Agent; Radiological/Contrast Media, Nonionic

Use Contrast medium for magnetic resonance imaging (MRI) of CNS lesions (brain, spine, and associated tissues); perfusion studies to diagnose stroke, or to detect focal cerebral ischemia or tumor perfusion; contrast-enhanced magnetic resonance angiography (CE-MRA)

Dosage Summary

I.V.:

Children: Dosage not established

Adults: 0.1-0.3 mL/kg (CNS imaging) **or** 7.5-20 mL (CE-MRA)

Dosage Forms - Canada

Injection, solution [preservative free]:

Gadovist®: 604.72 mg/mL (15 mL)

gadodiamide (gad oh DYE a mide)

Synonyms gadolinium-DTPA-BMA; Gd-DTPA-BMA

U.S./Canadian Brand Names Omniscan® [US]

Therapeutic Category Radiological/Contrast Media, Nonionic

Use Contrast medium for magnetic resonance imaging (MRI) to visualize CNS lesions with abnormal vascularity in the brain, spine, and associated tissues, and to visualize body lesions with abnormal vascularity within the thoracic (noncardiac), abdominal, pelvic cavities, and retroperitoneal space

Dosage Summary

I.V.:

Children <2 years: Dosage not established

Children ≥2 years:

CNS, intraabdominal, intrathoracic (noncardiac), pelvic cavities imaging: 0.1 mmol/kg (0.2 mL/kg)

Kidney imaging: 0.05 mmol/kg (0.1 mL/kg)

Adults:

CNS imaging: 0.1 mmol/kg (0.2 mL/kg); may repeat 0.2 mmol/kg (0.4 mL/kg) once if needed

Intraabdominal, intrathoracic (noncardiac), pelvic cavities imaging: 0.1 mmol/kg (0.2 mL/kg)

Kidney imaging: 0.05 mmol/kg (0.1 mL/kg)

Dosage Forms

Injection, solution [preservative free]:

Omniscan®: 287 mg/mL (5 mL, 10 mL, 15 mL, 20 mL, 50 mL)

gadofosveset (gad oh FOS ve set)

Sound-Alike/Look-Alike Issues

Vasovist® may be confused with Magnevist®, Gadovist®

Synonyms gadofosveset trisodium

U.S./Canadian Brand Names Ablavar™ [US]; Vasovist® [Can]

Therapeutic Category Gadolinium-Containing Contrast Agent; Radiological/Contrast Media, Paramagnetic Agent

Use Contrast medium used in magnetic resonance angiography (MRA) to evaluate or better define aortoiliac occlusive disease

Dosage Summary

I.V.:

Children: Dosage not established

Adults: 0.03 mmol/kg (MRA)

Dosage Forms

Injection, solution [preservative free]:

Ablavar™: 0.25 mmol/mL (10 mL, 15 mL)

Dosage Forms - Canada

Injection, solution [preservative free]:

Vasovist®: 0.25 mmoL/mL (10 mL, 15 mL, 20 mL)

gadofosveset trisodium *see* gadofosveset *on page 434*

gadolinium-DTPA *see* gadopentetate dimeglumine *on page 434*

gadolinium-DTPA-BMA *see* gadodiamide *on page 434*

gadolinium-DTPA-BMEA *see* gadoversetamide *on page 435*

gadolinium-HP-DO3A *see* gadoteridol *on page 435*

gadolinum-BOPTA *see* gadobenate dimeglumine *on page 433*

gadopentetate dimeglumine (gad oh PEN te tate dye MEG loo meen)

Synonyms gadolinium-DTPA; Gd-DTPA

U.S./Canadian Brand Names Magnevist® [US/Can]

Therapeutic Category Radiological/Contrast Media, Paramagnetic Agent

Use Contrast medium for magnetic resonance imaging (MRI) to visualize lesions with abnormal vascularity in the brain, spine and associated tissues, head and neck, and body (excluding the heart)

Dosage Summary Note: Dosing for patients >130 kg (286 pounds) has not been studied.

I.V.:

Children <2 years: Dosage not established
Children ≥2 years: 0.1 mmol/kg (0.2 mL/kg)
Adults: 0.1 mmol/kg (0.2 mL/kg)

Dosage Forms

Injection, solution [preservative free]:
Magnevist®: 469.01 mg/mL (5 mL, 10 mL, 15 mL, 20 mL, 50 mL, 100 mL)

gadoteridol (gad oh TER i dol)

Synonyms gadolinium-HP-DO3A; Gd-HP-DO3A

U.S./Canadian Brand Names ProHance® Multipack™ [US]; ProHance® [US]

Therapeutic Category Radiological/Contrast Media, Nonionic

Use Contrast medium for magnetic resonance imaging (MRI) to visualize CNS lesions with abnormal vascularity in the brain, spine, and associated tissues and to visualize extracranial/extraspinal tissues in the head and neck

Dosage Summary

I.V.:

Children <2 years: Dosage not established
Children ≥2 years: 0.1 mmol/kg (0.2 mL/kg)
Adults: 0.1 mmol/kg (0.2 mL/kg) [CNS or extracranial/extraspinal tissue imaging]; if needed, a second dose of 0.2 mmol/kg (0.4 mL/kg) may be repeated once within 30 minutes of the first dose [CNS imaging]

Dosage Forms

Injection, solution [preservative free]:
ProHance®: 279.3 mg/mL (5 mL, 10 mL, 15 mL, 17 mL, 20 mL)
ProHance® Multipack™: 279.3 mg/mL (50 mL)

gadoversetamide (gad oh ver SET a mide)

Synonyms gadolinium-DTPA-BMEA; Gd-DTPA-BMEA

U.S./Canadian Brand Names OptiMARK® [US]

Therapeutic Category Radiological/Contrast Media, Nonionic

Use Contrast medium for magnetic resonance imaging (MRI) to visualize lesions with abnormal vascularity in the liver or CNS (brain, spine, and associated tissues)

Dosage Summary

I.V.:

Children: Dosage not established
Adults: 0.1 mmol/kg (0.2 mL/kg)

Dosage Forms

Injection, solution [preservative free]:
OptiMARK®: 330.9 mg/mL (5 mL, 10 mL, 15 mL, 20 mL, 30 mL, 50 mL)

Gadovist® [Can] *see* gadobutrol *(Canada only) on page* 433
gadovist 1.0 *see* gadobutrol *(Canada only) on page* 433

gadoxetate (gad OX e tate)

Sound-Alike/Look-Alike Issues
Eovist® may be confused with Evista®

Synonyms gadoxetate disodium; Gd-EOB-DTPA

U.S./Canadian Brand Names Eovist® [US]; Primovist [Can]

Therapeutic Category Gadolinium-Containing Contrast Agent; Radiological/Contrast Media, Ionic (Low Osmolality); Radiological/Contrast Media, Paramagnetic Agent

Use Contrast medium for magnetic resonance imaging (MRI) to detect and characterize lesions within focal liver disease

Dosage Summary

I.V.:

Children: Dosage not established

Adults: 0.025 mmol/kg (0.1 mL/kg)

Dosage Forms

Injection, solution [preservative free]:

Eovist®: 181.43 mg/mL (10 mL)

gadoxetate disodium *see* gadoxetate *on page 435*

galantamine (ga LAN ta meen)

Sound-Alike/Look-Alike Issues

Razadyne® may be confused with Rozerem™

Reminyl® may be confused with Amaryl®, Robinul®

Synonyms galantamine hydrobromide

U.S./Canadian Brand Names Razadyne® ER [US]; Razadyne® [US]; Reminyl® ER [Can]; Reminyl® [Can]

Therapeutic Category Acetylcholinesterase Inhibitor (Central)

Use Treatment of mild-to-moderate dementia of Alzheimer disease

Dosage Summary

Oral:

Extended-release:

Children: Dosage not established

Adults: Initial: 8 mg once daily for 4 weeks; Maintenance: 16-24 mg once daily; **Note:** Titration is recommended

Immediate release:

Children: Dosage not established

Adults: Initial: 4 mg twice daily for 4 weeks; Maintenance: 16-24 mg/day in 2 divided doses; **Note:** Titration is recommended

Dosage Forms

Capsule, extended release, oral: 8 mg, 16 mg, 24 mg

Razadyne® ER: 8 mg, 16 mg, 24 mg

Solution, oral: 4 mg/mL (100 mL)

Razadyne®: 4 mg/mL (100 mL)

Tablet, oral: 4 mg, 8 mg, 12 mg

Razadyne®: 4 mg, 8 mg, 12 mg

galantamine hydrobromide *see* galantamine *on page 436*

galsulfase (gal SUL fase)

Synonyms recombinant N-acetylgalactosamine 4-sulfatase; rhASB

U.S./Canadian Brand Names Naglazyme™ [US]

Therapeutic Category Enzyme

Use Replacement therapy in mucopolysaccharidosis VI (MPS VI; Maroteaux-Lamy Syndrome) for improvement of walking and stair-climbing capacity

Dosage Summary Note: Premedicate with antihistamines with/without antipyretics 30-60 minutes prior to infusion.

I.V.:

Children <5 years: Dosage not established

Children >5 years: 1 mg/kg once weekly

Adults: 1 mg/kg once weekly

Dosage Forms

Injection, solution [preservative free]:

Naglazyme™: 5 mg/5 mL (5 mL)

Galzin® [US] *see* zinc acetate *on page 1001*

Gamimune® N [Can] *see* immune globulin (intravenous) *on page 502*

Gamimune® N Injection *(Discontinued)* *see* immune globulin (intravenous) *on page 502*

gamma benzene hexachloride *see* lindane *on page 567*

Gamma E-Gems® [US-OTC] *see* vitamin E *on page 988*

Gamma-E PLUS [US-OTC] *see* vitamin E *on page 988*

Gammagard® Liquid [US/Can] *see* immune globulin (intravenous) *on page 502*
Gammagard S/D® [US/Can] *see* immune globulin (intravenous) *on page 502*
gamma globulin *see* immune globulin (intramuscular) *on page 501*
gamma hydroxybutyric acid *see* sodium oxybate *on page 885*
gammaphos *see* amifostine *on page 63*
Gammar®-P I.V. ***(Discontinued)*** *see* immune globulin (intravenous) *on page 502*
GammaSTAN™ S/D [US] *see* immune globulin (intramuscular) *on page 501*
Gamulin® Rh ***(Discontinued)***
Gamunex® [US/Can] *see* immune globulin (intravenous) *on page 502*

ganciclovir (systemic) (gan SYE kloe veer)

Sound-Alike/Look-Alike Issues
ganciclovir may be confused with acyclovir
Cytovene® may be confused with Cytosar®, Cytosar-U®

Synonyms DHPG sodium; GCV sodium; nordeoxyguanosine

U.S./Canadian Brand Names Cytovene® [Can]; Cytovene®-IV [US]

Therapeutic Category Antiviral Agent

Use Treatment of CMV retinitis in immunocompromised individuals, including patients with acquired immunodeficiency syndrome; prophylaxis of CMV infection in transplant patients

Dosage Summary
I.V.:
Children: Induction: 5 mg/kg every 12 hours for 14-21 days; Maintenance: 30-35 mg/kg/week, given as once daily dose for 5-7 days per week
Adults: Induction: 5 mg/kg every 12 hours for 14-21 days; Maintenance: 30-35 mg/kg/week, given as once daily dose for 5-7 days per week

Dosage Forms
Injection, powder for reconstitution:
Cytovene®-IV: 500 mg

ganciclovir (ophthalmic) (gan SYE kloe veer)

Sound-Alike/Look-Alike Issues
ganciclovir may be confused with acyclovir

Synonyms nordeoxyguanosine

U.S./Canadian Brand Names Vitrasert™ [US/Can]; Zirgan™ [US]

Therapeutic Category Antiviral Agent

Use
Intravitreal implant: Treatment of CMV retinitis in patients with acquired immunodeficiency syndrome
Ophthalmic gel: Treatment of acute herpetic keratitis (dendritic ulcers)

Dosage Summary
Ocular implant:
Children <9 years: Dosage not established
Children ≥9 years: One implant for 5-8 month period
Adults: One implant for 5- to 8-month period
Ophthalmic gel:
Children <2 months: Dosage not established
Children ≥2 months: One drop in affected eye 5 times/day until corneal ulcer healed, then 1 drop 3 times/day for 7 days
Adults: One drop in affected eye 5 times/day until corneal ulcer healed, then 1 drop 3 times/day for 7 days

Dosage Forms
Gel, ophthalmic:
Zirgan®: 0.15% (5 g)
Implant, intravitreal:
Vitrasert®: 4.5 mg (1s)

Ganidin® NR [US-OTC] *see* guaifenesin *on page 454*

ganirelix (ga ni REL ix)

Synonyms antagon; ganirelix acetate

U.S./Canadian Brand Names Orgalutran® [Can]

Therapeutic Category Antigonadotropic Agent

Use Inhibits premature luteinizing hormone (LH) surges in women undergoing controlled ovarian hyperstimulation

Dosage Summary

SubQ:

Children: Dosage not established

Adults: 250 mcg/day during the mid-to-late phase after initiating follicle-stimulating hormone on day 2 or 3 of cycle.

Dosage Forms

Injection, solution: 250 mcg/0.5 mL (0.5 mL)

ganirelix acetate *see* ganirelix *on page 437*

Gani-Tuss DM NR [US] *see* guaifenesin and dextromethorphan *on page 455*

Gani-Tuss® NR [US] *see* guaifenesin and codeine *on page 455*

Gantrisin® ***(Discontinued)*** *see* sulfisoxazole *on page 903*

GAR-936 *see* tigecycline *on page 932*

Garamycin® [Can] *see* gentamicin (ophthalmic) *on page 443*

Garamycin® ***(Discontinued)*** *see* gentamicin (systemic) *on page 443*

Garasone [Can] *see* gentamicin (ophthalmic) *on page 443*

Gardasil® [US/Can] *see* papillomavirus (types 6, 11, 16, 18) vaccine (human, recombinant) *on page 727*

Gas-X® [US-OTC] *see* simethicone *on page 875*

Gas-X®, Children's Tongue Twisters™ [US-OTC] *see* simethicone *on page 875*

Gas-X® Extra Strength [US-OTC] *see* simethicone *on page 875*

Gas-X® Infant [US-OTC] *see* simethicone *on page 875*

Gas-X® Maximum Strength [US-OTC] *see* simethicone *on page 875*

Gas-X® Thin Strips™ [US-OTC] *see* simethicone *on page 875*

Gas Ban™ [US-OTC] *see* calcium carbonate and simethicone *on page 168*

Gas-Ban DS® ***(Discontinued)*** *see* aluminum hydroxide, magnesium hydroxide, and simethicone *on page 59*

Gas Free Extra Strength [US-OTC] *see* simethicone *on page 875*

Gas Relief Ultra Strength [US-OTC] *see* simethicone *on page 875*

Gastrocrom® [US] *see* cromolyn (systemic, oral inhalation) *on page 254*

Gastrografin® [US] *see* diatrizoate meglumine and diatrizoate sodium *on page 292*

Gastrosed™ ***(Discontinued)*** *see* hyoscyamine *on page 491*

gatifloxacin (gat i FLOKS a sin)

U.S./Canadian Brand Names Zymar® [US/Can]; Zymaxid™ [US]

Therapeutic Category Antibiotic, Quinolone

Use Treatment of bacterial conjunctivitis

Dosage Summary

Ophthalmic:

Children <1 year: Dosage not established

Children ≥1 year: One drop into affected eye(s) every 2 hours while awake (maximum: 8 times/day) for 1-2 days; followed by 1 drop into affected eye(s) 2-4 times/day through day 7

Adults: One drop into affected eye(s) every 2 hours while awake (maximum: 8 times/day) for 1-2 days; followed by 1 drop into affected eye(s) 2-4 times/day through day 7

Dosage Forms

Solution, ophthalmic:

Zymar®: 0.3% (5 mL)

Zymaxid™: 0.5% (2.5 mL)

Gaviscon® Extra Strength [US-OTC] *see* aluminum hydroxide and magnesium carbonate *on page 58*

Gaviscon® Liquid [US-OTC] *see* aluminum hydroxide and magnesium carbonate *on page 58*

Gaviscon® Tablet [US-OTC] *see* aluminum hydroxide and magnesium trisilicate *on page 59*

G-CSF *see* filgrastim *on page 403*

G-CSF (PEG conjugate) *see* pegfilgrastim *on page* 732
GCV sodium *see* ganciclovir (systemic) *on page* 437
GD-Amlodipine [Can] *see* amlodipine *on page* 68
GD-Atorvastatin [Can] *see* atorvastatin *on page* 104
Gd-BOPTA *see* gadobenate dimeglumine *on page* 433
Gd-DTPA *see* gadopentetate dimeglumine *on page* 434
Gd-DTPA-BMA *see* gadodiamide *on page* 434
Gd-DTPA-BMEA *see* gadoversetamide *on page* 435
Gd-EOB-DTPA *see* gadoxetate *on page* 435
Gd-HP-DO3A *see* gadoteridol *on page* 435
GD-Quinapril [Can] *see* quinapril *on page* 822
Gebauer's Ethyl Chloride® [US] *see* ethyl chloride *on page* 382
Gee Gee® *(Discontinued)* *see* guaifenesin *on page* 454

gefitinib (ge FI tye nib)

Sound-Alike/Look-Alike Issues
gefitinib may be confused with erlotinib

Synonyms NSC-715055; ZD1839

U.S./Canadian Brand Names Iressa® [US/Can]

Therapeutic Category Antineoplastic Agent, Tyrosine Kinase Inhibitor

Use

U.S. labeling: Treatment of locally advanced or metastatic nonsmall cell lung cancer after failure of platinum-based and docetaxel therapies. Treatment is limited to patients who are benefiting or have benefited from treatment with gefitinib.

Note: Due to the lack of improved survival data from clinical trials of gefitinib, and in response to positive survival data with another EGFR inhibitor, physicians are advised to use other treatment options in advanced nonsmall cell lung cancer patients following one or two prior chemotherapy regimens when they are refractory/intolerant to their most recent regimen.

Canada labeling: Approved indication is limited to NSCLC patients with epidermal growth factor receptor (EGFR) expression status positive or unknown.

Dosage Summary

Oral:
Children: Dosage not established
Adults: 250 mg once daily; **Note:** May need 500 mg/day in patients receiving effective CYP3A4 inducers

Dosage Forms

Tablet, oral:
Iressa®: 250 mg

gelatin (absorbable) (JEL a tin, ab SORB a ble)

Synonyms absorbable gelatin sponge

U.S./Canadian Brand Names Gelfilm® [US]; Gelfoam® [US]

Therapeutic Category Hemostatic Agent

Use Adjunct to provide hemostasis in surgery; open prostatic surgery

Dosage Summary

Topical:
Children: Apply packs or sponges dry or saturated with sodium chloride
Adults: Apply packs or sponges dry or saturated with sodium chloride

Dosage Forms

Film, ophthalmic:
Gelfilm®: (6s)

Film, topical:
Gelfilm®: (1s)

Powder, topical:
Gelfoam®: (1 g)

Sponge, oral, topical:
Gelfoam®: (12s)

Sponge, topical:
Gelfoam®: (1s, 4s, 6s, 12s)

gelatin, pectin, and methylcellulose (JEL a tin, PEK tin, & meth il SEL yoo lose)

Synonyms methylcellulose, gelatin, and pectin; pectin, gelatin, and methylcellulose
Therapeutic Category Protectant, Topical
Use Temporary relief from minor oral irritations
Dosage Summary
Topical:
Children: Press small dabs into place until the involved area is coated with a thin film as needed
Adults: Press small dabs into place until the involved area is coated with a thin film as needed

Gelclair® [US] *see* mucosal barrier gel, oral *on page* 648
Gelfilm® [US] *see* gelatin (absorbable) *on page* 439
Gelfoam® [US] *see* gelatin (absorbable) *on page* 439
Gel-Kam® [US-OTC] *see* fluoride *on page* 413
Gel-Kam® Rinse [US] *see* fluoride *on page* 413
Gelnique™ [US] *see* oxybutynin *on page* 713
GelRite™ [US-OTC] *see* alcohol (ethyl) *on page* 45
Gel-Stat™ [US-OTC] *see* alcohol (ethyl) *on page* 45
Gel-Tin® *(Discontinued)* *see* fluoride *on page* 413
Gelucast® [US] *see* zinc gelatin *on page* 1001
Gelusil® [US-OTC/Can] *see* aluminum hydroxide, magnesium hydroxide, and simethicone *on page* 59
Gelusil® Extra Strength [Can] *see* aluminum hydroxide and magnesium hydroxide *on page* 59

gemcitabine (jem SITE a been)

Sound-Alike/Look-Alike Issues
gemcitabine may be confused with gemtuzumab
Gemzar® may be confused with Zinecard®
Synonyms gemcitabine hydrochloride
U.S./Canadian Brand Names Gemcitabine For Injection, USP [Can]; Gemzar® [US/Can]
Therapeutic Category Antineoplastic Agent
Use Treatment of metastatic breast cancer; locally-advanced or metastatic nonsmall cell lung cancer (NSCLC) or pancreatic cancer; advanced, relapsed ovarian cancer
Dosage Summary
I.V.:
Children: Dosage not established
Adults: Initial: 1000 mg/m^2 once weekly for up to 7 weeks; 21-day cycle: 1250 mg/m^2 days 1and 8; repeat cycle every 21 days; 28-day cycle: 1000 mg/m^2 days 1, 8, and 15; repeat cycle every 28 days
Dosage Forms
Injection, powder for reconstitution:
Gemzar®: 200 mg, 1 g

Gemcitabine For Injection, USP [Can] *see* gemcitabine *on page* 440
gemcitabine hydrochloride *see* gemcitabine *on page* 440

gemfibrozil (jem FI broe zil)

Sound-Alike/Look-Alike Issues
Lopid® may be confused with Levbid®, Lipitor®, Lodine®, Lorabid®, Slo-bid™
Synonyms CI-719
U.S./Canadian Brand Names Apo-Gemfibrozil® [Can]; Gen-Gemfibrozil [Can]; GMD-Gemfibrozil [Can]; Lopid® [US/Can]; Mylan-Gemfibrozil [Can]; Novo-Gemfibrozil [Can]; Nu-Gemfibrozil [Can]; PMS-Gemfibrozil [Can]
Therapeutic Category Antihyperlipidemic Agent, Miscellaneous
Use Treatment of hypertriglyceridemia in Fredrickson types IV and V hyperlipidemia for patients who are at greater risk for pancreatitis and who have not responded to dietary intervention; to reduce the risk of CHD development in Fredrickson type IIb patients without a history or symptoms of existing CHD who have not responded to dietary and other interventions (including pharmacologic treatment) and who have decreased HDL, increased LDL, and increased triglycerides

Dosage Summary

Oral:

Children: Dosage not established

Adults: 600 mg twice daily

Dosage Forms

Tablet, oral: 600 mg

Lopid®: 600 mg

gemifloxacin (je mi FLOKS a sin)

Synonyms DW286; gemifloxacin mesylate; LA 20304a; SB-265805

U.S./Canadian Brand Names Factive® [US/Can]

Therapeutic Category Antibiotic, Quinolone

Use Treatment of acute exacerbation of chronic bronchitis; treatment of community-acquired pneumonia (CAP), including pneumonia caused by multidrug-resistant strains of *S. pneumoniae* (MDRSP)

Dosage Summary

Oral:

Children: Dosage not established

Adults: 320 mg once daily

Dosage Forms

Tablet, oral:

Factive®: 320 mg

gemifloxacin mesylate *see* gemifloxacin *on page* 441

gemtuzumab ozogamicin (gem TOO zoo mab oh zog a MY sin)

Sound-Alike/Look-Alike Issues

gemtuzumab may be confused with gemcitabine

Synonyms CMA-676

U.S./Canadian Brand Names Mylotarg® [US/Can]

Therapeutic Category Antineoplastic Agent, Natural Source (Plant) Derivative

Use Treatment of relapsed CD33 positive acute myeloid leukemia (AML) in patients ≥60 years of age who are not candidates for cytotoxic chemotherapy

Note: Due to safety concerns as well as lack of clinical benefit demonstrated in a post-approval clinical trial, gemtuzumab was withdrawn from the U.S. commercial market.

Dosage Summary

I.V.:

Adults ≥60 years: 9 mg/m^2 every 2 weeks for a total of 2 doses per treatment course

Product Availability As of June 2010, no longer commercially available in the U.S. market for new patients.

Dosage Forms

Injection, powder for reconstitution [preservative free]:

Mylotarg®: 5 mg

Gemzar® [US/Can] *see* gemcitabine *on page* 440

Genabid® *(Discontinued)*

Genac™ [US-OTC] *see* triprolidine and pseudoephedrine *on page* 961

Genaced™ *(Discontinued)* *see* acetaminophen, aspirin, and caffeine *on page* 27

Genacote™ *(Discontinued)* *see* aspirin *on page* 100

Gen-Acyclovir [Can] *see* acyclovir (systemic) *on page* 36

Genahist™ [US-OTC] *see* diphenhydramine (systemic) *on page* 310

Gen-Amilazide [Can] *see* amiloride and hydrochlorothiazide *on page* 64

Genamin® Expectorant *(Discontinued)*

Gen-Amoxicillin [Can] *see* amoxicillin *on page* 72

Genapap™ *(Discontinued)* *see* acetaminophen *on page* 21

Genapap™ Extra Strength *(Discontinued)* *see* acetaminophen *on page* 21

Genapap™ Infant *(Discontinued)* *see* acetaminophen *on page* 21

Genapap™ Sinus Maximum Strength *(Discontinued)* *see* acetaminophen and pseudoephedrine *on page* 26

Genaphed™ [US-OTC] *see* pseudoephedrine *on page 810*
Genasal *(Discontinued)* *see* oxymetazoline (nasal) *on page 716*
Genasec™ *(Discontinued)* *see* acetaminophen and phenyltoloxamine *on page 26*
Genasoft® *(Discontinued)* *see* docusate *on page 321*
Genasyme® *(Discontinued)* *see* simethicone *on page 875*
Genaton™ [US-OTC] *see* aluminum hydroxide and magnesium carbonate *on page 58*
Genaton Tablet *(Discontinued)* *see* aluminum hydroxide and magnesium trisilicate *on page 59*
Genatuss® *(Discontinued)* *see* guaifenesin *on page 454*
Genatuss DM® *(Discontinued)* *see* guaifenesin and dextromethorphan *on page 455*
Gen-Beclo [Can] *see* beclomethasone (nasal) *on page 120*
Gen-Bromazepam [Can] *see* bromazepam *(Canada only) on page 146*
Gen-Budesonide AQ [Can] *see* budesonide (nasal) *on page 151*
Gen-Buspirone [Can] *see* buspirone *on page 157*
Gencalc® 600 *(Discontinued)* *see* calcium carbonate *on page 167*
Gen-Captopril [Can] *see* captopril *on page 176*
Gen-Carbamazepine CR [Can] *see* carbamazepine *on page 177*
Gen-Clindamycin [Can] *see* clindamycin (systemic) *on page 232*
Gen-Clobetasol [Can] *see* clobetasol *on page 235*
Gen-Clomipramine [Can] *see* clomipramine *on page 237*
Gen-Clonazepam [Can] *see* clonazepam *on page 237*
Gen-Clozapine [Can] *see* clozapine *on page 241*
Gen-Combo Sterinebs [Can] *see* ipratropium and albuterol *on page 524*
Gen-Cyclobenzaprine [Can] *see* cyclobenzaprine *on page 258*
Gen-Cyproterone [Can] *see* cyproterone *(Canada only) on page 262*
Gen-Doxazosin [Can] *see* doxazosin *on page 328*
gene-activated human acid-beta-glucosidase *see* velaglucerase alfa *on page 980*
Genebs *(Discontinued)* *see* acetaminophen *on page 21*
Genebs Extra Strength *(Discontinued)* *see* acetaminophen *on page 21*
Generlac [US] *see* lactulose *on page 544*
Genexa™ LA *(Discontinued)* *see* guaifenesin and phenylephrine *on page 456*
Genfiber™ [US-OTC] *see* psyllium *on page 814*
Gen-Fluoxetine [Can] *see* fluoxetine *on page 415*
Gen-Gemfibrozil [Can] *see* gemfibrozil *on page 440*
Gengraf® [US] *see* cyclosporine (systemic) *on page 260*
Gen-Hydroxychloroquine [Can] *see* hydroxychloroquine *on page 488*
Gen-Hydroxyurea [Can] *see* hydroxyurea *on page 489*
Gen-Ipratropium [Can] *see* ipratropium (oral inhalation) *on page 523*
Gen-K® *(Discontinued)* *see* potassium chloride *on page 781*
Gen-Lovastatin [Can] *see* lovastatin *on page 579*
Gen-Medroxy [Can] *see* medroxyprogesterone *on page 597*
Gen-Metoprolol [Can] *see* metoprolol *on page 625*
Gen-Nabumetone [Can] *see* nabumetone *on page 654*
Gen-Nifedipine XL [Can] *see* nifedipine *on page 675*
Gen-Nitro [Can] *see* nitroglycerin *on page 679*
Gen-Nizatidine [Can] *see* nizatidine *on page 681*
Gen-Nortriptyline [Can] *see* nortriptyline *on page 684*
Genoptic® *(Discontinued)* *see* gentamicin (ophthalmic) *on page 443*
Genora® 0.5/35 *(Discontinued)* *see* ethinyl estradiol and norethindrone *on page 378*
Genora® 1/35 *(Discontinued)* *see* ethinyl estradiol and norethindrone *on page 378*
Genora® 1/50 *(Discontinued)* *see* norethindrone and mestranol *on page 683*
Genotropin® [US] *see* somatropin *on page 889*
Genotropin Miniquick® [US] *see* somatropin *on page 889*
Gen-Pindolol [Can] *see* pindolol *on page 761*

Gen-Piroxicam [Can] *see* piroxicam *on page* *764*
Genpril® ***(Discontinued)*** *see* ibuprofen *on page* *494*
Gen-Risperidone [Can] *see* risperidone *on page* *845*
Gen-Selegiline [Can] *see* selegiline *on page* *869*
Gen-Sumatriptan [Can] *see* sumatriptan *on page* *904*
Gentacidin® ***(Discontinued)*** *see* gentamicin (ophthalmic) *on page* *443*
Gentak® [US/Can] *see* gentamicin (ophthalmic) *on page* *443*

gentamicin (systemic) (jen ta MYE sin)

Sound-Alike/Look-Alike Issues
gentamicin may be confused with gentian violet, kanamycin, vancomycin

Synonyms gentamicin sulfate

U.S./Canadian Brand Names Gentamicin Injection, USP [Can]

Therapeutic Category Antibiotic, Aminoglycoside

Use Treatment of susceptible bacterial infections, normally gram-negative organisms, including *Pseudomonas*, *Proteus*, *Serratia*, and gram-positive *Staphylococcus*; treatment of bone infections, respiratory tract infections, skin and soft tissue infections, as well as abdominal and urinary tract infections, and septicemia; treatment of infective endocarditis

Dosage Summary Note: Use of ideal body weight (IBW) for determining the mg/kg/dose appears to be more accurate than dosing on the basis of total body weight (TBW). In morbid obesity, dosage requirement may best be estimated using a dosing weight of IBW + 0.4 (TBW - IBW).

I.M.:

Children <5 years: 2.5 mg/kg/dose every 8 hours; **Note:** Higher individual doses and/or more frequent intervals (eg, every 6 hours) may be required in selected clinical situations (cystic fibrosis) or if serum levels document the need

Children ≥5 years: 2-2.5 mg/kg/dose every 8 hours; **Note:** Higher individual doses and/or more frequent intervals (eg, every 6 hours) may be required in selected clinical situations (cystic fibrosis) or if serum levels document the need hours

Adults: 1-2.5 mg/kg/dose every 8-12 hours **or** 4-7 mg/kg once daily

I.V.:

Neonates 0-7 days and <2000 g: 2.5 mg/kg every 18-24 hours
Neonates 0-7 days and >2000 g: 2.5 mg/kg every 12 hours
Neonates 8-28 days and <2000 g: 2.5 mg/kg every 8-12 hours
Neonates 8-28 days and >2000 g: 2.5 mg/kg every 8 hours

Children <5 years: 2.5 mg/kg/dose every 8 hours; **Note:** Higher individual doses and/or more frequent intervals (eg, every 6 hours) may be required in selected clinical situations (cystic fibrosis) or if serum levels document the need

Children ≥5 years: 2-2.5 mg/kg/dose every 8 hours; **Note:** Higher individual doses and/or more frequent intervals (eg, every 6 hours) may be required in selected clinical situations (cystic fibrosis) or if serum levels document the need hours

Adults: 1-2.5 mg/kg/dose every 8-12 hours **or** 4-7 mg/kg once daily

Intrathecal:

Children: Dosage not established
Adults: 4-8 mg/day

Dosage Forms

Infusion, premixed in NS: 60 mg (50 mL, 100 mL); 80 mg (50 mL, 100 mL); 100 mg (50 mL, 100 mL); 120 mg (50 mL, 100 mL)

Injection, solution: 10 mg/mL (2 mL, 6 mL, 8 mL, 10 mL); 40 mg/mL (2 mL, 20 mL, 50 mL)

Injection, solution [preservative free]: 10 mg/mL (2 mL)

gentamicin (ophthalmic) (jen ta MYE sin)

Sound-Alike/Look-Alike Issues
gentamicin may be confused with gentian violet, kanamycin, vancomycin

Synonyms gentamicin sulfate

U.S./Canadian Brand Names Diogent® [Can]; Garamycin® [Can]; Garasone [Can]; Gentak® [US/Can]; Gentasol™ [US]; Gentocin [Can]; PMS-Gentamicin [Can]

Therapeutic Category Antibiotic, Aminoglycoside; Antibiotic, Ophthalmic

Use Treatment of ophthalmic infections caused by susceptible bacteria

Dosage Summary

Ophthalmic:

Ointment:

Children: Instill 1/2" (1.25 cm) 2-3 times/day to every 3-4 hours

Adults: Instill 1/2" (1.25 cm) 2-3 times/day to every 3-4 hours

Solution:

Children: Instill 1-2 drops every 2-4 hours, up to 2 drops every hour for severe infections

Adults: Instill 1-2 drops every 2-4 hours, up to 2 drops every hour for severe infections

Dosage Forms

Ointment, ophthalmic:

Gentak®: 0.3% [3 mg/g] (3.5 g)

Solution, ophthalmic: 0.3% (5 mL, 15 mL)

Gentak®: 0.3% (5 mL)

Gentasol™: 0.3% (5 mL)

gentamicin (topical) (jen ta MYE sin)

Sound-Alike/Look-Alike Issues

gentamicin may be confused with gentian violet, kanamycin, vancomycin

U.S./Canadian Brand Names PMS-Gentamicin [Can]; ratio-Gentamicin [Can]

Therapeutic Category Antibiotic, Aminoglycoside; Antibiotic, Topical

Use Used topically to treat superficial infections of the skin

Dosage Summary

Topical:

Children: Apply 3-4 times/day to affected area

Adults: Apply 3-4 times/day to affected area

Dosage Forms

Cream, topical: 0.1% (15 g, 30 g)

Ointment, topical: 0.1% (15 g, 30 g)

gentamicin and prednisolone *see* prednisolone and gentamicin *on page* 791

Gentamicin Injection, USP [Can] *see* gentamicin (systemic) *on page* 443

gentamicin sulfate *see* gentamicin (ophthalmic) *on page* 443

gentamicin sulfate *see* gentamicin (systemic) *on page* 443

Gentasol™ [US] *see* gentamicin (ophthalmic) *on page* 443

GenTeal® [US-OTC/Can] *see* hydroxypropyl methylcellulose *on page* 489

GenTeal® Mild [US-OTC] *see* hydroxypropyl methylcellulose *on page* 489

Gen-Temazepam [Can] *see* temazepam *on page* 914

Gentex HC *(Discontinued)*

Gentex LA *(Discontinued)* *see* guaifenesin and phenylephrine *on page* 456

Gentex LQ [US] *see* carbetapentane, guaifenesin, and phenylephrine *on page* 180

Gen-Ticlopidine [Can] *see* ticlopidine *on page* 932

Gen-Tizanidine [Can] *see* tizanidine *on page* 937

Gentlax® [Can] *see* bisacodyl *on page* 138

Gentlax® *(Discontinued)* *see* bisacodyl *on page* 138

Gentocin [Can] *see* gentamicin (ophthalmic) *on page* 443

Gentran® *(Discontinued)* *see* dextran *on page* 285

Gentrasul® *(Discontinued)* *see* gentamicin (ophthalmic) *on page* 443

Gen-Triazolam [Can] *see* triazolam *on page* 956

Gentuss-HC *(Discontinued)*

Gen-Verapamil [Can] *see* verapamil *on page* 981

Gen-Verapamil SR [Can] *see* verapamil *on page* 981

Geocillin® *(Discontinued)*

Geodon® [US] *see* ziprasidone *on page* 1002

Geref® Diagnostic *(Discontinued)* *see* sermorelin acetate *on page* 871

Geriation [US-OTC] *see* vitamins (multiple/oral) *on page* 990

Geridium® *(Discontinued)* *see* phenazopyridine *on page* 746

Geri-Freeda [US-OTC] *see* vitamins (multiple/oral) *on page* 990

Geri-Hydrolac™ [US-OTC] *see* lactic acid and ammonium hydroxide *on page 542*
Geri-Hydrolac™-12 [US-OTC] *see* lactic acid and ammonium hydroxide *on page 542*
Geritol Complete® [US-OTC] *see* vitamins (multiple/oral) *on page 990*
Geritol Extend® [US-OTC] *see* vitamins (multiple/oral) *on page 990*
Geritol® Tonic [US-OTC] *see* vitamins (multiple/oral) *on page 990*
German measles vaccine *see* rubella virus vaccine (live) *on page 855*
Gets-It® [US-OTC] *see* salicylic acid *on page 858*
GF196960 *see* tadalafil *on page 908*
GG *see* guaifenesin *on page 454*
GG-Cen® ***(Discontinued)*** *see* guaifenesin *on page 454*
GHB *see* sodium oxybate *on page 885*
GI87084B *see* remifentanil *on page 834*
Gianvi™ [US] *see* ethinyl estradiol and drospirenone *on page 375*
Gilphex TR® ***(Discontinued)*** *see* guaifenesin and phenylephrine *on page 456*
Giltuss® [US] *see* guaifenesin, dextromethorphan, and phenylephrine *on page 458*
Giltuss HC® ***(Discontinued)***
Giltuss Pediatric® [US] *see* guaifenesin, dextromethorphan, and phenylephrine *on page 458*
Giltuss TR® [US] *see* guaifenesin, dextromethorphan, and phenylephrine *on page 458*
glargine insulin *see* insulin glargine *on page 510*

glatiramer acetate (gla TIR a mer AS e tate)

Sound-Alike/Look-Alike Issues
Copaxone® may be confused with Compazine®

Synonyms copolymer-1

U.S./Canadian Brand Names Copaxone® [US/Can]

Therapeutic Category Biological, Miscellaneous

Use Management of relapsing-remitting type multiple sclerosis, including patients with a first clinical episode with MRI features consistent with multiple sclerosis

Dosage Summary
SubQ:
Children: Dosage not established
Adults: 20 mg daily

Dosage Forms
Injection, solution [preservative free]:
Copaxone®: 20 mg/mL (1 mL)

Glaucon® ***(Discontinued)*** *see* epinephrine (systemic, oral inhalation) *on page 352*
glcCerase *see* velaglucerase alfa *on page 980*
Gleevec® [US/Can] *see* imatinib *on page 499*
Gliadel® [US] *see* carmustine *on page 186*
Gliadel Wafer® [Can] *see* carmustine *on page 186*
glibenclamide *see* glyburide *on page 448*
Gliclazide-80 [Can] *see* gliclazide *(Canada only) on page 445*

gliclazide *(Canada only)* (GLYE kla zide)

U.S./Canadian Brand Names Apo-Gliclazide® MR [Can]; Apo-Gliclazide® [Can]; Diamicron® MR [Can]; Diamicron® [Can]; Gliclazide-80 [Can]; Mylan-Gliclazide [Can]; Novo-Gliclazide [Can]; PMS-Gliclazide [Can]

Therapeutic Category Antidiabetic Agent, Oral; Hypoglycemic Agent, Oral; Sulfonylurea Agent

Use Management of type 2 diabetes mellitus (noninsulin-dependent, NIDDM)

Dosage Summary
Oral:
Immediate release:
Children: Dosage not established
Adults: Initial: 80-160 mg/day; Maintenance: 80-320 mg/day in 1-2 (≥160 mg) divided doses (maximum: 320 mg/day)

Sustained release:
Children: Dosage not established
Adults: 30-120 mg once daily

Dosage Forms - Canada

Tablet:
Diamicron®: 80 mg

Tablet, sustained release:
Diamicron® MR: 30 mg

glimepiride (GLYE me pye ride)

Sound-Alike/Look-Alike Issues
glimepiride may be confused with glipiZIDE
Amaryl® may be confused with Altace®, Amerge®, Reminyl®

U.S./Canadian Brand Names Amaryl® [US/Can]; Apo-Glimepiride [Can]; CO Glimepiride [Can]; Novo-Glimepiride [Can]; PMS-Glimepiride [Can]; ratio-Glimepiride [Can]; Rhoxal-glimepiride [Can]; Sandoz-Glimepiride [Can]

Therapeutic Category Antidiabetic Agent, Oral

Use Management of type 2 diabetes mellitus (noninsulin-dependent, NIDDM) as an adjunct to diet and exercise to lower blood glucose; may be used in combination with metformin or insulin in patients whose hyperglycemia cannot be controlled by diet and exercise in conjunction with a single oral hypoglycemic agent

Dosage Summary

Oral:
Children <10 years: Dosage not established
Adults: Initial: 1-2 mg once daily; Maintenance: 1-4 mg once daily (maximum: 8 mg/day)
Elderly: Initial: 1 mg/day; dose titration and maintenance dosing should be conservative to avoid hypoglycemia

Dosage Forms

Tablet, oral: 1 mg, 2 mg, 4 mg
Amaryl®: 1 mg, 2 mg, 4 mg

glimepiride and pioglitazone *see* pioglitazone and glimepiride *on page 762*

glimepiride and pioglitazone hydrochloride *see* pioglitazone and glimepiride *on page 762*

glimepiride and rosiglitazone maleate *see* rosiglitazone and glimepiride *on page 853*

glipizide (GLIP i zide)

Sound-Alike/Look-Alike Issues
glipiZIDE may be confused with glimepiride, glyBURIDE
Glucotrol® may be confused with Glucophage®, Glucotrol® XL, glyBURIDE
Glucotrol XL® may be confused with Glucotrol®

Synonyms glydiazinamide

Tall-Man glipi**ZIDE**

U.S./Canadian Brand Names Glucotrol XL® [US]; Glucotrol® [US]

Therapeutic Category Antidiabetic Agent, Oral

Use Management of type 2 diabetes mellitus (noninsulin-dependent, NIDDM)

Dosage Summary

Oral:
Immediate release:
Children: Dosage not established
Adults: Initial: 5 mg/day; Maintenance: Adjust dosage at 2.5-5 mg daily increments as determined by blood glucose response at intervals of several days (maximum: 15 mg once-daily; 40 mg total daily). Doses >15 mg/day should be administered in divided doses.
Elderly: Initial: 2.5 mg/day; Maintenance: Increase by 2.5-5 mg/day at 1- to 2-week intervals (maximum: 15 mg once-daily; 40 mg total daily)
Extended release:
Children: Dosage not established
Adults: Initial: 5 mg/day; Maintenance: Adjust dosage at 2.5-5 mg daily increments as determined by blood glucose response at intervals of several days (maximum: 20 mg/day)
Elderly: Initial: 2.5 mg/day; Maintenance: Increase by 2.5-5 mg/day at 1- to 2-week intervals (maximum: 20 mg/day)

Dosage Forms

Tablet, oral: 5 mg, 10 mg

Glucotrol®: 5 mg, 10 mg

Tablet, extended release, oral: 2.5 mg, 5 mg, 10 mg

Glucotrol XL®: 2.5 mg, 5 mg, 10 mg

glipizide and metformin (GLIP i zide & met FOR min)

Synonyms glipizide and metformin hydrochloride; metformin and glipizide

U.S./Canadian Brand Names Metaglip™ [US]

Therapeutic Category Antidiabetic Agent (Biguanide); Antidiabetic Agent (Sulfonylurea)

Use Indicated as an adjunct to diet and exercise to improve glycemic control in adults with type 2 diabetes mellitus (noninsulin-dependent, NIDDM)

Dosage Summary

Oral:

Children: Dosage not established

Adults: Initial: Glipizide 2.5 mg and metformin 250 mg once daily; Maintenance: Increase dose by 1 tablet/day every 2 weeks up to a maximum of glipizide 20 mg/day and metformin 2000 mg/day in divided doses

Elderly ≥80 years: Do not use unless renal function verified as normal

Dosage Forms

Tablet: 2.5/250: Glipizide 2.5 mg and metformin 250 mg; 2.5/500: Glipizide 2.5 mg and metformin 500 mg; 5/500: Glipizide 5 mg and metformin 500 mg

Metaglip™: 2.5/500: Glipizide 2.5 mg and metformin 500 mg; 5/500: Glipizide 5 mg and metformin 500 mg

glipizide and metformin hydrochloride *see* glipizide and metformin *on page 447*

glivec *see* imatinib *on page 499*

GlucaGen® [US] *see* glucagon *on page 447*

GlucaGen® Diagnostic Kit [US] *see* glucagon *on page 447*

GlucaGen® HypoKit® [US] *see* glucagon *on page 447*

glucagon (GLOO ka gon)

Sound-Alike/Look-Alike Issues

glucagon may be confused with Glaucon®

Synonyms glucagon hydrochloride

U.S./Canadian Brand Names GlucaGen® Diagnostic Kit [US]; GlucaGen® HypoKit® [US]; GlucaGen® [US]; Glucagon Emergency Kit [US]

Therapeutic Category Antihypoglycemic Agent

Use Management of hypoglycemia; diagnostic aid in radiologic examinations to temporarily inhibit GI tract movement

Dosage Summary

I.M.:

Children <20 kg: 0.5 mg **or** 20-30 mcg/kg/dose, may repeat in 20 minutes as needed

Children ≥20 kg: 1 mg, may repeat in 20 minutes as needed

Adults: 1 mg, may repeat in 20 minutes as needed **or** (for diagnostic use) 0.25-2 mg 10 minutes prior to procedure

I.V.:

Children <20 kg: 0.5 mg **or** 20-30 mcg/kg/dose, may repeat in 20 minutes as needed

Children ≥20 kg: 1 mg, may repeat in 20 minutes as needed

Adults: 1 mg, may repeat in 20 minutes as needed **or** (for diagnostic use) 0.25-2 mg 10 minutes prior to procedure

SubQ:

Children <20 kg: 0.5 mg **or** 20-30 mcg/kg/dose, may repeat in 20 minutes as needed

Children ≥20 kg: 1 mg, may repeat in 20 minutes as needed

Adults: 1 mg, may repeat in 20 minutes as needed

Dosage Forms

Injection, powder for reconstitution:

GlucaGen®: 1 mg

GlucaGen® Diagnostic Kit: 1 mg

GlucaGen® HypoKit®: 1 mg

Glucagon Emergency Kit: 1 mg

Glucagon Diagnostic Kit ***(Discontinued)*** *see* glucagon *on page 447*
Glucagon Emergency Kit [US] *see* glucagon *on page 447*
glucagon hydrochloride *see* glucagon *on page 447*
Glucobay™ [Can] *see* acarbose *on page 20*
GlucoBurst® [US-OTC] *see* dextrose *on page 290*
glucocerebrosidase *see* alglucerase *on page 49*
GlucoNorm® [Can] *see* repaglinide *on page 835*
Glucophage® [US/Can] *see* metformin *on page 609*
Glucophage® XR [US] *see* metformin *on page 609*
glucose *see* dextrose *on page 290*
glucose monohydrate *see* dextrose *on page 290*

glucose polymers (GLOO kose POL i merz)

U.S./Canadian Brand Names Moducal® [US-OTC]; Polycose® [US-OTC]

Therapeutic Category Nutritional Supplement

Use Supplies calories for those persons not able to meet the caloric requirement with usual food intake

Dosage Summary

Oral:

Children: Add to foods or beverages or mix in water
Adults: Add to foods or beverages or mix in water

Dosage Forms

Powder for suspension, oral:
Moducal® [OTC]: 368 g
Polycose® [OTC]: 350 g

Glucotrol® [US] *see* glipizide *on page 446*
Glucotrol XL® [US] *see* glipizide *on page 446*
Glucovance® [US] *see* glyburide and metformin *on page 449*
glulisine insulin *see* insulin glulisine *on page 511*
Glumetza® [US/Can] *see* metformin *on page 609*

glutamic acid (gloo TAM ik AS id)

Synonyms glutamic acid hydrochloride

Therapeutic Category Gastrointestinal Agent, Miscellaneous

Use Treatment of hypochlorhydria and achlorhydria

Dosage Summary

Oral:

Children: Dosage not established
Adults: 500-1000 mg/day in 3 divided doses before meals

Dosage Forms

Tablet, oral: 500 mg

glutamic acid hydrochloride *see* glutamic acid *on page 448*
Glutofac®-MX [US] *see* vitamins (multiple/oral) *on page 990*
Glutofac®-ZX [US] *see* vitamins (multiple/oral) *on page 990*
Glutol™ [US-OTC] *see* dextrose *on page 290*
Glutose 15™ [US-OTC] *see* dextrose *on page 290*
Glutose 45™ [US-OTC] *see* dextrose *on page 290*
Glyate® ***(Discontinued)*** *see* guaifenesin *on page 454*
glybenclamide *see* glyburide *on page 448*
glybenzcyclamide *see* glyburide *on page 448*

glyburide (GLYE byoor ide)

Sound-Alike/Look-Alike Issues

glyBURIDE may be confused with glipiZIDE, Glucotrol®
Diaβeta® may be confused with Diabinese®, Zebeta®

Micronase® may be confused with microK®, miconazole, Micronor®, Microzide™

Synonyms glibenclamide; glybenclamide; glybenzcyclamide

Tall-Man gly**BURIDE**

U.S./Canadian Brand Names Apo-Glyburide® [Can]; Diaβeta® [US/Can]; Dom-Glyburide [Can]; Euglucon® [Can]; Glynase® PresTab® [US]; Med-Glybe [Can]; Mylan-Glybe [Can]; Novo-Glyburide [Can]; Nu-Glyburide [Can]; PMS-Glyburide [Can]; PRO-Glyburide [Can]; ratio-Glyburide [Can]; Riva-Glyburide [Can]; Sandoz-Glyburide [Can]

Therapeutic Category Antidiabetic Agent, Oral

Use Adjunct to diet and exercise for the management of type 2 diabetes mellitus (noninsulin-dependent, NIDDM)

Dosage Summary

Oral:

Regular tablets (Diaβeta®):

Children: Dosage not established

Adults: Initial: 1.25-5 mg once daily; Maintenance: 1.25-20 mg/day as single or divided doses (maximum: 20 mg/day); **Note:** Titration is recommended

Elderly: Initial: 1.25-2.5 mg once daily; Maintenance: Increase by 1.25-2.5 mg/day every 1-3 weeks (maximum: 20 mg/day)

Micronized tablets (Glynase® PresTab®):

Children: Dosage not established

Adults: Initial: 0.75-3 mg once daily; Maintenance: 0.75-12 mg/day as single or divided doses (maximum: 12 mg/day). **Note:** Titration is recommended

Dosage Forms

Tablet, oral: 1.25 mg, 1.5 mg, 2.5 mg, 3 mg, 5 mg, 6 mg

DiaBeta®: 1.25 mg, 2.5 mg, 5 mg

Glynase® PresTab®: 1.5 mg, 3 mg, 6 mg

glyburide and metformin (GLYE byoor ide & met FOR min)

Sound-Alike/Look-Alike Issues

Glucovance® may be confused with Vyvanse™

Synonyms glyburide and metformin hydrochloride; metformin and glyburide

U.S./Canadian Brand Names Glucovance® [US]

Therapeutic Category Antidiabetic Agent (Sulfonylurea); Antidiabetic Agent, Oral

Use Adjunct to diet and exercise for the management of type 2 diabetes mellitus (noninsulin-dependent, NIDDM)

Dosage Summary

Oral:

Children: Dosage not established

Adults: Initial: Glyburide 1.25-5 mg and metformin 250-500 mg once or twice daily; Maintenance: Up to glyburide 20 mg/day and metformin 2000 mg/day

Elderly ≥80 years: Do not use unless renal function verified as normal

Dosage Forms

Tablet: Glyburide 1.25 mg and metformin 250 mg; glyburide 2.5 mg and metformin 500 mg; glyburide 5 mg and metformin 500 mg

Glucovance®: 2.5 mg/500 mg: Glyburide 2.5 mg and metformin 500 mg; 5 mg/500 mg: Glyburide 5 mg and metformin 500 mg

glyburide and metformin hydrochloride *see* glyburide and metformin *on page 449*

glycerin (GLIS er in)

Synonyms glycerol

U.S./Canadian Brand Names Fleet® Glycerin Maximum Strength [US-OTC]; Fleet® Glycerin Suppositories [US-OTC]; Fleet® Liquid Glycerin [US-OTC]; Fleet® Pedia-Lax™ Glycerin Suppositories [US-OTC]; Fleet® Pedia-Lax™ Liquid Glycerin Suppositories [US-OTC]; Orajel® Dry Mouth [US-OTC]; Sani-Supp® [US-OTC]

Therapeutic Category Laxative; Ophthalmic Agent, Miscellaneous

Use Constipation; reduction of intraocular pressure; reduction of corneal edema; glycerin has been administered orally to reduce intracranial pressure

Dosage Summary

Ophthalmic:

Children: Instill 1-2 drops in eye(s) every 3-4 hours **or** prior to examination
Adults: Instill 1-2 drops in eye(s) every 3-4 hours **or** prior to examination

Oral:

Children: 1.5 g/kg/day divided every 4 hours **or** 1 g/kg/dose every 6 hours **or** 1-1.8 g/kg preoperatively
Adults: 1.5 g/kg/day divided every 4 hours **or** 1 g/kg/dose every 6 hours **or** 1-1.8 g/kg preoperatively

Rectal:

Children <6 years: 1 infant suppository 1-2 times/day as needed **or** 2-5 mL as an enema
Children ≥6 years: 1 adult suppository 1-2 times/day as needed **or** 5-15 mL as an enema
Adults: 1 adult suppository 1-2 times/day as needed **or** 5-15 mL as an enema

Dosage Forms

Gel, oral:
Orajel® Dry Mouth [OTC]: 18% (42 g)

Liquid, for prescription compounding: USP: 100% (3840 mL)

Liquid, topical: USP: 100% (120 mL, 180 mL, 480 mL, 3840 mL)

Solution, rectal:
Fleet® Liquid Glycerin [OTC]: 5.6 g/5.5 mL (7.5 mL)
Fleet® Pedia-Lax™ Liquid Glycerin Suppositories [OTC]: 2.3 g/2.3 mL (4 mL)

Suppository, rectal: 1.5 g (12s, 25s); 80.7% (25s, 50s, 100s); 82.5% (12s, 25s, 50s, 100s)
Fleet® Glycerin Maximum Strength [OTC]: 3 g (18s)
Fleet® Glycerin Suppositories [OTC]: 2 g (12s, 50s)
Fleet® Pedia-Lax™ Glycerin Suppositories [OTC]: 1 g (12s)
Sani-Supp® [OTC]: 82.5% (10s, 25s)

glycerol *see* glycerin *on page 449*

glycerol guaiacolate *see* guaifenesin *on page 454*

Glycerol-T® ***(Discontinued)***

glycerol triacetate *see* triacetin *on page 952*

glyceryl trinitrate *see* nitroglycerin *on page 679*

Glycofed® ***(Discontinued)*** *see* guaifenesin and pseudoephedrine *on page 457*

Glycon [Can] *see* metformin *on page 609*

glycopyrrolate (glye koe PYE roe late)

Sound-Alike/Look-Alike Issues
Robinul® may be confused with Reminyl®

Synonyms Cuvposa™; glycopyrronium bromide

U.S./Canadian Brand Names Glycopyrrolate Injection, USP [Can]; Robinul® Forte [US]; Robinul® [US]

Therapeutic Category Anticholinergic Agent

Use Inhibit salivation and excessive secretions of the respiratory tract preoperatively; control of upper airway secretions; adjunct in treatment of peptic ulcer (currently replaced by more effective agents); prevention and treatment of bradycardia

Dosage Summary

I.M.:

Children <2 years: 4-9 mcg/kg prior to procedure **or** 4-10 mcg/kg every 3-4 hours (maximum: 0.2 mg/dose; 0.8 mg/day)
Children ≥2 years: 4 mcg/kg prior to procedure **or** 4-10 mcg/kg every 3-4 hours (maximum: 0.2 mg/dose; 0.8 mg/day)
Adults: 4 mcg/kg prior to procedure **or** 0.1-0.2 mg 3-4 times/day

I.V.:

Children: 4-10 mcg/kg every 3-4 hours (maximum: 0.2 mg/dose; 0.8 mg/day) **or** 4 mcg/kg (maximum: 0.1 mg), repeat at 2- to 3-minute intervals as needed intraoperatively **or** 0.2 mg for each 1 mg of neostigmine or 5 mg of pyridostigmine (5-15 mcg/kg with 25-70 mcg/kg of neostigmine or 0.1-0.3 mg/kg of pyridostigmine)
Adults: 0.1-0.2 mg 3-4 times/day **or** 0.1 mg repeated as needed at 2- to 3-minute intervals intraoperatively **or** 0.2 mg for each 1 mg of neostigmine or 5 mg of pyridostigmine (5-15 mcg/kg with 25-70 mcg/kg of neostigmine or 0.1-0.3 mg/kg of pyridostigmine)

Oral:

Children: 40-100 mcg/kg/dose 3-4 times/day
Adults: 1-2 mg 2-3 times/day

Product Availability

Cuvposa™: FDA approved July 2010; expected availability is currently unknown; consult prescribing information for additional information

Cuvposa™ oral solution is approved for use in children (3-16 years of age) to reduce chronic severe drooling due to certain neurologic conditions (eg, cerebral palsy).

Dosage Forms

Injection, solution: 0.2 mg/mL (1 mL, 2 mL, 5 mL, 20 mL)

Robinul®: 0.2 mg/mL (1 mL, 2 mL, 5 mL)

Tablet, oral: 1 mg, 2 mg

Robinul®: 1 mg

Robinul® Forte: 2 mg

Glycopyrrolate Injection, USP [Can] *see* glycopyrrolate *on page 450*

glycopyrronium bromide *see* glycopyrrolate *on page 450*

glycosum *see* dextrose *on page 290*

Glycotuss® ***(Discontinued)*** *see* guaifenesin *on page 454*

Glycotuss-dM® ***(Discontinued)*** *see* guaifenesin and dextromethorphan *on page 455*

glydiazinamide *see* glipizide *on page 446*

Glynase® PresTab® [US] *see* glyburide *on page 448*

Gly-Oxide® [US-OTC] *see* carbamide peroxide *on page 178*

Glyquin® ***(Discontinued)*** *see* hydroquinone *on page 487*

Glyquin® XM [Can] *see* hydroquinone *on page 487*

Glyquin-XM™ ***(Discontinued)*** *see* hydroquinone *on page 487*

Glyset® [US/Can] *see* miglitol *on page 633*

GM-CSF *see* sargramostim *on page 865*

GMD-Gemfibrozil [Can] *see* gemfibrozil *on page 440*

G-myticin® ***(Discontinued)*** *see* gentamicin (topical) *on page 444*

Gold Bond® Antifungal ***(Discontinued)*** *see* tolnaftate *on page 940*

gold sodium thiomalate (gold SOW dee um thye oh MAL ate)

Synonyms sodium aurothiomalate

U.S./Canadian Brand Names Myochrysine® [US/Can]

Therapeutic Category Gold Compound

Use Treatment of progressive rheumatoid arthritis

Dosage Summary

I.M.:

Children: Test dose (recommended): 10 mg first week; Initial dosing: 1 mg/kg/week for 20 weeks; Maintenance: 1 mg/kg every 2-4 weeks

Adults: Test dose: 10 mg first week; Initial dosing: 25 mg second week, then 25-50 mg/week until 1 g cumulative dose has been given; Maintenance: 25-50 mg every 2-3 weeks for 2-20 weeks, then every 3-4 weeks

Dosage Forms

Injection, solution:

Myochrysine®: 50 mg/mL (1 mL, 10 mL)

golimumab (goe LIM ue mab)

Synonyms CNTO-148

U.S./Canadian Brand Names Simponi™ [US/Can]

Therapeutic Category Antipsoriatic Agent; Antirheumatic, Disease Modifying; Monoclonal Antibody; Tumor Necrosis Factor (TNF) Blocking Agent

Use Treatment of active rheumatoid arthritis (moderate-to-severe), active psoriatic arthritis, and active ankylosing spondylitis

Dosage Summary

SubQ:

Children: Dosage not established

Adults: 50 mg once per month

Dosage Forms

Injection, solution [preservative free]:

Simponi™: 50 mg/0.5 mL (0.5 mL)

GoLYTELY® [US] *see* polyethylene glycol-electrolyte solution *on page 775*

gonadorelin *(Discontinued)*

Gonak™ [US-OTC] *see* hydroxypropyl methylcellulose *on page 489*

Gonal-f® [US/Can] *see* follitropin alfa *on page 424*

Gonal-f® Pen [Can] *see* follitropin alfa *on page 424*

Gonal-f® RFF [US] *see* follitropin alfa *on page 424*

gonioscopic ophthalmic solution *see* hydroxypropyl methylcellulose *on page 489*

Goniosoft™ [US-OTC] *see* hydroxypropyl methylcellulose *on page 489*

Goniosol® *(Discontinued)* *see* hydroxypropyl methylcellulose *on page 489*

Goody's® Extra Strength Headache Powder [US-OTC] *see* acetaminophen, aspirin, and caffeine *on page 27*

Goody's® Extra Strength Pain Relief [US-OTC] *see* acetaminophen, aspirin, and caffeine *on page 27*

Goody's PM® [US-OTC] *see* acetaminophen and diphenhydramine *on page 24*

Gordofilm [US-OTC] *see* salicylic acid *on page 858*

Gordon Boro-Packs [US-OTC] *see* aluminum sulfate and calcium acetate *on page 60*

Gordon's® Urea [US-OTC] *see* urea *on page 970*

Gormel® [US-OTC] *see* urea *on page 970*

Gormel® Ten [US-OTC] *see* urea *on page 970*

goserelin (GOE se rel in)

Synonyms D-ser(bu^t)^6,Azgly^{10}-LHRH; goserelin acetate; ICI-118630

U.S./Canadian Brand Names Zoladex® LA [Can]; Zoladex® [US/Can]

Therapeutic Category Gonadotropin-Releasing Hormone Analog

Use Treatment (including palliative treatment) of prostate cancer; palliative treatment of advanced breast cancer; treatment of endometriosis, including pain relief and reduction of endometriotic lesions; endometrial thinning agent as part of treatment for dysfunctional uterine bleeding

Dosage Summary

SubQ:

Children: Dosage not established

Adults: 3.6 mg every 28 days **or** 10.8 mg every 12 weeks

Dosage Forms

Implant, subcutaneous:

Zoladex®: 3.6 mg (1s); 10.8 mg (1s)

goserelin acetate *see* goserelin *on page 452*

GP 47680 *see* oxcarbazepine *on page 712*

GPI 15715 *see* fospropofol *on page 429*

GR38032R *see* ondansetron *on page 704*

gramicidin, neomycin, and polymyxin B *see* neomycin, polymyxin B, and gramicidin *on page 667*

granisetron (gra NI se tron)

Sound-Alike/Look-Alike Issues

granisetron may be confused with dolasetron, ondansetron, palonosetron

Synonyms BRL 43694

U.S./Canadian Brand Names Apo-Granisetron® [Can]; Granisol™ [US]; Kytril® [US/Can]; Sancuso® [US]

Therapeutic Category Selective 5-HT$_3$ Receptor Antagonist

Use Prophylaxis of nausea and vomiting associated with emetogenic chemotherapy and radiation therapy; prophylaxis and treatment of postoperative nausea and vomiting (PONV)

Dosage Summary

I.V.:

Children <2 years: Dosage not established

Children ≥2 years: 10 mcg/kg/dose (maximum: 1 mg/dose) prior to chemotherapy **or** every 12 hours

Adults: 10 mcg/kg/dose (maximum: 1 mg/dose) prior to chemotherapy **or** every 12 hours or 1 mg as a single dose [PONV]

Oral:

Children: Dosage not established

Adults: 2 mg/day in 1-2 divided dose

Transdermal:

Children: Dosage not established

Adults: One patch applied ≥24 hours to ≤48 hours prior to chemotherapy regimen. Maximum duration: Patch may be worn up to 7 days

Dosage Forms

Injection, solution: 0.1 mg/mL (1 mL); 1 mg/mL (1 mL, 4 mL)

Kytril®: 1 mg/mL (4 mL)

Injection, solution [preservative free]: 0.1 mg/mL (1 mL); 1 mg/mL (1 mL)

Patch, transdermal:

Sancuso®: 3.1 mg/24 hours (1s)

Solution, oral:

Granisol™: 2 mg/10 mL (30 mL)

Tablet, oral: 1 mg

Kytril®: 1 mg

Granisol™ [US] *see* granisetron *on page 452*

Granulex® [US] *see* trypsin, balsam Peru, and castor oil *on page 964*

granulocyte colony-stimulating factor *see* filgrastim *on page 403*

granulocyte colony stimulating factor (PEG conjugate) *see* pegfilgrastim *on page 732*

granulocyte-macrophage colony-stimulating factor *see* sargramostim *on page 865*

Gravol® [Can] *see* dimenhydrinate *on page 307*

green tea extract *see* sinecatechins *on page 878*

Grifulvin V® [US] *see* griseofulvin *on page 453*

Grifulvin® V Tablet 250 mg and 500 mg *(Discontinued)* *see* griseofulvin *on page 453*

Grisactin® Ultra *(Discontinued)* *see* griseofulvin *on page 453*

griseofulvin (gri see oh FUL vin)

Synonyms griseofulvin microsize; griseofulvin ultramicrosize

U.S./Canadian Brand Names Grifulvin V® [US]; Gris-PEG® [US]

Therapeutic Category Antifungal Agent

Use Treatment of susceptible tinea infections of the skin, hair, and nails

Dosage Summary

Oral:

Microsize:

Children ≤2 years: Dosage not established

Children >2 years: 10-15 mg/kg/day in single or divided doses

Adults: 500-1000 mg/day in single or divided doses

Ultramicrosize:

Children ≤2 years: Dosage not established

Children >2 years: 5-15 mg/kg/day in single dose or 2 divided doses (maximum: 750 mg/day)

Adults: 375-750 mg/day in single or divided doses

Dosage Forms

Suspension, oral: 125 mg/5 mL (120 mL)

Tablet, oral:

Grifulvin V®: 500 mg

Gris-PEG®: 125 mg, 250 mg

griseofulvin microsize *see* griseofulvin *on page 453*

griseofulvin ultramicrosize *see* griseofulvin *on page 453*

Gris-PEG® [US] *see* griseofulvin *on page 453*

growth hormone, human *see* somatropin *on page 889*

Guaicon DM [US-OTC] *see* guaifenesin and dextromethorphan *on page 455*

Guaifed® [US] *see* guaifenesin and phenylephrine *on page 456*

Guaifed-PD® [US] *see* guaifenesin and phenylephrine *on page 456*

Guaifen™ DM ***(Discontinued)*** *see* guaifenesin, dextromethorphan, and phenylephrine *on page 458*

guaifenesin (gwye FEN e sin)

Sound-Alike/Look-Alike Issues

guaiFENesin may be confused with guanFACINE
Mucinex® may be confused with Mucomyst®
Naldecon® may be confused with Nalfon®

Synonyms cheratussin; GG; glycerol guaiacolate

Tall-Man guai**FEN**esin

U.S./Canadian Brand Names Allfen [US-OTC]; Balminil Expectorant [Can]; Benylin® E Extra Strength [Can]; Diabetic Siltussin DAS-Na [US-OTC]; Diabetic Tussin® EX [US-OTC]; Fenesin IR [US-OTC]; Ganidin® NR [US-OTC]; Humibid® Maximum Strength [US-OTC]; Koffex Expectorant [Can]; Mucinex® Kid's Mini-Melts™ [US-OTC]; Mucinex® Kid's [US-OTC]; Mucinex® Maximum Strength [US-OTC]; Mucinex® [US-OTC]; Mucus Relief [US-OTC]; Organidin® NR [US-OTC]; Refenesen™ 400 [US-OTC]; Refenesen™ [US-OTC]; Robafen [US-OTC]; Robitussin® Chest Congestion [US-OTC]; Robitussin® [Can]; Scot-Tussin® Expectorant [US-OTC]; Siltussin DAS [US-OTC]; Siltussin SA [US-OTC]; Vicks® Casero™ Chest Congestion Relief [US-OTC]; Vicks® DayQuil® Mucus Control [US-OTC]; Xpect™ [US-OTC]

Therapeutic Category Expectorant

Use Help loosen phlegm and thin bronchial secretions to make coughs more productive

Dosage Summary

Oral:

Extended release:
Children <12 years: Dosage not established
Children ≥12 years: 600-1200 mg every 12 hours (maximum: 2.4 g/day)
Adults: 600-1200 mg every 12 hours (maximum: 2.4 g/day)

Immediate release:
Children <6 months: Dosage not established
Children 6 months to 2 years: 25-50 mg every 4 hours (maximum: 300 mg/day)
Children 2-5 years: 50-100 mg every 4 hours (maximum: 600 mg/day)
Children 6-11 years: 100-200 mg every 4 hours (maximum: 1.2 g/day)
Children ≥12 years: 200-400 mg every 4 hours (maximum: 2.4 g/day)
Adults: 200-400 mg every 4 hours (maximum: 2.4 g/day)

Dosage Forms

Caplet, oral:
Fenesin IR [OTC]: 400 mg
Refenesen™ 400 [OTC]: 400 mg

Granules, oral:
Mucinex® Kid's Mini-Melts™ [OTC]: 50 mg/packet (12s); 100 mg/packet (12s)

Liquid, oral:
Diabetic Tussin® EX [OTC]: 100 mg/5 mL (118 mL)
Ganidin® NR [OTC]: 100 mg/5 mL (473 mL)
Mucinex® Kid's [OTC]: 100 mg/5 mL (118 mL)
Scot-Tussin® Expectorant [OTC]: 100 mg/5 mL (120 mL)
Vicks® Casero™ Chest Congestion Relief [OTC]: 100 mg/6.25 mL (120 mL, 240 mL)
Vicks® DayQuil® Mucus Control [OTC]: 200 mg/15 mL (295 mL)

Syrup, oral: 100 mg/5 mL (5 mL, 10 mL, 15 mL, 118 mL, 120 mL, 240 mL, 473 mL, 480 mL)
Diabetic Siltussin DAS-Na [OTC]: 100 mg/5 mL (118 mL)
Robafen [OTC]: 100 mg/5 mL (120 mL, 240 mL, 480 mL)
Siltussin SA [OTC]: 100 mg/5 mL (120 mL, 240 mL, 480 mL)

Tablet, oral: 200 mg
Allfen [OTC]: 400 mg
Mucus Relief [OTC]: 400 mg
Organidin® NR [OTC]: 200 mg
Refenesen™ [OTC]: 200 mg
Xpect™ [OTC]: 400 mg

Tablet, extended release, oral:
Humibid® Maximum Strength [OTC]: 1200 mg
Mucinex® [OTC]: 600 mg
Mucinex® Maximum Strength [OTC]: 1200 mg

guaifenesin and codeine (gwye FEN e sin & KOE deen)

Synonyms codeine and guaifenesin

U.S./Canadian Brand Names Dex-Tuss [US]; ExeClear-C [US]; Gani-Tuss® NR [US]; Mar-Cof® CG [US]; Robafen AC [US]; Tusso-C™ [US]

Therapeutic Category Antitussive/Expectorant

Controlled Substance C-V

Use Temporary control of cough due to minor throat and bronchial irritation

Dosage Summary

Oral: Also refer to specific product labeling; not all products indicated for each age group

Children <2 years: Dosage not established

Children 2-6 years: Dose based on codeine 1 mg/kg/day in 4 divided doses

Children 6-12 years: 5 mL every 4 hours (maximum: 30 mL/day)

Children ≥12 years: 1 tablet or 10 mL every 4 hours (maximum: 6 tablets or 60 mL per day)

Adults: 1 tablet or 10 mL every 4 hours (maximum: 6 tablets or 60 mL per day)

Dosage Forms

Liquid: Guaifenesin 300 mg and codeine 10 mg per 5 mL

Dex-Tuss: Guaifenesin 300 mg and codeine 10 mg per 5 mL

Gani-Tuss® NR: Guaifenesin 100 mg and codeine 10 mg per 5 mL

Solution, oral: Guaifenesin 100 mg and codeine 10 mg per 5 mL

Mar-Cof® CG: Guaifenesin 225 mg and codeine 7.5 mg per 5 mL

Syrup: Guaifenesin 100 mg and codeine 10 mg per 5 mL (473 mL)

Robafen AC: Guaifenesin 100 mg and codeine 10 mg per 5 mL

ExeClear-C,Tusso-C™: Guaifenesin 200 mg and codeine 10 mg per 5 mL

guaifenesin and dextromethorphan (gwye FEN e sin & deks troe meth OR fan)

Sound-Alike/Look-Alike Issues

Benylin® may be confused with Benadryl®, Ventolin®

Synonyms dextromethorphan and guaifenesin

U.S./Canadian Brand Names Allfen DM [US-OTC]; Balminil DM E [Can]; Benylin® DM-E [Can]; Cheracol® D [US-OTC]; Cheracol® Plus [US-OTC]; Coricidin HBP® Chest Congestion and Cough [US-OTC]; Diabetic Siltussin-DM DAS-Na Maximum Strength [US-OTC]; Diabetic Siltussin-DM DAS-Na [US-OTC]; Diabetic Tussin® DM Maximum Strength [US-OTC]; Diabetic Tussin® DM [US-OTC]; Double Tussin DM [US-OTC]; Fenesin DM IR [US]; Gani-Tuss DM NR [US]; Guaicon DM [US-OTC]; Guia-D [US]; Guiacon DMS [US-OTC]; Koffex DM-Expectorant [Can]; Kolephrin® GG/DM [US-OTC]; Mintab DM [US]; Mucinex® DM Maximum Strength [US-OTC]; Mucinex® DM [US-OTC]; Mucinex® Kid's Cough Mini-Melts™ [US-OTC]; Mucinex® Kid's Cough [US-OTC]; Phlemex [US]; Refenesen™ DM [US-OTC]; Respa-DM® [US]; Robafen DM Clear [US-OTC]; Robafen DM [US-OTC]; Robitussin® Cough and Congestion [US-OTC]; Robitussin® DM [US-OTC/Can]; Robitussin® Sugar Free Cough [US-OTC]; Safe Tussin® DM [US-OTC]; Scot-Tussin® Senior [US-OTC]; Silexin [US-OTC]; Siltussin DM DAS [US-OTC]; Siltussin DM [US-OTC]; Simuc-DM [US]; Tussi-Bid® [US]; Vicks® 44E [US-OTC]; Vicks® DayQuil® Mucus Control DM [US-OTC]; Vicks® Pediatric Formula 44E [US-OTC]; Z-Cof LA™ [US]

Therapeutic Category Antitussive/Expectorant

Use Temporary control of cough due to minor throat and bronchial irritation

Dosage Summary

Oral:

Children <2 years: Dosage not established

Children 2-6 years: Guaifenesin 50-100 mg and dextromethorphan 2.5-5 mg every 4 hours (maximum: Guaifenesin 600 mg/day; Dextromethorphan 30 mg/day)

Children 6-12 years: Guaifenesin 100-200 mg and dextromethorphan 5-10 mg every 4 hours (maximum: Guaifenesin 1200 mg/day; Dextromethorphan 60 mg/day)

Children ≥12 years: Guaifenesin 200-400 mg and dextromethorphan 10-20 mg every 4 hours (maximum: Guaifenesin 2400 mg/day; Dextromethorphan 120 mg/day)

Adults: Guaifenesin 200-400 mg and dextromethorphan 10-20 mg every 4 hours (maximum: Guaifenesin 2400 mg/day; Dextromethorphan 120 mg/day)

Dosage Forms

Caplet, oral:

Fenesin DM IR: Guaifenesin 400 mg and dextromethorphan 15 mg

Refenesen™ DM [OTC]: Guaifenesin 400 mg and dextromethorphan 20 mg

Capsule, softgel, oral:
Coricidin HBP® Chest Congestion and Cough [OTC]: Guaifenesin 200 mg and dextromethorphan 10 mg
Elixir, oral:
Simuc-DM: Guaifenesin 225 mg and dextromethorphan 25 mg per 5 mL
Granules, oral:
Mucinex® Kid's Cough Mini-Melts™: Guaifenesin 100 mg and dextromethorphan hydrobromide 5 mg per packet (12s)
Liquid, oral: Guaifenesin 100 mg and dextromethorphan 10 mg per 5 mL; guaifenesin 300 mg and dextromethorphan 10 mg per 5 mL
Diabetic Tussin® DM [OTC], Gani-Tuss DM NR: Guaifenesin 100 mg and dextromethorphan 10 mg per 5 mL
Diabetic Tussin® DM Maximum Strength [OTC]: Guaifenesin 200 mg and dextromethorphan 10 mg per 5 mL
Double Tussin DM [OTC]: Guaifenesin 300 mg and dextromethorphan 20 mg per 5 mL
Kolephrin® GG/DM [OTC]: Guaifenesin 150 mg and dextromethorphan 10 mg per 5 mL
Mucinex® Kid's Cough: Guaifenesin 100 mg and dextromethorphan 5 mg per 5 mL
Safe Tussin® DM [OTC]: Guaifenesin 100 mg and dextromethorphan 15 mg per 5 mL
Scot-Tussin® Senior [OTC]: Guaifenesin 200 mg and dextromethorphan 15 mg per 5 mL
Vicks® 44E [OTC]: Guaifenesin 200 mg and dextromethorphan hydrobromide 20 mg per 15 mL
Vicks® DayQuil® Mucus Control DM [OTC]: Guaifenesin 200 mg and dextromethorphan hydrobromide 10 mg per 15 mL
Vicks® Pediatric Formula 44E [OTC]: Guaifenesin 100 mg and dextromethorphan hydrobromide 10 mg per 15 mL
Syrup, oral: Guaifenesin 100 mg and dextromethorphan 10 mg per 5 mL
Cheracol® D [OTC], Cheracol® Plus [OTC], Diabetic Siltussin-DM DAS-Na [OTC], Diabetic Siltussin-DM DAS-Na Maximum Strength [OTC], Guaicon DM [OTC], Guaicon DMS [OTC], Robafen DM [OTC], Robafen DM Clear [OTC], Robitussin® Cough and Congestion [OTC], Robitussin® DM [OTC], Robitussin® Sugar Free Cough [OTC], Silexin [OTC], Siltussin DM [OTC], Siltussin DM DAS [OTC]: Guaifenesin 100 mg and dextromethorphan 10 mg per 5 mL
Mintab DM: Guaifenesin 200 mg and dextromethorphan hydrobromide 10 mg per 5 mL
Tablet, oral: Guaifenesin 1000 mg and dextromethorphan hydrobromide 60 mg; guaifenesin 1200 mg and dextromethorphan hydrobromide 60 mg
Allfen DM [OTC]: Guaifenesin 400 mg and dextromethorphan 20 mg
Silexin [OTC]: Guaifenesin 100 mg and dextromethorphan hydrobromide 10 mg
Tablet, extended release, oral: Guaifenesin 800 mg and dextromethorphan 30 mg; Guaifenesin 1200 mg and dextromethorphan 20 mg
Mucinex® DM [OTC], Respa-DM®: Guaifenesin 600 mg and dextromethorphan 30 mg
Mucinex® DM Maximum Strength [OTC]: Guaifenesin 1200 mg and dextromethorphan 60 mg
Phlemex: Guaifenesin 1200 mg and dextromethorphan 20 mg
Tablet, long-acting, oral: Guaifenesin 1000 mg and dextromethorphan 60 mg
Z-Cof LA™ [scored]: Guaifenesin 650 mg and dextromethorphan 30 mg
Tablet, sustained release, oral:
Tussi-Bid®: Guaifenesin 1200 mg and dextromethorphan 60 mg
Tablet, timed release, oral [scored]: Guaifenesin 1200 mg and dextromethorphan 60 mg
Guia-D: Guaifenesin 1000 mg and dextromethorphan 60 mg

guaifenesin and dyphylline *see* dyphylline and guaifenesin *on page* 339

guaifenesin and phenylephrine (gwye FEN e sin & fen il EF rin)

Sound-Alike/Look-Alike Issues
Entex® may be confused with Tenex®
Entex® LA brand name represents a different product in the U.S. than it does in Canada. In the U.S., Entex® LA contains guaifenesin and phenylephrine, while in Canada the product bearing this brand name contains guaifenesin and pseudoephedrine.

Synonyms guaifenesin and phenylephrine tannate; phenylephrine hydrochloride and guaifenesin

U.S./Canadian Brand Names Aldex™ [US]; Crantex LA [US]; D-Phen 1000 [US]; Deconsal® II [US]; Donatussin Drops [US]; Duomax [US]; Duratuss GP® [US]; Duratuss® [US]; ExeFen-PD [US]; ExeTuss-GP [US]; Fenesin PE IR [US]; Guaifed-PD® [US]; Guaifed® [US]; Guaiphen-D 1200 [US]; Guaiphen-D [US]; Guaiphen-PD [US]; Liquibid-D® [US]; Mucinex® Cold [US-OTC]; MyDex [US]; Nexphen PD [US]; norel® EX [US]; Pendex [US]; Refenesen™ PE [US-OTC]; Rescon GG [US-OTC]; Sil-Tex [US]; Sina-12X [US]; SINUvent® PE [US]

Therapeutic Category Cold Preparation

Use Temporary relief of nasal congestion, sinusitis, rhinitis, and hay fever; temporary relief of cough associated with upper respiratory tract conditions, especially when associated with dry, nonproductive cough

Dosage Summary **Note:** Dosage varies considerably by product, ranges listed are representative. Consult specific product labeling.

Oral:

Children 3-6 months: 0.3-0.6 mL; may repeat every 4-6 hours as needed (maximum: 4 doses/24 hours) [Donatussin liquid drops]

Children 6 months to 1 year: 0.6-1 mL; may repeat every 4-6 hours as needed (maximum: 4 doses/24 hours) [Donatussin liquid drops]

Children 1-2 years: 1-2 mL; may repeat every 4-6 hours as needed (maximum: 4 doses/24 hours) [Donatussin liquid drops]

Children 2-6 years: 2.5 mL every 4-6 hours (maximum: 10 mL/day) [Rescon GG] **or** 2.5-5 mL every 12 hours [Sina-12X suspension]

Children 6-12 years: One-half to 1 tablet every 12 hours [Liquibid-D®] **or** 1 capsule every 12 hours [Deconsal® II] **or** 5 mL every 4-6 hours (maximum: 20 mL/day) [Rescon GG] **or** 5-10 mL every 12 hours [Sina-12X suspension]

Children ≥12 years: 1-2 capsules/tablets every 12 hours [Prolex®-PD] **or** 5-10 mL every 4-6 hours (maximum: 40 mL/day) **or** 5-10 mL every 12 hours [Sina-12X suspension]

Adults: 1-2 capsules/tablets every 12 hours [Prolex®-PD] **or** 5-10 mL every 4-6 hours (maximum: 40 mL/day) **or** 5-10 mL every 12 hours [Sina-12X suspension]

Dosage Forms

Caplet, oral:

Fenesin PE IR, OneTab™ Congestion & Cold [OTC], Refenesen™ PE [OTC]: Guaifenesin 400 mg and phenylephrine 10 mg

Sudafed PE® Non-Drying Sinus [OTC]: Guaifenesin 200 mg and phenylephrine 5 mg

Liquid, oral:

Crantex®: Guaifenesin 100 mg and phenylephrine 7.5 mg per 5 mL (473 mL)

Mucinex® Cold [OTC]: Guaifenesin 100 mg and phenylephrine 2.5 mg per 5 mL (480 mL)

Rescon GG [OTC]: Guaifenesin 100 mg and phenylephrine 5 mg per 5 mL (120 mL, 480 mL)

Liquid, oral [drops]:

Donatussin Drops: Guaifenesin 20 mg and phenylephrine 1.5 mg per 1 mL (30 mL)

Suspension, oral:

Sina-12X®: Guaifenesin 100 mg and phenylephrine 5 mg per 5 mL

Syrup, oral:

Guiatex PE™: Guaifenesin 200 mg and phenylephrine 5 mg per 5 mL (473 mL)

Triaminic® Children's Chest & Nasal Congestion [OTC]: Guaifenesin 50 mg and phenylephrine 2.5 mg per 5 mL (118 mL)

Tablet, oral:

Ambi 10PEH/400GFN [OTC], Liquibid® D-R [OTC], Maxiphen [OTC], Medent®-PEI [OTC], Mucus Relief Sinus [OTC]: Guaifenesin 400 mg and phenylephrine 10 mg

Liquibid® PD-R [OTC]: Guaifenesin 200 mg and phenylephrine 5 mg

Sina-12X®: Guaifenesin 200 mg and phenylephrine tannate 25 mg

Tablet, long acting: Guaifenesin 900 mg and phenylephrine 25 mg; guaifenesin 1200 mg and phenylephrine 25 mg

Tablet, prolonged release: Guaifenesin 600 mg and phenylephrine 15 mg

guaifenesin and phenylephrine tannate *see* guaifenesin and phenylephrine *on page* 456

guaifenesin and potassium guaiacolsulfonate *(Discontinued)*

guaifenesin and pseudoephedrine (gwye FEN e sin & soo doe e FED rin)

Sound-Alike/Look-Alike Issues

Entex® may be confused with Tenex®

Entex® LA brand name represents a different product in the U.S. than it does in Canada. In the U.S., Entex® LA contains guaifenesin and phenylephrine, while in Canada the product bearing this brand name contains guaifenesin and pseudoephedrine.

Profen II® may be confused with Profen II DM®, Profen Forte®, Profen Forte™ DM

Profen Forte® may be confused with Profen II®, Profen II DM®, Profen Forte™ DM

Synonyms pseudoephedrine and guaifenesin

U.S./Canadian Brand Names Ambifed [US-OTC]; Ambifed-G [US-OTC]; Congestac® [US-OTC]; Contac® Cold-Chest Congestion, Non Drowsy, Regular Strength [Can]; Entex® LA [Can]; ExeFen-IR [US]; Maxifed [US-OTC]; Maxifed-G [US-OTC]; Mucinex® D Maximum Strength [US-OTC]; Mucinex® D [US-OTC]; Novahistex® Expectorant with Decongestant [Can]; Refenesen Plus [US-OTC]; Respaire®-30 [US]; SudaTex-G [US-OTC]; Tenar™ PSE [US]

Therapeutic Category Expectorant/Decongestant

Use Temporary relief of nasal congestion and to help loosen phlegm and thin bronchial secretions in the treatment of cough

Dosage Summary Note: Dosage varies considerably by product, ranges listed are representative. Consult specific product labeling.

Oral:

Children <2 years: Dosage not established

Children 2-6 years: One-third to 1/2 tablet every 12 hours (maximum: 1 tablet/12 hours) **or** 2.5 mg every 4-6 hours (maximum: 4 dose/day)

Children 6-12 years: One-half to 1 caplet/tablet every 12-24 hours (maximum: 1-2 caplets/tablets per day) **or** One-half caplet/tablet every 4-6 hours (maximum: 2 caplets/tablets per day) **or** 5 mL every 4-6 hours (maximum: 4 doses/day)

Children >12 years: 1-2 tablets or capsules every 12 hours **or** 1-2 capsules/tablets every 4-6 hours (maximum: 4 doses/day) **or** 10 mL every 4-6 hours (maximum: 4 doses/24 hours)

Adults: 1-2 tablets or capsules every 12 hours **or** 1-2 capsules/tablets every 4-6 hours (maximum: 4 doses/day) **or** 10 mL every 4-6 hours (maximum: 4 doses/24 hours)

Dosage Forms

Caplet, oral:

Congestac® [OTC], Refenesen Plus [OTC]: Guaifenesin 400 mg and pseudoephedrine 60 mg

Capsule, oral:

Respaire®-30: Guaifenesin 150 mg and pseudoephedrine 30 mg

Liquid, oral:

Tenar™ PSE: Guaifenesin 200 mg and pseudoephedrine 40 mg per 5 mL

Syrup, oral: Guaifenesin 200 mg and pseudoephedrine 40 mg per 5 mL

Tablet, oral:

Ambifed [OTC]: Guaifenesin 400 mg and pseudoephedrine 30 mg

Ambifed-G [OTC]: Guaifenesin 400 mg and pseudoephedrine 20 mg

ExeFen-IR, Maxifed [OTC]: Guaifenesin 400 mg and pseudoephedrine 60 mg

Maxifed-G [OTC], SudaTex-G [OTC]: Guaifenesin 400 mg and pseudoephedrine 40 mg

Tablet, extended release, oral:

Mucinex® D [OTC]: Guaifenesin 600 mg and pseudoephedrine 60 mg

Mucinex® D Maximum Strength [OTC]: Guaifenesin 1200 mg and pseudoephedrine 120 mg

guaifenesin, carbetapentane citrate, and phenylephrine hydrochloride *see* carbetapentane, guaifenesin, and phenylephrine *on page 180*

guaifenesin, chlorpheniramine, phenylephrine, and dextromethorphan *see* dextromethorphan, chlorpheniramine, phenylephrine, and guaifenesin *on page 290*

guaifenesin, dextromethorphan, and phenylephrine

(gwye FEN e sin, deks troe meth OR fan, & fen il EF rin)

Synonyms dextromethorphan hydrobromide, guaifenesin, and phenylephrine hydrochloride; guaifenesin, dextromethorphan hydrobromide, and phenylephrine hydrochloride; phenylephrine hydrochloride, guaifenesin, and dextromethorphan hydrobromide

U.S./Canadian Brand Names Certuss-D® [US]; Duraphen™ Forte [US]; Duraphen™ II DM [US]; ExeCof [US]; ExeTuss-DM [US]; Giltuss Pediatric® [US]; Giltuss TR® [US]; Giltuss® [US]; Maxiphen DM [US]; Robitussin® Cold and Cough CF [US-OTC]; Robitussin® Pediatric Cold and Cough CF [US-OTC]; SINUtuss® DM [US]; TriTuss® ER [US]; TriTuss® [US]; Tusso™-DMR [US]

Therapeutic Category Antitussive; Decongestant

Use Symptomatic relief of dry nonproductive coughs and upper respiratory symptoms associated with hay fever, colds, or the flu

Dosage Summary

Oral:

Children <6 years: Dosage not established

Children 6-12 years: Certuss-D®, Duraphen™ DM, Duraphen™ Forte, Duraphen™ II DM, Maxiphen DM: One-half tablet every 12 hours (maximum: 1 tablet/day)

Children ≥12 years:

Certuss-D®, Duraphen™ DM, Duraphen™ Forte, Maxiphen DM: One tablet every 12 hours (maximum: 2 tablets/day)

Duraphen™ II DM: 1-1½ tablets twice daily (maximum: 3 tablets/day)

Adults:

Certuss-D, Duraphen™ DM, Duraphen™ Forte, Maxiphen DM: One tablet every 12 hours (maximum: 2 tablets/day)

Duraphen™ II DM: 1-1½ tablets twice daily (maximum: 3 tablets/day)

Dosage Forms

Caplet, extended release:

TriTuss®-ER: Guaifenesin 600 mg, dextromethorphan 30 mg, and phenylephrine 10 mg

Capsule:

Tusso™-DMR: Guaifenesin 288 mg, dextromethorphan 14 mg, and phenylephrine 7 mg

Liquid:

Giltuss®: Guaifenesin 300 mg, dextromethorphan 15 mg, and phenylephrine 10 mg per 5 mL

Giltuss Pediatric®: Guaifenesin 50 mg, dextromethorphan 5 mg, and phenylephrine 2.5 mg per mL

Liquid, oral [drops]: Guaifenesin 50 mg, dextromethorphan 5 mg, and phenylephrine 2.5 mg per mL

Robitussin® Pediatric Cold and Cough CF [OTC]: Guaifenesin 100 mg, dextromethorphan 5 mg, and phenylephrine 2.5 mg per 2.5 mL

Syrup: Guaifenesin 200 mg, dextromethorphan 30 mg, and phenylephrine 10 mg

Robitussin® Cold and Cough CF [OTC]: Guaifenesin 100 mg, dextromethorphan 10 mg, and phenylephrine 5 mg per 5 mL

Tablet [scored]:

SINUtuss™ DM: Guaifenesin 600 mg, dextromethorphan hydrobromide 30 mg, and phenylephrine hydrochloride 15 mg

Tablet, extended release [scored]:

Duraphen™ II DM: Guaifenesin 800 mg, dextromethorphan 20 mg, and phenylephrine 20 mg

Duraphen™ Forte: Guaifenesin 1200 mg, dextromethorphan 30 mg, and phenylephrine 30 mg

Tablet, prolonged release [scored]:

Maxiphen DM: Guaifenesin 1000 mg, dextromethorphan 60 mg, and phenylephrine 40 mg

Tablet, sustained release: Guaifenesin 1200 mg, dextromethorphan 20 mg, and phenylephrine 40 mg

Certuss-D® [scored]: Guaifenesin 600 mg, dextromethorphan 60 mg, and phenylephrine 40 mg

ExeCof: Guaifenesin 100 mg, dextromethorphan 60 mg, and phenylephrine 40 mg

ExeTuss-DM: Guaifenesin 600 mg, dextromethorphan 25 mg, and phenylephrine 20 mg

Tablet, timed release [scored]:

Giltuss TR®: Guaifenesin 600 mg, dextromethorphan 30 mg, and phenylephrine 20 mg

guaifenesin, dextromethorphan hydrobromide, and phenylephrine hydrochloride *see* guaifenesin, dextromethorphan, and phenylephrine *on page 458*

guaifenesin, dihydrocodeine, and pseudoephedrine *see* dihydrocodeine, pseudoephedrine, and guaifenesin *on page 304*

guaifenesin, phenylephrine, and chlorpheniramine *see* chlorpheniramine, phenylephrine, and guaifenesin *on page 212*

guaifenesin, phenylephrine tannate, and pyrilamine tannate *see* phenylephrine, pyrilamine, and guaifenesin *on page 756*

guaifenesin, pseudoephedrine, and codeine

(gwye FEN e sin, soo doe e FED rin, & KOE deen)

Synonyms codeine, guaifenesin, and pseudoephedrine; pseudoephedrine, guaifenesin, and codeine

U.S./Canadian Brand Names Benylin® 3.3 mg-D-E [Can]; Calmylin with Codeine [Can]; Mytussin® DAC [US]

Therapeutic Category Antitussive/Decongestant/Expectorant

Controlled Substance C-III; C-V

Use Temporarily relieves nasal congestion and controls cough associated with upper respiratory infections and related conditions (common cold, sinusitis, bronchitis, influenza)

Dosage Summary

Oral:

Children 6-12 years: Guaituss DAC: 5 mL every 4 hours (maximum: 20 mL/24 hours)

Children >12 years: Guaituss DAC: 10 mL every 4 hours (maximum: 40 mL/24 hours)

Adults: Guaituss DAC: 10 mL every 4 hours (maximum: 40 mL/24 hours)

Dosage Forms

Syrup: Guaifenesin 100 mg, pseudoephedrine 30 mg, and codeine 10 mg per 5 mL (473 mL)

Mytussin® DAC: Guaifenesin 100 mg, pseudoephedrine 30 mg, and codeine 10 mg per 5 mL

guaifenesin, pseudoephedrine, and dextromethorphan

(gwye FEN e sin, soo doe e FED rin, & deks troe meth OR fan)

Sound-Alike/Look-Alike Issues

Profen II DM® may be confused with Profen II®, Profen Forte®, Profen Forte™ DM

Profen Forte™ DM may be confused with Profen II®, Profen II DM®, Profen Forte®

Synonyms dextromethorphan, guaifenesin, and pseudoephedrine; pseudoephedrine, dextromethorphan, and guaifenesin

U.S./Canadian Brand Names Ambifed-G DM [US]; Balminil DM + Decongestant + Expectorant [Can]; Benylin® DM-D-E [Can]; BP 8 [US]; ExeFen-DMX [US]; Koffex DM + Decongestant + Expectorant [Can]; Liquicough DM [US]; Maxifed DM [US]; Maxifed DMX [US]; Medent-DM [US]; Novahistex® DM Decongestant Expectorant [Can]; Novahistine® DM Decongestant Expectorant [Can]; Profen Forte™ DM [US]; Profen II DM® [US]; Pseudo DM GG [US]; Pseudo Max DMX [US]; Robitussin® Cough and Cold D [US-OTC]; Robitussin® Cough and Cold [Can]; Ru-Tuss DM [US]; SudaTex-DM [US]; Tenar™ DM [US]; Tusnel Pediatric® [US]; Tusnel-DM Pediatric® [US]; Tusnel® [US]

Therapeutic Category Cold Preparation

Use Temporarily relieves nasal congestion and controls cough due to minor throat and bronchial irritation; helps loosen phlegm and thin bronchial secretions to make coughs more productive

Dosage Summary **Note:** Dosage varies considerably by product, ranges listed are representative. Consult specific product labeling.

Oral:

Children <2 years: Dosage not established

Children 2-6 years: 1/3 to 1/2 tablet every 12 hours **or** 1.25-2.5 mL every 4-6 hours (2-4 times/day)

Children 6-12 years: 1/2 to 1 tablet every 12 hours **or** 1 caplet every 4-6 hours (maximum: 4 doses/day) **or** 2.5-5 mL every 4 hours (2-4 times/day)

Children ≥12 years: 1-2 tablets every 12 hours **or** 2 caplets every 4-6 hours (maximum: 4 doses/day) **or** 5-10 mL every 4 hours (2-4 times/day)

Adults: 1-2 tablets every 12 hours **or** 2 caplets every 4-6 hours (maximum: 4 doses/day) **or** 5-10 mL every 4 hours (2-4 times/day)

Dosage Forms

Caplet, prolonged release, oral:

Ambifed-G DM: Guaifenesin 1000 mg, pseudoephedrine 60 mg, and dextromethorphan 30 mg

Liquid, oral:

Liquicough™ DM, Tenar™ DM: Guaifenesin 200 mg, pseudoephedrine 32 mg, and dextromethorphan 15 mg per 5 mL

Profen II DM®: Guaifenesin 200 mg, pseudoephedrine 15 mg, and dextromethorphan 10 mg per 5 mL

Tusnel®: Guaifenesin 200 mg, pseudoephedrine 30 mg, and dextromethorphan 15 mg per 5 mL

Tusnel Pediatric®: Guaifenesin 50 mg, pseudoephedrine 15 mg, and dextromethorphan 5 mg per 5 mL

Liquid, oral [drops]:

Tusnel-DM Pediatric®: Guaifenesin 25 mg, pseudoephedrine 5 mg, and dextromethorphan 5 mg per 1 mL

Suspension, oral:

BP 8: Guaifenesin 175 mg, pseudoephedrine 30 mg, and dextromethorphan 15 mg per 5 mL

Syrup, oral:

Pseudo DM GG: Guaifenesin 100 mg, pseudoephedrine hydrochloride 40 mg, and dextromethorphan hydrobromide 15 mg per 5 mL

Robitussin® Cough and Cold D [OTC]: Guaifenesin 100 mg, pseudoephedrine 30 mg, and dextromethorphan 10 mg per 5 mL

Ru-Tuss DM: Guaifenesin 100 mg, pseudoephedrine 45 mg, and dextromethorphan 15 mg per 5 mL

Tablet, extended release, oral:

Profen Forte™ DM: Guaifenesin 800 mg, pseudoephedrine 90 mg, and dextromethorphan 60 mg

Profen II DM®: Guaifenesin 800 mg, pseudoephedrine 45 mg, and dextromethorphan 30 mg

Tablet, long acting, oral: Guaifenesin 800 mg, pseudoephedrine 60 mg, and dextromethorphan 30 mg

Medent-DM: Guaifenesin 800 mg, pseudoephedrine 60 mg, and dextromethorphan 30 mg

Tablet, sustained release, oral:
ExeFen-DMX, Maxifed DMX: Guaifenesin 780 mg, pseudoephedrine 80 mg, and dextromethorphan 40 mg
Maxifed DM, SudaTex-DM: Guaifenesin 580 mg, pseudoephedrine 60 mg, and dextromethorphan 30 mg
Pseudo Max DMX: Guaifenesin 700 mg, pseudoephedrine 80 mg, and dextromethorphan 40 mg

Guaifenex® *(Discontinued)*
Guaifenex® DM *(Discontinued)* *see* guaifenesin and dextromethorphan *on page 455*
Guaifenex® GP *(Discontinued)* *see* guaifenesin and pseudoephedrine *on page 457*
Guaifenex® PPA 75 *(Discontinued)*
Guaifenex® PSE *(Discontinued)* *see* guaifenesin and pseudoephedrine *on page 457*
Guaifenex™-Rx *(Discontinued)* *see* guaifenesin and pseudoephedrine *on page 457*
Guaifenex™-Rx DM *(Discontinued)* *see* guaifenesin, pseudoephedrine, and dextromethorphan *on page 460*
Guaimax-D® *(Discontinued)* *see* guaifenesin and pseudoephedrine *on page 457*
Guaipax® *(Discontinued)*
Guaiphen-D [US] *see* guaifenesin and phenylephrine *on page 456*
Guaiphen-D 1200 [US] *see* guaifenesin and phenylephrine *on page 456*
Guaiphen-PD [US] *see* guaifenesin and phenylephrine *on page 456*
Guaitab® *(Discontinued)* *see* guaifenesin and pseudoephedrine *on page 457*
Guaituss CF® *(Discontinued)*
Guaivent® *(Discontinued)* *see* guaifenesin and pseudoephedrine *on page 457*

guanabenz (GWAHN a benz)

Sound-Alike/Look-Alike Issues
guanabenz may be confused with guanadrel, guanfacine

Synonyms guanabenz acetate

U.S./Canadian Brand Names Wytensin® [Can]

Therapeutic Category Alpha-Adrenergic Agonist

Use Management of hypertension

Dosage Summary

Oral:
Children: Dosage not established
Adults: Initial: 4 mg twice daily; Maintenance: 4-32 mg twice daily; **Note:** Titration is recommended
Elderly: Initial: 4 mg once daily, increase every 1-2 weeks

Dosage Forms

Tablet, oral: 4 mg, 8 mg

guanabenz acetate *see* guanabenz *on page 461*

guanfacine (GWAHN fa seen)

Sound-Alike/Look-Alike Issues
guanFACINE may be confused with guaiFENesin, guanabenz, guanidine
Tenex® may be confused with Entex®, Ten-K®, Xanax®

Synonyms guanfacine hydrochloride

Tall-Man guan**FACINE**

U.S./Canadian Brand Names Intuniv™ [US]; Tenex® [US/Can]

Therapeutic Category Alpha-Adrenergic Agonist

Use
Tablet, immediate release: Management of hypertension
Tablet, extended release: Treatment of attention-deficit/hyperactivity disorder (ADHD)

Dosage Summary

Oral, immediate release:
Children <12 years: Dosage not established
Children ≥12 years: 0.5-2 mg once daily
Adults: 0.5-2 mg once daily

Oral, extended release:
Children <6 years: Dosage not established
Children ≥6 years and Adolescents: 1-4 mg once daily
Adults: Dosage not established

Dosage Forms

Tablet, oral: 1 mg, 2 mg
Tenex®: 1 mg, 2 mg
Tablet, extended release, oral:
Intuniv™: 1 mg, 2 mg, 3 mg, 4 mg

guanfacine hydrochloride *see* guanfacine *on page 461*

guanidine (GWAHN i deen)

Sound-Alike/Look-Alike Issues
guanidine may be confused with guanfacine, guanethidine

Synonyms guanidine hydrochloride

Therapeutic Category Cholinergic Agent

Use Reduction of the symptoms of muscle weakness associated with the myasthenic syndrome of Eaton-Lambert, not for myasthenia gravis

Dosage Summary

Oral:
Children: Dosage not established
Adults: Initial: 10-15 mg/kg/day in 3-4 divided doses; Maintenance: Up to 35 mg/kg/day; **Note:** Titration is recommended

Dosage Forms

Tablet, oral: 125 mg

guanidine hydrochloride *see* guanidine *on page 462*
Guia-D [US] *see* guaifenesin and dextromethorphan *on page 455*
Guiacon DMS [US-OTC] *see* guaifenesin and dextromethorphan *on page 455*
GuiaCough® *(Discontinued)* *see* guaifenesin and dextromethorphan *on page 455*
GuiaCough® Expectorant *(Discontinued)* *see* guaifenesin *on page 454*
Guiaplex™ HC *(Discontinued)*
Guiatex® *(Discontinued)*
Guiatuss DAC *(Discontinued)* *see* guaifenesin, pseudoephedrine, and codeine *on page 459*
Guiatuss™ *(Discontinued)* *see* guaifenesin *on page 454*
Guiatuss-DM® *(Discontinued)* *see* guaifenesin and dextromethorphan *on page 455*
gum benjamin *see* benzoin *on page 127*
GW506U78 *see* nelarabine *on page 664*
GW-1000-02 *see* tetrahydrocannabinol and cannabidiol *(Canada only) on page 923*
GW433908G *see* fosamprenavir *on page 426*
GW572016 *see* lapatinib *on page 550*
GW786034 *see* pazopanib *on page 730*
G-well® *(Discontinued)* *see* lindane *on page 567*
Gynazole-1® [US/Can] *see* butoconazole *on page 161*
Gyne-Lotrimin® 3 [US-OTC] *see* clotrimazole (topical) *on page 240*
Gyne-Lotrimin® 7 [US-OTC] *see* clotrimazole (topical) *on page 240*
Gyne-Sulf® *(Discontinued)* *see* sulfabenzamide, sulfacetamide, and sulfathiazole *on page 899*
Gynodiol® *(Discontinued)* *see* estradiol (systemic) *on page 366*
Gynogen L.A.® Injection *(Discontinued)* *see* estradiol (systemic) *on page 366*
Gynol II® [US-OTC] *see* nonoxynol 9 *on page 681*
Gynol II® Extra Strength [US-OTC] *see* nonoxynol 9 *on page 681*
Gynovite® Plus [US-OTC] *see* vitamins (multiple/oral) *on page 990*
H5N1 influenza vaccine *see* influenza virus vaccine (H5N1) *on page 507*
Habitrol® [Can] *see* nicotine *on page 674*

Haemophilus B conjugate and hepatitis B vaccine

(he MOF i lus bee KON joo gate & hep a TYE tis bee vak SEEN)

Sound-Alike/Look-Alike Issues

Comvax® may be confused with Recombivax [Recombivax HB®]

Synonyms *Haemophilus* b (meningococcal protein conjugate) conjugate vaccine; hepatitis B vaccine (recombinant); hib conjugate vaccine; hib-hepB

U.S./Canadian Brand Names Comvax® [US]

Therapeutic Category Vaccine, Inactivated Virus

Use

Immunization against invasive disease caused by *H. influenzae* type b and against infection caused by all known subtypes of hepatitis B virus in infants 6 weeks to 15 months of age born of hepatitis B surface antigen (HB_sAg)-negative mothers

Infants born of HB_sAg-positive mothers or mothers of unknown HB_sAg status should receive hepatitis B immune globulin and hepatitis B vaccine (recombinant) at birth and should complete the hepatitis B vaccination series given according to a particular schedule

Dosage Summary

I.M.

Infants <6 weeks: Dosage not established

Infants ≥6 weeks: 0.5 mL at 2, 4, and 12-15 months of age (total of 3 doses); Modified schedule: Children who receive one dose of hepatitis B vaccine at or shortly after birth may receive Comvax® on a schedule of 2, 4, and 12-15 months of age

Dosage Forms

Injection, suspension [preservative free]:

Comvax®: *Haemophilus* b capsular polysaccharide 7.5 mcg and hepatitis B surface antigen 5 mcg per 0.5 mL (0.5 mL)

***Haemophilus* B conjugate (Hib)** *see* diphtheria and tetanus toxoids, acellular pertussis, poliovirus and *Haemophilus* b conjugate vaccine *on page 314*

Haemophilus B conjugate vaccine (he MOF fi lus bee KON joo gate vak SEEN)

Synonyms *Haemophilus* b oligosaccharide conjugate vaccine; *Haemophilus* b polysaccharide vaccine; diphtheria toxoid conjugate; HbCV; hib; hib conjugate vaccine; hib polysaccharide conjugate; PRP-OMP; PRP-T

U.S./Canadian Brand Names ActHIB® [US/Can]; Hiberix® [US]; PedvaxHIB® [US/Can]

Therapeutic Category Vaccine, Inactivated Bacteria

Use Routine immunization of children against invasive disease caused by *H. influenzae* type b

The Advisory Committee on Immunization Practices (ACIP) recommends routine vaccination of all children through age 59 months. Efficacy data is not available for use in older children and adults with chronic conditions associated with an increased risk of Hib disease. However, a single dose may also be considered for older children, adolescents, and adults who did not receive the childhood series and who have had splenectomies or who have sickle cell disease, leukemia, or HIV infection.

Dosage Summary

I.M.

Children: 0.5 mL as a single dose administered according to one of the "brand-specific" schedules

ActHIB®: Age at first dose:

2 months of age: Immunization consists of 3 doses (0.5 mL/dose) administered at 2, 4 and 6 months of age (may reconstitute with provided diluent or DTP vaccine). A booster dose is given at 15-18 months of age (may reconstitute with provided diluent or Tripedia® vaccine).

7-11 months of age: Two doses (0.5 mL/dose) administered 8 months apart, with a booster dose at 15-18 months of age

12-14 months of age: One dose (0.5 mL) followed by a booster dose 2 months later

PedvaxHIB®: Age at first dose:

2-10 months of age: Two doses (0.5 mL/dose) administered 2 months apart; booster dose at 12-15 months of age

11-14 months of age: Two doses (0.5 mL/dose) administered 1 month apart

15-71 months of age: One 0.5 mL dose

Hiberix®: 15-59 months: One 0.5 mL dose (approved for booster dose only)

Dosage Forms

Injection, powder for reconstitution [preservative free]:

ActHIB® *Haemophilus* b capsular polysaccharide 10 mcg per 0.5 mL

Hiberix®: *Haemophilus* b capsular polysaccharide 10 mcg per 0.5 mL

Injection, suspension:

PedvaxHIB®: *Haemophilus* b capsular polysaccharide 7.5 mcg

***Haemophilus* b (meningococcal protein conjugate) conjugate vaccine** *see Haemophilus* B conjugate and hepatitis B vaccine *on page 463*

***Haemophilus* b oligosaccharide conjugate vaccine** *see Haemophilus* B conjugate vaccine *on page 463*

***Haemophilus* B polysaccharide** *see* diphtheria and tetanus toxoids, acellular pertussis, poliovirus and *Haemophilus* b conjugate vaccine *on page 314*

***Haemophilus* b polysaccharide vaccine** *see Haemophilus* B conjugate vaccine *on page 463*

***Haemophilus influenzae* b conjugate vaccine and diphtheria, tetanus toxoids, and acellular pertussis vaccine** *see* diphtheria, tetanus toxoids, and acellular pertussis vaccine and *Haemophilus influenzae* b conjugate vaccine *on page 317*

halcinonide (hal SIN oh nide)

Sound-Alike/Look-Alike Issues

halcinonide may be confused with Halcion®

Halog® may be confused with Haldol®, Mycolog®

U.S./Canadian Brand Names Halog® [US/Can]

Therapeutic Category Corticosteroid, Topical

Use Inflammation of corticosteroid-responsive dermatoses [high potency topical corticosteroid]

Dosage Summary

Topical:

Children: Apply sparingly 1-3 times/day

Adults: Apply sparingly 1-3 times/day

Dosage Forms

Cream, topical:

Halog®: 0.1% (30 g, 60 g)

Ointment, topical:

Halog®: 0.1% (30 g, 60 g)

Halcion® [US/Can] *see* triazolam *on page 956*

Haldol® [US] *see* haloperidol *on page 465*

Haldol® Decanoate [US] *see* haloperidol *on page 465*

Haley's M-O *see* magnesium hydroxide and mineral oil *on page 586*

HalfLytely® and Bisacodyl [US] *see* polyethylene glycol-electrolyte solution and bisacodyl *on page 776*

Halfprin® [US-OTC] *see* aspirin *on page 100*

halobetasol (hal oh BAY ta sol)

Sound-Alike/Look-Alike Issues

Ultravate® may be confused with Cutivate®

Synonyms halobetasol propionate

U.S./Canadian Brand Names Ultravate® [US/Can]

Therapeutic Category Corticosteroid, Topical

Use Relief of inflammatory and pruritic manifestations of corticosteroid-response dermatoses [super high potency topical corticosteroid]

Dosage Summary

Topical:

Children <12 years: Dosage not established

Children ≥12 years: Apply sparingly to lesion/skin twice daily (maximum: 50 g/week; 2 consecutive weeks)

Adults: Apply sparingly to lesion/skin twice daily (maximum: 50 g/week; 2 consecutive weeks)

Dosage Forms

Cream, topical: 0.05% (15 g, 50 g)

Ultravate®: 0.05% (15 g, 50 g)

Ointment, topical: 0.05% (15 g, 50 g)

Ultravate®: 0.05% (15 g, 50 g)

halobetasol propionate *see* halobetasol *on page 464*

Halog® [US/Can] *see* halcinonide *on page 464*

Halog®-E *(Discontinued)* *see* halcinonide *on page 464*

haloperidol (ha loe PER i dole)

Sound-Alike/Look-Alike Issues

haloperidol may be confused Halotestin®

Haldol® may be confused with Halcion®, Halenol®, Halog®, Halotestin®, Stadol®

Synonyms haloperidol decanoate; haloperidol lactate

U.S./Canadian Brand Names Apo-Haloperidol LA® [Can]; Apo-Haloperidol® [Can]; Haldol® Decanoate [US]; Haldol® [US]; Haloperidol Injection, USP [Can]; Haloperidol Long Acting [Can]; Haloperidol-LA Omega [Can]; Haloperidol-LA [Can]; Novo-Peridol [Can]; Peridol [Can]; PMS-Haloperidol LA [Can]

Therapeutic Category Antipsychotic Agent, Butyrophenone

Use Management of schizophrenia; control of tics and vocal utterances of Tourette disorder in children and adults; severe behavioral problems in children

Dosage Summary

I.M.:

Decanoate:

Children: Dosage not established

Adults: Initial: 10-20 times daily oral dose at 4-week intervals; Maintenance: 10-15 times initial oral dose

Lactate:

Children <6 years: Dosage not established

Children 6-12 years: 1-3 mg/dose every 4-8 hours (maximum: 0.15 mg/kg/day)

Adults: 2-5 mg every 4-8 hours as needed

Oral:

Children <3 years: Dosage not established

Children 3-12 years (15-40 kg): Initial: 0.05 mg/kg/day **or** 0.25-0.5 mg/day in 2-3 divided doses; Maintenance: 0.05-0.15 mg/kg/day in 2-3 divided doses **or** 0.01-0.03 mg/kg once daily (maximum: 0.15 mg/kg/day); **Note:** Titration is recommended

Adults: Initial: 0.5-5 mg 2-3 times/day; Maintenance: Up to 30 mg/day in 2-3 divided doses; **Note:** Titration is recommended

Dosage Forms

Injection, oil: 50 mg/mL (1 mL, 5 mL); 100 mg/mL (1 mL, 5 mL)

Haldol® Decanoate: 100 mg/mL (1 mL)

Injection, solution: 5 mg/mL (1 mL, 10 mL)

Haldol®: 5 mg/mL (1 mL)

Solution, oral: 2 mg/mL (5 mL, 15 mL, 120 mL)

Tablet, oral: 0.5 mg, 1 mg, 2 mg, 5 mg, 10 mg, 20 mg

haloperidol decanoate *see* haloperidol *on page 465*

Haloperidol Injection, USP [Can] *see* haloperidol *on page 465*

Haloperidol-LA [Can] *see* haloperidol *on page 465*

haloperidol lactate *see* haloperidol *on page 465*

Haloperidol-LA Omega [Can] *see* haloperidol *on page 465*

Haloperidol Long Acting [Can] *see* haloperidol *on page 465*

halothane *(Discontinued)*

Halotussin® *(Discontinued)* *see* guaifenesin *on page 454*

Halotussin® DM *(Discontinued)* *see* guaifenesin and dextromethorphan *on page 455*

Halotussin® PE *(Discontinued)* *see* guaifenesin and pseudoephedrine *on page 457*

Haltran® *(Discontinued)* *see* ibuprofen *on page 494*

hamamelis water *see* witch hazel *on page 994*

HandClens® [US-OTC] *see* benzalkonium chloride *on page 124*

harkoseride *see* lacosamide *on page 541*

Havrix® [US/Can] *see* hepatitis A vaccine *on page* 468
Havrix® and Engerix-B® *see* hepatitis A and hepatitis B recombinant vaccine *on page* 468
HbCV *see Haemophilus* B conjugate vaccine *on page* 463
HBIG *see* hepatitis B immune globulin (human) *on page* 469
hBNP *see* nesiritide *on page* 669
hCG *see* chorionic gonadotropin (human) *on page* 219
HD 200® Plus *(Discontinued)* *see* barium *on page* 117
HDA® Toothache [US-OTC] *see* benzocaine *on page* 124
HDCV *see* rabies vaccine *on page* 825
Head & Shoulders® Citrus Breeze [US-OTC] *see* pyrithione zinc *on page* 819
Head & Shoulders® Citrus Breeze 2-in-1 [US-OTC] *see* pyrithione zinc *on page* 819
Head & Shoulders® Classic Clean [US-OTC] *see* pyrithione zinc *on page* 819
Head & Shoulders® Classic Clean 2-In-1 [US-OTC] *see* pyrithione zinc *on page* 819
Head & Shoulders® Dry Scalp [US-OTC] *see* pyrithione zinc *on page* 819
Head & Shoulders® Dry Scalp 2-in-1 [US-OTC] *see* pyrithione zinc *on page* 819
Head & Shoulders® Dry Scalp Care [US-OTC] *see* pyrithione zinc *on page* 819
Head & Shoulders® Dry Scalp Care 2-in-1 [US-OTC] *see* pyrithione zinc *on page* 819
Head & Shoulders® Extra Volume [US-OTC] *see* pyrithione zinc *on page* 819
Head & Shoulders® intensive solutions 2-in-1 [US-OTC] *see* pyrithione zinc *on page* 819
Head & Shoulders® intensive solutions for dry/damaged hair [US-OTC] *see* pyrithione zinc *on page* 819
Head & Shoulders® intensive solutions for fine/oily hair [US-OTC] *see* pyrithione zinc *on page* 819
Head & Shoulders® intensive solutions for normal hair [US-OTC] *see* pyrithione zinc *on page* 819
Head & Shoulders® Intensive Treatment [US-OTC] *see* selenium sulfide *on page* 869
Head & Shoulders® Ocean Lift [US-OTC] *see* pyrithione zinc *on page* 819
Head & Shoulders® Ocean Lift 2-in-1 [US-OTC] *see* pyrithione zinc *on page* 819
Head & Shoulders® Refresh [US-OTC] *see* pyrithione zinc *on page* 819
Head & Shoulders® Refresh 2-in-1 [US-OTC] *see* pyrithione zinc *on page* 819
Head & Shoulders® Restoring Shine [US-OTC] *see* pyrithione zinc *on page* 819
Head & Shoulders® Restoring Shine 2-in-1 [US-OTC] *see* pyrithione zinc *on page* 819
Head & Shoulders® Sensitive Care [US-OTC] *see* pyrithione zinc *on page* 819
Head & Shoulders® Sensitive Care 2-in-1 [US-OTC] *see* pyrithione zinc *on page* 819
Head & Shoulders® Smooth & Silky [US-OTC] *see* pyrithione zinc *on page* 819
Head & Shoulders® Smooth & Silky 2-In-1 [US-OTC] *see* pyrithione zinc *on page* 819
Healon® [US/Can] *see* hyaluronate and derivatives *on page* 475
Healon®5 [US] *see* hyaluronate and derivatives *on page* 475
Healon GV® [US/Can] *see* hyaluronate and derivatives *on page* 475
Heartburn Relief [US-OTC] *see* famotidine *on page* 390
Heartburn Relief Maximum Strength [US-OTC] *see* famotidine *on page* 390
Hectorol® [US/Can] *see* doxercalciferol *on page* 329
Helidac® [US] *see* bismuth, metronidazole, and tetracycline *on page* 140
Helistat® [US] *see* collagen hemostat *on page* 248
Helitene® [US] *see* collagen hemostat *on page* 248
Helixate® FS [US/Can] *see* antihemophilic factor (recombinant) *on page* 81
Hemabate® [US/Can] *see* carboprost tromethamine *on page* 183
hematin *see* hemin *on page* 466
hemiacidrin *see* citric acid, magnesium carbonate, and glucono-delta-lactone *on page* 228

hemin (HEE min)

Synonyms hematin
U.S./Canadian Brand Names Panhematin® [US]
Therapeutic Category Blood Modifiers

Use Treatment of recurrent attacks of acute intermittent porphyria (AIP)

Dosage Summary

I.V.:

Children <16 years: Dosage not established

Children ≥16 years: 1-4 mg/kg/day repeated no earlier than every 12 hours (maximum: 6 mg/kg in any 24-hour period)

Adults: 1-4 mg/kg/day repeated no earlier than every 12 hours (maximum: 6 mg/kg/24-hour period)

Dosage Forms

Injection, powder for reconstitution:

Panhematin®: 313 mg

Hemocyte® [US-OTC] *see* ferrous fumarate *on page 398*

Hemocyte Plus® [US] *see* vitamins (multiple/oral) *on page 990*

Hemofil M [US/Can] *see* antihemophilic factor (human) *on page 81*

Hemorrhoidal HC *(Discontinued)* *see* hydrocortisone (topical) *on page 483*

Hemorrhoidal-HC Uniserts® [US] *see* hydrocortisone (topical) *on page 483*

Hemril®-30 [US] *see* hydrocortisone (topical) *on page 483*

HepA *see* hepatitis A vaccine *on page 468*

HepaGam B® [US/Can] *see* hepatitis B immune globulin (human) *on page 469*

HepA-HepB *see* hepatitis A and hepatitis B recombinant vaccine *on page 468*

Hepalean® [Can] *see* heparin *on page 467*

Hepalean® Leo [Can] *see* heparin *on page 467*

Hepalean®-LOK [Can] *see* heparin *on page 467*

heparin (HEP a rin)

Sound-Alike/Look-Alike Issues

heparin may be confused with Hespan®

Synonyms heparin calcium; heparin lock flush; heparin sodium

U.S./Canadian Brand Names Hep-Lock U/P [US]; Hep-Lock [US]; Hepalean® Leo [Can]; Hepalean® [Can]; Hepalean®-LOK [Can]; HepFlush®-10 [US]

Therapeutic Category Anticoagulant (Other)

Use Prophylaxis and treatment of thromboembolic disorders; as an anticoagulant for extracorporeal and dialysis procedures

Note: Heparin lock flush solution is intended only to maintain patency of I.V. devices and is **not** to be used for anticoagulant therapy.

Dosage Summary

I.V.:

Children: Bolus: 50 units/kg; Initial Infusion: 15-25 units/kg/hour; Maintenance: Increase dose by 2-4 units/kg/hour every 6-8 hours as needed **or** 50-100 units/kg every 4 hours intermittently

Adults: Bolus: 60-80 units/kg; Infusion: 10-30 units/kg/hour (weight-based institutional nomogram recommended) **or** 10,000 units (initially), then 50-70 units/kg (5000-10,000 units) every 4-6 hours intermittently

SubQ:

Children: Dosage not established

Adults: Thromboprophylaxis: 5000 units every 8-12 hours; Treatment: 17,500 units every 12 hours

Dosage Forms

Infusion, premixed in 1/2 NS: 25,000 units (250 mL, 500 mL)

Infusion, premixed in D_5W: 10,000 units (100 mL, 250 mL); 12,500 units (250 mL); 20,000 units (500 mL); 25,000 units (250 mL, 500 mL)

Infusion, premixed in D_5W [preservative free]: 20,000 units (500 mL); 25,000 units (250 mL, 500 mL)

Infusion, premixed in NS: 1000 units (500 mL); 2000 units (1000 mL)

Infusion, premixed in NS [preservative free]: 1000 units (500 mL); 2000 units (1000 mL)

Injection, solution: 10 units/mL (1 mL, 2 mL, 3 mL, 5 mL, 10 mL, 30 mL); 100 units/mL (1 mL, 2 mL, 3 mL, 5 mL, 10 mL, 30 mL); 1000 units/mL (1 mL, 10 mL, 30 mL); 5000 units/mL (1 mL, 10 mL); 10,000 units/mL (1 mL, 4 mL, 5 mL); 20,000 units/mL (1 mL)

Hep-Lock: 10 units/mL (1 mL, 2 mL, 10 mL, 30 mL); 100 units/mL (1 mL, 2 mL, 10 mL, 30 mL)

Injection, solution [preservative free]: 1 units/mL (2 mL, 3 mL, 5 mL); 2 units/mL (3 mL); 10 units/mL (1 mL, 2 mL, 2.5 mL, 3 mL, 5 mL, 6 mL, 10 mL); 100 units/mL (1 mL, 2 mL, 3 mL, 5 mL, 10 mL); 1000 units/mL (2 mL); 10,000 units/mL (0.5 mL)
Hep-Lock U/P: 10 units/mL (1 mL); 100 units/mL (1 mL)
HepFlush®-10: 10 units/mL (10 mL)

heparin calcium *see* heparin *on page 467*

heparin lock flush *see* heparin *on page 467*

heparin sodium *see* heparin *on page 467*

HepatAmine® [US] *see* amino acid injection *on page 64*

Hepatasol® [US] *see* amino acid injection *on page 64*

hepatitis A and hepatitis B recombinant vaccine

(hep a TYE tis aye & hep a TYE tis bee ree KOM be nant vak SEEN)

Synonyms Engerix-B® and Havrix®; Havrix® and Engerix-B®; HepA-HepB; hepatitis B and hepatitis A vaccine

U.S./Canadian Brand Names Twinrix® Junior [Can]; Twinrix® [US/Can]

Therapeutic Category Vaccine

Use Active immunization against disease caused by hepatitis A virus and hepatitis B virus (all known subtypes) in populations desiring protection against or at high risk of exposure to these viruses.

Populations include travelers or people living in or relocating to areas of intermediate/high endemicity for **both** HAV and HBV and are at increased risk of HBV infection due to behavioral or occupational factors; patients with chronic liver disease; laboratory workers who handle live HAV and HBV; healthcare workers, police, and other personnel who render first-aid or medical assistance; workers who come in contact with sewage; employees of day care centers and correctional facilities; patients/staff of hemodialysis units; male homosexuals; patients frequently receiving blood products; military personnel; users of injectable illicit drugs; close household contacts of patients with hepatitis A and hepatitis B infection; residents of drug and alcohol treatment centers

Dosage Summary

I.M.:

Children: Dosage not established

Adults: Three doses (1 mL each) given on a 0-, 1-, and 6-month schedule

Dosage Forms

Injection, suspension [preservative free]:

Twinrix®: Hepatitis A virus antigen 720 ELISA units and hepatitis B surface antigen 20 mcg per mL (1 mL)

Dosage Forms - Canada

Injection, suspension [preservative free]:

Twinrix® Junior: Hepatitis A virus antigen 360 ELISA units and hepatitis B surface antigen 10 mcg per 0.5 mL (0.5 mL)

hepatitis A vaccine (hep a TYE tis aye vak SEEN)

Synonyms HepA

U.S./Canadian Brand Names Avaxim® [Can]; Avaxim®-Pediatric [Can]; Havrix® [US/Can]; VAQTA® [US/Can]

Therapeutic Category Vaccine, Inactivated Virus

Use

Active immunization against disease caused by hepatitis A virus (HAV)

The Advisory Committee on Immunization Practices (ACIP) recommends routine vaccination for:

- All children ≥12 months of age
- Travelers to countries with intermediate to high endemicity of HAV (a list of countries is available at http://wwwn.cdc.gov/travel/contentdiseases.aspx)
- Persons who anticipate close personal contact with international adoptee from a country of intermediate to high endemicity of HAV, during their first 60 days of arrival into the United States (eg, household contacts, babysitters)
- Men who have sex with men
- Illegal drug users
- Patients with chronic liver disease
- Patients who receive clotting-factor concentrates
- Persons who work with HAV-infected primates or with HAV in a research laboratory setting

Dosage Summary

I.M.:

Children <12 months: Dosage not established

Children 12 months to 18 years:

HAVRIX®: 720 ELISA units (0.5 mL) with a booster dose of 720 ELISA units to be given 6-12 months following primary immunization

VAQTA®: 25 units (0.5 mL) with a booster dose of 25 units to be given 6-18 months after primary immunization

Adults:

HAVRIX®: 1440 ELISA units (1 mL) with a booster dose of 1400 ELISA units to be given 6-12 months following primary immunization

VAQTA®: 50 units (1 mL) with a booster dose of 50 units to be given 6-18 months after primary immunization

Dosage Forms

Injection, suspension [preservative free]:

Havrix®: Hepatitis A virus antigen 720 ELISA units/0.5 mL (0.5 mL); Hepatitis A virus antigen 1440 ELISA units/mL (1 mL)

VAQTA®: Hepatitis A virus antigen 25 units/0.5 mL (0.5 mL); Hepatitis A virus antigen 50 units/mL (1 mL)

hepatitis B and hepatitis A vaccine *see* hepatitis A and hepatitis B recombinant vaccine *on page 468*

hepatitis B immune globulin (human) (hep a TYE tis bee i MYUN GLOB yoo lin YU man)

Sound-Alike/Look-Alike Issues

HBIG may be confused with BabyBIG

Synonyms HBIG

U.S./Canadian Brand Names HepaGam B® [US/Can]; HyperHep B® [Can]; HyperHEP B™ S/D [US]; Nabi-HB® [US]

Therapeutic Category Immune Globulin

Use

Passive prophylactic immunity to hepatitis B following: Acute exposure to blood containing hepatitis B surface antigen (HBsAg); perinatal exposure of infants born to HBsAg-positive mothers; sexual exposure to HBsAg-positive persons; household exposure to persons with acute HBV infection

Prevention of hepatitis B virus recurrence after liver transplantation in HBsAg-positive transplant patients

Note: Hepatitis B immune globulin is not indicated for treatment of active hepatitis B infection and is ineffective in the treatment of chronic active hepatitis B infection.

Dosage Summary

I.M.:

Newborns: 0.5 mL within 12 hours of birth, and begin active vaccination program; may repeat at 3 months if vaccination is delayed

Infants <12 months: 0.5 mL as a single dose (if mother or primary caregiver has acute HBV infection)

Children ≥12 months: 0.06 mL/kg within 24 hours of needlestick, ocular or mucosal exposure and within 14 days of sexual exposure; repeat in 28-30 days if no response or if refuse vaccination

Adults: 0.06 mL/kg within 24 hours of needlestick, ocular or mucosal exposure and within 14 days of sexual exposure; repeat in 28-30 days if no response or if refuse vaccination

I.V.:

Adults: 20,000 int. units/dose according to the following schedule:

Anhepatic phase (Initial dose): One dose given with the liver transplant

Week 1 postop: One dose daily for 7 days (days 1-7)

Weeks 2-12 postop: One dose every 2 weeks starting day 14

Month 4 onward: One dose monthly starting on month 4

Dose adjustment: Adjust dose to reach anti-HBs levels of 500 int. units/L within the first week after transplantation. In patients with surgical bleeding, abdominal fluid drainage >500 mL or those undergoing plasmapheresis, administer 10,000 int. units/dose every 6 hours until target anti-HBs levels are reached.

Dosage Forms

Injection, solution [preservative free]:

HepaGam B®: Anti-HBs > 312 int. units/mL (1 mL, 5 mL)

HyperHEP B™ S/D: Anti-HBs ≥ 220 int. units/mL (0.5 mL, 1 mL, 5 mL)

Nabi-HB®: Anti-HBs > 312 int. units/mL (1 mL, 5 mL)

hepatitis B inactivated virus vaccine (recombinant DNA) *see* hepatitis B vaccine (recombinant) *on page 470*

hepatitis B vaccine (recombinant) (hep a TYE tis bee vak SEEN ree KOM be nant)

Sound-Alike/Look-Alike Issues

Engerix-B® adult may be confused with Engerix-B® pediatric/adolescent
Recombivax HB® may be confused with Comvax®

Synonyms hepatitis B inactivated virus vaccine (recombinant DNA); HepB

U.S./Canadian Brand Names Engerix-B® [US/Can]; Recombivax HB® [US/Can]

Therapeutic Category Vaccine, Inactivated Virus

Use Immunization against infection caused by all known subtypes of hepatitis B virus (HBV), in individuals seeking protection from HBV infection and/or in the following individuals considered at high risk of potential exposure to hepatitis B virus or HBsAg-positive materials:

Workplace Exposure:

- Healthcare workers[1] (including students, custodial staff, lab personnel, etc)
- Police and fire personnel
- Military personnel
- Morticians and embalmers
- Clients/staff of institutions for the developmentally disabled

Lifestyle Factors:

- Men who have sex with men
- Sexually-active persons with >1 partner in a 6-month period
- Persons with recently acquired sexually-transmitted disease
- Sex partners of persons who are HBsAG-positive
- Intravenous drug users

Specific Patient Groups:

- Those on hemodialysis[2], receiving transfusions[3], or in hematology/oncology units
- Adolescents
- Infants born of HBsAG-positive mothers
- Individuals with chronic liver disease
- Individuals with chronic hepatitis C
- Individuals with HIV infection

Others:

- Prison inmates and staff of correctional facilities
- Household and sexual contacts of HBV carriers
- Residents, immigrants, adoptees, and refugees from areas with endemic HBV infection (eg, Alaskan Eskimos, Pacific Islanders, Indochinese, and Haitian descent)
- International travelers to areas of endemic HBV
- Children born after 11/21/1991

[1]The risk of hepatitis B virus (HBV) infection for healthcare workers varies both between hospitals and within hospitals. Hepatitis B vaccination is recommended for all healthcare workers with blood exposure.
[2]Hemodialysis patients often respond poorly to hepatitis B vaccination; higher vaccine doses or increased number of doses are required. A special formulation of one vaccine is now available for such persons (Recombivax HB®, 40 mcg/mL). The anti-HB_s (antibody to hepatitis B surface antigen) response of such persons should be tested after they are vaccinated, and those who have not responded should be revaccinated with 1-3 additional doses. Patients with chronic renal disease should be vaccinated as early as possible, ideally before they require hemodialysis. In addition, their anti-HB_s levels should be monitored at 6- to 12-month intervals to assess the need for revaccination.
[3]Patients with hemophilia should be immunized subcutaneously, not intramuscularly.

The Advisory Committee on Immunization Practices (ACIP) recommends vaccination of all infants at birth, vaccination of all children and adolescents aged <19 years not previously vaccinated, and vaccination of all adults at high risk for HBV infection. In addition, the ACIP recommends vaccination for any persons who are wounded in bombings or similar mass casualty events who have penetrating injuries or nonintact skin exposure, or who have contact with mucous membranes (exception - superficial contact with intact skin), and who cannot confirm receipt of a hepatitis B vaccination.

Dosage Summary

I.M.:

Birth to 19 years: Initial: 0.5 mL (pediatric/adolescent formulation), then repeat 0.5 mL at 1 and 6 months after first dose

Adults ≥20 years: Initial: 1 mL (adult formulation), then repeat 1 mL at 1 and 6 months after first dose; **Note:** Dialysis or immunocompromised patients may require a higher dose

Dosage Forms

Injection, suspension [preservative free]:

Engerix-B®: Hepatitis B surface antigen 10 mcg/0.5 mL (0.5 mL); Hepatitis B surface antigen 20 mcg/mL (1 mL)

Recombivax HB®: Hepatitis B surface antigen 5 mcg/0.5 mL (0.5 mL); Hepatitis B surface antigen 10 mcg/mL (1 mL); Hepatitis B surface antigen 40 mcg/mL (1 mL)

hepatitis B vaccine (recombinant) *see Haemophilus* B conjugate and hepatitis B vaccine *on page 463*

HepB *see* hepatitis B vaccine (recombinant) *on page 470*

HepFlush®-10 [US] *see* heparin *on page 467*

Hep-Lock [US] *see* heparin *on page 467*

Hep-Lock U/P [US] *see* heparin *on page 467*

Hepsera® [US/Can] *see* adefovir *on page 38*

Heptalac® ***(Discontinued)*** *see* lactulose *on page 544*

Heptovir® [Can] *see* lamivudine *on page 545*

Herceptin® [US/Can] *see* trastuzumab *on page 948*

HES *see* hetastarch *on page 471*

HES *see* tetrastarch *on page 924*

HES 130/0.4 *see* tetrastarch *on page 924*

Hespan® [US] *see* hetastarch *on page 471*

hetastarch (HET a starch)

Sound-Alike/Look-Alike Issues

Hespan® may be confused with heparin

Synonyms HES; hydroxyethyl starch

U.S./Canadian Brand Names Hespan® [US]; Hextend® [US/Can]

Therapeutic Category Plasma Volume Expander

Use Blood volume expander used in treatment of hypovolemia; adjunct in leukapheresis to improve harvesting and increase the yield of granulocytes by centrifugation (Hespan®)

Dosage Summary

I.V.:

Children: Dosage not established

Adults: 500-1500 mL/day **or** 20 mL/kg/day (up to 1500 mL/day)

Leukapheresis: Hextend®:

Children: Dosage not established

Adults: 250-700 mL

Dosage Forms

Infusion:

Hextend®: 6% (500 mL)

Infusion, premixed in NS: 6% (500 mL)

Hespan®: 6% (500 mL)

Hexabrix™ [US] *see* ioxaglate meglumine and ioxaglate sodium *on page 522*

hexachlorocyclohexane *see* lindane *on page 567*

hexachlorophene (heks a KLOR oh feen)

Sound-Alike/Look-Alike Issues

pHisoHex® may be confused with Fostex®, pHisoDerm®

U.S./Canadian Brand Names pHisoHex® [US/Can]

Therapeutic Category Antibacterial, Topical

Use Surgical scrub and as a bacteriostatic skin cleanser; control an outbreak of gram-positive infection when other procedures have been unsuccessful

Dosage Summary

Topical:

Children: Apply 5 mL cleanser and water to area to be cleansed

Adults: Apply 5 mL cleanser and water to area to be cleansed

Dosage Forms

Liquid, topical:

pHisoHex®: 3% (150 mL, 480 mL)

Hexalen® [US/Can] *see* altretamine *on page 57*

hexamethylenetetramine *see* methenamine *on page 612*

hexamethylmelamine *see* altretamine *on page 57*

Hexit™ [Can] *see* lindane *on page 567*

HEXM *see* altretamine *on page 57*

Hextend® [US/Can] *see* hetastarch *on page 471*

hexylresorcinol (heks il re ZOR si nole)

U.S./Canadian Brand Names Sucrets® Original [US-OTC]

Therapeutic Category Local Anesthetic

Use Minor antiseptic and local anesthetic for sore throat; topical antiseptic for minor cuts or abrasions

Dosage Summary

Oral:

Children <2 years: Dosage not established

Children ≥2 years: Up to 10 lozenges/day **or** gargle/swish solution up to 4 times/day

Adults: Up to 10 lozenges/day **or** gargle/swish solution up to 4 times/day

Topical:

Children <2 years: Dosage not established

Children ≥2 years: Apply to affected area 1-3 times/day

Adults: Apply to affected area 1-3 times/day

Dosage Forms

Lozenge, oral:

Sucrets® Original [OTC]: 2.4 mg (18s)

hFSH *see* urofollitropin *on page 971*

hGH *see* somatropin *on page 889*

hib *see Haemophilus* B conjugate vaccine *on page 463*

hib conjugate vaccine *see Haemophilus* B conjugate and hepatitis B vaccine *on page 463*

hib conjugate vaccine *see Haemophilus* B conjugate vaccine *on page 463*

Hiberix® [US] *see Haemophilus* B conjugate vaccine *on page 463*

hib-hepB *see Haemophilus* B conjugate and hepatitis B vaccine *on page 463*

Hibiclens® [US-OTC] *see* chlorhexidine gluconate *on page 204*

Hibidil® 1:2000 [Can] *see* chlorhexidine gluconate *on page 204*

Hibistat® [US-OTC] *see* chlorhexidine gluconate *on page 204*

hib polysaccharide conjugate *see Haemophilus* B conjugate vaccine *on page 463*

HibTITER® ***(Discontinued)*** *see Haemophilus* B conjugate vaccine *on page 463*

High Gamma Vitamin E Complete™ [US-OTC] *see* vitamin E *on page 988*

high-molecular-weight iron dextran (DexFerrum®) *see* iron dextran complex *on page 525*

Hi-Kovite [US-OTC] *see* vitamins (multiple/oral) *on page 990*

Hiprex® [US/Can] *see* methenamine *on page 612*

hirulog *see* bivalirudin *on page 141*

Histacol™ BD [US] *see* brompheniramine, pseudoephedrine, and dextromethorphan *on page 149*

Histade™ ***(Discontinued)*** *see* chlorpheniramine and pseudoephedrine *on page 209*

Histalet® X ***(Discontinued)*** *see* guaifenesin and pseudoephedrine *on page 457*

Histantil [Can] *see* promethazine *on page 800*

Histaprin [US-OTC] *see* diphenhydramine (systemic) *on page 310*

Histatab PH [US] *see* chlorpheniramine, phenylephrine, and methscopolamine *on page 212*

Histatab® Plus ***(Discontinued)*** *see* chlorpheniramine and phenylephrine *on page 208*

Hista-Vent® DA ***(Discontinued)*** *see* chlorpheniramine, phenylephrine, and methscopolamine *on page* *212*

Hista-Vent® PSE ***(Discontinued)*** *see* chlorpheniramine, pseudoephedrine, and methscopolamine *on page* *215*

Histerone® Injection ***(Discontinued)*** *see* testosterone *on page* *919*

Histex™ I/E ***(Discontinued)*** *see* carbinoxamine *on page* *182*

Histex™ ***(Discontinued)*** *see* chlorpheniramine and pseudoephedrine *on page* *209*

Histex® SR [US] *see* brompheniramine and pseudoephedrine *on page* *148*

Histinex® D Liquid ***(Discontinued)***

Histinex® HC [US] *see* phenylephrine, hydrocodone, and chlorpheniramine *on page* *754*

Histinex® PV ***(Discontinued)***

Histor-D® Syrup ***(Discontinued)*** *see* chlorpheniramine and phenylephrine *on page* *208*

Histor-D® Timecelles® ***(Discontinued)*** *see* chlorpheniramine, phenylephrine, and methscopolamine *on page* *212*

Histrodrix® ***(Discontinued)*** *see* dexbrompheniramine and pseudoephedrine *on page* *282*

Histussin D® ***(Discontinued)***

Histussin® HC ***(Discontinued)*** *see* phenylephrine, hydrocodone, and chlorpheniramine *on page* *754*

Hi-Vegi-Lip [US-OTC] *see* pancreatin *on page* *723*

Hivid® ***(Discontinued)***

Hizentra™ [US] *see* immune globulin (subcutaneous) *on page* *503*

hMG *see* menotropins *on page* *602*

HMM *see* altretamine *on page* *57*

HMR 3647 *see* telithromycin *on page* *913*

HMS Liquifilm® ***(Discontinued)***

HN_2 *see* mechlorethamine *on page* *594*

Hold® DM [US-OTC] *see* dextromethorphan *on page* *287*

homatropine (hoe MA troe peen)

Sound-Alike/Look-Alike Issues

homatropine may be confused with Humatrope®, somatropin

Synonyms homatropine hydrobromide

U.S./Canadian Brand Names Isopto® Homatropine [US]

Therapeutic Category Anticholinergic Agent

Use Producing cycloplegia and mydriasis for refraction; treatment of acute inflammatory conditions of the uveal tract; optical aid in axial lens opacities

Dosage Summary

Ophthalmic:

Children: Instill 1 drop (2% solution) 2-3 times/day **or** immediately prior to procedure, repeat every 10 minutes intervals as needed

Adults: Instill 1-2 drops (2% or 5% solution) 2-3 times/day, up to every 3-4 hours as needed **or** 1-2 drops (2% solution) or 1 drop (5% solution) prior to procedure, repeat every 5-10 minutes as needed up to 3 doses

Dosage Forms

Solution, ophthalmic:

Isopto® Homatropine: 2% (5 mL); 5% (5 mL)

homatropine and hydrocodone *see* hydrocodone and homatropine *on page* *481*

homatropine hydrobromide *see* homatropine *on page* *473*

horse antihuman thymocyte gamma globulin *see* antithymocyte globulin (equine) *on page* *84*

12 Hour Nasal Relief [US-OTC] *see* oxymetazoline (nasal) *on page* *716*

H.P. Acthar® [US] *see* corticotropin *on page* *251*

hpAT *see* antithrombin III *on page* *83*

Hp-PAC® [Can] *see* lansoprazole, amoxicillin, and clarithromycin *on page* *549*

HPV2 *see* papillomavirus (types 16, 18) vaccine (human, recombinant) *on page* *726*

HPV4 *see* papillomavirus (types 6, 11, 16, 18) vaccine (human, recombinant) *on page* *727*

HPV vaccine *see* papillomavirus (types 6, 11, 16, 18) vaccine (human, recombinant) *on page* *727*

hyaluronate and derivatives (hye al yoor ON ate & dah RIV ah tives)

Sound-Alike/Look-Alike Issues

Healon® may be confused with Hyalgan®
Hyalgan® may be confused with Healon®
Synvisc® may be confused with Synagis®

Synonyms hyaluronan; hyaluronic acid; hylan G-F 20; hylan polymers; sodium hyaluronate

U.S./Canadian Brand Names Bionect® [US]; Cystistat® [Can]; Durolane® [Can]; Euflexxa™ [US]; Eyestil [Can]; Healon GV® [US/Can]; Healon® [US/Can]; Healon®5 [US]; Hyalgan® [US]; Hylaform® Plus [US]; Hylaform® [US]; Hylira™ [US]; IPM Wound Gel™ [US-OTC]; Juvederm™ 24HV [US]; Juvederm™ 30 [US]; Juvederm™ 30HV [US]; Orthovisc® [US/Can]; Perlane® [US]; Provisc® [US]; Restylane® [US]; Supartz™ [US]; Suplasyn® [Can]; Synvisc-One™ [US]; Synvisc® [US]; Vitrax® [US]

Therapeutic Category Antirheumatic Miscellaneous; Ophthalmic Agent, Viscoelastic; Skin and Mucous Membrane Agent

Use

Intraarticular injection: Treatment of pain in osteoarthritis in knee in patients who have failed nonpharmacologic treatment and simple analgesics
Intradermal: Correction of moderate-to-severe facial wrinkles or folds
Ophthalmic: Surgical aid in cataract extraction, intraocular implantation, corneal transplant, glaucoma filtration, and retinal attachment surgery
Topical cream, gel, spray: Management of skin ulcers and wounds
Topical lotion: Treatment of xerosis (dry, scaly skin)

Dosage Summary

Intra-articular:
Children: Dosage not established
Adults:
Euflexxa™; Hyalgan®: Inject 20 mg (2 mL) once weekly
Orthovisc®: Inject 30 mg (2 mL) once weekly
Supartz™: Inject 25 mg (2.5 mL) once weekly
Synvisc®: Inject 16 mg (2 mL) once weekly
Synvisc-One™: Inject 48 mg (6 mL) once per knee
Note: Maximum number of injections is 3-5 depending on product

Intradermal:
Children: Dosage not established
Adults:
Hylaform®, Hylaform® Plus: Inject as required for cosmetic effect; limit to ≤1.6 mL per injection site (maximum: 20 mL/60 kg/year)
Perlane®: Inject as required for cosmetic result; typical treatment regimen requires 1.9-4.6 mL (maximum: 6 mL/treatment)

Ophthalmic:
Children: Dosage not established
Adults: Depends upon procedure (slowly introduce a sufficient quantity into eye)

Topical Cream:
Children: Dosage not established
Adults: Apply to clean wound or ulcer 2-3 times daily

Topical Gel:
Children: Dosage not established
Adults: Apply to clean dry ulcer or wound once daily or apply to clean wound or ulcer 2-3 times daily

Topical Lotion:
Children: Dosage not established
Adults: Apply to affected area 2-3 times daily

Topical Spray:
Children: Dosage not established
Adults: Apply to clean wound or ulcer 2-3 times daily

Dosage Forms

Hylan B:
Injection, gel:
Hylaform® [500 micron particle]: 5.5 mg/mL (0.75 mL)
Hylaform® Plus [700 micron particle]: 5.5 mg/mL (0.75 mL)

Hylan Polymers A and B (Hylan G-F 20):
Injection, solution, intraarticular:
Synvisc®: 8 mg/mL (2 mL)

Hyaluronate:

Cream, topical:

Bionect®: 0.2% (25 g)

Gel, topical:

Bionect®: 0.2% (30 g, 60 g)

IPM Wound Gel™ [OTC]: 2.5% (10 g)

Lotion, topical: 0.1% (340 g, 1000 g)

Hylira™ Lotion: 0.1% (340 g, 1000 g)

Injection, gel, intradermal:

Juvederm™ 24HV, Juvederm™ 30, Juvederm™ 30HV: 24 mg/mL [prefilled syringe]

Perlane®: 20 mg/mL (1mL) [prefilled syringe]

Restylane®: 20 mg/mL

Injection, solution, intraarticular:

Euflexxa™, Hyalgan®: 10 mg/mL (2 mL)

Orthovisc®: 15 mg/mL (2 mL)

Supartz™: 10 mg/mL (2.5 mL)

Synvisc®: 8 mg/mL (2 mL)

Injection, solution, intraocular:

Healon®: 10 mg/mL (0.4 mL, 0.55 mL, 0.85 mL, 2 mL)

Healon®5: 23 mg/mL

Healon GV®: 14 mg/mL (0.55 mL, 0.85 mL)

Provisc®: 10 mg/mL (0.4 mL, 0.55 mL, 0.8 mL)

Vitrax®: 30 mg/mL (0.65 mL)

hyaluronic acid *see* hyaluronate and derivatives *on page 475*

hyaluronidase (hye al yoor ON i dase)

Sound-Alike/Look-Alike Issues

Wydase® may be confused with Lidex®, Wyamine®

U.S./Canadian Brand Names Amphadase™ [US]; Hylenex™ [US]; Vitrase® [US]

Therapeutic Category Enzyme

Use Increase the dispersion and absorption of other injected drugs; increase rate of absorption of parenteral fluids given by subcutaneous administration (hypodermoclysis)

Dosage Summary

Intradermal:

Children: 0.02 mL (3 units) of a 150 units/mL solution

Adults: 0.02 mL (3 units) of a 150 units/mL solution

SubQ:

Premature Infants and Neonates: Volume of a single clysis should not exceed 25 mL/kg; rate of administration should not exceed 2 mL/minute

Children <3 years: Volume of a single clysis should not exceed 200 mL **or** 75 units over each scapula followed by injection of contrast medium at the same site

Children ≥3 years: Rate and volume of a single clysis should not exceed those used for infusion of I.V. fluids **or** 75 units over each scapula followed by injection of contrast medium at the same site

Adults: Rate and volume of a single clysis should not exceed those used for infusion of I.V. fluids **or** 75 units over each scapula followed by injection of contrast medium at the same site

Dosage Forms

Injection, solution:

Amphadase™: 150 units/mL (1 mL)

Injection, solution [preservative free]:

Hylenex™: 150 units/mL (1 mL)

Vitrase®: 200 units/mL (2 mL)

hycamptamine *see* topotecan *on page 943*

Hycamtin® [US/Can] *see* topotecan *on page 943*

hycet® [US] *see* hydrocodone and acetaminophen *on page 479*

HycoClear Tuss® *(Discontinued)*

Hycodan® *(Discontinued)* *see* hydrocodone and homatropine *on page 481*

Hycomine® Compound *(Discontinued)*

Hycomine® *(Discontinued)*

Hycomine® Pediatric *(Discontinued)*

Hycort™ [Can] *see* hydrocortisone (topical) *on page 483*
Hycotuss® ***(Discontinued)***
Hydase™ ***(Discontinued)*** *see* hyaluronidase *on page 476*
Hydeltra T.B.A.® [Can] *see* prednisolone (systemic) *on page 790*
Hydergine® [Can] *see* ergoloid mesylates *on page 358*
Hydergine® ***(Discontinued)*** *see* ergoloid mesylates *on page 358*
Hyderm [Can] *see* hydrocortisone (topical) *on page 483*

hydralazine (hye DRAL a zeen)

Sound-Alike/Look-Alike Issues
hydrALAZINE may be confused with hydrOXYzine

Synonyms hydralazine hydrochloride

Tall-Man hydr**ALAZINE**

U.S./Canadian Brand Names Apo-Hydralazine® [Can]; Apresoline® [Can]; Novo-Hylazin [Can]; Nu-Hydral [Can]

Therapeutic Category Vasodilator

Use Management of moderate-to-severe hypertension

Dosage Summary

I.M.:

Children: 0.1-0.2 mg/kg/dose (not to exceed 20 mg) every 4-6 hours as needed (maximum: 3.5 mg/kg/day in 4-6 divided doses)

Adults: Initial: 10-20 mg/dose every 4-6 hours as needed; Maintenance: Up to 40 mg/dose every 4-6 hours **or** Eclampsia/Pre-eclampsia: 5 mg/dose then 5-10 mg every 20-30 minutes as needed

I.V.:

Children: 0.1-0.2 mg/kg/dose (not to exceed 20 mg) every 4-6 hours as needed (maximum: 3.5 mg/kg/day in 4-6 divided doses)

Adults: Initial: 10-20 mg/dose every 4-6 hours as needed; Maintenance: Up to 40 mg/dose every 4-6 hours **or** Eclampsia/Pre-eclampsia: 5 mg/dose then 5-10 mg every 20-30 minutes as needed

Oral:

Children: Initial: 0.75-1 mg/kg/day in 2-4 divided doses; Maintenance: Up to 7.5 mg/kg/day in 2-4 divided doses (maximum: 200 mg/day)

Adults: Initial: 10-25 mg 3-4 times/day; Maintenance: 25-300 mg/day (target dose: 225-300 mg/day for CHF) in 2-4 divided doses (maximum: 300 mg/day)

Elderly: Initial: 10 mg 2-3 times/day, increase by 10-25 mg/day every 2-5 days; Target dose: 225-300 mg/day for CHF

Dosage Forms

Injection, solution: 20 mg/mL (1 mL)
Tablet, oral: 10 mg, 25 mg, 50 mg, 100 mg

hydralazine and hydrochlorothiazide (hye DRAL a zeen & hye droe klor oh THYE a zide)

Synonyms hydrochlorothiazide and hydralazine

Therapeutic Category Antihypertensive Agent, Combination

Use Management of moderate-to-severe hypertension and treatment of congestive heart failure

Dosage Summary

Oral:

Children: Dosage not established

Adults: Hydralazine 25-100 mg/day and hydrochlorothiazide 25-50 mg/day in 2 divided doses (maximum: Hydrochlorothiazide: 50 mg/day)

hydralazine and isosorbide dinitrate *see* isosorbide dinitrate and hydralazine *on page 529*
hydralazine hydrochloride *see* hydralazine *on page 477*
Hydramine ***(Discontinued)*** *see* diphenhydramine (systemic) *on page 310*
hydrated chloral *see* chloral hydrate *on page 202*
Hydrate® ***(Discontinued)*** *see* dimenhydrinate *on page 307*
Hydrea® [US/Can] *see* hydroxyurea *on page 489*
Hydrisalic® [US-OTC] *see* salicylic acid *on page 858*
Hydro 40™ [US] *see* urea *on page 970*
Hydrocet® ***(Discontinued)*** *see* hydrocodone and acetaminophen *on page 479*

hydrochlorothiazide (hye droe klor oh THYE a zide)

Sound-Alike/Look-Alike Issues

hydrochlorothiazide may be confused with hydrocortisone, hydroflumethiazide, Viskazide®
Esidrix may be confused with Lasix®
HCTZ is an error-prone abbreviation (mistaken as hydrocortisone)
Microzide® may be confused with Maxzide®, Micronase®

U.S./Canadian Brand Names Apo-Hydro® [Can]; Bio-Hydrochlorothiazide [Can]; Dom-Hydrochlorothiazide [Can]; Microzide® [US]; Novo-Hydrazide [Can]; Nu-Hydro [Can]; PMS-Hydrochlorothiazide [Can]

Therapeutic Category Diuretic, Thiazide

Use Management of mild-to-moderate hypertension; treatment of edema in heart failure and nephrotic syndrome

Dosage Summary

Oral:

Children <6 months: 1-3 mg/kg/day in 2 divided doses
Children >6 months to 2 years: 1-3 mg/kg/day in 2 divided doses (maximum: 37.5 mg/day)
Children >2-17 years: Initial: 1 mg/kg/day (maximum: 3 mg/kg/day [50 mg/day])
Adults: 12.5-100 mg/day in 1-2 divided doses (maximum: 200 mg/day; exceptions occur [indication specific])
Elderly: 12.5-25 once daily

Dosage Forms

Capsule, oral: 12.5 mg
Microzide®: 12.5 mg
Tablet, oral: 12.5 mg, 25 mg, 50 mg

hydrochlorothiazide, amlodipine, and valsartan *see* amlodipine, valsartan, and hydrochlorothiazide *on page 71*
hydrochlorothiazide and aliskiren *see* aliskiren and hydrochlorothiazide *on page 50*
hydrochlorothiazide and amiloride *see* amiloride and hydrochlorothiazide *on page 64*
hydrochlorothiazide and benazepril *see* benazepril and hydrochlorothiazide *on page 122*
hydrochlorothiazide and bisoprolol *see* bisoprolol and hydrochlorothiazide *on page 141*
hydrochlorothiazide and captopril *see* captopril and hydrochlorothiazide *on page 176*
hydrochlorothiazide and cilazapril *see* cilazapril and hydrochlorothiazide *(Canada only) on page 222*
hydrochlorothiazide and enalapril *see* enalapril and hydrochlorothiazide *on page 348*
hydrochlorothiazide and eprosartan *see* eprosartan and hydrochlorothiazide *on page 357*
hydrochlorothiazide and fosinopril *see* fosinopril and hydrochlorothiazide *on page 428*
hydrochlorothiazide and hydralazine *see* hydralazine and hydrochlorothiazide *on page 477*
hydrochlorothiazide and irbesartan *see* irbesartan and hydrochlorothiazide *on page 525*
hydrochlorothiazide and lisinopril *see* lisinopril and hydrochlorothiazide *on page 570*
hydrochlorothiazide and losartan *see* losartan and hydrochlorothiazide *on page 577*
hydrochlorothiazide and methyldopa *see* methyldopa and hydrochlorothiazide *on page 619*
hydrochlorothiazide and metoprolol *see* metoprolol and hydrochlorothiazide *on page 626*
hydrochlorothiazide and metoprolol tartrate *see* metoprolol and hydrochlorothiazide *on page 626*
hydrochlorothiazide and moexipril *see* moexipril and hydrochlorothiazide *on page 640*
hydrochlorothiazide and olmesartan medoxomil *see* olmesartan and hydrochlorothiazide *on page 698*
hydrochlorothiazide and pindolol *see* pindolol and hydrochlorothiazide *(Canada only) on page 762*
hydrochlorothiazide and propranolol *see* propranolol and hydrochlorothiazide *on page 807*
hydrochlorothiazide and quinapril *see* quinapril and hydrochlorothiazide *on page 822*
hydrochlorothiazide and ramipril *see* ramipril and hydrochlorothiazide *(Canada only) on page 827*

hydrochlorothiazide and spironolactone

(hye droe klor oh THYE a zide & speer on oh LAK tone)

Sound-Alike/Look-Alike Issues

Aldactazide® may be confused with Aldactone®

Synonyms spironolactone and hydrochlorothiazide

U.S./Canadian Brand Names Aldactazide 25® [Can]; Aldactazide 50® [Can]; Aldactazide® [US]; Novo-Spirozine [Can]

Therapeutic Category Antihypertensive Agent, Combination

Use Management of mild-to-moderate hypertension; treatment of edema in congestive heart failure and nephrotic syndrome, and cirrhosis of the liver accompanied by edema and/or ascites

Dosage Summary

Oral:

Children: 1.5-3 mg/kg/day in 2-4 divided doses (maximum: 200 mg/day)

Adults: 12.5-50 mg hydrochlorothiazide and 12.5-50 mg spironolactone/day in 1-2 divided doses

Dosage Forms

Tablet: Hydrochlorothiazide 25 mg and spironolactone 25 mg

Aldactazide®: 25/25: Hydrochlorothiazide 25 mg and spironolactone 25 mg; 50/50: Hydrochlorothiazide 50 mg and spironolactone 50 mg

hydrochlorothiazide and telmisartan *see* telmisartan and hydrochlorothiazide *on page 914*

hydrochlorothiazide and triamterene (hye droe klor oh THYE a zide & trye AM ter een)

Sound-Alike/Look-Alike Issues

Dyazide® may be confused with diazoxide, Dynacin®

Maxzide® may be confused with Maxidex®, Microzide®

Synonyms triamterene and hydrochlorothiazide

U.S./Canadian Brand Names Apo-Triazide® [Can]; Dyazide® [US]; Maxzide® [US]; Maxzide®-25 [US]; Novo-Triamzide [Can]; Nu-Triazide [Can]; Penta-Triamterene HCTZ [Can]; Riva-Zide [Can]

Therapeutic Category Antihypertensive Agent, Combination

Use Treatment of hypertension or edema (not recommended for initial treatment) when hypokalemia has developed on hydrochlorothiazide alone or when the development of hypokalemia must be avoided

Dosage Summary

Oral:

Children: Dosage not established

Adults: 25-50 mg hydrochlorothiazide and 37.5-75 mg triamterene once daily

Dosage Forms

Capsule: Hydrochlorothiazide 25 mg and triamterene 37.5 mg; hydrochlorothiazide 25 mg and triamterene 50 mg

Dyazide®: Hydrochlorothiazide 25 mg and triamterene 37.5 mg

Tablet: Hydrochlorothiazide 25 mg and triamterene 37.5 mg; hydrochlorothiazide 50 mg and triamterene 75 mg

Maxzide®: Hydrochlorothiazide 50 mg and triamterene 75 mg [scored]

Maxzide®-25: Hydrochlorothiazide 25 mg and triamterene 37.5 mg [scored]

hydrochlorothiazide and valsartan *see* valsartan and hydrochlorothiazide *on page 976*

hydrochlorothiazide, olmesartan, and amlodipine *see* olmesartan, amlodipine, and hydrochlorothiazide *on page 698*

Hydrocil® Instant [US-OTC] *see* psyllium *on page 814*

hydrocodone and acetaminophen (hye droe KOE done & a seet a MIN oh fen)

Sound-Alike/Look-Alike Issues

Lorcet® may be confused with Fioricet®

Lortab® may be confused with Cortef®, Lorabid®, Luride®

Vicodin® may be confused with Hycodan®, Hycomine®, Indocin®, Uridon®

Zydone® may be confused with Vytone®

Synonyms acetaminophen and hydrocodone

U.S./Canadian Brand Names hycet® [US]; Lorcet® 10/650 [US]; Lorcet® Plus [US]; Lortab® [US]; Margesic® H [US]; Maxidone® [US]; Norco® [US]; Stagesic™ [US]; Vicodin® ES [US]; Vicodin® HP [US]; Vicodin® [US]; Xodol® 10/300 [US]; Xodol® 5/300 [US]; Xodol® 7.5/300 [US]; Zamicet™ [US]; Zydone® [US]

Therapeutic Category Analgesic, Narcotic

Controlled Substance C-III

Use Relief of moderate-to-severe pain

Dosage Summary

Oral:

Children <2 years: Dosage not established

Children 2-13 years or <50 kg: Hydrocodone 0.1-0.2 mg/kg/dose every 4-6 hours (maximum: 6 doses/day or maximum recommended dose of acetaminophen for age/weight)

Children ≥50 kg: Hydrocodone 2.5-10 mg every 4-6 hours (maximum: 4 g/day [acetaminophen])

Adults: Hydrocodone 2.5-10 mg every 4-6 hours (maximum: 4 g/day [acetaminophen])

Elderly: Hydrocodone 2.5-5 mg every 4-6 hours

Dosage Forms

Capsule, oral: Hydrocodone 5 mg and acetaminophen 500 mg

Margesic® H, Stagesic™: Hydrocodone 5 mg and acetaminophen 500 mg

Elixir, oral:

Lortab®: Hydrocodone 7.5 mg and acetaminophen 500 mg per 15 mL

Solution, oral: Hydrocodone 7.5 mg and acetaminophen 500 mg per 15 mL; hydrocodone 10 mg and acetaminophen 325 mg per 15 mL

hycet®: Hydrocodone 7.5 mg and acetaminophen 325 mg per 15 mL

Zamicet™: Hydrocodone 10 mg and acetaminophen 325 mg per 15 mL

Tablet, oral:

Generics:

Hydrocodone 2.5 mg and acetaminophen 500 mg
Hydrocodone 5 mg and acetaminophen 325 mg
Hydrocodone 5 mg and acetaminophen 500 mg
Hydrocodone 7.5 mg and acetaminophen 325 mg
Hydrocodone 7.5 mg and acetaminophen 500 mg
Hydrocodone 7.5 mg and acetaminophen 650 mg
Hydrocodone 7.5 mg and acetaminophen 750 mg
Hydrocodone 10 mg and acetaminophen 325 mg
Hydrocodone 10 mg and acetaminophen 500 mg
Hydrocodone 10 mg and acetaminophen 650 mg
Hydrocodone 10 mg and acetaminophen 660 mg
Hydrocodone 10 mg and acetaminophen 750 mg

Brands:

Lorcet® 10/650: Hydrocodone 10 mg and acetaminophen 650 mg

Lorcet® Plus: Hydrocodone 7.5 mg and acetaminophen 650 mg

Lortab®: 5/500: Hydrocodone 5 mg and acetaminophen 500 mg; 7.5/500: Hydrocodone 7.5 mg and acetaminophen 500 mg; 10/500: Hydrocodone 10 mg and acetaminophen 500 mg

Maxidone®: Hydrocodone 10 mg and acetaminophen 750 mg

Norco®: Hydrocodone 5 mg and acetaminophen 325 mg; hydrocodone 7.5 mg and acetaminophen 325 mg; hydrocodone 10 mg and acetaminophen 325 mg

Vicodin®: Hydrocodone 5 mg and acetaminophen 500 mg

Vicodin® ES: Hydrocodone 7.5 mg and acetaminophen 750 mg

Vicodin® HP: Hydrocodone 10 mg and acetaminophen 660 mg

Xodol®: 5/300: Hydrocodone 5 mg and acetaminophen 300 mg; 7.5/300: Hydrocodone 7.5 mg and acetaminophen 300 mg; 10/300: Hydrocodone 10 mg and acetaminophen 300 mg

Zydone®: Hydrocodone 5 mg and acetaminophen 400 mg; hydrocodone 7.5 mg and acetaminophen 400 mg; hydrocodone 10 mg and acetaminophen 400 mg

hydrocodone and aspirin *(Discontinued)*

hydrocodone and chlorpheniramine (hye droe KOE done & klor fen IR a meen)

Sound-Alike/Look-Alike Issues

Tussionex® represents a different product in the U.S. than it does in Canada. In the U.S., Tussionex® contains hydrocodone and chlorpheniramine, while in Canada the product bearing this name contains hydrocodone and phenyltoloxamine.

Synonyms chlorpheniramine maleate and hydrocodone bitartrate; hydrocodone polistirex and chlorpheniramine polistirex

U.S./Canadian Brand Names TussiCaps® [US]; Tussionex® [US]

Therapeutic Category Antihistamine/Antitussive

Controlled Substance C-III

Use Symptomatic relief of cough and upper respiratory symptoms associated with cold and allergy

Dosage Summary

Oral:

Children <6 years: Dosage not established

Children 6-12 years: TussiCaps® 5 mg/4 mg: One capsule every 12 hours (maximum: 2 capsules/24 hours); Tussionex®: 2.5 mL every 12 hours (maximum: 5 mL/24 hours)

Children >12 years: TussiCaps® 10 mg/8 mg: One capsule every 12 hours (maximum: 2 capsules/24 hours); Tussionex®: 5 mL every 12 hours (maximum: 10 mL/24 hours)

Adults: TussiCaps® 10 mg/8 mg: One capsule every 12 hours (maximum: 2 capsules/24 hours); Tussionex®: 5 mL every 12 hours (maximum: 10 mL/24 hours)

Dosage Forms

Capsule, extended release:

TussiCaps® 5/4: Hydrocodone bitartrate 5 mg and chlorpheniramine maleate 4 mg

TussiCaps® 10/8: Hydrocodone bitartrate 10 mg and chlorpheniramine maleate 8 mg

Suspension, extended release:

Tussionex®: Hydrocodone bitartrate 10 mg and chlorpheniramine maleate 8 mg per 5 mL

hydrocodone and guaifenesin *(Discontinued)*

hydrocodone and homatropine (hye droe KOE done & hoe MA troe peen)

Sound-Alike/Look-Alike Issues

Hycodan® may be confused with Hycomine®, Vicodin®

Synonyms homatropine and hydrocodone; hydrocodone bitartrate and homatropine methylbromide

U.S./Canadian Brand Names Hydromet® [US]; Tussigon® [US]

Therapeutic Category Antitussive

Controlled Substance C-III

Use Symptomatic relief of cough

Dosage Summary

Oral:

Children <6 years: Dosage not established

Children 6-11 years: 1/2 tablet or 2.5 mL every 4-6 hours as needed (maximum: 3 tablets or 15 mL/24 hours)

Children ≥12 years: 1 tablet or 5 mL every 4-6 hours as needed (maximum: 6 tablets/24 hours or 30 mL/24 hours)

Adults: 1 tablet or 5 mL every 4-6 hours as needed (maximum: 6 tablets/24 hours or 30 mL/24 hours)

Dosage Forms

Syrup: Hydrocodone 5 mg and homatropine 1.5 mg per 5 mL

Hydromet®: Hydrocodone 5 mg and homatropine 1.5 mg per 5 mL

Tablet:

Tussigon®: Hydrocodone 5 mg and homatropine 1.5 mg

hydrocodone and ibuprofen (hye droe KOE done & eye byoo PROE fen)

Sound-Alike/Look-Alike Issues

Reprexain™ may be confused with Zyprexa®

Synonyms hydrocodone bitartrate and ibuprofen; ibuprofen and hydrocodone

U.S./Canadian Brand Names Ibudone™ [US]; Reprexain™ [US]; Vicoprofen® [US/Can]

Therapeutic Category Analgesic, Narcotic

Controlled Substance C-III

Use Short-term (generally <10 days) management of moderate-to-severe acute pain; is not indicated for treatment of such conditions as osteoarthritis or rheumatoid arthritis

Dosage Summary

Oral:

Children: Dosage not established

Adults: 1 tablet every 4-6 hours (maximum: 5 tablets/day; <10 days total therapy)

Dosage Forms

Tablet: Hydrocodone 5 mg and ibuprofen 200 mg; hydrocodone 7.5 mg and ibuprofen 200 mg

Ibudone™: 5/200: Hydrocodone 5 mg and ibuprofen 200 mg; 10/200: Hydrocodone 10 mg and ibuprofen 200 mg

Reprexain™: 2.5/200: Hydrocodone 2.5 mg and ibuprofen 200 mg; 5/200: Hydrocodone 5 mg and ibuprofen 200 mg; 10/200: Hydrocodone 10 mg and ibuprofen 200 mg

Vicoprofen®: 7.5/200: Hydrocodone 7.5 mg and ibuprofen 200 mg

hydrocodone and pseudoephedrine ***(Discontinued)***

hydrocodone bitartrate and homatropine methylbromide *see* hydrocodone and homatropine *on page 481*

hydrocodone bitartrate and ibuprofen *see* hydrocodone and ibuprofen *on page 481*

hydrocodone, carbinoxamine, and pseudoephedrine ***(Discontinued)***

hydrocodone, chlorpheniramine, phenylephrine, acetaminophen, and caffeine ***(Discontinued)***

Hydrocodone PA® Syrup ***(Discontinued)***

hydrocodone, phenylephrine, and chlorpheniramine *see* phenylephrine, hydrocodone, and chlorpheniramine *on page 754*

hydrocodone, phenylephrine, and diphenhydramine ***(Discontinued)***

hydrocodone, phenylephrine, and guaifenesin ***(Discontinued)***

hydrocodone polistirex and chlorpheniramine polistirex *see* hydrocodone and chlorpheniramine *on page 480*

hydrocodone, pseudoephedrine, and guaifenesin ***(Discontinued)***

hydrocortisone (systemic) (hye droe KOR ti sone)

Sound-Alike/Look-Alike Issues

hydrocortisone may be confused with hydrocodone, hydroxychloroquine, hydrochlorothiazide

Cortef® may be confused with Coreg®, Lortab®

HCT (occasional abbreviation for hydrocortisone) is an error-prone abbreviation (mistaken as hydrochlorothiazide)

Solu-Cortef® may be confused with Solu-Medrol®

Synonyms A-hydroCort; compound F; cortisol; hydrocortisone sodium succinate

U.S./Canadian Brand Names A-Hydrocort® [US]; Cortef® [US/Can]; Solu-Cortef® [US/Can]

Therapeutic Category Corticosteroid, Systemic

Use Management of adrenocortical insufficiency

Dosage Summary

Intraarticular (Acetate):

Children: Dosage not established

Adults: Large joints 25-37.5 mg; Small joints: 10-25 mg; Tendon sheaths 5-12.5 mg

Intralesional or soft-tissue injection (Acetate):

Bursae:

Children: Dosage not established

Adults: 25-37.5 mg

Ganglia:

Children: Dosage not established

Adults: 12.5-25 mg

Soft tissue infiltration:

Children: Dosage not established

Adults: 25-50 mg (up to 75 mg)

I.M. (Succinate):

Children: 0.25-5 mg/kg/day divided every 12-24 hours **or** 12-150 mg/m^2/day divided every 12-24 hours **or** 50 mg/kg then repeat in 4 hours and/or every 24 hours as needed (shock) **or** 1-2 mg/kg bolus, then 25-150 mg/day divided every 6-8 hours

Adolescents: 15-240 mg every 12 hours **or** 0.25-0.35 mg/kg/day **or** 12-15 mg/m^2/day **or** 500 mg to 2 g every 2-6 hours (shock) **or** 1-2 mg/kg bolus, then 150-250 mg/day divided every 6-8 hours

Adults: 15-240 mg every 12 hours **or** 500 mg to 2 g every 2-6 hours (shock) **or** 100 mg bolus I.V., then 300 mg/day divided every 8 hours

I.V. (Succinate):

Children: 1-5 mg/kg/day divided every 12-24 hours **or** 30-150 mg/m^2/day divided every 12-24 hours **or** 50 mg/kg then repeat in 4 hours and/or every 24 hours as needed (shock) **or** 1-2 mg/kg/dose every 6 hours for 24 hours then 0.5-1 mg/kg every 6 hours (status asthmaticus) **or** 1-2 mg/kg bolus, then 25-150 mg/day divided every 6-8 hours

Adolescents: 15-240 mg every 12 hours **or** 500 mg to 2 g every 2-6 hours (shock) **or** 1-2 mg/kg/dose every 6 hours for 24 hours then 0.5-1 mg/kg every 6 hours (status asthmaticus) **or** 1-2 mg/kg bolus, then 150-250 mg/day divided every 6-8 hours

Adults: 15-240 mg every 12 hours **or** 50 mg every 6 hours (septic shock) **or** 500 mg to 2 g every 2-6 hours (shock) or 1-2 mg/kg every 6 hours for 24 hours, then 0.5-1 mg/kg every 6 hours (status asthmaticus) **or** 100 mg bolus, then 300 mg/day divided every 8 hours or as continuous infusion

Oral:

Children: 0.5-10 mg/kg/day **or** 10-300 mg/m^2/day divided every 6-8 hours

Adolescents: 0.5-10 mg/kg/day **or** 10-300 mg/m^2/day divided every 6-8 hours **or** 15-240 mg every 12 hours

Adults: 20-480 mg/day in divided doses every 8-12 hours **or** 10-20 mg/m^2/day in 3 divided doses

Dosage Forms

Injection, powder for reconstitution:

A-Hydrocort®: 100 mg

Solu-Cortef®: 100 mg, 250 mg, 500 mg, 1000 mg

Tablet, oral: 20 mg

Cortef®: 5 mg, 10 mg, 20 mg

hydrocortisone (topical) (hye droe KOR ti sone)

Sound-Alike/Look-Alike Issues

hydrocortisone may be confused with hydrocodone, hydroxychloroquine, hydrochlorothiazide

Anusol® may be confused with Anusol-HC®, Aplisol®, Aquasol®

Anusol-HC® may be confused with Anusol®

Cortizone® may be confused with cortisone

HCT (occasional abbreviation for hydrocortisone) is an error-prone abbreviation (mistaken as hydrochlorothiazide)

Hytone® may be confused with Vytone®

Proctocort® may be confused with ProctoCream®

ProctoCream® may be confused with Proctocort®

Synonyms A-hydroCort; compound F; cortisol; hydrocortisone acetate; hydrocortisone butyrate; hydrocortisone probutate; hydrocortisone valerate

U.S./Canadian Brand Names Anu-med HC [US]; Anucort-HC™ [US]; Anusol HC-1® [US-OTC]; Anusol-HC® [US]; Aquacort® [Can]; Aquanil HC® [US-OTC]; Beta-HC® [US-OTC]; Caldecort® [US-OTC]; Colocort® [US]; Cortaid® Intensive Therapy [US-OTC]; Cortaid® Maximum Strength [US-OTC]; Cortamed® [Can]; Cortenema® [US/Can]; CortiCool® [US-OTC]; Cortifoam® [US/Can]; Cortizone-10® Maximum Strength Cooling Relief [US-OTC]; Cortizone-10® Maximum Strength Easy Relief [US-OTC]; Cortizone-10® Maximum Strength Intensive Healing Formula [US-OTC]; Cortizone-10® Maximum Strength [US-OTC]; Cortizone-10® Plus Maximum Strength [US-OTC]; Delacort [US-OTC]; Dermarest® Psoriasis Medicated Lotion [US-OTC]; Dermtex® HC [US-OTC]; Emo-Cort® [Can]; Hemorrhoidal-HC Uniserts® [US]; Hemril®-30 [US]; Hycort™ [Can]; Hyderm [Can]; Hydrocortisone Plus [US-OTC]; Hydroskin® [US]; HydroVal® [Can]; Ivy Soothe® [US-OTC]; Locoid Lipocream® [US]; Locoid® [US/Can]; Nutracort® [US]; Pandel® [US]; Post-Peel Healing Balm® [US-OTC]; Preparation H® Hydrocortisone [US-OTC]; Prevex® HC [Can]; Procto-Kit™ [US]; Procto-Pak™ [US-OTC]; Proctocort® [US]; ProctoCream®-HC [US]; Proctosol-HC® [US]; Proctozone-HC™ [US-OTC]; Recort [US-OTC]; Sarna® HC [Can]; Sarnol®-HC [US]; Scalp Mycin [US-OTC]; Texacort® [US]; Tucks® Anti-Itch [US-OTC]; U-Cort™ [US]; Westcort® [US/Can]

Therapeutic Category Corticosteroid, Rectal; Corticosteroid, Topical

Use Relief of inflammation of corticosteroid-responsive dermatoses (low and medium potency topical corticosteroid); adjunctive treatment of ulcerative colitis

Dosage Summary

Rectal:

Children: Dosage not established

Adults: 10-100 mg 1-2 times/day

Topical:

Children ≤2 years: Dosage not established

Children >2 years: Apply to affected area 2-4 times/day

Adults: Apply to affected area 2-4 times/day

Dosage Forms

Aerosol, rectal:

Cortifoam®: 10% (15 g)

Cream, topical: 2% (43 g); 0.1% (15 g, 45 g); 0.2% (15 g, 45 g, 60 g); 0.5% (0.9 g, 15 g, 30 g, 60 g); 1% (0.9 g, 1 g, 1.5 g, 15 g, 20 g, 28.35 g, 28.4 g, 30 g, 114 g, 120 g, 454 g); 2.5% (20 g, 28 g, 28.35 g, 30 g, 454 g)

Anusol-HC®: 2.5% (30 g)

Caldecort® [OTC]: 1% (30 g)
Cortaid® Intensive Therapy [OTC]: 1% (60 g)
Cortaid® Maximum Strength [OTC]: 1% (15 g, 30 g, 40 g, 60 g)
Cortizone-10® Maximum Strength [OTC]: 1% (15 g, 28 g, 56 g)
Cortizone-10® Maximum Strength Intensive Healing Formula [OTC]: 1% (28 g, 56 g)
Cortizone-10® Plus Maximum Strength [OTC]: 1% (28 g, 56 g)
Dermtex® HC [OTC]: 1% (30 g)
Hydrocortisone Plus [OTC]: 1% (28.4 g)
Hydroskin®: 1% (30 g)
Ivy Soothe® [OTC]: 1% (28.4 g)
Locoid Lipocream®: 0.1% (15 g, 45 g, 60 g)
Locoid®: 0.1% (15 g, 45 g)
Pandel®: 0.1% (15 g, 45 g, 80 g)
Post-Peel Healing Balm® [OTC]: 1% (30 g)
Preparation H® Hydrocortisone [OTC]: 1% (27 g)
Procto-Kit™: 1% (30 g); 2.5% (30 g)
Procto-Pak™ [OTC]: 1% (28.4 g)
Proctocort®: 1% (28.35 g)
ProctoCream®-HC: 2.5% (30 g)
Proctosol-HC®: 2.5% (28.35 g)
Proctozone-HC™ [OTC]: 2.5% (30 g)
Recort [OTC]: 1% (30 g)
U-Cort™: 1% (28 g)

Gel, topical:
CortiCool® [OTC]: 1% (45 g)
Cortizone-10® Maximum Strength Cooling Relief [OTC]: 1% (28 g)

Liquid, topical:
Cortizone-10® Maximum Strength Easy Relief [OTC]: 1% (36 mL)
Scalp Mycin [OTC]: 1% (59 mL)

Lotion, topical: 1% (114 g, 118 mL, 120 mL); 2.5% (59 mL, 60 mL, 118 mL)
Aquanil HC® [OTC]: 1% (120 mL)
Beta-HC® [OTC]: 1% (60 mL)
Delacort [OTC]: 1% (120 mL)
Dermarest® Psoriasis Medicated Lotion [OTC]: 1% (120 mL)
Hydroskin®: 1% (120 mL)
Locoid®: 0.1% (60 mL)
Nutracort®: 1% (60 mL, 120 mL); 2.5% (60 mL, 120 mL)
Sarnol®-HC: 1% (59 mL)

Ointment, topical: 0.1% (15 g, 45 g); 0.2% (15 g, 45 g, 60 g); 0.5% (30 g); 1% (25 g, 28.4 g, 30 g, 110 g, 430 g, 454 g); 2.5% (20 g, 28.35 g, 30 g, 454 g)
Cortaid® Maximum Strength [OTC]: 1% (30 g, 39.9 g)
Cortizone-10® Maximum Strength [OTC]: 1% (28 g, 56 g)
Locoid®: 0.1% (15 g, 45 g)
Tucks® Anti-Itch [OTC]: 1% (19.8 g)
Westcort®: 0.2% (15 g, 45 g, 60 g)

Powder, for prescription compounding: USP: 100% (10 g, 25 g, 50 g, 100 g, 1000 g)

Solution, topical: 0.1% (20 mL, 60 mL)
Cortaid® Intensive Therapy [OTC]: 1% (59 mL)
Dermtex® HC [OTC]: 1% (52 mL)
Locoid®: 0.1% (20 mL, 60 mL)
Texacort®: 2.5% (30 mL)

Suppository, rectal: 25 mg (12s, 24s, 1000s); 30 mg (12s)
Anu-med HC: 25 mg (12s)
Anucort-HC™: 25 mg (12s, 24s, 100s)
Anusol-HC®: 25 mg (12s, 24s)
Hemorrhoidal-HC Uniserts®: 25 mg (12s)
Hemril® -30: 30 mg (12s, 24s)
Proctocort®: 30 mg (12s)
Proctosol-HC®: 25 mg (12s, 24s)

Suspension, rectal: 100 mg/60 mL (60 mL)
Colocort®: 100 mg/60 mL (60 mL)
Cortenema®: 100 mg/60 mL (60 mL)

hydrocortisone acetate *see* hydrocortisone (topical) *on page* 483
hydrocortisone, acetic acid, and propylene glycol diacetate *see* acetic acid, propylene glycol diacetate, and hydrocortisone *on page* 33
hydrocortisone and benzoyl peroxide *see* benzoyl peroxide and hydrocortisone *on page* 129
hydrocortisone and ciprofloxacin *see* ciprofloxacin and hydrocortisone *on page* 226
hydrocortisone and iodoquinol *see* iodoquinol and hydrocortisone *on page* 519
hydrocortisone and lidocaine *see* lidocaine and hydrocortisone *on page* 564
hydrocortisone and pramoxine *see* pramoxine and hydrocortisone *on page* 787
hydrocortisone and urea *see* urea and hydrocortisone *on page* 971
hydrocortisone, bacitracin, neomycin, and polymyxin B *see* bacitracin, neomycin, polymyxin B, and hydrocortisone *on page* 114
hydrocortisone butyrate *see* hydrocortisone (topical) *on page* 483
hydrocortisone, neomycin, and polymyxin B *see* neomycin, polymyxin B, and hydrocortisone *on page* 667
hydrocortisone, neomycin, colistin, and thonzonium *see* neomycin, colistin, hydrocortisone, and thonzonium *on page* 666
Hydrocortisone Plus [US-OTC] *see* hydrocortisone (topical) *on page* 483
hydrocortisone probutate *see* hydrocortisone (topical) *on page* 483
hydrocortisone sodium succinate *see* hydrocortisone (systemic) *on page* 482
hydrocortisone valerate *see* hydrocortisone (topical) *on page* 483
HydroDIURIL® *(Discontinued)* *see* hydrochlorothiazide *on page* 478
Hydro DP *(Discontinued)*
HydroFed *(Discontinued)*
Hydrogesic® *(Discontinued)* *see* hydrocodone and acetaminophen *on page* 479
Hydro-GP *(Discontinued)*
Hydromet® [US] *see* hydrocodone and homatropine *on page* 481
Hydromorph Contin® [Can] *see* hydromorphone *on page* 485
Hydromorph-IR® [Can] *see* hydromorphone *on page* 485

hydromorphone (hye droe MOR fone)

Sound-Alike/Look-Alike Issues

Dilaudid® may be confused with Demerol®, Dilantin®

HYDROmorphone may be confused with morphine; significant overdoses have occurred when hydromorphone products have been inadvertently administered instead of morphine sulfate. Commercially available prefilled syringes of both products looks similar and are often stored in close proximity to each other. **Note:** Hydromorphone 1 mg oral is approximately equal to morphine 4 mg oral; hydromorphone 1 mg I.V. is approximately equal to morphine 5 mg I.V.

Dilaudid®, Dilaudid-HP®: Extreme caution should be taken to avoid confusing the highly-concentrated (Dilaudid-HP®) injection with the less-concentrated (Dilaudid®) injectable product.

Synonyms dihydromorphinone; hydromorphone hydrochloride

Tall-Man **HYDRO**morphone

U.S./Canadian Brand Names Dilaudid-HP-Plus® [Can]; Dilaudid-HP® [US/Can]; Dilaudid-XP® [Can]; Dilaudid® Sterile Powder [Can]; Dilaudid® [US/Can]; Exalgo™ [US]; Hydromorph Contin® [Can]; Hydromorph-IR® [Can]; Hydromorphone HP [Can]; Hydromorphone HP® 10 [Can]; Hydromorphone HP® 20 [Can]; Hydromorphone HP® 50 [Can]; Hydromorphone HP® Forte [Can]; Hydromorphone Hydrochloride Injection, USP [Can]; Jurnista™ [Can]; PMS-Hydromorphone [Can]

Therapeutic Category Analgesic, Narcotic

Controlled Substance C-II

Use Management of moderate-to-severe pain

Exalgo™: Management of moderate-to-severe pain in opioid-tolerant patients (requiring around-the-clock analgesia for an extended period of time)

Dosage Summary

I.M.:

Children <50 kg: Dosage not established
Children >50 kg: 0.8-2 mg every 4-6 hours
Adults: 0.8-2 mg every 4-6 hours

I.V.:

Children <6 months: Dosage not established

Children ≥6 months and <50 kg: 0.015 mg/kg/dose every 3-6 hours as needed

Children >50 kg: 0.2-0.6 mg every 2-3 hours as needed

Adults: 0.2-0.6 mg every 2-3 hours as needed

Adults (mechanically-ventilated): 0.7-2 mg every 1-2 hours as needed; Infusion: 0.5-1 mg/hour (based on 70 kg patient)

Epidural:

Children <50 kg: Dosage not established

Children >50 kg: Concentration: 0.05-0.075 mg/mL; Bolus: 1-1.5 mg; Infusion: 0.04-0.4 mg/hour; Demand dose: 0.15 mg; Lockout interval: 30 minutes

Adults: Concentration: 0.05-0.075 mg/mL; Bolus: 1-1.5 mg; Infusion: 0.04-0.4 mg/hour; Demand dose: 0.15 mg; Lockout interval: 30 minutes

Oral:

Children <6 months: Dosage not established

Children ≥6 months and <50 kg: 0.03-0.08 mg/kg/dose every 3-4 hours as needed

Children >50 kg: 2-8 mg every 3-4 hours as needed

Adults: 2-8 mg every 3-4 hours as needed; Extended release: 8-64 mg every 24 hours

Elderly: 1-2 mg every 3-6 hours

PCA:

Children <50 kg: Usual concentration: 0.2 mg/mL; Demand dose: 0.003-0.005 mg/kg/dose; Lockout interval: 6-10 minutes; Usual basal rate: 0-0.004 mg/kg/hour

Children >50 kg: Usual concentration: 0.2 mg/mL; Demand dose: 0.05-0.4 mg; Lockout interval: 5-10 minutes

Adults: Usual concentration: 0.2 mg/mL; Demand dose: 0.05-0.4 mg; Lockout interval: 5-10 minutes

Rectal:

Children <50 kg: Dosage not established

Children >50 kg: 3 mg every 4-8 hours as needed

Adults: 3 mg every 4-8 hours as needed

SubQ:

Children <50 kg: Dosage not established

Children >50 kg: 0.8-2 mg every 4-6 hours

Adults: 0.8-2 mg every 4-6 hours

Dosage Forms

Injection, powder for reconstitution:

Dilaudid-HP®: 250 mg

Injection, solution: 1 mg/mL (1 mL); 2 mg/mL (1 mL, 20 mL); 4 mg/mL (1 mL)

Dilaudid-HP®: 10 mg/mL (1 mL, 5 mL, 50 mL)

Dilaudid®: 1 mg/mL (1 mL); 2 mg/mL (1 mL); 4 mg/mL (1 mL)

Injection, solution [preservative free]: 10 mg/mL (1 mL, 5 mL, 50 mL)

Liquid, oral:

Dilaudid®: 1 mg/mL (473 mL)

Powder, for prescription compounding: USP: 100% (972 mg)

Suppository, rectal: 3 mg (6s)

Tablet, oral: 2 mg, 4 mg, 8 mg

Dilaudid®: 2 mg, 4 mg, 8 mg

Tablet, extended release, oral:

Exalgo™: 8 mg, 12 mg, 16 mg

Dosage Forms - Canada

Capsule, controlled release:

Hydromorph Contin®: 3 mg, 6 mg, 12 mg, 18 mg, 24 mg, 30 mg [not available in U.S.]

Hydromorphone HP [Can] *see* hydromorphone *on page 485*

Hydromorphone HP® 10 [Can] *see* hydromorphone *on page 485*

Hydromorphone HP® 20 [Can] *see* hydromorphone *on page 485*

Hydromorphone HP® 50 [Can] *see* hydromorphone *on page 485*

Hydromorphone HP® Forte [Can] *see* hydromorphone *on page 485*

hydromorphone hydrochloride *see* hydromorphone *on page 485*

Hydromorphone Hydrochloride Injection, USP [Can] *see* hydromorphone *on page 485*

Hydromox® ***(Discontinued)***

Hydron CP [US] *see* phenylephrine, hydrocodone, and chlorpheniramine *on page 754*

Hydron PSC *(Discontinued)*

Hydro-Par® *(Discontinued)* *see* hydrochlorothiazide *on page 478*

Hydro-PC II [US] *see* phenylephrine, hydrocodone, and chlorpheniramine *on page 754*

Hydro PC II Plus [US] *see* phenylephrine, hydrocodone, and chlorpheniramine *on page 754*

hydroquinol *see* hydroquinone *on page 487*

hydroquinone (HYE droe kwin one)

Sound-Alike/Look-Alike Issues

Eldopaque® may be confused with Eldoquin®
Eldoquin® may be confused with Eldopaque®
Eldopaque Forte® may be confused with Eldoquin Forte®
Eldoquin Forte® may be confused with Eldopaque Forte®

Synonyms hydroquinol; quinol

U.S./Canadian Brand Names Aclaro PD™ [US]; Alphaquin HP® [US]; Dermarest® Skin Correcting Cream Plus [US-OTC]; Eldopaque Forte® [US]; Eldopaque® [US/Can]; Eldoquin Forte® [US]; Eldoquin® [US/Can]; EpiQuin™ Micro [US]; Esoterica® Daytime [US-OTC]; Esoterica® Nighttime [US-OTC]; Glyquin® XM [Can]; Lustra-AF® [US]; Lustra-Ultra™ [US]; Lustra® [US/Can]; Melanex® [US]; Melpaque HP® [US-OTC]; Melquin HP® [US-OTC]; Melquin-3® [US-OTC]; NeoStrata® AHA [US-OTC]; NeoStrata® HQ [Can]; Nuquin HP® [US]; Palmer's® Skin Success® Eventone® Fade Cream [US]; Solaquin Forte® [Can]; Solaquin® [Can]; Ultraquin™ [Can]

Therapeutic Category Topical Skin Product

Use Gradual bleaching of hyperpigmented skin conditions

Dosage Summary

Topical:

Children ≤12 years: Dosage not established
Children >12 years: Apply thin layer and rub in twice daily
Adults: Apply thin layer and rub in twice daily

Dosage Forms

Cream, topical: 4% (28 g); 4% (28 g, 28.35 g, 30 g, s); 5% (24s)

Alphaquin HP®: 4% (28.4 g, 56.7 g)
Dermarest® Skin Correcting Cream Plus [OTC]: 2% (85 g)
Eldopaque Forte®: 4% (28.35 g)
Eldopaque®: 2% (30 g)
Eldoquin Forte®: 4% (28.4 g)
Eldoquin®: 2% (28.35 g)
EpiQuin™ Micro: 4% (30 g)
Esoterica® Daytime [OTC]: 2% (70 g)
Esoterica® Nighttime [OTC]: 2% (70 g)
Lustra-AF®: 4% (56.8 g)
Lustra-Ultra™: 4% (56.8 g)
Lustra®: 4% (56.8 g)
Melpaque HP® [OTC]: 4% (14.2 g, 28.4 g)
Melquin HP® [OTC]: 4% (14.2 g, 28.4 g)
Nuquin HP®: 4% (14.2 g, 28.4 g, 56.7s)
Palmer's® Skin Success® Eventone® Fade Cream: 2% (81 g, 132 g)

Emulsion, topical:

Aclaro PD™: 4% (42.5 g)

Gel, topical: 4% (28 g, 30 g)

NeoStrata® AHA [OTC]: 2% (45 g)
Nuquin HP®: 4% (14.2 g, 28.4 g)

Solution, topical:

Melanex®: 3% (30 mL)
Melquin-3® [OTC]: 3% (29.57 mL)

hydroquinone, fluocinolone acetonide, and tretinoin *see* fluocinolone, hydroquinone, and tretinoin *on page 411*

HYDRO-Rx *(Discontinued)* *see* hydrocortisone (topical) *on page 483*

Hydroskin® [US] *see* hydrocortisone (topical) *on page 483*

Hydrotropine® *(Discontinued)* *see* hydrocodone and homatropine *on page 481*

Hydro-Tussin™-CBX *(Discontinued)*

Hydro-Tussin™ DHC ***(Discontinued)*** *see* pseudoephedrine, dihydrocodeine, and chlorpheniramine *on page 813*

Hydro-Tussin™ DM ***(Discontinued)*** *see* guaifenesin and dextromethorphan *on page 455*

Hydro-Tussin™ EXP ***(Discontinued)*** *see* dihydrocodeine, pseudoephedrine, and guaifenesin *on page 304*

Hydro-Tussin™ HC ***(Discontinued)***

Hydro-Tussin™ HD ***(Discontinued)***

Hydro-Tussin™ XP ***(Discontinued)***

HydroVal® [Can] *see* hydrocortisone (topical) *on page 483*

hydroxyamphetamine and tropicamide (hye droks ee am FET a meen & troe PIK a mide)

Synonyms hydroxyamphetamine hydrobromide and tropicamide; tropicamide and hydroxyamphetamine

U.S./Canadian Brand Names Paremyd® [US]

Therapeutic Category Adrenergic Agonist Agent, Ophthalmic

Use Short-term pupil dilation for diagnostic procedures and exams

Dosage Summary

Ophthalmic:

Children: Dosage not established

Adults: Instill 1-2 drops into conjunctival sac(s)

Dosage Forms

Solution, ophthalmic:

Paremyd®: Hydroxyamphetamine 1% and tropicamide 0.25% (15 mL)

hydroxyamphetamine hydrobromide and tropicamide *see* hydroxyamphetamine and tropicamide *on page 488*

4-hydroxybutyrate *see* sodium oxybate *on page 885*

hydroxycarbamide *see* hydroxyurea *on page 489*

hydroxychloroquine (hye droks ee KLOR oh kwin)

Sound-Alike/Look-Alike Issues

hydroxychloroquine may be confused with hydrocortisone

Plaquenil® may be confused with Platinol®

Synonyms hydroxychloroquine sulfate

U.S./Canadian Brand Names Apo-Hydroxyquine® [Can]; Gen-Hydroxychloroquine [Can]; Mylan-Hydroxychloroquine [Can]; Plaquenil® [US/Can]; PRO-Hydroxyquine [Can]

Therapeutic Category Aminoquinoline (Antimalarial)

Use Suppression and treatment of acute attacks of malaria; treatment of systemic lupus erythematosus (SLE) and rheumatoid arthritis

Dosage Summary Note: Hydroxychloroquine sulfate 200 mg is equivalent to 155 mg hydroxychloroquine base and 250 mg chloroquine phosphate. All doses below expressed as hydroxychloroquine sulfate.

Oral:

Children:

Malaria prophylaxis:

No pretreatment: 13 mg/kg in 2 divided doses 6 hours apart, followed by normal prophylactic regimen

Prior to exposure: 6.5 mg/kg once weekly (maximum: 400 mg/dose)

Malaria treatment: 13 mg/kg (maximum: 800 mg) initially, followed by 6.5 mg/kg at 6, 24, and 48 hours (maximum: 400 mg/dose)

Adults:

SLE: Initial: 400-800 mg/day divided 1-2 times/day; Maintenance: 200-400 mg/day

Malaria prophylaxis:

No pretreatment: 800 mg in 2 divided doses 6 hours apart, followed by normal prophylactic regimen

Prior to exposure: 400 mg once weekly

Malaria treatment: 800 mg initially, followed by 400 mg at 6, 24, and 48 hours

Rheumatoid arthritis: Initial: 400-600 mg/day; Maintenance: 200-400 mg/day

Dosage Forms

Tablet, oral: 200 mg

Plaquenil®: 200 mg

hydroxychloroquine sulfate *see* hydroxychloroquine *on page 488*

hydroxydaunomycin hydrochloride *see* doxorubicin *on page 330*

hydroxyethylcellulose *see* artificial tears *on page* 97
hydroxyethyl starch *see* hetastarch *on page* 471
hydroxyethyl starch *see* tetrastarch *on page* 924
hydroxyldaunorubicin hydrochloride *see* doxorubicin *on page* 330

hydroxypropyl cellulose (hye droks ee PROE pil SEL yoo lose)

U.S./Canadian Brand Names Lacrisert® [US/Can]

Therapeutic Category Ophthalmic Agent, Miscellaneous

Use Dry eyes (moderate-to-severe)

Dosage Summary

Ophthalmic:

Children: Dosage not established

Adults: Apply once daily into the inferior cul-de-sac beneath the base of tarsus

Dosage Forms

Insert, ophthalmic [preservative free]:

Lacrisert®: 5 mg (60s)

hydroxypropyl methylcellulose (hye droks ee PROE pil meth il SEL yoo lose)

Sound-Alike/Look-Alike Issues

Isopto® Tears may be confused with Isoptin®

Synonyms gonioscopic ophthalmic solution; hypromellose

U.S./Canadian Brand Names Cellugel® [US]; GenTeal® Mild [US-OTC]; GenTeal® [US-OTC/Can]; Gonak™ [US-OTC]; Goniosoft™ [US-OTC]; Isopto® Tears [US-OTC/Can]; Natural Balance Tears [US-OTC]; Nature's Tears [US-OTC]; Tears Again® MC Gel Drops™ [US-OTC]

Therapeutic Category Ophthalmic Agent, Miscellaneous

Use Relief of burning and minor irritation due to dry eyes; diagnostic agent in gonioscopic examination

Dosage Summary

Ophthalmic:

Children: Dosage not established

Adults: Instill 1-2 drops in affected eye(s) as needed

Dosage Forms

Gel, ophthalmic [preservative free]:

GenTeal® [OTC]: 0.3% (10 mL)

Injection, solution, ophthalmic:

Cellugel®: 2% (1 mL)

Solution, ophthalmic:

Gonak™: 2.5% (15 mL)
Goniosoft™ [OTC]: 2.5% (15 mL)
Isopto® Tears [OTC]: 0.5% (15 mL)
Natural Balance Tears [OTC]: 0.4% (15 mL)
Nature's Tears [OTC]: 0.4% (15 mL)
Tears Again® MC Gel Drops™ [OTC]: 0.3% (15 mL)

Solution, ophthalmic [preservative free]:

GenTeal® [OTC]: 0.3% (15 mL, 25 mL)
GenTeal® Mild [OTC]: 0.2% (15 mL, 25 mL)

9-hydroxy-risperidone *see* paliperidone *on page* 720

hydroxyurea (hye droks ee yoor EE a)

Sound-Alike/Look-Alike Issues

hydroxyurea may be confused with hydrOXYzine

Synonyms hydroxycarbamide

U.S./Canadian Brand Names Apo-Hydroxyurea® [Can]; Droxia® [US]; Gen-Hydroxyurea [Can]; Hydrea® [US/Can]; Mylan-Hydroxyurea [Can]

Therapeutic Category Antineoplastic Agent

Use Treatment of melanoma, refractory chronic myelocytic leukemia (CML); recurrent, metastatic, or inoperable ovarian cancer; radiosensitizing agent in the treatment of squamous cell head and neck cancer (excluding lip cancer); adjunct in the management of sickle cell patients who have had at least three painful crises in the previous 12 months (to reduce frequency of these crises and the need for blood transfusions)

Dosage Summary

Oral:

Adults: 15-35 mg/kg/day **or** 500-3000 mg/day as single or divided dose **or** 80 mg/kg as a single dose every third day

Dosage Forms

Capsule, oral: 500 mg

Droxia®: 200 mg, 300 mg, 400 mg

Hydrea®: 500 mg

hydroxyzine (hye DROKS i zeen)

Sound-Alike/Look-Alike Issues

hydrOXYzine may be confused with hydrALAZINE, hydroxyurea

Atarax® may be confused with Ativan®

Vistaril® may be confused with Restoril™, Versed, Zestril®

Synonyms hydroxyzine hydrochloride; hydroxyzine pamoate

Tall-Man hydr**OXY**zine

U.S./Canadian Brand Names Apo-Hydroxyzine® [Can]; Atarax® [Can]; Hydroxyzine Hydrochloride Injection, USP [Can]; Novo-Hydroxyzin [Can]; PMS-Hydroxyzine [Can]; Vistaril® [US/Can]

Therapeutic Category Antiemetic; Antihistamine

Use Treatment of anxiety; preoperative sedative; antipruritic

Dosage Summary

I.M.:

Children <6 years: 0.5-1 mg/kg/dose prior to procedure **or** 50 mg/day in divided doses

Children ≥6 years: 0.5-1 mg/kg/dose prior to procedure **or** 50-100 mg/day in divided doses

Adults: 25-100 mg every 4-6 hours as needed **or** 25-100 mg prior to procedure

Oral:

Children <6 years: 0.6 mg/kg/dose prior to procedure **or** 50 mg/day in divided doses

Children ≥6 years: 0.6 mg/kg/dose prior to procedure **or** 50-100 mg/day in divided doses

Adults: 25-100 mg 4 times/day or 50-100 mg prior to procedure

Elderly: Initial: 10 mg 3-4 times/day

Dosage Forms

Capsule, oral: 25 mg, 50 mg, 100 mg

Vistaril®: 25 mg, 50 mg

Injection, solution: 25 mg/mL (1 mL); 50 mg/mL (1 mL, 2 mL, 10 mL)

Solution, oral: 10 mg/5 mL (473 mL)

Syrup, oral: 10 mg/5 mL (118 mL, 473 mL, 480 mL)

Tablet, oral: 10 mg, 25 mg, 50 mg

hydroxyzine hydrochloride *see* hydroxyzine *on page* 490

Hydroxyzine Hydrochloride Injection, USP [Can] *see* hydroxyzine *on page* 490

hydroxyzine pamoate *see* hydroxyzine *on page* 490

HydroZone Plus *(Discontinued)* *see* hydrocortisone (topical) *on page* 483

Hyflex-DS® *(Discontinued)* *see* acetaminophen and phenyltoloxamine *on page* 26

Hygroton® *(Discontinued)* *see* chlorthalidone *on page* 217

Hylaform® [US] *see* hyaluronate and derivatives *on page* 475

Hylaform® Plus [US] *see* hyaluronate and derivatives *on page* 475

hylan G-F 20 *see* hyaluronate and derivatives *on page* 475

hylan polymers *see* hyaluronate and derivatives *on page* 475

Hylenex™ [US] *see* hyaluronidase *on page* 476

Hylira™ [US] *see* hyaluronate and derivatives *on page* 475

Hylutin Injection *(Discontinued)*

HyoMax™-DT [US] *see* hyoscyamine *on page* 491

HyoMax™-FT [US] *see* hyoscyamine *on page* 491

HyoMax® -SR [US] *see* hyoscyamine *on page* 491

Hyonatol [US] *see* hyoscyamine, atropine, scopolamine, and phenobarbital *on page* 492

hyoscine butylbromide *see* scopolamine derivatives (systemic) *on page* 866

hyoscine hydrobromide *see* scopolamine derivatives (ophthalmic) *on page* 867

hyoscyamine (hye oh SYE a meen)

Sound-Alike/Look-Alike Issues

Anaspaz® may be confused with Anaprox®, Antispas®
Levbid® may be confused with Enbrel®, Lithobid®, Lopid®, Lorabid®
Levsinex® may be confused with Lanoxin®
Levsin®/SL maybe confused with Levaquin®

Synonyms *l*-hyoscyamine sulfate; hyoscyamine sulfate

U.S./Canadian Brand Names Anaspaz® [US]; HyoMax® -SR [US]; HyoMax™-DT [US]; HyoMax™-FT [US]; Hyosyne [US]; Levbid® [US]; Levsin® [US/Can]; Levsin®/SL [US]; Symax® DuoTab [US]; Symax® FasTab [US]; Symax® SL [US]; Symax® SR [US]

Therapeutic Category Anticholinergic Agent

Use

Oral: Adjunctive therapy for peptic ulcers, irritable bowel, neurogenic bladder/bowel; treatment of infant colic, GI tract disorders caused by spasm; to reduce rigidity, tremors, sialorrhea, and hyperhidrosis associated with parkinsonism; as a drying agent in acute rhinitis

Injection: Preoperative antimuscarinic to reduce secretions and block cardiac vagal inhibitory reflexes; to improve radiologic visibility of the kidneys; symptomatic relief of biliary and renal colic; reduce GI motility to facilitate diagnostic procedures (ie, endoscopy, hypotonic duodenography); reduce pain and hypersecretion in pancreatitis, certain cases of partial heart block associated with vagal activity; reversal of neuromuscular blockade

Dosage Summary

I.M.:

Children: Dosage not established
Adults: 0.25-0.5 mg 4 times/day as needed

I.V.:

Children <2 years: Dosage not established
Children ≥2 years: 5 mcg/kg given 30-60 minutes prior to induction of anesthesia
Adults: 0.125-0.5 mg 4 times/day as needed **or** 0.25-0.5 mg 5-10 minutes prior to procedure **or** 5 mcg/kg given 30-60 minutes prior to induction of anesthesia **or** 0.2 mg for every 1 mg neostigmine

Oral:

Regular release:
Children <2 years and 3.4 kg: 4 drops every 4 hours as needed (maximum: 24 drops/day)
Children <2 years and 5 kg: 5 drops every 4 hours as needed (maximum: 30 drops/day)
Children <2 years and 7 kg: 6 drops every 4 hours as needed (maximum: 36 drops/day)
Children <2 years and 10 kg: 8 drops every 4 hours as needed (maximum: 48 drops/day)
Children ≥2 years and 10 kg: 0.031-0.033 mg every 4 hours as needed (maximum: 0.75 mg/day)
Children ≥2 years and 20 kg: 0.0625 mg every 4 hours as needed (maximum: 0.75 mg/day)
Children ≥2 years and 40 kg: 0.0938 mg every 4 hours as needed (maximum: 0.75 mg/day)
Children ≥2 years and 50 kg: 0.125 mg every 4 hours as needed (maximum: 0.75 mg/day)
Adults: 0.125-0.25 mg every 4 hours or as needed (maximum: 1.5 mg/day)

Timed release:
Children: Dosage not established
Adults: 0.375-0.75 mg every 12 hours (maximum: 1.5 mg/day)

S.L.:

Children <2 years: Dosage not established
Children ≥2 years and 10 kg: 0.031-0.033 mg every 4 hours as needed (maximum: 0.75 mg/day)
Children ≥2 years and 20 kg: 0.0625 mg every 4 hours as needed (maximum: 0.75 mg/day)
Children ≥2 years and 40 kg: 0.0938 mg every 4 hours as needed (maximum: 0.75 mg/day)
Children ≥2 years and 50 kg: 0.125 mg every 4 hours as needed (maximum: 0.75 mg/day)
Adults: 0.125-0.25 mg every 4 hours or as needed (maximum: 1.5 mg/day)

SubQ:

Children: Dosage not established
Adults: 0.25-0.5 mg 4 times/day as needed

Dosage Forms

Elixir, oral: 0.125 mg/5 mL (473 mL, 480 mL)
Hyosyne: 0.125 mg/5 mL (473 mL)

Injection, solution:
Levsin®: 0.5 mg/mL (1 mL)

Solution, oral: 0.125 mg/mL (15 mL)
Hyosyne: 0.125 mg/mL (15 mL)
Tablet, oral: 0.125 mg
Levsin®: 0.125 mg
Tablet, sublingual: 0.125 mg
Levsin®/SL: 0.125 mg
Symax® SL: 0.125 mg
Tablet, chewable/disintegrating, oral:
HyoMax™-FT: 0.125 mg
Symax® FasTab: 0.125 mg
Tablet, extended release, oral: 0.375 mg
Levbid®: 0.375 mg
Tablet, orally disintegrating, oral: 0.125 mg
Anaspaz®: 0.125 mg
Tablet, sustained release, oral: 0.375 mg
HyoMax® -SR: 0.375 mg
Symax® SR: 0.375 mg
Tablet, variable release, oral:
HyoMax™-DT: Hyoscyamine sulfate 0.125 mg [immediate release] and hyoscyamine sulfate 0.25 mg [sustained release]
Symax® DuoTab: Hyoscyamine sulfate 0.125 mg [immediate release] and hyoscyamine sulfate 0.25 mg [sustained release]

hyoscyamine, atropine, scopolamine, and phenobarbital

(hye oh SYE a meen, A troe peen, skoe POL a meen, & fee noe BAR bi tal)

Sound-Alike/Look-Alike Issues
Donnatal® may be confused with Donnagel®, Donnatal Extentabs®

Synonyms atropine, hyoscyamine, phenobarbital, and scopolamine; belladonna alkaloids with phenobarbital; phenobarbital, hyoscyamine, atropine, and scopolamine; scopolamine, hyoscyamine, atropine, and phenobarbital

U.S./Canadian Brand Names Donnatal Extentabs® [US]; Donnatal® [US]; Hyonatol [US]

Therapeutic Category Anticholinergic Agent

Use Adjunct in treatment of irritable bowel syndrome, acute enterocolitis, duodenal ulcer

Dosage Summary
Oral:
Extended release:
Children: Dosage not established
Adults: 1 tablet every 12 hours, may increase to every 8 hours
Regular release:
Children 4.5 kg: 0.5 mL every 4 hours **or** 0.75 mL every 6 hours
Children 10 kg: 1 mL every 4 hours **or** 1.5 mL every 6 hours
Children 14 kg: 1.5 mL every 4 hours **or** 2 mL every 6 hours
Children 23 kg: 2.5 mL every 4 hours **or** 3.8 mL every 6 hours
Children 34 kg: 3.8 mL every 4 hours **or** 5 mL every 6 hours
Children ≥45 kg: 5 mL every 4 hours **or** 7.5 mL every 6 hours
Adults: 1-2 tablets **or** 5-10 mL of elixir 3-4 times/day

Dosage Forms
Elixir:
Donnatal®: Hyoscyamine 0.1037 mg, atropine 0.0194 mg, scopolamine 0.0065 mg, and phenobarbital 16.2 mg per 5 mL
Tablet: Hyoscyamine 0.1037 mg, atropine 0.0194 mg, scopolamine 0.0065 mg, and phenobarbital 16.2 mg
Donnatal®: Hyoscyamine 0.1037 mg, atropine 0.0194 mg, scopolamine 0.0065 mg, and phenobarbital 16.2 mg
Hyonatol: Hyoscyamine 0.1037 mg, atropine 0.0194 mg, scopolamine 0.0065 mg, and phenobarbital 16.2 mg
Tablet, extended release:
Donnatal Extentabs®: Hyoscyamine 0.3111 mg, atropine 0.0582 mg, scopolamine 0.0195 mg, and phenobarbital 48.6 mg

hyoscyamine, methenamine, benzoic acid, phenyl salicylate, and methylene blue *see* methenamine, phenyl salicylate, methylene blue, benzoic acid, and hyoscyamine *on page 613*

hyoscyamine sulfate *see* hyoscyamine *on page 491*
Hyosyne [US] *see* hyoscyamine *on page 491*
Hy-Pam® Oral *(Discontinued)* *see* hydroxyzine *on page 490*
Hypaque™ Sodium [US] *see* diatrizoate sodium *on page 293*
Hyperab® *(Discontinued)* *see* rabies immune globulin (human) *on page 824*
hyperal *see* total parenteral nutrition *on page 944*
hyperalimentation *see* total parenteral nutrition *on page 944*
Hypercare™ [US] *see* aluminum chloride hexahydrate *on page 58*
HyperHep B® [Can] *see* hepatitis B immune globulin (human) *on page 469*
HyperHEP B™ S/D [US] *see* hepatitis B immune globulin (human) *on page 469*
HyperRAB™ S/D [US/Can] *see* rabies immune globulin (human) *on page 824*
HyperRHO™ S/D Full Dose [US] *see* Rh_o(D) immune globulin *on page 838*
HyperRHO™ S/D Mini Dose [US] *see* Rh_o(D) immune globulin *on page 838*
Hyper-Sal™ [US] *see* sodium chloride *on page 882*
Hyperstat® *(Discontinued)* *see* diazoxide *on page 295*
HyperTET™ S/D [US/Can] *see* tetanus immune globulin (human) *on page 920*
hypertonic saline *see* sodium chloride *on page 882*
Hyphed *(Discontinued)*
Hy-Phen® *(Discontinued)* *see* hydrocodone and acetaminophen *on page 479*
HypoTears [US-OTC] *see* artificial tears *on page 97*
HypoTears PF [US-OTC] *see* artificial tears *on page 97*
HypRho®-D *(Discontinued)*
HypRho®-D Mini-Dose *(Discontinued)*
Hyprogest® 250 *(Discontinued)*
hypromellose *see* hydroxypropyl methylcellulose *on page 489*
Hytakerol® *(Discontinued)*
HyTan™ *(Discontinued)* *see* hydrocodone and chlorpheniramine *on page 480*
Hytone® *(Discontinued)* *see* hydrocortisone (topical) *on page 483*
Hytrin® [Can] *see* terazosin *on page 917*
Hytrin® *(Discontinued)* *see* terazosin *on page 917*
Hyzaar® [US/Can] *see* losartan and hydrochlorothiazide *on page 577*
Hyzaar® DS [Can] *see* losartan and hydrochlorothiazide *on page 577*
Hyzine® *(Discontinued)* *see* hydroxyzine *on page 490*
I^{123} iobenguane *see* iobenguane I 123 *on page 517*
I-123 MIBG *see* iobenguane I 123 *on page 517*

ibandronate (eye BAN droh nate)

Synonyms ibandronate sodium; ibandronic acid

U.S./Canadian Brand Names Boniva® [US]

Therapeutic Category Bisphosphonate Derivative

Use Treatment and prevention of osteoporosis in postmenopausal females

Dosage Summary

I.V.:
Children: Dosage not established
Adults: 3 mg every 3 months

Oral:
Children: Dosage not established
Adults: 2.5 mg once daily **or** 150 mg once a month

Dosage Forms

Injection, solution:
Boniva®: 1 mg/mL (3 mL)

Tablet, oral:
Boniva®: 150 mg

ibandronate sodium *see* ibandronate *on page 493*
ibandronic acid *see* ibandronate *on page 493*

Iberet®-500 *(Discontinued)* *see* vitamins (multiple/oral) *on page 990*

ibidomide hydrochloride *see* labetalol *on page 541*

ibritumomab (ib ri TYOO mo mab)

Synonyms ibritumomab tiuxetan; IDEC-Y2B8; In-111 ibritumomab; In-111 zevalin; Y-90 ibritumomab; Y-90 zevalin

U.S./Canadian Brand Names Zevalin® [US/Can]

Therapeutic Category Antineoplastic Agent, Monoclonal Antibody; Radiopharmaceutical

Use Treatment of relapsed or refractory low-grade or follicular B-cell non-Hodgkin lymphoma (NHL); treatment of follicular NHL in patients who achieve a response (partial or complete) to first-line chemotherapy

Dosage Summary

I.V.:

Children: Dosage not established

Adults:

Day 1: In-111: Within 4 hours of the completion of rituximab, inject 5 mCi (1.6 mg total antibody dose)

Day 7, 8, or 9: Y-90: Within 4 hours of the completion of rituximab infusion, inject 0.3 mCi/kg (11.1 MBq/kg actual body weight) if platelet count 100,000-149,000 cell/mm^3 (in relapsed or refractory patients) **or** 0.4 mCi/kg (14.8 MBq/kg actual body weight) if platelet count ≥150,000 cell/mm^3 (maximum: 32 mCi [1184 MBq])

Dosage Forms

Injection, solution [preservative free]:

Zevalin®: 1.6 mg/mL (2 mL)

ibritumomab tiuxetan *see* ibritumomab *on page 494*

Ibu® [US] *see* ibuprofen *on page 494*

Ibu-200 [US-OTC] *see* ibuprofen *on page 494*

Ibudone™ [US] *see* hydrocodone and ibuprofen *on page 481*

Ibuprin® *(Discontinued)* *see* ibuprofen *on page 494*

ibuprofen (eye byoo PROE fen)

Sound-Alike/Look-Alike Issues

Haltran® may be confused with Halfprin®

Motrin® may be confused with Neurontin®

Synonyms *p*-isobutylhydratropic acid; ibuprofen lysine

U.S./Canadian Brand Names Addaprin [US-OTC]; Advil® Children's [US-OTC]; Advil® Infants' [US-OTC]; Advil® Migraine [US-OTC]; Advil® [US-OTC/Can]; Apo-Ibuprofen® [Can]; Caldolor™ [US]; I-Prin [US-OTC]; Ibu-200 [US-OTC]; Ibu® [US]; Midol® Cramps & Body Aches [US-OTC]; Motrin® Children's [US-OTC/Can]; Motrin® IB [US-OTC/Can]; Motrin® Infants' [US-OTC]; Motrin® Junior [US-OTC]; NeoProfen® [US]; Novo-Profen [Can]; Nu-Ibuprofen [Can]; Proprinal® [US-OTC]; Ultraprin [US-OTC]

Therapeutic Category Analgesic, Nonnarcotic; Antipyretic; Nonsteroidal Antiinflammatory Drug (NSAID)

Use

Oral: Inflammatory diseases and rheumatoid disorders including juvenile rheumatoid arthritis, mild-to-moderate pain, fever, dysmenorrhea, osteoarthritis

Ibuprofen injection (Caldolor™): Management of mild-to-moderate pain; management moderate-to-severe pain when used concurrently with an opioid analgesic; reduction of fever

Ibuprofen lysine injection (NeoProfen®): To induce closure of a clinically-significant patent ductus arteriosus (PDA) in premature infants weighing between 500-1500 g and who are ≤32 weeks gestational age (GA) when usual treatments are ineffective

Dosage Summary

I.V. (ibuprofen [Caldolor™]):

Children: Dosage not established

Adults: 100-400 mg every 4-6 hours or 400-800 mg every 6 hours (maximum: 3.2 g/day)

I.V. (ibuprofen lysine [NeoProfen®]):

Infants between 500-1500 g and ≤32 weeks GA: Initial: 10 mg/kg, followed by two doses of 5 mg/kg at 24 and 48 hours; **Note:** Dose should be based on birth weight.

Children: Dosage not established

Adults: Dosage not established

Oral:

Children <6 months: Dosage not established

Children 6-11 months and 12-17 lbs:

Analgesic/antipyretic: 50 mg every 6-8 hours (maximum: 4 doses/day) **or** 4-10 mg/kg every 6-8 hours (maximum: 40 mg/kg/day)

JRA: 30-50 mg/kg/day divided every 8 hours (maximum: 2.4 g/day)

Children 12-23 months and 18-23 lbs:

Analgesic/antipyretic: 75 mg every 6-8 hours (maximum: 4 doses/day) **or** 4-10 mg/kg every 6-8 hours (maximum: 40 mg/kg/day)

JRA: 30-50 mg/kg/day divided every 8 hours (maximum: 2.4 g/day)

Children 2-3 years and 24-35 lbs:

Analgesic/antipyretic: 100 mg every 6-8 hours (maximum: 4 doses/day) **or** 4-10 mg/kg every 6-8 hours (maximum: 40 mg/kg/day)

JRA: 30-50 mg/kg/day divided every 8 hours (maximum: 2.4 g/day)

Children 4-5 years and 36-47 lbs:

Analgesic/antipyretic: 150 mg every 6-8 hours (maximum: 4 doses/day) **or** 4-10 mg/kg every 6-8 hours (maximum: 40 mg/kg/day)

JRA: 30-50 mg/kg/day divided every 8 hours (maximum: 2.4 g/day)

Children 6-8 years and 48-59 lbs:

Analgesic/antipyretic: 200 mg every 6-8 hours (maximum: 4 doses/day) **or** 4-10 mg/kg every 6-8 hours (maximum: 40 mg/kg/day)

JRA: 30-50 mg/kg/day divided every 8 hours (maximum: 2.4 g/day)

Children 9-10 years and 60-71 lbs:

Analgesic/antipyretic: 250 mg every 6-8 hours (maximum: 4 doses/day) **or** 4-10 mg/kg every 6-8 hours (maximum: 40 mg/kg/day)

JRA: 30-50 mg/kg/day divided every 8 hours (maximum: 2.4 g/day)

Children 11-12 years and 72-95 lbs:

Analgesic/antipyretic: 300 mg every 6-8 hours (maximum: 4 doses/day) **or** 4-10 mg/kg every 6-8 hours (maximum: 40 mg/kg/day)

JRA: 30-50 mg/kg/day divided every 8 hours (maximum: 2.4 g/day)

Children >12 years:

Analgesic/antipyretic: 200 mg every 4-6 hours as needed (maximum: 1200 mg/day) **or** 4-10 mg/kg every 6-8 hours (maximum: 40 mg/kg/day)

JRA: 30-50 mg/kg/day divided every 8 hours (maximum: 2.4 g/day)

Adults:

Analgesic/antipyretic/dysmenorrhea: 200-400 mg every 4-6 hours

Inflammatory disease: 400-800 mg 3-4 times/day (maximum: 3200 mg/day)

Dosage Forms

Caplet, oral: 200 mg

Advil® [OTC]: 200 mg

Motrin® IB [OTC]: 200 mg

Motrin® Junior [OTC]: 100 mg

Capsule, liquid filled, oral:

Advil® [OTC]: 200 mg

Advil® Migraine [OTC]: 200 mg

Capsule, softgel, oral: 200 mg

Gelcap, oral:

Advil® [OTC]: 200 mg

Injection, solution:

Caldolor™: 100 mg/mL (4 mL, 8 mL)

Injection, solution [preservative free]:

NeoProfen®: 17.1 mg/mL (2 mL)

Suspension, oral: 100 mg/5 mL (5 mL, 10 mL, 120 mL, 240 mL, 480 mL); 40 mg/mL (15 mL)

Advil® Children's [OTC]: 100 mg/5 mL (120 mL)

Advil® Infants' [OTC]: 40 mg/mL (15 mL)

Motrin® Children's [OTC]: 100 mg/5 mL (60 mL, 120 mL)

Motrin® Infants' [OTC]: 40 mg/mL (15 mL)

Tablet, oral: 200 mg, 400 mg, 600 mg, 800 mg

Addaprin [OTC]: 200 mg

Advil® [OTC]: 200 mg

I-Prin [OTC]: 200 mg

Ibu-200 [OTC]: 200 mg

Ibu®: 400 mg, 600 mg, 800 mg
Midol® Cramps & Body Aches [OTC]: 200 mg
Motrin® IB [OTC]: 200 mg
Proprinal® [OTC]: 200 mg
Ultraprin [OTC]: 200 mg

Tablet, chewable, oral:
Motrin® Junior [OTC]: 100 mg

ibuprofen and hydrocodone *see* hydrocodone and ibuprofen *on page* *481*
ibuprofen and oxycodone *see* oxycodone and ibuprofen *on page* *716*
ibuprofen and pseudoephedrine *see* pseudoephedrine and ibuprofen *on page* *812*
ibuprofen lysine *see* ibuprofen *on page* *494*

ibuprofen, pseudoephedrine, and chlorpheniramine

(eye byoo PROE fen, soo doe e FED rin, & klor fen IR a meen)

Synonyms chlorpheniramine maleate, ibuprofen, and pseudoephedrine; ibuprofen, pseudoephedrine, and chlorpheniramine maleate; pseudoephedrine, chlorpheniramine, and ibuprofen

U.S./Canadian Brand Names Advil® Allergy Sinus [US]; Advil® Cold and Sinus Plus [Can]; Advil® Multi-Symptom Cold [US]

Therapeutic Category Antihistamine/Decongestant/Analgesic

Use Temporary relief of symptoms associated with the common cold, hay fever, or other respiratory allergies

Dosage Summary

Oral:
Children <12 years: Dosage not established
Children ≥12 years: One caplet every 4-6 hours (maximum: 6 caplets/day)
Adults: One caplet every 4-6 hours (maximum: 6 caplets/day)

Dosage Forms

Caplet:
Advil® Allergy Sinus, Advil® Multi-Symptom Cold: Ibuprofen 200 mg, pseudoephedrine 30 mg, and chlorpheniramine 2 mg

ibuprofen, pseudoephedrine, and chlorpheniramine maleate *see* ibuprofen, pseudoephedrine, and chlorpheniramine *on page* *496*

ibutilide (i BYOO ti lide)

Synonyms ibutilide fumarate

U.S./Canadian Brand Names Corvert® [US]

Therapeutic Category Antiarrhythmic Agent, Class III

Use Acute termination of atrial fibrillation or flutter of recent onset; the effectiveness of ibutilide has not been determined in patients with arrhythmias >90 days in duration

Dosage Summary

I.V.:
Children: Dosage not established
Adults <60 kg: 0.01 mg/kg, may repeat once
Adults ≥60 kg: 1 mg, may repeat once

Dosage Forms

Injection, solution: 0.1 mg/mL (10 mL)
Corvert®: 0.1 mg/mL (10 mL)

ibutilide fumarate *see* ibutilide *on page* *496*
IC51 *see* Japanese encephalitis virus vaccine (inactivated) *on page* *532*
IC-Green™ [US] *see* indocyanine green *on page* *505*
ICI-182,780 *see* fulvestrant *on page* *431*
ICI-204,219 *see* zafirlukast *on page* *996*
ICI-46474 *see* tamoxifen *on page* *909*
ICI-118630 *see* goserelin *on page* *452*
ICI-176334 *see* bicalutamide *on page* *137*
ICI-D1033 *see* anastrozole *on page* *78*
ICI-D1694 *see* raltitrexed *(Canada only) on page* *826*

ICL670 *see* deferasirox *on page 272*

icodextrin (eye KOE dex trin)

U.S./Canadian Brand Names Extraneal [US]

Therapeutic Category Adhesiolytic; Peritoneal Dialysate, Osmotic

Use

Adept®: Reduction of postsurgical adhesions in gynecologic laparoscopic procedures

Extraneal®: Daily exchange for the long dwell (8- to 16-hour) during continuous ambulatory peritoneal dialysis (CAPD) or automated peritoneal dialysis (APD) for the management of end-stage renal disease (ESRD); improvement of long-dwell ultrafiltration and clearance of creatinine and urea nitrogen (compared to 4.25% dextrose) in patients with high/average or greater transport characteristics as measured by peritoneal equilibration test (PET)

Dosage Summary

Intraperitoneal:

Children: Dosage not established

Adults:

CAPD or APD (Extraneal®): Intraperitoneal: Given as a single daily exchange in CAPD or APD; dwell time of 8-16 hours is suggested

Laparoscopic gynecologic surgery (Adept®): Intraperitoneal: Irrigate with at least 100 mL every 30 minutes during surgery; aspirate remaining fluid after surgery is completed, then instill 1 L into the cavity

Dosage Forms

Solution, intraperitoneal [preservative free]:

Extraneal: 7.5% (1.5 L, 2 L, 2.5 L)

ICRF-187 *see* dexrazoxane *on page 284*

Icy Hot® [US-OTC] *see* methyl salicylate and menthol *on page 623*

Idamycin® [Can] *see* idarubicin *on page 497*

Idamycin® *(Discontinued)* *see* idarubicin *on page 497*

Idamycin PFS® [US] *see* idarubicin *on page 497*

idarubicin (eye da ROO bi sin)

Sound-Alike/Look-Alike Issues

IDArubicin may be confused with DOXOrubicin, DAUNOrubicin, epirubicin

Idamycin PFS® may be confused with Adriamycin

Synonyms 4-demethoxydaunorubicin; 4-DMDR; idarubicin hydrochloride; IDR; IMI 30; SC 33428

Tall-Man **IDA**rubicin

U.S./Canadian Brand Names Idamycin PFS® [US]; Idamycin® [Can]

Therapeutic Category Antineoplastic Agent

Use Treatment of acute myeloid leukemia (AML)

Dosage Summary

I.V.:

Children: Dosage not established

Adults: Induction: 12 mg/m^2/day for 3 days; Consolidation: 10-12 mg/m^2/day for 2 days

Dosage Forms

Injection, solution [preservative free]: 1 mg/mL (5 mL, 10 mL, 20 mL)

Idamycin PFS®: 1 mg/mL (5 mL, 10 mL, 20 mL)

idarubicin hydrochloride *see* idarubicin *on page 497*

IDEC-C2B8 *see* rituximab *on page 846*

IDEC-Y2B8 *see* ibritumomab *on page 494*

IDR *see* idarubicin *on page 497*

idursulfase (eye dur SUL fase)

Sound-Alike/Look-Alike Issues

Elaprase™ may be confused with Elspar®

U.S./Canadian Brand Names Elaprase™ [US/Can]

Therapeutic Category Enzyme

Use Replacement therapy in mucopolysaccharidosis II (MPS II, Hunter syndrome) for improvement of walking capacity

Dosage Summary

I.V.:

Children <5 years: Dosage not established

Children ≥5 years: 0.5 mg/kg once weekly

Adults: 0.5 mg/kg once weekly

Elderly: Studies did not include patients ≥65 years

Dosage Forms

Injection, solution [preservative free]:

Elaprase™: 2 mg/mL (5 mL)

Ifex [US/Can] *see* ifosfamide *on page 498*

ifosfamide (eye FOSS fa mide)

Sound-Alike/Look-Alike Issues

ifosfamide may be confused with cyclophosphamide

Synonyms isophosphamide; Z4942

U.S./Canadian Brand Names Ifex [US/Can]

Therapeutic Category Antineoplastic Agent

Use Treatment of testicular cancer

Dosage Summary

I.V.:

Adults: 4000-5000 mg/m^2/day for 1 day every 14-28 days **or** 1000-3000 mg/m^2/day for 2-5 days every 21-28 days

Dosage Forms

Injection, powder for reconstitution: 1 g, 3 g

Ifex: 1 g, 3 g

Injection, solution: 50 mg/mL (20 mL, 60 mL)

IG *see* immune globulin (intramuscular) *on page 501*

IgG4-kappa monoclonal antibody *see* natalizumab *on page 662*

IGIM *see* immune globulin (intramuscular) *on page 501*

IGIV *see* immune globulin (intravenous) *on page 502*

IGIVnex® [Can] *see* immune globulin (intravenous) *on page 502*

IL-1Ra *see* anakinra *on page 77*

IL-2 *see* aldesleukin *on page 46*

IL-11 *see* oprelvekin *on page 706*

Ilaris® [US] *see* canakinumab *on page 173*

Ilopan-Choline® Oral *(Discontinued)* *see* dexpanthenol *on page 284*

Ilopan® Injection *(Discontinued)* *see* dexpanthenol *on page 284*

iloperidone (eye loe PER i done)

Sound-Alike/Look-Alike Issues

iloperidone may be confused with domperidone

U.S./Canadian Brand Names Fanapt™ [US]

Therapeutic Category Antipsychotic Agent, Atypical

Use Acute treatment of schizophrenia

Dosage Summary

Oral:

Children: Dosage not established

Adults: Initial: 1 mg twice daily; Dosage range: 6-12 mg twice daily (maximum: 24 mg/day); **Note:** Titration is recommended

Dosage Forms

Tablet, oral:

Fanapt™: 1 mg, 2 mg, 4 mg, 6 mg, 8 mg, 10 mg, 12 mg, 1 mg (2s), 2 mg (2s), 4 mg (2s), and 6 mg (2s)

iloprost (EYE loe prost)

Synonyms iloprost tromethamine; prostacyclin PGI_2

U.S./Canadian Brand Names Ventavis® [US]

Therapeutic Category Prostaglandin

Use Treatment of idiopathic pulmonary arterial hypertension in patients with NYHA Class III or IV symptoms

Dosage Summary

Inhalation:

Children: Dosage not established

Adults: Initial: 2.5 mcg/dose; Maintenance: 2.5-5 mcg/dose 6-9 times/day (maximum: 45 mcg/day)

Dosage Forms

Solution, for oral inhalation [preservative free]:

Ventavis®: 10 mcg/mL (1 mL); 20 mcg/mL (1 mL)

iloprost tromethamine *see* iloprost *on page* *499*

Ilozyme® ***(Discontinued)*** *see* pancrelipase *on page* *723*

imatinib (eye MAT eh nib)

Sound-Alike/Look-Alike Issues

imatinib may be confused with dasatinib, erlotinib, nilotinib, sorafenib, sunitinib

Synonyms CGP-57148B; glivec; imatinib mesylate; STI-571

U.S./Canadian Brand Names Gleevec® [US/Can]

Therapeutic Category Antineoplastic Agent, Tyrosine Kinase Inhibitor

Use Treatment of:

Gastrointestinal stromal tumors (GIST) kit-positive (CD117), including unresectable and/or metastatic malignant and adjuvant treatment following complete resection

Philadelphia chromosome-positive (Ph+) chronic myeloid leukemia (CML) in chronic phase (newly-diagnosed)

Ph+ CML in chronic phase in pediatric patients recurring following stem cell transplant or who are resistant to interferon-alpha therapy (**not** an approved use in Canada)

Ph+ CML in blast crisis, accelerated phase, or chronic phase after failure of interferon therapy

Ph+ acute lymphoblastic leukemia (ALL) (relapsed or refractory)

Aggressive systemic mastocytosis (ASM) without D816V c-Kit mutation (or c-Kit mutation status unknown)

Dermatofibrosarcoma protuberans (DFSP) (unresectable, recurrent and/or metastatic)

Hypereosinophilic syndrome (HES) and/or chronic eosinophilic leukemia (CEL)

Myelodysplastic/myeloproliferative disease (MDS/MPD) associated with platelet-derived growth factor receptor (PDGFR) gene rearrangements

Note: The following use is approved in Canada (not an approved indication in the U.S.):

Ph+ ALL induction therapy (newly diagnosed)

Dosage Summary

Oral:

Children <2 years: Dosage not established

Children ≥2 years: 260-340 mg/m^2/day in 1-2 divided doses (maximum: 600 mg/day)

Adults: 100-800 mg/day in 1-2 divided doses

Dosage Forms

Tablet, oral:

Gleevec®: 100 mg, 400 mg

imatinib mesylate *see* imatinib *on page* *499*

IMC-C225 *see* cetuximab *on page* *199*

Imdur® [US/Can] *see* isosorbide mononitrate *on page* *529*

123I-metaiodobenzylguanidine (MIBG) *see* iobenguane I 123 *on page* *517*

imferon *see* iron dextran complex *on page* *525*

IMI 30 *see* idarubicin *on page* *497*

IMid-1 *see* lenalidomide *on page* *552*

imidazole carboxamide *see* dacarbazine *on page* *265*

imidazole carboxamide dimethyltriazene *see* dacarbazine *on page* *265*

imiglucerase (i mi GLOO ser ace)

Sound-Alike/Look-Alike Issues

Cerezyme® may be confused with Cerebyx®, Ceredase®

U.S./Canadian Brand Names Cerezyme® [US/Can]

Therapeutic Category Enzyme

Use Long-term enzyme replacement therapy for patients with Type 1 Gaucher disease

Dosage Summary

I.V.:

Children <2 years: Dosage not established

Children ≥2 years: Initial: 30-60 units/kg every 2 weeks; Range: 2.5 units/kg 3 times/week to 60 units/kg once weekly; Average dose: 60 units/kg every 2 weeks

Adults: Initial: 30-60 units/kg every 2 weeks; Range: 2.5 units/kg 3 times/week to 60 units/kg once weekly; Average dose: 60 units/kg every 2 weeks

Dosage Forms

Injection, powder for reconstitution:

Cerezyme®: 200 units, 400 units

imipemide *see* imipenem and cilastatin *on page 500*

imipenem and cilastatin (i mi PEN em & sye la STAT in)

Sound-Alike/Look-Alike Issues

imipenem may be confused with ertapenem, meropenem

Primaxin® may be confused with Premarin®, Primacor®

Synonyms imipemide

U.S./Canadian Brand Names Primaxin® I.V. [Can]; Primaxin® [US/Can]

Therapeutic Category Carbapenem (Antibiotic)

Use Treatment of lower respiratory tract, urinary tract, intraabdominal, gynecologic, bone and joint, skin and skin structure, and polymicrobic infections as well as bacterial septicemia and endocarditis. Antibacterial activity includes resistant gram-negative bacilli (*Pseudomonas aeruginosa* and *Enterobacter* sp), gram-positive bacteria (methicillin-sensitive *Staphylococcus aureus* and *Streptococcus* sp) and anaerobes.

Dosage Summary

I.M.:

Children: Dosage not established

Adults: 500-750 mg every 12 hours

I.V.:

Neonates <1 week and ≥1500 g: 25 mg/kg every 12 hours

Neonates 1-4 weeks and ≥1500 g: 25 mg/kg every 8 hours

Neonates 4 weeks to 3 months and ≥1500 g: 25 mg/kg every 6 hours

Children >3 months: 15-25 mg/kg every 6 hours (maximum: 4 g/day)

Adults 30 to <70 kg: 125 mg every 12 hours up to 1000 mg every 8 hours (weight dependent)

Adults ≥70 kg: 250-1000 mg every 6-8 hours (maximum: 50 mg/kg/day; 4 g/day)

Dosage Forms

Injection, powder for reconstitution [I.M.]:

Primaxin®: Imipenem 500 mg and cilastatin 500 mg

Injection, powder for reconstitution [I.V.]:

Primaxin®: Imipenem 250 mg and cilastatin 250 mg; imipenem 500 mg and cilastatin 500 mg

imipramine (im IP ra meen)

Sound-Alike/Look-Alike Issues

imipramine may be confused with amitriptyline, desipramine, Norpramin®

Synonyms imipramine hydrochloride; imipramine pamoate

U.S./Canadian Brand Names Apo-Imipramine® [Can]; Novo-Pramine [Can]; Tofranil-PM® [US]; Tofranil® [US/Can]

Therapeutic Category Antidepressant, Tricyclic (Tertiary Amine)

Use Treatment of depression; treatment of nocturnal enuresis in children

Dosage Summary

Oral:

Children <6 years: Dosage not established

Children ≥6-12 years: Initial: 25 mg at bedtime, may increase to 50 mg at bedtime if no response (maximum: 2.5 mg/kg/day; 50 mg/day)

Children >12 years: Initial: 25 mg at bedtime, may increase to 75 mg at bedtime if not response (maximum: 75 mg/day) **or** 30-40 mg/day, increase gradually, to a maximum of 100 mg/day in single or divided doses

Adults: Initial: 75-150 mg/day, increase gradually to a maximum of 200 mg/day (outpatients) or 300 mg/day (inpatients) in divided doses or a single dose at bedtime

Elderly: Initial: 10-25 mg at bedtime; Maintenance: 50-150 mg/day **or** 10-50 mg at bedtime or twice daily; **Note:** Titration is recommended

Dosage Forms

Capsule, oral: 75 mg, 100 mg, 125 mg, 150 mg

Tofranil-PM®: 75 mg, 100 mg, 125 mg, 150 mg

Tablet, oral: 10 mg, 25 mg, 50 mg

Tofranil®: 10 mg, 25 mg, 50 mg

imipramine hydrochloride *see* imipramine *on page* *500*

imipramine pamoate *see* imipramine *on page* *500*

imiquimod (i mi KWI mod)

Sound-Alike/Look-Alike Issues

Aldara® may be confused with Alora®, Lialda™

U.S./Canadian Brand Names Aldara® [US/Can]; Zyclara™ [US/Can]

Therapeutic Category Immune Response Modifier

Use Treatment of external genital and perianal warts/condyloma acuminata; nonhyperkeratotic actinic keratosis on face or scalp; superficial basal cell carcinoma (sBCC) with a maximum tumor diameter of 2 cm located on the trunk, neck, or extremities (excluding hands or feet)

Dosage Summary

Topical:

Children <12 years: Dosage not established

Children ≥12 years: Apply a thin layer 3 times/week on alternate days, leave on for 6-10 hours

Adults:

Actinic keratosis: Apply twice weekly up to 16 weeks or once daily at bedtime for 2 treatment cycles (14 days each) separated by a 14-day rest period with no treatment, leave on for 8 hours

External genital and/or perianal warts/condyloma acuminata: Apply a thin layer 3 times/week on alternate days, leave on for 6-10 hours

Superficial basal cell carcinoma: Apply once daily at bedtime 5 days/week; leave on for 8 hours before washing

Dosage Forms

Cream, topical: 5% (24s)

Aldara®: 5% (24s)

Zyclara™: 3.75% (28s)

Imitrex® [US/Can] *see* sumatriptan *on page* *904*

Imitrex® DF [Can] *see* sumatriptan *on page* *904*

Imitrex® Nasal Spray [Can] *see* sumatriptan *on page* *904*

ImmuCyst® [Can] *see* BCG *on page* *118*

immune globulin (intramuscular) (i MYUN GLOB yoo lin, IN tra MUS kyoo ler)

Synonyms gamma globulin; IG; IGIM; immune serum globulin; ISG

U.S./Canadian Brand Names BayGam® [Can]; GammaSTAN™ S/D [US]

Therapeutic Category Immune Globulin

Use To provide passive immunity in susceptible individuals under the following circumstances:

Hepatitis A: Within 14 days of exposure and prior to manifestation of disease

Measles: For use within 6 days of exposure in an unvaccinated person, who has not previously had measles

Varicella: When Varicella Zoster Immune Globulin is not available

Rubella: Postexposure prophylaxis (within 72 hours) to reduce the risk of infection in exposed pregnant women who will not consider therapeutic abortion

Immunoglobulin deficiency: To help prevent serious infections

Dosage Summary

I.M.:

Children:

Hepatitis A:

Pre-exposure prophylaxis upon travel into endemic areas:

0.02 mL/kg for anticipated risk of exposure <3 months

0.06 mL/kg for anticipated risk of exposure ≥3 months

Postexposure prophylaxis: 0.02 mL/kg

Measles:

Prophylaxis, immunocompetent: 0.25 mL/kg/dose (maximum dose: 15 mL)

Prophylaxis, immunocompromised: 0.5 mL/kg (maximum dose: 15 mL)

Rubella: Prophylaxis during pregnancy: 0.55 mL/kg/dose

Varicella: Prophylaxis: 0.6-1.2 mL/kg

IgG deficiency: 0.66 mL/kg/dose; a double dose may be given at onset of therapy

Adults:

Hepatitis A:

Pre-exposure prophylaxis upon travel into endemic areas:

0.02 mL/kg for anticipated risk of exposure <3 months

0.06 mL/kg for anticipated risk of exposure ≥3 months

Postexposure prophylaxis: 0.02 mL/kg

Measles:

Prophylaxis, immunocompetent: 0.25 mL/kg/dose (maximum dose: 15 mL)

Prophylaxis, immunocompromised: 0.5 mL/kg (maximum dose: 15 mL)

Rubella: Prophylaxis during pregnancy: 0.55 mL/kg/dose

Varicella: Prophylaxis: 0.6-1.2 mL/kg

IgG deficiency: 0.66 mL/kg/dose; a double dose may be given at onset of therapy

Dosage Forms

Injection, solution [preservative free]:

GamaSTAN™ S/D: 15% to 18% (2 mL, 10 mL)

immune globulin (intravenous) (i MYUN GLOB yoo lin, IN tra VEE nus)

Sound-Alike/Look-Alike Issues

immune globulin (intravenous) may be confused with hepatitis B immune globulin

Gamimune® N may be confused with CytoGam®

Synonyms IGIV; IV immune globulin; IVIG; panglobulin

U.S./Canadian Brand Names Carimune® NF [US]; Flebogamma® DIF [US]; Flebogamma® [US]; Gamimune® N [Can]; Gammagard S/D® [US/Can]; Gammagard® Liquid [US/Can]; Gamunex® [US/Can]; IGIVnex® [Can]; Octagam® [US]; Privigen® [US/Can]

Therapeutic Category Immune Globulin

Use

Treatment of primary immunodeficiency syndromes (congenital agammaglobulinemia, severe combined immunodeficiency syndromes [SCIDS], common variable immunodeficiency, X-linked immunodeficiency, Wiskott-Aldrich syndrome) (Carimune® NF, Flebogamma®, Gammagard Liquid, Gammagard S/D, Gamunex®, Octagam®, Privigen®)

Treatment of immune (idiopathic) thrombocytopenic purpura (ITP) (Carimune® NF, Gammagard S/D, Gamunex®, Privigen®)

Treatment of chronic inflammatory demyelinating polyneuropathy (CIDP) (Gamunex®)

Prevention of coronary artery aneurysms associated with Kawasaki disease (in combination with aspirin) (Gammagard S/D)

Prevention of bacterial infection in B-cell chronic lymphocytic leukemia (CLL) (Gammagard S/D)

Dosage Summary

I.V.:

Children:

CLL: 400 mg/kg/dose every 3-4 weeks

HSCT: 400 mg/kg per month

ITP: 400 mg/kg/day for 2-5 days **or** 1000 mg/kg/day for 1-2 days

Kawasaki disease: 2000 mg/kg as a single dose **or** 1000 mg as a single dose **or** 400 mg/kg /day for 4 days

Pediatric HIV: 400 mg/kg every 2-4 weeks

Primary immunodeficiency disorders: 200-800 mg/kg every 3-4 weeks

Adolescents: HSCT: 500 mg/kg/week

Adults:
CLL: 400 mg/kg/dose every 3-4 weeks
CIDP: Loading dose: 2000 mg/kg divided over 2-4 consecutive days; Maintenance: 1000 mg/kg/day for 1 day every 3 weeks **or** 500 mg/kg/day for 2 consecutive days every 3 weeks
HSCT: 500 mg/kg/week
ITP: 400 mg/kg/day for 5 days **or** 1000 mg/kg/day for 1-2 days
Kawasaki disease: 2000 mg/kg as a single dose **or** 1000 mg/kg as a single dose **or** 400 mg/kg/day for 4 days
Primary immunodeficiency disorders: 200-800 mg/kg every 3-4 weeks

Dosage Forms
Injection, powder for reconstitution [preservative free]:
Carimune® NF: 3 g, 6 g, 12 g
Gammagard S/D®: 0.5 g, 2.5 g, 5 g, 10 g
Injection, solution [preservative free]:
Flebogamma®: 5% [50 mg/mL] (10 mL, 50 mL, 100 mL, 200 mL)
Flebogamma® DIF: 5% [50 mg/mL] (10 mL, 50 mL, 100 mL, 200 mL, 400 mL)
Gammagard® Liquid: 10% [100 mg/mL] (10 mL, 25 mL, 50 mL, 100 mL, 200 mL)
Gamunex®: 10% [100 mg/mL] (10 mL, 25 mL, 50 mL, 100 mL, 200 mL)
Octagam®: 5% [50 mg/mL] (20 mL, 50 mL, 100 mL, 200 mL)
Privigen®: 10% [100 mg/mL] (50 mL, 100 mL, 200 mL)

immune globulin (subcutaneous) (i MYUN GLOB yoo lin sub kyoo TAY nee us)

Synonyms immune globulin subcutaneous (human); SCIG
U.S./Canadian Brand Names Hizentra™ [US]; Vivaglobin® [US]
Therapeutic Category Immune Globulin
Use Treatment of primary humoral immunodeficiency (PI)
Dosage Summary
SubQ:
Hizentra™:
Children: Initial dose: Multiply previous I.V. dose (in grams) by 1.53, then divide by number of weeks between I.V. dose (eg, if the dosing interval was every 3 weeks, divide by 3); adjust dose based on clinical response and serum IgG trough concentration
Measles prevention: ≥200 mg/kg once weekly for 2 consecutive weeks
Adults: Initial dose: Multiply previous I.V. dose (in grams) by 1.53, then divide by number of weeks between I.V. dose (eg, if the dosing interval was every 3 weeks, divide by 3); adjust dose based on clinical response and serum IgG trough concentration
Measles prevention: ≥200 mg/kg once weekly for 2 consecutive weeks
Vivaglobin®:
Children: Initial dose: Multiply previous I.V. dose (in grams) by 1.37, then divide by number of weeks between I.V. dose (eg, if the dosing interval was every 3 weeks, divide by 3); adjust dose based on clinical response and serum IgG trough concentration
Adults: Initial dose: Multiply previous I.V. dose (in grams) by 1.37, then divide by number of weeks between I.V. dose (eg, if the dosing interval was every 3 weeks, divide by 3); adjust dose based on clinical response and serum IgG trough concentration

Dosage Forms
Injection, solution [preservative free]:
Hizentra™: 200 mg/mL (5 mL, 10 mL, 20 mL)
Vivaglobin®: 160 mg/mL (3 mL, 10 mL, 20 mL)

immune globulin subcutaneous (human) *see* immune globulin (subcutaneous) *on page* 503
immune serum globulin *see* immune globulin (intramuscular) *on page* 501
Immunine® VH [Can] *see* factor IX *on page* 389
Imodium® [Can] *see* loperamide *on page* 573
Imodium® A-D [US-OTC] *see* loperamide *on page* 573
Imodium® A-D for children [US-OTC] *see* loperamide *on page* 573
Imodium® Advanced *(Discontinued)* *see* loperamide and simethicone *on page* 574
Imodium® Advanced Multi-Symptom [Can] *see* loperamide and simethicone *on page* 574
Imodium® Multi-Symptom Relief [US-OTC] *see* loperamide and simethicone *on page* 574
Imogam® Rabies-HT [US] *see* rabies immune globulin (human) *on page* 824
Imogam® Rabies Pasteurized [Can] *see* rabies immune globulin (human) *on page* 824

Imovane® [Can] *see* zopiclone *(Canada only) on page 1005*
Imovax® Rabies [US/Can] *see* rabies vaccine *on page 825*
Implanon™ [US] *see* etonogestrel *on page 384*
Imuran® [US/Can] *see* azathioprine *on page 109*
In-111 ibritumomab *see* ibritumomab *on page 494*
In-111 zevalin *see* ibritumomab *on page 494*

inamrinone (eye NAM ri none)

Sound-Alike/Look-Alike Issues
amrinone may be confused with aMILoride, amiodarone

Synonyms amrinone lactate

Therapeutic Category Adrenergic Agonist Agent

Use Short-term therapy in patients with intractable heart failure

Dosage Summary

I.V.:
Adults: Bolus: 0.75 mg/kg, may repeat; Infusion: 5-10 mcg/kg/minute

Dosage Forms

Injection, solution: 5 mg/mL (20 mL)

I-Naphline® Ophthalmic ***(Discontinued)*** *see* naphazoline (ophthalmic) *on page 658*
Inapsine® ***(Discontinued)*** *see* droperidol *on page 334*

incobotulinumtoxinA (in kuh BOT yoo lin num TOKS in aye)

Synonyms botulinum toxin type A

U.S./Canadian Brand Names Xeomin® [US]

Therapeutic Category Neuromuscular Blocker Agent, Toxin; Ophthalmic Agent, Toxin

Use Treatment of blepharospasm in patients previously treated with onabotulinumtoxinA; treatment of cervical dystonia in botulinum toxin-naïve and previously-treated patients

Product Availability Xeomin®: FDA approved August 2010; availability expected late September 2010; consult prescribing information for additional information

Increlex™ [US] *see* mecasermin *on page 594*

indapamide (in DAP a mide)

Sound-Alike/Look-Alike Issues
indapamide may be confused with Iopidine®

U.S./Canadian Brand Names Apo-Indapamide® [Can]; Dom-Indapamide [Can]; Lozide® [Can]; Lozol® [Can]; Mylan-Indapamide [Can]; Novo-Indapamide [Can]; Nu-Indapamide [Can]; PHL-Indapamide [Can]; PMS-Indapamide [Can]; PRO-Indapamide [Can]; Riva-Indapamide [Can]

Therapeutic Category Diuretic, Miscellaneous

Use Management of mild-to-moderate hypertension; treatment of edema in heart failure and nephrotic syndrome

Dosage Summary

Oral:
Children: Dosage not established
Adults: 1.25-5 mg once daily

Dosage Forms

Tablet, oral: 1.25 mg, 2.5 mg

indapamide and perindopril erbumine *see* perindopril erbumine and indapamide *(Canada only) on page 744*
Inderal® [Can] *see* propranolol *on page 806*
Inderal® ***(Discontinued)*** *see* propranolol *on page 806*
Inderal® LA [US/Can] *see* propranolol *on page 806*
Inderide® ***(Discontinued)*** *see* propranolol and hydrochlorothiazide *on page 807*
indigo carmine *see* indigotindisulfonate sodium *on page 504*

indigotindisulfonate sodium (in di goe tin dye SUL foe nate SOW dee um)

Synonyms indigo carmine

Therapeutic Category Diagnostic Agent, Kidney Function

Use Localizing ureteral orifices during cystoscopy and ureteral catheterization

Dosage Summary

I.M.:

Infants: <5 mL
Children: <5 mL
Adults: 5 mL

I.V.:

Infants: <5 mL
Children: <5 mL
Adults: 5 mL

Dosage Forms

Injection, solution: 8 mg/mL (5 mL)

indinavir (in DIN a veer)

Sound-Alike/Look-Alike Issues

indinavir may be confused with Denavir™

Synonyms indinavir sulfate

U.S./Canadian Brand Names Crixivan® [US/Can]

Therapeutic Category Antiviral Agent

Use Treatment of HIV infection; should always be used as part of a multidrug regimen (at least three antirctroviral agents)

Dosage Summary

Oral:

Children: Dosage not established
Adults: 800 mg every 8 hours; Boosted regimen: 400-800 mg every 12 hours

Dosage Forms

Capsule, oral:

Crixivan®: 100 mg, 200 mg, 400 mg

indinavir sulfate *see* indinavir *on page 505*
Indocid® P.D.A. [Can] *see* indomethacin *on page 505*
Indocin® [US] *see* indomethacin *on page 505*
Indocin® I.V. [US] *see* indomethacin *on page 505*

indocyanine green (in doe SYE a neen green)

U.S./Canadian Brand Names IC-Green™ [US]

Therapeutic Category Diagnostic Agent

Use Determining hepatic function, cardiac output, and liver blood flow; ophthalmic angiography

Dosage Summary

Cardiac catheter:

Infants: 1.25 mg (maximum total dose: 2 mg/kg)
Children: 2.5 mg (maximum total dose: 2 mg/kg)
Adults: 5 mg (maximum total dose: 2 mg/kg)

I.V.:

Ophthalmic angiography:

Children: Dosage not established
Adults: ≤40 mg bolus

Hepatic function:

Children: Dosage not established
Adults: 0.5 mg/kg

Dosage Forms

Injection, powder for reconstitution: 25 mg

IC-Green™: 25 mg

indometacin *see* indomethacin *on page 505*

indomethacin (in doe METH a sin)

Sound-Alike/Look-Alike Issues

Indocin® may be confused with Imodium®, Lincocin®, Minocin®, Vicodin®

Synonyms indometacin; indomethacin sodium trihydrate

U.S./Canadian Brand Names Apo-Indomethacin® [Can]; Indocid® P.D.A. [Can]; Indocin® I.V. [US]; Indocin® [US]; Novo-Methacin [Can]; Nu-Indo [Can]; Pro-Indo [Can]; ratio-Indomethacin [Can]; Sandoz-Indomethacin [Can]

Therapeutic Category Analgesic, Nonnarcotic; Nonsteroidal Antiinflammatory Drug (NSAID)

Use Acute gouty arthritis, acute bursitis/tendonitis, moderate-to-severe osteoarthritis, rheumatoid arthritis, ankylosing spondylitis; I.V. form used as alternative to surgery for closure of patent ductus arteriosus in neonates

Dosage Summary

I.V.:

Neonates <48 hours old at time of first dose: Initial: 0.2 mg/kg, followed by 2 doses of 0.1 mg/kg at 12- to 24- hour intervals

Neonates 2-7 days old at time of first dose: Initial: 0.2 mg/kg, followed by 2 doses of 0.2 mg/kg at 12- to 24-hour intervals

Neonates >7 days old at time of first dose: Initial: 0.2 mg/kg, followed by 0.25 mg/kg at 12- to 24-hour intervals

Children: Dosage not established

Adults: Dosage not established

Oral:

Extended release:

Children ≤14 years: Dosage not established

Children >14 years: 75-150 mg/day in 1-2 divided doses (maximum: 150 mg/day)

Adults: 75-150 mg/day in 1-2 divided doses (maximum: 150 mg/day)

Immediate release:

Children ≥2 years: 1-2 mg/kg/day in 2-4 divided doses (maximum: 4 mg/kg/day; 200 mg/day)

Adults: 50-150 mg/day in 2-4 divided doses (maximum: 200 mg/day)

Dosage Forms

Caplet, extended release, oral: 75 mg

Capsule, oral: 25 mg, 50 mg

Capsule, extended release, oral: 75 mg

Injection, powder for reconstitution: 1 mg

Indocin® I.V.: 1 mg

Suppository, rectal: 50 mg (30s)

Suspension, oral:

Indocin®: 25 mg/5 mL (237 mL)

indomethacin sodium trihydrate *see* indomethacin *on page* 505

INF-alpha 2 *see* interferon alfa-2b *on page* 514

Infanrix® [US] *see* diphtheria, tetanus toxoids, and acellular pertussis vaccine *on page* 316

Infantaire [US-OTC] *see* acetaminophen *on page* 21

Infantaire Gas [US-OTC] *see* simethicone *on page* 875

Infants Gas Relief Drops [US-OTC] *see* simethicone *on page* 875

Infants' Tylenol® Cold Plus Cough Concentrated Drops *(Discontinued)*

Infasurf® [US] *see* calfactant *on page* 172

INFeD® [US] *see* iron dextran complex *on page* 525

Infergen® [US] *see* interferon alfacon-1 *on page* 515

infliximab (in FLIKS e mab)

Sound-Alike/Look-Alike Issues

inFLIXimab may be confused with riTUXimab

Remicade® may be confused with Renacidin®, Rituxan®

Synonyms avakine; infliximab, recombinant

Tall-Man in**FLIX**imab

U.S./Canadian Brand Names Remicade® [US/Can]

Therapeutic Category Monoclonal Antibody

Use

Treatment of moderately- to severely-active rheumatoid arthritis (with methotrexate)

Treatment of moderately- to severely-active Crohn disease with inadequate response to conventional therapy (to reduce signs/symptoms and induce and maintain clinical remission) or to reduce the number of draining enterocutaneous and rectovaginal fistulas and maintain fistula closure

Treatment of psoriatic arthritis (to reduce signs/symptoms of active arthritis and inhibit progression of structural damage and improve physical function)

Treatment of chronic severe plaque psoriasis

Treatment of active ankylosing spondylitis (reduce signs/symptoms)

Treatment of moderately- to severely-active ulcerative colitis with inadequate response to conventional therapy (reduce signs/symptoms and induce and maintain clinical remission, mucosal healing and eliminate corticosteroid use)

Dosage Summary

I.V.:

Children: U.S. labeling <6 years, Canadian labeling <9 years: Dosage not established

Children: U.S. labeling ≥6 years, Canadian labeling ≥9 years: Initial: 5 mg/kg at 0, 2, and 6 weeks; Maintenance: 5 mg/kg every 8 weeks (Crohn's disease)

Adults: Initial: 3-10 mg/kg (specific dose varies by indication) at 0, 2, and 6 weeks; Maintenance: 3-10 mg/kg every 8 weeks **or** 5 mg/kg every 6 weeks

Dosage Forms

Injection, powder for reconstitution:

Remicade®: 100 mg

infliximab, recombinant *see* infliximab *on page 506*

influenza vaccine *see* influenza virus vaccine (inactivated) *on page 507*

influenza vaccine *see* influenza virus vaccine (live/attenuated) *on page 508*

influenza virus vaccine (H1N1, inactivated) *(Discontinued)*

influenza virus vaccine (H1N1, live/attenuated) *(Discontinued)*

influenza virus vaccine (H5N1) (in floo EN za VYE rus vak SEEN H5N1)

Sound-Alike/Look-Alike Issues

influenza virus vaccine (H5N1) may be confused with the nonavian strain of influenza virus vaccine

Synonyms avian influenza virus vaccine; bird flu vaccine; H5N1 influenza vaccine; influenza virus vaccine (monovalent)

Therapeutic Category Vaccine

Use Active immunization of adults at increased risk of exposure to the H5N1 viral subtype of influenza

Dosage Summary

I.M.:

Children: Dosage not established

Adults 18-64 years: 1 mL, followed by second 1 mL dose given 28 days later

Dosage Forms

Injection, suspension: Hemagglutinin (H5N1strain) 90 mcg/mL (5 mL)

influenza virus vaccine (inactivated) (in floo EN za VYE rus vak SEEN, in ak ti VAY ted)

Sound-Alike/Look-Alike Issues

influenza virus vaccine may be confused with flumazenil

influenza virus vaccine may be confused with tetanus toxoid and tuberculin products. Medication errors have occurred when tuberculin skin tests (PPD) have been inadvertently administered instead of tetanus toxoid products and influenza virus vaccine. These products are refrigerated and often stored in close proximity to each other.

influenza virus vaccine (human strain) may be confused with the avian strain (H5N1) of influenza virus vaccine or the influenza A (H1N1) 2009 vaccine

Fluarix® may be confused with Flarex®

Synonyms influenza vaccine; influenza virus vaccine (purified surface antigen); influenza virus vaccine (split-virus); trivalent inactivated influenza vaccine (TIV)

U.S./Canadian Brand Names Afluria® [US]; Agriflu® [US]; Fluarix® [US]; FluLaval® [US]; Fluviral S/F® [Can]; Fluvirin® [US]; Fluzone® High-Dose [Can]; Fluzone® [US]; Vaxigrip® [Can]

Therapeutic Category Vaccine, Inactivated (Viral)

Use Provide active immunity to influenza virus strains contained in the vaccine

Advisory Committee on Immunization Practices (ACIP) recommends annual vaccination with the seasonal trivalent inactivated influenza vaccine (TIV) (injection) for all children (6 months to 18 years) and adults. Target groups for vaccination (those at higher risk of complications from influenza infection and their close contacts) include the following:

- Persons ≥50 years of age
- Residents of nursing homes and other chronic-care facilities that house persons of any age with chronic medical conditions
- Adults and children with chronic disorders of the pulmonary or cardiovascular systems (except hypertension), including asthma
- Adults and children who have chronic metabolic diseases (including diabetes mellitus), hepatic disease, renal dysfunction, hematologic disorders, hemoglobinopathies, or immunosuppression (including immunosuppression caused by medications or HIV)
- Adults and children with cognitive or neurologic/neuromuscular conditions (including conditions such as spinal cord injuries or seizure disorders) which may compromise respiratory function, the handling of respiratory secretions, or that can increase the risk of aspiration
- Children and adolescents (6 months to 18 years of age) who are receiving long-term aspirin therapy, and therefore, may be at risk for developing Reye syndrome after influenza
- Women who will be pregnant during the influenza season
- Children 6-59 months of age
- Healthcare personnel
- Household contacts and caregivers of children <5 years (particularly children <6 months) and adults ≥50 years
- Household contacts and caregivers of persons with medical conditions which put them at high risk of complications from influenza infection

The Advisory Committee on Immunization Practices (ACIP) states that healthy, nonpregnant persons aged 2-49 years may receive vaccination with either the seasonal live, attenuated influenza vaccine (LAIV) (nasal spray) or the seasonal trivalent inactivated influenza vaccine (TIV) (injection).

Dosage Summary Note: Children <9 years who are not previously vaccinated or who received only 1 dose of vaccine during the previous season should receive 2 doses separated by ≥ 4 weeks, in order to achieve satisfactory antibody response.

I.M.:

Children <6 months: Dosage not established
Children 6-35 months: Afluria®, Fluzone®: 0.25 mL/dose (1 or 2 doses per season; see **"Note"**)
Children 3-8 years: Afluria®, Fluarix®, Fluzone®: 0.5 mL/dose (1 or 2 doses per season; see **"Note"**)
Children 4-8 years: Fluvirin®: 0.5 mL/dose (1 or 2 doses per season; see **"Note"**)
Children ≥9 years: Afluria®, Fluarix®, Fluvirin®, Fluzone®: 0.5 mL/dose (1 dose per season)
Adults: Afluria®, Agriflu®, Fluarix®, FluLaval®, Fluvirin®, Fluzone®: 0.5 mL/dose (1 dose per season)
Adults ≥65 years: Afluria®, Agriflu®, Fluarix®, FluLaval®, Fluvirin®, Fluzone®, Fluzone® High-Dose: 0.5 mL/dose (1 dose per season)

Dosage Forms

Injection, suspension:
Afluria®: Hemagglutinin 45 mcg/0.5 mL (5 mL)
FluLaval®: Hemagglutinin 45 mcg/0.5 mL (5 mL)
Fluvirin®: Hemagglutinin 45 mcg/0.5 mL (5 mL)
Fluzone®: Hemagglutinin 45 mcg/0.5 mL (5 mL)

Injection, suspension [preservative free]:
Afluria®: Hemagglutinin 45 mcg/0.5 mL (0.5 mL)
Agriflu®: Hemagglutinin 45 mcg/0.5 mL (0.5 mL)
Fluarix®: Hemagglutinin 45 mcg/0.5 mL (0.5 mL)
Fluvirin®: Hemagglutinin 45 mcg/0.5 mL (0.5 mL)
Fluzone®: Hemagglutinin 22.5 mcg/0.25 mL (0.25 mL); Hemagglutinin 45 mcg/0.5 mL (0.5 mL)
Fluzone® High-Dose: Hemagglutinin 180 mcg/0.5 mL (0.5 mL)

influenza virus vaccine (live/attenuated) (in floo EN za VYE rus vak SEEN)

Sound-Alike/Look-Alike Issues

influenza virus vaccine may be confused with flumazenil
influenza virus vaccine (human strain) may be confused with the avian strain (H5N1) of influenza virus vaccine or the influenza A (H1N1) 2009 vaccine

Synonyms influenza vaccine; influenza virus vaccine (trivalent, live); live attenuated influenza vaccine (LAIV)

U.S./Canadian Brand Names FluMist® [US]

Therapeutic Category Vaccine, Live (Viral)

Use Provide active immunity to influenza virus strains contained in the vaccine

The Advisory Committee on Immunization Practices (ACIP) states that healthy, nonpregnant persons aged 2-49 years may receive vaccination with either the seasonal live, attenuated influenza vaccine (LAIV) (nasal spray) or the seasonal trivalent inactivated influenza vaccine (TIV) (injection).

Dosage Summary Note: Children <9 years who are not previously vaccinated or who received only 1 dose of vaccine during the previous season should receive 2 doses separated by ≥4 weeks, in order to achieve satisfactory antibody response. Refer to current guidelines.

Intranasal:

Children <2 years: Dosage not established

*Children 2-8 years (see **"Note"**):* Previously not vaccinated: Two doses (0.2 mL/dose) separated by at least 4 weeks; Previously vaccinated: 0.2 mL/dose (1 dose per season)

Children ≥9 years: 0.2 mL/dose (1 dose per season)

Adults ≤49 years: 0.2 mL/dose (1 dose per season)

Dosage Forms

Solution, intranasal [preservative free]:

FluMist®: (0.2 mL)

influenza virus vaccine (monovalent) *see* influenza virus vaccine (H5N1) *on page 507*

influenza virus vaccine (purified surface antigen) *see* influenza virus vaccine (inactivated) *on page 507*

influenza virus vaccine (split-virus) *see* influenza virus vaccine (inactivated) *on page 507*

influenza virus vaccine (trivalent, live) *see* influenza virus vaccine (live/attenuated) *on page 508*

Infufer® [Can] *see* iron dextran complex *on page 525*

Infumorph® 200 [US] *see* morphine (systemic) *on page 644*

Infumorph® 500 [US] *see* morphine (systemic) *on page 644*

Infuvite® Adult [US] *see* vitamins (multiple/injectable) *on page 989*

Infuvite® Pediatric [US] *see* vitamins (multiple/injectable) *on page 989*

INH *see* isoniazid *on page 527*

Inhibace® [Can] *see* cilazapril *(Canada only) on page 222*

Inhibace® Plus [Can] *see* cilazapril and hydrochlorothiazide *(Canada only) on page 222*

Innohep® [US/Can] *see* tinzaparin *on page 935*

InnoPran XL® [US] *see* propranolol *on page 806*

Inocor® ***(Discontinued)***

INOmax® [US/Can] *see* nitric oxide *on page 678*

Inova™ [US] *see* benzoyl peroxide *on page 128*

insect sting kit *see* epinephrine and chlorpheniramine *on page 354*

insoluble prussian blue *see* ferric hexacyanoferrate *on page 397*

Inspra™ [US] *see* eplerenone *on page 355*

Insta-Glucose® [US-OTC] *see* dextrose *on page 290*

Instat™ [US] *see* collagen hemostat *on page 248*

Instat™ MCH [US] *see* collagen hemostat *on page 248*

insulin aspart (IN soo lin AS part)

Sound-Alike/Look-Alike Issues

NovoLog® may be confused with Humalog®, Humulin® R, Novolin® N, Novolin® R, NovoLog® Mix 70/30

Synonyms aspart insulin

U.S./Canadian Brand Names NovoLog® [US]; NovoRapid® [Can]

Therapeutic Category Antidiabetic Agent, Insulin

Use Treatment of type 1 diabetes mellitus (insulin-dependent, IDDM) and type 2 diabetes mellitus (noninsulin-dependent, NIDDM) to improve glycemic control

Dosage Summary Note: When compared to insulin regular, insulin aspart has a more rapid onset and shorter duration of activity.

I.V.:

Children: Dosage not established.

Adults: Refer to Insulin Regular on page 513

SubQ:

Children <2 years: Dosage not established

Children ≥2 years: Refer to Insulin Regular on page 513

Adults: Refer to Insulin Regular on page 513

Dosage Forms

Injection, solution:

NovoLog®: 100 units/mL (3 mL, 10 mL)

insulin aspart and insulin aspart protamine *see* insulin aspart protamine and insulin aspart *on page 510*

insulin aspart protamine and insulin aspart

(IN soo lin AS part PROE ta meen & IN soo lin AS part)

Sound-Alike/Look-Alike Issues

NovoLog® Mix 70/30 may be confused with Humalog® Mix 75/25™, Humulin® 70/30, Novolin® 70/30, NovoLog®

Synonyms insulin aspart and insulin aspart protamine

U.S./Canadian Brand Names NovoLog® Mix 70/30 [US]; NovoMix® 30 [Can]

Therapeutic Category Antidiabetic Agent, Insulin

Use Treatment of type 1 diabetes mellitus (insulin-dependent, IDDM) and type 2 diabetes mellitus (noninsulin-dependent, NIDDM) to improve glycemic control

Dosage Summary Note: Insulin aspart protamine and insulin aspart combination products are approximately equipotent to insulin NPH and insulin regular combination products but with a more rapid onset and similar duration of activity. The proportion of rapid-acting to long-acting insulin is fixed in the combination products; basal versus prandial dose adjustments cannot be made.

SubQ:

Children: Dosage not established

Adults: Refer to Insulin Regular on page 513

Dosage Forms

Injection, suspension:

NovoLog® Mix 70/30: Insulin aspart protamine suspension 70% [intermediate acting] and insulin aspart solution 30% [rapid acting]: 100 units/mL (3 mL) [FlexPen® prefilled syringe]; (10 mL) [vial]

insulin detemir (IN soo lin DE te mir)

Synonyms detemir insulin

U.S./Canadian Brand Names Levemir® [US/Can]

Therapeutic Category Antidiabetic Agent, Insulin

Use Treatment of type 1 diabetes mellitus (insulin-dependent, IDDM) and type 2 diabetes mellitus (noninsulin-dependent, NIDDM) to improve glycemic control

Dosage Summary Note: When compared to insulin NPH, insulin detemir has a slower, more prolonged absorption; duration is dose-dependent. Insulin detemir may be given once or twice daily when used as the basal insulin component of therapy. Changing the basal insulin component from another insulin to insulin detemir can be done on a unit-to-unit basis.

SubQ:

Children <6 years: Dosage not established

Children ≥6 years: Refer to Insulin Regular on page 513

Adults: Refer to Insulin Regular on page 513; 0.1-0.2 units/kg once daily **or** 10 units once- or twice daily (manufacturer recommendations)

Dosage Forms

Injection, solution:

Levemir®: 100 units/mL (3 mL, 10 mL)

insulin glargine (IN soo lin GLAR jeen)

Sound-Alike/Look-Alike Issues

insulin glargine may be confused with insulin glulisine

Lantus® may be confused with latanoprost, Xalatan®

Synonyms glargine insulin

U.S./Canadian Brand Names Lantus® OptiSet® [Can]; Lantus® [US/Can]

Therapeutic Category Antidiabetic Agent, Insulin

Use Treatment of type 1 diabetes mellitus (insulin-dependent, IDDM) and type 2 diabetes mellitus (noninsulin-dependent, NIDDM) to improve glycemic control

Dosage Summary Note: Insulin glargine is approximately equipotent to human insulin, but has a slower onset, no pronounced peak, and a longer duration of activity. Changing the basal insulin component from another insulin to insulin glargine can be done on a unit-to-unit basis.

SubQ:

Children <6 years: Dosage not established

Children ≥6 years: Refer to Insulin Regular on page 513

Adults: Refer to Insulin Regular on page 513

Dosage Forms

Injection, solution:

Lantus®: 100 units/mL (3 mL, 10 mL)

insulin glulisine (IN soo lin gloo LIS een)

Sound-Alike/Look-Alike Issues

insulin glulisine may be confused with insulin glargine

Synonyms glulisine insulin

U.S./Canadian Brand Names Apidra® [US/Can]

Therapeutic Category Antidiabetic Agent, Insulin

Use Treatment of type 1 diabetes mellitus (insulin-dependent, IDDM) and type 2 diabetes mellitus (noninsulin-dependent, NIDDM) to improve glycemic control

Dosage Summary Note: Insulin glulisine is equipotent to insulin regular, but has a more rapid onset and shorter duration of activity.

I.V.:

Children: Dosage not established

Adults: Refer to Insulin Regular on page 513

SubQ:

Children <4 years: Dosage not established

Children ≥4 years: Refer to Insulin Regular on page 513

Adults: Refer to Insulin Regular on page 513

Dosage Forms

Injection, solution:

Apidra®: 100 units/mL (3 mL, 10 mL)

insulin lispro (IN soo lin LYE sproe)

Sound-Alike/Look-Alike Issues

Humalog® may be confused with Humalog® Mix 50/50, Humira®, Humulin® N, Humulin® R, NovoLog®

Synonyms lispro insulin

U.S./Canadian Brand Names Humalog® [US/Can]

Therapeutic Category Antidiabetic Agent, Insulin

Use Treatment of type 1 diabetes mellitus (insulin-dependent, IDDM) and type 2 diabetes mellitus (noninsulin-dependent, NIDDM) to improve glycemic control

Dosage Summary Note: Insulin lispro is equipotent to insulin regular, but has a more rapid onset and shorter duration of activity.

SubQ:

Children: Refer to Insulin Regular on page 513

Adults: Refer to Insulin Regular on page 513

Dosage Forms

Injection, solution:

Humalog®: 100 units/mL (3 mL, 10 mL)

insulin lispro and insulin lispro protamine *see* insulin lispro protamine and insulin lispro *on page 511*

insulin lispro protamine and insulin lispro

(IN soo lin LYE sproe PROE ta meen & IN soo lin LYE sproe)

Sound-Alike/Look-Alike Issues

Humalog® Mix 50/50™ may be confused with Humalog® and Humulin® 50/50

Humalog® Mix 75/25™ may be confused with Humulin® 70/30, Novolin® 70/30, and NovoLog® Mix 70/30

Synonyms insulin lispro and insulin lispro protamine

U.S./Canadian Brand Names Humalog® Mix 25 [Can]; Humalog® Mix 50/50™ [US]; Humalog® Mix 75/25™ [US]

Therapeutic Category Antidiabetic Agent, Insulin

Use Treatment of type 1 diabetes mellitus (insulin-dependent, IDDM) and type 2 diabetes mellitus (noninsulin-dependent, NIDDM) to improve glycemic control

Dosage Summary **Note:** Insulin lispro protamine and insulin lispro combination products are approximately equipotent to insulin NPH and insulin regular combination products but with a more rapid onset and similar duration of activity.

SubQ:

Children: Dosage not established

Adults: Refer to Insulin Regular on page 513

Dosage Forms

Injection, suspension:

Humalog® Mix 50/50™: Insulin lispro protamine suspension 50% [intermediate acting] and insulin lispro solution 50% [rapid acting]: 100 units/mL (3 mL) [disposable pen]; (10 mL) [vial]

Humalog® Mix 75/25™: Insulin lispro protamine suspension 75% [intermediate acting] and insulin lispro solution 25% [rapid acting]: 100 units/mL (3 mL) [disposable pen]; (10 mL) [vial]

insulin NPH (IN soo lin N P H)

Sound-Alike/Look-Alike Issues

Humulin® N may be confused with Humulin® R, Humalog®, Humira®

Novolin® N may be confused with Novolin® R, NovoLog®

Synonyms isophane insulin; NPH insulin

U.S./Canadian Brand Names Humulin® N [US/Can]; Novolin® ge NPH [Can]; Novolin® N [US]

Therapeutic Category Antidiabetic Agent, Insulin

Use Treatment of type 1 diabetes mellitus (insulin-dependent, IDDM) and type 2 diabetes mellitus (noninsulin-dependent, NIDDM) to improve glycemic control

Dosage Summary **Note:** When compared to insulin regular, insulin NPH has a slower onset and longer duration of activity.

SubQ:

Children: Refer to Insulin Regular on page 513

Adults: Refer to Insulin Regular on page 513

Dosage Forms

Injection, suspension:

Humulin® N: 100 units/mL (3 mL, 10 mL)

Novolin® N: 100 units/mL (10 mL)

Dosage Forms - Canada

Injection, suspension:

Novolin® ge NPH: 100 units/mL (3 mL, 10 mL)

insulin NPH and insulin regular (IN soo lin N P H & IN soo lin REG yoo ler)

Sound-Alike/Look-Alike Issues

Humulin® 50/50 may be confused with Humalog® Mix 50/50

Humulin® 70/30 may be confused with Humalog® Mix 75/25, Humulin® R, Novolin® 70/30, NovoLog® Mix 70/30

Novolin® 70/30 may be confused with Humalog® Mix 75/25, Humulin® 70/30, Humulin® R, Novolin® R, and NovoLog® Mix 70/30

Synonyms insulin regular and insulin NPH; isophane insulin and regular insulin; NPH insulin and regular insulin

U.S./Canadian Brand Names Humulin® 20/80 [Can]; Humulin® 70/30 [US/Can]; Novolin® 70/30 [US]; Novolin® ge 30/70 [Can]; Novolin® ge 40/60 [Can]; Novolin® ge 50/50 [Can]

Therapeutic Category Antidiabetic Agent, Insulin

Use Treatment of type 1 diabetes mellitus (insulin-dependent, IDDM) and type 2 diabetes mellitus (noninsulin-dependent, NIDDM) to improve glycemic control

Dosage Summary **Note:** When compared to insulin NPH, the combination product (insulin NPH and insulin regular) has a more rapid onset of action and a similar duration of action.

SubQ:

Children: Refer to Insulin Regular on page 513

Adults: Refer to Insulin Regular on page 513

Dosage Forms

Injection, suspension:

Humulin® 70/30: Insulin NPH suspension 70% [intermediate acting] and insulin regular solution 30% [short acting]: 100 units/mL (3 mL, 10 mL)

Novolin® 70/30: Insulin NPH suspension 70% [intermediate acting] and insulin regular solution 30% [short acting]: 100 units/mL (10 mL)

Dosage Forms - Canada

Injection, suspension:

Humulin® 20/80: Insulin regular solution 20% [short acting] and insulin NPH suspension 80% [intermediate acting]: 100 units/mL (3 mL)

Novolin® ge 30/70: Insulin regular solution 30% [short acting] and insulin NPH suspension 70% [intermediate acting]: 100 units/mL (3 mL)

Novolin® ge 40/60: Insulin regular solution 40% [short acting] and insulin NPH suspension 60% [intermediate acting]: 100 units/mL (3 mL)

Novolin® ge 50/50: Insulin regular solution 50% [short acting] and insulin NPH suspension 50% [intermediate acting]: 100 units/mL (3 mL)

insulin regular (IN soo lin REG yoo ler)

Sound-Alike/Look-Alike Issues

Humulin® R may be confused with Humalog®, Humira®, Humulin® 70/30, Humulin® N, Novolin® 70/30, Novolin® R, NovoLog®

Novolin® R may be confused with Humulin® R, Novolin® 70/30, Novolin® N, NovoLog®

Synonyms regular insulin

U.S./Canadian Brand Names Humulin® R U-500 [US]; Humulin® R [US/Can]; Novolin® ge Toronto [Can]; Novolin® R [US]

Therapeutic Category Antidiabetic Agent, Insulin; Antidote

Use Treatment of type 1 diabetes mellitus (insulin dependent, IDDM) and type 2 diabetes mellitus (noninsulin dependent, NIDDM) to improve glycemic control

Dosage Summary

I.V.:

Diabetes mellitus types 1 and 2:

Children: See SubQ administration

Adults: See SubQ administration

SubQ:

Diabetes mellitus: **Note:** Insulin requirements vary dramatically between patients and therapy requires dosage adjustments with careful medical supervision. Specific formulations may require distinct administration procedures; please see individual agents.

Children:

Diabetes mellitus, type 1: Initial: 0.5-1 unit/kg/day in divided doses; Usual maintenance: 0.5-1.2 units/kg/day in divided doses. Titration is usually required to achieve glycemic goals. **Note:** Generally, 50% to 75% of the total daily dose (TDD) is given as an intermediate- or long-acting form of insulin (1-2 daily injections) and the remaining portion is then divided and administered before or at mealtime (depending on the formulation) as a rapid-acting or short-acting form of insulin.

Diabetes mellitus, type 2: Initial basal insulin dose: 0.2 units/kg or 10 units/day given as an intermediate- or long-acting insulin at bedtime or long-acting insulin given in the morning; Titration is usually required to achieve glycemic goals.

Adults:

Diabetes mellitus, type 1: Initial: 0.5-1 unit/kg/day in divided doses; Usual maintenance: 0.5-1.2 units/kg/day in divided doses. Titration is usually required to achieve glycemic goals. **Note:** Generally, 50% to 75% of the total daily dose (TDD) is given as an intermediate- or long-acting form of insulin (1-2 daily injections) and the remaining portion is then divided and administered before or at mealtime (depending on the formulation) as a rapid-acting or short-acting form of insulin.

Diabetes mellitus, type 2: Initial basal insulin dose: 0.2 units/kg or 10 units/day given as an intermediate- or long-acting insulin at bedtime or long-acting insulin given in the morning; Titration is usually required to achieve glycemic goals.

Dosage Forms

Injection, solution:

Humulin® R: 100 units/mL (3 mL, 10 mL)

Humulin® R U-500: 500 units/mL (20 mL)

Novolin® R: 100 units/mL (10 mL)

insulin regular and insulin NPH *see* insulin NPH and insulin regular *on page* 512
Intal® [Can] *see* cromolyn (systemic, oral inhalation) *on page* 254
Intal® *(Discontinued)* *see* cromolyn (systemic, oral inhalation) *on page* 254
Integrilin® [US/Can] *see* eptifibatide *on page* 358
Intelence™ [US/Can] *see* etravirine *on page* 385
Intensol® Solution *(Discontinued)* *see* metoclopramide *on page* 624
α-2-interferon *see* interferon alfa-2b *on page* 514
interferon alfa-2a *(Discontinued)*
interferon alfa-2a (PEG conjugate) *see* peginterferon alfa-2a *on page* 733
interferon alfa-2b (PEG conjugate) *see* peginterferon alfa-2b *on page* 734

interferon alfa-2b (in ter FEER on AL fa too bee)

Sound-Alike/Look-Alike Issues

interferon alfa-2b may be confused with interferon alfa-2a, interferon alfa-n3, pegylated interferon alfa-2b

Intron® A may be confused with PEG-Intron®

Synonyms INF-alpha 2; interferon alpha-2b; rLFN-α2; α-2-interferon

U.S./Canadian Brand Names Intron® A [US/Can]

Therapeutic Category Biological Response Modulator

Use

Patients ≥1 year of age: Chronic hepatitis B

Patients ≥3 years of age: Chronic hepatitis C (in combination with ribavirin)

Patients ≥18 years of age: Condyloma acuminata, chronic hepatitis B, chronic hepatitis C, hairy cell leukemia, malignant melanoma, AIDS-related Kaposi sarcoma, follicular non-Hodgkin lymphoma

Dosage Summary

I.M.:

Children: Dosage not established

Adults:

AIDS-related Kaposi sarcoma: 30 million units/m^2 3 times/week

Chronic hepatitis B: 5 million units/day or 10 million units 3 times/week

Chronic hepatitis C: 3 million units 3 times/week

Hairy cell leukemia: 2 million units/m^2 3 times/week

I.V.:

Children: Dosage not established

Adults: 20 million units/m^2 for 5 consecutive days per week for 4 weeks

Intralesionally:

Children: Dosage not established

Adults: 1 million units/lesion 3 times/week, on alternate days (maximum: 5 lesions/treatment)

SubQ:

Children <1 year: Dosage not established

Children 1-17 years: Initial: 3 million units/m^2 3 times/week for 1 week; Maintenance: 6 million units/m^2 3 times/week (maximum: 10 million units 3 times/week)

Children 3-17 years: Initial: 3 million units/m^2 3 times/week (combination therapy) for up to 48 weeks

Adults:

AIDS-related Kaposi sarcoma: 30 million units/m^2 3 times/week

Chronic hepatitis B: 5 million units/day or 10 million units 3 times/week

Chronic hepatitis C: 3 million units 3 times/week

Hairy cell leukemia: 2 million units/m^2 3 times/week

Lymphoma (follicular): 5 million units 3 times/week

Malignant melanoma: 10 million units/m^2 3 times/week

Dosage Forms

Injection, powder for reconstitution [preservative free]:

Intron® A: 10 million int. units, 18 million int. units, 50 million int. units

Injection, solution:

Intron® A: 6 million int. units/mL (3 mL); 10 million int. units/mL (2.5 mL); 3 million int. units/0.2 mL (1.2 mL); 5 million int. units/0.2 mL (1.2 mL); 10 million int. units/0.2 mL (1.2 mL)

interferon alfacon-1 (in ter FEER on AL fa con one)

Sound-Alike/Look-Alike Issues

interferon alfacon-1 may be confused with interferon alfa-2a, interferon alfa-2b, interferon alfa-n3, peginterferon alfa-2b

U.S./Canadian Brand Names Infergen® [US]

Therapeutic Category Interferon

Use Treatment of chronic hepatitis C virus (HCV) infection in patients ≥18 years of age with compensated liver disease and anti-HCV serum antibodies or HCV RNA.

Dosage Summary

SubQ:

Children: Dosage not established

Adults: 9 mcg 3 times/week. Patients who do not respond or relapse after tolerating initial therapy may be increased to 15 mcg 3 times/week.

Dosage Forms

Injection, solution [preservative free]:

Infergen®: 30 mcg/mL (0.3 mL, 0.5 mL)

interferon alfa-n3 (in ter FEER on AL fa en three)

Sound-Alike/Look-Alike Issues

Alferon® may be confused with Alkeran®

U.S./Canadian Brand Names Alferon® N [US/Can]

Therapeutic Category Biological Response Modulator

Use Patients ≥18 years of age: Intralesional treatment of refractory or recurring genital or venereal warts (condylomata acuminata)

Dosage Summary

Intralesional:

Children: Dosage not established

Adults: Inject 250,000 units (0.05 mL) in each wart twice weekly (maximum: 8 weeks)

Dosage Forms

Injection, solution:

Alferon® N: 5 million int. units (1 mL)

interferon alpha-2b *see* interferon alfa-2b *on page* 514

interferon beta-1a (in ter FEER on BAY ta won aye)

Sound-Alike/Look-Alike Issues

Avonex® may be confused with Avelox®

Synonyms rIFN beta-1a

U.S./Canadian Brand Names Avonex® [US/Can]; Rebif® [US/Can]

Therapeutic Category Biological Response Modulator

Use Treatment of relapsing forms of multiple sclerosis (MS)

Dosage Summary

I.M.:

Children: Dosage not established

Adults: 30 mcg once weekly

SubQ:

Children: Dosage not established

Adults: Initial: 4.4 or 8.8 mcg 3 times/week for 2 weeks; Titration: 11 or 22 mcg 3 times/week for 2 weeks; Maintenance: 22 or 44 mcg 3 times/week

Dosage Forms

Combination package [preservative free]:

Rebif® Titration Pack:

Injection, solution: 8.8 mcg/0.2 mL (0.2 mL) [6 prefilled syringes]

Injection, solution: 22 mcg/0.5 mL (0.5 mL) [6 prefilled syringes]

Injection, powder for reconstitution:

Avonex®: 33 mcg [6.6 million units; provides 30 mcg/mL following reconstitution]

Injection, solution:
Avonex®: 30 mcg/0.5 mL (0.5 mL)
Injection, solution [preservative free]:
Rebif®: 22 mcg/0.5 mL (0.5 mL) [prefilled syringe]; 44 mcg/0.5 mL (0.5 mL) [prefilled syringe]

interferon beta-1b (in ter FEER on BAY ta won bee)

Synonyms rIFN beta-1b

U.S./Canadian Brand Names Betaseron® [US/Can]; Extavia® [US/Can]

Therapeutic Category Biological Response Modulator

Use Treatment of relapsing forms of multiple sclerosis (MS); treatment of first clinical episode with MRI features consistent with MS

Canadian labeling: Additional use (not in U.S. labeling): Treatment of secondary-progressive MS

Dosage Summary

SubQ:
Children: Use not recommended
Adults: 0.0625-0.25 mg (2-8 million units) every other day

Dosage Forms

Injection, powder for reconstitution:
Betaseron®: 0.3 mg [~9.6 million int. units]
Injection, powder for reconstitution [preservative free]:
Extavia®: 0.3 mg [~9.6 million int. units]

interferon gamma-1b (in ter FEER on GAM ah won bee)

U.S./Canadian Brand Names Actimmune® [US/Can]

Therapeutic Category Biological Response Modulator

Use Reduce frequency and severity of serious infections associated with chronic granulomatous disease; delay time to disease progression in patients with severe, malignant osteopetrosis

Dosage Summary

SubQ:
Children:
BSA ≤0.5 m^2: 1.5 mcg/kg/dose 3 times/week
BSA >0.5 m^2: 50 mcg/m^2 (1 million int. units/m^2) 3 times/week
Adults:
BSA ≤0.5 m^2: 1.5 mcg/kg/dose 3 times/week
BSA >0.5 m^2: 50 mcg/m^2 (1 million int. units/m^2) 3 times/week

Dosage Forms

Injection, solution [preservative free]:
Actimmune®: 100 mcg (0.5 mL)

interleukin-1 receptor antagonist *see* anakinra *on page* 77
interleukin 2 *see* aldesleukin *on page* 46
interleukin-11 *see* oprelvekin *on page* 706
Intralipid® [US/Can] *see* fat emulsion *on page* 391
intrapleural talc *see* talc (sterile) *on page* 908
intravenous fat emulsion *see* fat emulsion *on page* 391
intrifiban *see* eptifibatide *on page* 358
Intron® A [US/Can] *see* interferon alfa-2b *on page* 514
Intropaste *(Discontinued)* *see* barium *on page* 117
Intropin® *(Discontinued)* *see* dopamine *on page* 326
Intuniv™ [US] *see* guanfacine *on page* 461
Invanz® [US/Can] *see* ertapenem *on page* 360
Invega® [US/Can] *see* paliperidone *on page* 720
Invega® Sustenna™ [US] *see* paliperidone *on page* 720
Inversine® [Can] *see* mecamylamine *on page* 594
Inversine® *(Discontinued)* *see* mecamylamine *on page* 594
Invirase® [US/Can] *see* saquinavir *on page* 865

iobenguane I 123 (eye oh BEN gwane eye one TWEN tee three)

Synonyms 123 meta-iodobenzlyguanidine sulfate; 123I-metaiodobenzylguanidine (MIBG); I-123 MIBG; I^{123} iobenguane; iobenguane sulfate I 123

U.S./Canadian Brand Names AdreView™ [US]

Therapeutic Category Radiopharmaceutical

Use As an adjunct to other diagnostic tests, in the detection of primary or metastatic pheochromocytoma or neuroblastoma

Dosage Summary

I.V.:

Infants <1 month: Dosage not established
Children <16 years and 3 kg: 1 mCi (37 MBq)
Children <16 years and 4 kg: 1.4 mCi (52 MBq)
Children <16 years and 6 kg: 1.9 mCi (70 MBq)
Children <16 years and 8 kg: 2.3 mCi (85.1 MBq)
Children <16 years and 10 kg: 2.7 mCi (99.9 MBq)
Children <16 years and 12 kg: 3.2 mCi (118.4 MBq)
Children <16 years and 14 kg: 3.6 mCi (133.2 MBq)
Children <16 years and 16 kg: 4 mCi (148 MBq)
Children <16 years and 18 kg: 4.4 mCi (162.8 MBq)
Children <16 years and 20 kg: 4.6 mCi (170.2 MBq)
Children <16 years and 22 kg: 5 mCi (185 MBq)
Children <16 years and 24 kg: 5.3 mCi (196.1 MBq)
Children <16 years and 26 kg: 5.6 mCi (207.2 MBq)
Children <16 years and 28 kg: 5.8 mCi (214.6 MBq)
Children <16 years and 30 kg: 6.2 mCi (229.4 MBq)
Children <16 years and 32 kg: 6.5 mCi (240.5 MBq)
Children <16 years and 34 kg: 6.8 mCi (251.6 MBq)
Children <16 years and 36 kg: 7.1 mCi (262.7 MBq)
Children <16 years and 38 kg: 7.3 mCi (270.1 MBq)
Children <16 years and 40 kg: 7.6 mCi (281.2 MBq)
Children <16 years and 42 kg: 7.8 mCi (288.6 MBq)
Children <16 years and 44 kg: 8 mCi (296 MBq)
Children <16 years and 46 kg: 8.2 mCi (303.4 MBq)
Children <16 years and 48 kg: 8.5 mCi (314.5 MBq)
Children <16 years and 50 kg: 8.8 mCi (325.6 MBq)
Children <16 years and 52-54 kg: 9 mCi (333 MBq)
Children <16 years and 56-58 kg: 9.2 mCi (340.4 MBq)
Children <16 years and 60-62 kg: 9.6 mCi (355.2 MBq)
Children <16 years and 64-66 kg: 9.8 mCi (362.6 MBq)
Children <16 years and 68 kg: 9.9 mCi (366.3 MBq)
Children <16 years and ≥70 kg: 10 mCi (370 MBq)
Children ≥16 years: 10 mCi (370 MBq)
Adults: 10 mCi (370 MBq)

Dosage Forms

Injection, solution:

AdreView™: Iobenguane sulfate 0.08 mg and I 123 74 MBq (2 mCi) per mL (5 mL)

iobenguane sulfate I 123 *see* iobenguane I 123 *on page 517*
Iodex® [US-OTC] *see* iodine *on page 517*
Iodex-p® *(Discontinued)* *see* povidone-iodine (topical) *on page 784*

iodine (EYE oh dyne)

Sound-Alike/Look-Alike Issues

iodine may be confused with codeine, Iopidine®, Lodine®

U.S./Canadian Brand Names Iodex® [US-OTC]; Iodoflex™ [US-OTC]; Iodosorb® [US-OTC]

Therapeutic Category Topical Skin Product

Use Used topically as an antiseptic in the management of minor, superficial skin wounds and has been used to disinfect the skin preoperatively

Dosage Summary

Topical:

Children: Dosage not established

Adults:

Antiseptic: Apply to affected area 1-3 times/day

Ulcer/wound cleansing: apply to clean wound 3 times/week (maximum: 50 g/application; 150 g/week)

Dosage Forms

Dressing, topical:

Iodoflex™ [OTC]: 0.9% (3s, 5s)

Gel, topical:

Iodosorb® [OTC]: 0.9% (40 g)

Ointment, topical:

Iodex® [OTC]: 4.7% (30 g, 720 g)

Tincture, topical: 2% (30 mL, 59 mL, 473 mL); 7% (30 mL, 473 mL)

iodine *see* trace metals *on page 945*

iodine I 131 tositumomab and tositumomab *see* tositumomab and iodine I 131 tositumomab *on page 944*

iodipamide meglumine (eye oh DI pa mide MEG loo meen)

U.S./Canadian Brand Names Cholografin® Meglumine [US]

Therapeutic Category Iodinated Contrast Media; Radiological/Contrast Media, Ionic

Use Contrast medium for intravenous cholangiography and cholecystography

Dosage Summary

I.V.: Do not repeat for 24 hours

Infants: 0.3-0.6 mL/kg (maximum: 20 mL)

Children: 0.3-0.6 mL/kg (maximum: 20 mL)

Adults: 20 mL

Dosage Forms

Injection, solution:

Cholografin® Meglumine: 520 mg/mL (20 mL)

iodipamide meglumine and diatrizoate meglumine *see* diatrizoate meglumine and iodipamide meglumine *on page 293*

iodixanol (EYE oh dix an ole)

U.S./Canadian Brand Names Visipaque™ [US/Can]

Therapeutic Category Iodinated Contrast Media; Radiological/Contrast Media, Nonionic

Use

Intraarterial: Digital subtraction angiography, angiocardiography, peripheral arteriography, visceral arteriography, cerebral arteriography

Intravenous: Contrast enhanced computed tomography imaging, excretory urography, and peripheral venography

Dosage Summary

I.V.:

Children ≤1 year: Dosage not established

Children >1-12 years: Iodixanol 270 mg iodine/mL: 1-2 mL/kg (maximum: 2 mL/kg)

Children >12 years: Iodixanol 270 mg and 320 mg iodine/mL: concentration and dose vary based on study type; refer to product labeling (maximum total dose: 80 g iodine)

Adults: Iodixanol 270 mg and 320 mg iodine/mL: concentration and dose vary based on study type; refer to product labeling (maximum total dose: 80 g iodine)

Intra-arterial:

Children ≤1 year: Dosage not established

Children >1-12 years: Iodixanol 320 mg iodine/mL: 1-2 mL/kg (maximum: 4 mL/kg)

Children >12 years: Iodixanol 320 mg iodine/mL: Dose individualized based on injection site and study type; refer to product labeling (maximum total dose: 80 g iodine)

Adults: Iodixanol 320 mg iodine/mL: Dose individualized based on injection site and study type; refer to product labeling (maximum total dose: 80 g iodine)

Dosage Forms

Injection, solution [preservative free]:

Visipaque™: 270: 550 mg/mL (50 mL, 100 mL, 125 mL, 150 mL, 200 mL, 500 mL); 320: 652 mg/mL (50 mL, 100 mL, 125 mL, 150 mL, 200 mL, 500 mL)

iodochlorhydroxyquin and flumethasone *see* clioquinol and flumethasone *(Canada only) on page 234*

Iodoflex™ [US-OTC] *see* iodine *on page 517*

iodoquinol (eye oh doe KWIN ole)

Synonyms diiodohydroxyquin

U.S./Canadian Brand Names Diodoquin® [Can]; Yodoxin® [US]

Therapeutic Category Amebicide

Use Treatment of acute and chronic intestinal amebiasis; asymptomatic cyst passers; *Blastocystis hominis* infections; ineffective for amebic hepatitis or hepatic abscess

Dosage Summary

Oral:

Children: 30-40 mg/kg/day in 3 divided doses (maximum: 1.95 g/day)

Adults: 650 mg 3 times/day (maximum: 1.95 g/day)

Elderly: Only use if other therapy contraindicated or has failed; due to optic nerve damage use cautiously

Dosage Forms

Tablet, oral:

Yodoxin®: 210 mg, 650 mg

iodoquinol and hydrocortisone (eye oh doe KWIN ole & hye droe KOR ti sone)

Sound-Alike/Look-Alike Issues

Vytone® may be confused with Hytone®, Zydone®

Synonyms hydrocortisone and iodoquinol

U.S./Canadian Brand Names Alcortin™ [US]; Dermazene® [US]; Vytone® [US]

Therapeutic Category Antifungal/Corticosteroid

Use Treatment of eczema (including impetiginized, nuchal, and nummular); acne urticaria; anogenital pruritus, atopic dermatitis, chronic infectious dermatitis; chronic eczematoid otitis externa; folliculitis, intertrigo; lichen simplex chronicus; moniliasis; mycotic dermatoses; neurodermatitis (localized or systemic); pyoderma, stasis dermatitis

Dosage Summary

Topical:

Children <12 years: Dosage not established

Children ≥12 years: Apply 3-4 times/day

Adults: Apply 3-4 times/day

Dosage Forms

Cream, topical: Iodoquinol 1% and hydrocortisone 1% (30 g)

Dermazene®: Iodoquinol 1% and hydrocortisone 1% (30 g, 45 g)

Vytone®: Iodoquinol 1% and hydrocortisone 1% (30 g)

Gel, topical:

Alcortin™: Iodoquinol 1% and hydrocortisone 2% (2 g)

Iodosorb® [US-OTC] *see* iodine *on page 517*

iohexol (eye oh HEX ole)

U.S./Canadian Brand Names Omnipaque™ 140 [US]; Omnipaque™ 180 [US]; Omnipaque™ 240 [US]; Omnipaque™ 300 [US]; Omnipaque™ 350 [US]; Omnipaque™ [Can]

Therapeutic Category Polypeptide Hormone; Radiological/Contrast Media, Nonionic

Use

Intrathecal: Myelography; contrast enhancement for computerized tomography

Intravascular: Angiocardiography, aortography, digital subtraction angiography, peripheral arteriography, excretory urography; contrast enhancement for computed tomographic imaging

Oral/body cavity: Arthrography, GI tract examination, hysterosalpingography, pancreatography, cholangiopancreatography, herniography, cystourethrography; enhanced computed tomography of the abdomen

Dosage Forms
Injection, solution [preservative free]:
Omnipaque™ 140: 302 mg/mL (50 mL)
Omnipaque™ 180: 388 mg/mL (10 mL, 20 mL)
Omnipaque™ 240: 518 mg/mL (10 mL, 20 mL, 50 mL, 75 mL, 100 mL, 150 mL, 200 mL)
Omnipaque™ 300: 647 mg/mL (10 mL, 30 mL, 50 mL, 75 mL, 100 mL, 125 mL, 150 mL, 200 mL, 500 mL)
Omnipaque™ 350: 755 mg/mL (50 mL, 75 mL, 100 mL, 125 mL, 150 mL, 200 mL, 250 mL, 500 mL)
Injection, solution, oral [preservative free]:
Omnipaque™ 240: 518 mg/mL (50 mL)
Omnipaque™ 300: 647 mg/mL (50 mL)
Omnipaque™ 350: 755 mg/mL (50 mL)

Ionil® [US-OTC] *see* salicylic acid *on page 858*
Ionil Plus® [US-OTC] *see* salicylic acid *on page 858*
ionil-T® [US-OTC] *see* coal tar *on page 242*
ionil-T® Plus [US-OTC] *see* coal tar *on page 242*

iopamidol (eye oh PA mi dole)

U.S./Canadian Brand Names Isovue Multipack® [US]; Isovue-M® [US]; Isovue® 200 [US]; Isovue® 300 [US]; Isovue® 370 [US]; Isovue® [US]

Therapeutic Category Iodinated Contrast Media; Radiological/Contrast Media, Nonionic

Use
Intrathecal (Isovue-M®): Myelography contrast enhancement of computed tomographic cisternography and ventriculography; thoracolumbar myelography
Intravascular (Isovue®, Isovue Multipack®): Angiography (eg, coronary, cerebral, peripheral arteriogram), pediatric angiocardiography, excretory urography; contrast enhancement of computed tomographic imaging (in adults and children); evaluation of certain malignancies; image enhancement of non-neoplastic lesions

Dosage Summary Dosing is based numerous variables including: Type of examination, route of administration, patient age/weight, and product. Consult specific product information for detailed dosing.

Dosage Forms
Injection, solution:
Isovue Multipack®: 51% (200 mL); 61% (200 mL, 500 mL); 76% (200 mL, 500 mL)
Isovue® 200: 41% (50 mL, 200 mL)
Isovue®: 51% (50 mL, 100 mL, 150 mL, 200 mL)
Isovue® 300: 61% (30 mL, 50 mL, 75 mL, 100 mL, 125 mL, 150 mL)
Isovue® 370: 76% (50 mL, 75 mL, 100 mL, 125 mL, 150 mL)
Injection, solution, intrathecal:
Isovue-M®: 41% (10 mL, 20 mL); 61% (15 mL)

Iopidine® [US/Can] *see* apraclonidine *on page 91*

iopromide (eye oh PROE mide)

U.S./Canadian Brand Names Ultravist® [US]

Therapeutic Category Radiological/Contrast Media, Nonionic

Use Enhance imaging in cerebral arteriography and peripheral arteriography; coronary arteriography and left ventriculography, visceral angiography and aortography; contrast-enhanced computed tomographic imaging of the head and body, excretory urography, intraarterial digital subtraction angiography, peripheral venography

Dosage Summary
I.V.:
Children ≤2 years: Dosage not established
Children >2 years:
Cardiac chambers and related arteries (370 mg iodine/mL): 1-2 mL/kg (maximum: 4 mL/kg/procedure)
CT (300 mg iodine/mL): 1-2 mL/kg (maximum: 3 mL/kg/procedure)
Adults:
CT (300 mg iodine/mL): 50-200 mL (maximum: 200 mL)
Excretory urography (300 mg iodine/mL): 1 mL/kg (maximum: 100 mL)
Peripheral venography (240 mg iodine/mL): Minimum amount to clearly visualize the structure under examination (maximum: 250 mL)

Intravascular:

Children: Dosage not established

Adults:

Aortography and visceral angiography (370 mg iodine/mL): Up to 225 mL

Cerebral arteriography (300 mg iodine/mL): Aortic arch: 20-50 mL; Carotid artery: 3-12 mL; Vertebral artery: 4-12 mL (maximum: 150 mL/procedure)

Coronary arteriography and left ventriculography (370 mg iodine/mL): Left and right coronary: 3-14 mL; Left ventricle: 30-60 mL (maximum: 225 mL/procedure)

Intraarterial digital subtraction angiography (150 mg iodine/mL): Abdominal aorta major branches: 2-20 mL; Aorta: 20-50 mL; Carotid arteries: 6-10 mL; Vertebral: 4-8 mL (maximum: 250 mL/procedure)

Peripheral arteriography (300 mg iodine/mL): Aortic bifurcation for distal runoff: 25-50 mL; Subclavian or femoral artery: 5-40 mL (maximum: 250 mL/procedure)

Dosage Forms

Injection, solution:

Ultravist®: Iodine 150 mg/mL (50 mL); Iodine 240 mg/mL (50 mL, 100 mL, 150 mL, 200 mL); Iodine 300 mg/mL (50 mL, 75 mL, 100 mL, 125 mL, 150 mL, 200 mL, 500 mL); Iodine 370 mg/mL (50 mL, 75 mL, 100 mL, 125 mL, 150 mL, 200 mL, 250 mL, 500 mL)

iOSAT™ [US-OTC] *see* potassium iodide *on page 782*

iothalamate meglumine (eye oh thal A mate MEG loo meen)

U.S./Canadian Brand Names Conray® 30 [US]; Conray® 43 [US]; Conray® [US]; Cysto-Conray® II [US]

Therapeutic Category Iodinated Contrast Media; Radiological/Contrast Media, Ionic

Use

Solution for injection: Arthrography, cerebral angiography, cranial computerized angiotomography, digital subtraction angiography, direct cholangiography, endoscopic retrograde cholangiopancreatography, excretory urography, peripheral arteriography, urography, venography; contrast enhancement of computed tomographic images

Solution for instillation: Retrograde cystography and cystourethrography

Dosage Forms

Injection, solution:

Conray® 30: 30% (50 mL, 150 mL)

Conray® 43: 43% (50 mL, 100 mL, 200 mL, 250 mL)

Conray®: 60% (30 mL, 50 mL, 100 mL, 150 mL)

Injection, solution for instillation:

Cysto-Conray® II: 17.2% (250 mL, 500 mL)

iothalamate sodium *(Discontinued)*

iotrolan *(Canada only)* (eye OH troe lan)

Sound-Alike/Look-Alike Issues

Osmovist® may be confused with Gadovist®, Magnevist®, Vasovist®

U.S./Canadian Brand Names Osmovist® [Can]

Therapeutic Category Iodinated Contrast Media; Radiological/Contrast Media, Nonionic (Iso-Osmolality)

Use Myelography (lumbar, cervical, total columnar); computerized tomography (CT) of spinal and subarachnoid spaces

Dosage Summary

Intrathecal:

Children: Dosage not established

Adults:

Lumbar myelography: 7-12 mL

Radiculography: 7-10 mL

Thoracic myelography: 8-15 mL

Total columnar myelography: 10-15 mL

Cervical myelography: Direct instillation: 7-12 mL; Indirect instillation: 8-15 mL

Ventriculography: Indirect instillation: 3-5 mL

Cisternography: Indirect instillation: 4-12 mL

Dosage Forms - Canada

Injection, solution, intrathecal [preservative free]:

Osmovist®:

240 [contains iotrolan 513 mg equivalent to iodine 240 mg/mL] (10 mL)

300 [contains iotrolan 641 mg equivalent to iodine 300 mg /mL] (10 mL)

ioversol (EYE oh ver sole)

U.S./Canadian Brand Names Optiray® 160 [US]; Optiray® 240 [US]; Optiray® 300 [US]; Optiray® 320 [US]; Optiray® 350 [US]

Therapeutic Category Iodinated Contrast Media; Radiological/Contrast Media, Nonionic

Use Arteriography, angiography, angiocardiography, ventriculography, excretory urography, and venography procedures; contrast enhanced tomographic imaging; intraarterial digital substraction angiography (Optiray® 160)

Dosage Forms

Injection, solution [preservative free]:

Optiray® 160: 34% (50 mL, 100 mL)

Optiray® 240: 51% (50 mL, 100 mL, 125 mL, 150 mL, 200 mL)

Optiray® 300: 64% (50 mL, 100 mL, 125 mL, 150 mL, 200 mL)

Optiray® 320: 68% (20 mL, 30 mL, 50 mL, 75 mL, 100 mL, 125 mL, 150 mL, 200s)

Optiray® 350: 74% (30 mL, 50 mL, 75 mL, 100 mL, 125 mL, 150 mL, 200 mL)

ioxaglate meglumine and ioxaglate sodium

(eye ox AG late MEG loo meen & eye ox AG late SOW dee um)

Synonyms ioxaglate sodium and ioxaglate meglumine

U.S./Canadian Brand Names Hexabrix™ [US]

Therapeutic Category Iodinated Contrast Media; Radiological/Contrast Media, Ionic

Use Angiocardiography, arteriography, aortography, arthrography, angiography, hysterosalpingography, venography, and urography procedures; contrast enhancement of computed tomographic imaging

Dosage Forms

Injection, solution:

Hexabrix™: Ioxaglate meglumine 39.3% and ioxaglate sodium 19.6% (20 mL, 50 mL, 100 mL, 150 mL, 200 mL)

ioxaglate sodium and ioxaglate meglumine *see* ioxaglate meglumine and ioxaglate sodium *on page 522*

ioxilan (eye OKS ee lan)

U.S./Canadian Brand Names Oxilan® 300 [US/Can]; Oxilan® 350 [US/Can]

Therapeutic Category Iodinated Contrast Media; Radiological/Contrast Media, Nonionic

Use

Intraarterial: Ioxilan 300 mgI/mL is indicated for cerebral arteriography. Ioxilan 350 mgI/mL is indicated for coronary arteriography and left ventriculography, visceral angiography, aortography, and peripheral arteriography

Intravenous: Both products are indicated for excretory urography and contrast-enhanced computed tomographic (CECT) imaging of the head and body

Dosage Summary

Intraarterial:

Children: Dosage not established

Adults:

Cerebral arteriography (300 mg iodine/mL): 8-12 mL (2.4-3.6 g iodine); total dose should not exceed 150 mL

Coronary arteriography and left ventriculography (350 mg iodine/mL): Left and right coronary: 2-10 mL (0.7-3.5 g iodine); Left ventricle: 25-50 mL (8.75-17.5 g iodine); total doses should not exceed 250 mL

Dosage Forms

Injection, solution [preservative free]:

Oxilan® 300: 62% (50 mL, 100 mL, 150 mL, 200 mL)

Oxilan® 350: 73% (50 mL, 100 mL, 150 mL, 200 mL)

ipecac syrup (IP e kak SIR up)

Synonyms syrup of ipecac

Therapeutic Category Antidote

Use Treatment of acute oral drug overdosage and in certain poisonings

Dosage Summary

Oral:

Children <6 months: Dosage not established

Children 6-12 months: 5-10 mL followed by 10-20 mL/kg of water, may repeat if vomiting does not occur within 20 minutes

Children 1-12 years: 15 mL followed by 10-20 mL/kg of water, may repeat if vomiting does not occur within 20 minutes

Adults: 15-30 mL followed by 200-300 mL of water; may repeat if vomiting does not occur within 20 minutes

Dosage Forms

Syrup, oral: USP: 7% (30 mL)

I-Pentolate® *(Discontinued)* *see* cyclopentolate *on page* *258*

I-Phrine® Ophthalmic Solution *(Discontinued)* *see* phenylephrine (ophthalmic) *on page* *752*

I-Picamide® *(Discontinued)* *see* tropicamide *on page* *964*

Iplex™ *(Discontinued)* *see* mecasermin *on page* *594*

IPM Wound Gel™ [US-OTC] *see* hyaluronate and derivatives *on page* *475*

IPOL® [US/Can] *see* poliovirus vaccine (inactivated) *on page* *774*

ipratropium (oral inhalation) (i pra TROE pee um)

Sound-Alike/Look-Alike Issues

ipratropium may be confused with tiotropium

Atrovent® may be confused with Alupent®, Serevent®

Synonyms ipratropium bromide

U.S./Canadian Brand Names Atrovent® HFA [US/Can]; Gen-Ipratropium [Can]; Mylan-Ipratropium Sterinebs [Can]; Novo-Ipramide [Can]; Nu-Ipratropium [Can]; PMS-Ipratropium [Can]

Therapeutic Category Anticholinergic Agent

Use Anticholinergic bronchodilator used in bronchospasm associated with COPD, bronchitis, and emphysema

Dosage Summary

Inhalation:

Children ≤12 years: Dosage not established

Children >12 years: 2 inhalations 4 times/day (maximum: 12 inhalations/day)

Adults: 2 inhalations 4 times/day (maximum: 12 inhalations/day)

Nebulization:

Children ≤12 years: Dosage not established

Children >12 years: 500 mcg every 6-8 hours

Adults: 500 mcg every 6-8 hours

Dosage Forms

Aerosol, for oral inhalation:

Atrovent® HFA: 17 mcg/actuation (12.9 g)

Solution, for nebulization: 0.02% [500 mcg/2.5 mL] (25s, 30s, 60s)

Solution, for nebulization [preservative free]: 0.02% [500 mcg/2.5 mL] (25s, 30s, 60s)

ipratropium (nasal) (i pra TROE pee um)

Sound-Alike/Look-Alike Issues

ipratropium may be confused with tiotropium

Atrovent® may be confused with Alupent®, Serevent®

Synonyms ipratropium bromide

U.S./Canadian Brand Names Alti-Ipratropium [Can]; Apo-Ipravent® [Can]; Atrovent® [US/Can]; Mylan-Ipratropium Solution [Can]

Therapeutic Category Anticholinergic Agent

Use Symptomatic relief of rhinorrhea associated with the common cold and allergic and nonallergic rhinitis

Dosage Summary

Intranasal:

0.03% solution:

Children <6 years: Dosage not established

Children ≥6 years: 2 sprays in each nostril 2-3 times/day
Adults: 2 sprays in each nostril 2-3 times/day
0.06% solution:
Children <5 years: Dosage not established
Children 5-11 years: 2 sprays in each nostril 3-4 times/day
Children ≥12 years: 2 sprays in each nostril 3-4 times/day
Adults: 2 sprays in each nostril 3-4 times/day

Dosage Forms

Solution, intranasal: 0.03% (30 mL); 0.06% (15 mL)
Atrovent®: 0.03% (30 mL); 0.06% (15 mL)

ipratropium and albuterol (i pra TROE pee um & al BYOO ter ole)

Sound-Alike/Look-Alike Issues
Combivent® may be confused with Combivir®, Serevent®

Synonyms albuterol and ipratropium; salbutamol and ipratropium

U.S./Canadian Brand Names CO Ipra-Sal [Can]; Combivent UDV [Can]; Combivent® [US]; DuoNeb® [US]; Gen-Combo Sterinebs [Can]; ratio-Ipra Sal UDV [Can]

Therapeutic Category Bronchodilator

Use Treatment of COPD in those patients who are currently on a regular bronchodilator who continue to have bronchospasms and require a second bronchodilator

Dosage Summary

Inhalation:
Children: Dosage not established
Adults: 2 inhalations 4 times/day (maximum: 12 inhalations/day)

Nebulization:
Children: Dosage not established
Adults: 3 mL every 4-6 hours

Dosage Forms

Aerosol for oral inhalation:
Combivent®: Ipratropium bromide 18 mcg and albuterol (base) 90 mcg per inhalation (14.7 g) [200 metered actuations]

Solution for nebulization: Ipratropium 0.5 mg and albuterol (base) 2.5 mg per 3 mL (30s, 60s)
DuoNeb®: Ipratropium 0.5 mg and albuterol (base) 2.5 mg per 3 mL (30s, 60s)

ipratropium and fenoterol *(Canada only)* (i pra TROE pee um & fen oh TER ole)

Sound-Alike/Look-Alike Issues
Duovent® UDV may be confused with Combivent® UDV

Synonyms fenoterol and ipratropium; fenoterol hydrobromide and ipratropium bromide; ipratropium bromide and fenoterol hydrobromide

U.S./Canadian Brand Names Duovent® UDV [Can]

Therapeutic Category Anticholinergic Agent; $Beta_2$-Adrenergic Agonist

Use Treatment of bronchospasm associated with acute severe exacerbation of COPD or bronchial asthma

Dosage Summary

Nebulization:
Children <12 years: Dosage not established
Children ≥12 years and Adults: Usual dose: 4 mL; may repeat every 6 hours as needed
Adults: Usual dose: 4 mL; may repeat every 6 hours as needed

Dosage Forms - Canada

Solution for nebulization:
Duovent® UDV: Ipratropium bromide 0.5 mg and fenoterol 1.25 mg per 4 mL (20s)

ipratropium bromide *see* ipratropium (nasal) *on page* 523
ipratropium bromide *see* ipratropium (oral inhalation) *on page* 523
ipratropium bromide and fenoterol hydrobromide *see* ipratropium and fenoterol *(Canada only) on page* 524
I-Prin [US-OTC] *see* ibuprofen *on page* 494
Iprivask® [US] *see* desirudin *on page* 277
iproveratril hydrochloride *see* verapamil *on page* 981
IPV *see* poliovirus vaccine (inactivated) *on page* 774

Iquix® [US] *see* levofloxacin (ophthalmic) *on page 558*

irbesartan (ir be SAR tan)

Sound-Alike/Look-Alike Issues

Avapro® may be confused with Anaprox®

U.S./Canadian Brand Names Avapro® [US/Can]

Therapeutic Category Angiotensin II Receptor Antagonist

Use Treatment of hypertension alone or in combination with other antihypertensives; treatment of diabetic nephropathy in patients with type 2 diabetes mellitus (noninsulin-dependent, NIDDM) and hypertension

Dosage Summary

Oral:

Children <6 years: Dosage not established

Children 6-12 years: Initial: 75 mg once daily; Maintenance: May be titrated up to 150 mg once daily

Children ≥13 years: Initial: 75-150 mg once daily; Maintenance: May be titrated up to 300 mg once daily

Adults: Initial: 75-150 mg once daily; Maintenance: May be titrated up to 300 mg once daily

Dosage Forms

Tablet, oral:

Avapro®: 75 mg, 150 mg, 300 mg

irbesartan and hydrochlorothiazide (ir be SAR tan & hye droe klor oh THYE a zide)

Sound-Alike/Look-Alike Issues

Avalide® may be confused with Avandia®

Synonyms Avapro® HCT; hydrochlorothiazide and irbesartan

U.S./Canadian Brand Names Avalide® [US/Can]

Therapeutic Category Antihypertensive Agent, Combination

Use Combination therapy for the management of hypertension; may be used as initial therapy in patients likely to need multiple drugs to achieve blood pressure goals

Note: In Canada, this combination product is approved for initial therapy in severe, essential hypertension (sitting diastolic blood pressure [DBP] ≥110 mm Hg).

Dosage Summary

Oral:

Children: Dosage not established

Adults: Irbesartan 150-300 mg and hydrochlorothiazide 12.5-25 mg once daily

Dosage Forms

Tablet:

Avalide®: Irbesartan 150 mg and hydrochlorothiazide 12.5 mg; irbesartan 300 mg and hydrochlorothiazide 12.5 mg; irbesartan 300 mg and hydrochlorothiazide 25 mg

Ircon® [US-OTC] *see* ferrous fumarate *on page 398*

Iressa® [US/Can] *see* gefitinib *on page 439*

irinotecan (eye rye no TEE kan)

Synonyms camptothecin-11; CPT-11

U.S./Canadian Brand Names Camptosar® [US/Can]; Irinotecan Hydrochloride Trihydrate [Can]

Therapeutic Category Antineoplastic Agent

Use Treatment of metastatic carcinoma of the colon or rectum

Dosage Summary

I.V.:

Adults: Dosage varies greatly depending on indication

Dosage Forms

Injection, solution: 20 mg/mL (2 mL, 5 mL, 25 mL); (2 mL, 5 mL, 25 mL)

Camptosar®: 20 mg/mL (2 mL, 5 mL)

Irinotecan Hydrochloride Trihydrate [Can] *see* irinotecan *on page 525*

iron dextran *see* iron dextran complex *on page 525*

iron dextran complex (EYE ern DEKS tran KOM pleks)

Sound-Alike/Look-Alike Issues

iron dextran complex may be confused with ferumoxytol

Dexferrum® may be confused with Desferal®

Synonyms high-molecular-weight iron dextran (DexFerrum®); imferon; iron dextran; low-Molecular-weight iron dextran (INFeD®)

U.S./Canadian Brand Names Dexferrum® [US]; Dexiron™ [Can]; INFeD® [US]; Infufer® [Can]

Therapeutic Category Electrolyte Supplement, Oral

Use Treatment of iron deficiency in patients in whom oral administration is infeasible or ineffective

Dosage Summary **Note:** A 0.5 mL test dose (0.25 mL in infants) should be given prior to starting iron dextran therapy.

I.M.:

Children <4 months: Use not recommended

Children <5 kg: (INFeD®): Replacement iron (mg) = blood loss (mL) x Hct; **Note:** Total dose should be divided daily at not more than 25 mg/day

Children 5-15 kg: (INFeD®): Total Dose (mL) = 0.0442 (desired Hgb [usually 12 g/dL] - observed Hgb) x W (in kg) + (0.26 x W [in kg]) **or** replacement iron (mg) = blood loss (mL) x hematocrit; **Note:** Total dose should be divided daily at not more than 50 mg/day [5-10 kg] or 100 mg/day [10-15 kg]

Children >15 kg: (INFeD®): Total Dose (mL) = 0.0442 (desired Hgb [usually 14.8 g/dL] - observed Hgb) x LBW + (0.26 x LBW) **or** replacement iron (mg) = blood loss (mL) x Hct; **Note:** Total dose should be divided daily at not more than 100 mg/day

Adults: (INFeD®): Total Dose (mL) = 0.0442 (desired Hgb [usually 14.8 g/dL] - observed Hgb) x LBW + (0.26 x LBW) **or** replacement iron (mg) = blood loss (mL) x Hct; **Note:** Total dose should be divided daily at not more than 100 mg/day

I.V.:

Children <4 months: Use not recommended

Children <5 kg: Replacement iron (mg) = blood loss (mL) x Hct; **Note:** Total dose should be divided daily at not more than 100 mg/day

Children 5-15 kg: Total Dose (mL) = 0.0442 (desired Hgb [usually 12 g/dL] - observed Hgb) x W (in kg) + (0.26 x W [in kg]) **or** replacement iron (mg) = blood loss (mL) x hematocrit; **Note:** Total dose should be divided daily at not more than 100 mg/day

Children >15 kg: Total Dose (mL) = 0.0442 (desired Hgb [usually 14.8 g/dL] - observed Hgb) x LBW + (0.26 x LBW) **or** replacement iron (mg) = blood loss (mL) x Hct (maximum: 100 mg/day); **Note:** Total dose should be divided daily at not more than 100 mg/day

Adults: Total Dose (mL) = 0.0442 (desired Hgb [usually 14.8 g/dL] - observed Hgb) x LBW + (0.26 x LBW) **or** replacement iron (mg) = blood loss (mL) x Hct (maximum: 100 mg/day); **Note:** Total dose should be divided daily at not more than 100 mg/day

Dosage Forms

Injection, solution:

Dexferrum®: Elemental iron 50 mg/mL (1 mL, 2 mL)

INFeD®: Elemental iron 50 mg/mL (2 mL)

iron fumarate *see* ferrous fumarate *on page* 398

iron gluconate *see* ferrous gluconate *on page* 398

iron-polysaccharide complex *see* polysaccharide-iron complex *on page* 777

iron-polysaccharide complex, vitamin B12, and folic acid *see* polysaccharide-iron complex, vitamin B12, and folic acid *on page* 778

iron sucrose (EYE ern SOO krose)

Sound-Alike/Look-Alike Issues

iron sucrose may be confused with ferumoxytol

U.S./Canadian Brand Names Venofer® [US/Can]

Therapeutic Category Iron Salt

Use Treatment of iron-deficiency anemia in chronic renal failure, including nondialysis-dependent patients (with or without erythropoietin therapy) and dialysis-dependent patients receiving erythropoietin therapy

Dosage Summary

I.V.:

Children: Dosage not established

Adults: 100 mg (5 mL) 1-3 times/week during dialysis **or** 200 mg on 5 different occasions within a 14-day period **or** two 300 mg infusion 14 days apart, followed by a single 400 mg infusion 14 days later (maximum: 1000 mg cumulative total)

Dosage Forms

Injection, solution [preservative free]:

Venofer®: Elemental iron 20 mg/mL (5 mL, 10 mL)

iron sulfate *see* ferrous sulfate *on page* *398*

iron sulfate and vitamin C *see* ferrous sulfate and ascorbic acid *on page* *399*

Isagel® [US-OTC] *see* alcohol (ethyl) *on page* *45*

ISD *see* isosorbide dinitrate *on page* *529*

ISDN *see* isosorbide dinitrate *on page* *529*

Isentress® [US/Can] *see* raltegravir *on page* *826*

ISG *see* immune globulin (intramuscular) *on page* *501*

ISMN *see* isosorbide mononitrate *on page* *529*

Ismo® [US] *see* isosorbide mononitrate *on page* *529*

isoamyl nitrite *see* amyl nitrite *on page* *76*

isobamate *see* carisoprodol *on page* *185*

Isocal® [US-OTC] *see* nutritional formula, enteral/oral *on page* *692*

isocarboxazid (eye soe kar BOKS a zid)

U.S./Canadian Brand Names Marplan® [US]

Therapeutic Category Antidepressant, Monoamine Oxidase Inhibitor

Use Treatment of depression

Dosage Summary

Oral:

Children: Dosage not established

Adults: Initial: 10 mg 2-4 times/day; may increase to a maximum of 60 mg/day divided in 2-4 doses

Dosage Forms

Tablet, oral:

Marplan®: 10 mg

Isochron™ [US] *see* isosorbide dinitrate *on page* *529*

isoflurane (eye soe FLURE ane)

Sound-Alike/Look-Alike Issues

isoflurane may be confused with enflurane, isoflurophate

U.S./Canadian Brand Names Forane® [US/Can]; Terrell™ [US]

Therapeutic Category General Anesthetic

Use Maintenance of general anesthesia

Note: Use of isoflurane for induction of general anesthesia is an FDA labeled indication; however, it is not recommended clinically due to its irritant properties and unpleasant odor, which causes breath-holding or coughing.

Dosage Summary

Inhalation:

Children: Dosage not established

Adults: Maintenance: in nitrous oxide: 1% to 2.5%; in oxygen: 1.5% to 3.5%

Dosage Forms

Liquid, for inhalation: USP: ≥ 99.9 mL/100 mL (100 mL, 250 mL)

Forane®: USP: ≥ 99.9 mL/100 mL (100 mL, 250 mL)

Terrell™: USP: ≥ 99.9 mL/100 mL (100 mL, 250 mL)

isometheptene, acetaminophen, and dichloralphenazone *see* acetaminophen, isometheptene, and dichloralphenazone *on page* *31*

isometheptene, dichloralphenazone, and acetaminophen *see* acetaminophen, isometheptene, and dichloralphenazone *on page* *31*

IsonaRif™ [US] *see* rifampin and isoniazid *on page* *842*

isoniazid (eye soe NYE a zid)

Synonyms INH; isonicotinic acid hydrazide

U.S./Canadian Brand Names Isotamine® [Can]; PMS-Isoniazid [Can]

Therapeutic Category Antitubercular Agent

Use Treatment of susceptible tuberculosis infections; treatment of latent tuberculosis infection (LTBI)

Dosage Summary Note: Concomitant administration of 10-50 mg/day pyridoxine is recommended in malnourished patients or those prone to neuropathy (eg, alcoholics, patients with diabetes)

Oral, I.M.:

Children: 10-15 mg/kg/day once daily (maximum: 300 mg/day) **or** 20-40 mg/kg 2-3 times/week (maximum: 900 mg/dose)

Adults: 300 mg (5 mg/kg) once daily **or** 900 mg (15 mg/kg) 2-3 times/week

Dosage Forms

Injection, solution: 100 mg/mL (10 mL)

Solution, oral: 50 mg/5 mL (473 mL)

Tablet, oral: 100 mg, 300 mg

isoniazid and rifampin *see* rifampin and isoniazid *on page* *842*

isoniazid, pyrazinamide, and rifampin *see* rifampin, isoniazid, and pyrazinamide *on page* *842*

isonicotinic acid hydrazide *see* isoniazid *on page* *527*

isonipecaine hydrochloride *see* meperidine *on page* *603*

isophane insulin *see* insulin NPH *on page* *512*

isophane insulin and regular insulin *see* insulin NPH and insulin regular *on page* *512*

isophosphamide *see* ifosfamide *on page* *498*

isoproterenol (eye soe proe TER e nole)

Sound-Alike/Look-Alike Issues

Isuprel® may be confused with Disophrol®, Ismelin®, Isordil®

Synonyms isoproterenol hydrochloride

U.S./Canadian Brand Names Isuprel® [US]

Therapeutic Category Adrenergic Agonist Agent

Use Manufacturer's labeled indications (see **"Note"**): Mild or transient episodes of heart block that do not require electric shock or pacemaker therapy; serious episodes of heart block and Adams-Stokes attacks (except when caused by ventricular tachycardia or fibrillation); cardiac arrest until electric shock or pacemaker therapy is available; bronchospasm during anesthesia; adjunct to fluid and electrolyte replacement therapy and other drugs and procedures in the treatment of hypovolemic or septic shock and low cardiac output states (eg, decompensated heart failure, cardiogenic shock)

Note: The use of isoproterenol in advanced cardiac life support (ACLS) has largely been supplanted by the use of other adrenergic agents (eg, epinephrine and dopamine). The use of isoproterenol for bronchospasm during anesthesia and cardiogenic, hypovolemic, or septic shock is no longer recommended.

Dosage Summary

Continuous I.V. infusion:

Children: 0.05-2 mcg/kg/minute; titrate to patient response

Adults: 2-10 mcg/minute; titrate to patient response

Dosage Forms

Injection, solution:

Isuprel®: 0.2 mg/mL (1 mL, 5 mL)

isoproterenol hydrochloride *see* isoproterenol *on page* *528*

Isoptin® ***(Discontinued)*** *see* verapamil *on page* *981*

Isoptin® SR [US/Can] *see* verapamil *on page* *981*

Isopto® Atropine [US/Can] *see* atropine *on page* *105*

Isopto® Carbachol [US/Can] *see* carbachol *on page* *177*

Isopto® Carpine [US/Can] *see* pilocarpine (ophthalmic) *on page* *760*

Isopto® Cetapred® ***(Discontinued)***

Isopto® Eserine ***(Discontinued)*** *see* physostigmine *on page* *759*

Isopto® Frin Ophthalmic Solution ***(Discontinued)*** *see* phenylephrine (ophthalmic) *on page* *752*

Isopto® Homatropine [US] *see* homatropine *on page* *473*

Isopto® Hyoscine [US] *see* scopolamine derivatives (ophthalmic) *on page* *867*

Isopto® Plain Solution ***(Discontinued)*** *see* artificial tears *on page* *97*

Isopto® Tears [US-OTC/Can] *see* hydroxypropyl methylcellulose *on page* *489*

Isordil® [US] *see* isosorbide dinitrate *on page* *529*

isosorbide dinitrate (eye soe SOR bide dye NYE trate)

Sound-Alike/Look-Alike Issues

Isordil® may be confused with Inderal®, Isuprel®, Plendil®

Synonyms ISD; ISDN

U.S./Canadian Brand Names Dilatrate®-SR [US]; Isochron™ [US]; Isordil® [US]; Novo-Sorbide [Can]; PMS-Isosorbide [Can]

Therapeutic Category Vasodilator

Use Prevention and treatment of angina pectoris; for congestive heart failure; to relieve pain, dysphagia, and spasm in esophageal spasm with GE reflux

Dosage Summary

Oral:

Immediate release:

Children: Dosage not established

Adults: 5-40 mg 3-4 times/day

Sustained release:

Children: Dosage not established

Adults: 40 mg every 8-12 hours

Sublingual:

Children: Dosage not established

Adults: 2.5-5 mg every 5-10 minutes for maximum of 3 doses in 15-30 minutes

Dosage Forms

Capsule, sustained release, oral:

Dilatrate®-SR: 40 mg

Tablet, oral: 5 mg, 10 mg, 20 mg, 30 mg

Isordil®: 5 mg, 40 mg

Tablet, sublingual: 2.5 mg, 5 mg

Tablet, extended release, oral: 40 mg

Isochron™: 40 mg

isosorbide dinitrate and hydralazine

(eye soe SOR bide dye NYE trate & hye DRAL a zeen)

Synonyms hydralazine and isosorbide dinitrate

U.S./Canadian Brand Names BiDil® [US]

Therapeutic Category Vasodilator

Use Treatment of heart failure, adjunct to standard therapy, in self-identified African-Americans

Dosage Summary

Oral:

Children: Dosage not established

Adults: 1-2 tablets 3 times/day

Dosage Forms

Tablet:

BiDil®: Isosorbide 20 mg and hydralazine 37.5 mg

isosorbide mononitrate (eye soe SOR bide mon oh NYE trate)

Sound-Alike/Look-Alike Issues

Imdur® may be confused with Imuran®, Inderal LA®, K-Dur®

Monoket® may be confused with Monopril®

Synonyms ISMN

U.S./Canadian Brand Names Apo-ISMN® [Can]; Imdur® [US/Can]; Ismo® [US]; Monoket® [US]; PMS-ISMN [Can]; PRO-ISMN [Can]

Therapeutic Category Vasodilator

Use Long-acting metabolite of the vasodilator isosorbide dinitrate used for the prophylactic treatment of angina pectoris

Dosage Summary

Oral:

Extended release:

Children: Dosage not established

Adults: Initial: 30-60 mg once daily; Maintenance: 30-240 mg once daily (maximum: 240 mg/day); **Note:** Titration is recommended

Regular release:
Children: Dosage not established
Adults: 5-20 mg twice daily

Dosage Forms
Tablet, oral: 10 mg, 20 mg
Ismo®: 20 mg
Monoket®: 10 mg, 20 mg
Tablet, extended release, oral: 30 mg, 60 mg, 120 mg
Imdur®: 30 mg, 60 mg, 120 mg

isosulfan blue (eye soe SUL fan bloo)

U.S./Canadian Brand Names Lymphazurin™ [US]
Therapeutic Category Contrast Agent
Use Adjunct to lymphography for visualization of the lymphatic system; sentinel node identification
Dosage Summary
SubQ:
Children: Dosage not established
Adults: Inject 0.5 mL into 3 interdigital spaces of each extremity per study (maximum: 3 mL [30 mg])
Dosage Forms
Injection, solution [preservative free]:
Lymphazurin™: 1% (5 mL)

Isotamine® [Can] *see* isoniazid *on page* 527

isotretinoin (eye soe TRET i noyn)

Sound-Alike/Look-Alike Issues
isotretinoin may be confused with tretinoin
Accutane® may be confused with Accolate®, Accupril®
Claravis™ may be confused with Cleviprex™
Synonyms 13-*cis*-retinoic acid
U.S./Canadian Brand Names Accutane® [Can]; Amnesteem® [US]; Claravis™ [US]; Clarus™ [Can]; Isotrex® [Can]; Sotret® [US]
Therapeutic Category Retinoic Acid Derivative
Use Treatment of severe recalcitrant nodular acne unresponsive to conventional therapy
Dosage Summary
Oral:
Children <12 years: Dosage not established
Children 12-17 years: 0.5-1 mg/kg/day in 2 divided doses; doses as low as 0.05 mg/kg/day have been reported to be beneficial
Adults: 0.5-2 mg/kg/day in 2 divided doses; doses as low as 0.05 mg/kg/day have been reported to be beneficial
Dosage Forms
Capsule, oral:
Claravis™: 10 mg, 20 mg, 30 mg, 40 mg
Capsule, softgel, oral:
Amnesteem®: 10 mg, 20 mg, 40 mg
Sotret®: 10 mg, 20 mg, 30 mg, 40 mg

Isotrex® [Can] *see* isotretinoin *on page* 530
Isovue® [US] *see* iopamidol *on page* 520
Isovue® 200 [US] *see* iopamidol *on page* 520
Isovue® 300 [US] *see* iopamidol *on page* 520
Isovue® 370 [US] *see* iopamidol *on page* 520
Isovue-M® [US] *see* iopamidol *on page* 520
Isovue Multipack® [US] *see* iopamidol *on page* 520

isoxsuprine (eye SOKS syoo preen)

Sound-Alike/Look-Alike Issues
Vasodilan® may be confused with Vasocidin®
Synonyms isoxsuprine hydrochloride

Therapeutic Category Vasodilator

Use Treatment of peripheral vascular diseases, such as arteriosclerosis obliterans and Raynaud disease

Dosage Summary

Oral:

Children: Dosage not established

Adults: 10-20 mg 3-4 times/day

Dosage Forms

Tablet, oral: 10 mg, 20 mg

isoxsuprine hydrochloride *see* isoxsuprine *on page 530*

isradipine (iz RA di peen)

Sound-Alike/Look-Alike Issues

DynaCirc® may be confused with Dynabac®, Dynacin®

U.S./Canadian Brand Names DynaCirc CR® [US]; DynaCirc® [Can]

Therapeutic Category Calcium Channel Blocker

Use Treatment of hypertension

Dosage Summary

Oral:

Adults:

Capsule: Initial: 2.5 mg twice daily; titrate dose in 2- to 4-week intervals; usual range: 2.5-10 mg/day

Controlled release tablet: Initial: 5 mg once daily; Maintenance: 5-20 mg once daily (maximum: 20 mg/day)

Dosage Forms

Capsule, oral: 2.5 mg, 5 mg

Tablet, controlled release, oral:

DynaCirc CR®: 5 mg, 10 mg

Istalol® [US] *see* timolol (ophthalmic) *on page 933*

Istodax® [US] *see* romidepsin *on page 850*

Isuprel® [US] *see* isoproterenol *on page 528*

Itch-X® [US-OTC] *see* pramoxine *on page 787*

itraconazole (i tra KOE na zole)

Sound-Alike/Look-Alike Issues

itraconazole may be confused with fluconazole

Sporanox® may be confused with Suprax®, Topamax®

U.S./Canadian Brand Names Sporanox® [US/Can]

Therapeutic Category Antifungal Agent

Use

Oral capsules: Treatment of susceptible fungal infections in immunocompromised and immunocompetent patients including blastomycosis and histoplasmosis; indicated for aspergillosis (in patients intolerant/refractory to amphotericin B), and onychomycosis of the toenail and fingernail (in nonimmunocompromised patients)

Oral solution: Treatment of oral and esophageal candidiasis

Dosage Summary

Oral:

Children: Dosage not established

Adults: 100-800 mg/day; doses >200 mg/day are given in 2-3 divided doses

Dosage Forms

Capsule, oral: 100 mg

Sporanox®: 100 mg

Solution, oral:

Sporanox®: 10 mg/mL (150 mL)

I-Tropine® ***(Discontinued)*** *see* atropine *on page 105*

ivermectin (eye ver MEK tin)

U.S./Canadian Brand Names Stromectol® [US]

Therapeutic Category Antibiotic, Miscellaneous

Use Treatment of the following infections: Strongyloidiasis of the intestinal tract due to the nematode parasite *Strongyloides stercoralis*. Onchocerciasis due to the immature form of the nematode parasite *Onchocerca volvulus*.

Dosage Summary

Oral:

Children <15 kg: Dosage not established

Children ≥15 kg: 150-200 mcg/kg as a single dose

Adults: 150-200 mcg/kg as a single dose

Dosage Forms

Tablet, oral:

Stromectol®: 3 mg

IVIG *see* immune globulin (intravenous) *on page 502*

IV immune globulin *see* immune globulin (intravenous) *on page 502*

Ivy Block® [US-OTC] *see* bentoquatam *on page 123*

Ivy-Rid® [US-OTC] *see* benzocaine *on page 124*

Ivy Soothe® [US-OTC] *see* hydrocortisone (topical) *on page 483*

ixabepilone (ix ab EP i lone)

Synonyms azaepothilone B; BMS-247550; epothilone B lactam

U.S./Canadian Brand Names Ixempra® [US]

Therapeutic Category Antineoplastic Agent, Antimicrotubular; Antineoplastic Agent, Epothilone B Analog

Use Treatment of metastatic or locally-advanced breast cancer (refractory or resistant)

Dosage Summary

I.V.:

Children: Dosage not established

Adults: 40 mg/m^2 every 3 weeks (maximum dose: 88 mg)

Dosage Forms

Injection, powder for reconstitution:

Ixempra®: 15 mg, 45 mg

Ixempra® [US] *see* ixabepilone *on page 532*

Ixiaro® [US] *see* Japanese encephalitis virus vaccine (inactivated) *on page 532*

Jalyn™ [US] *see* dutasteride and tamsulosin *on page 337*

JAMP-Amlodipine [Can] *see* amlodipine *on page 68*

JAMP-Citalopram [Can] *see* citalopram *on page 227*

JAMP-Ondansetron [Can] *see* ondansetron *on page 704*

JAMP-Ramipril [Can] *see* ramipril *on page 826*

JAMP-Ropinirole [Can] *see* ropinirole *on page 851*

JAMP-Simvastatin [Can] *see* simvastatin *on page 877*

JAMP-Tamsulosin [Can] *see* tamsulosin *on page 909*

Janimine® ***(Discontinued)*** *see* imipramine *on page 500*

Jantoven® [US] *see* warfarin *on page 993*

Janumet® [US/Can] *see* sitagliptin and metformin *on page 879*

Januvia™ [US/Can] *see* sitagliptin *on page 879*

Japanese encephalitis virus vaccine (inactivated)

(jap a NEESE en sef a LYE tis VYE rus vak SEEN, in ak ti VAY ted)

Synonyms IC51; JE-MB (Je-Vax®); JE-VC (Ixiaro®)

U.S./Canadian Brand Names Ixiaro® [US]; JE-VAX® [Can]

Therapeutic Category Vaccine, Inactivated Virus

Use Active immunization against Japanese encephalitis

Japanese encephalitis vaccine is not recommended for all persons traveling to or residing in Asia. The Advisory Committee on Immunization Practices (ACIP) recommends vaccination for:

- Persons spending ≥1 month in endemic areas during transmission season
- Research laboratory workers who may be exposed to the Japanese encephalitis virus

Vaccination may also be considered for the following:

- Travelers to areas with an ongoing outbreak
- Travelers spending <30 days in endemic areas during the transmission season and planning to go outside of urban areas and have an increased risk of exposure. For example, high-risk activities include extensive outdoor activity in rural areas especially at night; extensive outdoor activities such as camping, hiking, etc; staying in accommodations without air conditioning, screens or bed nets.
- Travelers to endemic areas who are unsure of specific destination, activities, or duration of travel

Dosage Summary

I.M.:

Children <17 years: Ixiaro®: Dosage not established

Adults ≥17 years: Ixiaro®: 0.5 mL/dose; a total of 2 doses given on days 0 and 28

SubQ:

Children <1 year: Je-Vax®: Dosage not established

Children 1-2 years: Je-Vax®: 0.5 mL/dose; a total of 3 doses given on days 0, 7, and 30; booster dose given after 2 years

Children ≥3 years: Je-Vax®: 1 mL/dose; a total of 3 doses given on days 0, 7, and 30; booster dose given after 2 years

Adults: Je-Vax®: 1 mL/dose; a total of 3 doses given on days 0, 7, and 30; booster dose given after 2 years

Dosage Forms

Injection, suspension:

Ixiaro®: Inactivated JEV proteins 6 mcg/0.5 mL (0.5 mL)

JE-MB (Je-Vax®) *see* Japanese encephalitis virus vaccine (inactivated) *on page* 532

Jenamicin® ***(Discontinued)*** *see* gentamicin (systemic) *on page* 443

Jenest™-28 ***(Discontinued)*** *see* ethinyl estradiol and norethindrone *on page* 378

JE-VAX® [Can] *see* Japanese encephalitis virus vaccine (inactivated) *on page* 532

JE-VAX® ***(Discontinued)*** *see* Japanese encephalitis virus vaccine (inactivated) *on page* 532

JE-VC (Ixiaro®) *see* Japanese encephalitis virus vaccine (inactivated) *on page* 532

Jevtana® [US] *see* cabazitaxel *on page* 162

Jolessa™ [US] *see* ethinyl estradiol and levonorgestrel *on page* 376

Jolivette® [US] *see* norethindrone *on page* 682

Junel™ [US] *see* ethinyl estradiol and norethindrone *on page* 378

Junel™ Fe [US] *see* ethinyl estradiol and norethindrone *on page* 378

Jurnista™ [Can] *see* hydromorphone *on page* 485

Just for Kids™ [US-OTC] *see* fluoride *on page* 413

Just Tears® Solution ***(Discontinued)*** *see* artificial tears *on page* 97

Juvederm™ 24HV [US] *see* hyaluronate and derivatives *on page* 475

Juvederm™ 30 [US] *see* hyaluronate and derivatives *on page* 475

Juvederm™ 30HV [US] *see* hyaluronate and derivatives *on page* 475

K-10® [Can] *see* potassium chloride *on page* 781

Kabikinase® ***(Discontinued)***

Kadian® [US/Can] *see* morphine (systemic) *on page* 644

Kala® [US-OTC] *see* Lactobacillus *on page* 543

Kalbitor® [US] *see* ecallantide *on page* 340

Kalcinate® ***(Discontinued)*** *see* calcium gluconate *on page* 170

Kaletra® [US/Can] *see* lopinavir and ritonavir *on page* 574

Kalexate [US] *see* sodium polystyrene sulfonate *on page* 887

Kalmz [US-OTC] *see* fructose, dextrose, and phosphoric acid *on page* 430

kanamycin (kan a MYE sin)

Sound-Alike/Look-Alike Issues

kanamycin may be confused with Garamycin®, gentamicin

Synonyms kanamycin sulfate

U.S./Canadian Brand Names Kantrex® [Can]

Therapeutic Category Aminoglycoside (Antibiotic)

Use Treatment of serious infections caused by susceptible strains of *E. coli*, *Proteus* species, *Enterobacter aerogenes*, *Klebsiella pneumoniae*, *Serratia marcescens*, and *Acinetobacter* species; second-line treatment of *Mycobacterium tuberculosis*

Dosage Summary Note: Dosing should be based on ideal body weight

I.M.:

Children: 15 mg/kg/day divided every 8-12 hours
Adults: 5-7.5 mg/kg every 8-12 hours
Elderly: 5-7.5 mg/kg every 12-24 hours

I.V.:

Children: 15 mg/kg/day divided every 8-12 hours
Adults: 5-7.5 mg/kg every 8-12 hours
Elderly: 5-7.5 mg/kg every 12-24 hours

Inhalation: Aerosol:

Children: Dosage not established
Adults: 250 mg 2-4 times/day

Intraperitoneal:

Children: Dosage not established
Adults: 500 mg

Irrigation:

Children: Dosage not established
Adults: 0.25% (maximum: 1.5 g/day)

Dosage Forms

Injection, solution: 1 g/3 mL (3 mL)

kanamycin sulfate *see* kanamycin *on page* *533*
Kank-A® Soft Brush [US-OTC] *see* benzocaine *on page* *124*
Kantrex® [Can] *see* kanamycin *on page* *533*
Kantrex® ***(Discontinued)*** *see* kanamycin *on page* *533*
Kaochlor-Eff® ***(Discontinued)***
Kaochlor® SF ***(Discontinued)*** *see* potassium chloride *on page* *781*
Kaodene® ***(Discontinued)***
Kaodene® NN ***(Discontinued)***
Kaon-CL® 10 [US] *see* potassium chloride *on page* *781*
Kao-Paverin® ***(Discontinued)*** *see* loperamide *on page* *573*
Kaopectate® [US-OTC] *see* bismuth *on page* *139*
Kaopectate® II ***(Discontinued)*** *see* loperamide *on page* *573*
Kaopectate® Advanced Formula ***(Discontinued)***
Kaopectate® Extra Strength [US-OTC] *see* bismuth *on page* *139*
Kaopectate® Maximum Strength Caplets ***(Discontinued)***
Kaopectate® Stool Softener [US-OTC] *see* docusate *on page* *321*
Kao-Spen® ***(Discontinued)***
Kao-Tin [US-OTC] *see* bismuth *on page* *139*
Kapectolin ***(Discontinued)*** *see* bismuth *on page* *139*
Kapidex™ ***(Discontinued)*** *see* dexlansoprazole *on page* *283*
Karidium® ***(Discontinued)*** *see* fluoride *on page* *413*
Karigel® ***(Discontinued)*** *see* fluoride *on page* *413*
Karigel®-N ***(Discontinued)*** *see* fluoride *on page* *413*
Kariva™ [US] *see* ethinyl estradiol and desogestrel *on page* *374*
Kasof® ***(Discontinued)*** *see* docusate *on page* *321*
Kaybovite-1000® ***(Discontinued)*** *see* cyanocobalamin *on page* *257*
Kay Ciel® ***(Discontinued)*** *see* potassium chloride *on page* *781*
Kayexalate® [US/Can] *see* sodium polystyrene sulfonate *on page* *887*
K-Citra® [Can] *see* potassium citrate *on page* *782*
KCl *see* potassium chloride *on page* *781*
K-Dur® [Can] *see* potassium chloride *on page* *781*
kdur *see* potassium chloride *on page* *781*
Keflex® [US/Can] *see* cephalexin *on page* *197*

Keftab® [Can] *see* cephalexin *on page 197*
Kefurox® Injection *(Discontinued)* *see* cefuroxime *on page 194*
Kefzol® *(Discontinued)* *see* cefazolin *on page 189*
K-Electrolyte® Effervescent *(Discontinued)* *see* potassium bicarbonate *on page 780*
Kelnor™ [US] *see* ethinyl estradiol and ethynodiol diacetate *on page 376*
Kemadrin® *(Discontinued)* *see* procyclidine *(Canada only) on page 798*
Kemsol® [Can] *see* dimethyl sulfoxide *on page 308*
Kenacort® Oral *(Discontinued)*
Kenaject® Injection *(Discontinued)*
Kenalog® [US/Can] *see* triamcinolone (topical) *on page 954*
Kenalog®-10 [Can] *see* triamcinolone (systemic, oral inhalation) *on page 952*
Kenalog®-40 [Can] *see* triamcinolone (systemic, oral inhalation) *on page 952*
Kenonel® Topical *(Discontinued)*
keoxifene hydrochloride *see* raloxifene *on page 825*
Kepivance® [US] *see* palifermin *on page 720*
Keppra® [US/Can] *see* levetiracetam *on page 555*
Keppra XR™ [US] *see* levetiracetam *on page 555*
Kerafoam® [US] *see* urea *on page 970*
Keralac™ [US] *see* urea *on page 970*
Keralac™ Nailstik [US] *see* urea *on page 970*
Keralyt® [US-OTC] *see* salicylic acid *on page 858*
Keratol 40™ [US] *see* urea *on page 970*
Kerlone® [US] *see* betaxolol (systemic) *on page 135*
Kerol™ [US] *see* urea *on page 970*
Kerol™ Redi-Cloths [US] *see* urea *on page 970*
Kerol™ ZX [US] *see* urea *on page 970*
Kerr Insta-Char® [US-OTC] *see* charcoal *on page 200*
Ketalar® [US/Can] *see* ketamine *on page 535*

ketamine (KEET a meen)

Sound-Alike/Look-Alike Issues
Ketalar® may be confused with Kenalog®, ketorolac

Synonyms ketamine hydrochloride

U.S./Canadian Brand Names Ketalar® [US/Can]; Ketamine Hydrochloride Injection, USP [Can]

Therapeutic Category General Anesthetic

Controlled Substance C-III

Use Induction and maintenance of general anesthesia

Dosage Summary

I.M.:
Children: 4-5 mg/kg
Adults: 6.5-13 mg/kg

I.V.:
Children: 1-2 mg/kg **or** 5-20 mcg/kg/minute as a continuous infusion
Adults: 1-4.5 mg/kg **or** 1-2 mg/kg

Oral:
Children: 6-10 mg/kg for 1 dose given 30 minutes before the procedure
Adults: Dosage not established

Dosage Forms

Injection, solution: 10 mg/mL (20 mL); 50 mg/mL (10 mL); 100 mg/mL (5 mL, 10 mL)
Ketalar®: 10 mg/mL (20 mL); 50 mg/mL (10 mL); 100 mg/mL (5 mL)

ketamine hydrochloride *see* ketamine *on page 535*
Ketamine Hydrochloride Injection, USP [Can] *see* ketamine *on page 535*
Ketek® [US/Can] *see* telithromycin *on page 913*

ketoconazole (systemic) (kee toe KOE na zole)

U.S./Canadian Brand Names Apo-Ketoconazole® [Can]; Novo-Ketoconazole [Can]

Therapeutic Category Antifungal Agent, Oral

Use Treatment of susceptible fungal infections, including candidiasis, oral thrush, blastomycosis, histoplasmosis, paracoccidioidomycosis, coccidioidomycosis, chromomycosis, candiduria, chronic mucocutaneous candidiasis, as well as certain recalcitrant cutaneous dermatophytoses

Dosage Summary

Oral:

Children <2 years: Dosage not established
Children ≥2 years: 3.3-6.6 mg/kg/day as a single daily dose
Adults: 200-400 mg/day as a single daily dose

Dosage Forms

Tablet, oral: 200 mg

ketoconazole (topical) (kee toe KOE na zole)

Sound-Alike/Look-Alike Issues

Kuric™ may be confused with Carac®
Nizoral® may be confused with Nasarel®, Neoral®, Nitrol®

U.S./Canadian Brand Names Extina® [US]; Ketoderm® [Can]; Kuric™ [US]; Nizoral® A-D [US-OTC]; Nizoral® [US]; Xolegel® [US/Can]

Therapeutic Category Antifungal Agent, Topical

Use

Cream: Treatment of tinea corporis, tinea cruris, tinea versicolor, cutaneous candidiasis, seborrheic dermatitis
Foam, gel: Treatment of seborrheic dermatitis
Shampoo: Treatment of dandruff, seborrheic dermatitis, tinea versicolor

Dosage Summary

Topical:

Cream:
Children <12 years: Dosage not established
Children ≥12 years: Rub gently into the affected area 1-2 times daily
Adults: Rub gently into the affected area 1-2 times daily

Foam:
Children <12 years: Dosage not established
Children ≥12 years: Apply to affected area twice daily for 4 weeks
Adults: Apply to affected area twice daily for 4 weeks

Gel:
Children <12 years: Dosage not established
Children ≥12 years: Apply gently to affected area once daily
Adults: Apply gently to affected area once daily

Shampoo:
Children <12 years: Dosage not established
Children ≥12 years: Apply twice weekly with at least 3 days between each shampoo
Adults: Apply twice weekly with at least 3 days between each shampoo or once

Dosage Forms

Aerosol, topical:
Extina®: 2% (50 g, 100 g)

Cream, topical: 2% (15 g, 30 g, 60 g)
Kuric™: 2% (75 g)

Gel, topical:
Xolegel®: 2% (15 g, 45 g)

Shampoo, topical: 2% (120 mL)
Nizoral®: 2% (120 mL)
Nizoral® A-D [OTC]: 1% (6 mL, 120 mL, 210 mL)

Ketoderm® [Can] *see* ketoconazole (topical) *on page* 536

3-keto-desogestrel *see* etonogestrel *on page* 384

ketoprofen (kee toe PROE fen)

Sound-Alike/Look-Alike Issues

ketoprofen may be confused with ketotifen

U.S./Canadian Brand Names Apo-Keto SR® [Can]; Apo-Keto-E® [Can]; Apo-Keto® [Can]; Nu-Ketoprofen [Can]; Nu-Ketoprofen-E [Can]; PMS-Ketoprofen [Can]; PMS-Ketoprofen-E [Can]; Rhodis SR™ [Can]; Rhodis-EC™ [Can]; Rhodis™ [Can]

Therapeutic Category Analgesic, Nonnarcotic; Nonsteroidal Antiinflammatory Drug (NSAID)

Use Acute and long-term treatment of rheumatoid arthritis and osteoarthritis; primary dysmenorrhea; mild-to-moderate pain

Dosage Summary

Oral:

Extended release:

Children: Dosage not established

Adults: 200 mg once daily

Regular release:

Children: Dosage not established

Adults: 25-50 mg 4 times/day or 75 mg 3 times a day (maximum: 300 mg/day)

Elderly: Initial: 25-50 mg 3-4 times/day; Maintenance: 150-300 mg/day (maximum: 300 mg/day)

Dosage Forms

Capsule, oral: 50 mg, 75 mg

Capsule, extended release, oral: 200 mg

ketorolac (systemic) (KEE toe role ak)

Sound-Alike/Look-Alike Issues

ketorolac may be confused with Ketalar®

Toradol® may be confused with Foradil®, Inderal®, Tegretol®, Torecan®, traMADol, tromethamine

Synonyms ketorolac tromethamine

U.S./Canadian Brand Names Apo-Ketorolac Injectable® [Can]; Apo-Ketorolac® [Can]; Ketorolac Tromethamine Injection, USP [Can]; Novo-Ketorolac [Can]; Nu-Ketorolac [Can]; Toradol® IM [Can]; Toradol® [Can]

Therapeutic Category Nonsteroidal Antiinflammatory Drug (NSAID), Oral; Nonsteroidal Antiinflammatory Drug (NSAID), Parenteral

Use Short-term (≤5 days) management of moderate-to-severe acute pain requiring analgesia at the opioid level

Dosage Summary Note: The maximum combined duration of treatment (for parenteral and oral) is 5 days

I.M.:

Children <16 years: Dosage not established

Children ≥16 years and <50 kg: 30 mg as a single dose **or** 15 mg every 6 hours (maximum: 60 mg/day)

Children ≥16 years and ≥50 kg: 60 mg as a single dose **or** 30 mg every 6 hours (maximum: 120 mg/day)

Adults <50 kg: 30 mg as a single dose **or** 15 mg every 6 hours (maximum: 60 mg/day)

Adults ≥50 kg: 60 mg as a single dose **or** 30 mg every 6 hours (maximum: 120 mg/day)

Elderly ≥65 years: 30 mg as a single dose **or** 15 mg every 6 hours (maximum: 60 mg/day)

I.V.:

Children <16 years: Dosage not established

Children ≥16 years and <50 kg: 15 mg as a single dose **or** 15 mg every 6 hours (maximum: 60 mg/day)

Children ≥16 years and ≥50 kg: 30 mg as a single dose **or** 30 mg every 6 hours (maximum: 120 mg/day)

Adults <50 kg: 15 mg as a single dose **or** 15 mg every 6 hours (maximum: 60 mg/day)

Adults ≥50 kg: 30 mg as a single dose **or** 30 mg every 6 hours (maximum: 120 mg/day)

Elderly ≥65 years: 15 mg as a single dose **or** 15 mg every 6 hours (maximum: 60 mg/day)

Oral:

Children <17 years: Dosage not established

Children ≥17 years and <50 kg: 10 mg every 4-6 hours (maximum: 40 mg/day)

Children ≥17 years and ≥50 kg: 20 mg, followed by 10 mg every 4-6 hours (maximum: 40 mg/day)

Adults <50 kg: 10 mg every 4-6 hours (maximum: 40 mg/day)

Adults ≥50 kg: 20 mg, followed by 10 mg every 4-6 hours (maximum: 40 mg/day)

Elderly ≥65 years: 10 mg every 4-6 hours (maximum: 40 mg/day)

Dosage Forms

Injection, solution: 15 mg/mL (1 mL, 2 mL); 30 mg/mL (1 mL, 2 mL, 10 mL)

Tablet, oral: 10 mg

ketorolac (nasal) (KEE toe role ak)

Synonyms ketorolac tromethamine

U.S./Canadian Brand Names Sprix™ [US]

Therapeutic Category Nonsteroidal Antiinflammatory Drug (NSAID), Nasal

Use Short-term (≤5 days) management of moderate-to-moderately severe acute pain requiring analgesia at the opioid level

Product Availability Sprix™: FDA approved May 2010; availability expected in early 2011; consult prescribing information for additional information

ketorolac (ophthalmic) (KEE toe role ak)

Sound-Alike/Look-Alike Issues

ketorolac may be confused with Ketalar®

Acular® may be confused with Acthar®, Ocular®

Synonyms ketorolac tromethamine

U.S./Canadian Brand Names Acular LS® [US/Can]; Acular® [US/Can]; Acuvail™ [US]; ratio-Ketorolac [Can]

Therapeutic Category Nonsteroidal Antiinflammatory Drug (NSAID), Ophthalmic

Use Temporary relief of ocular itching due to seasonal allergic conjunctivitis; postoperative inflammation following cataract extraction; reduction of ocular pain and photophobia following incisional refractive surgery; reduction of ocular pain, burning, and stinging following corneal refractive surgery

Dosage Summary

Ophthalmic:

Children <3 years: Dosage not established

Children ≥3 years: Instill 1 drop (0.25 mg) 4 times/day to eye(s)

Adults: Instill 1 drop (0.25 mg) 4 times/day to eye(s)

Dosage Forms

Solution, ophthalmic: 0.4% (5 mL); 0.5% (3 mL, 5 mL, 10 mL)

Acular LS®: 0.4% (5 mL)

Acular®: 0.5% (3 mL, 5 mL, 10 mL)

Solution, ophthalmic [preservative free]:

Acuvail™: 0.45% (0.4 mL)

ketorolac tromethamine *see* ketorolac (nasal) *on page* 538

ketorolac tromethamine *see* ketorolac (ophthalmic) *on page* 538

ketorolac tromethamine *see* ketorolac (systemic) *on page* 537

Ketorolac Tromethamine Injection, USP [Can] *see* ketorolac (systemic) *on page* 537

ketotifen (kee toe TYE fen)

Sound-Alike/Look-Alike Issues

ketotifen may be confused with ketoprofen

Claritin™ Eye (ketotifen) may be confused with Claritin® (loratadine)

Zyrtec® Itchy Eye (ketotifen) may be confused with Zyrtec® (cetirizine)

Synonyms ketotifen fumarate

U.S./Canadian Brand Names Alaway™ [US-OTC]; Claritin™ Eye [US-OTC]; Novo-Ketotifen® [Can]; Nu-Ketotifen® [Can]; Zaditen® [Can]; Zaditor® [US-OTC/Can]; Zyrtec® Itchy Eye [US-OTC]

Therapeutic Category Antihistamine, H_1 Blocker, Ophthalmic

Use

Ophthalmic: Temporary relief of eye itching due to allergic conjunctivitis

Oral (Canadian use; not approved in U.S.): Adjunctive therapy in the chronic treatment of pediatric patients ≥6 months of age with mild, atopic asthma

Dosage Summary

Ophthalmic:

Children <3 years: Dosage not established

Children ≥3 years: Instill 1 drop into the affected eye(s) twice daily, every 8-12 hours

Adults: Instill 1 drop into the affected eye(s) twice daily, every 8-12 hours

Oral (not approved in U.S.):

Children 6 months to 3 years: Initial: 0.025 mg/kg once daily or in 2 divided doses for 5 days; Maintenance: 0.05 mg/kg twice daily

Children >3 years: Initial: 0.5 mg once daily or in 2 divided doses for 5 days; Maintenance: 1 mg twice daily

Adults: Dosage not established

Dosage Forms

Solution, ophthalmic: 0.025% (5 mL)

Alaway™ [OTC]: 0.025% (10 mL)

Claritin™ Eye [OTC]: 0.025% (5 mL)

Zaditor® [OTC]: 0.025% (5 mL)

Zyrtec® Itchy Eye [OTC]: 0.025% (5 mL)

Dosage Forms - Canada

Syrup: 1 mg/5 mL

Novo-Ketotifen®, Nu-Ketotifen®, Zaditen®: 1 mg/5 mL

Tablet: 1 mg

Novo-Ketotifen®, Zaditen®: 1 mg

ketotifen fumarate *see* ketotifen *on page* *538*

Key-E® [US-OTC] *see* vitamin E *on page* *988*

Key-E® Kaps [US-OTC] *see* vitamin E *on page* *988*

Key-E® Powder [US-OTC] *see* vitamin E *on page* *988*

Keygesic [US-OTC] *see* magnesium salicylate *on page* *587*

Key-Pred® *(Discontinued)*

Key-Pred-SP® *(Discontinued)*

K-G® *(Discontinued)* *see* potassium gluconate *on page* *782*

K-Gen® Effervescent *(Discontinued)* *see* potassium bicarbonate *on page* *780*

khloditan *see* mitotane *on page* *638*

KI *see* potassium iodide *on page* *782*

K-Ide® *(Discontinued)*

Kidkare Children's Cough and Cold [US-OTC] *see* chlorpheniramine, pseudoephedrine, and dextromethorphan *on page* *214*

Kidrolase® [Can] *see* asparaginase *on page* *99*

Kinerase® *(Discontinued)* *see* hyaluronidase *on page* *476*

Kineret® [US/Can] *see* anakinra *on page* *77*

Kinesed® *(Discontinued)* *see* hyoscyamine, atropine, scopolamine, and phenobarbital *on page* *492*

Kinevac® [US] *see* sincalide *on page* *877*

Kinrix™ [US] *see* diphtheria and tetanus toxoids, acellular pertussis, and poliovirus vaccine *on page* *314*

Kionex® [US] *see* sodium polystyrene sulfonate *on page* *887*

Kivexa™ [Can] *see* abacavir and lamivudine *on page* *18*

Klaron® [US] *see* sulfacetamide (topical) *on page* *900*

Klean-Prep® [Can] *see* polyethylene glycol-electrolyte solution *on page* *775*

K-Lease® *(Discontinued)* *see* potassium chloride *on page* *781*

Klerist-D® Tablet *(Discontinued)* *see* chlorpheniramine and pseudoephedrine *on page* *209*

Klonopin® [US/Can] *see* clonazepam *on page* *237*

Klonopin® Wafers *(Discontinued)* *see* clonazepam *on page* *237*

Klor-Con® [US] *see* potassium chloride *on page* *781*

Klor-Con® 8 [US] *see* potassium chloride *on page* *781*

Klor-Con® 10 [US] *see* potassium chloride *on page* *781*

Klor-Con®/25 [US] *see* potassium chloride *on page* *781*

Klor-Con®/EF [US] *see* potassium bicarbonate and potassium citrate *on page* *780*

Klor-Con® M10 [US] *see* potassium chloride *on page* *781*

Klor-Con® M15 [US] *see* potassium chloride *on page* *781*

Klor-Con® M20 [US] *see* potassium chloride *on page* *781*

Klorominr® Oral *(Discontinued)* *see* chlorpheniramine *on page* *207*

Klorvess® *(Discontinued)* *see* potassium chloride *on page* *781*

Klorvess® Effervescent *(Discontinued)*
K-Lyte® [US] *see* potassium bicarbonate and potassium citrate *on page* 780
K-Lyte® [Can] *see* potassium citrate *on page* 782
K-Lyte/Cl® 50 *(Discontinued)* *see* potassium bicarbonate and potassium chloride *on page* 780
K-Lyte®/Cl [Can] *see* potassium chloride *on page* 781
K-Lyte/Cl® *(Discontinued)* *see* potassium bicarbonate and potassium chloride *on page* 780
K-Lyte® DS [US] *see* potassium bicarbonate and potassium citrate *on page* 780
K-Lyte® Effervescent *(Discontinued)* *see* potassium bicarbonate *on page* 780
KMD 3213 *see* silodosin *on page* 874
K-Norm® *(Discontinued)* *see* potassium chloride *on page* 781
Koāte®-DVI [US] *see* antihemophilic factor (human) *on page* 81
Koāte®-HP *(Discontinued)* *see* antihemophilic factor (human) *on page* 81
Koffex DM-D [Can] *see* pseudoephedrine and dextromethorphan *on page* 812
Koffex DM + Decongestant + Expectorant [Can] *see* guaifenesin, pseudoephedrine, and dextromethorphan *on page* 460
Koffex DM-Expectorant [Can] *see* guaifenesin and dextromethorphan *on page* 455
Koffex Expectorant [Can] *see* guaifenesin *on page* 454
Kogenate® [Can] *see* antihemophilic factor (recombinant) *on page* 81
Kogenate® *(Discontinued)* *see* antihemophilic factor (recombinant) *on page* 81
Kogenate® FS [US/Can] *see* antihemophilic factor (recombinant) *on page* 81
Kolephrin® GG/DM [US-OTC] *see* guaifenesin and dextromethorphan *on page* 455
Konakion [Can] *see* phytonadione *on page* 759
Konakion® Injection *(Discontinued)* *see* phytonadione *on page* 759
Kondon's Nasal® *(Discontinued)* *see* ephedrine (systemic) *on page* 351
Konsyl® [US-OTC] *see* psyllium *on page* 814
Konsyl-D™ [US-OTC] *see* psyllium *on page* 814
Konsyl® Easy Mix™ [US-OTC] *see* psyllium *on page* 814
Konsyl® Fiber [US-OTC] *see* polycarbophil *on page* 774
Konsyl® Orange [US-OTC] *see* psyllium *on page* 814
Konsyl® Original [US-OTC] *see* psyllium *on page* 814
Kovia® *(Discontinued)*
K-Pek® *(Discontinued)*
K-Phos® MF [US] *see* potassium phosphate and sodium phosphate *on page* 783
K-Phos® Neutral [US] *see* potassium phosphate and sodium phosphate *on page* 783
K-Phos® No. 2 [US] *see* potassium phosphate and sodium phosphate *on page* 783
K-Phos® Original [US] *see* potassium acid phosphate *on page* 780
KPN Prenatal [US-OTC] *see* vitamins (multiple/prenatal) *on page* 991
Kristalose® [US] *see* lactulose *on page* 544
K-Tab® [US] *see* potassium chloride *on page* 781
K-Tan 4 *(Discontinued)* *see* phenylephrine and pyrilamine *on page* 753
K-Tan *(Discontinued)* *see* phenylephrine and pyrilamine *on page* 753
kunecatechins *see* sinecatechins *on page* 878
Kuric™ [US] *see* ketoconazole (topical) *on page* 536
kutrase® *(Discontinued)* *see* pancreatin *on page* 723
Kuvan™ [US] *see* sapropterin *on page* 864
ku-zyme® *(Discontinued)* *see* pancreatin *on page* 723
ku-zyme® HP *(Discontinued)* *see* pancrelipase *on page* 723
Kwelcof® *(Discontinued)*
Kwellada-P™ [Can] *see* permethrin *on page* 744
Kytril® [US/Can] *see* granisetron *on page* 452
L-749,345 *see* ertapenem *on page* 360
L-758,298 *see* fosaprepitant *on page* 427
L-M-X® 4 [US-OTC] *see* lidocaine (topical) *on page* 562

L-M-X® 5 [US-OTC] *see* lidocaine (topical) *on page* 562
L 754030 *see* aprepitant *on page* 92
LA 20304a *see* gemifloxacin *on page* 441

labetalol (la BET a lole)

Sound-Alike/Look-Alike Issues
labetalol may be confused with betaxolol, Hexadrol®, lamoTRIgine, Lipitor®
Normodyne® may be confused with Norpramin®
Trandate® may be confused with traMADol, Trendar®, Trental®, Tridrate®

Synonyms ibidomide hydrochloride; labetalol hydrochloride

U.S./Canadian Brand Names Apo-Labetalol® [Can]; Labetalol Hydrochloride Injection, USP [Can]; Normodyne® [Can]; Trandate® [US/Can]

Therapeutic Category Alpha-/Beta- Adrenergic Blocker

Use Treatment of mild-to-severe hypertension; I.V. for severe hypertension (eg, hypertensive emergencies)

Dosage Summary
I.V.:
Children: 0.3-1 mg/kg/dose intermittently **or** 0.4-1 mg/kg/hour infusion (maximum: 3 mg/kg/hour)
Adults: Bolus: 20 mg, may give 40-80 mg at 10-minute intervals; Infusion: 2 mg/minute (maximum: 300 mg total)
Oral:
Adults: Initial: 100 mg twice daily; Maintenance: 200-800 mg/day in 2 divided doses (maximum: 2.4 g/day); **Note:** Titration is recommended

Dosage Forms
Injection, solution: 5 mg/mL (4 mL, 8 mL, 20 mL, 40 mL)
Trandate®: 5 mg/mL (20 mL, 40 mL)
Tablet, oral: 100 mg, 200 mg, 300 mg
Trandate®: 100 mg, 200 mg, 300 mg

labetalol hydrochloride *see* labetalol *on page* 541
Labetalol Hydrochloride Injection, USP [Can] *see* labetalol *on page* 541
Lac-Dose® [US-OTC] *see* lactase *on page* 542
Lac-Hydrin® [US] *see* lactic acid and ammonium hydroxide *on page* 542
Lac-Hydrin® Five [US-OTC] *see* lactic acid and ammonium hydroxide *on page* 542
LAClotion™ [US] *see* lactic acid and ammonium hydroxide *on page* 542

lacosamide (la KOE sa mide)

Sound-Alike/Look-Alike Issues
lacosamide may be confused with zonisamide
Vimpat® may be confused with Vimovo™

Synonyms ADD 234037; harkoseride; LCM; SPM 927

U.S./Canadian Brand Names Vimpat® [US]

Therapeutic Category Anticonvulsant, Miscellaneous

Controlled Substance C-V

Use Adjunctive therapy in the treatment of partial-onset seizures

Dosage Summary
Oral:
Children <17 years: Dosage not established
Adolescents ≥17 years: Initial: 50 mg twice daily; Maintenance dose: 200-400 mg/day
Adults: Initial: 50 mg twice daily; Maintenance dose: 200-400 mg/day

Dosage Forms
Injection, solution:
Vimpat®: 10 mg/mL (20 mL)
Solution, oral:
Vimpat®: 10 mg/mL (20 mL)
Tablet, oral:
Vimpat®: 50 mg, 100 mg, 150 mg, 200 mg

Lacril® Ophthalmic Solution *(Discontinued)* *see* artificial tears *on page* 97

Lacrisert® [US/Can] *see* hydroxypropyl cellulose *on page* 489
LaCrosse Complete [US-OTC] *see* sodium phosphates *on page* 887
Lactaid® Extra Strength *(Discontinued)* *see* lactase *on page* 542
Lactaid® Fast Act [US-OTC] *see* lactase *on page* 542
Lactaid® Original [US-OTC] *see* lactase *on page* 542
Lactaid® Ultra *(Discontinued)* *see* lactase *on page* 542

lactase (LAK tase)

U.S./Canadian Brand Names Dairyaid® [Can]; Lac-Dose® [US-OTC]; Lactaid® Fast Act [US-OTC]; Lactaid® Original [US-OTC]; Lactose Intolerance [US-OTC]; Lactrase® [US-OTC]

Therapeutic Category Nutritional Supplement

Use Help digest lactose in milk for patients with lactose intolerance

Dosage Summary

Oral:

Children: Dosage not established

Adults: 1-2 capsules with milk or meals **or** 5-15 drops or 1-2 capsules/quart of milk **or** 1-3 tablets with meals

Dosage Forms

Caplet, oral: 3000 FCC lactase units

Lactaid® Fast Act [OTC]: 9000 FCC lactase units

Lactaid® Original [OTC]: 3000 FCC lactase units

Capsule, oral:

Lactrase® [OTC]: 250 mg standardized enzyme lactase

Capsule, softgel, oral:

Lactose Intolerance [OTC]: 250 mg standardized enzyme lactase

Tablet, oral:

Lac-Dose® [OTC]: 3000 FCC lactase units

Tablet, chewable, oral:

Lactaid® Fast Act [OTC]: 9000 FCC lactase units

lactic acid (LAK tik AS id)

Synonyms sodium-PCA and lactic acid

U.S./Canadian Brand Names LactiCare® [US-OTC]

Therapeutic Category Topical Skin Product

Use Lubricate and moisturize the skin counteracting dryness and itching

Dosage Summary

Topical:

Children: Dosage not established

Adults: Apply twice daily

Dosage Forms

Cream, topical: 10% (113 g, 113.4 g)

Lotion, topical: 10% (360 mL)

LactiCare® [OTC]: 5% (222 mL, 340 mL)

lactic acid and ammonium hydroxide (LAK tik AS id & a MOE nee um hye DROKS ide)

Synonyms ammonium hydroxide and lactic acid; ammonium lactate

U.S./Canadian Brand Names AmLactin® [US-OTC]; Geri-Hydrolac™ [US-OTC]; Geri-Hydrolac™-12 [US-OTC]; Lac-Hydrin® Five [US-OTC]; Lac-Hydrin® [US]; LAClotion™ [US]

Therapeutic Category Topical Skin Product

Use Treatment of moderate-to-severe xerosis and ichthyosis vulgaris

Dosage Summary

Topical:

Cream:

Children <2 years: Dosage not established

Children ≥2 years: Apply twice daily to affected area

Adults: Apply twice daily to affected area

Lotion:

Children: Apply twice daily to affected area

Adults: Apply twice daily to affected area

Dosage Forms

Cream, topical: Lactic acid 12% with ammonium hydroxide (140 g, 280 g, 385 g)
AmLactin® [OTC]: Lactic acid 12% with ammonium hydroxide (140 g)
Lac-Hydrin®: Lactic acid 12% with ammonium hydroxide (280 g, 385 g)

Lotion, topical: Lactic acid 12% with ammonium hydroxide (225 g, 400 g)
AmLactin® [OTC], Lac-Hydrin®, LAClotion™: Lactic acid 12% with ammonium hydroxide (225 g, 400 g)
Geri-Hydrolac™ [OTC], Lac-Hydrin® Five: Lactic acid 5% with ammonium hydroxide (120 mL, 240 mL)
Geri-Hydrolac™-12 [OTC]: Lactic acid 12% with ammonium hydroxide (120 mL, 240 mL)

LactiCare® [US-OTC] *see* lactic acid *on page* 542

Lactinex™ [US-OTC] *see* Lactobacillus *on page* 543

Lactinol® *(Discontinued)* *see* lactic acid *on page* 542

Lactinol-E® *(Discontinued)* *see* lactic acid *on page* 542

Lactobacillus (lak toe ba SIL us)

Synonyms *Lactobacillus acidophilus*; *Lactobacillus bifidus*; *Lactobacillus bulgaricus*; *Lactobacillus casei*; *Lactobacillus paracasei*; *Lactobacillus plantarum*; *Lactobacillus reuteri*; *Lactobacillus rhamnosus* GG

U.S./Canadian Brand Names Bacid® [US-OTC/Can]; Culturelle® [US-OTC]; Dofus [US-OTC]; Fermalac [Can]; Flora-Q™ [US-OTC]; Floranex™ [US-OTC]; Kala® [US-OTC]; Lactinex™ [US-OTC]; Lacto-Bifidus [US-OTC]; Lacto-Key [US-OTC]; Lacto-Pectin [US-OTC]; Lacto-TriBlend [US-OTC]; Megadophilus® [US-OTC]; MoreDophilus® [US-OTC]; RisaQuad™ [US-OTC]; Superdophilus® [US-OTC]; VSL #3® [US-OTC]; VSL #3®-DS [US]

Therapeutic Category Gastrointestinal Agent, Miscellaneous

Use Promote normal bacterial flora of the intestinal tract

Dosage Summary

Oral:

Children:
Culturelle®: 1 capsule daily

Adults:
Bacid®: 2 caplets/day
Culturelle®: 1 capsule once or twice daily
Flora-Q™: 1 capsule/day
Lactinex™: 1 packet **or** 4 tablets 3-4 times/day
Lacto-Key 100 or 600: 1-2 capsules/day
VSL #3®: 1-8 sachets or 2-32 capsules/day
VSL #3®-DS: 1-4 packets/day

Dosage Forms

Capsule:
Culturelle® [OTC]: *L. rhamnosus* GG 10 billion colony-forming units
Dofus [OTC]: *L. acidophilus* and *L. bifidus* 10:1 ratio
Flora-Q™ [OTC]: *L. acidophilus* and *L. paracasei* ≥8 billion colony-forming units
Lacto-Key [OTC]:
100: *L. acidophilus* 1 billion colony-forming units
600: *L. acidophilus* 6 billion colony-forming units
Lacto-Bifidus [OTC]:
100: *L. bifidus* 1 billion colony-forming units
600: *L. bifidus* 6 billion colony-forming units
Lacto-Pectin [OTC]: *L. acidophilus* and *L. casei* ≥5 billion colony-forming units
Lacto-TriBlend [OTC]:
100: *L. acidophilus, L. bifidus,* and *L. bulgaricus* 1 billion colony-forming units
600: *L. acidophilus, L. bifidus,* and *L. bulgaricus* 6 billion colony-forming units
Megadophilus® [OTC], Superdophilus® [OTC]: *L. acidophilus* 2 billion units
RisaQuad™ [OTC]: *L. acidophilus* and *L. paracasei* 8 billion colony-forming units
VSL #3® [OTC]: *L. acidophilus, L. plantarum, L. paracasei, L. bulgaricus* 112 billion live cells

Capsule, softgel: *L. acidophilus* 100 active units

Caplet:
Bacid® [OTC]: *L. acidophilus 80%* and *L. bulgaricus* 10%

Granules:
Lactinex™ [OTC]: *L. acidophilus* and *L. bulgaricus* 100 million live cells per 1 g packet (12s)

Powder:

Lacto-TriBlend [OTC]: *L. acidophilus, L. bifidus,* and *L. bulgaricus* 10 billion colony-forming units per ¼ teaspoon

Megadophilus® [OTC], Superdophilus® [OTC]: *L. acidophilus* 2 billion units per half-teaspoon

MoreDophilus® [OTC]: *L. acidophilus* 12.4 billion units per teaspoon

VSL #3® [OTC]: *L. acidophilus, L. plantarum, L. paracasei, L. bulgaricus* 450 billion live cells

VSL #3®-DS: *L. acidophilus, L. plantarum, L. paracasei, L. bulgaricus* 900 billion live cells

Tablet:

Kala® [OTC]: *L. acidophilus* 200 million units

Tablet, chewable: *L. reuteri* 100 million organisms

Floranex™ [OTC]: *L. acidophilus* and *L. bulgaricus* 1 million colony-forming units

Lactinex™ [OTC]: *L. acidophilus* and *L. bulgaricus* 1 million live cells

Wafer: *L. acidophilus* 90 mg and *L. bifidus* 25 mg (100s)

Lactobacillus acidophilus *see* Lactobacillus *on page 543*

Lactobacillus bifidus *see* Lactobacillus *on page 543*

Lactobacillus bulgaricus *see* Lactobacillus *on page 543*

Lactobacillus casei *see* Lactobacillus *on page 543*

Lactobacillus paracasei *see* Lactobacillus *on page 543*

Lactobacillus plantarum *see* Lactobacillus *on page 543*

Lactobacillus reuteri *see* Lactobacillus *on page 543*

***Lactobacillus rhamnosus* GG** *see* Lactobacillus *on page 543*

Lacto-Bifidus [US-OTC] *see* Lactobacillus *on page 543*

lactoflavin *see* riboflavin *on page 840*

Lacto-Key [US-OTC] *see* Lactobacillus *on page 543*

Lacto-Pectin [US-OTC] *see* Lactobacillus *on page 543*

Lactose Intolerance [US-OTC] *see* lactase *on page 542*

Lacto-TriBlend [US-OTC] *see* Lactobacillus *on page 543*

Lactrase® [US-OTC] *see* lactase *on page 542*

lactulose (LAK tyoo lose)

Sound-Alike/Look-Alike Issues

lactulose may be confused with lactose

U.S./Canadian Brand Names Acilac [Can]; Apo-Lactulose® [Can]; Constulose [US]; Enulose [US]; Generlac [US]; Kristalose® [US]; Laxilose [Can]; PMS-Lactulose [Can]

Therapeutic Category Ammonium Detoxicant; Laxative

Use Adjunct in the prevention and treatment of portal-systemic encephalopathy; treatment of chronic constipation

Dosage Summary

Oral:

Infants: PSE: 2.5-10 mL/day divided 3-4 times/day

Children:

Constipation: 5 g/day (7.5 mL) after breakfast

PSE: 40-90 mL divided 3-4 times/day [PSE]

Adults:

Constipation: 15-60 mL/day in 1-2 divided doses

PSE: Initial: 20-30 g (30-45 mL) every 1-2 hours to induce rapid laxation, then reduce dose; Usual daily dose: 60-100 g (90-150 mL) daily

Rectal:

Children: Dosage not established

Adults: Constipation: 200 g (300 mL) diluted with 700 mL of water or NS, retain for 30-60 minutes every 4-6 hours

Dosage Forms

Crystals for solution, oral:

Kristalose®: 10 g/packet (30s); 20 g/packet (30s)

Solution, oral: 10 g/15 mL (15 mL, 30 mL, 237 mL, 240 mL, 473 mL, 480 mL, 500 mL, 946 mL, 960 mL, 1000 mL, 1890 mL, 1920 mL)

Constulose: 10 g/15 mL (240 mL, 960 mL)

Enulose: 10 g/15 mL (480 mL)

Generlac: 10 g/15 mL (473 mL, 1892 mL)

Solution, oral/rectal: 10 g/15 mL (237 mL, 473 mL, 946 mL)

Lactulose PSE® *(Discontinued)* *see* lactulose *on page* *544*
ladakamycin *see* azacitidine *on page* *109*
Lagesic™ [US] *see* acetaminophen and phenyltoloxamine *on page* *26*
L-All 12 *(Discontinued)* *see* carbetapentane and phenylephrine *on page* *179*
L-AmB *see* amphotericin B liposomal *on page* *75*
Lamictal® [US/Can] *see* lamotrigine *on page* *546*
Lamictal® ODT™ [US] *see* lamotrigine *on page* *546*
Lamictal® XR™ [US] *see* lamotrigine *on page* *546*
Lamisil® [US/Can] *see* terbinafine (systemic) *on page* *917*
Lamisil® [Can] *see* terbinafine (topical) *on page* *917*
Lamisil AT® [US-OTC] *see* terbinafine (topical) *on page* *917*

lamivudine (la MI vyoo deen)

Sound-Alike/Look-Alike Issues

lamiVUDine may be confused with lamoTRIgine
Epivir® may be confused with Combivir®

Tall-Man lami**VUD**ine

U.S./Canadian Brand Names 3TC® [Can]; Epivir-HBV® [US]; Epivir® [US]; Heptovir® [Can]

Therapeutic Category Antiviral Agent

Use

Epivir®: Treatment of HIV infection when antiretroviral therapy is warranted; should always be used as part of a multidrug regimen (at least three antiretroviral agents)

Epivir-HBV®: Treatment of chronic hepatitis B associated with evidence of hepatitis B viral replication and active liver inflammation

Dosage Summary

Oral:

Neonates <30 days: HIV (AIDS*info* guidelines): 2 mg/kg/dose twice daily
Infants 1-3 months: HIV (AIDS*info* guidelines): 4 mg/kg/dose twice daily
Children 3 months to 2 years: HIV: 4 mg/kg/dose twice daily (maximum: 150 mg/dose twice daily)
Children 2-16 years:
Hepatitis B: 3 mg/kg/dose once daily (maximum: 100 mg/day)
HIV: 4 mg/kg/dose twice daily (maximum: 150 mg/dose twice daily)
Children >16 years and <50 kg:
Hepatitis B: 3 mg/kg/dose once daily (maximum: 100 mg/day)
HIV (AIDS*info* guidelines): 4 mg/kg/dose twice daily (maximum: 150 mg/dose twice daily)
Children >16 years and ≥50 kg:
Hepatitis B: 3 mg/kg/dose once daily (maximum: 100 mg/day)
HIV: 150 mg twice daily **or** 300 mg once daily
Adults <50 kg:
Hepatitis B: 100 mg/day
HIV (AIDS*info* guidelines): 4 mg/kg/dose twice daily (maximum: 150 mg/dose twice daily)
Adults ≥50 kg:
Hepatitis B: 100 mg/day
HIV: 150 mg twice daily **or** 300 mg once daily

Dosage Forms

Solution, oral:
Epivir-HBV®: 5 mg/mL (240 mL)
Epivir®: 10 mg/mL (240 mL)

Tablet, oral:
Epivir-HBV®: 100 mg
Epivir®: 150 mg, 300 mg

lamivudine, abacavir, and zidovudine *see* abacavir, lamivudine, and zidovudine *on page* *18*
lamivudine and abacavir *see* abacavir and lamivudine *on page* *18*
lamivudine and zidovudine *see* zidovudine and lamivudine *on page* *1000*

lamotrigine (la MOE tri jeen)

Sound-Alike/Look-Alike Issues
lamoTRIgine may be confused with labetalol, Lamisil®, lamiVUDine, levothyroxine, Lomotil®, ludiomil
Lamictal® may be confused with Lamisil®, Lomotil®, ludiomil

Synonyms BW-430C; LTG

Tall-Man lamo**TRI**gine

U.S./Canadian Brand Names Apo-Lamotrigine® [Can]; Lamictal® ODT™ [US]; Lamictal® XR™ [US]; Lamictal® [US/Can]; Mylan-Lamotrigine [Can]; Novo-Lamotrigine [Can]; PMS-Lamotrigine [Can]; ratio-Lamotrigine [Can]

Therapeutic Category Anticonvulsant

Use Adjunctive therapy in the treatment of generalized seizures of Lennox-Gastaut syndrome, primary generalized tonic-clonic seizures, and partial seizures in adults and children ≥2 years of age; conversion to monotherapy in adults (≥16 years of age) with partial seizures who are receiving treatment with valproic acid or a single enzyme-inducing antiepileptic drug (specifically carbamazepine, phenytoin, phenobarbital or primidone); maintenance treatment of bipolar I disorder in adults

Dosage Summary Note: Doses should be rounded down to the nearest whole tablet

Oral:

Bipolar disorder: Immediate release formulations:

Monotherapy:

Children: Dosage not established

Adults: 25-200 mg/day; **Note:** Titration is recommended

Patients receiving valproic acid:

Children: Dosage not established

Adults: Initial: 25 mg every other day for 2 weeks, followed by 25 mg/day for 2 weeks; Maintenance: 100 mg/day; **Note:** Titration is recommended

Patients receiving enzyme-inducing drugs (eg, carbamazepine):

Children: Dosage not established

Adults: 50-400 mg/day; Goal: 400 mg/day; **Note:** Titration is recommended

Lennox-Gastaut (adjunctive), primary generalized tonic-clonic seizures (adjunctive), or treatment of partial seizures (adjunctive): Immediate release formulations:

Conversion to monotherapy:

Children >16 years and Adults: Initiate and titrate as per recommendations to 200 mg (adjunct with valproic acid) or 500 mg (adjunct with enzyme-inducing AED), then continue titrating lamotrigine while titrating down drug discontinuing; Maintenance: 500 mg/day

Patients receiving AED regimens containing valproic acid:

Children <2 years: Dosage not established

Children 2-12 years:

Weeks 1 and 2: 0.15 mg/kg/day in 1-2 divided doses; **Note:** Patients >6.7 kg and <14 kg, dosing should be 2 mg every other day.

Weeks 3 and 4: 0.3 mg/kg/day in 1-2 divided doses; **Note:** Patients >6.7 kg and <14 kg, dosing should be 2 mg every other day.

Maintenance dose: 1-5 mg/kg/day (1-3 mg/kg/day in patients taking lamotrigine with valproic acid alone) in 1-2 divided doses (maximum: 200 mg/day); **Note:** Titration is recommended. Patients <30 kg may require maintenance dose to be increased as much as 50% based on clinical response.

Children >12 years: Initial: 25 mg every other day for 2 weeks, then every day for 2 weeks; Maintenance: 100-400 mg/day in 1-2 divided doses; **Note:** Titration is recommended

Adults: Initial: 25 mg every other day for 2 weeks, then every day for 2 weeks; Maintenance: 100-400 mg/day in 1-2 divided doses; **Note:** Titration is recommended

Patients receiving carbamazepine, phenytoin, phenobarbital, or primidone and not taking valproic acid:

Children <2 years: Dosage not established

Children 2-12 years:

Weeks 1 and 2: 0.6 mg/kg/day in 2 divided doses

Weeks 3 and 4: 1.2 mg/kg/day in 2 divided doses

Maintenance dose: 5-15 mg/kg/day in 2 divided doses (maximum: 400 mg/day); **Note:** Titration is recommended. Patients <30 kg may require maintenance dose to be increased as much as 50% based on clinical response.

Children >12 years: Initial: 50 mg/day for 2 weeks, then 100 mg in 2 doses for 2 weeks; Maintenance: 300-500 mg/day in 2 divided doses (maximum: 700 mg/day has been reported); **Note:** Titration is recommended

Adults: Initial: 50 mg/day for 2 weeks, then 100 mg in 2 doses for 2 weeks; Maintenance: 300-500 mg/day in 2 divided doses (maximum: 700 mg/day has been reported); **Note:** Titration is recommended

Patients receiving AED regimens other than carbamazepine, phenytoin, phenobarbital, primidone or valproic acid:

Children <2 years: Dosage not established

Children 2-12 years:

Weeks 1 and 2: 0.3 mg/kg/day in 1 or 2 divided doses

Weeks 3 and 4: 0.6 mg/kg/day in 2 divided dose

Maintenance dose: 4.5-7.5 mg/kg/day in 2 divided doses; maximum 300 mg/day. **Note:** Titration is recommended. Patients <30 kg may require maintenance dose to be increased as much as 50% based on clinical response.

Children >12 years: Initial: 25 mg/day for 2 weeks, then 50 mg/day for 2 weeks. Maintenance: 225-375 mg/day in 2 divided doses. **Note:** Titration is recommended.

Adults: Initial: 25 mg/day for 2 weeks, then 50 mg/day for 2 weeks. Maintenance: 225-375 mg/day in 2 divided doses. **Note:** Titration is recommended.

Partial seizures (adjunctive): Extended release formulation: **Note:** increases after week 8 should not exceed 100 mg/day at weekly intervals

Children ≤12 years: Dosage not established

Children ≥13 years:

Regimens containing valproic acid: Initial: Week 1 and 2: 25 mg every other day; Week 3 and 4: 25 mg once daily; Week 5: 50 mg once daily; Week 6: 100 mg once daily; Week 7: 150 mg once daily; Maintenance: 200-250 mg once daily

Regimens containing carbamazepine, phenytoin, phenobarbital, or primidone and without valproic acid: Initial: Week 1 and 2: 50 mg once daily; Week 3 and 4: 100 mg once daily; Week 5: 200 mg once daily; Week 6: 300 mg once daily; Week 7: 400 mg once daily; Maintenance: 400-600 mg once daily

Regimens not containing carbamazepine, phenytoin, phenobarbital, primidone, or valproic acid: Initial: Week 1 and 2: 25 mg once daily; Week 3 and 4: 50 mg once daily; Week 5: 100 mg once daily; Week 6: 150 mg once daily; Week 7: 200 mg once daily; Maintenance: 300-400 mg once daily

Adults:

Regimens containing valproic acid: Initial: Week 1 and 2: 25 mg every other day; Week 3 and 4: 25 mg once daily; Week 5: 50 mg once daily; Week 6: 100 mg once daily; Week 7: 150 mg once daily; Maintenance: 200-250 mg once daily

Regimens containing carbamazepine, phenytoin, phenobarbital, or primidone and without valproic acid: Initial: Week 1 and 2: 50 mg once daily; Week 3 and 4: 100 mg once daily; Week 5: 200 mg once daily; Week 6: 300 mg once daily; Week 7: 400 mg once daily; Maintenance: 400-600 mg once daily

Regimens not containing carbamazepine, phenytoin, phenobarbital, primidone, or valproic acid: Initial: Week 1 and 2: 25 mg once daily; Week 3 and 4: 50 mg once daily; Week 5: 100 mg once daily; Week 6: 150 mg once daily; Week 7: 200 mg once daily; Maintenance: 300-400 mg once daily

Dosage Forms

Tablet, oral: 25 mg, 100 mg, 150 mg, 200 mg

Lamictal®: 25 mg, 100 mg, 150 mg, 200 mg, 25 mg (42s) [white tablets] and 100 mg (7s) [peach tablets], 25 mg (84s) [white tablets] and 100 mg (14s) [peach tablets]

Tablet, chewable/dispersible, oral: 5 mg, 25 mg

Lamictal®: 2 mg, 5 mg, 25 mg

Tablet, extended release, oral:

Lamictal® XR™: 25 mg, 50 mg, 100 mg, 200 mg, 25 mg (21s) [yellow/white tablets] and 50 mg (7s) [green/white tablets], 50 mg (14s) [green/white tablets], 100 mg (14s) [orange/white tablets], and 200 mg (7s) [blue/white tablets], 25 mg (14s) [yellow/white tablets], 50 mg (14s) [green/white tablets], and 100 mg (7s) [orange/white tablets]

Tablet, orally disintegrating, oral:

Lamictal® ODT™: 25 mg, 50 mg, 100 mg, 200 mg, 25 mg (21s) and 50 mg (7s), 50 mg (42s) and 100 mg (14s), 25 mg (14s), 50 mg (14s), and 100 mg (7s)

Lanacane® [US-OTC] *see* benzocaine *on page 124*

Lanacane® Maximum Strength [US-OTC] *see* benzocaine *on page 124*

Lanaphilic® with Urea [US-OTC] *see* urea *on page 970*

lanolin, cetyl alcohol, glycerin, petrolatum, and mineral oil

(LAN oh lin, SEE til AL koe hol, GLIS er in, pe troe LAY tum, & MIN er al oyl)

Synonyms cetyl alcohol, glycerin, lanolin, mineral oil, and petrolatum; mineral oil, petrolatum, lanolin, cetyl alcohol, and glycerin

U.S./Canadian Brand Names Lubriderm® Fragrance Free [US-OTC]; Lubriderm® [US-OTC]

Therapeutic Category Topical Skin Product

Use Treatment of dry skin

Dosage Summary

Topical:

Children: Dosage not established

Adults: Apply to skin as necessary

Dosage Forms

Lotion, topical [bottle]: 180 mL, 300 mL, 480 mL

Lubriderm® Fragrance Free [OTC], Lubriderm® [OTC]: 180 mL, 300 mL, 480 mL

Lotion, topical [tube]: 100 mL

Lubriderm® Fragrance Free [OTC], Lubriderm® [OTC]: 100 mL

Lanorinal® *(Discontinued)*

Lanoxicaps® *(Discontinued)* *see* digoxin *on page* 302

Lanoxin® [US/Can] *see* digoxin *on page* 302

lanreotide (lan REE oh tide)

Sound-Alike/Look-Alike Issues

Somatuline® may be confused with somatropin, SUMAtriptan

Synonyms lanreotide acetate

U.S./Canadian Brand Names Somatuline® Autogel® [Can]; Somatuline® Depot [US]

Therapeutic Category Somatostatin Analog

Use Long-term treatment of acromegaly in patients who are not candidates for or are unresponsive to surgery and/or radiotherapy

Canadian labeling: Also approved in Canada for relief of symptoms of acromegaly

Dosage Summary

SubQ:

Children <18 years: Dosage not established.

Adults: 90 mg once every 4 weeks for 3 months; beyond 3 months adjust dose according to GH levels, IGF-1 levels, and clinical symptoms

Dosage Forms

Injection, solution:

Somatuline® Depot: 60 mg/0.4 mL (0.4 mL); 90 mg/0.4 mL (0.4 mL); 120 mg/0.5 mL (0.5 mL)

Dosage Forms - Canada

Injection, solution:

Somatuline® Autogel®: 60 mg/~0.3 mL (~0.3 mL); 90 mg/~0.4 mL (~0.4 mL); 120 mg/~0.5 mL (~0.5 mL)

lanreotide acetate *see* lanreotide *on page* 548

lansoprazole (lan SOE pra zole)

Sound-Alike/Look-Alike Issues

lansoprazole may be confused with aripiprazole, dexlansoprazole

Prevacid® may be confused with Pravachol®, Prevpac®, Prilosec®, Prinivil®

U.S./Canadian Brand Names Apo-Lansoprazole® [Can]; Mylan-Lansoprazole [Can]; Novo-Lansoprazole [Can]; Prevacid® 24 HR [US-OTC]; Prevacid® FasTab [Can]; Prevacid® SoluTab™ [US]; Prevacid® [US/Can]

Therapeutic Category Gastric Acid Secretion Inhibitor

Use Short-term treatment of active duodenal ulcers; maintenance treatment of healed duodenal ulcers; as part of a multidrug regimen for *H. pylori* eradication to reduce the risk of duodenal ulcer recurrence; short-term treatment of active benign gastric ulcer; treatment of NSAID-associated gastric ulcer; to reduce the risk of NSAID-associated gastric ulcer in patients with a history of gastric ulcer who require an NSAID; short-term treatment of symptomatic GERD; short-term treatment for all grades of erosive esophagitis; to maintain healing of erosive esophagitis; long-term treatment of pathological hypersecretory conditions, including Zollinger-Ellison syndrome

OTC labeling: Relief of frequent heartburn (≥2 days/week)

Dosage Summary

Oral:

Children <1 year: Dosage not established

Children 1-11 years and ≤30 kg: 15 mg once daily (maximum: 30 mg twice daily)

Children 1-11 years and >30 kg: 30 mg once daily (maximum: 30 mg twice daily)

Children 12-17 years: 15-30 mg once daily

Adults: 15-30 mg once daily **or** 60 mg/day in 2 divided doses **or** 60-90 mg once or twice daily [hypersecretory conditions]

Dosage Forms

Capsule, delayed release, oral: 15 mg, 30 mg

Prevacid®: 15 mg, 30 mg

Prevacid® 24 HR [OTC]: 15 mg

Tablet, delayed release, orally disintegrating, oral:

Prevacid® SoluTab™: 15 mg, 30 mg

lansoprazole, amoxicillin, and clarithromycin

(lan SOE pra zole, a moks i SIL in, & kla RITH roe mye sin)

Sound-Alike/Look-Alike Issues

Prevpac® may be confused with Prevacid®

Synonyms amoxicillin, clarithromycin, and lansoprazole; clarithromycin, lansoprazole, and amoxicillin; lansoprazole, amoxicillin, and clarithromycin

U.S./Canadian Brand Names Hp-PAC® [Can]; Prevpac® [US]

Therapeutic Category Antibiotic, Macrolide Combination; Antibiotic, Penicillin; Gastrointestinal Agent, Miscellaneous

Use Eradication of *H. pylori* to reduce the risk of recurrent duodenal ulcer

Dosage Summary

Oral:

Children: Dosage not established

Adults: Lansoprazole 30 mg, amoxicillin 1 g, and clarithromycin 500 mg taken together twice daily

Dosage Forms

Combination package [each administration card contains]:

Prevpac®:

Capsule: Amoxicillin 500 mg (4 capsules/day)

Capsule, delayed release (Prevacid®): Lansoprazole 30 mg (2 capsules/day)

Tablet (Biaxin®): Clarithromycin 500 mg (2 tablets/day)

lansoprazole, amoxicillin, and clarithromycin *see* lansoprazole, amoxicillin, and clarithromycin *on page 549*

lansoprazole and naproxen (lan SOE pra zole & na PROKS en)

Sound-Alike/Look-Alike Issues

Prevacid® may be confused with Pravachol®, Prevpac®, Prilosec®, Prinivil®

Synonyms NapraPAC®; naproxen and lansoprazole

U.S./Canadian Brand Names Prevacid® NapraPAC® [US]

Therapeutic Category Gastric Acid Secretion Inhibitor; Nonsteroidal Antiinflammatory Drug (NSAID)

Use Reduction of the risk of NSAID-associated gastric ulcers in patients with history of gastric ulcer who require an NSAID for the treatment of rheumatoid arthritis, osteoarthritis, and ankylosing spondylitis

Dosage Summary

Oral:

Children: Dosage not established

Adults: 15 mg once daily of lansoprazole and 500 mg twice daily of naproxen

Elderly: Naproxen dosing adjustment should be considered

Dosage Forms

Combination package:

Prevacid® NapraPAC® 500 [each administration card contains]:

Capsule, delayed release (Prevacid®): Lansoprazole 15 mg (7 capsules per card)

Tablet (Naprosyn®): Naproxen 500 mg (14 tablets per card)

lanthanum (LAN tha num)

Sound-Alike/Look-Alike Issues
lanthanum may be confused with lithium

Synonyms lanthanum carbonate

U.S./Canadian Brand Names Fosrenol® [US/Can]

Therapeutic Category Phosphate Binder

Use Reduction of serum phosphate in patients with stage 5 chronic kidney disease (end-stage renal disease [ESRD]; kidney failure: GFR <15 mL/minute/1.73 m^2 or dialysis)

Dosage Summary

Oral:

Children: Dosage not established

Adults: Initial: 1500 mg/day in divided doses with meals; Usual range: 1500-3000 mg/day; **Note:** Titration is recommended

Dosage Forms

Tablet, chewable, oral:

Fosrenol®: 500 mg, 750 mg, 1000 mg

lanthanum carbonate *see* lanthanum *on page* 550

Lantus® [US/Can] *see* insulin glargine *on page* 510

Lantus® OptiSet® [Can] *see* insulin glargine *on page* 510

Lanvis® [Can] *see* thioguanine *on page* 927

Lapase *(Discontinued)* *see* pancreatin *on page* 723

lapatinib (la PA ti nib)

Sound-Alike/Look-Alike Issues
lapatinib may be confused with dasatinib, erlotinib, imatinib

Synonyms GW572016; lapatinib ditosylate

U.S./Canadian Brand Names Tykerb® [US/Can]

Therapeutic Category Antineoplastic Agent, Tyrosine Kinase Inhibitor; Epidermal Growth Factor Receptor (EGFR) Inhibitor

Use Treatment of HER2 overexpressing advanced or metastatic breast cancer (in combination with capecitabine) in patients who have received prior therapy (with an anthracycline, a taxane, and trastuzumab) and HER2 overexpressing hormone receptor positive metastatic breast cancer in postmenopausal women (in combination with letrozole)

Dosage Summary

Oral:

Children: Dosage not established

Adults: 1250 mg or 1500 mg once daily

Dosage Forms

Tablet:

Tykerb®: 250 mg

lapatinib ditosylate *see* lapatinib *on page* 550

Largactil® [Can] *see* chlorpromazine *on page* 216

L-arginine *see* arginine *on page* 94

L-arginine hydrochloride *see* arginine *on page* 94

Lariam® [Can] *see* mefloquine *on page* 598

Lariam® *(Discontinued)* *see* mefloquine *on page* 598

laronidase (lair OH ni days)

Synonyms recombinant α-L-iduronidase (glycosaminoglycan α-L-iduronohydrolase)

U.S./Canadian Brand Names Aldurazyme® [US/Can]

Therapeutic Category Enzyme

Use Treatment of Hurler and Hurler-Scheie forms of mucopolysaccharidosis I (MPS I); treatment of Scheie form of MPS I in patients with moderate-to-severe symptoms

Dosage Summary Note: Dose should be rounded to nearest whole vial. Premedicate with antipyretic and/or antihistamines 1 hour prior to start of infusion.

I.V.:
Children <5 years: Dosage not established
Children ≥5 years: 0.58 mg/kg once weekly
Adults: 0.58 mg/kg once weekly

Dosage Forms
Injection, solution [preservative free]:
Aldurazyme®: 2.9 mg/5 mL (5 mL)

Lasix® [US/Can] *see* furosemide *on page 431*

Lasix® Special [Can] *see* furosemide *on page 431*

L-asparaginase *see* asparaginase *on page 99*

L-asparaginase with polyethylene glycol *see* pegaspargase *on page 732*

lassar's zinc paste *see* zinc oxide *on page 1001*

Lastacaft™ [US] *see* alcaftadine *on page 45*

latanoprost (la TA noe prost)

Sound-Alike/Look-Alike Issues
latanoprost may be confused with Lantus®
Xalatan® may be confused with Lantus®, Travatan®, Xalacom™, Zarontin®

U.S./Canadian Brand Names Xalatan® [US/Can]

Therapeutic Category Prostaglandin

Use Reduction of elevated intraocular pressure in patients with open-angle glaucoma or ocular hypertension

Dosage Summary
Ophthalmic:
Children: Dosage not established
Adults: 1 drop (1.5 mcg) in the affected eye(s) once daily in the evening

Dosage Forms
Solution, ophthalmic:
Xalatan®: 0.005% (2.5 mL)

latanoprost and timolol *(Canada only)* (la TA noe prost & TIM oh lol)

Sound-Alike/Look-Alike Issues
Xalacom™ may be confused with Xalatan®

Synonyms timolol maleate and latanoprost

U.S./Canadian Brand Names Xalacom™ [Can]

Therapeutic Category Beta Blocker, Nonselective; Ophthalmic Agent, Antiglaucoma; Prostaglandin, Ophthalmic

Use Reduction of intraocular pressure (IOP) in patients with open-angle glaucoma or ocular hypertension who are insufficiently responsive to topical beta-blockers, prostaglandin analogues, or other IOP-reducing agents and in whom combination therapy is appropriate

Dosage Summary
Ophthalmic:
Children: Dosage not established
Adults: Instill 1 drop once daily

Dosage Forms - Canada
Solution, ophthalmic:
Xalacom™: Latanoprost (0.005%) and timolol 0.5% (as base) (2.5 mL)

Latisse™ [US] *see* bimatoprost *on page 138*

***Latrodectus* antivenin** *see* antivenin *(Latrodectus mactans) on page 85*

***Latrodectus mactans* antivenin** *see* antivenin *(Latrodectus mactans) on page 85*

Lavacol® [US-OTC] *see* alcohol (ethyl) *on page 45*

Laxilose [Can] *see* lactulose *on page 544*

***l*-bunolol hydrochloride** *see* levobunolol *on page 556*

L-Carnitine® [US-OTC] *see* levocarnitine *on page 556*

L-carnitine *see* levocarnitine *on page 556*

LCD *see* coal tar *on page 242*

LCM *see* lacosamide *on page 541*

L-deoxythymidine *see* telbivudine *on page* *912*
L-deprenyl *see* selegiline *on page* *869*
LDP-341 *see* bortezomib *on page* *143*
LdT *see* telbivudine *on page* *912*
Lectopam® [Can] *see* bromazepam *(Canada only) on page* *146*
Leena™ [US] *see* ethinyl estradiol and norethindrone *on page* *378*

leflunomide (le FLOO noh mide)

U.S./Canadian Brand Names Apo-Leflunomide® [Can]; Arava® [US/Can]; Mylan-Leflunomide [Can]; Novo-Leflunomide [Can]; PHL-Leflunomide [Can]; PMS-Leflunomide [Can]; Sandoz-Leflunomide [Can]

Therapeutic Category Antiinflammatory Agent

Use Treatment of active rheumatoid arthritis; indicated to reduce signs and symptoms, and to inhibit structural damage and improve physical function

Dosage Summary

Oral:

Children: Dosage not established

Adults: Initial: 100 mg/day for 3 days followed by 20 mg/day (may decrease to 10 mg/day if necessary); Maintenance range: 10-20 mg/day

Dosage Forms

Tablet, oral: 10 mg, 20 mg

Arava®: 10 mg, 20 mg

Legatrin PM® [US-OTC] *see* acetaminophen and diphenhydramine *on page* *24*

lenalidomide (le na LID oh mide)

Sound-Alike/Look-Alike Issues

lenalidomide may be confused with thalidomide

Synonyms CC-5013; IMid-1

U.S./Canadian Brand Names Revlimid® [US/Can]

Therapeutic Category Angiogenesis Inhibitor; Immunosuppressant Agent; Tumor Necrosis Factor (TNF) Blocking Agent

Use Treatment of myelodysplastic syndrome (MDS) in patients with deletion 5q (del 5q) cytogenetic abnormality with transfusion-dependent anemia; treatment of multiple myeloma

Dosage Summary

Oral:

Children: Dosage not established

Adults: 10 once daily **or** 25 mg once daily for 21 of 28 days

Dosage Forms

Capsule, oral:

Revlimid®: 5 mg, 10 mg, 15 mg, 25 mg

Lente® Iletin® II *(Discontinued)*

lepirudin (leh puh ROO din)

Synonyms lepirudin (rDNA); recombinant hirudin

U.S./Canadian Brand Names Refludan® [US/Can]

Therapeutic Category Anticoagulant (Other)

Use Indicated for anticoagulation in patients with heparin-induced thrombocytopenia (HIT) and associated thromboembolic disease in order to prevent further thromboembolic complications

Dosage Summary Note: Dosing is weight-based; however, patients weighing >110 kg should not receive doses greater than the recommended dose for a patient weighing 110 kg (44 mg bolus and initial maximal infusion rate of 16.5 mg/hour).

I.V.:

Children: Dosage not established

Adults: Bolus: 0.2-0.4 mg/kg; Infusion: 0.1-0.15 mg/kg/hour (maximum: 0.21 mg/kg/hour); **Note:** Initial bolus dose may be omitted unless acute HITTS

Dosage Forms

Injection, powder for reconstitution:

Refludan®: 50 mg

lepirudin (rDNA) *see* lepirudin *on page* 552
Lescol® [US/Can] *see* fluvastatin *on page* 421
Lescol® XL [US/Can] *see* fluvastatin *on page* 421
Lessina™ [US] *see* ethinyl estradiol and levonorgestrel *on page* 376
Letairis® [US] *see* ambrisentan *on page* 62

letrozole (LET roe zole)

Sound-Alike/Look-Alike Issues
letrozole may be confused with anastrozole
Femara® may be confused with Famvir®, femhrt®, Provera®

Synonyms CGS-20267

U.S./Canadian Brand Names Femara® [US/Can]; PMS-Letrozole [Can]; Sandoz-Letrozole [Can]

Therapeutic Category Antineoplastic Agent, Hormone (Antiestrogen)

Use For use in postmenopausal women in the adjuvant treatment of hormone receptor positive early breast cancer, extended adjuvant treatment of early breast cancer after 5 years of tamoxifen, advanced breast cancer with disease progression following antiestrogen therapy, hormone receptor positive or hormone receptor unknown, locally-advanced, or metastatic breast cancer

Dosage Summary

Oral:
Children: Dosage not established
Adults (females): 2.5 mg once daily

Dosage Forms

Tablet, oral:
Femara®: 2.5 mg

leucovorin *see* leucovorin calcium *on page* 553

leucovorin calcium (loo koe VOR in KAL see um)

Sound-Alike/Look-Alike Issues
leucovorin may be confused with Leukeran®, Leukine®, LEVOleucovorin
folinic acid may be confused with folic acid
folinic acid is an error prone synonym and should not be used

Synonyms 5-formyl tetrahydrofolate; calcium leucovorin; citrovorum factor; leucovorin

Therapeutic Category Folic Acid Derivative

Use Antidote for folic acid antagonists (methotrexate, trimethoprim, pyrimethamine) and rescue therapy following high-dose methotrexate; in combination with fluorouracil in the treatment of colon cancer; treatment of megaloblastic anemias when folate is deficient as in infancy, sprue, pregnancy, and nutritional deficiency when oral folate therapy is not possible

Dosage Summary

I.M.:
Children: ≤1 mg/day [folate deficient megaloblastic anemia] **or** 15 mg (~10 mg/m^2) starting 24 hours after beginning methotrexate infusion, continue every 6 hours for 10 doses; adjust dose based on methotrexate level/elimination [methotrexate rescue dose]
Adults: ≤1 mg/day [folate deficient megaloblastic anemia] **or** 15 mg (~10 mg/m^2) starting 24 hours after beginning methotrexate infusion, continue every 6 hours for 10 doses; adjust dose based on methotrexate level/elimination [methotrexate rescue dose]

I.V.:
Children: 15 mg (~10 mg/m^2) starting 24 hours after beginning methotrexate infusion, continue every 6 hours for 10 doses; adjust dose based on methotrexate level/elimination [methotrexate rescue dose]
Adults: Initial: 15 mg (~10 mg/m^2) starting 24 hours after beginning methotrexate infusion, continue every 6 hours for 10 doses; adjust dose based on methotrexate level/elimination [methotrexate rescue dose] **or** 200 mg/m^2 over at least 3 minutes (used in combination with fluorouracil 370 mg/m^2) [colorectal cancer] **or** 20 mg/m^2 (used in combination with fluorouracil 425 mg/m^2) [colorectal cancer]

Oral:
Children: 5-15 mg/day [weak folic acid antagonist overdose] **or** 15 mg (~10 mg/m^2) starting 24 hours after beginning methotrexate infusion, continue every 6 hours for 10 doses; adjust dose based on methotrexate level/elimination [methotrexate rescue dose]
Adults: 5-15 mg/day [weak folic acid antagonist overdose] **or** 15 mg (~10 mg/m^2) starting 24 hours after beginning methotrexate infusion, continue every 6 hours for 10 doses; adjust dose based on methotrexate level/elimination [methotrexate rescue dose]

Dosage Forms

Injection, powder for reconstitution: 50 mg, 100 mg, 200 mg, 350 mg
Injection, solution [preservative free]: 10 mg/mL (50 mL)
Tablet, oral: 5 mg, 10 mg, 15 mg, 25 mg

Leukeran® [US/Can] *see* chlorambucil *on page 202*
Leukine® [US/Can] *see* sargramostim *on page 865*

leuprolide (loo PROE lide)

Sound-Alike/Look-Alike Issues

Lupron® may be confused with Nuprin®
Lupron Depot®-3 Month may be confused with Lupron Depot-Ped®

Synonyms abbott-43818; leuprolide acetate; leuprorelin acetate; TAP-144

U.S./Canadian Brand Names Eligard® [US/Can]; Lupron Depot-Ped® [US]; Lupron Depot® [US/Can]; Lupron Depot®-3 Month [US]; Lupron Depot®-4 Month [US]; Lupron® [US/Can]

Therapeutic Category Antineoplastic Agent; Luteinizing Hormone-Releasing Hormone Analog

Use Palliative treatment of advanced prostate cancer; management of endometriosis; treatment of anemia caused by uterine leiomyomata (fibroids); central precocious puberty

Dosage Summary

I.M.:

Children ≤25 kg: Lupron® Depot-Ped®: 0.3 mg/kg/dose **or** 7.5 mg every 28 days (minimum dose: 7.5 mg)

Children >25-37.5 kg: Lupron® Depot-Ped®: 0.3 mg/kg/dose **or** 11.25 mg every 28 days (minimum dose: 7.5 mg)

Children >37.5 kg: Lupron® Depot-Ped®: 0.3 mg/kg/dose **or** 15 mg every 28 days (minimum dose: 7.5 mg)

Adults:

Lupron Depot®: 3.75 **or** 7.5 mg/dose once monthly
Lupron Depot®-3: 11.25 mg **or** 22.5 mg once every 3 months **or** 11.25 as a single dose
Lupron Depot®-4: 30 mg every 4 months

SubQ:

Children: Lupron®: Initial: 50 mcg/kg/day; titrate dose upward by 10 mcg/kg/day if down-regulation is not achieved

Adults:

Eligard®: 7.5 mg monthly **or** 22.5 mg every 3 months **or** 30 mg every 4 months **or** 45 mg every 6 months
Lupron®: 1 mg/day

Dosage Forms

Injection, powder for reconstitution:
Eligard®: 7.5 mg, 22.5 mg, 30 mg, 45 mg
Lupron Depot-Ped®: 7.5 mg, 11.25 mg, 15 mg
Lupron Depot®: 3.75 mg, 7.5 mg
Lupron Depot®-3 Month: 11.25 mg, 22.5 mg
Lupron Depot®-4 Month: 30 mg

Injection, solution: 5 mg/mL (2.8 mL)
Lupron®: 5 mg/mL (2.8 mL)

leuprolide acetate *see* leuprolide *on page 554*
leuprorelin acetate *see* leuprolide *on page 554*
leurocristine sulfate *see* vincristine *on page 985*
Leustatin® [US/Can] *see* cladribine *on page 229*

levalbuterol (leve al BYOO ter ole)

Sound-Alike/Look-Alike Issues

Xopenex® may be confused with Xanax®

Synonyms levalbuterol hydrochloride; levalbuterol tartrate; R-albuterol

U.S./Canadian Brand Names Xopenex HFA™ [US]; Xopenex® [US/Can]

Therapeutic Category Adrenergic Agonist Agent; Beta$_2$-Adrenergic Agonist Agent; Bronchodilator

Use Treatment or prevention of bronchospasm in children and adults with reversible obstructive airway disease

Dosage Summary

Inhalation (metered-dose inhaler):

Children <4 years: Dosage not established

Children ≥4 years: 1-2 puffs every 4-6 hours

Adults: 1-2 puffs every 4-6 hours

Nebulization (solution):

Children <6 years: Dosage not established

Children 6-11 years: 0.31-0.63 mg 3 times/day

Children ≥12 years: 0.63-1.25 mg 3 times/day at 6-8 hour intervals

Adults: 0.63-1.25 mg 3 times/day at 6-8 hour intervals

Elderly: Initial: 0.63 mg 3 times/day

Dosage Forms

Aerosol, for oral inhalation:

Xopenex HFA™: 45 mcg/actuation (15 g)

Solution, for nebulization [preservative free]: 1.25 mg/0.5 mL (30s)

Xopenex®: 0.31 mg/3 mL (24s); 0.63 mg/3 mL (24s); 1.25 mg/3 mL (24s); 1.25 mg/0.5 mL (30s)

levalbuterol hydrochloride *see* levalbuterol *on page* 554

levalbuterol tartrate *see* levalbuterol *on page* 554

Levall 5.0 *(Discontinued)*

Levall™ *(Discontinued)* *see* carbetapentane, guaifenesin, and phenylephrine *on page* 180

Levaquin® [US/Can] *see* levofloxacin (systemic) *on page* 557

levarterenol bitartrate *see* norepinephrine *on page* 682

Levate® [Can] *see* amitriptyline *on page* 67

Levatol® [US/Can] *see* penbutolol *on page* 736

Levbid® [US] *see* hyoscyamine *on page* 491

Levemir® [US/Can] *see* insulin detemir *on page* 510

levetiracetam (lee va tye RA se tam)

Sound-Alike/Look-Alike Issues

levetiracetam may be confused with levocarnitine, levofloxacin

Keppra® may be confused with Keflex®, Keppra XR™

Potential for dispensing errors between Keppra® and Kaletra® (lopinavir/ritonavir)

U.S./Canadian Brand Names Apo-Levetiracetam® [Can]; CO Levetiracetam [Can]; Dom-Levetiracetam [Can]; Keppra XR™ [US]; Keppra® [US/Can]; PHL-Levetiracetam [Can]; PMS-Levetiracetam [Can]; PRO-Levetiracetam [Can]

Therapeutic Category Anticonvulsant

Use Adjunctive therapy in the treatment of partial-onset, myoclonic, and/or primary generalized tonic-clonic seizures

Dosage Summary

Oral:

Children <4 years: Dosage not established

Children 4-15 years: Immediate release: Initial: 10 mg/kg twice daily; Maintenance: 10-30 mg/kg twice daily (maximum: 60 mg/kg/day); **Note:** Titration is recommended every 2 weeks

Children ≥12 years: Immediate release: Initial: 500 mg twice daily; Maintenance: 500-1500 mg twice daily (maximum: 3000 mg/day); **Note:** Titration is recommended every 2 weeks

Children ≥16 years: Extended release: Initial: 1000 mg once daily; Maintenance: 1000-3000 mg once daily (maximum: 3000 mg/day); **Note:** Titration is recommended every 2 weeks

Adults: Initial: Immediate release: 500 mg twice daily; Maintenance: 500-1500 mg twice daily (maximum: 3000 mg/day) **or** Extended release: Initial: 1000 mg once daily; Maintenance: 1000-3000 mg once daily (maximum: 3000 mg/day); **Note:** Titration is recommended every 2 weeks

I.V.:

Children <16 years: Dosage not established

Children ≥16 years: Initial: 500 mg twice daily; Maintenance: 500-1500 mg twice daily (maximum: 3000 mg/day); **Note:** Titration is recommended every 2 weeks

Adults: Initial: 500 mg twice daily; Maintenance: 500-1500 mg twice daily (maximum: 3000 mg/day); **Note:** Titration is recommended every 2 weeks

Dosage Forms

Injection, solution: 100 mg/mL (5 mL)

Keppra®: 100 mg/mL (5 mL)

Solution, oral: 100 mg/mL (5 mL, 472 mL, 473 mL, 480 mL, 500 mL)
Keppra®: 100 mg/mL (480 mL)
Tablet, oral: 250 mg, 500 mg, 750 mg, 1000 mg
Keppra®: 250 mg, 500 mg, 750 mg
Tablet, extended release, oral:
Keppra XR™: 500 mg, 750 mg

Levitra® [US/Can] *see* vardenafil *on page 978*
Levlen® [US] *see* ethinyl estradiol and levonorgestrel *on page 376*
Levlite™ [US] *see* ethinyl estradiol and levonorgestrel *on page 376*

levobunolol (lee voe BYOO noe lole)

Sound-Alike/Look-Alike Issues
levobunolol may be confused with levocabastine
Betagan® may be confused with Betadine®, Betoptic® S

Synonyms *l*-bunolol hydrochloride; levobunolol hydrochloride

U.S./Canadian Brand Names Apo-Levobunolol® [Can]; Betagan® [US/Can]; Novo-Levobunolol [Can]; Optho-Bunolol® [Can]; PMS-Levobunolol [Can]; Sandoz-Levobunolol [Can]

Therapeutic Category Beta-Adrenergic Blocker

Use To lower intraocular pressure in chronic open-angle glaucoma or ocular hypertension

Dosage Summary
Ophthalmic:
Children: Dosage not established
Adults: Instill 1 drop in the affected eye(s) 1-2 times/day

Dosage Forms
Solution, ophthalmic: 0.25% (5 mL, 10 mL); 0.5% (5 mL, 10 mL, 15 mL)
Betagan®: 0.5% (5 mL, 10 mL, 15 mL)

levobunolol hydrochloride *see* levobunolol *on page 556*

levocarnitine (lee voe KAR ni teen)

Sound-Alike/Look-Alike Issues
levocarnitine may be confused with levetiracetam, levocabastine

Synonyms L-carnitine

U.S./Canadian Brand Names Carnitine-300 [US-OTC]; Carnitor® SF [US]; Carnitor® [US/Can]; L-Carnitine® [US-OTC]

Therapeutic Category Dietary Supplement

Use
Oral: Primary systemic carnitine deficiency; acute and chronic treatment of patients with an inborn error of metabolism which results in secondary carnitine deficiency
I.V.: Acute and chronic treatment of patients with an inborn error of metabolism which results in secondary carnitine deficiency; prevention and treatment of carnitine deficiency in patients with end-stage renal disease (ESRD) who are undergoing hemodialysis.

Dosage Summary
I.V.:
Children: 50 mg/kg/day in divided doses (maximum: 300 mg/kg/day); **Note:** Titration is recommended
Adults: 50 mg/kg/day (titration is recommended; maximum: 300 mg/kg/day) **or** 20 mg/kg after each hemodialysis session
Oral:
Infants: Initial: 50 mg/kg/day; Maintenance: 50-100 mg/kg/day in divided doses (maximum: 3 g/day); **Note:** Titration is recommended
Children: Initial: 50 mg/kg/day; Maintenance: 50-100 mg/kg/day in divided doses (maximum: 3 g/day); **Note:** Titration is recommended
Adults: 990 mg (tablet) 2-3 times/day **or** 1-3 g/day (solution)

Dosage Forms
Capsule, oral:
Carnitine-300 [OTC]: 300 mg
L-Carnitine® [OTC]: 250 mg
Injection, solution [preservative free]: 200 mg/mL (5 mL, 12.5 mL)
Carnitor®: 200 mg/mL (5 mL)

Solution, oral: 100 mg/mL (118 mL, 120 mL)
Carnitor®: 100 mg/mL (118 mL)
Carnitor® SF: 100 mg/mL (118 mL)
Tablet, oral: 330 mg
Carnitor®: 330 mg
L-Carnitine® [OTC]: 500 mg

levocetirizine (LEE vo se TI ra zeen)

Sound-Alike/Look-Alike Issues
levocetirizine may be confused with cetirizine

Synonyms levocetirizine dihydrochloride

U.S./Canadian Brand Names Xyzal® [US]

Therapeutic Category Antihistamine

Use Relief of symptoms of perennial and seasonal allergic rhinitis; treatment of skin manifestations (uncomplicated) of chronic idiopathic urticaria

Dosage Summary

Oral:
Children <6 months: Dosage not established
Children 6 months to 5 years: 1.25 mg once daily
Children 6-11 years: 2.5 mg once daily
Children ≥12 years: 2.5-5 mg once daily
Adults: 2.5-5 mg once daily

Dosage Forms

Solution, oral:
Xyzal®: 0.5 mg/mL (150 mL)
Tablet, oral: 250 mg
Xyzal®: 5 mg

levocetirizine dihydrochloride *see* levocetirizine *on page 557*
Levoclen™-4 [US] *see* benzoyl peroxide *on page 128*
Levoclen™-8 [US] *see* benzoyl peroxide *on page 128*
Levoclen® Acne Wash Kit [US] *see* benzoyl peroxide *on page 128*
levodopa and benserazide *see* benserazide and levodopa *(Canada only) on page 123*
levodopa and carbidopa *see* carbidopa and levodopa *on page 182*

levodopa, carbidopa, and entacapone (lee voe DOE pa, kar bi DOE pa, & en TA ka pone)

Synonyms carbidopa, entacapone, and levodopa; carbidopa, levodopa, and entacapone; entacapone, carbidopa, and levodopa

U.S./Canadian Brand Names Stalevo® [US/Can]

Therapeutic Category Anti-Parkinson Agent (Dopamine Agonist); Anti-Parkinson Agent, COMT Inhibitor

Use Treatment of idiopathic Parkinson disease

Dosage Summary

Oral:
Children: Dosage not established
Adults: 1 tablet at each dosing interval (maximum: 1600 mg entacapone or 300 mg of carbidopa)

Dosage Forms

Tablet:
Stalevo®: 50: Levodopa 50 mg, carbidopa 12.5 mg, and entacapone 200 mg; 75: Levodopa 75 mg, carbidopa 18.75 mg, and entacapone 200 mg; 100: Levodopa 100 mg, carbidopa 25 mg, and entacapone 200 mg; 125: Levodopa 125 mg, carbidopa 31.25 mg, and entacapone 200 mg; 150: Levodopa 150 mg, carbidopa 37.5 mg, and entacapone 200 mg; 200: Levodopa 200 mg, carbidopa 50 mg, and entacapone 200 mg

Levo-Dromoran® [US] *see* levorphanol *on page 559*

levofloxacin (systemic) (lee voe FLOKS a sin)

Sound-Alike/Look-Alike Issues
levofloxacin may be confused with levetiracetam, levodopa, Levophed®, levothyroxine
Levaquin® may be confused with Levoxyl®, Levsin/SL®, Lovenox®

U.S./Canadian Brand Names Levaquin® [US/Can]; Novo-Levofloxacin [Can]; PMS-Levofloxacin [Can]

Therapeutic Category Antibiotic, Quinolone; Respiratory Fluoroquinolone

Use Treatment of community-acquired pneumonia, including multidrug resistant strains of *S. pneumoniae* (MDRSP); nosocomial pneumonia; chronic bronchitis (acute bacterial exacerbation); acute bacterial sinusitis; prostatitis, urinary tract infection (uncomplicated or complicated); acute pyelonephritis; skin or skin structure infections (uncomplicated or complicated); reduce incidence or disease progression of inhalational anthrax (postexposure)

Dosage Summary

I.V.:

Children <6 months: Dosage not established

Children ≥6 months and ≤50 kg: 8 mg/kg every 12 hours (maximum: 250 mg/dose)

Children >50 kg: 500 mg every once daily

Adults: 250-750 mg once daily

Oral:

Children <6 months: Dosage not established

Children ≥6 months and ≤50 kg: 8 mg/kg every 12 hours (maximum: 250 mg/dose)

Children >50 kg: 500 mg every once daily

Adults: 250-750 mg once daily

Dosage Forms

Infusion, premixed in D_5W [preservative free]:

Levaquin®: 250 mg (50 mL); 500 mg (100 mL); 750 mg (150 mL)

Injection, solution [preservative free]:

Levaquin®: 25 mg/mL (30 mL)

Solution, oral:

Levaquin®: 25 mg/mL (480 mL)

Tablet, oral:

Levaquin®: 250 mg, 500 mg, 750 mg

levofloxacin (ophthalmic) (lee voe FLOKS a sin)

Sound-Alike/Look-Alike Issues

levofloxacin may be confused with levetiracetam, levodopa, levothyroxine

U.S./Canadian Brand Names Iquix® [US]; Quixin® [US]

Therapeutic Category Antibiotic, Ophthalmic; Antibiotic, Quinolone

Use Treatment of bacterial conjunctivitis caused by susceptible organisms (Quixin® 0.5% ophthalmic solution); treatment of corneal ulcer caused by susceptible organisms (Iquix® 1.5% ophthalmic solution)

Dosage Summary

Ophthalmic:

Children ≥1 year: 1-2 drops every 2-6 hours

Adults: 1-2 drops every 2-6 hours

Dosage Forms

Solution, ophthalmic:

Iquix®: 1.5% (5 mL)

Quixin®: 0.5% (5 mL)

levo-folinic acid *see* LEVOleucovorin *on page 558*

LEVOleucovorin (lee voe loo koe VOR in)

Sound-Alike/Look-Alike Issues

LEVOleucovorin may be confused with leucovorin calcium, Leukeran®, Leukine®

Synonyms 6S-leucovorin; calcium levoleucovorin; L-leucovorin; levo-folinic acid; levo-leucovorin; levoleucovorin calcium pentahydrate; S-leucovorin

U.S./Canadian Brand Names Fusilev™ [US]

Therapeutic Category Antidote; Rescue Agent (Chemotherapy)

Use Rescue agent after high-dose methotrexate therapy in osteosarcoma; antidote for impaired methotrexate elimination and for inadvertent overdosage of folic acid antagonists

Dosage Summary

I.V.:

Children: 7.5-75 mg every 3-6 hours or 50 mg/m^2 every 3 hours

Adults: 7.5-75 mg every 3-6 hours or 50 mg/m^2 every 3 hours

Dosage Forms

Injection, powder for reconstitution:

Fusilev™: 50 mg

levo-leucovorin *see* LEVOleucovorin *on page 558*

levoleucovorin calcium pentahydrate *see* LEVOleucovorin *on page 558*

levomepromazine *see* methotrimeprazine *(Canada only) on page 615*

levonordefrin and mepivacaine hydrochloride *see* mepivacaine and levonordefrin *on page 605*

levonorgestrel (LEE voe nor jes trel)

Synonyms LNg 20

U.S./Canadian Brand Names Mirena® [US/Can]; Next Choice™ [US]; Plan B® One Step [US]; Plan B® [Can]

Therapeutic Category Contraceptive, Implant (Progestin); Contraceptive, Progestin Only

Use

Intrauterine device (IUD): Prevention of pregnancy; treatment of heavy menstrual bleeding in women who also choose to use an IUD for contraception

Oral: Emergency contraception following unprotected intercourse or possible contraceptive failure

Dosage Summary

Intrauterine:

Children: Not for use prior to menarche

Adults: Insert into uterine cavity, releases 20 mcg/day over 5 years

Oral:

Children: Not for use prior to menarche

Adults: One 0.75 mg tablet as soon as possible within 72 hours of unprotected sexual intercourse, repeat once 12 hours after the first dose **or** one 1.5 mg tablet as soon as possible within 72 hours of unprotected sexual intercourse

Dosage Forms

Intrauterine device, intrauterine:

Mirena®: 52 mg/device

Tablet, oral:

Next Choice™: 0.75 mg

Plan B® One Step: 1.5 mg

levonorgestrel and estradiol *see* estradiol and levonorgestrel *on page 368*

levonorgestrel and ethinyl estradiol *see* ethinyl estradiol and levonorgestrel *on page 376*

Levophed® [US/Can] *see* norepinephrine *on page 682*

Levora® [US] *see* ethinyl estradiol and levonorgestrel *on page 376*

levorphanol (lee VOR fa nole)

Synonyms levorphan tartrate; levorphanol tartrate

U.S./Canadian Brand Names Levo-Dromoran® [US]

Therapeutic Category Analgesic, Narcotic

Controlled Substance C-II

Use Relief of moderate-to-severe pain; preoperative sedation/analgesia; management of chronic pain (eg, cancer) requiring opoid therapy

Dosage Summary

I.M.:

Children: Dosage not established

Adults: 1-2 mg every 6-8 hours as needed **or** 1-2 mg/dose 60-90 minutes prior to surgery

I.V.:

Children: Dosage not established

Adults: Up to 1 mg/dose every 3-6 hours as needed

Oral:

Children: Dosage not established

Adults: 2-4 mg every 6-8 hours as needed

SubQ:

Children: Dosage not established

Adults: 1-2 mg every 6-8 hours as needed **or** 1-2 mg/dose 60-90 minutes prior to surgery

Dosage Forms

Injection, solution:

Levo-Dromoran®: 2 mg/mL (1 mL, 10 mL)

Tablet, oral: 2 mg

levorphanol tartrate *see* levorphanol *on page 559*

levorphan tartrate *see* levorphanol *on page 559*

Levo-T™ *(Discontinued)* *see* levothyroxine *on page 560*

Levothroid® [US] *see* levothyroxine *on page 560*

levothyroxine (lee voe thye ROKS een)

Sound-Alike/Look-Alike Issues

levothyroxine may be confused with lamoTRIgine, Lanoxin®, levofloxacin, liothyronine
Levoxyl® may be confused with Lanoxin®, Levaquin®, Luvox®
Synthroid® may be confused with Symmetrel®

Synonyms *L*-thyroxine sodium; levothyroxine sodium; T_4

U.S./Canadian Brand Names Eltroxin® [Can]; Euthyrox [Can]; Levothroid® [US]; Levothyroxine Sodium [Can]; Levoxyl® [US]; Synthroid® [US/Can]; Unithroid® [US]

Therapeutic Category Thyroid Product

Use Replacement or supplemental therapy in hypothyroidism; pituitary TSH suppression

Dosage Summary **Note:** Doses should be adjusted based on clinical response and laboratory parameters.

I.M.:

Newborns: 50% of oral dose
Children: 50% of oral dose
Adults: 50% of oral dose

I.V.:

Newborns: 50% of oral dose
Children: 50% of oral dose
Adults: 50% of oral dose or 200-500 mcg, then 100-300 mcg the next day if necessary [myxedema coma or stupor]

Oral:

Newborns: Initial: 10-15 mcg/kg/day; **Note:** Special circumstances may warrant lower starting doses
Children 0-3 months: 10-15 mcg/kg/day; **Note:** Special circumstances may warrant lower starting doses
Children 3-6 months: 8-10 mcg/kg/day; **Note:** Special circumstances may warrant lower starting doses
Children 6-12 months: 6-8 mcg/kg/day; **Note:** Special circumstances may warrant lower starting doses
Children 1-5 years: 5-6 mcg/kg/day; **Note:** Special circumstances may warrant lower starting doses
Children 6-12 years: 4-5 mcg/kg/day; **Note:** Special circumstances may warrant lower starting doses
Children >12 years: 2-3 mcg/kg/day; **Note:** Special circumstances may warrant lower starting doses
Adults: Initial: 12.5-25 mcg/day ***or*** 1.7 mcg/kg/day; **Note:** Titration is recommended (usual doses are ≤200 mcg/day)
Elderly >50 years without cardiac disease ***or*** *<50 years with cardiac disease:* Initial: 25-50 mcg/day; **Note:** Titration is recommended
Elderly >50 years with cardiac disease: Initial: 12.5-25 mcg/day; **Note:** Titration is recommended

Dosage Forms

Injection, powder for reconstitution: 200 mcg, 500 mcg

Tablet, oral: 25 mcg, 50 mcg, 75 mcg, 88 mcg, 100 mcg, 112 mcg, 125 mcg, 137 mcg, 150 mcg, 175 mcg, 200 mcg, 300 mcg

Levothroid®: 25 mcg, 50 mcg, 75 mcg, 88 mcg, 100 mcg, 112 mcg, 125 mcg, 137 mcg, 150 mcg, 175 mcg, 200 mcg, 300 mcg

Levoxyl®: 25 mcg, 50 mcg, 75 mcg, 88 mcg, 100 mcg, 112 mcg, 125 mcg, 137 mcg, 150 mcg, 175 mcg, 200 mcg

Synthroid®: 25 mcg, 50 mcg, 75 mcg, 88 mcg, 100 mcg, 112 mcg, 125 mcg, 137 mcg, 150 mcg, 175 mcg, 200 mcg, 300 mcg

Unithroid®: 25 mcg, 50 mcg, 75 mcg, 88 mcg, 100 mcg, 112 mcg, 125 mcg, 150 mcg, 175 mcg, 200 mcg, 300 mcg

Levothyroxine Sodium [Can] *see* levothyroxine *on page 560*

levothyroxine sodium *see* levothyroxine *on page 560*

Levoxyl® [US] *see* levothyroxine *on page 560*

Levsin® [US/Can] *see* hyoscyamine *on page 491*

Levsin®/SL [US] *see* hyoscyamine *on page 491*
Levulan® Kerastick® [US/Can] *see* aminolevulinic acid *on page 65*
levulose, dextrose and phosphoric acid *see* fructose, dextrose, and phosphoric acid *on page 430*
Lexapro® [US] *see* escitalopram *on page 363*
Lexiscan™ [US] *see* regadenoson *on page 833*
Lexiva® [US] *see* fosamprenavir *on page 426*
Lexxel® [Can] *see* enalapril and felodipine *on page 348*
Lexxel® *(Discontinued)* *see* enalapril and felodipine *on page 348*
LFA-3/IgG(1) fusion protein, human *see* alefacept *on page 47*
***l*-hyoscyamine sulfate** *see* hyoscyamine *on page 491*
Lialda™ [US] *see* mesalamine *on page 607*
Librax® *[original formulation]* [US/Can] *see* clidinium and chlordiazepoxide *on page 231*
Librax® *[reformulation] (Discontinued)*
Librium® *(Discontinued)* *see* chlordiazepoxide *on page 203*
Lice-Enz® Shampoo *(Discontinued)*
Licide® [US-OTC] *see* pyrethrins and piperonyl butoxide *on page 816*
LidaMantle® [US] *see* lidocaine (topical) *on page 562*
LidaMantle HC® [US] *see* lidocaine and hydrocortisone *on page 564*
LidaMantle HC® Relief Pad™ [US] *see* lidocaine and hydrocortisone *on page 564*
Lidemol® [Can] *see* fluocinonide *on page 411*
Lidex® [Can] *see* fluocinonide *on page 411*
Lidex® *(Discontinued)* *see* fluocinonide *on page 411*
Lidex-E® *(Discontinued)* *see* fluocinonide *on page 411*

lidocaine (systemic) (LYE doe kane)

Synonyms lidocaine hydrochloride; lignocaine hydrochloride

U.S./Canadian Brand Names Xylocaine® Dental [US]; Xylocaine® MPF [US]; Xylocaine® [US]; Xylocard® [Can]

Therapeutic Category Antiarrhythmic Agent, Class Ib; Local Anesthetic

Use Local and regional anesthesia by infiltration, nerve block, epidural, or spinal techniques; acute treatment of ventricular arrhythmias from myocardial infarction or cardiac manipulation

Dosage Summary

E.T.:

Children: 2-3 mg/kg; flush with 5 mL of NS and follow with 5 assisted manual ventilations

Adults (loading dose only): 2-2.5 times the I.V. bolus dose

I.O.:

Children: Loading dose: 1 mg/kg, may repeat 0.5-1 mg/kg (maximum: 100 mg); Infusion: 20-50 mcg/kg/minute

Adults: Dosage not established

I.V.:

Children: Loading dose: 1 mg/kg (maximum: 100 mg), may repeat 0.5-1 mg/kg; Infusion: 20-50 mcg/kg/minute

Adults: Bolus: 1-1.5 mg/kg, may repeat 0.5-0.75 mg/kg up to a total of 3 mg/kg; Infusion: 1-4 mg/minute

Local injection:

Children: Varies with procedure, degree of anesthesia needed, vascularity of tissue, duration of anesthesia required, and physical condition of patient (maximum: 4.5 mg/kg/dose); do not repeat within 2 hours

Adults: Varies with procedure, degree of anesthesia needed, vascularity of tissue, duration of anesthesia required, and physical condition of patient (maximum: 4.5 mg/kg/dose); do not repeat within 2 hours

Dosage Forms

Infusion, premixed in D_5W: 0.4% [4 mg/mL] (250 mL, 500 mL); 0.8% [8 mg/mL] (250 mL, 500 mL)

Injection, solution: 0.5% [5 mg/mL] (50 mL); 1% [10 mg/mL] (2 mL, 10 mL, 20 mL, 30 mL, 50 mL); 2% [20 mg/mL] (2 mL, 5 mL, 20 mL, 50 mL)

Xylocaine®: 0.5% [5 mg/mL] (50 mL); 1% [10 mg/mL] (10 mL, 20 mL, 50 mL); 2% [20 mg/mL] (10 mL, 20 mL, 50 mL)

Xylocaine® Dental: 2% [20 mg/mL] (1.8 mL)

Injection, solution [preservative free]: 0.5% [5 mg/mL] (50 mL); 1% [10 mg/mL] (2 mL, 5 mL, 30 mL); 1.5% [15 mg/mL] (20 mL); 2% [20 mg/mL] (2 mL, 5 mL, 10 mL); 4% [40 mg/mL] (5 mL)
Xylocaine®: 2% [20 mg/mL] (5 mL)
Xylocaine® MPF: 0.5% [5 mg/mL] (50 mL); 1% [10 mg/mL] (2 mL, 5 mL, 10 mL, 30 mL); 1.5% [15 mg/mL] (10 mL, 20 mL); 2% [20 mg/mL] (2 mL, 5 mL, 10 mL); 4% [40 mg/mL] (5 mL)

lidocaine (ophthalmic) (LYE doe kane)

Synonyms lidocaine hydrochloride; lignocaine hydrochloride

U.S./Canadian Brand Names Akten™ [US]

Therapeutic Category Local Anesthetic; Local Anesthetic, Ophthalmic

Use To provide local anesthesia to ocular surface during ophthalmologic procedures

Dosage Summary

Ophthalmic:

Children: 2 drops to ocular surface; may repeat to maintain effect
Adults: 2 drops to ocular surface; may repeat to maintain effect

Dosage Forms

Gel, ophthalmic [preservative free]:
Akten™: 3.5% (5 mL)

lidocaine (topical) (LYE doe kane)

Synonyms lidocaine hydrochloride; lidocaine patch; lignocaine hydrochloride; viscous lidocaine

U.S./Canadian Brand Names Anestafoam™ [US-OTC]; Band-Aid® Hurt-Free™ Antiseptic Wash [US-OTC]; Betacaine® [Can]; Burn Jel Plus [US-OTC]; Burn Jel® [US-OTC]; L-M-X® 4 [US-OTC]; L-M-X® 5 [US-OTC]; LidaMantle® [US]; Lidodan™ [Can]; Lidoderm® [US/Can]; LTA® 360 [US]; Maxilene® [Can]; Premjact® [US]; Regenecare® HA [US-OTC]; Regenecare® [US]; Solarcaine® cool aloe Burn Relief [US-OTC]; Topicaine® [US-OTC]; Unburn® [US-OTC]; Xylocaine® [US/Can]

Therapeutic Category Analgesic, Topical; Local Anesthetic

Use

Rectal: Temporary relief of pain and itching due to anorectal disorders
Topical: Local anesthetic for oral muscous membrane; use in laser/cosmetic surgeries; minor burns, cuts, and abrasions of the skin
Oral solution (viscous): Topical anesthesia of irritated oral mucous membranes and pharyngeal tissue
Patch (Lidoderm®): Relief of allodynia (painful hypersensitivity) and chronic pain in postherpetic neuralgia

Dosage Summary Topical: Unless otherwise noted, the following traditional pediatric guideline for topical lidocaine dosage may be observed: Apply to affected area as needed; maximum dose: 3 mg/kg/dose; do not repeat within 2 hours (Benitz, 1988)

Cream:
Children <2 years: LidaMantle®: Apply to affected area 2-3 times/day as needed
Children 2-12 years:
LidaMantle®: Apply to affected area 2-3 times/day as needed
L-M-X® 4: Apply 1/4 inch thick layer to intact skin, remove once adequate anesthetic effect obtained
Children ≥12 years:
LidaMantle®: Apply to affected area 2-3 times/day as needed
L-M-X® 4: Apply 1/4 inch thick layer to intact skin, remove once adequate anesthetic effect obtained
L-M-X® 5: Apply to clean, dry area or using applicator, insert rectally, ≤6 times/day
Adults:
LidaMantle®: Apply to affected area 2-3 times/day as needed
L-M-X® 4: Apply 1/4 inch thick layer to intact skin, remove once adequate anesthetic effect obtained
L-M-X® 5: Apply to clean, dry area or using applicator, insert rectally, ≤6 times/day

Gel, ointment, solution:
Children: Dosage not established
Adults: Apply to affected area ≤3 times/day as needed (maximum: 4.5 mg/kg/dose; 300 mg/dose)

Jelly:
Children <10 years: Dosage not established
Children ≥10 years: Dose varies with age and weight (maximum: 4.5 mg/kg/dose)
Adults: 5-30 mL (maximum: 30 mL (600 mg)/12 hour period)
Adults: Apply to affected area every 6 hours as needed

Oral solution (viscous):

Infants and Children <3 years: 1.25 mL applied to area with a cotton-tipped applicator every 3-8 hours (maximum: 4 doses per 12-hour period)

Children ≥3 years: Should not exceed 4.5 mg/kg/dose (not to exceed 300 mg/dose); swished in the mouth and spit out every 3-8 hours; patient should not swallow viscous solution

Adults: 15 mL swished in the mouth and spit out every 3-8 hours (maximum: 8 doses per 24-hour period); patient should not swallow viscous solution

Patch:

Children: Dosage not established

Adults: Apply up to 3 patches in a single application for up to 12 hours in any 24-hour period.

Dosage Forms

Aerosol, topical:
Anestafoam™ [OTC]: 4% (30 g)
Solarcaine® cool aloe Burn Relief [OTC]: 0.5% (127 g)

Cream, rectal:
L-M-X® 5 [OTC]: 5% (15 g, 30 g)

Cream, topical: 0.5% (0.9 g)
AneCream™ [OTC]: 4% (5 g, 15 g, 30 g)
L-M-X® 4 [OTC]: 4% (5 g, 15 g, 30 g)
LidaMantle®: 3% (85 g)

Gel, topical:
Burn Jel Plus [OTC]: 2.5% (118 mL)
Burn Jel® [OTC]: 2% (59 mL, 118 mL); 2% (3.5 g)
Regenecare®: 2% (14 g, 85 g)
Regenecare® HA [OTC]: 2% (85 g)
Solarcaine® cool aloe Burn Relief [OTC]: 0.5% (113 g, 226 g)
Topicaine® [OTC]: 4% (10 g, 30 g, 113 g); 5% (10 g, 30 g, 113 g)
Unburn® [OTC]: 2.5% (59 mL)

Jelly, topical: 2% (5 mL, 30 mL)
Xylocaine®: 2% (5 mL, 30 mL)

Jelly, topical [preservative free]: 2% (5 mL, 10 mL, 20 mL)

Lotion, topical:
LidaMantle®: 3% (177 mL)

Ointment, topical: 5% (30 g, 35.4 g, 50 g)

Patch, transdermal:
Lidoderm®: 5% (30s)

Solution, topical: 4% [40 mg/mL] (50 mL)
Band-Aid® Hurt Free™ Antiseptic Wash [OTC]: 2% [20 mg/mL] (177 mL)
LTA® 360: 4% [40 mg/mL] (4 mL)
Premjact®: 9.6% (13 mL)
Xylocaine®: 4% [40 mg/mL] (50 mL)

Solution, topical [preservative free]: 4% [40 mg/mL] (4 mL)

Solution, viscous, oral: 2% [20 mg/mL] (20 mL, 100 mL, 500 mL)

lidocaine and bupivacaine *(Discontinued)*

lidocaine and epinephrine (LYE doe kane & ep i NEF rin)

Synonyms epinephrine and lidocaine

U.S./Canadian Brand Names Lignospan® Forte [US]; Lignospan® Standard [US]; Xylocaine® MPF With Epinephrine [US]; Xylocaine® With Epinephrine [US/Can]

Therapeutic Category Local Anesthetic

Use Local infiltration anesthesia; AVS for nerve block; topical local analgesia for superficial dermatologic procedures

Dosage Summary Note: Dosage varies with the anesthetic procedure, degree of anesthesia needed, vascularity of tissue, duration of anesthesia required, and physical condition of patient.

Conduction block or infiltration (dental):

Children <12 years: 20-30 mg (1-1.5 mL) of 2% lidocaine with epinephrine 1:100,000 (maximum: 4.5 mg/kg of lidocaine or 100-150 mg as a single dose)

Children ≥12 years: Do not exceed 7 mg/kg body weight up to a maximum range of 300 mg (usual dental practice) to 500 mg (approved product labeling) of lidocaine hydrochloride and 3 mcg (0.003 mg) of epinephrine/kg of body weight or 0.2 mg epinephrine per dental appointment.

Adults: Up to 7 mg/kg or 300 mg of lidocaine and 3 mcg/kg or 0.2 mg of epinephrine per dental appointment

Infiltration (local anesthetic):

Children: Up to 7 mg/kg/dose of 0.5% to 1% lidocaine; do not repeat within 2 hours

Adults: Dosage not established

Topical:

Children <5 years: Dosage not established

Children ≥5 years: Place 1 transdermal patch over area requiring analgesia for 10 minutes (maximum: 1 patch/30 minutes)

Adults: Place 1 transdermal patch over area requiring analgesia for 10 minutes (maximum: 1 patch/30 minutes)

Dosage Forms

Injection, solution:

Generics:

0.5% / 1:200,000: Lidocaine hydrochloride 0.5% and epinephrine 1:200,000 (50 mL)

1% / 1:100,000: Lidocaine hydrochloride 1% and epinephrine 1:100,000 (20 mL, 30 mL, 50 mL)

2% / 1:100,000: Lidocaine hydrochloride 2% and epinephrine 1:100,000 (30 mL, 50 mL)

Brands:

Xylocaine® with Epinephrine:

0.5% / 1:200,000: Lidocaine hydrochloride 0.5% and epinephrine 1:200,000 (50 mL)

1% / 1:100,000: Lidocaine hydrochloride 1% and epinephrine 1:100,000 (10 mL, 20 mL, 50 mL)

2% / 1:100,000: Lidocaine hydrochloride 2% and epinephrine 1:100,000 (10 mL, 20 mL, 50 mL)

Injection, solution [preservative free]

Generics:

1% / 1:200,000: Lidocaine hydrochloride 1% and epinephrine 1:200,000 (30 mL)

1.5% / 1:200,000: Lidocaine hydrochloride 1.5% and epinephrine 1:200,000 (5 mL, 30 mL)

2% / 1:200,000: Lidocaine hydrochloride 2% and epinephrine 1:200,000 (20 mL)

Brands:

Xylocaine®-MPF with Epinephrine:

1% / 1:200,000: Lidocaine hydrochloride 1% and epinephrine 1:200,000 (5 mL, 10 mL, 30 mL)

1.5% / 1:200,000: Lidocaine hydrochloride 1.5% and epinephrine 1:200,000 (5 mL, 10 mL, 30 mL)

2% / 1:200,000: Lidocaine hydrochloride 2% and epinephrine 1:200,000 (5 mL, 10 mL, 20 mL)

Injection, solution [for dental use]

Generics:

2% / 1:50,000: Lidocaine hydrochloride 2% and epinephrine 1:50,000 (1.7 mL, 1.8 mL)

2% / 1:100,000: Lidocaine hydrochloride 2% and epinephrine 1:100,000 (1.7 mL, 1.8 mL)

Brands:

Lignospan® Forte: 2% / 1:50,000: Lidocaine hydrochloride 2% and epinephrine 1:50,000 (1.7 mL)

Lignospan® Standard: 2% / 1:100,000: Lidocaine hydrochloride 2% and epinephrine 1:100,000 (1.7 mL)

lidocaine and hydrocortisone (LYE doe kane & hye droe KOR ti sone)

Synonyms hydrocortisone and lidocaine

U.S./Canadian Brand Names AnaMantle HC® Cream [US]; AnaMantle HC® Forte [US]; AnaMantle HC® Gel [US]; LidaMantle HC® Relief Pad™ [US]; LidaMantle HC® [US]; LidoCort™ [US]; Peranex™ HC Medi-Pad [US]; Peranex™ HC [US]; RectaGel™ HC [US]

Therapeutic Category Anesthetic/Corticosteroid

Use Topical antiinflammatory and anesthetic for skin disorders; rectal for the treatment of hemorrhoids, anal fissures, pruritus ani, or similar conditions

Dosage Summary

Rectal:

Children: Dosage not established

Adults: One applicatorful twice daily

Topical:

Children: Dosage not established

Adults: Apply 2-3 times/day

Dosage Forms

Cream, rectal: Lidocaine 3% and hydrocortisone 0.5% (7 g); lidocaine 3% and hydrocortisone 1% (7 g)

AnaMantle HC® Forte: Lidocaine 3% and hydrocortisone 1% (7 g)

AnaMantle HC®: Lidocaine 3% and hydrocortisone 0.5% (7 g)

Peranex™ HC: Lidocaine 2% and hydrocortisone 2% (7 g)

Cream, topical:
LidaMantle HC®: Lidocaine 3% and hydrocortisone 0.5% (85 g)
Gel, rectal: Lidocaine 3% and hydrocortisone 2.5% (7 g)
AnaMantle HC®, LidoCort™: Lidocaine 3% and hydrocortisone 2.5% (7 g)
RectaGel™ HC: Lidocaine 2.8% and hydrocortisone 0.55% (20 g)
Lotion, topical: Lidocaine 3% and hydrocortisone 0.5% (177 mL)
LidaMantle HC®: Lidocaine 3% and hydrocortisone 0.5% (177 mL)
Pad, topical:
LidaMantel HC® Relief Pad™: Lidocaine 2% and hydrocortisone 2% (60s)
Peranex™ HC Medi-Pad: Lidocaine 3% and hydrocortisone 1% (60s)

lidocaine and prilocaine (LYE doe kane & PRIL oh kane)

Synonyms prilocaine and lidocaine

U.S./Canadian Brand Names EMLA® [US/Can]; Oraquix® [US]

Therapeutic Category Analgesic, Topical

Use Topical anesthetic for use on normal intact skin to provide local analgesia for minor procedures such as I.V. cannulation or venipuncture; has also been used for painful procedures such as lumbar puncture and skin graft harvesting; for superficial minor surgery of genital mucous membranes and as an adjunct for local infiltration anesthesia in genital mucous membranes.

Dosage Summary

Periodontal:
Children: Dosage not established
Adults: Maximum recommended dose: One treatment session: 5 cartridges (8.5 g)

Topical, cream:
Children 0-3 months or <5 kg: Apply up to 1 g over no more than 10 cm^2 of skin for no longer than 1 hour; **Note:** Should not be used in neonates with a gestational age <37 weeks
Children 3-12 months and >5 kg: Apply up to 2 g total over no more than 20 cm^2 of skin for no longer than 4 hours
Children 1-6 years and >10 kg: Apply up to 10 g total over no more than 100 cm^2 of skin for no longer than 4 hours
Children 7-12 years and >20 kg: Apply up to 20 g total over no more than 200 cm^2 of skin for no longer than 4 hours
Adults: Apply 2-2.5 g per 10-25 cm^{2}of skin for at least 1-2 hours **or** 5-10 g for 5-10 minutes
Adults (males): Apply 1 g/10 cm^2 for 15 minutes

Topical, transdermal patch: Canadian labeling (not available in U.S.):
Children 0-3 months or <5 kg: Apply 1 patch and leave on for ~1 hour; maximum dose: 1 patch. **Note:** Should not be used in neonates with a gestational age <37 weeks.
Children 3 months to 12 months and >5 kg: Apply 1-2 patches for ~1 hour (maximum application time: 4 hours); maximum dose: 2 patches
Children 1-6 years and >10 kg: Apply 1or more patches for minimum of 1 hour (maximum application time: 5 hours); maximum dose: 10 patches
Children 7-12 years and >20 kg: Apply 1 or more patches for a minimum of 1 hour (maximum application time: 5 hours); maximum dose: 20 patches
Adults: Apply 1 or more patches to skin surface area <10 cm^2 for at least 1 hour (maximum application time: 5 hours)

Dosage Forms

Cream, topical: Lidocaine 2.5% and prilocaine 2.5% (5 g, 30 g)
EMLA®: Lidocaine 2.5% and prilocaine 2.5% (5 g, 30 g)
Gel, periodontal:
Oraqix®: Lidocaine 2.5% and prilocaine 2.5% (1.7 g)

Dosage Forms - Canada

Patch, transdermal:
EMLA® Patch: Lidocaine 2.5% and prilocaine 2.5% per patch (2s, 20s)

lidocaine and tetracaine (LYE doe kane & TET ra kane)

Synonyms tetracaine and lidocaine

U.S./Canadian Brand Names Pliaglis™ [US]; Synera™ [US]

Therapeutic Category Analgesic, Topical; Local Anesthetic

Use Topical anesthetic for use on normal intact skin for minor procedures (eg, I.V. cannulation or venipuncture) and superficial dermatologic procedures

Dosage Summary

Topical:

Children: <3 years: Dosage not established

Children ≥3 years: Apply patch to intact skin for 20-30 minutes, prior to procedure

Adults: Apply patch to intact skin for 20-30 minutes, prior to procedure

Dosage Forms

Cream, topical:

Pliaglis™: Lidocaine 7% and tetracaine 7% (30 g)

Patch, transdermal:

Synera™: Lidocaine 70 mg and tetracaine 70 mg (10s)

lidocaine hydrochloride *see* lidocaine (ophthalmic) *on page* 562

lidocaine hydrochloride *see* lidocaine (systemic) *on page* 561

lidocaine hydrochloride *see* lidocaine (topical) *on page* 562

lidocaine patch *see* lidocaine (topical) *on page* 562

LidoCort™ [US] *see* lidocaine and hydrocortisone *on page* 564

Lidodan™ [Can] *see* lidocaine (topical) *on page* 562

Lidoderm® [US/Can] *see* lidocaine (topical) *on page* 562

LidoPen® I.M. Injection Auto-Injector *(Discontinued)* *see* lidocaine (systemic) *on page* 561

LidoSite™ *(Discontinued)* *see* lidocaine and epinephrine *on page* 563

LID-Pack® [Can] *see* bacitracin and polymyxin B *on page* 113

lignocaine hydrochloride *see* lidocaine (ophthalmic) *on page* 562

lignocaine hydrochloride *see* lidocaine (systemic) *on page* 561

lignocaine hydrochloride *see* lidocaine (topical) *on page* 562

Lignospan® Forte [US] *see* lidocaine and epinephrine *on page* 563

Lignospan® Standard [US] *see* lidocaine and epinephrine *on page* 563

Limbitrol® [Can] *see* amitriptyline and chlordiazepoxide *on page* 68

Limbitrol® *(Discontinued)* *see* amitriptyline and chlordiazepoxide *on page* 68

Limbitrol® DS *(Discontinued)* *see* amitriptyline and chlordiazepoxide *on page* 68

Limbrel 250™ [US] *see* flavocoxid *on page* 404

Limbrel 500™ [US] *see* flavocoxid *on page* 404

Limbrel™ *(Discontinued)* *see* flavocoxid *on page* 404

Lin-Amox [Can] *see* amoxicillin *on page* 72

Lin-Buspirone [Can] *see* buspirone *on page* 157

Lincocin® [US/Can] *see* lincomycin *on page* 566

lincomycin (lin koe MYE sin)

Sound-Alike/Look-Alike Issues

Lincocin® may be confused with Cleocin®, Indocin®, Minocin®

Synonyms lincomycin hydrochloride

U.S./Canadian Brand Names Lincocin® [US/Can]

Therapeutic Category Antibiotic, Lincosamide

Use Treatment of serious susceptible bacterial infections, mainly those caused by streptococci, pneumococci, and staphylococci resistant to other agents

Dosage Summary

I.M.:

Children ≤1 month: Dosage not established

Children >1 month: 10 mg/kg every 12-24 hours

Adults: 600 mg every 12-24 hours

I.V.:

Children ≤1 month: Dosage not established

Children >1 month: 10-20 mg/kg/day divided every 8-12 hours

Adults: 600 mg to 1 g every 8-12 hours (maximum: 8 g/day)

Subconjunctival injection:

Children: Dosage not established

Adults: 75 mg

Dosage Forms

Injection, solution:

Lincocin®: 300 mg/mL (2 mL, 10 mL)

lincomycin hydrochloride *see* lincomycin *on page 566*

lindane (LIN dane)

Synonyms benzene hexachloride; gamma benzene hexachloride; hexachlorocyclohexane

U.S./Canadian Brand Names Hexit™ [Can]; PMS-Lindane [Can]

Therapeutic Category Scabicides/Pediculicides

Use Treatment of *Sarcoptes scabiei* (scabies), *Pediculus capitis* (head lice), and *Phthirus pubis* (crab lice); FDA recommends reserving lindane as a second-line agent or with inadequate response to other therapies

Dosage Summary

Topical:

Lotion:

Children: Apply a thin layer and massage onto skin from the neck to the toes; bathe and remove drug after 8-12 hours

Adults: Apply a thin layer and massage onto skin from the neck to the toes; bathe and remove drug after 8-12 hours

Shampoo:

Children: Apply to dry hair and massage for 4 minutes; add small quantities of water until lather forms, then rinse thoroughly and comb with a fine tooth comb to remove nits (maximum: 60 mL)

Adults: Apply to dry hair and massage for 4 minutes; add small quantities of water until lather forms, then rinse thoroughly and comb with a fine tooth comb to remove nits (maximum: 60 mL)

Dosage Forms

Lotion, topical: 1% (60 mL, 480 mL)

Shampoo, topical: 1% (60 mL, 480 mL)

Linessa® [Can] *see* ethinyl estradiol and desogestrel *on page 374*

linezolid (li NE zoh lid)

Sound-Alike/Look-Alike Issues

Zyvox® may be confused with Ziox™, Zosyn®, Zovirax®

U.S./Canadian Brand Names Zyvoxam® [Can]; Zyvox® [US]

Therapeutic Category Antibiotic, Oxazolidinone

Use Treatment of vancomycin-resistant *Enterococcus faecium* (VRE) infections, nosocomial pneumonia caused by *Staphylococcus aureus* (including MRSA) or *Streptococcus pneumoniae* (including multidrug-resistant strains [MDRSP]), complicated and uncomplicated skin and skin structure infections (including diabetic foot infections without concomitant osteomyelitis), and community-acquired pneumonia caused by susceptible gram-positive organisms

Dosage Summary

I.V.:

Preterm neonates (<34 weeks gestational age): 10 mg/kg every 8-12 hours

Children ≤11 years: 10 mg/kg every 8 hours

Children ≥12 years: 600 mg every 12 hours

Adults: 600 mg every 12 hours

Oral:

Preterm neonates (<34 weeks gestational age): 10 mg/kg every 8-12 hours

Children <5 years: 10 mg/kg every 8 hours

Children 5-11 years: 10 mg/kg every 8-12 hours

Children ≥12 years: 400-600 mg every 12 hours

Adults: 400-600 mg every 12 hours

Dosage Forms

Infusion, premixed:

Zyvox®: 200 mg (100 mL); 600 mg (300 mL)

Powder for suspension, oral:

Zyvox®: 100 mg/5 mL (150 mL)

Tablet, oral:

Zyvox®: 600 mg

Lioresal® [US/Can] *see* baclofen *on page 115*

Liotec [Can] *see* baclofen *on page 115*

liothyronine (lye oh THYE roe neen)

Sound-Alike/Look-Alike Issues

liothyronine may be confused with levothyroxine

T3 is an error-prone abbreviation (mistaken as acetaminophen and codeine [ie, Tylenol® #3])

Synonyms liothyronine sodium; sodium *L*-triiodothyronine

U.S./Canadian Brand Names Cytomel® [US/Can]; Triostat® [US]

Therapeutic Category Thyroid Product

Use

Oral: Replacement or supplemental therapy in hypothyroidism; management of nontoxic goiter; a diagnostic aid

I.V.: Treatment of myxedema coma/precoma

Dosage Summary

I.V.:

Children: Dosage not established

Adults: 10-50 mcg/dose, at least 4 hours between doses, but not more than 12 hours

Oral:

Infants: Initial: 5 mcg/day; Usual maintenance dose: 20 mcg/day; **Note:** Titration is recommended

Children 1-3 years: Initial: 5 mcg/day; Usual maintenance dose: 50 mcg/day; **Note:** Titration is recommended

Children >3 years: Initial: 5 mcg/day; Maintenance: Up to 100 mcg/day; **Note:** Titration is recommended

Adults: Initial 5-25 mcg/day; Maintenance range 5-100 mcg/day; **Note:** Titration is recommended

Elderly: 5 mcg/day; increase by 5 mcg/day every 2 weeks

Dosage Forms

Injection, solution: 10 mcg/mL (1 mL)

Triostat®: 10 mcg/mL (1 mL)

Tablet, oral: 5 mcg, 25 mcg, 50 mcg

Cytomel®: 5 mcg, 25 mcg, 50 mcg

liothyronine sodium *see* liothyronine *on page 568*

liotrix (LYE oh triks)

Sound-Alike/Look-Alike Issues

liotrix may be confused with Klotrix®

Thyrolar® may be confused with Thyrogen®, Thytropar®

Synonyms T_3/T_4 liotrix

U.S./Canadian Brand Names Thyrolar® [US/Can]

Therapeutic Category Thyroid Product

Use Replacement or supplemental therapy in hypothyroidism (uniform mixture of T_4:T_3 in 4:1 ratio by weight); little advantage to this product exists and cost is not justified

Dosage Summary

Oral:

Children 0-6 months: 8-10 mcg/kg **or** 25-50 mcg/day

Children 6-12 months: 6-8 mcg/kg **or** 50-75 mcg/day

Children 1-5 years: 5-6 mcg/kg **or** 75-100 mcg/day

Children 6-12 years: 4-5 mcg/kg **or** 100-150 mcg/day

Children >12 years: 2-3 mcg/kg **or** >150 mcg/day

Adults: Initial: 15-30 mg/day (lower dose in cardiovascualr impairment and elderly); Usual maintenance: 60-120 mg/day; **Note:** Titration is recommended

Elderly: Initial: 15 mg, adjust dose at 2- to 4-week intervals by increments of 15 mg

Dosage Forms

Tablet, oral:

Thyrolar®:

1/4 [levothyroxine 12.5 mcg and liothyronine 3.1 mcg]

1/2 [levothyroxine 25 mcg and liothyronine 6.25 mcg]

1 [levothyroxine 50 mcg and liothyronine 12.5 mcg]

2 [levothyroxine 100 mcg and liothyronine 25 mcg]

3 [levothyroxine 150 mcg and liothyronine 37.5 mcg]

lipancreatin *see* pancrelipase *on page 723*

lipase, protease, and amylase *see* pancrelipase *on page 723*
Lipidil EZ® [Can] *see* fenofibrate *on page 393*
Lipidil Micro® [Can] *see* fenofibrate *on page 393*
Lipidil Supra® [Can] *see* fenofibrate *on page 393*
Lipitor® [US/Can] *see* atorvastatin *on page 104*
Lipofen® [US] *see* fenofibrate *on page 393*
liposomal DAUNOrubicin *see* daunorubicin citrate (liposomal) *on page 271*
liposomal DOXOrubicin *see* doxorubicin (liposomal) *on page 330*
Liposyn® II [Can] *see* fat emulsion *on page 391*
Liposyn® II *(Discontinued)* *see* fat emulsion *on page 391*
Liposyn® III [US] *see* fat emulsion *on page 391*
Lipram 4500 *(Discontinued)* *see* pancrelipase *on page 723*
Lipram-CR *(Discontinued)* *see* pancrelipase *on page 723*
Lipram-PN *(Discontinued)* *see* pancrelipase *on page 723*
Lipram-UL *(Discontinued)* *see* pancrelipase *on page 723*
Liqua-Cal [US-OTC] *see* calcium and vitamin D *on page 166*
Liquaemin® *(Discontinued)* *see* heparin *on page 467*
Liquibid-D® [US] *see* guaifenesin and phenylephrine *on page 456*
Liquibid® 1200 *(Discontinued)* *see* guaifenesin *on page 454*
Liquibid® *(Discontinued)* *see* guaifenesin *on page 454*
Liquibid-PD 1200 *(Discontinued)* *see* guaifenesin and phenylephrine *on page 456*
Liquibid-PD *(Discontinued)* *see* guaifenesin and phenylephrine *on page 456*
Liqui-Char® *(Discontinued)* *see* charcoal *on page 200*
Liqui-Coat HD® *(Discontinued)* *see* barium *on page 117*
Liquicough DM [US] *see* guaifenesin, pseudoephedrine, and dextromethorphan *on page 460*
liquid antidote *see* charcoal *on page 200*
Liquid Barosperse® *(Discontinued)* *see* barium *on page 117*
Liquid Polibar® [US] *see* barium *on page 117*
Liquid Polibar Plus® [US] *see* barium *on page 117*
Liquid Pred® *(Discontinued)* *see* prednisone *on page 792*
Liquifilm® Forte Solution *(Discontinued)* *see* artificial tears *on page 97*
Liquifilm® Tears [US-OTC] *see* artificial tears *on page 97*
Liquifilm® Tears Solution *(Discontinued)* *see* artificial tears *on page 97*

liraglutide (lir a GLOO tide)

Synonyms NN2211
U.S./Canadian Brand Names Victoza® [US/Can]
Therapeutic Category Antidiabetic Agent, Glucagon-Like Peptide-1 (GLP-1) Receptor Agonist
Use Treatment of type 2 diabetes mellitus (noninsulin-dependent, NIDDM) to improve glycemic control
Dosage Summary
SubQ:
Children: Dosage not established.
Adults: Initial: 0.6 mg once daily; maintenance: 1.2-1.8 mg/day
Dosage Forms
Injection, solution:
Victoza®: 6 mg/mL (3 mL)

lisdexamfetamine (lis dex am FET a meen)

Sound-Alike/Look-Alike Issues
Vyvanse™ may be confused with Vytorin®, Glucovance®, Vivactil®
Synonyms lisdexamfetamine dimesylate; lisdexamphetamine; NRP104
U.S./Canadian Brand Names Vyvanse® [US/Can]
Therapeutic Category Stimulant
Controlled Substance C-II
Use Treatment of attention-deficit/hyperactivity disorder (ADHD)

Dosage Summary

Oral:

Children <6 years: Dosage not established

Children 6-12 years: Initial: 30 mg once daily; may increase in increments of 10 mg or 20 mg/day at weekly intervals until optimal response is obtained (maximum: 70 mg/day)

Children >12 years: Dosage not established

Adults: Initial: 30 mg once daily; may increase in increments of 10 mg or 20 mg/day at weekly intervals until optimal response is obtained (maximum: 70 mg/day)

Dosage Forms

Capsule, oral:

Vyvanse®: 20 mg, 30 mg, 40 mg, 50 mg, 60 mg, 70 mg

lisdexamfetamine dimesylate *see* lisdexamfetamine *on page 569*

lisdexamphetamine *see* lisdexamfetamine *on page 569*

lisinopril (lyse IN oh pril)

Sound-Alike/Look-Alike Issues

lisinopril may be confused with fosinopril, Lioresal®, Risperdal®

Prinivil® may be confused with Plendil®, Pravachol®, Prevacid®, Prilosec®, Proventil®

Zestril® may be confused with Desyrel®, Restoril™, Vistaril®, Zegerid®, Zerit®, Zetia®, Zostrix®, Zyprexa®

U.S./Canadian Brand Names Apo-Lisinopril® [Can]; CO Lisinopril [Can]; Dom-Lisinopril [Can]; Mint-Lisinopril [Can]; Mylan-Lisinopril [Can]; Novo-Lisinopril [Can]; PHL-Lisinopril [Can]; PMS-Lisinopril [Can]; Prinivil® [US/Can]; PRO-Lisinopril [Can]; RAN™-Lisinopril [Can]; ratio-Lisinopril [Can]; Riva-Lisinopril [Can]; Sandoz-Lisinopril [Can]; Zestril® [US/Can]; ZYM-Lisinopril [Can]

Therapeutic Category Angiotensin-Converting Enzyme (ACE) Inhibitor

Use Treatment of hypertension, either alone or in combination with other antihypertensive agents; adjunctive therapy in treatment of heart failure (afterload reduction); treatment of acute myocardial infarction within 24 hours in hemodynamically-stable patients to improve survival; treatment of left ventricular dysfunction after myocardial infarction

Dosage Summary

Oral:

Children <6 years: Dosage not established

Children ≥6 years: Initial: 0.07 mg/kg once daily (up to 5 mg); Maintenance: Increase at 1- to 2- week intervals (maximum: >0.61 mg/kg or >40 mg has not been evaluated)

Adults: Initial: 2.5-10 mg/day; Maintenance: 10-80 mg/day (lisinopril doses >40 mg may not provide additional efficacy)

Elderly: Initial: 2.5-5 mg/day (maximum: 40 mg/day)

Dosage Forms

Tablet, oral: 2.5 mg, 5 mg, 10 mg, 20 mg, 30 mg, 40 mg

Prinivil®: 5 mg, 10 mg, 20 mg

Zestril®: 2.5 mg, 5 mg, 10 mg, 20 mg, 30 mg, 40 mg

lisinopril and hydrochlorothiazide (lyse IN oh pril & hye droe klor oh THYE a zide)

Synonyms hydrochlorothiazide and lisinopril

U.S./Canadian Brand Names Apo-Lisinopril®/Hctz [Can]; Mylan-Lisinopril/Hctz [Can]; Novo-Lisinopril/Hctz [Can]; Prinzide® [US/Can]; Sandoz Lisinopril/Hctz [Can]; Zestoretic® [US/Can]

Therapeutic Category Antihypertensive Agent, Combination

Use Treatment of hypertension

Dosage Summary

Oral:

Children: Dosage not established

Adults: Lisinopril 10-80 mg and hydrochlorothiazide 12.5-50 mg once daily (lisinopril doses >40 mg may not provide additional efficacy)

Dosage Forms

Tablet, oral: 10/12.5: Lisinopril 10 mg and hydrochlorothiazide 12.5 mg; 20/12.5: Lisinopril 20 mg and hydrochlorothiazide 12.5 mg; 20/25: Lisinopril 20 mg and hydrochlorothiazide 25 mg

Prinzide®:

10/12.5: Lisinopril 10 mg and hydrochlorothiazide 12.5 mg

20/12.5: Lisinopril 20 mg and hydrochlorothiazide 12.5 mg

Zestoretic®:
10/12.5: Lisinopril 10 mg and hydrochlorothiazide 12.5 mg
20/12.5: Lisinopril 20 mg and hydrochlorothiazide 12.5 mg
20/25: Lisinopril 20 mg and hydrochlorothiazide 25 mg

lispro insulin *see* insulin lispro *on page 511*

Listermint® With Fluoride *(Discontinued)* *see* fluoride *on page 413*

Lithane™ [Can] *see* lithium *on page 571*

Lithane® *(Discontinued)* *see* lithium *on page 571*

lithium (LITH ee um)

Sound-Alike/Look-Alike Issues
lithium may be confused with lanthanum
Eskalith® may be confused with Estratest®
Lithobid® may be confused with Levbid®, Lithostat®

Synonyms lithium carbonate; lithium citrate

U.S./Canadian Brand Names Apo-Lithium® Carbonate SR [Can]; Apo-Lithium® Carbonate [Can]; Carbolith™ [Can]; Duralith® [Can]; Euro-Lithium [Can]; Lithane™ [Can]; Lithobid® [US]; PMS-Lithium Carbonate [Can]; PMS-Lithium Citrate [Can]

Therapeutic Category Antimanic Agent

Use Management of bipolar disorders; treatment of mania in individuals with bipolar disorder (maintenance treatment prevents or diminishes intensity of subsequent episodes)

Dosage Summary

Oral:

Immediate release:
Children <6 years: Dosage not established
Children 6-12 years: 15-60 mg/kg/day in 3-4 divided doses
Adults: 900-2400 mg/day in 3-4 divided doses
Elderly: Initial: 300 mg twice daily (maximum: >900-1200 mg/day rarely needed); **Note:** Titration is recommended

Extended release:
Children: Dosage not established
Adults: 900-1800 mg/day in 2 divided doses

Dosage Forms
Capsule, oral: 150 mg, 300 mg, 600 mg
Solution, oral: 300 mg/5 mL (5 mL, 473 mL, 500 mL)
Tablet, oral: 300 mg, 600 mg
Tablet, extended release, oral: 300 mg, 450 mg
Lithobid®: 300 mg

lithium carbonate *see* lithium *on page 571*

lithium citrate *see* lithium *on page 571*

Lithobid® [US] *see* lithium *on page 571*

Lithonate® *(Discontinued)* *see* lithium *on page 571*

Lithostat® [US/Can] *see* acetohydroxamic acid *on page 33*

Lithotabs® *(Discontinued)* *see* lithium *on page 571*

Little Colds® Multi-Symptom Cold Formula *(Discontinued)* *see* acetaminophen, dextromethorphan, and phenylephrine *on page 29*

Little Fevers™ [US-OTC] *see* acetaminophen *on page 21*

Little Noses® Decongestant [US-OTC] *see* phenylephrine (nasal) *on page 751*

Little Noses® Saline [US-OTC] *see* sodium chloride *on page 882*

Little Noses® Stuffy Nose Kit [US-OTC] *see* sodium chloride *on page 882*

Little Phillips'® Milk of Magnesia [US-OTC] *see* magnesium hydroxide *on page 585*

Little Teethers® [US-OTC] *see* benzocaine *on page 124*

Little Tummys® Gas Relief [US-OTC] *see* simethicone *on page 875*

Little Tummys® Laxative [US-OTC] *see* senna *on page 870*

Livalo® [US] *see* pitavastatin *on page 765*

live attenuated influenza vaccine (LAIV) *see* influenza virus vaccine (live/attenuated) *on page 508*

live smallpox vaccine *see* smallpox vaccine *on page 880*

Livostin® ***(Discontinued)***

L-leucovorin *see* LEVOleucovorin *on page* 558

l-lysine (el LYE seen)

Synonyms l-lysine hydrochloride

U.S./Canadian Brand Names Lysinyl [US-OTC]

Therapeutic Category Dietary Supplement

Use Improves utilization of vegetable proteins

Dosage Summary

Oral:

Children: Dosage not established

Adults: 334-1500 mg/day

Dosage Forms

Capsule, oral: 500 mg

Lysinyl [OTC]: 500 mg

Powder, oral: 100% (100 g)

Lysinyl [OTC]: 500 mg/0.25 teaspoon (150 g)

Tablet, oral: 500 mg, 1000 mg

l-lysine hydrochloride *see* l-lysine *on page* 572

LM3100 *see* plerixafor *on page* 766

LMD® [US] *see* dextran *on page* 285

L-methylfolate *see* methylfolate *on page* 620

L-methylfolate, methylcobalamin, and N-acetylcysteine *see* methylfolate, methylcobalamin, and acetylcysteine *on page* 620

LNg 20 *see* levonorgestrel *on page* 559

Locacorten® Vioform® [Can] *see* clioquinol and flumethasone *(Canada only) on page* 234

LoCHOLEST® ***(Discontinued)*** *see* cholestyramine resin *on page* 218

LoCHOLEST® Light ***(Discontinued)*** *see* cholestyramine resin *on page* 218

Locoid® [US/Can] *see* hydrocortisone (topical) *on page* 483

Locoid Lipocream® [US] *see* hydrocortisone (topical) *on page* 483

Lodine® XL ***(Discontinued)*** *see* etodolac *on page* 383

Lodine® ***(Discontinued)*** *see* etodolac *on page* 383

Lodosyn® [US] *see* carbidopa *on page* 181

lodoxamide (loe DOKS a mide)

Synonyms lodoxamide tromethamine

U.S./Canadian Brand Names Alomide® [US/Can]

Therapeutic Category Mast Cell Stabilizer

Use Treatment of vernal keratoconjunctivitis, vernal conjunctivitis, and vernal keratitis

Dosage Summary

Ophthalmic:

Children <2 years: Dosage not established

Children ≥2 years: Instill 1-2 drops in eye(s) 4 times/day

Adults: Instill 1-2 drops in eye(s) 4 times/day

Dosage Forms

Solution, ophthalmic:

Alomide®: 0.1% (10 mL)

lodoxamide tromethamine *see* lodoxamide *on page* 572

Lodrane® 12D [US] *see* brompheniramine and pseudoephedrine *on page* 148

Lodrane® 12 Hour [US] *see* brompheniramine *on page* 147

Lodrane® 24 [US] *see* brompheniramine *on page* 147

Lodrane® 24D [US] *see* brompheniramine and pseudoephedrine *on page* 148

Lodrane® D ***(Discontinued)*** *see* brompheniramine and pseudoephedrine *on page* 148

Lodrane® ***(Discontinued)*** *see* brompheniramine and pseudoephedrine *on page* 148

Lodrane® XR [US] *see* brompheniramine *on page* 147

Loestrin® [US] *see* ethinyl estradiol and norethindrone *on page 378*
Loestrin™ 1.5/30 [Can] *see* ethinyl estradiol and norethindrone *on page 378*
Loestrin® 24 Fe [US] *see* ethinyl estradiol and norethindrone *on page 378*
Loestrin® Fe [US] *see* ethinyl estradiol and norethindrone *on page 378*
Lofibra® [US] *see* fenofibrate *on page 393*
Logen® ***(Discontinued)*** *see* diphenoxylate and atropine *on page 313*
LoHist-12 [US] *see* brompheniramine *on page 147*
LoHist 12D [US] *see* brompheniramine and pseudoephedrine *on page 148*
LoHist-D [US] *see* chlorpheniramine and pseudoephedrine *on page 209*
LoHist LQ [US] *see* brompheniramine and pseudoephedrine *on page 148*
LoHist PD ***(Discontinued)*** *see* brompheniramine and pseudoephedrine *on page 148*
L-OHP *see* oxaliplatin *on page 711*
LoKara™ [US] *see* desonide *on page 279*
Lomanate® ***(Discontinued)*** *see* diphenoxylate and atropine *on page 313*
Lomine [Can] *see* dicyclomine *on page 299*
Lomotil® [US/Can] *see* diphenoxylate and atropine *on page 313*

lomustine (loe MUS teen)

Sound-Alike/Look-Alike Issues

lomustine may be confused with bendamustine, carmustine

Synonyms CCNU; lomustinum

U.S./Canadian Brand Names CeeNU® [US/Can]

Therapeutic Category Antineoplastic Agent

Use Treatment of primary and metastatic brain tumors (after surgery and/or radiation therapy); treatment of relapsed or refractory Hodgkin disease (as part of a combination chemotherapy regimen)

Dosage Summary

Oral:

Children: 100-130 mg/m^2 as a single dose once every 6 weeks
Adults: 100-130 mg/m^2 as a single dose once every 6 weeks

Dosage Forms

Capsule, oral:

CeeNU®: 10 mg, 40 mg, 100 mg

lomustinum *see* lomustine *on page 573*
longastatin *see* octreotide *on page 694*
Loniten® [Can] *see* minoxidil (systemic) *on page 636*
Loniten® 2.5 mg Tablet ***(Discontinued)*** *see* minoxidil (systemic) *on page 636*
Lo/Ovral®-28 [US] *see* ethinyl estradiol and norgestrel *on page 380*
Loperacap [Can] *see* loperamide *on page 573*

loperamide (loe PER a mide)

Sound-Alike/Look-Alike Issues

loperamide may be confused with furosemide
Imodium® A-D may be confused with Indocin®

Synonyms loperamide hydrochloride

U.S./Canadian Brand Names Anti-Diarrheal [US-OTC]; Apo-Loperamide® [Can]; Diamode [US-OTC]; Diarr-Eze [Can]; Dom-Loperamide [Can]; Imodium® A-D for children [US-OTC]; Imodium® A-D [US-OTC]; Imodium® [Can]; Loperacap [Can]; Novo-Loperamide [Can]; PMS-Loperamine [Can]; Rhoxal-loperamide [Can]; Rho®-Loperamine [Can]; Riva-Loperamine [Can]; Sandoz-Loperamide [Can]

Therapeutic Category Antidiarrheal

Use Treatment of chronic diarrhea associated with inflammatory bowel disease; acute nonspecific diarrhea; increased volume of ileostomy discharge

OTC labeling: Control of symptoms of diarrhea, including traveler's diarrhea

Dosage Summary

Oral:

Children <2 years: Dosage not established

Children 2-5 years (13-20 kg): Acute diarrhea: Initial: 1 mg 3 times/day for first 24 hours; Maintenance: 0.1 mg/kg after each loose stool

Children 6-8 years (20-30 kg):

Acute diarrhea: Initial: 2 mg twice daily for first 24 hours; Maintenance: 0.1 mg/kg after each loose stool

Traveler's diarrhea: 2 mg after first loose stool, followed by 1 mg after each subsequent stool (maximum: 4 mg/day)

Children 8-12 years (>30 kg): Acute diarrhea: Initial: 2 mg 3 times/day for first 24 hours; Maintenance: 0.1 mg/kg after each loose stool

Children 9-11 years: Traveler's diarrhea: 2 mg after first loose stool, followed by 1 mg after each subsequent stool (maximum: 6 mg/day)

Children ≥12 years: Traveler's diarrhea: Initial: 4 mg after first loose stool, followed by 2 mg after each subsequent stool (maximum: 8 mg/day)

Adults:

Acute diarrhea: Initial: 4 mg followed by 2 mg after each loose stool (maximum: 16 mg/day)

Chronic diarrhea: 4-8 mg/day in divided doses

Traveler's diarrhea: Initial: 4 mg after first loose stool, followed by 2 mg after each subsequent stool (maximum: 8 mg/day)

Dosage Forms

Caplet, oral: 2 mg

Anti-Diarrheal [OTC]: 2 mg

Diamode [OTC]: 2 mg

Imodium® A-D [OTC]: 2 mg

Capsule, oral: 2 mg

Liquid, oral: 1 mg/5 mL (120 mL)

Anti-Diarrheal [OTC]: 1 mg/5 mL (120 mL)

Imodium® A-D [OTC]: 1 mg/5 mL (60 mL, 120 mL); 1 mg/7.5 mL (120 mL)

Imodium® A-D for children [OTC]: 1 mg/7.5 mL (120 mL)

Solution, oral: 1 mg/5 mL (5 mL, 10 mL, 118 mL, 120 mL)

loperamide and simethicone (loe PER a mide & sye METH i kone)

Synonyms simethicone and loperamide hydrochloride

U.S./Canadian Brand Names Imodium® Advanced Multi-Symptom [Can]; Imodium® Multi-Symptom Relief [US-OTC]

Therapeutic Category Antidiarrheal; Antiflatulent

Use Control of symptoms of diarrhea and gas (bloating, pressure, and cramps)

Dosage Summary

Oral:

Children <6 years or <48 lbs: Dosage not established

Children 6-8 years (48-59 lbs): 1 caplet/tablet after first loose stool, followed by 1/2 caplet/tablet with each subsequent loose stool (maximum: 2 caplets or tablets/24 hours)

Children 9-11 years (60-95 lbs): 1 caplet/tablet after first loose stool, followed by 1/2 caplet/tablet with each subsequent loose stool (maximum: 3 caplets or tablets/24 hours)

Children ≥12 years: 1 caplet/tablet after each loose stool (maximum: 4 caplets or tablets/24 hours)

Adults: 1 caplet/tablet after each loose stool (maximum: 4 caplets or tablets/24 hours)

Dosage Forms

Caplet:

Imodium® Multi-Symptom Relief: Loperamide hydrochloride 2 mg and simethicone 125 mg

Tablet, chewable:

Imodium® Muliti-Symptom Relief: Loperamide hydrochloride 2 mg and simethicone 125 mg

loperamide hydrochloride *see* loperamide *on page* 573

Lopid® [US/Can] *see* gemfibrozil *on page* 440

lopinavir and ritonavir (loe PIN a veer & rit ON uh veer)

Sound-Alike/Look-Alike Issues

Potential for dispensing errors between Kaletra® and Keppra® (levetiracetam)

Synonyms ritonavir and lopinavir

U.S./Canadian Brand Names Kaletra® [US/Can]

Therapeutic Category Antiretroviral Agent, Nonnucleoside Reverse Transcriptase Inhibitor (NNRTI)

Use Treatment of HIV infection in combination with other antiretroviral agents

Dosage Summary

Oral:

Children <14 days: Dosage not established

Children 14 days to 6 months: Lopinavir 16 mg/kg or 300 mg/m^2 twice daily

Children 6 months to 18 years and <15 kg: 12 mg lopinavir/kg twice daily (maximum dose: Lopinavir 400 mg/ritonavir 100 mg)

Children 6 months to 18 years and 15-40 kg: 10 mg lopinavir/kg twice daily (maximum dose: Lopinavir 400 mg/ritonavir 100 mg)

Children 6 months to 18 years and >40 kg: Lopinavir 400 mg/ritonavir 100 mg twice daily

Adults: Lopinavir 400 mg/ritonavir 100 mg twice daily **or** lopinavir 800 mg/ritonavir 200 mg once daily

Dosage Forms

Solution, oral:

Kaletra®: Lopinavir 80 mg and ritonavir 20 mg per mL

Tablet:

Kaletra®:

Lopinavir 100 mg and ritonavir 25 mg

Lopinavir 200 mg and ritonavir 50 mg

Lopressor® [US/Can] *see* metoprolol *on page 625*

Lopressor HCT® [US] *see* metoprolol and hydrochlorothiazide *on page 626*

Loprox® [US/Can] *see* ciclopirox *on page 221*

Loradamed [US-OTC] *see* loratadine *on page 575*

loratadine (lor AT a deen)

Sound-Alike/Look-Alike Issues

Claritin® may be confused with clarithromycin

Claritin® (loratadine) may be confused with Claritin™ Eye (ketotifen)

U.S./Canadian Brand Names Alavert® Allergy 24 Hour [US-OTC]; Alavert® Children's Allergy [US-OTC]; Apo-Loratadine® [Can]; Claritin® 24 Hour Allergy [US-OTC]; Claritin® Children's Allergy [US-OTC]; Claritin® Kids [Can]; Claritin® Liqui-Gels® 24 Hour Allergy [US-OTC]; Claritin® RediTabs® 24 Hour Allergy [US-OTC]; Claritin® [Can]; Loradamed [US-OTC]; Tavist® ND Allergy [US-OTC]

Therapeutic Category Antihistamine

Use Relief of nasal and nonnasal symptoms of seasonal allergic rhinitis; treatment of chronic idiopathic urticaria

Dosage Summary

Oral:

Children <2 years: Dosage not established

Children 2-5 years: 5 mg once daily

Children ≥6 years: 10 mg once daily

Adults: 10 mg once daily

Dosage Forms

Capsule, liquid gel, oral:

Claritin® Liqui-Gels® 24 Hour Allergy [OTC]: 10 mg

Solution, oral: 5 mg/5 mL (120 mL)

Syrup, oral: 5 mg/5 mL (120 mL)

Claritin® Children's Allergy [OTC]: 5 mg/5 mL (60 mL, 120 mL)

Tablet, oral: 10 mg

Alavert® Allergy 24 Hour [OTC]: 10 mg

Claritin® 24 Hour Allergy [OTC]: 10 mg

Loradamed [OTC]: 10 mg

Tavist® ND Allergy [OTC]: 10 mg

Tablet, chewable, oral:

Claritin® Children's Allergy [OTC]: 5 mg

Tablet, orally disintegrating, oral: 10 mg

Alavert® Allergy 24 Hour [OTC]: 10 mg

Alavert® Children's Allergy [OTC]: 10 mg

Claritin® RediTabs® 24 Hour Allergy [OTC]: 10 mg

loratadine and pseudoephedrine (lor AT a deen & soo doe e FED rin)

Sound-Alike/Look-Alike Issues

Claritin-D® may be confused with Claritin-D® 24

Claritin-D® 24 may be confused with Claritin-D®

Synonyms pseudoephedrine and loratadine

U.S./Canadian Brand Names Alavert™ Allergy and Sinus [US-OTC]; Chlor-Tripolon ND® [Can]; Claritin-D® 12 Hour Allergy & Congestion [US-OTC]; Claritin-D® 24 Hour Allergy & Congestion [US-OTC]; Claritin® Extra [Can]; Claritin® Liberator [Can]

Therapeutic Category Antihistamine/Decongestant Combination

Use Temporary relief of symptoms of seasonal allergic rhinitis, other upper respiratory allergies, or the common cold

Dosage Summary

Oral:

Children <12 years: Dosage not established

Children ≥12 years:

Alavert™ Allergy and Sinus, Claritin-D® 24-Hour: 1 tablet every 24 hours

Claritin-D® 12-Hour: 1 tablet every 12 hours

Adults:

Alavert™ Allergy and Sinus, Claritin-D® 24-Hour: 1 tablet every 24 hours

Claritin-D® 12-Hour: 1 tablet every 12 hours

Dosage Forms

Tablet, extended release: Loratadine 10 mg and pseudoephedrine 240 mg

Alavert™ Allergy and Sinus [OTC]: Loratadine 5 mg and pseudoephedrine 120 mg

Claritin-D® 12 Hour Allergy & Congestion [OTC]: Loratadine 5 mg and pseudoephedrine 120 mg

Claritin-D® 24 Hour Allergy & Congestion [OTC]: Loratadine 10 mg and pseudoephedrine 240 mg

lorazepam (lor A ze pam)

Sound-Alike/Look-Alike Issues

LORazepam may be confused with ALPRAZolam, clonazePAM, diazepam, Lovaza®, temazepam, zolpidem

Ativan® may be confused with Ambien®, Atarax®, Atgam®, Avitene®

Tall-Man **LOR**azepam

U.S./Canadian Brand Names Apo-Lorazepam® [Can]; Ativan® [US/Can]; Dom-Lorazepam [Can]; Lorazepam Injection, USP [Can]; Lorazepam Intensol™ [US]; Novo-Lorazem [Can]; Nu-Loraz [Can]; PHL-Lorazepam [Can]; PMS-Lorazepam [Can]; PRO-Lorazepam [Can]

Therapeutic Category Benzodiazepine

Controlled Substance C-IV

Use

Oral: Management of anxiety disorders or short-term (≤4 months) relief of the symptoms of anxiety or anxiety associated with depressive symptoms

I.V.: Status epilepticus, amnesia, sedation

Dosage Summary

I.M.:

Children: 0.02-0.09 mg/kg prior to procedure

Adults: 0.5-1 mg every 30-60 minutes as needed or 0.05 mg/kg 2 hours prior to procedure (maximum: 4 mg/dose)

I.V.:

Children <2 years: 0.02-0.09 mg/kg every 4-8 hours or as a single dose prior to procedure **or** 0.01-0.03 mg/kg prior to procedure, may repeat every 20 minutes until desired effect **or** 0.05-0.1 mg/kg (maximum: 4 mg/dose); may repeat every 10-15 minutes as needed

Children 2-15 years: 0.02-0.09 mg/kg every 4-8 hours or as a single dose prior to procedure **or** 0.01-0.03 mg/kg prior to procedure, may repeat every 20 minutes until desired effect **or** 0.05-0.1 mg/kg (maximum: 4 mg/dose); may repeat every 10-15 minutes as needed **or** 0.05 mg/kg (up to 2 mg/dose) prior to chemotherapy

Adolescents: 0.02-0.09 mg/kg every 4-8 hours or as a single dose prior to procedure **or** 0.01-0.03 mg/kg prior to procedure, may repeat every 20 minutes until desired effect **or** 4 mg, then repeat in 10-15 minutes (maximum: 8 mg/dose)

Adults: 0.5-2 mg every 4-6 hours as needed **or** 4 mg, then repeat in 10-15 minutes (maximum: 8 mg/dose) **or** 0.044 mg/kg 15-20 minutes prior to procedure (maximum: 2 mg/dose) **or** up to 0.05 mg/kg for operative amnesia (maximum: 4 mg/dose)

Elderly: 0.5-4 mg/day **or** 0.5-2 mg every 4-6 hours as needed **or** 4 mg, then repeat in 10-15 minutes (maximum: 8 mg/dose) **or** 0.044 mg/kg 15-20 minutes prior to procedure (maximum: 2 mg/dose) **or** up to 0.05 mg/kg for operative amnesia (maximum: 4 mg/dose)

Oral:

Children: 0.02-0.09 mg/kg every 4-8 hours or as a single dose prior to procedure

Adults: 0.5-2 mg every 4-6 hours **or** 1-10 mg/day in 2-3 divided doses **or** 2-4 mg at bedtime **or** 1-2 mg every 30-60 minutes as needed

Elderly: 0.5-4 mg/day **or** 0.5-2 mg every 4-6 hours **or** 1-2 mg every 30-60 minutes as needed

Dosage Forms

Injection, solution: 2 mg/mL (1 mL, 10 mL); 4 mg/mL (1 mL, 10 mL)

Ativan®: 2 mg/mL (1 mL, 10 mL); 4 mg/mL (1 mL, 10 mL)

Injection, solution [preservative free]: 2 mg/mL (1 mL); 4 mg/mL (1 mL)

Solution, oral: 2 mg/mL (30 mL)

Lorazepam Intensol™: 2 mg/mL (30 mL)

Tablet, oral: 0.5 mg, 1 mg, 2 mg

Ativan®: 0.5 mg, 1 mg, 2 mg

Lorazepam Injection, USP [Can] *see* lorazepam *on page 576*

Lorazepam Intensol™ [US] *see* lorazepam *on page 576*

Lorcet® 10/650 [US] *see* hydrocodone and acetaminophen *on page 479*

Lorcet®-HD *(Discontinued)* *see* hydrocodone and acetaminophen *on page 479*

Lorcet® Plus [US] *see* hydrocodone and acetaminophen *on page 479*

Lorsin® *(Discontinued)* *see* acetaminophen, chlorpheniramine, and pseudoephedrine *on page 28*

Lortab® [US] *see* hydrocodone and acetaminophen *on page 479*

Lortab® ASA *(Discontinued)*

losartan (loe SAR tan)

Sound-Alike/Look-Alike Issues

losartan may be confused with valsartan

Cozaar® may be confused with Colace®, Coreg®, Hyzaar®, Zocor®

Synonyms DuP 753; losartan potassium; MK594

U.S./Canadian Brand Names Cozaar® [US/Can]

Therapeutic Category Angiotensin II Receptor Antagonist

Use Treatment of hypertension (HTN); treatment of diabetic nephropathy in patients with type 2 diabetes mellitus (noninsulin-dependent, NIDDM) and a history of hypertension; stroke risk reduction in patients with HTN and left ventricular hypertrophy (LVH)

Dosage Summary

Oral:

Children <6 years: Dosage not established

Children 6-16 years (U.S. labeling): Initial: 0.7 mg/kg once daily (maximum: 50 mg/day); Maintenance: Maximum: ≤1.4 mg/kg; 100 mg

Children 6-16 years (Canadian labeling): ≥20 kg to <50 kg: 25 mg once daily (maximum: 50 mg once daily); ≥50 kg: 50 mg once daily (maximum: 100 mg once daily)

Adults: Initial: 25-50 mg once daily; Maintenance: 25-100 mg/day in 1-2 divided doses (maximum: 100 mg/day)

Dosage Forms

Tablet, oral: 25 mg, 50 mg, 100 mg

Cozaar®: 25 mg, 50 mg, 100 mg

losartan and hydrochlorothiazide (loe SAR tan & hye droe klor oh THYE a zide)

Sound-Alike/Look-Alike Issues

Hyzaar® may be confused with Cozaar®

Synonyms hydrochlorothiazide and losartan

U.S./Canadian Brand Names Hyzaar® DS [Can]; Hyzaar® [US/Can]

Therapeutic Category Antihypertensive Agent, Combination

Use Treatment of hypertension; stroke risk reduction in patients with HTN and left ventricular hypertrophy (LVH)

Dosage Summary

Oral:

Children: Dosage not established

Adults: Losartan 50-100 mg and hydrochlorothiazide 12.5-50 mg once daily

Dosage Forms

Tablet: 50/12.5: Losartan 50 mg and hydrochlorothiazide 12.5 mg; 100/12.5: Losartan 100 mg and hydrochlorothiazide 12.5 mg; 100/25: Losartan 100 mg and hydrochlorothiazide 25 mg

Hyzaar®: 50/12.5: Losartan 50 mg and hydrochlorothiazide 12.5 mg; 100/12.5: Losartan 100 mg and hydrochlorothiazide 12.5 mg; 100/25: Losartan 100 mg and hydrochlorothiazide 25 mg

losartan potassium *see* losartan *on page 577*

LoSeasonique™ [US] *see* ethinyl estradiol and levonorgestrel *on page 376*

Losec® [Can] *see* omeprazole *on page 701*

Losec MUPS® [Can] *see* omeprazole *on page 701*

Losopan® *(Discontinued)* *see* magaldrate and simethicone *on page 583*

Lotemax® [US/Can] *see* loteprednol *on page 578*

Lotensin® [US/Can] *see* benazepril *on page 122*

Lotensin HCT® [US] *see* benazepril and hydrochlorothiazide *on page 122*

loteprednol (loe te PRED nol)

Synonyms loteprednol etabonate

U.S./Canadian Brand Names Alrex® [US/Can]; Lotemax® [US/Can]

Therapeutic Category Corticosteroid, Ophthalmic

Use

Suspension, 0.2% (Alrex®): Temporary relief of signs and symptoms of seasonal allergic conjunctivitis

Suspension, 0.5% (Lotemax®): Inflammatory conditions (treatment of steroid-responsive inflammatory conditions of the palpebral and bulbar conjunctiva, cornea, and anterior segment of the globe such as allergic conjunctivitis, acne rosacea, superficial punctate keratitis, herpes zoster keratitis, iritis, cyclitis, selected infective conjunctivitis, when the inherent hazard of steroid use is accepted to obtain an advisable diminution in edema and inflammation) and treatment of postoperative inflammation following ocular surgery

Dosage Summary

Ophthalmic:

Children: Dosage not established

Adults:

Suspension, 0.2% (Alrex®): Instill 1 drop into affected eye(s) 4 times/day

Suspension, 0.5% (Lotemax®): Instill 1-2 drop into affected eye(s) 4 times/day

Dosage Forms

Suspension, ophthalmic:

Alrex®: 0.2% (5 mL, 10 mL)

Lotemax®: 0.5% (2.5 mL, 5 mL, 10 mL, 15 mL)

loteprednol and tobramycin (loe te PRED nol & toe bra MYE sin)

Synonyms loteprednol etabonate and tobramycin; tobramycin and loteprednol etabonate

U.S./Canadian Brand Names Zylet™ [US]

Therapeutic Category Antibiotic/Corticosteroid, Ophthalmic

Use Treatment of steroid-responsive ocular inflammatory conditions where either a superficial bacterial ocular infection or the risk of a superficial bacterial ocular infection exists

Dosage Summary

Ophthalmic:

Children and Adults: Instill 1-2 drops into the affected eye(s) every 4-6 hours

Dosage Forms

Suspension, ophthalmic [drops]:

Zylet®: Loteprednol 0.5% and tobramycin 0.3% (2.5 mL, 5 mL, 10 mL)

loteprednol etabonate *see* loteprednol *on page 578*

loteprednol etabonate and tobramycin *see* loteprednol and tobramycin *on page 578*

Lotrel® [US] *see* amlodipine and benazepril *on page 69*

Lotriderm® [Can] *see* betamethasone and clotrimazole *on page 134*

Lotrimin AF® [US-OTC] *see* miconazole (topical) *on page* 630
Lotrimin® AF Athlete's Foot [US-OTC] *see* clotrimazole (topical) *on page* 240
Lotrimin® AF Cream *(Discontinued)* *see* clotrimazole (topical) *on page* 240
Lotrimin® AF for Her [US-OTC] *see* clotrimazole (topical) *on page* 240
Lotrimin® AF Jock Itch [US-OTC] *see* clotrimazole (topical) *on page* 240
Lotrimin® AF Lotion *(Discontinued)* *see* clotrimazole (topical) *on page* 240
Lotrimin® AF Solution *(Discontinued)* *see* clotrimazole (topical) *on page* 240
Lotrimin® ultra™ [US-OTC] *see* butenafine *on page* 160
Lotrisone® [US] *see* betamethasone and clotrimazole *on page* 134
Lotronex® [US] *see* alosetron *on page* 53

lovastatin (LOE va sta tin)

Sound-Alike/Look-Alike Issues

lovastatin may be confused with atorvastatin, Leustatin®, Livostin®, Lotensin®, nystatin, pitavastatin
Mevacor® may be confused with Benicar®, Lipitor®, Mivacron®

Synonyms mevinolin; monacolin K

U.S./Canadian Brand Names Altoprev® [US]; Apo-Lovastatin® [Can]; CO Lovastatin [Can]; Dom-Lovastatin [Can]; Gen-Lovastatin [Can]; Mevacor® [US/Can]; Mylan-Lovastatin [Can]; Novo-Lovastatin [Can]; Nu-Lovastatin [Can]; PHL-Lovastatin [Can]; PMS-Lovastatin [Can]; PRO-Lovastatin [Can]; RAN™-Lovastatin [Can]; ratio-Lovastatin [Can]; Riva-Lovastatin [Can]; Sandoz-Lovastatin [Can]

Therapeutic Category HMG-CoA Reductase Inhibitor

Use

Adjunct to dietary therapy to decrease elevated serum total and LDL-cholesterol concentrations in primary hypercholesterolemia

Primary prevention of coronary artery disease (patients without symptomatic disease with average to moderately elevated total and LDL-cholesterol and below average HDL-cholesterol); slow progression of coronary atherosclerosis in patients with coronary heart disease

Adjunct to dietary therapy in adolescent patients (10-17 years of age, females >1 year postmenarche) with heterozygous familial hypercholesterolemia having LDL >189 mg/dL, **or** LDL >160 mg/dL with positive family history of premature cardiovascular disease (CVD), **or** LDL >160 mg/dL with the presence of at least two other CVD risk factors

Dosage Summary

Oral:

Extended release:

Children: Dosage not established

Adults: Initial: 20 mg with evening meal; Maintenance: 20-60 mg with evening meal (maximum: 60 mg/day; may change depending upon concurrent medications)

Immediate release:

Children <10 years: Dosage not established

Children 10-17 years: Initial: 10-20 mg with evening meal; Maintenance: 10-40 mg with evening meal (maximum: 40 mg/day)

Adults: Initial: 20 mg with evening meal; Maintenance: 20-80 mg with evening meal (maximum: 80 mg/day; may change depending upon concurrent medications)

Dosage Forms

Tablet, oral: 10 mg, 20 mg, 40 mg

Mevacor®: 20 mg, 40 mg

Tablet, extended release, oral:

Altoprev®: 20 mg, 40 mg, 60 mg

lovastatin and niacin *see* niacin and lovastatin *on page* 672
Lovaza® [US] *see* omega-3-acid ethyl esters *on page* 701
Lovenox® [US/Can] *see* enoxaparin *on page* 350
Lovenox® HP [Can] *see* enoxaparin *on page* 350
low-Molecular-weight iron dextran (INFeD®) *see* iron dextran complex *on page* 525
Low-Ogestrel® [US] *see* ethinyl estradiol and norgestrel *on page* 380
Loxapac® IM [Can] *see* loxapine *on page* 580

loxapine (LOKS a peen)

Sound-Alike/Look-Alike Issues

Loxitane® may be confused with Lexapro®, Soriatane®

Synonyms loxapine succinate; oxilapine succinate

U.S./Canadian Brand Names Apo-Loxapine® [Can]; Loxapac® IM [Can]; Loxitane® [US]; Nu-Loxapine [Can]; PMS-Loxapine [Can]

Therapeutic Category Antipsychotic Agent, Dibenzoxazepine

Use Management of psychotic disorders

Dosage Summary

Oral:

Children: Dosage not established

Adults: Initial: 10 mg twice daily; Usual range: 20-100 mg/day in 2-4 divided doses (maximum: 250 mg/day)

Elderly: 20-60 mg/day

Dosage Forms

Capsule, oral: 5 mg, 10 mg, 25 mg, 50 mg

Loxitane®: 5 mg, 10 mg, 25 mg, 50 mg

loxapine succinate *see* loxapine *on page* *580*

Loxitane® [US] *see* loxapine *on page* *580*

Loxitane® I.M. *(Discontinued)* *see* loxapine *on page* *580*

Lozide® [Can] *see* indapamide *on page* *504*

Lozi-Flur™ [US] *see* fluoride *on page* *413*

Lozi-Tab® *(Discontinued)* *see* fluoride *on page* *413*

Lozol® [Can] *see* indapamide *on page* *504*

Lozol® *(Discontinued)* *see* indapamide *on page* *504*

L-PAM *see* melphalan *on page* *599*

L-phenylalanine mustard *see* melphalan *on page* *599*

L-sarcolysin *see* melphalan *on page* *599*

LTA® 360 [US] *see* lidocaine (topical) *on page* *562*

LTG *see* lamotrigine *on page* *546*

***L*-thyroxine sodium** *see* levothyroxine *on page* *560*

Lu-26-054 *see* escitalopram *on page* *363*

lubiprostone (loo bi PROS tone)

Synonyms RU 0211; SPI 0211

U.S./Canadian Brand Names Amitiza® [US]

Therapeutic Category Gastrointestinal Agent, Miscellaneous

Use Treatment of chronic idiopathic constipation; treatment of irritable bowel syndrome with constipation in adult women

Dosage Summary

Oral:

Children: Dosage not established

Adults (females): 8 mcg twice daily **or** 24 mcg twice daily

Adults (males): 24 mcg twice daily

Dosage Forms

Capsule, softgel, oral:

Amitiza®: 8 mcg, 24 mcg

Lubriderm® [US-OTC] *see* lanolin, cetyl alcohol, glycerin, petrolatum, and mineral oil *on page* *548*

Lubriderm® Fragrance Free [US-OTC] *see* lanolin, cetyl alcohol, glycerin, petrolatum, and mineral oil *on page* *548*

LubriTears® Solution *(Discontinued)* *see* artificial tears *on page* *97*

Lucentis® [US/Can] *see* ranibizumab *on page* *828*

Ludiomil® *(Discontinued)* *see* maprotiline *on page* *590*

Lufyllin® [US/Can] *see* dyphylline *on page* *339*

Lufyllin®-GG [US] *see* dyphylline and guaifenesin *on page* *339*

lumefantrine and artemether *see* artemether and lumefantrine *on page* 95
Lumigan® [US/Can] *see* bimatoprost *on page* 138
Lumigan® RC [Can] *see* bimatoprost *on page* 138
Luminal® Sodium *(Discontinued)* *see* phenobarbital *on page* 747
Lumitene™ [US-OTC] *see* beta-carotene *on page* 132
Lumizyme™ [US] *see* alglucosidase alfa *on page* 49
Lunesta® [US] *see* eszopiclone *on page* 372
LupiCare® Dandruff [US-OTC] *see* salicylic acid *on page* 858
LupiCare® Psoriasis [US-OTC] *see* salicylic acid *on page* 858
LupiCare® Psoriasis Scalp *(Discontinued)* *see* salicylic acid *on page* 858
Lupron® [US/Can] *see* leuprolide *on page* 554
Lupron Depot® [US/Can] *see* leuprolide *on page* 554
Lupron Depot®-3 Month [US] *see* leuprolide *on page* 554
Lupron Depot®-4 Month [US] *see* leuprolide *on page* 554
Lupron Depot-Ped® [US] *see* leuprolide *on page* 554
Luride® *(Discontinued)* *see* fluoride *on page* 413
Luride®-SF *(Discontinued)* *see* fluoride *on page* 413
Lusedra™ [US] *see* fospropofol *on page* 429
LuSonal™ [US] *see* phenylephrine (systemic) *on page* 751
Lustra® [US/Can] *see* hydroquinone *on page* 487
Lustra-AF® [US] *see* hydroquinone *on page* 487
Lustra-Ultra™ [US] *see* hydroquinone *on page* 487
Lutera™ [US] *see* ethinyl estradiol and levonorgestrel *on page* 376

lutropin alfa (LOO troe pin AL fa)

Synonyms r-hLH; recombinant human luteinizing hormone

U.S./Canadian Brand Names Luveris® [US]

Therapeutic Category Gonadotropin; Ovulation Stimulator

Use Stimulation of follicular development in infertile hypogonadotropic hypogonadal (HH) women with profound luteinizing hormone (LH) deficiency; to be used in combination with follitropin alfa

Dosage Summary

SubQ:

Children: Dosage not established

Adults (females): 75 int. units daily (maximum duration: 14 days)

Dosage Forms

Injection, powder for reconstitution:

Luveris®: 75 int. units

Luveris® [US] *see* lutropin alfa *on page* 581
Luvox® [Can] *see* fluvoxamine *on page* 422
Luvox® CR [US] *see* fluvoxamine *on page* 422
Luvox® *(Discontinued)* *see* fluvoxamine *on page* 422
Luxíq® [US] *see* betamethasone *on page* 133
LY139603 *see* atomoxetine *on page* 103
LY146032 *see* daptomycin *on page* 269
LY170053 *see* olanzapine *on page* 696
LY231514 *see* pemetrexed *on page* 735
LY246736 *see* alvimopan *on page* 60
LY248686 *see* duloxetine *on page* 336
LY303366 *see* anidulafungin *on page* 79
LY-640315 *see* prasugrel *on page* 788
LY2148568 *see* exenatide *on page* 387
Lybrel® [US] *see* ethinyl estradiol and levonorgestrel *on page* 376
Lycolan® Elixir *(Discontinued)* *see* l-lysine *on page* 572
Lyderm® [Can] *see* fluocinonide *on page* 411

LYMErix™ ***(Discontinued)***
Lymphazurin™ [US] *see* isosulfan blue *on page* 530
lymphocyte immune globulin *see* antithymocyte globulin (equine) *on page* 84
lymphocyte mitogenic factor *see* aldesleukin *on page* 46
Lyphocin® Injection ***(Discontinued)*** *see* vancomycin *on page* 977
Lyrica® [US/Can] *see* pregabalin *on page* 792
Lysinyl [US-OTC] *see* l-lysine *on page* 572
Lysodren® [US/Can] *see* mitotane *on page* 638
Lysteda™ [US] *see* tranexamic acid *on page* 947
Maalox® Advanced Maximum Strength [US-OTC] *see* calcium carbonate and simethicone *on page* 168
Maalox® Advanced Maximum Strength Liquid [US-OTC] *see* aluminum hydroxide, magnesium hydroxide, and simethicone *on page* 59
Maalox® Advanced Regular Strength [US-OTC] *see* aluminum hydroxide, magnesium hydroxide, and simethicone *on page* 59
Maalox® Anti-Gas ***(Discontinued)*** *see* aluminum hydroxide, magnesium hydroxide, and simethicone *on page* 59
Maalox® Anti-Gas Extra Strength ***(Discontinued)*** *see* aluminum hydroxide, magnesium hydroxide, and simethicone *on page* 59
Maalox® Children's [US-OTC] *see* calcium carbonate *on page* 167
Maalox® ***(Discontinued)*** *see* aluminum hydroxide, magnesium hydroxide, and simethicone *on page* 59
Maalox® Extra Strength ***(Discontinued)*** *see* aluminum hydroxide and magnesium hydroxide *on page* 59
Maalox® Junior Plus Antigas [US-OTC] *see* calcium carbonate and simethicone *on page* 168
Maalox® Max ***(Discontinued)*** *see* aluminum hydroxide, magnesium hydroxide, and simethicone *on page* 59
Maalox® Plus ***(Discontinued)*** *see* aluminum hydroxide, magnesium hydroxide, and simethicone *on page* 59
Maalox® Regular ***(Discontinued)*** *see* calcium carbonate *on page* 167
Maalox® Regular Strength [US-OTC] *see* calcium carbonate *on page* 167
Maalox® TC (Therapeutic Concentrate) ***(Discontinued)*** *see* aluminum hydroxide and magnesium hydroxide *on page* 59
Maalox® Total Relief® [US-OTC] *see* bismuth *on page* 139
MabCampath® [Can] *see* alemtuzumab *on page* 47
Macrobid® [US/Can] *see* nitrofurantoin *on page* 678
Macrodantin® [US/Can] *see* nitrofurantoin *on page* 678
Macrodex® ***(Discontinued)*** *see* dextran *on page* 285
Macugen® [US/Can] *see* pegaptanib *on page* 732

mafenide (MA fe nide)

Synonyms mafenide acetate

U.S./Canadian Brand Names Sulfamylon® [US]

Therapeutic Category Antibacterial, Topical

Use

Cream: Adjunctive antibacterial agent in the treatment of second- and third-degree burns

Solution: Adjunctive antibacterial agent for use under moist dressings over meshed autografts on excised burn wounds

Dosage Summary

Topical:

Children: Apply to a thickness of approximately 1/16 inch once or twice daily

Adults: Apply to a thickness of approximately 1/16 inch once or twice daily

Dosage Forms

Cream, topical:

Sulfamylon®: 85 mg/g (56.7 g, 113.4 g, 453.6 g)

Powder for solution, topical:

Sulfamylon®: 50 g/packet (5s)

mafenide acetate *see* mafenide *on page 582*
Mag 64™ [US-OTC] *see* magnesium chloride *on page 583*
Mag-Al [US-OTC] *see* aluminum hydroxide and magnesium hydroxide *on page 59*

magaldrate and simethicone (MAG al drate & sye METH i kone)

Sound-Alike/Look-Alike Issues
Riopan Plus® may be confused with Repan®

Synonyms simethicone and magaldrate

Therapeutic Category Antacid; Antiflatulent

Use Relief of hyperacidity associated with peptic ulcer, gastritis, peptic esophagitis, and hiatal hernia which are accompanied by symptoms of gas

Dosage Summary

Oral:

Children: Dosage not established
Adults: 5-10 mL (540-1080 mg magaldrate) between meals and at bedtime

Dosage Forms

Suspension, oral: Magaldrate 540 mg and simethicone 20 mg per 5 mL

Magalox Plus® *(Discontinued)* *see* aluminum hydroxide, magnesium hydroxide, and simethicone *on page 59*
Mag-Al Ultimate [US-OTC] *see* aluminum hydroxide and magnesium hydroxide *on page 59*
Magan® *(Discontinued)* *see* magnesium salicylate *on page 587*
mag citrate *see* magnesium citrate *on page 584*
Mag Delay [US-OTC] *see* magnesium chloride *on page 583*
Mag®-G [US-OTC] *see* magnesium gluconate *on page 585*
MagGel™ 600 [US-OTC] *see* magnesium oxide *on page 587*
Maginex™ [US-OTC] *see* magnesium L-aspartate hydrochloride *on page 586*
Maginex™ DS [US-OTC] *see* magnesium L-aspartate hydrochloride *on page 586*
Magnacal® [US-OTC] *see* nutritional formula, enteral/oral *on page 692*
Magnacet™ *(Discontinued)* *see* oxycodone and acetaminophen *on page 715*
MagneBind® 400 Rx [US] *see* magnesium carbonate, calcium carbonate, and folic acid *on page 583*
Magnelium® [Can] *see* magnesium glucoheptonate *on page 584*
magnesia magma *see* magnesium hydroxide *on page 585*
magnesium carbonate and aluminum hydroxide *see* aluminum hydroxide and magnesium carbonate *on page 58*

magnesium carbonate, calcium carbonate, and folic acid

(mag NEE zhum KAR bun ate, KAL see um KAR bun ate, & FOE lik AS id)

Synonyms calcium carbonate, folic acid, and magnesium carbonate; folic acid, magnesium carbonate, and calcium carbonate

U.S./Canadian Brand Names MagneBind® 400 Rx [US]

Therapeutic Category Calcium Salt; Electrolyte Supplement, Oral; Magnesium Salt; Vitamin; Vitamin, Water Soluble

Use Prevention or treatment of nutritional deficiencies

Dosage Summary

Oral:

Children: Dosing not established
Adults: 1-3 tablets 3 times/day with meals

Dosage Forms

Tablet, oral:

MagneBind® 400 Rx: Magnesium carbonate 400 mg, calcium carbonate 200 mg, and folic acid 1 mg

magnesium chloride (mag NEE zhum KLOR ide)

U.S./Canadian Brand Names Chloromag® [US]; Mag 64™ [US-OTC]; Mag Delay [US-OTC]; Slow-Mag® [US-OTC]

Therapeutic Category Electrolyte Supplement, Oral

Use Correction or prevention of hypomagnesemia; dietary supplement

Dosage Summary

I.V.:

Children <50 kg: 0.3-0.5 mEq/kg/day

Children >50 kg: 10-30 mEq/day

Adults: 8-24 mEq/day added to TPN

Oral: RDA (elemental magnesium):

Children:

1-3 years: 80 mg/day

4-8 years: 130 mg/day

9-13 years: 240 mg/day

14-18 years:

Female: 360 mg/day

Pregnant female: 400 mg/day

Male: 410 mg/day

Adults:

19-30 years:

Female: 310 mg/day

Pregnant female: 350 mg/day

Male: 400 mg/day

≥31 years:

Female: 320 mg/day

Pregnant female: 360 mg/day

Male: 420 mg/day

Dosage Forms

Injection, solution: 200 mg/mL (50 mL)

Chloromag®: 200 mg/mL (50 mL)

Tablet, delayed release, enteric coated, oral:

Mag 64™ [OTC]: Elemental magnesium 64 mg

Mag Delay [OTC]: Elemental magnesium 64 mg

Tablet, enteric coated, oral:

Slow-Mag® [OTC]: Elemental magnesium 64 mg

magnesium citrate (mag NEE zhum SIT rate)

Synonyms citrate of magnesia; mag citrate

U.S./Canadian Brand Names Citro-Mag® [Can]; Citroma® [US-OTC]

Therapeutic Category Laxative

Use Evacuation of bowel prior to certain surgical and diagnostic procedures or overdose situations

Dosage Summary

Oral:

Children <6 years: 2–4 mL/kg given once or in divided doses

Children 6-12 years: 100-150 mL given once or in divided doses

Children >12 years: 150-300 mL given once or in divided doses

Adults: 150-300 mL

Dosage Forms

Solution, oral: 290 mg/5 mL (296 mL, 300 mL)

Citroma® [OTC]: 290 mg/5 mL (296 mL, 340 mL)

Tablet, oral: Elemental magnesium 100 mg

magnesium gluceptate *see* magnesium glucoheptonate *on page 584*

magnesium glucoheptonate (mag NEE zhum gloo koh HEP toh nate)

Synonyms magnesium gluceptate

U.S./Canadian Brand Names Magnelium® [Can]; Magnolex® [Can]; Magnorol® Sirop [Can]; ratio-Magnesium [Can]

Therapeutic Category Electrolyte Supplement, Parenteral; Magnesium Salt

Use Treatment and prevention of hypomagnesemia

Dosage Summary

Oral:

Children: Dosage not established

Adults: 100-600 mg (5-30 mg elemental magnesium) 1-2 times/day with food

Dosage Forms - Canada

Capsule: 20 mg, 300 mg
Magnelium®, Magnorol®: 20 mg
Magnolex®: 300 mg
Solution, oral: 100 mg/mL
ratio-Magnesium: 100 mg/mL
Syrup: 90 mg/mL
Magnorol® Sirop: 90 mg/mL

magnesium gluconate (mag NEE zhum GLOO koe nate)

U.S./Canadian Brand Names Magonate® [US-OTC]; Magtrate® [US-OTC]; Mag®-G [US-OTC]

Therapeutic Category Electrolyte Supplement, Oral

Use Dietary supplement

Dosage Summary

Oral: RDA (elemental magnesium):
Children:
1-3 years: 80 mg/day
4-8 years: 130 mg/day
9-13 years: 240 mg/day
14-18 years:
Female: 360 mg/day
Pregnant female: 400 mg/day
Male: 410 mg/day
Adults:
19-30 years:
Female: 310 mg/day
Pregnant female: 350 mg/day
Male: 400 mg/day
≥31 years:
Female: 320 mg/day
Pregnant female: 360 mg/day
Male: 420 mg/day

Dosage Forms

Liquid, oral:
Magonate® [OTC]: 1000 mg/5 mL (355 mL)
Tablet, oral: 500 mg, 550 mg
Magonate® [OTC]: 500 mg
Magtrate® [OTC]: 500 mg
Mag®-G [OTC]: 500 mg

magnesium hydroxide (mag NEE zhum hye DROKS ide)

Synonyms magnesia magma; MOM

U.S./Canadian Brand Names Fleet® Pedia-Lax™ Chewable Tablet [US-OTC]; Little Phillips'® Milk of Magnesia [US-OTC]; Milk of Magnesia [US-OTC]; Phillips'® Milk of Magnesia [US-OTC]

Therapeutic Category Antacid; Electrolyte Supplement, Oral; Laxative

Use Short-term treatment of occasional constipation and symptoms of hyperacidity, laxative; dietary supplement

Dosage Summary

Oral:
Children <2 years: OTC laxative: Dosage not established; use not recommended
Children 2-5 years: OTC laxative: Magnesium hydroxide 400 mg/5 mL: 5-15 mL/day
Children 6-11 years: OTC laxative: Magnesium hydroxide 400 mg/5 mL: 15-30 mL/day
Children ≥12 years: OTC laxative: Magnesium hydroxide 400 mg/5 mL: 30-60 mL/day
Adults: OTC laxative: Magnesium hydroxide 400 mg/5 mL: 30-60 mL/day

Dosage Forms

Suspension, oral: 400 mg/5 mL (30 mL, 473 mL, 3840 mL); 2400 mg/10 mL (10 mL)
Little Phillips'® Milk of Magnesia [OTC]: 800 mg/5 mL (120 mL)
Milk of Magnesia [OTC]: 400 mg/5 mL (360 mL, 480 mL); 800 mg/5 mL (100 mL, 400 mL)
Phillips'® Milk of Magnesia [OTC]: 400 mg/5 mL (120 mL, 240 mL, 360 mL, 780 mL); 800 mg/5 mL (240 mL)

Tablet, chewable, oral:
Fleet® Pedia-Lax™ Chewable Tablet [OTC]: 400 mg
Phillips'® Milk of Magnesia [OTC]: 311 mg

magnesium hydroxide, aluminum hydroxide, and simethicone *see* aluminum hydroxide, magnesium hydroxide, and simethicone *on page 59*

magnesium hydroxide and aluminum hydroxide *see* aluminum hydroxide and magnesium hydroxide *on page 59*

magnesium hydroxide and calcium carbonate *see* calcium carbonate and magnesium hydroxide *on page 168*

magnesium hydroxide and mineral oil (mag NEE zhum hye DROKS ide & MIN er al oyl)

Synonyms Haley's M-O; MOM/mineral oil emulsion

U.S./Canadian Brand Names Phillips'® M-O [US-OTC]

Therapeutic Category Laxative

Use Short-term treatment of occasional constipation

Dosage Summary

Oral:
Children <6 years: Dosage not established
Children 6-11 years: 20-30 mL at bedtime
Children ≥12 years: 45-60 mL at bedtime
Adults: 45-60 mL at bedtime

Dosage Forms

Suspension, oral:
Phillips'® M-O [OTC]: Magnesium hydroxide 300 mg and mineral oil 1.25 mL per 5 mL

magnesium hydroxide, famotidine, and calcium carbonate *see* famotidine, calcium carbonate, and magnesium hydroxide *on page 391*

magnesium L-aspartate hydrochloride
(mag NEE zhum el as PAR tate hye droe KLOR ide)

Synonyms MAH

U.S./Canadian Brand Names Maginex™ DS [US-OTC]; Maginex™ [US-OTC]

Therapeutic Category Electrolyte Supplement, Oral

Use Dietary supplement

Dosage Summary

Oral: RDA (elemental magnesium):
Children:
1-3 years: 80 mg/day
4-8 years: 130 mg/day
9-13 years: 240 mg/day
14-18 years:
Female: 360 mg/day
Pregnant female: 400 mg/day
Male: 410 mg/day
Adults:
19-30 years:
Female: 310 mg/day
Pregnant female: 350 mg/day
Male: 400 mg/day
≥31 years:
Female: 320 mg/day
Pregnant female: 360 mg/day
Male: 420 mg/day

Dosage Forms

Granules for solution, oral [preservative free]:
Maginex™ DS [OTC]: 1230 mg/packet (30s)

Tablet, enteric coated, oral [preservative free]:
Maginex™ [OTC]: 615 mg

magnesium oxide (mag NEE zhum OKS ide)

Synonyms mag oxide

U.S./Canadian Brand Names Mag-Ox® 400 [US-OTC]; MagGel™ 600 [US-OTC]; MAGnesium-Oxide™ [US-OTC]; Phillips'® Laxative Dietary Supplement Cramp-Free [US-OTC]; Uro-Mag® [US-OTC]

Therapeutic Category Antacid; Electrolyte Supplement, Oral; Laxative

Use Electrolyte replacement

Dosage Summary

Oral: RDA (elemental magnesium):

Children:

1-3 years: 80 mg/day

4-8 years: 130 mg/day

9-13 years: 240 mg/day

14-18 years:

Female: 360 mg/day

Pregnant female: 400 mg/day

Male: 410 mg/day

Adults:

19-30 years:

Female: 310 mg/day

Pregnant female: 350 mg/day

Male: 400 mg/day

≥31 years:

Female: 320 mg/day

Pregnant female: 360 mg/day

Male: 420 mg/day

Dosage Forms

Caplet, oral: Elemental magnesium 250 mg

Phillips'® Laxative Dietary Supplement Cramp-Free [OTC]: Elemental magnesium 500 mg

Capsule, oral:

Uro-Mag® [OTC]: 140 mg

Capsule, softgel, oral:

MagGel™ 600 [OTC]: 600 mg

Tablet, oral: 400 mg, 500 mg, Elemental magnesium 500 mg

Mag-Ox® 400 [OTC]: 400 mg

MAGnesium-Oxide™ [OTC]: 400 mg

MAGnesium-Oxide™ [US-OTC] *see* magnesium oxide *on page 587*

magnesium salicylate (mag NEE zhum sa LIS i late)

U.S./Canadian Brand Names Doan's® Extra Strength [US-OTC]; Keygesic [US-OTC]; Momentum® [US-OTC]; MST 600 [US]

Therapeutic Category Nonsteroidal Antiinflammatory Drug (NSAID)

Use Mild-to-moderate pain, fever, various inflammatory conditions; relief of pain and inflammation of rheumatoid arthritis and osteoarthritis

Dosage Summary

Oral:

Children <12 years: Dosage not established

Children ≥12 years:

Doan's® Extra Strength, Momentum®: Two caplets every 6 hours as needed (maximum: 8 caplets/day)

Keygesic: One tablet every 4 hours as needed (maximum: 4 tablets/day)

Adults:

Doan's® Extra Strength, Momentum®: Two caplets every 6 hours as needed (maximum: 8 caplets/day)

Keygesic: One tablet every 4 hours as needed (maximum: 4 tablets/day)

Dosage Forms

Caplet, oral:

Doan's® Extra Strength [OTC]: 580 mg

Momentum® [OTC]: 580 mg

Tablet, oral:

Keygesic [OTC]: 650 mg

MST 600: 600 mg

magnesium sulfate (mag NEE zhum SUL fate)

Sound-Alike/Look-Alike Issues

magnesium sulfate may be confused with manganese sulfate, morphine sulfate

$MgSO_4$ is an error-prone abbreviation (mistaken as morphine sulfate)

Synonyms epsom salts

Therapeutic Category Anticonvulsant; Electrolyte Supplement, Oral; Laxative

Use Treatment and prevention of hypomagnesemia; prevention and treatment of seizures in severe preeclampsia or eclampsia, pediatric acute nephritis; torsade de pointes; treatment of cardiac arrhythmias (VT/VF) caused by hypomagnesemia; soaking aid

Dosage Summary

I.V.:

Children:

Hypomagnesemia: 25-50 mg/kg/dose; maximum single dose: 2000 mg; may also administer I.O.

TPN:

<50 kg: 0.3-0.5 mEq elemental magnesium/kg/day

>50 kg: 10-30 mEq elemental magnesium/day

Adults:

Hypomagnesemia, torsade de pointes: 1-2 g, followed by 0.5-1 g/hour continuous infusion

Eclampsia, pre-eclampsia (severe): 4-5 g infusion; followed by a 1-2 g/hour continuous infusion; or may follow with I.M. doses of 4-5 g in each buttock every 4 hours. **Note:** Initial infusion may be given over 3-4 minutes if eclampsia is severe; ACOG guidelines recommend infusion over 15-20 minutes. Maximum: 40 g/24 hours.

TPN: 8-24 mEq elemental magnesium/day

Oral:

Children:

RDA:

1-3 years: 80 mg elemental magnesium/day

4-8 years: 130 mg elemental magnesium/day

9-13 years: 240 mg elemental magnesium/day

14-18 years:

Female: 360 mg elemental magnesium/day

Pregnant female: 400 mg elemental magnesium/day

Male: 410 mg elemental magnesium/day

Adults:

RDA:

19-30 years:

Female: 310 mg elemental magnesium/day

Pregnant female: 350 mg elemental magnesium/day

Male: 400 mg elemental magnesium/day

≥31 years:

Female: 320 mg elemental magnesium/day

Pregnant female: 360 mg elemental magnesium/day

Male: 420 mg elemental magnesium/day

I.M.:

Children: Dosage not established

Adults: Hypomagnesemia: 1-4 g/day in divided doses

Topical:

Children: Dosage not established

Adults: Soaking aid: Dissolve 2 cupfuls of powder per gallon of warm water

Dosage Forms

Infusion, premixed in D_5W: 10 mg/mL (100 mL); 20 mg/mL (500 mL)

Infusion, premixed in water for injection: 40 mg/mL (50 mL, 100 mL, 500 mL, 1000 mL); 80 mg/mL (50 mL)

Injection, solution: 500 mg/mL (5 mL, 10 mL, 20 mL, 25 mL, 50 mL)

Injection, solution [preservative free]: 500 mg/mL (2 mL, 5 mL, 10 mL, 20 mL, 50 mL)

Powder, oral/topical: USP: 100% (227 g, 454 g, 1810 g, 2720 g)

magnesium trisilicate and aluminum hydroxide *see* aluminum hydroxide and magnesium trisilicate *on page 59*

Magnevist® [US/Can] *see* gadopentetate dimeglumine *on page 434*

Magnolex® [Can] *see* magnesium glucoheptonate *on page* *584*
Magnorol® Sirop [Can] *see* magnesium glucoheptonate *on page* *584*
Magonate® [US-OTC] *see* magnesium gluconate *on page* *585*
Magonate® Sport *(Discontinued)* *see* magnesium gluconate *on page* *585*
Mag-Ox® 400 [US-OTC] *see* magnesium oxide *on page* *587*
mag oxide *see* magnesium oxide *on page* *587*
Magsal® *(Discontinued)* *see* magnesium salicylate *on page* *587*
Mag-SR *(Discontinued)* *see* magnesium chloride *on page* *583*
Mag-SR with Calcium *(Discontinued)* *see* magnesium chloride *on page* *583*
Magtrate® [US-OTC] *see* magnesium gluconate *on page* *585*
MAH *see* magnesium L-aspartate hydrochloride *on page* *586*
Malarone® [US/Can] *see* atovaquone and proguanil *on page* *105*
Malarone® Pediatric [Can] *see* atovaquone and proguanil *on page* *105*

malathion (mal a THYE on)

U.S./Canadian Brand Names Ovide® [US]
Therapeutic Category Scabicides/Pediculicides
Use Treatment of head lice and their ova
Dosage Summary
Topical:
Neonates: Use contraindicated
Infants: Use contraindicated
Children: Sprinkle lotion on dry hair and allow to dry naturally, after 8-12 hours wash hair and use fine-toothed comb to remove dead lice and eggs; may repeat in 7-9 days
Adults: Sprinkle lotion on dry hair and allow to dry naturally, after 8-12 hours wash hair and use fine-toothed comb to remove dead lice and eggs; may repeat in 7-9 days
Dosage Forms
Lotion, topical: 0.5% (59 mL)
Ovide®: 0.5% (59 mL)

Mallisol® *(Discontinued)* *see* povidone-iodine (topical) *on page* *784*

maltodextrin (mal toe DEK strin)

U.S./Canadian Brand Names Carrington® Oral Wound Rinse [US-OTC]; Multidex® [US-OTC]
Therapeutic Category Skin and Mucous Membrane Agent
Use Topical: Treatment of infected or noninfected wounds
Dosage Summary
Oral:
Children: Dosage not established
Adults: 1 packet or tablespoonful 3-4 times/day or more if needed
Topical:
Children: Dosage not established
Adults: Apply to wounds with dressing changes
Dosage Forms
Gel, topical [preservative free]:
Multidex® [OTC]: 7.1 mL (7.1 mL); 14.2 mL (14.2 mL); 85.2 mL (85.2 mL)
Powder, topical [preservative free]:
Multidex® [OTC]: 6 g (6 g); 12 g (12 g); 25 g (25 g); 45 g (45 g)
Powder for suspension, oral:
Carrington® Oral Wound Rinse [OTC]: 23 g
Solution, topical [preservative free]:
Multidex® [OTC]: 45 mL (45 mL)

Mandelamine® [Can] *see* methenamine *on page* *612*
Mandelamine® *(Discontinued)* *see* methenamine *on page* *612*
mandrake *see* podophyllum resin *on page* *773*
Manerix® [Can] *see* moclobemide *(Canada only) on page* *639*
manganese *see* trace metals *on page* *945*

mannitol (MAN i tole)

Sound-Alike/Look-Alike Issues

Osmitrol® may be confused with esmolol

Synonyms *D*-mannitol

U.S./Canadian Brand Names Osmitrol® [US/Can]; Resectisol® [US]

Therapeutic Category Diuretic, Osmotic

Use Reduction of increased intracranial pressure associated with cerebral edema; promotion of diuresis in the prevention and/or treatment of oliguria or anuria due to acute renal failure; reduction of increased intraocular pressure; promoting urinary excretion of toxic substances; genitourinary irrigant in transurethral prostatic resection or other transurethral surgical procedures

Dosage Summary

I.V.:

Children: Initial: 0.25-1 g/kg; Maintenance: 0.25-0.5 g/kg every 4-6 hours

Adults:

Diuresis: Initial: 0.5-1 g/kg; Maintenance: 0.25-0.5 g/kg every 4-6 hours (usually 20-200 g/day)

Intracranial pressure/cerebral edema: 0.25-1.5 g/kg as 15-20% solution; maintain serum osmolality 310 to <320 mOsm/kg

Preoperative: 1.5-2 g/kg prior to surgery

Prevention/treatment oliguria: 50-100 g dose

Transurethral:

Children: Dosage not established

Adults: Use urogenital solution as required for irrigation

Dosage Forms

Injection, solution: 20% [200 mg/mL] (250 mL, 500 mL); 25% [250 mg/mL] (50 mL)

Osmitrol: 5% [50 mg/mL] (1000 mL); 10% [100 mg/mL] (500 mL); 15% [150 mg/mL] (500 mL); 20% [200 mg/mL] (250 mL, 500 mL)

Injection, solution [preservative free]: 25% [250 mg/mL] (50 mL)

Solution, genitourinary irrigation: 5% [50 mg/mL] (2000 mL)

mantoux *see* tuberculin tests *on page 965*

Maox® *(Discontinued)* *see* magnesium oxide *on page 587*

Mapap® Arthritis Pain [US-OTC] *see* acetaminophen *on page 21*

Mapap® Children's [US-OTC] *see* acetaminophen *on page 21*

Mapap® *(Discontinued)* *see* acetaminophen *on page 21*

Mapap® Extra Strength [US-OTC] *see* acetaminophen *on page 21*

Mapap® Infant's [US-OTC] *see* acetaminophen *on page 21*

Mapap® Junior Rapid Tabs [US-OTC] *see* acetaminophen *on page 21*

Mapap® Multi-Symptom Cold [US-OTC] *see* acetaminophen, dextromethorphan, and phenylephrine *on page 29*

Mapap PM [US-OTC] *see* acetaminophen and diphenhydramine *on page 24*

Mapap® Sinus Congestion and Pain Daytime [US-OTC] *see* acetaminophen and phenylephrine *on page 25*

Mapezine® [Can] *see* carbamazepine *on page 177*

maprotiline (ma PROE ti leen)

Sound-Alike/Look-Alike Issues

Ludiomil® may be confused with Lamictal®, lamotrigine, Lomotil®

Synonyms maprotiline hydrochloride

U.S./Canadian Brand Names Novo-Maprotiline [Can]

Therapeutic Category Antidepressant, Tetracyclic

Use Treatment of depression and anxiety associated with depression

Dosage Summary

Oral:

Children: Dosage not established

Adults: Initial: 75 mg once daily; Maintenance: 150-225 mg/day as a single dose or in 3 divided doses; **Note:** Titration is recommended

Elderly: Initial: 25 mg at bedtime; Maintenance: 50-75 mg/day; **Note:** Titration is recommended

Dosage Forms
Tablet, oral: 25 mg, 50 mg, 75 mg

maprotiline hydrochloride *see* maprotiline *on page* 590

maraviroc (mah RAV er rock)

Synonyms UK-427,857
U.S./Canadian Brand Names Celsentri™ [Can]; Selzentry™ [US]
Therapeutic Category Antiretroviral Agent, CCR5 Antagonist
Use Treatment of CCR5-tropic HIV-1 infection, in combination with other antiretroviral agents
Dosage Summary
Oral:
Children <16 years: Dosage not established
Children ≥16 years: 300 mg twice daily; adjusted dosage: 150 mg twice daily **or** 600 mg twice daily
Adults: 300 mg twice daily; adjusted dosage: 150 mg twice daily **or** 600 mg twice daily
Dosage Forms
Tablet, oral:
Selzentry™: 150 mg, 300 mg

Marcaine® [US/Can] *see* bupivacaine *on page* 153
Marcaine® Spinal [US] *see* bupivacaine *on page* 153
Marcaine® with Epinephrine [US] *see* bupivacaine and epinephrine *on page* 154
Mar-Cof® CG [US] *see* guaifenesin and codeine *on page* 455
Margesic [US] *see* butalbital, acetaminophen, and caffeine *on page* 159
Margesic® H [US] *see* hydrocodone and acetaminophen *on page* 479
Marinol® [US/Can] *see* dronabinol *on page* 333
Mark 1™ *see* atropine and pralidoxime *on page* 107
Marmine® Injection *(Discontinued)* *see* dimenhydrinate *on page* 307
Marmine® Oral *(Discontinued)* *see* dimenhydrinate *on page* 307
Marplan® [US] *see* isocarboxazid *on page* 527
Marthritic® *(Discontinued)* *see* salsalate *on page* 862
Marvelon® [Can] *see* ethinyl estradiol and desogestrel *on page* 374
Matulane® [US/Can] *see* procarbazine *on page* 797
3M™ Avagard® *(Discontinued)* *see* chlorhexidine gluconate *on page* 204
Mavik® [US/Can] *see* trandolapril *on page* 947
Maxair® Autohaler® [US] *see* pirbuterol *on page* 764
Maxalt® [US/Can] *see* rizatriptan *on page* 848
Maxalt-MLT® [US] *see* rizatriptan *on page* 848
Maxalt RPD™ [Can] *see* rizatriptan *on page* 848
Maxaquin® *(Discontinued)*
Maxaron® Forte [US] *see* polysaccharide-iron complex, vitamin B12, and folic acid *on page* 778
Maxidex® [US/Can] *see* dexamethasone (ophthalmic) *on page* 281
Maxidone® [US] *see* hydrocodone and acetaminophen *on page* 479
Maxifed [US-OTC] *see* guaifenesin and pseudoephedrine *on page* 457
Maxifed DM [US] *see* guaifenesin, pseudoephedrine, and dextromethorphan *on page* 460
Maxifed DMX [US] *see* guaifenesin, pseudoephedrine, and dextromethorphan *on page* 460
Maxifed-G [US-OTC] *see* guaifenesin and pseudoephedrine *on page* 457
Maxiflor® *(Discontinued)* *see* diflorasone *on page* 301
Maxilene® [Can] *see* lidocaine (topical) *on page* 562
Maximum D3® [US-OTC] *see* cholecalciferol *on page* 218
Maximum Strength Desenex® Antifungal Cream *(Discontinued)* *see* miconazole (topical) *on page* 630
Maximum Strength Dex-A-Diet® *(Discontinued)*
Maximum Strength Dexatrim® *(Discontinued)*
Maxiphen DM [US] *see* guaifenesin, dextromethorphan, and phenylephrine *on page* 458
Maxipime® [US/Can] *see* cefepime *on page* 190

Maxitrol® [US/Can] *see* neomycin, polymyxin B, and dexamethasone *on page 666*
Maxi-Tuss HC® [US] *see* phenylephrine, hydrocodone, and chlorpheniramine *on page 754*
Maxi-Tuss HCG ***(Discontinued)***
Maxi-Tuss HCX [US] *see* phenylephrine, hydrocodone, and chlorpheniramine *on page 754*
Maxolon® ***(Discontinued)*** *see* metoclopramide *on page 624*
Maxzide® [US] *see* hydrochlorothiazide and triamterene *on page 479*
Maxzide®-25 [US] *see* hydrochlorothiazide and triamterene *on page 479*
may apple *see* podophyllum resin *on page 773*
3M™ Cavilon™ Skin Cleanser ***(Discontinued)*** *see* benzalkonium chloride *on page 124*
MCH *see* collagen hemostat *on page 248*

m-cresyl acetate (em-KREE sil AS e tate)

U.S./Canadian Brand Names Cresylate® [US]

Therapeutic Category Otic Agent, Antiinfective

Use Provides an acid medium; for external otitis infections caused by susceptible bacteria or fungus

Dosage Summary

Otic:

Children: Instill 2-4 drops as required

Adults: Instill 2-4 drops as required

Dosage Forms

Solution, otic:

Cresylate™: 25% (15 mL)

MCT *see* medium chain triglycerides *on page 596*
MCT Oil® [US-OTC/Can] *see* medium chain triglycerides *on page 596*
MCV *see* meningococcal (groups A / C / Y and W-135) diphtheria conjugate vaccine *on page 601*
MCV4 *see* meningococcal (groups A / C / Y and W-135) diphtheria conjugate vaccine *on page 601*
MD-76®R [US] *see* diatrizoate meglumine and diatrizoate sodium *on page 292*
MD-Gastroview® [US] *see* diatrizoate meglumine and diatrizoate sodium *on page 292*
MDL 73,147EF *see* dolasetron *on page 323*

measles, mumps, and rubella virus vaccine

(MEE zels, mumpz & roo BEL a VYE rus vak SEEN)

Sound-Alike/Look-Alike Issues

MMR (measles, mumps, and rubella virus vaccine) may be confused with MMRV (measles, mumps, rubella and varicella) vaccine

Synonyms MMR; mumps, measles, and rubella vaccines; rubella, measles, and mumps vaccines

U.S./Canadian Brand Names M-M-R® II [US/Can]; Priorix™ [Can]

Therapeutic Category Vaccine, Live Virus

Use Measles, mumps, and rubella prophylaxis

The Advisory Committee on Immunization Practices (ACIP) recommends routine vaccination for the following:

- All children (first dose given at 12-15 months of age)
- Adults born 1957 or later (without evidence of immunity or documentation of vaccination).
- Adults at higher risk for exposure to and transmission of measles mumps and rubella should receive special consideration for vaccination, unless an acceptable evidence of immunity exists. This includes international travelers, persons attending colleges and other post-high school education, persons working in healthcare facilities.

Dosage Summary

SubQ:

Infants <12 months: If there is risk of exposure to measles, single-antigen measles vaccine should be administered at 6-11 months of age with a second dose (of MMR) at >12 months

Children ≥12 months: 0.5 mL at 12 months and then repeated at 4-6 years of age; minimum interval between doses is 28 days

Adults: Born ≥1957 without evidence of immunity: 1 or 2 doses (0.5 mL/dose); minimum interval between doses is 28 days

Dosage Forms

Injection, powder for reconstitution [preservative free]:

M-M-R® II: Measles virus ≥1000 $TCID_{50}$, mumps virus ≥20,000 $TCID_{50}$, and rubella virus ≥1000 $TCID_{50}$

measles, mumps, rubella, and varicella virus vaccine

(MEE zels, mumpz, roo BEL a, & var i SEL a VYE rus vak SEEN)

Synonyms MMR-V; MMRV; mumps, rubella, varicella, and measles vaccine; rubella, varicella, measles, and mumps vaccine; varicella, measles, mumps, and rubella vaccine

U.S./Canadian Brand Names Priorix-Tetra™ [Can]; ProQuad® [US]

Therapeutic Category Vaccine, Live Virus

Use To provide simultaneous active immunization against measles, mumps, rubella, and varicella

The Advisory Committee on Immunization Practices (ACIP) recommends routine vaccination against measles, mumps, rubella, and varicella in healthy children 12 months to 12 years of age. For children receiving their first dose at 12-47 months of age, either the MMRV combination vaccine or separate MMR and varicella vaccines can be used. (The ACIP prefers administration of separate MMR and varicella vaccines as the first dose in this age group unless the parent or caregiver expresses preference for the MMRV combination.) For children receiving the first dose at ≥48 months or their second dose at any age, use of MMRV is preferred.

Note: Canadian labeling (not in U.S. labeling): MMRV combination vaccine is approved for use in healthy children 9 months to 6 years; may consider use in healthy children ≤12 years of age based upon prior experience with the separate component (live-attenuated MMR or live-attenuated varicella [OKA-strain]) vaccines.

Dosage Summary

SubQ:

Children <12 months: Dosage not established

Children 12 months to 12 years: One dose (0.5 mL)

Children >12 years and Adults: Dosage not established

Dosage Forms

Injection, powder for reconstitution [preservative free]:

ProQuad®: Measles virus ≥3.00 log_{10} $TCID_{50}$, mumps virus ≥4.30 log_{10} $TCID_{50}$, rubella virus ≥3.00 log_{10} $TCID_{50}$, and varicella virus ≥3.99 log_{10} PFU

Dosage Forms - Canada

Injection, powder for reconstitution [preservative free]:

Priorix-Tetra™ (CAN): Measles virus ≥3.00 log_{10} $CCID_{50}$, mumps virus ≥4.4 log_{10} $CCID_{50}$, rubella virus ≥3.00 log_{10} $CCID_{50}$, and varicella virus ≥3.3 log_{10} PFU

measles virus vaccine (live) (MEE zels VYE rus vak SEEN, live)

Sound-Alike/Look-Alike Issues

Attenuvax® may be confused with Meruvax®

Synonyms more attenuated Enders strain; rubeola vaccine

Therapeutic Category Vaccine, Live Virus

Use Active immunization against measles (rubeola)

Note: Unless otherwise contraindicated, trivalent measles - mumps - rubella (MMR) is the vaccine of choice if recipients are likely to be susceptible to rubella and/or mumps as well as to measles.

The Advisory Committee on Immunization Practices (ACIP) recommends routine vaccination for the following:

- All children. For routine vaccination, the first dose given at 12-15 months of age
- Adults born 1957 or later (without evidence of immunity or documentation of vaccination)
- Adults at higher risk for exposure to and transmission of measles should receive special consideration for vaccination, unless an acceptable evidence of immunity exists. This includes international travelers, persons attending colleges and other post-high school education, persons working in healthcare facilities.

Dosage Summary

SubQ:

Children <6 months: Dosage not established

Children ≥6 months: 0.5 mL as a single dose; when 2 doses are needed, at least 28 days should elapse between doses

Adults: 0.5 mL as a single dose; when 2 doses are needed, at least 28 days should elapse between doses

Measurin® *(Discontinued)* *see* aspirin *on page 100*
Mebaral® [US/Can] *see* mephobarbital *on page 604*

mebendazole (me BEN da zole)

Sound-Alike/Look-Alike Issues
mebendazole may be confused with metroNIDAZOLE

U.S./Canadian Brand Names Vermox® [Can]

Therapeutic Category Anthelmintic

Use Treatment of pinworms (*Enterobius vermicularis*), whipworms (*Trichuris trichiura*), roundworms (*Ascaris lumbricoides*), and hookworms (*Ancylostoma duodenale*)

Dosage Summary

Oral:

Children <2 years: Dosage not established
Children ≥2 years: 100 mg as a single dose or twice daily **or** 200 mg twice daily
Adults: 100 mg as a single dose or twice daily **or** 200 mg twice daily

Dosage Forms

Tablet, chewable, oral: 100 mg

mecamylamine (mek a MIL a meen)

Sound-Alike/Look-Alike Issues
mecamylamine may be confused with mesalamine

Synonyms mecamylamine hydrochloride

U.S./Canadian Brand Names Inversine® [Can]

Therapeutic Category Ganglionic Blocking Agent

Use Treatment of moderately severe to severe hypertension and in uncomplicated malignant hypertension

Dosage Summary

Oral:

Children: Dosage not established
Adults: Initial: 2.5 mg twice daily; Average dose: 25 mg/day in 3 divided doses; **Note:** Titration is recommended

mecamylamine hydrochloride *see* mecamylamine *on page 594*

mecasermin (mek a SER min)

Synonyms mecasermin (rDNA origin); mecasermin rinfabate; recombinant human insulin-like growth factor-1; rhIGF-1 (mecasermin [Increlex™]); rhIGF-1/rhIGFBP-3 (mecasermin rinfabate [Iplex™])

U.S./Canadian Brand Names Increlex™ [US]

Therapeutic Category Growth Hormone

Use Treatment of growth failure in children with severe primary insulin-like growth factor-1 deficiency (IGF-1 deficiency; primary IGFD), or with growth hormone (GH) gene deletions who have developed neutralizing antibodies to GH

Dosage Summary

SubQ:

Children <2 years: Dosage not established
Children 2-<3 years: Increlex™: Initial: 0.04-0.08 mg/kg twice daily; Maintenance: 0.04-0.12 mg/kg twice daily
Children ≥3 years: Increlex™: Initial: 0.04-0.08 mg/kg twice daily; Maintenance: 0.04-0.12 mg/kg twice daily
Adults: Dosage not established

Dosage Forms

Injection, solution:
Increlex™: 10 mg/mL (4 mL)

mecasermin (rDNA origin) *see* mecasermin *on page 594*
mecasermin rinfabate *see* mecasermin *on page 594*

mechlorethamine (me klor ETH a meen)

Synonyms chlorethazine; chlorethazine mustard; HN_2; mechlorethamine hydrochloride; mustine; nitrogen mustard

U.S./Canadian Brand Names Mustargen® [US/Can]

Therapeutic Category Antineoplastic Agent

Use Hodgkin disease; non-Hodgkin lymphoma; intracavitary injection for treatment of metastatic tumors; pleural and other malignant effusions

Dosage Summary Note: Dosage should be based on ideal dry weight (evaluate the presence of edema or ascites so that dosage will be based on actual weight unaugmented by edema/ascites).

I.V.:

Adults: 0.4 mg/kg as a single dose **or** in divided doses of 0.1 mg/kg/day (for 4 days) or 0.2 mg/kg/day (for 2 days) per treatment course

Intracavitary:

Children: Dosage not established

Adults: 0.4 mg/kg as a single dose, although 0.2 mg/kg (10-20 mg) as a single dose has been used by the *intrapericardial* route

Topical:

Children: Dosage not established

Dosage Forms

Injection, powder for reconstitution:

Mustargen®: 10 mg

mechlorethamine hydrochloride *see* mechlorethamine *on page* 594

meclizine (MEK li zeen)

Sound-Alike/Look-Alike Issues

Antivert® may be confused with Anzemet®, Axert®

Synonyms meclizine hydrochloride; meclozine hydrochloride

U.S./Canadian Brand Names Antivert® [US]; Bonamine™ [Can]; Bonine® [US-OTC/Can]; Dramamine® Less Drowsy Formula [US-OTC]; Medi-Meclizine [US-OTC]; Trav-L-Tabs® [US-OTC]

Therapeutic Category Antihistamine

Use Prevention and treatment of symptoms of motion sickness; management of vertigo with diseases affecting the vestibular system

Dosage Summary

Oral:

Children ≤12 years: Dosage not established

Children >12 years: 12.5-50 mg 1 hour before travel, may repeat every 12-24 hours if needed **or** 25-100 mg/day in divided doses

Adults: 12.5-50 mg 1 hour before travel, may repeat every 12-24 hours if needed **or** 25-100 mg/day in divided doses

Dosage Forms

Caplet, oral: 12.5 mg

Tablet, oral: 12.5 mg, 25 mg

Antivert®: 12.5 mg, 25 mg, 50 mg

Dramamine® Less Drowsy Formula [OTC]: 25 mg

Medi-Meclizine [OTC]: 25 mg

Trav-L-Tabs® [OTC]: 25 mg

Tablet, chewable, oral: 25 mg

Bonine® [OTC]: 25 mg

meclizine hydrochloride *see* meclizine *on page* 595

meclofenamate (me kloe fen AM ate)

Synonyms meclofenamate sodium

U.S./Canadian Brand Names Meclomen® [Can]

Therapeutic Category Analgesic, Nonnarcotic; Nonsteroidal Antiinflammatory Drug (NSAID)

Use Treatment of inflammatory disorders, arthritis, mild-to-moderate pain, dysmenorrhea

Dosage Summary

Oral:

Children ≤14 years: Dosage not established

Children >14 years: 50-100 mg every 4-6 hours (maximum: 400 mg/day)

Adults: 50-100 mg every 4-6 hours (maximum: 400 mg/day)

Dosage Forms

Capsule, oral: 50 mg, 100 mg

meclofenamate sodium *see* meclofenamate *on page 595*
Meclomen® [Can] *see* meclofenamate *on page 595*
meclozine hydrochloride *see* meclizine *on page 595*
Med-Atenolol [Can] *see* atenolol *on page 102*
Med-Baclofen [Can] *see* baclofen *on page 115*
Med-Diltiazem [Can] *see* diltiazem *on page 306*
Medebar® Plus *(Discontinued)* *see* barium *on page 117*
Medent-DM [US] *see* guaifenesin, pseudoephedrine, and dextromethorphan *on page 460*
Med-Glybe [Can] *see* glyburide *on page 448*
medicinal carbon *see* charcoal *on page 200*
medicinal charcoal *see* charcoal *on page 200*
Medicone® Hemorrhoidal [US-OTC] *see* benzocaine *on page 124*
Medicone® Suppositories [US-OTC] *see* phenylephrine (topical) *on page 752*
Medidin® Liquid *(Discontinued)*
Medi-First® Sinus Decongestant [US-OTC] *see* phenylephrine (systemic) *on page 751*
Medihaler-Iso® *(Discontinued)* *see* isoproterenol *on page 528*
Medi-Meclizine [US-OTC] *see* meclizine *on page 595*
Medi Pads [US-OTC] *see* witch hazel *on page 994*
Medipain 5® *(Discontinued)* *see* hydrocodone and acetaminophen *on page 479*
Medi-Phenyl [US-OTC] *see* phenylephrine (systemic) *on page 751*
Medipren® *(Discontinued)* *see* ibuprofen *on page 494*
Mediproxen [US-OTC] *see* naproxen *on page 659*
Medi-Quick® Topical Ointment *(Discontinued)* *see* bacitracin, neomycin, and polymyxin B *on page 114*
Medispaz® *(Discontinued)* *see* hyoscyamine *on page 491*
Medi-Tuss® *(Discontinued)* *see* guaifenesin *on page 454*

medium chain triglycerides (mee DEE um chane trye GLIS er ides)

Synonyms MCT; triglycerides, medium chain

U.S./Canadian Brand Names MCT Oil® [US-OTC/Can]

Therapeutic Category Nutritional Supplement

Use Dietary supplement for those who cannot digest long chain fats; malabsorption associated with disorders such as pancreatic insufficiency, bile salt deficiency, short bowel syndrome, and bacterial overgrowth of the small bowel; induce ketosis as a prevention for seizures

Dosage Summary

Oral:

Infants: Initial: 0.5 mL every other feeding, then advance to every feeding, then increase in increments of 0.25-0.5 mL/feeding at intervals of 2-3 days as tolerated

Children:

Cystic fibrosis: 3 tablespoons/day in divided doses

Seizures: About 39 mL with each meal or 50% to 70% (800-1120 kcal) of total calories (1600 kcal)

Adults:

Cystic fibrosis: 3 tablespoons/day in divided doses

Dietary supplement: 15 mL 3-4 times/day

Dosage Forms

Oil, oral:

MCT Oil® [OTC]: 14 g/15 mL (960 mL)

Med-Metformin [Can] *see* metformin *on page 609*
Medralone® Injection *(Discontinued)* *see* methylprednisolone *on page 622*
Med-Ranitidine [Can] *see* ranitidine *on page 828*
Medrol® [US/Can] *see* methylprednisolone *on page 622*
medrol dose pack *see* methylprednisolone *on page 622*
Medrol® Dosepak™ [US] *see* methylprednisolone *on page 622*

medroxyprogesterone (me DROKS ee proe JES te rone)

Sound-Alike/Look-Alike Issues

medroxyPROGESTERone may be confused with hydroxyprogesterone, methylPREDNISolone, methylTESTOSTERone

Depo-Provera® may be confused with depo-subQ provera 104™

depo-subQ provera 104™ may be confused with Depo-Provera®

Provera® may be confused with Covera®, Femara®, Parlodel®, Premarin®, Proscar®, Prozac®

Synonyms acetoxymethylprogesterone; medroxyprogesterone acetate; methylacetoxyprogesterone; MPA

Tall-Man medroxy**PROGESTER**one

U.S./Canadian Brand Names Alti-MPA [Can]; Apo-Medroxy® [Can]; Depo-Prevera® [Can]; Depo-Provera® Contraceptive [US]; Depo-Provera® [US/Can]; depo-subQ provera 104™ [US]; Gen-Medroxy [Can]; Novo-Medrone [Can]; Provera-Pak [Can]; Provera® [US/Can]

Therapeutic Category Contraceptive, Progestin Only; Progestin

Use Secondary amenorrhea or abnormal uterine bleeding due to hormonal imbalance; reduction of endometrial hyperplasia in nonhysterectomized postmenopausal women receiving conjugated estrogens; prevention of pregnancy; management of endometriosis-associated pain

Dosage Summary

I.M.:

Children: Dosage not established
Adolescents: Contraceptive: 150 mg every 3 months
Adults: Contraceptive: 150 mg every 3 months

Oral:

Children: Dosage not established
Adolescents: 5-10 mg once daily
Adults: 5-10 mg once daily

SubQ:

Children: Dosage not established
Adolescents: 104 mg every 3 months (every 12-14 weeks)
Adults: 104 mg every 3 months (every 12-14 weeks)

Dosage Forms

Injection, suspension: 150 mg/mL (1 mL)
Depo-Provera®: 400 mg/mL (2.5 mL)
Depo-Provera® Contraceptive: 150 mg/mL (1 mL)
depo-subQ provera 104™: 104 mg/0.65 mL (0.65 mL)

Tablet, oral: 2.5 mg, 5 mg, 10 mg
Provera®: 2.5 mg, 5 mg, 10 mg

medroxyprogesterone acetate *see* medroxyprogesterone *on page* 597

medroxyprogesterone and estrogens (conjugated) *see* estrogens (conjugated/equine) and medroxyprogesterone *on page* 371

medrysone *(Discontinued)*

Med-Salbutamol [Can] *see* albuterol *on page* 43

Med-Sotalol [Can] *see* sotalol *on page* 892

Med-Timolol [Can] *see* timolol (ophthalmic) *on page* 933

Med-Verapamil [Can] *see* verapamil *on page* 981

Mefenamic-250 [Can] *see* mefenamic acid *on page* 597

mefenamic acid (me fe NAM ik AS id)

Sound-Alike/Look-Alike Issues

Ponstel® may be confused with Pronestyl®

U.S./Canadian Brand Names Apo-Mefenamic® [Can]; Dom-Mefenamic Acid [Can]; Mefenamic-250 [Can]; Nu-Mefenamic [Can]; PMS-Mefenamic Acid [Can]; Ponstan® [Can]; Ponstel® [US]

Therapeutic Category Analgesic, Nonnarcotic; Nonsteroidal Antiinflammatory Drug (NSAID)

Use Short-term relief of mild-to-moderate pain including primary dysmenorrhea

Dosage Summary

Oral:

Children ≤14 years: Dosage not established
Children >14 years: 500 mg to start then 250 mg every 4 hours as needed (maximum therapy: 1 week)
Adults: 500 mg to start then 250 mg every 4 hours as needed (maximum therapy: 1 week)

Dosage Forms
Capsule, oral:
Ponstel®: 250 mg

mefloquine (ME floe kwin)

Synonyms mefloquine hydrochloride
U.S./Canadian Brand Names Apo-Mefloquine® [Can]; Lariam® [Can]
Therapeutic Category Antimalarial Agent
Use Treatment of mild-to-moderate acute malarial infections (including treatment of chloroquine-resistant malaria) and prevention of malaria caused by *Plasmodium falciparum* or *P. vivax*
Dosage Summary
Oral:
Children <6 months: Dosage not established
Children ≥6 months: Prophylaxis: 5 mg/kg/once weekly (maximum: 250 mg/dose); Treatment: 20-25 mg/kg/day in 2 divided doses, taken 6-8 hours apart (maximum: 1250 mg)
Adults: Prophylaxis: 1 tablet (250 mg) once weekly; Treatment: 5 tablets (1250 mg) as a single dose
Dosage Forms
Tablet, oral: 250 mg

mefloquine hydrochloride *see* mefloquine *on page 598*
Mefoxin® [US] *see* cefoxitin *on page 191*
Megace® [US/Can] *see* megestrol *on page 598*
Megace® ES [US] *see* megestrol *on page 598*
Megace® OS [Can] *see* megestrol *on page 598*
Megadophilus® [US-OTC] *see* Lactobacillus *on page 543*

megestrol (me JES trole)

Sound-Alike/Look-Alike Issues
megestrol may be confused with mesalamine
Megace® may be confused with Reglan®
Synonyms 5071-1DL(6); megestrol acetate; NSC-71423
U.S./Canadian Brand Names Apo-Megestrol® [Can]; Megace® ES [US]; Megace® OS [Can]; Megace® [US/Can]; Nu-Megestrol [Can]
Therapeutic Category Antineoplastic Agent; Progestin
Use Palliative treatment of breast and endometrial carcinoma; treatment of anorexia, cachexia, or unexplained significant weight loss in patients with AIDS
Dosage Summary
Oral:
Children: Dosage not established
Adults (females): Tablet: 40-320 mg/day in divided doses
Adults (males/females): Suspension: 400-800 mg/day [Megace®] **or** 625 mg/day [Megace® ES]
Dosage Forms
Suspension, oral: 40 mg/mL (10 mL, 20 mL, 237 mL, 240 mL, 473 mL, 480 mL)
Megace®: 40 mg/mL (240 mL)
Megace® ES: 125 mg/mL (150 mL)
Tablet, oral: 20 mg, 40 mg

megestrol acetate *see* megestrol *on page 598*
Melanex® [US] *see* hydroquinone *on page 487*
Melfiat® *(Discontinued)* *see* phendimetrazine *on page 747*
Mellaril® (all products) *(Discontinued)* *see* thioridazine *on page 928*
Mellaril-S® *(Discontinued)* *see* thioridazine *on page 928*

meloxicam (mel OKS i kam)

U.S./Canadian Brand Names Apo-Meloxicam® [Can]; CO Meloxicam [Can]; Dom-Meloxicam [Can]; Mobicox® [Can]; Mobic® [US/Can]; Mylan-Meloxicam [Can]; Novo-Meloxicam [Can]; PHL-Meloxicam [Can]; PMS-Meloxicam [Can]; ratio-Meloxicam [Can]; Teva-Meloxicam [Can]
Therapeutic Category Nonsteroidal Antiinflammatory Drug (NSAID)

Use Relief of signs and symptoms of osteoarthritis, rheumatoid arthritis, and juvenile rheumatoid arthritis (JRA)

Dosage Summary

Oral:

Children <2 years: Dosage not established

Children ≥2 years: 0.125 mg/kg/day (maximum: 7.5 mg/day)

Adults: Initial: 7.5 mg once daily; Maintenance: 7.5-15 mg once daily (maximum: 15 mg/day)

Dosage Forms

Suspension, oral:

Mobic®: 7.5 mg/5 mL (100 mL)

Tablet, oral: 7.5 mg, 15 mg

Mobic®: 7.5 mg, 15 mg

Melpaque HP® [US-OTC] *see* hydroquinone *on page 487*

melphalan (MEL fa lan)

Sound-Alike/Look-Alike Issues

melphalan may be confused with Mephyton®, Myleran®

Alkeran® may be confused with Alferon®, Leukeran®, Myleran®

Synonyms L-PAM; L-phenylalanine mustard; L-sarcolysin; phenylalanine mustard

U.S./Canadian Brand Names Alkeran® [US/Can]

Therapeutic Category Antineoplastic Agent

Use Palliative treatment of multiple myeloma and nonresectable epithelial ovarian carcinoma

Dosage Summary

I.V.:

Adults: 16 mg/m^2 administered at 2-week intervals for 4 doses, then repeat at 4-week intervals

Oral:

Children: Dosage not established

Adults: 6 mg/day for 2-3 weeks (initially) then (after 4-week rest) 2 mg once daily **or** 10 mg/day for 7-10 days, then 2 mg once daily (after 4- to 8-week rest period) **or** 0.15 mg/kg/day for 7 days, then ≤0.05 mg/kg/day (after 2- to 6-week rest period) **or** 0.25 mg/kg/day for 4 days or 0.2 mg/kg/day for 5 days every 4-6 weeks **or** 6 mg/m^2/day for 7 days every 4 weeks **or** 0.25 mg/kg/day for 4 days every 6 weeks **or** 9 mg/m^2/day for 4 days every 6 weeks **or** 7 mg/m^2/day in 2 divided doses for 5 days every 4 weeks

Dosage Forms

Injection, powder for reconstitution: 50 mg

Alkeran®: 50 mg

Tablet, oral:

Alkeran®: 2 mg

Melquin-3® [US-OTC] *see* hydroquinone *on page 487*

Melquin HP® [US-OTC] *see* hydroquinone *on page 487*

memantine (me MAN teen)

Sound-Alike/Look-Alike Issues

memantine may be confused with mesalamine

Synonyms memantine hydrochloride

U.S./Canadian Brand Names CO Memantine [Can]; Ebixa® [Can]; Namenda® [US]; PMS-Memantine [Can]; ratio-Memantine [Can]; Riva-Memantine [Can]; Sandoz-Memantine [Can]

Therapeutic Category N-Methyl-D-Aspartate Receptor Antagonist

Use Treatment of moderate-to-severe dementia of the Alzheimer type

Dosage Summary

Oral:

Children: Dosage not established

Adults: Initial: 5 mg once daily; Target: 20 mg/day in 2 divided doses; **Note:** Titration is recommended on a weekly basis

Product Availability Namenda XR™: FDA approved in June 2010; anticipated availability is currently undetermined.

Dosage Forms

Combination package, oral:

Namenda®: Tablet: 5 mg (28s) and Tablet: 10 mg (21s)

Solution, oral:

Namenda®: 2 mg/mL (360 mL)

Tablet, oral:

Namenda®: 5 mg, 10 mg

memantine hydrochloride *see* memantine *on page 599*

Menactra® [US] *see* meningococcal (groups A / C / Y and W-135) diphtheria conjugate vaccine *on page 601*

menACWY-D (Menactra®) *see* meningococcal (groups A / C / Y and W-135) diphtheria conjugate vaccine *on page 601*

menACWY-CRM (Menveo®) *see* meningococcal (groups A / C / Y and W-135) diphtheria conjugate vaccine *on page 601*

Menadol® ***(Discontinued)*** *see* ibuprofen *on page 494*

menCC *see* meningococcal group C-CRM197 conjugate vaccine *(Canada only) on page 600*

menC-CRM197 *see* meningococcal group C-CRM197 conjugate vaccine *(Canada only) on page 600*

Menest® [US/Can] *see* estrogens (esterified) *on page 371*

Meni-D® ***(Discontinued)*** *see* meclizine *on page 595*

meningococcal conjugate vaccine *see* meningococcal (groups A / C / Y and W-135) diphtheria conjugate vaccine *on page 601*

meningococcal group C-CRM197 conjugate vaccine *(Canada only)*

(me NIN joe kok al groop see see ahr em wuhn nahyn tee sev uhn KON joo gate vak SEEN)

Synonyms menC-CRM197; menCC

U.S./Canadian Brand Names Menjugate® [Can]

Therapeutic Category Vaccine

Use To provide active immunization against invasive meningococcal disease caused by *N. meningitidis* serogroup C, in children ≥2 months and adults

The National Advisory Committee on Immunization (NACI) recommendations for persons considered at an increased risk for meningococcal disease:

Chemoprophylaxis and immunoprophylaxis: Selection of meningococcal vaccination to be based upon serogroup(s):

Individuals living in the same household or with close contact (eg, kissing, shared cigarettes, shared eating or drinking utensils) of infected patient

Employees and children of nursery schools or day care

Immunoprophylaxis: Selection of meningococcal vaccination to be based upon serogroup(s):

Adolescents and young adults

Laboratory workers routinely exposed to isolates of *N. meningitidis*

Military recruits

Persons traveling to or who reside in countries where *N. meningitidis* is hyperendemic or epidemic, particularly if contact with local population will be prolonged

Persons with terminal complement component deficiencies

Persons with anatomic or functional asplenia

Note: Use is also recommended during meningococcal outbreaks caused by serogroup C.

Chemoprophylaxis:

Healthcare workers with intensive unprotected contact with infected patients

Airline passengers sitting directly next to an infected patient for duration of at least 8 hours

See NACI guidelines for specific drug treatment at http://www.phac-aspc.gc.ca/naci-ccni

Dosage Summary

I.M.:

Infants ≥2-12 months: 0.5 mL as a single dose for a total of 3 doses administered at least 4 weeks apart

Infants ≥4-11 months without prior vaccination: 0.5 mL as a single dose for a total of 2 doses administered at least 4 weeks apart

Children ≥1 year: 0.5 mL as a single dose

Adults: 0.5 mL as a single dose

Dosage Forms - Canada

Injection, powder for reconstitution:

Menjugate®: 10 mcg of oligosaccharide antigen group C

meningococcal (groups A / C / Y and W-135) diphtheria conjugate vaccine

(me NIN joe kok al groops aye, see, why & dubl yoo won thur tee fyve dif THEER ee a KON joo gate vak SEEN)

Synonyms MCV; MCV4; menACWY-CRM (Menveo®); menACWY-D (Menactra®); meningococcal conjugate vaccine

U.S./Canadian Brand Names Menactra® [US]; Menveo® [US]

Therapeutic Category Vaccine

Use Provide active immunization of children and adults against invasive meningococcal disease caused by *N. meningitidis* serogroups A, C, Y, and W-135. (Menactra® is FDA approved for use in children and adults 2-55 years of age; Menveo® is FDA approved for use in children and adults 11-55 years of age.)

The Advisory Committee on Immunization Practices (ACIP) recommends routine vaccination of all persons 11-18 years of age at the earliest opportunity. Adolescents should be vaccinated at the 11-12 year visit. For adolescents not previously vaccinated, vaccine should be administered prior to high school entry (~15 years of age).

The ACIP also recommends vaccination for persons at increased risk for meningococcal disease. Meningococcal conjugate vaccine (MCV4 [Menactra®]) should be used in children 2-10 years of age; MenACWY-CRM (Menveo®) or MCV4 (Menactra®) is preferred for persons aged 11-55 years; meningococcal polysaccharide vaccine (MPSV4 [Menomune®]) may be used if the conjugate vaccine is not available. MPSV4 is preferred in adults ≥56 years of age. Persons at increased risk include:

College freshmen living in dormitories

Microbiologists routinely exposed to isolates of *N. meningitides*

Military recruits

Persons traveling to or who reside in countries where *N. meningitides* is hyperendemic or epidemic, particularly if contact with local population will be prolonged

Persons with terminal complement component deficiencies

Persons with anatomic or functional asplenia

Use is also recommended during meningococcal outbreaks caused by vaccine preventable serogroups.

Dosage Summary

I.M.:

Children <2 years: Dosage not established

Children ≥2 years: Menactra®: 0.5 mL as a single dose

Adolescents 11-18 years: Menactra®, Menveo®: 0.5 mL as a single dose

Adults ≤55 years: Menactra®, Menveo®: 0.5 mL as a single dose

Adults >55 years: Dosage not established

Dosage Forms

Injection, solution [preservative free]:

Menactra®: 4 mcg each of polysaccharide antigen groups A, C, Y, and W-135 [bound to diphtheria toxoid 48 mcg] per 0.5 mL

Menveo®: MenA oligosaccharide 10 mcg, MenC oligosaccharide 5 mcg, MenY oligosaccharide 5 mcg, and MenW-135 oligosaccharide 5 mcg [bound to CRM_{197} protein 32.7-64.1 mcg] per 0.5 mL

meningococcal polysaccharide vaccine *see* meningococcal polysaccharide vaccine (groups A / C / Y and W-135) *on page 601*

meningococcal polysaccharide vaccine (groups A / C / Y and W-135)

(me NIN joe kok al pol i SAK a ride vak SEEN groops aye, see, why & dubl yoo won thur tee fyve)

Synonyms meningococcal polysaccharide vaccine; MPSV; MPSV4

U.S./Canadian Brand Names Menomune®-A/C/Y/W-135 [US]

Therapeutic Category Vaccine, Live Bacteria

Use Provide active immunity to meningococcal serogroups contained in the vaccine

The Advisory Committee on Immunization Practices (ACIP) recommends routine vaccination for persons at increased risk for meningococcal disease. (Meningococcal polysaccharide vaccine [MPSV4; Menomune®] is preferred in adults ≥56 years of age; Meningococcal conjugate vaccine [MCV4; Menactra®] is preferred for persons aged 2-55 years; MPSV4 may be used if MCV4 is not available.)

Persons at increased risk include:

College freshmen living in dormitories

Microbiologists routinely exposed to isolates of *N. meningitides*

Military recruits

Persons traveling to or who reside in countries where *N. meningitides* is hyperendemic or epidemic, particularly if contact with local population will be prolonged

Persons with terminal complement component deficiencies

Persons with anatomic or functional asplenia

Use is also recommended during meningococcal outbreaks caused by vaccine preventable serogroups.

Dosage Summary

SubQ:

Children <2 years: Not usually recommended

Children ≥2 years: 0.5 mL as a single dose

Adults: 0.5 mL as a single dose

Dosage Forms

Injection, powder for reconstitution [MPSV4]:

Menomune®-A/C/Y/W-135: 50 mcg each of polysaccharide antigen groups A, C, Y, and W-135 per 0.5 mL dose

Menjugate® [Can] *see* meningococcal group C-CRM197 conjugate vaccine *(Canada only) on page 600*

Menomune®-A/C/Y/W-135 [US] *see* meningococcal polysaccharide vaccine (groups A / C / Y and W-135) *on page 601*

Menopur® [US/Can] *see* menotropins *on page 602*

Menostar® [US/Can] *see* estradiol (systemic) *on page 366*

menotropins (men oh TROE pins)

Sound-Alike/Look-Alike Issues

Repronex® may be confused with Regranex®

Synonyms hMG; human menopausal gonadotropin

U.S./Canadian Brand Names Menopur® [US/Can]; Repronex® [US/Can]

Therapeutic Category Gonadotropin

Use Female:

In conjunction with hCG to induce ovulation and pregnancy in infertile females experiencing oligoanovulation or anovulation when the cause of anovulation is functional and not caused by primary ovarian failure (Repronex®)

Stimulation of multiple follicle development in ovulatory patients as part of an assisted reproductive technology (ART) (Menopur®, Repronex®)

Dosage Summary

I.M.:

Children: Dosage not established

Adults: Repronex®: Initial: 150 int. units **or** 225 int. units daily, followed by hCG (maximum: 450 int. units/day; 12 days of therapy); **Note:** Titration is recommended

SubQ:

Children: Dosage not established

Adults:

Menopur®: Initial: 225 int. units daily, followed by hCG (maximum: 450 int. units/day; 20 days of therapy): **Note:** Titration is recommended

Repronex®: Initial: 150 int. units **or** 225 int. units daily, followed by hCG (maximum: 450 int. units/day; 12 days of therapy); **Note:** Titration is recommended

Dosage Forms

Injection, powder for reconstitution:

Menopur®, Repronex®: Follicle stimulating hormone activity 75 int. units and luteinizing hormone activity 75 int. units

Mentax® [US] *see* butenafine *on page 160*

menthol and methyl salicylate *see* methyl salicylate and menthol *on page 623*

menthol and zinc oxide (topical) (MEN thole & zink OKS ide)

U.S./Canadian Brand Names Calmoseptine® [US-OTC]; Risamine™ [US-OTC]

Therapeutic Category Protectant, Topical; Topical Skin Product

Use Provides a barrier to protect intact and/or injured skin from moisture, wound or fistula drainage, urine, or feces; diaper rash

Dosage Summary

Topical:

Children: Apply thin layer to clean, dry skin 2-4 times/day or after each incontinent episode/diaper change

Adults: Apply thin layer to clean, dry skin 2-4 times/day or after each incontinent episode/diaper change

Dosage Forms

Ointment, topical:

Calmoseptine®: Methanol 0.44% and zinc oxide 20.625% (3.5 g/packet, 75 g, 120 g)

Risamine™: Menthol 0.44% and zinc oxide 20.625% (113 g)

Menveo® [US] *see* meningococcal (groups A / C / Y and W-135) diphtheria conjugate vaccine *on page* 601

292 MEP® [Can] *see* meprobamate and aspirin *on page* 606

mepenzolate (me PEN zoe late)

Sound-Alike/Look-Alike Issues

Cantil® may be confused with Bentyl®

Synonyms mepenzolate bromide

U.S./Canadian Brand Names Cantil® [US/Can]

Therapeutic Category Anticholinergic Agent

Use Adjunctive treatment of peptic ulcer disease

Dosage Summary

Oral:

Children: Dosage not established

Adults: 25-50 mg 4 times/day with meals and at bedtime

Dosage Forms

Tablet, oral:

Cantil®: 25 mg

mepenzolate bromide *see* mepenzolate *on page* 603

meperidine (me PER i deen)

Sound-Alike/Look-Alike Issues

meperidine may be confused with meprobamate

Demerol® may be confused with Demulen®, Desyrel®, dicumarol, Dilaudid®, Dymelor®, Pamelor®

Synonyms isonipecaine hydrochloride; meperidine hydrochloride; pethidine hydrochloride

U.S./Canadian Brand Names Demerol® [US/Can]

Therapeutic Category Analgesic, Narcotic

Controlled Substance C-II

Use Management of moderate-to-severe pain; adjunct to anesthesia and preoperative sedation

Dosage Summary

I.M.:

Children: 1-1.5 mg/kg/dose every 3-4 hours as needed **or** 1-2 mg/kg as a single dose preoperatively (maximum: 100 mg/dose)

Adults: Initial: 50-75 mg every 3-4 hours as needed **or** 50-100 mg as a single dose preoperatively

Elderly: 25 mg every 4 hours

I.V.:

Children: 1-1.5 mg/kg/dose every 3-4 hours as needed **or** 1-2 mg as a single dose preoperatively (maximum: 100 mg/dose)

Adults: Initial: 5-10 mg every 5 minutes as needed

Oral:

Children: 1-1.5 mg/kg/dose every 3-4 hours as needed (maximum: 100 mg/dose)

Adults: Initial: 50 mg every 3-4 hours as needed; Maintenance: 50-150 mg every 2-4 hours as needed

Elderly: 50 mg every 4 hours

SubQ:

Children: 1-1.5 mg/kg/dose every 3-4 hours as needed **or** 1-2 mg as a single dose preoperatively (maximum: 100 mg/dose)

Adults: Initial: 50-75 mg every 3-4 hours as needed **or** 50-100 mg as a single dose preoperatively

Dosage Forms

Injection, solution: 10 mg/mL (30 mL, 50 mL, 60 mL); 25 mg/mL (1 mL); 50 mg/mL (1 mL); 100 mg/mL (1 mL)

Demerol®: 25 mg/mL (1 mL); 25 mg/0.5 mL (0.5 mL); 50 mg/mL (1 mL, 1.5 mL, 2 mL, 30 mL); 75 mg/mL (1 mL); 100 mg/mL (1 mL, 20 mL)

Solution, oral: 50 mg/5 mL (500 mL)

Tablet, oral: 50 mg, 100 mg

Demerol®: 50 mg, 100 mg

meperidine and promethazine *(Discontinued)*

meperidine hydrochloride *see* meperidine *on page* 603

mephobarbital (me foe BAR bi tal)

Sound-Alike/Look-Alike Issues

mephobarbital may be confused with methocarbamol

Mebaral® may be confused with Medrol®, Mellaril®, Tegretol®

Synonyms methylphenobarbital

U.S./Canadian Brand Names Mebaral® [US/Can]

Therapeutic Category Barbiturate

Controlled Substance C-IV

Use Sedative; treatment of grand mal and petit mal epilepsy

Dosage Summary

Oral:

Children <5 years: 6-12 mg/kg/day in 2-4 divided doses **or** 16-32 mg 3-4 times/day

Children ≥5 years: 6-12 mg/kg/day in 2-4 divided doses **or** 32-64 mg 3-4 times/day

Adults: 96-600 mg/day in 2-4 divided doses

Dosage Forms

Tablet, oral:

Mebaral®: 32 mg, 50 mg, 100 mg

Mephyton® [US/Can] *see* phytonadione *on page* 759

mepivacaine (me PIV a kane)

Sound-Alike/Look-Alike Issues

mepivacaine may be confused with bupivacaine

Polocaine® may be confused with prilocaine

Synonyms mepivacaine hydrochloride

U.S./Canadian Brand Names Carbocaine® [US/Can]; Polocaine® Dental [US]; Polocaine® MPF [US]; Polocaine® [US/Can]; Scandonest® 3% Plain [US]

Therapeutic Category Local Anesthetic

Use Local or regional analgesia; anesthesia by local infiltration, peripheral and central neural techniques (epidural and caudal); **not** for use in spinal anesthesia

Dosage Summary

Brachial, cervical, intercostal, pudendal nerve block:

Children: Dosage not established

Adults: 5-40 mL of 1% solution **or** 5-20 mL of 2% solution (maximum: 400 mg)

Caudal and epidural block (preservative free solutions only):

Children: Dosage not established

Adults: 15-30 mL of 1% solution (maximum: 300 mg) **or** 10-25 mL of 1.5% solution (maximum: 375 mg) **or** 10-20 mL of a 2% solution (maximum: 400 mg)

Dental anesthesia:

Children: Dosage not established

Adults: 54 mg (1.8 mL) as a 3% solution (single site) **or** 270 mg (9 mL) as a 3% solution (entire oral cavity) (maximum: 400 mg)

Infiltration:

Children: Dosage not established

Adults: Up to 40 mL of 1% solution (maximum: 400 mg)

Local injection:

Children <3 years or <14 kg: Dose varies; only concentrations less than 2% should be used (maximum: 5-6 mg/kg)

Children ≥3 years or ≥14 kg: Dose varies (maximum: 5-6 mg/kg)

Adults: Dose varies (maximum: 400 mg/dose; 1000 mg/day)

Paracervical block:

Children: Dosage not established

Adults: Up to 20 mL (both sides) of 1% solution (maximum: 200 mg)

Therapeutic block:

Children: Dosage not established

Adults: 1-5 mL of 1% solution (maximum: 50 mg) or 1-5 mL of 2% solution (maximum: 100 mg)

Transvaginal block:

Children: Dosage not established

Adults: Up to 30 mL (both sides) of a 1% solution (maximum: 300 mg)

Dosage Forms

Injection, solution: 3% [30 mg/mL] (1.8 mL)

Carbocaine®: 1% [10 mg/mL] (50 mL); 2% [20 mg/mL] (50 mL); 3% [30 mg/mL] (1.7 mL)

Polocaine®: 1% [10 mg/mL] (50 mL); 2% [20 mg/mL] (50 mL)

Polocaine® Dental: 3% [30 mg/mL] (1.7 mL)

Scandonest® 3% Plain: 3% [30 mg/mL] (1.7 mL)

Injection, solution [preservative free]:

Carbocaine®: 1% [10 mg/mL] (30 mL); 1.5% [15 mg/mL] (30 mL); 2% [20 mg/mL] (20 mL)

Polocaine® MPF: 1% [10 mg/mL] (30 mL); 1.5% [15 mg/mL] (30 mL); 2% [20 mg/mL] (20 mL)

mepivacaine and levonordefrin (me PIV a kane & lee voe nor DEF rin)

Synonyms levonordefrin and mepivacaine hydrochloride

U.S./Canadian Brand Names Carbocaine® 2% with Neo-Cobefrin® [US]; Polocaine® 2% and Levonordefrin 1:20,000 [Can]; Polocaine® Dental with Levonordefrin [US]; Scandonest® 2% L [US]

Therapeutic Category Local Anesthetic

Use Amide-type anesthetic used for local infiltration anesthesia; injection near nerve trunks to produce nerve block

Dosage Summary

Infiltration and nerve block (single site):

Children ≤10 years: Dosage not established

Children >10 years: 36 mg (1.8 mL) of mepivacaine hydrochloride as a 2% solution with levonordefrin 1:20,000

Adults: 36 mg (1.8 mL) of mepivacaine hydrochloride as a 2% solution with levonordefrin 1:20,000

Infiltration and nerve block (entire cavity):

Children ≤10 years: Carefully calculate on basis of patient's weight (maximum: 6.6 mg/kg; 180 mg of mepivacaine as 2% solution with levonordefrin 1:20,000)

Children >10 years: 180 mg (9 mL) of mepivacaine hydrochloride as 2% solution with levonordefrin 1:20,000 (maximum: 6.6 mg/kg; 400 mg of mepivacaine hydrochloride per appointment)

Adults: 180 mg (9 mL) of mepivacaine hydrochloride as 2% solution with levonordefrin 1:20,000 (maximum: 6.6 mg/kg; 400 mg of mepivacaine hydrochloride per appointment)

Dosage Forms

Injection, solution [for dental use]:

Carbocaine® 2% with Neo-Cobefrin®: Mepivacaine 2% and levonordefrin 1:20,000 (1.7 mL)

Polocaine® Dental with Levonordefrin: Mepivacaine 2% and levonordefrin 1:20,000 (1.7 mL)

Scandonest® 2% L: Mepivacaine 2% and levonordefrin 1:20,000 (1.7 mL)

mepivacaine hydrochloride *see* mepivacaine *on page 604*

meprobamate (me proe BA mate)

Sound-Alike/Look-Alike Issues

meprobamate may be confused with Mepergan, meperidine

U.S./Canadian Brand Names Novo-Mepro [Can]

Therapeutic Category Antianxiety Agent

Controlled Substance C-IV

Use Management of anxiety disorders

Dosage Summary

Oral:

Children <6 years: Dosage not established
Children 6-12 years: 100-200 mg 2-3 times/day
Adults: 400 mg 3-4 times/day (maximum: 2400 mg/day)
Elderly: Initial: 200 mg 2-3 times/day

Dosage Forms

Tablet, oral: 200 mg, 400 mg

meprobamate and aspirin (me proe BA mate & AS pir in)

Synonyms aspirin and meprobamate

U.S./Canadian Brand Names 292 MEP® [Can]; Equagesic® [US]

Therapeutic Category Skeletal Muscle Relaxant

Controlled Substance C-IV

Use Adjunct to the short-term treatment of pain in patients with skeletal-muscular disease exhibiting tension and/or anxiety

Dosage Summary

Oral:

Children <12 years: Dosage not established
Children ≥12 years: 1-2 tablets 3-4 times/day for up to 10 days
Adults: 1-2 tablet 3-4 times/day for up to 10 days

Dosage Forms

Tablet:

Equagesic®: Meprobamate 200 mg and aspirin 325 mg

Mepron® [US/Can] *see* atovaquone *on page 104*

mequinol and tretinoin (ME kwi nole & TRET i noyn)

Synonyms tretinoin and mequinol

U.S./Canadian Brand Names Solagé® [US/Can]

Therapeutic Category Retinoic Acid Derivative; Vitamin A Derivative; Vitamin, Topical

Use Treatment of solar lentigines; the efficacy of using Solagé® daily for >24 weeks has not been established

Dosage Summary

Topical:

Children: Dosage not established
Adults: Apply twice daily, separate application by at least 8 hours

mercaptoethane sulfonate *see* mesna *on page 608*

mercaptopurine (mer kap toe PYOOR een)

Sound-Alike/Look-Alike Issues

mercaptopurine may be confused with methotrexate
Purinethol® may be confused with propylthiouracil
6-Mercaptopurine (error-prone abbreviation)
6-MP (error-prone abbreviation)

Synonyms NSC-755

U.S./Canadian Brand Names Purinethol® [US/Can]

Therapeutic Category Antineoplastic Agent

Use Treatment (maintenance and induction) of acute lymphoblastic leukemia (ALL)

Dosage Summary

Oral:

Children: Induction: 2.5-5 mg/kg/day **or** 70-100 mg/m^2/day given once daily; Maintenance: 1.5-2.5 mg/kg/day **or** 50-75 mg/m^2/day given once daily
Adults: Induction: 2.5-5 mg/kg/day (100-200 mg); Maintenance: 1.5-2.5 mg/kg/day **or** 80-100 mg/m^2/day given once daily

Dosage Forms

Tablet, oral: 50 mg
Purinethol®: 50 mg

mercapturic acid *see* acetylcysteine *on page 34*
Meridia® [US/Can] *see* sibutramine *on page 873*

meropenem (mer oh PEN em)

Sound-Alike/Look-Alike Issues
meropenem may be confused with ertapenem, imipenem, metronidazole

U.S./Canadian Brand Names Merrem® I.V. [US]; Merrem® [Can]

Therapeutic Category Carbapenem (Antibiotic)

Use Treatment of intraabdominal infections (complicated appendicitis and peritonitis); treatment of bacterial meningitis in pediatric patients ≥3 months of age caused by *S. pneumoniae*, *H. influenzae*, and *N. meningitidis*; treatment of complicated skin and skin structure infections caused by susceptible organisms

Dosage Summary
I.V.:
Neonates (postnatal age 0-7 days): 20 mg/kg/dose every 12 hours
Neonates (postnatal age >7 days and 1200-2000 g): 20 mg/kg/dose every 12 hours
Neonates (postnatal age >7 days and >2000 g): 20 mg/kg/dose every 8 hours
Children ≥3 months and <50 kg: 10-40 mg/kg every 8 hours (maximum: 2 g every 8 hours)
Children ≥50 kg: 500 mg to 2 g every 8 hours
Adults: 500 mg to 2 g every 8 hours

Dosage Forms
Injection, powder for reconstitution: 500 mg, 1 g
Merrem® I.V.: 500 mg, 1 g

Merrem® [Can] *see* meropenem *on page 607*
Merrem® I.V. [US] *see* meropenem *on page 607*
Mersyndol® With Codeine [Can] *see* acetaminophen, codeine, and doxylamine *(Canada only) on page 28*
Meruvax® II *(Discontinued)* *see* rubella virus vaccine (live) *on page 855*

mesalamine (me SAL a meen)

Sound-Alike/Look-Alike Issues
mesalamine may be confused with mecamylamine, megestrol, memantine, metaxalone, methenamine
Apriso™ may be confused with Apri®
Asacol® may be confused with Ansaid®, Os-Cal®, Visicol®
Lialda™ may be confused with Aldara®
Pentasa® may be confused with Pancrease®, Pangestyme™

Synonyms 5-aminosalicylic acid; 5-ASA; fisalamine; mesalazine

U.S./Canadian Brand Names Apriso™ [US]; Asacol® 800 [Can]; Asacol® HD [US]; Asacol® [US/Can]; Canasa® [US]; Lialda™ [US]; Mesasal® [Can]; Mezavant® [Can]; Novo-5 ASA [Can]; Pentasa® [US/Can]; Rowasa® [US]; Salofalk® [Can]; sfRowasa™ [US]

Therapeutic Category 5-Aminosalicylic Acid Derivative

Use
Oral:
Asacol®, Pentasa®: Treatment and maintenance of remission of mildly- to moderately-active ulcerative colitis
Apriso™: Maintenance of remission of ulcerative colitis
Asacol® HD: Treatment of moderately-active ulcerative colitis
Lialda™: Treatment of mildly- to moderately-active ulcerative colitis
Rectal: Treatment of active mild-to-moderate distal ulcerative colitis, proctosigmoiditis, or proctitis

Dosage Summary
Oral:
Children: Dosage not established
Adults:
Capsule:
Apriso™: 1.5 g once daily
Pentasa®: 1 g 4 times/day
Tablet:
Asacol®: 800 mg 3 times/day or 1600 g/day in divided doses
Asacol® HD: 1.6 g 3 times/day
Lialda™, Mezavant®: 2.4-4.8 g once daily

Rectal:

Children: Dosage not established

Adults:

Retention enema: 60 mL (4 g) at bedtime, retained overnight (~8 hours)

Suppository: Insert 1000 mg at bedtime; **Note:** Suppositories should be retained for at least 1-3 hours to achieve maximum benefit

Dosage Forms

Capsule, controlled release, oral:

Pentasa®: 250 mg, 500 mg

Capsule, delayed and extended release, oral:

Apriso™: 0.375 g

Suppository, rectal:

Canasa®: 1000 mg (30s, 42s)

Suspension, rectal: 4 g/60 mL (7s, 28s)

Rowasa®: 4 g/60 mL (7s, 28s)

sfRowasa™: 4 g/60 mL (7s, 28s)

Tablet, delayed release, enteric coated, oral:

Asacol®: 400 mg

Asacol® HD: 800 mg

Lialda™: 1.2 g

Dosage Forms - Canada

Tablet, delayed and extended release:

Mezavant®: 1.2 g

mesalazine *see* mesalamine *on page 607*

Mesasal® [Can] *see* mesalamine *on page 607*

M-Eslon® [Can] *see* morphine (systemic) *on page 644*

mesna (MES na)

Synonyms mercaptoethane sulfonate; sodium 2-mercaptoethane sulfonate

U.S./Canadian Brand Names Mesnex® [US/Can]; Uromitexan [Can]

Therapeutic Category Antidote

Use Preventative agent to reduce the incidence of ifosfamide-induced hemorrhagic cystitis

Dosage Summary

I.V.:

Children: 60% of the ifosfamide dose given in 3 divided doses

Adults: 60% of the ifosfamide dose given in 3 divided doses

I.V./Oral:

Children: 100% of the ifosfamide dose, given as 20% I.V., followed by 2 (40% each) doses orally

Adults: 100% of the ifosfamide dose, given as 20% I.V., followed by 2 (40% each) doses orally

Dosage Forms

Injection, solution: 100 mg/mL (10 mL)

Mesnex®: 100 mg/mL (10 mL)

Tablet, oral:

Mesnex®: 400 mg

Mesnex® [US/Can] *see* mesna *on page 608*

Mestinon® [US/Can] *see* pyridostigmine *on page 817*

Mestinon® Injection *(Discontinued)* *see* pyridostigmine *on page 817*

Mestinon®-SR [Can] *see* pyridostigmine *on page 817*

Mestinon® Timespan® [US] *see* pyridostigmine *on page 817*

mestranol and norethindrone *see* norethindrone and mestranol *on page 683*

Metadate CD® [US] *see* methylphenidate *on page 621*

Metadate® ER [US] *see* methylphenidate *on page 621*

Metadol™ [Can] *see* methadone *on page 611*

Metadol-D™ [Can] *see* methadone *on page 611*

Metaglip™ [US] *see* glipizide and metformin *on page 447*

123 meta-iodobenzlyguanidine sulfate *see* iobenguane I 123 *on page 517*

Metamucil® [US-OTC/Can] *see* psyllium *on page 814*

Metamucil® Plus Calcium [US-OTC] *see* psyllium *on page 814*
Metamucil® Smooth Texture [US-OTC] *see* psyllium *on page 814*

metaproterenol (met a proe TER e nol)

Sound-Alike/Look-Alike Issues
metaproterenol may be confused with metipranolol, metoprolol
Alupent® may be confused with Atrovent®

Synonyms metaproterenol sulfate; orciprenaline sulfate

U.S./Canadian Brand Names Apo-Orciprenaline® [Can]; ratio-Orciprenaline® [Can]; Tanta-Orciprenaline® [Can]

Therapeutic Category Adrenergic Agonist Agent

Use Bronchodilator in reversible airway obstruction due to asthma or COPD

Dosage Summary

Inhalation:
Children ≤12 years: Dosage not established
Children >12 years: 2-3 inhalations every 3-4 hours (maximum: 12 inhalations/day)
Adults: 2-3 inhalations every 3-4 hours (maximum: 12 inhalations/day)

Nebulizer:
Infants: 0.01-0.02 mL/kg of 5% solution diluted in 2-3 mL normal saline every 4-6 hours (minimum: 0.1 mL/dose; maximum: 0.3 mL/dose)
Children: 0.01-0.02 mL/kg of 5% solution diluted in 2-3 mL normal saline every 4-6 hours (minimum: 0.1 mL/dose; maximum: 0.3 mL/dose)
Adolescents: 5-20 breaths of full strength 5% metaproterenol **or** 0.2 to 0.3 mL 5% metaproterenol in 2.5-3 mL normal saline every 4-6 hours
Adults: 5-20 breaths of full strength 5% metaproterenol **or** 0.2 to 0.3 mL 5% metaproterenol in 2.5-3 mL normal saline every 4-6 hours

Oral:
Children <2 years: 0.4 mg/kg/dose 3-4 times/day (every 8-12 hours for infants)
Children 2-6 years: 1-2.6 mg/kg/day divided every 6 hours
Children 6-9 years: 10 mg/dose 3-4 times/day
Children >9 years: 20 mg 3-4 times/day
Adults: 20 mg 3-4 times/day
Elderly: Initial: 10 mg 3-4 times/day, may increase to 20 mg 3-4 times/day

Dosage Forms
Syrup, oral: 10 mg/5 mL (473 mL)
Tablet, oral: 10 mg, 20 mg

metaproterenol sulfate *see* metaproterenol *on page 609*
Metasep® ***(Discontinued)***
Metastron® [US/Can] *see* strontium-89 *on page 896*

metaxalone (me TAKS a lone)

Sound-Alike/Look-Alike Issues
metaxalone may be confused with mesalamine, metolazone
Skelaxin® may be confused with Robaxin®

U.S./Canadian Brand Names Skelaxin® [US/Can]

Therapeutic Category Skeletal Muscle Relaxant

Use Relief of discomfort associated with acute, painful musculoskeletal conditions

Dosage Summary

Oral:
Children ≤12 years: Dosage not established
Children >12 years: 800 mg 3-4 times/day
Adults: 800 mg 3-4 times/day

Dosage Forms
Tablet, oral: 800 mg
Skelaxin®: 800 mg

metformin (met FOR min)

Sound-Alike/Look-Alike Issues
metFORMIN may be confused with metroNIDAZOLE

Glucophage® may be confused with Glucotrol®, Glutofac®

Synonyms metformin hydrochloride

Tall-Man met**FORMIN**

U.S./Canadian Brand Names Apo-Metformin® [Can]; CO Metformin [Can]; Dom-Metformin [Can]; Fortamet® [US]; Glucophage® XR [US]; Glucophage® [US/Can]; Glumetza® [US/Can]; Glycon [Can]; Med-Metformin [Can]; Mylan-Metformin [Can]; Novo-Metformin [Can]; Nu-Metformin [Can]; PHL-Metformin [Can]; PMS-Metformin [Can]; PRO-Metformin [Can]; RAN™-Metformin [Can]; ratio-Metformin [Can]; Riomet® [US]; Riva-Metformin [Can]; Sandoz-Metformin FC [Can]

Therapeutic Category Antidiabetic Agent, Oral

Use Management of type 2 diabetes mellitus (noninsulin-dependent, NIDDM) as monotherapy when hyperglycemia cannot be managed with diet and exercise alone. In adults, may be used concomitantly with a sulfonylurea or insulin to improve glycemic control.

Dosage Summary

Oral:

Extended release:

Children: Dosage not established

Adults: Initial: 500 mg once daily; Maintenance: Up to 2000-2500 mg/day (varies by product) in 1-2 divided doses; **Note:** Titration is recommended

Immediate release:

Children <10 years: Dosage not established

Children 10-16 years: Initial: 500 mg twice daily; Maintenance: Up to 2000 mg/day in divided doses; **Note:** Titration is recommended

Children >16 years: Initial: 500 mg twice daily **or** 850 mg once daily; Maintenance: Up to 2000 mg/day in 2 divided doses **or** 2550 mg/day in 3 divided doses; **Note:** Titration is recommended

Adults: Initial: 500 mg twice daily **or** 850 mg once daily; Maintenance: Up to 2000 mg/day in 2 divided doses **or** 2550 mg/day in 3 divided doses; **Note:** Titration is recommended

Dosage Forms

Solution, oral:

Riomet®: 100 mg/mL (118 mL, 473 mL)

Tablet, oral: 500 mg, 850 mg, 1000 mg

Glucophage®: 500 mg, 850 mg, 1000 mg

Tablet, extended release, oral: 500 mg, 750 mg

Fortamet®: 500 mg, 1000 mg

Glucophage® XR: 500 mg, 750 mg

Glumetza®: 500 mg, 1000 mg

metformin and glipizide *see* glipizide and metformin *on page 447*

metformin and glyburide *see* glyburide and metformin *on page 449*

metformin and repaglinide *see* repaglinide and metformin *on page 835*

metformin and rosiglitazone *see* rosiglitazone and metformin *on page 853*

metformin and sitagliptin *see* sitagliptin and metformin *on page 879*

metformin hydrochloride *see* metformin *on page 609*

metformin hydrochloride and pioglitazone hydrochloride *see* pioglitazone and metformin *on page 763*

metformin hydrochloride and rosiglitazone maleate *see* rosiglitazone and metformin *on page 853*

methacholine (meth a KOLE leen)

Synonyms methacholine chloride

U.S./Canadian Brand Names Methacholine Omega [Can]; Provocholine® [US/Can]

Therapeutic Category Diagnostic Agent

Use Diagnosis of bronchial airway hyperactivity

Dosage Summary

Inhalation:

Children <5 years: Dosage not established

Children ≥5 years: 5 breaths of each of the following concentrations 0.025 mg/mL, 0.25 mg/mL, 2.5 mg/mL, 10 mg/mL and 25 mg/mL

Adults: 5 breaths of each of the following concentrations 0.025 mg/mL, 0.25 mg/mL, 2.5 mg/mL, 10 mg/mL and 25 mg/mL

Dosage Forms

Powder for reconstitution, for oral inhalation:
Provocholine®: 100 mg

methacholine chloride *see* methacholine *on page* 610
Methacholine Omega [Can] *see* methacholine *on page* 610

methadone (METH a done)

Sound-Alike/Look-Alike Issues

methadone may be confused with dexmethylphenidate, Mephyton®, methylphenidate, Metadate® CD, Metadate® ER, morphine

Synonyms methadone hydrochloride

U.S./Canadian Brand Names Dolophine® [US]; Metadol-D™ [Can]; Metadol™ [Can]; Methadone Diskets® [US]; Methadone Intensol™ [US]; Methadose® [US]

Therapeutic Category Analgesic, Narcotic

Controlled Substance C-II

Use Management of moderate-to-severe pain; detoxification and maintenance treatment of opioid addiction as part of an FDA-approved program

Dosage Summary

I.M.:
Children: Dosage not established
Adults: Initial: 2.5-10 mg every 8-12 hours; Titrate slowly to effect
Elderly: 2.5 mg every 8-12 hours

I.V.:
Adults: Initial: 2.5-10 mg every 8-12 hours; Titrate slowly to effect

Oral:
Adults:
Detoxification: Initial: Up to 40 mg/day; Maintenance: 80-120 mg/day
Pain: 2.5-10 mg every 4-12 hours as needed
Elderly: 2.5 mg every 8-12 hours

SubQ:
Children: Dosage not established
Adults: Initial: 2.5-10 mg every 8-12 hours; Titrate slowly to effect

Dosage Forms

Injection, solution: 10 mg/mL (20 mL)
Solution, oral: 5 mg/5 mL (500 mL); 10 mg/5 mL (500 mL); 10 mg/mL (946 mL, 960 mL, 1000 mL)
Methadone Intensol™: 10 mg/mL (30 mL)
Methadose®: 10 mg/mL (1000 mL)
Tablet, oral: 5 mg, 10 mg
Dolophine®: 5 mg, 10 mg
Tablet, dispersible, oral: 40 mg
Methadone Diskets®: 40 mg
Methadose®: 40 mg

Methadone Diskets® [US] *see* methadone *on page* 611
methadone hydrochloride *see* methadone *on page* 611
Methadone Intensol™ [US] *see* methadone *on page* 611
Methadose® [US] *see* methadone *on page* 611
methaminodiazepoxide hydrochloride *see* chlordiazepoxide *on page* 203

methamphetamine (meth am FET a meen)

Sound-Alike/Look-Alike Issues

Desoxyn® may be confused with digoxin

Synonyms desoxyephedrine hydrochloride; methamphetamine hydrochloride

U.S./Canadian Brand Names Desoxyn® [US/Can]

Therapeutic Category Amphetamine

Controlled Substance C-II

Use Treatment of attention-deficit/hyperactivity disorder (ADHD); exogenous obesity (short-term adjunct)

Dosage Summary

Oral:

Children <6 years: Dosage not established

Children ≥6-11 years: Initial: 5 mg 1-2 times/day; Maintenance: 20-25 mg/day; **Note:** Titration is recommended

Children ≥12 years:

ADHD: Initial: 5 mg 1-2 times/day; Maintenance: 20-25 mg/day; **Note:** Titration is recommended

Obesity: 5 mg before each meal

Adults:

ADHD: Initial: 5 mg 1-2 times/day; Maintenance: 20-25 mg/day; **Note:** Titration is recommended

Obesity: 5 mg before each meal

Dosage Forms

Tablet, oral: 5 mg

Desoxyn®: 5 mg

methamphetamine hydrochloride *see* methamphetamine *on page 611*

methazolamide (meth a ZOE la mide)

Sound-Alike/Look-Alike Issues

methazolamide may be confused with methenamine, metolazone

Neptazane™ may be confused with Nesacaine®

U.S./Canadian Brand Names Apo-Methazolamide® [Can]; Neptazane™ [US]

Therapeutic Category Carbonic Anhydrase Inhibitor

Use Treatment of chronic open-angle or secondary glaucoma; short-term therapy of acute angle-closure glaucoma prior to surgery

Dosage Summary

Oral:

Children: Dosage not established

Adults: 50-100 mg 2-3 times/day

Dosage Forms

Tablet, oral: 25 mg, 50 mg

Neptazane™: 25 mg, 50 mg

methenamine (meth EN a meen)

Sound-Alike/Look-Alike Issues

methenamine may be confused with mesalamine, methazolamide, methionine

Hiprex® may be confused with Mirapex®

Urex® may be confused with Eurax®, Serax®

Synonyms hexamethylenetetramine; methenamine hippurate; methenamine mandelate

U.S./Canadian Brand Names Dehydral® [Can]; Hiprex® [US/Can]; Mandelamine® [Can]; Urasal® [Can]; Urex™ [Can]

Therapeutic Category Antibiotic, Miscellaneous

Use Prophylaxis or suppression of recurrent urinary tract infections; urinary tract discomfort secondary to hypermotility

Dosage Summary

Oral:

Hippurate:

Children <6 years: Dosage not established

Children ≥6 years: 0.5-1 g twice daily

Adults: 1 g twice daily

Mandelate:

Children ≤2 years: Dosage not established

Children >2-6 years: 50-75 mg/kg/day in 3-4 divided doses **or** 0.25 g/30 lb 4 times/day

Children 6-12 years: 50-75 mg/kg/day in 3-4 divided doses or 0.5 g 4 times/day

Children >12 years: 1 g 4 times/day

Adults: 1 g 4 times/day

Dosage Forms

Tablet, oral: 500 mg, 1 g

Hiprex®: 1 g

methenamine hippurate *see* methenamine *on page 612*

methenamine mandelate *see* methenamine *on page 612*

methenamine, phenyl salicylate, methylene blue, benzoic acid, and hyoscyamine

(meth EN a meen, fen nil sa LIS i late, METH i leen bloo, ben ZOE ik AS id & hye oh SYE a meen)

Synonyms benzoic acid, hyoscyamine, methenamine, methylene blue, and phenyl salicylate; benzoic acid, methenamine, methylene blue, phenyl salicylate, and hyoscyamine; hyoscyamine, methenamine, benzoic acid, phenyl salicylate, and methylene blue; methylene blue, methenamine, benzoic acid, phenyl salicylate, and hyoscyamine; phenyl salicylate, methenamine, methylene blue, benzoic acid, and hyoscyamine

U.S./Canadian Brand Names Prosed®/DS [US]

Therapeutic Category Antibiotic, Miscellaneous

Use Urinary tract discomfort secondary to hypermotility resulting from infection or diagnostic procedures

Dosage Summary

Oral:

Children ≤12 years: Dosage not established

Children >12 years: Must be individualized

Adults: One tablet 4 times/day

Dosage Forms

Tablet, oral:

Prosed®/DS: Methenamine 81.6 mg, phenyl salicylate 36.2 mg, methylene blue 10.8 mg, benzoic acid 9 mg, hyoscyamine sulfate 0.12 mg

Methergine® [US/Can] *see* methylergonovine *on page 619*

methimazole (meth IM a zole)

Sound-Alike/Look-Alike Issues

methimazole may be confused with metolazone

Synonyms thiamazole

U.S./Canadian Brand Names Dom-Methimazole [Can]; PHL-Methimazole [Can]; Tapazole® [US/Can]

Therapeutic Category Antithyroid Agent

Use Treatment of hyperthyroidism; improve hyperthyroidism prior to thyroidectomy or radioactive iodine therapy

Dosage Summary

Oral:

Children: Initial: 0.4 mg/kg/day in 3 divided doses (approximately every 8 hours); Maintenance: 0.2 mg/kg/day i n 3 divided doses (approximately every 8 hours)

Adults: Initial: 15-60 mg/day in 3 divided doses (approximately every 8 hours); Maintenance: 5-15 mg/day in 1-3 divided doses (approximately every 8 hours)

Dosage Forms

Tablet, oral: 5 mg, 10 mg

Tapazole®: 5 mg, 10 mg

Methitest™ [US] *see* methyltestosterone *on page 624*

methocarbamol (meth oh KAR ba mole)

Sound-Alike/Look-Alike Issues

methocarbamol may be confused with mephobarbital

Robaxin® may be confused with ribavirin, Rubex®, Skelaxin®

U.S./Canadian Brand Names Robaxin® [US/Can]; Robaxin®-750 [US]

Therapeutic Category Skeletal Muscle Relaxant

Use Adjunctive treatment of muscle spasm associated with acute painful musculoskeletal conditions (eg, tetanus)

Dosage Summary **Note:** Dosing and route are indication specific.

I.M.:

Children: Dosage not established

Adults: 1 g every 8 hours (maximum dose: 3 g/day for 3 consecutive days)

I.V.:

Children: 15 mg/kg/dose **or** 500 mg/m^2/dose every 6 hours as needed (maximum dose: 1.8 g/m^2/day for 3 consecutive days)

Adults: 1-3 g every 6 hours **or** 1 g every 8 hours (maximum dose: 3 g/day for 3 consecutive days)

Oral:

Children <16 years: Dosage not established

Children ≥16 years: Initial: 1.5 g 4 times/day for 2-3 days (maximum: 8 g/day); Maintenance: 4-4.5 g/day in 3-6 divided doses

Adults: Initial: 1.5 g 4 times/day for 2-3 days (maximum: 8 g/day); Maintenance: 4-4.5 g/day in 3-6 divided doses

Dosage Forms

Injection, solution:

Robaxin®: 100 mg/mL (10 mL)

Tablet, oral: 500 mg, 750 mg

Robaxin®: 500 mg

Robaxin®-750: 750 mg

methohexital (meth oh HEKS i tal)

Sound-Alike/Look-Alike Issues

Brevital® may be confused with Brevibloc®

Synonyms methohexital sodium

U.S./Canadian Brand Names Brevital® Sodium [US]; Brevital® [Can]

Therapeutic Category Barbiturate

Controlled Substance C-IV

Use For induction of anesthesia prior to the use of other general anesthetic agents; as an adjunct to subpotent inhalational anesthetic agents for short surgical procedures; for short surgical, diagnostic, or therapeutic procedures associated with minimal painful stimuli

Additional indications for adults: For use with other parenteral agents, usually narcotic analgesics, to supplement subpotent inhalational anesthetic agents for longer surgical procedures; as an agent to induce a hypnotic state

Dosage Summary

I.M.:

Infants <1 month: Dosage not established

Infants ≥1 month: Induction: 6.6-10 mg/kg of a 5% solution

Children: Induction: 6.6-10 mg/kg of a 5% solution

Adults: Use not indicated

I.V.:

Infants <1 month: Dosage not established

Adults: Induction: 1-1.5 mg/kg; Maintenance: 50-120 mcg/kg/minute (or 20-40 mg every 4-7 minutes)

Rectal:

Infants <1 month: Dosage not established

Infants ≥1 month: Induction: 25 mg/kg of a 1% solution or 25 mg/kg of a 10% (100 mg/mL) solution; maximum dose: 500 mg

Children: Induction: 25 mg/kg of a 1% solution or 25 mg/kg of a 10% (100 mg/mL) solution; maximum dose: 500 mg

Adults: Use not indicated

Dosage Forms

Injection, powder for reconstitution:

Brevital® Sodium: 500 mg, 2.5 g

methohexital sodium *see* methohexital *on page* 614

methotrexate (meth oh TREKS ate)

Sound-Alike/Look-Alike Issues

methotrexate may be confused with mercaptopurine, methylPREDNISolone sodium succinate, metolazone, metroNIDAZOLE, mitoxantrone, pralatrexate

MTX is an error-prone abbreviation (mistaken as mitoxantrone)

Synonyms amethopterin; methotrexate sodium; methotrexatum

U.S./Canadian Brand Names Apo-Methotrexate® [Can]; ratio-Methotrexate [Can]; Rheumatrex® [US]; Trexall™ [US]

Therapeutic Category Antineoplastic Agent

Use

Oncology-related uses: Treatment of trophoblastic neoplasms (gestational choriocarcinoma, chorioadenoma destruens and hydatidiform mole), acute lymphocytic leukemia (ALL), meningeal leukemia, breast cancer, head and neck cancer (epidermoid), cutaneous T-Cell lymphoma (advanced mycosis fungoides), lung cancer (squamous cell and small cell), advanced non-Hodgkin lymphomas (NHL), osteosarcoma

Nononcology uses: Treatment of psoriasis (severe, recalcitrant, disabling) and severe rheumatoid arthritis (RA), including polyarticular-course juvenile rheumatoid arthritis (JRA)

Dosage Summary Note: Doses between 100-500 mg/m^2 may require leucovorin calcium rescue in some patients

I.M.:

Children: 5-30 mg/m^2 once weekly or every 2 weeks

Adults: 15-30 mg/day for 5 days **or** 25-50 mg/m^2 once weekly **or** 5-50 mg once weekly **or** 15-37.5 mg twice weekly **or** 50 mg/m^2 as a single dose

I.V.:

Children: 10-18,000 mg/m^2 bolus dosing or continuous infusion over 6-42 hours

Adults: 11-1500 mg/m^2 on a specified number of days every 3-4 weeks **or** 25-50 mg/m^2 once weekly **or** 8-12 g/m^2 weekly for 2-4 weeks **or** 50 mg/m^2 as a single dose

Intrathecal:

Children <1 year: 6 mg/dose

Children 1 year: 8 mg/dose

Children 2 years: 10 mg/dose

Children ≥3 years: 12 mg/dose

Adults: 12 mg/dose

Oral:

Children: 5-30 mg/m^2 once weekly or every 2 weeks

Adults: 15-30 mg/day for 5 days **or** 25-50 mg/m^2 once weekly **or** 5-50 mg once weekly **or** 15-37.5 mg twice weekly

Dosage Forms

Injection, powder for reconstitution: 1 g

Injection, solution: 25 mg/mL (2 mL, 10 mL)

Injection, solution [preservative free]: 25 mg/mL (2 mL, 4 mL, 8 mL, 10 mL, 20 mL, 40 mL, 100 mL)

Tablet, oral: 2.5 mg

Rheumatrex®: 2.5 mg

Trexall™: 5 mg, 7.5 mg, 10 mg, 15 mg

methotrexate sodium *see* methotrexate *on page 614*

methotrexatum *see* methotrexate *on page 614*

methotrimeprazine *(Canada only)* (meth oh trye MEP ra zeen)

Synonyms levomepromazine; methotrimeprazine hydrochloride

U.S./Canadian Brand Names Apo-Methoprazine® [Can]; Novo-Meprazine [Can]; Nozinan® [Can]; PMS-Methotrimeprazine [Can]

Therapeutic Category Neuroleptic Agent

Use Treatment of schizophrenia or psychosis; management of pain, including pain caused by neuralgia or cancer; adjunct to general anesthesia; management of nausea and vomiting; sedation

Dosage Summary

I.M.:

Children ≤2 years: Dosage not established

Children >2 years: 0.06-0.125 mg/kg/day in 1-3 divided doses

Adults: 10-25 mg every 8 hours **or** 75-100 mg as a single dose

I.V.:

Children: Dosage not established

Adults: 20-100 mcg/minute

Oral:

Children ≤2 years: Dosage not established

Children >2 years: 0.25 mg/kg/day in 2-3 divided doses (maximum: 40 mg/day [children <12 years])

Adults: 6-75 mg/day in 2-3 divided doses (maximum: doses up to 1000 mg/day have been used) **or** 10-25 mg at bedtime

SubQ:

Children: Dosage not established.

Adults: 25-200 mg/day via continuous infusion

Dosage Forms - Canada

Injection, solution:

Nozinan®: 25 mg/mL (1 mL)

Solution, oral:

Nozinan®: 5 mg/mL

Solution, oral drops:

Nozinan®: 40 mg/mL

Tablet:

Apo-Methoprazine®: 2 mg, 5 mg, 25 mg, 50 mg

Nozinan®: 5 mg, 25 mg, 50 mg

methotrimeprazine hydrochloride *see* methotrimeprazine *(Canada only) on page* 615

methoxsalen (systemic) (meth OKS a len)

Sound-Alike/Look-Alike Issues

methoxsalen soft gelatin capsules (Oxsoralen-Ultra®) may be confused with methoxsalen hard gelatin capsules (8-MOP®, Oxsoralen®); bioavailability and photosensitization onset differ between the two products.

Synonyms 8-methoxypsoralen; methoxypsoralen

U.S./Canadian Brand Names 8-MOP® [US]; Oxsoralen-Ultra® [US/Can]; Oxsoralen® Capsule [Can]; Ultramop™ [Can]; Uvadex® [US]

Therapeutic Category Psoralen

Use

Oral: Symptomatic control of severe, recalcitrant disabling psoriasis; repigmentation of idiopathic vitiligo; palliative treatment of skin manifestations of cutaneous T-cell lymphoma (CTCL)

Extracorporeal: Palliative treatment of skin manifestations of CTCL

Dosage Summary

Extracorporeal:

Children: Dosage not established

Adults: 200 mcg injected into photoactivation bag for 2 consecutive days every 4 weeks for a minimum of 7 treatment cycles; may accelerate to 2 consecutive days every 2 weeks if skin score worsens (eg, increases from baseline) after assessment during the fourth treatment cycle. If skin score improves by 25% after 4 consecutive weeks of accelerated therapy, may resume regular treatment schedule. Maximum: 20 accelerated therapy cycles.

Oral:

Children: Dosage not established

Adults:

Psoriasis: Initial: 10-70 mg 1.5-2 hours prior to UVA light exposure, may repeat 2-3 times/week (48 hours between doses); dose based on patient's weight. **Note:** Dosage may be increased (one time) by 10 mg after 15th treatment if minimal or no response. Maintenance: When 95% psoriasis clearing achieved, may begin 1 treatment every week for at least 2 treatments; followed by 1 treatment every 2 weeks for at least 2 treatments; then every 3 weeks for at least 2 treatments then as needed to maintain response while minimizing UVA exposure.

Vitiligo: 20 mg 2-4 hours prior to UVA light exposure, may repeat based on erythema and tenderness of skin; do not give on 2 consecutive days

Dosage Forms

Capsule, oral:

8-MOP®: 10 mg

Oxsoralen-Ultra®: 10 mg

Solution, for extracorporeal administration:

Uvadex®: 20 mcg/mL (10 mL)

methoxsalen (topical) (meth OKS a len)

Synonyms methoxypsoralen

U.S./Canadian Brand Names Oxsoralen® Lotion [Can]; Oxsoralen® [US]

Therapeutic Category Psoralen

Use Repigmentation of idiopathic vitiligo

Dosage Summary

Topical:

Children <12 years: Dosage not established

Children ≥12 years: Lotion is applied by healthcare provider prior to UVA light exposure, usually no more than once weekly; frequency is determined by erythema response

Adults: Lotion is applied by healthcare provider prior to UVA light exposure, usually no more than once weekly; frequency is determined by erythema response

Dosage Forms

Lotion, topical:

Oxsoralen®: 1% (29.57 mL)

methoxypsoralen *see* methoxsalen (systemic) *on page 616*

methoxypsoralen *see* methoxsalen (topical) *on page 616*

8-methoxypsoralen *see* methoxsalen (systemic) *on page 616*

methscopolamine (meth skoe POL a meen)

Synonyms methscopolamine bromide

U.S./Canadian Brand Names Pamine® Forte [US]; Pamine® [US/Can]

Therapeutic Category Anticholinergic Agent

Use Adjunctive therapy in the treatment of peptic ulcer

Dosage Summary

Oral:

Children: Dosage not established

Adults: 2.5-5 mg twice daily

Dosage Forms

Tablet, oral: 2.5 mg, 5 mg

Pamine®: 2.5 mg

Pamine® Forte: 5 mg

methscopolamine and pseudoephedrine *see* pseudoephedrine and methscopolamine *on page 813*

methscopolamine bromide *see* methscopolamine *on page 617*

methscopolamine, chlorpheniramine, and pseudoephedrine *see* chlorpheniramine, pseudoephedrine, and methscopolamine *on page 215*

methscopolamine nitrate, chlorpheniramine maleate, and phenylephrine hydrochloride *see* chlorpheniramine, phenylephrine, and methscopolamine *on page 212*

methscopolamine, pseudoephedrine, and chlorpheniramine *see* chlorpheniramine, pseudoephedrine, and methscopolamine *on page 215*

methsuximide (meth SUKS i mide)

Sound-Alike/Look-Alike Issues

methsuximide may be confused with ethosuximide

U.S./Canadian Brand Names Celontin® [US/Can]

Therapeutic Category Anticonvulsant

Use Control of absence (petit mal) seizures that are refractory to other drugs

Dosage Summary

Oral:

Children: Dosage not established

Adults: Initial: 300 mg/day for 1 week; Maintenance: Up to 1.2 g/day in 2-4 divided doses; **Note:** Titration is recommended on a weekly basis (300 mg/week)

Dosage Forms

Capsule, oral:

Celontin®: 150 mg, 300 mg

methyclothiazide (meth i kloe THYE a zide)

Sound-Alike/Look-Alike Issues

Enduron® may be confused with Empirin®, Imuran®, Inderal®

Therapeutic Category Diuretic, Thiazide

Use Management of mild-to-moderate hypertension; treatment of edema in congestive heart failure and nephrotic syndrome

Dosage Summary

Oral:

Children: Dosage not established

Adults: 2.5-10 mg once daily

Dosage Forms

Tablet, oral: 5 mg

methylacetoxyprogesterone *see* medroxyprogesterone *on page 597*

methylcellulose (meth il SEL yoo lose)

Sound-Alike/Look-Alike Issues

Citrucel® may be confused with Citracal®

U.S./Canadian Brand Names Citrucel® [US-OTC]; Soluble Fiber Therapy [US-OTC]

Therapeutic Category Laxative

Use Adjunct in treatment of constipation

Dosage Summary

Oral:

Caplet:

Children <6 years: Dosage not established

Children 6-12 years: 1 caplet up to 6 times/day

Children ≥12 years: 2-4 caplets 1-3 times/day

Adults: 2-4 caplets 1-3 times/day

Powder:

Children <6 years: Dosage not established

Children 6-12 years: Half the adult dose 1-3 times/day

Children ≥12 years: 2 g (1 scoop [rounded tablespoon]) 1-3 times/day

Adults: 2 g (1 scoop [rounded tablespoon]) 1-3 times/day

Dosage Forms

Caplet, oral:

Citrucel® [OTC]: 500 mg

Powder, oral:

Citrucel® [OTC]: 2 g/scoop (454 g, 479 g, 850 g, 907 g, 1190 g, 1843 g)

Soluble Fiber Therapy [OTC]: 2 g/scoop (454 g)

methylcellulose, gelatin, and pectin *see* gelatin, pectin, and methylcellulose *on page 440*

methylcobalamin, acetylcysteine, and methylfolate *see* methylfolate, methylcobalamin, and acetylcysteine *on page 620*

methyldopa (meth il DOE pa)

Sound-Alike/Look-Alike Issues

methyldopa may be confused with L-dopa, levodopa

Synonyms methyldopate hydrochloride

U.S./Canadian Brand Names Apo-Methyldopa® [Can]; Nu-Medopa [Can]

Therapeutic Category Alpha-Adrenergic Blocking Agent

Use Management of moderate-to-severe hypertension

Dosage Summary

I.V.:

Children: 5-10 mg/kg/dose every 6-8 hours (maximum: 65 mg/kg/day; 3 g/day)

Adults: 250-500 mg every 6-8 hours (maximum: 1 g every 6 hours)

Oral:

Children: Initial: 10 mg/kg/day in 2-4 divided doses; Maintenance: Up to 65 mg/kg/day (maximum: 3 g/day)

Adults: Initial: 250 mg 2-3 times/day; Maintenance: 250-1000 mg/day in 2 divided doses (maximum: 3 g/day)

Elderly: Initial: 125 mg 1-2 times/day; increase by 125 mg every 2-3 days as needed

Dosage Forms

Injection, solution: 50 mg/mL (5 mL)

Tablet, oral: 250 mg, 500 mg

methyldopa and hydrochlorothiazide (meth il DOE pa & hye droe klor oh THYE a zide)

Sound-Alike/Look-Alike Issues

Aldoril® may be confused with Aldoclor®, Aldomet®, Elavil®

Synonyms hydrochlorothiazide and methyldopa

U.S./Canadian Brand Names Apo-Methazide® [Can]

Therapeutic Category Antihypertensive Agent, Combination

Use Management of moderate-to-severe hypertension

Dosage Summary

Oral:

Children: Dosage not established

Adults: 1 tablet 2-3 times/day (maximum: 50 mg/day [hydrochlorothiazide]; 3 g/day [methyldopa])

Dosage Forms

Tablet: Methyldopa 250 mg and hydrochlorothiazide 15 mg; methyldopa 250 mg and hydrochlorothiazide 25 mg

methyldopate hydrochloride *see* methyldopa *on page 618*

methylene blue (METH i leen bloo)

Synonyms methylthionine chloride

Therapeutic Category Antidote

Use Antidote for cyanide poisoning and drug-induced methemoglobinemia, indicator dye

Dosage Summary

I.V.:

Children: 1-2 mg/kg **or** 25-50 mg/m^2 as a single dose, may repeat in 1 hour

Adults: 1-2 mg/kg **or** 25-50 mg/m^2 as a single dose, may repeat in 1 hour

Dosage Forms

Injection, solution: 10 mg/mL (1 mL, 10 mL)

methylene blue, methenamine, benzoic acid, phenyl salicylate, and hyoscyamine *see* methenamine, phenyl salicylate, methylene blue, benzoic acid, and hyoscyamine *on page 613*

methylergometrine maleate *see* methylergonovine *on page 619*

methylergonovine (meth il er goe NOE veen)

Sound-Alike/Look-Alike Issues

methylergonovine and terbutaline parenteral dosage forms look similar. Due to their contrasting indications, use care when administering these agents.

Methergine® may be confused with Brethine

Synonyms methylergometrine maleate; methylergonovine maleate

U.S./Canadian Brand Names Methergine® [US/Can]

Therapeutic Category Ergot Alkaloid and Derivative

Use Prevention and treatment of postpartum and postabortion hemorrhage caused by uterine atony or subinvolution

Dosage Summary

I.M.:

Children: Dosage not established

Adults: 0.2 mg after delivery of anterior shoulder, after delivery of placenta, or during puerperium; may repeat every 2-4 hours

I.V.:

Children: Dosage not established

Adults: 0.2 mg after delivery of anterior shoulder, after delivery of placenta, or during puerperium; may repeat every 2-4 hours

Oral:

Children: Dosage not established

Adults: 0.2 mg 3-4 times/day in the puerperium for 2-7 days

Dosage Forms

Injection, solution: 0.2 mg/mL (1 mL)

Methergine®: 0.2 mg/mL (1 mL)

Tablet, oral:

Methergine®: 0.2 mg

methylergonovine maleate *see* methylergonovine *on page 619*

methylfolate (meth il FO late)

Synonyms 6(S)-5-methyltetrahydrofolate; 6(S)-5-MTHF; L-methylfolate

U.S./Canadian Brand Names Deplin™ [US]

Therapeutic Category Dietary Supplement

Use Medicinal food for management of patients with low plasma and/or low red blood cell folate

Dosage Summary

Oral:

Children: Dosage not established

Adults: 7.5 mg daily

Dosage Forms

Tablet, oral: 7.5 mg

Deplin™: L-methylfolate 7.5 mg

methylfolate, methylcobalamin, and acetylcysteine

(meth il FO late meth il koe BAL a min & a se teel SIS teen)

Synonyms acetylcysteine, methylcobalamin, and methylfolate; acetylcysteine, methylfolate, and methylcobalamin; L-methylfolate, methylcobalamin, and N-acetylcysteine; methylcobalamin, acetylcysteine, and methylfolate

U.S./Canadian Brand Names Cerefolin® NAC [US]

Therapeutic Category Dietary Supplement

Use Medicinal food for use in patients with neurovascular oxidative stress and/or hyperhomocysteinemia

Dosage Summary

Oral:

Children <12 years: Dosage not established

Children ≥12 years: One caplet daily

Adults: One caplet daily

Dosage Forms

Caplet, oral:

Cerefolin® NAC: L-methylfolate 5.6 mg, methylcobalamin 2 mg, and N-acetylcysteine 600 mg [gluten free, sugar free]

Methylin® [US] *see* methylphenidate *on page 621*

Methylin® ER [US] *see* methylphenidate *on page 621*

methylmorphine *see* codeine *on page 244*

methylnaltrexone (meth il nal TREKS one)

Sound-Alike/Look-Alike Issues

methylnaltrexone may be confused with naltrexone

Synonyms methylnaltrexone bromide; N-methylnaltrexone bromide

U.S./Canadian Brand Names Relistor® [US/Can]

Therapeutic Category Gastrointestinal Agent, Miscellaneous; Opioid Antagonist, Peripherally-Acting

Use Treatment of opioid-induced constipation in patients with advanced illness receiving palliative care with inadequate response to conventional laxative regimens

Dosage Summary

SubQ:

Children: Dosage not established

Adults <38 kg: 0.15 mg/kg (round dose up to nearest 0.1 mL of volume) every other day as needed (maximum: 1 dose/24 hours)

Adults 38 to <62 kg: 8 mg every other day as needed (maximum: 1 dose/24 hours)

Adults 62-114 kg: 12 mg every other day as needed (maximum: 1 dose/24 hours)

Adults >114 kg: 0.15 mg/kg (round dose up to nearest 0.1 mL of volume) every other day as needed (maximum: 1 dose/24 hours)

Dosage Forms

Injection, solution:

Relistor®: 12 mg/0.6 mL (0.6 mL)

methylnaltrexone bromide *see* methylnaltrexone *on page 620*

methylphenidate (meth il FEN i date)

Sound-Alike/Look-Alike Issues

methylphenidate may be confused with methadone
Metadate CD® may be confused with Metadate® ER
Metadate® ER may be confused with Metadate CD®, methadone
Ritalin® may be confused with Ismelin®, Rifadin®, ritodrine
Ritalin LA® may be confused with Ritalin-SR®
Ritalin-SR® may be confused with Ritalin LA®

Synonyms methylphenidate hydrochloride

U.S./Canadian Brand Names Apo-Methylphenidate® SR [Can]; Apo-Methylphenidate® [Can]; Biphentin® [Can]; Concerta® [US/Can]; Daytrana™ [US]; Metadate CD® [US]; Metadate® ER [US]; Methylin® ER [US]; Methylin® [US]; Novo-Methylphenidate ER-C [Can]; PHL-Methylphenidate [Can]; PMS-Methylphenidate [Can]; ratio-Methylphenidate [Can]; Ritalin LA® [US]; Ritalin-SR® [US/Can]; Ritalin® [US/Can]; Sandoz-Methylphenidate SR [Can]

Therapeutic Category Central Nervous System Stimulant, Nonamphetamine

Controlled Substance C-II

Use Treatment of attention-deficit/hyperactivity disorder (ADHD); symptomatic management of narcolepsy

Dosage Summary

Oral:

Immediate release:

Children <6 years: Dosage not established

Children ≥6 years: Initial: 5 mg twice daily; may increase by 5-10 mg/day at weekly intervals (maximum: 60 mg/day)

Adults:

ADHD: Initial: 5 mg twice daily; may increase by 5-10 mg/day at weekly intervals (maximum: 60 mg/day)

Narcolepsy: 10 mg 2-3 times/day (maximum: 60 mg/day)

Extended release:

Children <6 years: Dosage not established

Children 6-12 years:

Concerta®: 18-54 mg once every morning (maximum: 54 mg/day); **Note:** Dosage based on current regimen

Metadate® ER, Methylin® ER, Ritalin® SR: May be given in place of regular tablets, once the daily dose is titrated using the regular tablets and the titrated 8-hour dosage corresponds to sustained or extended release tablet size (maximum: 60 mg/day)

Metadate CD®, Ritalin LA®: Initial: 20 mg once daily (maximum: 60 mg/day); **Note:** Titration is recommended

Children 13-17 years:

Concerta®: 18-72 mg once every morning (maximum: 72 mg/day); **Note:** Dosage based on current regimen

Metadate® ER, Methylin® ER, Ritalin® SR: May be given in place of regular tablets, once the daily dose is titrated using the regular tablets and the titrated 8-hour dosage corresponds to sustained or extended release tablet size

Metadate CD®, Ritalin LA®: Initial: 20 mg once daily (maximum: 60 mg/day); **Note:** Titration is recommended

Adults:

Concerta®: 18-72 mg once every morning (maximum: 72 mg/day); **Note:** Dosage based on current regimen

Metadate® ER, Methylin® ER, Ritalin® SR: May be given in place of regular tablets, once the daily dose is titrated using the regular tablets and the titrated 8-hour dosage corresponds to sustained or extended release tablet size

Metadate CD®, Ritalin LA®: Initial: 20 mg once daily (maximum: 60 mg/day); **Note:** Titration is recommended

Transdermal:

Children <6 years: Dosage not established

Children 6-17 years: Initial: 10 mg patch once daily; remove up to 9 hours after application; **Note:** Titration is recommended

Dosage Forms

Capsule, extended release, oral:

Metadate CD®: 10 mg, 20 mg, 30 mg, 40 mg, 50 mg, 60 mg

Ritalin LA®: 10 mg, 20 mg, 30 mg, 40 mg

Patch, transdermal:

Daytrana™: 10 mg/9 hours (30s); 15 mg/9 hours (30s); 20 mg/9 hours (30s); 30 mg/9 hours (30s)

Solution, oral:

Methylin®: 5 mg/5 mL (500 mL); 10 mg/5 mL (500 mL)

Tablet, oral:

Methylin®: 5 mg, 10 mg, 20 mg

Ritalin®: 5 mg, 10 mg, 20 mg

Tablet, chewable, oral:

Methylin®: 2.5 mg, 5 mg, 10 mg

Tablet, extended release, oral:

Concerta®: 18 mg, 27 mg, 36 mg, 54 mg

Metadate® ER: 20 mg

Methylin® ER: 10 mg, 20 mg

Tablet, sustained release, oral:

Ritalin-SR®: 20 mg

methylphenidate hydrochloride *see* methylphenidate *on page 621*

methylphenobarbital *see* mephobarbital *on page 604*

methylphenoxy-benzene propanamine *see* atomoxetine *on page 103*

methylphenyl isoxazolyl penicillin *see* oxacillin *on page 710*

methylphytyl napthoquinone *see* phytonadione *on page 759*

methylprednisolone (meth il pred NIS oh lone)

Sound-Alike/Look-Alike Issues

methylPREDNISolone may be confused with medroxyPROGESTERone, methotrexate, predniSONE

Depo-Medrol® may be confused with Solu-Medrol®

Medrol® may be confused with Mebaral®

Solu-Medrol® may be confused with Depo-Medrol®, salmeterol, Solu-Cortef®

Synonyms 6-α-methylprednisolone; medrol dose pack; methylprednisolone acetate; methylprednisolone sodium succinate; solumedrol

Tall-Man methyl**PREDNIS**olone

U.S./Canadian Brand Names A-Methapred® [US]; Depo-Medrol® [US/Can]; Medrol® Dosepak™ [US]; Medrol® [US/Can]; Methylprednisolone Acetate [Can]; Solu-Medrol® [US/Can]

Therapeutic Category Adrenal Corticosteroid

Use Primarily as an antiinflammatory or immunosuppressant agent in the treatment of a variety of diseases including those of hematologic, allergic, inflammatory, neoplastic, and autoimmune origin. Prevention and treatment of graft-versus-host disease following allogeneic bone marrow transplantation.

Dosage Summary Note: Dosing should be based on the lesser of ideal body weight or actual body weight. Only sodium succinate may be given I.V.

I.M.:

Acetate:

Children: Dosage not established

Adults: 10-120 mg every 1-2 weeks

Sodium succinate:

Children: 0.5-1.7 mg/kg/day **or** 5-25 mg/m^2/day divided every 6-12 hours; "Pulse" therapy: 15-30 mg/kg/dose over ≥30 minutes given once daily for 3 days

Adults: 10-80 mg once daily

I.V. (sodium succinate):

Note: Dosage varies considerably by indication; ranges listed are representative.

Children: 0.5-4 mg/kg/day **or** 5-25 mg/m^2/day divided every 6-12 hours; "Pulse" therapy: 15-30 mg/kg/dose over ≥30 minutes given once daily for 3 days or every other day for 6 doses.

Adults: 10-60 mg/dose at intervals depending on clinical response **or** 2 mg/kg/dose, then 0.5-1 mg/kg/dose every 6 hours **or** 1 g/day for 3 days **or** 1 mg/kg/day or 40 mg/day (whichever dose is higher), for 4 days **or** 30 mg/kg every 4-6 hours for 48 hours

Intraarticular (acetate):
Children: Dosage not established
Adults: Administer every 1-5 weeks
Large joints (eg, knee, ankle): 20-80 mg
Medium joints (eg, elbow, wrist): 10-40 mg
Small joints: 4-10 mg
Intralesional (acetate):
Children: Dosage not established
Adults: 20-60 mg every 1-5 weeks
Oral:
Children: 0.5-1.7 mg/kg/day **or** 5-25 mg/m^2/day divided every 6-12 hours; "Pulse" therapy: 15-30 mg/kg/dose once daily for 3 days
Adults: 2-60 mg/day in 1-4 divided doses

Dosage Forms
Injection, powder for reconstitution: 40 mg, 125 mg, 500 mg, 1 g
A-Methapred®: 40 mg
Solu-Medrol®: 500 mg, 1 g, 2 g
Injection, powder for reconstitution [preservative free]:
Solu-Medrol®: 40 mg, 125 mg, 500 mg, 1 g
Injection, suspension: 40 mg/mL (1 mL, 5 mL, 10 mL); 80 mg/mL (1 mL, 5 mL)
Depo-Medrol®: 20 mg/mL (5 mL); 40 mg/mL (1 mL, 5 mL, 10 mL); 80 mg/mL (1 mL, 5 mL)
Tablet, oral: 4 mg, 8 mg, 16 mg, 32 mg
Medrol®: 2 mg, 4 mg, 8 mg, 16 mg, 32 mg
Medrol® Dosepak™: 4 mg

6-α-methylprednisolone *see* methylprednisolone *on page 622*
Methylprednisolone Acetate [Can] *see* methylprednisolone *on page 622*
methylprednisolone acetate *see* methylprednisolone *on page 622*
methylprednisolone sodium succinate *see* methylprednisolone *on page 622*
4-methylpyrazole *see* fomepizole *on page 425*

methyl salicylate and menthol (METH il sa LIS i late & MEN thol)

Synonyms menthol and methyl salicylate

U.S./Canadian Brand Names BenGay® [US-OTC]; Icy Hot® [US-OTC]; Salonpas® Arthritis Pain® [US-OTC]; Salonpas® Pain Relief Patch® [US-OTC]; Salonpas® [US-OTC]; Thera-Gesic® Plus [US-OTC]; Thera-Gesic® [US-OTC]

Therapeutic Category Analgesic, Topical; Salicylate; Topical Skin Product

Use Temporary relief of minor aches and pains of muscle and joints associated with arthritis, bruises, simple backache, sprains, and strains

Dosage Summary
Topical:
Balm, cream, stick:
Children <12 years of age: Dosage not established
Children ≥12 years of age: Apply up to 3-4 times/day
Adults: Apply up to 3-4 times/day
Gel:
Children <2 years of age: Dosage not established
Children ≥2 years of age: Apply up to 3-4 times/day
Adults: Apply up to 3-4 times/day
Patch:
Children: Dosage not established
Adults: Apply 1 patch for up to 8-12 hours (maximum: 1 patch/application; 2 patches/24 hours; 3 days of consecutive use)

Dosage Forms
Balm, topical:
Icy Hot® Balm [OTC]: Methyl salicylate 29% and menthol 7.6% (99.2 g)
Cream, topical:
BenGay® Arthritis Formula [OTC]: Methyl salicylate 30% and menthol 8% (57 g, 113 g)
BenGay® Greaseless [OTC]: Methyl salicylate 15% and menthol 10% (57 g, 113 g)
Icy Hot® [OTC]: Methyl salicylate 30% and menthol 10% (35.4 g, 85 g)
Thera-Gesic® [OTC]: Methyl salicylate 15% and menthol 1% (85 g, 142 g)

Thera-Gesic® Plus [OTC]: Methyl salicylate 15% and menthol 4% (85 g) [contains aloe]

Gel, topical:

Salonpas® [OTC]: Methyl salicylate 15% and menthol 7% (40 g) [contains ethanol]

Patch, topical:

Salonpas® Arthritis Pain® [OTC], Salonpas® Pain Relief Patch® [OTC]: Methyl salicylate 10% and menthol 3% (5s)

Stick, topical:

Icy Hot® [OTC]: Methyl salicylate 30% and menthol 10% (49 g)

methyltestosterone (meth il tes TOS te rone)

Sound-Alike/Look-Alike Issues

methylTESTOSTERone may be confused with medroxyPROGESTERone

Tall-Man methyl**TESTOSTER**one

U.S./Canadian Brand Names Android® [US]; Methitest™ [US]; Testred® [US]

Therapeutic Category Androgen

Controlled Substance C-III

Use

Male: Hypogonadism; delayed puberty; impotence and climacteric symptoms

Female: Palliative treatment of metastatic breast cancer

Dosage Summary

Buccal:

Children: Dosage not established

Adults: 5-100 mg/day

Oral:

Children: Dosage not established

Adults: 10-200 mg/day

Dosage Forms

Capsule, oral:

Android®: 10 mg

Testred®: 10 mg

Tablet, oral:

Methitest™: 10 mg

methylthionine chloride *see* methylene blue *on page* 619

Meticorten® *(Discontinued)* *see* prednisone *on page* 792

Metimyd Ophthalmic Ointment *(Discontinued)*

metipranolol (met i PRAN oh lol)

Sound-Alike/Look-Alike Issues

metipranolol may be confused with metaproterenol

Synonyms metipranolol hydrochloride

U.S./Canadian Brand Names OptiPranolol® [US/Can]

Therapeutic Category Beta-Adrenergic Blocker

Use Agent for lowering intraocular pressure in patients with chronic open-angle glaucoma

Dosage Summary

Ophthalmic:

Children: Dosage not established

Adults: Instill 1 drop into affected eye(s) twice daily

Dosage Forms

Solution, ophthalmic: 0.3% (5 mL, 10 mL)

OptiPranolol®: 0.3% (5 mL, 10 mL)

metipranolol hydrochloride *see* metipranolol *on page* 624

metoclopramide (met oh KLOE pra mide)

Sound-Alike/Look-Alike Issues

metoclopramide may be confused with metolazone, metoprolol, metroNIDAZOLE

Reglan® may be confused with Megace®, Regonol®, Renagel®

U.S./Canadian Brand Names Apo-Metoclop® [Can]; Metoclopramide Hydrochloride Injection [Can]; Metoclopramide Omega [Can]; Metozolv™ ODT [US]; Nu-Metoclopramide [Can]; PMS-Metoclopramide [Can]; Reglan® [US]

Therapeutic Category Gastrointestinal Agent, Prokinetic

Use

Oral: Symptomatic treatment of diabetic gastroparesis; gastroesophageal reflux

I.V., I.M.: Symptomatic treatment of diabetic gastroparesis; postpyloric placement of enteral feeding tubes; prevention and/or treatment of nausea and vomiting associated with chemotherapy, or postsurgery; to stimulate gastric emptying and intestinal transit of barium during radiological examination of the stomach/small intestine

Dosage Summary

I.M.:

Children: Dosage not established

Adults: 10-20 mg near end of surgery **or** 10 mg before each meal and at bedtime

I.V.:

Children <6 years: 0.1 mg/kg as a single dose for feeding tube placement

Children 6-14 years: 2.5-5 mg as a single dose for feeding tube placement

Children >14 years: 10 mg as a single dose for feeding tube placement

Adults: 10 mg before each meal and at bedtime **or** 1-2 mg/kg every 2-3 hours (maximum: 5 doses/day) **or** 10 mg as a single dose for feeding tube placement

Oral:

Adults: 10-15 mg up to 4 times/day

Dosage Forms

Injection, solution [preservative free]: 5 mg/mL (2 mL, 10 mL, 20 mL, 30 mL)

Reglan®: 5 mg/mL (2 mL, 10 mL, 30 mL)

Solution, oral: 5 mg/5 mL (10 mL, 473 mL, 480 mL)

Tablet, oral: 5 mg, 10 mg

Reglan®: 5 mg, 10 mg

Tablet, orally disintegrating, oral:

Metozolv™ ODT: 5 mg, 10 mg

Metoclopramide Hydrochloride Injection [Can] *see* metoclopramide *on page* 624

Metoclopramide Omega [Can] *see* metoclopramide *on page* 624

metolazone (me TOLE a zone)

Sound-Alike/Look-Alike Issues

metolazone may be confused with metaxalone, methazolamide, methimazole, methotrexate, metoclopramide, metoprolol, minoxidil

Zaroxolyn® may be confused with Zarontin®

U.S./Canadian Brand Names Zaroxolyn® [US/Can]

Therapeutic Category Diuretic, Miscellaneous

Use Management of mild-to-moderate hypertension; treatment of edema in heart failure and nephrotic syndrome, impaired renal function

Dosage Summary

Oral:

Children: Dosage not established

Adults: 2.5-20 mg every 24 hours

Dosage Forms

Tablet, oral: 2.5 mg, 5 mg, 10 mg

Zaroxolyn®: 2.5 mg, 5 mg

Metopirone® [US] *see* metyrapone *on page* 628

metoprolol (me toe PROE lole)

Sound-Alike/Look-Alike Issues

metoprolol may be confused with metaproterenol, metoclopramide, metolazone, misoprostol

metoprolol succinate may be confused with metoprolol tartrate

Lopressor® may be confused with Lyrica®

Toprol-XL® may be confused with Tegretol®, Tegretol®-XR, Topamax®

Synonyms metoprolol succinate; metoprolol tartrate

U.S./Canadian Brand Names Apo-Metoprolol SR® [Can]; Apo-Metoprolol® [Can]; Betaloc® [Can]; Dom-Metoprolol [Can]; Gen-Metoprolol [Can]; Lopressor® [US/Can]; Metoprolol Tartrate Injection, USP [Can]; Metoprolol-25 [Can]; Metoprolol-L [Can]; Mylan-Metoprolol (Type L) [Can]; Novo-Metoprolol [Can]; Nu-Metop [Can]; PHL-Metoprolol [Can]; PMS-Metoprolol [Can]; Riva-Metoprolol [Can]; Sandoz-Metoprolol [Can]; Toprol-XL® [US]

Therapeutic Category Beta-Adrenergic Blocker

Use Treatment of angina pectoris, hypertension, or hemodynamically-stable acute myocardial infarction

Extended release: Treatment of angina pectoris or hypertension; to reduce mortality/hospitalization in patients with heart failure (stable NYHA Class II or III) already receiving ACE inhibitors, diuretics, and/or digoxin

Dosage Summary

I.V.:

Children: Dosage not established

Adults: 1.25-5 mg every 6-12 hours (maximum: 15 mg every 3 hours) **or** 5 mg every 2 minutes for 3 doses (acute MI)

Oral:

Extended release:

Children <6 years: Dosage not established

Children ≥6 years: 1-2 mg/kg once daily (maximum: 2 mg/kg/day or 200 mg/day)

Adults: 12.5-200 mg/day (maximum: 400 mg/day; exceptions occur [indication specific])

Immediate release:

Children >1 year: 1-6 mg/kg/day divided twice daily (maximum: 200 mg/day)

Adults: 50-450 mg/day in 2-3 divided doses

Dosage Forms

Injection, solution: 1 mg/mL (5 mL)

Lopressor®: 1 mg/mL (5 mL)

Tablet, oral: 25 mg, 50 mg, 100 mg

Lopressor®: 50 mg, 100 mg

Tablet, extended release, oral: 25 mg, 50 mg, 100 mg, 200 mg

Toprol-XL®: 25 mg, 50 mg, 100 mg, 200 mg

Metoprolol-25 [Can] *see* metoprolol *on page 625*

Metoprolol-L [Can] *see* metoprolol *on page 625*

metoprolol and hydrochlorothiazide (me toe PROE lole & hye droe klor oh THYE a zide)

Synonyms hydrochlorothiazide and metoprolol; hydrochlorothiazide and metoprolol tartrate; metoprolol tartrate and hydrochlorothiazide

U.S./Canadian Brand Names Lopressor HCT® [US]

Therapeutic Category Beta Blocker, Beta-1 Selective; Diuretic, Thiazide

Use Treatment of hypertension (not recommended for initial treatment)

Dosage Summary

Oral:

Children: Dosage not established

Adults: Metoprolol 50-100 mg and hydrochlorothiazide 25-50 mg administered daily as single or 2 divided doses (maximum: 50 mg/day [hydrochlorothiazide])

Dosage Forms

Tablet: 50/25: Metoprolol 50 mg and hydrochlorothiazide 25 mg; 100/25: Metoprolol 100 mg and hydrochlorothiazide 25 mg; 100/50: Metoprolol 100 mg and hydrochlorothiazide 50 mg

Lopressor HCT®: 50/25: Metoprolol 50 mg and hydrochlorothiazide 25 mg; 100/25: Metoprolol 100 mg and hydrochlorothiazide 25 mg; 100/50: Metoprolol 100 mg and hydrochlorothiazide 50 mg

metoprolol succinate *see* metoprolol *on page 625*

metoprolol tartrate *see* metoprolol *on page 625*

metoprolol tartrate and hydrochlorothiazide *see* metoprolol and hydrochlorothiazide *on page 626*

Metoprolol Tartrate Injection, USP [Can] *see* metoprolol *on page 625*

Metozolv™ ODT [US] *see* metoclopramide *on page 624*

Metreton® ***(Discontinued)***

MetroCream® [US/Can] *see* metronidazole (topical) *on page 627*

MetroGel® [US/Can] *see* metronidazole (topical) *on page 627*

MetroGel® 1% Kit [US] *see* metronidazole (topical) *on page 627*

MetroGel-Vaginal® [US] *see* metronidazole (topical) *on page* 627
Metro I.V.® Injection ***(Discontinued)*** *see* metronidazole (systemic) *on page* 627
MetroLotion® [US/Can] *see* metronidazole (topical) *on page* 627

metronidazole (systemic) (met roe NYE da zole)

Sound-Alike/Look-Alike Issues
metroNIDAZOLE may be confused with mebendazole, meropenem, metFORMIN, methotrexate, metoclopramide, miconazole

Synonyms metronidazole hydrochloride

Tall-Man metro**NIDAZOLE**

U.S./Canadian Brand Names Apo-Metronidazole® [Can]; Flagyl® 375 [US]; Flagyl® ER [US]; Flagyl® [US/Can]; Florazole® ER [Can]

Therapeutic Category Amebicide; Antibiotic, Miscellaneous; Antiprotozoal, Nitroimidazole

Use Treatment of susceptible anaerobic bacterial and protozoal infections in the following conditions: Amebiasis, symptomatic and asymptomatic trichomoniasis; skin and skin structure infections, bone and joint infections, CNS infections, endocarditis, gynecologic infections, intraabdominal infections (as part of combination regimen), respiratory tract infections (lower), systemic anaerobic infections; treatment of antibiotic-associated pseudomembranous colitis (AAPC); as part of a multidrug regimen for *H. pylori* eradication to reduce the risk of duodenal ulcer recurrence; surgical prophylaxis (colorectal)

Dosage Summary

I.V.:
Infants: 30 mg/kg/day divided every 6 hours
Children: 30 mg/kg/day divided every 6 hours
Adults: 500 mg every 6-8 hours (maximum: 4 g/day)

Oral:
Extended release:
Children: Dosage not established
Adults: 750 mg once daily
Regular release:
Infants: 15-50 mg/kg/day divided every 8 hours **or** 20 mg/kg/day divided every 6 hours (maximum: 2 g/day)
Children: 15-50 mg/kg/day divided every 8 hours **or** 20 mg/kg/day divided every 6 hours (maximum: 2 g/day)
Adults: 250-750 mg every 6-12 hours (maximum: 4 g/day) **or** 2 g as a single dose

Dosage Forms
Capsule, oral: 375 mg
Flagyl® 375: 375 mg
Infusion, premixed iso-osmotic sodium chloride solution: 500 mg (100 mL)
Tablet, oral: 250 mg, 500 mg
Flagyl®: 250 mg, 500 mg
Tablet, extended release, oral:
Flagyl® ER: 750 mg

metronidazole (topical) (met roe NYE da zole)

Synonyms metronidazole hydrochloride

Tall-Man metro**NIDAZOLE**

U.S./Canadian Brand Names MetroCream® [US/Can]; MetroGel-Vaginal® [US]; MetroGel® 1% Kit [US]; MetroGel® [US/Can]; MetroLotion® [US/Can]; Nidagel™ [Can]; Noritate® [US/Can]; Rosasol® [Can]; Vandazole® [US]

Therapeutic Category Antibiotic, Topical

Use
Topical: Treatment of inflammatory lesions and erythema of rosacea
Vaginal gel: Bacterial vaginosis

Dosage Summary

Intravaginal:
Children: Dosage not established
Adults: One applicatorful (~37.5 mg metronidazole) intravaginally once or twice daily

Topical:
Children: Dosage not established
Adults: Apply a thin film to affected area once [1%] or twice [0.75%] daily

Dosage Forms

Cream, topical: 0.75% (45 g)
MetroCream®: 0.75% (45 g)
Noritate®: 1% (60 g)
Gel, topical: 0.75% (45 g)
MetroGel®: 1% (60 g)
MetroGel® 1% Kit: 1% (60 g)
Gel, vaginal: 0.75% (70 g)
MetroGel-Vaginal®: 0.75% (70 g)
Vandazole®: 0.75% (70 g)
Lotion, topical: 0.75% (59 mL, 60 mL)
MetroLotion®: 0.75% (59 mL)

metronidazole and nystatin *(Canada only)* (met roe NYE da zole & nye STAT in)

Synonyms nystatin and metronidazole

U.S./Canadian Brand Names Flagystatin® [Can]

Therapeutic Category Antifungal Agent, Vaginal; Antiprotozoal, Nitroimidazole

Use Treatment of mixed vaginal infection due to *T. vaginalis* and *C. albicans*

Dosage Summary

Intravaginal:
Children: Dosage not established
Adults: Insert 1 applicatorful or tablet daily at bedtime

Dosage Forms - Canada

Cream, vaginal:
Flagystatin®: Metronidazole 500 mg and nystatin 100,000 units per applicatorful (55 g)
Tablet, vaginal:
Flagystatin® Ovule: Metronidazole 500 mg and nystatin 100,000 units (10s)

metronidazole, bismuth subcitrate potassium, and tetracycline *see* bismuth, metronidazole, and tetracycline *on page 140*

metronidazole, bismuth subsalicylate, and tetracycline *see* bismuth, metronidazole, and tetracycline *on page 140*

metronidazole hydrochloride *see* metronidazole (systemic) *on page 627*

metronidazole hydrochloride *see* metronidazole (topical) *on page 627*

metyrapone (me TEER a pone)

Sound-Alike/Look-Alike Issues
metyrapone may be confused with metyrosine

U.S./Canadian Brand Names Metopirone® [US]

Therapeutic Category Diagnostic Agent

Use Diagnostic test for hypothalamic-pituitary ACTH function

Dosage Summary

Oral:
Children: 15 mg/kg every 4 hours for 6 doses (minimum: 250 mg/dose)
Adults: 750 mg every 4 hours for 6 doses

Dosage Forms

Capsule, oral:
Metopirone®: 250 mg

metyrosine (me TYE roe seen)

Sound-Alike/Look-Alike Issues
metyrosine may be confused with metyrapone

Synonyms AMPT; OGMT

U.S./Canadian Brand Names Demser® [US/Can]

Therapeutic Category Tyrosine Hydroxylase Inhibitor

Use Short-term management of pheochromocytoma before surgery, long-term management when surgery is contraindicated or when chronic malignant pheochromocytoma exists

Dosage Summary

Oral:

Children ≤12 years: Dosage not established

Children >12 years: Initial: 250 mg 4 times/day; Maintenance: 2-3 g/day in 4 divided doses (maximum: 4 g/day)

Adults: Initial: 250 mg 4 times/day; Maintenance: 2-3 g/day in 4 divided doses (maximum: 4 g/day)

Dosage Forms

Capsule, oral:

Demser®: 250 mg

Mevacor® [US/Can] *see* lovastatin *on page 579*

mevinolin *see* lovastatin *on page 579*

Mexar™ ***(Discontinued)*** *see* sulfacetamide (topical) *on page 900*

mexiletine (meks IL e teen)

U.S./Canadian Brand Names Novo-Mexiletine [Can]

Therapeutic Category Antiarrhythmic Agent, Class I-B

Use Management of serious ventricular arrhythmias; suppression of PVCs

Dosage Summary

Oral:

Children: Dosage not established

Adults: Initial: 200 mg every 8 hours; Maintenance: 200-300 mg every 8 hours (maximum: 1.2 g/day)

Dosage Forms

Capsule, oral: 150 mg, 200 mg, 250 mg

Mexitil® ***(Discontinued)*** *see* mexiletine *on page 629*

Mezavant® [Can] *see* mesalamine *on page 607*

MG217® Medicated Tar [US-OTC] *see* coal tar *on page 242*

MG217® Medicated Tar Extra Strength [US-OTC] *see* coal tar *on page 242*

MG217® Medicated Tar Intensive Strength [US-OTC] *see* coal tar *on page 242*

MG217® Sal-Acid [US-OTC] *see* salicylic acid *on page 858*

Miacalcin® [US] *see* calcitonin *on page 165*

Miacalcin® NS [Can] *see* calcitonin *on page 165*

Mi-Acid [US-OTC] *see* aluminum hydroxide, magnesium hydroxide, and simethicone *on page 59*

Mi-Acid™ Double Strength [US-OTC] *see* calcium carbonate and magnesium hydroxide *on page 168*

Mi-Acid Gas Relief [US-OTC] *see* simethicone *on page 875*

Mi-Acid Maximum Strength ***(Discontinued)*** *see* aluminum hydroxide, magnesium hydroxide, and simethicone *on page 59*

Micaderm® [US-OTC] *see* miconazole (topical) *on page 630*

micafungin (mi ka FUN gin)

Synonyms micafungin sodium

U.S./Canadian Brand Names Mycamine® [US/Can]

Therapeutic Category Antifungal Agent, Parenteral; Drug-induced Neuritis, Treatment Agent

Use Treatment of esophageal candidiasis; *Candida* prophylaxis in patients undergoing hematopoietic stem cell transplant (HSCT); treatment of candidemia, acute disseminated candidiasis, and other *Candida* infections (peritonitis and abscesses)

Dosage Summary

I.V.:

Children: Dosage not established

Adults: Prophylaxis: 50 mg daily; Treatment: 100-150 mg daily

Dosage Forms

Injection, powder for reconstitution:

Mycamine®: 50 mg, 100 mg

micafungin sodium *see* micafungin *on page 629*

Micanol® [Can] *see* anthralin *on page 79*

Micardis® [US/Can] *see* telmisartan *on page 913*

Micardis® HCT [US] *see* telmisartan and hydrochlorothiazide *on page 914*
Micardis® Plus [Can] *see* telmisartan and hydrochlorothiazide *on page 914*
Micatin® [US-OTC/Can] *see* miconazole (topical) *on page 630*

miconazole (oral) (mi KON a zole)

Sound-Alike/Look-Alike Issues

miconazole may be confused with metroNIDAZOLE, Micronase®, Micronor®

Synonyms miconazole nitrate

U.S./Canadian Brand Names Oravig™ [US]

Therapeutic Category Antifungal Agent, Oral Nonabsorbed

Use Treatment of oropharyngeal candidiasis

Dosage Summary

Buccal tablet:

Children <16 years: Dosage not established
Children ≥16 years: 50 mg (1 tablet) once daily for 14 days
Adults: 50 mg (1 tablet) once daily for 14 days

Dosage Forms

Tablet, for buccal application:
Oravig™: 50 mg

miconazole (topical) (mi KON a zole)

Sound-Alike/Look-Alike Issues

miconazole may be confused with metroNIDAZOLE, Micronase®, Micronor®
Lotrimin® may be confused with Lotrisone®, Otrivin®
Micatin® may be confused with Miacalcin®

Synonyms miconazole nitrate

U.S./Canadian Brand Names Aloe Vesta® Antifungal [US-OTC]; Baza® Antifungal [US-OTC]; Carrington® Antifungal [US-OTC]; Critic-Aid® Clear AF [US-OTC]; DermaFungal [US-OTC]; Dermagran® AF [US-OTC]; Dermazole [Can]; DiabetAid® Antifungal Foot Bath [US-OTC]; Fungoid® [US-OTC]; Lotrimin AF® [US-OTC]; Micaderm® [US-OTC]; Micatin® [US-OTC/Can]; Micozole [Can]; Micro-Guard® [US-OTC]; Miranel AF™ [US-OTC]; Mitrazol® [US-OTC]; Monistat® 1 Day or Night [US-OTC]; Monistat® 1 [US-OTC]; Monistat® 3 [US-OTC/Can]; Monistat® 7 [US-OTC]; Monistat® [Can]; Neosporin® AF [US-OTC]; Podactin Cream [US-OTC]; Secura® Antifungal Extra Thick [US-OTC]; Secura® Antifungal Greaseless [US-OTC]; Ting® Spray Powder [US-OTC]; Zeasorb®-AF [US-OTC]

Therapeutic Category Antifungal Agent

Use Treatment of vulvovaginal candidiasis and a variety of skin and mucous membrane fungal infections

Dosage Summary

Intravaginal:

Children <12 years: Dosage not established
Children ≥12 years: Insert 1 applicatorful or suppository (100 mg or 200 mg) once daily at bedtime **or** insert 1 (1200 mg) suppository as a single dose. **Note:** Not for OTC use in children <12 years.
Adults: Insert 1 applicatorful or suppository (100 mg or 200 mg) once daily at bedtime **or** insert 1 (1200 mg) suppository as a single dose

Topical:

Children: **Note:** Not for OTC use in children <2 years. Apply twice daily **or** dissolve 1 effervescent tablet in ~1 gallon of water and soak feet for 15-30 minutes
Adults: Apply twice daily **or** dissolve 1 effervescent tablet in ~1 gallon of water and soak feet for 15-30 minutes

Dosage Forms

Aerosol, topical:
Lotrimin AF® [OTC]: 2% (133 g)
Micatin® [OTC]: 2% (90 g, 105 mL); 2% (90 g)
Neosporin® AF [OTC]: 2% (105 mL); 2% (85 g)
Ting® Spray Powder [OTC]: 2% (128 g)

Combination package, topical/vaginal: Cream, topical: 2% (9 g) and Suppository, vaginal: 200 mg (3s)
Monistat® 1 [OTC]: Cream, topical: 2% (9 g) and Insert, vaginal: 1200 mg (1)
Monistat® 3 [OTC]: Cream, topical: 2% (9 g) and Cream, vaginal: 4% (25 g), Cream, topical: 2% (9 g) and Cream, vaginal: 4% (3 x 5 g), Cream, topical: 2% (9 g) and Insert, vaginal: 200 mg (3s)

Monistat® 7 [OTC]: Cream, topical: 2% (9 g) and Cream, vaginal: 2% (45 g), Cream, topical: 2% (9 g) and Cream, vaginal: 2% (7 x 5 g), Cream, topical: 2% (9 g) and Suppository, vaginal: 100 mg (7s)
Monistat® 1 Day or Night [OTC]: Cream, topical: 2% (9 g) and Insert, vaginal: 1200 mg (1)

Cream, topical: 2% (15 g, 30 g, 45 g)
Baza® Antifungal [OTC]: 2% (4 g, 57 g, 142 g)
Carrington® Antifungal [OTC]: 2% (150 g)
Micaderm® [OTC]: 2% (30 g)
Micatin® [OTC]: 2% (14 g)
Micro-Guard® [OTC]: 2% (60 g)
Miranel AF™ [OTC]: 2% (28 g)
Neosporin® AF [OTC]: 2% (14 g, 15 g)
Podactin Cream [OTC]: 2% (30 g)
Secura® Antifungal Extra Thick [OTC]: 2% (97.5 g)
Secura® Antifungal Greaseless [OTC]: 2% (60 g)

Cream, vaginal: 2% (45 g); 4% (25 g)
Monistat® 7 [OTC]: 2% (45 g)
Monistat® 3 [OTC]: 4% (15 g, 25 g)

Gel, topical:
Zeasorb®-AF [OTC]: 2% (24 g)

Liquid, topical:
Lotrimin AF® [OTC]: 2% (150 g)

Ointment, topical:
Aloe Vesta® Antifungal [OTC]: 2% (60 g, 150 g)
Critic-Aid® Clear AF [OTC]: 2% (57 g, 142 g, 300s)
DermaFungal [OTC]: 2% (120 g)
Dermagran® AF [OTC]: 2% (120 g)

Powder, topical:
Lotrimin AF® [OTC]: 2% (90 g)
Micro-Guard® [OTC]: 2% (90 g)
Mitrazol® [OTC]: 2% (30 g)
Zeasorb®-AF [OTC]: 2% (70 g)

Suppository, vaginal: 100 mg (7s); 200 mg (3s)

Tablet for solution, topical:
DiabetAid® Antifungal Foot Bath [OTC]: 2% (10s)

Tincture, topical:
Fungoid® [OTC]: 2% (7.39 mL, 30 mL)

miconazole and zinc oxide (mi KON a zole & zink OKS ide)

Synonyms zinc oxide and miconazole nitrate

U.S./Canadian Brand Names Vusion® [US]

Therapeutic Category Antifungal Agent, Topical

Use Adjunctive treatment of diaper dermatitis complicated by *Candida albicans* infection

Dosage Summary

Topical:
Children <4 weeks: Dosage not established
Children ≥4 weeks: Apply to affected area with each diaper change (maximum therapy: 7 days)
Adults: Dosage not established

Dosage Forms

Ointment, topical:
Vusion®: Miconazole 0.25% and zinc oxide 15% (50 g)

miconazole nitrate *see* miconazole (oral) *on page* 630
miconazole nitrate *see* miconazole (topical) *on page* 630
Micozole [Can] *see* miconazole (topical) *on page* 630
MICRhoGAM® [US] *see* Rh_o(D) immune globulin *on page* 838
microfibrillar collagen hemostat *see* collagen hemostat *on page* 248
Microgestin™ [US] *see* ethinyl estradiol and norethindrone *on page* 378
Microgestin™ Fe [US] *see* ethinyl estradiol and norethindrone *on page* 378
Micro-Guard® [US-OTC] *see* miconazole (topical) *on page* 630
microK® [US] *see* potassium chloride *on page* 781

microK® 10 [US] *see* potassium chloride *on page 781*
Micro-K Extencaps® [Can] *see* potassium chloride *on page 781*
Micro-K® LS *(Discontinued)* *see* potassium chloride *on page 781*
Microlipid™ [US-OTC] *see* nutritional formula, enteral/oral *on page 692*
Micronase® *(Discontinued)* *see* glyburide *on page 448*
microNefrin® *(Discontinued)* *see* epinephrine (systemic, oral inhalation) *on page 352*
Micronor® [Can] *see* norethindrone *on page 682*
Microzide® [US] *see* hydrochlorothiazide *on page 478*
***Micrurus fulvius* antivenin** *see* antivenin *(Micrurus fulvius) on page 85*
Midamor® *(Discontinued)* *see* amiloride *on page 63*

midazolam (MID aye zoe lam)

Sound-Alike/Look-Alike Issues
Versed® may be confused with VePesid®, Vistaril®

Synonyms midazolam hydrochloride

U.S./Canadian Brand Names Apo-Midazolam® [Can]; Midazolam Injection [Can]

Therapeutic Category Benzodiazepine

Controlled Substance C-IV

Use Preoperative sedation; moderate sedation prior to diagnostic or radiographic procedures; ICU sedation (continuous infusion); induction and maintenance of general anesthesia

Dosage Summary Note: The dose of midazolam needs to be individualized based on the patient's age, underlying diseases, and concurrent medications. Decrease dose (by ~30%) if narcotics or other CNS depressants are administered concomitantly. Children <6 years may require higher doses and closer monitoring than older children; calculate dose on ideal body weight

I.M.:

Children: 0.05-0.15 mg/kg 30-60 minutes prior to procedure (maximum: 10 mg total)

Adults: 0.07-0.08 mg/kg 30-60 minutes prior to procedure; Usual dose: 5 mg

I.V.:

Infants <6 months: 0.05-0.2 mg/kg loading dose followed by 0.4-6 mcg/kg/minute infusion; Limited information on dosing prior to a procedure; **Note:** Titration is recommended

Infants 6 months to Children 5 years: Initial: 0.05-0.1 mg/kg prior to procedure (maximum: 6 mg or 0.6 mg/kg total) **or** 0.05-0.2 mg/kg loading dose followed by 0.4-6 mcg/kg/minute infusion; **Note:** Titration is recommended

Children 6-12 years: 0.025-0.05 mg/kg prior to procedure (maximum: 10 mg or 0.4 mg/kg total) **or** 0.05-0.2 mg/kg loading dose followed by 0.4-6 mcg/kg/minute infusion; **Note:** Titration is recommended

Children 12-16 years: 0.02-0.2 mg/kg prior to procedure (maximum: 10 mg total) **or** 0.05-0.2 mg/kg loading dose followed by 0.4-6 mcg/kg/minute infusion; **Note:** Titration is recommended

Adults:

Anesthesia: Induction: 0.15-0.35 mg/kg (premedicated) **or** 0.3-0.35 mg/kg (not premedicated), up to 0.6 mg/kg in resistant cases; Maintenance: 0.05-0.3 mg/kg as needed **or** 0.25-1.5 mcg/kg/minute as continuous infusion

Conscious sedation: Initial: 0.5-2 mg, may repeat every 2-3 minutes if needed (usual total dose: 2.5-5 mg); Maintenance: 25% of dose used to reach sedation

Preoperative sedation: 0.02-0.04 mg/kg, may repeat every 5 minutes to desired effect or up to 0.2 mg/kg

Adults (mechanically-ventilated): Initial: 0.02-0.08 mg/kg as a single dose or repeated every 5-15 minutes; Infusion: 0.04-0.2 mg/kg/hour; **Note:** Titration is recommended

Elderly: Initial: 0.5 mg as a single dose prior to procedure; may give no more than 1.5 mg in a 2-minute period, if additional needed give <1 mg at a time (total dose >3.5 mg is rarely necessary)

Oral:

Children <6 years: 0.25-0.5 mg/kg as single dose prior to procedure; may require as much as 1 mg/kg (maximum: 20 mg total)

Children 6-16 years: 0.25-0.5 mg/kg as a single dose prior to procedure (maximum: 20 mg total)

Dosage Forms

Injection, solution: 1 mg/mL (2 mL, 5 mL, 10 mL); 5 mg/mL (1 mL, 2 mL, 5 mL, 10 mL)

Injection, solution [preservative free]: 1 mg/mL (2 mL, 5 mL); 5 mg/mL (1 mL, 2 mL)

Syrup, oral: 2 mg/mL (2.5 mL, 118 mL)

midazolam hydrochloride *see* midazolam *on page 632*

Midazolam Injection [Can] *see* midazolam *on page* 632

midodrine (MI doe dreen)

Sound-Alike/Look-Alike Issues

midodrine may be confused with Midrin®, minoxidil
ProAmatine® may be confused with protamine

Synonyms midodrine hydrochloride

U.S./Canadian Brand Names Amatine® [Can]; Apo-Midodrine® [Can]; ProAmatine® [US]

Therapeutic Category Alpha-Adrenergic Agonist

Use **Orphan drug:** Treatment of symptomatic orthostatic hypotension

Dosage Summary

Oral:

Children: Dosage not established
Adults: 10 mg 3 times/day (maximum: 40 mg/day)

Dosage Forms

Tablet, oral: 2.5 mg, 5 mg, 10 mg
ProAmatine®: 2.5 mg, 5 mg, 10 mg

midodrine hydrochloride *see* midodrine *on page* 633
Midol® Cramps & Body Aches [US-OTC] *see* ibuprofen *on page* 494
Midol® Extended Relief [US-OTC] *see* naproxen *on page* 659
Midol® Teen Formula [US-OTC] *see* acetaminophen and pamabrom *on page* 25
Midrin® [US] *see* acetaminophen, isometheptene, and dichloralphenazone *on page* 31
Mifeprex® [US] *see* mifepristone *on page* 633

mifepristone (mi FE pris tone)

Sound-Alike/Look-Alike Issues

mifepristone may be confused with misoprostol
Mifeprex® may be confused with Mirapex®

Synonyms RU-38486; RU-486

U.S./Canadian Brand Names Mifeprex® [US]

Therapeutic Category Abortifacient; Antineoplastic Agent, Hormone Antagonist; Antiprogestin

Use Medical termination of intrauterine pregnancy, through day 49 of pregnancy. Patients may need treatment with misoprostol and possibly surgery to complete therapy

Dosage Summary

Oral:

Children: Not for use prior to menarche
Adults:
Day 1: 600 mg (three 200 mg tablets) taken as a single dose under physician supervision
Day 3: 400 mcg (two 200 mcg tablets) of misoprostol if abortion had not occurred
Elderly: Dosage not established

Dosage Forms

Tablet, oral:
Mifeprex®: 200 mg

Migergot [US] *see* ergotamine and caffeine *on page* 359

miglitol (MIG li tol)

Sound-Alike/Look-Alike Issues

Glyset® may be confused with Cycloset®

U.S./Canadian Brand Names Glyset® [US/Can]

Therapeutic Category Antidiabetic Agent, Oral

Use Type 2 diabetes mellitus (noninsulin-dependent, NIDDM):

Monotherapy as an adjunct to diet to improve glycemic control in patients with type 2 diabetes mellitus (noninsulin-dependent, NIDDM) whose hyperglycemia cannot be managed with diet alone

Combination therapy with a sulfonylurea when diet plus either miglitol or a sulfonylurea alone do not result in adequate glycemic control. The effect of miglitol to enhance glycemic control is additive to that of sulfonylureas when used in combination.

Dosage Summary

Oral:

Children: Dosage not established

Adults: Initial: 25 mg 3 times/day; Maintenance: 25-100 mg 3 times/day (maximum: 300 mg/day)

Dosage Forms

Tablet, oral:

Glyset®: 25 mg, 50 mg, 100 mg

miglustat (MIG loo stat)

Sound-Alike/Look-Alike Issues

International issues:

Zavesca®: Brand name for miglustat [Canada, U.S., and multiple international markets], but also brand name for escitalopram [in multiple international markets; ISMP April 21, 2010]

Synonyms OGT-918

U.S./Canadian Brand Names Zavesca® [US/Can]

Therapeutic Category Enzyme Inhibitor

Use Treatment of mild-to-moderate type 1 Gaucher disease when enzyme replacement therapy is not a therapeutic option

Dosage Summary

Oral:

Children: Dosage not established

Adults: 100 mg 3 times/day; may be reduced to 1-2 times/day in patients who cannot tolerate due to adverse effects

Dosage Forms

Capsule, oral:

Zavesca®: 100 mg

Migquin ***(Discontinued)*** *see* acetaminophen, isometheptene, and dichloralphenazone *on page 31*

Migranal® [US/Can] *see* dihydroergotamine *on page 305*

Migrapap® ***(Discontinued)*** *see* acetaminophen, isometheptene, and dichloralphenazone *on page 31*

Migratine [US] *see* acetaminophen, isometheptene, and dichloralphenazone *on page 31*

Migrazone® ***(Discontinued)*** *see* acetaminophen, isometheptene, and dichloralphenazone *on page 31*

Migrin-A ***(Discontinued)*** *see* acetaminophen, isometheptene, and dichloralphenazone *on page 31*

Mild-C® [US-OTC] *see* ascorbic acid *on page 98*

Milk of Magnesia [US-OTC] *see* magnesium hydroxide *on page 585*

Millipred™ [US] *see* prednisolone (systemic) *on page 790*

milnacipran (mil NAY ci pran)

Sound-Alike/Look-Alike Issues

Savella® may be confused with cevimeline, sevelamer

U.S./Canadian Brand Names Savella® [US]

Therapeutic Category Antidepressant, Serotonin/Norepinephrine Reuptake Inhibitor

Use Management of fibromyalgia

Dosage Summary

Oral:

Children <17 years: Dosage not established

Adults: 50 mg twice daily (maximum dose: 200 mg/day)

Dosage Forms

Combination package, oral:

Savella®: Tablet: 12.5 mg (5s), Tablet: 25 mg (8s), and Tablet: 50 mg (42s)

Tablet, oral:

Savella®: 12.5 mg, 25 mg, 50 mg, 100 mg

Milontin® ***(Discontinued)***

Milophene® [Can] *see* clomiphene *on page 236*

Milophene® ***(Discontinued)*** *see* clomiphene *on page 236*

milrinone (MIL ri none)

Sound-Alike/Look-Alike Issues

Primacor® may be confused with Primaxin®

Synonyms milrinone lactate

U.S./Canadian Brand Names Milrinone Lactate Injection [Can]; Primacor® [Can]

Therapeutic Category Cardiovascular Agent, Other

Use Short-term I.V. therapy of acutely-decompensated heart failure

Dosage Summary

I.V.:

Children: Dosage not established

Adults: Loading dose (optional): 50 mcg/kg; Maintenance: 0.375-0.75 mcg/kg/minute

Dosage Forms

Infusion, premixed in D_5W: 200 mcg/mL (100 mL, 200 mL)

Injection, solution: 1 mg/mL (10 mL, 20 mL, 50 mL)

Injection, solution [preservative free]: 1 mg/mL (10 mL, 20 mL)

milrinone lactate *see* milrinone *on page* 635

Milrinone Lactate Injection [Can] *see* milrinone *on page* 635

Miltown® *(Discontinued)* *see* meprobamate *on page* 605

Mimvey™ [US] *see* estradiol and norethindrone *on page* 368

Mindal DM *(Discontinued)* *see* guaifenesin and dextromethorphan *on page* 455

mineral oil, petrolatum, lanolin, cetyl alcohol, and glycerin *see* lanolin, cetyl alcohol, glycerin, petrolatum, and mineral oil *on page* 548

Minestrin™ 1/20 [Can] *see* ethinyl estradiol and norethindrone *on page* 378

Mini-Gamulin® Rh *(Discontinued)*

Mini-Prenatal [US-OTC] *see* vitamins (multiple/prenatal) *on page* 991

Minipress® [US/Can] *see* prazosin *on page* 789

Minirin® [Can] *see* desmopressin acetate *on page* 278

Minitran™ [US/Can] *see* nitroglycerin *on page* 679

Minizide® *(Discontinued)*

Minocin® [US/Can] *see* minocycline *on page* 635

Minocin® PAC [US] *see* minocycline *on page* 635

minocycline (mi noe SYE kleen)

Sound-Alike/Look-Alike Issues

Dynacin® may be confused with Dyazide®, Dynabac®, DynaCirc®, Dynapen®

Minocin® may be confused with Indocin®, Lincocin®, Minizide®, Mithracin®, niacin

Synonyms minocycline hydrochloride

U.S./Canadian Brand Names Apo-Minocycline® [Can]; Arestin Microspheres [Can]; Dom-Minocycline [Can]; Dynacin® [US]; Minocin® PAC [US]; Minocin® [US/Can]; Mylan-Minocycline [Can]; Novo-Minocycline [Can]; PHL-Minocycline [Can]; PMS-Minocycline [Can]; ratio-Minocycline [Can]; Riva-Minocycline [Can]; Sandoz-Minocycline [Can]; Solodyn® [US]

Therapeutic Category Tetracycline Derivative

Use Treatment of susceptible bacterial infections of both gram-negative and gram-positive organisms; treatment of anthrax (inhalational, cutaneous, and gastrointestinal); moderate-to-severe acne; meningococcal (asymptomatic) carrier state; Rickettsial diseases (including Rocky Mountain spotted fever, Q fever); nongonococcal urethritis, gonorrhea; acute intestinal amebiasis; respiratory tract infection; skin/soft tissue infections; chlamydial infections

Extended release (Solodyn®): Only indicated for treatment of inflammatory lesions of non-nodular moderate-to-severe acne

Dosage Summary

I.V.:

Children ≤8 years: Dosage not established

Children >8 years: 4 mg/kg initially, followed by 2 mg/kg/dose every 12 hours (maximum: 400 mg/day)

Adults: 200 mg initially, followed by 100 mg every 12 hours (maximum: 400 mg/day)

Oral:

Children ≤8 years: Dosage not established

Children >8 years: 4 mg/kg initially, followed by 2 mg/kg/dose every 12 hours

Children ≥12 years: Solodyn®: 45-135 mg once daily (weight based)
Adults: 200 mg initially, followed by 100 mg every 12 hours **or** 50-100 mg twice daily (acne)
Solodyn®: 45-135 mg once daily (weight based)

Dosage Forms

Capsule, oral: 50 mg, 75 mg, 100 mg
Capsule, pellet filled, oral:
Minocin®: 50 mg, 100 mg
Minocin® PAC: 50 mg, 100 mg
Injection, powder for reconstitution:
Minocin®: 100 mg
Tablet, oral: 50 mg, 75 mg, 100 mg
Dynacin®: 50 mg, 75 mg, 100 mg
Tablet, extended release, oral:
Solodyn®: 45 mg, 65 mg, 90 mg, 115 mg, 135 mg

minocycline hydrochloride *see* minocycline *on page 635*
Min-Ovral® [Can] *see* ethinyl estradiol and levonorgestrel *on page 376*

minoxidil (systemic) (mi NOKS i dil)

Sound-Alike/Look-Alike Issues
minoxidil may be confused with metolazone, midodrine, Minipress®, Minocin®, Monopril®, Noxafil®
Loniten® may be confused with Lipitor®

U.S./Canadian Brand Names Loniten® [Can]

Therapeutic Category Vasodilator, Direct-Acting

Use Management of severe hypertension (usually in combination with a diuretic and beta-blocker)

Dosage Summary

Oral:
Children <12 years: Initial: 0.1-0.2 mg/kg once daily (maximum: 5 mg/day); Usual dosage range: 0.25-1 mg/kg/day in 1-2 divided doses (maximum: 50 mg/day); **Note:** Titration is recommended
Children ≥12 years: Initial: 5 mg once daily; Usual dosage range: 2.5-80 mg/day in 1-2 divided doses (maximum: 100 mg/day); **Note:** Titration is recommended
Adults: Initial: 5 mg once daily; Usual dosage range: 2.5-80 mg/day in 1-2 divided doses (maximum: 100 mg/day); **Note:** Titration is recommended
Elderly: Initial: 2.5 mg once daily; increase gradually

Dosage Forms

Tablet, oral: 2.5 mg, 10 mg

minoxidil (topical) (mi NOKS i dil)

U.S./Canadian Brand Names Apo-Gain® [Can]; Rogaine® Extra Strength for Men [US-OTC]; Rogaine® for Men [US-OTC]; Rogaine® for Women [US-OTC]; Rogaine® [Can]

Therapeutic Category Topical Skin Product

Use Treatment of alopecia androgenetica in males and females

Dosage Summary

Topical:
Children: Dosage not established
Adults: Apply twice daily

Dosage Forms

Aerosol, topical:
Rogaine® for Men [OTC]: 5% (60 g)
Solution, topical: 2% (60 mL); 5% (60 mL)
Rogaine® Extra Strength for Men [OTC]: 5% (60 mL)
Rogaine® for Women [OTC]: 2% (60 mL)

Mintab DM [US] *see* guaifenesin and dextromethorphan *on page 455*
Mint-Cefprozil [Can] *see* cefprozil *on page 192*
Mint-Ciprofloxacin [Can] *see* ciprofloxacin (systemic) *on page 224*
Mint-Citalopram [Can] *see* citalopram *on page 227*
Mintezol® *(Discontinued)*
Mint-Lisinopril [Can] *see* lisinopril *on page 570*
Mint-Ondansetron [Can] *see* ondansetron *on page 704*

Mintox Extra Strength [US-OTC] *see* aluminum hydroxide, magnesium hydroxide, and simethicone *on page* 59
Mintox Plus [US-OTC] *see* aluminum hydroxide, magnesium hydroxide, and simethicone *on page* 59
Mint-Pioglitazone [Can] *see* pioglitazone *on page* 762
Mint-Topiramate [Can] *see* topiramate *on page* 942
Mintuss DR [US] *see* chlorpheniramine, phenylephrine, and dextromethorphan *on page* 211
Mintuss G *(Discontinued)*
Mintuss HC [US] *see* phenylephrine, hydrocodone, and chlorpheniramine *on page* 754
Mintuss MS [US] *see* phenylephrine, hydrocodone, and chlorpheniramine *on page* 754
Minute-Gel® *(Discontinued)* *see* fluoride *on page* 413
Miochol®-E [US/Can] *see* acetylcholine *on page* 33
Miostat® [US/Can] *see* carbachol *on page* 177
MiraLAX® [US-OTC] *see* polyethylene glycol 3350 *on page* 775
Miranel AF™ [US-OTC] *see* miconazole (topical) *on page* 630
Mirapex® [US/Can] *see* pramipexole *on page* 786
Mirapex® ER™ [US] *see* pramipexole *on page* 786
Mircette® [US] *see* ethinyl estradiol and desogestrel *on page* 374
Mirena® [US/Can] *see* levonorgestrel *on page* 559

mirtazapine (mir TAZ a peen)

Sound-Alike/Look-Alike Issues

Remeron® may be confused with Premarin®, ramelteon, Rozerem®, Zemuron®

U.S./Canadian Brand Names Apo-Mirtazapine [Can]; CO Mirtazapine [Can]; Dom-Mirtazapine [Can]; Mylan-Mirtazapine [Can]; Novo-Mirtazapine [Can]; PHL-Mirtazapine [Can]; PMS-Mirtazapine [Can]; PRO-Mirtazapine [Can]; ratio-Mirtazapine [Can]; Remeron SolTab® [US]; Remeron® RD [Can]; Remeron® [US/Can]; Riva-Mirtazapine [Can]; Sandoz-Mirtazapine FC [Can]; Sandoz-Mirtazapine [Can]; ZYM-Mirtazapine [Can]

Therapeutic Category Antidepressant, Alpha-2 Antagonist

Use Treatment of depression

Dosage Summary

Oral:

Children: Dosage not established

Adults: Initial: 15 mg nightly; Maintenance: 15-45 mg nightly; **Note:** Titration is recommended every 1-2 weeks

Dosage Forms

Tablet, oral: 7.5 mg, 15 mg, 30 mg, 45 mg

Remeron®: 15 mg, 30 mg, 45 mg

Tablet, orally disintegrating, oral: 15 mg, 30 mg, 45 mg

Remeron SolTab®: 15 mg, 30 mg, 45 mg

misoprostol (mye soe PROST ole)

Sound-Alike/Look-Alike Issues

misoprostol may be confused with metoprolol, mifepristone

Cytotec® may be confused with Cytoxan®, Sytobex®

U.S./Canadian Brand Names Apo-Misoprostol® [Can]; Cytotec® [US]; Novo-Misoprostol [Can]; PMS-Misoprostol [Can]

Therapeutic Category Prostaglandin

Use Prevention of NSAID-induced gastric ulcers; medical termination of pregnancy of ≤49 days (in conjunction with mifepristone)

Dosage Summary

Intravaginal:

Children: Not for use prior to menarche

Oral:

Children <8 years: Dosage not established

Adults: 100-200 mcg 4 times/day with food

Elderly: May initiate at 100 mcg/day and increase by 100 mcg/day at 3-day intervals until desired dose is achieved

Dosage Forms
Tablet, oral: 100 mcg, 200 mcg
Cytotec®: 100 mcg, 200 mcg

misoprostol and diclofenac *see* diclofenac and misoprostol *on page* 298
Mito-Carn® ***(Discontinued)*** *see* levocarnitine *on page* 556

mitomycin (mye toe MYE sin)

Sound-Alike/Look-Alike Issues
mitomycin may be confused with mithramycin, mitotane, mitoxantrone
Synonyms mitomycin-C; mitomycin-X; MTC
U.S./Canadian Brand Names Mutamycin® [Can]
Therapeutic Category Antineoplastic Agent
Use Treatment of adenocarcinoma of stomach or pancreas
Dosage Summary
I.V.:
Adults: 20 mg/m^2 every 6-8 weeks as a single agent **or** 10 mg/m^2 every 6-8 weeks as combination therapy
Dosage Forms
Injection, powder for reconstitution: 5 mg, 20 mg, 40 mg

mitomycin-X *see* mitomycin *on page* 638
mitomycin-C *see* mitomycin *on page* 638

mitotane (MYE toe tane)

Sound-Alike/Look-Alike Issues
mitotane may be confused with mitomycin, mitoxantrone
Synonyms chloditan; chlodithane; khloditan; mytotan; o,p′-DDD; ortho,para-DDD
U.S./Canadian Brand Names Lysodren® [US/Can]
Therapeutic Category Antineoplastic Agent
Use Treatment of inoperable adrenocortical carcinoma
Dosage Summary
Oral:
Adults: Initial: 2-6 g/day in divided doses, then increase incrementally to 9-10 g/day in 3-4 divided doses (maximum: 18 g/day)
Dosage Forms
Tablet, oral:
Lysodren®: 500 mg

mitoxantrone (mye toe ZAN trone)

Sound-Alike/Look-Alike Issues
mitoxantrone may be confused with methotrexate, mitomycin, mitotane, Mutamycin®
Synonyms CL-232315; DHAD; DHAQ; dihydroxyanthracenedione; dihydroxyanthracenedione dihydrochloride; mitoxantrone dihydrochloride; mitoxantrone HCl; mitoxantrone hydrochloride; mitozantrone
U.S./Canadian Brand Names Mitoxantrone Injection® [Can]; Novantrone® [US/Can]
Therapeutic Category Antineoplastic Agent
Use Treatment of acute nonlymphocytic leukemias (ANLL [includes myelogenous, promyelocytic, monocytic and erythroid leukemias]); advanced hormone-refractory prostate cancer; secondary progressive or relapsing-remitting multiple sclerosis (MS)
Dosage Summary
I.V.:
Children: Dosage not established
Adults: 12 mg/m^2/day once daily for 2-3 days **or** 12-14 mg/m^2 every 3 weeks **or** 12 mg/m^2 every 3 months (multiple sclerosis; maximum lifetime cumulative dose: 140 mg/m^2)
Dosage Forms
Injection, solution [preservative free]: 2 mg/mL (10 mL, 12.5 mL, 15 mL, 20 mL)
Novantrone®: 2 mg/mL (10 mL)

mitoxantrone dihydrochloride *see* mitoxantrone *on page* 638
mitoxantrone HCl *see* mitoxantrone *on page* 638

mitoxantrone hydrochloride *see* mitoxantrone *on page 638*
Mitoxantrone Injection® [Can] *see* mitoxantrone *on page 638*
mitozantrone *see* mitoxantrone *on page 638*
Mitran® Oral *(Discontinued)* *see* chlordiazepoxide *on page 203*
Mitrazol® [US-OTC] *see* miconazole (topical) *on page 630*
Mivacron® *(Discontinued)*
mivacurium *(Discontinued)*
MK-217 *see* alendronate *on page 47*
MK383 *see* tirofiban *on page 936*
MK-0431 *see* sitagliptin *on page 879*
MK462 *see* rizatriptan *on page 848*
MK 0517 *see* fosaprepitant *on page 427*
MK-0518 *see* raltegravir *on page 826*
MK594 *see* losartan *on page 577*
MK0826 *see* ertapenem *on page 360*
MK 869 *see* aprepitant *on page 92*
MLN341 *see* bortezomib *on page 143*
MMF *see* mycophenolate *on page 650*
MMR *see* measles, mumps, and rubella virus vaccine *on page 592*
M-M-R® II [US/Can] *see* measles, mumps, and rubella virus vaccine *on page 592*
MMR-V *see* measles, mumps, rubella, and varicella virus vaccine *on page 593*
MMRV *see* measles, mumps, rubella, and varicella virus vaccine *on page 593*
MOAB ABX-EGF *see* panitumumab *on page 724*
MOAB anti-tac *see* daclizumab *on page 265*
MOAB C225 *see* cetuximab *on page 199*
MoAb CD52 *see* alemtuzumab *on page 47*
MOAB HER2 *see* trastuzumab *on page 948*
Moban® [Can] *see* molindone *on page 640*
Moban® *(Discontinued)* *see* molindone *on page 640*
Mobic® [US/Can] *see* meloxicam *on page 598*
Mobicox® [Can] *see* meloxicam *on page 598*
Mobidin® *(Discontinued)* *see* magnesium salicylate *on page 587*
Mobisyl® [US-OTC] *see* trolamine *on page 963*

moclobemide *(Canada only)* (moe KLOE be mide)

U.S./Canadian Brand Names Apo-Moclobemide® [Can]; Dom-Moclobemide [Can]; Manerix® [Can]; Novo-Moclobemide [Can]; Nu-Moclobemide [Can]; PMS-Moclobemide [Can]

Therapeutic Category Antidepressant, Monoamine Oxidase Inhibitor

Use Symptomatic relief of depressive illness

Dosage Summary

Oral:

Children: Dosage not established

Adults: Initial: 300 mg/day in 2 divided doses; Maintenance: Increase gradually up to 600 mg/day

Dosage Forms - Canada

Tablet:

Apo-Moclobemide®, Dom-Moclobemide, Manerix®, Novo-Moclobemide, Nu-Moclobemide, PMS-Moclobemide: 150 mg, 300 mg

modafinil (moe DAF i nil)

U.S./Canadian Brand Names Alertec® [Can]; Apo-Modafinil [Can]; Provigil® [US]

Therapeutic Category Central Nervous System Stimulant, Nonamphetamine

Controlled Substance C-IV

Use Improve wakefulness in patients with excessive daytime sleepiness associated with narcolepsy and shift work sleep disorder (SWSD); adjunctive therapy for obstructive sleep apnea/hypopnea syndrome (OSAHS)

Dosage Summary

Oral:

Children: Dosage not established

Adults: 200 mg once daily; **Note:** Doses of 400 mg/day, have been well tolerated, but there is no consistent evidence that this dose confers additional benefit

Dosage Forms

Tablet, oral:

Provigil®: 100 mg, 200 mg

Modane® Soft *(Discontinued)* *see* docusate *on page* 321

Modecate® [Can] *see* fluphenazine *on page* 417

Modecate® Concentrate [Can] *see* fluphenazine *on page* 417

Modicon® [US] *see* ethinyl estradiol and norethindrone *on page* 378

modified Dakin's solution *see* sodium hypochlorite solution *on page* 884

Moducal® [US-OTC] *see* glucose polymers *on page* 448

Modulon® [Can] *see* trimebutine *(Canada only) on page* 959

Moduret [Can] *see* amiloride and hydrochlorothiazide *on page* 64

Moduretic® *(Discontinued)* *see* amiloride and hydrochlorothiazide *on page* 64

moexipril (mo EKS i pril)

Sound-Alike/Look-Alike Issues

moexipril may be confused with Monopril®

Synonyms moexipril hydrochloride

U.S./Canadian Brand Names Univasc® [US]

Therapeutic Category Angiotensin-Converting Enzyme (ACE) Inhibitor

Use Treatment of hypertension, alone or in combination with thiazide diuretics

Dosage Summary

Oral:

Children: Dosage not established

Adults: Initial: 3.75-7.5 mg once daily; Maintenance: 7.5-30 mg/day in 1 or 2 divided doses

Dosage Forms

Tablet, oral: 7.5 mg, 15 mg

Univasc®: 7.5 mg, 15 mg

moexipril and hydrochlorothiazide (mo EKS i pril & hye droe klor oh THYE a zide)

Synonyms hydrochlorothiazide and moexipril

U.S./Canadian Brand Names Uniretic® [US/Can]

Therapeutic Category Angiotensin-Converting Enzyme (ACE) Inhibitor; Diuretic, Thiazide

Use Treatment of hypertension; not indicated for initial treatment of hypertension

Dosage Summary

Oral:

Children: Dosage not established

Adults: 7.5-30 mg of moexipril/day and ≤50 mg hydrochlorothiazide/day in a single or divided dose

Dosage Forms

Tablet, oral: 7.5/12.5: Moexipril 7.5 mg and hydrochlorothiazide 12.5; 15/12.5: Moexipril 15 mg and hydrochlorothiazide 12.5; 15/25: Moexipril 15 mg and hydrochlorothiazide 25

Uniretic®: 7.5/12.5: Moexipril 7.5 mg and hydrochlorothiazide 12.5 mg [scored]; 15/12.5: Moexipril 15 mg and hydrochlorothiazide 12.5 mg [scored]; 15/25: Moexipril 15 mg and hydrochlorothiazide 25 mg [scored]

moexipril hydrochloride *see* moexipril *on page* 640

Mogadon [Can] *see* nitrazepam *(Canada only) on page* 678

Moi-Stir® [US-OTC] *see* saliva substitute *on page* 861

Moisture® Eyes [US-OTC] *see* artificial tears *on page* 97

Moisture® Eyes PM [US-OTC] *see* artificial tears *on page* 97

molindone (moe LIN done)

Sound-Alike/Look-Alike Issues

molindone may be confused with Mobidin®

Moban® may be confused with Mobidin®

Synonyms molindone hydrochloride

U.S./Canadian Brand Names Moban® [Can]

Therapeutic Category Antipsychotic Agent, Dihydroindoline

Use Management of schizophrenia

Dosage Summary

Oral:

Children <3 years: Dosage not established

Children 3-5 years: 1-2.5 mg/day in 4 divided doses

Children 5-12 years: 0.5-1 mg/kg/day in 4 divided doses

Adults: Initial: 50-75 mg/day; titrate gradually every 3-4 days to maximum: 225 mg/day; Maintenance: 5-25 mg 3-4 times/day (maximum: 225 mg/day); **Note:** Titration is recommended every 3-4 days

Elderly: Initial: 5-10 mg 1-2 times/day; Maintenance: Up to 112 mg/day; **Note:** Titration is recommended every 4-7 days (5-10 mg/day)

molindone hydrochloride *see* molindone *on page 640*

molybdenum *see* trace metals *on page 945*

MOM *see* magnesium hydroxide *on page 585*

Momentum® [US-OTC] *see* magnesium salicylate *on page 587*

mometasone (oral inhalation) (moe MET a sone)

Synonyms mometasone furoate

U.S./Canadian Brand Names Asmanex® Twisthaler® [US]

Therapeutic Category Corticosteroid, Inhalant (Oral)

Use Maintenance treatment of asthma as prophylactic therapy or as a supplement in asthma patients requiring oral corticosteroids for the purpose of decreasing or eliminating the oral corticosteroid requirement

Dosage Summary

Inhalation:

Children <4 years: Dosage not established

Children 4-11 years: 110 mcg once daily in the evening (maximum: 110 mcg/day)

Children ≥12 years: 1-4 inhalations (220-880 mcg) in 1-2 divided doses (maximum: 880 mcg/day); **Note:** Dosage depends on previous therapy

Adults: 1-4 inhalations (220-880 mcg) in 1-2 divided doses (maximum: 880 mcg/day); **Note:** Dosage depends on previous therapy

Dosage Forms

Powder, for oral inhalation:

Asmanex® Twisthaler®: 110 mcg (30 units); 220 mcg (14 units, 30 units, 60 units, 120 units)

mometasone (nasal) (moe MET a sone)

Synonyms mometasone furoate

U.S./Canadian Brand Names Nasonex® [US/Can]

Therapeutic Category Corticosteroid, Nasal

Use Treatment of nasal symptoms of seasonal and perennial allergic rhinitis; prevention of nasal symptoms associated with seasonal allergic rhinitis; treatment of nasal polyps in adults

Dosage Summary

Intranasal:

Children <2 years: Dosage not established

Children 2-11 years: 1 spray (50 mcg) in each nostril daily

Children ≥12 years: 2 sprays (100 mcg) in each nostril daily

Adults: 2 sprays (100 mcg) in each nostril daily

Dosage Forms

Suspension, intranasal:

Nasonex®: 50 mcg/spray (17 g)

mometasone (topical) (moe MET a sone)

Sound-Alike/Look-Alike Issues

Elocon® lotion may be confused with ophthalmic solutions. Manufacturer's labeling emphasizes the product is **NOT** for use in the eyes.

Synonyms mometasone furoate

U.S./Canadian Brand Names Elocom® [Can]; Elocon® [US]; PMS-Mometasone [Can]; ratio-Mometasone [Can]; Taro-Mometasone [Can]

Therapeutic Category Corticosteroid, Topical

Use Relief of the inflammatory and pruritic manifestations of corticosteroid-responsive dermatoses (medium potency topical corticosteroid)

Dosage Summary

Topical:

Cream, ointment:

Children <2 years: Dosage not established

Children ≥2 years: Apply a thin film to affected area once daily

Adults: Apply a thin film to affected area once daily

Lotion:

Children <12 years: Dosage not established

Children ≥12 years: Apply a few drops to affected area once daily

Adults: Apply a few drops to affected area once daily

Dosage Forms

Cream, topical: 0.1% (15 g, 45 g)

Elocon®: 0.1% (15 g, 45 g)

Lotion, topical: 0.1% (30 mL, 60 mL)

Elocon®: 0.1% (30 mL, 60 mL)

Ointment, topical: 0.1% (15 g, 45 g)

Elocon®: 0.1% (15 g, 45 g)

mometasone and formoterol (moe MET a sone & for MOH te rol)

Synonyms formoterol and mometasone; formoterol and mometasone furoate; formoterol fumarate dihydrate and mometasone

U.S./Canadian Brand Names Dulera® [US]

Therapeutic Category $Beta_2$-Adrenergic Agonist; $Beta_2$-Adrenergic Agonist, Long-Acting; Corticosteroid, Inhalant (Oral)

Use Treatment of asthma where combination therapy is indicated

Dosage Summary

Inhalation:

Children ≤11 years: Dosage not established

Children ≥12 years: Two inhalations twice daily (maximum: 4 inhalations/day)

Adults: Two inhalations twice daily (maximum: 4 inhalations/day)

Dosage Forms

Aerosol, for oral inhalation:

Dulera®: Mometasone 100 mcg and formoterol 5 mcg per inhalation (13 g) [120 metered actuations]

Dulera®: Mometasone 200 mcg and formoterol 5 mcg per inhalation (13 g) [120 metered actuations]

mometasone furoate *see* mometasone (nasal) *on page 641*

mometasone furoate *see* mometasone (oral inhalation) *on page 641*

mometasone furoate *see* mometasone (topical) *on page 641*

MOM/mineral oil emulsion *see* magnesium hydroxide and mineral oil *on page 586*

monacolin K *see* lovastatin *on page 579*

Monafed® ***(Discontinued)*** *see* guaifenesin *on page 454*

Monafed® DM ***(Discontinued)*** *see* guaifenesin and dextromethorphan *on page 455*

Monarc-M™ [US] *see* antihemophilic factor (human) *on page 81*

Monilia **skin test** *see Candida albicans (Monilia) on page 174*

Monistat® [Can] *see* miconazole (topical) *on page 630*

Monistat® 1 [US-OTC] *see* miconazole (topical) *on page 630*

Monistat® 1 Day or Night [US-OTC] *see* miconazole (topical) *on page 630*

Monistat® 3 [US-OTC/Can] *see* miconazole (topical) *on page 630*

Monistat® 7 [US-OTC] *see* miconazole (topical) *on page 630*

Monistat-Derm® ***(Discontinued)*** *see* miconazole (topical) *on page 630*

Monistat i.v.™ Injection ***(Discontinued)*** *see* miconazole (oral) *on page 630*

monobenzone (mon oh BEN zone)

Therapeutic Category Topical Skin Product

Use Final depigmentation in extensive vitiligo

Dosage Summary

Topical:

Children <12 years: Dosage not established

Children ≥12 years: Initial: Apply 2-3 times/day; once depigmentation obtained apply as needed (usually 2 times/week)

Adults: Initial: Apply 2-3 times/day; once desired degree of pigmentation obtained apply as needed (usually 2 times/week)

Monocaps [US-OTC] *see* vitamins (multiple/oral) *on page 990*

Monoclate-P® [US] *see* antihemophilic factor (human) *on page 81*

monoclonal antibody *see* muromonab-CD3 *on page 649*

monoclonal antibody ABX-EGF *see* panitumumab *on page 724*

monoclonal antibody campath-1H *see* alemtuzumab *on page 47*

monoclonal antibody CD52 *see* alemtuzumab *on page 47*

Monodox® [US] *see* doxycycline *on page 331*

monoethanolamine *see* ethanolamine oleate *on page 374*

Monoket® [US] *see* isosorbide mononitrate *on page 529*

MonoNessa® [US] *see* ethinyl estradiol and norgestimate *on page 380*

Mononine® [US/Can] *see* factor IX *on page 389*

Monopril® [Can] *see* fosinopril *on page 428*

Monopril® *(Discontinued)* *see* fosinopril *on page 428*

Monopril-HCT® [Can] *see* fosinopril and hydrochlorothiazide *on page 428*

Monopril-HCT® *(Discontinued)* *see* fosinopril and hydrochlorothiazide *on page 428*

montelukast (mon te LOO kast)

Sound-Alike/Look-Alike Issues

Singulair® may be confused with Sinequan®

Synonyms montelukast sodium

U.S./Canadian Brand Names Singulair® [US/Can]

Therapeutic Category Leukotriene Receptor Antagonist

Use Prophylaxis and chronic treatment of asthma; relief of symptoms of seasonal allergic rhinitis and perennial allergic rhinitis; prevention of exercise-induced bronchospasm

Dosage Summary

Oral:

Children <6 months: Dosage not established

Children 6-23 months: 4 mg (oral granules) once daily

Children 2-5 years: 4 mg (chewable tablet or oral granules) once daily

Children 6-14 years: 5 mg (chewable tablet) once daily

Children ≥15 years: 10 mg once daily **or** 10 mg 2 hours prior to exercise

Adults: 10 mg once daily **or** 10 mg 2 hours prior to exercise

Dosage Forms

Granules, oral:

Singulair®: 4 mg/packet (30s)

Tablet, oral:

Singulair®: 10 mg

Tablet, chewable, oral:

Singulair®: 4 mg, 5 mg

montelukast sodium *see* montelukast *on page 643*

Monurol® [US/Can] *see* fosfomycin *on page 428*

8-MOP® [US] *see* methoxsalen (systemic) *on page 616*

more attenuated Enders strain *see* measles virus vaccine (live) *on page 593*

MoreDophilus® [US-OTC] *see* Lactobacillus *on page 543*

moricizine *(Discontinued)*

morning after pill *see* ethinyl estradiol and norgestrel *on page 380*

morphine (systemic) (MOR feen)

Sound-Alike/Look-Alike Issues

morphine may be confused with HYDROmorphone, methadone

morphine sulfate may be confused with magnesium sulfate

Avinza® may be confused with Evista®, Invanz®

Kadian® may be confused with Kapidex™ [DSC]

MS Contin® may be confused with Oxycontin®

MS (error-prone abbreviation and should not be used)

MSO_4 and MS are error-prone abbreviations (mistaken as magnesium sulfate)

Roxanol™ may be confused with OxyFast®, Roxicet™, Roxicodone®

U.S./Canadian Brand Names Astramorph/PF™ [US]; Avinza® [US]; Doloral [Can]; Duramorph® [US]; Infumorph® 200 [US]; Infumorph® 500 [US]; Kadian® [US/Can]; M-Eslon® [Can]; M.O.S.-SR® [Can]; M.O.S.-Sulfate® [Can]; M.O.S.® 10 [Can]; M.O.S.® 20 [Can]; M.O.S.® 30 [Can]; Morphine HP® [Can]; Morphine LP® Epidural [Can]; MS Contin® [US/Can]; MS-IR® [Can]; Novo-Morphine SR [Can]; Oramorph® SR [US]; PMS-Morphine Sulfate SR [Can]; ratio-Morphine SR [Can]; ratio-Morphine [Can]; Statex® [Can]

Therapeutic Category Analgesic, Opioid

Controlled Substance C-II

Use Relief of moderate-to-severe acute and chronic pain; relief of pain of myocardial infarction; relief of dyspnea of acute left ventricular failure and pulmonary edema; preanesthetic medication

Infumorph®: Used in continuous microinfusion devices for intrathecal or epidural administration in treatment of intractable chronic pain

Controlled-, extended-, or sustained-release products: Only intended/indicated for use when repeated doses for an extended period of time are required. The 100 mg and 200 mg tablets or capsules of Kadian®, MS Contin®, and morphine sulfate controlled-release tablets and the 60 mg, 90 mg, and 120 mg capsules of Avinza® should only be used in opioid-tolerant patients.

Dosage Summary

Epidural:

Children: Dosage not established

Adults: 5 mg [Astromorph/PF™, Duramorph®] as a single dose **or** 1-6 mg bolus followed by 0.1-0.2 mg/hour (maximum: 10 mg/day) **or** continuous microinfusion [Infumorph®] opioid-naive patients: 3.5-7.5 mg/day, opioid-tolerant patients: 4.5-30 mg/day

I.M.:

Children ≤6 months: Dosage not established

Children >6 months and <50 kg: 0.1-0.2 mg/kg every 3-4 hours as needed

Adults: 5-20 mg every 4 hours as needed

I.T. (I.T. dose is usually 1/10 that of epidural dose):

Children: Dosage not established

Adults:

Single dose: Opioid-naive: 0.2-1 mg/dose as single dose (repeat doses not recommended); Opioid-tolerant: 1-10 mg/day

Microinfusion (Infumorph®): Initial: Opioid-naive: 0.2-1 mg/day; Opioid-tolerant: 1-10 mg/day (titrate to effect)

I.V.:

Children ≤6 months: Dosage not established

Children >6 months and <50 kg: 0.1-0.2 mg/kg every 3-4 hours as needed **or** 10-60 mcg/kg/**hour** as a continuous infusion

Adults: 2.5-5 mg every 3-4 hours **or** 0.8-10 mg/hour; Usual range: Up to 80 mg/hour

Adults (mechanically-ventilated): 0.7-10 mg every 1-2 hours as needed **or** 5-35 mg/hour infusion

Oral:

Controlled, extended or sustained release:

Children: Dosage not established

Adults:

Capsules: Established daily dose on prompt-release formulations administered in 1-2 divided doses (every 12 hours)

Tablets: Established daily dose on prompt-release formulations administered in divided doses every 8-12 hours

Immediate release:

Children ≤6 months: Dosage not established

Children >6 months and <50 kg: 0.15-0.3 mg/kg every 3-4 hours as needed

Adults: 10-30 mg every 4 hours as needed; **Note:** Much higher doses may be necessary for chronic pain

PCA:

Children: Dosage not established

Adults: Concentration: 1 mg/mL; Demand dose: 0.5-2.5 mg; Lockout interval: 5-10 minutes

Rectal:

Children: Dosage not established

Adults: 10-20 mg every 3-4 hours

SubQ:

Children: Dosage not established

Adults: 5-20 mg every 3-4 hours as needed **or** 0.8-10 mg/hour (up to 80 mg/hour) as continuous infusion

Adults (mechanically-ventilated): 0.7-10 mg every 1-2 hours as needed **or** 5-35 mg/hour infusion

Dosage Forms

Capsule, extended release, oral:

Avinza®: 30 mg, 45 mg, 60 mg, 75 mg, 90 mg, 120 mg

Kadian®: 10 mg, 20 mg, 30 mg, 50 mg, 60 mg, 80 mg, 200 mg

Injection, solution: 1 mg/mL (10 mL, 30 mL, 50 mL); 2 mg/mL (1 mL); 4 mg/mL (1 mL); 5 mg/mL (1 mL, 30 mL, 50 mL); 8 mg/mL (1 mL); 10 mg/mL (1 mL, 10 mL); 10 mg/0.7 mL (0.7 mL); 15 mg/mL (1 mL, 20 mL); 25 mg/mL (4 mL, 10 mL, 20 mL); 50 mg/mL (20 mL, 40 mL, 50 mL)

Injection, solution [preservative free]: 0.5 mg/mL (10 mL, 30 mL); 1 mg/mL (10 mL, 30 mL); 5 mg/mL (30 mL); 25 mg/mL (4 mL, 10 mL, 20 mL)

Astramorph/PF™: 0.5 mg/mL (2 mL, 10 mL); 1 mg/mL (2 mL, 10 mL)

Duramorph®: 0.5 mg/mL (10 mL); 1 mg/mL (10 mL)

Infumorph® 200: 10 mg/mL (20 mL)

Infumorph® 500: 25 mg/mL (20 mL)

Solution, oral: 10 mg/5 mL (5 mL, 10 mL, 100 mL, 500 mL); 20 mg/5 mL (100 mL, 500 mL); 100 mg/5 mL (1 mL, 15 mL, 30 mL, 120 mL, 240 mL)

Suppository, rectal: 5 mg (12s); 10 mg (12s); 20 mg (12s); 30 mg (12s)

Tablet, oral: 15 mg, 30 mg

Tablet, controlled release, oral:

MS Contin®: 15 mg, 30 mg, 60 mg, 100 mg, 200 mg

Tablet, extended release, oral: 15 mg, 30 mg, 60 mg, 100 mg, 200 mg

Tablet, sustained release, oral:

Oramorph® SR: 15 mg, 30 mg, 60 mg, 100 mg

Dosage Forms - Canada

Solution, oral:

Doloral: 1 mg/mL; 5 mg/mL [not available in U.S.]

morphine (liposomal) (MOR feen)

Sound-Alike/Look-Alike Issues

morphine may be confused with HYDROmorphone

morphine sulfate may be confused with magnesium sulfate

MS (error-prone abbreviation and should not be used)

MSO_4 and MS are error-prone abbreviations (mistaken as magnesium sulfate)

Synonyms extended release epidural morphine

U.S./Canadian Brand Names DepoDur® [US]

Therapeutic Category Analgesic, Opioid

Controlled Substance C-II

Use Epidural (lumbar) single-dose management of surgical pain

Dosage Summary Epidural:

Children: Dosage not established

Adults: 10-15 mg as a single dose depending on surgery

Dosage Forms

Injection, extended release liposomal suspension [preservative free]:

DepoDur®: 10 mg/mL (1 mL, 1.5 mL)

morphine and naltrexone (MOR feen & nal TREKS one)

Sound-Alike/Look-Alike Issues

morphine may be confused with HYDROmorphone
morphine sulfate may be confused with magnesium sulfate
naltrexone may be confused with methylnaltrexone, naloxone
MS (error-prone abbreviation and should not be used)
MSO_4 and MS are error-prone abbreviations (mistaken as magnesium sulfate)

Synonyms morphine sulfate and naltrexone hydrochloride; naltrexone and morphine

U.S./Canadian Brand Names Embeda™ [US]

Therapeutic Category Analgesic, Opioid; Opioid Antagonist

Controlled Substance C-II

Use Relief of moderate-to-severe pain when continual, around-the-clock therapy is needed for an extended period of time

Dosage Summary

Oral:

Children: Dosage not established
Adults: Initial: 20 mg/0.8 mg once or twice daily; Maintenance: Adjust based on individual patient requirement

Dosage Forms

Capsule, extended release, oral:

Embeda™ 20/0.8: Morphine 20 mg and naltrexone 0.8 mg
Embeda™ 30/1.2: Morphine 30 mg and naltrexone 1.2 mg
Embeda™ 50/2: Morphine 50 mg and naltrexone 2 mg
Embeda™ 80/3.2: Morphine 80 mg and naltrexone 3.2 mg
Embeda™ 100/4: Morphine 100 mg and naltrexone 4 mg

Morphine HP® [Can] *see* morphine (systemic) *on page 644*
Morphine LP® Epidural [Can] *see* morphine (systemic) *on page 644*
morphine sulfate and naltrexone hydrochloride *see* morphine and naltrexone *on page 646*

morrhuate sodium (MOR yoo ate SOW dee um)

U.S./Canadian Brand Names Scleromate® [US]

Therapeutic Category Sclerosing Agent

Use Treatment of small, uncomplicated varicose veins of the lower extremities

Dosage Summary

I.V.:

Children: Dosage not established
Adults: 50-250 mg, repeated at 5- to 7-day intervals

Dosage Forms

Injection, solution: 50 mg/mL (30 mL)
Scleromate®: 50 mg/mL (30 mL)

M.O.S.® 10 [Can] *see* morphine (systemic) *on page 644*
M.O.S.® 20 [Can] *see* morphine (systemic) *on page 644*
M.O.S.® 30 [Can] *see* morphine (systemic) *on page 644*
Mosco® Callus & Corn Remover [US-OTC] *see* salicylic acid *on page 858*
Mosco® One Step Corn Remover [US-OTC] *see* salicylic acid *on page 858*
M.O.S.-SR® [Can] *see* morphine (systemic) *on page 644*
M.O.S.-Sulfate® [Can] *see* morphine (systemic) *on page 644*
Motofen® [US] *see* difenoxin and atropine *on page 300*
Motrin® Children's [US-OTC/Can] *see* ibuprofen *on page 494*
Motrin® *(Discontinued)* *see* ibuprofen *on page 494*
Motrin® IB [US-OTC/Can] *see* ibuprofen *on page 494*
Motrin® IB Sinus *(Discontinued)* *see* pseudoephedrine and ibuprofen *on page 812*
Motrin® Infants' [US-OTC] *see* ibuprofen *on page 494*
Motrin® Junior [US-OTC] *see* ibuprofen *on page 494*
Mouthkote® [US-OTC] *see* saliva substitute *on page 861*
MoviPrep® [US] *see* polyethylene glycol-electrolyte solution *on page 775*

Moxatag™ [US] *see* amoxicillin *on page* 72

moxifloxacin (systemic) (moxs i FLOKS a sin)

Sound-Alike/Look-Alike Issues

Avelox® may be confused with Avonex®

Synonyms moxifloxacin hydrochloride

U.S./Canadian Brand Names Avelox® ABC Pack [US]; Avelox® I.V. [US/Can]; Avelox® [US/Can]

Therapeutic Category Antibiotic, Quinolone; Respiratory Fluoroquinolone

Use Treatment of mild-to-moderate community-acquired pneumonia, including multidrug-resistant *Streptococcus pneumoniae* (MDRSP); acute bacterial exacerbation of chronic bronchitis; acute bacterial sinusitis; complicated and uncomplicated skin and skin structure infections; complicated intraabdominal infections

Dosage Summary

I.V.:

Children: Dosage not established

Adults: 400 mg every 24 hours

Oral:

Children: Dosage not established

Adults: 400 mg every 24 hours

Dosage Forms

Infusion, premixed in sodium chloride 0.8% [preservative free]:

Avelox® I.V.: 400 mg (250 mL)

Tablet, oral:

Avelox®: 400 mg

Avelox® ABC Pack: 400 mg

moxifloxacin (ophthalmic) (moxs i FLOKS a sin)

Synonyms moxifloxacin hydrochloride

U.S./Canadian Brand Names Vigamox® [US/Can]

Therapeutic Category Antibiotic, Ophthalmic; Antibiotic, Quinolone

Use Treatment of bacterial conjunctivitis caused by susceptible organisms

Dosage Summary

Ophthalmic:

Children <1 year: Dosage not established

Children ≥1 year: Instill 1 drop into affected eye(s) 3 times/day

Adults: Instill 1 drop into affected eye(s) 3 times/day

Dosage Forms

Solution, ophthalmic:

Vigamox®: 0.5% (3 mL)

moxifloxacin hydrochloride *see* moxifloxacin (ophthalmic) *on page* 647

moxifloxacin hydrochloride *see* moxifloxacin (systemic) *on page* 647

Mozobil™ [US] *see* plerixafor *on page* 766

4-MP *see* fomepizole *on page* 425

MPA *see* medroxyprogesterone *on page* 597

MPA *see* mycophenolate *on page* 650

MPA and estrogens (conjugated) *see* estrogens (conjugated/equine) and medroxyprogesterone *on page* 371

M-Prednisol® Injection *(Discontinued)* *see* methylprednisolone *on page* 622

MPSV *see* meningococcal polysaccharide vaccine (groups A / C / Y and W-135) *on page* 601

MPSV4 *see* meningococcal polysaccharide vaccine (groups A / C / Y and W-135) *on page* 601

MRA *see* tocilizumab *on page* 939

MS Contin® [US/Can] *see* morphine (systemic) *on page* 644

MS-IR® [Can] *see* morphine (systemic) *on page* 644

MST 600 [US] *see* magnesium salicylate *on page* 587

MTC *see* mitomycin *on page* 638

Mucinex® [US-OTC] *see* guaifenesin *on page* 454

Mucinex® D [US-OTC] *see* guaifenesin and pseudoephedrine *on page* 457

Mucinex® D Maximum Strength [US-OTC] *see* guaifenesin and pseudoephedrine *on page 457*
Mucinex® Children's Cough *(Discontinued)* *see* guaifenesin and dextromethorphan *on page 455*
Mucinex® Cold [US-OTC] *see* guaifenesin and phenylephrine *on page 456*
Mucinex® DM [US-OTC] *see* guaifenesin and dextromethorphan *on page 455*
Mucinex® DM Maximum Strength [US-OTC] *see* guaifenesin and dextromethorphan *on page 455*
Mucinex® Full force™ *(Discontinued)* *see* oxymetazoline (nasal) *on page 716*
Mucinex® Kid's [US-OTC] *see* guaifenesin *on page 454*
Mucinex® Kid's Mini-Melts™ [US-OTC] *see* guaifenesin *on page 454*
Mucinex® Kid's Cough [US-OTC] *see* guaifenesin and dextromethorphan *on page 455*
Mucinex® Kid's Cough Mini-Melts™ [US-OTC] *see* guaifenesin and dextromethorphan *on page 455*
Mucinex® Maximum Strength [US-OTC] *see* guaifenesin *on page 454*
Mucinex® moisture smart™ *(Discontinued)* *see* oxymetazoline (nasal) *on page 716*
Mucomyst® [Can] *see* acetylcysteine *on page 34*

mucosal barrier gel, oral (myoo KOH sul BAR ee er GEL, OR al)

Synonyms mucosal bioadherent gel

U.S./Canadian Brand Names Gelclair® [US]

Therapeutic Category Gastrointestinal Agent, Miscellaneous

Use Management of oral mucosal pain caused by oral mucositis/stomatitis (resulting from chemotherapy or radiation therapy), irritation due to oral surgery, traumatic ulcers caused by braces/ill-fitting dentures or disease, diffuse aphthous ulcers (canker sores)

Dosage Forms

Gel, oral:

Gelclair®: 15 mL/packet (15s)

mucosal bioadherent gel *see* mucosal barrier gel, oral *on page 648*
Mucosil™ *(Discontinued)* *see* acetylcysteine *on page 34*
Mucus Relief [US-OTC] *see* guaifenesin *on page 454*
Multaq® [US/Can] *see* dronedarone *on page 333*
Multidex® [US-OTC] *see* maltodextrin *on page 589*
Multihance® [US] *see* gadobenate dimeglumine *on page 433*
Multihance® Multipak™ [US] *see* gadobenate dimeglumine *on page 433*
multiple vitamins *see* vitamins (multiple/oral) *on page 990*
Multitest CMI® *(Discontinued)*
Multitrace®-4 [US] *see* trace metals *on page 945*
Multitrace®-4 Concentrate [US] *see* trace metals *on page 945*
Multitrace®-4 Neonatal [US] *see* trace metals *on page 945*
Multitrace®-4 Pediatric [US] *see* trace metals *on page 945*
Multitrace®-5 [US] *see* trace metals *on page 945*
Multitrace®-5 Concentrate [US] *see* trace metals *on page 945*
multivitamins/fluoride *see* vitamins (multiple/pediatric) *on page 990*
mumps, measles, and rubella vaccines *see* measles, mumps, and rubella virus vaccine *on page 592*
mumps, rubella, varicella, and measles vaccine *see* measles, mumps, rubella, and varicella virus vaccine *on page 593*
Mumpsvax® *(Discontinued)* *see* mumps virus vaccine *on page 648*

mumps virus vaccine (mumpz VYE rus vak SEEN)

Therapeutic Category Vaccine, Live Virus

Use Mumps prophylaxis by promoting active immunity

Note: Unless contraindicated, trivalent measles - mumps - rubella (MMR) is the vaccine of choice if recipients are likely to be susceptible to rubella and/or measles as well as to mumps.

The Advisory Committee on Immunization Practices (ACIP) recommends routine vaccination for the following:

- All children (first dose given at 12-15 months of age)

- Adults born 1957 or later (without evidence of immunity or documentation of vaccination)
- Adults at higher risk for exposure to and transmission of mumps should receive special consideration for vaccination, unless an acceptable evidence of immunity exists. This includes international travelers, persons attending colleges and other post-high school education, persons working in healthcare facilities.

Dosage Summary

SubQ:

Children <12 months: Dosage not established

Children ≥12-15 months: 0.5 mL; when 2 doses are needed, at least 28 days should elapse between dose

Adults: 0.5 mL; when 2 doses are needed, at least 28 days should elapse between dose

mupirocin (myoo PEER oh sin)

Sound-Alike/Look-Alike Issues

Bactroban® may be confused with bacitracin, baclofen, Bactrim™

Synonyms mupirocin calcium; pseudomonic acid A

U.S./Canadian Brand Names Bactroban Cream® [US]; Bactroban Nasal® [US]; Bactroban® [US/Can]

Therapeutic Category Antibiotic, Topical

Use

Intranasal: Eradication of nasal colonization with MRSA in adult patients and healthcare workers

Topical: Treatment of impetigo or secondary infected traumatic skin lesions due to *S. aureus* and *S. pyogenes*

Dosage Summary

Intranasal:

Children <12 years: Dosage not established

Children ≥12 years: Approximately one-half of the ointment from the single-use tube should be applied into one nostril and the other half into the other nostril twice daily

Adults: Approximately one-half of the ointment from the single-use tube should be applied into one nostril and the other half into the other nostril twice daily

Topical:

Children ≥2 months: Ointment: Apply to affected area 3 times/day [impetigo]

Children ≥ 3 months: Cream: Apply to affected area 3 times/day for 10 days [secondary skin infections]

Adults: Apply to affected area 3 times/day

Dosage Forms

Cream, topical:

Bactroban Cream®: 2% (15 g, 30 g)

Ointment, intranasal:

Bactroban Nasal®: 2% (1 g)

Ointment, topical: 2% (0.9 g, 15 g, 22 g, 30 g)

Bactroban®: 2% (22 g)

mupirocin calcium *see* mupirocin *on page* 649

Murine® Ear [US-OTC] *see* carbamide peroxide *on page* 178

Murine® Ear Wax Removal Kit [US-OTC] *see* carbamide peroxide *on page* 178

Murine® Tears [US-OTC] *see* artificial tears *on page* 97

Murine® Tears Plus [US-OTC] *see* tetrahydrozoline (ophthalmic) *on page* 923

Muro 128® [US-OTC] *see* sodium chloride *on page* 882

Murocel® [US-OTC] *see* artificial tears *on page* 97

Murocoll-2® *(Discontinued)* *see* phenylephrine and scopolamine *on page* 753

muromonab-CD3 (myoo roe MOE nab see dee three)

Synonyms monoclonal antibody; OKT3

Therapeutic Category Immunosuppressant Agent

Use Treatment of acute allograft rejection in renal transplant patients; treatment of steroid-resistant acute allograft rejection in cardiac or hepatic transplantation

Dosage Summary

I.V.:

Children ≤30 kg: 2.5 mg once daily

Children >30 kg: 5 mg once daily

Adults: 5 mg once daily

Product Availability Orthoclone OKT® 3: Due to diminishing use, the manufacturer of muromonab is discontinuing production; supplies are expected to be available through the end of 2010.

Muroptic-5® ***(Discontinued)*** *see* sodium chloride *on page* *882*
Muse® [US] *see* alprostadil *on page* *55*
Muse® Pellet [Can] *see* alprostadil *on page* *55*
Mustargen® [US/Can] *see* mechlorethamine *on page* *594*
mustine *see* mechlorethamine *on page* *594*
Mutamycin® [Can] *see* mitomycin *on page* *638*
M.V.I.®-12 [US] *see* vitamins (multiple/injectable) *on page* *989*
M.V.I. Adult™ [US] *see* vitamins (multiple/injectable) *on page* *989*
M.V.I® Pediatric [US] *see* vitamins (multiple/injectable) *on page* *989*
Myadec® [US-OTC] *see* vitamins (multiple/oral) *on page* *990*
Myambutol® [US] *see* ethambutol *on page* *373*
Mycamine® [US/Can] *see* micafungin *on page* *629*
Mycelex® [US] *see* clotrimazole (oral) *on page* *240*
Mycelex *see* clotrimazole (oral) *on page* *240*
Mycelex®-G ***(Discontinued)*** *see* clotrimazole (topical) *on page* *240*
Mycifradin® Sulfate ***(Discontinued)*** *see* neomycin *on page* *665*
Mycinaire™ ***(Discontinued)*** *see* sodium chloride *on page* *882*
Mycinettes® [US-OTC] *see* benzocaine *on page* *124*
Mycobutin® [US/Can] *see* rifabutin *on page* *841*
Mycocide® NS [US-OTC] *see* tolnaftate *on page* *940*
Mycolog®-II ***(Discontinued)*** *see* nystatin and triamcinolone *on page* *693*
Myco-Nail [US-OTC] *see* triacetin *on page* *952*
Myconel® Topical ***(Discontinued)*** *see* nystatin and triamcinolone *on page* *693*

mycophenolate (mye koe FEN oh late)

Synonyms MMF; MPA; mycophenolate mofetil; mycophenolate sodium; mycophenolic acid

U.S./Canadian Brand Names CellCept® [US/Can]; Myfortic® [US/Can]

Therapeutic Category Immunosuppressant Agent

Use Prophylaxis of organ rejection concomitantly with cyclosporine and corticosteroids in patients receiving allogeneic renal (CellCept®, Myfortic®), cardiac (CellCept®), or hepatic (CellCept®) transplants

Dosage Summary

I.V.:

Children: Dosage not established
Adults: 1-1.5 g twice daily

Oral:

Cellcept®:

Children (suspension): 600 mg/m^2/dose twice daily (maximum: 1 g twice daily)
Children with BSA 1.25-1.5 m^2: 750 mg capsule twice daily
Children with BSA >1.5 m^2: 1 g capsule or tablet twice daily
Adults: 1-1.5 g twice daily

Myfortic®:

Children with BSA <1.19 m^2: Use of this formulation is not recommended
Children with BSA 1.19-1.58 m^2: 540 mg twice daily (maximum: 1080 mg/day)
Children with BSA >1.58 m^2: 720 mg twice daily (maximum: 1440 mg/day)
Adults: 720 mg twice daily

Dosage Forms

Capsule, oral: 250 mg
CellCept®: 250 mg

Injection, powder for reconstitution:
CellCept®: 500 mg

Powder for suspension, oral:
CellCept®: 200 mg/mL (175 mL)

Tablet, oral: 500 mg
CellCept®: 500 mg

Tablet, delayed release, oral:
Myfortic®: 180 mg, 360 mg

mycophenolate mofetil *see* mycophenolate *on page* *650*
mycophenolate sodium *see* mycophenolate *on page* *650*
mycophenolic acid *see* mycophenolate *on page* *650*
MyDex [US] *see* guaifenesin and phenylephrine *on page* *456*
Mydfrin® [US/Can] *see* phenylephrine (ophthalmic) *on page* *752*
Mydral™ [US] *see* tropicamide *on page* *964*
Mydriacyl® [US/Can] *see* tropicamide *on page* *964*
My First Flintstones™ [US-OTC] *see* vitamins (multiple/pediatric) *on page* *990*
Myfortic® [US/Can] *see* mycophenolate *on page* *650*
MyHist-DM [US] *see* phenylephrine, pyrilamine, and dextromethorphan *on page* *755*
MyHist-PD [US] *see* chlorpheniramine, pyrilamine, and phenylephrine *on page* *215*
MyKidz Iron™ [US-OTC] *see* vitamins (multiple/pediatric) *on page* *990*
MyKidz Iron 10™ [US-OTC] *see* ferrous sulfate *on page* *398*
MyKidz Iron FL™ [US] *see* vitamins (multiple/pediatric) *on page* *990*
Mykrox® *(Discontinued)* *see* metolazone *on page* *625*
Mylan-Acebutolol [Can] *see* acebutolol *on page* *21*
Mylan-Acyclovir [Can] *see* acyclovir (systemic) *on page* *36*
Mylan-Alendronate [Can] *see* alendronate *on page* *47*
Mylan-Alprazolam [Can] *see* alprazolam *on page* *55*
Mylan-Amantadine [Can] *see* amantadine *on page* *61*
Mylan-Amilazide [Can] *see* amiloride *on page* *63*
Mylan-Amiodarone [Can] *see* amiodarone *on page* *67*
Mylan-Amlodipine [Can] *see* amlodipine *on page* *68*
Mylan-Amoxicillin [Can] *see* amoxicillin *on page* *72*
Mylan-Anagrelide [Can] *see* anagrelide *on page* *77*
Mylan-Atenolol [Can] *see* atenolol *on page* *102*
Mylan-Azathioprine [Can] *see* azathioprine *on page* *109*
Mylan-Azithromycin [Can] *see* azithromycin (systemic) *on page* *111*
Mylan-Baclofen [Can] *see* baclofen *on page* *115*
Mylan-Bicalutamide [Can] *see* bicalutamide *on page* *137*
Mylan-Budesonide AQ [Can] *see* budesonide (nasal) *on page* *151*
Mylan-Buspirone [Can] *see* buspirone *on page* *157*
Mylan-Captopril [Can] *see* captopril *on page* *176*
Mylan-Carbamazepine CR [Can] *see* carbamazepine *on page* *177*
Mylan-Carvedilol [Can] *see* carvedilol *on page* *186*
Mylan-Cilazapril [Can] *see* cilazapril *(Canada only) on page* *222*
Mylan-Cimetidine [Can] *see* cimetidine *on page* *223*
Mylan-Ciprofloxacin [Can] *see* ciprofloxacin (systemic) *on page* *224*
Mylan-Citalopram [Can] *see* citalopram *on page* *227*
Mylan-Clarithromycin [Can] *see* clarithromycin *on page* *229*
Mylan-Clobetasol Cream [Can] *see* clobetasol *on page* *235*
Mylan-Clobetasol Ointment [Can] *see* clobetasol *on page* *235*
Mylan-Clobetasol Scalp Application [Can] *see* clobetasol *on page* *235*
Mylan-Clonazepam [Can] *see* clonazepam *on page* *237*
Mylan-Cyclobenzaprine [Can] *see* cyclobenzaprine *on page* *258*
Mylan-Cyproterone [Can] *see* cyproterone *(Canada only) on page* *262*
Mylan-Divalproex [Can] *see* divalproex *on page* *319*
Mylan-Domperidone [Can] *see* domperidone *(Canada only) on page* *325*
Mylan-Doxazosin [Can] *see* doxazosin *on page* *328*
Mylan-Enalapril [Can] *see* enalapril *on page* *348*
Mylan-Eti-Cal Carepac [Can] *see* etidronate and calcium carbonate *(Canada only) on page* *383*

nabumetone (na BYOO me tone)

U.S./Canadian Brand Names Apo-Nabumetone® [Can]; Gen-Nabumetone [Can]; Mylan-Nabumetone [Can]; Novo-Nabumetone [Can]; Relafen® [Can]; Rhoxal-nabumetone [Can]; Sandoz-Nabumetone [Can]

Therapeutic Category Analgesic, Nonnarcotic; Nonsteroidal Antiinflammatory Drug (NSAID)

Use Management of osteoarthritis and rheumatoid arthritis

Dosage Summary **Note:** Patients <50 kg are less likely to require doses >1000 mg/day.

Oral:

Children: Dosage not established

Adults: 1000 mg/day in 1-2 divided doses (maximum: 2000 mg/day)

Dosage Forms

Tablet, oral: 500 mg, 750 mg

NAC *see* acetylcysteine *on page 34*

***N*-acetyl-L-cysteine** *see* acetylcysteine *on page 34*

***N*-acetylcysteine** *see* acetylcysteine *on page 34*

n-acetyl-p-aminophenol *see* acetaminophen *on page 21*

NaCl *see* sodium chloride *on page 882*

nadolol (NAY doe lol)

Sound-Alike/Look-Alike Issues

nadolol may be confused with Mandol®

Corgard® may be confused with Cognex®, Coreg®

U.S./Canadian Brand Names Alti-Nadolol [Can]; Apo-Nadol® [Can]; Corgard® [US/Can]; Novo-Nadolol [Can]

Therapeutic Category Beta-Adrenergic Blocker

Use Treatment of hypertension and angina pectoris; prophylaxis of migraine headaches

Dosage Summary

Oral:

Children: Dosage not established

Adults: Initial: 40 mg once daily; Maintenance: 40-320 mg once daily; **Note:** Titration is recommended

Elderly: Initial: 20 mg once daily; Maintenance: 20-240 mg once daily; **Note:** Titration is recommended

Dosage Forms

Tablet, oral: 20 mg, 40 mg, 80 mg

Corgard®: 20 mg, 40 mg, 80 mg

nadolol and bendroflumethiazide (NAY doe lol & ben droe floo meth EYE a zide)

Synonyms bendroflumethiazide and nadolol

U.S./Canadian Brand Names Corzide® [US]

Therapeutic Category Antihypertensive Agent, Combination; Beta-Adrenergic Blocker, Nonselective; Diuretic, Thiazide

Use Treatment of hypertension; combination product should not be used for initial therapy

Dosage Summary

Oral:

Children: Dosage not established

Adults: Initial: Nadolol 40 mg and bendroflumethiazide 5 mg once daily; Maintenance: Nadolol 40-80 mg and bendroflumethiazide 5 mg once daily

Dosage Forms

Tablet: Nadolol 40 mg and bendroflumethiazide 5 mg; nadolol 80 mg and bendroflumethiazide 5 mg

Corzide® 40/5: Nadolol 40 mg and bendroflumethiazide 5 mg [scored]

Corzide® 80/5: Nadolol 80 mg and bendroflumethiazide 5 mg [scored]

nadroparin calcium *see* nadroparin *(Canada only) on page 654*

nadroparin *(Canada only)* (nad roe PA rin)

Synonyms nadroparin calcium

U.S./Canadian Brand Names Fraxiparine™ Forte [Can]; Fraxiparine™ [Can]

Therapeutic Category Low Molecular Weight Heparin

Use Prophylaxis of thromboembolic disorders (particularly deep venous thrombosis and pulmonary embolism) in general and orthopedic surgery; treatment of deep venous thrombosis; prevention of clotting during hemodialysis

Dosage Summary

SubQ:

Children: Dosage not established

Adults:

Prophylaxis: 2850 anti-Xa int. units once daily **or** 38 anti-Xa int. units/kg 12 hours before and 12 hours after surgery, followed by 38 anti-Xa int. units/kg/day up to and including day 3, then 57 anti-Xa int. units/kg/day **or** 65 anti-Xa int. units/kg as a single dose into arterial line at start of each dialysis session

Treatment: 171 anti-Xa int. units/kg/day (maximum of 17,100 int. units/day) **or** 86 anti-Xa int. units/kg twice daily

Dosage Forms - Canada

Injection, solution:

Fraxiparine™: 9500 anti-Xa int. units/mL (0.2 mL, 0.3 mL, 0.4 mL, 0.6 mL, 0.8 mL, 1 mL)

Fraxiparine™ Forte: 19,000 anti-Xa int. units/mL (0.6 mL, 0.8 mL, 1 mL)

nafarelin (naf a REL in)

Sound-Alike/Look-Alike Issues

nafarelin may be confused with Anafranil®, enalapril

Synonyms nafarelin acetate

U.S./Canadian Brand Names Synarel® [US/Can]

Therapeutic Category Hormone, Posterior Pituitary

Use Treatment of endometriosis, including pain and reduction of lesions; treatment of central precocious puberty (CPP; gonadotropin-dependent precocious puberty) in children of both sexes

Dosage Summary

Nasal:

Children: 2 sprays (400 mcg) into each nostril in the morning and evening, may increase to 3 sprays (600 mcg) into alternating nostrils 3 times/day

Adults: 1 spray (200 mcg) in 1 nostril each morning and the other nostril each evening starting on days 2-4 of menstrual cycle for 6 month

Dosage Forms

Solution, intranasal:

Synarel®: 2 mg/mL (8 mL)

nafarelin acetate *see* nafarelin *on page 655*

Nafazair® Ophthalmic *(Discontinued)* *see* naphazoline (ophthalmic) *on page 658*

nafcillin (naf SIL in)

Synonyms ethoxynaphthamido penicillin sodium; nafcillin sodium; sodium nafcillin

U.S./Canadian Brand Names Nallpen® [Can]; Unipen® [Can]

Therapeutic Category Penicillin

Use Treatment of infections such as osteomyelitis, septicemia, endocarditis, and CNS infections caused by susceptible strains of staphylococci species

Dosage Summary

I.M.:

Neonates 1200-2000 g, <7 days: 50 mg/kg/day divided every 12 hours

Neonates >2000 g, <7 days: 75 mg/kg/day divided every 8 hours

Neonates 1200-2000 g, ≥7 days: 75 mg/kg/day divided every 8 hours

Neonates >2000 g, ≥7 days: 100-140 mg/kg/day divided every 6 hours

Children: 25 mg/kg twice daily

Adults: 500 mg every 4-6 hours

I.V.:

Neonates 1200-2000 g, <7 days: 50 mg/kg/day divided every 12 hours

Neonates >2000 g, <7 days: 75 mg/kg/day divided every 8 hours

Neonates 1200-2000 g, ≥7 days: 75 mg/kg/day divided every 8 hours

Neonates >2000 g, ≥7 days: 100-140 mg/kg/day divided every 6 hours

Children: 50-200 mg/kg/day in divided every 4-6 hours (maximum: 12 g/day)

Adults: 500-2000 mg every 4-6 hours

Dosage Forms
Infusion, premixed iso-osmotic dextrose solution: 1 g (50 mL); 2 g (100 mL)
Injection, powder for reconstitution: 1 g, 2 g, 10 g
Powder, for prescription compounding: 200 g

nafcillin sodium *see* nafcillin *on page 655*

naftifine (NAF ti feen)

Synonyms naftifine hydrochloride
U.S./Canadian Brand Names Naftin® [US]
Therapeutic Category Antifungal Agent
Use Topical treatment of tinea cruris (jock itch), tinea corporis (ringworm), and tinea pedis (athlete's foot)
Dosage Summary
Topical:
Children: Dosage not established
Adults: Apply cream once daily and gel twice daily
Dosage Forms
Cream, topical:
Naftin®: 1% (30 g, 60 g, 90 g)
Gel, topical:
Naftin®: 1% (40 g, 60 g, 90 g)

naftifine hydrochloride *see* naftifine *on page 656*
Naftin® [US] *see* naftifine *on page 656*
Naglazyme™ [US] *see* galsulfase *on page 436*
NaHCO$_3$ *see* sodium bicarbonate *on page 882*

nalbuphine (NAL byoo feen)

Sound-Alike/Look-Alike Issues
Nubain® may be confused with Navane®, Nebcin®
Synonyms nalbuphine hydrochloride
U.S./Canadian Brand Names Nubain® [US]
Therapeutic Category Analgesic, Narcotic
Use Relief of moderate-to-severe pain; preoperative analgesia, postoperative and surgical anesthesia, and obstetrical analgesia during labor and delivery
Dosage Summary
I.M.:
Children <1 year: Dosage not established
Adults: 10 mg/70 kg every 3-6 hours (maximum: 20 mg/dose; 160 mg/day)
I.V.:
Children <1 year: Dosage not established
Adults: 10 mg/70 kg every 3-6 hours (maximum: 20 mg/dose; 160 mg/day) **or** 0.3-3 mg/kg over 10-15 minutes, then 0.25-0.5 mg/kg as required for anesthesia **or** 2.5-5 mg (1-2 doses)
SubQ:
Children <1 year: Dosage not established
Adults: 10 mg/70 kg every 3-6 hours (maximum: 20 mg/dose; 160 mg/day)
Dosage Forms
Injection, solution: 10 mg/mL (10 mL); 20 mg/mL (10 mL)
Nubain®: 20 mg/mL (10 mL)
Injection, solution [preservative free]: 10 mg/mL (1 mL); 20 mg/mL (1 mL)
Nubain®: 10 mg/mL (1 mL); 20 mg/mL (1 mL)

nalbuphine hydrochloride *see* nalbuphine *on page 656*
Nalcrom® [Can] *see* cromolyn (systemic, oral inhalation) *on page 254*
Naldecon® DX Adult Liquid *(Discontinued)*
Naldecon-EX® Children's Syrup *(Discontinued)*
Naldecon Senior EX® *(Discontinued)* *see* guaifenesin *on page 454*
Nalex®-A [US] *see* chlorpheniramine, phenylephrine, and phenyltoloxamine *on page 213*
Nalex A 12 [US] *see* chlorpheniramine, pyrilamine, and phenylephrine *on page 215*
Nalfon® [US/Can] *see* fenoprofen *on page 395*

Nallpen® [Can] *see* nafcillin *on page 655*
Nallpen® *(Discontinued)* *see* nafcillin *on page 655*
***N*-allylnoroxymorphine hydrochloride** *see* naloxone *on page 657*
nalmefene *(Discontinued)*

naloxone (nal OKS one)

Sound-Alike/Look-Alike Issues
naloxone may be confused with Lanoxin®, naltrexone
Narcan® may be confused with Marcaine®, Norcuron®

Synonyms *N*-allylnoroxymorphine hydrochloride; naloxone hydrochloride

U.S./Canadian Brand Names Naloxone Hydrochloride Injection® [Can]

Therapeutic Category Antidote

Use Complete or partial reversal of opioid drug effects, including respiratory depression; management of known or suspected opioid overdose; diagnosis of suspected opioid dependence or acute opioid overdose

Dosage Summary

I.M.:

Birth (including premature infants) to 5 years or <20 kg: 0.1 mg/kg (maximum dose: 2 mg) every 2-3 minutes if needed **or** 0.01 mg/kg every 2-3 minutes as needed postoperatively

Children >5 years or ≥20 kg: 2 mg/dose, if no response repeat every 2-3 minutes **or** 0.01 mg/kg every 2-3 minutes as needed postoperatively

Adults: 0.4-2 mg every 2-3 minutes as needed (maximum: 10 mg) or 0.1-0.2 mg every 2-3 minutes

I.V.:

Birth (including premature infants) to 5 years or <20 kg: 0.1 mg/kg (maximum dose: 2 mg) every 2-3 minutes if needed **or** 0.01 mg/kg every 2-3 minutes as needed postoperatively; Infusion: Calculate dosage/hour based on effective intermittent dose used and duration of adequate response seen

Children >5 years or ≥20 kg: 2 mg/dose, if no response repeat every 2-3 minutes **or** 0.01 mg/kg every 2-3 minutes as needed postoperatively; Infusion: Calculate dosage/hour based on effective intermittent dose used and duration of adequate response seen

Adults: 0.4-2 mg every 2-3 minutes as needed (maximum: 10 mg) **or** 0.1-0.2 mg every 2-3 minutes; Infusion: Calculate dosage/hour based on effective intermittent dose used and duration of adequate response seen; typically 0.25-6.25 mg/hour

Intratracheal:

Birth (including premature infants) to 5 years or <20 kg: 0.1 mg/kg (maximum dose: 2 mg) every 2-3 minutes if needed **or** 0.01 mg/kg every 2-3 minutes as needed postoperatively

Children >5 years or ≥20 kg: 2 mg/dose, if no response repeat every 2-3 minutes **or** 0.01 mg/kg every 2-3 minutes as needed postoperatively

Adults: 0.4-2 mg every 2-3 minutes as needed (maximum: 10 mg)

SubQ:

Birth (including premature infants) to 5 years or <20 kg: 0.1 mg/kg (maximum dose: 2 mg) every 2-3 minutes if needed or 0.01 mg/kg every 2-3 minutes as needed postoperatively **or** 0.01 mg/kg every 2-3 minutes as needed postoperatively

Children >5 years or ≥20 kg: 2 mg/dose, if no response repeat every 2-3 minutes **or** 0.01 mg/kg every 2-3 minutes as needed postoperatively

Adults: 0.4-2 mg every 2-3 minutes as needed (maximum: 10 mg) **or** 0.1-0.2 mg every 2-3 minutes

Dosage Forms

Injection, solution: 0.4 mg/mL (1 mL, 10 mL)
Injection, solution [preservative free]: 0.4 mg/mL (1 mL); 1 mg/mL (2 mL)

naloxone and buprenorphine *see* buprenorphine and naloxone *on page 155*
naloxone hydrochloride *see* naloxone *on page 657*
naloxone hydrochloride and pentazocine *see* pentazocine and naloxone *on page 740*
naloxone hydrochloride dihydrate and buprenorphine hydrochloride *see* buprenorphine and naloxone *on page 155*
Naloxone Hydrochloride Injection® [Can] *see* naloxone *on page 657*

naltrexone (nal TREKS one)

Sound-Alike/Look-Alike Issues
naltrexone may be confused with methylnaltrexone, naloxone
ReVia® may be confused with Revatio®, Revex®

Synonyms naltrexone hydrochloride

U.S./Canadian Brand Names Depade® [US]; ReVia® [US/Can]; Vivitrol™ [US]

Therapeutic Category Antidote

Use Treatment of ethanol dependence; blockade of the effects of exogenously administered opioids

Dosage Summary Note: Dosage is variable and individualized

I.M.:

Children: Dosage not established

Adults: 380 mg once every 4 weeks

Oral:

Children: Dosage not established

Adults: Initial: 25 mg; if no withdrawal signs within 1 hour give another 25 mg; Maintenance: 50 mg/day to 100-150 mg 3 times/week (maximum: 800 mg/day)

Dosage Forms

Injection, microspheres for suspension, extended release:

Vivitrol™: 380 mg

Tablet, oral: 50 mg

Depade®: 25 mg, 50 mg, 100 mg

ReVia®: 50 mg

naltrexone and morphine *see* morphine and naltrexone *on page 646*

naltrexone hydrochloride *see* naltrexone *on page 657*

Namenda® [US] *see* memantine *on page 599*

nandrolone *(Canada only)* (NAN droe lone)

Synonyms nandrolone decanoate; nandrolone phenpropionate

U.S./Canadian Brand Names Deca-Durabolin® [Can]

Therapeutic Category Androgen

Use Adjunctive treatment in aplastic or sickle cell anemia, osteoporosis (senile and postmenopausal), pituitary dwarfism. Also demonstrates anabolic effects in chronic disease, inoperable breast cancer, decubitus ulcers, burns, corticoid-induced catabolic states, and myopathies.

Dosage Forms - Canada

Injection, solution:

Deca-Durabolin®: 100 mg/mL (2 mL)

nandrolone decanoate *see* nandrolone *(Canada only) on page 658*

nandrolone phenpropionate *see* nandrolone *(Canada only) on page 658*

nanoparticle albumin-bound paclitaxel *see* paclitaxel (protein bound) *on page 720*

NAPA and NABZ *see* sodium phenylacetate and sodium benzoate *on page 886*

naphazoline (nasal) (naf AZ oh leen)

Synonyms naphazoline hydrochloride

U.S./Canadian Brand Names Privine® [US-OTC]

Therapeutic Category Alpha$_1$ Agonist

Use Temporary relief of nasal congestion associated with the common cold, upper respiratory allergies, or sinusitis

Dosage Summary

Intranasal:

Children <12 years: Dosage not established

Children ≥12 years: Instill 1-2 drops or sprays of 0.05% every 6 hours if needed (maximum duration: 3 days)

Adults: Instill 1-2 drops or sprays of 0.05% every 6 hours if needed (maximum duration: 3 days)

Dosage Forms

Solution, intranasal:

Privine® [OTC]: 0.05% (20 mL, 25 mL)

naphazoline (ophthalmic) (naf AZ oh leen)

Synonyms naphazoline hydrochloride

U.S./Canadian Brand Names AK-Con™ [US]; Clear eyes® for Dry Eyes Plus ACR Relief [US-OTC]; Clear eyes® for Dry Eyes plus Redness Relief [US-OTC]; Clear eyes® Redness Relief [US-OTC]; Clear eyes® Seasonal Relief [US-OTC]; Naphcon Forte® [Can]; Vasocon® [Can]

Therapeutic Category Alpha$_1$ Agonist; Ophthalmic Agent, Vasoconstrictor

Use Topical ocular vasoconstrictor; relief of redness of the eye due to minor irritation

Dosage Summary

Ophthalmic:

Children: Dosage not established

Adults:

0.1% solution (prescription): 1-2 drops into conjuctival sac every 3-4 hours as needed

0.012% or 0.025% solution (OTC): 1-2 drops into affected eye(s) up to 4 times a day (maximum duration: 3 days)

Dosage Forms

Solution, ophthalmic:

AK-Con™: 0.1% (15 mL)
Clear eyes® for Dry Eyes Plus ACR Relief [OTC]: 0.025% (15 mL)
Clear eyes® for Dry Eyes plus Redness Relief [OTC]: 0.012% (15 mL)
Clear eyes® Redness Relief [OTC]: 0.012% (6 mL, 15 mL, 30 mL)
Clear eyes® Seasonal Relief [OTC]: 0.012% (15 mL, 30 mL)

naphazoline and pheniramine (naf AZ oh leen & fen NIR a meen)

Sound-Alike/Look-Alike Issues

Visine® may be confused with Visken®

Synonyms pheniramine and naphazoline

U.S./Canadian Brand Names Naphcon-A® [US-OTC/Can]; Opcon-A® [US-OTC]; Visine-A® [US-OTC]; Visine® Advanced Allergy [Can]

Therapeutic Category Antihistamine/Decongestant Combination

Use Treatment of ocular congestion, irritation, and itching

Dosage Summary

Ophthalmic:

Children <6 years: Dosage not established
Children ≥6 years: 1-2 drops up to 4 times/day
Adults: 1-2 drops up to 4 times/day

Dosage Forms

Solution, ophthalmic:

Naphcon-A® [OTC]: Naphazoline 0.025% and pheniramine 0.3%
Opcon-A® [OTC]: Naphazoline 0.027% and pheniramine 0.3%
Visine-A® [OTC]: Naphazoline 0.025% and pheniramine 0.3%

naphazoline hydrochloride *see* naphazoline (nasal) *on page* 658
naphazoline hydrochloride *see* naphazoline (ophthalmic) *on page* 658
Naphcon-A® [US-OTC/Can] *see* naphazoline and pheniramine *on page* 659
Naphcon® *(Discontinued)* *see* naphazoline (ophthalmic) *on page* 658
Naphcon Forte® [Can] *see* naphazoline (ophthalmic) *on page* 658
Naphcon Forte® Ophthalmic *(Discontinued)* *see* naphazoline (ophthalmic) *on page* 658
NapraPAC® *see* lansoprazole and naproxen *on page* 549
Naprelan® [US/Can] *see* naproxen *on page* 659
Naprosyn® [US/Can] *see* naproxen *on page* 659

naproxen (na PROKS en)

Sound-Alike/Look-Alike Issues

naproxen may be confused with Natacyn®, Nebcin®
Aleve® may be confused with Alesse®
Anaprox® may be confused with Anaspaz®, Avapro®
Naprelan® may be confused with Naprosyn®
Naprosyn® may be confused with Naprelan®, Natacyn®, Nebcin®

Synonyms naproxen sodium

U.S./Canadian Brand Names Aleve® [US-OTC]; Anaprox® DS [US/Can]; Anaprox® [US/Can]; Apo-Napro-Na DS® [Can]; Apo-Napro-Na® [Can]; Apo-Naproxen EC® [Can]; Apo-Naproxen SR® [Can]; Apo-Naproxen® [Can]; EC-Naprosyn® [US]; Mediproxen [US-OTC]; Midol® Extended Relief [US-OTC]; Mylan-Naproxen EC [Can]; Naprelan® [US/Can]; Naprosyn® [US/Can]; Novo-Naproc EC [Can]; Novo-Naprox Sodium DS [Can]; Novo-Naprox Sodium [Can]; Novo-Naprox SR [Can]; Novo-Naprox [Can]; Nu-Naprox [Can]; Pamprin® Maximum Strength All Day Relief [US-OTC]; PMS-Naproxen EC [Can]; PRO-Naproxen EC [Can]; Riva-Naproxen [Can]; Teva-Naproxen Sodium DS [Can]; Teva-Naproxen Sodium [Can]

Therapeutic Category Analgesic, Nonnarcotic; Antipyretic; Nonsteroidal Antiinflammatory Drug (NSAID)

Use Management of ankylosing spondylitis, osteoarthritis, and rheumatoid disorders (including juvenile rheumatoid arthritis); acute gout; mild-to-moderate pain; tendonitis, bursitis; dysmenorrhea; fever

Dosage Summary Note: Dosage expressed as naproxen base; 200 mg naproxen base is equivalent to 220 mg naproxen sodium

Oral:

Children ≤2 years: Dosage not established

Children >2-11 years: 2.5-10 mg/kg/dose **or** 10 mg/kg/day in 2 divided doses (maximum: 10 mg/kg/day)

Children ≥12 years: 2.5-10 mg/kg/dose **or** 10 mg/kg/day in 2 divided doses (maximum: 10 mg/kg/day) **or** 200 mg every 8-12 hours (maximum: 600 mg/day)

Adults ≤65 kg: Initial: 200-750 mg as a single dose Maintenance: 200-500 mg every 6-12 hours (maximum: 1500 mg/day; exceptions occur [indication specific])

Elderly >65 years: Initial: 500-750 mg as a single dose; Maintenance: 200-500 mg every 6-12 hours (maximum: 1500 mg/day; exceptions occur [indication specific])

Dosage Forms

Caplet, oral: 220 mg

Aleve® [OTC]: 220 mg

Midol® Extended Relief [OTC]: 220 mg

Pamprin® Maximum Strength All Day Relief [OTC]: 220 mg

Capsule, liquid gel, oral:

Aleve® [OTC]: 220 mg

Combination package, oral:

Naprelan®: Day 1-3: Tablet, controlled release: 825 mg [equivalent to naproxen base 750 mg] (6s) [contains sodium 75 mg] and Day 4-10: Tablet, controlled release: 550 mg [equivalent to naproxen base 500 mg] (14s) [contains sodium 50 mg]

Gelcap, oral:

Aleve® [OTC]: 220 mg

Suspension, oral: 125 mg/5 mL (500 mL)

Naprosyn®: 125 mg/5 mL (473 mL)

Tablet, oral: 220 mg, 250 mg, 275 mg, 375 mg, 500 mg, 550 mg

Aleve® [OTC]: 220 mg

Anaprox®: 275 mg

Anaprox® DS: 550 mg

Mediproxen [OTC]: 220 mg

Naprosyn®: 250 mg, 375 mg, 500 mg

Tablet, controlled release, oral:

Naprelan®: 412.5 mg, 550 mg, 825 mg

Tablet, delayed release, enteric coated, oral: 375 mg, 500 mg

EC-Naprosyn®: 375 mg, 500 mg

naproxen and esomeprazole (na PROKS en & es oh ME pray zol)

Sound-Alike/Look-Alike Issues

Vimovo™ may be confused with Vimpat®

Synonyms esomeprazole and naproxen

U.S./Canadian Brand Names Vimovo™ [US]

Therapeutic Category Nonsteroidal Antiinflammatory Drug (NSAID); Proton Pump Inhibitor

Use Reduction of the risk of NSAID-associated gastric ulcers in patients at risk of developing gastric ulcers who require an NSAID for the treatment of rheumatoid arthritis, osteoarthritis, and ankylosing spondylitis

Dosage Summary

Oral:

Children: Dosage not established

Adults: One tablet twice daily; maximum daily dose of esomeprazole: 40 mg/day

Elderly: Naproxen: dosing adjustment should be considered; use lowest effective dose

Dosage Forms

Tablet, variable release, oral:

Vimovo™: Naproxen [delayed release] 375 mg and esomeprazole [immediate release] 20 mg, Naproxen [delayed release] 500 mg and esomeprazole [immediate release] 20 mg

naproxen and lansoprazole *see* lansoprazole and naproxen *on page 549*

naproxen and pseudoephedrine (na PROKS en & soo doe e FED rin)

Synonyms naproxen sodium and pseudoephedrine; pseudoephedrine and naproxen

U.S./Canadian Brand Names Aleve®-D Sinus & Cold [US-OTC]; Aleve®-D Sinus & Headache [US-OTC]; Sudafed® 12 Hour Pressure + Pain [US-OTC]

Therapeutic Category Decongestant/Analgesic

Use Temporary relief of cold, sinus, and flu symptoms (including nasal congestion, sinus congestion/ pressure, headache, minor body aches and pains, and fever)

Dosage Summary

Oral:

Children <12 years: Dosage not established

Children ≥12 years: One caplet every 12 hours (maximum: 2 caplets/day)

Adults: One caplet every 12 hours (maximum: 2 caplets/day)

Dosage Forms

Caplet, extended release:

Aleve®-D Sinus & Cold [OTC], Aleve®-D Sinus & Headache [OTC], Sudafed® 12 Hour Pressure + Pain [OTC]: Naproxen sodium 220 mg [equivalent to naproxen 200 mg and sodium 20 mg] and pseudoephedrine hydrochloride 120 mg

naproxen and sumatriptan *see* sumatriptan and naproxen *on page 905*
naproxen sodium *see* naproxen *on page 659*
naproxen sodium and pseudoephedrine *see* naproxen and pseudoephedrine *on page 661*
naproxen sodium and sumatriptan *see* sumatriptan and naproxen *on page 905*
naproxen sodium and sumatriptan succinate *see* sumatriptan and naproxen *on page 905*

naratriptan (NAR a trip tan)

Sound-Alike/Look-Alike Issues

Amerge® may be confused with Altace®, Amaryl®

Synonyms naratriptan hydrochloride

U.S./Canadian Brand Names Amerge® [US/Can]

Therapeutic Category Antimigraine Agent; Serotonin Agonist

Use Treatment of acute migraine headache with or without aura

Dosage Summary

Oral:

Children: Dosage not established

Adults: 1-2.5 mg, may repeat after 4 hours (maximum: 5 mg/day)

Elderly: Use not recommended

Dosage Forms

Tablet, oral: 1 mg, 2.5 mg

Amerge®: 1 mg, 2.5 mg

naratriptan hydrochloride *see* naratriptan *on page 661*
Narcan® *(Discontinued)* *see* naloxone *on page 657*
Nardil® [US/Can] *see* phenelzine *on page 747*
Naropin® [US/Can] *see* ropivacaine *on page 852*
Nasacort® AQ [US/Can] *see* triamcinolone (nasal) *on page 953*
Nasahist B® *(Discontinued)* *see* brompheniramine *on page 147*
NāSal™ [US-OTC] *see* sodium chloride *on page 882*
NasalCrom® [US-OTC] *see* cromolyn (nasal) *on page 255*
Nasalide® [Can] *see* flunisolide (nasal) *on page 410*
Nasal Moist® Saline [US-OTC] *see* sodium chloride *on page 882*
Nasal Spray [US-OTC] *see* sodium chloride *on page 882*
Nasarel® *(Discontinued)* *see* flunisolide (nasal) *on page 410*

Nasatab® LA *(Discontinued)* *see* guaifenesin and pseudoephedrine *on page* 457
Nascobal® [US] *see* cyanocobalamin *on page* 257
Nasofed™ *(Discontinued)* *see* pseudoephedrine *on page* 810
Nasonex® [US/Can] *see* mometasone (nasal) *on page* 641
NāSop™ *(Discontinued)* *see* phenylephrine (systemic) *on page* 751
Nasop12™ *(Discontinued)* *see* phenylephrine (systemic) *on page* 751
Natabec® *(Discontinued)*
Natabec® FA *(Discontinued)*
Natabec® Rx *(Discontinued)*
NataCaps™ [US] *see* vitamins (multiple/prenatal) *on page* 991
NataChew® [US-OTC] *see* vitamins (multiple/prenatal) *on page* 991
Natacyn® [US/Can] *see* natamycin *on page* 662
NataFort® [US-OTC] *see* vitamins (multiple/prenatal) *on page* 991
NatalCare® CFe 60 *(Discontinued)* *see* vitamins (multiple/prenatal) *on page* 991
NatalCare® GlossTabs™ [US] *see* vitamins (multiple/prenatal) *on page* 991
NatalCare® PIC [US] *see* vitamins (multiple/prenatal) *on page* 991
NatalCare® PIC Forte [US] *see* vitamins (multiple/prenatal) *on page* 991
NatalCare® Plus [US] *see* vitamins (multiple/prenatal) *on page* 991
NatalCare® Rx [US] *see* vitamins (multiple/prenatal) *on page* 991
NatalCare® Three [US] *see* vitamins (multiple/prenatal) *on page* 991
Natalins® Rx *(Discontinued)*

natalizumab (na ta LIZ u mab)

Synonyms AN100226; anti-4 alpha integrin; IgG4-kappa monoclonal antibody

U.S./Canadian Brand Names Tysabri® [US/Can]

Therapeutic Category Monoclonal Antibody, Selective Adhesion-Molecule Inhibitor

Use

U.S. labeling: Monotherapy for the treatment of relapsing forms of multiple sclerosis; treatment of moderately- to severely-active Crohn disease

Canada labeling: Treatment of relapsing forms of multiple sclerosis

Dosage Summary

I.V.:

Children: Dosage not established

Adults: 300 mg every 4 weeks (infused over 1 hour)

Dosage Forms

Injection, solution [preservative free]:

Tysabri®: 300 mg/15 mL (15 mL)

natamycin (na ta MYE sin)

Sound-Alike/Look-Alike Issues

Natacyn® may be confused with Naprosyn®

Synonyms pimaricin

U.S./Canadian Brand Names Natacyn® [US/Can]

Therapeutic Category Antifungal Agent

Use Treatment of blepharitis, conjunctivitis, and keratitis caused by susceptible fungi (*Aspergillus*, *Candida*, *Cephalosporium*, *Fusarium*, and *Penicillium*)

Dosage Summary

Ophthalmic:

Children: Dosage not established

Adults: Initial: Instill 1 drop in conjunctival sac every 1-2 hours for 3-4 days; Maintenance: 1 drop 4-8 times/day

Dosage Forms

Suspension, ophthalmic:

Natacyn®: 5% (15 mL)

NataTab™ CFe [US] *see* vitamins (multiple/prenatal) *on page* 991
NataTab™ FA [US] *see* vitamins (multiple/prenatal) *on page* 991

NataTab™ Rx [US] *see* vitamins (multiple/prenatal) *on page 991*
Natazia™ [US] *see* estradiol and dienogest *on page 367*

nateglinide (na te GLYE nide)

U.S./Canadian Brand Names Starlix® [US/Can]
Therapeutic Category Antidiabetic Agent, Oral
Use Management of type 2 diabetes mellitus (noninsulin-dependent, NIDDM) as monotherapy when hyperglycemia cannot be managed by diet and exercise alone; in combination with metformin or a thiazolidinedione to lower blood glucose in patients whose hyperglycemia cannot be controlled by exercise, diet, or a single agent alone
Dosage Summary
Oral:
Children: Dosage not established
Adults: 60-120 mg 3 times/day before meals
Dosage Forms
Tablet, oral: 60 mg, 120 mg
Starlix®: 60 mg, 120 mg

Natrecor® [US/Can] *see* nesiritide *on page 669*
natriuretic peptide *see* nesiritide *on page 669*
Natulan® [Can] *see* procarbazine *on page 797*
Natural Balance Tears [US-OTC] *see* hydroxypropyl methylcellulose *on page 489*
Natural Fiber Therapy [US-OTC] *see* psyllium *on page 814*
Natural Fiber Therapy Smooth Texture [US-OTC] *see* psyllium *on page 814*
natural lung surfactant *see* beractant *on page 131*
Nature's Tears® [US-OTC] *see* artificial tears *on page 97*
Nature's Tears [US-OTC] *see* hydroxypropyl methylcellulose *on page 489*
Nature-Throid™ [US] *see* thyroid, desiccated *on page 930*
Naus-A-Way® *(Discontinued)*
Nausea Relief [US-OTC] *see* fructose, dextrose, and phosphoric acid *on page 430*
Nauseatol [Can] *see* dimenhydrinate *on page 307*
Nausetrol® [US-OTC] *see* fructose, dextrose, and phosphoric acid *on page 430*
Navane® [US/Can] *see* thiothixene *on page 929*
Navelbine® [US/Can] *see* vinorelbine *on page 986*
Navstel® [US] *see* balanced salt solution *on page 116*
Na-Zone® [US-OTC] *see* sodium chloride *on page 882*
N-carbamoyl-L-glutamic acid *see* carglumic acid *on page 184*
N-carbamylglutamate *see* carglumic acid *on page 184*
***n*-docosanol** *see* docosanol *on page 321*
Nebcin® *(Discontinued)* *see* tobramycin (systemic, oral inhalation) *on page 937*

nebivolol (ne BIV oh lole)

Synonyms nebivolol hydrochloride
U.S./Canadian Brand Names Bystolic® [US]
Therapeutic Category Beta Blocker, Beta-1 Selective
Use Treatment of hypertension, alone or in combination with other agents
Dosage Summary
Oral:
Children ≤18 years: Dosage not established
Adults: Initial: 5 mg once daily; Maintenance: 5-40 mg once daily
Dosage Forms
Tablet, oral:
Bystolic®: 2.5 mg, 5 mg, 10 mg, 20 mg

nebivolol hydrochloride *see* nebivolol *on page 663*
Nebupent® [US] *see* pentamidine *on page 739*
Necon® 0.5/35 [US] *see* ethinyl estradiol and norethindrone *on page 378*

Necon® 1/35 [US] *see* ethinyl estradiol and norethindrone *on page 378*
Necon® 1/50 [US] *see* norethindrone and mestranol *on page 683*
Necon® 7/7/7 [US] *see* ethinyl estradiol and norethindrone *on page 378*
Necon® 10/11 [US] *see* ethinyl estradiol and norethindrone *on page 378*

nedocromil (ne doe KROE mil)

Synonyms nedocromil sodium
U.S./Canadian Brand Names Alocril® [US/Can]; Tilade® [Can]
Therapeutic Category Mast Cell Stabilizer
Use
Aerosol: Maintenance therapy in patients with mild-to-moderate bronchial asthma
Ophthalmic: Treatment of itching associated with allergic conjunctivitis
Dosage Summary
Inhalation:
Children <6 years: Dosage not established
Children ≥6 years: 2 inhalations 2-4 times/day
Adults: 2 inhalations 2-4 times/day
Ophthalmic:
Children <3 years: Dosage not established
Children ≥3 years: 1-2 drops in each eye twice daily
Adults: 1-2 drops in each eye twice daily
Dosage Forms
Solution, ophthalmic:
Alocril®: 2% (5 mL)

nedocromil sodium *see* nedocromil *on page 664*
Néevo® [US] *see* vitamins (multiple/prenatal) *on page 991*
Néevo® DHA [US] *see* vitamins (multiple/prenatal) *on page 991*

nefazodone (nef AY zoe done)

Sound-Alike/Look-Alike Issues
Serzone® may be confused with selegiline, Serentil®, Seroquel®, sertraline
Synonyms nefazodone hydrochloride
Therapeutic Category Antidepressant, Miscellaneous
Use Treatment of depression
Dosage Summary
Oral:
Adults: Initial: 200 mg/day in 2 divided doses; Maintenance: 300-600 mg/day in 2 divided doses
Elderly: Initial: 50 mg twice daily; Maintenance: 200-400 mg/day in 2 divided doses
Dosage Forms
Tablet, oral: 50 mg, 100 mg, 150 mg, 200 mg, 250 mg

nefazodone hydrochloride *see* nefazodone *on page 664*
NegGram® ***(Discontinued)***

nelarabine (nel AY re been)

Synonyms 2-amino-6-methoxypurine arabinoside; 506U78; GW506U78
U.S./Canadian Brand Names Arranon® [US]; Atriance™ [Can]
Therapeutic Category Antineoplastic Agent, Antimetabolite
Use Treatment of relapsed or refractory T-cell acute lymphoblastic leukemia (ALL) and T-cell lymphoblastic lymphoma
Dosage Summary
I.V.:
Children: 650 mg/m^2/dose on days 1 through 5; repeat every 21 days
Adults: 1500 mg/m^2/dose on days 1, 3, and 5; repeat every 21 days
Dosage Forms
Injection, solution:
Arranon®: 5 mg/mL (50 mL)

Dosage Forms - Canada

Injection, solution:

Atriance™: 5 mg/mL (50 mL)

nelfinavir (nel FIN a veer)

Sound-Alike/Look-Alike Issues

nelfinavir may be confused with nevirapine

Viracept® may be confused with Viramune®

Synonyms NFV

U.S./Canadian Brand Names Viracept® [US/Can]

Therapeutic Category Antiviral Agent

Use In combination with other antiretroviral therapy in the treatment of HIV infection

Dosage Summary

Oral:

Children <2 years: Dosage not established

Children 2-13 years: 45-55 mg/kg twice daily **or** 25-35 mg/kg 3 times/day (maximum: 2500 mg/day)

Adults: 750 mg 3 times/day **or** 1250 mg twice daily with meals

Dosage Forms

Powder, oral:

Viracept®: 50 mg/g (144 g)

Tablet, oral:

Viracept®: 250 mg, 625 mg

Nelova™ 0.5/35E *(Discontinued)* *see* ethinyl estradiol and norethindrone *on page 378*

Nelova™ 1/35E *(Discontinued)* *see* ethinyl estradiol and norethindrone *on page 378*

Nelova™ 1/50M *(Discontinued)* *see* norethindrone and mestranol *on page 683*

Nelova™ 10/11 *(Discontinued)* *see* ethinyl estradiol and norethindrone *on page 378*

Nembutal® [US] *see* pentobarbital *on page 741*

Nembutal® Sodium [Can] *see* pentobarbital *on page 741*

NeoBenz® Micro *(Discontinued)* *see* benzoyl peroxide *on page 128*

NeoBenz® Micro SD *(Discontinued)* *see* benzoyl peroxide *on page 128*

NeoBenz® Micro Wash *(Discontinued)* *see* benzoyl peroxide *on page 128*

Neo-Calglucon® *(Discontinued)* *see* calcium glubionate *on page 170*

Neo-Dexameth® Ophthalmic *(Discontinued)*

Neo DM [US] *see* chlorpheniramine, phenylephrine, and dextromethorphan *on page 211*

Neo-Durabolic® *(Discontinued)* *see* nandrolone *(Canada only) on page 658*

Neofed® *(Discontinued)* *see* pseudoephedrine *on page 810*

Neo-Fradin™ [US] *see* neomycin *on page 665*

Neofrin [US] *see* phenylephrine (ophthalmic) *on page 752*

Neomixin® Topical *(Discontinued)* *see* bacitracin, neomycin, and polymyxin B *on page 114*

neomycin (nee oh MYE sin)

Synonyms neomycin sulfate

U.S./Canadian Brand Names Neo-Fradin™ [US]

Therapeutic Category Aminoglycoside (Antibiotic); Antibiotic, Topical

Use Orally to prepare GI tract for surgery; topically to treat minor skin infections; treatment of diarrhea caused by *E. coli*; adjunct in the treatment of hepatic encephalopathy; bladder irrigation; ocular infections

Dosage Summary

Oral:

Children: Encephalopathy: 50-100 mg/kg/day divided every 6-8 hours **or** 2.5-7 g/m^2/day divided every 4-6 hours (maximum: 12 g/day); Preoperative GI preparation: 75-90 mg/kg/day given at specific times or in divided doses every 4hours in combination with erythromycin.

Adults: Encephalopathy/hepatic insufficiency: 500 mg to 12 g/day in divided doses every 4-8 hours; Preoperative GI preparation: 1 g each hour for 4 doses then 1 g every 4 hours for 5 doses **or** 1 g at 1 PM, 2 PM, and 11 PM on day preceding surgery

Topical:

Children: Solutions containing 0.1% to 1% neomycin have been used for irrigation

Adults: Solutions containing 0.1% to 1% neomycin have been used for irrigation

Dosage Forms

Solution, oral:

Neo-Fradin™: 125 mg/5 mL (480 mL)

Tablet, oral: 500 mg

neomycin and polymyxin B (nee oh MYE sin & pol i MIKS in bee)

Synonyms polymyxin B and neomycin

U.S./Canadian Brand Names Neosporin® G.U. Irrigant [US]; Neosporin® Irrigating Solution [Can]

Therapeutic Category Antibiotic, Topical; Genitourinary Irrigant

Use Short-term as a continuous irrigant or rinse in the urinary bladder to prevent bacteriuria and gram-negative rod septicemia associated with the use of indwelling catheters

Dosage Summary

Irrigation (bladder):

Children: Add 1 mL irrigant to 1 L isotonic saline solution, continuously irrigate or rinse in the urinary bladder for up to a maximum of 10 days (maximum: usually no more than 1 L of irrigant/day)

Adults: Add 1 mL irrigant to 1 L isotonic saline solution, continuously irrigate or rinse in the urinary bladder for up to a maximum of 10 days (maximum: usually no more than 1 L of irrigant/day)

Dosage Forms

Solution, irrigation: Neomycin 40 mg and polymyxin B 200,000 units per mL (1 mL, 20 mL)

Neosporin® G.U. Irrigant: Neomycin 40 mg and polymyxin B 200,000 units per mL (1 mL, 20 mL)

neomycin, bacitracin, and polymyxin B *see* bacitracin, neomycin, and polymyxin B *on page 114*

neomycin, bacitracin, polymyxin B, and hydrocortisone *see* bacitracin, neomycin, polymyxin B, and hydrocortisone *on page 114*

neomycin, bacitracin, polymyxin B, and pramoxine *see* bacitracin, neomycin, polymyxin B, and pramoxine *on page 115*

neomycin, colistin, hydrocortisone, and thonzonium

(nee oh MYE sin, koe LIS tin, hye droe KOR ti sone, & thon ZOE nee um)

Synonyms colistin, hydrocortisone, neomycin, and thonzonium; hydrocortisone, neomycin, colistin, and thonzonium; thonzonium, neomycin, colistin, and hydrocortisone

U.S./Canadian Brand Names Coly-Mycin® S [US]; Cortisporin®-TC [US]

Therapeutic Category Antibiotic/Corticosteroid, Otic

Use Treatment of superficial and susceptible bacterial infections of the external auditory canal; for treatment of susceptible bacterial infections of mastoidectomy and fenestration cavities

Dosage Summary

Otic:

Children: 3-4 drops in affected ear 3-4 times/day

Adults: 4-5 drops in affected ear 3-4 times/day

Dosage Forms

Suspension, otic [drops]:

Coly-Mycin® S: Neomycin 0.33%, colistin 0.3%, hydrocortisone 1%, and thonzonium 0.05% (5 mL)

Cortisporin®-TC: Neomycin 0.33%, colistin 0.3%, hydrocortisone 1%, and thonzonium 0.05% (10 mL)

neomycin, polymyxin B, and dexamethasone

(nee oh MYE sin, pol i MIKS in bee, & deks a METH a sone)

Synonyms dexamethasone, neomycin, and polymyxin B; polymyxin B, neomycin, and dexamethasone

U.S./Canadian Brand Names Dioptrol® [Can]; Maxitrol® [US/Can]; Poly-Dex™ [US]

Therapeutic Category Antibiotic/Corticosteroid, Ophthalmic

Use Steroid-responsive inflammatory ocular conditions in which a corticosteroid is indicated and where bacterial infection or a risk of bacterial infection exists

Dosage Summary

Ophthalmic:

Ointment:

Children: Place a small amount (~1/2") in the affected eye 3-4 times/day **or** apply at bedtime as an adjunct with drops

Adults: Place a small amount (~1/2") in the affected eye 3-4 times/day **or** apply at bedtime as an adjunct with drops

Suspension:

Children: Instill 1-2 drops into affected eye(s) every 3-4 hours

Adults: Instill 1-2 drops into affected eye(s) every 3-4 hours

Dosage Forms

Ointment, ophthalmic: Neomycin 3.5 mg, polymyxin B 10,000 units, and dexamethasone 0.1% per g (3.5 g)

Maxitrol®, Poly-Dex™: Neomycin 3.5 mg, polymyxin B 10,000 units, and dexamethasone 0.1% per g (3.5 g)

Suspension, ophthalmic: Neomycin 3.5 mg, polymyxin B 10,000 units, and dexamethasone 0.1% per mL (5 mL)

Maxitrol®, Poly-Dex™: Neomycin 3.5 mg, polymyxin B10,000 units, and dexamethasone 0.1% per mL (5 mL)

neomycin, polymyxin B, and gramicidin

(nee oh MYE sin, pol i MIKS in bee, & gram i SYE din)

Synonyms gramicidin, neomycin, and polymyxin B; polymyxin B, neomycin, and gramicidin

U.S./Canadian Brand Names Neosporin® Ophthalmic Solution [US]; Neosporin® [Can]; Optimyxin Plus® [Can]

Therapeutic Category Antibiotic, Ophthalmic

Use Treatment of superficial ocular infection

Dosage Summary

Ophthalmic:

Children: Instill 1-2 drops 4-6 times/day

Adults: Instill 1-2 drops 4-6 times/day

Dosage Forms

Solution, ophthalmic: Neomycin 1.75 mg, polymyxin B 10,000 units, and gramicidin 0.025 mg per 1 mL (10 mL)

Neosporin® Ophthalmic Solution: Neomycin 1.75 mg, polymyxin B 10,000 units, and gramicidin 0.025 mg per 1 mL (10 mL)

neomycin, polymyxin B, and hydrocortisone

(nee oh MYE sin, pol i MIKS in bee, & hye droe KOR ti sone)

Synonyms hydrocortisone, neomycin, and polymyxin B; polymyxin B, neomycin, and hydrocortisone

U.S./Canadian Brand Names Cortimyxin® [Can]; Cortisporin® Cream [US]; Cortisporin® Otic [US/Can]

Therapeutic Category Antibiotic/Corticosteroid, Ophthalmic; Antibiotic/Corticosteroid, Otic; Antibiotic/Corticosteroid, Topical

Use Steroid-responsive inflammatory condition for which a corticosteroid is indicated and where bacterial infection or a risk of bacterial infection exists

Dosage Summary

Ophthalmic:

Adults: Instill 1-2 drops every 3-4 hours, or more frequently as required for severe infections

Otic:

Children <2 years: Dosage not established

Children ≥2 years: Instill 3 drops into affected ear 3-4 times/day

Children ≥12 years: Instill 4 drops into affected ear 3-4 times/day

Adults: Instill 4 drops into affected ear 3-4 times/day

Topical:

Adults: Apply a thin layer 1-4 times/day

Dosage Forms

Cream, topical: Neomycin 3.5 mg, polymyxin B 10,000 units, and hydrocortisone 5 mg per g (7.5 g)

Cortisporin®: Neomycin 3.5 mg, polymyxin B 10,000 units, and hydrocortisone 5 mg per g (7.5 g)

Solution, otic: Neomycin 3.5 mg, polymyxin B 10,000 units, and hydrocortisone 10 mg per mL (10 mL)

Cortisporin®: Neomycin 3.5 mg, polymyxin B 10,000 units, and hydrocortisone 10 mg per mL (10 mL)

Suspension, ophthalmic: Neomycin 3.5 mg, polymyxin B 10,000 units, and hydrocortisone 10 mg per mL (7.5 mL)

Suspension, otic: Neomycin 3.5 mg, polymyxin B 10,000 units, and hydrocortisone 10 mg per mL (10 mL)

Cortisporin®: Neomycin 3.5 mg, polymyxin B 10,000 units, and hydrocortisone 10 mg per mL (10 mL)

neomycin, polymyxin B, and prednisolone

(nee oh MYE sin, pol i MIKS in bee, & pred NIS oh lone)

Synonyms polymyxin B, neomycin, and prednisolone; prednisolone, neomycin, and polymyxin B

U.S./Canadian Brand Names Poly-Pred® [US]

Therapeutic Category Antibiotic/Corticosteroid, Ophthalmic

Use Steroid-responsive inflammatory ocular condition in which bacterial infection or a risk of bacterial ocular infection exists

Dosage Summary

Ophthalmic:

Children: Initial (acute): 1-2 drops every 30 minutes until infection is under control; Maintenance: Instill 1-2 drops every 3-4 hours

Adults: Initial (acute): 1-2 drops every 30 minutes until infection is under control; Maintenance: Instill 1-2 drops every 3-4 hours

Dosage Forms

Suspension, ophthalmic:

Poly-Pred®: Neomycin 0.35%, polymyxin B 10,000 units per mL, and prednisolone 0.5% (5 mL)

neomycin sulfate *see* neomycin *on page 665*

neonatal trace metals *see* trace metals *on page 945*

NeoProfen® [US] *see* ibuprofen *on page 494*

Neoral® [US/Can] *see* cyclosporine (systemic) *on page 260*

Neo-Rx *(Discontinued)* *see* neomycin *on page 665*

neosar *see* cyclophosphamide *on page 259*

Neosporin® [Can] *see* neomycin, polymyxin B, and gramicidin *on page 667*

Neosporin® AF [US-OTC] *see* miconazole (topical) *on page 630*

Neosporin® G.U. Irrigant [US] *see* neomycin and polymyxin B *on page 666*

Neosporin® Irrigating Solution [Can] *see* neomycin and polymyxin B *on page 666*

Neosporin® Neo To Go® [US-OTC] *see* bacitracin, neomycin, and polymyxin B *on page 114*

Neosporin® Ophthalmic Ointment *(Discontinued)* *see* bacitracin, neomycin, and polymyxin B *on page 114*

Neosporin® Ophthalmic Solution [US] *see* neomycin, polymyxin B, and gramicidin *on page 667*

Neosporin® + Pain Relief Ointment [US-OTC] *see* bacitracin, neomycin, polymyxin B, and pramoxine *on page 115*

Neosporin® Topical [US-OTC] *see* bacitracin, neomycin, and polymyxin B *on page 114*

neostigmine (nee oh STIG meen)

Sound-Alike/Look-Alike Issues

Prostigmin® may be confused with physostigmine

Synonyms neostigmine bromide; neostigmine methylsulfate

U.S./Canadian Brand Names Prostigmin® [US/Can]

Therapeutic Category Cholinergic Agent

Use Reversal of the effects of nondepolarizing neuromuscular-blocking agents; treatment of myasthenia gravis; prevention and treatment of postoperative bladder distention and urinary retention

Dosage Summary

I.M.:

Children: Myasthenia gravis: Diagnosis: 0.04 mg/kg as a single dose; Treatment: 0.01-0.04 mg/kg every 2-4 hours

Adults:

Bladder atony: Prevention: 0.25 mg every 4-6 hours; Treatment: 0.5-1 mg every 3 hours for 5 doses after bladder emptied

Myasthenia gravis: Diagnosis: 0.02 mg/kg as a single dose; Treatment: 0.5-2.5 mg every 1-3 hours (maximum: 10 mg/day)

I.V.:

Infants: 0.025-0.1 mg/kg/dose to reverse nondepolarizing neuromuscular blockade after surgery

Children: Myasthenia gravis: 0.01-0.04 mg/kg every 2-4 hours **or** 0.025-0.08 mg/kg/dose to reverse nondepolarizing neuromuscular blockade after surgery

Adults: Myasthenia gravis: 0.5-2.5 mg every 1-3 hours (maximum: 10 mg/day) **or** 0.5-2.5 mg to reverse nondepolarizing neuromuscular blockade after surgery (maximum dose: 5 mg)

Oral:

Children: 2 mg/kg/day divided every 3-4 hours

Adults: 15 mg/dose every 3-4 hours (maximum: 375 mg/day)

SubQ:

Children: 0.01-0.04 mg/kg every 2-4 hours

Adults:

Bladder atony: Prevention: 0.25 mg every 4-6 hours; Treatment: 0.5-1 mg every 3 hours for 5 doses after bladder emptied

Myasthenia gravis: 0.5-2.5 mg every 1-3 hours (maximum: 10 mg/day)

Dosage Forms

Injection, solution: 0.5 mg/mL (1 mL, 10 mL); 1 mg/mL (10 mL)

Prostigmin®: 0.5 mg/mL (1 mL, 10 mL); 1 mg/mL (10 mL)

Tablet, oral:

Prostigmin®: 15 mg

neostigmine bromide *see* neostigmine *on page 668*

neostigmine methylsulfate *see* neostigmine *on page 668*

NeoStrata® AHA [US-OTC] *see* hydroquinone *on page 487*

NeoStrata® HQ [Can] *see* hydroquinone *on page 487*

Neo-Synephrine® [Can] *see* phenylephrine (nasal) *on page 751*

Neo-Synephrine® 12-Hour [US-OTC] *see* oxymetazoline (nasal) *on page 716*

Neo-Synephrine® 12-Hour Extra Moisturizing [US-OTC] *see* oxymetazoline (nasal) *on page 716*

Neo-Synephrine® Extra Strength [US-OTC] *see* phenylephrine (nasal) *on page 751*

Neo-Synephrine® Injection *(Discontinued)* *see* phenylephrine (systemic) *on page 751*

Neo-Synephrine® Mild Formula [US-OTC] *see* phenylephrine (nasal) *on page 751*

Neo-Synephrine® Ophthalmic *(Discontinued)* *see* phenylephrine (ophthalmic) *on page 752*

Neo-Synephrine® Regular Strength [US-OTC] *see* phenylephrine (nasal) *on page 751*

Neo-Tabs® *(Discontinued)* *see* neomycin *on page 665*

NeoVadrin® *(Discontinued)*

nepafenac (ne pa FEN ak)

U.S./Canadian Brand Names Nevanac™ [US/Can]

Therapeutic Category Nonsteroidal Antiinflammatory Drug (NSAID), Ophthalmic

Use Treatment of pain and inflammation associated with cataract surgery

Dosage Summary

Ophthalmic:

Children <10 years: Dosage not established

Children ≥10 years: Instill 1 drop into affected eye(s) 3 times/day

Adults: Instill 1 drop into affected eye(s) 3 times/day

Dosage Forms

Suspension, ophthalmic:

Nevanac™: 0.1% (3 mL)

NephrAmine® [US] *see* amino acid injection *on page 64*

Nephro-Calci® [US-OTC] *see* calcium carbonate *on page 167*

Nephro-Fer® *(Discontinued)* *see* ferrous fumarate *on page 398*

Nephrox Suspension *(Discontinued)* *see* aluminum hydroxide *on page 58*

Neptazane™ [US] *see* methazolamide *on page 612*

nerve agent antidote kit *see* atropine and pralidoxime *on page 107*

Nervocaine® Injection *(Discontinued)* *see* lidocaine (systemic) *on page 561*

Nesacaine® [US] *see* chloroprocaine *on page 206*

Nesacaine®-CE [Can] *see* chloroprocaine *on page 206*

Nesacaine®-MPF [US] *see* chloroprocaine *on page 206*

nesiritide (ni SIR i tide)

Synonyms B-type natriuretic peptide (human); hBNP; natriuretic peptide

U.S./Canadian Brand Names Natrecor® [US/Can]

Therapeutic Category Natriuretic Peptide, B-type, Human; Vasodilator

Use Treatment of acutely decompensated heart failure (HF) with dyspnea at rest or with minimal activity

Dosage Summary

I.V.:

Children: Dosage not established

Adults: Bolus: 2 mcg/kg; Infusion: Initial: 0.01 mcg/kg/minute (maximum: 0.03 mcg/kg/minute); **Note:** Titration is recommended

Dosage Forms

Injection, powder for reconstitution:

Natrecor®: 1.5 mg

NESP *see* darbepoetin alfa *on page* 269

Nestrex® ***(Discontinued)*** *see* pyridoxine *on page* 818

Netromycin® ***(Discontinued)***

Neucalm-50® Injection ***(Discontinued)*** *see* hydroxyzine *on page* 490

Neulasta® [US/Can] *see* pegfilgrastim *on page* 732

Neuleptil® [Can] *see* periciazine *(Canada only) on page* 743

Neumega® [US] *see* oprelvekin *on page* 706

Neupogen® [US/Can] *see* filgrastim *on page* 403

Neupro® ***(Discontinued)***

Neuramate® ***(Discontinued)*** *see* meprobamate *on page* 605

Neurontin® [US/Can] *see* gabapentin *on page* 433

Neut® [US] *see* sodium bicarbonate *on page* 882

NeutraCare® [US-OTC] *see* fluoride *on page* 413

NeutraGard® [US-OTC] *see* fluoride *on page* 413

NeutraGard® Advanced [US] *see* fluoride *on page* 413

NeutraGard® Plus [US] *see* fluoride *on page* 413

Neutra-Phos® ***(Discontinued)*** *see* potassium phosphate and sodium phosphate *on page* 783

Neutra-Phos®-K ***(Discontinued)*** *see* potassium phosphate *on page* 783

NeuTrexin® ***(Discontinued)***

Neutrogena® Acne Stress Control [US-OTC] *see* salicylic acid *on page* 858

Neutrogena® Advanced Solutions™ [US-OTC] *see* salicylic acid *on page* 858

Neutrogena® Blackhead Eliminating™ 2-in-1 Foaming Pads [US-OTC] *see* salicylic acid *on page* 858

Neutrogena® Blackhead Eliminating™ Astringent ***(Discontinued)*** *see* salicylic acid *on page* 858

Neutrogena® Blackhead Eliminating™ Daily Scrub [US-OTC] *see* salicylic acid *on page* 858

Neutrogena® Blackhead Eliminating™ Treatment Mask ***(Discontinued)*** *see* salicylic acid *on page* 858

Neutrogena® Blackhead Elinimating™ [US-OTC] *see* salicylic acid *on page* 858

Neutrogena® Body Clear® [US-OTC] *see* salicylic acid *on page* 858

Neutrogena® Clear Pore™ [US-OTC] *see* benzoyl peroxide *on page* 128

Neutrogena® Clear Pore™ Oil-Controlling Astringent [US-OTC] *see* salicylic acid *on page* 858

Neutrogena® Maximum Strength T/Sal® [US-OTC] *see* salicylic acid *on page* 858

Neutrogena® Oil-Free Acne [US-OTC] *see* salicylic acid *on page* 858

Neutrogena® Oil-Free Acne Stress Control [US-OTC] *see* salicylic acid *on page* 858

Neutrogena® Oil-Free Acne Wash [US-OTC] *see* salicylic acid *on page* 858

Neutrogena® Oil-Free Acne Wash 60 Second Mask Scrub [US-OTC] *see* salicylic acid *on page* 858

Neutrogena® Oil-Free Acne Wash Cream Cleanser [US-OTC] *see* salicylic acid *on page* 858

Neutrogena® Oil-Free Acne Wash Foam Cleanser [US-OTC] *see* salicylic acid *on page* 858

Neutrogena® Oil-Free Anti-Acne [US-OTC] *see* salicylic acid *on page* 858

Neutrogena® On The Spot® Acne Treatment [US-OTC] *see* benzoyl peroxide *on page* 128

Neutrogena® Rapid Clear® [US-OTC] *see* salicylic acid *on page* 858

Neutrogena® Rapid Clear® Acne Defense [US-OTC] *see* salicylic acid *on page* 858

Neutrogena® Rapid Clear® Acne Eliminating [US-OTC] *see* salicylic acid *on page* 858

Neutrogena® T/Gel® [US-OTC] *see* coal tar *on page* 242

Neutrogena® T/Gel® Extra Strength [US-OTC] *see* coal tar *on page* *242*
Neutrogena® T/Gel® Stubborn Itch Control [US-OTC] *see* coal tar *on page* *242*
Nevanac™ [US/Can] *see* nepafenac *on page* *669*

nevirapine (ne VYE ra peen)

Sound-Alike/Look-Alike Issues
nevirapine may be confused with nelfinavir
Viramune® may be confused with Viracept®

Synonyms NVP

U.S./Canadian Brand Names Viramune® [US/Can]

Therapeutic Category Antiviral Agent

Use In combination therapy with other antiretroviral agents for the treatment of HIV-1

Dosage Summary

Oral:

Infants (AIDS*info* guidelines): 2 mg/kg as a single dose between birth and 72 hours if mother received intrapartum dose of nevirapine. If maternal dose was given ≤2 hours prior to delivery or not received, administer infant dose as soon as possible following birth

Infants ≥15 days and Children: 150 mg/m^2 once daily for first 14 days (maximum dose: 200 mg/day); increase dose to 150 mg/m^2 twice daily if no rash or untoward effects (maximum dose: ≤400 mg/day). Children ≤8 years of age: May require 200 mg/m^2 twice daily.

Adolescents: Initial: 200 mg once daily for first 14 days; Maintenance: 200 mg twice daily with other antiretrovirals

Adults: Initial: 200 mg once daily for first 14 days; Maintenance: 200 mg twice daily with other antiretrovirals

Pregnant women: 200 mg as a single dose at onset of labor

Dosage Forms

Suspension, oral:
Viramune®: 50 mg/5 mL (240 mL)

Tablet, oral:
Viramune®: 200 mg

Nexavar® [US/Can] *see* sorafenib *on page* *892*
Nexium® [US/Can] *see* esomeprazole *on page* *364*
Nexium® I.V. [US] *see* esomeprazole *on page* *364*
Nexphen PD [US] *see* guaifenesin and phenylephrine *on page* *456*
Next Choice™ [US] *see* levonorgestrel *on page* *559*
NFV *see* nelfinavir *on page* *665*
N.G.A.® Topical *(Discontinued)* *see* nystatin and triamcinolone *on page* *693*
NG-Citalopram [Can] *see* citalopram *on page* *227*
NGX-4010 *see* capsaicin *on page* *175*

niacin (NYE a sin)

Sound-Alike/Look-Alike Issues
niacin may be confused with Minocin®, Niaspan®, Nispan®
Niaspan® may be confused with niacin
Nicobid® may be confused with Nitro-Bid®

Synonyms nicotinic acid; vitamin B_3

U.S./Canadian Brand Names Niacin-Time® [US-OTC]; Niacor® [US]; Niaspan® [US/Can]; Slo-Niacin® [US-OTC]

Therapeutic Category Vitamin, Water Soluble

Use Treatment of dyslipidemias (Fredrickson types IIa and IIb or primary hypercholesterolemia) as mono- or adjunctive therapy; to lower the risk of recurrent MI in patients with a history of MI and hyperlipidemia; to slow progression or promote regression of coronary artery disease; treatment of hypertriglyceridemia in patients at risk of pancreatitis

Dosage Summary Note: Formulations of niacin (regular release versus extended release) are not interchangeable.

Oral:

Extended release:

Children: Dosage not established

Adults: 500 mg to 2 g once daily at bedtime; Niaspan®: Initial: 500 mg at bedtime; Maintenance: 500 mg to 2 g/day at bedtime; **Note:** Titration is recommended

Regular release:

Adults:

Dietary supplement (OTC labeling): 50 mg twice daily or 100 mg once daily

Hyperlipidemia: 1.5-6 g/day in 3 divided doses; Niacor®: Initial: 250 mg once daily; Maintenance: 1.5-2 g/day in 2-3 divided doses **or** 3 g/day in 3 divided doses (maximum dose: 6 g/day in 3 divided doses); **Note:** Titration is recommended

Sustained release:

Children: Dosage not established

Adults: Hyperlipidemia: Usual daily dose after titration (NCEP, 2002): 1-2 g/day

Dosage Forms

Caplet, timed release, oral: 500 mg

Capsule, oral: 50 mg, 250 mg

Capsule, extended release, oral: 250 mg, 500 mg

Capsule, timed release, oral: 250 mg, 400 mg, 500 mg

Tablet, oral: 50 mg, 100 mg, 250 mg, 500 mg

Niacor®: 500 mg

Tablet, controlled release, oral:

Slo-Niacin® [OTC]: 250 mg, 500 mg, 750 mg

Tablet, extended release, oral:

Niaspan®: 500 mg, 750 mg, 1000 mg

Tablet, timed release, oral: 250 mg, 500 mg, 750 mg, 1000 mg

Niacin-Time® [OTC]: 500 mg

niacinamide (nye a SIN a mide)

Sound-Alike/Look-Alike Issues

niacinamide may be confused with niCARdipine

Synonyms nicotinamide; nicotinic acid amide; vitamin B_3

U.S./Canadian Brand Names Nicomide-T™ [US-OTC]

Therapeutic Category Vitamin, Water Soluble

Use

Oral: Prophylaxis and treatment of pellagra

Topical: Improve the appearance of acne and decrease visible inflammation and irritation caused by acne medications

Dosage Summary

Oral:

Children: Pellagra: 10-50 mg every 6 hours until resolution of signs and symptoms

Adults: Pellagra: 100 mg every 6 hours for several days (or until resolution of major signs and symptoms), followed by 50 mg every 8-12 hours until skin lesions heal

Topical:

Children: Dosage not established

Adults: Apply to affected area on face twice daily

Dosage Forms

Cream, topical:

Nicomide-T™ [OTC]: 4% (30 g)

Gel, topical:

Nicomide-T™ [OTC]: 4% (30 g)

Tablet, oral: 100 mg, 250 mg, 500 mg

niacin and lovastatin (NYE a sin & LOE va sta tin)

Sound-Alike/Look-Alike Issues

Advicor® may be confused with Adcirca™, Advair, Altocor™

Synonyms lovastatin and niacin

U.S./Canadian Brand Names Advicor® [US/Can]

Therapeutic Category HMG-CoA Reductase Inhibitor; Vitamin, Water Soluble

Use For use when treatment with both extended-release niacin and lovastatin is appropriate in combination with a standard cholesterol-lowering diet:

Extended-release niacin: Adjunctive treatment of dyslipidemias (types IIa and IIb or primary hypercholesterolemia) to lower the risk of recurrent MI and/or slow progression of coronary artery disease, including combination therapy with other antidyslipidemic agents when additional triglyceride-lowering or HDL-increasing effects are desired; treatment of hypertriglyceridemia in patients at risk of pancreatitis

Lovastatin: Treatment of primary hypercholesterolemia (Frederickson types IIa and IIb); primary and secondary prevention of cardiovascular disease

Dosage Summary

Oral:

Children: Dosage not established

Adults: Initial: Niacin 500 mg/lovastatin 20 mg at bedtime; Maintenance: Up to niacin 2000 mg/lovastatin 40 mg at bedtime; **Note:** Titration is recommended

Dosage Forms

Tablet, variable release:

Advicor®: 500/20: Niacin 500 mg [extended release] and lovastatin 20 mg [immediate release]; 750/20: Niacin 750 mg [extended release] and lovastatin 20 mg [immediate release]; 1000/20: Niacin 1000 mg [extended release] and lovastatin 20 mg [immediate release]; 1000/40: Niacin 1000 mg [extended release] and lovastatin 40 mg [immediate release]

niacin and simvastatin (NYE a sin & sim va STAT in)

Synonyms simvastatin and niacin

U.S./Canadian Brand Names Simcor® [US]

Therapeutic Category Antilipemic Agent, HMG-CoA Reductase Inhibitor; Antilipemic Agent, Miscellaneous

Use Reduce total cholesterol, LDL, Apo B, non-HDL, TG, and/or increase HDL in patients with primary hypercholesterolemia, mixed dyslipidemia, or hypertriglyceridemia in combination with standard cholesterol-lowering diet when simvastatin or niacin monotherapy is inadequate

Dosage Summary

Oral: Note: Dosage forms are a fixed combination of niacin extended-release and simvastatin.

Children: Dosage not established

Adults: Niacin 500-2000 mg/ simvastatin 20-40 mg once daily

Dosage Forms

Tablet, variable release, oral:

Simcor®: 500/20: Niacin 500 mg [extended release] and simvastatin 20 mg [immediate release]; 500/40: Niacin 500 mg [extended release] and simvastatin 40 mg [immediate release]; 750/20: Niacin 750 mg [extended release] and simvastatin 20 mg [immediate release]; 1000/20: Niacin 1000 mg [extended release] and simvastatin 20 mg [immediate release]; 1000/40: Niacin 1000 mg [extended release] and simvastatin 40 mg [immediate release]

Niacin-Time® [US-OTC] *see* niacin *on page 671*

Niacor® [US] *see* niacin *on page 671*

Niaspan® [US/Can] *see* niacin *on page 671*

Niastase® [Can] *see* factor VIIa (recombinant) *on page 388*

nicardipine (nye KAR de peen)

Sound-Alike/Look-Alike Issues

niCARdipine may be confused with niacinamide, NIFEdipine, niMODipine

Cardene® may be confused with Cardizem®, Cardura®, codeine

Synonyms nicardipine hydrochloride

Tall-Man ni**CAR**dipine

U.S./Canadian Brand Names Cardene® I.V. [US]; Cardene® SR [US]; Cardene® [US]

Therapeutic Category Calcium Channel Blocker

Use Chronic stable angina (immediate-release product only); management of hypertension (immediate and sustained release products); parenteral only for short-term use when oral treatment is not feasible

Dosage Summary

I.V.:

Children: Dosage not established

Adults: Initial: 5 mg/hour; Maintenance: 3-15 mg/hour; **Note:** Titration is recommended

Oral:

Immediate release:

Children: Dosage not established

Adults: Initial: 20 mg 3 times/day; Maintenance: 20-40 mg 3 times/day; **Note:** Titration is recommended

Sustained release:

Children: Dosage not established

Adults: Initial: 30 mg twice daily; Maintenance: Up to 60 mg twice daily; **Note:** Titration is recommended

Dosage Forms

Capsule, oral: 20 mg, 30 mg

Cardene®: 20 mg, 30 mg

Capsule, sustained release, oral:

Cardene® SR: 30 mg, 45 mg, 60 mg

Infusion, premixed iso-osmotic dextrose solution:

Cardene® I.V.: 20 mg (200 mL); 40 mg (200 mL)

Infusion, premixed iso-osmotic sodium chloride solution:

Cardene® I.V.: 20 mg (200 mL); 40 mg (200 mL)

Injection, solution: 2.5 mg/mL (10 mL)

Cardene® I.V.: 2.5 mg/mL (10 mL)

nicardipine hydrochloride *see* nicardipine *on page 673*

N'ice® *(Discontinued)* *see* ascorbic acid *on page 98*

Nicobid® *(Discontinued)* *see* niacin *on page 671*

Nicoderm® [Can] *see* nicotine *on page 674*

NicoDerm® CQ® [US-OTC] *see* nicotine *on page 674*

Nicolar® *(Discontinued)* *see* niacin *on page 671*

Nicomide-T™ [US-OTC] *see* niacinamide *on page 672*

Nicorelief [US-OTC] *see* nicotine *on page 674*

Nicorette® [US-OTC/Can] *see* nicotine *on page 674*

Nicorette® Plus [Can] *see* nicotine *on page 674*

nicotinamide *see* niacinamide *on page 672*

nicotine (nik oh TEEN)

Sound-Alike/Look-Alike Issues

NicoDerm® may be confused with Nitroderm

Nicorette® may be confused with Nordette®

Synonyms nicotine patch

U.S./Canadian Brand Names Commit® [US-OTC]; Habitrol® [Can]; NicoDerm® CQ® [US-OTC]; Nicoderm® [Can]; Nicorelief [US-OTC]; Nicorette® Plus [Can]; Nicorette® [US-OTC/Can]; Nicotrol® Inhaler [US]; Nicotrol® NS [US]; Nicotrol® [Can]; Thrive™ [US-OTC]

Therapeutic Category Smoking Deterrent

Use Treatment to aid smoking cessation for the relief of nicotine withdrawal symptoms (including nicotine craving)

Dosage Summary

Inhalation:

Nasal:

Children: Dosage not established

Adults: 1-2 sprays/hour (maximum: 10 sprays/hour; 80 sprays/day)

Oral:

Children: Dosage not established

Adults: Usually 6 to 16 cartridges per day; best effect was achieved by frequent continuous puffing (20 minutes)

Oral:

Gum:

Children: Dosage not established

Adults: 2 mg or 4 mg piece of gum every 1-2 hours (weeks 1-6); every 2-4 hours (weeks 7-9); and every 4-8 hours (weeks 10-12) (maximum: 24 pieces/day)

Lozenge:

Children: Dosage not established

Adults: 2 mg or 4 mg lozenge every 1-2 hours (weeks 1-6); every 2-4 hours (weeks 7-9); and every 4-8 hours (weeks 10-12) (maximum: 5 lozenges every 6 hours; 20 lozenges/day)

Topical:

Children: Dosage not established

Adults: Apply one patch daily; strength dependent on smoking history

Dosage Forms

Gum, chewing, oral: 2 mg (20s, 40s, 50s, 100s, 108s, 110s); 4 mg (20s, 40s, 48s, 50s, 100s, 108s, 110s)

Nicorelief [OTC]: 2 mg (50s, 110s); 4 mg (50s, 110s)

Nicorette® [OTC]: 2 mg (40s, 48s, 50s, 100s, 108s, 110s, 168s, 170s, 192s, 200s, 216s); 4 mg (40s, 48s, 50s, 100s, 108s, 110s, 168s, 170s, 192s, 200s, 216s)

Thrive™ [OTC]: 2 mg (40s); 4 mg (40s)

Lozenge, oral:

Commit® [OTC]: 2 mg (48s, 72s); 4 mg (48s, 72s)

Nicorette® [OTC]: 4 mg (50s)

Oral inhalation system, for oral inhalation:

Nicotrol® Inhaler: 10 mg (168s)

Patch, transdermal: 7 mg/24 hours (7s, 14s, 30s); 14 mg/24 hours (7s, 14s, 30s); 21 mg/24 hours (7s, 14s, 30s)

NicoDerm® CQ® [OTC]: 7 mg/24 hours (14s); 14 mg/24 hours (14s); 21 mg/24 hours (7s, 14s)

Solution, intranasal:

Nicotrol® NS: 10 mg/mL (10 mL)

nicotine patch *see* nicotine *on page* *674*

nicotinic acid *see* niacin *on page* *671*

nicotinic acid amide *see* niacinamide *on page* *672*

Nicotrol® [Can] *see* nicotine *on page* *674*

Nicotrol® Inhaler [US] *see* nicotine *on page* *674*

Nicotrol® NS [US] *see* nicotine *on page* *674*

Nico-Vert® ***(Discontinued)*** *see* meclizine *on page* *595*

Nidagel™ [Can] *see* metronidazole (topical) *on page* *627*

Nifediac CC® [US] *see* nifedipine *on page* *675*

Nifedical XL® [US] *see* nifedipine *on page* *675*

nifedipine (nye FED i peen)

Sound-Alike/Look-Alike Issues

NIFEdipine may be confused with niCARdipine, niMODipine, nisoldipine

Procardia XL® may be confused with Cartia® XT

Tall-Man **NIFE**dipine

U.S./Canadian Brand Names Adalat® CC [US]; Adalat® XL® [Can]; Afeditab® CR [US]; Apo-Nifed PA® [Can]; Apo-Nifed® [Can]; Gen-Nifedipine XL [Can]; Mylan-Nifedipine Extended Release [Can]; Nifediac CC® [US]; Nifedical XL® [US]; Nifedipine PA [Can]; Nu-Nifed [Can]; Nu-Nifedipine-PA [Can]; PMS-Nifedipine [Can]; Procardia XL® [US]; Procardia® [US]

Therapeutic Category Calcium Channel Blocker

Use Management of chronic stable or vasospastic angina; treatment of hypertension (sustained release products only)

Dosage Summary

Oral:

Immediate release:

Children: Dosage not established

Adults: Initial: 10 mg 3-4 times/day; maximum: 180 mg/day

Extended release:

Adults: Initial: 30 mg once daily; Maintenance: 30-60 mg once daily (maximum: 120-180 mg/day)

Dosage Forms

Capsule, softgel, oral: 10 mg, 20 mg

Procardia®: 10 mg

Tablet, extended release, oral: 30 mg, 60 mg, 90 mg
Adalat® CC: 30 mg, 60 mg, 90 mg
Afeditab® CR: 30 mg, 60 mg
Nifediac CC®: 30 mg, 60 mg, 90 mg
Nifedical XL®: 30 mg, 60 mg
Procardia XL®: 30 mg, 60 mg, 90 mg

Nifedipine PA [Can] *see* nifedipine *on page 675*
Niferex® [US-OTC] *see* polysaccharide-iron complex *on page 777*
niftolid *see* flutamide *on page 418*
Nilandron® [US] *see* nilutamide *on page 676*

nilotinib (nye LOE ti nib)

Sound-Alike/Look-Alike Issues
nilotinib may be confused with dasatinib, imatinib, nilutamide
Synonyms AMN107; nilotinib hydrochloride monohydrate
U.S./Canadian Brand Names Tasigna® [US/Can]
Therapeutic Category Antineoplastic Agent, Tyrosine Kinase Inhibitor
Use Treatment of newly-diagnosed Philadelphia chromosome-positive chronic myelogenous leukemia (Ph+ CML) in chronic phase; treatment of chronic and accelerated phase Ph+ CML (refractory or intolerant to prior therapy, including imatinib)
Dosage Summary
Oral:
Children: Dosage not established
Adults: 300-400 mg twice daily
Dosage Forms
Capsule, oral:
Tasigna®: 150 mg, 200 mg

nilotinib hydrochloride monohydrate *see* nilotinib *on page 676*
Nilstat® ***(Discontinued)*** *see* nystatin (topical) *on page 693*

nilutamide (ni LOO ta mide)

Sound-Alike/Look-Alike Issues
nilutamide may be confused with nilotinib
Synonyms NSC-684588; RU-23908
U.S./Canadian Brand Names Anandron® [Can]; Nilandron® [US]
Therapeutic Category Antineoplastic Agent
Use Treatment of metastatic prostate cancer
Dosage Summary
Oral:
Children: Dosage not established
Adults: Initial: 300 mg once daily for 30 days; Maintenance: 150 mg once daily
Dosage Forms
Tablet, oral:
Nilandron®: 150 mg

Nimbex® [US/Can] *see* cisatracurium *on page 226*

nimodipine (nye MOE di peen)

Sound-Alike/Look-Alike Issues
niMODipine may be confused with niCARdipine, NIFEdipine, nisoldipine
Tall-Man ni**MOD**ipine
U.S./Canadian Brand Names Nimotop® [Can]
Therapeutic Category Calcium Channel Blocker
Use Vasospasm following subarachnoid hemorrhage from ruptured intracranial aneurysms
Dosage Summary
Oral:
Children: Dosage not established
Adults: 60 mg every 4 hours

Dosage Forms

Capsule, liquid filled, oral: 30 mg

Capsule, softgel, oral: 30 mg

Nimotop® [Can] *see* nimodipine *on page 676*

Nimotop® *(Discontinued)* *see* nimodipine *on page 676*

Nipent® [US/Can] *see* pentostatin *on page 742*

Niravam™ [US] *see* alprazolam *on page 55*

nisoldipine (nye SOL di peen)

Sound-Alike/Look-Alike Issues

nisoldipine may be confused with NIFEdipine, niMODipine

U.S./Canadian Brand Names Sular® [US]

Therapeutic Category Calcium Channel Blocker

Use Management of hypertension, alone or in combination with other antihypertensive agents

Dosage Summary

Oral:

Children: Dosage not established

Adults:

Sular® (Geomatrix® delivery system): Initial: 17 mg once daily; Maintenance: 17-34 mg once daily (maximum: 34 mg/day)

Nisoldipine extended-release (original formulation): Initial: 20 mg once daily; Maintenance: 10-40 mg once daily (maximum: 60 mg/day)

Elderly:

Sular® (Geomatrix® delivery system): Initial: 8.5 mg once daily; Maintenance: 17-34 mg once daily (maximum: 34 mg/day)

Nisoldipine extended-release (original formulation): Initial: 10 mg once daily; Maintenance: 10-40 mg once daily (maximum: 60 mg/day)

Dosage Forms

Tablet, extended release, oral: 8.5 mg, 17 mg, 20 mg, 25.5 mg, 30 mg, 34 mg, 40 mg

Sular®: 8.5 mg, 17 mg, 25.5 mg, 34 mg

nitalapram *see* citalopram *on page 227*

nitazoxanide (nye ta ZOX a nide)

Synonyms NTZ

U.S./Canadian Brand Names Alinia® [US]

Therapeutic Category Antiprotozoal

Use Treatment of diarrhea caused by *Cryptosporidium parvum* or *Giardia lamblia*

Dosage Summary

Oral:

Children <1 year: Dosage not established

Children 1-3 years: 100 mg every 12 hours

Children 4-11 years: 200 mg every 12 hours

Children ≥12 years: 500 mg every 12 hours

Adults: 500 mg every 12 hours

Dosage Forms

Powder for suspension, oral:

Alinia®: 100 mg/5 mL (60 mL)

Tablet, oral:

Alinia®: 500 mg

nitisinone (ni TIS i known)

Synonyms NTBC

U.S./Canadian Brand Names Orfadin® [US]

Therapeutic Category 4-Hydroxyphenylpyruvate Dioxygenase Inhibitor

Use Treatment of hereditary tyrosinemia type 1 (HT-1) as an adjunct to dietary restriction of tyrosine and phenylalanine

Dosage Summary Note: Must be used in conjunction with a low-protein diet restricted in tyrosine and phenylalanine

Oral:

Infants: 1-2 mg/kg/day in 2 divided doses

Children: 1-2 mg/kg/day in 2 divided doses

Adults: 1-2 mg/kg/day in 2 divided doses

Dosage Forms

Capsule, oral:

Orfadin®: 2 mg, 5 mg, 10 mg

Nitoman™ [Can] *see* tetrabenazine *on page 921*

Nitrazadon [Can] *see* nitrazepam *(Canada only) on page 678*

nitrazepam *(Canada only)* (nye TRA ze pam)

Synonyms nitrozepamum

U.S./Canadian Brand Names Apo-Nitrazepam® [Can]; Mogadon [Can]; Nitrazadon [Can]; Nitrazepam (Pro-Doc) [Can]; Sandoz-Nitrazepam [Can]

Therapeutic Category Benzodiazepine

Controlled Substance CDSA IV

Use Short-term management of insomnia; treatment of myoclonic seizures

Dosage Summary

Oral:

Children ≤30 kg: Myoclonic seizures: 0.3-1 mg/kg/day in 3 divided doses

Adults: Insomnia: 5-10 mg once daily at bedtime (maximum: 10 consecutive days)

Elderly: Insomnia: 2.5-5 mg once daily at bedtime

Dosage Forms - Canada

Tablet:

Apo-Nitrazepam®, Mogadon, Nitrazadon, Nitrazepam (Pro-Doc), Sandoz-Nitrazepam: 5 mg, 10 mg

Nitrazepam (Pro-Doc) [Can] *see* nitrazepam *(Canada only) on page 678*

Nitrek® *(Discontinued)* *see* nitroglycerin *on page 679*

nitric oxide (NYE trik OKS ide)

U.S./Canadian Brand Names INOmax® [US/Can]

Therapeutic Category Vasodilator, Pulmonary

Use Treatment of term and near-term (>34 weeks) neonates with hypoxic respiratory failure associated with pulmonary hypertension; used concurrently with ventilatory support and other agents

Dosage Summary

Inhalation:

Neonates (up to 14 days old): 20 ppm for up to 14 days or until underlying oxygen desaturation has resolved

Children: Dosage not established

Adults: Dosage not established

Dosage Forms

Gas, for inhalation:

INOmax®: 100 ppm (353 L, 1963 L); 800 ppm (353 L, 1963 L)

Nitro-Bid® [US] *see* nitroglycerin *on page 679*

Nitrodisc® Patch *(Discontinued)* *see* nitroglycerin *on page 679*

Nitro-Dur® [US/Can] *see* nitroglycerin *on page 679*

nitrofurantoin (nye troe fyoor AN toyn)

Sound-Alike/Look-Alike Issues

nitrofurantoin may be confused with Neurontin®, nitroglycerin

Macrobid® may be confused with microK®, Nitro-Bid®

U.S./Canadian Brand Names Apo-Nitrofurantoin® [Can]; Furadantin® [US]; Macrobid® [US/Can]; Macrodantin® [US/Can]; Novo-Furantoin [Can]

Therapeutic Category Antibiotic, Miscellaneous

Use Prevention and treatment of urinary tract infections caused by susceptible strains of *E. coli*, *S. aureus*, *Enterococcus*, *Klebsiella*, and *Enterobacter*

Dosage Summary

Oral:

Children ≤1 month: Dosage not established

Children >1 month: Furadantin®, Macrodantin®: 5-7 mg/kg/day divided every 6 hours (maximum: 400 mg/day) (treatment) **or** 1-2 mg/kg/day divided every 12-24 hours (maximum: 100 mg/day) (prophylaxis)

Children >12 years: Macrobid®: 100 mg twice daily for 7 days

Adults: Furadantin®, Macrodantin®: 50-100 mg/dose every 6 hours (treatment) **or** 50-100 mg/dose at bedtime (prophylaxis); Macrobid®: 100 mg twice daily (treatment)

Dosage Forms

Capsule, oral: 50 mg, 100 mg

Macrobid®: 100 mg

Macrodantin®: 25 mg, 50 mg, 100 mg

Suspension, oral:

Furadantin®: 25 mg/5 mL (230 mL)

nitrogen mustard *see* mechlorethamine *on page 594*

nitroglycerin (nye troe GLI ser in)

Sound-Alike/Look-Alike Issues

nitroglycerin may be confused with nitrofurantoin, nitroprusside

Nitro-Bid® may be confused with Macrobid®, Nicobid®

Nitrol® may be confused with Nizoral®

Nitrostat® may be confused with Nilstat®, nystatin

Synonyms glyceryl trinitrate; nitroglycerol; NTG

U.S./Canadian Brand Names Gen-Nitro [Can]; Minitran™ [US/Can]; Mylan-Nitro Sublingual Spray [Can]; Nitro-Bid® [US]; Nitro-Dur® [US/Can]; Nitro-Time® [US]; Nitroglycerin Injection, USP [Can]; Nitrolingual® [US]; Nitrol® [Can]; Nitrostat® [US/Can]; Rho®-Nitro [Can]; Transderm-Nitro® [Can]; Trinipatch® 0.2 [Can]; Trinipatch® 0.4 [Can]; Trinipatch® 0.6 [Can]

Therapeutic Category Vasodilator

Use Treatment of angina pectoris; I.V. for congestive heart failure (especially when associated with acute myocardial infarction); pulmonary hypertension; perioperative hypertension (especially during cardiovascular surgery); induction of intraoperative hypotension

Dosage Summary

I.V.:

Children: Initial: 0.25-0.5 mcg/kg/minute Maintenance: 1-3 mcg/kg/minute (maximum: 5 mcg/kg/minute); **Note:** Titration is recommended

Adults: Initial: 5 mcg/minute; Maintenance: 20-200 mcg/minute; **Note:** Titration is recommended

Oral:

Children: Dosage not established

Adults: 2.5-9 mg 2-4 times/day (maximum: 104 mg/day)

Sublingual:

Children: Dosage not established

Adults: 0.2-0.6 mg every 5 minutes for maximum of 3 doses in 15 minutes **or** 5-10 minutes prior to activities which may provoke an attack

Topical:

Children: Dosage not established

Adults:

Ointment: Apply 0.5" to 2" every 6 hours with a nitrate free interval of ~10-12 hours

Patch: Initial: 0.2-0.4 mg/hour for 12-14 hours; Maintenance: 0.2-0.8 mg/hour for 12-14 hours; **Note:** Titration is recommended

Translingual:

Children: Dosage not established

Adults: 1-2 sprays under tongue every 3-5 minutes for maximum of 3 doses in 15 minutes **or** 5-10 minutes prior to activities which may provoke an attack

Dosage Forms

Capsule, extended release, oral: 2.5 mg, 6.5 mg

Nitro-Time®: 2.5 mg, 6.5 mg, 9 mg

Capsule, sustained release, oral: 2.5 mg, 6.5 mg, 9 mg

Infusion, premixed in D_5W: 25 mg (250 mL); 50 mg (250 mL, 500 mL); 100 mg (250 mL)

Injection, solution: 5 mg/mL (5 mL, 10 mL)

Ointment, topical:
Nitro-Bid®: 2% (1 g, 30 g, 60 g)
Patch, transdermal: 0.1 mg/hr (30s); 0.2 mg/hr (30s); 0.4 mg/hr (30s); 0.6 mg/hr (30s)
Minitran™: 0.1 mg/hr (30s); 0.2 mg/hr (30s); 0.4 mg/hr (30s); 0.6 mg/hr (30s)
Nitro-Dur®: 0.1 mg/hr (30s); 0.2 mg/hr (30s); 0.3 mg/hr (30s); 0.4 mg/hr (30s); 0.6 mg/hr (30s); 0.8 mg/hr (30s)
Solution, translingual:
Nitrolingual®: 0.4 mg/spray (4.9 g, 12 g)
Tablet, sublingual:
Nitrostat®: 0.3 mg, 0.4 mg, 0.6 mg

Nitroglycerin Injection, USP [Can] *see* nitroglycerin *on page 679*
nitroglycerol *see* nitroglycerin *on page 679*
Nitrol® [Can] *see* nitroglycerin *on page 679*
Nitrol® *(Discontinued)* *see* nitroglycerin *on page 679*
Nitrolingual® [US] *see* nitroglycerin *on page 679*
Nitrong® Oral Tablet *(Discontinued)* *see* nitroglycerin *on page 679*
Nitropress® [US] *see* nitroprusside *on page 680*

nitroprusside (nye troe PRUS ide)

Sound-Alike/Look-Alike Issues
nitroprusside may be confused with nitroglycerin
Synonyms nitroprusside sodium; sodium nitroferricyanide; sodium nitroprusside
U.S./Canadian Brand Names Nitropress® [US]
Therapeutic Category Vasodilator
Use Management of hypertensive crises; acute decompensated heart failure (HF); used for controlled hypotension to reduce bleeding during surgery
Dosage Summary
I.V.:
Children: Infusion: Initial: 1 mcg/kg/minute; Usual dose: 3 mcg/kg/minute (maximum: 5 mcg/kg/minute); **Note:** Titration is recommended
Adults: Infusion: Initial: 0.3-0.5 mcg/kg/minute; Usual dose: 3 mcg/kg/minute (maximum: 10 mcg/kg/minute); **Note:** Titration is recommended
Dosage Forms
Injection, solution:
Nitropress®: 25 mg/mL (2 mL)

nitroprusside sodium *see* nitroprusside *on page 680*
NitroQuick® *(Discontinued)* *see* nitroglycerin *on page 679*
Nitrostat® [US/Can] *see* nitroglycerin *on page 679*
Nitro-Time® [US] *see* nitroglycerin *on page 679*
4′-nitro-3′-trifluoromethylisobutyrantide *see* flutamide *on page 418*

nitrous oxide (NYE trus OKS ide)

Therapeutic Category Anesthetic, Gas
Use Sedation, analgesia, and amnesia; principal adjunct to inhalation and intravenous general anesthesia
Dosage Summary
Inhalation:
Children: Dental: Concentrations of 25% to 50% nitrous oxide with oxygen; Surgical: Concentrations of 25% to 70% nitrous oxide with oxygen
Adults: Dental: Concentrations of 25% to 50% nitrous oxide with oxygen; Surgical: Concentrations of 25% to 70% nitrous oxide with oxygen
Dosage Forms
Supplied in blue cylinders

nitrozepamum *see* nitrazepam *(Canada only) on page 678*
Nix® [Can] *see* permethrin *on page 744*
Nix® Complete Lice Treatment System [US-OTC] *see* permethrin *on page 744*
Nix® Creme Rinse [US-OTC] *see* permethrin *on page 744*
Nix® Creme Rinse Lice Treatment [US-OTC] *see* permethrin *on page 744*

Nix® Lice Control Spray [US-OTC] *see* permethrin *on page 744*

nizatidine (ni ZA ti deen)

Sound-Alike/Look-Alike Issues

Axid® may be confused with Ansaid®

U.S./Canadian Brand Names Apo-Nizatidine® [Can]; Axid® AR [US-OTC]; Axid® [US/Can]; Gen-Nizatidine [Can]; Novo-Nizatidine [Can]; Nu-Nizatidine [Can]; PMS-Nizatidine [Can]

Therapeutic Category Histamine H_2 Antagonist

Use Treatment and maintenance of duodenal ulcer; treatment of benign gastric ulcer; treatment of gastroesophageal reflux disease (GERD)

OTC labeling: Prevention of meal-induced heartburn, acid indigestion, and sour stomach

Dosage Summary

Oral:

Children ≥12 years: 150 mg twice daily

Adults: 150 mg twice daily **or** 300 mg at bedtime **or** 75 mg twice daily (OTC dosing)

Dosage Forms

Capsule, oral: 150 mg, 300 mg

Solution, oral: 15 mg/mL (473 mL)

Axid®: 15 mg/mL (480 mL)

Tablet, oral:

Axid® AR [OTC]: 75 mg

Nizoral® [US] *see* ketoconazole (topical) *on page 536*

Nizoral® A-D [US-OTC] *see* ketoconazole (topical) *on page 536*

N-methylhydrazine *see* procarbazine *on page 797*

N-methylnaltrexone bromide *see* methylnaltrexone *on page 620*

NN2211 *see* liraglutide *on page 569*

No Doz® Maximum Strength [US-OTC] *see* caffeine *on page 163*

NoHist [US] *see* chlorpheniramine and phenylephrine *on page 208*

NoHist-A [US] *see* chlorpheniramine, phenylephrine, and phenyltoloxamine *on page 213*

Nolahist® *(Discontinued)*

Nolex® LA *(Discontinued)*

Nolvadex®-D [Can] *see* tamoxifen *on page 909*

Nolvadex® *(Discontinued)* *see* tamoxifen *on page 909*

nonoxynol 9 (non OKS i nole nine)

Sound-Alike/Look-Alike Issues

Delfen® may be confused with Delsym®

Synonyms N-9

U.S./Canadian Brand Names Conceptrol® [US-OTC]; Delfen® [US-OTC]; Encare® [US-OTC]; Gynol II® Extra Strength [US-OTC]; Gynol II® [US-OTC]; Today® [US-OTC]; VCF® [US-OTC]

Therapeutic Category Spermicide

Use Prevention of pregnancy

Dosage Summary

Intravaginal:

Children: Dosage not established

Adolescents: Insert 1 applicatorful, film, suppository or sponge 10 minutes to 3 hours prior to intercourse (formulation-dependent)

Adults: Insert 1 applicatorful, film, suppository or sponge 10 minutes to 3 hours prior to intercourse (formulation-dependent)

Dosage Forms

Aerosol, vaginal:

Delfen® [OTC]: 12.5% (18 g)

VCF® [OTC]: 12.5% (40 g)

Film, vaginal:

VCF® [OTC]: 28% (3s, 6s, 12s)

Gel, vaginal:
Conceptrol® [OTC]: 4% (2.7 g)
Encare® [OTC]: 4% (2.7 g)
Gynol II® [OTC]: 2% (108 g)
Gynol II® Extra Strength [OTC]: 3% (81 g)
Sponge, vaginal:
Today® [OTC]: 1 g (3s, 12s)
Suppository, vaginal:
Encare® [OTC]: 100 mg (12s, 18s)

No Pain-HP® ***(Discontinued)*** *see* capsaicin *on page 175*
Nora-BE® [US] *see* norethindrone *on page 682*
noradrenaline *see* norepinephrine *on page 682*
noradrenaline acid tartrate *see* norepinephrine *on page 682*
Norcet® ***(Discontinued)*** *see* hydrocodone and acetaminophen *on page 479*
Norco® [US] *see* hydrocodone and acetaminophen *on page 479*
Norcuron® [Can] *see* vecuronium *on page 980*
Norcuron® ***(Discontinued)*** *see* vecuronium *on page 980*
nordeoxyguanosine *see* ganciclovir (ophthalmic) *on page 437*
nordeoxyguanosine *see* ganciclovir (systemic) *on page 437*
Nordette® [US] *see* ethinyl estradiol and levonorgestrel *on page 376*
Norditropin® [US] *see* somatropin *on page 889*
Norditropin® NordiFlex® [US] *see* somatropin *on page 889*
Nordryl® Injection ***(Discontinued)*** *see* diphenhydramine (systemic) *on page 310*
Nordryl® Oral ***(Discontinued)*** *see* diphenhydramine (systemic) *on page 310*
Norel DM™ [US] *see* chlorpheniramine, phenylephrine, and dextromethorphan *on page 211*
norel® EX [US] *see* guaifenesin and phenylephrine *on page 456*
norelgestromin and ethinyl estradiol *see* ethinyl estradiol and norelgestromin *on page 378*

norepinephrine (nor ep i NEF rin)

Sound-Alike/Look-Alike Issues
Levophed® may be confused with levofloxacin

Synonyms levarterenol bitartrate; noradrenaline; noradrenaline acid tartrate; norepinephrine bitartrate

U.S./Canadian Brand Names Levophed® [US/Can]

Therapeutic Category Adrenergic Agonist Agent

Use Treatment of shock which persists after adequate fluid volume replacement

Dosage Summary Note: Norepinephrine dosage is stated in terms of norepinephrine base.
I.V.:
Children: Initial: 0.05-0.1 mcg/kg/minute; Maintenance: Titrate to desired effect (maximum: 2 mcg/kg/minute)
Adults: Initial: 0.5-1 mcg/minute; Maintenance: 0.5-30 mcg/minute; **Note:** Titration is recommended

Dosage Forms
Injection, solution: 1 mg/mL (4 mL)
Levophed®: 1 mg/mL (4 mL)

norepinephrine bitartrate *see* norepinephrine *on page 682*
Norethin™ 1/35E ***(Discontinued)*** *see* ethinyl estradiol and norethindrone *on page 378*

norethindrone (nor ETH in drone)

Sound-Alike/Look-Alike Issues
Micronor® may be confused with miconazole, Micronase®

Synonyms norethindrone acetate; norethisterone

U.S./Canadian Brand Names Aygestin® [US]; Camila® [US]; Errin® [US]; Jolivette® [US]; Micronor® [Can]; Nor-QD® [US]; Nora-BE® [US]; Norlutate® [Can]; Ortho Micronor® [US]

Therapeutic Category Contraceptive, Progestin Only; Progestin

Use Treatment of amenorrhea; abnormal uterine bleeding; endometriosis; prevention of pregnancy

Dosage Summary

Oral:

Norethindrone:

Children (premenarche): Dosage not established

Children (postmenarche): Contraception: 0.35 mg every day

Adults: Contraception: 0.35 mg every day

Norethindrone acetate:

Children: Dosage not established

Adolescents:

Amenorrhea and abnormal uterine bleeding: 2.5-10 mg once daily for 5-10 days during the second half of the menstrual cycle

Endometriosis: Initial: 5 mg/day for 14 days; Maintenance: 15 mg/day; **Note:** Titration is recommended

Adults:

Amenorrhea and abnormal uterine bleeding: 2.5-10 mg once daily for 5-10 days during the second half of the menstrual cycle

Endometriosis: Initial: 5 mg/day for 14 days; Maintenance: 15 mg/day; **Note:** Titration is recommended

Dosage Forms

Tablet, oral: 5 mg

Aygestin®: 5 mg

Camila®: 0.35 mg

Errin®: 0.35 mg

Jolivette®: 0.35 mg

Nor-QD®: 0.35 mg

Nora-BE®: 0.35 mg

Ortho Micronor®: 0.35 mg

norethindrone acetate *see* norethindrone *on page 682*

norethindrone acetate and ethinyl estradiol *see* ethinyl estradiol and norethindrone *on page 378*

norethindrone and estradiol *see* estradiol and norethindrone *on page 368*

norethindrone and mestranol (nor eth IN drone & MES tra nole)

Sound-Alike/Look-Alike Issues

Norinyl® may be confused with Nardil®

Synonyms mestranol and norethindrone

U.S./Canadian Brand Names Necon® 1/50 [US]; Norinyl® 1+50 [US]; Ortho-Novum® 1/50 [Can]

Therapeutic Category Contraceptive, Oral

Use Prevention of pregnancy

Dosage Summary

Oral:

21 tablet package:

Children prior to menarche: Dosage not established

Children (menarche): 1 tablet daily for 21 days, followed by 7 days off

Adults: 1 tablet daily for 21 days, followed by 7 days off

28 tablet package:

Children prior to menarche: Dosage not established

Children (menarche): 1 tablet daily without interruption

Adults: 1 tablet daily without interruption

Dosage Forms

Tablet, monophasic formulations:

Necon® 1/50: Norethindrone 1 mg and mestranol 0.05 mg [21 light blue tablets and 7 white inactive tablets] (28s)

Norinyl® 1+50: Norethindrone 1 mg and mestranol 0.05 mg [21 white tablets and 7 orange inactive tablets] (28s)

norethisterone *see* norethindrone *on page 682*

Norflex™ [US/Can] *see* orphenadrine *on page 708*

norfloxacin (nor FLOKS a sin)

Sound-Alike/Look-Alike Issues

norfloxacin may be confused with Norflex™, Noroxin®
Noroxin® may be confused with Neurontin®, Norflex™, norfloxacin

U.S./Canadian Brand Names Apo-Norflox® [Can]; CO Norfloxacin [Can]; Norfloxacine® [Can]; Noroxin® [US]; Novo-Norfloxacin [Can]; PMS-Norfloxacin [Can]; Riva-Norfloxacin [Can]

Therapeutic Category Quinolone

Use Uncomplicated and complicated urinary tract infections caused by susceptible gram-negative and gram-positive bacteria; sexually-transmitted disease (eg, uncomplicated urethral and cervical gonorrhea) caused by *N. gonorrhoeae*; prostatitis due to *E. coli*

Note: As of April 2007, the CDC no longer recommends the use of fluoroquinolones for the treatment of gonococcal disease.

Dosage Summary

Oral:

Children: Dosage not established
Adults: 400 mg every 12 hours **or** 800 mg as a single dose

Dosage Forms

Tablet, oral:

Noroxin®: 400 mg

Norfloxacine® [Can] *see* norfloxacin *on page 684*
Norgesic™ *(Discontinued)* *see* orphenadrine, aspirin, and caffeine *on page 708*
Norgesic™ Forte *(Discontinued)* *see* orphenadrine, aspirin, and caffeine *on page 708*
norgestimate and estradiol *see* estradiol and norgestimate *on page 369*
norgestimate and ethinyl estradiol *see* ethinyl estradiol and norgestimate *on page 380*
norgestrel and ethinyl estradiol *see* ethinyl estradiol and norgestrel *on page 380*
Norinyl® 1+35 [US] *see* ethinyl estradiol and norethindrone *on page 378*
Norinyl® 1+50 [US] *see* norethindrone and mestranol *on page 683*
Noritate® [US/Can] *see* metronidazole (topical) *on page 627*
Norlutate® [Can] *see* norethindrone *on page 682*
normal human serum albumin *see* albumin *on page 43*
normal saline *see* sodium chloride *on page 882*
normal serum albumin (human) *see* albumin *on page 43*
Normiflo® *(Discontinued)*
Normocarb HF™ [US] *see* electrolyte solution, renal replacement *on page 345*
Normodyne® [Can] *see* labetalol *on page 541*
Noroxin® [US] *see* norfloxacin *on page 684*
Norpace® [US/Can] *see* disopyramide *on page 318*
Norpace® CR [US] *see* disopyramide *on page 318*
Norplant® Implant *(Discontinued)* *see* levonorgestrel *on page 559*
Norpramin® [US/Can] *see* desipramine *on page 277*
Nor-QD® [US] *see* norethindrone *on page 682*
Nortemp Children's [US-OTC] *see* acetaminophen *on page 21*
North American antisnake-bite serum, FAB (ovine) *see* crotalidae polyvalent immune FAB (ovine) *on page 255*
North American coral snake antivenin *see* antivenin *(Micrurus fulvius) on page 85*
Northyx™ *(Discontinued)* *see* methimazole *on page 613*
Nortrel™ [US] *see* ethinyl estradiol and norethindrone *on page 378*
Nortrel™ 7/7/7 [US] *see* ethinyl estradiol and norethindrone *on page 378*

nortriptyline (nor TRIP ti leen)

Sound-Alike/Look-Alike Issues

nortriptyline may be confused with amitriptyline, desipramine, Norpramin®
Aventyl® HCl may be confused with Bentyl®
Pamelor® may be confused with Demerol®, Dymelor®, Panlor® DC, Tambocor™

Synonyms nortriptyline hydrochloride

U.S./Canadian Brand Names Alti-Nortriptyline [Can]; Apo-Nortriptyline® [Can]; Aventyl® [Can]; Gen-Nortriptyline [Can]; Norventyl [Can]; Novo-Nortriptyline [Can]; Nu-Nortriptyline [Can]; Pamelor® [US]; PMS-Nortriptyline [Can]

Therapeutic Category Antidepressant, Tricyclic (Secondary Amine)

Use Treatment of symptoms of depression

Dosage Summary

Oral:

Adults: 25 mg 3-4 times/day (maximum: 150 mg/day); **Note:** Titration is recommended

Elderly: Initial: 10-25 mg at bedtime; Maintenance: 75 mg/day at bedtime or in 2 divided doses; **Note:** Titration is recommended every 3 days (inpatients) or every 7 days (outpatients)

Dosage Forms

Capsule, oral: 10 mg, 25 mg, 50 mg, 75 mg

Pamelor®: 10 mg, 25 mg, 50 mg, 75 mg

Solution, oral: 10 mg/5 mL (473 mL, 480 mL)

Pamelor®: 10 mg/5 mL (480 mL)

nortriptyline hydrochloride *see* nortriptyline *on page 684*

Norvasc® [US/Can] *see* amlodipine *on page 68*

Norventyl [Can] *see* nortriptyline *on page 684*

Norvir® [US/Can] *see* ritonavir *on page 846*

Norvir® SEC [Can] *see* ritonavir *on page 846*

Nostrilla® [US-OTC] *see* oxymetazoline (nasal) *on page 716*

Notuss®-DC [US] *see* pseudoephedrine and codeine *on page 811*

Novacet® *(Discontinued)* *see* sulfur and sulfacetamide *on page 903*

Novafed® A *(Discontinued)* *see* chlorpheniramine and pseudoephedrine *on page 209*

Novahistex® DM Decongestant [Can] *see* pseudoephedrine and dextromethorphan *on page 812*

Novahistex® DM Decongestant Expectorant [Can] *see* guaifenesin, pseudoephedrine, and dextromethorphan *on page 460*

Novahistex® Expectorant with Decongestant [Can] *see* guaifenesin and pseudoephedrine *on page 457*

Novahistine DH [US] *see* dihydrocodeine, chlorpheniramine, and phenylephrine *on page 304*

Novahistine® DM Decongestant [Can] *see* pseudoephedrine and dextromethorphan *on page 812*

Novahistine® DM Decongestant Expectorant [Can] *see* guaifenesin, pseudoephedrine, and dextromethorphan *on page 460*

Novamilor [Can] *see* amiloride and hydrochlorothiazide *on page 64*

Novamoxin® [Can] *see* amoxicillin *on page 72*

Novantrone® [US/Can] *see* mitoxantrone *on page 638*

Novarel® [US] *see* chorionic gonadotropin (human) *on page 219*

Novasen [Can] *see* aspirin *on page 100*

Nove-Desmopressin [Can] *see* desmopressin acetate *on page 278*

novel erythropoiesis-stimulating protein *see* darbepoetin alfa *on page 269*

Novo-5 ASA [Can] *see* mesalamine *on page 607*

Novo-Acebutolol [Can] *see* acebutolol *on page 21*

Novo-Acyclovir [Can] *see* acyclovir (systemic) *on page 36*

Novo-Alendronate [Can] *see* alendronate *on page 47*

Novo-Alprazol [Can] *see* alprazolam *on page 55*

Novo-Amiodarone [Can] *see* amiodarone *on page 67*

Novo-Amlodipine [Can] *see* amlodipine *on page 68*

Novo-Ampicillin [Can] *see* ampicillin *on page 75*

Novo-Atenolthalidone [Can] *see* atenolol and chlorthalidone *on page 103*

Novo-Atorvastatin [Can] *see* atorvastatin *on page 104*

Novo-Azithromycin [Can] *see* azithromycin (systemic) *on page 111*

Novo-AZT [Can] *see* zidovudine *on page 999*

Novo-Baclofen [Can] *see* baclofen *on page 115*

Novo-Benzydamine [Can] *see* benzydamine *(Canada only) on page 130*

Novo-Betahistine [Can] *see* betahistine *(Canada only) on page 133*

Novo-Rythro Estolate [Can] *see* erythromycin (systemic) *on page 361*
Novo-Rythro Ethylsuccinate [Can] *see* erythromycin (systemic) *on page 361*
Novo-Salbutamol [Can] *see* albuterol *on page 43*
Novo-Selegiline [Can] *see* selegiline *on page 869*
Novo-Semide [Can] *see* furosemide *on page 431*
Novo-Sertraline [Can] *see* sertraline *on page 872*
NovoSeven *(Discontinued)* *see* factor VIIa (recombinant) *on page 388*
NovoSeven® RT [US] *see* factor VIIa (recombinant) *on page 388*
Novo-Sorbide [Can] *see* isosorbide dinitrate *on page 529*
Novo-Sotalol [Can] *see* sotalol *on page 892*
Novo-Soxazole [Can] *see* sulfisoxazole *on page 903*
Novo-Spiroton [Can] *see* spironolactone *on page 894*
Novo-Spirozine [Can] *see* hydrochlorothiazide and spironolactone *on page 478*
Novo-Sucralate [Can] *see* sucralfate *on page 897*
Novo-Sumatriptan [Can] *see* sumatriptan *on page 904*
Novo-Sundac [Can] *see* sulindac *on page 904*
Novo-Tamoxifen [Can] *see* tamoxifen *on page 909*
Novo-Tamsulosin [Can] *see* tamsulosin *on page 909*
Novo-Temazepam [Can] *see* temazepam *on page 914*
Novo-Terbinafine [Can] *see* terbinafine (systemic) *on page 917*
Novo-Theophyl SR [Can] *see* theophylline *on page 925*
Novo-Tiaprofenic [Can] *see* tiaprofenic acid *(Canada only) on page 931*
Novo-Ticlopidine [Can] *see* ticlopidine *on page 932*
Novo-Topiramate [Can] *see* topiramate *on page 942*
Novo-Trazodone [Can] *see* trazodone *on page 950*
Novo-Triamzide [Can] *see* hydrochlorothiazide and triamterene *on page 479*
Novo-Trifluzine [Can] *see* trifluoperazine *on page 957*
Novo-Trimel [Can] *see* sulfamethoxazole and trimethoprim *on page 901*
Novo-Trimel D.S. [Can] *see* sulfamethoxazole and trimethoprim *on page 901*
Novo-Triptyn [Can] *see* amitriptyline *on page 67*
Novo-Veramil [Can] *see* verapamil *on page 981*
Novo-Veramil SR [Can] *see* verapamil *on page 981*
Novo-Warfarin [Can] *see* warfarin *on page 993*
Novoxapram® [Can] *see* oxazepam *on page 712*
Novo-Zopiclone [Can] *see* zopiclone *(Canada only) on page 1005*
Noxafil® [US] *see* posaconazole *on page 779*
Nozinan® [Can] *see* methotrimeprazine *(Canada only) on page 615*
NP-27® *(Discontinued)* *see* tolnaftate *on page 940*
NPH Iletin® II *(Discontinued)*
NPH Iletin® Insulin *(Discontinued)*
NPH insulin *see* insulin NPH *on page 512*
NPH insulin and regular insulin *see* insulin NPH and insulin regular *on page 512*
Nplate™ [US/Can] *see* romiplostim *on page 851*
NRP104 *see* lisdexamfetamine *on page 569*
NRS® [US-OTC] *see* oxymetazoline (nasal) *on page 716*
NSC-750 *see* busulfan *on page 158*
NSC-755 *see* mercaptopurine *on page 606*
NSC-13875 *see* altretamine *on page 57*
NSC-71423 *see* megestrol *on page 598*
NSC-89199 *see* estramustine *on page 369*
NSC-105014 *see* cladribine *on page 229*
NSC-106977 (*Erwinia*) *see* asparaginase *on page 99*
NSC-109229 (*E. coli*) *see* asparaginase *on page 99*

Nu-Pravastatin [Can] *see* pravastatin *on page* 789
Nu-Prazo [Can] *see* prazosin *on page* 789
Nuprin® *(Discontinued)* *see* ibuprofen *on page* 494
Nu-Prochlor [Can] *see* prochlorperazine *on page* 797
Nu-Propranolol [Can] *see* propranolol *on page* 806
Nuquin HP® [US] *see* hydroquinone *on page* 487
Nu-Ranit [Can] *see* ranitidine *on page* 828
Nuromax® *(Discontinued)*
Nu-Salbutamol [Can] *see* albuterol *on page* 43
Nu-Selegiline [Can] *see* selegiline *on page* 869
Nu-Sertraline [Can] *see* sertraline *on page* 872
Nu-Simvastatin [Can] *see* simvastatin *on page* 877
Nu-Sotalol [Can] *see* sotalol *on page* 892
Nu-Sucralate [Can] *see* sucralfate *on page* 897
Nu-Sundac [Can] *see* sulindac *on page* 904
Nu-Tears® [US-OTC] *see* artificial tears *on page* 97
Nu-Tears® II [US-OTC] *see* artificial tears *on page* 97
Nu-Temazepam [Can] *see* temazepam *on page* 914
Nu-Terazosin [Can] *see* terazosin *on page* 917
Nu-Tetra [Can] *see* tetracycline *on page* 922
Nu-Tiaprofenic [Can] *see* tiaprofenic acid *(Canada only) on page* 931
Nu-Ticlopidine [Can] *see* ticlopidine *on page* 932
Nu-Timolol [Can] *see* timolol (systemic) *on page* 933
Nutracort® [US] *see* hydrocortisone (topical) *on page* 483
Nutralox® [US-OTC] *see* calcium carbonate *on page* 167
Nutraplus® [US-OTC] *see* urea *on page* 970
Nu-Trazodone [Can] *see* trazodone *on page* 950
Nu-Triazide [Can] *see* hydrochlorothiazide and triamterene *on page* 479
Nutrimin-Plus [US-OTC] *see* vitamins (multiple/oral) *on page* 990
Nu-Trimipramine [Can] *see* trimipramine *on page* 960
NutriNate® [US] *see* vitamins (multiple/prenatal) *on page* 991
NutriSpire™ [US] *see* vitamins (multiple/prenatal) *on page* 991

nutritional formula, enteral/oral (noo TRISH un al FOR myoo la, EN ter al/OR al)

Synonyms dietary supplements

U.S./Canadian Brand Names Carnation Instant Breakfast® [US-OTC]; Citrotein® [US-OTC]; Criticare HN® [US-OTC]; Ensure Plus® [US-OTC]; Ensure® [US-OTC]; Isocal® [US-OTC]; Magnacal® [US-OTC]; Microlipid™ [US-OTC]; Osmolite® HN [US-OTC]; Pedialyte® [US-OTC]; Portagen® [US-OTC]; Pregestimil® [US-OTC]; Propac™ [US-OTC]; Soyalac® [US-OTC]; Vital HN® [US-OTC]; Vitaneed™ [US-OTC]; Vivonex® T.E.N. [US-OTC]; Vivonex® [US-OTC]

Therapeutic Category Nutritional Supplement

Dosage Forms

Liquid: Calcium and sodium caseinate, maltodextrin, sucrose, partially hydrogenated soy oil, soy lecithin
Powder: Amino acids, predigested carbohydrates, safflower oil

Nutropin® [US/Can] *see* somatropin *on page* 889
Nutropin AQ® [US/Can] *see* somatropin *on page* 889
NuvaRing® [US/Can] *see* ethinyl estradiol and etonogestrel *on page* 376
Nu-Verap [Can] *see* verapamil *on page* 981
Nu-Verap SR [Can] *see* verapamil *on page* 981
Nuvigil™ [US] *see* armodafinil *on page* 95
Nu-Zopiclone [Can] *see* zopiclone *(Canada only) on page* 1005
NVP *see* nevirapine *on page* 671
Nyaderm [Can] *see* nystatin (topical) *on page* 693
Nyamyc® [US] *see* nystatin (topical) *on page* 693

Nycoff [US-OTC] *see* dextromethorphan *on page* 287
Nydrazid® *(Discontinued)* *see* isoniazid *on page* 527

nystatin (oral) (nye STAT in)

Sound-Alike/Look-Alike Issues

nystatin may be confused with HMG-CoA reductase inhibitors (also known as "statins"; eg, atorvastatin, fluvastatin, lovastatin, pitavastatin, pravastatin, rosuvastatin, simvastatin), Nitrostat®

U.S./Canadian Brand Names Nystat-Rx [US]; PMS-Nystatin [Can]

Therapeutic Category Antifungal Agent, Oral Nonabsorbed

Use Treatment of susceptible cutaneous, mucocutaneous, and oral cavity fungal infections normally caused by the *Candida* species

Dosage Summary

Oral:

Premature infants: 100,000 units 4 times/day; paint suspension into recesses of the mouth

Infants: 200,000 units 4 times/day **or** 100,000 units to each side of mouth 4 times/day; paint suspension into recesses of the mouth

Children: 400,000-600,000 units 4 times/day; swish in the mouth and retain for as long as possible (several minutes) before swallowing

Adults: 400,000-1,000,000 units/day in 3-4 divided doses; swish in the mouth and retain for as long as possible (several minutes) before swallowing

Dosage Forms

Powder, for prescription compounding: 50 million units (10 g); 150 million units (30 g); 500 million units (100 g)

Nystat-Rx: 50 million units (10 g); 150 million units (30 g); 1 billion units (190 g); 2 billion units (350 g)

Suspension, oral: 100,000 units/mL (5 mL, 60 mL, 240 mL, 473 mL, 480 mL, 3785 mL)

Tablet, oral: 500,000 units

nystatin (topical) (nye STAT in)

Sound-Alike/Look-Alike Issues

nystatin may be confused with HMG-CoA reductase inhibitors (also known as "statins"; eg, atorvastatin, fluvastatin, lovastatin, pitavastatin, pravastatin, rosuvastatin, simvastatin), Nitrostat®

U.S./Canadian Brand Names Candistatin® [Can]; Nyaderm [Can]; Nyamyc® [US]; Nystop® [US]; Pedi-Dri® [US]

Therapeutic Category Antifungal Agent, Topical; Antifungal Agent, Vaginal

Use Treatment of susceptible cutaneous and mucocutaneous fungal infections normally caused by the *Candida* species

Dosage Summary

Intravaginal:

Children: Dosage not established

Adults: Insert 1 vaginal tablet/day at bedtime

Topical:

Children: Apply 2-3 times/day to affected areas

Adults: Apply 2-3 times/day to affected areas

Dosage Forms

Cream, topical: 100,000 units/g (15 g, 30 g)

Ointment, topical: 100,000 units/g (15 g, 30 g)

Powder, topical: 100,000 units/g (15 g, 30 g, 60 g)

Nyamyc®: 100,000 units/g (15 g, 30 g, 60 g)

Nystop®: 100,000 units/g (15 g, 30 g, 60 g)

Pedi-Dri®: 100,000 units/g (56.7 g)

Tablet, vaginal: 100,000 units

nystatin and metronidazole *see* metronidazole and nystatin *(Canada only) on page* 628

nystatin and triamcinolone (nye STAT in & trye am SIN oh lone)

Synonyms triamcinolone and nystatin

Therapeutic Category Antifungal/Corticosteroid

Use Treatment of cutaneous candidiasis

Dosage Summary

Topical:

Children: Apply sparingly 2-4 times/day

Adults: Apply sparingly 2-4 times/day

Dosage Forms

Cream: Nystatin 100,000 units and triamcinolone 0.1% (15 g, 30 g, 60 g)

Ointment: Nystatin 100,000 units and triamcinolone 0.1% (15 g, 30 g, 60 g)

Nystat-Rx [US] *see* nystatin (oral) *on page* 693

Nystex® ***(Discontinued)*** *see* nystatin (topical) *on page* 693

Nystop® [US] *see* nystatin (topical) *on page* 693

Nytol® [Can] *see* diphenhydramine (systemic) *on page* 310

Nytol® Extra Strength [Can] *see* diphenhydramine (systemic) *on page* 310

Nytol® Quick Caps [US-OTC] *see* diphenhydramine (systemic) *on page* 310

Nytol® Quick Gels [US-OTC] *see* diphenhydramine (systemic) *on page* 310

O-V Staticin® ***(Discontinued)*** *see* nystatin (oral) *on page* 693

Oasis® [US] *see* saliva substitute *on page* 861

Obezine® ***(Discontinued)*** *see* phendimetrazine *on page* 747

OCBZ *see* oxcarbazepine *on page* 712

Occlusal™-HP [Can] *see* salicylic acid *on page* 858

Occlusal®-HP ***(Discontinued)*** *see* salicylic acid *on page* 858

Ocean® [US-OTC] *see* sodium chloride *on page* 882

Ocean® for Kids [US-OTC] *see* sodium chloride *on page* 882

Ocella™ [US] *see* ethinyl estradiol and drospirenone *on page* 375

OCL® ***(Discontinued)*** *see* polyethylene glycol-electrolyte solution *on page* 775

Octagam® [US] *see* immune globulin (intravenous) *on page* 502

Octamide® ***(Discontinued)*** *see* metoclopramide *on page* 624

Octaplex® [Can] *see* prothrombin complex (human) [(factors II, VII, IX, X), protein C, and protein S] *(Canada only) on page* 809

Octicair® Otic ***(Discontinued)*** *see* neomycin, polymyxin B, and hydrocortisone *on page* 667

Octocaine® ***(Discontinued)*** *see* lidocaine and epinephrine *on page* 563

Octostim® [Can] *see* desmopressin acetate *on page* 278

octreotide (ok TREE oh tide)

Sound-Alike/Look-Alike Issues

Sandostatin® may be confused with Sandimmune®, Sandostatin LAR®, sargramostim, simvastatin

Synonyms longastatin; octreotide acetate

U.S./Canadian Brand Names Octreotide Acetate Injection [Can]; Octreotide Acetate Omega [Can]; Sandostatin LAR® [US/Can]; Sandostatin® [US/Can]

Therapeutic Category Somatostatin Analog

Use Control of symptoms (diarrhea and flushing) in patients with metastatic carcinoid tumors; treatment of watery diarrhea associated with vasoactive intestinal peptide-secreting tumors (VIPomas); treatment of acromegaly

Dosage Summary

I.M.:

Children: Dosage not established

Adults: Depot: 20 mg every 4 weeks (maximum: 40 mg every 2 weeks)

I.V.:

Adults: 50-1500 mcg/day in 2-4 divided doses

SubQ:

Adults: 50-1500 mcg/day in 2-4 divided doses

Dosage Forms

Injection, microspheres for suspension:

Sandostatin LAR®: 10 mg, 20 mg, 30 mg

Injection, solution: 0.2 mg/mL (5 mL); 1 mg/mL (5 mL)

Sandostatin®: 0.2 mg/mL (5 mL); 1 mg/mL (5 mL)

Injection, solution [preservative free]: 0.05 mg/mL (1 mL); 0.1 mg/mL (1 mL); 0.5 mg/mL (1 mL)

Sandostatin®: 0.05 mg/mL (1 mL); 0.1 mg/mL (1 mL); 0.5 mg/mL (1 mL)

octreotide acetate *see* octreotide *on page 694*
Octreotide Acetate Injection [Can] *see* octreotide *on page 694*
Octreotide Acetate Omega [Can] *see* octreotide *on page 694*
OcuClear® *(Discontinued)* *see* oxymetazoline (ophthalmic) *on page 717*
Ocufen® [US/Can] *see* flurbiprofen (ophthalmic) *on page 418*
Ocuflox® [US/Can] *see* ofloxacin (ophthalmic) *on page 696*
OcuNefrin™ [US-OTC] *see* phenylephrine (ophthalmic) *on page 752*
Ocupress® *(Discontinued)* *see* carteolol (ophthalmic) *on page 186*
Ocusert Pilo-20® *(Discontinued)* *see* pilocarpine (ophthalmic) *on page 760*
Ocusert Pilo-40® *(Discontinued)* *see* pilocarpine (ophthalmic) *on page 760*
Ocu-Sul® *(Discontinued)* *see* sulfacetamide (ophthalmic) *on page 899*
Ocutricin® Topical Ointment *(Discontinued)* *see* bacitracin, neomycin, and polymyxin B *on page 114*
Ocuvite® [US-OTC] *see* vitamins (multiple/oral) *on page 990*
Ocuvite® Adult 50+ [US-OTC] *see* vitamins (multiple/oral) *on page 990*
Ocuvite® Extra® [US-OTC] *see* vitamins (multiple/oral) *on page 990*
Ocuvite® Lutein [US-OTC] *see* vitamins (multiple/oral) *on page 990*
O-desmethylvenlafaxine *see* desvenlafaxine *on page 280*
ODV *see* desvenlafaxine *on page 280*
Oesclim® [Can] *see* estradiol (systemic) *on page 366*

ofatumumab (oh fa TOOM yoo mab)

Sound-Alike/Look-Alike Issues
ofatumumab may be confused with omalizumab

Synonyms huMax-CD20

U.S./Canadian Brand Names Arzerra™ [US]

Therapeutic Category Antineoplastic Agent, Monoclonal Antibody; Monoclonal Antibody

Use Treatment of refractory chronic lymphocytic leukemia (CLL)

Dosage Summary

I.V.:

Children: Dosage not established

Adults: 300 mg week 1, followed 1 week later by 2000 mg once weekly for 7 doses (doses 2-8), followed 4 weeks later by 2000 mg once every 4 weeks for 4 doses (doses 9-12; for a total of 12 doses)

Dosage Forms

Injection, solution [preservative free]:

Arzerra™: 20 mg/mL (5 mL)

Off-Ezy® Wart Remover *(Discontinued)* *see* salicylic acid *on page 858*

ofloxacin (systemic) (oh FLOKS a sin)

U.S./Canadian Brand Names Apo-Oflox® [Can]; Novo-Ofloxacin [Can]

Therapeutic Category Antibiotic, Quinolone

Use Quinolone antibiotic for the treatment of acute exacerbations of chronic bronchitis, community-acquired pneumonia, skin and skin structure infections (uncomplicated), urethral and cervical gonorrhea (acute, uncomplicated), urethritis and cervicitis (nongonococcal), mixed infections of the urethra and cervix, pelvic inflammatory disease (acute), cystitis (uncomplicated), urinary tract infections (complicated), prostatitis

Note: As of April 2007, the CDC no longer recommends the use of fluoroquinolones for the treatment of gonococcal disease.

Dosage Summary

Oral:

Children: Dosage not established

Adults: 200-400 mg every 12 hours

Dosage Forms

Tablet, oral: 200 mg, 300 mg, 400 mg

ofloxacin (ophthalmic) (oh FLOKS a sin)

Sound-Alike/Look-Alike Issues

Ocuflox® may be confused with Occlusal®-HP, Ocufen®

U.S./Canadian Brand Names Ocuflox® [US/Can]

Therapeutic Category Antibiotic, Ophthalmic; Antibiotic, Quinolone

Use Treatment of superficial ocular infections involving the conjunctiva or cornea due to strains of susceptible organisms

Dosage Summary

Ophthalmic:

Children ≤1 year: Dosage not established

Children >1 year: Initial: 1-2 drops every 30 minutes to 4 hours; Maintenance: 1-2 drops every 4-6 hours

Adults: Initial: 1-2 drops every 30 minutes to 4 hours; Maintenance: 1-2 drops every 4-6 hours

Dosage Forms

Solution, ophthalmic: 0.3% (5 mL, 10 mL)

Ocuflox®: 0.3% (5 mL)

ofloxacin (otic) (oh FLOKS a sin)

Sound-Alike/Look-Alike Issues

Floxin® may be confused with Flexeril®

Synonyms floxin otic singles

U.S./Canadian Brand Names Floxin® [Can]

Therapeutic Category Antibiotic, Quinolone

Use Otitis externa, chronic suppurative otitis media, acute otitis media

Dosage Summary

Otic:

Children <6 months: Dosage not established

Children ≥6 months to 12 years: 5 drops daily

Children >12 years: 10 drops once or twice daily

Adults: 10 drops once or twice daily

Dosage Forms

Solution, otic: 0.3% (5 mL, 10 mL)

Oforta™ [US] *see* fludarabine *on page 408*

Ogen® [Can] *see* estropipate *on page 372*

Ogen® *(Discontinued)* *see* estropipate *on page 372*

Ogestrel® [US] *see* ethinyl estradiol and norgestrel *on page 380*

OGMT *see* metyrosine *on page 628*

OGT-918 *see* miglustat *on page 634*

9-OH-risperidone *see* paliperidone *on page 720*

OKT3 *see* muromonab-CD3 *on page 649*

olanzapine (oh LAN za peen)

Sound-Alike/Look-Alike Issues

OLANZapine may be confused with olsalazine, QUEtiapine

Zyprexa® may be confused with Celexa®, Reprexain™, Zestril®, Zyrtec®

Zyprexa® Zydis® may be confused with Zelapar™

Zyprexa® Relprevv™ may be confused with Zyprexa® IntraMuscular

Synonyms LY170053; olanzapine pamoate

Tall-Man OLANZapine

U.S./Canadian Brand Names Apo-Olanzapine® [Can]; CO Olanzapine ODT [Can]; CO Olanzapine [Can]; Novo-Olanzapine [Can]; Olanzapine ODT [Can]; PHL-Olanzapine ODT [Can]; PHL-Olanzapine [Can]; PMS-Olanzapine ODT [Can]; PMS-Olanzapine [Can]; Sandoz-Olanzapine ODT [Can]; Teva-Olanzapine OD [Can]; Teva-Olanzapine [Can]; Zyprexa® IntraMuscular [US/Can]; Zyprexa® Relprevv™ [US]; Zyprexa® Zydis® [US/Can]; Zyprexa® [US/Can]

Therapeutic Category Antipsychotic Agent

Use

Oral: Treatment of the manifestations of schizophrenia; treatment of acute or mixed mania episodes associated with bipolar I disorder (as monotherapy or in combination with lithium or valproate); maintenance treatment of bipolar disorder; acute agitation (patients with schizophrenia or bipolar mania); in combination with fluoxetine for treatment-resistant or bipolar I depression

I.M., extended-release (Zyprexa® Relprevv™): Treatment of schizophrenia

I.M., short-acting (Zyprexa® IntraMuscular): Treatment of acute agitation associated with schizophrenia and bipolar I mania

Dosage Summary

I.M.:

Children: Dosage not established

Adults:

Extended-release: 150-300 mg every 2 weeks or 300-405 mg every 4 weeks (maximum: 405 mg every 4 weeks; 300 mg every 2 weeks)

Short-acting: Initial: 10 mg/dose, 2-4 hours between doses (maximum: 30 mg/day)

Oral:

Adolescents ≥13 years: Initial: 2.5-5 mg once daily; dosing range: 2.5-20 mg/day; **Note:** Titration is recommended

Adults: Initial: 5-15 mg once daily; Maintenance: 5-20 mg once daily; **Note:** Titration is recommended

Elderly: Initial: 2.5-5 mg/day; **Note:** Titration is recommended

Dosage Forms

Injection, powder for reconstitution:

Zyprexa® IntraMuscular: 10 mg

Injection, powder for suspension, extended release:

Zyprexa® Relprevv™: 210 mg, 300 mg, 405 mg

Tablet, oral:

Zyprexa®: 2.5 mg, 5 mg, 7.5 mg, 10 mg, 15 mg, 20 mg

Tablet, orally disintegrating, oral:

Zyprexa® Zydis®: 5 mg, 10 mg, 15 mg, 20 mg

olanzapine and fluoxetine (oh LAN za peen & floo OKS e teen)

Sound-Alike/Look-Alike Issues

Symbyax® may be confused with Cymbalta®

Synonyms fluoxetine and olanzapine; olanzapine and fluoxetine hydrochloride

U.S./Canadian Brand Names Symbyax® [US]

Therapeutic Category Antidepressant, Selective Serotonin Reuptake Inhibitor; Antipsychotic Agent, Thienobenzodiaepine

Use Treatment of depressive episodes associated with bipolar I disorder; treatment-resistant depression (unresponsive to 2 trials of different antidepressants in the current episode)

Dosage Summary

Oral:

Children: Dosage not established

Adults: Initial: Olanzapine 6 mg and fluoxetine 25 mg once daily in the evening; Maintenance: Olanzapine 6-12 mg and fluoxetine 25-50 mg once daily in the evening

Elderly >65 years: Initial: Olanzapine 3-6 mg and fluoxetine 25 mg once daily in the evening; safety and efficacy has not been established

Dosage Forms

Capsule:

Symbyax®:

3/25: Olanzapine 3 mg and fluoxetine 25 mg

6/25: Olanzapine 6 mg and fluoxetine 25 mg

6/50: Olanzapine 6 mg and fluoxetine 50 mg

12/25: Olanzapine 12 mg and fluoxetine 25 mg

12/50: Olanzapine 12 mg and fluoxetine 50 mg

olanzapine and fluoxetine hydrochloride *see* olanzapine and fluoxetine *on page* 697

Olanzapine ODT [Can] *see* olanzapine *on page* 696

olanzapine pamoate *see* olanzapine *on page* 696

oleovitamin A *see* vitamin A *on page* 987

Oleptro™ [US] *see* trazodone *on page* 950

Oleptro™ *see* trazodone *on page 950*

oleum ricini *see* castor oil *on page 187*

olmesartan (ole me SAR tan)

Sound-Alike/Look-Alike Issues

Benicar® may be confused with Mevacor®

Synonyms olmesartan medoxomil

U.S./Canadian Brand Names Benicar® [US]; Olmetec® [Can]

Therapeutic Category Angiotensin II Receptor Antagonist

Use Treatment of hypertension with or without concurrent use of other antihypertensive agents

Dosage Summary

Oral:

Children <6 years: Dosage not established

Children 6-16 years:

20 kg to <35 kg: Initial: 10 mg once daily (maximum: 20 mg once daily)

≥35 kg: Initial: 20 mg once daily (maximum: 40 mg once daily)

Adolescents >16 years: Initial: 20 mg once daily; Maintenance: 20-40 mg once daily

Adults: Initial: 20 mg once daily; Maintenance: 20-40 mg once daily

Elderly: Initial: 5-20 mg once daily; Maintenance: 5-40 mg once daily

Dosage Forms

Tablet, oral:

Benicar®: 5 mg, 20 mg, 40 mg

olmesartan, amlodipine, and hydrochlorothiazide

(ole me SAR tan, am LOE di peen, & hye droe klor oh THYE a zide)

Synonyms amlodipine besylate, olmesartan medoxomil, and hydrochlorothiazide; amlodipine, hydrochlorothiazide, and olmesartan; hydrochlorothiazide, olmesartan, and amlodipine; olmesartan, amlodipine, and hydrochlorothiazide

U.S./Canadian Brand Names Tribenzor™ [US]

Therapeutic Category Angiotensin II Receptor Blocker; Calcium Channel Blocker; Calcium Channel Blocker, Dihydropyridine; Diuretic, Thiazide

Use Treatment of hypertension (not for initial therapy)

Dosage Summary

Oral:

Children: Dosage not established

Adults: Amlodipine 5-10 mg and olmesartan 20-40 mg and hydrochlorothiazide 12.5-25 mg once daily (maximum: 10 mg/day [amlodipine]; 25 mg/day [hydrochlorothiazide]; 40 mg/day [olmesartan]); **Note:** Titration is recommended

Elderly: Patients ≥75 years should start amlodipine at 2.5 mg (combination product dosage form not available in this strength)

Dosage Forms

Tablet, oral:

Tribenzor™: Olmesartan 40 mg, amlodipine 5 mg, and hydrochlorothiazide 25 mg, Olmesartan 40 mg, amlodipine 10 mg, and hydrochlorothiazide 25 mg, Olmesartan 20 mg, amlodipine 5 mg, and hydrochlorothiazide 12.5 mg, Olmesartan 40 mg, amlodipine 5 mg, and hydrochlorothiazide 12.5 mg, Olmesartan 40 mg, amlodipine 10 mg, and hydrochlorothiazide 12.5 mg

olmesartan, amlodipine, and hydrochlorothiazide *see* olmesartan, amlodipine, and hydrochlorothiazide *on page 698*

olmesartan and amlodipine *see* amlodipine and olmesartan *on page 70*

olmesartan and hydrochlorothiazide (ole me SAR tan & hye droe klor oh THYE a zide)

Synonyms hydrochlorothiazide and olmesartan medoxomil; olmesartan medoxomil and hydrochlorothiazide

U.S./Canadian Brand Names Benicar HCT® [US]; Olmetec Plus® [Can]

Therapeutic Category Angiotensin II Receptor Antagonist; Diuretic, Thiazide

Use Treatment of hypertension (not recommended for initial treatment)

Dosage Summary

Oral:

Children: Dosage not established

Adults: Olmesartan 20-40 mg and hydrochlorothiazide 12.5-25 mg once daily (maximum: 25 mg/day [hydrochlorothiazide]; 40 mg/day [olmesartan])

Dosage Forms

Tablet:

Benicar HCT®: 20/12.5: Olmesartan 20 mg and hydrochlorothiazide 12.5 mg; 40/12.5: Olmesartan 40 mg and hydrochlorothiazide 12.5 mg; 40/25: Olmesartan 40 mg and hydrochlorothiazide 25 mg

olmesartan medoxomil *see* olmesartan *on page* 698

olmesartan medoxomil and hydrochlorothiazide *see* olmesartan and hydrochlorothiazide *on page* 698

Olmetec® [Can] *see* olmesartan *on page* 698

Olmetec Plus® [Can] *see* olmesartan and hydrochlorothiazide *on page* 698

olopatadine (nasal) (oh la PAT a deen)

Synonyms olopatadine hydrochloride

U.S./Canadian Brand Names Patanase® [US]

Therapeutic Category Histamine H_1 Antagonist; Histamine H_1 Antagonist, Second Generation

Use Treatment of the symptoms of seasonal allergic rhinitis

Dosage Summary Intranasal:

Children <12 years: Dosage not established

Children ≥12 years: 2 sprays into each nostril twice daily

Adults: 2 sprays into each nostril twice daily

Dosage Forms

Solution, intranasal:

Patanase®: 0.6% (30.5 g)

olopatadine (ophthalmic) (oh la PAT a deen)

Sound-Alike/Look-Alike Issues

Patanol® may be confused with Platinol®

Synonyms olopatadine hydrochloride

U.S./Canadian Brand Names Pataday™ [US]; Patanol® [US/Can]

Therapeutic Category Histamine H_1 Antagonist; Histamine H_1 Antagonist, Second Generation

Use Treatment of the signs and symptoms of allergic conjunctivitis

Dosage Summary

Ophthalmic:

Children <3 years: Dosage not established

Children ≥3 years:

Patanol®: Instill 1 drop into affected eye(s) twice daily

Pataday™: Instill 1 drop into affected eye(s) once daily

Adults:

Patanol®: Instill 1 drop into affected eye(s) twice daily

Pataday™: Instill 1 drop into affected eye(s) once daily

Dosage Forms

Solution, ophthalmic:

Pataday™: 0.2% (2.5 mL)

Patanol®: 0.1% (5 mL)

olopatadine hydrochloride *see* olopatadine (nasal) *on page* 699

olopatadine hydrochloride *see* olopatadine (ophthalmic) *on page* 699

olsalazine (ole SAL a zeen)

Sound-Alike/Look-Alike Issues

olsalazine may be confused with OLANZapine

Dipentum® may be confused with Dilantin®

Synonyms olsalazine sodium

U.S./Canadian Brand Names Dipentum® [US/Can]

Therapeutic Category 5-Aminosalicylic Acid Derivative
Use Maintenance of remission of ulcerative colitis in patients intolerant to sulfasalazine
Dosage Summary
Oral:
Children: Dosage not established
Adults: 1 g/day in 2 divided doses
Dosage Forms
Capsule, oral:
Dipentum®: 250 mg

olsalazine sodium *see* olsalazine *on page 699*
Olux® [US] *see* clobetasol *on page 235*
Olux-E™ [US] *see* clobetasol *on page 235*
Olux®/Olux-E™ CP [US] *see* clobetasol *on page 235*
Omacor® *(Discontinued)* *see* omega-3-acid ethyl esters *on page 701*

omalizumab (oh mah lye ZOO mab)

Sound-Alike/Look-Alike Issues
omalizumab may be confused with ofatumumab
Synonyms rhuMAb-E25
U.S./Canadian Brand Names Xolair® [US/Can]
Therapeutic Category Monoclonal Antibody
Use Treatment of moderate-to-severe, persistent allergic asthma not adequately controlled with inhaled corticosteroids
Dosage Summary
SubQ: Dose is based on pretreatment IgE serum levels and body weight.
IgE ≥30-100 int. units/mL:
Children <12 years: Dosage not established
Children ≥12 years and 30-90 kg: 150 mg every 4 weeks
Children ≥12 years and >90-150 kg: 300 mg every 4 weeks
Adults 30-90 kg: 150 mg every 4 weeks
Adults >90-150 kg: 300 mg every 4 weeks
IgE >100-200 int. units/mL:
Children <12 years: Dosage not established
Children ≥12 years and 30-90 kg: 300 mg every 4 weeks
Children ≥12 years and >90-150 kg: 225 mg every 2 weeks
Adults 30-90 kg: 300 mg every 4 weeks
Adults >90-150 kg: 225 mg every 2 weeks
IgE >200-300 int. units/mL:
Children <12 years: Dosage not established
Children ≥12 years and 30-60 kg: 300 mg every 4 weeks
Children ≥12 years and >60-90 kg: 225 mg every 2 weeks
Children ≥12 years and >90-150 kg: 300 mg every 2 weeks
Adults 30-60 kg: 300 mg every 4 weeks
Adults >60-90 kg: 225 mg every 2 weeks
Adults >90-150 kg: 300 mg every 2 weeks
IgE >300-400 int. units/mL:
Children <12 years: Dosage not established
Children ≥12 years and 30-70 kg: 225 mg every 2 weeks
Children ≥12 years and >70-90 kg: 300 mg every 2 weeks
Children ≥12 years and >90 kg: Do not administer dose
Adults 30-70 kg: 225 mg every 2 weeks
Adults >70-90 kg: 300 mg every 2 weeks
Adults >90 kg: Do not administer dose
IgE >400-500 int. units/mL:
Children <12 years: Dosage not established
Children ≥12 years and 30-70 kg: 300 mg every 2 weeks
Children ≥12 years and >70-90 kg: 375 mg every 2 weeks
Children ≥12 years and >90 kg: Do not administer dose
Adults 30-70 kg: 300 mg every 2 weeks

Adults >70-90 kg: 375 mg every 2 weeks
Adults >90 kg: Do not administer
IgE >500-600 int. units/mL:
Children <12 years: Dosage not established
Children ≥12 years and 30-60 kg: 300 mg every 2 weeks
Children ≥12 years and >60-70 kg: 375 mg every 2 weeks
Children ≥12 years and >70 kg: Do not administer dose
Adults 30-60 kg: 300 mg every 2 weeks
Adults >60-70 kg: 375 mg every 2 weeks
Adults >70 kg: Do not administer dose
IgE >600-700 int. units/mL:
Children <12 years: Dosage not established
Children ≥12 years and 30-60 kg: 375 mg every 2 weeks
Children ≥12 years and >60 kg: Do not administer dose
Adults 30-60 kg: 375 mg every 2 weeks
Adults >60 kg: Do not administer dose

Dosage Forms

Injection, powder for reconstitution:
Xolair®: 150 mg

omega 3 *see* omega-3-acid ethyl esters *on page 701*

omega-3-acid ethyl esters (oh MEG a three AS id ETH il ES ters)

Sound-Alike/Look-Alike Issues
Lovaza® may be confused with LORazepam
Omacor® may be confused with Amicar®

Synonyms ethyl esters of omega-3 fatty acids; fish oil; omega 3

U.S./Canadian Brand Names Lovaza® [US]

Therapeutic Category Antilipemic Agent, Miscellaneous

Use Lovaza®: Adjunct to diet therapy in the treatment of hypertriglyceridemia (≥500 mg/dL)

Note: A number of OTC formulations containing omega-3 fatty acids are marketed as nutritional supplements; these do not have FDA-approved indications and may not contain the same amounts of the active ingredient.

Dosage Summary

Oral:
Children: Dosage not established
Adults: 4 g/day in 1-2 divided doses

Dosage Forms

Capsule, liquid gel, oral:
Lovaza®: 1 g

omeprazole (oh MEP ra zole)

Sound-Alike/Look-Alike Issues
omeprazole may be confused with aripiprazole, fomepizole
Prilosec® may be confused with Plendil®, Prevacid®, predniSONE, prilocaine, Prinivil®, Proventil®, Prozac®

Synonyms omeprazole magnesium

U.S./Canadian Brand Names Apo-Omeprazole® [Can]; Losec MUPS® [Can]; Losec® [Can]; Mylan-Omeprazole [Can]; PMS-Omeprazole DR [Can]; PMS-Omeprazole [Can]; Prilosec OTC® [US-OTC]; Prilosec® [US]; ratio-Omeprazole [Can]; Sandoz Omeprazole [Can]

Therapeutic Category Gastric Acid Secretion Inhibitor

Use Short-term (4-8 weeks) treatment of active duodenal ulcer disease or active benign gastric ulcer; treatment of heartburn and other symptoms associated with gastroesophageal reflux disease (GERD); short-term (4-8 weeks) treatment of endoscopically-diagnosed erosive esophagitis; maintenance healing of erosive esophagitis; long-term treatment of pathological hypersecretory conditions; as part of a multidrug regimen for *H. pylori* eradication to reduce the risk of duodenal ulcer recurrence

OTC labeling: Short-term treatment of frequent, uncomplicated heartburn occurring ≥2 days/week

Dosage Summary

Oral:

Children <1 year: Dosage not established

Children 1-16 years and 5 kg to <10 kg: 5 mg once daily

Children 1-16 years and 10 kg to <20 kg: 10 mg once daily

Children 1-16 years and ≥20 kg: 20 mg once daily

Adults: 20-40 mg/day (may be given in 2 divided doses); doses up to 360 mg/day have been reported for pathological hypersecretory syndrome

Dosage Forms

Capsule, oral: 20 mg

Capsule, delayed release, oral: 10 mg, 20 mg, 40 mg

Prilosec®: 10 mg, 20 mg, 40 mg

Granules for suspension, delayed release, enteric coated, oral:

Prilosec®: 2.5 mg/packet (30s); 10 mg/packet (30s)

Tablet, delayed release, oral: 20 mg, 40 mg

Prilosec OTC® [OTC]: 20 mg

omeprazole and sodium bicarbonate (oh MEP ra zole & SOW dee um bye KAR bun ate)

Sound-Alike/Look-Alike Issues

Zegerid® may be confused with Zestril®

Synonyms sodium bicarbonate and omeprazole

U.S./Canadian Brand Names Zegerid OTC™ [US-OTC]; Zegerid® [US]

Therapeutic Category Proton Pump Inhibitor; Substituted Benzimidazole

Use Short-term (4-8 weeks) treatment of active duodenal ulcer disease or active benign gastric ulcer; treatment of heartburn and other symptoms associated with gastroesophageal reflux disease (GERD); short-term (4-8 weeks) treatment of endoscopically-diagnosed erosive esophagitis; maintenance healing of erosive esophagitis; reduction of risk of upper gastrointestinal bleeding in critically-ill patients

OTC labeling: Short-term treatment of frequent (2 days/week), uncomplicated heartburn

Dosage Summary

Oral: Both strengths of Zegerid® capsule and powder for oral suspension have identical sodium bicarbonate content, respectively. Do not substitute two 20 mg capsules/packets for one 40 mg dose.

Children: Dosage not established

Adults: 20-40 mg/day (may be given in 2 divided doses)

Dosage Forms

Capsule, immediate release:

Zegerid®: Omeprazole 20 mg and sodium bicarbonate 1100 mg

Zegerid®: Omeprazole 40 mg and sodium bicarbonate 1100 mg

Zegerid OTC™ [OTC]: Omeprazole 20 mg and sodium bicarbonate 1100 mg

Powder for oral suspension:

Zegerid®: Omeprazole 20 mg and sodium bicarbonate 1680 mg per packet

Zegerid®: Omeprazole 40 mg and sodium bicarbonate 1680 mg per packet

omeprazole magnesium *see* omeprazole *on page* 701

Omnaris™ [US/Can] *see* ciclesonide (nasal) *on page* 221

Omnicef® [US/Can] *see* cefdinir *on page* 189

OMNIhist® II L.A. [US] *see* chlorpheniramine, phenylephrine, and methscopolamine *on page* 212

Omnii Gel™ [US-OTC] *see* fluoride *on page* 413

Omnipaque™ [Can] *see* iohexol *on page* 519

Omnipaque™ 140 [US] *see* iohexol *on page* 519

Omnipaque™ 180 [US] *see* iohexol *on page* 519

Omnipaque™ 240 [US] *see* iohexol *on page* 519

Omnipaque™ 300 [US] *see* iohexol *on page* 519

Omnipaque™ 350 [US] *see* iohexol *on page* 519

Omnipen® *(Discontinued)* *see* ampicillin *on page* 75

Omnipen®-N *(Discontinued)* *see* ampicillin *on page* 75

Omnipred™ [US] *see* prednisolone (ophthalmic) *on page* 791

Omniscan® [US] *see* gadodiamide *on page* 434

Omnitrope® [US/Can] *see* somatropin *on page* 889

onabotulinumtoxinA (oh nuh BOT yoo lin num TOKS in aye)

Synonyms botulinum toxin type A; BTX-A

U.S./Canadian Brand Names Botox® Cosmetic [US/Can]; Botox® [US/Can]

Therapeutic Category Ophthalmic Agent, Toxin

Use Treatment of strabismus and blepharospasm associated with dystonia (including benign essential blepharospasm or VII nerve disorders) in patients ≥12 years of age; cervical dystonia (spasmodic torticollis) in patients ≥16 years of age; temporary improvement in the appearance of lines/wrinkles of the face (moderate-to-severe glabellar lines associated with corrugator and/or procerus muscle activity) in adult patients ≤65 years of age; treatment of severe primary axillary hyperhidrosis in adults not adequately controlled with topical treatments; focal spasticity (specifically upper limb spasticity) in adults

Canadian labeling: Additional use (not in U.S. labeling): Dynamic equinus foot deformity in pediatric cerebral palsy patients; treatment of forehead, lateral canthus, and glabellar lines in adults >65 years of age

Dosage Summary

I.M.:

Blepharospasm:

Children <12 years: Dosage not established

Children ≥12 years: Initial: 1.25-2.5 units into upper and lower lid, may increase up to twice the previous dose if response from initial dose ≤2 months (maximum: 5 units/site; 200 units/30 days)

Adults: Initial: 1.25-2.5 units into upper and lower lid, may increase up to twice the previous dose if response from initial dose ≤2 months (maximum: 5 units/site; 200 units/30 days)

Cervical dystonia:

Children <16 years: Dosage not established

Children ≥16 years: 198-300 units divided among the affected muscles, decrease dose in patients previously untreated

Adults: 198-300 units divided among the affected muscles, decrease dose in patients previously untreated

Reduction of glabellar lines:

Children: Dosage not established

Adults ≤65 years: 0.1 mL (4 units) dose into each of five sites, two in each corrugator muscle and one in the procerus muscle [total dose 0.5 mL (20 units)]

Adults >65 years: Use not indicated

Strabismus:

Children <12 years: Dosage not established

Children ≥12 years: Initial: 1.25-5 units in any one muscle; Subsequent dose: May increase to up to twice previous dose (maximum: 25 units/single muscle)

Adults: Initial: 1.25-5 units in any one muscle; Subsequent dose: May increase to up to twice previous dose (maximum: 25 units/single muscle)

Spasticity (focal):

Children: Dosage not established

Adults: 12.5-50 units/site (maximum: 200 units)

Intradermal:

Children: Dosage not established

Adults: 50 units/axilla evenly distributed into multiple sites (10-15), in 0.1-0.2 mL aliquots, ~1-2 cm apart

Dosage Forms

Injection, powder for reconstitution [preservative free]:

Botox®: *Clostridium botulinum* type A neurotoxin complex 100 units, *Clostridium botulinum* type A neurotoxin complex 200 units

Botox® Cosmetic: *Clostridium botulinum* type A neurotoxin complex 100 units

Powder for reconstitution, for injection [preservative free]:

Botox® Cosmetic: *Clostridium botulinum* type A neurotoxin complex 50 units

Dosage Forms - Canada

Injection, powder for reconstitution [preservative free]:

Botox®: Botulinum toxin A 50 units, 100 units, 200 units

Botox Cosmetic®: Botulinum toxin A 50 unit, 100 units, 200 units

Oncaspar® [US] *see* pegaspargase *on page* 732

Oncet® *(Discontinued)* *see* hydrocodone and homatropine *on page* 481

Oncotice™ [Can] *see* BCG *on page* 118

Oncovin® *(Discontinued)* *see* vincristine *on page* 985

ondansetron (on DAN se tron)

Sound-Alike/Look-Alike Issues

ondansetron may be confused with dolasetron, granisetron, palonosetron

Zofran® may be confused with Zantac®, Zosyn®

Synonyms GR38032R; ondansetron hydrochloride; Zuplenz®

U.S./Canadian Brand Names Apo-Ondansetron® [Can]; CO Ondansetron [Can]; Dom-Ondansetron [Can]; JAMP-Ondansetron [Can]; Mint-Ondansetron [Can]; Mylan-Ondansetron [Can]; Novo-Ondansetron [Can]; Ondansetron Injection [Can]; Ondansetron-Omega [Can]; PHL-Ondansetron [Can]; PMS-Ondansetron [Can]; RAN™-Ondansetron [Can]; ratio-Ondansetron [Can]; Sandoz-Ondansetron [Can]; Zofran® ODT [US/Can]; Zofran® [US/Can]; ZYM-Ondansetron [Can]

Therapeutic Category Selective 5-HT_3 Receptor Antagonist

Use Prevention of nausea and vomiting associated with moderately- to highly-emetogenic cancer chemotherapy; radiotherapy; prevention of postoperative nausea and vomiting (PONV); treatment of PONV if no prophylactic dose of ondansetron received

Dosage Summary **Note:** Studies in adults have shown a single daily dose of 8-12 mg I.V. or 8-24 mg orally to be as effective as mg/kg dosing, and should be considered for all patients whose mg/kg dose exceeds 8-12 mg I.V.; oral solution and ODT formulations are bioequivalent to corresponding doses of tablet formulation

I.M.:

Children: Dosage not established

Adults: 4 mg as a single dose postoperatively

I.V.:

Infants <1 month: Dosage not established

Infants 1-6 months: 0.1 mg/kg as a single dose postoperatively

Children 6 months to 12 years and ≤40 kg: 0.1 mg/kg as a single dose postoperatively **or** 0.15 mg/kg/dose administered 30 minutes prior to chemotherapy, 4 and 8 hours after the first dose **or** 0.45 mg/kg/day as a single dose

Children 6 months to 12 years and >40 kg: 4 mg as a single dose postoperatively **or** 0.15 mg/kg/dose administered 30 minutes prior to chemotherapy, 4 and 8 hours after the first dose **or** 0.45 mg/kg/day as a single dose

Children >12 years to 18 years: 4 mg as a single dose postoperatively **or** 0.15 mg/kg/dose administered 30 minutes prior to chemotherapy, 4 and 8 hours after the first dose **or** 0.45 mg/kg/day as a single dose

Adults: 4 mg as a single dose postoperatively **or** 0.15 mg/kg 3 times/day beginning 30 minutes prior to chemotherapy **or** 0.45 mg/kg once daily **or** 8-10 mg 1-2 times/day **or** 24 mg or 32 mg once daily

Oral:

Children <4 years: Dosage not established

Children 4-11 years: 4 mg 30 minutes before chemotherapy; repeat 4 and 8 hours after initial dose, then 4 mg every 8 hours for 1-2 days after chemotherapy completed

Children ≥12 years: 24 mg given 30 minutes prior to the start of therapy **or** 8 mg every 8-12 hours

Adults: 16 mg given 1 hour prior to induction of anesthesia **or** 24 mg given 30 minutes prior to the start of therapy **or** 8 mg every 8-12 hours **or** 8 mg 1-2 hours before irradiation

Product Availability Zuplenz® oral soluble film: FDA approved July 2010; availability expected during the third quarter of 2010

Dosage Forms

Infusion, premixed in D_5W [preservative free]: 32 mg (50 mL)

Infusion, premixed in NS [preservative free]: 32 mg (50 mL)

Injection, solution: 2 mg/mL (2 mL, 20 mL)

Zofran®: 2 mg/mL (2 mL, 20 mL)

Injection, solution [preservative free]: 2 mg/mL (2 mL)

Solution, oral: 4 mg/5 mL (5 mL, 50 mL)

Zofran®: 4 mg/5 mL (50 mL)

Tablet, oral: 4 mg, 8 mg, 24 mg

Zofran®: 4 mg, 8 mg

Tablet, orally disintegrating, oral: 4 mg, 8 mg

Zofran® ODT: 4 mg, 8 mg

ondansetron hydrochloride *see* ondansetron *on page* 704

Ondansetron Injection [Can] *see* ondansetron *on page* 704

Ondansetron-Omega [Can] *see* ondansetron *on page* 704

One A Day® Cholesterol Plus [US-OTC] *see* vitamins (multiple/oral) *on page* 990

One A Day® Energy [US-OTC] *see* vitamins (multiple/oral) *on page 990*
One A Day® Essential [US-OTC] *see* vitamins (multiple/oral) *on page 990*
One A Day® Kids Bugs Bunny and Friends Complete [US-OTC] *see* vitamins (multiple/pediatric) *on page 990*
One-A-Day® Kids Scooby-Doo!™ Complete [US-OTC] *see* vitamins (multiple/pediatric) *on page 990*
One A Day® Kids Scooby-Doo!™ Gummies [US-OTC] *see* vitamins (multiple/pediatric) *on page 990*
One-A-Day® Kids Scooby-Doo!™ Plus Calcium [US-OTC] *see* vitamins (multiple/pediatric) *on page 990*
One A Day® Maximum [US-OTC] *see* vitamins (multiple/oral) *on page 990*
One A Day® Men's 50+ Advantage [US-OTC] *see* vitamins (multiple/oral) *on page 990*
One A Day® Men's Health Formula [US-OTC] *see* vitamins (multiple/oral) *on page 990*
One A Day® Teen Advantage for Her [US-OTC] *see* vitamins (multiple/oral) *on page 990*
One A Day® Teen Advantage for Him [US-OTC] *see* vitamins (multiple/oral) *on page 990*
One A Day® Weight Smart® Advanced [US-OTC] *see* vitamins (multiple/oral) *on page 990*
One A Day® Women's 50+ Advantage [US-OTC] *see* vitamins (multiple/oral) *on page 990*
One A Day® Women's [US-OTC] *see* vitamins (multiple/oral) *on page 990*
One A Day® Women's Active Mind & Body [US-OTC] *see* vitamins (multiple/oral) *on page 990*
One A Day® Women's Prenatal [US-OTC] *see* vitamins (multiple/prenatal) *on page 991*
One Gram C [US-OTC] *see* ascorbic acid *on page 98*
One Tab™ Allergy & Sinus [US-OTC] *see* acetaminophen, diphenhydramine, and phenylephrine *on page 30*
One Tab™ Cold & Flu [US-OTC] *see* acetaminophen, diphenhydramine, and phenylephrine *on page 30*
Onglyza™ [US/Can] *see* saxagliptin *on page 866*
Onsolis™ [US] *see* fentanyl *on page 395*
ONTAK® [US] *see* denileukin diftitox *on page 275*
Onxol® *(Discontinued)* *see* paclitaxel *on page 719*
Ony-Clear *(Discontinued)* *see* benzalkonium chloride *on page 124*
Opana® [US] *see* oxymorphone *on page 718*
Opana® ER [US] *see* oxymorphone *on page 718*
OPC-13013 *see* cilostazol *on page 222*
OPC-14597 *see* aripiprazole *on page 94*
OPC-41061 *see* tolvaptan *on page 941*
OP-CCK *see* sincalide *on page 877*
Opcon-A® [US-OTC] *see* naphazoline and pheniramine *on page 659*
Opcon® Ophthalmic *(Discontinued)* *see* naphazoline (ophthalmic) *on page 658*
o,p'-DDD *see* mitotane *on page 638*
Operand® Chlorhexidine Gluconate [US-OTC] *see* chlorhexidine gluconate *on page 204*
Operand® Povidone-Iodine [US-OTC] *see* povidone-iodine (topical) *on page 784*
Ophthalgan® Ophthalmic *(Discontinued)* *see* glycerin *on page 449*
Ophthetic® *(Discontinued)* *see* proparacaine *on page 803*
Ophthifluor® *(Discontinued)* *see* fluorescein *on page 412*
Ophthochlor® Ophthalmic *(Discontinued)* *see* chloramphenicol *on page 203*
Ophtho-Dipivefrin™ [Can] *see* dipivefrin *on page 317*
Ophtho-Tate® [Can] *see* prednisolone (ophthalmic) *on page 791*
opium and belladonna *see* belladonna and opium *on page 121*

opium tincture (OH pee um TING chur)

Sound-Alike/Look-Alike Issues

opium tincture may be confused with camphorated tincture of opium (paregoric)

DTO is an error-prone abbreviation (mistaken as Diluted Tincture of Opium; dose equivalency of paregoric)

Synonyms opium tincture, deodorized; tincture of opium

Therapeutic Category Analgesic, Narcotic

Controlled Substance C-II

Use Treatment of diarrhea or relief of pain

Dosage Summary

Oral: Note: Opium tincture 10% contains morphine 10 mg/mL. Use caution in ordering, dispensing, and/or administering.

Children: 0.005-0.02 mL/kg/dose every 3-4 hours (maximum: 0.06 mL/kg/day [diarrhea])

Adults: 0.3-1.5 mL/dose every 2-6 hours (maximum: 6 mL/day [diarrhea])

Dosage Forms

Tincture, oral: Anhydrous morphine 10 mg/mL (120 mL, 480 mL)

opium tincture, deodorized *see* opium tincture *on page 705*

oprelvekin (oh PREL ve kin)

Sound-Alike/Look-Alike Issues

oprelvekin may be confused with aldesleukin, Proleukin®

Neumega® may be confused with Neulasta®, Neupogen®

Synonyms IL-11; interleukin-11; recombinant human interleukin-11; recombinant interleukin-11; rhIL-11

U.S./Canadian Brand Names Neumega® [US]

Therapeutic Category Platelet Growth Factor

Use Prevention of severe thrombocytopenia; reduce the need for platelet transfusions following myelosuppressive chemotherapy for nonmyeloid malignancy

Dosage Summary

SubQ:

Adults: 50 mcg/kg once daily

Dosage Forms

Injection, powder for reconstitution:

Neumega®: 5 mg

Optase™ [US] *see* trypsin, balsam Peru, and castor oil *on page 964*

Optho-Bunolol® [Can] *see* levobunolol *on page 556*

Opti-Clear [US-OTC] *see* tetrahydrozoline (ophthalmic) *on page 923*

Opticrom® [Can] *see* cromolyn (ophthalmic) *on page 255*

Optigene® 3 *(Discontinued)* *see* tetrahydrozoline (ophthalmic) *on page 923*

OptiMARK® [US] *see* gadoversetamide *on page 435*

Optimine® *(Discontinued)*

Optimoist® Solution *(Discontinued)* *see* saliva substitute *on page 861*

Optimyxin® [Can] *see* bacitracin and polymyxin B *on page 113*

Optimyxin Plus® [Can] *see* neomycin, polymyxin B, and gramicidin *on page 667*

OptiNate® [US] *see* vitamins (multiple/prenatal) *on page 991*

OptiPranolol® [US/Can] *see* metipranolol *on page 624*

Optiray® 160 [US] *see* ioversol *on page 522*

Optiray® 240 [US] *see* ioversol *on page 522*

Optiray® 300 [US] *see* ioversol *on page 522*

Optiray® 320 [US] *see* ioversol *on page 522*

Optiray® 350 [US] *see* ioversol *on page 522*

Optivar® [US] *see* azelastine (ophthalmic) *on page 110*

Optive™ [US-OTC] *see* carboxymethylcellulose *on page 184*

Optivite® P.M.T. [US-OTC] *see* vitamins (multiple/oral) *on page 990*

Orabase® with Benzocaine [US-OTC] *see* benzocaine *on page 124*

Oracea® [US] *see* doxycycline *on page 331*

Oracort [Can] *see* triamcinolone (topical) *on page 954*

Oradex-C® *(Discontinued)* *see* dyclonine *on page 338*

Orajel® Baby Daytime and Nighttime [US-OTC] *see* benzocaine *on page 124*

Orajel® Baby Teething [US-OTC] *see* benzocaine *on page 124*

Orajel® Baby Teething Nighttime [US-OTC] *see* benzocaine *on page 124*

Orajel® Brace-Aid Oral Anesthetic *(Discontinued)* *see* benzocaine *on page 124*

Orajel® Cold Sore [US-OTC] *see* benzocaine *on page 124*
Orajel® Denture Plus [US-OTC] *see* benzocaine *on page 124*
Orajel® Dry Mouth [US-OTC] *see* glycerin *on page 449*
Orajel® Maximum Strength [US-OTC] *see* benzocaine *on page 124*
Orajel® Maximum Strength Overnight Cold Sore [US-OTC] *see* dyclonine *on page 338*
Orajel® Medicated Mouth Sore [US-OTC] *see* benzocaine *on page 124*
Orajel® Medicated Toothache [US-OTC] *see* benzocaine *on page 124*
Orajel® Mouth Sore [US-OTC] *see* benzocaine *on page 124*
Orajel® Multi-Action Cold Sore [US-OTC] *see* benzocaine *on page 124*
Orajel® PM Maximum Strength [US-OTC] *see* benzocaine *on page 124*
Orajel® Ultra Mouth Sore [US-OTC] *see* benzocaine *on page 124*
Oral Balance® [US-OTC] *see* saliva substitute *on page 861*
oral cholera vaccine *see* traveler's diarrhea and cholera vaccine *(Canada only) on page 949*
Oralone® [US] *see* triamcinolone (topical) *on page 954*
Oramorph® SR [US] *see* morphine (systemic) *on page 644*
Oranyl [US-OTC] *see* pseudoephedrine *on page 810*
Orap® [US/Can] *see* pimozide *on page 761*
Orapred® [US] *see* prednisolone (systemic) *on page 790*
Orapred ODT® [US] *see* prednisolone (systemic) *on page 790*
Oraquix® [US] *see* lidocaine and prilocaine *on page 565*
Orasone® *(Discontinued)* *see* prednisone *on page 792*
OraVerse™ [US] *see* phentolamine *on page 750*
Oravig™ [US] *see* miconazole (oral) *on page 630*
Oraxyl™ [US] *see* doxycycline *on page 331*
Orazinc® 110 [US-OTC] *see* zinc sulfate *on page 1002*
Orazinc® 220 [US-OTC] *see* zinc sulfate *on page 1002*
Orbivan™ [US] *see* butalbital, acetaminophen, and caffeine *on page 159*
orciprenaline sulfate *see* metaproterenol *on page 609*
Orencia® [US/Can] *see* abatacept *on page 19*
Oreton® Methyl *(Discontinued)* *see* methyltestosterone *on page 624*
Orfadin® [US] *see* nitisinone *on page 677*
ORG 946 *see* rocuronium *on page 850*
Orgalutran® [Can] *see* ganirelix *on page 437*
Organidin® NR [US-OTC] *see* guaifenesin *on page 454*
Orgaran® [Can] *see* danaparoid *(Canada only) on page 267*
Orgaran® *(Discontinued)* *see* danaparoid *(Canada only) on page 267*
ORG NC 45 *see* vecuronium *on page 980*
Orinase Diagnostic® *(Discontinued)* *see* tolbutamide *on page 939*
Orinase® Oral *(Discontinued)* *see* tolbutamide *on page 939*
ORLAAM® *(Discontinued)*

orlistat (OR li stat)

Sound-Alike/Look-Alike Issues
Xenical® may be confused with Xeloda®

U.S./Canadian Brand Names Alli™ [US-OTC]; Xenical® [US/Can]

Therapeutic Category Lipase Inhibitor

Use Management of obesity, including weight loss and weight management, when used in conjunction with a reduced-calorie and low-fat diet; reduce the risk of weight regain after prior weight loss; indicated for obese patients with an initial body mass index (BMI) ≥30 kg/m^2 or ≥27 kg/m^2 in the presence of other risk factors (eg, diabetes, dyslipidemia, hypertension)

Dosage Summary

Oral:

Children <12 years: Dosage not established
Children ≥12 years: Xenical®: 120 mg 3 times/day with meals

Adults:
Alli™ (OTC labeling): 60 mg 3 times/day with meals
Xenical®: 120 mg 3 times/day with meals

Dosage Forms

Capsule, oral:
Alli™ [OTC]: 60 mg
Xenical®: 120 mg

Ormazine® *(Discontinued)* *see* chlorpromazine *on page* 216
Ornex® [US-OTC] *see* acetaminophen and pseudoephedrine *on page* 26
Ornex® Maximum Strength [US-OTC] *see* acetaminophen and pseudoephedrine *on page* 26
Ornidyl® Injection *(Discontinued)* *see* eflornithine *on page* 344
ORO-Clense [Can] *see* chlorhexidine gluconate *on page* 204
Orphenace® [Can] *see* orphenadrine *on page* 708

orphenadrine (or FEN a dreen)

Sound-Alike/Look-Alike Issues
Norflex™ may be confused with norfloxacin, Noroxin®

Synonyms orphenadrine citrate

U.S./Canadian Brand Names Norflex™ [US/Can]; Orphenace® [Can]; Rhoxal-orphendrine [Can]

Therapeutic Category Skeletal Muscle Relaxant

Use Treatment of muscle spasm associated with acute painful musculoskeletal conditions

Dosage Summary

I.M.:
Children: Dosage not established
Adults: 60 mg every 12 hours
Elderly: Dosage not established

I.V.:
Children: Dosage not established
Adults: 60 mg every 12 hours
Elderly: Dosage not established

Oral:
Children: Dosage not established
Adults: 100 mg twice daily
Elderly: Dosage not established

Dosage Forms

Injection, solution: 30 mg/mL (2 mL)
Norflex™: 30 mg/mL (2 mL)

Tablet, extended release, oral: 100 mg

orphenadrine, aspirin, and caffeine (or FEN a dreen, AS pir in, & KAF een)

Sound-Alike/Look-Alike Issues
Norgesic™ Forte may be confused with Norgesic 40®

Synonyms aspirin, caffeine, and orphenadrine; aspirin, orphenadrine, and caffeine; caffeine, orphenadrine, and aspirin

Therapeutic Category Analgesic, Nonnarcotic; Skeletal Muscle Relaxant

Use Relief of discomfort associated with skeletal muscular conditions

Dosage Summary

Oral:
Children: Dosage not established
Adults: 1-2 tablets 3-4 times/day
Elderly: Use not recommended

Dosage Forms

Tablet: Orphenadrine 25 mg, aspirin 385 mg, and caffeine 30 mg; orphenadrine 50 mg, aspirin 770 mg, and caffeine 60 mg

orphenadrine citrate *see* orphenadrine *on page* 708
Orphengesic *(Discontinued)* *see* orphenadrine, aspirin, and caffeine *on page* 708
Orphengesic Forte *(Discontinued)* *see* orphenadrine, aspirin, and caffeine *on page* 708
Ortho® 0.5/35 [Can] *see* ethinyl estradiol and norethindrone *on page* 378

Ortho® 1/35 [Can] *see* ethinyl estradiol and norethindrone *on page 378*
Ortho® 7/7/7 [Can] *see* ethinyl estradiol and norethindrone *on page 378*
Ortho-Cept® [US/Can] *see* ethinyl estradiol and desogestrel *on page 374*
Orthoclone OKT® 3 *(Discontinued)* *see* muromonab-CD3 *on page 649*
Ortho-Cyclen® [US] *see* ethinyl estradiol and norgestimate *on page 380*
Ortho Evra® [US] *see* ethinyl estradiol and norelgestromin *on page 378*
Ortho Micronor® [US] *see* norethindrone *on page 682*
Ortho-Novum® [US] *see* ethinyl estradiol and norethindrone *on page 378*
Ortho-Novum® 1/50 [Can] *see* norethindrone and mestranol *on page 683*
Ortho-Novum® 1/50 *(Discontinued)* *see* norethindrone and mestranol *on page 683*
Ortho-Novum® 7/7/7 [US] *see* ethinyl estradiol and norethindrone *on page 378*
ortho,para-DDD *see* mitotane *on page 638*
ortho prefest *see* estradiol and norgestimate *on page 369*
Ortho Tri-Cyclen® [US] *see* ethinyl estradiol and norgestimate *on page 380*
Ortho Tri-Cyclen® Lo [US] *see* ethinyl estradiol and norgestimate *on page 380*
Orthovisc® [US/Can] *see* hyaluronate and derivatives *on page 475*
Or-Tyl® Injection *(Discontinued)* *see* dicyclomine *on page 299*
Orudis® KT *(Discontinued)* *see* ketoprofen *on page 537*
Os-Cal® [Can] *see* calcium carbonate *on page 167*
oscal *see* calcium carbonate *on page 167*
Os-Cal® 500+D [US-OTC] *see* calcium and vitamin D *on page 166*
Os-Cal® 500 *(Discontinued)* *see* calcium carbonate *on page 167*

oseltamivir (oh sel TAM i vir)

Sound-Alike/Look-Alike Issues

Tamiflu® may be confused with Tambocor™, Thera-Flu®

U.S./Canadian Brand Names Tamiflu® [US/Can]

Therapeutic Category Antiviral Agent, Oral

Use Treatment of uncomplicated acute illness due to influenza (A or B) infection in children ≥1 year of age and adults who have been symptomatic for no more than 2 days; prophylaxis against influenza (A or B) infection in children ≥1 year of age and adults

The Advisory Committee on Immunization Practices (ACIP) recommends that **treatment** be considered for the following:

- Persons hospitalized with laboratory-confirmed influenza (may also have benefit if started >48 hours after onset of illness).
- Persons with laboratory-confirmed influenza pneumonia.
- Persons with laboratory-confirmed influenza and bacterial infections.
- Persons with laboratory-confirmed influenza and who are at higher risk for influenza complications.
- Persons presenting for care within 48 hours of laboratory-confirmed influenza onset and who want to decrease duration and/or severity of their symptoms or decrease the risk of transmission to those at high risk for complications.

The ACIP recommends that **prophylaxis** be considered for the following:

- Persons at high risk for influenza infection during the first 2 weeks following vaccination (eg, children <9 years and not previously vaccinated) if the virus is circulating in the community.
- Persons at high risk for influenza infection, but the vaccination is contraindicated.
- Unvaccinated family members or healthcare providers with prolonged exposure to or close contact with high-risk persons, unvaccinated persons, or infants <6 months of age.
- Persons at high risk for influenza infection, their family members and close contacts, and healthcare workers when the circulating strain of influenza is not matched with the vaccine.
- Persons with immune deficiency or those who may not respond to vaccination.
- Unvaccinated staff and persons during response to an outbreak in a closed institutional setting that has patients at high risk for infection (eg, extended care facilities).

Dosage Summary

Oral:

Children 1-12 years and ≤15 kg: 30 mg twice daily (treatment) **or** 30 mg once daily (prophylaxis)
Children 1-12 years and >15 to ≤23 kg: 45 mg twice daily (treatment) **or** 45 mg once daily (prophylaxis)
Children 1-12 years and >23 to ≤40 kg: 60 mg twice daily (treatment) **or** 60 mg once daily (prophylaxis) ▶

Children 1-12 years and >40 kg: 75 mg twice daily (treatment) **or** 75 mg once daily (prophylaxis)
Children ≥13 years: 75 mg twice daily (treatment) **or** 75 mg once daily (prophylaxis)
Adults: 75 mg twice daily (treatment) **or** 75 mg once daily (prophylaxis)

Dosage Forms

Capsule:
Tamiflu®: 30 mg, 45 mg, 75 mg

Powder for oral suspension:
Tamiflu®: 12 mg/mL

OSI-774 *see* erlotinib *on page 360*
Osmitrol® [US/Can] *see* mannitol *on page 590*
Osmoglyn® ***(Discontinued)*** *see* glycerin *on page 449*
Osmolite® HN [US-OTC] *see* nutritional formula, enteral/oral *on page 692*
OsmoPrep® [US] *see* sodium phosphates *on page 887*
Osmovist® [Can] *see* iotrolan *(Canada only) on page 521*
Osteocalcin® ***(Discontinued)*** *see* calcitonin *on page 165*
Osteocit® [Can] *see* calcium citrate *on page 169*
Ostoforte® [Can] *see* ergocalciferol *on page 358*
OTFC (oral transmucosal fentanyl citrate) *see* fentanyl *on page 395*
Otic-Care® Otic ***(Discontinued)*** *see* neomycin, polymyxin B, and hydrocortisone *on page 667*
Otix® [US-OTC] *see* carbamide peroxide *on page 178*
Otobiotic Otic Solution ***(Discontinued)***
Otocort® Otic ***(Discontinued)*** *see* neomycin, polymyxin B, and hydrocortisone *on page 667*
Otosporin® Otic ***(Discontinued)*** *see* neomycin, polymyxin B, and hydrocortisone *on page 667*
Otrivin® ***(Discontinued)***
Otrivin® Pediatric ***(Discontinued)***
Outgro® [US-OTC] *see* benzocaine *on page 124*
Ovace® [US] *see* sulfacetamide (topical) *on page 900*
Ovace® Plus [US] *see* sulfacetamide (topical) *on page 900*
Ovcon® [US] *see* ethinyl estradiol and norethindrone *on page 378*
Ovide® [US] *see* malathion *on page 589*
Ovidrel® [US/Can] *see* chorionic gonadotropin (recombinant) *on page 219*
ovine corticotrophin-releasing hormone *see* corticorelin *on page 251*
Ovol® [Can] *see* simethicone *on page 875*
Ovral® [Can] *see* ethinyl estradiol and norgestrel *on page 380*
Ovral® ***(Discontinued)*** *see* ethinyl estradiol and norgestrel *on page 380*
Ovrette® ***(Discontinued)***

oxacillin (oks a SIL in)

Synonyms methylphenyl isoxazolyl penicillin; oxacillin sodium

Therapeutic Category Penicillin

Use Treatment of infections such as osteomyelitis, septicemia, endocarditis, and CNS infections caused by susceptible strains of *Staphylococcus*

Dosage Summary

I.M.:
Children: 100-200 mg/kg/day in divided doses every 6 hours (maximum: 12 g/day)
Adults: 250-2000 mg every 4-6 hours

I.V.:
Children: 100-200 mg/kg/day in divided doses every 6 hours (maximum: 12 g/day)
Adults: 250-2000 mg every 4-6 hours

Dosage Forms

Infusion, premixed iso-osmotic solution: 1 g (50 mL); 2 g (50 mL)
Injection, powder for reconstitution: 1 g, 2 g, 10 g

oxacillin sodium *see* oxacillin *on page 710*
oxalatoplatin *see* oxaliplatin *on page 711*
oxalatoplatinum *see* oxaliplatin *on page 711*

oxaliplatin (ox AL i pla tin)

Sound-Alike/Look-Alike Issues

oxaliplatin may be confused with Aloxi®, carboplatin, cisplatin

Synonyms diaminocyclohexane oxalatoplatinum; L-OHP; oxalatoplatin; oxalatoplatinum

U.S./Canadian Brand Names Eloxatin® [US/Can]

Therapeutic Category Antineoplastic Agent, Alkylating Agent

Use Treatment of stage III colon cancer (adjuvant) and advanced colorectal cancer

Dosage Summary

I.V.:

Children: Dosage not established

Adults: 85 mg/m^2 every 2 weeks

Dosage Forms

Injection, powder for reconstitution: 50 mg, 100 mg

Injection, solution: 5 mg/mL (10 mL, 20 mL)

Injection, solution [preservative free]:

Eloxatin®: 5 mg/mL (10 mL, 20 mL, 40 mL)

Dosage Forms - Canada

Injection, powder for reconstitution:

Eloxatin®: 50 mg, 100 mg

Oxandrin® [US] *see* oxandrolone *on page* 711

oxandrolone (oks AN droe lone)

U.S./Canadian Brand Names Oxandrin® [US]

Therapeutic Category Androgen

Controlled Substance C-III

Use Adjunctive therapy to promote weight gain after weight loss following extensive surgery, chronic infections, or severe trauma, and in some patients who, without definite pathophysiologic reasons, fail to gain or to maintain normal weight; to offset protein catabolism with prolonged corticosteroid administration; relief of bone pain associated with osteoporosis

Dosage Summary

Oral:

Children: ≤0.1 mg/kg/day or ≤0.045 mg/lb/day

Adults: 2.5-20 mg/day in 2-4 divided doses

Elderly: 5 mg twice daily

Dosage Forms

Tablet, oral: 2.5 mg, 10 mg

Oxandrin®: 2.5 mg, 10 mg

oxaprozin (oks a PROE zin)

Sound-Alike/Look-Alike Issues

oxaprozin may be confused with oxazepam

Daypro® may be confused with Diupres®

U.S./Canadian Brand Names Apo-Oxaprozin® [Can]; Daypro® [US/Can]

Therapeutic Category Analgesic, Nonnarcotic; Nonsteroidal Antiinflammatory Drug (NSAID)

Use Acute and long-term use in the management of signs and symptoms of osteoarthritis and rheumatoid arthritis; juvenile rheumatoid arthritis

Dosage Summary

Oral:

Children <6 years: Dosage not established

Children 6-16 years and 22-31 kg: 600 mg once daily

Children 6-16 years and 32-54 kg: 900 mg once daily

Children 6-16 years and ≥55 kg: 1200 mg once daily

Adults: 600-1200 mg once daily (maximum: 1200 mg/day [<50 kg]; 1800 mg/day or 26 mg/kg/day (whichever lower) [>50 kg])

Dosage Forms

Caplet, oral:

Daypro®: 600 mg

Tablet, oral: 600 mg

oxazepam (oks A ze pam)

Sound-Alike/Look-Alike Issues

oxazepam may be confused with oxaprozin, quazepam
Serax® may be confused with Eurax®, Urex®, Zyrtec®

U.S./Canadian Brand Names Apo-Oxazepam® [Can]; Bio-Oxazepam [Can]; Novoxapram® [Can]; Oxpam® [Can]; Oxpram® [Can]; PMS-Oxazepam [Can]; Riva-Oxazepam [Can]; Serax® [US]

Therapeutic Category Anticonvulsant; Benzodiazepine

Controlled Substance C-IV

Use Treatment of anxiety; management of ethanol withdrawal

Dosage Summary

Oral:

Adults: 10-30 mg 3-4 times/day
Elderly: Initial: 10 mg 2-3 times/day; Maintenance: 30-45 mg/day; **Note:** Titration is recommended

Dosage Forms

Capsule, oral: 10 mg, 15 mg, 30 mg
Serax®: 10 mg, 15 mg, 30 mg

Tablet, oral:
Serax®: 15 mg

oxcarbazepine (ox car BAZ e peen)

Sound-Alike/Look-Alike Issues

OXcarbazepine may be confused with carBAMazepine
Trileptal® may be confused with TriLipix™

Synonyms GP 47680; OCBZ

Tall-Man **OX**carbazepine

U.S./Canadian Brand Names Apo-Oxcarbazepine® [Can]; Trileptal® [US/Can]

Therapeutic Category Anticonvulsant

Use Monotherapy or adjunctive therapy in the treatment of partial seizures in adults and children ≥4 years of age with epilepsy; adjunctive therapy in the treatment of partial seizures in children ≥2 years of age with epilepsy

Dosage Summary

Oral:

Children <2 years: Dosage not established
Children 2-3 years and <20 kg: Initial: 8-20 mg/kg/day (maximum: 600 mg/day) in 2 divided doses; maintenance: maximum of 60 mg/kg/day in 2 divided doses; **Note:** Titration recommended
Children 2-3 years and ≥20 kg: Initial: 8-10 mg/kg/day (maximum: 600 mg/day) in 2 divided doses; maintenance: maximum of 60 mg/kg/day in 2 divided doses; **Note:** Titration is recommended
Children 4-16 years and <25 kg: Initial: 8-10 mg/kg/day (maximum: 600 mg/day) in 2 divided doses; maintenance: up to 900 mg/day; **Note:** Titration is recommended
Children 4-16 years and 25-30 kg: Initial: 8-10 mg/kg/day (maximum: 600 mg/day) in 2 divided doses; maintenance: up to 1200 mg/day; **Note:** Titration is recommended
Children 4-16 years and 31-39 kg: Initial: 8-10 mg/kg/day (maximum: 600 mg/day) in 2 divided doses; maintenance: up to 1500 mg/day; **Note:** Titration is recommended
Children 4-16 years and 40-55 kg: Initial: 8-10 mg/kg/day (maximum: 600 mg/day) in 2 divided doses; maintenance: up to 1800 mg/day; **Note:** Titration is recommended
Children 4-16 years and >55 kg: Initial: 8-10 mg/kg/day (maximum: 600 mg/day) in 2 divided doses; maintenance: up to 2100 mg/day; **Note:** Titration is recommended
Children >16 years: Initial: 300 mg twice daily; Maintenance: 1200-2400 mg/day in 2 divided doses (maximum: 2400 mg/day); **Note:** Titration is recommended
Adults: Initial: 300 mg twice daily; Maintenance: 1200-2400 mg/day in 2 divided doses (maximum: 2400 mg/day); **Note:** Titration is recommended

Dosage Forms

Suspension, oral: 300 mg/5 mL (250 mL)
Trileptal®: 300 mg/5 mL (250 mL)

Tablet, oral: 150 mg, 300 mg, 600 mg
Trileptal®: 150 mg, 300 mg, 600 mg

Oxeze® Turbuhaler® [Can] *see* formoterol *on page* 425

oxiconazole (oks i KON a zole)

Synonyms oxiconazole nitrate

U.S./Canadian Brand Names Oxistat® [US/Can]

Therapeutic Category Antifungal Agent

Use Treatment of tinea pedis (athlete's foot), tinea cruris (jock itch), tinea corporis (ringworm), and tinea (pityriasis) versicolor

Dosage Summary

Topical:

Children: Apply to affected areas 1-2 times daily

Adults: Apply to affected areas 1-2 times daily

Dosage Forms

Cream, topical:

Oxistat®: 1% (30 g, 60 g)

Lotion, topical:

Oxistat®: 1% (30 mL)

oxiconazole nitrate *see* oxiconazole *on page 713*

oxidized regenerated cellulose *see* cellulose, oxidized regenerated *on page 195*

Oxilan® 300 [US/Can] *see* ioxilan *on page 522*

Oxilan® 350 [US/Can] *see* ioxilan *on page 522*

oxilapine succinate *see* loxapine *on page 580*

Oxipor® VHC [US-OTC] *see* coal tar *on page 242*

Oxistat® [US/Can] *see* oxiconazole *on page 713*

Oxpam® [Can] *see* oxazepam *on page 712*

oxpentifylline *see* pentoxifylline *on page 742*

Oxpram® [Can] *see* oxazepam *on page 712*

Oxsoralen® [US] *see* methoxsalen (topical) *on page 616*

Oxsoralen® Capsule [Can] *see* methoxsalen (systemic) *on page 616*

Oxsoralen® Lotion [Can] *see* methoxsalen (topical) *on page 616*

Oxsoralen-Ultra® [US/Can] *see* methoxsalen (systemic) *on page 616*

OXY® [US-OTC] *see* benzoyl peroxide *on page 128*

Oxy-5® ***(Discontinued)*** *see* benzoyl peroxide *on page 128*

OXY® Body Wash [US-OTC] *see* salicylic acid *on page 858*

Oxybutyn [Can] *see* oxybutynin *on page 713*

oxybutynin (oks i BYOO ti nin)

Sound-Alike/Look-Alike Issues

oxybutynin may be confused with OxyContin®

Ditropan® may be confused with Detrol®, diazepam, Diprivan®, dithranol

Synonyms oxybutynin chloride

U.S./Canadian Brand Names Apo-Oxybutynin® [Can]; Ditropan XL® [US/Can]; Ditropan® [US/Can]; Dom-Oxybutynin [Can]; Gelnique™ [US]; Mylan-Oxybutynin [Can]; Novo-Oxybutynin [Can]; Nu-Oxybutyn [Can]; Oxybutyn [Can]; Oxybutynine [Can]; Oxytrol® [US/Can]; PHL-Oxybutynin [Can]; PMS-Oxybutynin [Can]; Riva-Oxybutynin [Can]; Uromax® [Can]

Therapeutic Category Antispasmodic Agent, Urinary

Use Antispasmodic for neurogenic bladder (urgency, frequency, leakage, urge incontinence, dysuria); extended release formulation also indicated for treatment of symptoms associated with detrusor overactivity due to a neurological condition (eg, spina bifida)

Dosage Summary

Oral:

Extended release:

Children ≤6 years: Dosage not established

Children >6 years: 5 mg once daily (maximum: 20 mg/day)

Adults: Initial: 5-10 mg once daily; Maintenance: 5-30 mg once daily (maximum: 30 mg/day)

Regular release:

Children <1 years: Dosage not established

Children >5 years: 5 mg 2-3 times/day (maximum: 15 mg/day)

Adults: 5 mg 2-4 times/day (maximum: 20 mg/day)

Elderly: 2.5 mg 2-3 times/day

Topical gel:
Children: Dosage not established
Adults: Apply contents of 1 sachet (100 mg/g) once daily
Transdermal:
Children: Dosage not established
Adults: Apply one 3.9 mg/day patch twice weekly

Dosage Forms
Gel, topical:
Gelnique™: 10% (1 g)
Patch, transdermal:
Oxytrol®: 3.9 mg/24 hours (8s)
Syrup, oral: 5 mg/5 mL (5 mL, 473 mL, 480 mL)
Tablet, oral: 5 mg
Tablet, extended release, oral: 5 mg, 10 mg, 15 mg
Ditropan XL®: 5 mg, 10 mg, 15 mg

oxybutynin chloride *see* oxybutynin *on page 713*
Oxybutynine [Can] *see* oxybutynin *on page 713*
OXY® Chill Factor® [US-OTC] *see* benzoyl peroxide *on page 128*

oxychlorosene (oks i KLOR oh seen)

Synonyms oxychlorosene sodium
U.S./Canadian Brand Names Clorpactin® WCS-90 [US-OTC]
Therapeutic Category Antibiotic, Topical
Use Treatment of localized infections

Dosage Summary
Topical:
Children: Dosage not established
Adults: Apply by irrigation, instillation, spray, soaks, or wet compresses

Dosage Forms
Powder for solution, topical:
Clorpactin® WCS-90 [OTC]: 2 g/bottle

oxychlorosene sodium *see* oxychlorosene *on page 714*
Oxycocet® [Can] *see* oxycodone and acetaminophen *on page 715*
Oxycodan® [Can] *see* oxycodone and aspirin *on page 716*

oxycodone (oks i KOE done)

Sound-Alike/Look-Alike Issues
oxyCODONE may be confused with HYDROcodone, OxyContin®, oxymorphone
OxyContin® may be confused with MS Contin®, oxybutynin, oxycodone
Roxicodone® may be confused with Roxanol™

Synonyms dihydrohydroxycodeinone; oxycodone hydrochloride
Tall-Man oxy**CODONE**
U.S./Canadian Brand Names Oxy.IR® [Can]; OxyContin® [US/Can]; PMS-Oxycodone [Can]; Roxicodone® [US]; Supeudol® [Can]
Therapeutic Category Analgesic, Narcotic
Controlled Substance C-II
Use Management of moderate-to-severe pain, normally used in combination with nonopioid analgesics

OxyContin® is indicated for around-the-clock management of moderate-to-severe pain when an analgesic is needed for an extended period of time.

Dosage Summary
Oral:
Controlled release:
Children: Dosage not established
Adults: 10-160 mg every 12 hours; **Note:** 60 mg, 80 mg, or 160 mg tablets are for use only in opioid-tolerant patients

Immediate release:

Children <6 years: Dosage not established

Children 6-18 years: 0.1-0.2 mg/kg/dose every 6 hours as needed (maximum initial dose: 5 mg for moderate pain; 10 mg for severe pain)

Adults: 2.5-15 mg every 4-6 hours as needed

Dosage Forms

Capsule, immediate release, oral: 5 mg

Liquid, oral:

Roxicodone®: 20 mg/mL (30 mL)

Solution, oral: 5 mg/5 mL (100 mL, 500 mL); 20 mg/mL (30 mL)

Roxicodone®: 5 mg/5 mL (5 mL, 500 mL)

Tablet, oral: 5 mg, 10 mg, 15 mg, 20 mg, 30 mg

Roxicodone®: 5 mg, 15 mg, 30 mg

Tablet, controlled release, oral:

OxyContin®: 10 mg, 15 mg, 20 mg, 30 mg, 40 mg, 60 mg, 80 mg

oxycodone and acetaminophen (oks I KOE done & a seet a MIN oh fen)

Sound-Alike/Look-Alike Issues

Endocet® may be confused with Indocid®

Percocet® may be confused with Darvocet®, Fioricet®, Percodan®

Roxicet™ may be confused with Roxanol™

Tylox® may be confused with Trimox®, Tylenol®, Wymox®, Xanax®

Synonyms acetaminophen and oxycodone

U.S./Canadian Brand Names Endocet® [US/Can]; Novo-Oxycodone Acet [Can]; Oxycocet® [Can]; Percocet® [US/Can]; Percocet®-Demi [Can]; PMS-Oxycodone-Acetaminophen [Can]; Roxicet™ 5/500 [US]; Roxicet™ [US]; Tylox® [US]

Therapeutic Category Analgesic, Narcotic

Controlled Substance C-II

Use Management of moderate-to-severe pain

Dosage Summary Note: Initial dose is based on the oxycodone content; however, the maximum daily dose is based on the acetaminophen content.

Oral:

Acetaminophen:

Children <45 kg: 10-15 mg/kg every 4-6 hours as needed (maximum: 90 mg/kg/day)

Children ≥45 kg: 10-15 mg/kg every 4-6 hours (maximum: 4 g/day)

Adults: 325-650 mg every 4-6 hours (maximum: 4 g/day)

Oxycodone:

Children: 0.05-0.3 mg/kg every 4-6 hours as needed

Adults: 2.5-30 mg/dose every 4-6 hours as needed

Elderly: Initial: 2.5-5 mg every 6 hours as needed

Dosage Forms

Caplet: Oxycodone 5 mg and acetaminophen 500 mg

Roxicet™ 5/500: Oxycodone 5 mg and acetaminophen 500 mg

Capsule: Oxycodone 5 mg and acetaminophen 500 mg

Tylox®: Oxycodone 5 mg and acetaminophen 500 mg

Solution, oral: Oxycodone 5 mg and acetaminophen 325 mg per 5 mL

Roxicet™: Oxycodone 5 mg and acetaminophen 325 mg per 5 mL

Tablet:

Generics:

Oxycodone 2.5 mg and acetaminophen 325 mg

Oxycodone 5 mg and acetaminophen 325 mg

Oxycodone 7.5 mg and acetaminophen 325 mg

Oxycodone 7.5 mg and acetaminophen 500 mg

Oxycodone 10 mg and acetaminophen 325 mg

Oxycodone 10 mg and acetaminophen 650 mg

Brands:

Endocet®:

5/325 [scored]: Oxycodone 5 mg and acetaminophen 325 mg

7.5/325: Oxycodone 7.5 mg and acetaminophen 325 mg

7.5/500: Oxycodone 7.5 mg and acetaminophen 500 mg

10/325: Oxycodone 10 mg and acetaminophen 325 mg

10/650: Oxycodone 10 mg and acetaminophen 650 mg
Percocet®:
2.5/325: Oxycodone 2.5 mg and acetaminophen 325 mg
5/325 [scored]: Oxycodone 5 mg and acetaminophen 325 mg
7.5/325: Oxycodone 7.5 mg and acetaminophen 325 mg
7.5/500: Oxycodone 7.5 mg and acetaminophen 500 mg
10/325: Oxycodone 10 mg and acetaminophen 325 mg
10/650: Oxycodone 10 mg and acetaminophen 650 mg
Primlev™:
5/300: Oxycodone 5 mg and acetaminophen 300 mg
7.5/300: Oxycodone 7.5 mg and acetaminophen 300 mg
10/300: Oxycodone 10 mg and acetaminophen 300 mg
Roxicet™ [scored]: Oxycodone 5 mg and acetaminophen 325 mg

oxycodone and aspirin (oks i KOE done & AS pir in)

Sound-Alike/Look-Alike Issues
Percodan® may be confused with Decadron®, Percocet®, Percogesic®, Periactin®
Synonyms aspirin and oxycodone
U.S./Canadian Brand Names Endodan® [US/Can]; Oxycodan® [Can]; Percodan® [US/Can]
Therapeutic Category Analgesic, Narcotic
Controlled Substance C-II
Use Management of moderate- to moderately-severe pain
Dosage Summary
Oral:
Children: 0.1-0.2 mg/kg/dose (based on oxycodone content) every 4-6 hours as needed (maximum: 5 mg/dose [oxycodone]; 4 g/day [aspirin])
Adults: One tablet every 6 hours as needed (maximum: 4 g/day [aspirin])
Dosage Forms
Tablet: Oxycodone hydrochloride 4.5 mg, oxycodone terephthalate 0.38 mg, and aspirin 325 mg
Endodan®, Percodan®: Oxycodone hydrochloride 4.8355 mg and aspirin 325 mg

oxycodone and ibuprofen (oks i KOE done & eye byoo PROE fen)

Synonyms ibuprofen and oxycodone
Therapeutic Category Analgesic, Opioid; Nonsteroidal Antiinflammatory Drug (NSAID), Oral
Controlled Substance C-II
Use Short-term (≤7 days) management of acute, moderate-to-severe pain
Dosage Summary
Oral:
Children: Dosage not established
Adults: 1 tablet every 6 hours as needed (maximum: 4 tablets/day; 7 days)
Dosage Forms
Tablet: Oxycodone 5 mg and ibuprofen 400 mg

oxycodone hydrochloride *see* oxycodone *on page 714*
OxyContin® [US/Can] *see* oxycodone *on page 714*
OXY® Daily [US-OTC] *see* salicylic acid *on page 858*
OXY® Daily Cleansing [US-OTC] *see* salicylic acid *on page 858*
Oxyderm™ [Can] *see* benzoyl peroxide *on page 128*
OXY® Face Wash [US-OTC] *see* salicylic acid *on page 858*
Oxy.IR® [Can] *see* oxycodone *on page 714*
OxyIR® ***(Discontinued)*** *see* oxycodone *on page 714*
OXY® Maximum [US-OTC] *see* salicylic acid *on page 858*
OXY® Maximum Daily Cleansing [US-OTC] *see* salicylic acid *on page 858*

oxymetazoline (nasal) (oks i met AZ oh leen)

Sound-Alike/Look-Alike Issues
oxymetazoline may be confused with oxymetholone
Afrin® may be confused with aspirin
Afrin® (oxymetazoline) may be confused with Afrin® (saline)

Neo-Synephrine® (oxymetazoline) may be confused with Neo-Synephrine® (phenylephrine)

Synonyms oxymetazoline hydrochloride

U.S./Canadian Brand Names 12 Hour Nasal Relief [US-OTC]; 4-Way® 12 Hour [US-OTC]; Afrin® Extra Moisturizing [US-OTC]; Afrin® Original [US-OTC]; Afrin® Severe Congestion [US-OTC]; Afrin® Sinus [US-OTC]; Claritin® Allergic Decongestant [Can]; Dristan® Long Lasting Nasal [Can]; Dristan® [US-OTC]; Drixoral® Nasal [Can]; Duramist Plus [US-OTC]; Neo-Synephrine® 12-Hour Extra Moisturizing [US-OTC]; Neo-Synephrine® 12-Hour [US-OTC]; Nostrilla® [US-OTC]; NRS® [US-OTC]; Sudafed OM® Sinus Congestion [US-OTC]; Vicks® Early Defense™ [US-OTC]; Vicks® Sinex® VapoSpray 12-Hour UltraFine Mist [US-OTC]; Vicks® Sinex® VapoSpray 12-Hour [US]; Vicks® Sinex® VapoSpray Moisturizing 12-Hour UltraFine Mist [US-OTC]

Therapeutic Category Adrenergic Agonist Agent; Imidazoline Derivative

Use Adjunctive therapy for nasal congestion, associated with acute or chronic rhinitis, the common cold, sinusitis, hay fever, or other allergies

Dosage Summary

Intranasal:

Children <6 years: Dosage not established

Children ≥6 years: Instill 2-3 sprays into each nostril twice daily

Adults: Instill 2-3 sprays into each nostril twice daily

Dosage Forms

Gel, intranasal:

Vicks® Early Defense™ [OTC]: 0.05% (14.7 mL)

Solution, intranasal: 0.05% (15 mL, 30 mL)

12 Hour Nasal Relief [OTC]: 0.05% (15 mL, 30 mL)
4-Way® 12 Hour [OTC]: 0.05% (15 mL)
Afrin® Extra Moisturizing [OTC]: 0.05% (15 mL)
Afrin® Original [OTC]: 0.05% (15 mL, 30 mL)
Afrin® Severe Congestion [OTC]: 0.05% (15 mL)
Afrin® Sinus [OTC]: 0.05% (15 mL)
Dristan® [OTC]: 0.05% (15 mL)
Duramist Plus [OTC]: 0.05% (15 mL)
Neo-Synephrine® 12-Hour [OTC]: 0.05% (15 mL)
Neo-Synephrine® 12-Hour Extra Moisturizing [OTC]: 0.05% (15 mL)
Nostrilla® [OTC]: 0.05% (15 mL)
NRS® [OTC]: 0.05% (15 mL, 30 mL)
Sudafed OM® Sinus Congestion [OTC]: 0.05% (15 mL)
Vicks® Sinex® VapoSpray 12-Hour: 0.05% (15 mL)
Vicks® Sinex® VapoSpray 12-Hour UltraFine Mist [OTC]: 0.05% (15 mL)
Vicks® Sinex® VapoSpray Moisturizing 12-Hour UltraFine Mist [OTC]: 0.05% (15 mL)

oxymetazoline (ophthalmic) (oks i met AZ oh leen)

Sound-Alike/Look-Alike Issues

oxymetazoline may be confused with oxymetholone
Visine® may be confused with Visken®

Synonyms oxymetazoline hydrochloride

U.S./Canadian Brand Names Visine L.R.® [US-OTC]

Therapeutic Category Vasoconstrictor

Use Relief of redness of eye due to minor eye irritations

Dosage Summary

Ophthalmic:

Children <6 years: Dosage not established

Children ≥6 years: Instill 1-2 drops in affected eye(s) every 6 hours as needed

Adults: Instill 1-2 drops in affected eye(s) every 6 hours as needed

Dosage Forms

Solution, ophthalmic:

Visine L.R.® [OTC]: 0.025% (15 mL, 30 mL)

oxymetazoline hydrochloride *see* oxymetazoline (nasal) *on page* 716

oxymetazoline hydrochloride *see* oxymetazoline (ophthalmic) *on page* 717

oxymetholone (oks i METH oh lone)

Sound-Alike/Look-Alike Issues

oxymetholone may be confused with oxymetazoline, oxymorphone

U.S./Canadian Brand Names Anadrol®-50 [US]

Therapeutic Category Anabolic Steroid

Controlled Substance C-III

Use Treatment of anemias caused by deficient red cell production

Dosage Summary

Oral:

Children: 1-5 mg/kg once daily

Adults: 1-5 mg/kg once daily

Dosage Forms

Tablet, oral:

Anadrol®-50: 50 mg

oxymorphone (oks i MOR fone)

Sound-Alike/Look-Alike Issues

oxymorphone may be confused with oxycodone, oxymetholone

Synonyms oxymorphone hydrochloride

U.S./Canadian Brand Names Opana® ER [US]; Opana® [US]

Therapeutic Category Analgesic, Narcotic

Controlled Substance C-II

Use

Parenteral: Management of moderate-to-severe pain

Oral, regular release: Management of moderate-to-severe pain

Oral, extended release: Management of moderate-to-severe pain in patients requiring around-the-clock opioid treatment for an extended period of time

Dosage Summary

I.M.:

Children: Dosage not established

Adults: Initial: 0.5 mg; Maintenance: 1-1.5 mg every 4-6 hours as needed

I.V.:

Children: Dosage not established

Adults: Initial: 0.5 mg

Oral:

Extended release:

Children: Dosage not established

Adults (opioid-naive): Initial: 5 mg every 12 hours; Maintenance: Titrate upward with 5-10 mg every 12 hours at 3-7 day intervals until desired response.

Note: Initial dosage in the opioid-tolerant patient may be extremely variable; must be evaluated in context of prior requirements and tolerance.

Immediate release:

Children: Dosage not established

Adults (opioid-naive): Initial: 5-20 mg every 4-6 hours; Maintenance: Titrate upward to desired response

SubQ:

Children: Dosage not established

Adults: Initial: 0.5 mg; Maintenance: 1-1.5 mg every 4-6 hours as needed

Dosage Forms

Injection, solution:

Opana®: 1 mg/mL (1 mL)

Tablet, oral:

Opana®: 5 mg, 10 mg

Tablet, extended release, oral:

Opana® ER: 5 mg, 7.5 mg, 10 mg, 15 mg, 20 mg, 30 mg, 40 mg

oxymorphone hydrochloride *see* oxymorphone *on page 718*

OXY® Post-Shave [US-OTC] *see* salicylic acid *on page 858*

OXY® Spot Treatment [US-OTC] *see* salicylic acid *on page 858*

oxytetracycline *(Discontinued)*

oxytocin (oks i TOE sin)

Synonyms pit

U.S./Canadian Brand Names Pitocin® [US/Can]; Syntocinon® [Can]

Therapeutic Category Oxytocic Agent

Use Induction of labor at term; control of postpartum bleeding; adjunctive therapy in management of abortion

Dosage Summary

I.M.:

Children: Not for use prior to menarche

Adults: Total dose of 10 units after delivery

I.V.:

Children: Not for use prior to menarche

Adults:

Abortion adjunctive treatment: 10-20 milliunits/minute (maximum: 30 units/12 hours)

Labor induction: Initial: 0.5-1 milliunit/minute; Titration is recommended (rates >9-10 milliunits/minute rarely required)

Postpartum bleeding: 10-40 units in 1000 mL at a rate sufficient to control uterine atony

Dosage Forms

Injection, solution: 10 units/mL (1 mL, 10 mL, 30 mL)

Pitocin®: 10 units/mL (1 mL, 10 mL)

Oxytrol® [US/Can] *see* oxybutynin *on page 713*

Oysco D [US-OTC] *see* calcium and vitamin D *on page 166*

Oysco 500 [US-OTC] *see* calcium carbonate *on page 167*

Oysco 500+D [US-OTC] *see* calcium and vitamin D *on page 166*

Oyst-Cal-D [US-OTC] *see* calcium and vitamin D *on page 166*

Oyst-Cal-D 500 [US-OTC] *see* calcium and vitamin D *on page 166*

Oyst-Cal 500 *(Discontinued)* *see* calcium carbonate *on page 167*

Oystercal™ 500 [US-OTC] *see* calcium carbonate *on page 167*

Ozurdex™ [US] *see* dexamethasone (ophthalmic) *on page 281*

P2E1 *(Discontinued)*

P-V-Tussin® Syrup *(Discontinued)*

P-V Tussin Tablet *(Discontinued)*

P32 *see* chromic phosphate P 32 *on page 220*

P-071 *see* cetirizine *on page 198*

Pacerone® [US] *see* amiodarone *on page 67*

Pacis™ [Can] *see* BCG *on page 118*

paclitaxel (pac li TAKS el)

Sound-Alike/Look-Alike Issues

paclitaxel may be confused with paroxetine, Paxil®

paclitaxel (conventional) may be confused with paclitaxel (protein-bound)

Taxol® may be confused with Abraxane®, Paxil®, Taxotere®

U.S./Canadian Brand Names Abraxane® For Injectable Suspension [Can]; Apo-Paclitaxel® [Can]; Taxol® [Can]

Therapeutic Category Antineoplastic Agent

Use Treatment of breast, nonsmall cell lung, and ovarian cancers; treatment of AIDS-related Kaposi sarcoma (KS)

Dosage Summary

I.V.:

Children: Dosage not established

Adults: 135-250 mg/m^2 over 3 hours every 3 weeks **or** 135 mg/m^2 over 24 hours every 3 weeks **or** 50-80 mg/m^2 over 1-3 hours weekly **or** 1.4-4 mg/m^2/day continuous infusion for 14 days every 4 weeks **or** 100 mg/m^2 over 3 hours every 2 weeks

Dosage Forms

Injection, solution: 6 mg/mL (5 mL, 16.7 mL, 25 mL, 50 mL)

paclitaxel, albumin-bound *see* paclitaxel (protein bound) *on page 720*

paclitaxel (protein bound) (pac li TAKS el PROE teen bownd)

Sound-Alike/Look-Alike Issues

paclitaxel (protein bound) may be confused with paclitaxel (conventional)
Abraxane® may be confused with Paxil®, Taxol®, Taxotere®

Synonyms ABI-007; albumin-bound paclitaxel; albumin-stabilized nanoparticle paclitaxel; nab-paclitaxel; nanoparticle albumin-bound paclitaxel; paclitaxel, albumin-bound; protein-bound paclitaxel

U.S./Canadian Brand Names Abraxane® [US]

Therapeutic Category Antineoplastic Agent, Antimicrotubular; Antineoplastic Agent, Natural Source (Plant) Derivative

Use Treatment of refractory (metastatic) or relapsed (within 6 months of adjuvant therapy) breast cancer

Dosage Summary

I.V.:

Children: Dosage not established
Adults: 260 mg/m^2 every 3 weeks

Dosage Forms

Injection, powder for reconstitution:
Abraxane®: 100 mg

Pacnex™ [US] *see* benzoyl peroxide *on page 128*
Pain-A-Lay® [US-OTC] *see* phenol *on page 748*
Pain Eze [US-OTC] *see* acetaminophen *on page 21*
Pain-Off [US-OTC] *see* acetaminophen, aspirin, and caffeine *on page 27*
Palafer® [Can] *see* ferrous fumarate *on page 398*
Palcaps *(Discontinued)* *see* pancrelipase *on page 723*
Palgic® [US] *see* carbinoxamine *on page 182*
Palgic®-D *(Discontinued)*
Palgic®-DS *(Discontinued)*

palifermin (pal ee FER min)

Synonyms AMJ 9701; rhKGF; rhu keratinocyte growth factor; rHu-KGF

U.S./Canadian Brand Names Kepivance® [US]

Therapeutic Category Keratinocyte Growth Factor

Use Decrease the incidence and severity of severe oral mucositis associated with hematologic malignancies in patients receiving myelotoxic therapy requiring hematopoietic stem cell support

Dosage Summary

I.V.:

Children: Dosage not established
Adults: 60 mcg/kg/day for 3 consecutive days before and after myelotoxic therapy; total of 6 doses

Dosage Forms

Injection, powder for reconstitution [preservative free]:
Kepivance®: 6.25 mg

paliperidone (pal ee PER i done)

Synonyms 9-hydroxy-risperidone; 9-OH-risperidone; paliperidone palmitate

U.S./Canadian Brand Names Invega® Sustenna™ [US]; Invega® [US/Can]

Therapeutic Category Antipsychotic Agent, Atypical

Use

Oral: Acute and maintenance treatment of schizophrenia; acute treatment of schizoaffective disorder (monotherapy or adjunctive therapy to mood stabilizers and/or antidepressants)
Injection: Acute and maintenance treatment of schizophrenia

Dosage Summary

I.M.:

Children: Dosage not established
Adults: Initial: 234 mg, then 156 mg one week later; Maintenance: 39-234 mg/month

Oral:

Children: Dosage not established
Adults: 3-12 mg once daily (maximum: 12 mg/day)

Dosage Forms

Injection, suspension, extended release:

Invega® Sustenna®: 39 mg/0.25 mL (0.25 mL); 78 mg/0.5 mL (0.5 mL); 117 mg/0.75 mL (0.75 mL); 156 mg/mL (1 mL); 234 mg/1.5 mL (1.5 mL)

Tablet, extended release, oral:

Invega®: 1.5 mg, 3 mg, 6 mg, 9 mg

paliperidone palmitate *see* paliperidone *on page* 720

palivizumab (pah li VIZ u mab)

Sound-Alike/Look-Alike Issues

Synagis® may be confused with Synalgos®-DC, Synvisc®

U.S./Canadian Brand Names Synagis® [US/Can]

Therapeutic Category Monoclonal Antibody

Use Prevention of serious lower respiratory tract disease caused by respiratory syncytial virus (RSV) in infants and children at high risk of RSV disease

The American Academy of Pediatrics recommends RSV prophylaxis with palivizumab during RSV season for:

- Infants <3 months of age who were born between 32 and 34 6/7 weeks gestational age and have one of the following:
  - Day-care attendance
  - One or more siblings <5 years of age living in the same household
- Infants <6 months of age who were born between 29 and 31 6/7 weeks gestational age
- Infants <12 months of age who were born <28 weeks gestational age
- Infants <12 months of age with congenital airway abnormality or neuromuscular disorder that decreases the ability to manage airway secretions
- Infants and children <24 months of age with chronic lung disease (CLD) necessitating medical therapy within 6 month prior to the beginning of RSV season
- Infants and children ≤24 months of age with congenital heart disease and one of the following:
  - Receiving medication to treat congestive heart failure
  - Moderate-to-severe pulmonary hypertension
  - Cyanotic heart disease

Dosage Summary

I.M.:

Children <2 years: 15 mg/kg monthly throughout RSV season

Children >2 years: Dosage not established

Adults: Dosage not established

Dosage Forms

Injection, solution [preservative free]:

Synagis®: 100 mg/mL (0.5 mL, 1 mL)

Palladone™ *(Discontinued)* *see* hydromorphone *on page* 485

Palmer's® Skin Success Acne Cleanser [US-OTC] *see* salicylic acid *on page* 858

Palmer's® Skin Success® Eventone® Fade Cream [US] *see* hydroquinone *on page* 487

Palmer's® Skin Success Invisible Acne [US-OTC] *see* benzoyl peroxide *on page* 128

palonosetron (pal oh NOE se tron)

Sound-Alike/Look-Alike Issues

palonosetron may be confused with dolasetron, granisetron, ondansetron

Aloxi® may be confused with Eloxatin®, oxaliplatin

Synonyms palonosetron hydrochloride; RS-25259; RS-25259-197

U.S./Canadian Brand Names Aloxi® [US]

Therapeutic Category Antiemetic; Selective $5\text{-}HT_3$ Receptor Antagonist

Use Prevention of chemotherapy-associated nausea and vomiting; indicated for prevention of acute (highly-emetogenic therapy) as well as acute and delayed (moderately-emetogenic therapy) nausea and vomiting; prevention of postoperative nausea and vomiting (PONV)

Dosage Summary

I.V.:

Children: Dosage not established

Adults: 0.25 mg 30 minutes prior to the start of chemotherapy **or** 0.075 mg immediately prior to anesthesia induction

Dosage Forms

Injection, solution:

Aloxi®: 0.05 mg/mL (1.5 mL, 5 mL)

palonosetron hydrochloride *see* palonosetron *on page 721*

2-PAM *see* pralidoxime *on page 785*

pamabrom (PAM a brom)

U.S./Canadian Brand Names Aqua-Ban® Maximum Strength [US-OTC]; diurex® Aquagels® [US-OTC]; diurex® Maximum Relief [US-OTC]; diurex® [US-OTC]

Therapeutic Category Diuretic

Use Temporary relief of symptoms associated with premenstrual and menstrual periods (eg, bloating, water-weight gain, swelling, full feeling)

Dosage Summary

Oral:

Children: Dosage not established

Adults: 50 mg every 6 hours as needed (maximum: 200 mg/day)

Dosage Forms

Caplet, oral:

diurex® Maximum Relief [OTC]: 50 mg

Capsule, oral:

diurex® [OTC]: 50 mg

Capsule, softgel, oral:

diurex® Aquagels® [OTC]: 50 mg

Tablet, oral:

Aqua-Ban® Maximum Strength [OTC]: 50 mg

pamabrom and acetaminophen *see* acetaminophen and pamabrom *on page 25*

Pamelor® [US] *see* nortriptyline *on page 684*

pamidronate (pa mi DROE nate)

Sound-Alike/Look-Alike Issues

pamidronate may be confused with papaverine

Aredia® may be confused with adriamycin, Meridia®

Synonyms pamidronate disodium

U.S./Canadian Brand Names Aredia® [US/Can]; Pamidronate Disodium Omega [Can]; Pamidronate Disodium® [Can]; PMS-Pamidronate [Can]; Rhoxal-pamidronate [Can]

Therapeutic Category Bisphosphonate Derivative

Use Treatment of moderate or severe hypercalcemia associated with malignancy; treatment of osteolytic bone lesions associated with multiple myeloma or metastatic breast cancer; moderate-to-severe Paget disease of bone

Dosage Summary

I.V.:

Children: Dosage not established

Adults: 60-90 mg as a single dose, may repeat every 3-4 weeks **or** 30 mg daily for 3 consecutive days

Dosage Forms

Injection, powder for reconstitution: 30 mg, 90 mg

Aredia®: 30 mg, 90 mg

Injection, solution: 3 mg/mL (10 mL); 6 mg/mL (10 mL); 9 mg/mL (10 mL)

Injection, solution [preservative free]: 3 mg/mL (10 mL); 9 mg/mL (10 mL)

Pamidronate Disodium® [Can] *see* pamidronate *on page 722*

pamidronate disodium *see* pamidronate *on page 722*

Pamidronate Disodium Omega [Can] *see* pamidronate *on page 722*

Pamine® [US/Can] *see* methscopolamine *on page 617*

Pamine® Forte [US] *see* methscopolamine *on page 617*

p-amino-benzenesulfonamide *see* sulfanilamide *on page 902*

p-aminoclonidine *see* apraclonidine *on page 91*

Pamprin IB® *(Discontinued)* *see* ibuprofen *on page 494*
Pamprin® Maximum Strength All Day Relief [US-OTC] *see* naproxen *on page 659*
Pan-2400™ [US-OTC] *see* pancreatin *on page 723*
Panadol® *(Discontinued)* *see* acetaminophen *on page 21*
Panafil® *(Discontinued)*
Panafil® SE *(Discontinued)*
Panasal® 5/500 *(Discontinued)*
Pancof® *(Discontinued)* *see* pseudoephedrine, dihydrocodeine, and chlorpheniramine *on page 813*
Pancof®-EXP [US] *see* dihydrocodeine, pseudoephedrine, and guaifenesin *on page 304*
Pancof-HC *(Discontinued)*
Pancof-XP *(Discontinued)*
Pancrease® [Can] *see* pancrelipase *on page 723*
Pancrease® MT [Can] *see* pancrelipase *on page 723*
Pancrease® MT *(Discontinued)* *see* pancrelipase *on page 723*
pancreatic enzymes *see* pancrelipase *on page 723*

pancreatin (PAN kree a tin)

Sound-Alike/Look-Alike Issues
pancreatin may be confused with Panretin®

U.S./Canadian Brand Names Hi-Vegi-Lip [US-OTC]; Pan-2400™ [US-OTC]

Therapeutic Category Enzyme

Use Relief of functional indigestion due to enzyme deficiency or imbalance

Dosage Summary
Oral:
Children: Dosage not established
Adults: 1-2 capsules with each meal or snack

Dosage Forms
Capsule: Lipase 8500 units, protease 50,000 units, amylase 50,000 units
Pan-2400™ [OTC]: Lipase 9816 units, protease 60,214 units, amylase 75,900 units
Tablet: Lipase 565 units, protease 8200 units, amylase 8200 units [pancreatin 325 mg]; lipase 2400 units, protease 30,000 units, amylase 30,000 units
Hi-Vegi-Lip [OTC]: Lipase 4800 units, protease 60,000 units, amylase 60,000 units

Pancreaze™ [US] *see* pancrelipase *on page 723*
Pancrecarb MS® *(Discontinued)* *see* pancrelipase *on page 723*

pancrelipase (pan kre LYE pase)

Sound-Alike/Look-Alike Issues
pancrelipase may be confused with pancreatin

Synonyms amylase, lipase, and protease; lipancreatin; lipase, protease, and amylase; pancreatic enzymes; protease, lipase, and amylase

U.S./Canadian Brand Names Cotazym® [Can]; Creon® [US/Can]; Pancrease® MT [Can]; Pancrease® [Can]; Pancreaze™ [US]; Pancrelipase™ [US]; Ultrase® MT [Can]; Ultrase® [Can]; Viokase® [Can]; Zenpep™ [US]

Therapeutic Category Enzyme

Use Treatment of exocrine pancreatic insufficiency (EPI) due to conditions such as cystic fibrosis (Creon®, Pancreaze™, Zenpep™); chronic pancreatitis (Creon®); or pancreatectomy (Creon®)

Dosage Summary
Oral:
Children ≤1 year: Lipase 2000-4000 units per 120 mL of formula or breast milk
Children >1 and <4 years: Lipase 1000-2500 units/kg/meal. Maximum dose: Lipase 10,000 units/kg/day **or** lipase 4000 units/g of fat per day
Children ≥4 years: Lipase 500-2500 units/kg/meal. Maximum dose: Lipase 10,000 units/kg/day **or** lipase 4000 units/g of fat per day
Adults: Lipase 500-2500 units/kg/meal **or** lipase 72,000 units/meal (while consuming ≥100 g of fat per day). Maximum dose: Lipase 10,000 units/kg/day **or** lipase 4000 units/g of fat per day

Dosage Forms

Capsule, delayed release, enteric coated beads [porcine derived]:

Pancrelipase™: Lipase 5000 units, protease 17,000 units, amylase 27,000 units
Zenpep™: Lipase 5000 units, protease 17,000 units, amylase 27,000 units
Zenpep™: Lipase 10,000 units, protease 34,000 units, amylase 55,000 units
Zenpep™: Lipase 15,000 units, protease 51,000 units, amylase 82,000 units
Zenpep™: Lipase 20,000 units, protease 68,000 units, amylase 109,000 units

Capsule, delayed release, enteric coated microspheres [new formulation; porcine derived]:

Creon®: Lipase 6000 units, protease 19,000 units, and amylase 30,000 units
Creon®: Lipase 12000 units, protease 38,000 units, and amylase 60,000 units
Creon®: Lipase 24,000 units, protease 76,000 units, and amylase 120,000 units

Capsule, delayed release, enteric coated microtablets [porcine derived]:

Pancreaze™: Lipase 4200 units, protease 10,000 units, and amylase 17,500 units
Pancreaze™: Lipase 10,500 units, protease 25,000 units, and amylase 43,750 units
Pancreaze™: Lipase 16,800 units, protease 40,000 units, and amylase 70,000 units
Pancreaze™: Lipase 21,000 units, protease 37,000 units, and amylase 61,000 units

Capsule, enteric coated microspheres [porcine derived]:

Ultrase®: Lipase 4500 units, protease 25,000 units, and amylase 20,000 units

Pancrelipase™ [US] *see* pancrelipase *on page 723*

pancuronium (pan kyoo ROE nee um)

Sound-Alike/Look-Alike Issues

pancuronium may be confused with pipecuronium

Synonyms pancuronium bromide

U.S./Canadian Brand Names Pancuronium Bromide® [Can]

Therapeutic Category Skeletal Muscle Relaxant

Use Facilitation of endotracheal intubation and relaxation of skeletal muscles during surgery; facilitation of mechanical ventilation in ICU patients; does not relieve pain or produce sedation

Dosage Summary

I.V.:

Neonates ≤1 month: Test dose: 0.02 mg/kg; Initial: 0.03 mg/kg/dose repeated twice at 5- to 10-minute intervals as needed; Maintenance: 0.03-0.09 mg/kg/dose every 30 minutes to 4 hours as needed

Children >1 month:

ICU: 0.05-0.1 mg/kg bolus followed by 0.8-1.7 mcg/kg/minute infusion **or** 0.1-0.2 mg/kg every 1-3 hours

Surgery: Intubation: Initial: 0.06-1 mg/kg **or** 0.05 mg/kg after succinylcholine; Maintenance: 0.01 mg/kg 60-100 minutes after initial dose and then every 25-60 minutes

Adults:

ICU: 0.05-0.1 mg/kg bolus followed by 0.8-1.7 mcg/kg/minute infusion **or** 0.1-0.2 mg/kg every 1-3 hours

Surgery; Intubation: Initial: 0.06-1 mg/kg **or** 0.05 mg/kg after succinylcholine; Maintenance: 0.01 mg/kg 60-100 minutes after initial dose and then every 25-60 minutes

Dosage Forms

Injection, solution: 1 mg/mL (10 mL); 2 mg/mL (2 mL, 5 mL)

Pancuronium Bromide® [Can] *see* pancuronium *on page 724*
pancuronium bromide *see* pancuronium *on page 724*
Pandel® [US] *see* hydrocortisone (topical) *on page 483*
Pangestyme™ CN *(Discontinued)* *see* pancrelipase *on page 723*
Pangestyme™ EC *(Discontinued)* *see* pancrelipase *on page 723*
Pangestyme™ MT *(Discontinued)* *see* pancrelipase *on page 723*
Pangestyme™ UL *(Discontinued)* *see* pancrelipase *on page 723*
panglobulin *see* immune globulin (intravenous) *on page 502*
Panglobulin® NF *(Discontinued)* *see* immune globulin (intravenous) *on page 502*
Panhematin® [US] *see* hemin *on page 466*

panitumumab (pan i TOOM yoo mab)

Synonyms ABX-EGF; MOAB ABX-EGF; monoclonal antibody ABX-EGF; rHuMAb-EGFr

U.S./Canadian Brand Names Vectibix® [US/Can]

Therapeutic Category Antineoplastic Agent, Monoclonal Antibody; Epidermal Growth Factor Receptor (EGFR) Inhibitor

Use Monotherapy in treatment of refractory metastatic colorectal cancer

Note: Subset analyses (retrospective) in metastatic colorectal cancer trials have not shown a benefit with EGFR inhibitor treatment in patients whose tumors have codon 12 or 13 *KRAS* mutations; use is not recommended in these patients.

Dosage Summary

I.V.:

Children: Dosage not established

Adults: 6 mg/kg every 2 weeks

Dosage Forms

Injection, solution [preservative free]:

Vectibix®: 20 mg/mL (5 mL, 20 mL)

Panixine DisperDose™ ***(Discontinued)*** *see* cephalexin *on page* *197*

Panlor® DC ***(Discontinued)*** *see* acetaminophen, caffeine, and dihydrocodeine *on page* *28*

Panlor® SS [US] *see* acetaminophen, caffeine, and dihydrocodeine *on page* *28*

Panocaps ***(Discontinued)*** *see* pancrelipase *on page* *723*

Panocaps MT ***(Discontinued)*** *see* pancrelipase *on page* *723*

Panokase® 16 ***(Discontinued)*** *see* pancrelipase *on page* *723*

Panokase® ***(Discontinued)*** *see* pancrelipase *on page* *723*

PanOxyl® [Can] *see* benzoyl peroxide *on page* *128*

PanOxyl® Aqua Gel [US-OTC] *see* benzoyl peroxide *on page* *128*

PanOxyl® Bar [US-OTC] *see* benzoyl peroxide *on page* *128*

Panretin® [US/Can] *see* alitretinoin *on page* *51*

Panscol® Lotion ***(Discontinued)*** *see* salicylic acid *on page* *858*

Panscol® Ointment ***(Discontinued)*** *see* salicylic acid *on page* *858*

Panto-250 [US-OTC] *see* pantothenic acid *on page* *726*

Panto™ I.V. [Can] *see* pantoprazole *on page* *725*

Pantoloc® [Can] *see* pantoprazole *on page* *725*

Pantopon® ***(Discontinued)***

pantoprazole (pan TOE pra zole)

Sound-Alike/Look-Alike Issues

pantoprazole may be confused with aripiprazole

Protonix® may be confused with Lotronex®, Lovenox®, protamine

U.S./Canadian Brand Names Apo-Pantoprazole® [Can]; CO Pantoprazole [Can]; Mylan-Pantoprazole [Can]; Novo-Pantoprazole [Can]; Pantoloc® [Can]; Panto™ I.V. [Can]; PHL-Pantoprazole [Can]; PMS-Pantoprazole [Can]; Protonix® [US/Can]; RAN™-Pantoprazole [Can]; ratio-Pantoprazole [Can]; Riva-Pantoprazole [Can]; Sandoz-Pantoprazole [Can]; Tecta™ [Can]; ZYM-Pantoprazole [Can]

Therapeutic Category Proton Pump Inhibitor

Use

Oral: Treatment and maintenance of healing of erosive esophagitis associated with GERD; reduction in relapse rates of daytime and nighttime heartburn symptoms in GERD; hypersecretory disorders associated with Zollinger-Ellison syndrome or other GI hypersecretory disorders

I.V.: Short-term treatment (7-10 days) of patients with gastroesophageal reflux disease (GERD) and a history of erosive esophagitis; hypersecretory disorders associated with Zollinger-Ellison syndrome or other neoplastic disorders

Dosage Summary

I.V.:

Children: Dosage not established

Adults: Wide variation in dose based on indication:

Erosive gastritis: 40 mg once daily

Hypersecretory disorders: 160-240 mg/day in divided doses

Oral:

Children <5 years: Dosage not established

Adults: 20-40 mg once or twice daily (maximum: 240 mg/day normally reserved for treatment of hypersecretory conditions)

Dosage Forms

Granules for suspension, delayed release, enteric coated, oral:

Protonix®: 40 mg/packet (30s)

Injection, powder for reconstitution:

Protonix®: 40 mg

Tablet, delayed release, oral: 20 mg, 40 mg

Protonix®: 20 mg, 40 mg

Dosage Forms - Canada

Tablet, enteric coated:

Pantoloc®: 40 mg

pantothenic acid (pan toe THEN ik AS id)

Synonyms calcium pantothenate; vitamin B_5

U.S./Canadian Brand Names Panto-250 [US-OTC]

Therapeutic Category Vitamin, Water Soluble

Use Pantothenic acid deficiency

Dosage Summary

Oral:

Children: Dosage not established

Adults: 4-7 mg/day

Dosage Forms

Capsule, oral:

Panto-250 [OTC]: 250 mg

Liquid, oral: 200 mg/5 mL (240 mL)

Tablet, oral: 100 mg, 200 mg, 250 mg, 500 mg

Tablet, sustained release, oral: 500 mg

pantothenyl alcohol *see* dexpanthenol *on page* 284

papain and urea *(Discontinued)*

papaverine (pa PAV er een)

Sound-Alike/Look-Alike Issues

papaverine may be confused with pamidronate

Synonyms papaverine hydrochloride

Therapeutic Category Vasodilator

Use Oral: Relief of peripheral and cerebral ischemia associated with arterial spasm and myocardial ischemia complicated by arrhythmias

Dosage Summary

I.M.:

Children: 6 mg/kg/day in 4 divided doses

Adults: 30-65 mg, may repeat every 3 hours

I.V.:

Children: 6 mg/kg/day in 4 divided doses

Adults: 30-65 mg, may repeat every 3 hours

Oral:

Children: Dosage not established

Adults: 150-300 mg every 12 hours **or** 150 mg every 8 hours

Dosage Forms

Injection, solution: 30 mg/mL (2 mL, 10 mL)

papaverine hydrochloride *see* papaverine *on page* 726

Papfyll™ *(Discontinued)*

papillomavirus (types 16, 18) vaccine (human, recombinant)

(pap ih LO ma VYE rus typs SIX teen AYE teen vak SEEN YU man ree KOM be nant)

Sound-Alike/Look-Alike Issues

papillomavirus vaccine types 16, 18 (Cervarix®) may be confused with Papillomavirus vaccine types 6, 11, 16, 18 (Gardasil®)

Cervarix® may be confused with Cerebyx®, Celebrex®

Synonyms bivalent human papillomavirus vaccine; HPV vaccine; HPV2; human papillomavirus vaccine; papillomavirus vaccine, recombinant

U.S./Canadian Brand Names Cervarix® [US/Can]

Therapeutic Category Vaccine, Inactivated (Viral)

Use Females 10 through 25 years of age: Prevention of cervical cancer, cervical adenocarcinoma *in situ*, and cervical intraepithelial neoplasia caused by human papillomavirus (HPV) types 16, 18

The Advisory Committee on Immunization Practices (ACIP) recommends routine vaccination for females 11-12 years of age; catch-up vaccination is recommended for females 13-25 years of age.

Dosage Summary

I.M.:

Children ≥10 years (females): 0.5 mL initial dose, followed by 0.5 mL 1 and 6 months later

Adults ≤25 years (females): 0.5 mL initial dose, followed by 0.5 mL 1 and 6 months later

Dosage Forms

Injection, suspension [preservative free]:

Cervarix®: HPV 16 L1 protein 20 mcg and HPV 18 L1 protein 20 mcg per 0.5 mL (0.5 mL)

papillomavirus (types 6, 11, 16, 18) vaccine (human, recombinant)

(pap ih LO ma VYE rus typs six e LEV en SIX teen AYE teen vak SEEN YU man ree KOM be nant)

Sound-Alike/Look-Alike Issues

papillomavirus vaccine types 6, 11, 16, 18 (Gardasil®) may be confused with Papillomavirus vaccine types 16, 18 (Cervarix®)

Synonyms HPV vaccine; HPV4; human papillomavirus vaccine; papillomavirus vaccine, recombinant; quadrivalent human papillomavirus vaccine

U.S./Canadian Brand Names Gardasil® [US/Can]

Therapeutic Category Vaccine

Use

Males ≥9 years and ≤26 years of age: Prevention of genital warts caused by human papillomavirus (HPV) types 6 and 11

Note: Canadian labeling: Approved for use in males ≥9 years of age and ≤17 years

Females ≥9 years and ≤26 years of age: Prevention of cervical, vulvar, and vaginal cancer caused by HPV types 16 and 18, genital warts caused by HPV types 6 and 11, cervical adenocarcinoma *in situ*, and vulvar, vaginal, or cervical intraepithelial neoplasia caused by HPV types 6, 11, 16, 18

The Advisory Committee on Immunization Practices (ACIP) recommends routine vaccination for females 11-12 years of age; catch-up vaccination is recommended for females 13-26 years of age; ACIP does not recommend routine use among males

Dosage Summary

I.M.:

Children <9 years: Dosage not established

Children ≥9 years: 0.5 mL initial dose, followed by 0.5 mL 2 and 6 months later

Adults ≤26 years: 0.5 mL initial dose, followed by 0.5 mL 2 and 6 months later

Adults >26 years: Dosage not established

Dosage Forms

Injection, suspension [preservative free]:

Gardasil®: HPV 6 L1 protein 20 mcg, HPV 11 L1 protein 40 mcg, HPV 16 L1 protein 40 mcg, and HPV 18 L1 protein 20 mcg per 0.5 mL (0.5 mL)

papillomavirus vaccine, recombinant *see* papillomavirus (types 6, 11, 16, 18) vaccine (human, recombinant) *on page* 727

papillomavirus vaccine, recombinant *see* papillomavirus (types 16, 18) vaccine (human, recombinant) *on page* 726

Paptase™ *(Discontinued)*

para-aminosalicylate sodium *see* aminosalicylic acid *on page* 66

paracetamol *see* acetaminophen *on page* 21

Paraflex® *(Discontinued)* *see* chlorzoxazone *on page* 217

Parafon Forte® [Can] *see* chlorzoxazone *on page* 217

Parafon Forte® *(Discontinued)* *see* chlorzoxazone *on page* 217

Parafon Forte® DSC [US] *see* chlorzoxazone *on page* 217

Paraplatin-AQ [Can] *see* carboplatin *on page* 183

Paraplatin® *(Discontinued)* *see* carboplatin *on page* 183
parathyroid hormone (1-34) *see* teriparatide *on page* 919
Para-Time SR® *(Discontinued)* *see* papaverine *on page* 726
Parcaine™ [US] *see* proparacaine *on page* 803
Parcopa® [US] *see* carbidopa and levodopa *on page* 182
Paredrine® *(Discontinued)*

paregoric (par e GOR ik)

Sound-Alike/Look-Alike Issues
paregoric may be confused with Percogesic®
camphorated tincture of opium is an error-prone synonym (mistaken as opium tincture)

Therapeutic Category Analgesic, Narcotic

Controlled Substance C-III

Use Treatment of diarrhea or relief of pain; neonatal opiate withdrawal

Dosage Summary

Oral:
Neonates: 3-6 drops every 3-6 hours as needed **or** 0.2-0.7 mL every 3 hours; **Note:** Titration is recommended
Children: 0.25-0.5 mL/kg 1-4 times/day
Adults: 5-10 mL 1-4 times/day

Dosage Forms

Liquid, oral: Morphine equivalent 2 mg/5 mL (473 mL)

Paremyd® [US] *see* hydroxyamphetamine and tropicamide *on page* 488
parenteral nutrition *see* total parenteral nutrition *on page* 944
Parepectolin® *(Discontinued)*

paricalcitol (pah ri KAL si tole)

Sound-Alike/Look-Alike Issues
paricalcitol may be confused with calcitriol

U.S./Canadian Brand Names Zemplar® [US/Can]

Therapeutic Category Vitamin D Analog

Use
I.V.: Prevention and treatment of secondary hyperparathyroidism associated with stage 5 chronic kidney disease (CKD)
Oral: Prevention and treatment of secondary hyperparathyroidism associated with stage 3 and 4 CKD and stage 5 CKD patients on hemodialysis or peritoneal dialysis

Dosage Summary

I.V.:
Children <5 years: Dosage not established
Children ≥5 years: 0.04-0.24 mcg/kg (2.8-16.8 mcg) every other day during dialysis
Adults: 0.04-0.24 mcg/kg (2.8-16.8 mcg) every other day during dialysis

Oral:
Children: Dosage not established
Adults: 1-2 mcg/day **or** 2-4 mcg 3 times/week

Dosage Forms

Capsule, soft gelatin, oral:
Zemplar®: 1 mcg, 2 mcg, 4 mcg

Injection, solution:
Zemplar®: 2 mcg/mL (1 mL); 5 mcg/mL (1 mL, 2 mL)

Pariet® [Can] *see* rabeprazole *on page* 824
pariprazole *see* rabeprazole *on page* 824
Parlodel® [US/Can] *see* bromocriptine *on page* 146
Parlodel® SnapTabs® [US] *see* bromocriptine *on page* 146
Parnate® [US/Can] *see* tranylcypromine *on page* 948

paromomycin (par oh moe MYE sin)

Synonyms paromomycin sulfate

U.S./Canadian Brand Names Humatin® [Can]

Therapeutic Category Amebicide

Use Treatment of acute and chronic intestinal amebiasis; hepatic coma

Dosage Summary

Oral:

Children: 11 mg/kg every 15 minutes for 4 doses **or** 25-35 mg/kg/day in 3 divided doses **or** 45 mg/kg once daily

Adults: 25-35 mg/kg/day in 3 divided doses **or** 4 g/day in 2-4 divided doses **or** 45 mg/kg once daily

Dosage Forms

Capsule, oral: 250 mg

paromomycin sulfate *see* paromomycin *on page* 728

paroxetine (pa ROKS e teen)

Sound-Alike/Look-Alike Issues

PARoxetine may be confused with FLUoxetine, paclitaxel, pyridoxine

Paxil® may be confused with Doxil®, paclitaxel, Plavix®, Prozac®, Taxol®

Synonyms paroxetine hydrochloride; paroxetine mesylate

Tall-Man **PAR**oxetine

U.S./Canadian Brand Names Apo-Paroxetine® [Can]; CO Paroxetine [Can]; Dom-Paroxetine [Can]; Mylan-Paroxetine [Can]; Novo-Paroxetine [Can]; Paxil CR® [US/Can]; Paxil® [US/Can]; Pexeva® [US]; PHL-Paroxetine [Can]; PMS-Paroxetine [Can]; ratio-Paroxetine [Can]; Riva-paroxetine [Can]; Sandoz-Paroxetine [Can]; Teva-Paroxetine [Can]

Therapeutic Category Antidepressant, Selective Serotonin Reuptake Inhibitor

Use Treatment of major depressive disorder (MDD); treatment of panic disorder with or without agoraphobia; obsessive-compulsive disorder (OCD); social anxiety disorder (social phobia); generalized anxiety disorder (GAD); posttraumatic stress disorder (PTSD); premenstrual dysphoric disorder (PMDD)

Dosage Summary

Oral:

Controlled release:

Children: Dosage not established

Adults: Initial: 12.5-25 mg once daily; Maintenance: 12.5-75 mg once daily (maximum: 75 mg/day; exceptions occur [indication specific]); **Note:** Titration is recommended

Elderly: Initial: 12.5 mg once daily; Maintenance: 12.5-50 mg/day (maximum: 50 mg/day); **Note:** Titration is recommended

Immediate release:

Adults: Initial: 10-20 mg once daily: Maintenance: 10-60 mg once daily (maximum: 60 mg/day); **Note:** Titration is recommended

Elderly: Initial: 10 mg once daily; Maintenance: 10-40 mg once daily (maximum: 40 mg/day); **Note:** Titration is recommended

Dosage Forms

Suspension, oral:

Paxil®: 10 mg/5 mL (250 mL)

Tablet, oral: 10 mg, 20 mg, 30 mg, 40 mg

Paxil®: 10 mg, 20 mg, 30 mg, 40 mg

Pexeva®: 10 mg, 20 mg, 30 mg, 40 mg

Tablet, controlled release, enteric coated, oral: 37.5 mg

Paxil CR®: 12.5 mg, 25 mg, 37.5 mg

Tablet, extended release, enteric coated, oral: 12.5 mg, 25 mg

paroxetine hydrochloride *see* paroxetine *on page* 729

paroxetine mesylate *see* paroxetine *on page* 729

Partuss® LA *(Discontinued)*

Parvolex® [Can] *see* acetylcysteine *on page* 34

PAS *see* aminosalicylic acid *on page* 66

Paser® [US] *see* aminosalicylic acid *on page* 66

Pataday™ [US] *see* olopatadine (ophthalmic) *on page* 699

Patanase® [US] *see* olopatadine (nasal) *on page* 699

Patanol® [US/Can] *see* olopatadine (ophthalmic) *on page* 699

Pathilon® *(Discontinued)*

Pathocil® [Can] *see* dicloxacillin *on page 298*
Pathocil® *(Discontinued)* *see* dicloxacillin *on page 298*
Pavabid® *(Discontinued)* *see* papaverine *on page 726*
Pavatine® *(Discontinued)*
Pavulon® *(Discontinued)* *see* pancuronium *on page 724*
Paxene® *(Discontinued)* *see* paclitaxel *on page 719*
Paxil® [US/Can] *see* paroxetine *on page 729*
Paxil CR® [US/Can] *see* paroxetine *on page 729*

pazopanib (paz OH pa nib)

Sound-Alike/Look-Alike Issues
Votrient™ may be confused with vorinostat

Synonyms GW786034; pazopanib hydrochloride

U.S./Canadian Brand Names Votrient™ [US]

Therapeutic Category Antineoplastic Agent, Tyrosine Kinase Inhibitor; Vascular Endothelial Growth Factor (VEGF) Inhibitor

Use Treatment of advanced renal cell cancer (RCC)

Dosage Summary
Oral: Note: Avoid use with concurrent CYP3A4 interacting agents; dosage adjustment recommended with hepatic impairment or for toxicity.
Adults: 800 mg once daily

Dosage Forms
Tablet, oral:
Votrient™: 200 mg

pazopanib hydrochloride *see* pazopanib *on page 730*
PCC *see* factor IX complex (human) *on page 389*
PCE® [US/Can] *see* erythromycin (systemic) *on page 361*
PCEC *see* rabies vaccine *on page 825*
P Chlor GG [US] *see* chlorpheniramine, phenylephrine, and guaifenesin *on page 212*
PCM Allergy *(Discontinued)* *see* chlorpheniramine, phenylephrine, and methscopolamine *on page 212*
PCM *(Discontinued)* *see* chlorpheniramine, phenylephrine, and methscopolamine *on page 212*
PCV *see* pneumococcal conjugate vaccine (7-valent) *on page 771*
PCV-7 *see* pneumococcal conjugate vaccine (7-valent) *on page 771*
PCV-13 *see* pneumococcal conjugate vaccine (13-valent) *on page 770*
PCV13-CRM(197) *see* pneumococcal conjugate vaccine (13-valent) *on page 770*
PD-Cof [US] *see* chlorpheniramine, phenylephrine, and dextromethorphan *on page 211*
PD-Hist-D [US] *see* chlorpheniramine and phenylephrine *on page 208*
PDX *see* pralatrexate *on page 785*
pectin, gelatin, and methylcellulose *see* gelatin, pectin, and methylcellulose *on page 440*
Pedameth® *(Discontinued)*
PediaCare® Children's Decongestant [US-OTC] *see* phenylephrine (systemic) *on page 751*
PediaCare® Children's Long-Acting Cough [US-OTC] *see* dextromethorphan *on page 287*
Pediacare® Children's Long Acting Cough Plus Cold *(Discontinued)* *see* pseudoephedrine and dextromethorphan *on page 812*
PediaCare® Children's Medicated Freezer Pops Long Acting Cough *(Discontinued)* *see* dextromethorphan *on page 287*
PediaCare® Children's Allergy [US-OTC] *see* diphenhydramine (systemic) *on page 310*
PediaCare® Children's Multi-Symptom Cold [US-OTC] *see* dextromethorphan and phenylephrine *on page 289*
PediaCare® Children's NightTime Cough [US-OTC] *see* diphenhydramine (systemic) *on page 310*
PediaCare® Cold and Allergy *(Discontinued)* *see* chlorpheniramine and pseudoephedrine *on page 209*
PediaCare® Decongestant Infants *(Discontinued)* *see* pseudoephedrine *on page 810*

Pediacare® Infants' Decongestant & Cough ***(Discontinued)*** *see* pseudoephedrine and dextromethorphan *on page* *812*

PediaCare® Infants' Long-Acting Cough ***(Discontinued)*** *see* dextromethorphan *on page* *287*

PediaCare® Multi-Symptom Cold ***(Discontinued)*** *see* chlorpheniramine, pseudoephedrine, and dextromethorphan *on page* *214*

PediaCare® NightRest Cough and Cold ***(Discontinued)*** *see* chlorpheniramine, pseudoephedrine, and dextromethorphan *on page* *214*

Pediacel® [Can] *see* diphtheria and tetanus toxoids, acellular pertussis, poliovirus and *Haemophilus* b conjugate vaccine *on page* *314*

Pediacof® ***(Discontinued)***

Pediaflor® ***(Discontinued)*** *see* fluoride *on page* *413*

PediaHist DM [US] *see* brompheniramine, pseudoephedrine, and dextromethorphan *on page* *149*

Pedialyte® [US-OTC] *see* nutritional formula, enteral/oral *on page* *692*

PediaPatch Transdermal Patch ***(Discontinued)*** *see* salicylic acid *on page* *858*

Pediapred® [US/Can] *see* prednisolone (systemic) *on page* *790*

Pedia-Profen™ ***(Discontinued)*** *see* ibuprofen *on page* *494*

Pedia Relief™ [US-OTC] *see* chlorpheniramine, pseudoephedrine, and dextromethorphan *on page* *214*

Pedia Relief Cough and Cold [US-OTC] *see* pseudoephedrine and dextromethorphan *on page* *812*

Pedia Relief Infants [US-OTC] *see* pseudoephedrine and dextromethorphan *on page* *812*

Pediarix® [US/Can] *see* diphtheria, tetanus toxoids, acellular pertussis, hepatitis B (recombinant), and poliovirus (inactivated) vaccine *on page* *315*

PediaTan™ D [US] *see* chlorpheniramine and phenylephrine *on page* *208*

PediaTan™ ***(Discontinued)*** *see* chlorpheniramine *on page* *207*

Pediatex™ 12 ***(Discontinued)*** *see* carbinoxamine *on page* *182*

Pediatex™-D ***(Discontinued)***

Pediatex™ ***(Discontinued)*** *see* carbinoxamine *on page* *182*

Pediatex™ DM ***(Discontinued)***

Pediatex® TD [US] *see* triprolidine and pseudoephedrine *on page* *961*

Pediatric Digoxin CSD [Can] *see* digoxin *on page* *302*

Pediatric Triban® ***(Discontinued)***

Pediatrix [Can] *see* acetaminophen *on page* *21*

Pediazole® [Can] *see* erythromycin and sulfisoxazole *on page* *363*

Pediazole® ***(Discontinued)*** *see* erythromycin and sulfisoxazole *on page* *363*

Pedi-Boro® [US-OTC] *see* aluminum sulfate and calcium acetate *on page* *60*

Pedi-Dri® [US] *see* nystatin (topical) *on page* *693*

PediOtic® ***(Discontinued)*** *see* neomycin, polymyxin B, and hydrocortisone *on page* *667*

Pedi-Pro® [US] *see* benzalkonium chloride *on page* *124*

PedvaxHIB® [US/Can] *see* *Haemophilus* B conjugate vaccine *on page* *463*

PEG *see* polyethylene glycol 3350 *on page* *775*

PEG-L-asparaginase *see* pegaspargase *on page* *732*

pegademase (bovine) (peg A de mase BOE vine)

U.S./Canadian Brand Names Adagen® [US/Can]

Therapeutic Category Enzyme

Use Enzyme replacement therapy for adenosine deaminase (ADA) deficiency in patients with severe combined immunodeficiency disease (SCID) who are not candidates for or who have failed bone marrow transplant

Dosage Summary

I.M.:

Children: First dose: 10 units/kg; Second dose: 15 units/kg 7 days after first dose; Third dose: 20 units/kg 7 days after second dose; Maintenance: 20 units/kg/week (maximum: 30 units/kg/week)

Adults: Dosage not established

Dosage Forms

Injection, solution [preservative free]:

Adagen®: 250 units/mL (1.5 mL)

Peganone® [US/Can] *see* ethotoin *on page* 382

pegaptanib (peg AP ta nib)

Synonyms EYE001; pegaptanib sodium

U.S./Canadian Brand Names Macugen® [US/Can]

Therapeutic Category Ophthalmic Agent; Vaccine, Recombinant

Use Treatment of neovascular (wet) age-related macular degeneration (AMD)

Dosage Summary

Intravitreous:

Children: Dosage not established
Adults: 0.3 mg into affected eye every 6 weeks

Dosage Forms

Injection, solution [preservative free]:
Macugen®: 0.3 mg/0.09 mL (0.09 mL)

pegaptanib sodium *see* pegaptanib *on page* 732
PEG-ASP *see* pegaspargase *on page* 732
PEG-asparaginase *see* pegaspargase *on page* 732

pegaspargase (peg AS par jase)

Sound-Alike/Look-Alike Issues

pegaspargase may be confused with asparaginase
Oncaspar® may be confused with Elspar®

Synonyms L-asparaginase with polyethylene glycol; PEG-ASP; PEG-asparaginase; PEG-L-asparaginase; PEGLA; polyethylene glycol-L-asparaginase

U.S./Canadian Brand Names Oncaspar® [US]

Therapeutic Category Antineoplastic Agent

Use Treatment of acute lymphocytic leukemia (ALL); treatment of ALL with previous hypersensitivity to native L-asparaginase

Dosage Summary

I.M.:

Children: 2500 units/m^2 every 14 days
Adults: 2500 units/m^2 every 14 days

I.V.:

Children: 2500 units/m^2 every 14 days
Adults: 2500 units/m^2 every 14 days

Dosage Forms

Injection, solution [preservative free]:
Oncaspar®: 750 int. units/mL (5 mL)

Pegasys® [US/Can] *see* peginterferon alfa-2a *on page* 733
Pegasys® RBV [Can] *see* peginterferon alfa-2a and ribavirin *(Canada only) on page* 733
Pegetron® [Can] *see* peginterferon alfa-2b and ribavirin *(Canada only) on page* 734
Pegetron® Redipen [Can] *see* peginterferon alfa-2b and ribavirin *(Canada only) on page* 734

pegfilgrastim (peg fil GRA stim)

Sound-Alike/Look-Alike Issues

Neulasta® may be confused with Neumega®, Neupogen®, and Lunesta®

Synonyms G-CSF (PEG conjugate); granulocyte colony stimulating factor (PEG conjugate); NSC-725961; pegylated G-CSF; SD/01

U.S./Canadian Brand Names Neulasta® [US/Can]

Therapeutic Category Colony-Stimulating Factor

Use To decrease the incidence of infection, by stimulation of granulocyte production, in patients with nonmyeloid malignancies receiving myelosuppressive therapy associated with a significant risk of febrile neutropenia

Dosage Summary

SubQ:

Children: 100 mcg/kg (maximum dose: 6 mg) once per chemotherapy cycle
Adolescents >45 kg: 6 mg once per chemotherapy cycle
Adults: 6 mg once per chemotherapy cycle

Dosage Forms

Injection, solution [preservative free]:

Neulasta®: 10 mg/mL (0.6 mL)

peginterferon alfa-2a (peg in ter FEER on AL fa too aye)

Synonyms interferon alfa-2a (PEG conjugate); pegylated interferon alfa-2a

U.S./Canadian Brand Names Pegasys® [US/Can]

Therapeutic Category Interferon

Use Treatment of chronic hepatitis C (CHC), alone or in combination with ribavirin, in patients with compensated liver disease and not previously treated with alfa interferons (includes patients with histological evidence of cirrhosis [Child-Pugh class A] and patients with clinically-stable HIV disease); treatment of patients with HBeAg positive and HBeAg negative chronic hepatitis B with compensated liver disease and evidence of viral replication and liver inflammation

Dosage Summary

SubQ:

Children: Dosage not established

Adults: 180 mcg once weekly

Dosage Forms

Injection, solution:

Pegasys®: 180 mcg/mL (1 mL); 180 mcg/0.5 mL (0.5 mL)

peginterferon alfa-2a and ribavirin *(Canada only)*

(peg in ter FEER on AL fa too aye & rye ba VYE rin)

Synonyms ribavirin and peginterferon alfa-2a

U.S./Canadian Brand Names Pegasys® RBV [Can]

Therapeutic Category Antiviral Agent; Interferon

Use Combination therapy for the treatment of chronic hepatitis C (HCV) in patients without cirrhosis and patients with compensated cirrhosis; includes patients coinfected with stable HIV disease

Dosage Forms - Canada

Combination package:

Pegasys RBV® [1-week package]:

Tablet, oral: Ribavirin 200 mg (28s)
Injection, solution: Peginterferon alfa-2a: 180 mcg/0.5 mL (0.5 mL) (1s)

Tablet, oral: Ribavirin 200 mg (35s)
Injection, solution: Peginterferon alfa-2a: 180 mcg/0.5 mL (0.5 mL) (1s)

Tablet, oral: Ribavirin 200 mg (42s)
Injection, solution: Peginterferon alfa-2a: 180 mcg/0.5 mL (0.5 mL) (1s

Pegasys RBV® [1-week package]:

Tablet, oral: Ribavirin 200 mg (28s)
Injection, solution: Peginterferon alfa-2a: 180 mcg/mL (1 mL) (1s)

Tablet, oral: Ribavirin 200 mg (35s)
Injection, solution: Peginterferon alfa-2a: 180 mcg/mL (1 mL) (1s)

Tablet, oral: Ribavirin 200 mg (42s)
Injection, solution: Peginterferon alfa-2a: 180 mcg/mL (1 mL) (1s)

Pegasys RBV® [4-week package]:

Tablet, oral: Ribavirin 200 mg (112s)
Injection, solution: Peginterferon alfa-2a: 180 mcg/0.5 mL (0.5 mL) (4s)

Tablet, oral: Ribavirin 200 mg (140s)
Injection, solution: Peginterferon alfa-2a: 180 mcg/0.5 mL (0.5 mL) (4s)

Tablet, oral: Ribavirin 200 mg (168s)
Injection, solution: Peginterferon alfa-2a: 180 mcg/0.5 mL (0.5 mL) (4s)

Tablet, oral: Ribavirin 200 mg (168s + 28s)
Injection, solution: Peginterferon alfa-2a: 180 mcg/0.5 mL (0.5 mL) (4s)

Pegasys RBV® [4-week package]:
Tablet, oral: Ribavirin 200 mg (112s)
Injection, solution: Peginterferon alfa-2a: 180 mcg/mL (1 mL) (4s)

Tablet, oral: Ribavirin 200 mg (140s)
Injection, solution: Peginterferon alfa-2a: 180 mcg/mL (1 mL) (4s)

Tablet, oral: Ribavirin 200 mg (168s)
Injection, solution: Peginterferon alfa-2a: 180 mcg/mL (1 mL) (4s)

peginterferon alfa-2b (peg in ter FEER on AL fa too bee)

Sound-Alike/Look-Alike Issues

peginterferon alfa-2b may be confused with interferon alfa-2a, interferon alfa-2b, interferon alfa-n3, peginterferon alfa-2a
PegIntron® may be confused with Intron® A

Synonyms interferon alfa-2b (PEG conjugate); pegylated interferon alfa-2b

U.S./Canadian Brand Names PegIntron® [US/Can]; PegIntron™ Redipen® [US]

Therapeutic Category Interferon

Use Treatment of chronic hepatitis C (in combination with ribavirin) in patients who have compensated liver disease; treatment of chronic hepatitis C (as monotherapy) in adult patients with compensated liver disease who have never received alfa interferons

Dosage Summary

SubQ:

Children <3 years: Dosage not established
Children ≥3 years: 60 mcg/m^2/week (in combination with ribavirin)
Adults: Peginterferon monotherapy: 1 mcg/kg/week
Adults ≤45 kg: 40 mcg once weekly
Adults 46-56 kg: 50 mcg once weekly
Adults 57-72 kg: 64 mcg once weekly
Adults 73-88 kg: 80 mcg once weekly
Adults 89-106 kg: 96 mcg once weekly
Adults 107-136 kg: 120 mcg once weekly
Adults 137-160 kg: 150 mcg once weekly
Adults: Combination therapy with ribavirin: 1.5 mcg/kg/week
Adults <40 kg: 50 mcg once weekly (with ribavirin 800 mg/day)
Adults 40-50 kg: 64 mcg once weekly (with ribavirin 800 mg/day)
Adults 51-60 kg: 80 mcg once weekly (with ribavirin 800 mg/day)
Adults 61-65 kg: 96 mcg once weekly (with ribavirin 800 mg/day)
Adults 66-75 kg: 96 mcg once weekly (with ribavirin 1000 mg/day)
Adults 76-80 kg: 120 mcg once weekly (with ribavirin 1000 mg/day)
Adults 81-85 kg: 120 mcg once weekly (with ribavirin 1200 mg/day)
Adults 86-105 kg: 150 mcg once weekly (with ribavirin 1200 mg/day)
Adults >105 kg: 1.5 mcg/kg once weekly (with ribavirin 1400 mg/day)

Dosage Forms

Injection, powder for reconstitution:
PegIntron®: 50 mcg, 80 mcg, 120 mcg, 150 mcg
PegIntron™ Redipen®: 50 mcg, 80 mcg, 120 mcg, 150 mcg

peginterferon alfa-2b and ribavirin *(Canada only)*

(peg in ter FEER on AL fa too bee & rye ba VYE rin)

Synonyms ribavirin and peginterferon alfa-2b

U.S./Canadian Brand Names Pegetron® Redipen [Can]; Pegetron® [Can]

Therapeutic Category Antiviral Agent; Interferon

Use Combination therapy for the treatment of chronic hepatitis C in patients with compensated liver disease

Dosage Summary

SubQ:

Peginterferon Alfa-2b:
Children: Dosage not established
Adults: 1.5 mcg/kg/week

Oral:

Ribavirin:

Children: Dosage not established

Adults ≤64 kg: 800 mg/day in 2 divided doses

Adults 64-84 kg: 1000 mg/day in 2 divided doses

Adults ≥85 kg: 1200 mg/day in 2 divided doses

Dosage Forms - Canada

Combination package:

Pegetron®:

Capsules: Ribavirin 200 mg (56s)

Injection, powder for reconstitution: Peginterferon alfa-2b: 50 mcg/0.5 mL

Pegetron®:

Capsules: Ribavirin 200 mg (56s)

Injection, powder for reconstitution: Peginterferon alfa-2b: 80 mcg/0.5 mL

Pegetron®:

Capsules: Ribavirin 200 mg (70s)

Injection, powder for reconstitution: Peginterferon alfa-2b: 100 mcg/0.5 mL

Pegetron®:

Capsules: Ribavirin 200 mg (70s)

Injection, powder for reconstitution: Peginterferon alfa-2b: 120 mcg/0.5 mL

Pegetron®:

Capsules: Ribavirin 200 mg (84s)

Injection, powder for reconstitution: Peginterferon alfa-2b: 150 mcg/0.5 mL

PegIntron® [US/Can] *see* peginterferon alfa-2b *on page 734*

PegIntron™ Redipen® [US] *see* peginterferon alfa-2b *on page 734*

PEGLA *see* pegaspargase *on page 732*

PegLyte® [Can] *see* polyethylene glycol-electrolyte solution *on page 775*

pegvisomant (peg VI soe mant)

Synonyms B2036-PEG

U.S./Canadian Brand Names Somavert® [US/Can]

Therapeutic Category Growth Hormone Receptor Antagonist

Use Treatment of acromegaly in patients resistant to or unable to tolerate other therapies

Dosage Summary

SubQ:

Children: Dosage not established

Adults: Initial loading dose: 40 mg; Maintenance: 10-30 mg/day (maximum: 30 mg/day). **Note:** Titration is recommended

Dosage Forms

Injection, powder for reconstitution:

Somavert®: 10 mg, 15 mg, 20 mg

pegylated DOXOrubicin liposomal *see* doxorubicin (liposomal) *on page 330*

pegylated G-CSF *see* pegfilgrastim *on page 732*

pegylated interferon alfa-2a *see* peginterferon alfa-2a *on page 733*

pegylated interferon alfa-2b *see* peginterferon alfa-2b *on page 734*

pegylated liposomal DOXOrubicin *see* doxorubicin (liposomal) *on page 330*

PE-Hist DM [US] *see* chlorpheniramine, phenylephrine, and dextromethorphan *on page 211*

pemetrexed (pem e TREKS ed)

Synonyms LY231514; pemetrexed disodium

U.S./Canadian Brand Names Alimta® [US/Can]

Therapeutic Category Antineoplastic Agent, Antimetabolite; Antineoplastic Agent, Antimetabolite (Antifolate)

Use Treatment of unresectable malignant pleural mesothelioma (in combination with cisplatin); treatment of locally advanced or metastatic nonsquamous nonsmall cell lung cancer (NSCLC; as initial treatment in combination with cisplatin, as single-agent maintenance treatment after 4 cycles of initial platinum-based double therapy, and single-agent treatment after prior chemotherapy)

Dosage Summary

I.V.:

Children: Dosage not established

Adults: 500 mg/m^2 on day 1 of each 21-day cycle

Dosage Forms

Injection, powder for reconstitution:

Alimta®: 500 mg

pemetrexed disodium *see* pemetrexed *on page 735*

pemirolast (pe MIR oh last)

U.S./Canadian Brand Names Alamast® [US/Can]

Therapeutic Category Mast Cell Stabilizer; Ophthalmic Agent, Miscellaneous

Use Prevention of itching of the eye due to allergic conjunctivitis

Dosage Summary

Ophthalmic:

Children ≤3 years: Dosage not established

Children >3 years: Instill 1-2 drops in affected eye(s) 4 times/day

Adults: Instill 1-2 drops in affected eye(s) 4 times/day

Dosage Forms

Solution, ophthalmic:

Alamast®: 0.1% (10 mL)

pemoline ***(Discontinued)***

penbutolol (pen BYOO toe lole)

Sound-Alike/Look-Alike Issues

Levatol® may be confused with Lipitor®

Synonyms penbutolol sulfate

U.S./Canadian Brand Names Levatol® [US/Can]

Therapeutic Category Beta-Adrenergic Blocker

Use Treatment of mild-to-moderate arterial hypertension

Dosage Summary

Oral:

Children: Dosage not established

Adults: Initial: 20 mg once daily; Maintenance: 10-40 mg once daily (maximum: 80 mg/day)

Dosage Forms

Tablet, oral:

Levatol®: 20 mg

penbutolol sulfate *see* penbutolol *on page 736*

penciclovir (pen SYE kloe veer)

Sound-Alike/Look-Alike Issues

Denavir® may be confused with indinavir

U.S./Canadian Brand Names Denavir® [US]

Therapeutic Category Antiviral Agent

Use Topical treatment of herpes simplex labialis (cold sores)

Dosage Summary

Topical:

Children <12 years: Dosage not established

Children ≥12 years: Apply every 2 hours during waking hours

Adults: Apply every 2 hours during waking hours

Dosage Forms

Cream, topical:

Denavir®: 1% (1.5 g)

Pendex [US] *see* guaifenesin and phenylephrine *on page 456*

Penetrex® ***(Discontinued)***

penicillamine (pen i SIL a meen)

Sound-Alike/Look-Alike Issues

penicillamine may be confused with penicillin

Synonyms D-3-mercaptovaline; D-penicillamine; β,β-dimethylcysteine

U.S./Canadian Brand Names Cuprimine® [US/Can]; Depen® [US/Can]

Therapeutic Category Chelating Agent

Use Treatment of Wilson disease, cystinuria; adjunctive treatment of rheumatoid arthritis

Dosage Summary

Oral:

Children (manufacturer labeling): 30 mg/kg/day in 4 divided doses

Adults: 125-4000 mg/day divided in 4 divided doses

Dosage Forms

Capsule, oral:

Cuprimine®: 250 mg

Tablet, oral:

Depen®: 250 mg

penicillin G benzathine (pen i SIL in jee BENZ a theen)

Sound-Alike/Look-Alike Issues

penicillin may be confused with penicillamine

Bicillin® may be confused with Wycillin®

Bicillin® C-R (penicillin G benzathine and penicillin G procaine) may be confused with Bicillin® L-A (penicillin G benzathine). Penicillin G benzathine is the only product currently approved for the treatment of syphilis. Administration of penicillin G benzathine and penicillin G procaine combination instead of Bicillin® L-A may result in inadequate treatment response.

Synonyms benzathine benzylpenicillin; benzathine penicillin G; benzylpenicillin benzathine

U.S./Canadian Brand Names Bicillin® L-A [US/Can]

Therapeutic Category Penicillin

Use Active against some gram-positive organisms, few gram-negative organisms such as *Neisseria gonorrhoeae*, and some anaerobes and spirochetes; used in the treatment of syphilis; used only for the treatment of mild to moderately-severe upper respiratory tract infections caused by organisms susceptible to low concentrations of penicillin G or for prophylaxis of infections caused by these organisms; primary and secondary prevention of rheumatic fever

Dosage Summary

I.M.:

Neonates >1200 g: 50,000 units/kg as a single dose

Children ≤27 kg: 600,000 units/dose; >27 kg: 1.2 million units/dose

Adults: 1.2-2.4 million units as a single dose

Dosage Forms

Injection, suspension:

Bicillin® L-A: 600,000 units/mL (1 mL, 2 mL, 4 mL)

penicillin G benzathine and penicillin G procaine

(pen i SIL in jee BENZ a theen & pen i SIL in jee PROE kane)

Sound-Alike/Look-Alike Issues

penicillin may be confused with penicillamine

Bicillin® may be confused with Wycillin®

Bicillin® C-R (penicillin G benzathine and penicillin G procaine) may be confused with Bicillin® L-A (penicillin G benzathine). Penicillin G benzathine is the only product currently approved for the treatment of syphilis. Administration of penicillin G benzathine and penicillin G procaine combination instead of Bicillin® L-A may result in inadequate treatment response.

Synonyms penicillin G procaine and benzathine combined

U.S./Canadian Brand Names Bicillin® C-R 900/300 [US]; Bicillin® C-R [US]

Therapeutic Category Penicillin

Use May be used in specific situations in the treatment of streptococcal infections; primary prevention of rheumatic fever

Dosage Summary

I.M.:

Children <14 kg: 600,000 units as a single dose
Children 14-27 kg: 900,000 units to 1.2 million units as a single dose
Children >27 kg: 2.4 million units as a single dose
Adults: 2.4 million units as a single dose

Dosage Forms

Injection, suspension [prefilled syringe]:

Bicillin® C-R: 1,200,000 units: Penicillin G benzathine 600,000 units and penicillin G procaine 600,000 units per 2 mL (2 mL)

Bicillin® C-R 900/300: 1,200,000 units: Penicillin G benzathine 900,000 units and penicillin G procaine 300,000 units per 2 mL (2 mL)

penicillin G (parenteral/aqueous) (pen i SIL in jee, pa REN ter al, AYE kwee us)

Sound-Alike/Look-Alike Issues

penicillin may be confused with penicillamine

Synonyms benzylpenicillin potassium; benzylpenicillin sodium; crystalline penicillin; penicillin G potassium; penicillin G sodium

U.S./Canadian Brand Names Crystapen® [Can]; Pfizerpen® [US]

Therapeutic Category Penicillin

Use Treatment of infections (including sepsis, pneumonia, pericarditis, endocarditis, meningitis, anthrax) caused by susceptible organisms; active against some gram-positive organisms, generally not *Staphylococcus aureus*; some gram-negative organisms such as *Neisseria gonorrhoeae*, and some anaerobes and spirochetes

Dosage Summary

I.M.:

Infants >1 month: 100,000-400,000 units/kg/day in divided doses every 4-6 hours (maximum: 24 million units/day)
Children: 100,000-400,000 units/kg/day in divided doses every 4-6 hours (maximum: 24 million units/day)
Adults: 2-30 million units/day in divided doses every 4-6 hours

I.V.:

Infants >1 month: 100,000-400,000 units/kg/day in divided doses every 4-6 hours (maximum: 24 million units/day)
Children: 100,000-400,000 units/kg/day in divided doses every 4-6 hours (maximum: 24 million units/day)
Adults: 2-30 million units/day in divided doses every 4-6 hours

Dosage Forms

Infusion, premixed iso-osmotic dextrose solution: 1 million units (50 mL); 2 million units (50 mL); 3 million units (50 mL)

Injection, powder for reconstitution: 5 million units, 20 million units

Pfizerpen®: 5 million units, 20 million units

penicillin G potassium *see* penicillin G (parenteral/aqueous) *on page 738*

penicillin G procaine (pen i SIL in jee PROE kane)

Sound-Alike/Look-Alike Issues

penicillin G procaine may be confused with penicillin V potassium
Wycillin® may be confused with Bicillin®

Synonyms APPG; aqueous procaine penicillin G; procaine benzylpenicillin; procaine penicillin G

U.S./Canadian Brand Names Pfizerpen-AS® [Can]; Wycillin® [Can]

Therapeutic Category Penicillin

Use Treatment of moderately-severe infections due to *Treponema pallidum* and other penicillin G-sensitive microorganisms that are susceptible to low, but prolonged serum penicillin concentrations; anthrax due to *Bacillus anthracis* (postexposure) to reduce the incidence or progression of disease following exposure to aerolized *Bacillus anthracis*

Dosage Summary

I.M.:

Children: 25,000-50,000 units/kg/day in divided doses 1-2 times/day; (maximum: 4.8 million units/day)
Adults: 0.6-4.8 million units/day in divided doses every 12-24 hours

Dosage Forms

Injection, suspension: 600,000 units/mL (1 mL, 2 mL)

penicillin G procaine and benzathine combined *see* penicillin G benzathine and penicillin G procaine *on page 737*

penicillin G sodium *see* penicillin G (parenteral/aqueous) *on page 738*

penicillin V potassium (pen i SIL in vee poe TASS ee um)

Sound-Alike/Look-Alike Issues

penicillin V procaine may be confused with penicillin G potassium

Synonyms pen VK; phenoxymethyl penicillin

U.S./Canadian Brand Names Apo-Pen VK® [Can]; Novo-Pen-VK [Can]; Nu-Pen-VK [Can]

Therapeutic Category Penicillin

Use Treatment of infections caused by susceptible organisms involving the respiratory tract, otitis media, sinusitis, skin, and urinary tract; prophylaxis in rheumatic fever

Dosage Summary

Oral:

Children <12 years: 25-50 mg/kg/day divided every 6-8 hours (maximum: 3 g/day)

Children ≥12 years: 125-500 mg every 6-8 hours

Adults: 125-500 mg every 6-8 hours

Dosage Forms

Powder for solution, oral: 125 mg/5 mL (100 mL, 200 mL); 250 mg/5 mL (100 mL, 200 mL)

Tablet, oral: 250 mg, 500 mg

Penlac® [US/Can] *see* ciclopirox *on page 221*

Pennsaid® [Can] *see* diclofenac (systemic) *on page 296*

Pennsaid® [US] *see* diclofenac (topical) *on page 297*

Pentacarinat® Injection *(Discontinued)* *see* pentamidine *on page 739*

Pentacel® [US/Can] *see* diphtheria and tetanus toxoids, acellular pertussis, poliovirus and *Haemophilus* b conjugate vaccine *on page 314*

pentahydrate *see* sodium thiosulfate *on page 888*

Pentam® 300 [US] *see* pentamidine *on page 739*

pentamidine (pen TAM I deen)

Synonyms pentamidine isethionate

U.S./Canadian Brand Names Nebupent® [US]; Pentam® 300 [US]

Therapeutic Category Antiprotozoal

Use Treatment and prevention of pneumonia caused by *Pneumocystis jiroveci* pneumonia (PCP)

Dosage Summary

I.M.:

Children: 4 mg/kg once daily for 14-21 days

Adults: 4 mg/kg once daily for 14-21 days

I.V.:

Children: 4 mg/kg once daily for 7-21 days **or** 3-4 mg/kg once daily for 21 days

Adults: 4 mg/kg once daily for 14-21 days or 3-4 mg once daily for 21 days

Inhalation:

Children <5 years: Dosage not established

Children ≥5 years: 300 mg/dose given every 4 weeks

Adults: 300 mg every 4 weeks

Dosage Forms

Injection, powder for reconstitution:

Pentam® 300: 300 mg

Powder for solution, for nebulization [preservative free]:

Nebupent®: 300 mg

pentamidine isethionate *see* pentamidine *on page 739*

Pentamycetin® [Can] *see* chloramphenicol *on page 203*

Pentasa® [US/Can] *see* mesalamine *on page 607*

pentasodium colistin methanesulfonate *see* colistimethate *on page 247*

Pentaspan® [US/Can] *see* pentastarch *on page 740*

pentastarch (PEN ta starch)

U.S./Canadian Brand Names Pentaspan® [US/Can]

Therapeutic Category Blood Modifiers

Use Orphan drug: Adjunct in leukapheresis to improve harvesting and increase yield of leukocytes by centrifugal means

Dosage Summary

Leukapheresis:

Children: Dosage not established

Adults: 250-700 mL to which citrate anticoagulant has been added is administered by adding to the input line of the centrifugation apparatus at a ratio of 1:8-1:13 to venous whole blood

Dosage Forms

Infusion, premixed in NS:

Pentaspan®: 10% (500 mL)

Penta-Triamterene HCTZ [Can] *see* hydrochlorothiazide and triamterene *on page 479*

pentavalent human-bovine reassortant rotavirus vaccine (PRV) *see* rotavirus vaccine *on page 854*

pentazocine (pen TAZ oh seen)

Synonyms pentazocine lactate

U.S./Canadian Brand Names Talwin® [US/Can]

Therapeutic Category Analgesic, Narcotic

Controlled Substance C-IV

Use Relief of moderate-to-severe pain; has also been used as a sedative prior to surgery and as a supplement to surgical anesthesia

Dosage Summary

I.M.:

Children <1 years: Dosage not established

Children 1-16 years: 0.5 mg/kg preoperatively

Adults: 30-60 mg every 3-4 hours (maximum: 360 mg/day; 60 mg/dose) **or** 30 mg once

Elderly: Use with caution; may be more sensitive to analgesic and sedative effects; decrease initial dose and monitor closely

I.V.:

Children: Dosage not established

Adults: 30 mg every 3-4 hours (maximum: 360 mg/day; 30 mg/dose) **or** 20 mg every 2-3 hours as needed (maximum total dose: 60 mg)

SubQ:

Children: Dosage not established

Adults: 30 mg every 3-4 hours (maximum: 360 mg/day; 60 mg/dose)

Dosage Forms

Injection, solution:

Talwin®: 30 mg/mL (1 mL, 10 mL)

pentazocine and acetaminophen (pen TAZ oh seen & a seet a MIN oh fen)

Synonyms acetaminophen and pentazocine; pentazocine hydrochloride and acetaminophen

Therapeutic Category Analgesic Combination (Opioid)

Controlled Substance C-IV

Use Relief of mild-to-moderate pain

Dosage Summary

Oral:

Children: Dosage not established

Adults: 1 caplet every 4 hours (maximum: 6 caplets/day)

Dosage Forms

Tablet: Pentazocine 25 mg and acetaminophen 650 mg

pentazocine and naloxone (pen TAZ oh seen & nal OKS one)

Synonyms naloxone hydrochloride and pentazocine; pentazocine hydrochloride and naloxone hydrochloride

Therapeutic Category Analgesic, Opioid

Controlled Substance C-IV

Use Relief of moderate-to-severe pain; indicated for oral use only

Dosage Summary

Oral:

Children <12 years: Dosage not established

Children ≥12 years: Based upon pentazocine: 50-100 mg every 3-4 hours; maximum: 600 mg/day

Adults: Based upon pentazocine: 50-100 mg every 3-4 hours; maximum: 600 mg/day

Dosage Forms

Tablet: Pentazocine 50 mg and naloxone 0.5 mg

pentazocine hydrochloride and acetaminophen *see* pentazocine and acetaminophen *on page 740*

pentazocine hydrochloride and naloxone hydrochloride *see* pentazocine and naloxone *on page 740*

pentazocine lactate *see* pentazocine *on page 740*

pentetate calcium trisodium *see* diethylene triamine penta-acetic acid *on page 300*

pentetate zinc trisodium *see* diethylene triamine penta-acetic acid *on page 300*

Penthrane® *(Discontinued)*

pentobarbital (pen toe BAR bi tal)

Sound-Alike/Look-Alike Issues

PENTobarbital may be confused with PHENobarbital

Nembutal® may be confused with Myambutol®

Synonyms pentobarbital sodium

Tall-Man **PENT**obarbital

U.S./Canadian Brand Names Nembutal® Sodium [Can]; Nembutal® [US]

Therapeutic Category Barbiturate

Controlled Substance C-II

Use Sedative/hypnotic; refractory status epilepticus

Dosage Summary

I.M.:

Children: 2-6 mg/kg (maximum: 100 mg/dose)

Adults: 150-200 mg

Elderly: Use not recommended

I.V.:

Children:

Hypnotic/sedative: 1-6 mg/kg

Refractory status epilepticus: Loading dose: 5-15 mg/kg; Maintenance infusion: 0.5-5 mg/kg/hour

Adults:

Hypnotic/sedative: 100 mg; may repeat (maximum total dose: 500 mg)

Refractory status epilepticus: Loading dose: 10-15 mg/kg; Maintenance infusion: 0.5-10 mg/kg/hour

Elderly: Use not recommended

Dosage Forms

Injection, solution:

Nembutal®: 50 mg/mL (20 mL, 50 mL)

pentobarbital sodium *see* pentobarbital *on page 741*

pentosan polysulfate sodium (PEN toe san pol i SUL fate SOW dee um)

Sound-Alike/Look-Alike Issues

pentosan may be confused with pentostatin

Elmiron® may be confused with Imuran®

Synonyms PPS

U.S./Canadian Brand Names Elmiron® [US/Can]

Therapeutic Category Analgesic, Urinary

Use Relief of bladder pain or discomfort due to interstitial cystitis

Dosage Summary

Oral:

Children <16 years: Dosage not established

Children ≥16 years: 100 mg 3 times/day
Adults: 100 mg 3 times/day

Dosage Forms

Capsule, oral:
Elmiron®: 100 mg

pentostatin (pen toe STAT in)

Sound-Alike/Look-Alike Issues
pentostatin may be confused with pentamidine, pentosan

Synonyms 2′-deoxycoformycin; co-vidarabine; dCF; deoxycoformycin; NSC-218321

U.S./Canadian Brand Names Nipent® [US/Can]

Therapeutic Category Antineoplastic Agent

Use Treatment of hairy cell leukemia

Dosage Summary

I.V.:
Children: Dosage not established
Adults: 4 mg/m^2 every 2 weeks

Dosage Forms

Injection, powder for reconstitution:
Nipent®: 10 mg
Injection, powder for reconstitution [preservative free]: 10 mg

Pentothal® [US/Can] *see* thiopental *on page 928*
Pentothal® Sodium Rectal Suspension *(Discontinued)* *see* thiopental *on page 928*

pentoxifylline (pen toks IF i lin)

Sound-Alike/Look-Alike Issues
pentoxifylline may be confused with tamoxifen
Trental® may be confused with Bentyl®, Tegretol®, Trandate®

Synonyms oxpentifylline

U.S./Canadian Brand Names Albert® Pentoxifylline [Can]; Apo-Pentoxifylline SR® [Can]; Nu-Pentoxifylline SR [Can]; ratio-Pentoxifylline [Can]; Trental® [US/Can]

Therapeutic Category Blood Viscosity Reducer Agent

Use Treatment of intermittent claudication on the basis of chronic occlusive arterial disease of the limbs; may improve function and symptoms, but not intended to replace more definitive therapy

Dosage Summary

Oral:
Children: Dosage not established
Adults: 400 mg 2-3 times/day with meals

Dosage Forms

Tablet, controlled release, oral:
Trental®: 400 mg
Tablet, extended release, oral: 400 mg

Pentoxil® *(Discontinued)* *see* pentoxifylline *on page 742*
Pentrax® [US-OTC] *see* coal tar *on page 242*
Pen.Vee® K *(Discontinued)* *see* penicillin V potassium *on page 739*
pen VK *see* penicillin V potassium *on page 739*
Pepcid® [US/Can] *see* famotidine *on page 390*
Pepcid® AC [US-OTC/Can] *see* famotidine *on page 390*
Pepcid® AC Maximum Strength [US-OTC] *see* famotidine *on page 390*
Pepcid® Complete® [US-OTC/Can] *see* famotidine, calcium carbonate, and magnesium hydroxide *on page 391*
Pepcid® I.V. [Can] *see* famotidine *on page 390*
Pepcid RPD® *(Discontinued)* *see* famotidine *on page 390*
Peptic Relief [US-OTC] *see* bismuth *on page 139*
Pepto-Bismol® [US-OTC] *see* bismuth *on page 139*
Pepto-Bismol® Maximum Strength [US-OTC] *see* bismuth *on page 139*
Pepto® Diarrhea Control *(Discontinued)* *see* loperamide *on page 573*

Pepto Relief [US-OTC] *see* bismuth *on page 139*

peramivir (pe RA mi veer)

Synonyms BCX-1812; RWJ-270201

Therapeutic Category Antiviral Agent; Neuraminidase Inhibitor

Dosage Summary

I.V.:

Infants ≤30 days of age: 6 mg/kg once daily
Infants 31-90 days: 8 mg/kg once daily
Infants 91-180 days: 10 mg/kg once daily
Infants >180 days to Children ≤5 years: 12 mg/kg once daily
Children 6-17 years: 10 mg/kg once daily
Adults: 600 mg once daily

Dosage Forms

Injection, solution: 10 mg/mL (20 mL)

Peranex™ HC [US] *see* lidocaine and hydrocortisone *on page 564*
Peranex™ HC Medi-Pad [US] *see* lidocaine and hydrocortisone *on page 564*
Perchloracap® *(Discontinued)*
Percocet® [US/Can] *see* oxycodone and acetaminophen *on page 715*
Percocet®-Demi [Can] *see* oxycodone and acetaminophen *on page 715*
Percodan® [US/Can] *see* oxycodone and aspirin *on page 716*
Percodan®-Demi *(Discontinued)* *see* oxycodone and aspirin *on page 716*
Percogesic® *(Discontinued)* *see* acetaminophen and phenyltoloxamine *on page 26*
Percogesic® Extra Strength [US-OTC] *see* acetaminophen and diphenhydramine *on page 24*
Percolone® *(Discontinued)* *see* oxycodone *on page 714*
Perdiem® Overnight Relief [US-OTC] *see* senna *on page 870*
Perfectoderm® Gel *(Discontinued)* *see* benzoyl peroxide *on page 128*

perflutren lipid microspheres (per FLOO tren LIP id MIKE roe sfeers)

U.S./Canadian Brand Names Definity® [US/Can]

Therapeutic Category Diagnostic Agent

Use Opacification of left ventricular chamber and improvement of delineation of the left ventricular endocardial border in patients with suboptimal echocardiograms

Dosage Summary

I.V.: Note: Maximum dose is either two I.V. bolus doses or one single I.V. infusion.

Children: Dosage not established
Adults: Bolus: 10 microliters (µL)/kg of activated product, followed by 10 mL saline flush; may repeat in 30 minutes if needed. Infusion: Initial: 4 mL/minute (or 240 mL/hour) of prepared infusion; titrate to achieve optimal image; maximum rate: 10 mL/minute (or 600 mL/hour)

Dosage Forms

Injection, solution [preservative free]:
Definity®: OFP 6.52 mg/mL and lipid blend 0.75 mg/mL (2 mL)

Perforomist™ [US] *see* formoterol *on page 425*
Pergonal® *(Discontinued)* *see* menotropins *on page 602*
Periactin® *(Discontinued)* *see* cyproheptadine *on page 261*

periciazine *(Canada only)* (per ee CYE ah zeen)

Synonyms pericyazine

U.S./Canadian Brand Names Neuleptil® [Can]

Therapeutic Category Phenothiazine Derivative

Use Adjunctive therapy in selected psychotic patients to control prevailing hostility, impulsivity, or aggression

Dosage Summary

Oral:

Children ≤5 years: Dosage not established
Children >5 years: 2.5-10 mg in the morning, followed by 5-30 mg in the evening
Adults: 5-20 mg in the morning, followed by 10-40 mg in the evening
Elderly: Initial: 5 mg/day

Dosage Forms - Canada

Capsule:

Neuleptil®: 5 mg, 10 mg, 20 mg

Solution, oral drops:

Neuleptil®: 10 mg/mL

Peri-Colace® [US-OTC] *see* docusate and senna *on page* 322

pericyazine *see* periciazine *(Canada only) on page* 743

Peridex® [US] *see* chlorhexidine gluconate *on page* 204

Peridex® Oral Rinse [Can] *see* chlorhexidine gluconate *on page* 204

Peridol [Can] *see* haloperidol *on page* 465

perindopril and indapamide *see* perindopril erbumine and indapamide *(Canada only) on page* 744

perindopril erbumine (per IN doe pril er BYOO meen)

U.S./Canadian Brand Names Aceon® [US]; Apo-Perindopril® [Can]; Coversyl® [Can]

Therapeutic Category Miscellaneous Product

Use Treatment of hypertension; reduction of cardiovascular mortality or nonfatal myocardial infarction in patients with stable coronary artery disease

Dosage Summary

Oral:

Children: Dosage not established

Adults: Initial: 2-4 mg once daily; Maintenance: 4-8 mg/day in 1-2 divided doses (maximum: 16 mg/day)

Elderly >65 to 70 years: Initial: 4 mg/day; Maintenance: 8 mg/day

Elderly >70 years: Initial: 2-4 mg/day; Maintenance: 8 mg/day

Dosage Forms

Tablet, oral: 2 mg, 4 mg, 8 mg

Aceon®: 2 mg, 4 mg, 8 mg

perindopril erbumine and indapamide *(Canada only)*

(per IN doe pril er BYOO meen & in DAP a mide)

Synonyms indapamide and perindopril erbumine; perindopril and indapamide

U.S./Canadian Brand Names Coversyl® Plus [Can]

Therapeutic Category Angiotensin-Converting Enzyme (ACE) Inhibitor; Antihypertensive Agent, Combination; Diuretic, Thiazide-Related

Use Treatment of hypertension; not indicated for initial treatment of hypertension

Dosage Summary

Oral:

Children: Dosage not established

Adults: Perindopril 4 mg/indapamide 1.25 mg once daily

Dosage Forms - Canada

Tablet:

Coversyl® Plus: Perindopril erbumine 4 mg and indapamide 1.25 mg

PerioChip® [US] *see* chlorhexidine gluconate *on page* 204

PerioGard® [US-OTC] *see* chlorhexidine gluconate *on page* 204

PerioMed™ [US] *see* fluoride *on page* 413

Periostat® [US/Can] *see* doxycycline *on page* 331

Perlane® [US] *see* hyaluronate and derivatives *on page* 475

permethrin (per METH rin)

U.S./Canadian Brand Names A200® Lice [US-OTC]; Acticin® [US]; Elimite® [US]; Kwellada-P™ [Can]; Nix® Complete Lice Treatment System [US-OTC]; Nix® Creme Rinse Lice Treatment [US-OTC]; Nix® Creme Rinse [US-OTC]; Nix® Lice Control Spray [US-OTC]; Nix® [Can]; Rid® [US-OTC]

Therapeutic Category Scabicides/Pediculicides

Use Single-application treatment of infestation with *Pediculus humanus capitis* (head louse) and its nits or *Sarcoptes scabiei* (scabies); indicated for prophylactic use during epidemics of lice

Dosage Summary

Topical:

Cream:

Neonates: 5% cream was shown to be safe and effective when applied to an infant <1 month of age with neonatal scabies; time of application was limited to 6 hours before rinsing with soap and water

Children: Apply from head to toe, leave on 8-14 hours before washing off with water; May reapply in 1 week if live mites appear

Adults: Apply from head to toe, leave on 8-14 hours before washing off with water; May reapply in 1 week if live mites appear

Liquid (lotion or cream rinse):

Children ≤2 months: Dosage not established

Children >2 months: Apply a sufficient volume to saturate the hair and scalp, leave on for 10 minutes before rinsing off with water; May reapply in 1 week if lice or nits still present

Adults: Apply a sufficient volume to saturate the hair and scalp, leave on for 10 minutes before rinsing off with water; May reapply in 1 week if lice or nits still present

Dosage Forms

Cream, topical: 5% (60 g)

Acticin®: 5% (60 g)

Elimite®: 5% (60 g)

Liquid, topical:

Nix® Complete Lice Treatment System [OTC]: 1% (1s)

Nix® Creme Rinse [OTC]: 1% (60 mL)

Nix® Creme Rinse Lice Treatment [OTC]: 1% (60 mL)

Nix® Lice Control Spray [OTC]: 0.25% (150 mL)

Lotion, topical: 1% (60 mL)

Solution, topical:

A200® Lice [OTC]: 0.5% (170.1 g)

Rid® [OTC]: 0.5% (150 mL)

Permitil® Oral *(Discontinued)* *see* fluphenazine *on page* 417

Peroxin A5® *(Discontinued)* *see* benzoyl peroxide *on page* 128

Peroxin A10® *(Discontinued)* *see* benzoyl peroxide *on page* 128

perphenazine (per FEN a zeen)

Sound-Alike/Look-Alike Issues

Trilafon® may be confused with Tri-Levlen®

U.S./Canadian Brand Names Apo-Perphenazine® [Can]

Therapeutic Category Phenothiazine Derivative

Use Treatment of schizophrenia; severe nausea and vomiting

Dosage Summary

Oral:

Children: Dosage not established

Adults: 4-16 mg 2-4 times/day (maximum: 64 mg/day; exceptions occur [indication specific])

Dosage Forms

Tablet, oral: 2 mg, 4 mg, 8 mg, 16 mg

perphenazine and amitriptyline hydrochloride *see* amitriptyline and perphenazine *on page* 68

Persa-Gel® *(Discontinued)* *see* benzoyl peroxide *on page* 128

Persantine® [US/Can] *see* dipyridamole *on page* 318

Pertussin® CS *(Discontinued)* *see* dextromethorphan *on page* 287

Pertussin® ES *(Discontinued)* *see* dextromethorphan *on page* 287

pertussis, acellular (adsorbed) *see* diphtheria and tetanus toxoids, acellular pertussis, poliovirus and *Haemophilus* b conjugate vaccine *on page* 314

pethidine hydrochloride *see* meperidine *on page* 603

Pexeva® [US] *see* paroxetine *on page* 729

PFA *see* foscarnet *on page* 427

Pfizerpen® [US] *see* penicillin G (parenteral/aqueous) *on page* 738

Pfizerpen-AS® [Can] *see* penicillin G procaine *on page* 738

PGE_1 *see* alprostadil *on page* 55

PGE_2 *see* dinoprostone *on page* 308

PGI_2 *see* epoprostenol *on page 357*
PGX *see* epoprostenol *on page 357*
Phanasin® Diabetic Choice *(Discontinued)* *see* guaifenesin *on page 454*
Phanasin® *(Discontinued)* *see* guaifenesin *on page 454*
Phanatuss® DM *(Discontinued)* *see* guaifenesin and dextromethorphan *on page 455*
Phanatuss® HC *(Discontinued)*
Pharmaflur® 1.1 *(Discontinued)* *see* fluoride *on page 413*
Pharmaflur® *(Discontinued)* *see* fluoride *on page 413*
Pharmorubicin® [Can] *see* epirubicin *on page 355*
Phazyme™ [Can] *see* simethicone *on page 875*
Phazyme® *(Discontinued)* *see* simethicone *on page 875*
Phazyme® Ultra Strength [US-OTC] *see* simethicone *on page 875*
Phenabid® [US] *see* chlorpheniramine and phenylephrine *on page 208*
Phenabid DM® [US] *see* chlorpheniramine, phenylephrine, and dextromethorphan *on page 211*
Phenadex® Senior *(Discontinued)* *see* guaifenesin and dextromethorphan *on page 455*
Phenadoz® [US] *see* promethazine *on page 800*
Phenagesic [US-OTC] *see* acetaminophen and phenyltoloxamine *on page 26*
Phenameth® DM *(Discontinued)* *see* promethazine and dextromethorphan *on page 801*
Phenaphen® *(Discontinued)* *see* acetaminophen *on page 21*
Phenaseptic [US-OTC] *see* phenol *on page 748*
PhenaVent™ D *(Discontinued)* *see* guaifenesin and phenylephrine *on page 456*
PhenaVent™ *(Discontinued)* *see* guaifenesin and phenylephrine *on page 456*
PhenaVent™ LA *(Discontinued)* *see* guaifenesin and phenylephrine *on page 456*
PhenaVent™ Ped *(Discontinued)* *see* guaifenesin and phenylephrine *on page 456*
Phenazine® Injection *(Discontinued)* *see* promethazine *on page 800*
Phenazo™ [Can] *see* phenazopyridine *on page 746*

phenazopyridine (fen az oh PEER i deen)

Sound-Alike/Look-Alike Issues
phenazopyridine may be confused with phenoxybenzamine
Pyridium® may be confused with Dyrenium®, Perdiem®, pyridoxine, pyrithione

Synonyms phenazopyridine hydrochloride; phenylazo diamino pyridine hydrochloride

U.S./Canadian Brand Names AZO Standard® Maximum Strength [US-OTC]; AZO Standard® [US-OTC]; Azo-Gesic™ [US-OTC]; Baridium [US-OTC]; Phenazo™ [Can]; Pyridium® [US]; ReAzo [US-OTC]; UTI Relief® [US-OTC]

Therapeutic Category Analgesic, Urinary

Use Symptomatic relief of urinary burning, itching, frequency, and urgency in association with urinary tract infection or following urologic procedures

Dosage Summary
Oral:
Children: 12 mg/kg/day in 3 divided doses after meals
Adults: 100-200 mg 3 times/day after meals

Dosage Forms
Tablet, oral: 100 mg, 200 mg
AZO Standard® [OTC]: 95 mg
AZO Standard® Maximum Strength [OTC]: 97.5 mg
Azo-Gesic™ [OTC]: 95 mg
Baridium [OTC]: 97.2 mg
Pyridium®: 100 mg, 200 mg
ReAzo [OTC]: 95 mg
UTI Relief® [OTC]: 97.2 mg

phenazopyridine hydrochloride *see* phenazopyridine *on page 746*
Phencarb GG [US] *see* carbetapentane, guaifenesin, and phenylephrine *on page 180*

phendimetrazine (fen dye ME tra zeen)

Sound-Alike/Look-Alike Issues
Bontril® PDM may be confused with Bentyl®

Synonyms phendimetrazine tartrate

U.S./Canadian Brand Names Bontril® PDM [US]; Bontril® Slow-Release [US]; Bontril® [Can]; Plegine® [Can]; Statobex® [Can]

Therapeutic Category Anorexiant

Controlled Substance C-III

Use Short-term (few weeks) adjunct in exogenous obesity

Dosage Summary

Oral:

Capsule:

Children: Dosage not established

Adults: 105 mg once daily before breakfast

Tablet:

Children: Dosage not established

Adults: 17.5-35 mg 2 or 3 times daily, 1 hour before meals (maximum: 70 mg 3 times/day)

Dosage Forms

Capsule, slow release, oral: 105 mg

Bontril® Slow-Release: 105 mg

Tablet, oral: 35 mg

Bontril® PDM: 35 mg

phendimetrazine tartrate *see* phendimetrazine *on page* 747

Phendry® Oral *(Discontinued)* *see* diphenhydramine (systemic) *on page* 310

phenelzine (FEN el zeen)

Sound-Alike/Look-Alike Issues
phenelzine may be confused with phenytoin
Nardil® may be confused with Norinyl®

Synonyms phenelzine sulfate

U.S./Canadian Brand Names Nardil® [US/Can]

Therapeutic Category Antidepressant, Monoamine Oxidase Inhibitor

Use Symptomatic treatment of atypical, nonendogenous, or neurotic depression

Dosage Summary

Oral:

Adults: 45-90 mg/day in 3 divided doses; **Note:** Titration is recommended

Elderly: Initial: 7.5 mg/day; Maintenance: 15-60 mg/day in 3-4 divided doses; **Note:** Titrations is recommended

Dosage Forms

Tablet, oral:

Nardil®: 15 mg

phenelzine sulfate *see* phenelzine *on page* 747

Phenerbel-S® *(Discontinued)*

Phenergan® [US/Can] *see* promethazine *on page* 800

Phenergan® VC With Codeine *(Discontinued)* *see* promethazine, phenylephrine, and codeine *on page* 802

Phenergan® With Dextromethorphan *(Discontinued)* *see* promethazine and dextromethorphan *on page* 801

pheniramine and naphazoline *see* naphazoline and pheniramine *on page* 659

phenobarbital (fee noe BAR bi tal)

Sound-Alike/Look-Alike Issues
PHENobarbital may be confused with PENTobarbital, Phenergan®, phenytoin
Luminal® may be confused with Tuinal®

Synonyms phenobarbital sodium; phenobarbitone; phenylethylmalonylurea

Tall-Man PHENobarbital

U.S./Canadian Brand Names PMS-Phenobarbital [Can]

Therapeutic Category Anticonvulsant; Barbiturate

Controlled Substance C-IV

Use Management of generalized tonic-clonic (grand mal), status epilepticus, and partial seizures; sedative/hypnotic

Dosage Summary

I.M.:

Children: 3-5 mg/kg at bedtime or 1-3 mg/kg 1-1.5 hours before procedure

Adults: 30-120 mg/day in 2-3 divided doses **or** 100-320 mg at bedtime **or** 100-200 mg 1-1.5 hours before procedure

I.V.:

Infants: Loading dose: 10-20 mg/kg in a single or divided dose; Maintenance: 5-8 mg/kg/day in 1-2 divided doses

Children 1-5 years: Loading dose: 15-20 mg/kg in a single or divided dose; Maintenance: 6-8 mg/kg/day in 1-2 divided doses **or** 1-3 mg/kg 1-1.5 hours before procedure **or** 3-5 mg/kg at bedtime

Children 5-12 years: Loading dose: 15-20 mg/kg in a single or divided dose; Maintenance: 4-6 mg/kg/day in 1-2 divided doses **or** 1-3 mg/kg 1-1.5 hours before procedure **or** 3-5 mg/kg at bedtime

Children >12 years: Loading dose: 15-20 mg/kg in a single or divided dose; Maintenance: 1-3 mg/kg/day in divided doses **or** 50-100 mg 2-3 times/day **or** 1-3 mg/kg 1-1.5 hours before procedure **or** 3-5 mg/kg at bedtime

Adults: Loading dose: 10-20 mg/kg; may repeat dose in 20-minute intervals as needed (maximum total dose: 30 mg/kg); Maintenance: 1-3 mg/kg/day in divided doses **or** 50-100 mg 2-3 times/day **or** 100-320 mg at bedtime

Oral:

Infants: 5-8 mg/kg/day in 1-2 divided doses

Children 1-5 years: 6-8 mg/kg/day in 1-2 divided doses **or** 2 mg/kg 3 times/day **or** 1-3 mg/kg 1-1.5 hours before procedure

Children 5-12 years: 4-6 mg/kg/day in 1-2 divided doses **or** 2 mg/kg 3 times/day **or** 1-3 mg/kg 1-1.5 hours before procedure

Children >12 years: 1-3 mg/kg/day in divided doses **or** 50-100 mg 2-3 times/day **or** 2 mg/kg 3 times/day **or** 1-3 mg/kg 1-1.5 hours before procedure

Adults: 1-3 mg/kg/day in divided doses **or** 50-100 mg 2-3 times/day **or** 100-320 mg at bedtime **or** 30-120 mg/day in 2-3 divided doses

Dosage Forms

Elixir, oral: 20 mg/5 mL (5 mL, 7.5 mL, 15 mL)

Injection, solution: 65 mg/mL (1 mL); 130 mg/mL (1 mL)

Tablet, oral: 15 mg, 30 mg, 60 mg, 100 mg

phenobarbital, hyoscyamine, atropine, and scopolamine *see* hyoscyamine, atropine, scopolamine, and phenobarbital *on page 492*

phenobarbital sodium *see* phenobarbital *on page 747*

phenobarbitone *see* phenobarbital *on page 747*

phenol (FEE nol)

Sound-Alike/Look-Alike Issues

Cēpastat® may be confused with Capastat®

Synonyms carbolic acid

U.S./Canadian Brand Names Castellani Paint Modified [US-OTC]; Cepastat® Extra Strength [US-OTC]; Cepastat® [US-OTC]; Cheracol® Spray [US-OTC]; Chloraseptic® Kids Sore Throat Spray [US-OTC]; Chloraseptic® Mouth Pain [US-OTC]; Chloraseptic® Sore Throat Gargle [US-OTC]; Chloraseptic® Sore Throat Spray [US-OTC]; P & S™ Liquid Phenol [Can]; Pain-A-Lay® [US-OTC]; Phenaseptic [US-OTC]; Phenol EZ® [US-OTC]; Ulcerease® [US-OTC]; Vicks® Formula 44® Sore Throat [US-OTC]

Therapeutic Category Pharmaceutical Aid

Use Relief of sore throat pain, mouth, gum, and throat irritations; antiseptic; topical anesthetic

Dosage Summary

Oral:

Children <2 years: Dosage not established

Children 2-12 years:

Chloraseptic®: Three sprays onto throat or affected area; may repeat every 2 hours

Chloraseptic® for Kids: Five sprays onto throat or affected area; may repeat every 2 hours

Children >3 years: (Ulcerease®): Gargle or swish for 15 seconds, then expectorate; may repeat every 2 hours

Children 6-12 years:

Cēpastat® Extra Strength: Up to 1 lozenge every 2 hours as needed (maximum: 10 lozenges/24 hours)

Cēpastat®: Up to 1 lozenge every 2 hours as needed (maximum: 18 lozenges/24 hours)

Pain-A-Lay® Gargle: Using gauze pad, apply 10 mL to affected area, or gargle or swish for 15 seconds, then expectorate

Children ≥12 years:

Cēpastat® Extra Strength, Cēpastat®: Up to 2 lozenges every 2 hours as needed

Cheracol®, Pain-A-Lay® Spray: Spray directly in throat; rinse for 15 seconds then expectorate; may repeat every 2 hours

Chloraseptic®: Five sprays onto throat or affected area; may repeat every 2 hours

Chloraseptic® Gargle, Cēpastat® Mouth Pain, Pain-A-Lay® Gargle, Ulcerease®: Gargle or swish for 15 seconds, then expectorate; may repeat every 2 hours

Adults:

Cēpastat® Extra Strength, Cēpastat®: Up to 2 lozenges every 2 hours as needed

Cheracol®, Pain-A-Lay® Spray: Spray directly in throat; rinse for 15 seconds then expectorate; may repeat every 2 hours

Chloraseptic®: Five sprays onto throat or affected area; may repeat every 2 hours

Chloraseptic® Gargle, Cēpastat® Mouth Pain, Pain-A-Lay® Gargle, Ulcerease®: Gargle or swish for 15 seconds, then expectorate; may repeat every 2 hours

Topical:

Children: Dosage not established

Adults: Apply small amount to affected area 1-3 times/day

Dosage Forms

Lozenge, oral:

Cepastat® [OTC]: 14.5 mg (18s)

Cepastat® Extra Strength [OTC]: 29 mg (18s)

Solution, oral: 1.4% (177 mL)

Cheracol® Spray [OTC]: 1.4% (177 mL)

Chloraseptic® Kids Sore Throat Spray [OTC]: 0.5% (177 mL)

Chloraseptic® Mouth Pain [OTC]: 1.4% (29 mL)

Chloraseptic® Sore Throat Gargle [OTC]: 1.4% (296 mL)

Chloraseptic® Sore Throat Spray [OTC]: 1.4% (20 mL, 177 mL)

Pain-A-Lay® [OTC]: 1.4% (177 mL, 236 mL, 532 mL)

Phenaseptic [OTC]: 1.4% (177 mL)

Ulcerease® [OTC]: 0.6% (30 mL, 180 mL)

Vicks® Formula 44® Sore Throat [OTC]: 1.4% (177 mL)

Solution, topical:

Castellani Paint Modified [OTC]: 1.5% (30 mL)

Swab, topical:

Phenol EZ® [OTC]: 89% (30s)

phenol and camphor *see* camphor and phenol *on page 173*

Phenol EZ® [US-OTC] *see* phenol *on page 748*

phenoptin *see* sapropterin *on page 864*

Phenoxine® ***(Discontinued)***

phenoxybenzamine (fen oks ee BEN za meen)

Sound-Alike/Look-Alike Issues

phenoxybenzamine may be confused with phenazopyridine

Synonyms phenoxybenzamine hydrochloride

U.S./Canadian Brand Names Dibenzyline® [US/Can]

Therapeutic Category Alpha-Adrenergic Blocking Agent

Use Symptomatic management of pheochromocytoma

Dosage Summary

Oral:

Adults: Initial: 10 mg twice daily; Maintenance: 10-40 mg 1-3 times/day (maximum: 240 mg/day)

Dosage Forms

Capsule, oral:

Dibenzyline®: 10 mg

phenoxybenzamine hydrochloride *see* phenoxybenzamine *on page 749*
phenoxymethyl penicillin *see* penicillin V potassium *on page 739*

phentermine (FEN ter meen)

Sound-Alike/Look-Alike Issues
phentermine may be confused with phentolamine, phenytoin

Synonyms phentermine hydrochloride

U.S./Canadian Brand Names Adipex-P® [US]

Therapeutic Category Anorexiant

Controlled Substance C-IV

Use Short-term (few weeks) adjunct therapy in obese patients with an initial body mass index (BMI) ≥30 kg/m^2 or ≥27 kg/m^2 in the presence of other risk factors (eg, diabetes, hyperlipidemia, hypertension)

Dosage Summary

Oral:

Children ≤16 years: Dosage not established
Children >16 years: 15-37.5 mg/ day
Adults: 15-37.5 mg/ day

Dosage Forms

Capsule, oral: 15 mg, 30 mg, 37.5 mg
Adipex-P®: 37.5 mg
Tablet, oral: 37.5 mg
Adipex-P®: 37.5 mg

phentermine hydrochloride *see* phentermine *on page 750*

phentolamine (fen TOLE a meen)

Sound-Alike/Look-Alike Issues
phentolamine may be confused with phentermine, Ventolin®

Synonyms phentolamine mesylate

U.S./Canadian Brand Names OraVerse™ [US]; Regitine® [Can]; Rogitine® [Can]

Therapeutic Category Alpha-Adrenergic Blocking Agent; Diagnostic Agent

Use Diagnosis of pheochromocytoma and treatment of hypertension associated with pheochromocytoma or other forms of hypertension caused by excess sympathomimetic amines; treatment of dermal necrosis after extravasation of drugs with alpha-adrenergic effects (ie, dopamine, epinephrine, norepinephrine, phenylephrine)

OraVerse™: Reversal of soft tissue anesthesia and the associated functional deficits resulting from a local dental anesthetic containing a vasoconstrictor

Dosage Summary

I.M.:

Children: 0.05-0.1 mg/kg/dose as a single dose 1-2 hours before procedure, repeat as needed every 2-4 hours (maximum: 5 mg/dose)
Adults: 5 mg as a single dose 1-2 hours before procedure, may repeat as needed every 2-4 hours

I.V.:

Children: 0.05-0.1 mg/kg/dose as a single dose 1-2 hours before procedure, repeat as needed every 2-4 hours (maximum: 5 mg/dose)
Adults: 5 mg as a single dose 1-2 hours before procedure, may repeat as needed every 2-4 hours **or** 5-20 mg (hypertensive crisis)

Submucosal injection:

Children <15 kg and <12 years: Dosage not established
Children 15-30 kg and <12 years: 0.2 mg (maximum)
Children >30 kg and <12 years: 0.4 mg (maximum)
Children >30 kg and ≥12 years: 0.2 mg to 0.8 mg (depending on number of cartridges of anesthesia)
Adults: 0.2 mg to 0.8 mg (depending on number of cartridges of anesthesia)

SubQ:

Children: Infiltrate area with a small amount (eg, 1 mL) of solution (made by diluting 5-10 mg in 10 mL of NS) within 12 hours of extravasation; maximum: 0.1-0.2 mg/kg (5 mg total)
Adults: Infiltrate area with a small amount (eg, 1 mL) of solution (made by diluting 5-10 mg in 10 mL of NS) within 12 hours of extravasation; in general, do not exceed 0.1-0.2 mg/kg (5 mg total); typically doses of ≤5 mg are effective; a case using 50 mg for a large extravasation has been reported.

Dosage Forms

Injection, powder for reconstitution: 5 mg

Injection, solution [preservative free]:

OraVerse™: 0.4 mg/1.7 mL (1.7 mL)

phentolamine mesylate *see* phentolamine *on page 750*

phenylalanine mustard *see* melphalan *on page 599*

phenylazo diamino pyridine hydrochloride *see* phenazopyridine *on page 746*

Phenyldrine® *(Discontinued)*

Phenylephrine CM [US] *see* chlorpheniramine, phenylephrine, and methscopolamine *on page 212*

phenylephrine (systemic) (fen il EF rin)

Sound-Alike/Look-Alike Issues

Neo-Synephrine® (phenylephrine) may be confused with Neo-Synephrine® (oxymetazoline)

Sudafed PE™ may be confused with Sudafed®

Synonyms phenylephrine hydrochloride

U.S./Canadian Brand Names LuSonal™ [US]; Medi-First® Sinus Decongestant [US-OTC]; Medi-Phenyl [US-OTC]; PediaCare® Children's Decongestant [US-OTC]; Sudafed PE® Children's [US-OTC]; Sudafed PE® Congestion [US-OTC]; Sudafed PE™ Nasal Decongestant [US-OTC]; Sudogest™ PE [US-OTC]; Triaminic Thin Strips® Children's Cold with Stuffy Nose [US-OTC]

Therapeutic Category Alpha/Beta Agonist

Use Treatment of hypotension, vascular failure in shock; as a vasoconstrictor in regional analgesia; supraventricular tachycardia (**Note:** Not for routine use in treatment of supraventricular tachycardias); as a decongestant [OTC]

Dosage Summary

I.V.:

Children: Bolus: 5-20 mcg/kg/dose every 10-15 minutes as needed; Infusion: 0.1-0.5 mcg/kg/minute

Adults: Bolus: 0.1-0.5 mg/dose every 10-15 minutes as needed (maximum: 0.5 mg); Infusion: Initial: 100-180 mcg/minute; **Note:** Titration is recommended

Oral:

Children 4 to <6 years: 2.5 mg every 4 hours as needed for ≤7 days

Children 6 to <12 years: 5 mg every 4 hours as needed for ≤7 days

Children ≥12 years and Adults: 10-20 mg every 4 hours as needed for ≤7 days

Dosage Forms

Injection, solution: 1% [10 mg/mL] (1 mL, 2 mL, 5 mL, 10 mL)

Liquid, oral:

LuSonal™: 7.5 mg/5 mL (473 mL)

PediaCare® Children's Decongestant [OTC]: 2.5 mg/5 mL (118 mL)

Sudafed PE® Children's [OTC]: 2.5 mg/5 mL (118 mL)

Strip, orally disintegrating, oral:

Triaminic Thin Strips® Children's Cold with Stuffy Nose [OTC]: 2.5 mg (14s)

Tablet, oral:

Medi-First® Sinus Decongestant [OTC]: 10 mg

Medi-Phenyl [OTC]: 5 mg

Sudafed PE® Congestion [OTC]: 10 mg

Sudafed PE™ Nasal Decongestant [OTC]: 10 mg

Sudogest™ PE [OTC]: 10 mg

phenylephrine (nasal) (fen il EF rin)

Synonyms phenylephrine hydrochloride

U.S./Canadian Brand Names 4 Way® Fast Acting [US-OTC]; 4 Way® Menthol [US-OTC]; Little Noses® Decongestant [US-OTC]; Neo-Synephrine® Extra Strength [US-OTC]; Neo-Synephrine® Mild Formula [US-OTC]; Neo-Synephrine® Regular Strength [US-OTC]; Neo-Synephrine® [Can]; Rhinall® [US-OTC]; Vicks® Sinex® VapoSpray™ 4 Hour Decongestant [US-OTC]

Therapeutic Category Alpha/Beta Agonist

Use For OTC use as symptomatic relief of nasal and nasopharyngeal mucosal congestion

Dosage Summary

Intranasal:

Children <2 years: Dosage not established

Children 2-6 years: 0.125% solution: Instill 1 drop in each nostril every 2-4 hours as needed for ≤3 days

Children 6-12 years: 0.25% solution: Instill 2-3 sprays in each nostril every 4 hours as needed for ≤3 days

Children >12 years: 0.25% to 0.5% solution: Instill 2-3 sprays or 2-3 drops in each nostril every 4 hours as needed for ≤3 days

Adults: 0.25% to 1% solution: Instill 2-3 sprays or 2-3 drops in each nostril every 4 hours as needed for ≤3 days

Dosage Forms

Solution, intranasal:

4 Way® Fast Acting [OTC]: 1% (15 mL, 30 mL, 37 mL)
4 Way® Menthol [OTC]: 1% (15 mL, 30 mL)
Little Noses® Decongestant [OTC]: 0.125% (15 mL)
Neo-Synephrine® Extra Strength [OTC]: 1% (15 mL)
Neo-Synephrine® Mild Formula [OTC]: 0.25% (15 mL)
Neo-Synephrine® Regular Strength [OTC]: 0.5% (15 mL)
Rhinall® [OTC]: 0.25% (30 mL, 40 mL)
Vicks® Sinex® VapoSpray™ 4 Hour Decongestant [OTC]: 0.5% (15 mL)

phenylephrine (ophthalmic) (fen il EF rin)

Sound-Alike/Look-Alike Issues

Mydfrin® may be confused with Midrin®

Synonyms phenylephrine hydrochloride

U.S./Canadian Brand Names AK-Dilate™ [US]; Altafrin [US]; Dionephrine® [Can]; Mydfrin® [US/Can]; Neofrin [US]; OcuNefrin™ [US-OTC]

Therapeutic Category Alpha/Beta Agonist; Ophthalmic Agent, Antiglaucoma; Ophthalmic Agent, Mydriatic

Use Used as a mydriatic in ophthalmic procedures and treatment of wide-angle glaucoma; OTC use as symptomatic relief of redness of the eye due to irritation

Dosage Summary

Ophthalmic:

Infants <1 year: Instill 1 drop of 2.5% solution 15-30 minutes before procedures

Children ≥1 year: Instill 1 drop of 2.5% or 10% solution; may repeat in 10-60 minutes as needed

Adults: Instill 1 drop of 2.5% or 10% solution; may repeat in 10-60 minutes as needed **or** 1-2 drops of 0.12% solution up to 4 times/day [OTC dosing] (maximum: 72 hours)

Dosage Forms

Solution, ophthalmic: 2.5% (2 mL, 3 mL, 5 mL, 15 mL)

AK-Dilate™: 2.5% (2 mL, 15 mL); 10% (5 mL)
Altafrin: 2.5% (15 mL); 10% (5 mL)
Mydfrin®: 2.5% (3 mL, 5 mL)
Neofrin: 2.5% (15 mL); 10% (5 mL)
OcuNefrin™ [OTC]: 0.12% (15 mL)

phenylephrine (topical) (fen il EF rin)

Synonyms phenylephrine hydrochloride

U.S./Canadian Brand Names Anu-Med [US-OTC]; Formulation R™ [US-OTC]; Medicone® Suppositories [US-OTC]; Preparation H® [US-OTC]; Rectacaine [US-OTC]; Tronolane® Suppository [US-OTC]

Therapeutic Category Alpha/Beta Agonist

Use For OTC use as treatment of hemorrhoids

Dosage Summary

Rectal:

Children ≤12 years: Dosage not established

Children >12 years: Ointment: Apply up to 4 times/day; Suppository: Insert 1 up to 4 times/day

Adults: Ointment: Apply up to 4 times/day; Suppository: Insert 1 up to 4 times/day

Dosage Forms

Ointment, rectal:

Formulation R™ [OTC]: 0.25% (30 g, 60 g)
Preparation H® [OTC]: 0.25% (30 g, 60 g)

Suppository, rectal: 0.25% (12s)
Anu-Med [OTC]: 0.25% (12s)
Medicone® Suppositories [OTC]: 0.25% (12s, 24s)
Preparation H® [OTC]: 0.25% (12s, 24s, 48s)
Rectacaine [OTC]: 0.25% (12s)
Tronolane® Suppository [OTC]: 0.25% (12s, 24s)

phenylephrine, acetaminophen, and dextromethorphan *see* acetaminophen, dextromethorphan, and phenylephrine *on page 29*
phenylephrine and brompheniramine *see* brompheniramine and phenylephrine *on page 148*
phenylephrine and chlorpheniramine *see* chlorpheniramine and phenylephrine *on page 208*
phenylephrine and cyclopentolate *see* cyclopentolate and phenylephrine *on page 259*
phenylephrine and dextromethorphan *see* dextromethorphan and phenylephrine *on page 289*
phenylephrine and diphenhydramine *see* diphenhydramine and phenylephrine *on page 312*
phenylephrine and promethazine *see* promethazine and phenylephrine *on page 802*

phenylephrine and pyrilamine (fen il EF rin & peer IL a meen)

Synonyms pyrilamine tannate and phenylephrine tannate

U.S./Canadian Brand Names Aldex®D [US]; Ryna-12 S® [US]; Ryna®-12 [US]

Therapeutic Category Antihistamine; Antihistamine/Decongestant Combination; Sympathomimetic

Use Symptomatic relief of nasal congestion and discharge associated with the common cold, sinusitis, allergic rhinitis, and other respiratory tract conditions

Dosage Summary

Oral:
Children <2 years: Dosage not established
Children 2-6 years: 2.5 mL of the suspension or 1/2 tablet every 12 hours
Children 6-12 years: 5 mL of the suspension or 1/2 to 1 tablet every 12 hours
Children >12 years: 5-10 mL of the suspension or 1-2 tablets every 12 hours
Adults: 5-10 mL of the suspension or 1-2 tablets every 12 hours

Dosage Forms

Suspension:
Aldex®D: Phenylephrine 5 mg and pyrilamine 16 mg
Ryna-12 S®: Phenylephrine 5 mg and pyrilamine 30 mg per 5 mL

Tablet:
Ryna®-12: Phenylephrine 25 mg and pyrilamine 60 mg

phenylephrine and scopolamine (fen il EF rin & skoe POL a meen)

Sound-Alike/Look-Alike Issues
Murocoll-2® may be confused with Murocel®

Synonyms scopolamine and phenylephrine

Therapeutic Category Anticholinergic/Adrenergic Agonist

Use Mydriasis, cycloplegia, and to break posterior synechiae in iritis

Dosage Summary

Ophthalmic:
Children: Dosage not established
Adults: Instill 1-2 drops into eye(s), repeat in 5 minutes

phenylephrine and zinc sulfate *(Canada only)* (fen il EF rin & zingk SUL fate)

Synonyms zinc sulfate and phenylephrine

U.S./Canadian Brand Names Zincfrin® [Can]

Therapeutic Category Adrenergic Agonist Agent

Use Soothe, moisturize, and remove redness due to minor eye irritation

Dosage Summary

Ophthalmic:
Children: Dosage not established
Adults: Instill 1-2 drops in eye(s) 2-4 times/day as needed

Dosage Forms - Canada

Solution, ophthalmic:
Zincfrin® [OTC]: Phenylephrine 0.12% and zinc sulfate 0.25% (15 mL)

phenylephrine, chlorpheniramine, and carbetapentane *see* carbetapentane, phenylephrine, and chlorpheniramine *on page 180*

phenylephrine, chlorpheniramine, and dextromethorphan *see* chlorpheniramine, phenylephrine, and dextromethorphan *on page 211*

phenylephrine, chlorpheniramine, and dihydrocodeine *see* dihydrocodeine, chlorpheniramine, and phenylephrine *on page 304*

phenylephrine, chlorpheniramine, and guaifenesin *see* chlorpheniramine, phenylephrine, and guaifenesin *on page 212*

phenylephrine, chlorpheniramine, and phenyltoloxamine *see* chlorpheniramine, phenylephrine, and phenyltoloxamine *on page 213*

phenylephrine, chlorpheniramine, and pyrilamine *see* chlorpheniramine, pyrilamine, and phenylephrine *on page 215*

phenylephrine, dextromethorphan, and acetaminophen *see* acetaminophen, dextromethorphan, and phenylephrine *on page 29*

phenylephrine, ephedrine, chlorpheniramine, and carbetapentane *see* chlorpheniramine, ephedrine, phenylephrine, and carbetapentane *on page 210*

phenylephrine hydrochloride *see* phenylephrine (nasal) *on page 751*

phenylephrine hydrochloride *see* phenylephrine (ophthalmic) *on page 752*

phenylephrine hydrochloride *see* phenylephrine (systemic) *on page 751*

phenylephrine hydrochloride *see* phenylephrine (topical) *on page 752*

phenylephrine hydrochloride, acetaminophen, and diphenhydramine *see* acetaminophen, diphenhydramine, and phenylephrine *on page 30*

phenylephrine hydrochloride and acetaminophen *see* acetaminophen and phenylephrine *on page 25*

phenylephrine hydrochloride and diphenhydramine hydrochloride *see* diphenhydramine and phenylephrine *on page 312*

phenylephrine hydrochloride and guaifenesin *see* guaifenesin and phenylephrine *on page 456*

phenylephrine hydrochloride, carbetapentane citrate, and guaifenesin *see* carbetapentane, guaifenesin, and phenylephrine *on page 180*

phenylephrine hydrochloride, chlorpheniramine maleate, dextromethorphan hydrobromide, and guaifenesin *see* dextromethorphan, chlorpheniramine, phenylephrine, and guaifenesin *on page 290*

phenylephrine hydrochloride, guaifenesin, and dextromethorphan hydrobromide *see* guaifenesin, dextromethorphan, and phenylephrine *on page 458*

phenylephrine hydrochloride, hydrocodone bitartrate, and chlorpheniramine Maleate *see* phenylephrine, hydrocodone, and chlorpheniramine *on page 754*

phenylephrine, hydrocodone, and chlorpheniramine

(fen il EF rin, hye droe KOE done, & klor fen IR a meen)

Synonyms chlorpheniramine, hydrocodone, and phenylephrine; dihydrocodeine bitartrate, phenylephrine hydrochloride, and chlorpheniramine maleate; hydrocodone, phenylephrine, and chlorpheniramine; phenylephrine hydrochloride, hydrocodone bitartrate, and chlorpheniramine Maleate

U.S./Canadian Brand Names B-Tuss™ [US]; Coughtuss [US]; Cytuss HC [US]; De-Chlor HC [US]; DroTuss-CP [US]; ED-TLC [US]; ED-Tuss HC [US]; Histinex® HC [US]; Hydro PC II Plus [US]; Hydro-PC II [US]; Hydron CP [US]; Maxi-Tuss HCX [US]; Maxi-Tuss HC® [US]; Mintuss HC [US]; Mintuss MS [US]; PolyTussin HD [US]; Rindal HD Plus [US]; Triant-HC™ [US]

Therapeutic Category Antihistamine; Antihistamine/Decongestant/Antitussive; Antitussive; Decongestant

Controlled Substance C-III

Use Symptomatic relief of cough and congestion associated with the common cold, sinusitis, or acute upper respiratory tract infections

Dosage Summary Note: Dosing is product specific; consult specific product labeling.

Oral:

Children <2 years: Dosage not established

Children 2-6 years: 1.25-2.5 mL every 6 hours (maximum: 10 mL/day)

Children 6-12 years:

2.5 mL every 4 hours (maximum: 15 mL/24 hours) **or** 5 mL every 4 hours (maximum: 20 mL/24 hours) or 2.5-5 mL every 6 hours

Children >12 years: 5-10 mL every 4-6 hours (maximum: 40 mL/day)

Adults: 5-10 mL every 4-6 hours (maximum: 40 mL/day)

Dosage Forms

Liquid:

B-Tuss™: Phenylephrine 5 mg, hydrocodone 5 mg, and chlorpheniramine 2 mg per 5 mL

Coughtuss, DroTuss-CP: Phenylephrine 5 mg, hydrocodone 5 mg, and chlorpheniramine 2 mg per 5 mL

De-Chlor HC: Phenylephrine 10 mg, hydrocodone 2.5 mg, and chlorpheniramine 2 mg per 5 mL

ED-Tuss HC: Phenylephrine 10 mg, hydrocodone 3.5 mg, and chlorpheniramine 4 mg per 5 mL

ED-TLC: Phenylephrine 5 mg, hydrocodone 1.67 mg, and chlorpheniramine 2 mg per 5 mL

Hydro PC II Plus: Phenylephrine 7.5 mg, hydrocodone 3.5 mg, and chlorpheniramine 2 mg per 5 mL

Hydron CP: Phenylephrine 10 mg, hydrocodone 5 mg, and chlorpheniramine 2 mg per 5 mL

Maxi-Tuss HCX: Phenylephrine 12 mg, hydrocodone 6 mg and chlorpheniramine 2 mg per 5 mL

Triant-HC™: Phenylephrine 5 mg, hydrocodone 1.67 mg, and chlorpheniramine 2 mg per 5 mL

Syrup:

Cytuss HC, Histinex® HC: Phenylephrine 5 mg, hydrocodone 2.5 mg, and chlorpheniramine 2 mg per 5 mL

Hydro-PC II: Phenylephrine 7.5 mg, hydrocodone 2 mg, and chlorpheniramine 2 mg per 5 mL

Maxi-Tuss HC®, Mintuss HD: Phenylephrine 10 mg, hydrocodone 2.5 mg, and chlorpheniramine 4 mg per 5 mL

Mintuss HC: Phenylephrine 10 mg, hydrocodone 2.5 mg, and chlorpheniramine 2 mg per 5 mL

Mintuss MS: Phenylephrine 10 mg, hydrocodone 5 mg, and chlorpheniramine 2 mg per 5 mL

PolyTussin HD: Phenylephrine 5 mg, hydrocodone 6 mg, and chlorpheniramine 2 mg per 5 mL

Rindal HD Plus: Phenylephrine 7.5 mg, hydrocodone 3.5 mg, and chlorpheniramine 2 mg per 5 mL

phenylephrine, promethazine, and codeine *see* promethazine, phenylephrine, and codeine *on page 802*

phenylephrine, pyrilamine, and dextromethorphan

(fen il EF rin, peer IL a meen, & deks troe meth OR fan)

Synonyms dextromethorphan tannate, pyrilamine tannate, and phenylephrine tannate; pyrilamine maleate, dextromethorphan hydrobromide, and phenylephrine hydrochloride

U.S./Canadian Brand Names Aldex® DM [US]; Codal-DM [US-OTC]; MyHist-DM [US]; Poly-Hist DM [US]; ViraTan™-DM [US]

Therapeutic Category Antihistamine; Antihistamine/Decongestant/Antitussive; Antitussive; Sympathomimetic

Use Symptomatic relief of cough, nasal congestion, and discharge associated with the common cold, sinusitis, allergic rhinitis, and other respiratory tract conditions

Dosage Summary

Oral:

Children <2 years: Dosage not established

Children 2-6 years: Viravan®-DM: 2.5 mL of the suspension **or** 1/2 tablet every 12 hours

Children 6-12 years:

codimal® DM: 5 mL every 4 hours (maximum: 30 mL/day)

ViraTan™-DM: 5 mL of the suspension **or** 1/2 to 1 tablet every 12 hours

Children >12 years:

codimal® DM: 10 mL every 4 hours (maximum: 60 mL/day)

ViraTan™-DM: 5-10 mL of the suspension **or** 1-2 tablets every 12 hours

Adults:

codimal® DM: 10 mL every 4 hours (maximum: 60 mL/day)

ViraTan™-DM: 5-10 mL of the suspension **or** 1-2 tablets every 12 hours

Dosage Forms

Liquid:

MyHist-DM: Phenylephrine 7.5 mg, pyrilamine 12.5 mg, and dextromethorphan 15 mg per 5 mL

Suspension:

Aldex® DM: Phenylephrine 5 mg, pyrilamine 16 mg, and dextromethorphan 15 mg per 5 mL

ViraTan™-DM: Phenylephrine 12.5 mg, pyrilamine 30 mg, and dextromethorphan 25 mg per 5 mL

Syrup:

Codal-DM [OTC]: Phenylephrine 5 mg, pyrilamine 8.33 mg, and dextromethorphan 10 mg

Tablet, chewable [scored]:

ViraTan™-DM: Phenylephrine 25 mg, pyrilamine 30 mg, and dextromethorphan 25 mg

phenylephrine, pyrilamine, and guaifenesin

(fen il EF rin, peer IL a meen, & gwye FEN e sin)

Synonyms guaifenesin, phenylephrine tannate, and pyrilamine tannate; pyrilamine tannate, guaifenesin, and phenylephrine tannate

U.S./Canadian Brand Names Ryna-12X® [US]

Therapeutic Category Alpha/Beta Agonist; Decongestant; Expectorant; Histamine H_1 Antagonist; Histamine H_1 Antagonist, First Generation

Use Symptomatic relief of cough, nasal congestion, and discharge associated with the common cold, sinusitis, allergic rhinitis, and other respiratory tract conditions

Dosage Summary

Oral:

Children <2 years: Dosage not established
Children 2-6 years: 2.5-5 mL of the suspension every 12 hours
Children 6-11 years: 5-10 mL of the suspension **or** 1/2 to 1 tablet every 12 hours
Children ≥12 years: 1-2 tablets every 12 hours
Adults: 1-2 tablets every 12 hours

Dosage Forms

Suspension:

Ryna-12X®: Phenylephrine 5 mg, pyrilamine 30 mg, and guaifenesin 100 mg per 5 mL

Tablet [scored]:

Ryna-12X®: Phenylephrine 25 mg, pyrilamine 60 mg, and guaifenesin 200 mg

phenylephrine tannate and carbetapentane tannate *see* carbetapentane and phenylephrine *on page 179*

phenylephrine tannate and diphenhydramine tannate *see* diphenhydramine and phenylephrine *on page 312*

phenylephrine tannate, carbetapentane tannate, and pyrilamine tannate *see* carbetapentane, phenylephrine, and pyrilamine *on page 181*

phenylephrine tannate, chlorpheniramine tannate, and methscopolamine nitrate *see* chlorpheniramine, phenylephrine, and methscopolamine *on page 212*

phenylethylmalonylurea *see* phenobarbital *on page 747*

Phenylfenesin® L.A. *(Discontinued)*

Phenylgesic *(Discontinued)* *see* acetaminophen and phenyltoloxamine *on page 26*

phenyl salicylate, methenamine, methylene blue, benzoic acid, and hyoscyamine *see* methenamine, phenyl salicylate, methylene blue, benzoic acid, and hyoscyamine *on page 613*

phenyltoloxamine, chlorpheniramine, and phenylephrine *see* chlorpheniramine, phenylephrine, and phenyltoloxamine *on page 213*

phenyltoloxamine citrate and acetaminophen *see* acetaminophen and phenyltoloxamine *on page 26*

Phenytek® [US] *see* phenytoin *on page 756*

phenytoin (FEN i toyn)

Sound-Alike/Look-Alike Issues

phenytoin may be confused with phenelzine, phentermine, PHENobarbital
Dilantin® may be confused with Dilaudid®, diltiazem, Dipentum®

Synonyms diphenylhydantoin; DPH; phenytoin sodium; phenytoin sodium, extended; phenytoin sodium, prompt

U.S./Canadian Brand Names Dilantin-125® [US]; Dilantin® [US/Can]; Phenytek® [US]

Therapeutic Category Antiarrhythmic Agent, Class I-B; Hydantoin

Use Management of generalized tonic-clonic (grand mal), complex partial seizures; prevention of seizures following head trauma/neurosurgery

Dosage Summary Note: Phenytoin base (eg, oral suspension, chewable tablets) contains ~8% more drug than phenytoin sodium (~92 mg base is equivalent to 100 mg phenytoin sodium). Dosage adjustments and closer serum monitoring may be necessary when switching dosage forms.

I.V.:

Infants <6 months: Dosage not established
Children 6 months to 3 years: Loading dose: 15-20 mg/kg in a single or divided dose; Maintenance: 5-10 mg/kg/day in 2 divided doses

Children 4-6 years: Loading dose: 15-20 mg/kg in a single or divided dose; Maintenance: 5-9 mg/kg/day in 2 divided doses

Children 7-9 years: Loading dose: 15-20 mg/kg in a single or divided dose; Maintenance: 5-8 mg/kg/day in 2 divided doses

Children 10-16 years: Loading dose: 15-20 mg/kg in a single or divided dose; Maintenance: 5-7 mg/kg/day in 2 divided doses

Adolescents >16 years: Loading dose: 10-25 mg/kg in a single or divided dose; Maintenance: 300 mg/day **or** 5-6 mg/kg/day in 3 divided doses

Adults: Loading dose: 10-25 mg/kg in a single or divided dose; Maintenance: 300 mg/day **or** 5-6 mg/kg/day in 3 divided doses

Oral:

Children: Loading dose: 15-20 mg/kg in 3 divided doses every 2-4 hours; Maintenance: 300 mg/day in 1-3 divided doses **or** 5-6 mg/kg/day in 1-3 divided doses (range: 200-1200 mg/day)

Adults: Loading dose: 15-20 mg/kg in 3 divided doses every 2-4 hours; Maintenance: 300 mg/day in 1-3 divided doses **or** 5-6 mg/kg/day in 1-3 divided doses (range: 200-1200 mg/day)

Dosage Forms

Capsule, extended release, oral: 100 mg, 200 mg, 300 mg

Dilantin®: 100 mg

Phenytek®: 200 mg, 300 mg

Injection, solution: 50 mg/mL (2 mL, 5 mL)

Suspension, oral: 100 mg/4 mL (4 mL); 125 mg/5 mL (4 mL, 120 mL, 237 mL, 240 mL)

Dilantin-125®: 125 mg/5 mL (240 mL)

Tablet, chewable, oral:

Dilantin®: 50 mg

phenytoin sodium *see* phenytoin *on page 756*

phenytoin sodium, extended *see* phenytoin *on page 756*

phenytoin sodium, prompt *see* phenytoin *on page 756*

Pherazine® VC With Codeine *(Discontinued)* *see* promethazine, phenylephrine, and codeine *on page 802*

Pherazine® With Codeine *(Discontinued)* *see* promethazine and codeine *on page 801*

Pherazine® With DM *(Discontinued)* *see* promethazine and dextromethorphan *on page 801*

Phillips'® M-O [US-OTC] *see* magnesium hydroxide and mineral oil *on page 586*

Phillips'® Laxative Dietary Supplement Cramp-Free [US-OTC] *see* magnesium oxide *on page 587*

Phillips'® Liquid-Gels® [US-OTC] *see* docusate *on page 321*

Phillips'® Milk of Magnesia [US-OTC] *see* magnesium hydroxide *on page 585*

Phillips'® Stool Softener Laxative [US-OTC] *see* docusate *on page 321*

pHisoHex® [US/Can] *see* hexachlorophene *on page 471*

PHL-Alendronate [Can] *see* alendronate *on page 47*

PHL-Amiodarone [Can] *see* amiodarone *on page 67*

PHL-Amlodipine [Can] *see* amlodipine *on page 68*

PHL-Amoxicillin [Can] *see* amoxicillin *on page 72*

PHL-Atenolol [Can] *see* atenolol *on page 102*

PHL-Azithromycin [Can] *see* azithromycin (systemic) *on page 111*

PHL-Baclofen [Can] *see* baclofen *on page 115*

PHL-Bicalutamide [Can] *see* bicalutamide *on page 137*

PHL-Bisoprolol [Can] *see* bisoprolol *on page 141*

PHL-Carbamazepine [Can] *see* carbamazepine *on page 177*

PHL-Carvedilol [Can] *see* carvedilol *on page 186*

PHL-Cilazapril [Can] *see* cilazapril *(Canada only) on page 222*

PHL-Ciprofloxacin [Can] *see* ciprofloxacin (systemic) *on page 224*

PHL-Citalopram [Can] *see* citalopram *on page 227*

PHL-Cyclobenzaprine [Can] *see* cyclobenzaprine *on page 258*

PHL-Divalproex [Can] *see* divalproex *on page 319*

PHL-Domperidone [Can] *see* domperidone *(Canada only) on page 325*

PHL-Doxycycline [Can] *see* doxycycline *on page 331*

Phlemex [US] *see* guaifenesin and dextromethorphan *on page 455*

PHL-Fenofibrate Supra [Can] *see* fenofibrate *on page 393*
PHL-Fluconazole [Can] *see* fluconazole *on page 407*
PHL-Fluoxetine [Can] *see* fluoxetine *on page 415*
PHL-Gabapentin [Can] *see* gabapentin *on page 433*
PHL-Indapamide [Can] *see* indapamide *on page 504*
PHL-Leflunomide [Can] *see* leflunomide *on page 552*
PHL-Levetiracetam [Can] *see* levetiracetam *on page 555*
PHL-Lisinopril [Can] *see* lisinopril *on page 570*
PHL-Lorazepam [Can] *see* lorazepam *on page 576*
PHL-Lovastatin [Can] *see* lovastatin *on page 579*
PHL-Meloxicam [Can] *see* meloxicam *on page 598*
PHL-Metformin [Can] *see* metformin *on page 609*
PHL-Methimazole [Can] *see* methimazole *on page 613*
PHL-Methylphenidate [Can] *see* methylphenidate *on page 621*
PHL-Metoprolol [Can] *see* metoprolol *on page 625*
PHL-Minocycline [Can] *see* minocycline *on page 635*
PHL-Mirtazapine [Can] *see* mirtazapine *on page 637*
PHL-Olanzapine [Can] *see* olanzapine *on page 696*
PHL-Olanzapine ODT [Can] *see* olanzapine *on page 696*
PHL-Ondansetron [Can] *see* ondansetron *on page 704*
PHL-Oxybutynin [Can] *see* oxybutynin *on page 713*
PHL-Pantoprazole [Can] *see* pantoprazole *on page 725*
PHL-Paroxetine [Can] *see* paroxetine *on page 729*
PHL-Pioglitazone [Can] *see* pioglitazone *on page 762*
PHL-Pramipexole [Can] *see* pramipexole *on page 786*
PHL-Pravastatin [Can] *see* pravastatin *on page 789*
PHL-Procyclidine [Can] *see* procyclidine *(Canada only) on page 798*
PHL-Ramipril [Can] *see* ramipril *on page 826*
PHL-Ranitidine [Can] *see* ranitidine *on page 828*
PHL-Risperidone [Can] *see* risperidone *on page 845*
PHL-Salbutamol [Can] *see* albuterol *on page 43*
PHL-Sertraline [Can] *see* sertraline *on page 872*
PHL-Simvastatin [Can] *see* simvastatin *on page 877*
PHL-Sotalol [Can] *see* sotalol *on page 892*
PHL-Sumatriptan [Can] *see* sumatriptan *on page 904*
PHL-Temazepam [Can] *see* temazepam *on page 914*
PHL-Terazosin [Can] *see* terazosin *on page 917*
PHL-Terbinafine [Can] *see* terbinafine (systemic) *on page 917*
PHL-Topiramate [Can] *see* topiramate *on page 942*
PHL-Trazodone [Can] *see* trazodone *on page 950*
PHL-Ursodiol C [Can] *see* ursodiol *on page 972*
PHL-Valacyclovir [Can] *see* valacyclovir *on page 973*
PHL-Valproic Acid [Can] *see* valproic acid *on page 974*
PHL-Valproic Acid E.C. [Can] *see* valproic acid *on page 974*
PHL-Verapamil SR [Can] *see* verapamil *on page 981*
PHL-Zopiclone [Can] *see* zopiclone *(Canada only) on page 1005*
Phos-Flur® [US] *see* fluoride *on page 413*
Phos-Flur® Rinse [US-OTC] *see* fluoride *on page 413*
PhosLo® [US/Can] *see* calcium acetate *on page 166*
Phos-NaK [US] *see* potassium phosphate and sodium phosphate *on page 783*
Phospha 250™ Neutral [US] *see* potassium phosphate and sodium phosphate *on page 783*
phosphate, potassium *see* potassium phosphate *on page 783*
phosphates, sodium *see* sodium phosphates *on page 887*

Phosphocol® P 32 [US] *see* chromic phosphate P 32 *on page 220*
Phospholine Iodide® [US] *see* echothiophate iodide *on page 340*
phosphonoformate *see* foscarnet *on page 427*
phosphonoformic acid *see* foscarnet *on page 427*
phosphorated carbohydrate solution *see* fructose, dextrose, and phosphoric acid *on page 430*
phosphoric acid, levulose and dextrose *see* fructose, dextrose, and phosphoric acid *on page 430*
phosphorus p32 *see* chromic phosphate P 32 *on page 220*
Photofrin® [US/Can] *see* porfimer *on page 779*
Phrenilin® [US] *see* butalbital and acetaminophen *on page 159*
Phrenilin® Forte [US] *see* butalbital and acetaminophen *on page 159*
Phrenilin® with Caffeine and Codeine *(Discontinued)* *see* butalbital, acetaminophen, caffeine, and codeine *on page 159*
***p*-hydroxyampicillin** *see* amoxicillin *on page 72*
Phyllocontin® [Can] *see* aminophylline *on page 66*
Phyllocontin®-350 [Can] *see* aminophylline *on page 66*
phylloquinone *see* phytonadione *on page 759*

physostigmine (fye zoe STIG meen)

Sound-Alike/Look-Alike Issues

physostigmine may be confused with Prostigmin®, pyridostigmine

Synonyms eserine salicylate; physostigmine salicylate; physostigmine sulfate

Therapeutic Category Cholinesterase Inhibitor

Use Reverse toxic, life-threatening delirium caused by atropine, diphenhydramine, dimenhydrinate, *Atropa belladonna* (deadly nightshade), or jimsonweed (*Datura* spp)

Dosage Summary

I.M.:

Children: Dosage not established

Adults: Initial: 0.5-2 mg, repeat every 20 minutes until response or adverse effects occur; repeat 1-4 mg every 30-60 minutes as life-threatening symptoms recur

I.V.: Note: Administer slowly over 5 minutes to prevent respiratory distress and seizures. Continuous infusions of physostigmine should never be used.

Children: 0.01-0.03 mg/kg/dose, may repeat after 5-10 minutes (maximum total dose: 2 mg)

Adults: Initial: 0.5-2 mg, repeat every 20 minutes until response or adverse effects occur; repeat 1-4 mg every 30-60 minutes as life-threatening symptoms recur

Dosage Forms

Injection, solution: 1 mg/mL (2 mL)

physostigmine salicylate *see* physostigmine *on page 759*
physostigmine sulfate *see* physostigmine *on page 759*
phytomenadione *see* phytonadione *on page 759*

phytonadione (fye toe na DYE one)

Sound-Alike/Look-Alike Issues

Mephyton® may be confused with melphalan, methadone

Synonyms methylphytyl napthoquinone; phylloquinone; phytomenadione; vitamin K_1

U.S./Canadian Brand Names AquaMEPHYTON® [Can]; Konakion [Can]; Mephyton® [US/Can]

Therapeutic Category Vitamin, Fat Soluble

Use Prevention and treatment of hypoprothrombinemia caused by coumarin derivative-induced or other drug-induced vitamin K deficiency, hypoprothrombinemia caused by malabsorption or inability to synthesize vitamin K; hemorrhagic disease of the newborn

Dosage Summary

I.M.:

Newborns: Prophylaxis: 0.5-1 mg within 1 hour of birth; Treatment: 1 mg/dose/day

Children: Dosage not established

Adults: Initial: 2.5-25 mg per dose (usual: 5-10 mg; maximum: 50 mg)

I.V.:

Children: Dosage not established

Adults: Initial: 2.5-25 mg per dose (usual: 5-10 mg; maximum: 50 mg)

Oral:
Children <1 years: Dosage not established
Children 1-3 years: RDA: 30 mcg/day
Children 4-8 years: RDA: 55 mcg/day
Children 9-13 years: RDA: 60 mcg/day
Children 14-18 years: RDA: 75 mcg/day
Adults: Initial: 2.5-25 mg per dose (usual: 5-10 mg; maximum: 50 mg)

SubQ:
Newborns: 1 mg/dose/day
Children: Dosage not established
Adults: Initial: 2.5-25 mg per dose (usual: 5-10 mg; maximum: 50 mg)

Dosage Forms
Injection, aqueous colloidal: 1 mg/0.5 mL (0.5 mL); 10 mg/mL (1 mL)
Injection, aqueous colloidal [preservative free]: 1 mg/0.5 mL (0.5 mL)
Tablet, oral: 100 mcg
Mephyton®: 5 mg

pidorubicin *see* epirubicin *on page 355*
pidorubicin hydrochloride *see* epirubicin *on page 355*
Pilagan® Ophthalmic *(Discontinued)* *see* pilocarpine (ophthalmic) *on page 760*

pilocarpine (systemic) (pye loe KAR peen)

Sound-Alike/Look-Alike Issues
Salagen® may be confused with Salacid®, selegiline
Synonyms pilocarpine hydrochloride
U.S./Canadian Brand Names Salagen® [US/Can]
Therapeutic Category Cholinergic Agonist
Use Symptomatic treatment of xerostomia caused by salivary gland hypofunction resulting from radiotherapy for cancer of the head and neck or Sjögren syndrome
Dosage Summary
Oral:
Children: Dosage not established
Adults: 5 mg 3-4 times/day (maximum: 30 mg/day)
Dosage Forms
Tablet, oral: 5 mg, 7.5 mg
Salagen®: 5 mg, 7.5 mg

pilocarpine (ophthalmic) (pye loe KAR peen)

Sound-Alike/Look-Alike Issues
Isopto® Carpine may be confused with Isopto® Carbachol
Synonyms pilocarpine hydrochloride
U.S./Canadian Brand Names Diocarpine [Can]; Isopto® Carpine [US/Can]; Pilopine HS® [US/Can]
Therapeutic Category Ophthalmic Agent, Antiglaucoma; Ophthalmic Agent, Miotic
Use Management of chronic simple glaucoma, chronic and acute angle-closure glaucoma
Dosage Summary
Ophthalmic:
Children: Dosage not established
Adults:
Gel: Instill 0.5" ribbon once daily at bedtime
Solution: Instill 1-2 drops up to 6 times/day
Dosage Forms
Gel, ophthalmic:
Pilopine HS®: 4% (4 g)
Solution, ophthalmic: 1% (2 mL, 15 mL); 2% (2 mL, 15 mL); 4% (2 mL, 15 mL)
Isopto® Carpine: 1% (15 mL); 2% (15 mL); 4% (15 mL)

pilocarpine hydrochloride *see* pilocarpine (ophthalmic) *on page 760*
pilocarpine hydrochloride *see* pilocarpine (systemic) *on page 760*
Pilopine HS® [US/Can] *see* pilocarpine (ophthalmic) *on page 760*
Pilostat® Ophthalmic *(Discontinued)* *see* pilocarpine (ophthalmic) *on page 760*

pimaricin *see* natamycin *on page 662*

pimecrolimus (pim e KROE li mus)

Sound-Alike/Look-Alike Issues

pimecrolimus may be confused with tacrolimus

U.S./Canadian Brand Names Elidel® [US/Can]

Therapeutic Category Immunosuppressant Agent; Topical Skin Product

Use Short-term and intermittent long-term treatment of mild-to-moderate atopic dermatitis in patients not responsive to conventional therapy or when conventional therapy is not appropriate

Dosage Summary

Topical:

Children <2 years: Dosage not established
Children >2 years: Apply thin layer to affected area twice daily
Adults: Apply thin layer to affected area twice daily

Dosage Forms

Cream, topical:

Elidel®: 1% (30 g, 60 g, 100 g)

pimozide (PI moe zide)

U.S./Canadian Brand Names Apo-Pimozide® [Can]; Orap® [US/Can]; PMS-Pimozide [Can]

Therapeutic Category Neuroleptic Agent

Use Suppression of severe motor and phonic tics in patients with Tourette disorder who have failed to respond satisfactorily to standard treatment

Dosage Summary

Oral:

Children ≤12 years: Initial: 0.05 mg/kg once daily (preferably bedtime); Maintenance: 2-4 mg once daily (maximum: 10 mg/day [0.2 mg/kg/day]); **Note:** Titration is recommended
Children >12 years: Initial: 1-2 mg in divided doses; Maintenance: 7-10 mg/day in divided doses (maximum: 10 mg/day [0.2 mg/kg/day]); **Note:** Titration is recommended
Adults: Initial: 1-2 mg in divided doses; Maintenance: 7-10 mg/day in divided doses (maximum: 10 mg/day [0.2 mg/kg/day]); **Note:** Titration is recommended
Elderly: Initial: 1 mg/day

Dosage Forms

Tablet, oral:

Orap®: 1 mg, 2 mg

Pin-X® [US-OTC] *see* pyrantel pamoate *on page 816*
pinaverium bromide *see* pinaverium *(Canada only) on page 761*

pinaverium *(Canada only)* (pin ah VEER ee um)

Synonyms pinaverium bromide

U.S./Canadian Brand Names Dicetel® [Can]

Therapeutic Category Calcium Antagonist; Gastrointestinal Agent, Miscellaneous

Use Treatment and relief of symptoms associated with irritable bowel syndrome (IBS); treatment of symptoms related to functional disorders of the biliary tract

Dosage Summary

Oral:

Children: Dosage not established
Adults: 50 mg 3 times/day with meals/snack (maximum: 300 mg/day)

Dosage Forms - Canada

Tablet:

Dicetel®: 50 mg, 100 mg

pindolol (PIN doe lole)

Sound-Alike/Look-Alike Issues

pindolol may be confused with Parlodel®, Plendil®
Visken® may be confused with Visine®, Viskazide®

U.S./Canadian Brand Names Apo-Pindol® [Can]; Gen-Pindolol [Can]; Novo-Pindol [Can]; Nu-Pindol [Can]; PMS-Pindolol [Can]; Visken® [Can]

Therapeutic Category Beta-Adrenergic Blocker

Use Treatment of hypertension, alone or in combination with other agents

Dosage Summary

Oral:

Children: Dosage not established

Adults: Initial: 5 mg twice daily; Maintenance: 10-40 mg twice daily (maximum: 60 mg/day)

Elderly: Initial: 5 mg once daily

Dosage Forms

Tablet, oral: 5 mg, 10 mg

pindolol and hydrochlorothiazide *(Canada only)*

(PIN doe lole & hye droe klor oh THYE a zide)

Sound-Alike/Look-Alike Issues

Viskazide® may be confused with hydrochlorothiazide, Visken®

Synonyms hydrochlorothiazide and pindolol

U.S./Canadian Brand Names Viskazide® [Can]

Therapeutic Category Beta Blocker With Intrinsic Sympathomimetic Activity; Diuretic, Thiazide

Use Treatment of hypertension; not for initial therapy

Dosage Forms - Canada

Tablet:

Viskazide® 10/25: Pindolol 10 mg and hydrochlorothiazide 25 mg

Viskazide® 10/50: Pindolol 10 mg and hydrochlorothiazide 50 mg

pink bismuth *see* bismuth *on page 139*

Pin-Rid® ***(Discontinued)*** *see* pyrantel pamoate *on page 816*

pioglitazone (pye oh GLI ta zone)

Sound-Alike/Look-Alike Issues

Actos® may be confused with Actidose®, Actonel®

U.S./Canadian Brand Names Actos® [US/Can]; Apo-Pioglitazone® [Can]; CO Pioglitazone [Can]; Dom-Pioglitazone [Can]; Mint-Pioglitazone [Can]; Mylan-Pioglitazone [Can]; Novo-Pioglitazone [Can]; PHL-Pioglitazone [Can]; PMS-Pioglitazone [Can]; PRO-Pioglitazone [Can]; ratio-Pioglitazone [Can]; Sandoz-Pioglitazone [Can]; ZYM-Pioglitazone [Can]

Therapeutic Category Antidiabetic Agent, Oral; Thiazolidinedione Derivative

Use

Type 2 diabetes mellitus (noninsulin-dependent, NIDDM), monotherapy: Adjunct to diet and exercise, to improve glycemic control

Type 2 diabetes mellitus (noninsulin-dependent, NIDDM), combination therapy with sulfonylurea, metformin, or insulin: When diet, exercise, and a single agent alone does not result in adequate glycemic control

Dosage Summary

Oral:

Children: Dosage not established

Adults: Initial: 15-30 mg once daily; Maintenance: 15-45 mg once daily (maximum: 45 mg/day)

Dosage Forms

Tablet, oral:

Actos®: 15 mg, 30 mg, 45 mg

pioglitazone and glimepiride (pye oh GLI ta zone & GLYE me pye ride)

Synonyms glimepiride and pioglitazone; glimepiride and pioglitazone hydrochloride

U.S./Canadian Brand Names Duetact™ [US]

Therapeutic Category Antidiabetic Agent, Sulfonylurea; Antidiabetic Agent, Thiazolidinedione; Hypoglycemic Agent, Oral

Use Management of type 2 diabetes mellitus (noninsulin-dependent, NIDDM) as an adjunct to diet and exercise

Dosage Summary

Oral:

Children: Dosage not established

Adults:
Patients inadequately controlled on **glimepiride** alone: Initial dose: Pioglitazone 30 mg and glimepiride 2-4 mg once daily (maximum: 45 mg/day [pioglitazone]; 8 mg/day [glimepiride])
Patients inadequately controlled on **pioglitazone** alone: Initial dose: Pioglitazone 30 mg and glimepiride 2 mg once daily (maximum: 45 mg/day [pioglitazone]; 8 mg/day [glimepiride])
Elderly: Initial: Glimepiride 1 mg/day prior to initiating Duetact™

Dosage Forms
Tablet:
Duetact™: 30 mg/2 mg: Pioglitazone 30 mg and glimepiride 2 mg; 30 mg/4 mg: Pioglitazone 30 mg and glimepiride 4 mg

pioglitazone and metformin (pye oh GLI ta zone & met FOR min)

Synonyms metformin hydrochloride and pioglitazone hydrochloride
U.S./Canadian Brand Names Actoplus Met® XR [US]; Actoplus Met® [US]
Therapeutic Category Antidiabetic Agent, Biguanide; Antidiabetic Agent, Thiazolidinedione
Use Management of type 2 diabetes mellitus (noninsulin-dependent, NIDDM)
Dosage Summary
Oral:
Children: Dosage not established
Adults:
Immediate release tablet: Pioglitazone 15-45 mg/day and metformin 500-2550 mg/day (maximum: 45 mg/day [pioglitazone]; 2550 mg/day [metformin])
Variable release tablet: Pioglitazone 15-45 mg/day and metformin 1000-2000 mg/day (maximum: 45 mg/day [pioglitazone]; 2000 mg/day [metformin])
Elderly ≥80 years: Do not use unless normal renal function has been established

Dosage Forms
Tablet, oral:
Actoplus Met®: 15/500: Pioglitazone 15 mg and metformin 500 mg; 15/850: Pioglitazone 15 mg and metformin 850 mg
Tablet, variable release, oral:
Actoplus Met® XR: 15/1000: Pioglitazone 15 mg and metformin 1000 mg; 30/1000: Pioglitazone 30 mg and metformin 1000 mg

piperacillin (pi PER a sil in)

Synonyms piperacillin sodium
U.S./Canadian Brand Names Piperacillin for Injection, USP [Can]
Therapeutic Category Penicillin
Use Treatment of susceptible infections such as septicemia, acute and chronic respiratory tract infections, skin and soft tissue infections, and urinary tract infections due to susceptible strains of *Pseudomonas*, *Proteus*, and *Escherichia coli* and *Enterobacter*; active against some streptococci and some anaerobic bacteria; febrile neutropenia (as part of combination regimen)
Dosage Summary
I.M.:
Neonates: 100 mg/kg every 12 hours
Children: 200-300 mg/kg/day in divided doses every 4-6 hours
Adults: 2-4 g/dose every 4-6 hours (maximum: 24 g/day)
I.V.:
Neonates: 100 mg/kg every 12 hours
Children: 200-300 mg/kg/day in divided doses every 4-6 hours
Adults: 2-4 g/dose every 4-6 hours (maximum: 24 g/day)
Dosage Forms
Injection, powder for reconstitution: 2 g, 3 g, 4 g, 40 g

piperacillin and tazobactam sodium (pi PER a sil in & ta zoe BAK tam SOW dee um)

Sound-Alike/Look-Alike Issues
Zosyn® may be confused with Zofran®, Zyvox®
Synonyms piperacillin sodium and tazobactam sodium; tazobactam and piperacillin
U.S./Canadian Brand Names Tazocin® [Can]; Zosyn® [US]
Therapeutic Category Penicillin

Use Treatment of moderate-to-severe infections caused by susceptible organisms, including infections of the lower respiratory tract (community-acquired pneumonia, nosocomial pneumonia); urinary tract; uncomplicated and complicated skin and skin structures; gynecologic (endometritis, pelvic inflammatory disease); bone and joint infections; intraabdominal infections (appendicitis with rupture/abscess, peritonitis); and septicemia. Tazobactam expands activity of piperacillin to include beta-lactamase producing strains of *S. aureus*, *H. influenzae*, *Bacteroides*, and other gram-negative bacteria.

Dosage Summary

I.V.:

Children 2-8 months: 80 mg/kg every 8 hours (appendicitis, peritonitis; dosing based on piperacillin component)

Children ≥9 months and ≤40 kg: 100 mg/kg every 8 hours (appendicitis, peritonitis; dosing based on piperacillin component)

Children >40 kg: 4.5 g every 8 hour **or** 3.375 every 6 hours (appendicitis, peritonitis)

Adults: 3.375 g every 6 hours **or** 4.5 g every 6-8 hours; maximum: 18 g/day

Dosage Forms 8:1 ratio of piperacillin sodium/tazobactam sodium

Infusion [premixed iso-osmotic solution, frozen]:

Zosyn®:

2.25 g: Piperacillin 2 g and tazobactam 0.25 g (50 mL)
3.375 g: Piperacillin 3 g and tazobactam 0.375 g (50 mL)
4.5 g: Piperacillin 4 g and tazobactam 0.5 g (100 mL)

Injection, powder for reconstitution: 2.25 g: Piperacillin 2 g and tazobactam 0.25 g; 3.375 g: Piperacillin 3 g and tazobactam 0.375 g; 4.5 g: Piperacillin 4 g and tazobactam 0.5 g; 40.5 g: Piperacillin 36 g and tazobactam 4.5 g

Zosyn®:

2.25 g: Piperacillin 2 g and tazobactam 0.25 g
3.375 g: Piperacillin 3 g and tazobactam 0.375 g
4.5 g: Piperacillin 4 g and tazobactam 0.5 g
40.5 g: Piperacillin 36 g and tazobactam 4.5 g

Piperacillin for Injection, USP [Can] *see* piperacillin *on page 763*

piperacillin sodium *see* piperacillin *on page 763*

piperacillin sodium and tazobactam sodium *see* piperacillin and tazobactam sodium *on page 763*

piperazine estrone sulfate *see* estropipate *on page 372*

piperonyl butoxide and pyrethrins *see* pyrethrins and piperonyl butoxide *on page 816*

Pipracil® *(Discontinued)* *see* piperacillin *on page 763*

pirbuterol (peer BYOO ter ole)

Synonyms pirbuterol acetate

U.S./Canadian Brand Names Maxair® Autohaler® [US]

Therapeutic Category Adrenergic Agonist Agent

Use Prevention and treatment of reversible bronchospasm including asthma

Dosage Summary

Inhalation:

Children <12 years: Dosage not established

Children ≥12 years: Prevention: 2 inhalations every 4-6 hours; Treatment: 2 inhalations at an interval of at least 1-3 minutes, followed by a third inhalation (maximum: 12 inhalations/day)

Adults: Prevention: 2 inhalations every 4-6 hours; Treatment: 2 inhalations at an interval of at least 1-3 minutes, followed by a third inhalation (maximum: 12 inhalations/day)

Dosage Forms

Aerosol, for oral inhalation:

Maxair® Autohaler®: 200 mcg/actuation (14 g)

pirbuterol acetate *see* pirbuterol *on page 764*

piroxicam (peer OKS i kam)

Sound-Alike/Look-Alike Issues

Feldene® may be confused with FLUoxetine

U.S./Canadian Brand Names Apo-Piroxicam® [Can]; Dom-Piroxicam [Can]; Feldene® [US]; Gen-Piroxicam [Can]; Novo-Pirocam [Can]; Nu-Pirox [Can]; PMS-Piroxicam [Can]; PRO-Piroxicam [Can]

Therapeutic Category Analgesic, Nonnarcotic; Nonsteroidal Antiinflammatory Drug (NSAID)

Use Symptomatic treatment of acute and chronic rheumatoid arthritis and osteoarthritis

Dosage Summary

Oral:

Adults: 10-20 mg once daily (maximum: 20 mg/day: higher doses used with increased frequency of adverse effects)

Elderly: Initial: 10 mg every other day has been used (maximum: 20 mg/day)

Dosage Forms

Capsule, oral: 10 mg, 20 mg

Feldene®: 10 mg, 20 mg

p-isobutylhydratropic acid *see* ibuprofen *on page 494*

pit *see* oxytocin *on page 719*

pitavastatin (pi TA va sta tin)

Sound-Alike/Look-Alike Issues

pitavastatin may be confused with atorvastatin, fluvastatin, lovastatin, nystatin, pravastatin, rosuvastatin, simvastatin

Synonyms pitavastatin calcium

U.S./Canadian Brand Names Livalo® [US]

Therapeutic Category Antilipemic Agent, HMG-CoA Reductase Inhibitor

Use Adjunct to dietary therapy to reduce elevations in total cholesterol (TC), LDL-C, apolipoprotein B (Apo B), and triglycerides (TG), and to increase low HDL-C in patients with primary hyperlipidemia and mixed dyslipidemia

Dosage Summary Note: Doses should be individualized according to the baseline LDL-cholesterol levels, the recommended goal of therapy, and patient response; adjustments should be made at intervals of 4 weeks.

Oral:

Children: Dosage not established

Adults: Initial: 2 mg once daily; Maintenance: 2-4 mg once daily (maximum: 4 mg/day)

Dosage Forms

Tablet, oral:

Livalo®: 1 mg, 2 mg, 4 mg

pitavastatin calcium *see* pitavastatin *on page 765*

Pitocin® [US/Can] *see* oxytocin *on page 719*

Pitressin® [US] *see* vasopressin *on page 980*

Pitrex [Can] *see* tolnaftate *on page 940*

pix carbonis *see* coal tar *on page 242*

pizotifen *(Canada only)* (pi ZOE ti fen)

Synonyms pizotifen malate

U.S./Canadian Brand Names Sandomigran DS® [Can]; Sandomigran® [Can]

Therapeutic Category Antimigraine Agent

Use Migraine prophylaxis

Dosage Summary Note: Therapeutic response may require several weeks of therapy. Do not discontinue abruptly (reduce gradually over 2-week period).

Oral:

Children <12 years: Dosage not established

Children ≥12 years: Initial: 0.5 mg at bedtime; Maintenance: 1-6 mg/day in 1-3 divided doses

Adults: Initial: 0.5 mg at bedtime; Maintenance: 1-6 mg/day in 1-3 divided doses

Dosage Forms - Canada

Tablet:

Sandomigran®: 0.5 mg

Tablet, double strength:

Sandomigran® DS: 1 mg

pizotifen malate *see* pizotifen *(Canada only) on page 765*

Plan B® [Can] *see* levonorgestrel *on page 559*

Plan B® *(Discontinued)* *see* levonorgestrel *on page 559*

Plan B® One Step [US] *see* levonorgestrel *on page 559*

plantago seed *see* psyllium *on page 814*
plantain seed *see* psyllium *on page 814*
Plaquase® *(Discontinued)* *see* collagenase (systemic) *on page 247*
Plaquenil® [US/Can] *see* hydroxychloroquine *on page 488*
Plaretase® 8000 *(Discontinued)* *see* pancrelipase *on page 723*
Plasbumin®-5 [US/Can] *see* albumin *on page 43*
Plasbumin®-25 [US/Can] *see* albumin *on page 43*
Plasmanate® [US] *see* plasma protein fraction *on page 766*
Plasma-Plex® *(Discontinued)* *see* plasma protein fraction *on page 766*

plasma protein fraction (PLAS mah PROE teen FRAK shun)

U.S./Canadian Brand Names Plasmanate® [US]

Therapeutic Category Blood Product Derivative

Use Plasma volume expansion and maintenance of cardiac output in the treatment of certain types of shock or impending shock

Dosage Summary

I.V.:

Children: Dosage not established

Adults: Usual minimum dose: 250-500 mL; adjust dose based on response

Dosage Forms

Injection, solution [preservative free]:

Plasmanate®: 5% (50 mL, 250 mL)

Plasmatein® *(Discontinued)* *see* plasma protein fraction *on page 766*
Platinol®-AQ *(Discontinued)* *see* cisplatin *on page 227*
Plavix® [US/Can] *see* clopidogrel *on page 239*
Plegine® [Can] *see* phendimetrazine *on page 747*
Plegine® *(Discontinued)* *see* phendimetrazine *on page 747*
Plenaxis™ *(Discontinued)*
Plendil® [Can] *see* felodipine *on page 393*
Plendil® *(Discontinued)* *see* felodipine *on page 393*

plerixafor (pler IX a fore)

Synonyms AMD3100; LM3100

U.S./Canadian Brand Names Mozobil™ [US]

Therapeutic Category Hematopoietic Stem Cell Mobilizer

Use Mobilization of hematopoietic stem cells (HSC) for collection and subsequent autologous transplantation (in combination with filgrastim) in patients with non-Hodgkin lymphoma (NHL) and multiple myeloma (MM)

Dosage Summary

SubQ:

Children: Dosage not established

Adults: 0.24 mg/kg/day for up to 4 days; maximum dose: 40 mg/day

Dosage Forms

Injection, solution [preservative free]:

Mozobil™: 20 mg/mL (1.2 mL)

Pletal® [US/Can] *see* cilostazol *on page 222*
Plexion® [US] *see* sulfur and sulfacetamide *on page 903*
Plexion SCT® [US] *see* sulfur and sulfacetamide *on page 903*
Plexion TS® *(Discontinued)* *see* sulfur and sulfacetamide *on page 903*
Pliaglis™ [US] *see* lidocaine and tetracaine *on page 565*
PMPA *see* tenofovir *on page 916*
PMS-Alendronate [Can] *see* alendronate *on page 47*
PMS-Alendronate-FC [Can] *see* alendronate *on page 47*
PMS-Amantadine [Can] *see* amantadine *on page 61*
PMS-Amiodarone [Can] *see* amiodarone *on page 67*

PMS-Metoclopramide [Can] *see* metoclopramide *on page 624*
PMS-Metoprolol [Can] *see* metoprolol *on page 625*
PMS-Minocycline [Can] *see* minocycline *on page 635*
PMS-Mirtazapine [Can] *see* mirtazapine *on page 637*
PMS-Misoprostol [Can] *see* misoprostol *on page 637*
PMS-Moclobemide [Can] *see* moclobemide *(Canada only) on page 639*
PMS-Mometasone [Can] *see* mometasone (topical) *on page 641*
PMS-Morphine Sulfate SR [Can] *see* morphine (systemic) *on page 644*
PMS-Naproxen EC [Can] *see* naproxen *on page 659*
PMS-Nifedipine [Can] *see* nifedipine *on page 675*
PMS-Nizatidine [Can] *see* nizatidine *on page 681*
PMS-Norfloxacin [Can] *see* norfloxacin *on page 684*
PMS-Nortriptyline [Can] *see* nortriptyline *on page 684*
PMS-Nystatin [Can] *see* nystatin (oral) *on page 693*
PMS-Olanzapine [Can] *see* olanzapine *on page 696*
PMS-Olanzapine ODT [Can] *see* olanzapine *on page 696*
PMS-Omeprazole [Can] *see* omeprazole *on page 701*
PMS-Omeprazole DR [Can] *see* omeprazole *on page 701*
PMS-Ondansetron [Can] *see* ondansetron *on page 704*
PMS-Oxazepam [Can] *see* oxazepam *on page 712*
PMS-Oxybutynin [Can] *see* oxybutynin *on page 713*
PMS-Oxycodone [Can] *see* oxycodone *on page 714*
PMS-Oxycodone-Acetaminophen [Can] *see* oxycodone and acetaminophen *on page 715*
PMS-Pamidronate [Can] *see* pamidronate *on page 722*
PMS-Pantoprazole [Can] *see* pantoprazole *on page 725*
PMS-Paroxetine [Can] *see* paroxetine *on page 729*
PMS-Phenobarbital [Can] *see* phenobarbital *on page 747*
PMS-Pimozide [Can] *see* pimozide *on page 761*
PMS-Pindolol [Can] *see* pindolol *on page 761*
PMS-Pioglitazone [Can] *see* pioglitazone *on page 762*
PMS-Piroxicam [Can] *see* piroxicam *on pagc 764*
PMS-Polytrimethoprim [Can] *see* trimethoprim and polymyxin B *on page 960*
PMS-Pramipexole [Can] *see* pramipexole *on page 786*
PMS-Pravastatin [Can] *see* pravastatin *on page 789*
PMS-Procyclidine [Can] *see* procyclidine *(Canada only) on page 798*
PMS-Promethazine [Can] *see* promethazine *on page 800*
PMS-Propafenone [Can] *see* propafenone *on page 803*
PMS-Propranolol [Can] *see* propranolol *on page 806*
PMS-Pseudoephedrine [Can] *see* pseudoephedrine *on page 810*
PMS-Quetiapine [Can] *see* quetiapine *on page 821*
PMS-Rabeprazole EC [Can] *see* rabeprazole *on page 824*
PMS-Ramipril [Can] *see* ramipril *on page 826*
PMS-Ramipril HCTZ [Can] *see* ramipril and hydrochlorothiazide *(Canada only) on page 827*
PMS-Ranitidine [Can] *see* ranitidine *on page 828*
PMS-Risedronate [Can] *see* risedronate *on page 844*
PMS-Risperidone ODT [Can] *see* risperidone *on page 845*
PMS-Rivastigmine [Can] *see* rivastigmine *on page 848*
PMS-Ropinirole [Can] *see* ropinirole *on page 851*
PMS-Salbutamol [Can] *see* albuterol *on page 43*
PMS-Sertraline [Can] *see* sertraline *on page 872*
PMS-Simvastatin [Can] *see* simvastatin *on page 877*
PMS-Sodium Cromoglycate [Can] *see* cromolyn (systemic, oral inhalation) *on page 254*
PMS-Sodium Polystyrene Sulfonate [Can] *see* sodium polystyrene sulfonate *on page 887*

pneumococcal conjugate vaccine (13-valent)

(noo moe KOK al KON ju gate vak SEEN, thur TEEN vay lent)

Sound-Alike/Look-Alike Issues

pneumococcal 13-valent conjugate vaccine (Prevnar 13™) may be confused with pneumococcal 7-valent conjugate vaccine (Prevnar®) or with pneumococcal 23-valent polysaccharide vaccine (Pneumovax® 23)

Synonyms diphtheria CRM_{197} protein; PCV-13; PCV13; PCV13-CRM(197); pneumococcal 13-valent conjugate vaccine

U.S./Canadian Brand Names Prevnar 13™ [US]

Therapeutic Category Vaccine, Inactivated (Bacterial)

Use

Immunization of infants and children against *Streptococcus pneumoniae* infection caused by serotypes included in the vaccine

Immunization of infants and children against otitis media caused by *Streptococcus pneumoniae* serotypes 4, 6B, 9V, 14, 18C, 19F, and 23F

The Advisory Committee on Immunization Practices (ACIP) recommends routine vaccination for the following:

All children age 2-59 months; ACIP recommends using 13-valent pneumococcal conjugate vaccine (PCV13; Prevnar 13™) as a replacement for the previously recommended 7-valent pneumococcal conjugate vaccine (PCV7; Prevnar®) for the immunization schedule

Children age 24-71 months who have underlying medical conditions increasing their risk of pneumococcal disease or complications including: cochlear implants, sickle cell disease (including other sickle cell hemoglobinopathies, asplenia, splenic dysfunction), HIV infection, immunocompromising conditions (congenital immunodeficiencies excluding chronic granulomatous disease, renal failure, nephrotic syndrome, diseases associated with immunosuppressive or radiation therapy, solid organ transplant), chronic illnesses (cardiac disease, cerebrospinal fluid leaks, diabetes mellitus, pulmonary disease excluding asthma unless on high dose corticosteroids)

Children 6-18 years of age at increased risk for invasive pneumococcal disease due to sickle cell disease, HIV infection or other immunocompromising condition, cochlear implant, or cerebrospinal fluid leaks (regardless of prior receipt of PCV7 or PPSV23)

Dosage Summary

I.M.:

Infants <6 weeks: Dosage not established

Infants 2-6 months: 0.5 mL at approximately 2-month intervals for 3 consecutive doses, followed by a fourth dose of 0.5 mL at 12-15 months of age

Infants 7-11 months (previously unvaccinated): 0.5 mL for a total of 3 doses, 2 doses at least 4 weeks apart, followed by a third dose at 12-15 months (at least 2 months after second dose)

Children 12-23 months (previously unvaccinated): 0.5 mL for a total of 2 doses, separated by at least 2 months

Children 24-59 months (previously unvaccinated): Healthy Children: 0.5 mL as a single dose

Children 24-71 months (previously unvaccinated): Children with underlying conditions: 0.5 mL for a total of 2 doses, separated by at least 2 months

Children 14 months-71 months (previously completing vaccination with PCV7): 0.5 mL supplemental dose

Children 6-18 years at high risk for invasive pneumococcal disease: 0.5 mL as a single dose

Adults: Dosage not established

Dosage Forms

Injection, suspension:

Prevnar 13™: 2 mcg of each capsular saccharide for serotypes 1, 3, 4, 5, 6A, 7F, 9V, 14, 18C, 19A, 19F, and 23F, and 4 mcg of serotype 6B [bound to diphtheria CRM_{197} protein ~34 mcg] per 0.5 mL (0.5 mL)

pneumococcal conjugate vaccine (7-valent)

(noo moe KOK al KON ju gate vak SEEN, seven vay lent)

Sound-Alike/Look-Alike Issues

pneumococcal 7-valent conjugate vaccine (Prevnar®) may be confused with pneumococcal 13-valent conjugate vaccine (Prevnar 13™) or with pneumococcal 23-valent polysaccharide vaccine (Pneumovax® 23)

Synonyms diphtheria CRM_{197} protein; PCV; PCV-7; PCV7; pneumococcal 7-valent conjugate vaccine

U.S./Canadian Brand Names Prevnar® [US/Can]

Therapeutic Category Vaccine

Use

Immunization of infants and toddlers against *Streptococcus pneumoniae* infection caused by serotypes included in the vaccine

Immunization of infants and toddlers against otitis media caused by serotypes included in the vaccine

The Advisory Committee on Immunization Practices (ACIP) recommends routine vaccination for the following:

All children 2-23 months

Children ≥2-59 months with cochlear implants

Children ages 24-59 months with: Sickle cell disease (including other sickle cell hemoglobinopathies, asplenia, splenic dysfunction), HIV infection, immunocompromising conditions (congenital immunodeficiencies excluding chronic granulomatous disease, renal failure, nephrotic syndrome, diseases associated with immunosuppressive or radiation therapy, solid organ transplant), chronic illnesses (cardiac disease, cerebrospinal fluid leaks, diabetes mellitus, pulmonary disease excluding asthma unless on high-dose corticosteroids)

Consider use in all children 24-59 months with priority given to:

Children 24-35 months

Children 24-59 months who are of Alaska native, American Indian, or African-American descent

Children 24-59 months who attend group daycare centers

Dosage Summary

I.M.:

Infants <6 weeks: Dosage not established

Infants 2-6 months: 0.5 mL at approximately 2-month intervals for 3 consecutive doses, followed by a fourth dose of 0.5 mL at 12-15 months of age

Infants 7-11 months (previously unvaccinated): 0.5 mL for a total of 3 doses, 2 doses at least 4 weeks apart, followed by a third dose at 12-15 months (at least 2 months after second dose)

Children 12-23 months (previously unvaccinated): 0.5 mL for a total of 2 doses, separated by at least 2 months

Children 24-59 months (previously unvaccinated): Healthy: 0.5 mL as a single dose; Chronic illness: 0.5 mL for a total of 2 doses, separated by 2 months

Children >59 months: Dosage not established

Adults: Dosage not established

Dosage Forms

Injection, suspension:

Prevnar®: 2 mcg of each capsular saccharide for serotypes 4, 9V, 14, 18C, 19F, and 23F, and 4 mcg of serotype 6B per 0.5 mL (0.5 mL)

pneumococcal polysaccharide vaccine (polyvalent)

(noo moe KOK al pol i SAK a ride vak SEEN, pol i VAY lent)

Sound-Alike/Look-Alike Issues

pneumococcal 23-valent polysaccharide vaccine (Pneumovax® 23) may be confused with pneumococcal 7-valent conjugate vaccine (Prevnar®) or with pneumococcal 13-valent conjugate vaccine (Prevnar 13™)

Synonyms 23-valent pneumococcal polysaccharide vaccine; 23PS; PPSV; PPSV23; PPV23

U.S./Canadian Brand Names Pneumo 23™ [Can]; Pneumovax® 23 [US/Can]

Therapeutic Category Vaccine, Inactivated Bacteria

Use Immunization against pneumococcal disease caused by serotypes included in the vaccine. Routine vaccination is recommended for persons ≥50 years of age and persons ≥2 years in certain situations.

The Advisory Committee on Immunization Practices (ACIP) recommends routine vaccination for the following:

1) All immunocompetent patients ≥65 years of age

2) Patients 2-64 years of age with certain high-risk condition(s):

- Chronic cardiovascular disease (heart failure and cardiomyopathies)
- Chronic pulmonary disease (including COPD and emphysema)
- Diabetes mellitus
- Alcoholism
- Chronic liver disease (including cirrhosis)
- Cerebrospinal fluid leaks
- Functional or anatomic asplenia (including sickle cell disease and splenectomy)
- Immunocompromising conditions (including HIV infection, leukemia, lymphoma, Hodgkin disease, multiple myeloma, generalized malignancy, chronic renal failure, nephrotic syndrome; patients receiving immunosuppressive chemotherapy, including corticosteroids; patients who have received an organ or bone marrow transplant)

3) Adults aged 19-64 years of age who smoke cigarettes or have asthma

4) Persons aged 2-64 years with cochlear implants

Routine vaccination is not recommended for Alaska Natives or American Indian persons unless they have underlying conditions which are indications for vaccination; in special situations, vaccination may be recommended when living in an area at increased risk of invasive pneumococcal disease.

Dosage Summary

I.M.:

Children <2 years: Dosage not established

Children ≥2 years: 0.5 mL

Adults: 0.5 mL

SubQ:

Children <2 years: Dosage not established

Children ≥2 years: 0.5 mL

Adults: 0.5 mL

Dosage Forms

Injection, solution:

Pneumovax® 23: 25 mcg each of 23 capsular polysaccharide isolates/0.5 mL (0.5 mL, 2.5 mL)

Pneumomist® *(Discontinued)* *see* guaifenesin *on page* 454

Pneumotussin® *(Discontinued)*

Pneumovax® 23 [US/Can] *see* pneumococcal polysaccharide vaccine (polyvalent) *on page* 772

PNU-140690E *see* tipranavir *on page* 936

Pnu-Imune® 23 *(Discontinued)*

Podactin Cream [US-OTC] *see* miconazole (topical) *on page* *630*
Podactin Powder [US-OTC] *see* tolnaftate *on page* *940*
Pod-Ben-25® *(Discontinued)* *see* podophyllum resin *on page* *773*
Podocon-25® [US] *see* podophyllum resin *on page* *773*
Podofilm® [Can] *see* podophyllum resin *on page* *773*

podofilox (poe DOF il oks)

U.S./Canadian Brand Names Condyline™ [Can]; Condylox® [US]; Wartec® [Can]

Therapeutic Category Keratolytic Agent

Use Treatment of external genital warts

Dosage Summary

Topical:

Children: Dosage not established

Adults: Apply twice daily for 3 consecutive days, then withhold use for 4 consecutive days; May repeat cycle up to 4 times

Dosage Forms

Gel, topical:

Condylox®: 0.5% (3.5 g)

Solution, topical: 0.5% (3.5 mL)

Condylox®: 0.5% (3.5 mL)

Podofin® *(Discontinued)* *see* podophyllum resin *on page* *773*
podophyllin *see* podophyllum resin *on page* *773*

podophyllum resin (po DOF fil um REZ in)

Synonyms mandrake; may apple; podophyllin

U.S./Canadian Brand Names Podocon-25® [US]; Podofilm® [Can]

Therapeutic Category Keratolytic Agent

Use Topical treatment of benign growths including external genital and perianal warts, papillomas, fibroids; compound benzoin tincture generally is used as the medium for topical application

Dosage Summary

Topical:

Children: 10-25% solution applied 1-5 times/day

Adults: 10-25% solution applied 1-5 times/day

Dosage Forms

Liquid, topical:

Podocon-25®: 25% (15 mL)

Point-Two® *(Discontinued)* *see* fluoride *on page* *413*
Poladex® *(Discontinued)* *see* dexchlorpheniramine *on page* *282*
Polaramine® *(Discontinued)* *see* dexchlorpheniramine *on page* *282*

polidocanol (pol i DOE kuh nol)

U.S./Canadian Brand Names Asclera™ [US]

Therapeutic Category Sclerosing Agent

Use Treatment of small, uncomplicated varicose veins of the lower extremities

Dosage Summary

I.V.:

Children: Dosage not established

Adults: 0.1-0.3 mL injection (0.5% or 1% solution) per session (maximum: 10 mL/session)

Dosage Forms

Injection, solution [preservative free]:

Asclera™: 0.5% (2 mL); 1% (2 mL)

poliovirus, inactivated (IPV) *see* diphtheria and tetanus toxoids, acellular pertussis, and poliovirus vaccine *on page* *314*

poliovirus, inactivated (IPV) *see* diphtheria and tetanus toxoids, acellular pertussis, poliovirus and *Haemophilus* b conjugate vaccine *on page* *314*

poliovirus vaccine (inactivated) (POE lee oh VYE rus vak SEEN, in ak ti VAY ted)

Synonyms enhanced-potency inactivated poliovirus vaccine; IPV; salk vaccine

U.S./Canadian Brand Names IPOL® [US/Can]

Therapeutic Category Vaccine, Live Virus and Inactivated Virus

Use Active immunization against poliomyelitis caused by poliovirus types 1, 2 and 3. **Note:** Combination products containing polio vaccine are also available and may be preferred in certain age groups if recipients are likely to be susceptible to the agents contained within each vaccine.

The Advisory Committee on Immunization Practices (ACIP) recommends routine vaccination for the following:

- All children (first dose given at 2 months of age)

Routine immunization of adults in the United States is generally not recommended. Adults with previous wild poliovirus disease, who have never been immunized, or those who are incompletely immunized may receive inactivated poliovirus vaccine if they fall into one of the following categories:

- Travelers to regions or countries where poliomyelitis is endemic or epidemic
- Healthcare workers in close contact with patients who may be excreting poliovirus
- Laboratory workers handling specimens that may contain poliovirus
- Members of communities or specific population groups with diseases caused by wild poliovirus
- Incompletely vaccinated or unvaccinated adults in a household or with other close contact with children receiving oral poliovirus (may be at increased risk of vaccine associated paralytic poliomyelitis)

Dosage Summary

I.M.:

Children: Primary immunization: Administer three 0.5 mL doses at 2, 4, and 6-18 months of age; do not administer more frequently than 4 weeks apart (preferably given more than 8 weeks apart). Booster dose: 0.5 mL at 4-6 years of age; Minimum interval between booster and previous dose is 6 months

Adults (previously unvaccinated): Two 0.5 mL doses administered at 1- to 2-month intervals followed by a third dose 6-12 months later. **Note:** Refer to CDC guidelines for incompletely vaccinated or already vaccinated adult guidelines.

SubQ:

Children: Primary immunization: Administer three 0.5 mL doses, preferably 8 or more weeks apart at 2, 4, and 6-18 months of age; Booster dose: 0.5 mL at 4-6 years of age

Adults (previously unvaccinated): Two 0.5 mL doses administered at 1- to 2-month intervals followed by a third dose 6-12 months later. **Note:** Refer to CDC guidelines for incompletely vaccinated or already vaccinated adult guidelines.

Dosage Forms

Injection, suspension:

IPOL®: Type 1 poliovirus 40 D-antigen units, type 2 poliovirus 8 D-antigen units, and type 3 poliovirus 32 D-antigen units per 0.5 mL (0.5 mL, 5 mL)

Polocaine® [US/Can] *see* mepivacaine *on page 604*

Polocaine® 2% and Levonordefrin 1:20,000 [Can] *see* mepivacaine and levonordefrin *on page 605*

Polocaine® Dental [US] *see* mepivacaine *on page 604*

Polocaine® Dental with Levonordefrin [US] *see* mepivacaine and levonordefrin *on page 605*

Polocaine® MPF [US] *see* mepivacaine *on page 604*

polycarbophil (pol i KAR boe fil)

U.S./Canadian Brand Names Equalactin® [US-OTC]; Fiber-Lax [US-OTC]; Fiber-Tabs™ [US-OTC]; FiberCon® [US-OTC]; Konsyl® Fiber [US-OTC]

Therapeutic Category Gastrointestinal Agent, Miscellaneous; Laxative

Use Treatment of constipation or diarrhea

Dosage Summary

Oral:

Children <6 years: Dosage not established

Children 6-12 years: 625 mg calcium polycarbophil 1-4 times/day

Children ≥12 years: 1250 mg calcium polycarbophil 1-4 times/day

Adults: 1250 mg calcium polycarbophil 1-4 times/day

Dosage Forms

Caplet, oral: Calcium polycarbophil 625 mg

FiberCon® [OTC]: Calcium polycarbophil 625 mg

Konsyl® Fiber [OTC]: Calcium polycarbophil 625 mg

Captab, oral:

Fiber-Lax [OTC]: Calcium polycarbophil 625 mg

Tablet, oral:

Fiber-Tabs™ [OTC]: Calcium polycarbophil 625 mg

Tablet, chewable, oral:

Equalactin® [OTC]: Calcium polycarbophil 625 mg

polycitra *see* citric acid, sodium citrate, and potassium citrate *on page* 228

Polycitra®-K [Can] *see* potassium citrate *on page* 782

Polycose® [US-OTC] *see* glucose polymers *on page* 448

Poly-Dex™ [US] *see* neomycin, polymyxin B, and dexamethasone *on page* 666

polyethylene glycol-L-asparaginase *see* pegaspargase *on page* 732

polyethylene glycol 3350 (pol i ETH i leen GLY kol 3350)

Sound-Alike/Look-Alike Issues

polyethylene glycol 3350 may be confused with polyethylene glycol electrolyte solution

MiraLAX® may be confused with Mirapex®

Synonyms PEG

U.S./Canadian Brand Names Dulcolax Balance® [US-OTC]; MiraLAX® [US-OTC]

Therapeutic Category Laxative, Osmotic

Use Treatment of occasional constipation in adults

Dosage Summary

Oral:

Adults: 17 g of powder (~1 heaping tablespoon) dissolved in 4-8 ounces of beverage once daily (maximum use: 1 week)

Dosage Forms

Powder for solution, oral: 17 g/dose (119 g, 238 g, 255 g, 510 g, 527 g); 17 g/packet (14s, 30s)

Dulcolax Balance® [OTC]: 17 g/dose (119 g, 238 g, 510 g)

MiraLAX® [OTC]: 17 g/dose (119 g, 238 g, 510 g); 17 g/packet (10s)

polyethylene glycol-electrolyte solution

(pol i ETH i leen GLY kol ee LEK troe lite soe LOO shun)

Sound-Alike/Look-Alike Issues

GoLYTELY® may be confused with NuLYTELY®

NuLYTELY® may be confused with GoLYTELY®

TriLyte® may be confused with TriLipix™

Synonyms electrolyte lavage solution

U.S./Canadian Brand Names Colyte® [US/Can]; GoLYTELY® [US]; Klean-Prep® [Can]; MoviPrep® [US]; NuLYTELY® [US]; PegLyte® [Can]; TriLyte® [US]

Therapeutic Category Laxative

Use Bowel cleansing prior to GI examination

Dosage Summary

Nasogastric tube:

Children <6 months: Dosage not established

Children ≥6 months: 25 mL/kg/hour until rectal effluent is clear

Adults: 20-30 mL/minute (1.2-1.8 L/hour) until rectal effluent is clear

Oral:

Children <6 months: Dosage not established

Children ≥6 months: (CoLyte®, GoLYTELY®, NuLYTELY®, TriLyte®): 25 mL/kg/hour (some studies have used up to 40 mL/kg/hour) for 4-10 hours until rectal effluent is clear (maximum total dose: 4 L)

Adults:

CoLyte®, GoLYTELY®, NuLYTELY®, TriLyte®: 240 mL (8 oz) every 10 minutes, until 4 L are consumed or the rectal effluent is clear

MoviPrep®: 240 mL (8 oz) every 15 minutes until 1 L consumed; repeat 1 time

Dosage Forms

Powder, for oral solution: PEG 3350 240 g, sodium sulfate 22.72 g, sodium bicarbonate 6.72 g, sodium chloride 5.84 g, and potassium 2.98 g; PEG 3350 236 g, sodium sulfate 22.74 g, sodium bicarbonate 6.74 g, sodium chloride 5.86 g, and potassium chloride 2.97 g; PEG 3350 240 g, sodium bicarbonate 5.72 g, sodium chloride 11.2 g, and potassium chloride 1.48 g

Colyte®: PEG 3350 240 g, sodium sulfate 22.72 g, sodium bicarbonate 6.72 g, sodium chloride 5.84 g, and potassium 2.98 g

GoLYTELY®:

PEG 3350 236 g, sodium sulfate 22.74 g, sodium bicarbonate 6.74 g, sodium chloride 5.86 g, and potassium 2.97 g

PEG 3350 227.1 g, sodium sulfate 21.5 g, sodium bicarbonate 6.36 g, sodium chloride 5.53 g, and potassium 2.82 g per packet (1s)

MoviPrep®: Pouch A: PEG 3350 100g, sodium sulfate 7.5 g, sodium chloride 2.69 g, potassium chloride 1.015 g; Pouch B: Ascorbic acid 4.7 g, sodium ascorbate 5.9 g

NuLYTELY®: PEG 3350 420 g, sodium bicarbonate 5.72 g, sodium chloride 11.2 g, and potassium 1.48 g

TriLyte®: PEG 3350 420 g, sodium bicarbonate 5.72 g, sodium chloride 11.2 g, and potassium 1.48 g

polyethylene glycol-electrolyte solution and bisacodyl

(pol i ETH i leen GLY kol ee LEK troe lite soe LOO shun & bis a KOE dil)

Synonyms electrolyte lavage solution

U.S./Canadian Brand Names HalfLytely® and Bisacodyl [US]

Therapeutic Category Laxative, Bowel Evacuant; Laxative, Stimulant

Use Bowel cleansing prior to colonoscopy

Dosage Summary

Oral:

Children: Dosage not established

Adults: 5 mg of bisacodyl as a single dose, after bowel movement or 6 hours (whichever occurs first) initiate 8 ounces of polyethylene glycol-electrolyte solution every 10 minutes until 2 L are consumed

Dosage Forms

Kit [each kit contains]:

HalfLytely® and Bisacodyl:

Powder for solution, oral (HalfLytely®): PEG 3350 210 g, sodium bicarbonate 2.86 g, sodium chloride 5.6 g, potassium chloride 0.74 g (2000 mL) [contains 4 flavor packs (each 1 g) cherry, lemon-lime, orange, pineapple flavors]

Tablet, delayed release (Bisacodyl): 5 mg (1s)

Polygam® S/D *(Discontinued)* *see* immune globulin (intravenous) *on page* 502

Poly-Hist DM [US] *see* phenylephrine, pyrilamine, and dextromethorphan *on page* 755

Poly Hist Forte® [US] *see* chlorpheniramine, pyrilamine, and phenylephrine *on page* 215

Poly-Histine-D® Capsule *(Discontinued)*

Poly Hist PD [US] *see* chlorpheniramine, pyrilamine, and phenylephrine *on page* 215

Poly-Iron 150 [US-OTC] *see* polysaccharide-iron complex *on page* 777

Poly-Iron 150 Forte [US] *see* polysaccharide-iron complex, vitamin B12, and folic acid *on page* 778

polymyxin B (pol i MIKS in bee)

Synonyms polymyxin B sulfate

U.S./Canadian Brand Names Poly-Rx [US]

Therapeutic Category Antibiotic, Irrigation; Antibiotic, Miscellaneous

Use Treatment of acute infections caused by susceptible strains of *Pseudomonas aeruginosa*; used occasionally for gut decontamination; parenteral use of polymyxin B has mainly been replaced by less toxic antibiotics, reserved for life-threatening infections caused by organisms resistant to the preferred drugs (eg, pseudomonal meningitis - intrathecal administration)

Dosage Summary

I.M.:

Children <2 years: Up to 40,000 units/kg/day divided every 6 hours

Children ≥2 years: 25,000-30,000 units/kg/day divided every 4-6 hours (maximum: 2,000,000 units/day)

Adults: 25,000-30,000 units/kg/day divided every 4-6 hours (maximum: 2,000,000 units/day)

I.V.:

Children <2 years: Up to 40,000 units/kg/day divided every 12 hours

Children ≥2 years: 15,000-25,000 units/kg/day divided every 12 hours (maximum: 2,000,000 units/day)

Adults: 15,000-25,000 units/kg/day divided every 12 hours (maximum: 2,000,000 units/day)

Intrathecal:

Children <2 years: 20,000 units/day for 3-4 days, then 25,000 units every other day

Children ≥2 years: 50,000 units/day for 3-4 days, then every other day

Adults: 50,000 units/day for 3-4 days, then every other day

Irrigation:
Children: Dosage not established
Adults:
Bladder: 20 mg (equal to 200,000 units) added to 1 L of normal saline as continuous irrigant or rinse
Topical: 500,000 units/L of normal saline (maximum: 2 million units/day)
Ophthalmic:
Children ≥2 years: Initial: 1-3 drops/hour; Reduce to 1-2 drops 4-6 times/day based on response
Adults: Initial: 1-3 drops/hour; Reduce to 1-2 drops 4-6 times/day based on response
Otic:
Children: 1-2 drops 3-4 times/day
Adults: 1-2 drops 3-4 times/day

Dosage Forms
Injection, powder for reconstitution: 500,000 units
Powder, for prescription compounding:
Poly-Rx: 100 million units (13 g)

polymyxin B and bacitracin *see* bacitracin and polymyxin B *on page 113*
polymyxin B and neomycin *see* neomycin and polymyxin B *on page 666*
polymyxin B and trimethoprim *see* trimethoprim and polymyxin B *on page 960*
polymyxin B, bacitracin, and neomycin *see* bacitracin, neomycin, and polymyxin B *on page 114*
polymyxin B, bacitracin, neomycin, and hydrocortisone *see* bacitracin, neomycin, polymyxin B, and hydrocortisone *on page 114*
polymyxin B, neomycin, and dexamethasone *see* neomycin, polymyxin B, and dexamethasone *on page 666*
polymyxin B, neomycin, and gramicidin *see* neomycin, polymyxin B, and gramicidin *on page 667*
polymyxin B, neomycin, and hydrocortisone *see* neomycin, polymyxin B, and hydrocortisone *on page 667*
polymyxin B, neomycin, and prednisolone *see* neomycin, polymyxin B, and prednisolone *on page 667*
polymyxin B, neomycin, bacitracin, and pramoxine *see* bacitracin, neomycin, polymyxin B, and pramoxine *on page 115*
polymyxin B sulfate *see* polymyxin B *on page 776*
polyphenols *see* sinecatechins *on page 878*
polyphenon E *see* sinecatechins *on page 878*
Poly-Pred® [US] *see* neomycin, polymyxin B, and prednisolone *on page 667*
Poly-Rx [US] *see* polymyxin B *on page 776*
Polysaccharide Iron 150 Forte [US] *see* polysaccharide-iron complex, vitamin B12, and folic acid *on page 778*

polysaccharide-iron complex (pol i SAK a ride-EYE ern KOM pleks)

Sound-Alike/Look-Alike Issues
Niferex® may be confused with Nephrox®

Synonyms iron-polysaccharide complex

U.S./Canadian Brand Names Ferrex™ 150 Plus [US-OTC]; Ferrex™ 150 [US-OTC]; Niferex® [US-OTC]; Nu-Iron® 150 [US-OTC]; Poly-Iron 150 [US-OTC]; ProFe [US-OTC]

Therapeutic Category Electrolyte Supplement, Oral

Use Prevention and treatment of iron-deficiency anemias

Dosage Summary
Oral:
Children <6 years: Dosage not established
Children ≥6 years: 50-100 mg once daily or in divided doses
Adults: 100-300 mg/day in 1-2 divided doses

Dosage Forms
Capsule, oral: Elemental iron 150 mg
Ferrex™ 150 [OTC]: Elemental iron 150 mg
Ferrex™ 150 Plus [OTC]: Elemental iron 150 mg (50 mg as ferrous asparto glycinate)
Niferex® [OTC]: Elemental iron 60 mg
Nu-Iron® 150 [OTC]: Elemental iron 150 mg

Poly-Iron 150 [OTC]: Elemental iron 150 mg
ProFe [OTC]: Elemental iron 180 mg

Elixir, oral:

Niferex® [OTC]: Elemental iron 100 mg/5 mL (236 mL)

polysaccharide-iron complex, vitamin B12, and folic acid

(pol i SAK a ride-EYE ern KOM pleks, VYE ta min bee twelve & FOE lik AS id)

Synonyms iron-polysaccharide complex, vitamin B12, and folic acid

U.S./Canadian Brand Names Ferrex™ 150 Forte Plus [US]; Ferrex™ 150 Forte [US]; Maxaron® Forte [US]; Poly-Iron 150 Forte [US]; Polysaccharide Iron 150 Forte [US]

Therapeutic Category Iron Salt

Use Prevention and treatment of iron-deficiency anemias and/or nutritional megaloblastic anemias

Dosage Summary

Oral:

Children: Dosage not established
Adults: 1-2 capsules daily

Dosage Forms

Capsule, oral:

Ferrex™ 150 Forte: Elemental iron 150 mg, cyanocobalamin 25 mcg, and folic acid 1 mg
Ferrex™ 150 Forte Plus: Elemental iron 150 mg (50 mg as ferrous asparto glycinate), cyanocobalamin 25 mcg, and folic acid 1 mg
Maxaron® Forte: Elemental iron 150 mg (80 mg as ferrous bisglycinate), cyanocobalamin 25 mcg, and folic acid 1 mg
Poly-Iron 150 Forte: Elemental iron 150 mg, cyanocobalamin 25 mcg, and folic acid 1 mg
Polysaccharide Iron 150 Forte: Elemental iron 150 mg, cyanocobalamin 25 mcg, and folic acid 1 mg

Polysporin® [US-OTC] *see* bacitracin and polymyxin B *on page 113*
Polytar® *(Discontinued)* *see* coal tar *on page 242*
Polytrim® [US/Can] *see* trimethoprim and polymyxin B *on page 960*
Poly Tussin DM [US] *see* chlorpheniramine, phenylephrine, and dextromethorphan *on page 211*
PolyTussin HD [US] *see* phenylephrine, hydrocodone, and chlorpheniramine *on page 754*
Poly-Vi-Flor® *(Discontinued)* *see* vitamins (multiple/pediatric) *on page 990*
polyvinyl alcohol *see* artificial tears *on page 97*
polyvinylpyrrolidone with iodine *see* povidone-iodine (ophthalmic) *on page 784*
polyvinylpyrrolidone with iodine *see* povidone-iodine (topical) *on page 784*
Poly-Vi-Sol® [US-OTC] *see* vitamins (multiple/pediatric) *on page 990*
Poly-Vi-Sol® with Iron [US-OTC] *see* vitamins (multiple/pediatric) *on page 990*
Ponstan® [Can] *see* mefenamic acid *on page 597*
Ponstel® [US] *see* mefenamic acid *on page 597*
Pontocaine® [Can] *see* tetracaine (ophthalmic) *on page 922*
Pontocaine® [Can] *see* tetracaine (systemic) *on page 921*
Pontocaine® [US/Can] *see* tetracaine (topical) *on page 922*
Pontocaine® Injection *(Discontinued)* *see* tetracaine (systemic) *on page 921*
Pontocaine® Niphanoid® *(Discontinued)* *see* tetracaine (systemic) *on page 921*

poractant alfa (por AKT ant AL fa)

U.S./Canadian Brand Names Curosurf® [US/Can]

Therapeutic Category Lung Surfactant

Use Treatment of respiratory distress syndrome (RDS) in premature infants

Dosage Summary

Intratracheal:

Premature infants: Initial: 2.5 mL/kg of birth weight, up to 2 subsequent doses of 1.25 mL/kg birth weight can be administered at 12-hour intervals if needed; Maximum total dose: 5 mL/kg
Children: Dosage not established
Adults: Dosage not established

Dosage Forms

Suspension, intratracheal [preservative free]:

Curosurf®: 80 mg/mL (1.5 mL, 3 mL)

Porcelana® Sunscreen *(Discontinued)* *see* hydroquinone *on page 487*

porfimer (POR fi mer)

Synonyms CL-184116; dihematoporphyrin ether; porfimer sodium

U.S./Canadian Brand Names Photofrin® [US/Can]

Therapeutic Category Antineoplastic Agent

Use Palliation in patients with obstructing (partial or complete) esophageal cancer; treatment of microinvasive endobronchial nonsmall cell lung cancer (NSCLC); reduction of obstruction and palliation in patients with obstructing (partial or complete) NSCLC; ablation of high-grade dysplasia in Barrett esophagus

Dosage Summary

I.V.:

Children: Dosage not established

Adults: 2 mg/kg, followed by exposure to the appropriate laser light

Dosage Forms

Injection, powder for reconstitution:

Photofrin®: 75 mg

porfimer sodium *see* porfimer *on page 779*

Portagen® [US-OTC] *see* nutritional formula, enteral/oral *on page 692*

Portia™ [US] *see* ethinyl estradiol and levonorgestrel *on page 376*

posaconazole (poe sa KON a zole)

Sound-Alike/Look-Alike Issues

Noxafil® may be confused with minoxidil

Synonyms SCH 56592

U.S./Canadian Brand Names Noxafil® [US]; Posanol™ [Can]

Therapeutic Category Antifungal Agent, Oral

Use Prophylaxis of invasive *Aspergillus* and *Candida* infections in severely-immunocompromised patients [eg, hematopoietic stem cell transplant (HSCT) recipients with graft-versus-host disease (GVHD) or those with prolonged neutropenia secondary to chemotherapy for hematologic malignancies]; treatment of oropharyngeal candidiasis (including patients refractory to itraconazole and/or fluconazole)

Dosage Summary

Oral:

Children <13 years: Dosage not established

Children ≥13 years: 100-800 mg/day; doses >100 mg/day are given in 2-3 divided doses

Adults: 100-800 mg/day; doses >100 mg/day are given in 2-3 divided doses

Dosage Forms

Suspension, oral:

Noxafil®: 40 mg/mL (123 mL)

Posanol™ [Can] *see* posaconazole *on page 779*

Post-Peel Healing Balm® [US-OTC] *see* hydrocortisone (topical) *on page 483*

Posture® [US-OTC] *see* calcium phosphate (tribasic) *on page 171*

Potasalan® *(Discontinued)* *see* potassium chloride *on page 781*

potassium acetate (poe TASS ee um AS e tate)

Therapeutic Category Electrolyte Supplement, Oral

Use Potassium deficiency; to avoid chloride when high concentration of potassium is needed, source of bicarbonate

Dosage Summary

I.V.:

Children: 2-5 mEq/kg/day; Intermittent infusion: 0.5-1 mEq/kg/dose (maximum: 30 mEq/dose) to infuse at 0.3-0.5 mEq/kg/hour (maximum: 1 mEq/kg/hour)

Adults: 40-100 mEq/day; Intermittent infusion: 5-10 mEq/dose (maximum: 40 mEq/dose) to infuse over 2-3 hours (maximum: 40 mEq over 1 hour)

Dosage Forms

Injection, solution: 2 mEq/mL (20 mL, 50 mL, 100 mL)

Injection, solution [preservative free]: 2 mEq/mL (20 mL, 50 mL, 100 mL); 4 mEq/mL (50 mL)

potassium acid phosphate (poe TASS ee um AS id FOS fate)

U.S./Canadian Brand Names K-Phos® Original [US]

Therapeutic Category Urinary Acidifying Agent

Use Acidifies urine and lowers urinary calcium concentration; reduces odor and rash caused by ammoniacal urine; increases the antibacterial activity of methenamine

Dosage Summary

Oral:

Children: Dosage not established

Adults: 1000 mg dissolved in 6-8 oz of water 4 times/day with meals and at bedtime

Dosage Forms

Tablet, oral:

K-Phos® Original: 500 mg

potassium bicarbonate (poe TASS ee um bye KAR bun ate)

Therapeutic Category Electrolyte Supplement, Oral

Use Potassium deficiency, hypokalemia

Dosage Summary

Oral:

Children: 1-4 mEq/kg/day

Adults: 25 mEq 2-4 times/day

Dosage Forms

Tablet for solution, oral: Potassium 25 mEq

potassium bicarbonate and potassium chloride
(poe TASS ee um bye KAR bun ate & poe TASS ee um KLOR ide)

Synonyms potassium bicarbonate and potassium chloride (effervescent)

Therapeutic Category Electrolyte Supplement, Oral

Use Treatment or prevention of hypokalemia

Dosage Summary

Oral:

Children: 1-4 mEq/kg/day in divided doses

Adults: Prevention: 16-24 mEq/day in 2-4 divided doses; Treatment: 40-100 mEq/day in 2-4 divided doses

Dosage Forms

Tablet for solution, oral [effervescent]: Potassium chloride 25 mEq

potassium bicarbonate and potassium chloride (effervescent) *see* potassium bicarbonate and potassium chloride *on page 780*

potassium bicarbonate and potassium citrate
(poe TASS ee um bye KAR bun ate & poe TASS ee um SIT rate)

Sound-Alike/Look-Alike Issues

Klor-Con® may be confused with Klaron®

Synonyms potassium bicarbonate and potassium citrate (effervescent)

U.S./Canadian Brand Names Effer-K® [US]; K-Lyte® DS [US]; K-Lyte® [US]; Klor-Con®/EF [US]

Therapeutic Category Electrolyte Supplement, Oral

Use Treatment or prevention of hypokalemia

Dosage Summary

Oral:

Children: 1-4 mEq/kg/day in divided doses

Adults: Prevention: 16-24 mEq/day in 2-4 divided doses; Treatment: 40-100 mEq/day in 2-4 divided doses

Dosage Forms

Tablet for solution, oral [effervescent]:

Effer-K®: Potassium 10 mEq; potassium 20 mEq; potassium 25 mEq

Klor-Con®/EF, K-Lyte®: Potassium 25 mEq

K-Lyte® DS: Potassium 50 mEq

potassium bicarbonate and potassium citrate (effervescent) *see* potassium bicarbonate and potassium citrate *on page 780*

potassium chloride (poe TASS ee um KLOR ide)

Sound-Alike/Look-Alike Issues

Kaon-CL 10® may be confused with kaolin
KCl may be confused with HCl
Klor-Con® may be confused with Klaron®
microK® may be confused with Macrobid®, Micronase®

Synonyms KCl; kdur

U.S./Canadian Brand Names Apo-K® [Can]; Epiklor™ [US]; Epiklor™/25 [US]; K-10® [Can]; K-Dur® [Can]; K-Lyte®/Cl [Can]; K-Tab® [US]; Kaon-CL® 10 [US]; Klor-Con® 10 [US]; Klor-Con® 8 [US]; Klor-Con® M10 [US]; Klor-Con® M15 [US]; Klor-Con® M20 [US]; Klor-Con® [US]; Klor-Con®/25 [US]; Micro-K Extencaps® [Can]; microK® 10 [US]; microK® [US]; Roychlor® [Can]; Slo-Pot [Can]; Slow-K® [Can]

Therapeutic Category Electrolyte Supplement, Oral

Use Treatment or prevention of hypokalemia

Dosage Summary

I.V.:

Children: Initial: 0.5-1 mEq/kg/dose (maximum dose: 40 mEq); repeat as needed based on lab values

Adults: Intermittent infusion: ≤10 mEq/hour; repeat as needed based on lab values (maximum: 200 mEq/day)

Oral:

Children: 1-2 mEq/kg/day in 1-2 divided doses or as needed based on lab values

Adults: 40-100 mEq/day in divided doses or as needed based on lab values

Dosage Forms

Caplet, extended release, oral: 10 mEq

Capsule, extended release, microencapsulated, oral: 8 mEq, 10 mEq

microK®: 8 mEq
microK® 10: 10 mEq

Infusion, premixed in 1/2 NS: 20 mEq (1000 mL)

Infusion, premixed in D_{10} 1/4 NS: 5 mEq (250 mL)

Infusion, premixed in D_5 1/2 NS: 10 mEq (500 mL, 1000 mL); 20 mEq (1000 mL); 30 mEq (1000 mL); 40 mEq (1000 mL)

Infusion, premixed in D_5 1/3 NS: 10 mEq (500 mL); 20 mEq (1000 mL)

Infusion, premixed in D_5 1/4 NS: 5 mEq (250 mL); 10 mEq (500 mL, 1000 mL); 20 mEq (1000 mL); 30 mEq (1000 mL); 40 mEq (1000 mL)

Infusion, premixed in D_5LR: 20 mEq (1000 mL); 40 mEq (1000 mL)

Infusion, premixed in D_5NS: 20 mEq (1000 mL); 40 mEq (1000 mL)

Infusion, premixed in D_5W: 20 mEq (500 mL, 1000 mL); 30 mEq (1000 mL); 40 mEq (1000 mL)

Infusion, premixed in NS: 20 mEq (1000 mL); 40 mEq (1000 mL)

Infusion, premixed in water for injection: 10 mEq (50 mL, 100 mL); 20 mEq (50 mL, 100 mL); 30 mEq (100 mL); 40 mEq (100 mL)

Injection, solution: 2 mEq/mL (5 mL, 10 mL, 15 mL, 20 mL, 30 mL, 250 mL, 500 mL)

Injection, solution [preservative free]: 2 mEq/mL (5 mL, 10 mL, 15 mL, 20 mL)

Powder for solution, oral:

Epiklor™: 20 mEq/packet (30s, 100s)
Epiklor™/25: 25 mEq/packet (30s, 100s)
Klor-Con®: 20 mEq/packet (30s, 100s)
Klor-Con®/25: 25 mEq/packet (30s, 100s)

Solution, oral: 20 mEq/15 mL (15 mL, 30 mL, 473 mL, 480 mL); 40 mEq/15 mL (15 mL, 473 mL)

Tablet, extended release, microencapsulated, oral: 8 mEq, 10 mEq, 20 mEq

Klor-Con® M10: 10 mEq
Klor-Con® M15: 15 mEq
Klor-Con® M20: 20 mEq

Tablet, extended release, wax matrix, oral: 8 mEq, 10 mEq

K-Tab®: 10 mEq
Kaon-CL® 10: 10 mEq
Klor-Con® 8: 8 mEq
Klor-Con® 10: 10 mEq

potassium citrate (poe TASS ee um SIT rate)

Sound-Alike/Look-Alike Issues
Urocit®-K may be confused with Urised®

U.S./Canadian Brand Names K-Citra® [Can]; K-Lyte® [Can]; Polycitra®-K [Can]; Urocit®-K [US]

Therapeutic Category Alkalinizing Agent

Use Prevention of uric acid nephrolithiasis; prevention of calcium renal stones in patients with hypocitraturia; urinary alkalinizer when sodium citrate is contraindicated

Dosage Summary
Oral:
Children: Dosage not established
Adults: 10-20 mEq 3 times/day with meals (maximum: 100 mEq/day)

Dosage Forms
Tablet, oral: 540 mg, 1080 mg
Urocit®-K: 540 mg, 1080 mg
Tablet, extended release, oral: 540 mg, 1080 mg

potassium citrate and citric acid (poe TASS ee um SIT rate & SI trik AS id)

Synonyms citric acid and potassium citrate

U.S./Canadian Brand Names Cytra-K [US]

Therapeutic Category Alkalinizing Agent

Use Treatment of metabolic acidosis; alkalinizing agent in conditions where long-term maintenance of an alkaline urine is desirable

Dosage Summary
Oral:
Children: 5-15 mL after meals and at bedtime
Adults: 15-30 mL **or** one packet dissolved in water after meals and at bedtime

Dosage Forms Equivalent to potassium 2 mEq/mL and bicarbonate 2 mEq/mL
Powder for solution, oral:
Cytra-K: Potassium citrate 3300 mg and citric acid 1002 mg per packet (100s)
Solution:
Cytra-K: Potassium citrate 1100 mg and citric acid 334 mg per 5 mL

potassium citrate, citric acid, and sodium citrate *see* citric acid, sodium citrate, and potassium citrate *on page 228*

potassium gluconate (poe TASS ee um GLOO coe nate)

Therapeutic Category Electrolyte Supplement, Oral

Use Treatment or prevention of hypokalemia

Dosage Summary Note: Doses listed as mEq of potassium
Oral:
Children: 1-5 mEq/kg/day in 1-4 divided doses
Adults: 16-100 mEq/day in 1-4 divided doses

Dosage Forms
Caplet, oral: 595 mg
Capsule, oral: 99 mg
Tablet, oral: 99 mg, 550 mg, 595 mg
Tablet, timed release, oral: 95 mg

potassium iodide (poe TASS ee um EYE oh dide)

Sound-Alike/Look-Alike Issues
potassium iodide products, including saturated solution of potassium iodide (SSKI®) may be confused with potassium iodide and iodine (Strong Iodide Solution or Lugol's solution)

Synonyms KI

U.S./Canadian Brand Names iOSAT™ [US-OTC]; SSKI® [US]; ThyroSafe™ [US]; Thyroshield™ [US-OTC]

Therapeutic Category Antithyroid Agent; Expectorant

Use Expectorant for the symptomatic treatment of chronic pulmonary diseases complicated by mucous; block thyroidal uptake of radioactive isotopes of iodine in a radiation emergency

Dosage Summary

Oral:

Neonates:

iOSAT™, ThyroSafe™, ThyroShield™: 16.25 mg once daily

Infants 1-12 month:

iOSAT™, ThyroSafe™, ThyroShield™: 32.5 mg once daily

Children 1-3 years:

iOSAT™, ThyroSafe™, ThyroShield™: 32.5 mg once daily

Children 3-18 years:

iOSAT™, ThyroSafe™, ThyroShield™: 65-130 mg once daily

Adults:

iOSAT™, ThyroSafe™, ThyroShield™: 130 mg once daily

SSKI®: 300-600 mg (6-12 drops) 3-4 times/day

Dosage Forms

Solution, oral:

SSKI®: 1 g/mL (30 mL, 237 mL)

Thyroshield™ [OTC]: 65 mg/mL (30 mL)

Tablet, oral:

iOSAT™ [OTC]: 130 mg

ThyroSafe™: 65 mg

potassium phosphate (poe TASS ee um FOS fate)

Sound-Alike/Look-Alike Issues

Neutra-Phos®-K may be confused with K-Phos Neutral®

Synonyms phosphate, potassium

Therapeutic Category Electrolyte Supplement, Oral

Use Treatment and prevention of hypophosphatemia; **Note:** The concomitant amount of potassium must be calculated into the total electrolyte content. For each 1 mmol of phosphate, ~1.5 mEq of potassium will be administered. Therefore, if ordering 30 mmol of potassium phosphate, the patient will receive ~45 mEq of potassium.

Dosage Summary

I.V.:

Children: 0.25-0.5 mmol/kg over 4-6 hours, may repeat if needed; Infusion: 0.5-2 mmol/kg/24 hours

Adults: Acute replacement in critically-ill patients: 0.32-0.64 mmol/kg over 6-12 hours (based on severity; doses up to 1 mmol/kg documented in extreme cases); Parenteral nutrition: Infusion: 10-40 mmol/day

Oral:

Children <4 years: 250 mg phosphorus (8 mmol) 4 times/day

Children ≥4 years: 250-500 mg phosphorus (8-16 mmol) 4 times/day

Adults: 250-500 mg phosphorus (8-16 mmol) 4 times/day

Dosage Forms

Injection, solution: Potassium 4.4 mEq and phosphorus 3 mmol per mL (5 mL, 15 mL, 50 mL)

potassium phosphate and sodium phosphate

(poe TASS ee um FOS fate & SOW dee um FOS fate)

Sound-Alike/Look-Alike Issues

K-Phos® Neutral may be confused with Neutra-Phos-K®

Synonyms sodium phosphate and potassium phosphate

U.S./Canadian Brand Names K-Phos® MF [US]; K-Phos® Neutral [US]; K-Phos® No. 2 [US]; Phos-NaK [US]; Phospha 250™ Neutral [US]; Uro-KP-Neutral® [US]

Therapeutic Category Electrolyte Supplement, Oral

Use Treatment of conditions associated with excessive renal phosphate loss or inadequate GI absorption of phosphate; to acidify the urine to lower calcium concentrations; to increase the antibacterial activity of methenamine; reduce odor and rash caused by ammonia in urine

Dosage Summary

Oral:

Children <4 years: Dosage not established

Children ≥4 years: Elemental phosphorus 250 mg 4 times/day after meals and at bedtime

Adults: Elemental phosphorus 250-500 mg 4 times/day after meals and at bedtime

Dosage Forms

Caplet:

Uro-KP-Neutral®: Dipotassium phosphate, disodium phosphate, and monobasic sodium phosphate

Powder, for oral solution:

Phos-NaK: Dibasic potassium phosphate, monobasic potassium phosphate, dibasic sodium phosphate, and monobasic sodium phosphate per packet (100s)

Tablet:

K-Phos® MF: Potassium phosphate 155 mg and sodium phosphate 350 mg

K-Phos® Neutral: Monobasic potassium phosphate 155 mg, dibasic sodium phosphate 852 mg, and monobasic sodium phosphate 130 mg

K-Phos® No. 2: Potassium phosphate 305 mg and sodium phosphate 700 mg

Phospha 250™ Neutral: Monobasic potassium phosphate 155 mg, dibasic sodium phosphate 852 mg, and monobasic sodium phosphate 130 mg

Povidine™ [US-OTC] *see* povidone-iodine (topical) *on page 784*

povidone-iodine (ophthalmic) (POE vi done EYE oh dyne)

Sound-Alike/Look-Alike Issues

Betadine® may be confused with Betagan®, betaine

Synonyms polyvinylpyrrolidone with iodine; PVP-I

U.S./Canadian Brand Names Betadine® [US]

Therapeutic Category Antiseptic, Ophthalmic

Use Prepping the periocular region (lids, brows, and cheeks) and irrigation of the ocular surface

Dosage Summary

Topical:

Children: Dosage not established

Adults: Ophthalmic solution: Eyelids: Apply to area (repeat once); Periocular area: Apply to area (repeat 3 times); Ocular area: Irrigate once

Dosage Forms

Solution, ophthalmic:

Betadine®: 5% (30 mL)

povidone-iodine (topical) (POE vi done EYE oh dyne)

Sound-Alike/Look-Alike Issues

Betadine® may be confused with Betagan®, betaine

Synonyms polyvinylpyrrolidone with iodine; PVP-I

U.S./Canadian Brand Names Betadine® Swab Aids [US-OTC]; Betadine® [US-OTC/Can]; Operand® Povidone-Iodine [US-OTC]; Povidine™ [US-OTC]; Proviodine [Can]; Summer's Eve® Medicated Douche [US-OTC]; Vagi-Gard® [US-OTC]

Therapeutic Category Antiseptic, Topical; Antiseptic, Vaginal; Topical Skin Product

Use External antiseptic with broad microbicidal spectrum for the prevention or treatment of topical infections associated with surgery, burns, minor cuts/scrapes; relief of minor vaginal irritation

Dosage Summary

Intravaginal:

Children: Dosage not established

Adults: Insert 0.3% solution vaginally once daily

Topical:

Children: Dosage not established

Adults: Apply to affected area as needed **or** apply to wet skin or hands, scrub for ~5 minutes, then rinse

Dosage Forms

Gel, topical: 10% (120 mL)

Operand® Povidone-Iodine [OTC]: 10% (118 mL)

Liquid, topical: 10% (0.65 mL)

Ointment, topical: 10% (1 g, 28 g)

Povidine™ [OTC]: 10% (30 g)

Pad, topical: 10% (200s)

Betadine® Swab Aids [OTC]: 10% (100s)

Solution, perineal:

Operand® Povidone-Iodine [OTC]: 10% (240 mL)

Solution, topical: 7.5% (60 mL, 120 mL); 10% (22 mL, 30 mL, 59 mL, 60 mL, 90 mL, 120 mL, 237 mL, 473 mL, 480 mL, 50s)
Betadine® [OTC]: 5% (88.7 mL); 10% (15 mL, 120 mL, 237 mL, 473 mL, 960 mL, 3840 mL); 7.5% (118 mL, 473 mL, 960 mL, 3840 mL)
Operand® Povidone-Iodine [OTC]: 10% (59 mL, 118 mL, 237 mL, 473 mL, 946 mL, 3785 mL); 7.5% (59 mL, 118 mL, 237 mL, 473 mL, 946 mL, 3785 mL)
Povidine™ [OTC]: 10% (240 mL)
Solution, vaginal:
Operand® Povidone-Iodine [OTC]: 10% (240 mL)
Summer's Eve® Medicated Douche [OTC]: 0.3% (135 mL)
Vagi-Gard® [OTC]: 10% (180 mL, 240 mL)
Swabsticks, topical: 7.5% (50s, 75s, 1000s); 10% (50s, 75s, 1000s)
Betadine® [OTC]: 10% (150s, 200s)

PPD *see* tuberculin tests *on page 965*
PPS *see* pentosan polysulfate sodium *on page 741*
PPSV *see* pneumococcal polysaccharide vaccine (polyvalent) *on page 772*
PPSV23 *see* pneumococcal polysaccharide vaccine (polyvalent) *on page 772*
PPV23 *see* pneumococcal polysaccharide vaccine (polyvalent) *on page 772*
Pradax™ [Can] *see* dabigatran etexilate *(Canada only) on page 265*

pralatrexate (pral a TREX ate)

Sound-Alike/Look-Alike Issues
pralatrexate may be confused with methotrexate, pemetrexed
Folotyn™ may be confused with Focalin®

Synonyms PDX

U.S./Canadian Brand Names Folotyn™ [US]

Therapeutic Category Antineoplastic Agent, Antimetabolite (Antifolate)

Use Treatment of relapsed or refractory peripheral T-cell lymphoma (PTCL)

Dosage Summary
I.V.:
Children: Dosage not established
Adults: 30 mg/m^2 once weekly for 6 weeks of a 7-week treatment cycle

Dosage Forms
Injection, solution [preservative free]:
Folotyn™: 20 mg/mL (1 mL)

pralidoxime (pra li DOKS eem)

Sound-Alike/Look-Alike Issues
pralidoxime may be confused with pramoxine, pyridoxine
Protopam® may be confused with protamine, Protropin®

Synonyms 2-PAM; 2-pyridine aldoxime methochloride; pralidoxime chloride

U.S./Canadian Brand Names Protopam® [US/Can]

Therapeutic Category Antidote

Use Reverse muscle paralysis caused by toxic exposure to organophosphate acetylcholinesterase-inhibiting pesticides and chemicals; control of overdose of acetylcholinesterase medications used to treat myasthenia gravis (ambenonium, neostigmine, pyridostigmine)

Dosage Summary
I.M.:
Children: 20-50 mg/kg/dose, repeat in 1-2 hours if muscle weakness has not been relieved, then at 8- to 12-hour intervals if cholinergic signs recur
Adults: 1-2 g; repeat in 1 hour if muscle weakness has not been relieved, then at 8- to 12-hour intervals if cholinergic signs recur **or** 1-2 g followed by increments of 250 mg every 5 minutes until response is observed
I.V.:
Children: 20-50 mg/kg/dose; repeat in 1-2 hours if muscle weakness has not been relieved, then at 8- to 12-hour intervals if cholinergic signs recur
Adults: 1-2 g; repeat in 1 hour if muscle weakness has not been relieved, then at 8- to 12-hour intervals if cholinergic signs recur **or** 1-2 g followed by increments of 250 mg every 5 minutes until response is observed

Dosage Forms

Injection, powder for reconstitution:

Protopam®: 1 g

Injection, solution: 300 mg/mL (2 mL)

pralidoxime and atropine *see* atropine and pralidoxime *on page 107*

pralidoxime chloride *see* pralidoxime *on page 785*

Pramet® FA *(Discontinued)*

Pramilet® FA *(Discontinued)*

pramipexole (pra mi PEKS ole)

Sound-Alike/Look-Alike Issues

Mirapex® may be confused with Hiprex®, Mifeprex®, MiraLax™

Synonyms pramipexole dihydrochloride monohydrate

U.S./Canadian Brand Names Apo-Pramipexole® [Can]; CO Pramipexole [Can]; Mirapex® ER™ [US]; Mirapex® [US/Can]; Novo-Pramipexole [Can]; PHL-Pramipexole [Can]; PMS-Pramipexole [Can]; Sandoz-Pramipexole [Can]

Therapeutic Category Anti-Parkinson Agent (Dopamine Agonist)

Use

Immediate release: Treatment of the signs and symptoms of idiopathic Parkinson disease; treatment of moderate-to-severe primary Restless Legs Syndrome (RLS)

Extended release: Treatment of the signs and symptoms of idiopathic Parkinson disease

Dosage Summary

Oral, immediate release:

Children: Dosage not established

Adults: Initial: 0.375 mg/day given in 3 divided doses **or** 0.125 mg once daily before bedtime; Maintenance: 1.5-4.5 mg/day in 3 divided doses **or** 0.125-0.5 mg/day; **Note:** Titration is recommended

Oral, extended release:

Children: Dosage not established

Adults: Initial: 0.375 mg to 4.5 mg once daily.

Dosage Forms

Tablet, oral: 0.125 mg, 0.25 mg, 0.5 mg, 1 mg, 1.5 mg

Mirapex®: 0.125 mg, 0.25 mg, 0.5 mg, 0.75 mg, 1 mg, 1.5 mg

Tablet, extended release, oral:

Mirapex® ER™: 0.375 mg, 0.75 mg, 1.5 mg, 3 mg, 4.5 mg

pramipexole dihydrochloride monohydrate *see* pramipexole *on page 786*

pramlintide (PRAM lin tide)

Synonyms pramlintide acetate

U.S./Canadian Brand Names Symlin® [US]

Therapeutic Category Antidiabetic Agent, Oral

Use

Adjunctive treatment with mealtime insulin in type 1 diabetes mellitus (insulin-dependent, IDDM) patients who have failed to achieve desired glucose control despite optimal insulin therapy

Adjunctive treatment with mealtime insulin in type 2 diabetes mellitus (noninsulin-dependent, NIDDM) patients who have failed to achieve desired glucose control despite optimal insulin therapy, with or without concurrent sulfonylurea and/or metformin

Dosage Summary

SubQ:

Children: Dosage not established

Adults:

Type 1 diabetes mellitus (insulin-dependent, IDDM): Initial: 15 mcg immediately prior to meals; Target dose: 30-60 mcg prior to meals; **Note:** Titration is recommended

Type 2 diabetes mellitus (noninsulin-dependent, NIDDM): Initial: 60 mcg immediately prior to meals, after 3-7 days increase to 120 mcg prior to meals

Dosage Forms

Injection, solution:

Symlin®: 600 mcg/mL (5 mL); 1000 mcg/mL (1.5 mL, 2.7 mL)

pramlintide acetate *see* pramlintide *on page 786*

Pramosone® [US] *see* pramoxine and hydrocortisone *on page* *787*
Pramox® HC [Can] *see* pramoxine and hydrocortisone *on page* *787*

pramoxine (pra MOKS een)

Sound-Alike/Look-Alike Issues

pramoxine may be confused with pralidoxime

Synonyms pramoxine hydrochloride

U.S./Canadian Brand Names Caladryl® Clear™ [US-OTC]; Callergy Clear [US-OTC]; Curasore® [US-OTC]; Itch-X® [US-OTC]; Prax® [US-OTC]; Proctofoam® NS [US-OTC]; Sarna® Sensitive [US-OTC]; Sarna® Ultra [US-OTC]; Soothing Care™ Itch Relief [US-OTC]; Summer's Eve® Anti-Itch Maximum Strength [US-OTC]; Tronolane® Cream [US-OTC]; Tucks® Hemorrhoidal [US-OTC]

Therapeutic Category Local Anesthetic

Use Temporary relief of pain and itching associated with anogenital pruritus or irritation; dermatosis, minor burns, or hemorrhoids

Dosage Summary

Topical:

Children: Dosage not established
Adults: Apply 3-5 times daily to affected area

Dosage Forms

Aerosol, topical: 1% (15 g)
Proctofoam® NS [OTC]: 1% (15 g)

Cloth, topical:
Summer's Eve® Anti-Itch Maximum Strength [OTC]: 1% (12s)

Cream, topical:
Sarna® Ultra [OTC]: 1% (56.6 g)
Tronolane® Cream [OTC]: 1% (30 g, 57 g)

Gel, topical:
Itch-X® [OTC]: 1% (35.4 g)
Summer's Eve® Anti-Itch Maximum Strength [OTC]: 1% (30 mL)

Liquid, topical:
Curasore® [OTC]: 1% (15 mL)

Lotion, topical:
Caladryl® Clear™ [OTC]: 1% (177 mL)
Callergy Clear [OTC]: 1% (177 mL)
Prax® [OTC]: 1% (15 mL, 120 mL, 240 mL)
Sarna® Sensitive [OTC]: 1% (222 mL)

Ointment, rectal:
Tucks® Hemorrhoidal [OTC]: 1% (28.3 g)

Solution, topical:
Itch-X® [OTC]: 1% (60 mL)
Soothing Care™ Itch Relief [OTC]: 1% (74 mL)

pramoxine and hydrocortisone (pra MOKS een & hye droe KOR ti sone)

Sound-Alike/Look-Alike Issues

Pramosone® may be confused with predniSONE

Synonyms hydrocortisone and pramoxine; pramoxine hydrochloride and hydrocortisone acetate

U.S./Canadian Brand Names Analpram E™ [US]; Analpram-HC® [US]; Epifoam® [US]; Pramosone® [US]; Pramox® HC [Can]; ProctoFoam®-HC [US/Can]

Therapeutic Category Anesthetic/Corticosteroid

Use Relief of inflammatory and pruritic manifestations of corticosteroid-responsive dermatoses

Dosage Summary

Rectal:

Children: Dosage not established
Adults: Apply to affected areas 3-4 times/day

Topical:

Children: Dosage not established
Adults: Apply to affected areas 3-4 times/day

Dosage Forms

Cream, topical: Pramoxine 1% and hydrocortisone 1% (30 g); pramoxine 1% and hydrocortisone 2.5% (4 g, 30 g)

Analpram E™: Pramoxine 1% and hydrocortisone 2.5% (4 g, 30 g)

Analpram HC®: Pramoxine 1% and hydrocortisone 1% (4 g, 30 g); pramoxine 1% and hydrocortisone 2.5% (4 g, 30 g)

Pramosone®: Pramoxine 1% and hydrocortisone 1% (30 g, 60 g); pramoxine 1% and hydrocortisone 2.5% (30 g, 60 g)

Pramosone E™: Pramoxine 1% and hydrocortisone 2.5% (30 g, 60 g)

Zypram™: Pramoxine 1% and hydrocortisone 2.35% (30 g)

Foam, rectal:

ProctoFoam® HC: Pramoxine 1% and hydrocortisone 1% (10 g)

Foam, topical:

Epifoam®: Pramoxine 1% and hydrocortisone 1% (10 g)

Lotion, topical:

Analpram HC®: Pramoxine 1% and hydrocortisone 2.5% (60 mL)

Pramosone®: Pramoxine 1% and hydrocortisone 1% (60 mL, 120 mL, 240 mL); pramoxine 1% and hydrocortisone 2.5% (60 mL, 120 mL)

Ointment, topical:

Pramosone®: Pramoxine 1% and hydrocortisone 1% (30 g); pramoxine 1% and hydrocortisone 2.5% (30 g)

pramoxine hydrochloride *see* pramoxine *on page 787*

pramoxine hydrochloride and hydrocortisone acetate *see* pramoxine and hydrocortisone *on page 787*

pramoxine, neomycin, bacitracin, and polymyxin B *see* bacitracin, neomycin, polymyxin B, and pramoxine *on page 115*

PrandiMet® [US] *see* repaglinide and metformin *on page 835*

Prandin® [US/Can] *see* repaglinide *on page 835*

Prascion® [US] *see* sulfur and sulfacetamide *on page 903*

Prascion® AV *(Discontinued)* *see* sulfur and sulfacetamide *on page 903*

Prascion® FC [US] *see* sulfur and sulfacetamide *on page 903*

Prascion® RA [US] *see* sulfur and sulfacetamide *on page 903*

Prascion® TS *(Discontinued)* *see* sulfur and sulfacetamide *on page 903*

prasugrel (PRA soo grel)

Sound-Alike/Look-Alike Issues

prasugrel may be confused with pravastatin, propranolol

Effient™ may be confused with EtheDent™

Synonyms CS-747; LY-640315; prasugrel hydrochloride

U.S./Canadian Brand Names Effient™ [US]

Therapeutic Category Antiplatelet Agent

Use Reduces rate of thrombotic cardiovascular events (eg, stent thrombosis) in patients with unstable angina, non-ST-segment elevation MI (NSTEMI), or ST-elevation MI (STEMI) managed with percutaneous coronary intervention (PCI)

Dosage Summary

Oral:

Children: Dosage not established

Adults: Loading dose: 60 mg; Maintenance dose: 10 mg once daily (in combination with aspirin 81-325 mg/day); **Note:** In patients weighing <60 kg, consider decreasing maintenance dose to 5 mg once daily.

Dosage Forms

Tablet, oral:

Effient™: 5 mg, 10 mg

prasugrel hydrochloride *see* prasugrel *on page 788*

Pravachol® [US/Can] *see* pravastatin *on page 789*

pravastatin (prav a STAT in)

Sound-Alike/Look-Alike Issues

pravastatin may be confused with nystatin, pitavastatin, prasugrel

Pravachol® may be confused with atorvastatin, Prevacid®, Prinivil®, propranolol

Synonyms pravastatin sodium

U.S./Canadian Brand Names Apo-Pravastatin® [Can]; CO Pravastatin [Can]; Dom-Pravastatin [Can]; Mylan-Pravastatin [Can]; Novo-Pravastatin [Can]; Nu-Pravastatin [Can]; PHL-Pravastatin [Can]; PMS-Pravastatin [Can]; Pravachol® [US/Can]; RAN™-Pravastatin [Can]; ratio-Pravastatin [Can]; Riva-Pravastatin [Can]; Sandoz-Pravastatin [Can]; ZYM-Pravastatin [Can]

Therapeutic Category HMG-CoA Reductase Inhibitor

Use Use with dietary therapy for the following:

Primary prevention of coronary events: In hypercholesterolemic patients without established coronary heart disease to reduce cardiovascular morbidity (myocardial infarction, coronary revascularization procedures) and mortality.

Secondary prevention of cardiovascular events in patients with established coronary heart disease: To slow the progression of coronary atherosclerosis; to reduce cardiovascular morbidity (myocardial infarction, coronary vascular procedures) and to reduce mortality; to reduce the risk of stroke and transient ischemic attacks

Hyperlipidemias: Reduce elevations in total cholesterol, LDL-C, apolipoprotein B, and triglycerides (elevations of 1 or more components are present in Fredrickson type IIa, IIb, III, and IV hyperlipidemias)

Heterozygous familial hypercholesterolemia (HeFH): In pediatric patients, 8-18 years of age, with HeFH having LDL-C ≥190 mg/dL **or** LDL ≥160 mg/dL with positive family history of premature cardiovascular disease (CVD) or 2 or more CVD risk factors in the pediatric patient

Dosage Summary

Oral:

Children <8 years: Dosage not established

Children 8-13 years: 20 mg once daily

Children 14-18 years: 40 mg once daily

Adults: Initial: 10-40 mg once daily; Maintenance: 10-80 mg once daily (maximum: 80 mg/day) **Note:** Titration is recommended

Dosage Forms

Tablet, oral: 10 mg, 20 mg, 40 mg, 80 mg

Pravachol®: 10 mg, 20 mg, 40 mg, 80 mg

pravastatin sodium *see* pravastatin *on page* *789*

Pravigard™ PAC *(Discontinued)*

Prax® [US-OTC] *see* pramoxine *on page* *787*

Praxis ASA EC 81 Mg Daily Dose [Can] *see* aspirin *on page* *100*

praziquantel (pray zi KWON tel)

U.S./Canadian Brand Names Biltricide® [US/Can]

Therapeutic Category Anthelmintic

Use Treatment of all stages of schistosomiasis caused by all *Schistosoma* species; treatment of infection (clonorchiasis and opisthorchiasis) due to liver flukes

Dosage Summary

Oral:

Children ≥4 years and Adults: 20 mg/kg/dose or 25 mg/kg/dose 3 times/day for 1 day

Dosage Forms

Tablet, oral:

Biltricide®: 600 mg

prazosin (PRAZ oh sin)

Sound-Alike/Look-Alike Issues

prazosin may be confused with predniSONE

Synonyms furazosin; prazosin hydrochloride

U.S./Canadian Brand Names Apo-Prazo® [Can]; Minipress® [US/Can]; Novo-Prazin [Can]; Nu-Prazo [Can]

Therapeutic Category Alpha-Adrenergic Blocking Agent

Use Treatment of hypertension

Dosage Summary

Oral:

Adults: Initial: 1 mg/dose 2-3 times/day; Maintenance: 3-15 mg/day in divided doses 2-4 times/day (maximum: 20 mg/day) **or** 10-20 mg once, may repeat in 30 minutes

Elderly: Initial: 1 mg 1-2 times/day

Dosage Forms

Capsule, oral: 1 mg, 2 mg, 5 mg

Minipress®: 1 mg, 2 mg, 5 mg

prazosin and polythiazide *(Discontinued)*

prazosin hydrochloride *see* prazosin *on page 789*

PreCare® [US] *see* vitamins (multiple/prenatal) *on page 991*

PreCare Conceive® [US] *see* vitamins (multiple/prenatal) *on page 991*

PreCare Premier® [US] *see* vitamins (multiple/prenatal) *on page 991*

Precedex® [US/Can] *see* dexmedetomidine *on page 283*

Precose® [US] *see* acarbose *on page 20*

Pred Forte® [US/Can] *see* prednisolone (ophthalmic) *on page 791*

Pred-G® [US] *see* prednisolone and gentamicin *on page 791*

Pred Mild® [US/Can] *see* prednisolone (ophthalmic) *on page 791*

prednicarbate (pred ni KAR bate)

Sound-Alike/Look-Alike Issues

Dermatop® may be confused with Dimetapp®

U.S./Canadian Brand Names Dermatop® [US/Can]

Therapeutic Category Corticosteroid, Topical

Use Relief of the inflammatory and pruritic manifestations of corticosteroid-responsive dermatoses (medium-potency topical corticosteroid)

Dosage Summary

Topical:

Children: Dosage not established

Adults: Apply a thin film to affected area twice daily.

Dosage Forms

Cream, topical:

Dermatop®: 0.1% (60 g)

Ointment, topical: 0.1% (15 g, 60 g)

Dermatop®: 0.1% (60 g)

Prednicen-M® *(Discontinued)* *see* prednisone *on page 792*

prednisolone (systemic) (pred NISS oh lone)

Sound-Alike/Look-Alike Issues

prednisoLONE may be confused with predniSONE

Pediapred® may be confused with Pediazole®

Prelone® may be confused with Prozac®

Synonyms prednisolone sodium phosphate

Tall-Man predniso**LONE**

U.S./Canadian Brand Names Hydeltra T.B.A.® [Can]; Millipred™ [US]; Novo-Prednisolone [Can]; Orapred ODT® [US]; Orapred® [US]; Pediapred® [US/Can]; Prelone® [US]; Veripred™ 20 [US]

Therapeutic Category Corticosteroid, Systemic

Use Treatment of endocrine disorders, rheumatic disorders, collagen diseases, allergic states, respiratory diseases, hematologic disorders, neoplastic diseases, edematous states, and gastrointestinal diseases; resolution of acute exacerbations of multiple sclerosis; management of fulminating or disseminated tuberculosis and trichinosis; acute or chronic solid organ rejection

Dosage Summary

Oral: Note: Oral dosage expressed in terms of prednisolone base.

Children: 1-2 mg/kg/day divided 1-2 times/day **or** 0.1-2 mg/kg/day divided 1-4 times/day **or** Nephrotic syndrome: Initial: 2 mg/kg/day **or** 60 mg/m^2/day (maximum: 80 mg/day) in divided doses 3-4 times/day until urine is protein free for 3 consecutive days (maximum: 28 days); followed by 1-1.5 mg/kg/dose **or** 40 mg/m^2/dose given every other day for 4 weeks; Maintenance (frequent relapses: 0.5-1 mg/kg/dose given every other day for 3-6 months

Adults: 5-60 mg/day **or** 200 mg/day for 1 week followed by 80 mg every other day for 1 month

Dosage Forms

Solution, oral: 5 mg/5 mL (5 mL, 10 mL, 20 mL, 118 mL, 120 mL); 15 mg/5 mL (237 mL, 240 mL, 473 mL, 480 mL)

Millipred™: 10 mg/5 mL (237 mL)

Orapred®: 15 mg/5 mL (20 mL, 237 mL)

Pediapred®: 5 mg/5 mL (120 mL)

Veripred™ 20: 20 mg/5 mL (237 mL)

Syrup, oral: 5 mg/5 mL (120 mL); 15 mg/5 mL (5 mL, 236 mL, 237 mL, 240 mL, 473 mL, 480 mL)

Prelone®: 15 mg/5 mL (240 mL, 480 mL)

Tablet, orally disintegrating, oral:

Orapred ODT®: 10 mg, 15 mg, 30 mg

prednisolone (ophthalmic) (pred NISS oh lone)

Sound-Alike/Look-Alike Issues

prednisoLONE may be confused with predniSONE

Synonyms prednisolone acetate, ophthalmic; prednisolone sodium phosphate, ophthalmic

Tall-Man predniso**LONE**

U.S./Canadian Brand Names Diopred® [Can]; Omnipred™ [US]; Ophtho-Tate® [Can]; Pred Forte® [US/Can]; Pred Mild® [US/Can]

Therapeutic Category Corticosteroid, Ophthalmic

Use Treatment of palpebral and bulbar conjunctivitis; corneal injury from chemical, radiation, thermal burns, or foreign body penetration; steroid-responsive inflammatory ophthalmic diseases

Dosage Summary

Ophthalmic:

Children: Instill 1-2 drops in the eye 2-4 times daily

Adults: Instill 1-2 drops in the eye 2-4 times daily

Dosage Forms

Solution, ophthalmic: 1% (5 mL, 10 mL, 15 mL)

Suspension, ophthalmic: 1% (5 mL, 10 mL, 15 mL)

Omnipred™: 1% (5 mL, 10 mL)

Pred Forte®: 1% (1 mL, 5 mL, 10 mL, 15 mL)

Pred Mild®: 0.12% (5 mL, 10 mL)

prednisolone acetate, ophthalmic *see* prednisolone (ophthalmic) *on page 791*

prednisolone and gentamicin (pred NIS oh lone & jen ta MYE sin)

Synonyms gentamicin and prednisolone

U.S./Canadian Brand Names Pred-G® [US]

Therapeutic Category Antibiotic/Corticosteroid, Ophthalmic

Use Treatment of steroid responsive inflammatory conditions and superficial ocular infections due to microorganisms susceptible to gentamicin

Dosage Summary

Ophthalmic:

Children: Ointment: Apply 1/2 inch ribbon in the conjunctival sac 1-3 times/day; Suspension: Initial: 1 drop every hour for 1-2 days; Maintenance: 1 drop 2-4 times/day

Adults: Ointment: Apply 1/2 inch ribbon in the conjunctival sac 1-3 times/day; Suspension: Initial: 1 drop every hour for 1-2 days; Maintenance: 1 drop 2-4 times/day

Dosage Forms

Ointment, ophthalmic:

Pred-G®: Prednisolone 0.6% and gentamicin 0.3% (3.5 g)

prednisolone and sulfacetamide *see* sulfacetamide and prednisolone *on page 900*

prednisolone, neomycin, and polymyxin B *see* neomycin, polymyxin B, and prednisolone *on page 667*

prednisolone sodium phosphate *see* prednisolone (systemic) *on page 790*

prednisolone sodium phosphate, ophthalmic *see* prednisolone (ophthalmic) *on page 791*

prednisone (PRED ni sone)

Sound-Alike/Look-Alike Issues

predniSONE may be confused with methylPREDNISolone, Pramosone®, prazosin, prednisoLONE, Prilosec®, primidone, promethazine

Synonyms deltacortisone; deltadehydrocortisone

Tall-Man predni**SONE**

U.S./Canadian Brand Names Apo-Prednisone® [Can]; Novo-Prednisone [Can]; PredniSONE Intensol™ [US]; Winpred™ [Can]

Therapeutic Category Adrenal Corticosteroid

Use Treatment of a variety of diseases, including:

Allergic states (including adjunctive treatment of anaphylaxis)
Autoimmune disorders (including systemic lupus erythematosus [SLE])
Collagen diseases
Dermatologic conditions/diseases
Edematous states (including nephrotic syndrome)
Endocrine disorders
Gastrointestinal diseases
Hematologic disorders (including idiopathic thrombocytopenia purpura [ITP])
Multiple sclerosis exacerbations
Neoplastic diseases
Ophthalmic diseases
Respiratory diseases (including acute asthma exacerbation)
Rheumatic disorders (including rheumatoid arthritis)
Trichinosis with neurologic or myocardial involvement
Tuberculous meningitis

Dosage Summary

Oral:

Children: General dosing range: Initial: 5-60 mg/day

Adults: General dosing range: Initial: 5-60 mg/day

Dosage Forms

Solution, oral: 1 mg/mL (5 mL, 120 mL, 500 mL)

PredniSONE Intensol™: 5 mg/mL (30 mL)

Tablet, oral: 1 mg, 2.5 mg, 5 mg, 10 mg, 20 mg, 50 mg

PredniSONE Intensol™ [US] *see* prednisone *on page 792*

Prefest™ [US] *see* estradiol and norgestimate *on page 369*

Prefrin™ *(Discontinued)* *see* phenylephrine (ophthalmic) *on page 752*

pregabalin (pre GAB a lin)

Sound-Alike/Look-Alike Issues

Lyrica® may be confused with Lopressor®

Synonyms CI-1008; S-(+)-3-isobutylgaba

U.S./Canadian Brand Names Lyrica® [US/Can]

Therapeutic Category Analgesic, Miscellaneous; Anticonvulsant, Miscellaneous

Controlled Substance C-V

Use Management of pain associated with diabetic peripheral neuropathy; management of postherpetic neuralgia; adjunctive therapy for partial-onset seizure disorder in adults; management of fibromyalgia

Dosage Summary

Oral:

Children: Dosage not established

Adults: Initial: 150 mg/day in 2-3 divided doses; Maintenance: 150-600 mg/day in 2-3 divided doses (maximum: 600 mg/day)

Product Availability Lyrica® oral solution: FDA approved December 2009; anticipated availability is currently undetermined

Dosage Forms

Capsule, oral:

Lyrica®: 25 mg, 50 mg, 75 mg, 100 mg, 150 mg, 200 mg, 225 mg, 300 mg

Pregestimil® [US-OTC] *see* nutritional formula, enteral/oral *on page* 692
pregnenedione *see* progesterone *on page* 799
Pregnyl® [US/Can] *see* chorionic gonadotropin (human) *on page* 219
Prelone® [US] *see* prednisolone (systemic) *on page* 790
Prelu-2® ***(Discontinued)*** *see* phendimetrazine *on page* 747
Premarin® [US/Can] *see* estrogens (conjugated/equine, systemic) *on page* 370
Premarin® [US/Can] *see* estrogens (conjugated/equine, topical) *on page* 371
Premarin® With Methyltestosterone ***(Discontinued)***
Premasol™ [US] *see* amino acid injection *on page* 64
PremesisRx® [US] *see* vitamins (multiple/prenatal) *on page* 991
Premjact® [US] *see* lidocaine (topical) *on page* 562
Premphase® [US/Can] *see* estrogens (conjugated/equine) and medroxyprogesterone *on page* 371
Premplus® [Can] *see* estrogens (conjugated/equine) and medroxyprogesterone *on page* 371
Prempro® [US/Can] *see* estrogens (conjugated/equine) and medroxyprogesterone *on page* 371
Prenatal 19 [US-OTC] *see* vitamins (multiple/prenatal) *on page* 991
Prenatal AD [US-OTC] *see* vitamins (multiple/prenatal) *on page* 991
Prenatal MR 90 Fe™ ***(Discontinued)*** *see* vitamins (multiple/prenatal) *on page* 991
Prenatal MTR With Selenium ***(Discontinued)*** *see* vitamins (multiple/prenatal) *on page* 991
Prenatal One Daily [US-OTC] *see* vitamins (multiple/prenatal) *on page* 991
Prenatal Rx 1 [US] *see* vitamins (multiple/prenatal) *on page* 991
Prenatal U [US-OTC] *see* vitamins (multiple/prenatal) *on page* 991
prenatal vitamins *see* vitamins (multiple/prenatal) *on page* 991
Prenatal Z Advanced Formula ***(Discontinued)*** *see* vitamins (multiple/prenatal) *on page* 991
Prenate DHA™ [US] *see* vitamins (multiple/prenatal) *on page* 991
Prenate Elite® [US] *see* vitamins (multiple/prenatal) *on page* 991
Preparation H® [US-OTC] *see* phenylephrine (topical) *on page* 752
Preparation H® Cleansing Pads [Can] *see* witch hazel *on page* 994
Preparation H® Hydrocortisone [US-OTC] *see* hydrocortisone (topical) *on page* 483
Preparation H® Medicated Wipes [US-OTC] *see* witch hazel *on page* 994
Prepcat ***(Discontinued)*** *see* barium *on page* 117
Pre-Pen® ***(Discontinued)***
Prepidil® [US/Can] *see* dinoprostone *on page* 308
Prescription Strength Desenex® ***(Discontinued)*** *see* miconazole (topical) *on page* 630
PreserVision® AREDS [US-OTC] *see* vitamins (multiple/oral) *on page* 990
PreserVision® Lutein [US-OTC] *see* vitamins (multiple/oral) *on page* 990
Pressyn® [Can] *see* vasopressin *on page* 980
Pressyn® AR [Can] *see* vasopressin *on page* 980
Pretz® [US-OTC] *see* sodium chloride *on page* 882
Prevacare® [US-OTC] *see* alcohol (ethyl) *on page* 45
Prevacid® [US/Can] *see* lansoprazole *on page* 548
Prevacid® 24 HR [US-OTC] *see* lansoprazole *on page* 548
Prevacid® FasTab [Can] *see* lansoprazole *on page* 548
Prevacid® NapraPAC® [US] *see* lansoprazole and naproxen *on page* 549
Prevacid® SoluTab™ [US] *see* lansoprazole *on page* 548
Prevalite® [US] *see* cholestyramine resin *on page* 218
Prevex® B [Can] *see* betamethasone *on page* 133
Prevex® HC [Can] *see* hydrocortisone (topical) *on page* 483
PreviDent® [US] *see* fluoride *on page* 413
PreviDent® 5000 Plus® [US] *see* fluoride *on page* 413
Previfem® ***(Discontinued)*** *see* ethinyl estradiol and norgestimate *on page* 380

Prevnar® [US/Can] *see* pneumococcal conjugate vaccine (7-valent) *on page 771*
Prevnar 13™ [US] *see* pneumococcal conjugate vaccine (13-valent) *on page 770*
Prevpac® [US] *see* lansoprazole, amoxicillin, and clarithromycin *on page 549*
Prezista® [US/Can] *see* darunavir *on page 270*
Prialt® [US] *see* ziconotide *on page 999*
Priftin® [US/Can] *see* rifapentine *on page 842*

prilocaine (PRIL oh kane)

Sound-Alike/Look-Alike Issues
prilocaine may be confused with Polocaine®, Prilosec®

U.S./Canadian Brand Names Citanest® Plain Dental [US]; Citanest® Plain [Can]

Therapeutic Category Local Anesthetic

Use Amide-type anesthetic used for local infiltration anesthesia; injection near nerve trunks to produce nerve block

Dosage Summary

Dental (infiltration or conduction block):

Children <10 years: Doses >40 mg (1 mL) as a 4% solution per procedure rarely needed

Children ≥10 years: Initial: 40-80 mg (1-2 mL) as a 4% solution, up to a maximum of 400 mg (10 mL) as a 4% solution within a 2-hour period (maximum: 600 mg/dose [per manufacturer])

Adults: Initial: 40-80 mg (1-2 mL) as a 4% solution, up to a maximum of 400 mg (10 mL) as a 4% solution within a 2-hour period (maximum: 600 mg/dose [per manufacturer])

Dosage Forms

Injection, solution:
Citanest® Plain Dental: 4% [40 mg/mL] (1.8 mL)

prilocaine and lidocaine *see* lidocaine and prilocaine *on page 565*
Prilosec® [US] *see* omeprazole *on page 701*
Prilosec OTC® [US-OTC] *see* omeprazole *on page 701*
PrimaCare® [US] *see* vitamins (multiple/prenatal) *on page 991*
PrimaCare® One [US] *see* vitamins (multiple/prenatal) *on page 991*
primaclone *see* primidone *on page 795*
Primacor® [Can] *see* milrinone *on page 635*
Primacor® *(Discontinued)* *see* milrinone *on page 635*
Primalev™ *(Discontinued)* *see* oxycodone and acetaminophen *on page 715*

primaquine (PRIM a kween)

Sound-Alike/Look-Alike Issues
primaquine may be confused with primidone

Synonyms primaquine phosphate; prymaccone

Therapeutic Category Aminoquinoline (Antimalarial)

Use Prevention of relapse of *P. vivax* malaria

Dosage Summary **Note:** Dosage expressed as mg of base (15 mg base = 26.3 mg primaquine phosphate)

Oral:

Children: 0.5 mg/kg once daily for 14 days (maximum dose: 30 mg/day); alternative regimen (recommended for mild G6PD deficiency): 45 mg once weekly for 8 weeks

Adults: 30 mg once daily for 14 days; alternative regimen (recommended for mild G6PD deficiency): 45 mg once weekly for 8 weeks

Dosage Forms

Tablet, oral: 26.3 mg

primaquine phosphate *see* primaquine *on page 794*
Primatene® Mist [US-OTC] *see* epinephrine (systemic, oral inhalation) *on page 352*
Primaxin® [US/Can] *see* imipenem and cilastatin *on page 500*
Primaxin® I.V. [Can] *see* imipenem and cilastatin *on page 500*
Primene® [Can] *see* amino acid injection *on page 64*

primidone (PRI mi done)

Sound-Alike/Look-Alike Issues

primidone may be confused with predniSONE, primaquine, pyridoxine

Synonyms desoxyphenobarbital; primaclone

U.S./Canadian Brand Names Apo-Primidone® [Can]; Mysoline® [US]

Therapeutic Category Anticonvulsant; Barbiturate

Use Management of grand mal, psychomotor, and focal seizures

Dosage Summary

Oral:

Children <8 years: Initial: 50 mg once daily at bedtime; Maintenance: 375-750 mg/day (10-25 mg/kg/day) in 3-4 divided doses; **Note:** Titration is recommended

Children ≥8 years: Initial: 100-125 mg/day at bedtime; Maintenance: 750-1500 mg/day in 3-4 divided doses (maximum: 2 g/day); **Note:** Titration is recommended

Adults: Initial: 100-125 mg/day at bedtime; Maintenance: 750-1500 mg/day in 3-4 divided doses (maximum: 2 g/day); **Note:** Titration is recommended

Dosage Forms

Tablet, oral: 50 mg, 250 mg

Mysoline®: 50 mg, 250 mg

Dosage Forms - Canada

Tablet:

Apo-Primidone®: 125 mg, 250 mg

Primovist [Can] *see* gadoxetate *on page* *435*

Primsol® [US] *see* trimethoprim *on page* *959*

Prinivil® [US/Can] *see* lisinopril *on page* *570*

Prinzide® [US/Can] *see* lisinopril and hydrochlorothiazide *on page* *570*

Priorix™ [Can] *see* measles, mumps, and rubella virus vaccine *on page* *592*

Priorix-Tetra™ [Can] *see* measles, mumps, rubella, and varicella virus vaccine *on page* *593*

Priscoline® ***(Discontinued)***

PrismaSol [US] *see* electrolyte solution, renal replacement *on page* *345*

pristinamycin *see* quinupristin and dalfopristin *on page* *823*

Pristiq® [US/Can] *see* desvenlafaxine *on page* *280*

Privigen® [US/Can] *see* immune globulin (intravenous) *on page* *502*

Privine® [US-OTC] *see* naphazoline (nasal) *on page* *658*

ProAir® HFA [US] *see* albuterol *on page* *43*

ProAmatine® [US] *see* midodrine *on page* *633*

PRO-Amiodarone [Can] *see* amiodarone *on page* *67*

PRO-Azithromycin [Can] *see* azithromycin (systemic) *on page* *111*

Pro-Banthine® ***(Discontinued)*** *see* propantheline *on page* *803*

probenecid (proe BEN e sid)

Sound-Alike/Look-Alike Issues

probenecid may be confused with Procanbid®

U.S./Canadian Brand Names Benuryl™ [Can]

Therapeutic Category Uricosuric Agent

Use Prevention of hyperuricemia associated with gout or gouty arthritis; prolongation and elevation of beta-lactam plasma levels

Dosage Summary

Oral:

Children <2 years: Contraindicated

Children 2-14 years: Prolong penicillin serum levels: Initial: 25 mg/kg then 40 mg/kg/day given 4 times/day (maximum: 500 mg/dose)

Children >45 kg: Gonorrhea: 1 g as a single dose

Adults:

Gonorrhea, PID: 1 g as a single dose

Gout: Initial: 250 mg twice daily (maximum: 2-3 g/day)

Neurosyphilis: 500 mg 4 times/day for 10-14 days

Prolong PCN levels: 500 mg 4 times/day

Dosage Forms

Tablet, oral: 500 mg

probenecid and colchicine *see* colchicine and probenecid *on page* 245
PRO-Bicalutamide [Can] *see* bicalutamide *on page* 137
Pro-Bionate® *(Discontinued)*
PRO-Bisoprolol [Can] *see* bisoprolol *on page* 141

procainamide (pro KANE a mide)

Sound-Alike/Look-Alike Issues

PCA (error-prone abbreviation)
Procanbid® may be confused with probenecid, Procan SR®
Procan SR® may be confused with procanbid
Pronestyl® may be confused with Ponstel®

Synonyms procainamide hydrochloride; procaine amide hydrochloride

U.S./Canadian Brand Names Apo-Procainamide® [Can]; Procainamide Hydrochloride Injection, USP [Can]; Procan SR® [Can]

Therapeutic Category Antiarrhythmic Agent, Class I-A

Use

Intravenous: Treatment of ventricular arrhythmias (eg, sustained ventricular tachycardia [VT]); **Note:** Due to proarrhythmic effects, use should be reserved for life-threatening arrhythmias

Oral (Canadian labeling; not available in U.S.): Treatment of supraventricular arrhythmias. **Note:** In the treatment of atrial fibrillation, use only when preferred treatment is ineffective or cannot be used. Use in paroxysmal atrial tachycardia when reflex stimulation or other measures are ineffective.

Dosage Summary

I.M.:

Children: 20-30 mg/kg/day divided every 4-6 hours (maximum: 4 g/day)

Adults: 50 mg/kg/day divided every 3-6 hours **or** 0.5-1 g every 4-8 hours

I.V.:

Children: Loading dose: 3-6 mg/kg/dose over 5 minutes (maximum: 100 mg/dose), may repeat every 5-10 minutes to maximum of 15 mg/kg/load; Infusion: 20-80 mcg/kg/minute (maximum: 2 g/day)

Adults: Loading dose: 15-18 mg/kg administered as slow infusion over 25-30 minutes **or** 100 mg/dose at a rate not to exceed 50 mg/minute repeated every 5 minutes as needed (maximum total dose: 1 g); Infusion: 1-4 mg/minute

Dosage Forms

Injection, solution: 100 mg/mL (10 mL); 500 mg/mL (2 mL)

Dosage Forms - Canada

Tablet, sustained release, oral:

Procan SR®: 250 mg, 500 mg, 750 mg

procainamide hydrochloride *see* procainamide *on page* 796
Procainamide Hydrochloride Injection, USP [Can] *see* procainamide *on page* 796

procaine (PROE kane)

Synonyms procaine hydrochloride

Therapeutic Category Local Anesthetic

Use Produces spinal anesthesia

Dosage Summary

Injection:

Children: Dosage not established

Adults: Dose varies with procedure, desired depth, and duration of anesthesia, desired muscle relaxation, vascularity of tissues, physical condition, and age of patient. Total dose (range): 50-200 mg

procaine amide hydrochloride *see* procainamide *on page* 796
procaine benzylpenicillin *see* penicillin G procaine *on page* 738
procaine hydrochloride *see* procaine *on page* 796
procaine penicillin G *see* penicillin G procaine *on page* 738
PRO-Calcitonin [Can] *see* calcitonin *on page* 165
Pro-Cal-Sof® *(Discontinued)* *see* docusate *on page* 321

Procanbid® *(Discontinued)* *see* procainamide *on page 796*

Procan SR® [Can] *see* procainamide *on page 796*

procarbazine (proe KAR ba zeen)

Sound-Alike/Look-Alike Issues

procarbazine may be confused with dacarbazine

Matulane® may be confused with Materna®

Synonyms benzmethyzin; N-methylhydrazine; procarbazine hydrochloride

U.S./Canadian Brand Names Matulane® [US/Can]; Natulan® [Can]

Therapeutic Category Antineoplastic Agent

Use Treatment of Hodgkin disease

Dosage Summary Note: Manufacturer states that the dose is based on patient's ideal weight if the patient is obese or has abnormal fluid retention. Other studies suggest that ideal body weight may not be necessary

Oral:

Children: 100 mg/m^2/day for 14 days and repeated every 4 weeks

Adults: Initial: 2-4 mg/kg/day in single or divided doses for 7 days then increase dose to 4-6 mg/kg/day; Maintenance: 1-2 mg/kg/day

Dosage Forms

Capsule, oral:

Matulane®: 50 mg

procarbazine hydrochloride *see* procarbazine *on page 797*

Procardia® [US] *see* nifedipine *on page 675*

Procardia XL® [US] *see* nifedipine *on page 675*

PRO-Cefadroxil [Can] *see* cefadroxil *on page 189*

PRO-Cefuroxime [Can] *see* cefuroxime *on page 194*

procetofene *see* fenofibrate *on page 393*

Prochieve® [US] *see* progesterone *on page 799*

prochlorperazine (proe klor PER a zeen)

Sound-Alike/Look-Alike Issues

prochlorperazine may be confused with chlorproMAZINE

Compazine® may be confused with Copaxone®, Coumadin®

CPZ (occasional abbreviation for Compazine®) is an error-prone abbreviation (mistaken as chlorpromazine)

Synonyms chlormeprazine; prochlorperazine edisylate; prochlorperazine maleate

U.S./Canadian Brand Names Apo-Prochlorperazine® [Can]; Compro® [US]; Nu-Prochlor [Can]; Stemetil® [Can]

Therapeutic Category Phenothiazine Derivative

Use Management of nausea and vomiting; psychotic disorders, including schizophrenia and anxiety

Dosage Summary

I.M.:

Children <2 years or <9 kg: Use not recommended

Children ≥2 years and ≥9 kg: 0.13 mg/kg/dose; change to oral as soon as possible

Adults:

Antiemetic: 5-10 mg every 3-4 hours **or** 5-10 mg as a single dose with surgery, may repeat (maximum: 40 mg/day)

Antipsychotic: Initial: 10-20 mg every 1-4 hours to gain control (rarely more than 3-4 doses are needed); Maintenance: 10-20 mg every 4-6 hours

I.V.:

Children: Dosage not established

Adults: 2.5-10 mg every 3-4 hours as needed (maximum: 40 mg/day) **or** 5-10 mg as a single dose with surgery, may repeat

Oral:

Children <2 years or <9 kg: Use not recommended

Children ≥2 years and ≥9 kg:

Antiemetic:

>9 kg: 0.4 mg/kg/day in 3-4 divided doses **or**

9-13 kg: 2.5 mg every 12-24 hours as needed (maximum: 7.5 mg/day)

13.1-17 kg: 2.5 mg every 8-12 hours as needed (maximum: 10 mg/day)

17.1-37 kg: 2.5 mg every 8 hours or 5 mg every 12 hours as needed (maximum: 15 mg/day)

Children 2-12 years:

Antipsychotic: Initial: 2.5 mg 2-3 times/day; Maintenance: Increase as needed to maximum of 20 mg/day for 2-5 years and 25 mg/day for 6-12 years

Adults:

Antiemetic: 5-10 mg 3-4 times/day (maximum: 40 mg/day)

Antipsychotic: Initial: 5-10 mg 3-4 times/day; Maintenance: Up to 150 mg/day; **Note:** Titration is recommended

Nonpsychotic anxiety: 15-20 mg/day in divided doses; do not give doses >20 mg/day or for longer than 12 weeks

Rectal:

Children <2 years or <9 kg: Use not recommended

Children ≥2 years and ≥9 kg:

Antiemetic:

>9 kg: 0.4 mg/kg/day in 3-4 divided doses **or**

9-13 kg: 2.5 mg every 12-24 hours as needed (maximum: 7.5 mg/day)

13.1-17 kg: 2.5 mg every 8-12 hours as needed (maximum: 10 mg/day)

17.1-37 kg: 2.5 mg every 8 hours or 5 mg every 12 hours as needed (maximum: 15 mg/day)

Children 2-12 years:

Antipsychotic: Initial: 2.5 mg 2-3 times/day; Maintenance: Increase as needed to maximum of 20 mg/day for 2-5 years and 25 mg/day for 6-12 years

Adults: 25 mg twice daily

Dosage Forms

Injection, solution: 5 mg/mL (2 mL, 10 mL)

Suppository, rectal: 25 mg (12s)

Compro®: 25 mg (12s)

Tablet, oral: 5 mg, 10 mg

prochlorperazine edisylate *see* prochlorperazine *on page 797*

prochlorperazine maleate *see* prochlorperazine *on page 797*

PRO-Ciprofloxacin [Can] *see* ciprofloxacin (systemic) *on page 224*

PRO-Clonazepam [Can] *see* clonazepam *on page 237*

Procrit® [US] *see* epoetin alfa *on page 356*

Proctocort® [US] *see* hydrocortisone (topical) *on page 483*

ProctoCream®-HC [US] *see* hydrocortisone (topical) *on page 483*

proctofene *see* fenofibrate *on page 393*

ProctoFoam®-HC [US/Can] *see* pramoxine and hydrocortisone *on page 787*

Proctofoam® NS [US-OTC] *see* pramoxine *on page 787*

Procto-Kit™ [US] *see* hydrocortisone (topical) *on page 483*

Procto-Pak™ [US-OTC] *see* hydrocortisone (topical) *on page 483*

Proctosol-HC® [US] *see* hydrocortisone (topical) *on page 483*

Proctozone-HC™ [US-OTC] *see* hydrocortisone (topical) *on page 483*

procyclidine *(Canada only)* (proe SYE kli deen)

Synonyms procyclidine hydrochloride

U.S./Canadian Brand Names PHL-Procyclidine [Can]; PMS-Procyclidine [Can]

Therapeutic Category Anti-Parkinson Agent; Anticholinergic Agent

Use Relieves symptoms of parkinsonian syndrome and drug-induced extrapyramidal symptoms

Dosage Forms - Canada

Tablet: 2.5 mg, 5 mg

Elixir: 2.5 mg/5 mL

procyclidine hydrochloride *see* procyclidine *(Canada only) on page 798*
Procytox® [Can] *see* cyclophosphamide *on page 259*
PRO-Diclo-Rapide [Can] *see* diclofenac (systemic) *on page 296*
PRO-Doc Limitee Bromazepam [Can] *see* bromazepam *(Canada only) on page 146*
PRO-Enalapril [Can] *see* enalapril *on page 348*
ProFe [US-OTC] *see* polysaccharide-iron complex *on page 777*
Profen II® ***(Discontinued)*** *see* guaifenesin and pseudoephedrine *on page 457*
Profen II DM® [US] *see* guaifenesin, pseudoephedrine, and dextromethorphan *on page 460*
Profen Forte™ DM [US] *see* guaifenesin, pseudoephedrine, and dextromethorphan *on page 460*
Profen LA® ***(Discontinued)***
PRO-Feno-Super [Can] *see* fenofibrate *on page 393*
Profilnine® SD [US] *see* factor IX complex (human) *on page 389*
Proflavanol C™ [Can] *see* ascorbic acid *on page 98*
PRO-Fluconazole [Can] *see* fluconazole *on page 407*
PRO-Fluoxetine [Can] *see* fluoxetine *on page 415*
PRO-Gabapentin [Can] *see* gabapentin *on page 433*

progesterone (proe JES ter one)

Synonyms pregnenedione; progestin

U.S./Canadian Brand Names Crinone® [US/Can]; Endometrin® [US]; First™-Progesterone VGS 100 [US]; First™-Progesterone VGS 200 [US]; First™-Progesterone VGS 25 [US]; First™-Progesterone VGS 400 [US]; First™-Progesterone VGS 50 [US]; Prochieve® [US]; Prometrium® [US/Can]

Therapeutic Category Progestin

Use

Oral: Prevention of endometrial hyperplasia in nonhysterectomized, postmenopausal women who are receiving conjugated estrogen tablets; secondary amenorrhea

I.M.: Amenorrhea; abnormal uterine bleeding due to hormonal imbalance

Intravaginal gel: Part of assisted reproductive technology (ART) for infertile women with progesterone deficiency; secondary amenorrhea

Vaginal tablet: Part of ART for infertile women with progesterone deficiency

Dosage Summary

I.M.:

Children: Dosage not established

Adults (females): 5-10 mg/day for 6 doses

Intravaginal:

Children: Dosage not established

Adults (females):

ART: 90 mg (8% gel) once or twice daily or 100 mg (vaginal tablet) 2-3 times/day

Secondary amenorrhea: 45 mg (4% gel) every other day, may increase to 90 mg (8% gel) every other day if needed (maximum: 6 doses)

Oral:

Children: Dosage not established

Adults (females):

Amenorrhea: 400 mg once daily in the evening for 10 days

Endometrial hyperplasia prevention: 200 mg once daily in the evening for 12 days sequentially per 28-day cycle

Dosage Forms

Capsule, oral:

Prometrium®: 100 mg, 200 mg

Gel, vaginal:

Crinone®: 8% (1.45 g)

Prochieve®: 4% (1.45 g); 8% (1.45 g)

Injection, oil: 50 mg/mL (10 mL)

Powder, for prescription compounding: USP: 100% (10 g, 25 g, 50 g, 100 g, 1000 g)

Suppository, vaginal:
First™-Progesterone VGS 25: 25 mg (30s)
First™-Progesterone VGS 50: 50 mg (30s)
First™-Progesterone VGS 100: 100 mg (30s)
First™-Progesterone VGS 200: 200 mg (30s)
First™-Progesterone VGS 400: 400 mg (30s)
Tablet, vaginal:
Endometrin®: 100 mg

progestin *see* progesterone *on page* 799
PRO-Glyburide [Can] *see* glyburide *on page* 448
Proglycem® [US/Can] *see* diazoxide *on page* 295
Prograf® [US/Can] *see* tacrolimus (systemic) *on page* 907
proguanil and atovaquone *see* atovaquone and proguanil *on page* 105
proguanil hydrochloride and atovaquone *see* atovaquone and proguanil *on page* 105
ProHance® [US] *see* gadoteridol *on page* 435
ProHance® Multipack™ [US] *see* gadoteridol *on page* 435
ProHIBiT® ***(Discontinued)***
PRO-Hydroxyquine [Can] *see* hydroxychloroquine *on page* 488
PRO-Indapamide [Can] *see* indapamide *on page* 504
Pro-Indo [Can] *see* indomethacin *on page* 505
PRO-ISMN [Can] *see* isosorbide mononitrate *on page* 529
Prolastin® [Can] *see* alpha$_1$-proteinase inhibitor *on page* 54
Prolastin®-C [US/Can] *see* alpha$_1$-proteinase inhibitor *on page* 54
Prolastin® ***(Discontinued)*** *see* alpha$_1$-proteinase inhibitor *on page* 54
Proleukin® [US/Can] *see* aldesleukin *on page* 46
PRO-Levetiracetam [Can] *see* levetiracetam *on page* 555
PRO-Levocarb [Can] *see* carbidopa and levodopa *on page* 182
Prolex®-D ***(Discontinued)*** *see* guaifenesin and phenylephrine *on page* 456
Prolex®-PD ***(Discontinued)*** *see* guaifenesin and phenylephrine *on page* 456
Prolia™ [US] *see* denosumab *on page* 275
PRO-Lisinopril [Can] *see* lisinopril *on page* 570
Prolixin® ***(Discontinued)*** *see* fluphenazine *on page* 417
Prolixin Enanthate® ***(Discontinued)*** *see* fluphenazine *on page* 417
Prolopa® [Can] *see* benserazide and levodopa *(Canada only) on page* 123
PRO-Lorazepam [Can] *see* lorazepam *on page* 576
PRO-Lovastatin [Can] *see* lovastatin *on page* 579
Promacet [US] *see* butalbital and acetaminophen *on page* 159
Promacta® [US] *see* eltrombopag *on page* 346
Prometa® ***(Discontinued)***
PRO-Metformin [Can] *see* metformin *on page* 609

promethazine (proe METH a zeen)

Sound-Alike/Look-Alike Issues
promethazine may be confused with chlorproMAZINE, predniSONE, promazine
Phenergan® may be confused with Phenaphen®, PHENobarbital, Phrenilin®, Theragran®

Synonyms promethazine hydrochloride

U.S./Canadian Brand Names Bioniche Promethazine [Can]; Histantil [Can]; Phenadoz® [US]; Phenergan® [US/Can]; PMS-Promethazine [Can]; Promethegan™ [US]

Therapeutic Category Antiemetic; Phenothiazine Derivative

Use Symptomatic treatment of various allergic conditions; antiemetic; motion sickness; sedative; adjunct to postoperative analgesia and anesthesia

Dosage Summary
I.M.:
Children <2 years: Dosage not established
Children ≥2 years: 0.25-1 mg/kg 4-6 times/day as needed (maximum: 25 mg/dose; sedation: 50 mg/dose)

Adults: 12.5-75 mg/dose as a single dose **or** 12.5-50 mg every 4-6 hours as needed

I.V.:

Children <2 years: Dosage not established

Children ≥2 years: 0.25-1 mg/kg 4-6 times/day as needed (maximum: 25 mg/dose; sedation: 50 mg/dose)

Adults: 12.5-75 mg/dose as a single dose **or** 12.5-50 mg every 4-6 hours as needed

Oral:

Children <2 years: Dosage not established

Children ≥2 years:

Allergic reactions: 0.1 mg/kg every 6 hours (maximum: 12.5 mg) during the day and 0.5 mg/kg (maximum: 25 mg/dose) at bedtime as needed

Antiemetic: 0.25-1 mg/kg 4-6 times/day as needed (maximum: 25 mg/dose)

Motion sickness: 0.5 mg/kg 30 minutes to 1 hour before departure, then every 12 hours as needed (maximum: 25 mg twice daily)

Sedation: 0.5-1 mg/kg every 6 hours as needed (maximum: 50 mg/dose)

Adults: 6.25-25 mg every 4-8 hours as needed **or** 12.5-50 mg as a single dose **or** 25 mg 30-60 minutes before departure, then every 12 hours as needed

Rectal:

Children <2 years: Dosage not established

Children ≥2 years:

Allergic reactions: 0.1 mg/kg every 6 hours (maximum: 12.5 mg) during the day and 0.5 mg/kg (maximum: 25 mg/dose) at bedtime as needed

Antiemetic: 0.25-1 mg/kg 4-6 times/day as needed (maximum: 25 mg/dose)

Motion sickness: 0.5 mg/kg 30 minutes to 1 hour before departure, then every 12 hours as needed (maximum: 25 mg twice daily)

Sedation: 0.5-1 mg/kg every 6 hours as needed (maximum: 50 mg/dose)

Adults: 6.25-25 mg every 4-8 hours as needed **or** 12.5-50 mg as a single dose **or** 25 mg 30-60 minutes before departure, then every 12 hours as needed

Dosage Forms

Injection, solution: 25 mg/mL (1 mL, 10 mL); 50 mg/mL (1 mL)

Phenergan®: 25 mg/mL (1 mL); 50 mg/mL (1 mL)

Suppository, rectal: 12.5 mg (12s); 25 mg (12s)

Phenadoz®: 12.5 mg (12s); 25 mg (12s)

Promethegan™: 12.5 mg (12s); 25 mg (12s); 50 mg (12s)

Syrup, oral: 6.25 mg/5 mL (118 mL, 473 mL)

Tablet, oral: 12.5 mg, 25 mg, 50 mg

promethazine and codeine (proe METH a zeen & KOE deen)

Synonyms codeine and promethazine

Therapeutic Category Antihistamine/Antitussive

Controlled Substance C-V

Use Temporary relief of coughs and upper respiratory symptoms associated with allergy or the common cold

Dosage Summary

Oral:

Children <6 years: Dosage not established

Children 6-11 years: 2.5-5 mL every 4-6 hours (maximum: 30 mL/day)

Children ≥12 years: 5 mL every 4-6 hours (maximum: 30 mL/day)

Adults: 5 mL every 4-6 hours (maximum: 30 mL/24 hours)

Dosage Forms

Syrup: Promethazine 6.25 mg and codeine 10 mg per 5 mL

promethazine and dextromethorphan (proe METH a zeen & deks troe meth OR fan)

Synonyms dextromethorphan and promethazine

Therapeutic Category Antihistamine/Antitussive

Use Temporary relief of coughs and upper respiratory symptoms associated with allergy or the common cold

Dosage Summary

Oral:

Children <2 years: Dosage not established

Children 2-6 years: 1.25-2.5 mL every 4-6 hours (maximum: 10 mL/day)

Children 6-12 years: 2.5-5 mL every 4-6 hours (maximum: 20 mL/day)
Adults: 5 mL every 4-6 hours (maximum: 30 mL/day)

Dosage Forms

Syrup: Promethazine 6.25 mg and dextromethorphan 15 mg per 5 mL

promethazine and phenylephrine (proe METH a zeen & fen il EF rin)

Synonyms phenylephrine and promethazine

Therapeutic Category Antihistamine/Decongestant Combination

Use Temporary relief of upper respiratory symptoms associated with allergy or the common cold

Dosage Summary

Oral:

Children <2 years: Dosage not established
Children 2-6 years: 1.25-2.5 mL every 4-6 hours (maximum: 7.5 mL/day)
Children 6-12 years: 2.5-5 mL every 4-6 hours (maximum: 30 mL/day)
Children >12 years: 5 mL every 4-6 hours (maximum: 30 mL/day)
Adults: 5 mL every 4-6 hours (maximum: 30 mL/day)

Dosage Forms

Syrup: Promethazine 6.25 mg and phenylephrine 5 mg per 5 mL

promethazine hydrochloride *see* promethazine *on page 800*

promethazine, phenylephrine, and codeine
(proe METH a zeen, fen il EF rin, & KOE deen)

Synonyms codeine, phenylephrine, and promethazine; phenylephrine, promethazine, and codeine

Therapeutic Category Antihistamine/Decongestant/Antitussive

Controlled Substance C-V

Use Temporary relief of coughs and upper respiratory symptoms including nasal congestion associated with allergy or the common cold

Dosage Summary

Oral:

Children <6 years: Dosage not established
Children 6-11 years: 2.5-5 mL every 4-6 hours (maximum: 30 mL/day)
Children ≥12 years: 5 mL every 4-6 hours (maximum: 30 mL/day)
Adults: 5 mL every 4-6 hours (maximum: 30 mL/day)

Dosage Forms

Syrup: Promethazine 6.25 mg, phenylephrine 5 mg, and codeine 10 mg per 5 mL

Promethegan™ [US] *see* promethazine *on page 800*

Promethist® With Codeine *(Discontinued)* *see* promethazine, phenylephrine, and codeine *on page 802*

Prometh® VC Plain Liquid *(Discontinued)* *see* promethazine and phenylephrine *on page 802*

Prometh® VC With Codeine *(Discontinued)* *see* promethazine, phenylephrine, and codeine *on page 802*

Prometrium® [US/Can] *see* progesterone *on page 799*

PRO-Mirtazapine [Can] *see* mirtazapine *on page 637*

Promit® *(Discontinued)*

PRO-Naproxen EC [Can] *see* naproxen *on page 659*

Pronestyl® *(Discontinued)* *see* procainamide *on page 796*

Pronto® Complete Lice Removal System [US-OTC] *see* pyrethrins and piperonyl butoxide *on page 816*

Pronto® Lice Control [Can] *see* pyrethrins and piperonyl butoxide *on page 816*

Pronto® Plus Hair and Scalp Masque *(Discontinued)* *see* pyrethrins and piperonyl butoxide *on page 816*

Pronto® Plus Lice Egg Remover Kit [US-OTC] *see* benzalkonium chloride *on page 124*

Pronto® Plus Lice Killing Mousse Plus Vitamin E [US-OTC] *see* pyrethrins and piperonyl butoxide *on page 816*

Pronto® Plus Lice Killing Mousse Shampoo Plus Natural Extracts and Oils [US-OTC] *see* pyrethrins and piperonyl butoxide *on page 816*

Pronto® Plus Warm Oil Treatment and Conditioner [US-OTC] *see* pyrethrins and piperonyl butoxide *on page 816*

Propac™ [US-OTC] *see* nutritional formula, enteral/oral *on page 692*

Propacet® *(Discontinued)* *see* propoxyphene and acetaminophen *on page 805*

propafenone (pro PAF en one)

Synonyms propafenone hydrochloride

U.S./Canadian Brand Names Apo-Propafenone® [Can]; Mylan-Propafenone [Can]; PMS-Propafenone [Can]; Rythmol® Gen-Propafenone [Can]; Rythmol® SR [US]; Rythmol® [US]

Therapeutic Category Antiarrhythmic Agent, Class I-C

Use Treatment of life-threatening ventricular arrhythmias

Rythmol® SR: Maintenance of normal sinus rhythm in patients with symptomatic atrial fibrillation

Dosage Summary

Oral:

Extended release:

Children: Dosage not established

Adults: Initial: 225 mg every 12 hours; Maintenance: 225-425 mg every 12 hours

Immediate release:

Children: Dosage not established

Adults: Initial: 150 mg every 8 hours; Maintenance: 150-300 mg every 8 hours

Dosage Forms

Capsule, extended release, oral:

Rythmol® SR: 225 mg, 325 mg, 425 mg

Tablet, oral: 150 mg, 225 mg, 300 mg

Rythmol®: 150 mg, 225 mg

propafenone hydrochloride *see* propafenone *on page 803*

Propagest® *(Discontinued)*

propantheline (proe PAN the leen)

Synonyms propantheline bromide

Therapeutic Category Anticholinergic Agent

Use Adjunctive treatment of peptic ulcer, irritable bowel syndrome, pancreatitis, ureteral and urinary bladder spasm; reduce duodenal motility during diagnostic radiologic procedures

Dosage Summary

Oral:

Children: 1-3 mg/kg/day in 3-6 divided doses

Adults: 15 mg 3 times/day before meals or food and 30 mg at bedtime

Dosage Forms

Tablet, oral: 15 mg

propantheline bromide *see* propantheline *on page 803*

proparacaine (proe PAR a kane)

Sound-Alike/Look-Alike Issues

proparacaine may be confused with propoxyphene

Synonyms proparacaine hydrochloride; proxymetacaine

U.S./Canadian Brand Names Alcaine® [US/Can]; Diocaine® [Can]; Parcaine™ [US]

Therapeutic Category Local Anesthetic

Use Anesthesia for tonometry, gonioscopy; suture removal from cornea; removal of corneal foreign body; cataract extraction, glaucoma surgery; short operative procedure involving the cornea and conjunctiva

Dosage Summary

Ophthalmic:

Children: Instill 1-2 drops of 0.5% solution in eye just prior to procedure **or** instill 1 drop of 0.5% solution in eye every 5-10 minutes for 5-7 doses

Adults: Instill 1-2 drops of 0.5% solution in eye just prior to procedure **or** instill 1 drop of 0.5% solution in eye every 5-10 minutes for 5-7 doses

Dosage Forms

Solution, ophthalmic: 0.5% (15 mL)

Alcaine®: 0.5% (15 mL)

Parcaine™: 0.5% (15 mL)

proparacaine and fluorescein (proe PAR a kane & FLURE e seen)

Synonyms fluorescein and proparacaine

U.S./Canadian Brand Names Flucaine® [US]

Therapeutic Category Diagnostic Agent; Local Anesthetic

Use Anesthesia for tonometry, gonioscopy; suture removal from cornea; removal of corneal foreign body; cataract extraction, glaucoma surgery

Dosage Summary

Ophthalmic:

Children: Instill 1 drop in each eye every 5-10 minutes for 5-7 doses **or** instill 1-2 drops in each eye just prior to procedure

Adults: Instill 1 drop in each eye every 5-10 minutes for 5-7 doses **or** instill 1-2 drops in each eye just prior to procedure

Dosage Forms

Solution, ophthalmic: Proparacaine 0.5% and fluorescein 0.25% (5 mL)

Flucaine®: Proparacaine 0.5% and fluorescein 0.25% (5 mL)

proparacaine hydrochloride *see* proparacaine *on page* 803

Propecia® [US/Can] *see* finasteride *on page* 403

Propine® [Can] *see* dipivefrin *on page* 317

Propine® *(Discontinued)* *see* dipivefrin *on page* 317

PRO-Pioglitazone [Can] *see* pioglitazone *on page* 762

PRO-Piroxicam [Can] *see* piroxicam *on page* 764

Proplex® T *(Discontinued)* *see* factor IX complex (human) *on page* 389

propofol (PROE po fole)

Sound-Alike/Look-Alike Issues

propofol may be confused with fospropofol

Diprivan® may be confused with Diflucan®, Ditropan®

U.S./Canadian Brand Names Diprivan® [US/Can]

Therapeutic Category General Anesthetic

Use Induction of anesthesia in patients ≥3 years of age; maintenance of anesthesia in patients >2 months of age; in adults, for monitored anesthesia care sedation during procedures; sedation in intubated, mechanically-ventilated ICU patients

Dosage Summary

I.V.:

Children <2 months: Dosage not established

Children:

Induction (3-16 years):

ASA-PS 1 or 2: 2.5-3.5 mg/kg over 20-30 seconds

ASA-PS 3 or 4: Use lower dose

Maintenance (2 months to 16 years):

ASA-PS 1 or 2: Initial: 200-300 mcg/kg/minute, decrease after 30 minutes; Infusion: 125-300 mcg/kg/minute; **Note:** Children ≤5 years may require higher infusion rates compared to older children

Adults:

Induction:

ASA-PS 1 or 2, <55 years:

General anesthesia: 2-2.5 mg/kg (~40 mg every 10 seconds)

Monitored anesthesia care sedation: 100-150 mcg/kg/minute for 3-5 minutes **or** 0.5 mg/kg over 3-5 minutes

Elderly, debilitated, ASA-PS 3 or 4:

General anesthesia: 1-1.5 mg/kg (~20 mg every 10 seconds until onset of induction); do not use rapid bolus dose (single or repeated)

Monitored anesthesia care sedation: Use 80% of healthy adult dose; do not use rapid bolus doses (single or repeated)

Maintenance:
ASA-PS 1 or 2, <55 years:
General anesthesia: 100-200 mcg/kg/minute for 10-15 minutes, then decrease by 30% to 50%; Usual rate: 50-100 mcg/kg/minute **or** 25-50 mg increments as needed
Monitored anesthesia care sedation: 25-75 mcg/kg/minute **or** 10-20 mg incremental boluses
Elderly, debilitated, ASA-PS 3 or 4:
General anesthesia: 50-100 mcg/kg/minute
Monitored anesthesia care sedation: Use 80% of healthy adult dose; do not use rapid bolus doses (single or repeated)
Adults (mechanically-ventilated): ICU sedation: Initial: 5 mcg/kg/minute; Maintenance: 5-80 mcg/kg/minute; **Note:** Titration is recommended
Elderly, debilitated, ASA-PS 3 or 4 (mechanically-ventilated): ICU sedation: Use 80% of healthy adult dose; do not use rapid bolus doses (single or repeated)

Dosage Forms
Injection, emulsion: 10 mg/mL (10 mL, 20 mL, 50 mL, 100 mL)
Diprivan®: 10 mg/mL (20 mL, 50 mL, 100 mL)

Propoxacet-N® ***(Discontinued)*** *see* propoxyphene and acetaminophen *on page 805*

propoxyphene (proe POKS i feen)

Sound-Alike/Look-Alike Issues
propoxyphene may be confused with proparacaine
Darvon® may be confused with Devrom®, Diovan®
Darvon-N® may be confused with Darvocet-N®

Synonyms dextropropoxyphene; propoxyphene hydrochloride; propoxyphene napsylate

U.S./Canadian Brand Names 642® Tablet [Can]; Darvon-N® [US/Can]; Darvon® [US]

Therapeutic Category Analgesic, Narcotic

Controlled Substance C-IV

Use Management of mild-to-moderate pain

Dosage Summary
Oral:
Hydrochloride:
Children: Dosage not established
Adults: 65 mg every 4 hours as needed (maximum: 390 mg/day)
Napsylate:
Children: Dosage not established
Adults: 100 mg every 4 hours as needed (maximum: 600 mg/day)

Dosage Forms
Capsule, oral: 65 mg
Darvon®: 65 mg
Tablet, oral:
Darvon-N®: 100 mg

propoxyphene and acetaminophen (proe POKS i feen & a seet a MIN oh fen)

Sound-Alike/Look-Alike Issues
Darvocet® may be confused with Percocet®
Darvocet-N® may be confused with Darvon-N®

Synonyms acetaminophen and propoxyphene; propoxyphene hydrochloride and acetaminophen; propoxyphene napsylate and acetaminophen

U.S./Canadian Brand Names Balacet 325™ [US]; Darvocet A500® [US]; Darvocet-N® 100 [US/Can]; Darvocet-N® 50 [US/Can]

Therapeutic Category Analgesic, Narcotic

Controlled Substance C-IV

Use Management of mild-to-moderate pain

Dosage Summary
Oral:
Propoxyphene hydrochloride and acetaminophen 65/650 mg:
Children: Dosage not established
Adults: 1 tablet every 4 hours as needed (maximum: 4 g/day [acetaminophen]; 390 mg/day propoxyphene hydrochloride])

Propoxyphene napsylate and acetaminophen:

Children: Dosage not established

Adults:

Darvocet A500™, Darvocet-N® 100: 1 tablet every 4 hours as needed (maximum: 4 g/day [acetaminophen]; 600 mg/day [propoxyphene napsylate])

Darvocet-N® 50: 1-2 tablets every 4 hours as needed (maximum: 4 g/day [acetaminophen]; 600 mg/day [propoxyphene napsylate])

Dosage Forms

Tablet:

65/650: Propoxyphene 65 mg and acetaminophen 650 mg; 100/325: Propoxyphene 100 mg and acetaminophen 325 mg; 100/500: Propoxyphene 100 mg and acetaminophen 500 mg; 100/650: Propoxyphene 100 mg and acetaminophen 650 mg

Balacet 325™: Propoxyphene 100 mg and acetaminophen 325 mg

Darvocet A500®: Propoxyphene 100 mg and acetaminophen 500 mg

Darvocet-N® 50: Propoxyphene 50 mg and acetaminophen 325 mg

Darvocet-N® 100: Propoxyphene 100 mg and acetaminophen 650 mg

propoxyphene, aspirin, and caffeine *(Discontinued)*

propoxyphene hydrochloride *see* propoxyphene *on page 805*

propoxyphene hydrochloride and acetaminophen *see* propoxyphene and acetaminophen *on page 805*

propoxyphene napsylate *see* propoxyphene *on page 805*

propoxyphene napsylate and acetaminophen *see* propoxyphene and acetaminophen *on page 805*

propranolol (proe PRAN oh lole)

Sound-Alike/Look-Alike Issues

propranolol may be confused with prasugrel, Pravachol®, Propulsid®

Inderal® may be confused with Adderall®, Enduron®, Enduronyl®, Imdur®, Imuran®, Inderide®, Isordil®, Toradol®

Inderal® 40 may be confused with Enduronyl® Forte

Synonyms propranolol hydrochloride

U.S./Canadian Brand Names Apo-Propranolol® [Can]; Dom-Propranolol [Can]; Inderal® LA [US/Can]; Inderal® [Can]; InnoPran XL® [US]; Novo-Pranol [Can]; Nu-Propranolol [Can]; PMS-Propranolol [Can]; Propranolol Hydrochloride Injection, USP [Can]

Therapeutic Category Antiarrhythmic Agent, Class II; Beta-Adrenergic Blocker

Use Management of hypertension; angina pectoris; pheochromocytoma; essential tremor; supraventricular arrhythmias (such as atrial fibrillation and flutter, AV nodal reentrant tachycardias), ventricular tachycardias (catecholamine-induced arrhythmias, digoxin toxicity); prevention of myocardial infarction; migraine headache prophylaxis; symptomatic treatment of hypertrophic subaortic stenosis (hypertrophic obstructive cardiomyopathy)

Dosage Summary

I.V.:

Children: Dosage not established

Adults: 1-3 mg, repeat every 2-5 minutes up to a total of 5 mg **or** 1-3 mg as a single dose **or** 0.1 mg/kg divided into 3 equal doses given at 2-3 minute intervals; may repeat total dose in 2 minutes if necessary [ACLS guidelines, 2005]

Oral:

Extended release:

Children: Dosage not established

Adults: Initial: 80 mg once daily; Maintenance: 60-320 mg once daily (maximum: 640 mg/day; exceptions occur [indication specific])

Regular release:

Children: Dosage not established

Adults: 30-320 mg/day in 2-4 divided doses (maximum: 640 mg/day; exceptions occur [indication specific])

Elderly: Tachyarrhythmias: Initial: 10 mg twice daily; Maintenance: 10-320 mg/day in 1-2 divided doses; Other indications: 30-320 mg/day in 2-4 divided doses (maximum: 640 mg/day; exceptions occur [indication specific]) **Note:** Titration is recommended.

Dosage Forms

Capsule, extended release, oral: 60 mg, 80 mg, 120 mg, 160 mg
InnoPran XL®: 80 mg, 120 mg

Capsule, sustained release, oral:
Inderal® LA: 60 mg, 80 mg, 120 mg, 160 mg

Injection, solution: 1 mg/mL (1 mL)

Injection, solution [preservative free]: 1 mg/mL (1 mL)

Solution, oral: 4 mg/mL (500 mL); 8 mg/mL (500 mL)

Tablet, oral: 10 mg, 20 mg, 40 mg, 60 mg, 80 mg

propranolol and hydrochlorothiazide (proe PRAN oh lole & hye droe klor oh THYE a zide)

Sound-Alike/Look-Alike Issues

Inderide® may be confused with Inderal®

Synonyms hydrochlorothiazide and propranolol

Therapeutic Category Antihypertensive Agent, Combination

Use Management of hypertension

Dosage Summary

Oral:

Children: Dosage not established

Adults: Propranolol 80-160 mg/day and hydrochlorothiazide 12.5-50 mg/day in 2 divided doses

Dosage Forms

Tablet: Propranolol 40 mg and hydrochlorothiazide 25 mg; propranolol 80 mg and hydrochlorothiazide 25 mg

propranolol hydrochloride *see* propranolol *on page 806*

Propranolol Hydrochloride Injection, USP [Can] *see* propranolol *on page 806*

Proprinal® [US-OTC] *see* ibuprofen *on page 494*

Proprinal® Cold and Sinus [US-OTC] *see* pseudoephedrine and ibuprofen *on page 812*

Propulsid® [US] *see* cisapride *on page 226*

propylene glycol diacetate, acetic acid, and hydrocortisone *see* acetic acid, propylene glycol diacetate, and hydrocortisone *on page 33*

propylhexedrine (proe pil HEKS e dreen)

U.S./Canadian Brand Names Benzedrex® [US-OTC]

Therapeutic Category Adrenergic Agonist Agent

Use Topical nasal decongestant

Dosage Summary

Oral:

Children <6 years: Dosage not established

Children 6-12 years: Two inhalations in each nostril, not more frequently than every 2 hours

Children >12 years: Two inhalations in each nostril, not more frequently than every 2 hours

Adults: Two inhalations in each nostril, not more frequently than every 2 hours

Dosage Forms

Inhaler, nasal:
Benzedrex® [OTC]: 0.4-0.5 mg/inhalation (1s)

2-propylpentanoic acid *see* valproic acid *on page 974*

propylthiouracil (proe pil thye oh YOOR a sil)

Sound-Alike/Look-Alike Issues

propylthiouracil may be confused with Purinethol®
PTU is an error-prone abbreviation (mistaken as mercaptopurine [Purinethol®; 6-MP])

U.S./Canadian Brand Names Propyl-Thyracil® [Can]

Therapeutic Category Antithyroid Agent

Use Adjunctive therapy in patients intolerant of methimazole to ameliorate hyperthyroidism symptoms in preparation for surgical treatment or radioactive iodine therapy; treatment of hyperthyroidism in patients intolerant of methimazole and not candidates for surgical/radiotherapy

Dosage Summary

Oral:

Children <6 years: Dosage not established

Children 6-10 years: 50-150 mg/day

Children >10 years: 150-300 mg/day

Adults: Initial: 300-900 mg/day in 3 divided doses; Maintenance: 100-150 mg/day

Dosage Forms

Tablet, oral: 50 mg

Propyl-Thyracil® [Can] *see* propylthiouracil *on page 807*
2-propylvaleric acid *see* valproic acid *on page 974*
ProQuad® [US] *see* measles, mumps, rubella, and varicella virus vaccine *on page 593*
PRO-Quetiapine [Can] *see* quetiapine *on page 821*
Proquin® XR [US] *see* ciprofloxacin (systemic) *on page 224*
PRO-Rabeprazole [Can] *see* rabeprazole *on page 824*
PRO-Risperidone [Can] *see* risperidone *on page 845*
Proscar® [US/Can] *see* finasteride *on page 403*
Prosed®/DS [US] *see* methenamine, phenyl salicylate, methylene blue, benzoic acid, and hyoscyamine *on page 613*
Prosol [US] *see* amino acid injection *on page 64*
ProSom® *(Discontinued)* *see* estazolam *on page 365*
PRO-Sotalol [Can] *see* sotalol *on page 892*
prostacyclin *see* epoprostenol *on page 357*
prostacyclin PGI_2 *see* iloprost *on page 499*
prostaglandin E_1 *see* alprostadil *on page 55*
prostaglandin E_2 *see* dinoprostone *on page 308*
prostaglandin F_2 *see* carboprost tromethamine *on page 183*
ProStep® Patch *(Discontinued)* *see* nicotine *on page 674*
Prostigmin® [US/Can] *see* neostigmine *on page 668*
Prostin E2® [US/Can] *see* dinoprostone *on page 308*
Prostin F_2 Alpha® *(Discontinued)*
Prostin® VR [Can] *see* alprostadil *on page 55*
Prostin VR Pediatric® [US] *see* alprostadil *on page 55*

protamine sulfate (PROE ta meen SUL fate)

Sound-Alike/Look-Alike Issues

protamine may be confused with ProAmatine®, Protonix®, Protopam®, Protropin®

Therapeutic Category Antidote

Use Treatment of heparin overdosage; neutralize heparin during surgery or dialysis procedures

Dosage Summary

I.V.:

Children: 1 mg of protamine neutralizes 90 USP units of heparin (lung) and 115 USP units of heparin (intestinal) (maximum dose: 50 mg); **Note:** Dosage should be adjusted depending on the duration since heparin administration

Adults: 1 mg of protamine neutralizes 90 USP units of heparin (lung) and 115 USP units of heparin (intestinal) (maximum dose: 50 mg); **Note:** Dosage should be adjusted depending on the duration since heparin administration

Dosage Forms

Injection, solution [preservative free]: 10 mg/mL (5 mL, 25 mL)

protease, lipase, and amylase *see* pancrelipase *on page 723*
Protection Plus® [US-OTC] *see* alcohol (ethyl) *on page 45*
protein C *see* protein C concentrate (human) *on page 809*
protein C (activated), human, recombinant *see* drotrecogin alfa *on page 334*
protein-bound paclitaxel *see* paclitaxel (protein bound) *on page 720*

protein C concentrate (human) (PROE teen cee KON suhn trate HYU man)

Sound-Alike/Look-Alike Issues

protein C concentrate (human) may be confused with activated protein C (human, recombinant) which refers to drotrecogin alfa

Ceprotin may be confused with aprotinin, Cipro®

Synonyms protein C

U.S./Canadian Brand Names Ceprotin [US]

Therapeutic Category Anticoagulant

Use Replacement therapy for severe congenital protein C deficiency for the prevention and/or treatment of venous thromboembolism and purpura fulminans

Dosage Summary

I.V.:

Children: Initial: 100-120 int. units, followed by 60-80 int. units every 6 hours for 3 doses; maintenance: 45-60 int. units every 6 hours (short-term) or every 12 hours (short-to-long term)

Adults: Initial: 100-120 int. units, followed by 60-80 int. units every 6 hours for 3 doses; maintenance: 45-60 int. units every 6 hours (short-term) or every 12 hours (short-to-long term)

Dosage Forms

Injection, powder for reconstitution:

Ceprotin: ~500 int. units, ~1000 int. units

Protenate® ***(Discontinued)*** *see* plasma protein fraction *on page* 766

Prothazine-DC® ***(Discontinued)*** *see* promethazine and codeine *on page* 801

prothrombin complex concentrate *see* factor IX complex (human) *on page* 389

prothrombin complex concentrate *see* prothrombin complex (human) [(factors II, VII, IX, X), protein C, and protein S] *(Canada only) on page* 809

prothrombin complex (human) [(factors II, VII, IX, X), protein C, and protein S] *(Canada only)*

(PRO throm bin KOM pleks HYU man FAK ters too SEV en nyne ten PROE teen cee & PROE teen ess)

Synonyms prothrombin complex concentrate

U.S./Canadian Brand Names Octaplex® [Can]

Therapeutic Category Hemostatic Agent

Use Prophylaxis (perioperative) and treatment of bleeding due to acquired deficiency (eg, overdose of vitamin K antagonist) of one or more of the prothrombin complex coagulation factors II, VII, IX, and X, when rapid correction of factor deficiency is necessary

Dosage Summary

I.V.:

Children <17 years: Dosage not established

Adults: Maximum dose not to exceed 120 mL. Approximate doses required for normalization of INR (≤1.2 within 1 hour):

Initial INR: 2-2.5: Administer 0.9-1.3 mL/kg

2.5-3: Administer 1.3-1.6 mL/kg

3-3.5: Administer 1.6-1.9 mL/kg

>3.5: Administer >1.9 mL/kg

With the correction of vitamin K antagonist-induced impairment of hemostasis in patients who have been treated concomitantly with an appropriate vitamin K dose, repeat dosing with PCC is usually not necessary.

Dosage Forms - Canada

Injection, powder for reconstitution:

Octaplex®: Human coagulation factor II: 11-38 int. units/mL; factor VII: 9-24 int. units/mL; factor IX: 20-31 int. units/mL; factor X: 18-30 int. units/mL: protein C: 7-31 int. units/mL; protein S: 7-32 int. units/mL (20 mL)

Protilase® ***(Discontinued)*** *see* pancrelipase *on page* 723

Protonix® [US/Can] *see* pantoprazole *on page* 725

Protopam® [US/Can] *see* pralidoxime *on page* 785

Protopic® [US/Can] *see* tacrolimus (topical) *on page* 908

PRO-Topiramate [Can] *see* topiramate *on page* 942

Protostat® Oral ***(Discontinued)*** *see* metronidazole (systemic) *on page* 627

protriptyline (proe TRIP ti leen)

Sound-Alike/Look-Alike Issues

Vivactil® may be confused with Vyvanse™

Synonyms protriptyline hydrochloride

U.S./Canadian Brand Names Vivactil® [US]

Therapeutic Category Antidepressant, Tricyclic (Secondary Amine)

Use Treatment of depression

Dosage Summary

Oral:

Children: Dosage not established

Adolescents: 15-20 mg/day

Adults: 15-60 mg/day in 3-4 divided doses

Elderly: Initial: 5-10 mg/day; Maintenance: 15-20 mg/day; **Note:** Titration is recommended

Dosage Forms

Tablet, oral: 5 mg, 10 mg

Vivactil®: 5 mg, 10 mg

protriptyline hydrochloride *see* protriptyline *on page* 810

Protuss®-DM ***(Discontinued)*** *see* guaifenesin, pseudoephedrine, and dextromethorphan *on page* 460

PRO-Valacyclovir [Can] *see* valacyclovir *on page* 973

Provenge® [US] *see* sipuleucel-T *on page* 878

Proventil® ***(Discontinued)*** *see* albuterol *on page* 43

Proventil® HFA [US] *see* albuterol *on page* 43

Proventil® Inhaler ***(Discontinued)*** *see* albuterol *on page* 43

Proventil® Solution ***(Discontinued)*** *see* albuterol *on page* 43

Proventil® Tablet ***(Discontinued)*** *see* albuterol *on page* 43

Provera® [US/Can] *see* medroxyprogesterone *on page* 597

Provera-Pak [Can] *see* medroxyprogesterone *on page* 597

PRO-Verapamil SR [Can] *see* verapamil *on page* 981

Provigil® [US] *see* modafinil *on page* 639

Proviodine [Can] *see* povidone-iodine (topical) *on page* 784

Provisc® [US] *see* hyaluronate and derivatives *on page* 475

Provocholine® [US/Can] *see* methacholine *on page* 610

proxymetacaine *see* proparacaine *on page* 803

Prozac® [US/Can] *see* fluoxetine *on page* 415

Prozac® Weekly™ [US] *see* fluoxetine *on page* 415

PRO-Zopiclone [Can] *see* zopiclone *(Canada only) on page* 1005

PRP-OMP *see Haemophilus* B conjugate vaccine *on page* 463

PRP-T *see Haemophilus* B conjugate vaccine *on page* 463

Prudoxin™ [US] *see* doxepin (topical) *on page* 329

prussian blue *see* ferric hexacyanoferrate *on page* 397

prymaccone *see* primaquine *on page* 794

P&S® [US-OTC] *see* salicylic acid *on page* 858

23PS *see* pneumococcal polysaccharide vaccine (polyvalent) *on page* 772

PS-341 *see* bortezomib *on page* 143

Pseudacarb™ [US] *see* carbetapentane and pseudoephedrine *on page* 180

Pseudo DM GG [US] *see* guaifenesin, pseudoephedrine, and dextromethorphan *on page* 460

pseudoephedrine (soo doe e FED rin)

Sound-Alike/Look-Alike Issues

Sudafed® may be confused with sotalol, Sudafed PE™, Sufenta®

Synonyms *d*-isoephedrine hydrochloride; pseudoephedrine hydrochloride; pseudoephedrine sulfate

U.S./Canadian Brand Names Balminil Decongestant [Can]; Benylin® D for Infants [Can]; Children's Nasal Decongestant [US-OTC]; Contac® Cold 12 Hour Relief Non Drowsy [Can]; Drixoral® ND [Can]; Eltor® [Can]; Genaphed™ [US-OTC]; Oranyl [US-OTC]; PMS-Pseudoephedrine [Can]; Pseudofrin [Can];

Robidrine® [Can]; Silfedrine Children's [US-OTC]; Sudafed® 12 Hour [US-OTC]; Sudafed® 24 Hour [US-OTC]; Sudafed® Children's [US-OTC]; Sudafed® Decongestant [Can]; Sudafed® Maximum Strength Nasal Decongestant [US-OTC]; Sudo-Tab® [US-OTC]; Sudogest 12 Hour [US-OTC]; SudoGest Children's [US-OTC]; SudoGest [US-OTC]

Therapeutic Category Adrenergic Agonist Agent

Use Temporary symptomatic relief of nasal congestion due to common cold, upper respiratory allergies, and sinusitis; also promotes nasal or sinus drainage

Dosage Summary

Oral:

Immediate release:

Children <4 years: Dosage not established

Children 4-5 years: 15 mg every 4-6 hours (maximum: 60 mg/day)

Children 6-12 years: 30 mg every 4-6 hours (maximum: 120 mg/day)

Adults: 60 mg every 4-6 hours (maximum: 240 mg/day)

Extended release:

Children: Dosage not established

Adults: 120 mg every 12 hours or 240 mg every 24 hours (maximum: 240 mg/day)

Dosage Forms

Caplet, extended release, oral:

Sudafed® 12 Hour [OTC]: 120 mg

Liquid, oral: 30 mg/5 mL (473 mL)

Children's Nasal Decongestant [OTC]: 30 mg/5 mL (118 mL)

Silfedrine Children's [OTC]: 15 mg/5 mL (118 mL, 237 mL)

Sudafed® Children's [OTC]: 15 mg/5 mL (118 mL)

Syrup, oral: 30 mg/5 mL (118 mL)

SudoGest Children's [OTC]: 15 mg/5 mL (118 mL)

Tablet, oral: 30 mg

Genaphed™ [OTC]: 30 mg

Oranyl [OTC]: 30 mg

Sudafed® Maximum Strength Nasal Decongestant [OTC]: 30 mg

Sudo-Tab® [OTC]: 30 mg

SudoGest [OTC]: 30 mg, 60 mg

Tablet, extended release, oral:

Sudafed® 24 Hour [OTC]: 240 mg

Sudogest 12 Hour [OTC]: 120 mg

pseudoephedrine, acetaminophen, and chlorpheniramine *see* acetaminophen, chlorpheniramine, and pseudoephedrine *on page 28*

pseudoephedrine and acetaminophen *see* acetaminophen and pseudoephedrine *on page 26*

pseudoephedrine and brompheniramine *see* brompheniramine and pseudoephedrine *on page 148*

pseudoephedrine and carbetapentane *see* carbetapentane and pseudoephedrine *on page 180*

pseudoephedrine and chlorpheniramine *see* chlorpheniramine and pseudoephedrine *on page 209*

pseudoephedrine and codeine (soo doe e FED rin & KOE deen)

Synonyms codeine and pseudoephedrine; codeine phosphate and pseudoephedrine hydrochloride; pseudoephedrine hydrochloride and codeine phosphate

U.S./Canadian Brand Names Notuss®-DC [US]

Therapeutic Category Antitussive/Decongestant

Controlled Substance Capsule: C-III; Liquid: C-V

Use Temporary symptomatic relief of congestion and cough due to upper respiratory infections including common cold, bronchitis, sinusitis, and influenza

Dosage Summary

Oral:

Children <6 years: Dosage not established

Children 6-11 years: 2.5-5 mL every 4-6 hours as needed (maximum: 20 mL/24 hours)

Children ≥12 years: One capsule every 6 hours as needed (maximum: 4 capsules/24 hours) **or** 5-10 mL every 4-6 hours as needed (maximum: 40 mL/24 hours)

Adults: One capsule every 6 hours as needed (maximum: 4 capsules/24 hours) **or** 5-10 mL every 4-6 hours as needed (maximum: 40 mL/24 hours)

Dosage Forms

Liquid, oral:

Notuss®-DC: Pseudoephedrine 30 mg and codeine 10 mg per 5 mL

pseudoephedrine and desloratadine *see* desloratadine and pseudoephedrine *on page 278*

pseudoephedrine and dexbrompheniramine *see* dexbrompheniramine and pseudoephedrine *on page 282*

pseudoephedrine and dextromethorphan (soo doe e FED rin & deks troe meth OR fan)

Synonyms dextromethorphan and pseudoephedrine

U.S./Canadian Brand Names Balminil DM D [Can]; Benylin® DM-D [Can]; Koffex DM-D [Can]; Novahistex® DM Decongestant [Can]; Novahistine® DM Decongestant [Can]; Pedia Relief Cough and Cold [US-OTC]; Pedia Relief Infants [US-OTC]; Robitussin® Childrens Cough & Cold [Can]; Sudafed® Children's Cold & Cough [US-OTC]

Therapeutic Category Antitussive/Decongestant

Use Temporary symptomatic relief of nasal congestion and cough due to common cold, hay fever, upper respiratory allergies

Dosage Summary

Oral:

Children <2 years: Dosage not established

Children 2-6 years: 15 mg (based on pseudoephedrine) every 4-6 hours (maximum: 60 mg/day)

Children 6-12 years: 30 mg (based on pseudoephedrine) every 4-6 hours (maximum: 120 mg/day)

Children ≥12 years: 60 mg (based on pseudoephedrine) every 4-6 hours (maximum: 240 mg/day)

Adults: 60 mg (based on pseudoephedrine) every 4-6 hours (maximum: 240 mg/day)

Dosage Forms

Liquid:

Sudafed® Children's Cold & Cough [OTC]: Pseudoephedrine 15 mg and dextromethorphan 5 mg per 5 mL

Liquid, oral [drops]:

Pedia Relief Infants [OTC]: Pseudoephedrine 7.5 mg and dextromethorphan 2.5 mg per 0.8 mL

Syrup:

Pedia Relief Cough and Cold [OTC]: Pseudoephedrine 15 mg and dextromethorphan 7.5 mg per 5 mL

pseudoephedrine and fexofenadine *see* fexofenadine and pseudoephedrine *on page 400*

pseudoephedrine and guaifenesin *see* guaifenesin and pseudoephedrine *on page 457*

pseudoephedrine and ibuprofen (soo doe e FED rin & eye byoo PROE fen)

Synonyms ibuprofen and pseudoephedrine

U.S./Canadian Brand Names Advil® Cold & Sinus [US-OTC/Can]; Children's Advil® Cold [Can]; Proprinal® Cold and Sinus [US-OTC]; Sudafed® Sinus Advance [Can]

Therapeutic Category Decongestant/Analgesic

Use For temporary relief of cold, sinus, and flu symptoms (including nasal congestion, sinus pressure, headache, minor body aches and pains, and fever)

Dosage Summary

Oral:

Children <12 years: Dosage not established

Children ≥12 years: 1-2 doses (ibuprofen 200 mg and pseudoephedrine 30 mg per dose) every 4-6 hours as needed (maximum: 6 doses/day)

Adults: 1-2 doses (ibuprofen 200 mg and pseudoephedrine 30 mg per dose) every 4-6 hours as needed (maximum: 6 doses/day)

Dosage Forms

Caplet:

Advil® Cold & Sinus [OTC], Proprinal® Cold and Sinus [OTC]: Pseudoephedrine 30 mg and ibuprofen 200 mg

Capsule, liquid filled:

Advil® Cold & Sinus [OTC]: Pseudoephedrine 30 mg and ibuprofen 200 mg

pseudoephedrine and loratadine *see* loratadine and pseudoephedrine *on page 576*

pseudoephedrine and methscopolamine (soo doe e FED rin & meth skoe POL a meen)

Synonyms methscopolamine and pseudoephedrine; pseudoephedrine hydrochloride and methscopolamine nitrate

U.S./Canadian Brand Names AlleRx™-D [US]; Extendryl PSE [US]

Therapeutic Category Decongestant/Anticholingeric Combination

Use Relief of symptoms of allergic rhinitis, vasomotor rhinitis, sinusitis, and the common cold

Dosage Summary

Oral:

Children <12 years: Dosage not established

Children ≥12 years: One tablet every 12 hours (maximum: 2 tablets/24 hours)

Adults: One tablet every 12 hours (maximum: 2 tablets/24 hours)

Dosage Forms

Tablet: Pseudoephedrine hydrochloride 120 mg and methscopolamine nitrate 2.5 mg

Allerx™-D: Pseudoephedrine 120 mg and methscopolamine 2.5 mg

Tablet, extended release:

Extendryl PSE: Pseudoephedrine 120 mg and methscopolamine 2.5 mg

pseudoephedrine and naproxen *see* naproxen and pseudoephedrine *on page 661*

pseudoephedrine and triprolidine *see* triprolidine and pseudoephedrine *on page 961*

pseudoephedrine, chlorpheniramine, and acetaminophen *see* acetaminophen, chlorpheniramine, and pseudoephedrine *on page 28*

pseudoephedrine, chlorpheniramine, and codeine *see* chlorpheniramine, pseudoephedrine, and codeine *on page 214*

pseudoephedrine, chlorpheniramine, and dextromethorphan *see* chlorpheniramine, pseudoephedrine, and dextromethorphan *on page 214*

pseudoephedrine, chlorpheniramine, and dihydrocodeine *see* pseudoephedrine, dihydrocodeine, and chlorpheniramine *on page 813*

pseudoephedrine, chlorpheniramine, and ibuprofen *see* ibuprofen, pseudoephedrine, and chlorpheniramine *on page 496*

pseudoephedrine, codeine, and triprolidine *see* triprolidine, pseudoephedrine, and codeine *(Canada only) on page 961*

pseudoephedrine, dextromethorphan, and guaifenesin *see* guaifenesin, pseudoephedrine, and dextromethorphan *on page 460*

pseudoephedrine, dextromethorphan, doxylamine, and acetaminophen *see* acetaminophen, dextromethorphan, doxylamine, and pseudoephedrine *on page 30*

pseudoephedrine, dihydrocodeine, and chlorpheniramine
(soo doe e FED rin, dye hye droe KOE deen, & klor fen IR a meen)

Synonyms chlorpheniramine, dihydrocodeine, and pseudoephedrine; dihydrocodeine bitartrate, pseudoephedrine hydrochloride, and chlorpheniramine maleate; pseudoephedrine, chlorpheniramine, and dihydrocodeine

U.S./Canadian Brand Names Coldcough [US]; DiHydro-CP [US]

Therapeutic Category Antihistamine/Decongestant/Antitussive

Controlled Substance C-III

Use Temporary relief of cough, congestion, and sneezing due to colds, respiratory infections, or hay fever

Dosage Summary

Oral:

Children <2 years: Dosage not established

Children 2-6 years: 1.25-2.5 mL every 4-6 hours (maximum: 4 doses/day)

Children 6-12 years: 2.5-5 mL every 4-6 hours (maximum: 4 doses/day)

Children >12 years: 5-10 mL every 4-6 hours (maximum: 4 doses/day)

Adults: 5-10 mL every 4-6 hours (maximum: 4 doses/day)

Dosage Forms

Syrup:

Coldcough, DiHydro-CP: Pseudoephedrine 15 mg, dihydrocodeine 7.5 mg, and chlorpheniramine 2 mg per 5 mL

pseudoephedrine, guaifenesin, and codeine *see* guaifenesin, pseudoephedrine, and codeine *on page 459*

pseudoephedrine hydrochloride *see* pseudoephedrine *on page 810*

pseudoephedrine hydrochloride and acetaminophen *see* acetaminophen and pseudoephedrine *on page 26*

pseudoephedrine hydrochloride and acrivastine *see* acrivastine and pseudoephedrine *on page 35*

pseudoephedrine hydrochloride and cetirizine hydrochloride *see* cetirizine and pseudoephedrine *on page 198*

pseudoephedrine hydrochloride and codeine phosphate *see* pseudoephedrine and codeine *on page 811*

pseudoephedrine hydrochloride and methscopolamine nitrate *see* pseudoephedrine and methscopolamine *on page 813*

pseudoephedrine hydrochloride, guaifenesin, and dihydrocodeine bitartrate *see* dihydrocodeine, pseudoephedrine, and guaifenesin *on page 304*

pseudoephedrine hydrochloride, methscopolamine nitrate, and chlorpheniramine maleate *see* chlorpheniramine, pseudoephedrine, and methscopolamine *on page 215*

pseudoephedrine, hydrocodone, and chlorpheniramine *(Discontinued)*

pseudoephedrine, methscopolamine, and chlorpheniramine *see* chlorpheniramine, pseudoephedrine, and methscopolamine *on page 215*

pseudoephedrine sulfate *see* pseudoephedrine *on page 810*

pseudoephedrine tannate and dexchlorpheniramine tannate *see* dexchlorpheniramine and pseudoephedrine *on page 283*

pseudoephedrine tannate, dextromethorphan tannate, and brompheniramine tannate *see* brompheniramine, pseudoephedrine, and dextromethorphan *on page 149*

pseudoephedrine, triprolidine, and codeine *see* triprolidine, pseudoephedrine, and codeine *(Canada only) on page 961*

Pseudofrin [Can] *see* pseudoephedrine *on page 810*

Pseudo-Gest Plus® Tablet *(Discontinued)* *see* chlorpheniramine and pseudoephedrine *on page 209*

Pseudo Max DMX [US] *see* guaifenesin, pseudoephedrine, and dextromethorphan *on page 460*

pseudomonic acid A *see* mupirocin *on page 649*

Pseudovent™ 400 *(Discontinued)* *see* guaifenesin and pseudoephedrine *on page 457*

Pseudovent™ *(Discontinued)* *see* guaifenesin and pseudoephedrine *on page 457*

Pseudovent™ DM *(Discontinued)* *see* guaifenesin, pseudoephedrine, and dextromethorphan *on page 460*

Pseudovent™-Ped *(Discontinued)* *see* guaifenesin and pseudoephedrine *on page 457*

P & S™ Liquid Phenol [Can] *see* phenol *on page 748*

Psorcon® *(Discontinued)* *see* diflorasone *on page 301*

Psorcon® e™ *(Discontinued)* *see* diflorasone *on page 301*

Psoriatec™ *(Discontinued)* *see* anthralin *on page 79*

PsoriGel® *(Discontinued)* *see* coal tar *on page 242*

Psorion® Topical *(Discontinued)*

psyllium (SIL i yum)

Sound-Alike/Look-Alike Issues

Fiberall® may be confused with Feverall®

Hydrocil® may be confused with Hydrocet®

Synonyms plantago seed; plantain seed; psyllium husk; psyllium hydrophilic mucilloid

U.S./Canadian Brand Names Bulk-K [US-OTC]; Fiberall® [US-OTC]; Fibro-Lax [US-OTC]; Fibro-XL [US-OTC]; Genfiber™ [US-OTC]; Hydrocil® Instant [US-OTC]; Konsyl-D™ [US-OTC]; Konsyl® Easy Mix™ [US-OTC]; Konsyl® Orange [US-OTC]; Konsyl® Original [US-OTC]; Konsyl® [US-OTC]; Metamucil® Plus Calcium [US-OTC]; Metamucil® Smooth Texture [US-OTC]; Metamucil® [US-OTC/Can]; Natural Fiber Therapy Smooth Texture [US-OTC]; Natural Fiber Therapy [US-OTC]; Reguloid [US-OTC]

Therapeutic Category Laxative

Use OTC labeling: Dietary fiber supplement; treatment of occasional constipation; reduce risk of coronary heart disease (CHD)

Dosage Summary

Oral:

Children <6 years: Dosage not established
Children 6-11 years: Psyllium 1.25-15 g per day in divided doses
Children ≥12 years: Psyllium 2.5-30 g per day in divided doses
Adults: Psyllium 2.5-30 g per day in divided doses

Dosage Forms

Capsule, oral: 500 mg
Fibro-XL [OTC]: 0.675 g
Genfiber™ [OTC]: 0.52 g
Konsyl® [OTC]: 0.52 g
Metamucil® [OTC]: 0.52 g
Metamucil® Plus Calcium [OTC]: 0.52 g
Reguloid [OTC]: 0.52 g

Powder, oral: 4.1 g/teaspoon (454 g)
Bulk-K [OTC]: 4.7 g/teaspoon (392 g)
Fiberall® [OTC]: 0.05 g/tablespoon (454 g)
Fibro-Lax [OTC]: 4.7 g/teaspoon (140 g, 392 g)
Genfiber™ [OTC]: 3.4 g/teaspoon (397 g); 3.4 g/tablespoon (397 g)
Hydrocil® Instant [OTC]: 3.5 g/teaspoon (300 g); 3.5 g/packet (30s, 500s)
Konsyl-D™ [OTC]: 3.4 g/teaspoon (325 g, 397 g, 500 g); 3.4 g/packet (100s, 500s)
Konsyl® Easy Mix™ [OTC]: 6 g/teaspoon (250 g); 6 g/packet (500s)
Konsyl® Orange [OTC]: 3.4 g/teaspoon (425 g); 3.4 g/tablespoon (538 g); 3.4 g/packet (30s)
Konsyl® Original [OTC]: 6 g/teaspoon (300 g, 450 g); 6 g/packet (30s, 100s, 500s)
Metamucil® [OTC]: 3.4 g/teaspoon (390 g, 570 g, 870 g); 3.4 g/tablespoon (570 g, 870 g, 1254 g)
Metamucil® Smooth Texture [OTC]: 3.3 g/teaspoon (288 g, 432 g, 684 g); 3.4 g/teaspoon (173 g, 283 g, 300 g, 425 g, 450 g, 660 g, 690 g, 1020 g); 3.4 g/tablespoon (609 g, 912 g, 1368 g); 3.4 g/packet (30s)
Natural Fiber Therapy [OTC]: 3.4 g/tablespoon (390 g, 539 g)
Natural Fiber Therapy Smooth Texture [OTC]: 3.4 g/teaspoon (300 g)
Reguloid [OTC]: 3.4 g/teaspoon (284 g, 426 g); 3.4 g/tablespoon (369 g, 540 g)

Wafer, oral:
Metamucil® [OTC]: 3.4 g/2 wafers (24s)

psyllium husk *see* psyllium *on page 814*
psyllium hydrophilic mucilloid *see* psyllium *on page 814*
P-Tann [US] *see* chlorpheniramine *on page 207*
pteroylglutamic acid *see* folic acid *on page 423*
PTG *see* teniposide *on page 916*
Pulmicort® [Can] *see* budesonide (systemic, oral inhalation) *on page 151*
Pulmicort Flexhaler® [US] *see* budesonide (systemic, oral inhalation) *on page 151*
Pulmicort Respules® [US] *see* budesonide (systemic, oral inhalation) *on page 151*
Pulmicort Turbuhaler® *(Discontinued)* *see* budesonide (systemic, oral inhalation) *on page 151*
Pulmophylline [Can] *see* theophylline *on page 925*
Pulmozyme® [US/Can] *see* dornase alfa *on page 327*
Puralube® Tears *(Discontinued)* *see* artificial tears *on page 97*
Puregon® [Can] *see* follitropin beta *on page 424*
Purell® [US-OTC] *see* alcohol (ethyl) *on page 45*
Purell® 2 in 1 [US-OTC] *see* alcohol (ethyl) *on page 45*
Purell® Lasting Care [US-OTC] *see* alcohol (ethyl) *on page 45*
Purell® Moisture Therapy [US-OTC] *see* alcohol (ethyl) *on page 45*
Purell® with Aloe [US-OTC] *see* alcohol (ethyl) *on page 45*
purified chick embryo cell *see* rabies vaccine *on page 825*
Purinethol® [US/Can] *see* mercaptopurine *on page 606*
PVP-I *see* povidone-iodine (ophthalmic) *on page 784*
PVP-I *see* povidone-iodine (topical) *on page 784*
Pylera™ [US] *see* bismuth, metronidazole, and tetracycline *on page 140*

pyrantel pamoate (pi RAN tel PAM oh ate)

U.S./Canadian Brand Names Combantrin™ [Can]; Pin-X® [US-OTC]; Reese's Pinworm Medicine [US-OTC]

Therapeutic Category Anthelmintic

Use Treatment of pinworms (*Enterobius vermicularis*) and roundworms (*Ascaris lumbricoides*)

Dosage Summary

Oral:

Children: 11 mg/kg as a single dose (maximum: 1 g/dose); repeat in 2 weeks for pinworm (dose is expressed as pyrantel base)

Adults: 11 mg/kg as a single dose (maximum: 1 g/dose); repeat in 2 weeks for pinworm (dose is expressed as pyrantel base)

Dosage Forms

Suspension, oral:

Pin-X® [OTC]: 144 mg/mL (30 mL, 60 mL)

Reese's Pinworm Medicine [OTC]: 144 mg/mL (30 mL, 60 mL, 240 mL)

Tablet, chewable, oral:

Pin-X® [OTC]: 720.5 mg

pyrazinamide (peer a ZIN a mide)

Synonyms pyrazinoic acid amide

U.S./Canadian Brand Names Tebrazid™ [Can]

Therapeutic Category Antitubercular Agent

Use Adjunctive treatment of tuberculosis in combination with other antituberculosis agents

Dosage Summary Note: Dosing in adults is based on lean body weight.

Oral:

Children: 15-30 mg/kg once daily (maximum: 2 g/day) **or** 50 mg/kg/dose twice weekly (maximum: 4 g/dose)

Adults 40-55 kg: 1000 mg once daily **or** 2000 mg twice weekly **or** 1500 mg three times/week

Adults: 56-75 kg: 1500 mg once daily **or** 3000 mg twice weekly **or** 2500 mg three times/week

Adults 76-90 kg: 2000 mg once daily (maximum dose regardless of weight) **or** 4000 mg twice weekly (maximum dose regardless of weight) **or** 3000 mg 3 times/week (maximum dose regardless of weight)

Elderly: Start with a lower daily dose (15 mg/kg) and increase as tolerated

Dosage Forms

Tablet, oral: 500 mg

pyrazinamide, rifampin, and isoniazid *see* rifampin, isoniazid, and pyrazinamide *on page 842*

pyrazinoic acid amide *see* pyrazinamide *on page 816*

pyrethrins and piperonyl butoxide (pye RE thrins & pi PER oh nil byo TOKS ide)

Synonyms piperonyl butoxide and pyrethrins

U.S./Canadian Brand Names A-200® Lice Treatment Kit [US-OTC]; A-200® Maximum Strength [US-OTC]; Licide® [US-OTC]; Pronto® Complete Lice Removal System [US-OTC]; Pronto® Lice Control [Can]; Pronto® Plus Lice Killing Mousse Plus Vitamin E [US-OTC]; Pronto® Plus Lice Killing Mousse Shampoo Plus Natural Extracts and Oils [US-OTC]; Pronto® Plus Warm Oil Treatment and Conditioner [US-OTC]; R & C™ II [Can]; R & C™ Shampoo/Conditioner [Can]; RID® Maximum Strength [US-OTC]; RID® Mousse [Can]

Therapeutic Category Scabicides/Pediculicides

Use Treatment of *Pediculus humanus* infestations (head lice, body lice, pubic lice, and their eggs)

Dosage Summary

Topical:

Children: Apply enough to completely wet infested area, allow to remain on for 10 minutes, wash and rinse; use fine-toothed comb to remove lice and eggs; may repeat once in a 24-hour period and then again in 7-10 days

Adults: Apply enough to completely wet infested area, allow to remain on for 10 minutes, wash and rinse; use fine-toothed comb to remove lice and eggs; may repeat once in a 24-hour period and then again in 7-10 days

Dosage Forms

Kit:

A-200® Lice Treatment Kit [OTC]:

Shampoo: Pyrethrins 0.33% and piperonyl butoxide 4% (120 mL)

Solution: Permethrin 0.5% (180 mL)

Pronto® Complete Lice Removal System [OTC]:

Shampoo: Pyrethrins 0.33% and piperonyl butoxide 4% (60 mL)

Solution, topical: Benzalkonium chloride 0.1% (60 mL)

Oil, topical:

Pronto® Plus Warm Oil Treatment and Conditioner [OTC]: Pyrethrins 0.33% and piperonyl butoxide 4% (36 mL)

Shampoo: Pyrethrins 0.33% and piperonyl butoxide 4% (60 mL, 120 mL)

A-200® Maximum Strength [OTC]: Pyrethrins 0.33% and piperonyl butoxide 4% (60 mL, 120 mL)

Licide® [OTC], Pronto® Plus Lice Killing Mousse Shampoo Plus Vitamin E [OTC]: Pyrethrins 0.33% and piperonyl butoxide 4% (120 mL)

Pronto® Plus Lice Killing Mousse Shampoo Plus Natural Extracts and Oils [OTC]: Pyrethrins 0.33% and piperonyl butoxide 4% (60 mL)

Pronto® Plus Lice Killing Mousse Shampoo Plus Vitamin E [OTC]: Pyrethrins 0.33% and piperonyl butoxide 4% (120 mL)

RID® Maximum Strength [OTC]: Pyrethrins 0.33% and piperonyl butoxide 4% (60 mL, 120 mL, 180 mL, 240 mL)

Pyri-500 [US-OTC] *see* pyridoxine *on page* *818*

2-pyridine aldoxime methochloride *see* pralidoxime *on page* *785*

Pyridium® [US] *see* phenazopyridine *on page* *746*

pyridostigmine (peer id oh STIG meen)

Sound-Alike/Look-Alike Issues

pyridostigmine may be confused with physostigmine

Mestinon® may be confused with Metatensin®

Regonol® may be confused with Reglan®, Renagel®

Synonyms pyridostigmine bromide

U.S./Canadian Brand Names Mestinon® Timespan® [US]; Mestinon® [US/Can]; Mestinon®-SR [Can]; Regonol® [US]

Therapeutic Category Cholinergic Agent

Use Symptomatic treatment of myasthenia gravis; antagonism of nondepolarizing neuromuscular blockers

Military use: Pretreatment for soman nerve gas exposure

Dosage Summary

I.M.:

Children: 0.05-0.15 mg/kg/dose

Adults: ~1/30th of oral dose

I.V.:

Children: 0.05-0.25 mg/kg/dose; **Note:** Atropine sulfate (0.6-1.2 mg) I.V. immediately prior to pyridostigmine to minimize side effects if used for reversal of nondepolarizing muscle relaxants

Adults: IVP: ~1/30th of oral dose **or** 0.1-0.25 mg/kg/dose (usual: 10-20 mg); Infusion: 2 mg/hour with gradual titration in increments of 0.5-1 mg/hour (maximum: 4 mg/hour); **Note:** Atropine sulfate (0.6-1.2 mg) I.V. immediately prior to pyridostigmine to minimize side effects is used for reversal of nondepolarizing muscle relaxants

Oral:

Immediate release:

Children: 7 mg/kg/day divided into 5-6 doses

Adults: 60-1500 mg/day in 5-6 divided doses (usual: 600 mg/day); **Note:** Dosing highly individualized

Sustained release:

Children: Dosage not established

Adults: 180-540 mg once or twice daily (doses separated by at least 6 hours); **Note:** Dosing highly individualized; Most clinicians reserve sustained release dosage form for bedtime dose only

Dosage Forms

Injection, solution:

Regonol®: 5 mg/mL (2 mL)

Syrup, oral:

Mestinon®: 60 mg/5 mL (480 mL)

Tablet, oral: 60 mg
Mestinon®: 60 mg
Tablet, sustained release, oral:
Mestinon® Timespan®: 180 mg

pyridostigmine bromide *see* pyridostigmine *on page* 817

pyridoxine (peer i DOKS een)

Sound-Alike/Look-Alike Issues
pyridoxine may be confused with paroxetine, pralidoxime, Pyridium®

Synonyms B6; B_6; pyridoxine hydrochloride; vitamin B_6

U.S./Canadian Brand Names Aminoxin® [US-OTC]; Pyri-500 [US-OTC]

Therapeutic Category Vitamin, Water Soluble

Use Prevention and treatment of vitamin B_6 deficiency, pyridoxine-dependent seizures in infants

Dosage Summary

I.M.:
Infants: Deficiency: 10-100 mg
Children: Dosage not established
Adults: Dosage not established

I.V.:
Infants: Deficiency: 10-100 mg

Oral:
Infants: Deficiency: 2-100 mg/day
Children:
Deficiency: 1.5-25 mg/day
Neuritis: Prophylaxis: 1-2 mg/kg/day; Treatment: 10-50 mg/day
Adults:
Deficiency: 10-20 mg/day
Neuritis: Prophylaxis: 25-100 mg/day; Treatment: 100-200 mg/day

SubQ:
Infants: Deficiency: 10-100 mg
Children: Dosage not established
Adults: Dosage not established

Dosage Forms
Capsule, oral: 50 mg, 250 mg
Aminoxin® [OTC]: 20 mg
Injection, solution: 100 mg/mL (1 mL)
Liquid, oral: 200 mg/5 mL (120 mL)
Tablet, oral: 25 mg, 50 mg, 100 mg, 250 mg, 500 mg
Tablet, sustained release, oral:
Pyri-500 [OTC]: 500 mg

pyridoxine and doxylamine *see* doxylamine and pyridoxine *(Canada only) on page* 332

pyridoxine, folic acid, and cyanocobalamin *see* folic acid, cyanocobalamin, and pyridoxine *on page* 423

pyridoxine hydrochloride *see* pyridoxine *on page* 818

Pyrilafen Tannate-12™ *(Discontinued)* *see* phenylephrine and pyrilamine *on page* 753

pyrilamine, chlorpheniramine, and phenylephrine *see* chlorpheniramine, pyrilamine, and phenylephrine *on page* 215

pyrilamine maleate, dextromethorphan hydrobromide, and phenylephrine hydrochloride *see* phenylephrine, pyrilamine, and dextromethorphan *on page* 755

pyrilamine, phenylephrine, and carbetapentane *see* carbetapentane, phenylephrine, and pyrilamine *on page* 181

pyrilamine tannate and phenylephrine tannate *see* phenylephrine and pyrilamine *on page* 753

pyrilamine tannate, guaifenesin, and phenylephrine tannate *see* phenylephrine, pyrilamine, and guaifenesin *on page* 756

pyrimethamine (peer i METH a meen)

Sound-Alike/Look-Alike Issues
Daraprim® may be confused with Dantrium®, Daranide®

U.S./Canadian Brand Names Daraprim® [US/Can]

Therapeutic Category Folic Acid Antagonist (Antimalarial)

Use Prophylaxis of malaria due to susceptible strains of plasmodia; used in conjunction with quinine and sulfadiazine for the treatment of uncomplicated attacks of chloroquine-resistant *P. falciparum* malaria; used in conjunction with fast-acting schizonticide to initiate transmission control and suppression cure; synergistic combination with sulfonamide in treatment of toxoplasmosis

Dosage Summary

Oral:

Infants: 1 mg/kg once daily for 6 months with sulfadiazine then every other month with sulfa, alternating with spiramycin

Children:

Malaria prophylaxis:

<4 years: 6.25mg or 0.5 mg/kg once weekly (maximum: 25 mg/dose)

4-10 years: 12.5 mg or 0.5 mg/kg once weekly (maximum: 25 mg/dose)

>10 years: 25 mg once weekly

Malaria treatment:

<10 kg: 6.25 mg once daily

10-20 kg: 12.5 mg once daily

20-40 kg: 25 mg once daily

Prophylaxis for first episode of *Toxoplasma gondii*:

Children <1 month: Dosage not established

Children ≥1 month of age: 1 mg/kg/day once daily with dapsone, plus oral leucovorin calcium 5 mg every 3 days

Prophylaxis to prevent recurrence of *Toxoplasma gondii*:

Children <1 month: Dosage not established

Children ≥1 month of age: 1 mg/kg/day once daily given with sulfadiazine or clindamycin, plus oral leucovorin calcium 5 mg every 3 days

Toxoplasmosis: Loading dose: 2 mg/kg/day divided into 2 equal doses for 1-3 days (maximum: 100 mg/day); Maintenance: 1 mg/kg/day divided into 2 doses (maximum: 25 mg/day)

Adults: 25-75 mg/day in 1-2 divided doses **or** 25 mg or 50 mg once weekly

Dosage Forms

Tablet, oral:

Daraprim®: 25 mg

pyrimethamine and sulfadoxine *see* sulfadoxine and pyrimethamine *on page 901*

pyrithione zinc (peer i THYE one zingk)

Sound-Alike/Look-Alike Issues

pyrithione may be confused with Pyridium®

U.S./Canadian Brand Names BetaMed™ [US-OTC]; DermaZinc™ [US-OTC]; DHS™ Zinc [US-OTC]; Head & Shoulders® Citrus Breeze 2-in-1 [US-OTC]; Head & Shoulders® Citrus Breeze [US-OTC]; Head & Shoulders® Classic Clean 2-In-1 [US-OTC]; Head & Shoulders® Classic Clean [US-OTC]; Head & Shoulders® Dry Scalp 2-in-1 [US-OTC]; Head & Shoulders® Dry Scalp Care 2-in-1 [US-OTC]; Head & Shoulders® Dry Scalp Care [US-OTC]; Head & Shoulders® Dry Scalp [US-OTC]; Head & Shoulders® Extra Volume [US-OTC]; Head & Shoulders® intensive solutions 2-in-1 [US-OTC]; Head & Shoulders® intensive solutions for dry/damaged hair [US-OTC]; Head & Shoulders® intensive solutions for fine/oily hair [US-OTC]; Head & Shoulders® intensive solutions for normal hair [US-OTC]; Head & Shoulders® Ocean Lift 2-in-1 [US-OTC]; Head & Shoulders® Ocean Lift [US-OTC]; Head & Shoulders® Refresh 2-in-1 [US-OTC]; Head & Shoulders® Refresh [US-OTC]; Head & Shoulders® Restoring Shine 2-in-1 [US-OTC]; Head & Shoulders® Restoring Shine [US-OTC]; Head & Shoulders® Sensitive Care 2-in-1 [US-OTC]; Head & Shoulders® Sensitive Care [US-OTC]; Head & Shoulders® Smooth & Silky 2-In-1 [US-OTC]; Head & Shoulders® Smooth & Silky [US-OTC]; Selsun® Salon™ Classic [US-OTC]; Selsun® Salon™ Dandruff 2-in-1 [US-OTC]; Selsun® Salon™ Dandruff Moisturizing [US-OTC]; Selsun® Salon™ Dandruff Volumizing [US-OTC]; Skin Care™ [US-OTC]; T/Gel® Daily Control 2 in 1 Dandruff Shampoo Plus Conditioner [US-OTC]; T/Gel® Daily Control Dandruff Shampoo [US-OTC]; Zincon® [US-OTC]; ZNP® [US-OTC]

Therapeutic Category Antiseborrheic Agent, Topical

Use Relieves the itching, irritation, and scalp flaking associated with dandruff and/or seborrheal dermatitis

Dosage Summary

Topical:

Children: Dosage not established

Adults: Apply to wet area or hair, massage in, and rinse at least twice weekly

Dosage Forms

Bar, topical:
DermaZinc™ [OTC]: 2% (112.5 g)
ZNP® [OTC]: 2% (119 g)

Conditioner, topical:
Head & Shoulders® Classic Clean [OTC]: 0.5% (400 mL)
Head & Shoulders® Dry Scalp Care [OTC]: 0.5% (400 mL)

Cream, topical:
DermaZinc™ [OTC]: 0.25% (120 g)

Lotion, topical:
Skin Care™ [OTC]: 0.25% (120 mL)

Shampoo, topical:
BetaMed™ [OTC]: 2% (480 mL)
DermaZinc™ [OTC]: 2% (240 mL)
DHS™ Zinc [OTC]: 2% (240 mL, 360 mL)
Head & Shoulders® Citrus Breeze [OTC]: 1% (420 mL, 700 mL)
Head & Shoulders® Citrus Breeze 2-in-1 [OTC]: 1% (420 mL)
Head & Shoulders® Classic Clean [OTC]: 1% (50 mL, 420 mL, 700 mL, 1000 mL, 1200 mL)
Head & Shoulders® Classic Clean 2-in-1 [OTC]: 1% (420 mL, 700 mL)
Head & Shoulders® Dry Scalp [OTC]: 1% (420 mL)
Head & Shoulders® Dry Scalp 2-in-1 [OTC]: 1% (420 mL)
Head & Shoulders® Dry Scalp Care [OTC]: 1% (340 mL, 700 mL, 1200 mL)
Head & Shoulders® Dry Scalp Care 2-in-1 [OTC]: 1% (700 mL)
Head & Shoulders® Extra Volume [OTC]: 1% (420 mL, 700 mL)
Head & Shoulders® intensive solutions 2 in 1 [OTC]: 2% (241 mL)
Head & Shoulders® intensive solutions for dry/damaged hair [OTC]: 2% (251 mL)
Head & Shoulders® intensive solutions for fine/oily hair [OTC]: 2% (251 mL)
Head & Shoulders® intensive solutions for normal hair [OTC]: 2% (251 mL)
Head & Shoulders® Ocean Lift [OTC]: 1% (420 mL, 700 mL)
Head & Shoulders® Ocean Lift 2-in-1 [OTC]: 1% (420 mL, 700 mL)
Head & Shoulders® Refresh [OTC]: 1% (420 mL, 700 mL, 1000 mL, 1200 mL)
Head & Shoulders® Refresh 2-in-1 [OTC]: 1% (420 mL)
Head & Shoulders® Restoring Shine [OTC]: 1% (420 mL, 700 mL)
Head & Shoulders® Restoring Shine 2 in 1 [OTC]: 1% (420 mL)
Head & Shoulders® Sensitive Care [OTC]: 1% (420 mL, 700 mL)
Head & Shoulders® Sensitive Care 2 in 1 [OTC]: 1% (420 mL, 700 mL)
Head & Shoulders® Smooth & Silky [OTC]: 1% (420 mL, 700 mL)
Head & Shoulders® Smooth & Silky 2-in-1 [OTC]: 1% (420 mL)
Selsun® Salon™ Classic [OTC]: 1% (384 mL)
Selsun® Salon™ Dandruff 2-in-1 [OTC]: 1% (384 mL)
Selsun® Salon™ Dandruff Moisturizing [OTC]: 1% (384 mL)
Selsun® Salon™ Dandruff Volumizing [OTC]: 1% (384 mL)
T/Gel® Daily Control 2 in 1 Dandruff Shampoo Plus Conditioner [OTC]: 1% (250 mL)
T/Gel® Daily Control Dandruff Shampoo [OTC]: 1% (250 mL)
Zincon® [OTC]: 1% (120 mL, 240 mL)

Solution, topical:
DermaZinc™ [OTC]: 0.25% (120 mL)

QDALL® ***(Discontinued)*** *see* chlorpheniramine and pseudoephedrine *on page 209*

quadrivalent human papillomavirus vaccine *see* papillomavirus (types 6, 11, 16, 18) vaccine (human, recombinant) *on page 727*

Quad Tann® [US] *see* chlorpheniramine, ephedrine, phenylephrine, and carbetapentane *on page 210*

Qualaquin® [US] *see* quinine *on page 823*

Quartuss™ [US] *see* dextromethorphan, chlorpheniramine, phenylephrine, and guaifenesin *on page 290*

Quasense™ [US] *see* ethinyl estradiol and levonorgestrel *on page 376*

quaternium-18 bentonite *see* bentoquatam *on page 123*

quazepam (KWAZ e pam)

Sound-Alike/Look-Alike Issues

quazepam may be confused with oxazepam

U.S./Canadian Brand Names Doral® [US/Can]
Therapeutic Category Benzodiazepine
Controlled Substance C-IV
Use Treatment of insomnia
Dosage Summary
Oral:
Children: Dosage not established
Adults: 7.5-15 mg at bedtime
Elderly: Initial: 7.5 mg at bedtime; may increase to 15 mg at bedtime with caution
Dosage Forms
Tablet, oral:
Doral®: 15 mg

Quelicin® [US/Can] *see* succinylcholine *on page 897*
Queltuss® *(Discontinued)* *see* guaifenesin and dextromethorphan *on page 455*
Questran® [US/Can] *see* cholestyramine resin *on page 218*
Questran® Light [US] *see* cholestyramine resin *on page 218*
Questran® Light Sugar Free [Can] *see* cholestyramine resin *on page 218*

quetiapine (kwe TYE a peen)

Sound-Alike/Look-Alike Issues
QUEtiapine may be confused with OLANZapine
Seroquel® may be confused with Serentil®, Serzone®, Sinequan®
Synonyms quetiapine fumarate
Tall-Man QUEtiapine
U.S./Canadian Brand Names Apo-Quetiapine® [Can]; CO Quetiapine [Can]; Mylan-Quetiapine [Can]; Novo-Quetiapine [Can]; PMS-Quetiapine [Can]; PRO-Quetiapine [Can]; ratio-Quetiapine [Can]; Riva-Quetiapine [Can]; Sandoz-Quetiapine [Can]; Seroquel XR® [US/Can]; Seroquel® [US/Can]
Therapeutic Category Antipsychotic Agent
Use Treatment of schizophrenia; treatment of acute manic or mixed episodes associated with bipolar I disorder (as monotherapy or in combination with lithium or divalproex); maintenance treatment of bipolar I disorder (in combination with lithium or divalproex); treatment of acute depressive episodes associated with bipolar disorder; adjunctive treatment of major depressive disorder
Dosage Summary
Oral:
Children <10 years: Dosage not established
Children ≥10 years:
Immediate release tablet: Initial: 25 mg twice daily; Maintenance: 50-800 mg/day; **Note:** Titration is recommended
Extended release tablet: Dosage not established
Adults:
Immediate release tablet: Initial: 25-50 mg twice daily; Maintenance: 150-800 mg/day in 2-3 divided doses; **Note:** Titration is recommended
Extended-release tablets: Initial 50-300 mg once daily; Maintenance: 150-800 mg/day; **Note:** Titration is recommended
Elderly: Immediate release: Initial: 25 mg/day; Extended release: Initial: 50 mg/day; **Note**: Slow titration is recommended
Dosage Forms
Tablet, oral:
Seroquel®: 25 mg, 50 mg, 100 mg, 200 mg, 300 mg, 400 mg
Tablet, extended release, oral:
Seroquel XR®: 50 mg, 150 mg, 200 mg, 300 mg, 400 mg

quetiapine fumarate *see* quetiapine *on page 821*
Quibron® *(Discontinued)*
Quibron®-T *(Discontinued)* *see* theophylline *on page 925*
Quibron®-T/SR *(Discontinued)* *see* theophylline *on page 925*
Quiess® Injection *(Discontinued)* *see* hydroxyzine *on page 490*
Quinaglute® Dura-Tabs® *(Discontinued)* *see* quinidine *on page 822*

quinagolide *(Discontinued)*

Quinalan® *(Discontinued)* *see* quinidine *on page 822*

quinalbarbitone sodium *see* secobarbital *on page 868*

quinapril (KWIN a pril)

Sound-Alike/Look-Alike Issues

Accupril® may be confused with Accolate®, Accutane®, AcipHex®, Monopril®

Synonyms quinapril hydrochloride

U.S./Canadian Brand Names Accupril® [US/Can]; GD-Quinapril [Can]

Therapeutic Category Angiotensin-Converting Enzyme (ACE) Inhibitor

Use Treatment of hypertension; treatment of heart failure

Dosage Summary

Oral:

Adults: Initial: 5-20 mg/day in 1-2 divided doses; Maintenance: 10-40 mg/day in 1-2 divided doses

Elderly: Initial: 2.5-5 mg/day; Maintenance: 10-40 mg/day

Dosage Forms

Tablet, oral: 5 mg, 10 mg, 20 mg, 40 mg

Accupril®: 5 mg, 10 mg, 20 mg, 40 mg

quinapril and hydrochlorothiazide (KWIN a pril & hye droe klor oh THYE a zide)

Synonyms hydrochlorothiazide and quinapril

U.S./Canadian Brand Names Accuretic® [US/Can]; Quinaretic [US]

Therapeutic Category Antihypertensive Agent, Combination

Use Treatment of hypertension (not for initial therapy)

Dosage Summary

Oral:

Children: Dosage not established

Adults: Initial: 10-20 mg quinapril and 12.5 mg hydrochlorothiazide once daily; Maintenance: 5-40 mg quinapril and 6.25-25 mg hydrochlorothiazide once daily

Dosage Forms

Tablet: 10/12.5: Quinapril 10 mg and hydrochlorothiazide 12.5 mg; 20/12.5: Quinapril 20 mg and hydrochlorothiazide 12.5 mg; 20/25: Quinapril 20 mg and hydrochlorothiazide 25 mg

Accuretic®, Quinaretic: 10/12.5: Quinapril 10 mg and hydrochlorothiazide 12.5 mg; 20/12.5: Quinapril 20 mg and hydrochlorothiazide 12.5 mg; 20/25: Quinapril 20 mg and hydrochlorothiazide 25 mg

quinapril hydrochloride *see* quinapril *on page 822*

Quinaretic [US] *see* quinapril and hydrochlorothiazide *on page 822*

Quinate® [Can] *see* quinidine *on page 822*

quinidine (KWIN i deen)

Sound-Alike/Look-Alike Issues

quiNIDine may be confused with cloNIDine, quiNINE, Quinora®

Synonyms quinidine gluconate; quinidine polygalacturonate; quinidine sulfate

Tall-Man qui**NID**ine

U.S./Canadian Brand Names Apo-Quinidine® [Can]; BioQuin® Durules™ [Can]; Novo-Quinidin [Can]; Quinate® [Can]

Therapeutic Category Antiarrhythmic Agent, Class I-A

Use

Quinidine gluconate and sulfate salts: Conversion and prevention of relapse into atrial fibrillation and/or flutter; suppression of ventricular arrhythmias. **Note:** Due to proarrhythmic effects, use should be reserved for life-threatening arrhythmias. Moreover, the use of quinidine has largely been replaced by more effective/safer antiarrhythmic agents and/or nonpharmacologic therapies (eg, radiofrequency ablation).

Quinidine gluconate (I.V. formulation): Conversion of atrial fibrillation/flutter and ventricular tachycardia. **Note:** The use of I.V. quinidine gluconate for these indications has been replaced by more effective/ safer antiarrhythmic agents (eg, amiodarone and procainamide).

Quinidine gluconate (I.V. formulation) and quinidine sulfate: Treatment of malaria (*Plasmodium falciparum*)

Dosage Summary Note: Dosage expressed in terms of the salt: 267 mg of quinidine gluconate = 200 mg of quinidine sulfate.

I.M.:

Children: Test dose: 2 mg/kg **or** 60 mg/m^2

Adults: Test dose: 200 mg, then 400 mg every 4-6 hours

I.V.:

Children: 2-10 mg/kg/dose every 3-6 hours as needed; **Note:** This route not recommended

Adults: 200-400 mg/dose

Oral:

Gluconate:

Children: Dosage not established

Adults: 324-972 mg every 8-12 hours

Sulfate:

Children: Initial: 6 mg/kg every 4-6 hours **or** 15-60 mg/kg/day in 4-5 divided doses; Usual: 30 mg/kg/day in 5 divided doses **or** 900 mg/m^2/day in 5 divided doses

Adults: 100-600 mg/dose every 4-6 hours (maximum: 4 g/day)

Dosage Forms

Injection, solution: 80 mg/mL (10 mL)

Tablet, oral: 200 mg, 300 mg

Tablet, extended release, oral: 300 mg, 324 mg

quinidine gluconate *see* quinidine *on page 822*

quinidine polygalacturonate *see* quinidine *on page 822*

quinidine sulfate *see* quinidine *on page 822*

quinine (KWYE nine)

Sound-Alike/Look-Alike Issues

quiNINE may be confused with quiNIDine

Synonyms quinine sulfate

Tall-Man qui**NINE**

U.S./Canadian Brand Names Apo-Quinine® [Can]; Novo-Quinine [Can]; Qualaquin® [US]; Quinine-Odan [Can]

Therapeutic Category Antimalarial Agent

Use In conjunction with other antimalarial agents, treatment of uncomplicated chloroquine-resistant *P. falciparum* malaria

Dosage Summary

Oral:

Children: 30 mg/kg/day divided every 8 hours

Adults: 648 mg every 8 hours

Dosage Forms

Capsule, oral:

Qualaquin®: 324 mg

Quinine-Odan [Can] *see* quinine *on page 823*

quinine sulfate *see* quinine *on page 823*

quinol *see* hydroquinone *on page 487*

Quinora® ***(Discontinued)*** *see* quinidine *on page 822*

Quintabs [US-OTC] *see* vitamins (multiple/oral) *on page 990*

Quintabs-M [US-OTC] *see* vitamins (multiple/oral) *on page 990*

Quintabs-M Iron-Free [US-OTC] *see* vitamins (multiple/oral) *on page 990*

quinupristin and dalfopristin (kwi NYOO pris tin & dal FOE pris tin)

Synonyms dalfopristin and quinupristin; pristinamycin; RP-59500

U.S./Canadian Brand Names Synercid® [US/Can]

Therapeutic Category Antibiotic, Streptogramin

Use Treatment of serious or life-threatening infections associated with vancomycin-resistant *Enterococcus faecium* bacteremia; treatment of complicated skin and skin structure infections caused by methcillin-susceptible *Staphylococcus aureus* or *Streptococcus pyogenes*

Has been studied in the treatment of a variety of infections caused by *Enterococcus faecium* (not *E. fecalis*) including vancomycin-resistant strains. May also be effective in the treatment of serious infections caused by *Staphylococcus* species including those resistant to methicillin.

Dosage Summary

I.V.:

Children (limited information): 7.5 mg/kg/dose every 8 hours

Adults: 7.5 mg/kg every 8-12 hours

Dosage Forms

Injection, powder for reconstitution:

Synercid®: 500 mg: Quinupristin 150 mg and dalfopristin 350 mg

Quixin® [US] *see* levofloxacin (ophthalmic) *on page 558*

Qutenza™ [US] *see* capsaicin *on page 175*

QVAR® [US/Can] *see* beclomethasone (oral inhalation) *on page 120*

R & C™ II [Can] *see* pyrethrins and piperonyl butoxide *on page 816*

R & C® Lice *(Discontinued)* *see* permethrin *on page 744*

R & C™ Shampoo/Conditioner [Can] *see* pyrethrins and piperonyl butoxide *on page 816*

R-1569 *see* tocilizumab *on page 939*

RabAvert® [US/Can] *see* rabies vaccine *on page 825*

rabeprazole (ra BEP ra zole)

Sound-Alike/Look-Alike Issues

rabeprazole may be confused with aripiprazole,donepezil, lansoprazole, omeprazole, raloxifene

Aciphex® may be confused with Acephen®, Accupril®, Aricept®, pHisoHex®

Synonyms pariprazole

U.S./Canadian Brand Names AcipHex® [US]; Novo-Rabeprazole EC [Can]; Pariet® [Can]; PMS-Rabeprazole EC [Can]; PRO-Rabeprazole [Can]; Rabeprazole EC [Can]; RAN™-Rabeprazole [Can]; Riva-Rabeprazole EC [Can]; Sandoz-Rabeprazole [Can]

Therapeutic Category Gastric Acid Secretion Inhibitor

Use Short-term (4-8 weeks) treatment and maintenance of erosive or ulcerative gastroesophageal reflux disease (GERD); symptomatic GERD; short-term (up to 4 weeks) treatment of duodenal ulcers; long-term treatment of pathological hypersecretory conditions, including Zollinger-Ellison syndrome; *H. pylori* eradication (in combination therapy)

Canadian labeling: Additional uses (not in U.S. labeling): Treatment of nonerosive reflux disease (NERD); treatment of gastric ulcers

Dosage Summary

Oral:

Children <12 years: Dosage not established

Children ≥12 years: 20 mg/day

Adults: 10-20 mg once to twice daily **or** 60 mg once daily

Dosage Forms

Tablet, delayed release, enteric coated, oral:

AcipHex®: 20 mg

Dosage Forms - Canada

Tablet, delayed release, enteric coated:

Pariet®: 10 mg, 20 mg

Rabeprazole EC [Can] *see* rabeprazole *on page 824*

rabies immune globulin (human) (RAY beez i MYUN GLOB yoo lin, HYU man)

Synonyms HRIG; RIG

U.S./Canadian Brand Names HyperRAB™ S/D [US/Can]; Imogam® Rabies Pasteurized [Can]; Imogam® Rabies-HT [US]

Therapeutic Category Immune Globulin

Use Part of postexposure prophylaxis of persons with rabies exposure. Provides passive immunity until active immunity with rabies vaccine is established. Not for use in persons with a history of preexposure vaccination, history of postexposure prophylaxis, or previous vaccination with rabies vaccine and documentation of antibody response.

Dosage Summary

Local Wound Infiltration/I.M.:

Children: 20 units/kg in a single dose

Adults: 20 units/kg in a single dose

Dosage Forms

Injection, solution [preservative free]:

HyperRAB™ S/D: 150 int. units/mL (2 mL, 10 mL)

Imogam® Rabies-HT: 150 int. units/mL (2 mL, 10 mL)

rabies vaccine (RAY beez vak SEEN)

Synonyms HDCV; human diploid cell cultures rabies vaccine; PCEC; purified chick embryo cell

U.S./Canadian Brand Names Imovax® Rabies [US/Can]; RabAvert® [US/Can]

Therapeutic Category Vaccine, Inactivated Virus

Use Preexposure and postexposure vaccination against rabies

The Advisory Committee on Immunization Practices (ACIP) recommends a primary course of prophylactic immunization (preexposure vaccination) for the following:

- Persons with continuous risk of infection, including rabies research laboratory and biologics production workers
- Persons with frequent risk of infection in areas where rabies is enzootic, including rabies diagnostic laboratory workers, cavers, veterinarians and their staff, and animal control and wildlife workers; persons who frequently handle bats
- Persons with infrequent risk of infection, including veterinarians and animal control staff with terrestrial animals in areas where rabies infection is rare, veterinary students, and travelers visiting areas where rabies is enzootic and immediate access to medical care and biologicals is limited

The ACIP recommends the use of postexposure vaccination for a particular person be assessed by the severity and likelihood versus the actual risk of acquiring rabies. Consideration should include the type of exposure, epidemiology of rabies in the area, species of the animal, circumstances of the incident, and the availability of the exposing animal for observation or rabies testing. Postexposure vaccination is used in both previously vaccinated and previously unvaccinated individuals.

Dosage Summary

I.M.:

Children: Preexposure: 1 mL on days 0, 7, and 21-28; Postexposure: 1 mL on days 0, 3, 7, 14, 28; Previous rabies vaccination: Booster: 1 mL based on antibody titers

Adults: Preexposure: 1 mL on days 0, 7, and 21-28; Postexposure: 1 mL on days 0, 3, 7, 14, 28; Previous rabies vaccination: 1 mL on days 0 and 3; Booster: 1 mL based on antibody titers

Dosage Forms

Injection, powder for reconstitution [preservative free]:

Imovax® Rabies: ≥ 2.5 int. units

RabAvert®: ≥ 2.5 int. units

racemic epinephrine *see* epinephrine (systemic, oral inhalation) *on page* 352

racepinephrine *see* epinephrine (systemic, oral inhalation) *on page* 352

RAD001 *see* everolimus *on page* 385

Radiogardase® [US] *see* ferric hexacyanoferrate *on page* 397

rAHF *see* antihemophilic factor (recombinant) *on page* 81

R-albuterol *see* levalbuterol *on page* 554

Ralivia™ ER [Can] *see* tramadol *on page* 946

Ralix *(Discontinued)* *see* chlorpheniramine, phenylephrine, and methscopolamine *on page* 212

raloxifene (ral OKS i feen)

Sound-Alike/Look-Alike Issues

Evista® may be confused with Avinza™, Eovist®

Synonyms keoxifene hydrochloride; raloxifene hydrochloride

U.S./Canadian Brand Names Apo-Raloxifene® [Can]; Evista® [US/Can]; Novo-Raloxifene [Can]

Therapeutic Category Selective Estrogen Receptor Modulator (SERM)

Use Prevention and treatment of osteoporosis in postmenopausal women; risk reduction for invasive breast cancer in postmenopausal women with osteoporosis and in postmenopausal women with high risk for invasive breast cancer

Dosage Summary

Oral:

Children: Dosage not established
Adults (females): 60 mg/day

Dosage Forms

Tablet, oral:

Evista®: 60 mg

raloxifene hydrochloride *see* raloxifene *on page 825*

raltegravir (ral TEG ra vir)

Synonyms MK-0518

U.S./Canadian Brand Names Isentress® [US/Can]

Therapeutic Category Antiretroviral Agent, Integrase Inhibitor

Use Treatment of HIV-1 infection in combination with other antiretroviral agents

Dosage Summary

Oral:

Children <16 years: Dosage not established
Adolescents ≥16 years: 400 mg twice daily; rifampin coadministration: 800 mg twice daily
Adults: 400 mg twice daily; rifampin coadministration: 800 mg twice daily

Dosage Forms

Tablet, oral:

Isentress®: 400 mg

raltitrexed *(Canada only)* (ral ti TREX ed)

Synonyms ICI-D1694; raltitrexed disodium; ZD1694

U.S./Canadian Brand Names Tomudex® [Can]

Therapeutic Category Antineoplastic Agent

Use Treatment of advanced colorectal neoplasms

Dosage Summary

I.V.:

Children: Dosage not established
Adults: 3 mg/m^2 every 3 weeks

Dosage Forms

Injection, powder for reconstitution:

2 mg [not available in the U.S.; investigational]

raltitrexed disodium *see* raltitrexed *(Canada only) on page 826*

ramelteon (ra MEL tee on)

Sound-Alike/Look-Alike Issues

ramelteon may be confused with Remeron®
Rozerem™ may be confused with Razadyne®, Remeron®

Synonyms TAK-375

U.S./Canadian Brand Names Rozerem™ [US]

Therapeutic Category Hypnotic, Nonbenzodiazepine

Use Treatment of insomnia characterized by difficulty with sleep onset

Dosage Summary

Oral:

Children: Dosage not established
Adults: 8 mg within 30 minutes of bedtime

Dosage Forms

Tablet, oral:

Rozerem™: 8 mg

ramipril (RA mi pril)

Sound-Alike/Look-Alike Issues

ramipril may be confused with enalapril, Monopril®
Altace® may be confused with alteplase, Amaryl®, Amerge®, Artane®

U.S./Canadian Brand Names Altace® [US/Can]; Apo-Ramipril® [Can]; CO Ramipril [Can]; JAMP-Ramipril [Can]; Mylan-Ramipril [Can]; PHL-Ramipril [Can]; PMS-Ramipril [Can]; RAN™-Ramipril [Can]; ratio-Ramipril [Can]; Sandoz-Ramipril [Can]; Teva-Ramipril [Can]

Therapeutic Category Angiotensin-Converting Enzyme (ACE) Inhibitor

Use Treatment of hypertension, alone or in combination with thiazide diuretics; treatment of left ventricular dysfunction after MI; to reduce risk of MI, stroke, and death in patients at increased risk for these events

Dosage Summary

Oral:

Children: Dosage not established

Adults: 2.5-20 mg/day (maximum: 20 mg/day)

Dosage Forms

Capsule, oral: 1.25 mg, 2.5 mg, 5 mg, 10 mg

Altace®: 1.25 mg, 2.5 mg, 5 mg, 10 mg

ramipril and felodipine *(Canada only)* (RA mi pril & fe LOE di peen)

Synonyms felodipine and ramipril; ramipril and felodipine ER

U.S./Canadian Brand Names Altace® Plus Felodipine [Can]

Therapeutic Category Antihypertensive Agent, Combination

Use Treatment of hypertension when combination therapy is appropriate (not for initial therapy)

Dosage Summary

Oral: Note: Not for initial therapy; titration of individual agents to an appropriate clinical response is required before patient is converted over to an equivalent dose of the combination product.

Children: Dosage not established

Adults (dose is individualized): Ramipril 2.5-10 mg and felodipine ER 2.5-10 mg once daily

Elderly: Initial: 2.5 mg daily based on felodipine ER component.

Dosage Forms - Canada

Tablet, variable release:

Altace® Plus Felodipine 2.5/2.5: Ramipril 2.5 mg [immediate release] and felodipine 2.5 mg [extended release]

Altace® Plus Felodipine 5/5: Ramipril 5 mg [immediate release] and felodipine 5 mg [extended release]

ramipril and felodipine ER *see* ramipril and felodipine *(Canada only) on page* 827

ramipril and hydrochlorothiazide *(Canada only)*

(RA mi pril & hye droe klor oh THYE a zide)

Sound-Alike/Look-Alike Issues

Altace® HCT may be confused with alteplase, Artane®, Altace®

Synonyms hydrochlorothiazide and ramipril

U.S./Canadian Brand Names Altace® HCT [Can]; PMS-Ramipril HCTZ [Can]

Therapeutic Category Angiotensin-Converting Enzyme (ACE) Inhibitor; Antihypertensive Agent, Combination; Diuretic, Thiazide

Use Treatment of essential hypertension (not for initial therapy)

Dosage Summary

Oral:

Children: Dosage not established

Adults: Ramipril 2.5 mg/hydrochlorothiazide 12.5 mg once daily (maximum: ramipril 10 mg/hydrochlorothiazide 50 mg once daily)

Dosage Forms - Canada

Tablet:

Altace® HCT: 2.5/12.5: Ramipril 2.5 mg and hydrochlorothiazide 12.5 mg; 5/12.5: Ramipril 5 mg and hydrochlorothiazide 12.5 mg; 5/25: Ramipril 5 mg and hydrochlorothiazide 25 mg; 10/12.5: Ramipril 10 mg and hydrochlorothiazide 12.5 mg; 10/25: Ramipril 10 mg and hydrochlorothiazide 25 mg

RAN™-Amlodipine [Can] *see* amlodipine *on page* 68

RAN™-Atenolol [Can] *see* atenolol *on page* 102

RAN™-Atorvastatin [Can] *see* atorvastatin *on page* 104

RAN™-Carvedilol [Can] *see* carvedilol *on page* 186

RAN™-Cefprozil [Can] *see* cefprozil *on page* 192

RAN™-Ciprofloxacin [Can] *see* ciprofloxacin (systemic) *on page* 224

RAN™-Citalopram [Can] *see* citalopram *on page 227*
RAN™-Domperidone [Can] *see* domperidone *(Canada only) on page 325*
RAN™-Enalapril [Can] *see* enalapril *on page 348*
Ranexa® [US] *see* ranolazine *on page 829*
RAN™-Fentanyl Matrix Patch [Can] *see* fentanyl *on page 395*
RAN™-Fentanyl Transdermal System [Can] *see* fentanyl *on page 395*
RAN™-Fosinopril [Can] *see* fosinopril *on page 428*
RAN™-Gabapentin [Can] *see* gabapentin *on page 433*

ranibizumab (ra ni BIZ oo mab)

Synonyms rhuFabV2

U.S./Canadian Brand Names Lucentis® [US/Can]

Therapeutic Category Monoclonal Antibody; Ophthalmic Agent; Vascular Endothelial Growth Factor (VEGF) Inhibitor

Use Treatment of neovascular (wet) age-related macular degeneration (AMD); treatment of macular edema following retinal vein occlusion (RVO)

Dosage Summary

Intravitreal:

Children: Dosage not established

Adults: 0.5 mg once a month; may reduce to once every 3 months after first 3-4 injections, although not as effective

Dosage Forms

Injection, solution [preservative free]:

Lucentis®: 10 mg/mL (0.2 mL)

Dosage Forms - Canada

Injection, solution [preservative free]:

Lucentis®: 10 mg/mL (0.3 mL)

Raniclor™ [US] *see* cefaclor *on page 188*

ranitidine (ra NI ti deen)

Sound-Alike/Look-Alike Issues

ranitidine may be confused with amantadine, rimantadine

Zantac® may be confused with Xanax®, Zarontin®, Zofran®, Zyrtec®

Synonyms ranitidine hydrochloride

U.S./Canadian Brand Names Acid Reducer Maximum Strength Non Prescription [Can]; Acid Reducer [Can]; Apo-Ranitidine® [Can]; CO Ranitidine [Can]; Dom-Ranitidine [Can]; Med-Ranitidine [Can]; Mylan-Ranitidine [Can]; Novo-Ranidine [Can]; Nu-Ranit [Can]; PHL-Ranitidine [Can]; PMS-Ranitidine [Can]; Ranitidine Injection, USP [Can]; ratio-Ranitidine [Can]; Riva-Ranitidine [Can]; Sandoz-Ranitidine [Can]; ScheinPharm Ranitidine [Can]; Zantac 150® [US-OTC]; Zantac 75® [US-OTC/Can]; Zantac Maximum Strength Non-Prescription [Can]; Zantac® EFFERdose® [US]; Zantac® [US/Can]; ZYM-Ranitidine [Can]

Therapeutic Category Histamine H_2 Antagonist

Use

Zantac®: Short-term and maintenance therapy of duodenal ulcer, gastric ulcer, gastroesophageal reflux disease (GERD), active benign ulcer, erosive esophagitis, and pathological hypersecretory conditions; as part of a multidrug regimen for *H. pylori* eradication to reduce the risk of duodenal ulcer recurrence

Zantac 75® [OTC]: Relief of heartburn, acid indigestion, and sour stomach

Dosage Summary

I.M.:

Children ≤16 years: Dosage not established

Children >16 years: 50 mg every 6-8 hours

Adults: 50 mg every 6-8 hours

I.V.:

Infants <1 month: Dosage not established

Children 1 month to 16 years: 2-4 mg/kg/day divided every 6-8 hours (maximum: 200 mg/day) **or** 1 mg/kg/dose for one dose followed by infusion of 0.08-0.17 mg/kg/hour

Children >16 years: 50 mg every 6-8 hours **or** Infusion: 6.25 mg/hour **or** 1-2.5 mg/kg/hour

Adults: 50 mg every 6-8 hours **or** Infusion: 6.25 mg/hour **or** 1-2.5 mg/kg/hour

Oral:

Infants <1 month: Dosage not established

Children 1 month to 11 years: 2-4 mg/kg/dose once or twice daily **or** 5-10 mg/kg/day in 2 divided doses (maximum: 300 mg/day; exceptions occur [indication specific])

Children ≥12 to 16 years: 2-4 mg/kg once or twice daily **or** 5-10 mg/kg/day in 2 divided doses (maximum: 300 mg/day; exceptions occur [indication specific])

OTC dosing: 75 mg 30-60 minutes before eating food or drinking beverages which cause heartburn (maximum: 150 mg/day)

Children >16 years: 150 mg 1-4 times/day **or** 300 mg once daily **or** 75 mg 30-60 minutes before eating food or drinking beverages which cause heartburn (maximum: 150 mg/day)

Adults: 150 mg 1-4 times/day **or** 300 mg once daily

OTC dosing: 75 mg 30-60 minutes before eating food or drinking beverages which cause heartburn (maximum: 150 mg/day)

Dosage Forms

Capsule, oral: 150 mg, 300 mg

Infusion, premixed in 1/2 NS [preservative free]:

Zantac®: 50 mg (50 mL)

Injection, solution: 25 mg/mL (2 mL, 6 mL, 40 mL)

Zantac®: 25 mg/mL (2 mL, 6 mL, 40 mL)

Syrup, oral: 15 mg/mL (5 mL, 10 mL, 473 mL, 480 mL)

Zantac®: 15 mg/mL (480 mL)

Tablet, oral: 75 mg, 150 mg, 300 mg

Zantac 150® [OTC]: 150 mg

Zantac 75® [OTC]: 75 mg

Zantac®: 150 mg, 300 mg

Tablet for solution, oral:

Zantac® EFFERdose®: 25 mg

ranitidine hydrochloride *see* ranitidine *on page* 828

Ranitidine Injection, USP [Can] *see* ranitidine *on page* 828

RAN™-Lisinopril [Can] *see* lisinopril *on page* 570

RAN™-Lovastatin [Can] *see* lovastatin *on page* 579

RAN™-Metformin [Can] *see* metformin *on page* 609

ranolazine (ra NOE la zeen)

Sound-Alike/Look-Alike Issues

Ranexa® may be confused with Celexa®

U.S./Canadian Brand Names Ranexa® [US]

Therapeutic Category Cardiovascular Agent, Miscellaneous

Use Treatment of chronic angina

Dosage Summary

Oral:

Children: Dosage not established

Adults: Initial: 500 mg twice daily; Maintenance: 500-1000 mg twice daily (maximum: 2000 mg/day)

Dosage Forms

Tablet, extended release, oral:

Ranexa®: 500 mg, 1000 mg

RAN™-Ondansetron [Can] *see* ondansetron *on page* 704

RAN™-Pantoprazole [Can] *see* pantoprazole *on page* 725

RAN™-Pravastatin [Can] *see* pravastatin *on page* 789

RAN™-Rabeprazole [Can] *see* rabeprazole *on page* 824

RAN™-Ramipril [Can] *see* ramipril *on page* 826

RAN™-Risperidone [Can] *see* risperidone *on page* 845

RAN™-Ropinirole [Can] *see* ropinirole *on page* 851

RAN™-Simvastatin [Can] *see* simvastatin *on page* 877

RAN™-Tamsulosin [Can] *see* tamsulosin *on page* 909

RAN™-Zopiclone [Can] *see* zopiclone *(Canada only) on page* 1005

Rapaflo™ [US] *see* silodosin *on page* 874

Rapamune® [US/Can] *see* sirolimus *on page* 878

rapamycin *see* sirolimus *on page 878*
Raphon ***(Discontinued)*** *see* epinephrine (systemic, oral inhalation) *on page 352*
Raplon® ***(Discontinued)***
Raptiva® ***(Discontinued)***

rasagiline (ra SA ji leen)

Sound-Alike/Look-Alike Issues
Azilect® may be confused with Aricept®

Synonyms AGN 1135; rasagiline mesylate; TVP-1012

U.S./Canadian Brand Names Azilect® [US]

Therapeutic Category Anti-Parkinson Agent, MAO Type B Inhibitor

Use Treatment of idiopathic Parkinson disease (initial monotherapy or as adjunct to levodopa)

Dosage Summary

Oral:
Children: Dosage not established
Adults: 0.5-1 mg once daily

Dosage Forms

Tablet, oral:
Azilect®: 0.5 mg, 1 mg

rasagiline mesylate *see* rasagiline *on page 830*

rasburicase (ras BYOOR i kayse)

Synonyms recombinant urate oxidase; urate oxidase

U.S./Canadian Brand Names Elitek™ [US]; Fasturtec® [Can]

Therapeutic Category Enzyme

Use Initial management of uric acid levels in patients with leukemia, lymphoma, and solid tumor malignancies receiving chemotherapy expected to result in tumor lysis and elevation of plasma uric acid

Dosage Summary

I.V.:
Children: 0.2 mg/kg once daily for up to 5 days
Adults: 0.2 mg/kg once daily for up to 5 days

Dosage Forms

Injection, powder for reconstitution:
Elitek™: 1.5 mg, 7.5 mg

Rasilez® [Can] *see* aliskiren *on page 50*
rATG *see* antithymocyte globulin (rabbit) *on page 84*
ratio-Aclavulanate [Can] *see* amoxicillin and clavulanate potassium *on page 73*
ratio-Acyclovir [Can] *see* acyclovir (systemic) *on page 36*
ratio-Alendronate [Can] *see* alendronate *on page 47*
ratio-Amcinonide [Can] *see* amcinonide *on page 62*
ratio-Amiodarone [Can] *see* amiodarone *on page 67*
ratio-Amiodarone I.V. [Can] *see* amiodarone *on page 67*
ratio-Amlodipine [Can] *see* amlodipine *on page 68*
ratio-Atenolol [Can] *see* atenolol *on page 102*
ratio-Azithromycin [Can] *see* azithromycin (systemic) *on page 111*
ratio-Baclofen [Can] *see* baclofen *on page 115*
ratio-Benzydamine [Can] *see* benzydamine *(Canada only) on page 130*
ratio-Bicalutamide [Can] *see* bicalutamide *on page 137*
ratio-Brimonidine [Can] *see* brimonidine *on page 144*
ratio-Bupropion SR [Can] *see* bupropion *on page 156*
ratio-Buspirone [Can] *see* buspirone *on page 157*
ratio-Carvedilol [Can] *see* carvedilol *on page 186*
ratio-Cefuroxime [Can] *see* cefuroxime *on page 194*
ratio-Ciprofloxacin [Can] *see* ciprofloxacin (systemic) *on page 224*
ratio-Citalopram [Can] *see* citalopram *on page 227*

ratio-Clarithromycin [Can] *see* clarithromycin *on page 229*
ratio-Clindamycin [Can] *see* clindamycin (systemic) *on page 232*
ratio-Clobazam [Can] *see* clobazam *(Canada only) on page 234*
ratio-Clobetasol [Can] *see* clobetasol *on page 235*
ratio-Cotridin [Can] *see* triprolidine, pseudoephedrine, and codeine *(Canada only) on page 961*
ratio-Cyclobenzaprine [Can] *see* cyclobenzaprine *on page 258*
ratio-Diltiazem CD [Can] *see* diltiazem *on page 306*
ratio-Domperidone [Can] *see* domperidone *(Canada only) on page 325*
ratio-Emtec [Can] *see* acetaminophen and codeine *on page 23*
ratio-Enalapril [Can] *see* enalapril *on page 348*
ratio-Fenofibrate MC [Can] *see* fenofibrate *on page 393*
ratio-Fentanyl [Can] *see* fentanyl *on page 395*
ratio-Finasteride [Can] *see* finasteride *on page 403*
ratio-Fluoxetine [Can] *see* fluoxetine *on page 415*
ratio-Fluticasone [Can] *see* fluticasone (nasal) *on page 419*
ratio-Gabapentin [Can] *see* gabapentin *on page 433*
ratio-Gentamicin [Can] *see* gentamicin (topical) *on page 444*
ratio-Glimepiride [Can] *see* glimepiride *on page 446*
ratio-Glyburide [Can] *see* glyburide *on page 448*
ratio-Indomethacin [Can] *see* indomethacin *on page 505*
ratio-Inspra-Sal [Can] *see* albuterol *on page 43*
ratio-Ipra Sal UDV [Can] *see* ipratropium and albuterol *on page 524*
ratio-Ketorolac [Can] *see* ketorolac (ophthalmic) *on page 538*
ratio-Lamotrigine [Can] *see* lamotrigine *on page 546*
ratio-Lenoltec [Can] *see* acetaminophen and codeine *on page 23*
ratio-Lisinopril [Can] *see* lisinopril *on page 570*
ratio-Lovastatin [Can] *see* lovastatin *on page 579*
ratio-Magnesium [Can] *see* magnesium glucoheptonate *on page 584*
ratio-Meloxicam [Can] *see* meloxicam *on page 598*
ratio-Memantine [Can] *see* memantine *on page 599*
ratio-Metformin [Can] *see* metformin *on page 609*
ratio-Methotrexate [Can] *see* methotrexate *on page 614*
ratio-Methylphenidate [Can] *see* methylphenidate *on page 621*
ratio-Minocycline [Can] *see* minocycline *on page 635*
ratio-Mirtazapine [Can] *see* mirtazapine *on page 637*
ratio-Mometasone [Can] *see* mometasone (topical) *on page 641*
ratio-Morphine [Can] *see* morphine (systemic) *on page 644*
ratio-Morphine SR [Can] *see* morphine (systemic) *on page 644*
ratio-Omeprazole [Can] *see* omeprazole *on page 701*
ratio-Ondansetron [Can] *see* ondansetron *on page 704*
ratio-Orciprenaline® [Can] *see* metaproterenol *on page 609*
ratio-Pantoprazole [Can] *see* pantoprazole *on page 725*
ratio-Paroxetine [Can] *see* paroxetine *on page 729*
ratio-Pentoxifylline [Can] *see* pentoxifylline *on page 742*
ratio-Pioglitazone [Can] *see* pioglitazone *on page 762*
ratio-Pravastatin [Can] *see* pravastatin *on page 789*
ratio-Quetiapine [Can] *see* quetiapine *on page 821*
ratio-Ramipril [Can] *see* ramipril *on page 826*
ratio-Ranitidine [Can] *see* ranitidine *on page 828*
ratio-Risperidone [Can] *see* risperidone *on page 845*
ratio-Rivastigmine [Can] *see* rivastigmine *on page 848*
ratio-Salbutamol [Can] *see* albuterol *on page 43*
ratio-Sertraline [Can] *see* sertraline *on page 872*

Redisol® *(Discontinued)* *see* cyanocobalamin *on page 257*
Reese's Pinworm Medicine [US-OTC] *see* pyrantel pamoate *on page 816*
ReFacto® [Can] *see* antihemophilic factor (recombinant) *on page 81*
ReFacto® *(Discontinued)* *see* antihemophilic factor (recombinant) *on page 81*
Refenesen™ [US-OTC] *see* guaifenesin *on page 454*
Refenesen™ 400 [US-OTC] *see* guaifenesin *on page 454*
Refenesen™ DM [US-OTC] *see* guaifenesin and dextromethorphan *on page 455*
Refenesen™ PE [US-OTC] *see* guaifenesin and phenylephrine *on page 456*
Refenesen Plus [US-OTC] *see* guaifenesin and pseudoephedrine *on page 457*
Refissa™ [US] *see* tretinoin (topical) *on page 951*
Refludan® [US/Can] *see* lepirudin *on page 552*
Refresh® [US-OTC] *see* artificial tears *on page 97*
Refresh Liquigel™ [US-OTC] *see* carboxymethylcellulose *on page 184*
Refresh Plus® [US-OTC] *see* artificial tears *on page 97*
Refresh Plus® [US-OTC/Can] *see* carboxymethylcellulose *on page 184*
Refresh Tears® [US-OTC] *see* artificial tears *on page 97*
Refresh Tears® [US-OTC/Can] *see* carboxymethylcellulose *on page 184*

regadenoson (re ga DEN of son)

Synonyms CVT-3146

U.S./Canadian Brand Names Lexiscan™ [US]

Therapeutic Category Diagnostic Agent

Use Radionuclide myocardial perfusion imaging (MPI) in patients unable to undergo adequate exercise stress testing

Dosage Summary

I.V.:
Children: Dosage not established
Adults: 0.4 mg (5 mL)

Dosage Forms

Injection, solution [preservative free]:
Lexiscan™: 0.08 mg/mL (5 mL)

Regenecare® [US] *see* lidocaine (topical) *on page 562*
Regenecare® HA [US-OTC] *see* lidocaine (topical) *on page 562*
Regitine® [Can] *see* phentolamine *on page 750*
Regitine *(Discontinued)* *see* phentolamine *on page 750*
Reglan® [US] *see* metoclopramide *on page 624*
Reglan® Syrup *(Discontinued)* *see* metoclopramide *on page 624*
Regonol® [US] *see* pyridostigmine *on page 817*
Regranex® [US/Can] *see* becaplermin *on page 119*
Regular Iletin® II *(Discontinued)*
regular insulin *see* insulin regular *on page 513*
Regulax SS® *(Discontinued)* *see* docusate *on page 321*
Regulex® [Can] *see* docusate *on page 321*
Reguloid [US-OTC] *see* psyllium *on page 814*
Rejuva-A® [Can] *see* tretinoin (topical) *on page 951*
Relacon-DM NR *(Discontinued)* *see* guaifenesin, pseudoephedrine, and dextromethorphan *on page 460*
Relafen® [Can] *see* nabumetone *on page 654*
Relafen® *(Discontinued)* *see* nabumetone *on page 654*
Relenza® [US/Can] *see* zanamivir *on page 997*
Reliable Gentle Laxative *(Discontinued)* *see* bisacodyl *on page 138*
Relief® *(Discontinued)* *see* phenylephrine (ophthalmic) *on page 752*
Relief® Ophthalmic Solution *(Discontinued)* *see* phenylephrine (ophthalmic) *on page 752*
Relief-SF® [US] *see* acetaminophen, chlorpheniramine, and pseudoephedrine *on page 28*

Relistor® [US/Can] *see* methylnaltrexone *on page* 620
Relpax® [US/Can] *see* eletriptan *on page* 345
Remeron® [US/Can] *see* mirtazapine *on page* 637
Remeron® RD [Can] *see* mirtazapine *on page* 637
Remeron SolTab® [US] *see* mirtazapine *on page* 637
Remicade® [US/Can] *see* infliximab *on page* 506

remifentanil (rem i FEN ta nil)

Sound-Alike/Look-Alike Issues
remifentanil may be confused with alfentanil

Synonyms GI87084B

U.S./Canadian Brand Names Ultiva® [US/Can]

Therapeutic Category Analgesic, Narcotic

Controlled Substance C-II

Use Analgesic for use during the induction and maintenance of general anesthesia; for continued analgesia into the immediate postoperative period; analgesic component of monitored anesthesia

Dosage Summary **Note:** Dose should be based on ideal body weight (IBW) in obese patients (>30% over IBW)

I.V.:

Infants Birth to 2 months: With nitrous oxide 70%: Infusion: 0.4-1 mcg/kg/minute; Supplemental bolus dose: ≤1 mcg/kg

Children 1-12 years: Anesthesia (with halothane, sevoflurane, or isoflurane): Infusion: 0.05-1.3 mcg/kg/minute; Bolus: 1 mcg/kg every 2-5 minutes; **Note:** Titration is recommended

Adults:

Induction of anesthesia: 0.5-1 mcg/kg/minute (1 mcg/kg/minute for coronary bypass)

Maintenance of anesthesia: **Note:** Supplemental boluses of 0.5-1 mcg/kg every 2-5 minutes may be given

Coronary bypass: 0.125-4 mcg/kg/minute
With isoflurane or propofol: 0.05-2 mcg/kg/minute
With nitrous oxide (66%): 0.1-2 mcg/kg/minute

Postoperative: 0.025-0.2 mcg/kg/minute; Coronary bypass or ICU: 0.05-1 mcg/kg/minute

Analgesic component of monitored anesthesia care: Alone: Bolus: 1 mcg/kg; Infusion: 0.025-0.2 mcg/kg/minute; With midazolam: Bolus: 0.5 mcg/kg; Infusion: 0.025-0.2 mcg/kg/minute; **Note:** Supplemental oxygen is recommended

Elderly: Doses should be decreased by 50% and titrated.

Dosage Forms

Injection, powder for reconstitution:
Ultiva®: 1 mg, 2 mg, 5 mg

Reminyl® [Can] *see* galantamine *on page* 436
Reminyl® *(Discontinued)* *see* galantamine *on page* 436
Reminyl® ER [Can] *see* galantamine *on page* 436
Remodulin® [US/Can] *see* treprostinil *on page* 951
Renacidin® [US] *see* citric acid, magnesium carbonate, and glucono-delta-lactone *on page* 228
Renagel® [US/Can] *see* sevelamer *on page* 872
renal replacement solution *see* electrolyte solution, renal replacement *on page* 345
RenAmin® [US] *see* amino acid injection *on page* 64
Renax® [US] *see* vitamins (multiple/oral) *on page* 990
Renax® 5.5 [US] *see* vitamins (multiple/oral) *on page* 990
Renedil® [Can] *see* felodipine *on page* 393
Reno-30® *(Discontinued)* *see* diatrizoate meglumine *on page* 292
Reno-60® *(Discontinued)* *see* diatrizoate meglumine *on page* 292
RenoCal-76® *(Discontinued)* *see* diatrizoate meglumine and diatrizoate sodium *on page* 292
Reno-Dip® *(Discontinued)* *see* diatrizoate meglumine *on page* 292
Renografin®-60 *(Discontinued)* *see* diatrizoate meglumine and diatrizoate sodium *on page* 292
Renoquid® *(Discontinued)*
Renova® [US/Can] *see* tretinoin (topical) *on page* 951
Renvela® [US] *see* sevelamer *on page* 872

Reopro® [US/Can] *see* abciximab *on page 19*

repaglinide (re PAG li nide)

Sound-Alike/Look-Alike Issues

Prandin® may be confused with Avandia®

U.S./Canadian Brand Names GlucoNorm® [Can]; Prandin® [US/Can]

Therapeutic Category Hypoglycemic Agent, Oral

Use Management of type 2 diabetes mellitus (noninsulin-dependent, NIDDM) as an adjunct to diet and exercise; may be used in combination with metformin or thiazolidinediones

Dosage Summary

Oral:

Children: Dosage not established

Adults: Initial: 0.5-2 mg before each meal; Maintenance: 0.5-4 mg before each meal (maximum: 16 mg/day)

Dosage Forms

Tablet, oral:

Prandin®: 0.5 mg, 1 mg, 2 mg

repaglinide and metformin (re PAG li nide & met FOR min)

Sound-Alike/Look-Alike Issues

PrandiMet® may be confused with Avandamet®, Prandin®

Synonyms metformin and repaglinide; repaglinide and metformin hydrochloride

U.S./Canadian Brand Names PrandiMet® [US]

Therapeutic Category Antidiabetic Agent, Biguanide; Antidiabetic Agent, Meglitinide Derivative; Hypoglycemic Agent, Oral

Use Management of type 2 diabetes mellitus (noninsulin-dependent, NIDDM), as an adjunct to diet and exercise, in patients currently receiving or not adequately controlled on metformin and/or a meglitinide

Dosage Summary

Oral:

Children: Dosage not established

Adults: Repaglinide 1-2 mg and metformin 500 mg 2-3 times daily with meals (maximum single dose: 4 mg/dose [repaglinide], 1000 mg/dose [metformin]; maximum daily dose: 10 mg/day [repaglinide], 2500 mg/day [metformin])

Dosage Forms

Tablet:

PrandiMet®: 1/500: Repaglinide 1 mg and metformin hydrochloride 500 mg; 2/500: Repaglinide 2 mg and metformin hydrochloride 500 mg

repaglinide and metformin hydrochloride *see* repaglinide and metformin *on page 835*

Repan® [US] *see* butalbital, acetaminophen, and caffeine *on page 159*

Replace [US-OTC] *see* vitamins (multiple/oral) *on page 990*

Replace Without Iron [US-OTC] *see* vitamins (multiple/oral) *on page 990*

Replagal™ [Can] *see* agalsidase alfa *(Canada only) on page 40*

Repliva 21/7® [US] *see* vitamins (multiple/oral) *on page 990*

Reposans-10® Oral *(Discontinued)* *see* chlordiazepoxide *on page 203*

Reprexain™ [US] *see* hydrocodone and ibuprofen *on page 481*

Repronex® [US/Can] *see* menotropins *on page 602*

Requa® Activated Charcoal [US-OTC] *see* charcoal *on page 200*

Requip® [US/Can] *see* ropinirole *on page 851*

Requip® XL™ [US] *see* ropinirole *on page 851*

Resa® *(Discontinued)* *see* reserpine *on page 836*

Rescon® [US] *see* chlorpheniramine, phenylephrine, and methscopolamine *on page 212*

Rescon DM [US-OTC] *see* chlorpheniramine, pseudoephedrine, and dextromethorphan *on page 214*

Rescon GG [US-OTC] *see* guaifenesin and phenylephrine *on page 456*

Rescon-Jr® *(Discontinued)* *see* chlorpheniramine and phenylephrine *on page 208*

Rescriptor® [US/Can] *see* delavirdine *on page 274*

Rescula® *(Discontinued)*

Resectisol® [US] *see* mannitol *on page 590*

reserpine (re SER peen)

Sound-Alike/Look-Alike Issues

reserpine may be confused with Risperdal®, risperidone

Therapeutic Category Rauwolfia Alkaloid

Use Management of mild-to-moderate hypertension; treatment of agitated psychotic states (schizophrenia)

Dosage Summary

Oral:

Children: 0.01-0.02 mg/kg/day divided every 12 hours (maximum: 0.25 mg/day); **Note:** Use not recommended in children

Adults: Initial: 0.5 mg once daily; Maintenance: 0.05-0.5 mg once daily; **Note:** May give 0.1 mg every other day to achieve 0.05 mg/day

Elderly: 0.05 mg once daily, increasing by 0.05 mg every week as needed

Dosage Forms

Tablet, oral: 0.1 mg, 0.25 mg

Resonium Calcium® [Can] *see* calcium polystyrene sulfonate *(Canada only) on page 172*

Respa-DM® [US] *see* guaifenesin and dextromethorphan *on page 455*

Respa-GF® ***(Discontinued)*** *see* guaifenesin *on page 454*

Respahist® [US] *see* brompheniramine and pseudoephedrine *on page 148*

Respaire®-30 [US] *see* guaifenesin and pseudoephedrine *on page 457*

Respaire®-60 SR ***(Discontinued)*** *see* guaifenesin and pseudoephedrine *on page 457*

Respaire®-120 SR ***(Discontinued)*** *see* guaifenesin and pseudoephedrine *on page 457*

Respa® PE ***(Discontinued)*** *see* guaifenesin and phenylephrine *on page 456*

Respbid® ***(Discontinued)*** *see* theophylline *on page 925*

Respi-Tann™ ***(Discontinued)*** *see* carbetapentane and pseudoephedrine *on page 180*

Resporal® ***(Discontinued)*** *see* dexbrompheniramine and pseudoephedrine *on page 282*

Restall® ***(Discontinued)*** *see* hydroxyzine *on page 490*

Restasis® [US] *see* cyclosporine (ophthalmic) *on page 260*

Restoril™ [US/Can] *see* temazepam *on page 914*

Restylane® [US] *see* hyaluronate and derivatives *on page 475*

retapamulin (re te PAM ue lin)

U.S./Canadian Brand Names Altabax™ [US]

Therapeutic Category Antibiotic, Pleuromutilin; Antibiotic, Topical

Use Treatment of impetigo caused by susceptible strains of *S. pyogenes* or methicillin-susceptible *S. aureus*

Dosage Summary

Topical:

Children <9 months: Dosage not established

Children ≥9 months: Apply to affected area twice daily for 5 days. Total treatment area should not exceed 2% of total body surface area.

Adults: Apply to affected area twice daily for 5 days. Total treatment area should not exceed 100 cm^2 total body surface area.

Dosage Forms

Ointment, topical:

Altabax™: 1% (15 g)

Retavase® [US/Can] *see* reteplase *on page 836*

reteplase (RE ta plase)

Synonyms r-PA; recombinant plasminogen activator

U.S./Canadian Brand Names Retavase® [US/Can]

Therapeutic Category Fibrinolytic Agent

Use Management of ST-elevation myocardial infarction (STEMI); improvement of ventricular function; reduction of the incidence of CHF and the reduction of mortality following AMI

Recommended criteria for treatment: STEMI: Chest pain ≥20 minutes duration, onset of chest pain within 12 hours of treatment (or within prior 12-24 hours in patients with continuing ischemic symptoms), and ST-segment elevation >0.1 mV in at least two contiguous precordial leads or two adjacent limb leads on ECG or new or presumably new left bundle branch block (LBBB)

Dosage Summary

I.V.:

Children: Dosage not established

Adults: 10 units over 2 minutes, repeat after 30 minutes

Dosage Forms

Injection, powder for reconstitution [preservative free]:

Retavase®: 10.4 units

Retin-A® [US/Can] *see* tretinoin (topical) *on page 951*

Retin-A Micro® [US/Can] *see* tretinoin (topical) *on page 951*

retinoic acid *see* tretinoin (topical) *on page 951*

Retinova® [Can] *see* tretinoin (topical) *on page 951*

Retisert® [US] *see* fluocinolone (ophthalmic) *on page 410*

Retrovir® [US/Can] *see* zidovudine *on page 999*

Retrovir® (AZT™) [Can] *see* zidovudine *on page 999*

Revatio® [US/Can] *see* sildenafil *on page 874*

Revex® *(Discontinued)*

Rēv-Eyes™ *(Discontinued)*

ReVia® [US/Can] *see* naltrexone *on page 657*

Revitalose C-1000® [Can] *see* ascorbic acid *on page 98*

Revlimid® [US/Can] *see* lenalidomide *on page 552*

Revolade® *see* eltrombopag *on page 346*

Revonto™ [US] *see* dantrolene *on page 268*

Rexigen Forte® *(Discontinued)* *see* phendimetrazine *on page 747*

Reyataz® [US/Can] *see* atazanavir *on page 102*

Rezulin® *(Discontinued)*

rFSH-alpha *see* follitropin alfa *on page 424*

rFSH-beta *see* follitropin beta *on page 424*

rFVIIa *see* factor VIIa (recombinant) *on page 388*

R-Gel® *(Discontinued)* *see* capsaicin *on page 175*

R-Gene® 10 [US] *see* arginine *on page 94*

rGM-CSF *see* sargramostim *on page 865*

rhAPC *see* drotrecogin alfa *on page 334*

rhASB *see* galsulfase *on page 436*

rhAT *see* antithrombin III *on page 83*

rhATIII *see* antithrombin III *on page 83*

r-hCG *see* chorionic gonadotropin (recombinant) *on page 219*

rhDNase *see* dornase alfa *on page 327*

Rheaban® *(Discontinued)*

Rheomacrodex® *(Discontinued)* *see* dextran *on page 285*

Rheumatrex® [US] *see* methotrexate *on page 614*

rhFSH-alpha *see* follitropin alfa *on page 424*

rhFSH-beta *see* follitropin beta *on page 424*

rhGAA *see* alglucosidase alfa *on page 49*

r-h α-GAL *see* agalsidase beta *on page 41*

RhIG *see* Rh_o(D) immune globulin *on page 838*

rhIGF-1 (mecasermin [Increlex™]) *see* mecasermin *on page 594*

rhIGF-1/rhIGFBP-3 (mecasermin rinfabate [Iplex™]) *see* mecasermin *on page 594*

rhIL-11 *see* oprelvekin *on page 706*

Rhinacon A [US] *see* chlorpheniramine, phenylephrine, and phenyltoloxamine *on page 213*

Rhinalar® [Can] *see* flunisolide (nasal) *on page 410*

Rhinall® [US-OTC] *see* phenylephrine (nasal) *on page 751*

Rhinaris-CS Anti-Allergic Nasal Mist [Can] *see* cromolyn (nasal) *on page 255*
Rhinocort Aqua® [US/Can] *see* budesonide (nasal) *on page 151*
Rhinocort® Nasal Inhaler *(Discontinued)* *see* budesonide (nasal) *on page 151*
Rhinocort® Turbuhaler® [Can] *see* budesonide (nasal) *on page 151*
RhinoFlex™ [US] *see* acetaminophen and phenyltoloxamine *on page 26*
RhinoFlex™-650 [US] *see* acetaminophen and phenyltoloxamine *on page 26*
r-hirudin *see* desirudin *on page 277*
rhKGF *see* palifermin *on page 720*
r-hLH *see* lutropin alfa *on page 581*
Rho(D) immune globulin (human) *see* Rh_o(D) immune globulin *on page 838*
Rho®-Clonazepam [Can] *see* clonazepam *on page 237*

Rh_o(D) immune globulin (ar aych oh (dee) i MYUN GLOB yoo lin)

Synonyms RhIG; Rho(D) immune globulin (human); RhoIGIV; RhoIVIM

U.S./Canadian Brand Names HyperRHO™ S/D Full Dose [US]; HyperRHO™ S/D Mini Dose [US]; MICRhoGAM® [US]; RhoGAM® [US]; Rhophylac® [US]; WinRho® SDF [US/Can]

Therapeutic Category Immune Globulin

Use

Suppression of Rh isoimmunization: Use in the following situations when an Rh_o(D)-negative individual is exposed to Rh_o(D)-positive blood: During delivery of an Rh_o(D)-positive infant; abortion; amniocentesis; chorionic villus sampling; ruptured tubal pregnancy; abdominal trauma; hydatidiform mole; transplacental hemorrhage. Used when the mother is Rh_o(D)-negative, the father of the child is either Rh_o(D)-positive or Rh_o(D)-unknown, or the baby is either Rh_o(D)-positive or Rh_o(D)-unknown.

Transfusion: Suppression of Rh isoimmunization in Rh_o(D)-negative individuals transfused with Rh_o(D) antigen-positive RBCs or blood components containing Rh_o(D) antigen-positive RBCs

Treatment of idiopathic thrombocytopenic purpura (ITP): Used intravenously in the following non-splenectomized Rh_o(D)-positive individuals: Children with acute or chronic ITP, adults with chronic ITP, and children and adults with ITP secondary to HIV infection

Dosage Summary

I.M.:

Children:

Transfusion: 12 mcg/mL Rho(D)-positive whole blood **or** 24 mcg/mL Rho(D)-positive red blood cell exposure; administer 1200 mcg every 12 hours until the total dose is received.

Adults:

Rho(D) suppression: 50 mcg, 120 mcg, or 300 mcg as a single dose

Transfusion: 12 mcg/mL Rho(D)-positive whole blood **or** 24 mcg/mL Rho(D)-positive red blood cell exposure; administer 1200 mcg every 12 hours until the total dose is received.

I.V.:

Children:

ITP: Initial: 25-50 mcg/kg as a single injection, or can be given as a divided dose on separate days; Maintenance: 25-60 mcg/kg based on platelet and hemoglobin levels

Transfusion: 9 mcg/mL Rho(D)-positive whole blood **or** 18 mcg/mL Rho(D)-positive red blood cell exposure; administer 600 mcg every 8 hours until the total dose is received.

Adults:

ITP: Initial: 25-50 mcg/kg as a single injection, or can be given as a divided dose on separate days; Maintenance: 25-60 mcg/kg based on platelet and hemoglobin levels

Rho(D) suppression: 50 mcg, 120 mcg, or 300 mcg as a single dose

Transfusion: 9 mcg/mL Rho(D)-positive whole blood **or** 18 mcg/mL Rho(D)-positive red blood cell exposure; administer 600 mcg every 8 hours until the total dose is received.

Dosage Forms

Injection, solution [preservative free]:

HyperRHO™ S/D Full Dose: ≥300 mcg/mL (1s)
HyperRHO™ S/D Mini-Dose: ≥50 mcg/0.17 mL (1s)
MICRhoGAM® UF Plus: ~50 mcg/0.75 mL (1s, 5s, 25s)
RhoGAM® UF Plus: ~300 mcg/0.75 mL (1s, 5s, 25s)
Rhophylac®: ≥ 300 mcg/2 mL (2 mL)
WinRho® SDF: 300 mcg/~1.3 mL; 500 mcg/~2.2 mL; 1000 mcg/~4.4 mL; 3000 mcg/~13 mL

Rhodis™ [Can] *see* ketoprofen *on page 537*
Rhodis-EC™ [Can] *see* ketoprofen *on page 537*

Rhodis SR™ [Can] *see* ketoprofen *on page 537*
RhoGAM® [US] *see* Rh_o(D) immune globulin *on page 838*
RhoIGIV *see* Rh_o(D) immune globulin *on page 838*
RhoIVIM *see* Rh_o(D) immune globulin *on page 838*
Rho®-Loperamine [Can] *see* loperamide *on page 573*
Rho®-Nitro [Can] *see* nitroglycerin *on page 679*
Rhophylac® [US] *see* Rh_o(D) immune globulin *on page 838*
Rhotral [Can] *see* acebutolol *on page 21*
Rhotrimine® [Can] *see* trimipramine *on page 960*
Rhovane® [Can] *see* zopiclone *(Canada only) on page 1005*
Rhoxal-cyclosporine [Can] *see* cyclosporine (systemic) *on page 260*
Rhoxal-fluvoxamine [Can] *see* fluvoxamine *on page 422*
Rhoxal-glimepiride [Can] *see* glimepiride *on page 446*
Rhoxal-loperamide [Can] *see* loperamide *on page 573*
Rhoxal-nabumetone [Can] *see* nabumetone *on page 654*
Rhoxal-orphendrine [Can] *see* orphenadrine *on page 708*
Rhoxal-pamidronate [Can] *see* pamidronate *on page 722*
Rhoxal-sotalol [Can] *see* sotalol *on page 892*
Rhoxal-sumatriptan [Can] *see* sumatriptan *on page 904*
Rhoxal-ticlopidine [Can] *see* ticlopidine *on page 932*
Rhoxal-Timolol [Can] *see* timolol (ophthalmic) *on page 933*
Rhoxal-valproic [Can] *see* valproic acid *on page 974*
rhPTH(1-34) *see* teriparatide *on page 919*
Rh-TSH *see* thyrotropin alpha *on page 930*
***r*HuEPO-α** *see* epoetin alfa *on page 356*
rhuFabV2 *see* ranibizumab *on page 828*
rhu keratinocyte growth factor *see* palifermin *on page 720*
rHu-KGF *see* palifermin *on page 720*
Rhulicaine® *(Discontinued)* *see* benzocaine *on page 124*
rhuMAb-E25 *see* omalizumab *on page 700*
rHuMAb-EGFr *see* panitumumab *on page 724*
rhuMAb HER2 *see* trastuzumab *on page 948*
rhuMAb-VEGF *see* bevacizumab *on page 136*
RiaSTAP™ [US] *see* fibrinogen concentrate (human) *on page 401*
RibaPak™ *(Discontinued)* *see* ribavirin *on page 839*
Ribasphere® [US] *see* ribavirin *on page 839*
Ribasphere® RibaPak® [US] *see* ribavirin *on page 839*

ribavirin (rye ba VYE rin)

Sound-Alike/Look-Alike Issues

ribavirin may be confused with riboflavin, rifampin, Robaxin®

Synonyms RTCA; tribavirin

U.S./Canadian Brand Names Copegus® [US]; Rebetol® [US]; Ribasphere® RibaPak® [US]; Ribasphere® [US]; Virazole® [US/Can]

Therapeutic Category Antiviral Agent

Use

Inhalation: Treatment of patients with respiratory syncytial virus (RSV) infections; specially indicated for treatment of severe lower respiratory tract RSV infections in patients with an underlying compromising condition (prematurity, bronchopulmonary dysplasia and other chronic lung conditions, congenital heart disease, immunodeficiency, immunosuppression), and recent transplant recipients

Oral capsule:

In combination with interferon alfa-2b (Intron® A) injection for the treatment of chronic hepatitis C in patients with compensated liver disease who have relapsed after alpha interferon therapy or were previously untreated with alpha interferons

In combination with peginterferon alfa-2b (PEG-Intron®) injection for the treatment of chronic hepatitis C in patients with compensated liver disease who were previously untreated with alpha interferons

Oral solution: In combination with interferon alfa 2b (Intron® A) injection for the treatment of chronic hepatitis C in patients with compensated liver disease who were previously untreated with alpha interferons or patients who have relapsed after alpha interferon therapy

Oral tablet: In combination with peginterferon alfa-2a (Pegasys®) injection for the treatment of chronic hepatitis C in patients with compensated liver disease who were previously untreated with alpha interferons (includes patients with histological evidence of cirrhosis [Child-Pugh class A] and patients with clinically-stable HIV disease)

Dosage Summary

Inhalation:

Children: RSV: 20 mg/mL (6 g in 300 mL) solution administered with Viratek® small particle aerosol generator; continuous: 12-18 hours/day

Adults: Dosage not established

Oral:

Children <3 years: Dosage not established

Children ≥3 years and ≤25 kg: 15 mg/kg/day in 2 divided doses in combination with interferon alfa-2b

Children ≥3 years and 26-36 kg: 400 mg/day in 2 divided doses in combination with interferon alfa-2b

Children ≥3 years and 37-49 kg: 600 mg/day (200 mg in the morning and 400 mg in the evening) in combination with interferon alfa-2b

Children ≥3 years and 50-61 kg: 800 mg/day (400 mg in the morning and evening) in combination with interferon alfa-2b

Children ≥3 years and >61 kg but <75 kg: 1000 mg/day (400 mg in the morning and 600 mg in the evening) in combination with interferon alfa-2b

Adults ≤75 kg: 400 mg in the morning, then 600 mg in the evening in combination with interferon alfa-2b **or** 800 mg/day **or** 1000 mg/day in 2 divided doses in combination with peginterferon alfa-2a

Adults >75 kg: 600 mg in the morning, then 600 mg in the evening in combination with interferon alfa-2b **or** 800 mg/day **or** 1200 mg/day in 2 divided doses in combination with peginterferon alfa-2a

Dosage Forms

Capsule, oral: 200 mg

Rebetol®: 200 mg

Ribasphere®: 200 mg

Combination package, oral:

Ribasphere® RibaPak®: Tablet: 400 mg (7s) [medium blue tablets] and Tablet: 600 mg (7s) [dark blue tablets] (14s, 56s)

Powder for solution, for nebulization:

Virazole®: 6 g

Solution, oral:

Rebetol®: 40 mg/mL (100 mL)

Tablet, oral: 200 mg

Copegus®: 200 mg

Ribasphere®: 200 mg, 400 mg, 600 mg

Ribasphere® RibaPak®: 400 mg, 600 mg

ribavirin and peginterferon alfa-2a *see* peginterferon alfa-2a and ribavirin *(Canada only)* *on page 733*

ribavirin and peginterferon alfa-2b *see* peginterferon alfa-2b and ribavirin *(Canada only)* *on page 734*

Ribo-100 [US-OTC] *see* riboflavin *on page 840*

riboflavin (RYE boe flay vin)

Sound-Alike/Look-Alike Issues

riboflavin may be confused with ribavirin

Synonyms lactoflavin; vitamin B_2; vitamin G

U.S./Canadian Brand Names Ribo-100 [US-OTC]

Therapeutic Category Vitamin, Water Soluble

Use Prevention of riboflavin deficiency and treatment of ariboflavinosis

Dosage Summary

Oral:

Children: 2.5-10 mg/day in divided doses

Adults: 5-30 mg/day in divided doses

Dosage Forms

Tablet, oral: 25 mg, 50 mg, 100 mg
Ribo-100 [OTC]: 100 mg

Rid® [US-OTC] *see* permethrin *on page 744*
Rid-A-Pain Dental [US-OTC] *see* benzocaine *on page 124*
Ridaura® [US/Can] *see* auranofin *on page 107*
RID® *(Discontinued)* *see* pyrethrins and piperonyl butoxide *on page 816*
RID® Maximum Strength [US-OTC] *see* pyrethrins and piperonyl butoxide *on page 816*
RID® Mousse [Can] *see* pyrethrins and piperonyl butoxide *on page 816*

rifabutin (rif a BYOO tin)

Sound-Alike/Look-Alike Issues
rifabutin may be confused with rifampin

Synonyms ansamycin

U.S./Canadian Brand Names Mycobutin® [US/Can]

Therapeutic Category Antibiotic, Miscellaneous

Use Prevention of disseminated *Mycobacterium avium* complex (MAC) in patients with advanced HIV infection

Dosage Summary

Oral:
Children ≤1 year: Dosage not established
Children <6 years: 5 mg/kg once daily
Children ≥6 years: 300 mg once daily
Adults: 300 mg once daily

Dosage Forms

Capsule, oral:
Mycobutin®: 150 mg

Rifadin® [US/Can] *see* rifampin *on page 841*
Rifamate® [US/Can] *see* rifampin and isoniazid *on page 842*
rifampicin *see* rifampin *on page 841*

rifampin (rif AM pin)

Sound-Alike/Look-Alike Issues
rifampin may be confused with ribavirin, rifabutin, Rifamate®, rifapentine, rifaximin
Rifadin® may be confused with Rifater®, Ritalin®

Synonyms rifampicin

U.S./Canadian Brand Names Rifadin® [US/Can]; Rofact™ [Can]

Therapeutic Category Antibiotic, Miscellaneous

Use Management of active tuberculosis in combination with other agents; elimination of meningococci from the nasopharynx in asymptomatic carriers

Dosage Summary

I.V.:
Children <12 years: 10-20 mg/kg/day in 1-2 divided doses **or** 10-20 mg/kg twice weekly (maximum: 600 mg/day)
Children ≥12 years: 10-20 mg/kg/day in 1-2 divided doses
Adults: 10 mg/kg/day **or** 10 mg/kg 2-3 times/week **or** 600 mg every 12-24 hours

Oral:
Children <12 years: 10-20 mg/kg/day in 1-2 divided doses **or** 10-20 mg/kg twice weekly (maximum: 600 mg/day)
Children ≥12 years: 10 mg/kg/day **or** 10 mg/kg 2-3 times/week **or** 600 mg every 12-24 hours
Adults: 10 mg/kg/day **or** 10 mg/kg 2-3 times/week **or** 600 mg every 12-24 hours

Dosage Forms

Capsule, oral: 150 mg, 300 mg
Rifadin®: 150 mg, 300 mg

Injection, powder for reconstitution: 600 mg
Rifadin®: 600 mg

rifampin and isoniazid (rif AM pin & eye soe NYE a zid)

Sound-Alike/Look-Alike Issues
Rifamate® may be confused with rifampin

Synonyms isoniazid and rifampin

U.S./Canadian Brand Names IsonaRif™ [US]; Rifamate® [US/Can]

Therapeutic Category Antibiotic, Miscellaneous

Use Management of active tuberculosis; see individual agents for additional information

Dosage Summary

Oral:

Children: Dosage not established
Adults: 2 capsules/day

Dosage Forms

Capsule:

IsonaRif™, Rifamate®: 300/150: Rifampin 300 mg and isoniazid 150 mg

rifampin, isoniazid, and pyrazinamide

(rif AM pin, eye soe NYE a zid, & peer a ZIN a mide)

Sound-Alike/Look-Alike Issues
Rifater® may be confused with Rifadin®

Synonyms isoniazid, pyrazinamide, and rifampin; pyrazinamide, rifampin, and isoniazid

U.S./Canadian Brand Names Rifater® [US/Can]

Therapeutic Category Antibiotic, Miscellaneous

Use Initial phase, short-course treatment of pulmonary tuberculosis; see individual agents for additional information

Dosage Summary

Oral:

Children <15 years: Dosage not established
Children ≥15 years and ≤44 kg: 4 tablets once daily
Children ≥15 years and 45-54 kg: 5 tablets once daily
Children ≥15 years and ≥55 kg: 6 tablets once daily
Adults ≤44 kg: 4 tablets once daily
Adults 45-54 kg: 5 tablets once daily
Adults ≥55 kg: 6 tablets once daily

Dosage Forms

Tablet:

Rifater®: Rifampin 120 mg, isoniazid 50 mg, and pyrazinamide 300 mg

rifapentine (rif a PEN teen)

Sound-Alike/Look-Alike Issues
rifapentine may be confused with rifampin

U.S./Canadian Brand Names Priftin® [US/Can]

Therapeutic Category Antitubercular Agent

Use Treatment of pulmonary tuberculosis; rifapentine must always be used in conjunction with at least one other antituberculosis drug to which the isolate is susceptible; it may also be necessary to add a third agent (either streptomycin or ethambutol) until susceptibility is known.

Dosage Summary Note: Rifapentine should not be used alone; initial phase should include a 3- to 4-drug regimen.

Oral:

Children: Dosage not established
Adults: 600 mg once or twice weekly

Dosage Forms

Tablet, oral:

Priftin®: 150 mg

Rifater® [US/Can] *see* rifampin, isoniazid, and pyrazinamide *on page 842*

rifaximin (rif AX i min)

Sound-Alike/Look-Alike Issues
rifaximin may be confused with rifampin

U.S./Canadian Brand Names Xifaxan® [US]

Therapeutic Category Antibiotic, Miscellaneous

Use Treatment of traveler's diarrhea caused by noninvasive strains of *E. coli*; reduction in the risk of overt hepatic encephalopathy recurrence

Dosage Summary

Oral:

Children <12 years: Dosage not established

Children ≥12 years: Traveler's diarrhea: 200 mg 3 times/day

Adults: 200 mg 3 times/day **or** 550 mg 2 times/day

Dosage Forms

Tablet, oral:

Xifaxan®: 200 mg, 550 mg

rIFN beta-1a *see* interferon beta-1a *on page 515*

rIFN beta-1b *see* interferon beta-1b *on page 516*

RIG *see* rabies immune globulin (human) *on page 824*

rilonacept (ri LON a sept)

U.S./Canadian Brand Names Arcalyst™ [US]

Therapeutic Category Interleukin-1 Inhibitor

Use **Orphan drug:** Treatment of cryopyrin-associated periodic syndromes (CAPS) including familial cold autoinflammatory syndrome (FCAS) and Muckle-Wells syndrome (MWS)

Dosage Summary

SubQ: Note: Do not administer more frequently than once weekly.

Children <12 years: Dosage not established

Children ≥12 years: Loading dose 4.4 mg/kg (maximum dose: 320 mg); Maintenance dose: 2.2 mg/kg once weekly (maximum dose: 160 mg)

Adults: Loading dose: 320 mg; Maintenance dose: 160 mg once weekly.

Dosage Forms

Injection, powder for reconstitution:

Arcalyst™: 220 mg

Rilutek® [US/Can] *see* riluzole *on page 843*

riluzole (RIL yoo zole)

Synonyms 2-amino-6-trifluoromethoxy-benzothiazole; RP-54274

U.S./Canadian Brand Names Rilutek® [US/Can]

Therapeutic Category Miscellaneous Product

Use Treatment of amyotrophic lateral sclerosis (ALS); riluzole can extend survival or time to tracheostomy

Dosage Summary

Oral:

Children: Dosage not established

Adults: 50 mg every 12 hours

Dosage Forms

Tablet, oral:

Rilutek®: 50 mg

rimabotulinumtoxinB (rime uh BOT yoo lin num TOKS in bee)

Synonyms botulinum toxin type B

U.S./Canadian Brand Names Myobloc® [US]

Therapeutic Category Neuromuscular Blocker Agent, Toxin

Use Treatment of cervical dystonia (spasmodic torticollis)

Dosage Summary

I.M.:

Children: Dosage not established

Adults: Initial: 2500-5000 units divided among the affected muscles, lower doses in previously untreated patients; Subsequent doses: Optimize according to patient's response

Dosage Forms

Injection, solution [preservative free]:

Myobloc®: 5000 units/mL (0.5 mL, 1 mL, 2 mL)

rimantadine (ri MAN ta deen)

Sound-Alike/Look-Alike Issues

rimantadine may be confused with amantadine, ranitidine, Rimactane®

Flumadine® may be confused with fludarabine, flunisolide, flutamide

Synonyms rimantadine hydrochloride

U.S./Canadian Brand Names Flumadine® [US/Can]

Therapeutic Category Antiviral Agent

Use Prophylaxis (adults and children >1 year of age) and treatment (adults) of influenza A viral infection (per manufacturer labeling; also refer to current ACIP guidelines for recommendations during current flu season)

Note: In certain circumstances, the ACIP recommends use of rimantadine in combination with oseltamivir for the treatment or prophylaxis of influenza A infection when resistance to oseltamivir is suspected.

Dosage Summary

Oral:

Children <1 year: Dosage not established

Children 1-9 years: 5 mg/kg/day in 1-2 divided doses (maximum: 150 mg/day)

Children ≥10 years and <40 kg: 5 mg/kg/day in 2 divided doses

Children ≥10 years: 100 mg twice daily

Adults: 100 mg twice daily

Elderly: 100 mg daily

Dosage Forms

Tablet, oral: 100 mg

Flumadine®: 100 mg

rimantadine hydrochloride *see* rimantadine *on page 844*

rimexolone (ri MEKS oh lone)

Sound-Alike/Look-Alike Issues

Vexol® may be confused with VoSol®

U.S./Canadian Brand Names Vexol® [US/Can]

Therapeutic Category Adrenal Corticosteroid

Use Treatment of inflammation after ocular surgery and the treatment of anterior uveitis

Dosage Summary

Ophthalmic:

Children: Dosage not established

Adults: Instill 1 drop 2-4 times/day (maximum: every 4 hours; exceptions occur [indication specific])

Dosage Forms

Suspension, ophthalmic:

Vexol®: 1% (5 mL, 10 mL)

Rimso-50® [US/Can] *see* dimethyl sulfoxide *on page 308*

Rinate™ Pediatric [US] *see* chlorpheniramine and phenylephrine *on page 208*

Rindal HD Plus [US] *see* phenylephrine, hydrocodone, and chlorpheniramine *on page 754*

Rindal HPD *(Discontinued)*

Riobin® *(Discontinued)* *see* riboflavin *on page 840*

Riomet® [US] *see* metformin *on page 609*

Riopan® Plus *(Discontinued)* *see* magaldrate and simethicone *on page 583*

Riopan® Plus Double Strength *(Discontinued)* *see* magaldrate and simethicone *on page 583*

Risamine™ [US-OTC] *see* menthol and zinc oxide (topical) *on page 603*

RisaQuad™ [US-OTC] *see* Lactobacillus *on page 543*

risedronate (ris ED roe nate)

Sound-Alike/Look-Alike Issues

risedronate may be confused with alendronate

Actonel® may be confused with Actos®

Synonyms risedronate sodium

U.S./Canadian Brand Names Actonel® [US/Can]; Novo-Risedronate [Can]; PMS-Risedronate [Can]; Sandoz-Risedronate [Can]

Therapeutic Category Bisphosphonate Derivative

Use Treatment of Paget disease of the bone; treatment and prevention of glucocorticoid-induced osteoporosis; treatment and prevention of osteoporosis in postmenopausal women; treatment of osteoporosis in men

Dosage Summary

Oral:

Children: Dosage not established

Adults: 5 mg once daily **or** 35 mg once weekly **or** 150 mg once a month **or** 30 mg once daily (Paget disease)

Dosage Forms

Tablet, oral:

Actonel®: 5 mg, 30 mg, 35 mg, 150 mg

risedronate and calcium (ris ED roe nate & KAL see um)

Sound-Alike/Look-Alike Issues

Actonel® may be confused with Actos®

Synonyms calcium and risedronate; risedronate sodium and calcium carbonate

U.S./Canadian Brand Names Actonel Plus Calcium [Can]; Actonel® and Calcium [US]

Therapeutic Category Bisphosphonate Derivative; Calcium Salt

Use Treatment and prevention of osteoporosis in postmenopausal women

Dosage Summary

Oral:

Children: Dosage not established

Adults: Calcium carbonate: 1250 mg (500 mg elemental calcium) once daily on days 2-7 of 7-day treatment cycle; Risedronate: 35 mg once weekly on day 1 or 7 day treatment cycle

Dosage Forms

Combination package [each package contains]:

Actonel® and Calcium:

Tablet (Actonel®): Risedronate 35 mg (4s)

Tablet: Calcium 1250 mg (24s)

risedronate sodium *see* risedronate *on page 844*

risedronate sodium and calcium carbonate *see* risedronate and calcium *on page 845*

Risperdal® [US/Can] *see* risperidone *on page 845*

Risperdal® M-Tab® [US/Can] *see* risperidone *on page 845*

Risperdal® Consta® [US/Can] *see* risperidone *on page 845*

risperidone (ris PER i done)

Sound-Alike/Look-Alike Issues

risperidone may be confused with reserpine, ropinirole

Risperdal® may be confused with lisinopril, reserpine, Restoril™

U.S./Canadian Brand Names Apo-Risperidone® [Can]; CO Risperidone [Can]; Dom-Risperidone [Can]; Gen-Risperidone [Can]; Mylan-Risperidone [Can]; Novo-Risperidone [Can]; PHL-Risperidone [Can]; PMS-Risperidone ODT [Can]; PRO-Risperidone [Can]; RAN™-Risperidone [Can]; ratio-Risperidone [Can]; Risperdal® Consta® [US/Can]; Risperdal® M-Tab® [US/Can]; Risperdal® [US/Can]; Riva-Risperidone [Can]; Sandoz-Risperidone [Can]; ZYM-Risperidone [Can]

Therapeutic Category Antipsychotic Agent, Benzisoxazole

Use

Oral: Treatment of schizophrenia; treatment of acute mania or mixed episodes associated with bipolar I disorder (as monotherapy in children or adults, or in combination with lithium or valproate in adults); treatment of irritability/aggression associated with autistic disorder

Injection: Treatment of schizophrenia; maintenance treatment of bipolar I disorder in adults as monotherapy or in combination with lithium or valproate

Dosage Summary

I.M.:

Children: Dosage not established

Adults: 25 mg every 2 weeks (range: 12.5-50 mg every 2 weeks; maximum: 50 mg every 2 weeks); **Note:** Titration is recommended

Elderly: 25 mg every 2 weeks

Oral:

Children <5 years: Dosage not established

Children ≥5 years: Autism: Initial: 0.25 mg/day (<20 kg) or 0.5 mg/day (≥20 kg); Maximum dose: <20 kg: 1 mg/day; ≥20 kg: 2.5 mg/day (3 mg/day in children >45 kg); **Note:** Titration is recommended

Children 10-17 years: Bipolar disorder: Initial: 0.5 mg once daily; Recommended target dose: 2.5 mg/day; dosing range 0.5-6 mg/day; **Note:** Titration is recommended

Children: 13-17 years: Schizophrenia Initial: 0.5 mg once daily; Recommended target dose: 3 mg/day; dosing range 1-6 mg/day; **Note:** Titration is recommended

Adults: Initial: 2-3 mg/day in 1-2 divided doses; Maintenance: 1-8 mg/day in 1-2 divided doses; **Note:** Titration is recommended

Elderly: Initial: 0.5 mg twice daily; **Note:** Titration is recommended

Dosage Forms

Injection, microspheres for reconstitution, extended release:

Risperdal® Consta®: 12.5 mg, 25 mg, 37.5 mg, 50 mg

Solution, oral: 1 mg/mL (30 mL)

Risperdal®: 1 mg/mL (30 mL)

Tablet, oral: 0.25 mg, 0.5 mg, 1 mg, 2 mg, 3 mg, 4 mg

Risperdal®: 0.25 mg, 0.5 mg, 1 mg, 2 mg, 3 mg, 4 mg

Tablet, orally disintegrating, oral: 0.25 mg, 0.5 mg, 1 mg, 2 mg, 3 mg, 4 mg

Risperdal® M-Tab®: 0.5 mg, 1 mg, 2 mg, 3 mg, 4 mg

Ritalin® [US/Can] *see* methylphenidate *on page 621*

Ritalin LA® [US] *see* methylphenidate *on page 621*

Ritalin-SR® [US/Can] *see* methylphenidate *on page 621*

ritonavir (ri TOE na veer)

Sound-Alike/Look-Alike Issues

ritonavir may be confused with Retrovir®

Norvir® may be confused with Norvasc®

U.S./Canadian Brand Names Norvir® SEC [Can]; Norvir® [US/Can]

Therapeutic Category Antiviral Agent

Use Treatment of HIV infection; should always be used as part of a multidrug regimen (at least three antiretroviral agents); may be used as a pharmacokinetic "booster" for other protease inhibitors

Dosage Summary

Oral:

Children <1 month: Dosage not established

Children >1 month: Initial: 250 mg/m^2 twice daily; Maintenance: 350-400 mg/m^2 twice daily (maximum dose: 1200 mg/day); **Note:** Titration is recommended

Adults: 600 mg twice daily; Booster with other protease inhibitors: 100-400 mg/day; **Note:** Dosage titration is recommended

Dosage Forms

Capsule, soft gelatin, oral:

Norvir®: 100 mg

Solution, oral:

Norvir®: 80 mg/mL (240 mL)

Tablet, oral:

Norvir®: 100 mg

ritonavir and lopinavir *see* lopinavir and ritonavir *on page 574*

Rituxan® [US/Can] *see* rituximab *on page 846*

rituximab (ri TUK si mab)

Sound-Alike/Look-Alike Issues

riTUXimab may be confused with bevacizumab, inFLIXimab

Rituxan® may be confused with Remicade®

Synonyms anti-CD20 monoclonal antibody; C2B8 monoclonal antibody; IDEC-C2B8

Tall-Man riTUXimab

U.S./Canadian Brand Names Rituxan® [US/Can]

Therapeutic Category Antineoplastic Agent

Use Treatment of low-grade or follicular CD20-positive, B-cell non-Hodgkin lymphoma (NHL); treatment of diffuse large B-cell CD20-positive NHL; treatment of CD20-positive chronic lymphocytic leukemia (CLL), in combination with cyclophosphamide and fludarabine; treatment of moderately- to severely-active rheumatoid arthritis (RA) in combination with methotrexate in patients with inadequate response to one or more TNF antagonists

Dosage Summary **Note:** Pretreatment with acetaminophen and an antihistamine is recommended.

I.V.:

Adults: Infusion: 375 mg/m^2 once weekly for 4 or 8 doses **or** 375 mg/m^2 on day 1 of each chemotherapy cycle for up to 8 doses **or** 375 mg/m^2, then 500 mg/m^2 every 28 days for 6 doses (total) **or** 250 mg/m^2 I.V. day 1, repeat in 7-9 days with ibritumomab **or** 1000 mg on days 1 and 15 in combination with methotrexate

Dosage Forms

Injection, solution [preservative free]:

Rituxan®: 10 mg/mL (10 mL, 50 mL)

Riva-Alendronate [Can] *see* alendronate *on page* 47
Riva-Amiodarone [Can] *see* amiodarone *on page* 67
Riva-Amlodipine [Can] *see* amlodipine *on page* 68
Riva-Atenolol [Can] *see* atenolol *on page* 102
Riva-Azithromycin [Can] *see* azithromycin (systemic) *on page* 111
Riva-Baclofen [Can] *see* baclofen *on page* 115
Riva-Buspirone [Can] *see* buspirone *on page* 157
Riva-Ciprofloxacin [Can] *see* ciprofloxacin (systemic) *on page* 224
Riva-Citalopram [Can] *see* citalopram *on page* 227
Riva-Clarithromycin [Can] *see* clarithromycin *on page* 229
Riva-Clindamycin [Can] *see* clindamycin (systemic) *on page* 232
Riva-Cycloprine [Can] *see* cyclobenzaprine *on page* 258
Riva-Dicyclomine [Can] *see* dicyclomine *on page* 299
Riva-Enalapril [Can] *see* enalapril *on page* 348
Riva-Fenofibrate Micro [Can] *see* fenofibrate *on page* 393
Riva-Fluconazole [Can] *see* fluconazole *on page* 407
Riva-Fluoxetine [Can] *see* fluoxetine *on page* 415
Riva-Fluvox [Can] *see* fluvoxamine *on page* 422
Riva-Fosinopril [Can] *see* fosinopril *on page* 428
Riva-Gabapentin [Can] *see* gabapentin *on page* 433
Riva-Glyburide [Can] *see* glyburide *on page* 448
Riva-Indapamide [Can] *see* indapamide *on page* 504
Riva-Lisinopril [Can] *see* lisinopril *on page* 570
Riva-Loperamine [Can] *see* loperamide *on page* 573
Riva-Lovastatin [Can] *see* lovastatin *on page* 579
Riva-Memantine [Can] *see* memantine *on page* 599
Riva-Metformin [Can] *see* metformin *on page* 609
Riva-Metoprolol [Can] *see* metoprolol *on page* 625
Riva-Minocycline [Can] *see* minocycline *on page* 635
Riva-Mirtazapine [Can] *see* mirtazapine *on page* 637
Riva-Naproxen [Can] *see* naproxen *on page* 659
Rivanase AQ [Can] *see* beclomethasone (nasal) *on page* 120
Riva-Norfloxacin [Can] *see* norfloxacin *on page* 684
Riva-Oxazepam [Can] *see* oxazepam *on page* 712
Riva-Oxybutynin [Can] *see* oxybutynin *on page* 713
Riva-Pantoprazole [Can] *see* pantoprazole *on page* 725
Riva-paroxetine [Can] *see* paroxetine *on page* 729
Riva-Pravastatin [Can] *see* pravastatin *on page* 789
Riva-Quetiapine [Can] *see* quetiapine *on page* 821
Riva-Rabeprazole EC [Can] *see* rabeprazole *on page* 824

Riva-Ranitidine [Can] *see* ranitidine *on page 828*
Riva-Risperidone [Can] *see* risperidone *on page 845*

rivaroxaban *(Canada only)* (riv a ROX a ban)

Synonyms BAY 59-7939

U.S./Canadian Brand Names Xarelto® [Can]

Therapeutic Category Factor Xa Inhibitor

Use Postoperative thromboprophylaxis in patients who have undergone elective total hip or knee replacement procedures

Dosage Summary

Oral:

Children: Dosage not established

Adults: 10 mg /day

Dosage Forms - Canada

Tablet:

Xarelto®: 10 mg

Riva-Sertraline [Can] *see* sertraline *on page 872*
Riva-Simvastatin [Can] *see* simvastatin *on page 877*
Rivasol [Can] *see* zinc sulfate *on page 1002*
Riva-Sotalol [Can] *see* sotalol *on page 892*

rivastigmine (ri va STIG meen)

Synonyms ENA 713; rivastigmine tartrate; SDZ ENA 713

U.S./Canadian Brand Names Exelon® [US/Can]; Mylan-Rivastigmine [Can]; Novo-Rivastigmine [Can]; PMS-Rivastigmine [Can]; ratio-Rivastigmine [Can]; Sandoz-Rivastigmine [Can]

Therapeutic Category Acetylcholinesterase Inhibitor; Cholinergic Agent

Use Treatment of mild-to-moderate dementia associated with Alzheimer disease or Parkinson disease

Dosage Summary

Oral:

Children: Dosage not established

Adults: Initial: 1.5 mg twice daily; Maintenance: 1.5-6 mg twice daily (maximum: 12 mg/day); **Note:** Titration is recommended

Transdermal patch:

Children: Dosage not established

Adults: Initial: 4.6 mg/24 hours; if well tolerated, may be increased (after at least 4 weeks) to 9.5 mg/24 hours (recommended effective dose). Maintenance: 9.5 mg/24 hours (maximum dose: 9.5 mg/24 hours)

Dosage Forms

Capsule, oral: 1.5 mg, 3 mg, 4.5 mg, 6 mg

Exelon®: 1.5 mg, 3 mg, 4.5 mg, 6 mg

Patch, transdermal:

Exelon®: 4.6 mg/24 hours (30s); 9.5 mg/24 hours (30s)

Solution, oral:

Exelon®: 2 mg/mL (120 mL)

rivastigmine tartrate *see* rivastigmine *on page 848*
Riva-Sumatriptan [Can] *see* sumatriptan *on page 904*
Riva-Terbinafine [Can] *see* terbinafine (systemic) *on page 917*
Riva-Valacyclovir [Can] *see* valacyclovir *on page 973*
Riva-Venlafaxine XR [Can] *see* venlafaxine *on page 981*
Riva-Verapamil SR [Can] *see* verapamil *on page 981*
Riva-Zide [Can] *see* hydrochlorothiazide and triamterene *on page 479*
Riva-Zopiclone [Can] *see* zopiclone *(Canada only) on page 1005*
Rivotril® [Can] *see* clonazepam *on page 237*

rizatriptan (rye za TRIP tan)

Synonyms MK462

U.S./Canadian Brand Names Maxalt RPD™ [Can]; Maxalt-MLT® [US]; Maxalt® [US/Can]

Therapeutic Category Antimigraine Agent; Serotonin Agonist
Use Acute treatment of migraine with or without aura
Dosage Summary
Oral:
Children: Dosage not established
Adults: 5-10 mg once, repeat after 2 hours if needed (maximum: 30 mg/day)
Dosage Forms
Tablet, oral:
Maxalt®: 5 mg, 10 mg
Tablet, orally disintegrating, oral:
Maxalt-MLT®: 5 mg, 10 mg

rLFN-α2 *see* interferon alfa-2b *on page 514*
R-modafinil *see* armodafinil *on page 95*
RMS® ***(Discontinued)*** *see* morphine (systemic) *on page 644*
Ro 5488 *see* tretinoin (systemic) *on page 951*
RoActemra® *see* tocilizumab *on page 939*
Robafen [US-OTC] *see* guaifenesin *on page 454*
Robafen AC [US] *see* guaifenesin and codeine *on page 455*
Robafen® CF ***(Discontinued)***
Robafen Cough [US-OTC] *see* dextromethorphan *on page 287*
Robafen DM [US-OTC] *see* guaifenesin and dextromethorphan *on page 455*
Robafen DM Clear [US-OTC] *see* guaifenesin and dextromethorphan *on page 455*
Robaxin® [US/Can] *see* methocarbamol *on page 613*
Robaxin®-750 [US] *see* methocarbamol *on page 613*
Robidrine® [Can] *see* pseudoephedrine *on page 810*
Robinul® [US] *see* glycopyrrolate *on page 450*
Robinul® Forte [US] *see* glycopyrrolate *on page 450*
Robitussin® [Can] *see* guaifenesin *on page 454*
Robitussin® A-C ***(Discontinued)*** *see* guaifenesin and codeine *on page 455*
Robitussin® Chest Congestion [US-OTC] *see* guaifenesin *on page 454*
Robitussin® Childrens Cough & Cold [Can] *see* pseudoephedrine and dextromethorphan *on page 812*
Robitussin® Children's Cough Long Acting [US-OTC] *see* dextromethorphan *on page 287*
Robitussin® Children's Cough & Cold Long-Acting [US-OTC] *see* dextromethorphan and chlorpheniramine *on page 288*
Robitussin® Cold and Cough CF [US-OTC] *see* guaifenesin, dextromethorphan, and phenylephrine *on page 458*
Robitussin® Cough and Allergy ***(Discontinued)*** *see* chlorpheniramine, phenylephrine, and dextromethorphan *on page 211*
Robitussin® Cough and Cold [Can] *see* guaifenesin, pseudoephedrine, and dextromethorphan *on page 460*
Robitussin® Cough and Cold D [US-OTC] *see* guaifenesin, pseudoephedrine, and dextromethorphan *on page 460*
Robitussin® Cough and Cold Nighttime [US-OTC] *see* chlorpheniramine, phenylephrine, and dextromethorphan *on page 211*
Robitussin® Cough and Congestion [US-OTC] *see* guaifenesin and dextromethorphan *on page 455*
Robitussin® Cough & Cold Long-Acting [US-OTC] *see* dextromethorphan and chlorpheniramine *on page 288*
Robitussin® CoughGels™ Long-Acting [US-OTC] *see* dextromethorphan *on page 287*
Robitussin® Cough Long-Acting [US-OTC] *see* dextromethorphan *on page 287*
Robitussin®-DAC ***(Discontinued)*** *see* guaifenesin, pseudoephedrine, and codeine *on page 459*
Robitussin® DM [US-OTC/Can] *see* guaifenesin and dextromethorphan *on page 455*
Robitussin® DM Infant ***(Discontinued)*** *see* guaifenesin and dextromethorphan *on page 455*
Robitussin® Maximum Strength Cough & Cold ***(Discontinued)*** *see* pseudoephedrine and dextromethorphan *on page 812*

Robitussin® Night Time Cough & Cold [US-OTC] *see* diphenhydramine and phenylephrine *on page* *312*

Robitussin® Pediatric Cold and Cough CF [US-OTC] *see* guaifenesin, dextromethorphan, and phenylephrine *on page* *458*

Robitussin® Pediatric Cough and Cold Nighttime [US-OTC] *see* chlorpheniramine, phenylephrine, and dextromethorphan *on page* *211*

Robitussin® Pediatric Cough & Cold *(Discontinued)* *see* pseudoephedrine and dextromethorphan *on page* *812*

Robitussin® Pediatric Cough *(Discontinued)* *see* dextromethorphan *on page* *287*

Robitussin® Pediatric Night Relief *(Discontinued)* *see* chlorpheniramine, pseudoephedrine, and dextromethorphan *on page* *214*

Robitussin-PE® *(Discontinued)* *see* guaifenesin and pseudoephedrine *on page* *457*

Robitussin® Severe Congestion *(Discontinued)* *see* guaifenesin and pseudoephedrine *on page* *457*

Robitussin® Sugar Free Cough [US-OTC] *see* guaifenesin and dextromethorphan *on page* *455*

Rocaltrol® [US/Can] *see* calcitriol *on page* *165*

Rocephin® [US/Can] *see* ceftriaxone *on page* *194*

rocuronium (roe kyoor OH nee um)

Sound-Alike/Look-Alike Issues

Zemuron® may be confused with Remeron®

Synonyms ORG 946; rocuronium bromide

U.S./Canadian Brand Names Rocuronium Bromide Injection [Can]; Zemuron® [US/Can]

Therapeutic Category Skeletal Muscle Relaxant

Use Facilitate both rapid sequence and routine endotracheal intubation and to relax skeletal muscles during surgery; to facilitate mechanical ventilation in ICU patients

Dosage Summary

I.V.:

Neonates <28 days: Initial: 0.45-0.6 mg/kg; Maintenance: 0.15 mg/kg **or** 7-10 **mcg**/kg/minute
Infants 28 days to 3 months: Initial: 0.45-0.6 mg/kg; Maintenance: 0.15 mg/kg **or** 7-10 **mcg**/kg/minute
Children ≥3 months: Initial: 0.45-0.6 mg/kg; Maintenance: 0.15 mg/kg **or** 7-10 **mcg**/kg/minute
Adults: 0.1-1.2 mg/kg; Infusion: 8-12 **mcg**/kg/minute

Dosage Forms

Injection, solution: 10 mg/mL (5 mL, 10 mL)
Zemuron®: 10 mg/mL (5 mL, 10 mL)

rocuronium bromide *see* rocuronium *on page* *850*

Rocuronium Bromide Injection [Can] *see* rocuronium *on page* *850*

Rofact™ [Can] *see* rifampin *on page* *841*

Roferon®-A *(Discontinued)*

Rogaine® [Can] *see* minoxidil (topical) *on page* *636*

Rogaine® Extra Strength for Men [US-OTC] *see* minoxidil (topical) *on page* *636*

Rogaine® for Men [US-OTC] *see* minoxidil (topical) *on page* *636*

Rogaine® for Women [US-OTC] *see* minoxidil (topical) *on page* *636*

Rogitine® [Can] *see* phentolamine *on page* *750*

Rolaids® [US-OTC] *see* calcium carbonate and magnesium hydroxide *on page* *168*

Rolaids® Extra Strength [US-OTC] *see* calcium carbonate *on page* *167*

Rolaids® Extra Strength [US-OTC] *see* calcium carbonate and magnesium hydroxide *on page* *168*

Rolatuss® Plain Liquid *(Discontinued)* *see* chlorpheniramine and phenylephrine *on page* *208*

Romazicon® [US/Can] *see* flumazenil *on page* *409*

romidepsin (roe mi DEP sin)

Sound-Alike/Look-Alike Issues

romidepsin may be confused with romiplostim

Synonyms depsipeptide; FK228; FR901228

U.S./Canadian Brand Names Istodax® [US]

Therapeutic Category Antineoplastic Agent, Histone Deacetylase Inhibitor

Use Treatment of cutaneous T-cell lymphoma (CTCL)

Dosage Summary

I.V.:

Children: Dosage not established

Adults: 14 mg/m^2 days 1, 8, and 15 of a 28-day treatment cycle

Dosage Forms

Injection, powder for reconstitution:

Istodax®: 10 mg

Romilar® AC ***(Discontinued)*** *see* guaifenesin and codeine *on page 455*

romiplostim (roe mi PLOE stim)

Sound-Alike/Look-Alike Issues

romiplostim may be confused with romidepsin

Synonyms AMG 531

U.S./Canadian Brand Names Nplate™ [US/Can]

Therapeutic Category Colony-Stimulating Factor; Thrombopoietic Agent

Use Treatment of thrombocytopenia in patients with chronic immune (idiopathic) thrombocytopenia purpura (ITP) who have had insufficient response to corticosteroids, immune globulin, or splenectomy

Dosage Summary

SubQ:

Children: Dosage not established

Adults: Initial: 1 mcg/kg once weekly; adjust dose by 1 mcg/kg/week to achieve platelet count ≥50,000/mm^3 and reduce the risk of bleeding; Maximum: 10 mcg/kg

Dosage Forms

Injection, powder for reconstitution:

Nplate™: 250 mcg, 500 mcg

Romycin® ***(Discontinued)*** *see* erythromycin (ophthalmic) *on page 362*

Rondec® [US] *see* chlorpheniramine and phenylephrine *on page 208*

Rondec®-DM [US] *see* chlorpheniramine, phenylephrine, and dextromethorphan *on page 211*

Rondec®-DM Drops ***(Discontinued)***

Rondec®-DM Syrup ***(Discontinued)*** *see* brompheniramine, pseudoephedrine, and dextromethorphan *on page 149*

Rondec® Drops ***(Discontinued)***

Rondec® Syrup ***(Discontinued)*** *see* brompheniramine and pseudoephedrine *on page 148*

Rondomycin® Capsule ***(Discontinued)***

ropinirole (roe PIN i role)

Sound-Alike/Look-Alike Issues

ropinirole may be confused with risperidone, ropivacaine

Requip® may be confused with Reglan®

Synonyms ropinirole hydrochloride

U.S./Canadian Brand Names CO Ropinirole [Can]; JAMP-Ropinirole [Can]; PMS-Ropinirole [Can]; RAN™-Ropinirole [Can]; Requip® XL™ [US]; Requip® [US/Can]

Therapeutic Category Anti-Parkinson Agent (Dopamine Agonist)

Use Treatment of idiopathic Parkinson disease; in patients with early Parkinson disease who were not receiving concomitant levodopa therapy as well as in patients with advanced disease on concomitant levodopa; treatment of moderate-to-severe primary restless legs syndrome (RLS)

Dosage Summary

Oral:

Children: Dosage not established

Adults:

Parkinson: Immediate release: Initial: 0.25 mg 3 times/day; Maintenance: 0.75-24 mg/day in 3 divided doses. Extended-release: Initial: 2 mg once daily; Maintenance: 2-24 mg once daily (maximum: 24 mg/day); **Note:** Titration is recommended

Restless legs: Immediate release: Initial: 0.25 mg prior to bedtime; Maintenance: 0.25-4 mg prior to bedtime; **Note:** Titration is recommended

Dosage Forms

Tablet, oral: 0.25 mg, 0.5 mg, 1 mg, 2 mg, 3 mg, 4 mg, 5 mg

Requip®: 0.25 mg, 0.5 mg, 1 mg, 2 mg, 3 mg, 4 mg, 5 mg

Tablet, extended release, oral:

Requip® XL™: 2 mg, 4 mg, 6 mg, 8 mg, 12 mg

ropinirole hydrochloride *see* ropinirole *on page 851*

ropivacaine (roe PIV a kane)

Sound-Alike/Look-Alike Issues

ropivacaine may be confused with bupivacaine, ropinirole

Synonyms ropivacaine hydrochloride

U.S./Canadian Brand Names Naropin® [US/Can]

Therapeutic Category Local Anesthetic

Use Local anesthetic for use in surgery, postoperative pain management, and obstetrical procedures when local or regional anesthesia is needed

Dosage Summary

Epidural:

Lumbar:

Children: Dosage not established

Adults: 10-30 mL of 0.2% to 1% solution **or** 15-20 mL of 0.75% solution; Infusion: 6-14 mL/hour of 0.2% solution, with incremental injections of 10-15 mL/hour of 0.2% solution

Thoracic:

Children: Dosage not established

Adults: 5-15 mL of 0.5% to 0.75% solution; Infusion: 6-14 mL/hour of 0.2% solution

Field Block:

Children: Dosage not established

Adults: 1-40 mL (5-200 mg) of 0.5% solution

Infiltration:

Children: Dosage not established

Adults: 1-100 mL of 0.2% solution **or** 1-40 mL of 0.5% solution

Nerve Block:

Children: Dosage not established

Adults: Major: 35-50 mL (175-250 mg) of 0.5% solution **or** 10-40 mL (75-300 mg) of 0.75% solution; Minor: 1-100 mL of 0.2% solution **or** 1-40 mL of 0.5% solution

Dosage Forms

Injection, solution [preservative free]:

Naropin®: 2 mg/mL (10 mL, 20 mL, 100 mL, 200 mL); 5 mg/mL (20 mL, 30 mL); 7.5 mg/mL (20 mL); 10 mg/mL (10 mL, 20 mL)

ropivacaine hydrochloride *see* ropivacaine *on page 852*

Rosac® *(Discontinued)* *see* sulfur and sulfacetamide *on page 903*

Rosanil® [US] *see* sulfur and sulfacetamide *on page 903*

Rosasol® [Can] *see* metronidazole (topical) *on page 627*

rosiglitazone (roh si GLI ta zone)

Sound-Alike/Look-Alike Issues

Avandia® may be confused with Avalide®, Coumadin®, Prandin®

U.S./Canadian Brand Names Avandia® [US/Can]

Therapeutic Category Hypoglycemic Agent, Oral; Thiazolidinedione Derivative

Use Type 2 diabetes mellitus (noninsulin-dependent, NIDDM):

Monotherapy: Improve glycemic control as an adjunct to diet and exercise

Note: Canadian labeling approves use as monotherapy only when metformin is contraindicated or not tolerated.

Combination therapy: **Note:** Use when diet, exercise, and a single agent do not result in adequate glycemic control.

U.S. labeling: In combination with a sulfonylurea, metformin, or sulfonylurea plus metformin

Canadian labeling: In combination with metformin; in combination with a sulfonylurea only when metformin use is contraindicated or not tolerated

Dosage Summary

Oral:

Children: Dosage not established

Adults: Initial: 4 mg/day in 1-2 divided doses; Maintenance: 4-8 mg/day in 1-2 divided doses. **Note:** All patients should be initiated at the lowest recommended dose.

Dosage Forms

Tablet, oral:

Avandia®: 2 mg, 4 mg, 8 mg

rosiglitazone and glimepiride (roh si GLI ta zone & GLYE me pye ride)

Synonyms glimepiride and rosiglitazone maleate

U.S./Canadian Brand Names Avandaryl® [US]

Therapeutic Category Antidiabetic Agent, Sulfonylurea; Antidiabetic Agent, Thiazolidinedione

Use Management of type 2 diabetes mellitus (noninsulin-dependent, NIDDM) as an adjunct to diet and exercise

Dosage Summary

Oral:

Children: Dosage not established

Adults: Initial: Rosiglitazone 4 mg and glimepiride 1-2 mg once daily; Maintenance: Rosiglitazone 4-8 mg and glimepiride 1-4 mg once daily; **Note:** Titration is recommended

Elderly: Initial: Rosiglitazone 4 mg and glimepiride 1 mg once daily; **Note:** Titration is recommended

Dosage Forms

Tablet:

Avandaryl®: 4 mg/1 mg: Rosiglitazone 4 mg and glimepiride 1 mg; 4 mg/2 mg: Rosiglitazone 4 mg and glimepiride 2 mg; 4 mg/4 mg: Rosiglitazone 4 mg and glimepiride 4 mg; 8 mg/2 mg: Rosiglitazone 8 mg and glimepiride 2 mg; 8 mg/4 mg: Rosiglitazone 8 mg and glimepiride 4 mg

rosiglitazone and metformin (roh si GLI ta zone & met FOR min)

Sound-Alike/Look-Alike Issues

Avandamet® may be confused with Anzemet®

Synonyms metformin and rosiglitazone; metformin hydrochloride and rosiglitazone maleate; rosiglitazone maleate and metformin hydrochloride

U.S./Canadian Brand Names Avandamet® [US/Can]

Therapeutic Category Antidiabetic Agent (Biguanide); Antidiabetic Agent (Thiazolidinedione)

Use Management of type 2 diabetes mellitus (noninsulin-dependent, NIDDM) as an adjunct to diet and exercise in patients where dual rosiglitazone and metformin therapy is appropriate

Dosage Summary

Oral:

Children: Dosage not established

Adults: Initial: Rosiglitazone 2 mg and metformin 500 mg once or twice daily; may increase by 2 mg/500 mg per day after 4 weeks (maximum: rosiglitazone 8 mg/day; metformin 2000 mg/day)

Elderly ≥80 years: Do not use unless normal renal function has been established

Dosage Forms

Tablet:

Avandamet®: 2/500: Rosiglitazone 2 mg and metformin 500 mg; 4/500: Rosiglitazone 4 mg and metformin 500 mg; 2/1000: Rosiglitazone 2 mg and metformin 1000 mg; 4/1000: Rosiglitazone 4 mg and metformin 1000 mg

rosiglitazone maleate and metformin hydrochloride *see* rosiglitazone and metformin *on page 853*

Rosula® [US] *see* sulfur and sulfacetamide *on page 903*

Rosula® Clarifying [US] *see* sulfur and sulfacetamide *on page 903*

Rosula® NS [US] *see* sulfacetamide (topical) *on page 900*

rosuvastatin (roe soo va STAT in)

Sound-Alike/Look-Alike Issues

rosuvastatin may be confused with atorvastatin, nystatin, pitavastatin

Synonyms rosuvastatin calcium

U.S./Canadian Brand Names Crestor® [US/Can]

Therapeutic Category Antilipemic Agent, HMG-CoA Reductase Inhibitor

Use

Treatment of dyslipidemias:

Used with dietary therapy for hyperlipidemias to reduce elevations in total cholesterol (TC), LDL-C, apolipoprotein B, nonHDL-C, and triglycerides (TG) in patients with primary hypercholesterolemia (elevations of 1 or more components are present in Fredrickson type IIa, IIb, and IV hyperlipidemias); increase HDL-C; treatment of primary dysbetalipoproteinemia (Fredrickson type III hyperlipidemia); treatment of homozygous familial hypercholesterolemia (FH); to slow progression of atherosclerosis as an adjunct to diet to lower TC and LDL-C

Heterozygous familial hypercholesterolemia (HeFH): In adolescent patients (10-17 years of age, females >1 year postmenarche) with HeFH having LDL-C >190 mg/dL or LDL >160 mg/dL with positive family history of premature cardiovascular disease (CVD), or ≥2 other CVD risk factors.

Primary prevention of cardiovascular disease: To reduce the risk of stroke, myocardial infarction, or arterial revascularization procedures in patients without clinically evident coronary heart disease or lipid abnormalities but with all of the following: 1) an increased risk of cardiovascular disease based on age ≥50 years old in men and ≥60 years old in women, 2) hsCRP ≥2 mg/L, and 3) the presence of at least one additional cardiovascular disease risk factor such as hypertension, low HDL-C, smoking, or a family history of premature coronary heart disease.

Secondary prevention of cardiovascular disease: To slow progression of atherosclerosis

Dosage Summary

Oral:

Children <10 years: Dosage not established

Children 10-17 years (females >1 year postmenarche): Initial: 5-20 mg once daily (maximum: 20 mg/day)

Adults: Initial: 5-20 mg once daily; Maintenance: 5-40 mg once daily (maximum: 40 mg/day); **Note:** Titration is recommended

Dosage Forms

Tablet, oral:

Crestor®: 5 mg, 10 mg, 20 mg, 40 mg

rosuvastatin calcium *see* rosuvastatin *on page 853*

Rotarix® [US/Can] *see* rotavirus vaccine *on page 854*

RotaShield® ***(Discontinued)***

RotaTeq® [US/Can] *see* rotavirus vaccine *on page 854*

rotavirus vaccine (ROE ta vye rus vak SEEN)

Synonyms human rotavirus vaccine, attenuated (HRV); pentavalent human-bovine reassortant rotavirus vaccine (PRV); rotavirus vaccine, pentavalent; RV1 (RotaTeq®); RV5 (Rotarix®)

U.S./Canadian Brand Names Rotarix® [US/Can]; RotaTeq® [US/Can]

Therapeutic Category Vaccine

Use Prevention of rotavirus gastroenteritis in infants and children

The Advisory Committee on Immunization Practices (ACIP) recommends routine vaccination of all infants.

Dosage Summary

Oral:

Infants <6 weeks: Dosage not established

Infants 6-24 weeks: Rotarix®: A total of two 1 mL doses, the first dose given at 6 weeks of age. The first and second dose should be separated by ≥4 weeks. The 2-dose series should be completed by 24 weeks of age.

Infants 6-32 weeks: RotaTeq®: A total of three 2 mL doses; the first given at 2-, 4-, and 6 months of age, given at 6-12 weeks of age, followed by subsequent doses at 4-10 week intervals

Children >24 weeks: Rotarix®: Dosage not established

Children >32 weeks: RotaTeq®: Dosage not established

Adults: Dosage not established

Dosage Forms

Powder, for suspension, oral [preservative free; human derived]:

Rotarix®: G1P[8] ≥10^6 infectious units per 1 mL [oral applicator contains natural latex/natural rubber]

Suspension, oral [preservative free]:

RotaTeq®: G1 ≥2.2 10^6 infectious units, G2 ≥2.8 10^6 infectious units, G3 ≥2.2 10^6 infectious units, G4 ≥2 10^6 infectious units, and P1 [8] ≥2.3 10^6 infectious units per 2 mL (2 mL)

rotavirus vaccine, pentavalent *see* rotavirus vaccine *on page 854*
rotigotine *(Discontinued)*
Rowasa® [US] *see* mesalamine *on page 607*
Roxanol™ *(Discontinued)* *see* morphine (systemic) *on page 644*
Roxanol SR™ Oral *(Discontinued)* *see* morphine (systemic) *on page 644*
Roxanol™-T *(Discontinued)* *see* morphine (systemic) *on page 644*
Roxicet™ [US] *see* oxycodone and acetaminophen *on page 715*
Roxicet™ 5/500 [US] *see* oxycodone and acetaminophen *on page 715*
Roxicodone® [US] *see* oxycodone *on page 714*
Roxiprin® *(Discontinued)* *see* oxycodone and aspirin *on page 716*
Roychlor® [Can] *see* potassium chloride *on page 781*
Rozerem™ [US] *see* ramelteon *on page 826*
RP-6976 *see* docetaxel *on page 321*
RP-54274 *see* riluzole *on page 843*
RP-59500 *see* quinupristin and dalfopristin *on page 823*
r-PA *see* reteplase *on page 836*
rPDGF-BB *see* becaplermin *on page 119*
RPR-116258A *see* cabazitaxel *on page 162*
(R,R)-formoterol L-tartrate *see* arformoterol *on page 93*
RS-25259 *see* palonosetron *on page 721*
RS-25259-197 *see* palonosetron *on page 721*
R-Tanna [US] *see* chlorpheniramine and phenylephrine *on page 208*
R-Tanna Pediatric [US] *see* chlorpheniramine and phenylephrine *on page 208*
RTCA *see* ribavirin *on page 839*
RU 0211 *see* lubiprostone *on page 580*
RU-486 *see* mifepristone *on page 633*
RU-23908 *see* nilutamide *on page 676*
RU-38486 *see* mifepristone *on page 633*
rubella, measles, and mumps vaccines *see* measles, mumps, and rubella virus vaccine *on page 592*
rubella, varicella, measles, and mumps vaccine *see* measles, mumps, rubella, and varicella virus vaccine *on page 593*

rubella virus vaccine (live) (rue BEL a VYE rus vak SEEN, live)

Sound-Alike/Look-Alike Issues

Meruvax® II may be confused with Attenuvax®

Synonyms German measles vaccine

Therapeutic Category Vaccine, Live Virus

Use Active immunization against rubella

Note: Unless otherwise contraindicated, trivalent measles - mumps - rubella (MMR) is the vaccine of choice if recipients are likely to be susceptible to mumps and/or measles as well as to rubella.

The Advisory Committee on Immunization Practices (ACIP) recommends routine vaccination for the following:

- All children (first dose given at 12-15 months of age)
- Adults born 1957 or later (without evidence of immunity or documentation of vaccination)
- Adults at higher risk for exposure to and transmission of rubella should receive special consideration for vaccination, unless an acceptable evidence of immunity exists. This includes international travelers, persons attending colleges and other post-high school education, persons working in healthcare facilities.

Dosage Summary

SubQ:

Children <12 months: Dosage not established

Children ≥12 months: 0.5 mL as a single dose at 12-15 months of age; revaccinate prior to elementary school (at least 28 days should elapse between doses)

Adults: 0.5 mL as a single dose

rubeola vaccine *see* measles virus vaccine (live) *on page 593*

Rubex® ***(Discontinued)*** *see* doxorubicin *on page* *330*
rubidomycin hydrochloride *see* daunorubicin hydrochloride *on page* *271*
Rubramin-PC® ***(Discontinued)*** *see* cyanocobalamin *on page* *257*
RUF 331 *see* rufinamide *on page* *856*

rufinamide (roo FIN a mide)

Synonyms CGP 33101; E 2080; RUF 331; xilep
U.S./Canadian Brand Names Banzel™ [US]
Therapeutic Category Anticonvulsant, Triazole Derivative
Use Adjunctive therapy in the treatment of generalized seizures of Lennox-Gastaut syndrome

Dosage Summary

Oral:

Children <4 years: Dosage not established

Children ≥4 years: Initial: 10 mg/kg/day in 2 equally divided doses (maximum: 45 mg/kg/day or 3200 mg/day); **Note:** Titration is recommended

Adults: Initial: 400-800 mg/day in 2 equally divided doses (maximum: 3200 mg/day); **Note:** Titration is recommended

Dosage Forms

Tablet, oral:
Banzel™: 200 mg, 400 mg

Ru-Hist Forte [US] *see* chlorpheniramine, pyrilamine, and phenylephrine *on page* *215*
Rulox [US-OTC] *see* aluminum hydroxide, magnesium hydroxide, and simethicone *on page* *59*
Rulox No. 1 ***(Discontinued)*** *see* aluminum hydroxide and magnesium hydroxide *on page* *59*
Ru-Tuss DM [US] *see* guaifenesin, pseudoephedrine, and dextromethorphan *on page* *460*
Ru-Tuss® Liquid ***(Discontinued)*** *see* chlorpheniramine and phenylephrine *on page* *208*
Ru-Vert-M® ***(Discontinued)*** *see* meclizine *on page* *595*
RV1 (RotaTeq®) *see* rotavirus vaccine *on page* *854*
RV5 (Rotarix®) *see* rotavirus vaccine *on page* *854*
RWJ-270201 *see* peramivir *on page* *743*
Rybix™ ODT [US] *see* tramadol *on page* *946*
Rylosol [Can] *see* sotalol *on page* *892*
Rymed® ***(Discontinued)*** *see* guaifenesin and pseudoephedrine *on page* *457*
Rymed-TR® ***(Discontinued)***
Ryna®-12 [US] *see* phenylephrine and pyrilamine *on page* *753*
Ryna-12 S® [US] *see* phenylephrine and pyrilamine *on page* *753*
Ryna-12X® [US] *see* phenylephrine, pyrilamine, and guaifenesin *on page* *756*
Ryna-C® ***(Discontinued)*** *see* chlorpheniramine, pseudoephedrine, and codeine *on page* *214*
Ryna® ***(Discontinued)*** *see* chlorpheniramine, pseudoephedrine, and codeine *on page* *214*
Rynatan® [US] *see* chlorpheniramine and phenylephrine *on page* *208*
Rynatan® Pediatric [US] *see* chlorpheniramine and phenylephrine *on page* *208*
Rynatuss® [US] *see* chlorpheniramine, ephedrine, phenylephrine, and carbetapentane *on page* *210*
Rynatuss® Pediatric ***(Discontinued)*** *see* chlorpheniramine, ephedrine, phenylephrine, and carbetapentane *on page* *210*
Rynesa 12S ***(Discontinued)*** *see* phenylephrine and pyrilamine *on page* *753*
Ry-T-12 ***(Discontinued)*** *see* phenylephrine and pyrilamine *on page* *753*
Rythmodan® [Can] *see* disopyramide *on page* *318*
Rythmodan®-LA [Can] *see* disopyramide *on page* *318*
Rythmol® [US] *see* propafenone *on page* *803*
Rythmol® Gen-Propafenone [Can] *see* propafenone *on page* *803*
Rythmol® SR [US] *see* propafenone *on page* *803*
Ryzolt™ [US] *see* tramadol *on page* *946*
S2® [US-OTC] *see* epinephrine (systemic, oral inhalation) *on page* *352*
S-(+)-3-isobutylgaba *see* pregabalin *on page* *792*
6(S)-5-methyltetrahydrofolate *see* methylfolate *on page* *620*

6(S)-5-MTHF *see* methylfolate *on page* *620*

S-4661 *see* doripenem *on page* *326*

Sabril® [US/Can] *see* vigabatrin *on page* *984*

Saccharomyces boulardii (sak roe MYE sees boo LAR dee)

Synonyms *S. boulardii; Saccharomyces boulardii lyo*

U.S./Canadian Brand Names Florastor® Kids [US-OTC]; Florastor® [US-OTC]

Therapeutic Category Dietary Supplement; Probiotic

Use Promote maintenance of normal microflora in the gastrointestinal tract; used in management of bloating, gas, and diarrhea, particularly to decrease the incidence of diarrhea associated with antibiotic use

Dosage Summary

Oral:

Children: Florastor® Kids: 250 mg twice daily

Adults: Florastor®: 250 mg twice daily

Dosage Forms

Capsule, oral:

Florastor® [OTC]: S. boulardii lyo 250 mg

Powder, oral:

Florastor® Kids [OTC]: S. boulardii lyo 250 mg/packet (10s)

Saccharomyces boulardii lyo *see Saccharomyces boulardii on page* *857*

sacrosidase (sak ROE si dase)

U.S./Canadian Brand Names Sucraid® [US/Can]

Therapeutic Category Enzyme

Use **Orphan drug:** Oral replacement therapy in sucrase deficiency, as seen in congenital sucrase-isomaltase deficiency (CSID)

Dosage Summary

Oral:

Infants <5 months: Dosage not established

Infants ≥5 and <15 kg: 8500 int. units (1 mL) per meal or snack

Children <15 kg: 8500 int. units (1 mL) per meal or snack

Children >15 kg: 17,000 int. units (2 mL) per meal or snack

Adults: 17,000 int. units (2 mL) per meal or snack

Dosage Forms

Solution, oral:

Sucraid®: 8500 int. units/mL (118 mL)

Safetussin® CD [US-OTC] *see* dextromethorphan and phenylephrine *on page* *289*

Safe Tussin® DM [US-OTC] *see* guaifenesin and dextromethorphan *on page* *455*

SAHA *see* vorinostat *on page* *992*

Saizen® [US/Can] *see* somatropin *on page* *889*

SalAc® *(Discontinued)* *see* salicylic acid *on page* *858*

Sal-Acid® *(Discontinued)* *see* salicylic acid *on page* *858*

Salacid® Ointment *(Discontinued)* *see* salicylic acid *on page* *858*

Salactic® [US-OTC] *see* salicylic acid *on page* *858*

Salagen® [US/Can] *see* pilocarpine (systemic) *on page* *760*

Salazopyrin® [Can] *see* sulfasalazine *on page* *902*

Salazopyrin En-Tabs® [Can] *see* sulfasalazine *on page* *902*

salbutamol *see* albuterol *on page* *43*

salbutamol and ipratropium *see* ipratropium and albuterol *on page* *524*

salbutamol sulphate *see* albuterol *on page* *43*

Saleto-200® *(Discontinued)* *see* ibuprofen *on page* *494*

Saleto-400® *(Discontinued)* *see* ibuprofen *on page* *494*

Salex® [US] *see* salicylic acid *on page* *858*

Salflex® [Can] *see* salsalate *on page* *862*

Salgesic® *(Discontinued)* *see* salsalate *on page* *862*

salicylazosulfapyridine *see* sulfasalazine *on page* 902

salicylic acid (sal i SIL ik AS id)

Sound-Alike/Look-Alike Issues

Occlusal®-HP may be confused with Ocuflox®

U.S./Canadian Brand Names Aliclen™ [US]; Beta Sal® [US-OTC]; Clean & Clear® Advantage® Acne Cleanser [US-OTC]; Clean & Clear® Advantage® Acne Spot Treatment [US-OTC]; Clean & Clear® Advantage® Invisible Acne Patch [US-OTC]; Clean & Clear® Advantage® Oil-Free Acne [US-OTC]; Clean & Clear® Blackhead Clearing Daily Cleansing [US-OTC]; Clean & Clear® Blackhead Clearing Scrub [US-OTC]; Clean & Clear® Continuous Control® Acne Wash [US-OTC]; Clean & Clear® Deep Cleaning [US-OTC]; Clean & Clear® Dual Action Moisturizer [US-OTC]; Clean & Clear® Invisible Blemish Treatment [US-OTC]; Compound W® One Step Invisible Strip [US-OTC]; Compound W® One Step Wart Remover for Feet [US-OTC]; Compound W® One Step Wart Remover for Kids [US-OTC]; Compound W® One Step Wart Remover [US-OTC]; Compound W® [US-OTC]; Curad® Mediplast® [US-OTC]; Denorex® Extra Strength Protection 2-in-1 [US-OTC]; Denorex® Extra Strength Protection [US-OTC]; Dermarest® Psoriasis Medicated Moisturizer [US-OTC]; Dermarest® Psoriasis Medicated Scalp Treatment [US-OTC]; Dermarest® Psoriasis Medicated Shampoo/Conditioner [US-OTC]; Dermarest® Psoriasis Medicated Skin Treatment [US-OTC]; Dermarest® Psoriasis Overnight Treatment [US-OTC]; DHS™ Sal [US-OTC]; Dr. Scholl's® Callus Removers [US-OTC]; Dr. Scholl's® Clear Away® One Step Wart Remover [US-OTC]; Dr. Scholl's® Clear Away® Plantar Wart Remover For Feet [US-OTC]; Dr. Scholl's® Clear Away® Wart Remover Fast-Acting [US-OTC]; Dr. Scholl's® Clear Away® Wart Remover Invisible Strips [US-OTC]; Dr. Scholl's® Clear Away® Wart Remover [US-OTC]; Dr. Scholl's® Corn Removers [US-OTC]; Dr. Scholl's® Corn/Callus Remover [US-OTC]; Dr. Scholl's® Extra Thick Corn Removers [US-OTC]; Dr. Scholl's® Extra-Thick Callus Removers [US-OTC]; Dr. Scholl's® For Her Corn Removers [US-OTC]; Dr. Scholl's® OneStep Callus Removers [US-OTC]; Dr. Scholl's® OneStep Corn Removers [US-OTC]; Dr. Scholl's® Small Corn Removers [US-OTC]; Dr. Scholl's® Ultra-Thin Corn Removers [US-OTC]; DuoFilm® [US-OTC/Can]; Duoforte® 27 [Can]; Durasal™ [US]; Freezone® [US-OTC]; Fung-O® [US-OTC]; Gets-It® [US-OTC]; Gordofilm [US-OTC]; Hydrisalic® [US-OTC]; Ionil Plus® [US-OTC]; Ionil® [US-OTC]; Keralyt® [US-OTC]; Keralyt® [US]; LupiCare® Dandruff [US-OTC]; LupiCare® Psoriasis [US-OTC]; MG217® Sal-Acid [US-OTC]; Mosco® Callus & Corn Remover [US-OTC]; Mosco® One Step Corn Remover [US-OTC]; Neutrogena® Acne Stress Control [US-OTC]; Neutrogena® Advanced Solutions™ [US-OTC]; Neutrogena® Blackhead Eliminating™ 2-in-1 Foaming Pads [US-OTC]; Neutrogena® Blackhead Eliminating™ Daily Scrub [US-OTC]; Neutrogena® Blackhead Elinimating™ [US-OTC]; Neutrogena® Body Clear® [US-OTC]; Neutrogena® Clear Pore™ Oil-Controlling Astringent [US-OTC]; Neutrogena® Maximum Strength T/Sal® [US-OTC]; Neutrogena® Oil-Free Acne Stress Control [US-OTC]; Neutrogena® Oil-Free Acne Wash 60 Second Mask Scrub [US-OTC]; Neutrogena® Oil-Free Acne Wash Cream Cleanser [US-OTC]; Neutrogena® Oil-Free Acne Wash Foam Cleanser [US-OTC]; Neutrogena® Oil-Free Acne Wash [US-OTC]; Neutrogena® Oil-Free Acne [US-OTC]; Neutrogena® Oil-Free Anti-Acne [US-OTC]; Neutrogena® Rapid Clear® Acne Defense [US-OTC]; Neutrogena® Rapid Clear® Acne Eliminating [US-OTC]; Neutrogena® Rapid Clear® [US-OTC]; Occlusal™-HP [Can]; OXY® Body Wash [US-OTC]; OXY® Daily Cleansing [US-OTC]; OXY® Daily [US-OTC]; OXY® Face Wash [US-OTC]; OXY® Maximum Daily Cleansing [US-OTC]; OXY® Maximum [US-OTC]; OXY® Post-Shave [US-OTC]; OXY® Spot Treatment [US-OTC]; P&S® [US-OTC]; Palmer's® Skin Success Acne Cleanser [US-OTC]; Sal-Plant® [US-OTC]; Salactic® [US-OTC]; Salex® [US]; Salitop™ [US]; Salvax [US]; Scalpicin® Anti-Itch [US-OTC]; Sebcur® [Can]; Soluver® Plus [Can]; Soluver® [Can]; Stridex® Essential Care® [US-OTC]; Stridex® Facewipes To Go® [US-OTC]; Stridex® Maximum Strength [US-OTC]; Stridex® Sensitive Skin [US-OTC]; Thera-Sal [US-OTC]; Tinamed® Corn and Callus Remover [US-OTC]; Tinamed® Wart Remover [US-OTC]; Trans-Plantar® [Can]; Trans-Ver-Sal® [US-OTC/Can]; Wart-Off® Maximum Strength [US-OTC]; Zapzyt® Acne Wash [US-OTC]; Zapzyt® Pore Treatment [US-OTC]

Therapeutic Category Keratolytic Agent

Use Topically for its keratolytic effect in controlling seborrheic dermatitis or psoriasis of body and scalp, dandruff, and other scaling dermatoses; also used to remove warts, corns, and calluses; acne

Dosage Summary

Topical:

Children <12 years: Consult specific product labeling

Children ≥12 years: Apply 1-4 times/day as directed; Consult specific product labeling

Adults: Apply 1-4 times/day as directed; Consult specific product labeling

Dosage Forms

Aerosol, topical: 6% (70 g)

Salvax: 6% (70 g, 200 g)

Bar, topical: 2% (113 g)
OXY® [OTC]: 0.5% (119 g)
Cloth, topical:
Neutrogena® Oil-Free Acne Wash [OTC]: 2% (30s)
Cream, topical: 6% (400 g)
Clean & Clear® Advantage® Acne Cleanser [OTC]: 2% (148 mL)
Clean & Clear® Advantage® Acne Spot Treatment [OTC]: 2% (22 g)
Clean & Clear® Blackhead Clearing Scrub [OTC]: 2% (141 g, 226 g)
Clean & Clear® Dual Action Moisturizer [OTC]: 0.5% (120 mL)
LupiCare® Psoriasis [OTC]: 2% (227 g)
Neutrogena® Acne Stress Control [OTC]: 2% (125 g)
Neutrogena® Oil-Free Acne [OTC]: 2% (125 mL)
Neutrogena® Oil-Free Acne Stress Control [OTC]: 2% (172 g)
Neutrogena® Oil-Free Acne Wash Cream Cleanser [OTC]: 2% (200 mL)
Neutrogena® Oil-Free Anti-Acne [OTC]: 0.5% (50 g)
Salex®: 6% (454 g)
Salitop™: 6% (400 g)
Gel, topical:
Clean & Clear® Advantage® Invisible Acne Patch [OTC]: 2% (1.9 mL)
Clean & Clear® Invisible Blemish Treatment [OTC]: 2% (22 mL)
Compound W® [OTC]: 17.6% (7 g)
Dermarest® Psoriasis Medicated Scalp Treatment [OTC]: 3% (118 mL)
Dermarest® Psoriasis Medicated Skin Treatment [OTC]: 3% (118 mL)
Dermarest® Psoriasis Overnight Treatment [OTC]: 3% (56.7 g)
Hydrisalic® [OTC]: 6% (28 g)
Keralyt® [OTC]: 3% (30 g); 6% (40 g, 100 g)
Neutrogena® Advanced Solutions™ [OTC]: 2% (40 g)
Neutrogena® Oil-Free Acne Wash [OTC]: 2% (177 mL, 296 mL)
Neutrogena® Rapid Clear® Acne Eliminating [OTC]: 2% (15 mL)
OXY® [OTC]: 2% (355 mL)
OXY® Body Wash [OTC]: 2% (355 mL)
OXY® Chill Factor® [OTC]: 2% (142 g)
OXY® Face Wash [OTC]: 2% (177 mL)
OXY® Maximum [OTC]: 2% (142 g)
OXY® Spot Treatment [OTC]: 1% (14.7 g)
Sal-Plant® [OTC]: 17% (14 g)
Zapzyt® Acne Wash [OTC]: 2% (188.5 g)
Zapzyt® Pore Treatment [OTC]: 2% (22 mL)
Liquid, topical:
Clean & Clear® Advantage® Oil-Free Acne [OTC]: 0.5% (120 mL)
Clean & Clear® Continuous Control® Acne Wash [OTC]: 2% (177 mL)
Clean & Clear® Deep Cleaning [OTC]: 2% (240 mL)
Compound W® [OTC]: 17.6% (9 mL)
Dr. Scholl's® Clear Away® Wart Remover Fast-Acting [OTC]: 17% (9.8 mL)
Dr. Scholl's® Corn/Callus Remover [OTC]: 12.6% (9.8 mL)
DuoFilm® [OTC]: 17% (9.8 mL)
Durasal™: 26% (10 mL)
Freezone® [OTC]: 17.6% (9.3 mL)
Fung-O® [OTC]: 17% (15 mL)
Gets-It® [OTC]: 13.9% (15 mL)
Gordofilm [OTC]: 16.7% (15 mL)
Mosco® Callus & Corn Remover [OTC]: 17.6% (9 mL)
Neutrogena® Blackhead Eliminating™ Daily Scrub [OTC]: 2% (125 mL)
Neutrogena® Body Clear® [OTC]: 2% (250 mL)
Neutrogena® Clear Pore™ Oil-Controlling Astringent [OTC]: 2% (236 mL)
Neutrogena® Oil-Free Acne Stress Control [OTC]: 0.5% (177 mL); 2% (50 mL)
Neutrogena® Oil-Free Acne Wash 60 Second Mask Scrub [OTC]: 1% (170 g)
Neutrogena® Oil-Free Acne Wash Foam Cleanser [OTC]: 2% (150 mL)
Palmer's® Skin Success Acne Cleanser [OTC]: 0.5% (240 mL)
Salactic® [OTC]: 17% (15 mL)
Scalpicin® Anti-Itch [OTC]: 3% (44 mL, 74 mL)
Tinamed® Corn and Callus Remover [OTC]: 17% (15 mL)

Tinamed® Wart Remover [OTC]: 17% (15 mL)
Wart-Off® Maximum Strength [OTC]: 17.5% (14.8 mL)

Lotion, topical: 6% (414 mL, 420 mL)
Dermarest® Psoriasis Medicated Moisturizer [OTC]: 2% (118 mL)
Neutrogena® Rapid Clear® Acne Defense [OTC]: 2% (50 mL)
OXY® Post-Shave [OTC]: 0.5% (50 g)
Salex®: 6% (237 mL)
Salitop™: 6% (414 mL)

Ointment, topical:
MG217® Sal-Acid [OTC]: 3% (57 g)

Pad, topical:
Clean & Clear® Blackhead Clearing Daily Cleansing [OTC]: 1% (70s)
Curad® Mediplast® [OTC]: 40% (25s)
Neutrogena® Blackhead Eliminating™ 2-in-1 Foaming Pads [OTC]: 0.5% (28s)
Neutrogena® Blackhead Elinimating™ [OTC]: 0.5% (28s)
Neutrogena® Rapid Clear® [OTC]: 2% (60s)
OXY® Chill Factor® [OTC]: 2% (90s)
OXY® Daily [OTC]: 0.2% (90s)
OXY® Daily Cleansing [OTC]: 0.5% (90s)
OXY® Maximum Daily Cleansing [OTC]: 2% (55s, 90s)
Stridex® Essential Care® [OTC]: 1% (55s)
Stridex® Facewipes To Go® [OTC]: 0.5% (32s)
Stridex® Maximum Strength [OTC]: 2% (55s, 90s)
Stridex® Sensitive Skin [OTC]: 0.5% (55s, 90s)

Patch, topical:
Compound W® One Step Invisible Strip [OTC]: 14% (14s)
Compound W® One Step Wart Remover for Feet [OTC]: 40% (20s)
Compound W® One-Step Wart Remover [OTC]: 40% (14s)
Compound W® One-Step Wart Remover for Kids [OTC]: 40% (12s)
Dr. Scholl's® Callus Removers [OTC]: 40% (4s)
Dr. Scholl's® Clear Away® One Step Wart Remover [OTC]: 40% (14s)
Dr. Scholl's® Clear Away® Plantar Wart Remover For Feet [OTC]: 40% (24s)
Dr. Scholl's® Clear Away® Wart Remover [OTC]: 40% (18s)
Dr. Scholl's® Clear Away® Wart Remover Invisible Strips [OTC]: 40% (18s)
Dr. Scholl's® Corn Removers [OTC]: 40% (9s)
Dr. Scholl's® Extra Thick Corn Removers [OTC]: 40% (9s)
Dr. Scholl's® Extra-Thick Callus Removers [OTC]: 40% (4s)
Dr. Scholl's® For Her Corn Removers [OTC]: 40% (6s)
Dr. Scholl's® OneStep Callus Removers [OTC]: 40% (4s)
Dr. Scholl's® OneStep Corn Removers [OTC]: 40% (6s)
Dr. Scholl's® Small Corn Removers [OTC]: 40% (9s)
Dr. Scholl's® Ultra-Thin Corn Removers [OTC]: 40% (9s)
Mosco® One Step Corn Remover [OTC]: 40% (8s)
Trans-Ver-Sal® [OTC]: 15% (10s, 12s, 15s, 25s, 40s)

Shampoo, topical: 6% (177 mL)
Aliclen™: 6% (177 mL)
Beta Sal® [OTC]: 3% (480 mL)
Denorex® Extra Strength Protection [OTC]: 3% (118 mL, 355 mL)
DHS™ Sal [OTC]: 3% (120 mL)
Ionil Plus® [OTC]: 2% (240 mL)
Ionil® [OTC]: 2% (120 mL)
LupiCare® Dandruff [OTC]: 2% (237 mL)
LupiCare® Psoriasis [OTC]: 2% (237 mL)
Neutrogena® Maximum Strength T/Sal® [OTC]: 3% (135 mL)
P&S® [OTC]: 2% (118 mL, 236 mL)
Salex®: 6% (177 mL)
Thera-Sal [OTC]: 3% (180 mL)

Shampoo/Conditioner, topical:
Denorex® Extra Strength Protection 2-in-1 [OTC]: 3% (118 mL, 355 mL)
Dermarest® Psoriasis Medicated Shampoo/Conditioner [OTC]: 3% (236 mL)

salicylic acid and coal tar *see* coal tar and salicylic acid *on page* 243

salicylsalicylic acid *see* salsalate *on page* 862

saline *see* sodium chloride *on page 882*
Saline Mist [US-OTC] *see* sodium chloride *on page 882*
SalineX® *(Discontinued)* *see* sodium chloride *on page 882*
Salitop™ [US] *see* salicylic acid *on page 858*
Salivart® *(Discontinued)* *see* saliva substitute *on page 861*

saliva substitute (sa LYE va SUB stee tute)

Synonyms artificial saliva

U.S./Canadian Brand Names Aquoral™ [US]; Caphosol® [US]; Entertainer's Secret® [US-OTC]; Moi-Stir® [US-OTC]; Mouthkote® [US-OTC]; Numoisyn™ [US]; Oasis® [US]; Oral Balance® [US-OTC]; SalivaSure™ [US-OTC]

Therapeutic Category Gastrointestinal Agent, Miscellaneous

Use Relief of dry mouth and throat in xerostomia or hyposalivation; adjunct to standard oral care in relief of symptoms associated with chemotherapy or radiation therapy-induced mucositis

Dosage Summary

Oral:

Children: Dosage not established

Adults: Use as needed or 2-10 doses/day (Caphosol®) or 2 mL as needed (Numoisyn™ liquid) or 1 lozenge as needed; maximum 16 lozenges/day (Numoisyn™ lozenges) or 30 mL 2 times a day and as needed (Oasis® mouthwash) or 1-2 sprays as needed; maximum 60 sprays/day (Oasis® Spray) or 4 times a day and as needed (Oral Balance®)

Dosage Forms

Liquid:

Numoisyn™: Water, sorbitol, linseed extract, *Chondrus crispus*, methylparaben, sodium benzoate, potassium sorbate, dipotassium phosphate, propylparaben

Oral Balance® [OTC]: Water, starch, sunflower oil, propylene glycol, xylitol, glycerine, purified milk extract

Lozenge:

Numoisyn™: Sorbitol 0.3 g/lozenge, polyethylene glycol, malic acid, sodium citrate, calcium phosphate dibasic, hydrogenated cottonseed oil, citric acid, magnesium stearate, silicon dioxide

SalivaSure™ [OTC]: Xylitol, citric acid, apple acid, sodium citrate dihydrate, sodium carboxymethylcellulose, dibasic calcium phosphate, silica colloidal, magnesium stearate, stearic acid

Solution, oral:

Caphosol®: Dibasic sodium phosphate 0.032%, monobasic sodium phosphate 0.009%, calcium chloride 0.052%, sodium chloride 0.569%, purified water

Entertainer's Secret® [OTC]: Sodium carboxymethylcellulose, aloe vera gel, glycerin (60 mL)

Solution, oral [mouthwash/gargle]:

Oasis®: Water, glycerin, sorbitol, poloxamer 338, PEG-60, hydrogenated castor oil, copovidone, sodium benzoate, carboxymethycellulose

Solution, oral [spray]:

Aquoral™: Oxidized glycerol triesters and silicon dioxide

Moi-Stir® [OTC]: Water, sorbitol, sodium carboxymethylcellulose, methylparaben, propylparaben, potassium chloride, dibasic sodium phosphate, calcium chloride, magnesium chloride, sodium chloride

Mouthkote® [OTC]: Water, xylitol, sorbitol, yerba santa, citric acid, ascorbic acid, sodium saccharin, sodium benzoate

Oasis®: Glycerin, cetylpyridinium, copovidone

Saliva Substitute® *(Discontinued)* *see* saliva substitute *on page 861*
SalivaSure™ [US-OTC] *see* saliva substitute *on page 861*
salk vaccine *see* poliovirus vaccine (inactivated) *on page 774*

salmeterol (sal ME te role)

Sound-Alike/Look-Alike Issues

salmeterol may be confused with Salbutamol, Solu-Medrol®

Serevent® may be confused with Atrovent®, Combivent®, Serentil®, sertraline, Sinemet®, Spiriva®, Zoloft®

Synonyms salmeterol xinafoate

U.S./Canadian Brand Names Serevent® Diskhaler® Disk [Can]; Serevent® Diskus® [US/Can]

Therapeutic Category Adrenergic Agonist Agent

Use Maintenance treatment of asthma; prevention of bronchospasm with reversible obstructive airway disease, including patients with symptoms of nocturnal asthma; prevention of exercise-induced bronchospasm; maintenance treatment of bronchospasm associated with COPD

Dosage Summary

Inhalation:

Children <4 years: Dosage not established

Children ≥4 years: One inhalation (50 mcg) twice daily

Adults: One inhalation (50 mcg) twice daily

Dosage Forms

Powder, for oral inhalation:

Serevent® Diskus®: 50 mcg (28s, 60s)

Dosage Forms - Canada

Powder for oral inhalation:

Serevent® Diskhaler® Disk: 50 mcg (60s)

salmeterol and fluticasone *see* fluticasone and salmeterol *on page 420*

salmeterol xinafoate *see* salmeterol *on page 861*

Salmonine® *(Discontinued)* *see* calcitonin *on page 165*

Salofalk® [Can] *see* mesalamine *on page 607*

Salonpas® [US-OTC] *see* methyl salicylate and menthol *on page 623*

Salonpas® Arthritis Pain® [US-OTC] *see* methyl salicylate and menthol *on page 623*

Salonpas® Hot [US-OTC] *see* capsaicin *on page 175*

Salonpas® Pain Relief Patch® [US-OTC] *see* methyl salicylate and menthol *on page 623*

Sal-Plant® [US-OTC] *see* salicylic acid *on page 858*

salsalate (SAL sa late)

Sound-Alike/Look-Alike Issues

salsalate may be confused with sucralfate, sulfasalazine

Synonyms disalicylic acid; salicylsalicylic acid

U.S./Canadian Brand Names Amigesic® [Can]; Salflex® [Can]

Therapeutic Category Analgesic, Nonnarcotic; Antipyretic; Nonsteroidal Antiinflammatory Drug (NSAID)

Use Treatment of minor pain or fever; arthritis

Dosage Summary

Oral:

Children: Dosage not established

Adults: 3 g/day in 2-3 divided doses

Dosage Forms

Tablet, oral: 500 mg, 750 mg

Salsitab® *(Discontinued)* *see* salsalate *on page 862*

salt *see* sodium chloride *on page 882*

salt-poor albumin *see* albumin *on page 43*

Sal-Tropine™ [US] *see* atropine *on page 105*

Salvax [US] *see* salicylic acid *on page 858*

Samsca™ [US] *see* tolvaptan *on page 941*

Sanctura® [US] *see* trospium *on page 964*

Sanctura® XR [US/Can] *see* trospium *on page 964*

Sancuso® [US] *see* granisetron *on page 452*

Sandimmune® [US] *see* cyclosporine (systemic) *on page 260*

Sandimmune® I.V. [Can] *see* cyclosporine (systemic) *on page 260*

Sandomigran® [Can] *see* pizotifen *(Canada only) on page 765*

Sandomigran DS® [Can] *see* pizotifen *(Canada only) on page 765*

Sandostatin® [US/Can] *see* octreotide *on page 694*

Sandostatin LAR® [US/Can] *see* octreotide *on page 694*

Sandoz-Acebutolol [Can] *see* acebutolol *on page 21*

Sandoz Alendronate [Can] *see* alendronate *on page 47*

Sandoz-Alfuzosin [Can] *see* alfuzosin *on page 49*

sapropterin (sap roe TER in)

Sound-Alike/Look-Alike Issues
sapropterin may be confused with cyproterone

Synonyms 6R-BH4; phenoptin; sapropterin dihydrochloride

U.S./Canadian Brand Names Kuvan™ [US]

Therapeutic Category Enzyme Cofactor

Use Adjunct to dietary management in the treatment of tetrahydrobiopterin (BH4) responsive phenylketonuria (PKU)

Dosage Summary

Oral:

Children <4 years: Dosage not established
Children ≥4 years: 10 mg/kg once daily; Maintenance range: 5-20 mg/kg/day
Adults: 10 mg/kg once daily; Maintenance range: 5-20 mg/kg/day

Dosage Forms

Tablet:

Kuvan™: 100 mg

saquinavir (sa KWIN a veer)

Sound-Alike/Look-Alike Issues

saquinavir may be confused with Sinequan®

Synonyms saquinavir mesylate

U.S./Canadian Brand Names Invirase® [US/Can]

Therapeutic Category Antiviral Agent

Use Treatment of HIV infection; used in combination with at least two other antiretroviral agents

Dosage Summary

Oral:

Children ≤16 years: Dosage not established

Children >16 years: 1000 mg (with ritonavir 100 mg) twice daily; **Note:** Saquinavir (Invirase®) should not be used in "unboosted regimens."

Adults: 1000 mg (with ritonavir 100 mg) twice daily; **Note:** Saquinavir (Invirase®) should not be used in "unboosted regimens."

Dosage Forms

Capsule, oral:

Invirase®: 200 mg

Tablet, oral:

Invirase®: 500 mg

saquinavir mesylate *see* saquinavir *on page* *865*

Sarafem® [US] *see* fluoxetine *on page* *415*

sargramostim (sar GRAM oh stim)

Sound-Alike/Look-Alike Issues

Leukine® may be confused with Leukeran®, leucovorin

Synonyms GM-CSF; granulocyte-macrophage colony-stimulating factor; NSC-613795; rGM-CSF

U.S./Canadian Brand Names Leukine® [US/Can]

Therapeutic Category Colony-Stimulating Factor

Use

Acute myelogenous leukemia (AML) following induction chemotherapy in older adults (≥55 years of age) to shorten time to neutrophil recovery and to reduce the incidence of severe and life-threatening infections and infections resulting in death

Bone marrow transplant (allogeneic or autologous) failure or engraftment delay

Myeloid reconstitution after allogeneic bone marrow transplantation

Myeloid reconstitution after autologous bone marrow transplantation: Non-Hodgkin lymphoma (NHL), acute lymphoblastic leukemia (ALL), Hodgkin lymphoma

Peripheral stem cell transplantation: Mobilization and myeloid reconstitution following autologous peripheral stem cell transplantation

Dosage Summary

I.V.:

Children: Infusion: 250 mcg/m^2/day (maximum: 500 mcg/m^2 /day)

Adults: Infusion: 250 mcg/m^2/day (maximum: 500 mcg/m^2/day)

SubQ:

Children: 250 mcg/m^2 once daily

Adults: 250 mcg/m^2 once daily

Dosage Forms

Injection, powder for reconstitution:

Leukine®: 250 mcg

Injection, solution:

Leukine®: 500 mcg/mL (1 mL)

Sarna® HC [Can] *see* hydrocortisone (topical) *on page* *483*

Sarna® Sensitive [US-OTC] *see* pramoxine *on page* *787*

Sarna® Ultra [US-OTC] *see* pramoxine *on page* *787*

Sarnol®-HC [US] *see* hydrocortisone (topical) *on page* *483*

Sativex® [Can] *see* tetrahydrocannabinol and cannabidiol *(Canada only) on page* *923*

Savella® [US] *see* milnacipran *on page* *634*

saxagliptin (sax a GLIP tin)

Sound-Alike/Look-Alike Issues
saxagliptin may be confused with sitaGLIPtin, SUMAtriptan

Synonyms BMS-477118

U.S./Canadian Brand Names Onglyza™ [US/Can]

Therapeutic Category Antidiabetic Agent, Dipeptidyl Peptidase IV (DPP-IV) Inhibitor

Use Treatment of type 2 diabetes mellitus (noninsulin-dependent, NIDDM) as an adjunct to diet and exercise as monotherapy or in combination therapy with other antidiabetic agents to improve glycemic control

Dosage Summary

Oral:

Children: Dosage not established

Adults: 2.5-5 mg once daily

Dosage Forms

Tablet, oral:

Onglyza™: 2.5 mg, 5 mg

SB-265805 *see* gemifloxacin *on page 441*

SB-497115 *see* eltrombopag *on page 346*

SB-497115-GR *see* eltrombopag *on page 346*

S. boulardii *see Saccharomyces boulardii on page 857*

SC 33428 *see* idarubicin *on page 497*

Scalpicin® Anti-Itch [US-OTC] *see* salicylic acid *on page 858*

Scalp Mycin [US-OTC] *see* hydrocortisone (topical) *on page 483*

Scandonest® 2% L [US] *see* mepivacaine and levonordefrin *on page 605*

Scandonest® 3% Plain [US] *see* mepivacaine *on page 604*

SCH 13521 *see* flutamide *on page 418*

SCH 56592 *see* posaconazole *on page 779*

ScheinPharm Ranitidine [Can] *see* ranitidine *on page 828*

SCIG *see* immune globulin (subcutaneous) *on page 503*

S-citalopram *see* escitalopram *on page 363*

Scleromate® [US] *see* morrhuate sodium *on page 646*

Sclerosol® [US] *see* talc (sterile) *on page 908*

Scopace™ [US] *see* scopolamine derivatives (systemic) *on page 866*

scopolamine and phenylephrine *see* phenylephrine and scopolamine *on page 753*

scopolamine base *see* scopolamine derivatives (systemic) *on page 866*

scopolamine butylbromide *see* scopolamine derivatives (systemic) *on page 866*

scopolamine derivatives (systemic) (skoe POL a meen dah RIV ah tives)

Synonyms hyoscine butylbromide; scopolamine base; scopolamine butylbromide; scopolamine hydrobromide

U.S./Canadian Brand Names Buscopan® [Can]; Scopace™ [US]; Transderm Scōp® [US]; Transderm-V® [Can]

Therapeutic Category Anticholinergic Agent

Use

Scopolamine base: Transdermal: Prevention of nausea/vomiting associated with motion sickness and recovery from anesthesia and surgery

Scopolamine hydrobromide:

Injection: Preoperative medication to produce amnesia, sedation, tranquilization, antiemetic effects, and decrease salivary and respiratory secretions

Oral: Symptomatic treatment of postencephalitic parkinsonism and paralysis agitans; in spastic states; inhibits excessive motility and hypertonus of the gastrointestinal tract in such conditions as the irritable colon syndrome, mild dysentery, diverticulitis, pylorospasm, and cardiospasm

Scopolamine butylbromide [not available in the U.S.]: Oral/injection: Treatment of smooth muscle spasm of the genitourinary or gastrointestinal tract; injection may also be used to prior to radiological/diagnostic procedures to prevent spasm

Dosage Summary

I.M.:

Children <6 months: Dosage not established
Children 6 months to 3 years: 0.1-0.15 mg
Children 3-6 years: 0.2-0.3 mg
Adults: 0.3-0.65 mg (single dose) **or** 0.6 mg 3-4 times/day

I.V.:

Children <6 months: Dosage not established
Children 6 months to 3 years: 0.1-0.15 mg
Children 3-6 years: 0.2-0.3 mg
Adults: 0.3-0.65 mg (single dose) **or** 0.6 mg 3-4 times/day

Oral:

Children: Dosage not established
Adults: 0.4-0.8 mg as a single dose or every 8-12 hours as needed.

SubQ:

Children <6 months: Dosage not established
Children 6 months to 3 years: 0.1-0.15 mg
Children 3-6 years: 0.2-0.3 mg
Adults: 0.3-0.65 mg (single dose) **or** 0.6 mg 3-4 times/day

Transdermal:

Children: Dosage not established
Adults: Apply 1 patch behind ear at least 4 hours prior to exposure and every 3 days as needed

Dosage Forms

Injection, solution: 0.4 mg/mL (1 mL)

Patch, transdermal:
Transderm Scōp®: 1.5 mg (4s, 10s, 24s)

Tablet, soluble, oral:
Scopace™: 0.4 mg

Dosage Forms - Canada

Injection, solution:
Buscopan®: 20 mg/mL

Tablet:
Buscopan®: 10 mg

scopolamine derivatives (ophthalmic) (skoe POL a meen dah RIV ah tives)

Synonyms hyoscine hydrobromide; scopolamine hydrobromide

U.S./Canadian Brand Names Isopto® Hyoscine [US]

Therapeutic Category Anticholinergic Agent; Anticholinergic Agent, Ophthalmic; Ophthalmic Agent, Mydriatic

Use **Scopolamine hydrobromide:** Produce cycloplegia and mydriasis; treatment of iridocyclitis

Dosage Summary

Ophthalmic:

Children: Instill 1 drop (0.25%) to eye(s) up to 3 times/day
Adults: Instill 1-2 drops (0.25%) eye(s) up to 4 times/day

Dosage Forms

Solution, ophthalmic:
Isopto® Hyoscine: 0.25% (5 mL)

scopolamine hydrobromide *see* scopolamine derivatives (ophthalmic) *on page* 867
scopolamine hydrobromide *see* scopolamine derivatives (systemic) *on page* 866
scopolamine, hyoscyamine, atropine, and phenobarbital *see* hyoscyamine, atropine, scopolamine, and phenobarbital *on page* 492
Scot-Tussin® Diabetes [US-OTC] *see* dextromethorphan *on page* 287
Scot-Tussin DM® Cough Chasers *(Discontinued)* *see* dextromethorphan *on page* 287
Scot-Tussin® DM Maximum Strength [US-OTC] *see* dextromethorphan and chlorpheniramine *on page* 288
Scot-Tussin® Expectorant [US-OTC] *see* guaifenesin *on page* 454
Scot-Tussin® Senior [US-OTC] *see* guaifenesin and dextromethorphan *on page* 455
Scytera™ [US-OTC] *see* coal tar *on page* 242
SD/01 *see* pegfilgrastim *on page* 732

SDX-105 *see* bendamustine *on page 122*
SDZ ENA 713 *see* rivastigmine *on page 848*
Seasonale® [US/Can] *see* ethinyl estradiol and levonorgestrel *on page 376*
Seasonique™ [US] *see* ethinyl estradiol and levonorgestrel *on page 376*
Sebcur® [Can] *see* salicylic acid *on page 858*
Sebcur/T® [Can] *see* coal tar and salicylic acid *on page 243*
Sebivo® [Can] *see* telbivudine *on page 912*
Sebizon® ***(Discontinued)*** *see* sulfacetamide (topical) *on page 900*
Seb-Prev™ [US] *see* sulfacetamide (topical) *on page 900*

secobarbital (see koe BAR bi tal)

Sound-Alike/Look-Alike Issues
Seconal® may be confused with Sectral®
Synonyms quinalbarbitone sodium; secobarbital sodium
U.S./Canadian Brand Names Seconal® [US]
Therapeutic Category Barbiturate
Controlled Substance C-II
Use Preanesthetic agent; short-term treatment of insomnia
Dosage Summary
Oral:
Children: 2-6 mg/kg 1-2 hours before procedure (maximum: 100 mg/dose) **or** 6 mg/kg/day divided every 8 hours
Adults: 100-200 mg at bedtime **or** 100-300 mg 1-2 hours before procedure
Elderly: Not recommended
Dosage Forms
Capsule, oral:
Seconal®: 100 mg

secobarbital sodium *see* secobarbital *on page 868*
Seconal® [US] *see* secobarbital *on page 868*
Secran® ***(Discontinued)***
SecreFlo™ ***(Discontinued)*** *see* secretin *on page 868*

secretin (SEE kr tin)

Synonyms secretin, human; secretin, porcine
U.S./Canadian Brand Names ChiRhoStim® [US]
Therapeutic Category Diagnostic Agent
Use Secretin-stimulation testing to aid in diagnosis of pancreatic exocrine dysfunction; diagnosis of gastrinoma (Zollinger-Ellison syndrome); facilitation of endoscopic retrograde cholangiopancreatography (ERCP) visualization
Dosage Summary
I.V.:
Children: Dosage not established
Adults:
Test dose: 0.1 mL (0.2-0.4 mcg)
Diagnostic dose: 0.2-0.4 mcg/kg over 1 minute
Dosage Forms
Injection, powder for reconstitution:
ChiRhoStim®: 16 mcg

secretin, human *see* secretin *on page 868*
secretin, porcine *see* secretin *on page 868*
Sectral® [US/Can] *see* acebutolol *on page 21*
Secura® Antifungal Extra Thick [US-OTC] *see* miconazole (topical) *on page 630*
Secura® Antifungal Greaseless [US-OTC] *see* miconazole (topical) *on page 630*
Sedapap® [US] *see* butalbital and acetaminophen *on page 159*
Selax® [Can] *see* docusate *on page 321*
Select™ 1/35 [Can] *see* ethinyl estradiol and norethindrone *on page 378*

Select-OB™ [US-OTC] *see* vitamins (multiple/prenatal) *on page 991*

selegiline (se LE ji leen)

Sound-Alike/Look-Alike Issues

selegiline may be confused with Salagen®, Serentil®, sertraline, Serzone®, Stelazine®
Eldepryl® may be confused with Elavil®, enalapril
Zelapar™ may be confused with zaleplon, Zemplar®, Zyprexa® Zydis®

Synonyms deprenyl; L-deprenyl; selegiline hydrochloride

U.S./Canadian Brand Names Apo-Selegiline® [Can]; Eldepryl® [US]; Emsam® [US]; Gen-Selegiline [Can]; Mylan-Selegiline [Can]; Novo-Selegiline [Can]; Nu-Selegiline [Can]; Zelapar™ [US]

Therapeutic Category Anti-Parkinson Agent; Dopaminergic Agent (Anti-Parkinson)

Use Adjunct in the management of parkinsonian patients in which levodopa/carbidopa therapy is deteriorating (oral products); treatment of major depressive disorder (transdermal product)

Dosage Summary

Oral:

Capsule/Tablet:

Adults: 5 mg twice daily with breakfast and lunch **or** 10 mg in the morning

Elderly: Initial: 5 mg in the morning; Maintenance: 5-10 mg in the morning

Disintegrating tablet:

Children: Dosage not established

Adults: Initial 1.25 mg daily for at least 6 weeks; may increase to 2.5 mg daily based on clinical response (maximum: 2.5 mg daily)

Elderly: Dosage not established

Transdermal:

Children: Dosage not established

Adults: Initial: 6 mg once daily; Maintenance: 6-12 mg once daily (maximum: 12 mg/day); **Note:** Titration is recommended

Elderly: 6 mg once daily

Dosage Forms

Capsule, oral: 5 mg

Eldepryl®: 5 mg

Patch, transdermal:

Emsam®: 6 mg/24 hours (30s); 9 mg/24 hours (30s); 12 mg/24 hours (30s)

Tablet, oral: 5 mg

Tablet, orally disintegrating, oral:

Zelapar™: 1.25 mg

selegiline hydrochloride *see* selegiline *on page 869*

selenium *see* trace metals *on page 945*

selenium sulfide (se LEE nee um SUL fide)

U.S./Canadian Brand Names Dandrex [US]; Head & Shoulders® Intensive Treatment [US-OTC]; Selseb® [US]; Selsun blue® 2-in-1 Treatment [US-OTC]; Selsun blue® Daily Treatment [US-OTC]; Selsun blue® Medicated Treatment [US-OTC]; Selsun blue® Moisturizing Treatment [US-OTC]; Tersi [US]; Versel® [Can]

Therapeutic Category Antiseborrheic Agent, Topical

Use Treatment of itching and flaking of the scalp associated with dandruff, to control scalp seborrheic dermatitis; treatment of tinea versicolor

Dosage Summary

Topical:

Children: Dosage not established

Adults:

Foam: Rub into affected skin twice daily

Lotion: Apply to affected area daily, leave on for 10 minutes then rinse

Shampoo: Massage 5-10 mL into wet scalp, leave on 2-3 minutes then rinse

Dosage Forms

Aerosol, topical:

Tersi: 2.25% (70 g)

Lotion, topical: 2.5% (118 mL, 120 mL)

Shampoo, topical: 1% (210 mL)
Dandrex: 1% (240 mL)
Head & Shoulders® Intensive Treatment [OTC]: 1% (400 mL, 420 mL)
Selseb®: 2.25% (180 mL)
Selsun blue® 2-in-1 Treatment [OTC]: 1% (207 mL, 325 mL)
Selsun blue® Daily Treatment [OTC]: 1% (207 mL, 325 mL)
Selsun blue® Medicated Treatment [OTC]: 1% (120 mL, 207 mL, 325 mL)
Selsun blue® Moisturizing Treatment [OTC]: 1% (207 mL, 325 mL)

Selfemra® [US] *see* fluoxetine *on page* *415*
Selpak® ***(Discontinued)*** *see* selegiline *on page* *869*
Selseb® [US] *see* selenium sulfide *on page* *869*
Selsun blue® 2-in-1 Treatment [US-OTC] *see* selenium sulfide *on page* *869*
Selsun blue® Daily Treatment [US-OTC] *see* selenium sulfide *on page* *869*
Selsun blue® Medicated Treatment [US-OTC] *see* selenium sulfide *on page* *869*
Selsun blue® Moisturizing Treatment [US-OTC] *see* selenium sulfide *on page* *869*
Selsun Gold® for Women ***(Discontinued)*** *see* selenium sulfide *on page* *869*
Selsun® Salon™ Classic [US-OTC] *see* pyrithione zinc *on page* *819*
Selsun® Salon™ Dandruff 2-in-1 [US-OTC] *see* pyrithione zinc *on page* *819*
Selsun® Salon™ Dandruff Moisturizing [US-OTC] *see* pyrithione zinc *on page* *819*
Selsun® Salon™ Dandruff Volumizing [US-OTC] *see* pyrithione zinc *on page* *819*
Selzentry™ [US] *see* maraviroc *on page* *591*
Semprex®-D [US] *see* acrivastine and pseudoephedrine *on page* *35*
Senatec HC ***(Discontinued)*** *see* lidocaine and hydrocortisone *on page* *564*
Senexon [US-OTC] *see* senna *on page* *870*

senna (SEN na)

Sound-Alike/Look-Alike Issues
Perdiem® may be confused with Pyridium®
Senexon® may be confused with Cenestin®
Senokot® may be confused with Depakote®

Synonyms sennosides

U.S./Canadian Brand Names Black Draught® [US-OTC]; Evac-U-Gen® [US-OTC]; ex-lax® Maximum Strength [US-OTC]; ex-lax® [US-OTC]; Fleet® Pedia-Lax™ Quick Dissolve [US-OTC]; Fletcher's® [US-OTC]; Little Tummys® Laxative [US-OTC]; Perdiem® Overnight Relief [US-OTC]; Senexon [US-OTC]; SennaGen [US-OTC]; Senokot® [US-OTC]

Therapeutic Category Laxative

Use Short-term treatment of constipation; evacuate the colon for bowel or rectal examinations

Dosage Summary

Oral:
Children <2 years: Dosage not established
Children 2-6 years: Initial: 3.75 mg once daily; Maintenance: 3.75-15 mg/day in 1-2 divided doses (maximum: 15 mg/day) **or** 5-10 mL (33.3 mg/mL) up to twice daily
Children 6-12 years: Initial: 8.6 mg once daily; Maintenance: 8.6-50 mg/day in 1-2 divided doses (maximum: 50 mg/day) **or** 10-30 mL (33.3 mg/mL) up to twice daily
Children ≥12 years: Initial: 15 mg once daily; Maintenance: 15-100 mg/day in 1-2 divided doses (maximum: 100 mg/day) **or** 130 mg the afternoon of day prior to surgery
Adults: Initial: 15 mg once daily; Maintenance: 15-100 mg/day in 1-2 divided doses (maximum: 100 mg/day) **or** 130 mg the afternoon of day prior to surgery

Dosage Forms

Liquid, oral:
Fletcher's® [OTC]: Senna concentrate 33.3 mg/mL (75 mL)
Little Tummys® Laxative [OTC]: Sennosides 8.8 mg/mL (30 mL)
Senexon [OTC]: Sennosides 8.8 mg/5 mL (237 mL)

Strip, orally disintegrating, oral:
Fleet® Pedia-Lax™ Quick Dissolve [OTC]: Sennosides 8.6 mg (12s)

Syrup, oral: Sennosides 8.8 mg/5 mL (237 mL, 240 mL)

Tablet, oral: Sennosides 8.6 mg
ex-lax® [OTC]: Sennosides USP 15 mg
ex-lax® Maximum Strength [OTC]: Sennosides USP 25 mg
Perdiem® Overnight Relief [OTC]: Sennosides USP 15 mg
Senexon [OTC]: Sennosides 8.6 mg
SennaGen [OTC]: Sennosides 8.6 mg
Senokot® [OTC]: Sennosides 8.6 mg

Tablet, chewable, oral:
Black Draught® [OTC]: Sennosides 10 mg
Evac-U-Gen® [OTC]: Sennosides 10 mg
ex-lax® [OTC]: Sennosides USP 15 mg

senna and docusate *see* docusate and senna *on page* *322*
SennaGen [US-OTC] *see* senna *on page* *870*
senna-S *see* docusate and senna *on page* *322*
sennosides *see* senna *on page* *870*
Senokot® [US-OTC] *see* senna *on page* *870*
Senokot-S® [US-OTC] *see* docusate and senna *on page* *322*
SenoSol™-X *(Discontinued)* *see* senna *on page* *870*
SenoSol™ *(Discontinued)* *see* senna *on page* *870*
SenoSol™-SS [US-OTC] *see* docusate and senna *on page* *322*
Sensipar® [US/Can] *see* cinacalcet *on page* *223*
Sensorcaine® [US/Can] *see* bupivacaine *on page* *153*
Sensorcaine®-MPF [US] *see* bupivacaine *on page* *153*
Sensorcaine®-MPF Spinal [US] *see* bupivacaine *on page* *153*
Sensorcaine®-MPF with Epinephrine [US] *see* bupivacaine and epinephrine *on page* *154*
Sensorcaine® with Epinephrine [US/Can] *see* bupivacaine and epinephrine *on page* *154*
Sepasoothe® [US-OTC] *see* benzocaine *on page* *124*
Septanest® N [Can] *see* articaine and epinephrine *on page* *96*
Septanest® SP [Can] *see* articaine and epinephrine *on page* *96*
Septa® Topical Ointment *(Discontinued)* *see* bacitracin, neomycin, and polymyxin B *on page* *114*
Septisol® *(Discontinued)* *see* hexachlorophene *on page* *471*
Septocaine® with epinephrine 1:100,000 [US] *see* articaine and epinephrine *on page* *96*
Septocaine® with epinephrine 1:200,000 [US] *see* articaine and epinephrine *on page* *96*
Septra® [US] *see* sulfamethoxazole and trimethoprim *on page* *901*
Septra® DS [US] *see* sulfamethoxazole and trimethoprim *on page* *901*
Septra® Injection [Can] *see* sulfamethoxazole and trimethoprim *on page* *901*
Serax® [US] *see* oxazepam *on page* *712*
Serc® [Can] *see* betahistine *(Canada only) on page* *133*
Serevent® *(Discontinued)* *see* salmeterol *on page* *861*
Serevent® Diskhaler® Disk [Can] *see* salmeterol *on page* *861*
Serevent® Diskus® [US/Can] *see* salmeterol *on page* *861*

sermorelin acetate (ser moe REL in AS e tate)

Therapeutic Category Diagnostic Agent

Use Geref® Diagnostic: For evaluation of the ability of the pituitary gland to secrete growth hormone (GH)

Dosage Summary

I.V.:
Children: 1 mcg/kg as a single dose
Adults: 1 mcg/kg as a single dose

Seromycin® [US] *see* cycloserine *on page* *259*
Serophene® [US/Can] *see* clomiphene *on page* *236*
Seroquel® [US/Can] *see* quetiapine *on page* *821*
Seroquel XR® [US/Can] *see* quetiapine *on page* *821*
Serostim® [US/Can] *see* somatropin *on page* *889*
Serpalan® *(Discontinued)* *see* reserpine *on page* *836*

Serpatabs® *(Discontinued)* *see* reserpine *on page 836*

sertaconazole (ser ta KOE na zole)

Synonyms sertaconazole nitrate

U.S./Canadian Brand Names Ertaczo® [US]

Therapeutic Category Antifungal Agent, Topical

Use Topical treatment of tinea pedis (athlete's foot)

Dosage Summary

Topical:

Children <12 years: Dosage not established
Children ≥12 years: Apply twice daily
Adults: Apply twice daily

Dosage Forms

Cream, topical:

Ertaczo®: 2% (30 g, 60 g)

sertaconazole nitrate *see* sertaconazole *on page 872*

sertraline (SER tra leen)

Sound-Alike/Look-Alike Issues

sertraline may be confused with selegiline, Serentil®, Serevent®, Soriatane®
Zoloft® may be confused with Zocor®

Synonyms sertraline hydrochloride

U.S./Canadian Brand Names Apo-Sertraline® [Can]; CO Sertraline [Can]; Dom-Sertraline [Can]; Mylan-Sertraline [Can]; Novo-Sertraline [Can]; Nu-Sertraline [Can]; PHL-Sertraline [Can]; PMS-Sertraline [Can]; ratio-Sertraline [Can]; Riva-Sertraline [Can]; Sandoz-Sertraline [Can]; Zoloft® [US/Can]

Therapeutic Category Antidepressant, Selective Serotonin Reuptake Inhibitor

Use Treatment of major depression; obsessive-compulsive disorder (OCD); panic disorder; posttraumatic stress disorder (PTSD); premenstrual dysphoric disorder (PMDD); social anxiety disorder

Dosage Summary

Oral:

Children <6 years: Dosage not established
Children 6-12 years: Initial: 25 mg once daily; Maintenance: 25-200 mg once daily (maximum: 200 mg/day); **Note:** Titration is recommended
Children 13-17 years: Initial: 50 mg once daily; Maintenance: 25-200 mg once daily (maximum: 200 mg/day); **Note:** Titration is recommended
Adults: Initial: 25-50 mg once daily; Maintenance: 50-200 mg once daily (maximum: 200 mg/day); **Note:** Titration is recommended
Elderly: Initial: 25 mg once daily in the morning; Maintenance: 50-100 mg once daily (maximum: 200 mg/day); **Note:** Titration is recommended

Dosage Forms

Solution, oral: 20 mg/mL (60 mL)
Zoloft®: 20 mg/mL (60 mL)

Tablet, oral: 25 mg, 50 mg, 100 mg
Zoloft®: 25 mg, 50 mg, 100 mg

sertraline hydrochloride *see* sertraline *on page 872*

Serzone® *(Discontinued)* *see* nefazodone *on page 664*

sevelamer (se VEL a mer)

Sound-Alike/Look-Alike Issues

sevelamer may be confused with Savella™
Renagel® may be confused with Reglan®, Regonol®, Renal Caps, Renvela®
Renvela® may be confused with Reglan®, Regonol®, Renagel®, Renal Caps

Synonyms sevelamer carbonate; sevelamer hydrochloride

U.S./Canadian Brand Names Renagel® [US/Can]; Renvela® [US]

Therapeutic Category Phosphate Binder

Use Reduction or control of serum phosphorous in patients with chronic kidney disease on hemodialysis

Dosage Summary

Oral:

Adults: Initial: 800-1600 mg 3 times/day with meals; Maintenance: Up to 2400-14,000 mg/day in 3 divided doses with meals

Dosage Forms

Powder for suspension, oral:

Renvela®: 0.8 g/packet (90s); 2.4 g/packet (90s)

Tablet, oral:

Renagel®: 400 mg, 800 mg

Renvela®: 800 mg

sevelamer carbonate *see* sevelamer *on page 872*

sevelamer hydrochloride *see* sevelamer *on page 872*

sevoflurane (see voe FLOO rane)

Sound-Alike/Look-Alike Issues

Ultane® may be confused with Ultram®

U.S./Canadian Brand Names Sevorane® AF [Can]; Sojourn Sevoflurane [Can]; Sojourn™ [US]; Ultane® [US]

Therapeutic Category General Anesthetic

Use Induction and maintenance of general anesthesia

Dosage Summary

Inhalation:

Neonates 0-1 month (full-term): 3.3% in O_2

Infants 1-<6 months: 3% in O_2

Children 6 months to <3 years: 2.8% in O_2; 2% in 60% N_20/40% O_2

Children 3-12 years: 2.5% in O_2

Adults 25 years: 2.6% in O_2; 1.4% in 65% N_20/35% O_2

Adults 40 years: 2.1% in O_2; 1.1% in 65% N_20/35% O_2

Adults 60 years: 1.7% in O_2; 0.9% in 65% N_20/35% O_2

Adults 80 years: 1.4% in O_2; 0.7% in 65% N_20/35% O_2

Dosage Forms

Liquid, for inhalation: 100% (250 mL)

Sojourn™: 100% (250 mL)

Ultane®: 100% (250 mL)

Sevorane® AF [Can] *see* sevoflurane *on page 873*

sfRowasa™ [US] *see* mesalamine *on page 607*

shingles vaccine *see* zoster vaccine *on page 1006*

Shur-Seal® ***(Discontinued)*** *see* nonoxynol 9 *on page 681*

Sibelium® [Can] *see* flunarizine *(Canada only) on page 409*

sibutramine (si BYOO tra meen)

Sound-Alike/Look-Alike Issues

Meridia® may be confused with Aredia®

Synonyms sibutramine hydrochloride monohydrate

U.S./Canadian Brand Names Apo-Sibutramine® [Can]; Meridia® [US/Can]

Therapeutic Category Anorexiant

Controlled Substance C-IV

Use Management of obesity in patients with an initial body mass index (BMI) ≥30 kg/m^2 or ≥27 kg/m^2 in the presence of other risk factors (eg, diabetes, hyperlipidemia, hypertension)

Dosage Summary

Oral:

Children <16 years: Dosage not established

Children ≥16 years: Initial: 10 mg once daily; Maintenance: 5-15 mg once daily; **Note:** Titration is recommended

Adults: Initial: 10 mg once daily; Maintenance: 5-15 mg once daily; **Note:** Titration is recommended

Dosage Forms

Capsule, oral:

Meridia®: 5 mg, 10 mg, 15 mg

sibutramine hydrochloride monohydrate *see* sibutramine *on page* 873
Sig-Enalapril [Can] *see* enalapril *on page* 348
Silace [US-OTC] *see* docusate *on page* 321
Siladryl Allergy [US-OTC] *see* diphenhydramine (systemic) *on page* 310
Silafed [US-OTC] *see* triprolidine and pseudoephedrine *on page* 961
Silain® *(Discontinued)* *see* simethicone *on page* 875
Silaminic® Expectorant *(Discontinued)*
Silapap Children's [US-OTC] *see* acetaminophen *on page* 21
Silapap Infant's [US-OTC] *see* acetaminophen *on page* 21
Sildec *(Discontinued)*
Sildec-DM *(Discontinued)*
Sildec PE *(Discontinued)* *see* chlorpheniramine and phenylephrine *on page* 208
Sildec PE-DM *(Discontinued)* *see* chlorpheniramine, phenylephrine, and dextromethorphan *on page* 211
Sildec Syrup [US] *see* brompheniramine and pseudoephedrine *on page* 148

sildenafil (sil DEN a fil)

Sound-Alike/Look-Alike Issues
sildenafil may be confused with silodosin, tadalafil, vardenafil
Revatio® may be confused with ReVia®, Revonto™
Viagra® may be confused with Allegra®, Vaniqa®

Synonyms sildenafil citrate; UK92480

U.S./Canadian Brand Names ratio-Sildenafil R [Can]; Revatio® [US/Can]; Viagra® [US/Can]

Therapeutic Category Phosphodiesterase (Type 5) Enzyme Inhibitor

Use
Revatio®: Treatment of pulmonary arterial hypertension (WHO Group I) to improve exercise ability and delay clinical worsening
Viagra®: Treatment of erectile dysfunction (ED)

Dosage Summary
I.V.:
Children: Dosage not established
Adults: Revatio®: 10 mg 3 times/day
Oral:
Children <1 month: Dosage not established
Adults:
Revatio®: 20 mg 3 times/day
Viagra®: 25-100 mg 30 minutes to 4 hours before sexual activity once daily
Elderly: Use with caution
Revatio®: 20 mg 3 times/day
Viagra®: Initial: 25 mg 30 minutes to 4 hours before sexual activity once daily

Dosage Forms
Injection, solution:
Revatio®: 0.8 mg/mL (12.5 mL)
Tablet, oral:
Revatio®: 20 mg
Viagra®: 25 mg, 50 mg, 100 mg

sildenafil citrate *see* sildenafil *on page* 874
Sildicon-E® *(Discontinued)*
Silexin [US-OTC] *see* guaifenesin and dextromethorphan *on page* 455
Silfedrine Children's [US-OTC] *see* pseudoephedrine *on page* 810

silodosin (SI lo doe sin)

Sound-Alike/Look-Alike Issues
silodosin may be confused with sildenafil
Rapaflo™ may be confused with Rapamune®, Raptiva®

Synonyms KMD 3213

U.S./Canadian Brand Names Rapaflo™ [US]

Therapeutic Category Alpha$_1$ Blocker

Use Treatment of signs and symptoms of benign prostatic hyperplasia (BPH)

Dosage Summary

Oral:

Children: Dosage not established

Adults: Males: 8 mg once daily

Dosage Forms

Capsule, oral:

Rapaflo™: 4 mg, 8 mg

Silphen [US-OTC] *see* diphenhydramine (systemic) *on page 310*

Silphen DM® [US-OTC] *see* dextromethorphan *on page 287*

Sil-Tex [US] *see* guaifenesin and phenylephrine *on page 456*

Siltussin-CF® ***(Discontinued)***

Siltussin DAS [US-OTC] *see* guaifenesin *on page 454*

Siltussin DM [US-OTC] *see* guaifenesin and dextromethorphan *on page 455*

Siltussin DM DAS [US-OTC] *see* guaifenesin and dextromethorphan *on page 455*

Siltussin SA [US-OTC] *see* guaifenesin *on page 454*

Silvadene® [US] *see* silver sulfadiazine *on page 875*

silver nitrate (SIL ver NYE trate)

Synonyms $AgNO_3$

Therapeutic Category Topical Skin Product

Use Cauterization of wounds and sluggish ulcers, removal of granulation tissue and warts; aseptic prophylaxis of burns

Dosage Summary

Topical:

Solution:

Children: Apply a cotton applicator dipped in solution on affected area 2-3 times/day

Adults: Apply a cotton applicator dipped in solution on affected area 2-3 times/day

Sticks:

Children: Apply to area to be treated 2-3 times/week

Adults: Apply to area to be treated 2-3 times/week

Dosage Forms

Applicator sticks, topical: Silver nitrate 75% and potassium 25% (6", 12", 18")

Solution, topical: 0.5% (960 mL); 10% (30 mL); 25% (30 mL); 50% (30 mL)

silver sulfadiazine (SIL ver sul fa DYE a zeen)

U.S./Canadian Brand Names Flamazine® [Can]; Silvadene® [US]; SSD AF® [US]; SSD® [US]; Thermazene® [US]

Therapeutic Category Antibacterial, Topical

Use Prevention and treatment of infection in second and third degree burns

Dosage Summary

Topical:

Children: Apply to a thickness of 1/16" once or twice daily

Adults: Apply to a thickness of 1/16" once or twice daily

Dosage Forms

Cream, topical: 1% (20 g, 25 g, 50 g, 85 g, 400 g)

Silvadene®: 1% (20 g, 50 g, 85 g, 400 g, 1000 g)

SSD AF®: 1% (50 g, 400 g)

SSD®: 1% (25 g, 50 g, 85 g, 400 g)

Thermazene®: 1% (20 g, 50 g, 85 g, 400 g, 1000 g)

Simcor® [US] *see* niacin and simvastatin *on page 673*

simethicone (sye METH i kone)

Sound-Alike/Look-Alike Issues

simethicone may be confused with cimetidine

Mylanta® may be confused with Mynatal®

Mylicon® may be confused with Modicon®, Myleran®
Phazyme® may be confused with Pherazine®

Synonyms activated dimethicone; activated methylpolysiloxane

U.S./Canadian Brand Names Equalizer Gas Relief [US-OTC]; Gas Free Extra Strength [US-OTC]; Gas Relief Ultra Strength [US-OTC]; Gas-X® Extra Strength [US-OTC]; Gas-X® Infant [US-OTC]; Gas-X® Maximum Strength [US-OTC]; Gas-X® Thin Strips™ [US-OTC]; Gas-X® [US-OTC]; Gas-X®, Children's Tongue Twisters™ [US-OTC]; Infantaire Gas [US-OTC]; Infants Gas Relief Drops [US-OTC]; Little Tummys® Gas Relief [US-OTC]; Mi-Acid Gas Relief [US-OTC]; Mylanta® Gas Maximum Strength [US-OTC]; Mylicon® Infants' [US-OTC]; Ovol® [Can]; Phazyme® Ultra Strength [US-OTC]; Phazyme™ [Can]

Therapeutic Category Antiflatulent

Use Postoperative gas pain or for use in endoscopic examination; relief of bloating, pressure, and discomfort of gas

Dosage Summary

Oral:

Infants: 20 mg 4 times/day, as needed
Children <2 years or <11 kg: 20 mg 4 times/day, as needed
Children >2 years or >11 kg: 40 mg 4 times/day, as needed
Children >12 years: 40-360 mg after meals and at bedtime, as needed
Adults: 40-360 mg after meals and at bedtime, as needed

Dosage Forms

Capsule, softgel, oral:
Gas Free Extra Strength [OTC]: 125 mg
Gas Relief Ultra Strength [OTC]: 180 mg
Gas-X® Extra Strength [OTC]: 125 mg
Gas-X® Maximum Strength [OTC]: 166 mg
Mylanta® Gas Maximum Strength [OTC]: 125 mg
Phazyme® Ultra Strength [OTC]: 180 mg

Strip, orally disintegrating, oral:
Gas-X® Children's Tongue Twisters™ [OTC]: 40 mg (16s)
Gas-X® Thin Strips™ [OTC]: 62.5 mg (18s, 32s)

Suspension, oral: 40 mg/0.6 mL (30 mL)
Equalizer Gas Relief [OTC]: 40 mg/0.6 mL (30 mL)
Gax-X® Infant [OTC]: 40 mg/0.6 mL (30 mL)
Infantaire Gas [OTC]: 40 mg/0.6 mL (30 mL)
Infants Gas Relief Drops [OTC]: 40 mg/0.6 mL (30 mL)
Little Tummys® Gas Relief [OTC]: 40 mg/0.6 mL (30 mL, 45 mL)
Mylicon® Infants' [OTC]: 40 mg/0.6 mL (15 mL, 30 mL)

Tablet, chewable, oral: 80 mg, 125 mg
Gas-X® [OTC]: 80 mg
Gas-X® Extra Strength [OTC]: 125 mg
Mi-Acid Gas Relief [OTC]: 80 mg
Mylanta® Gas Maximum Strength [OTC]: 125 mg

simethicone, aluminum hydroxide, and magnesium hydroxide *see* aluminum hydroxide, magnesium hydroxide, and simethicone *on page 59*

simethicone and calcium carbonate *see* calcium carbonate and simethicone *on page 168*

simethicone and loperamide hydrochloride *see* loperamide and simethicone *on page 574*

simethicone and magaldrate *see* magaldrate and simethicone *on page 583*

Similac® Glucose [US-OTC] *see* dextrose *on page 290*

Simply Cough® *(Discontinued)* *see* dextromethorphan *on page 287*

Simply Saline® [US-OTC] *see* sodium chloride *on page 882*

Simply Saline® Baby [US-OTC] *see* sodium chloride *on page 882*

Simply Saline® Nasal Moist® [US-OTC] *see* sodium chloride *on page 882*

Simply Sleep® [US-OTC/Can] *see* diphenhydramine (systemic) *on page 310*

Simply Stuffy™ *(Discontinued)* *see* pseudoephedrine *on page 810*

Simponi™ [US/Can] *see* golimumab *on page 451*

Simuc *(Discontinued)* *see* guaifenesin and phenylephrine *on page 456*

Simuc-DM [US] *see* guaifenesin and dextromethorphan *on page 455*

Simulect® [US/Can] *see* basiliximab *on page 118*

simvastatin (sim va STAT in)

Sound-Alike/Look-Alike Issues

simvastatin may be confused with atorvastatin, nystatin, pitavastatin

Zocor® may be confused with Cozaar®, Lipitor®, Yocon®, Zoloft®, Zyrtec®

U.S./Canadian Brand Names Apo-Simvastatin® [Can]; CO Simvastatin [Can]; Dom-Simvastatin [Can]; JAMP-Simvastatin [Can]; Mylan-Simvastatin [Can]; Nu-Simvastatin [Can]; PHL-Simvastatin [Can]; PMS-Simvastatin [Can]; RAN™-Simvastatin [Can]; ratio-Simvastatin [Can]; Riva-Simvastatin [Can]; Sandoz-Simvastatin [Can]; Taro-Simvastatin [Can]; Teva-Simvastatin [Can]; Zocor® [US/Can]; ZYM-Simvastatin [Can]

Therapeutic Category HMG-CoA Reductase Inhibitor

Use Used with dietary therapy for the following:

Secondary prevention of cardiovascular events in hypercholesterolemic patients with established coronary heart disease (CHD) or at high risk for CHD: To reduce cardiovascular morbidity (myocardial infarction, coronary/noncoronary revascularization procedures) and mortality; to reduce the risk of stroke

Hyperlipidemias: To reduce elevations in total cholesterol (total-C), LDL-C, apolipoprotein B, triglycerides, and VLDL-C, and to increase HDL-C in patients with primary hypercholesterolemia (elevations of 1 or more components are present in Fredrickson type IIa, IIb, III, and IV hyperlipidemias); treatment of homozygous familial hypercholesterolemia

Heterozygous familial hypercholesterolemia (HeFH): In adolescent patients (10-17 years of age, females >1 year postmenarche) with HeFH having LDL-C ≥190 mg/dL **or** LDL-C ≥160 mg/dL with positive family history of premature cardiovascular disease (CVD), or 2 or more CVD risk factors in the adolescent patient

Dosage Summary Note: Doses should be individualized according to the baseline LDL-cholesterol levels

Oral:

Children <10 years: Dosage not established

Children 10-17 years (females >1 year postmenarche): Initial: 10 mg once daily in the evening; Maintenance: 10-40 mg once daily in the evening (maximum: 40 mg/day)

Adults: Initial: 20-40 mg once daily in the evening; Maintenance: 5-80 mg once daily in the evening (maximum: 80 mg/day)

Elderly: Maximum reductions in LDL-cholesterol may be achieved with daily dose ≤20 mg

Dosage Forms

Tablet, oral: 5 mg, 10 mg, 20 mg, 40 mg, 80 mg

Zocor®: 5 mg, 10 mg, 20 mg, 40 mg, 80 mg

simvastatin and ezetimibe *see* ezetimibe and simvastatin *on page 388*

simvastatin and niacin *see* niacin and simvastatin *on page 673*

Sina-12X [US] *see* guaifenesin and phenylephrine *on page 456*

sincalide (SIN ka lide)

Synonyms C8-CCK; OP-CCK

U.S./Canadian Brand Names Kinevac® [US]

Therapeutic Category Diagnostic Agent

Use Postevacuation cholecystography; gallbladder bile sampling; stimulate pancreatic secretion for analysis; accelerate the transit of barium through the small bowel

Dosage Summary

I.M.:

Children: Dosage not established

Adults: 0.1 mcg/kg

I.V.:

Children: Dosage not established

Adults: 0.02-0.04 mcg/kg over 30-60 seconds, may repeat **or** 0.02 mcg/kg over 30 minutes **or** 0.12 mcg/kg in 30 or 100 mL of NS over 30-50 minutes

Dosage Forms

Injection, powder for reconstitution:

Kinevac®: 5 mcg

Sine-Aid® IB *(Discontinued)* *see* pseudoephedrine and ibuprofen *on page 812*

sinecatechins (sin e KAT e kins)

Synonyms catechins; green tea extract; kunecatechins; polyphenols; polyphenon E

U.S./Canadian Brand Names Veregen™ [US]

Therapeutic Category Immunomodulator, Topical; Topical Skin Product

Use Treatment of external genital and perianal warts secondary to *Condylomata acuminata*

Dosage Summary

Topical:

Children: Dosage not established

Adults: Apply a thin layer (~0.5 cm strand) 3 times/day

Dosage Forms

Ointment, topical:

Veregen™: 15% (15 g)

Sinemet® [US/Can] *see* carbidopa and levodopa *on page 182*

Sinemet® CR [US/Can] *see* carbidopa and levodopa *on page 182*

Sinequan® [Can] *see* doxepin (systemic) *on page 329*

Sinequan® *(Discontinued)* *see* doxepin (systemic) *on page 329*

Singulair® [US/Can] *see* montelukast *on page 643*

Sinografin® [US] *see* diatrizoate meglumine and iodipamide meglumine *on page 293*

Sinubid® *(Discontinued)*

Sinufed® Timecelles® *(Discontinued)* *see* guaifenesin and pseudoephedrine *on page 457*

Sinumed® *(Discontinued)* *see* acetaminophen, chlorpheniramine, and pseudoephedrine *on page 28*

Sinumist®-SR Capsulets® *(Discontinued)* *see* guaifenesin *on page 454*

Sinus Pain & Pressure [US-OTC] *see* acetaminophen and phenylephrine *on page 25*

Sinus-Relief *(Discontinued)* *see* acetaminophen and pseudoephedrine *on page 26*

Sinutab® Non Drowsy [Can] *see* acetaminophen and pseudoephedrine *on page 26*

Sinutab® Sinus [US-OTC] *see* acetaminophen and phenylephrine *on page 25*

SINUtuss® DM [US] *see* guaifenesin, dextromethorphan, and phenylephrine *on page 458*

SINUvent® PE [US] *see* guaifenesin and phenylephrine *on page 456*

sipuleucel-T (si pu LOO sel tee)

Synonyms APC8015

U.S./Canadian Brand Names Provenge® [US]

Therapeutic Category Cellular Immunotherapy, Autologous

Use Treatment of metastatic hormone-refractory prostate cancer in patients who are asymptomatic or minimally symptomatic

Dosage Summary

I.V.:

Children: Dosage not established

Adults: Males: ≥50 million autologous CD54+ cells activated with PAP-GM-CSF; dose administered at ~2 week intervals for a total of 3 doses

Dosage Forms

Infusion, premixed in LR [preservative free]:

Provenge®: ≥50 million autologous $CD54^+$ cells activated with PAP-GM-CSF (250 mL)

Sirdalud® *(Discontinued)* *see* tizanidine *on page 937*

sirolimus (sir OH li mus)

Sound-Alike/Look-Alike Issues

sirolimus may be confused with everolimus, tacrolimus, temsirolimus

Rapamune® may be confused with Rapaflo™

Synonyms rapamycin

U.S./Canadian Brand Names Rapamune® [US/Can]

Therapeutic Category Immunosuppressant Agent

Use Prophylaxis of organ rejection in patients receiving renal transplants

Dosage Summary

Oral:

Children <13 years: Dosage not established

Children ≥13 years and <40 kg: Low-to-moderate immunologic risk: Loading dose: 3 mg/m^2 on day 1; Maintenance: 1 mg/m^2/day; titrate to therapeutic dose based on levels

Children ≥13 years and ≥40 kg: Low-to-moderate immunologic risk: Loading dose: 6 mg on day 1; Maintenance: 2 mg/day; titrate to therapeutic dose based on levels; maximum daily dose: 40 mg; may divide larger doses (including loading dose) over 2 days

Adults <40 kg: Low-to-moderate immunologic risk: Loading dose: 3 mg/m^2 on day 1; Maintenance: 1 mg/m^2/day; titrate to therapeutic dose based on levels; maximum dose in 1 day: 40 mg; if required dose is >40 mg (due to loading dose), divide over 2 days

Adults ≥40 kg: Low-to-moderate immunologic risk: Loading dose: 6 mg on day 1; Maintenance: 2 mg/day; titrate to therapeutic dose based on levels; maximum daily dose: 40 mg; may divide larger doses (including loading dose) over 2 days; High risk: Loading dose: Up to 15 mg on day 1; maintenance: 5 mg/day; titrate to therapeutic dose based on levels; maximum dose in 1 day: 40 mg; if required dose is >40 mg (due to loading dose) divide over 2 days

Dosage Forms

Solution, oral:

Rapamune®: 1 mg/mL (60 mL)

Tablet, oral:

Rapamune®: 0.5 mg, 1 mg, 2 mg

sitagliptin (sit a GLIP tin)

Sound-Alike/Look-Alike Issues

sitaGLIPtin may be confused with saxagliptin, SUMAtriptan

Januvia™ may be confused with Enjuvia™, Janumet™, Jantoven™

Synonyms MK-0431; sitagliptin phosphate

Tall-Man sita**GLIP**tin

U.S./Canadian Brand Names Januvia™ [US/Can]

Therapeutic Category Antidiabetic Agent, Dipeptidyl Peptidase IV (DPP-IV) Inhibitor

Use Management of type 2 diabetes mellitus (noninsulin-dependent, NIDDM) as an adjunct to diet and exercise as monotherapy or in combination therapy with other antidiabetic agents

Dosage Summary

Oral:

Children: Dosage not established

Adults: 100 mg once daily

Dosage Forms

Tablet, oral:

Januvia™: 25 mg, 50 mg, 100 mg

sitagliptin and metformin (sit a GLIP tin & met FOR min)

Sound-Alike/Look-Alike Issues

Janumet® may be confused with Jantoven™, Januvia®

Synonyms metformin and sitagliptin; sitagliptin phosphate and metformin hydrochloride

U.S./Canadian Brand Names Janumet® [US/Can]

Therapeutic Category Antidiabetic Agent, Biguanide; Antidiabetic Agent, Dipeptidyl Peptidase IV (DPP-IV) Inhibitor; Hypoglycemic Agent, Oral

Use Management of type 2 diabetes mellitus (noninsulin-dependent, NIDDM) as an adjunct to diet and exercise in patients not adequately controlled on metformin or sitagliptin monotherapy

Dosage Summary

Oral:

Children: Dosage not established

Adults: Sitagliptin 50 mg and metformin 500-1000 mg twice daily (maximum: 100 mg/day [sitagliptin], 2000 mg/day [metformin])

Elderly <80 years: Initial and maintenance dosing should be conservative, due to the potential for decreased renal function

Elderly ≥80 years: Do not use unless normal renal function has been established

Dosage Forms

Tablet, oral:

Janumet®:

50/500: Sitagliptin 50 mg and metformin 500 mg

50/1000: Sitagliptin 50 mg and metformin 1000 mg

sitagliptin phosphate *see* sitagliptin *on page 879*

sitagliptin phosphate and metformin hydrochloride *see* sitagliptin and metformin *on page 879*

sitaxsentan *(Canada only)* (sye TACKS en tan)

Synonyms sitaxsentan sodium

U.S./Canadian Brand Names Thelin™ [Can]

Therapeutic Category Endothelin Antagonist

Use Treatment of primary pulmonary arterial hypertension (PAH) or pulmonary hypertension secondary to connective tissue disease, in World Health Organization (WHO) class III patients unresponsive to conventional therapy; treatment of PAH in WHO class II patients who are unresponsive to conventional therapy and have no alternative treatment options

Dosage Summary

Children: Dosing not established

Adults: 100 mg once daily; **Note:** Doses above 100 mg/day are not recommended; higher doses have not been shown to provide additional benefit and may increase risk of hepatic toxicity

Dosage Forms - Canada

Tablet:

Thelin™: 100 mg

sitaxsentan sodium *see* sitaxsentan *(Canada only) on page 880*

Skeeter Stik® [US-OTC] *see* benzocaine *on page 124*

Skelaxin® [US/Can] *see* metaxalone *on page 609*

Skelid® [US] *see* tiludronate *on page 933*

SKF 104864 *see* topotecan *on page 943*

SKF 104864-A *see* topotecan *on page 943*

Skin Care™ [US-OTC] *see* pyrithione zinc *on page 819*

Sleep-ettes D [US-OTC] *see* diphenhydramine (systemic) *on page 310*

Sleep-eze 3® Oral *(Discontinued)* *see* diphenhydramine (systemic) *on page 310*

Sleepinal® [US-OTC] *see* diphenhydramine (systemic) *on page 310*

Sleep-Tabs [US-OTC] *see* diphenhydramine (systemic) *on page 310*

Sleepwell 2-nite® *(Discontinued)* *see* diphenhydramine (systemic) *on page 310*

S-leucovorin *see* LEVOleucovorin *on page 558*

6S-leucovorin *see* LEVOleucovorin *on page 558*

Slim-Mint® *(Discontinued)* *see* benzocaine *on page 124*

Slo-bid™ *(Discontinued)* *see* theophylline *on page 925*

Slo-Niacin® [US-OTC] *see* niacin *on page 671*

Slo-Phyllin® (all products) *(Discontinued)* *see* theophylline *on page 925*

Slo-Phyllin® GG *(Discontinued)*

Slo-Pot [Can] *see* potassium chloride *on page 781*

Slow FE® [US-OTC] *see* ferrous sulfate *on page 398*

Slow-K® [Can] *see* potassium chloride *on page 781*

Slow-K® *(Discontinued)* *see* potassium chloride *on page 781*

Slow-Mag® [US-OTC] *see* magnesium chloride *on page 583*

smallpox vaccine (SMAL poks vak SEEN)

Synonyms live smallpox vaccine; vaccinia vaccine

U.S./Canadian Brand Names ACAM2000™ [US]

Therapeutic Category Vaccine

Use Active immunization against vaccinia virus, the causative agent of smallpox in persons determined to be at risk for smallpox infection.

The Advisory Committee on Immunization Practices (ACIP) recommends routine vaccination for the following:
- Laboratory workers at risk of exposure from cultures or contaminated animals which may be a source of vaccinia or related Orthopoxviruses capable of causing infections in humans (monkeypox, cowpox, or variola).
- Consideration may also be given for vaccination of healthcare workers having contact with clinical specimens, contaminated material, or patients receiving vaccinia or recombinant vaccinia viruses.

In a Pre-Event Vaccination Program, the ACIP recommends vaccination for the following:
- Persons designated by authorities to investigate smallpox cases with the likelihood of direct patient contact
- Persons responsible for administering smallpox vaccine

In the event of an intentional release of smallpox virus, the ACIP recommends vaccination for the following:
- Persons exposed to the initial release of the virus
- Persons who had close contact with a confirmed or suspected smallpox patient at any time from the onset of the patient's fever until all scabs have separated
- Healthcare providers involved in evaluation, care, or transport of confirmed or suspected smallpox patients
- Laboratory personnel involved in processing specimens of confirmed or suspected smallpox patients
- Persons likely to have increased contact with infectious materials from smallpox patients

Dosage Summary

Percutaneous:

Children <12 months: Dosage not established

Children ≥12 months: ACAM2000™: Emergency conditions only: A single drop of vaccine suspension and 15 needle punctures into superficial skin for both primary vaccination and revaccination.

Adults: ACAM2000™: A single drop of vaccine suspension and 15 needle punctures into superficial skin for both primary vaccination and revaccination

Dosage Forms

Injection, powder for reconstitution [purified monkey cell source]:

ACAM2000™: 1-5 x 10^8 plaque-forming units per mL

smelling salts *see* ammonia spirit (aromatic) *on page 71*

SMZ-TMP *see* sulfamethoxazole and trimethoprim *on page 901*

snake antivenin, FAB (ovine) *see* crotalidae polyvalent immune FAB (ovine) *on page 255*

Snaplets-EX® *(Discontinued)*

(+)-(*S*)-*N*-methyl-γ-(1-naphthyloxy)-2-thiophenepropylamine hydrochloride *see* duloxetine *on page 336*

sodium 2-mercaptoethane sulfonate *see* mesna *on page 608*

sodium 4-hydroxybutyrate *see* sodium oxybate *on page 885*

sodium *L*-triiodothyronine *see* liothyronine *on page 568*

sodium acetate (SOW dee um AS e tate)

Therapeutic Category Alkalinizing Agent; Electrolyte Supplement, Oral

Use Sodium source in large volume I.V. fluids to prevent or correct hyponatremia in patients with restricted intake; used to counter acidosis through conversion to bicarbonate

Dosage Summary

I.V.:

Children: Maintenance electrolyte requirements of sodium in parenteral nutrition solutions: 3-4 mEq/kg/24 hours

Adults: Maintenance electrolyte requirements of sodium in parenteral nutrition solutions: 3-4 mEq/kg/24 hours **or** 25-40 mEq/1000 kcal/24 hours (maximum: 100-150 mEq/24 hours)

Dosage Forms

Injection, solution [preservative free]: 2 mEq/mL (20 mL, 50 mL, 100 mL, 250 mL); 4 mEq/mL (50 mL, 100 mL)

sodium acid carbonate *see* sodium bicarbonate *on page 882*

sodium aurothiomalate *see* gold sodium thiomalate *on page 451*

sodium benzoate and caffeine *see* caffeine *on page 163*

sodium benzoate and sodium phenylacetate *see* sodium phenylacetate and sodium benzoate *on page 886*

sodium bicarbonate (SOW dee um bye KAR bun ate)

Synonyms baking soda; $NaHCO_3$; sodium acid carbonate; sodium hydrogen carbonate

U.S./Canadian Brand Names Brioschi® [US-OTC]; Neut® [US]

Therapeutic Category Alkalinizing Agent; Antacid; Electrolyte Supplement, Oral

Use Management of metabolic acidosis; gastric hyperacidity; as an alkalinization agent for the urine; treatment of hyperkalemia; management of overdose of certain drugs, including tricyclic antidepressants and aspirin

Dosage Summary

I.V.:

Children: 0.5-1 mEq/kg/dose repeated every 10 minutes or as indicated by arterial blood gases **or** HCO_3^- (mEq) = 0.3 x weight (kg) x base deficit (mEq/L), administer 1/2 dose initially, then remaining 1/2 dose over the next 24 hours **or** 2-5 mEq/kg I.V. infusion over 4-8 hours

Adults: Initial: 1 mEq/kg/dose or 50 mEq one time; Maintenance: 0.5 mEq/kg/dose every 10 minutes or as indicated by arterial blood gases **or** HCO_3^- (mEq) = 0.3 x weight (kg) x base deficit (mEq/L), administer 1/2 dose initially, then remaining 1/2 dose over the next 24 hours **or** 2-5 mEq/kg I.V. infusion over 4-8 hours

Oral:

Children: 1-10 mEq/kg/day as a single dose **or** divided every 4-6 hours

Adults <60 years: 0.5-200 mEq/kg/day in 4-5 divided doses **or** 325 mg to 2 g 1-4 times/day (maximum: 16 g [200 mEq] day)

Adults ≥60 years: 0.5-100 mEq/kg/day in 4-6 divided doses **or** 325 mg to 2 g 1-4 times/day (maximum: 8 g [100 mEq] day)

Dosage Forms

Granules for solution, oral:

Brioschi® [OTC]: 2.69 g/capful (120 g, 240 g); 2.69 g/packet (12s)

Infusion, premixed in water for injection: 5% (500 mL)

Injection, solution: 4.2% (10 mL); 7.5% (50 mL); 8.4% (10 mL, 50 mL, 250 mL, 500 mL)

Neut®: 4% (5 mL)

Injection, solution [preservative free]: 4.2% (5 mL, 10 mL); 7.5% (50 mL); 8.4% (10 mL, 50 mL)

Powder, oral: USP: 100% (120 g, 454 g, 480 g)

Tablet, oral: 325 mg, 650 mg

sodium bicarbonate and omeprazole *see* omeprazole and sodium bicarbonate *on page 702*

sodium chloride (SOW dee um KLOR ide)

Synonyms hypertonic saline; NaCl; normal saline; saline; salt

U.S./Canadian Brand Names 4-Way® Saline Moisturizing Mist [US-OTC]; Altachlore [US-OTC]; Altamist [US-OTC]; Ayr® Allergy Sinus [US-OTC]; Ayr® Baby Saline [US-OTC]; Ayr® Saline No-Drip [US-OTC]; Ayr® Saline [US-OTC]; Breathe Free® [US-OTC]; Deep Sea [US-OTC]; Entsol® [US-OTC]; HuMist® for Kids [US-OTC]; HuMist® [US-OTC]; Hyper-Sal™ [US]; Little Noses® Saline [US-OTC]; Little Noses® Stuffy Nose Kit [US-OTC]; Muro 128® [US-OTC]; Na-Zone® [US-OTC]; Nasal Moist® Saline [US-OTC]; Nasal Spray [US-OTC]; NāSal™ [US-OTC]; Ocean® for Kids [US-OTC]; Ocean® [US-OTC]; Pretz® [US-OTC]; Saline Mist [US-OTC]; Simply Saline® Baby [US-OTC]; Simply Saline® Nasal Moist® [US-OTC]; Simply Saline® [US-OTC]; Syrex [US]; Wound Wash Saline™ [US-OTC]

Therapeutic Category Electrolyte Supplement, Oral; Lubricant, Ocular

Use

Parenteral: Restores sodium ion in patients with restricted oral intake (especially hyponatremia states or low salt syndrome).

Concentrated sodium chloride: Additive for parenteral fluid therapy

Hypertonic sodium chloride: For severe hyponatremia and hypochloremia

Hypotonic sodium chloride: Hydrating solution

Normal saline: Restores water/sodium losses

Ophthalmic: Reduces corneal edema

Inhalation: Restores moisture to pulmonary system; loosens and thins congestion caused by colds or allergies; diluent for bronchodilator solutions that require dilution before inhalation

Intranasal: Restores moisture to nasal membranes

Irrigation: Wound cleansing, irrigation, and flushing

Dosage Summary

I.V.:

Children: 3-4 mEq/kg/day (maximum: 150 mEq/day) **or** sodium deficiency (mEq/kg) = [% dehydration (L/kg)/100 x 70 (mEq/L)] + [0.6 (L/kg) x (140 - serum sodium) (mEq/L)]

Adults: Sodium deficiency (mEq/kg) = [% dehydration (L/kg)/100 x 70 (mEq/L)] + [0.6 (L/kg) x (140 - serum sodium) (mEq/L) **or** mEq sodium = [desired sodium (mEq/L) - actual sodium (mEq/L)] x [0.6 x wt (kg)]] or 3-4 mEq/kg/24 hours or 25-40 mEq/1000 kcals/24 hours in parenteral nutrition (maximum: 150 mEq/day)

Inhalation:

Children <2 years: Dosage not established

Children ≥2 years: 1-3 sprays (1-3 mL) to dilute bronchodilator solution in nebulizer before administration

Adults: 1-3 sprays (1-3 mL) to dilute bronchodilator solution in nebulizer before administration

Intranasal:

Children <2 years: Dosage not established

Children ≥2 years: 2-3 sprays in each nostril as needed

Adults: 2-3 sprays in each nostril as needed

Irrigation:

Children <2 years: Dosage not established

Children ≥2 years: 1-3 L/day **or** spray affected area

Adults: 1-3 L/day **or** spray affected area

Ophthalmic:

Children: Dosage not established

Adults: Ointment: Apply once or more daily; Solution: Instill 1-2 drops into affected eye(s) every 3-4 hours

Dosage Forms

Aerosol, intranasal [preservative free]:
Entsol® [OTC]: 3% (100 mL)

Gel, intranasal:
Ayr® Saline [OTC]: < 0.5% (14 g)
Ayr® Saline No-Drip [OTC]: < 0.5% (22 mL)
Entsol® [OTC]: 3% (20 g)
Simply Saline® Nasal Moist® [OTC]: 0.65% (30 g)

Injection, solution: 0.45% (25 mL, 50 mL, 100 mL, 250 mL, 500 mL, 1000 mL); 0.9% (10 mL, 20 mL, 25 mL, 30 mL, 50 mL, 100 mL, 150 mL, 250 mL, 500 mL, 1000 mL, 1s); 3% (500 mL); 5% (500 mL); 14.6% (20 mL, 40 mL, 250 mL); 23.4% (50 mL, 100 mL, 250 mL)

Injection, solution [preservative free]: 0.9% (1 mL, 2 mL, 2.5 mL, 3 mL, 5 mL, 6 mL, 10 mL, 20 mL, 50 mL, 100 mL, 125 mL); 14.6% (20 mL, 40 mL); 23.4% (30 mL, 100 mL, 200 mL)
Syrex: 0.9% (2.5 mL, 3 mL, 5 mL, 10 mL)

Ointment, ophthalmic: 5% (3.5 g)
Altachlore [OTC]: 5% (3.5 g)

Ointment, ophthalmic [preservative free]:
Muro 128® [OTC]: 5% (3.5 g)

Powder for solution, intranasal [preservative free]:
Entsol® [OTC]: 3% (10s)

Solution, for blood processing: 0.9% (3000 mL)

Solution, for inhalation [preservative free]: 0.9% (3 mL, 5 mL, 15 mL)

Solution, for irrigation: 0.45% (2000 mL); 0.9% (250 mL, 500 mL, 1000 mL, 1500 mL, 2000 mL, 3000 mL, 4000 mL, 5000 mL)

Solution, for irrigation [preservative free]: 0.9% (250 mL, 500 mL, 1000 mL, 1500 mL, 2000 mL, 3000 mL)

Solution, for nebulization [preservative free]:
Hyper-Sal™: 7% (4 mL)

Solution, intranasal:
4-Way® Saline Moisturizing Mist [OTC]: 0.74% (29.6 mL)
Altamist [OTC]: 0.65% (60 mL)
Ayr® Allergy Sinus [OTC]: 2.65% (50 mL)
Ayr® Baby Saline [OTC]: 0.65% (30 mL)
Ayr® Saline [OTC]: 0.65% (50 mL)
Breathe Free® [OTC]: 0.65% (44.3 mL)
Deep Sea [OTC]: 0.65% (45 mL)
Entsol® [OTC]: 3% (30 mL)

HuMist® [OTC]: 0.65% (45 mL)
HuMist® for Kids [OTC]: 0.65% (30 mL)
Little Noses® Saline [OTC]: 0.65% (30 mL)
Little Noses® Stuffy Nose Kit [OTC]: 0.65% (15 mL)
Na-Zone® [OTC]: 0.65% (60 mL)
Nasal Moist® Saline [OTC]: 0.65% (45 mL)
Nasal Spray [OTC]: 0.65% (45 mL)
NāSal™ [OTC]: 0.65% (30 mL)
Ocean® [OTC]: 0.65% (45 mL, 473 mL)
Ocean® for Kids [OTC]: 0.65% (37.5 mL)
Pretz® [OTC]: 0.75% (50 mL, 237 mL, 960 mL)
Saline Mist [OTC]: 0.65% (45 mL)

Solution, intranasal [preservative free]:
Entsol® [OTC]: 3% (240 mL)
Simply Saline® [OTC]: 0.9% (44 mL, 90 mL); 3% (44 mL)
Simply Saline® Baby [OTC]: 0.9% (45 mL)

Solution, ophthalmic: 5% (15 mL)
Altachlore [OTC]: 5% (15 mL, 30 mL)
Muro 128® [OTC]: 2% (15 mL); 5% (15 mL, 30 mL)

Solution, topical [preservative free]:
Wound Wash Saline™ [OTC]: 0.9% (90 mL, 210 mL)

Swab, intranasal:
Ayr® Saline [OTC]: < 0.5% (20s)

Tablet, oral: 1 g

Tablet for solution, topical: 1000 mg

sodium chondroitin sulfate and sodium hyaluronate

(SOW de um kon DROY tin SUL fate & SOW de um hye al yoor ON ate)

Synonyms chondroitin sulfate and sodium hyaluronate; sodium hyaluronate and chondroitin sulfate

U.S./Canadian Brand Names DisCoVisc® [US]; Viscoat® [US]

Therapeutic Category Ophthalmic Agent, Viscoelastic

Use Ophthalmic surgical aid in the anterior segment during cataract extraction and intraocular lens implantation

Dosage Summary

Ophthalmic:
Children: Dosage not established
Adults: Carefully introduce into anterior chamber during surgery

Dosage Forms

Injection, solution, intraocular:
DisCoVisc®: Sodium chondroitin sulfate ≤4% and sodium hyaluronate ≤1.7% (0.5 mL, 1 mL)
Viscoat®: Sodium chondroitin sulfate ≤4% and sodium hyaluronate ≤3% (0.5 mL, 0.75 mL)

sodium citrate, citric acid, and potassium citrate *see* citric acid, sodium citrate, and potassium citrate *on page* 228

Sodium Diuril® [US] *see* chlorothiazide *on page* 207

Sodium Edecrin® [US] *see* ethacrynic acid *on page* 373

sodium edetate *see* edetate disodium *on page* 342

sodium etidronate *see* etidronate *on page* 383

sodium ferric gluconate *see* ferric gluconate *on page* 397

sodium fluorescein *see* fluorescein *on page* 412

sodium fluoride *see* fluoride *on page* 413

sodium fusidate *see* fusidic acid *(Canada only) on page* 432

sodium hyaluronate *see* hyaluronate and derivatives *on page* 475

sodium hyaluronate and chondroitin sulfate *see* sodium chondroitin sulfate and sodium hyaluronate *on page* 884

sodium hydrogen carbonate *see* sodium bicarbonate *on page* 882

sodium hypochlorite solution (SOW dee um hye poe KLOR ite soe LOO shun)

Synonyms modified Dakin's solution

U.S./Canadian Brand Names Dakin's Solution [US]; Di-Dak-Sol [US]

Therapeutic Category Disinfectant

Use Treatment of athlete's foot (0.5%); wound irrigation (0.5%); disinfection of utensils and equipment (5%)

Dosage Summary

Topical:

Children: Via irrigation

Adults: Via irrigation

Dosage Forms

Solution, topical:

Dakin's Solution: 0.125% (473 mL); 0.25% (473 mL); 0.5% (473 mL, 3840 mL)

Di-Dak-Sol: 0.0125% (473 mL)

sodium hyposulfate *see* sodium thiosulfate *on page* 888

sodium lactate (SOW dee um LAK tate)

Therapeutic Category Alkalinizing Agent

Use Source of bicarbonate for prevention and treatment of mild-to-moderate metabolic acidosis

Dosage Summary

I.V.:

Children: Dosage not established

Adults: Dosage depends on degree of acidosis

Dosage Forms

Infusion: 18.7 g (1000 mL)

Injection, solution [preservative free]: 560 mg/mL (10 mL)

sodium nafcillin *see* nafcillin *on page* 655

sodium nitrite, sodium thiosulfate, and amyl nitrite

(SOW dee um NYE trite, SOW dee um thye oh SUL fate, & AM il NYE trite)

Synonyms amyl nitrite, sodium nitrite, and sodium thiosulfate; cyanide antidote kit; sodium thiosulfate, sodium nitrite, and amyl nitrite

U.S./Canadian Brand Names Cyanide Antidote Package [US]

Therapeutic Category Antidote

Use Treatment of cyanide poisoning

Dosage Summary

I.V.:

Sodium nitrite: Prior to sodium thiosulfate:

Children: 10 mg/kg (0.33 mL/kg or 6-8 mL/m^2 of a 3% solution [maximum: 10 mL]); may repeat at 1/2 the original dose if needed

Adults: 300 mg or 10 mg/kg; may repeat at 1/2 the original dose if needed

Sodium thiosulfate: Given after sodium nitrite:

Children: 7 g/m^2 (maximum: 12.5 g) over ~10 minutes; may repeat at 1/2 the original dose if needed

Adults: 12.5 g over ~10 minutes; may repeat at 1/2 the original dose if needed

Inhalation:

Amyl nitrite:

Children: 0.3 mL ampul crushed every minute and vapor inhaled for 15-30 seconds until I.V. sodium nitrite infusion available

Adults: 0.3 mL ampul crushed every minute and vapor inhaled for 15-30 seconds until I.V. sodium nitrite infusion available

Dosage Forms Kit [each kit contains]:

Cyanide Antidote Package:

Injection, solution:

Sodium nitrite 300 mg/10 mL (2)

Sodium thiosulfate 12.5 g/50 mL (2)

Inhalant: Amyl nitrite 0.3 mL (12)

sodium nitroferricyanide *see* nitroprusside *on page* 680
sodium nitroprusside *see* nitroprusside *on page* 680

sodium oxybate (SOW dee um ox i BATE)

Synonyms 4-hydroxybutyrate; gamma hydroxybutyric acid; GHB; sodium 4-hydroxybutyrate

U.S./Canadian Brand Names Xyrem® [US/Can]

Therapeutic Category Central Nervous System Depressant

Controlled Substance C-I (illicit use); C-III (medical use)

Use Treatment of cataplexy and daytime sleepiness in patients with narcolepsy

Dosage Summary

Oral:

Children <16 years: Dosage not established

Children ≥16 years: Initial: 4.5 g/day in 2 equal doses given at bedtime and 2.5-4 hours later; Maintenance: 4.5-9 g/day (maximum: 9 g/day); **Note:** Titration is recommended

Adults: Initial: 4.5 g/day in 2 equal doses given at bedtime and 2.5-4 hours later; Maintenance: 4.5-9 g/day (maximum: 9 g/day); **Note:** Titration is recommended

Elderly >65 years: Dosage not established

Dosage Forms

Solution, oral:

Xyrem®: 500 mg/mL (180 mL)

sodium PAS *see* aminosalicylic acid *on page 66*

sodium-PCA and lactic acid *see* lactic acid *on page 542*

sodium phenylacetate and sodium benzoate

(SOW dee um fen il AS e tate & SOW dee um BENZ oh ate)

Synonyms NAPA and NABZ; sodium benzoate and sodium phenylacetate

U.S./Canadian Brand Names Ammonul® [US]

Therapeutic Category Ammonium Detoxicant

Use Adjunct to treatment of acute hyperammonemia and encephalopathy in patients with urea cycle disorders involving partial or complete deficiencies of carbamyl-phosphate synthetase (CPS), ornithine transcarbamoylase (OTC), argininosuccinate lysase (ASL), or argininosuccinate synthetase (ASS); for use with hemodialysis in acute neonatal hyperammonemic coma, moderate-to-severe hyperammonemic encephalopathy and hyperammonemia which fails to respond to initial therapy

Dosage Summary

I.V:

Children ≤20 kg: Loading dose: Ammonul® 2.5 mL/kg (sodium phenylacetate 250 mg/kg and sodium benzoate 250 mg/kg) with arginine 10% 2-6 mL/kg over 90-120 minutes; Maintenance: Repeat same loading dose over 24 hours

Children >20 kg: Loading dose: Ammonul® 55 mL/m^2 (sodium phenylacetate 5.5 g/m^2 and sodium benzoate 5.5 g/m^2) with arginine 10% 2-6 mL/kg over 90-120 minutes; Maintenance: Repeat same loading dose over 24 hours

Adults: Loading dose: Ammonul® 55 mL/m^2 (sodium phenylacetate 5.5 g/m^2 and sodium benzoate 5.5 g/m^2) with arginine 10% 2-6 mL/kg over 90-120 minutes; Maintenance: Repeat same loading dose over 24 hours

Dosage Forms

Injection, solution [concentrate]:

Ammonul®: Sodium phenylacetate 100 mg and sodium benzoate 100 mg per 1 mL (50 mL)

sodium phenylbutyrate (SOW dee um fen il BYOO ti rate)

Synonyms ammonapse

U.S./Canadian Brand Names Buphenyl® [US]

Therapeutic Category Miscellaneous Product

Use Adjunctive therapy in the chronic management of patients with urea cycle disorder involving deficiencies of carbamoylphosphate synthetase, ornithine transcarbamylase, or argininosuccinic acid synthetase

Dosage Summary

Oral:

Children <20 kg: Powder: 450-600 mg/kg/day administered in equally divided amounts with each meal or feeding, 3-6 times daily (maximum: 20 g/day)

Children ≥20 kg: 9.9-13 g/m^2/day, administered in equally divided amounts with each meal, 3-6 times daily (maximum: 20 g/day)

Adults: 9.9-13 g/m^2/day, administered in equally divided amounts with each meal, 3-6 times daily (maximum: 20 g/day)

Dosage Forms

Powder for solution, oral:

Buphenyl®: 3 g/teaspoon (250 g)

Tablet, oral:

Buphenyl®: 500 mg

sodium phosphate and potassium phosphate *see* potassium phosphate and sodium phosphate *on page 783*

sodium phosphates (SOW dee um FOS fates)

Sound-Alike/Look-Alike Issues

Visicol® may be confused with Asacol®, VESIcare®

Synonyms phosphates, sodium

U.S./Canadian Brand Names Fleet® Enema Extra® [US-OTC]; Fleet® Enema [US-OTC/Can]; Fleet® Pedia-Lax™ Enema [US-OTC]; LaCrosse Complete [US-OTC]; OsmoPrep® [US]; Visicol® [US]

Therapeutic Category Electrolyte Supplement, Oral; Laxative

Use

Oral, rectal: Short-term treatment of constipation and to evacuate the colon for rectal and bowel exams

I.V.: Source of phosphate in large volume I.V. fluids and parenteral nutrition; treatment and prevention of hypophosphatemia

Dosage Summary Note: Doses listed as millimoles (mmol) of phosphate

I.V.:

Children: 0.08-0.36 mmol/kg over 4-6 hours **or** 0.5-1.5 mmol/kg/day

Adults: 0.15-0.64 mmol/kg over 4-12 hours

Oral:

Children <5 years: Dosage not established

Children 5-9 years: 7.5 mL as a single dose (maximum daily dose: 7.5 mL)

Children 10-12 years: 15 mL as a single dose (maximum daily dose: 15 mL)

Children ≥12 years: 15 mL as a single dose (maximum daily dose: 45 mL)

Adults: 15-45 mL as a single dose (maximum daily dose: 45 mL)

Rectal:

Children <2 years: Dosage not established

Children 2-<5 years: One-half contents of one 2.25 oz pediatric enema

Children 5-12 years: Contents of one 2.25 oz pediatric enema, may repeat

Children ≥12 years: Contents of one 4.5-ounce enema as a single dose, may repeat

Adults: Contents of one 4.5-ounce enema as a single dose, may repeat

Dosage Forms

Injection, solution [concentrate; preservative free]: Phosphorus 3 mmol and sodium 4 mEq per 1 mL (5 mL, 15 mL, 50 mL)

Solution, oral: Monobasic sodium phosphate 2.4 g and dibasic sodium phosphate 0.9 g per 5 mL (45 mL)

Solution, rectal [enema]: Monobasic sodium phosphate 19 g and dibasic sodium phosphate 7 g per 118 mL delivered dose (133 mL)

Fleet® Enema [OTC], LaCrosse Complete [OTC]: Monobasic sodium phosphate 19 g and dibasic sodium phosphate 7 g per 118 mL delivered dose (133 mL)

Fleet® Enema Extra® [OTC]: Monobasic sodium phosphate 19 g and dibasic sodium phosphate 7 g per 197 mL delivered dose (230 mL)

Fleet® Pedia-Lax™ Enema [OTC]: Monobasic sodium phosphate 9.5 g and dibasic sodium phosphate 3.5 g per 59 mL delivered dose (66 mL)

Tablet, oral [scored]:

OsmoPrep®, Visicol®: Monobasic sodium phosphate 1.102 g and dibasic sodium phosphate 0.398 g

sodium polystyrene sulfonate (SOW dee um pol ee STYE reen SUL fon ate)

Sound-Alike/Look-Alike Issues

sodium polystyrene sulfonate may be confused with calcium polystyrene sulfonate

Kayexalate® may be confused with Kaopectate®

U.S./Canadian Brand Names Kalexate [US]; Kayexalate® [US/Can]; Kionex® [US]; PMS-Sodium Polystyrene Sulfonate [Can]; SPS® [US]

Therapeutic Category Antidote

Use Treatment of hyperkalemia

Dosage Summary

Oral:

Children: 1 g/kg/dose every 6 hours

Adults: 15 g 1-4 times/day

Rectal:

Children: 1 g/kg/dose every 2-6 hours

Adults: 30-50 g every 6 hours

Dosage Forms

Powder for suspension, oral/rectal: 15 g/4 teaspoon (454 g)

Kalexate: 15 g/4 teaspoon (454 g)

Kayexalate®: 15 g/4 teaspoon (454 g)

Kionex®: 15 g/4 teaspoon (454 g)

Suspension, oral/rectal:

SPS®: 15 g/60 mL (60 mL, 120 mL, 473 mL)

Sodium Sulamyd [Can] *see* sulfacetamide (ophthalmic) *on page 899*

sodium sulfacetamide *see* sulfacetamide (ophthalmic) *on page 899*

sodium sulfacetamide *see* sulfacetamide (topical) *on page 900*

sodium sulfacetamide and sulfur *see* sulfur and sulfacetamide *on page 903*

sodium tetradecyl (SOW dee um tetra DEK il)

Synonyms sodium tetradecyl sulfate

U.S./Canadian Brand Names Sotradecol® [US]; Trombovar® [Can]

Therapeutic Category Sclerosing Agent

Use Treatment of small, uncomplicated varicose veins of the lower extremities

Dosage Summary

I.V.:

Children: Dosage not established

Adults: 0.5-2 mL in each vein (maximum: 10 mL per treatment session)

Dosage Forms

Injection, solution:

Sotradecol®: 1% (2 mL); 3% (2 mL)

sodium tetradecyl sulfate *see* sodium tetradecyl *on page 888*

sodium thiosulfate (SOW dee um thye oh SUL fate)

Synonyms disodium thiosulfate pentahydrate; pentahydrate; sodium hyposulfate; sodium thiosulphate; thiosulfuric acid disodium salt

U.S./Canadian Brand Names Versiclear™ [US]

Therapeutic Category Antidote; Antifungal Agent

Use

Parenteral: Used alone or with sodium nitrite or amyl nitrite in cyanide poisoning; reduce the risk of nephrotoxicity associated with cisplatin therapy; treatment of cyanide poisoning due to nitroprusside

Topical: Treatment of tinea versicolor

Dosage Summary

I.V.:

Children: 7 g/m^2 (maximum dose: 12.5 g) given over 10 minutes; may repeat at 1/2 the original dose if symptoms return **or** 12 g/m^2 over 6 hours or 9 g/m^2 I.V. push followed by 1.2 g/m^2 continuous infusion for 6 hours

Adults: 12.5 g, may repeat at half dose if needed **or** 0.95-1.95 mL/kg (maximum: 50 mL) **or** 12 g/m^2 over 6 hours or 9 g/m^2 I.V. push followed by 1.2 g/m^2 continuous infusion for 6 hours

Topical:

Children: Apply a thin layer (20% to 25%) to affected areas twice daily

Adults: Apply a thin layer (20% to 25%) to affected areas twice daily

Dosage Forms

Injection, solution [preservative free]: 100 mg/mL (10 mL); 250 mg/mL (50 mL)

Versiclear™: 100 mg/mL (10 mL); 250 mg/mL (50 mL)

Lotion:

Versiclear™: Sodium thiosulfate 25% and salicylic acid 1% (120 mL)

sodium thiosulfate, sodium nitrite, and amyl nitrite *see* sodium nitrite, sodium thiosulfate, and amyl nitrite *on page 885*
sodium thiosulphate *see* sodium thiosulfate *on page 888*
Soflax™ [Can] *see* docusate *on page 321*
Sojourn™ [US] *see* sevoflurane *on page 873*
Sojourn Sevoflurane [Can] *see* sevoflurane *on page 873*
Solagé® [US/Can] *see* mequinol and tretinoin *on page 606*
Solaquin® [Can] *see* hydroquinone *on page 487*
Solaquin® ***(Discontinued)*** *see* hydroquinone *on page 487*
Solaquin Forte® [Can] *see* hydroquinone *on page 487*
Solaquin Forte® ***(Discontinued)*** *see* hydroquinone *on page 487*
Solaraze® [US] *see* diclofenac (topical) *on page 297*
Solarcaine® Aloe Extra Burn Relief ***(Discontinued)*** *see* lidocaine (topical) *on page 562*
Solarcaine® cool aloe Burn Relief [US-OTC] *see* lidocaine (topical) *on page 562*
Solfoton® ***(Discontinued)*** *see* phenobarbital *on page 747*
Solia™ [US] *see* ethinyl estradiol and desogestrel *on page 374*

solifenacin (sol i FEN a sin)

Sound-Alike/Look-Alike Issues
VESIcare® may be confused with Vesinoid®,Visicol®
Synonyms solifenacin succinate; YM905
U.S./Canadian Brand Names VESIcare® [US]
Therapeutic Category Anticholinergic Agent
Use Treatment of overactive bladder with symptoms of urinary frequency, urgency, or urge incontinence
Dosage Summary
Oral:
Children: Dosage not established
Adults: 5-10 mg/day
Dosage Forms
Tablet, oral:
VESIcare®: 5 mg, 10 mg

solifenacin succinate *see* solifenacin *on page 889*
Soliris® [US/Can] *see* eculizumab *on page 341*
Solodyn® [US] *see* minocycline *on page 635*
Soltamox™ ***(Discontinued)*** *see* tamoxifen *on page 909*
Soluble Fiber Therapy [US-OTC] *see* methylcellulose *on page 618*
soluble fluorescein *see* fluorescein *on page 412*
Solu-Cortef® [US/Can] *see* hydrocortisone (systemic) *on page 482*
Solugel® [Can] *see* benzoyl peroxide *on page 128*
Solu-Medrol® [US/Can] *see* methylprednisolone *on page 622*
solumedrol *see* methylprednisolone *on page 622*
Soluver® [Can] *see* salicylic acid *on page 858*
Soluver® Plus [Can] *see* salicylic acid *on page 858*
Soma® [US] *see* carisoprodol *on page 185*
Soma® Compound [US] *see* carisoprodol and aspirin *on page 185*
Soma® Compound w/Codeine ***(Discontinued)*** *see* carisoprodol, aspirin, and codeine *on page 185*

somatropin (soe ma TROE pin)

Sound-Alike/Look-Alike Issues
somatropin may be confused with homatropine, somatrem, sumatriptan
Humatrope® may be confused with homatropine
somatrem may be confused with somatropin
Synonyms growth hormone, human; hGH; human growth hormone

U.S./Canadian Brand Names Genotropin Miniquick® [US]; Genotropin® [US]; Humatrope® [US/Can]; Norditropin® NordiFlex® [US]; Norditropin® [US]; Nutropin AQ® [US/Can]; Nutropin® [US/Can]; Omnitrope® [US/Can]; Saizen® [US/Can]; Serostim® [US/Can]; Tev-Tropin® [US]; Zorbtive® [US]

Therapeutic Category Growth Hormone

Use

Children:

Treatment of growth failure due to inadequate endogenous growth hormone secretion (Genotropin®, Humatrope®, Norditropin®, Nutropin®, Nutropin AQ®, Omnitrope®, Saizen®, Tev-Tropin®)

Treatment of short stature associated with Turner syndrome (Genotropin®, Humatrope®, Norditropin®, Nutropin®, Nutropin AQ®)

Treatment of Prader-Willi syndrome (Genotropin®)

Treatment of growth failure associated with chronic renal insufficiency (CRI) up until the time of renal transplantation (Nutropin®, Nutropin AQ®)

Treatment of growth failure in children born small for gestational age who fail to manifest catch-up growth by 2 years of age (Genotropin®) or by 2-4 years of age (Humatrope®, Norditropin®)

Treatment of idiopathic short stature (nongrowth hormone-deficient short stature) defined by height standard deviation score (SDS) ≤-2.25 and growth rate not likely to attain normal adult height (Genotropin®, Humatrope®, Nutropin®, Nutropin AQ®)

Treatment of short stature or growth failure associated with short stature homeobox gene (SHOX) deficiency (Humatrope®)

Treatment of short stature associated with Noonan syndrome (Norditropin®)

Adults:

HIV patients with wasting or cachexia with concomitant antiviral therapy (Serostim®)

Replacement of endogenous growth hormone in patients with adult growth hormone deficiency who meet both of the following criteria (Genotropin®, Humatrope®, Norditropin®, Nutropin®, Nutropin AQ®, Omnitrope®, Saizen®):

Biochemical diagnosis of adult growth hormone deficiency by means of a subnormal response to a standard growth hormone stimulation test (peak growth hormone ≤5 mcg/L). Confirmatory testing may not be required in patients with congenital/genetic growth hormone deficiency or multiple pituitary hormone deficiencies due to organic diseases.

and

Adult-onset: Patients who have adult growth hormone deficiency whether alone or with multiple hormone deficiencies (hypopituitarism) as a result of pituitary disease, hypothalamic disease, surgery, radiation therapy, or trauma

or

Childhood-onset: Patients who were growth hormone deficient during childhood, confirmed as an adult before replacement therapy is initiated

Treatment of short-bowel syndrome (Zorbtive®)

Dosage Summary Note: Use caution: Dosage is indication and formulation specific; individualize dose

I.M.:

Children:

Growth hormone deficiency: Saizen®: Weekly dosage: 0.18 mg/kg divided into equal daily doses **or** as 0.06 mg/kg/dose administered 3 days per week **or** as 0.03 mg/kg/dose administered 6 days per week

Adults: Dosage not established

SubQ:

Children:

Chronic renal insufficiency: Nutropin®, Nutropin® AQ: Weekly dosage: 0.35 mg/kg divided into daily injections; continue until the time of renal transplantation

Growth hormone deficiency:

Genotropin®, Omnitrope®: Weekly dosage: 0.16-0.24 mg/kg divided into equal doses 6-7 days per week

Humatrope®: Weekly dosage: 0.18-0.3 mg/kg divided into equal doses 6-7 days per week

Norditropin®: 0.024-0.034 mg/kg/day, 6-7 days per week

Nutropin®, Nutropin® AQ: Weekly dosage: 0.3 mg/kg divided into equal daily doses; pubertal patients: ≤0.7 mg/kg divided into equal daily doses

Tev-Tropin®: Up to 0.1 mg/kg administered 3 days per week

Saizen®: Weekly dosage: 0.18 mg/kg divided into equal daily doses **or** as 0.06 mg/kg/dose administered 3 days per week **or** as 0.03 mg/kg/dose administered 6 days per week

Idiopathic short stature:

Gentropin®: SubQ: Weekly dosage: 0.47 mg/kg divided into equal doses 6-7 days per week

Humatrope®: Weekly dosage: 0.37 mg/kg divided into equal doses 6-7 days per week

Nutropin®, Nutropin AQ®: Weekly dosage: Up to 0.3 mg/kg divided into equal daily doses

Prader-Willi syndrome: Genotropin®: Weekly dosage: 0.24 mg/kg divided into equal doses 6-7 days per week

Small for gestational age:

Genotropin®: Weekly dosage: 0.48 mg/kg divided into equal doses 6-7 days per week

Humatrope®: SubQ: Weekly dosage: 0.47 mg/kg divided into equal doses 6-7 days per week

Norditropin®: SubQ: Up to 0.067 mg/kg/day

Turner syndrome:

Genotropin®: Weekly dosage: 0.33 mg/kg divided into equal doses 6-7 days per week

Humatrope®: Weekly dosage: 0.375 mg/kg divided into equal doses 6-7 days per week

Norditropin®: Up to 0.067 mg/kg/day

Nutropin®, Nutropin® AQ: Weekly dosage: ≤0.375 mg/kg divided into equal doses 3-7 days per week

SHOX deficiency: Humatrope®: Weekly dosage: 0.35 mg/kg/week divided into equal doses 6-7 days per week

Noonan syndrome: Norditropin®: SubQ: Up to 0.066 mg/kg/day

Adults:

Growth hormone deficiency: **Note:** To minimize adverse events in older or overweight patients, reduced dosages may be necessary. During therapy, dosage should be decreased if required by the occurrence of side effects or excessive IGF-I levels.

Weight-based dosing:

Genotropin®, Omnitrope®: Weekly dosage: ≤0.04 mg/kg divided into equal doses 6-7 days per week; dose may be increased at 4- to 8-week intervals according to individual requirements, to a maximum of 0.08 mg/kg/week

Humatrope®: ≤0.006 mg/kg/day; dose may be increased according to individual requirements, up to a maximum of 0.0125 mg/kg/day

Norditropin®: Initial dose ≤0.004 mg/kg/day; after 6 weeks of therapy, may increase dose to 0.016 mg/kg/day

Nutropin®, Nutropin® AQ: ≤0.006 mg/kg/day; dose may be increased according to individual requirements, up to a maximum of 0.025 mg/kg/day in patients <35 years of age, or up to a maximum of 0.0125 mg/kg/day in patients ≥35 years of age

Saizen®: ≤0.005 mg/kg/day; dose may be increased to not more than 0.01 mg/kg/day after 4 weeks, based on individual requirements.

Nonweight-based dosing: SubQ: Initial: 0.2 mg/day (range: 0.15-0.3 mg/day); may increase every 1-2 months by 0.1-0.2 mg/day based on response and/or serum IGF-I levels

HIV patients with wasting or cachexia (Serostim®): SubQ: 0.1 mg/kg once daily at bedtime (maximum: 6 mg/day)

Short-bowel syndrome (Zorbtive®): 0.1 mg/kg once daily for 4 weeks (maximum: 8 mg/day)

Dosage Forms

Injection, powder for reconstitution:

Genotropin Miniquick®: 0.2 mg, 0.4 mg, 0.6 mg, 0.8 mg, 1 mg, 1.2 mg, 1.4 mg, 1.6 mg, 1.8 mg, 2 mg

Genotropin®: 5.8 mg, 13.8 mg

Humatrope®: 5 mg, 6 mg, 12 mg, 24 mg

Nutropin®: 5 mg, 10 mg

Omnitrope®: 5.8 mg

Saizen®: 5 mg, 8.8 mg

Serostim®: 4 mg, 5 mg, 6 mg

Tev-Tropin®: 5 mg

Zorbtive®: 8.8 mg

Injection, solution:

Norditropin®: 5 mg/1.5 mL (1.5 mL); 15 mg/1.5 mL (1.5 mL)

Norditropin® NordiFlex®: 5 mg/1.5 mL (1.5 mL); 10 mg/1.5 mL (1.5 mL); 15 mg/1.5 mL (1.5 mL); 30 mg/3 mL (3 mL)

Nutropin AQ®: 5 mg/mL (2 mL)

Omnitrope®: 5 mg/1.5 mL (1.5 mL); 10 mg/1.5 mL (1.5 mL)

Somatuline® Autogel® [Can] *see* lanreotide *on page* *548*

Somatuline® Depot [US] *see* lanreotide *on page* *548*

Somavert® [US/Can] *see* pegvisomant *on page* *735*

Sominex® [US-OTC/Can] *see* diphenhydramine (systemic) *on page* *310*

Sominex® Maximum Strength [US-OTC] *see* diphenhydramine (systemic) *on page* *310*

Somnote® [US] *see* chloral hydrate *on page* *202*

Som Pam [Can] *see* flurazepam *on page* *417*

Sonata® [US] *see* zaleplon *on page 997*
Soothe® [US-OTC] *see* artificial tears *on page 97*
Soothing Care™ Itch Relief [US-OTC] *see* pramoxine *on page 787*

sorafenib (sor AF e nib)

Sound-Alike/Look-Alike Issues
sorafenib may be confused with imatinib, sunitinib
Nexavar® may be confused with Nexium®

Synonyms BAY 43-9006; sorafenib tosylate

U.S./Canadian Brand Names Nexavar® [US/Can]

Therapeutic Category Antineoplastic Agent, Tyrosine Kinase Inhibitor; Vascular Endothelial Growth Factor (VEGF) Inhibitor

Use Treatment of advanced renal cell cancer (RCC), unresectable hepatocellular cancer (HCC)

Dosage Summary

Oral:
Children: Dosage not established
Adults: 400 mg twice daily

Dosage Forms

Tablet, oral:
Nexavar®: 200 mg

sorafenib tosylate *see* sorafenib *on page 892*

sorbitol (SOR bi tole)

Therapeutic Category Genitourinary Irrigant; Laxative

Use Genitourinary irrigant in transurethral prostatic resection or other transurethral resection or other transurethral surgical procedures; diuretic; humectant; sweetening agent; hyperosmotic laxative; facilitate the passage of sodium polystyrene sulfonate through the intestinal tract

Dosage Summary

Oral:
Children <2 years: Dosage not established
Children 2-11 years: 2 mL/kg (70% solution) as a single dose
Children ≥12 years: 30-150 mL (70% solution) as a single dose
Adults: 30-150 mL (70% solution) as a single dose

Rectal:
Children <2 years: Dosage not established
Children 2-11 years: 30-60 mL (25% to 30% solution) as a single dose
Children ≥12 years: 120 mL (25% to 30% solution) as a single dose
Adults: 120 mL (25% to 30% solution) as a single dose

Topical:
Children: Dosage not established
Adults: 3% to 3.3% as a transurethral irrigation

Dosage Forms

Solution, genitourinary irrigation [preservative free]: 3% (3000 mL, 5000 mL); 3.3% (2000 mL, 4000 mL)
Solution, oral: 70% (30 mL, 473 mL, 480 mL, 3840 mL)

Sorbitrate® *(Discontinued)* *see* isosorbide dinitrate *on page 529*
Sore Throat Relief [US-OTC] *see* benzocaine *on page 124*
Soriatane® [Can] *see* acitretin *on page 35*
Soriatane® CK Convenience Kit™ *(Discontinued)* *see* acitretin *on page 35*
Soriatane® *(Discontinued)* *see* acitretin *on page 35*
Sorine® [US] *see* sotalol *on page 892*

sotalol (SOE ta lole)

Sound-Alike/Look-Alike Issues
sotalol may be confused with Stadol®, Sudafed®
Betapace® may be confused with Betapace AF®
Betapace AF® may be confused with Betapace®

Synonyms sotalol hydrochloride

U.S./Canadian Brand Names Apo-Sotalol® [Can]; Betapace AF® [US]; Betapace® [US]; CO Sotalol [Can]; Dom-Sotalol [Can]; Med-Sotalol [Can]; Mylan-Sotalol [Can]; Novo-Sotalol [Can]; Nu-Sotalol [Can]; PHL-Sotalol [Can]; PMS-Sotalol [Can]; PRO-Sotalol [Can]; ratio-Sotalol [Can]; Rhoxal-sotalol [Can]; Riva-Sotalol [Can]; Rylosol [Can]; Sandoz-Sotalol [Can]; Sorine® [US]; ZYM-Sotalol [Can]

Therapeutic Category Antiarrhythmic Agent, Class II; Antiarrhythmic Agent, Class III; Beta-Adrenergic Blocker, Nonselective

Use Treatment of documented ventricular arrhythmias (ie, sustained ventricular tachycardia), that in the judgment of the physician are life-threatening; maintenance of normal sinus rhythm in patients with symptomatic atrial fibrillation and atrial flutter who are currently in sinus rhythm. Manufacturer states substitutions should not be made for Betapace AF® since Betapace AF® is distributed with a patient package insert specific for atrial fibrillation/flutter.

Injection: Substitution for oral sotalol in those who are unable to take sotalol orally

Dosage Summary

I.V.:

Children: Dosage not established

Adults: Initial: 75 mg twice daily; Maintenance: 75-150 mg twice daily (maximum: 300 mg/day; exceptions occur [indication specific])

Oral:

Children ≤2 years: Dosage should be adjusted (decreased) by plotting of the child's age on a logarithmic scale; **Note:** Refer to manufacturer's package labeling

Children >2 years: Initial: 90 mg/m^2/day in 3 divided doses; Maintenance: 90-180 mg/m^2/day in 3 divided doses (maximum: 180 mg/m^2/day)

Adults: Initial: 80 mg twice daily; Maintenance: 240-320 mg/day in 2-3 divided doses (maximum: 320 mg/day; exceptions occur [indication specific])

Dosage Forms

Injection, solution [preservative free]: 15 mg/mL (10 mL)

Tablet, oral: 80 mg, 120 mg, 160 mg, 240 mg

Betapace AF®: 80 mg, 120 mg, 160 mg

Betapace®: 80 mg, 120 mg, 160 mg, 240 mg

Sorine®: 80 mg, 120 mg, 160 mg, 240 mg

sotalol hydrochloride *see* sotalol *on page* *892*

Sotradecol® [US] *see* sodium tetradecyl *on page* *888*

Sotret® [US] *see* isotretinoin *on page* *530*

SourceCF® [US] *see* vitamins (multiple/oral) *on page* *990*

SourceCF® [US-OTC] *see* vitamins (multiple/pediatric) *on page* *990*

Soyacal® *(Discontinued)* *see* fat emulsion *on page* *391*

Soyalac® [US-OTC] *see* nutritional formula, enteral/oral *on page* *692*

SPA *see* albumin *on page* *43*

Spacol *(Discontinued)* *see* hyoscyamine *on page* *491*

Spacol T/S *(Discontinued)* *see* hyoscyamine *on page* *491*

Span-FF® *(Discontinued)* *see* ferrous fumarate *on page* *398*

Spasmolin® *(Discontinued)* *see* hyoscyamine, atropine, scopolamine, and phenobarbital *on page* *492*

Spastrin® *(Discontinued)*

SPD417 *see* carbamazepine *on page* *177*

Spectazole® *(Discontinued)* *see* econazole *on page* *340*

Spec-T® *(Discontinued)* *see* benzocaine *on page* *124*

spectinomycin *(Discontinued)*

Spectracef® [US] *see* cefditoren *on page* *190*

Spectrocin Plus™ *(Discontinued)* *see* bacitracin, neomycin, polymyxin B, and pramoxine *on page* *115*

SPI 0211 *see* lubiprostone *on page* *580*

Spiriva® [Can] *see* tiotropium *on page* *936*

Spiriva® HandiHaler® [US] *see* tiotropium *on page* *936*

Spironazide® *(Discontinued)* *see* hydrochlorothiazide and spironolactone *on page* *478*

spironolactone (speer on oh LAK tone)

Sound-Alike/Look-Alike Issues

Aldactone® may be confused with Aldactazide®

U.S./Canadian Brand Names Aldactone® [US/Can]; Novo-Spiroton [Can]

Therapeutic Category Diuretic, Potassium Sparing

Use Management of edema associated with excessive aldosterone excretion; hypertension; primary hyperaldosteronism; hypokalemia; cirrhosis of liver accompanied by edema or ascites; nephritic syndrome; severe heart failure (NYHA class III-IV) to increase survival and reduce hospitalization when added to standard therapy

Dosage Summary

Oral:

Children <1 year: Dosage not established

Adults: 12.5-400 mg/day in 1-2 divided doses

Elderly: Initial: 25-50 mg/day in 1-2 divided doses; Maintenance: 12.5-400 mg/day in 1-2 divided doses

Dosage Forms

Tablet, oral: 25 mg, 50 mg, 100 mg

Aldactone®: 25 mg, 50 mg, 100 mg

spironolactone and hydrochlorothiazide *see* hydrochlorothiazide and spironolactone *on page 478*

Spirozide® ***(Discontinued)*** *see* hydrochlorothiazide and spironolactone *on page 478*

SPM 927 *see* lacosamide *on page 541*

Sporanox® [US/Can] *see* itraconazole *on page 531*

Sportscreme® [US-OTC] *see* trolamine *on page 963*

SPP100 *see* aliskiren *on page 50*

Sprayzoin™ [US-OTC] *see* benzoin *on page 127*

Sprintec® [US] *see* ethinyl estradiol and norgestimate *on page 380*

Sprix™ [US] *see* ketorolac (nasal) *on page 538*

Sprycel® [US/Can] *see* dasatinib *on page 270*

SPS® [US] *see* sodium polystyrene sulfonate *on page 887*

SR33589 *see* dronedarone *on page 333*

SRC® Expectorant ***(Discontinued)***

Sronyx™ [US] *see* ethinyl estradiol and levonorgestrel *on page 376*

SS734 *see* besifloxacin *on page 132*

SSD® [US] *see* silver sulfadiazine *on page 875*

SSD AF® [US] *see* silver sulfadiazine *on page 875*

SSKI® [US] *see* potassium iodide *on page 782*

Stadol® ***(Discontinued)*** *see* butorphanol *on page 161*

Stadol® NS ***(Discontinued)*** *see* butorphanol *on page 161*

Staflex [US] *see* acetaminophen and phenyltoloxamine *on page 26*

Stagesic™ [US] *see* hydrocodone and acetaminophen *on page 479*

Stalevo® [US/Can] *see* levodopa, carbidopa, and entacapone *on page 557*

StanGard® [US] *see* fluoride *on page 413*

StanGard® Perio [US] *see* fluoride *on page 413*

stannous fluoride *see* fluoride *on page 413*

stanozolol ***(Discontinued)***

Starlix® [US/Can] *see* nateglinide *on page 663*

Statex® [Can] *see* morphine (systemic) *on page 644*

Staticin® ***(Discontinued)*** *see* erythromycin (topical) *on page 362*

Statobex® [Can] *see* phendimetrazine *on page 747*

Statuss™ DM [US] *see* chlorpheniramine, phenylephrine, and dextromethorphan *on page 211*

stavudine (STAV yoo deen)

Sound-Alike/Look-Alike Issues

Zerit® may be confused with Zestril®, Ziac®, Zyrtec®

Synonyms d4T

U.S./Canadian Brand Names Zerit® [US/Can]

Therapeutic Category Antiviral Agent

Use Treatment of HIV infection in combination with other antiretroviral agents

Dosage Summary

Oral:

Newborns (Birth to 13 days): 0.5 mg/kg every 12 hours
Children ≥14 days and <30 kg: 1 mg/kg every 12 hours
Children 30-59 kg: 30 mg every 12 hours
Children ≥60 kg: 40 mg every 12 hours
Adults <60 kg: 30 mg every 12 hours
Adults ≥60 kg: 40 mg every 12 hours

Dosage Forms

Capsule, oral: 15 mg, 20 mg, 30 mg, 40 mg
Zerit®: 15 mg, 20 mg, 30 mg, 40 mg

Powder for solution, oral:
Zerit®: 1 mg/mL (200 mL)

Stavzor™ [US] *see* valproic acid *on page 974*
Staxyn™ *see* vardenafil *on page 978*
Stelara™ [US/Can] *see* ustekinumab *on page 972*
Stelazine® ***(Discontinued)*** *see* trifluoperazine *on page 957*
Stemetil® [Can] *see* prochlorperazine *on page 797*
Sterapred® ***(Discontinued)*** *see* prednisone *on page 792*
Sterapred® DS ***(Discontinued)*** *see* prednisone *on page 792*
sterile talc *see* talc (sterile) *on page 908*
Sterile Talc Powder™ [US] *see* talc (sterile) *on page 908*
STI-571 *see* imatinib *on page 499*
Stieprox® [Can] *see* ciclopirox *on page 221*
Stieva-A [Can] *see* tretinoin (topical) *on page 951*
Stimate® [US] *see* desmopressin acetate *on page 278*
Sting-Kill® [US-OTC] *see* benzocaine *on page 124*
St. Joseph® Adult Aspirin [US-OTC] *see* aspirin *on page 100*
St. Joseph® Cough Suppressant ***(Discontinued)*** *see* dextromethorphan *on page 287*
St. Joseph® Measured Dose Nasal Solution ***(Discontinued)*** *see* phenylephrine (nasal) *on page 751*
Stop® [US] *see* fluoride *on page 413*
Strattera® [US/Can] *see* atomoxetine *on page 103*
Streptase® ***(Discontinued)***
streptokinase ***(Discontinued)***

streptomycin (strep toe MYE sin)

Sound-Alike/Look-Alike Issues
streptomycin may be confused with streptozocin

Synonyms streptomycin sulfate

Therapeutic Category Antibiotic, Aminoglycoside; Antitubercular Agent

Use Part of combination therapy of active tuberculosis; used in combination with other agents for treatment of streptococcal or enterococcal endocarditis, mycobacterial infections, plague, tularemia, and brucellosis

Dosage Summary

I.M.:

Children: 20-40 mg/kg given daily or 2-3 times/week (maximum: 1 g/day)
Adults: Tuberculosis: 15 mg/kg/day **or** 25-30 mg/kg 2-3 times/week; Other indications: 1-4 g/day in 2 divided doses
Elderly: 10 mg/kg/day (maximum: 750 mg/day)

I.V.:

Children: 20-40 mg/kg/day **or** 20-40 mg/kg twice weekly **or** 25-30 mg/kg 3 times/week (maximum: 1 g/day)
Adults: 1-4 g/day in 2 divided doses

Dosage Forms

Injection, powder for reconstitution: 1 g

streptomycin sulfate *see* streptomycin *on page 895*

streptozocin (strep toe ZOE sin)

Sound-Alike/Look-Alike Issues

streptozocin may be confused with streptomycin

U.S./Canadian Brand Names Zanosar® [US/Can]

Therapeutic Category Antineoplastic Agent

Use Treatment of metastatic islet cell carcinoma of the pancreas

Dosage Summary

I.V.:

Children: 1-1.5 g/m^2 weekly for 6 weeks followed by a 4-week rest period **or** 0.5-1 g/m^2 for 5 consecutive days as combination therapy followed by a 4- to 6-week rest period

Adults: 1-1.5 g/m^2 weekly for 6 weeks followed by a 4-week rest period **or** 0.5-1 g/m^2 for 5 consecutive days as combination therapy followed by a 4- to 6-week rest period

Dosage Forms

Injection, powder for reconstitution:

Zanosar®: 1 g

Striant® [US] *see* testosterone *on page 919*
Stridex® Essential Care® [US-OTC] *see* salicylic acid *on page 858*
Stridex® Facewipes To Go® [US-OTC] *see* salicylic acid *on page 858*
Stridex® Maximum Strength [US-OTC] *see* salicylic acid *on page 858*
Stridex® Sensitive Skin [US-OTC] *see* salicylic acid *on page 858*
Strifon Forte® [Can] *see* chlorzoxazone *on page 217*
Stromectol® [US] *see* ivermectin *on page 531*
strontium-89 chloride *see* strontium-89 *on page 896*

strontium-89 (STRON shee um atey nine)

Synonyms strontium-89 chloride

U.S./Canadian Brand Names Metastron® [US/Can]

Therapeutic Category Radiopharmaceutical

Use Relief of bone pain in patients with skeletal metastases

Dosage Summary

I.V.:

Children: Dosage not established

Adults: 148 megabecquerel (4 millicurie) over 1-2 minutes **or** 1.5-2.2 megabecquerel (40-60 microcurie)/kg

Dosage Forms

Injection, solution [preservative free]:

Metastron®: 1 mCi/mL (4 mL)

Strovite® [US] *see* vitamins (multiple/oral) *on page 990*
Strovite® Advance [US] *see* vitamins (multiple/oral) *on page 990*
Strovite® Forte [US] *see* vitamins (multiple/oral) *on page 990*
Strovite® Plus [US] *see* vitamins (multiple/oral) *on page 990*
Stuartnatal® Plus 3™ *(Discontinued)* *see* vitamins (multiple/prenatal) *on page 991*
Stuart Prenatal® [US-OTC] *see* vitamins (multiple/prenatal) *on page 991*
SU011248 *see* sunitinib *on page 906*
suberoylanilide hydroxamic acid *see* vorinostat *on page 992*
Sublimaze® *(Discontinued)* *see* fentanyl *on page 395*
Suboxone® [US] *see* buprenorphine and naloxone *on page 155*
Subutex® [US/Can] *see* buprenorphine *on page 155*

succimer (SUKS si mer)

Synonyms DMSA

U.S./Canadian Brand Names Chemet® [US/Can]

Therapeutic Category Chelating Agent

Use Treatment of lead poisoning in children with serum lead levels >45 mcg/dL

Dosage Summary

Oral:

Children: 10 mg/kg (or 350 mg/m^2/dose) every 8-12 hours (maximum: 500 mg/dose)

Dosage Forms

Capsule, oral:

Chemet®: 100 mg

succinylcholine (suks in il KOE leen)

Synonyms succinylcholine chloride; suxamethonium chloride

U.S./Canadian Brand Names Anectine® [US]; Quelicin® [US/Can]

Therapeutic Category Skeletal Muscle Relaxant

Use To facilitate both rapid sequence and routine endotracheal intubation and to relax skeletal muscles during surgery; to reduce the intensity of muscle contractions of pharmacologically- or electrically-induced convulsions; does not relieve pain or produce sedation

Dosage Summary

I.M.:

Children: Up to 3-4 mg/kg (maximum: 150 mg total dose)

Adults: Up to 3-4 mg/kg (maximum: 150 mg total dose)

I.V.:

Smaller Children: Intermittent: Initial: 2 mg/kg/dose one time; Maintenance: 0.3-0.6 mg/kg/dose every 5-10 minutes as needed

Older Children and Adolescents: Intermittent: Initial: 1 mg/kg/dose one time; Maintenance: 0.3-0.6 mg/kg every 5-10 minutes as needed

Adults: Short surgical procedures: 0.6 mg/kg (range: 0.3-1.1 mg/kg); Long surgical procedures: 2.5-4.3 mg/minute continuous infusion, adjust dose based on response **or** 0.3-1.1 mg/kg followed by 0.04-0.07 mg/kg/dose as required

Dosage Forms

Injection, solution:

Anectine®: 20 mg/mL (10 mL)

Quelicin®: 20 mg/mL (10 mL)

Injection, solution [preservative free]:

Quelicin®: 100 mg/mL (10 mL)

succinylcholine chloride *see* succinylcholine *on page* 897

Suclor™ [US] *see* chlorpheniramine and pseudoephedrine *on page* 209

Sucraid® [US/Can] *see* sacrosidase *on page* 857

sucralfate (soo KRAL fate)

Sound-Alike/Look-Alike Issues

sucralfate may be confused with salsalate

Carafate® may be confused with Cafergot®

Synonyms aluminum sucrose sulfate, basic

U.S./Canadian Brand Names Carafate® [US]; Novo-Sucralate [Can]; Nu-Sucralate [Can]; PMS-Sucralate [Can]; Sulcrate® Suspension Plus [Can]; Sulcrate® [Can]

Therapeutic Category Gastrointestinal Agent, Gastric or Duodenal Ulcer Treatment

Use Short-term (≤8 weeks) management of duodenal ulcers; maintenance therapy for duodenal ulcers

Dosage Summary

Oral:

Children: Dosage not established

Adults: 1 g 2-4 times/day

Dosage Forms

Suspension, oral: 1 g/10 mL (10 mL)

Carafate®: 1 g/10 mL (420 mL)

Tablet, oral: 1 g

Carafate®: 1 g

Sucrets® Children's [US-OTC] *see* dyclonine *on page* 338

Sucrets® Cough Calmers *(Discontinued)* *see* dextromethorphan *on page* 287

Sucrets® Maximum Strength [US-OTC] *see* dyclonine *on page* 338

Sucrets® Original [US-OTC] *see* hexylresorcinol *on page* 472

Sucrets® Regular Strength [US-OTC] *see* dyclonine *on page 338*
Sudafed® 12 Hour [US-OTC] *see* pseudoephedrine *on page 810*
Sudafed® 12 Hour Pressure + Pain [US-OTC] *see* naproxen and pseudoephedrine *on page 661*
Sudafed® 24 Hour [US-OTC] *see* pseudoephedrine *on page 810*
Sudafed® Children's [US-OTC] *see* pseudoephedrine *on page 810*
Sudafed® Children's Cold & Cough [US-OTC] *see* pseudoephedrine and dextromethorphan *on page 812*
Sudafed® Decongestant [Can] *see* pseudoephedrine *on page 810*
Sudafed® Head Cold and Sinus Extra Strength [Can] *see* acetaminophen and pseudoephedrine *on page 26*
Sudafed® Maximum Strength Nasal Decongestant [US-OTC] *see* pseudoephedrine *on page 810*
Sudafed® Maximum Strength Sinus Nighttime *(Discontinued)* *see* triprolidine and pseudoephedrine *on page 961*
Sudafed® Non-Drying Sinus *(Discontinued)* *see* guaifenesin and pseudoephedrine *on page 457*
Sudafed OM® Sinus Congestion [US-OTC] *see* oxymetazoline (nasal) *on page 716*
Sudafed PE® Children's [US-OTC] *see* phenylephrine (systemic) *on page 751*
Sudafed PE® Children's Cold & Cough [US-OTC] *see* dextromethorphan and phenylephrine *on page 289*
Sudafed PE® Congestion [US-OTC] *see* phenylephrine (systemic) *on page 751*
Sudafed PE™ Nasal Decongestant [US-OTC] *see* phenylephrine (systemic) *on page 751*
Sudafed PE® Nighttime Cold [US-OTC] *see* acetaminophen, diphenhydramine, and phenylephrine *on page 30*
Sudafed PE® Pressure + Pain [US-OTC] *see* acetaminophen and phenylephrine *on page 25*
Sudafed PE® Severe Cold [US-OTC] *see* acetaminophen, diphenhydramine, and phenylephrine *on page 30*
Sudafed PE® Sinus + Allergy [US-OTC] *see* chlorpheniramine and phenylephrine *on page 208*
Sudafed PE® Sinus Headache *(Discontinued)* *see* acetaminophen and phenylephrine *on page 25*
Sudafed® Sinus Advance [Can] *see* pseudoephedrine and ibuprofen *on page 812*
Sudafed® Sinus & Allergy [US-OTC] *see* chlorpheniramine and pseudoephedrine *on page 209*
SudaHist® [US] *see* chlorpheniramine and pseudoephedrine *on page 209*
Sudal® 12 [US] *see* chlorpheniramine and pseudoephedrine *on page 209*
SudaTex-DM [US] *see* guaifenesin, pseudoephedrine, and dextromethorphan *on page 460*
SudaTex-G [US-OTC] *see* guaifenesin and pseudoephedrine *on page 457*
Sudex® *(Discontinued)* *see* guaifenesin and pseudoephedrine *on page 457*
SudoGest [US-OTC] *see* pseudoephedrine *on page 810*
Sudogest 12 Hour [US-OTC] *see* pseudoephedrine *on page 810*
SudoGest Children's [US-OTC] *see* pseudoephedrine *on page 810*
Sudogest™ PE [US-OTC] *see* phenylephrine (systemic) *on page 751*
Sudo-Tab® [US-OTC] *see* pseudoephedrine *on page 810*
Sufedrin® *(Discontinued)* *see* pseudoephedrine *on page 810*
Sufenta® [US/Can] *see* sufentanil *on page 898*

sufentanil (soo FEN ta nil)

Sound-Alike/Look-Alike Issues
SUFentanil may be confused with alfentanil, fentaNYL
Sufenta® may be confused with Alfenta®, Sudafed®, Survanta®

Synonyms sufentanil citrate

Tall-Man SUFentanil

U.S./Canadian Brand Names Sufentanil Citrate Injection, USP [Can]; Sufenta® [US/Can]

Therapeutic Category Analgesic, Narcotic; General Anesthetic

Controlled Substance C-II

Use Analgesic supplement in maintenance of general anesthesia; epidural analgesic in conjunction with a local anesthetic

Dosage Summary Note: In obese patients (ie, >20% above ideal body weight), use lean body weight to determine dosage

I.V.:

Children <2 years: Dosage not established

Children 2-12 years: 10-25 mcg/kg with 100% O_2; Maintenance: Up to 1-2 mcg/kg total dose

Adults: 1-2 mcg/kg with N_2O/O_2; Maintenance: 5-20 mcg/kg as needed

Epidural:

Children: Dosage not established

Adults: 10-15 mcg (maximum: 3 doses)

Dosage Forms

Injection, solution [preservative free]: 50 mcg/mL (1 mL, 2 mL, 5 mL)

Sufenta®: 50 mcg/mL (1 mL, 2 mL, 5 mL)

sufentanil citrate *see* sufentanil *on page 898*

Sufentanil Citrate Injection, USP [Can] *see* sufentanil *on page 898*

sulamyd *see* sulfacetamide (ophthalmic) *on page 899*

sulamyd *see* sulfacetamide (topical) *on page 900*

Sular® [US] *see* nisoldipine *on page 677*

sulbactam and ampicillin *see* ampicillin and sulbactam *on page 76*

sulconazole (sul KON a zole)

Synonyms sulconazole nitrate

U.S./Canadian Brand Names Exelderm® [US/Can]

Therapeutic Category Antifungal Agent

Use Treatment of superficial fungal infections of the skin, including tinea cruris (jock itch), tinea corporis (ringworm), tinea versicolor, and possibly tinea pedis (athlete's foot, cream only)

Dosage Summary

Topical:

Children: Dosage not established

Adults: Apply a small amount to affected area once or twice daily

Dosage Forms

Cream, topical:

Exelderm®: 1% (15 g, 30 g, 60 g)

Solution, topical:

Exelderm®: 1% (30 mL)

sulconazole nitrate *see* sulconazole *on page 899*

Sulcrate® [Can] *see* sucralfate *on page 897*

Sulcrate® Suspension Plus [Can] *see* sucralfate *on page 897*

sulfabenzamide, sulfacetamide, and sulfathiazole

(sul fa BENZ a mide, sul fa SEE ta mide, & sul fa THYE a zole)

Synonyms triple sulfa

U.S./Canadian Brand Names V.V.S.® [US]

Therapeutic Category Antibiotic, Vaginal

Use Treatment of *Haemophilus vaginalis* vaginitis

Dosage Summary

Intravaginal:

Children: Dosage not established

Adults: Insert 1/4 to 1 applicatorful twice daily

Dosage Forms

Cream, vaginal: Sulfabenzamide 3.7%, sulfacetamide 2.86%, and sulfathiazole 3.42% (78 g with applicator)

V.V.S.®: Sulfabenzamide 3.7%, sulfacetamide 2.86%, and sulfathiazole 3.42% (78 g with applicator)

sulfacetamide (ophthalmic) (sul fa SEE ta mide)

Sound-Alike/Look-Alike Issues

Bleph®-10 may be confused with Blephamide®

Synonyms sodium sulfacetamide; sulamyd

U.S./Canadian Brand Names AK Sulf Liq [Can]; Bleph 10 DPS [Can]; Bleph®-10 [US]; Diosulf™ [Can]; PMS-Sulfacetamide [Can]; Sodium Sulamyd [Can]; Sulfamide [US]

Therapeutic Category Antibiotic, Ophthalmic

Use Treatment and prophylaxis of conjunctivitis due to susceptible organisms; corneal ulcers; adjunctive treatment with systemic sulfonamides for therapy of trachoma

Dosage Summary

Ophthalmic:

Children ≤2 months: Dosage not established
Children >2 months: Solution: Instill 1-2 drops up to every 2-3 hours
Adults: Solution: Instill 1-2 drops up to every 2-3 hours

Dosage Forms

Solution, ophthalmic: 10% (15 mL)
Bleph®-10: 10% (5 mL)
Sulfamide: 10% (15 mL)

sulfacetamide (topical) (sul fa SEE ta mide)

Sound-Alike/Look-Alike Issues

Klaron® may be confused with Klor-Con®

Synonyms sodium sulfacetamide; sulamyd; sulfacetamide sodium

U.S./Canadian Brand Names Carmol® Scalp Treatment [US]; Klaron® [US]; Ovace® Plus [US]; Ovace® [US]; Rosula® NS [US]; Seb-Prev™ [US]; Sulfacet-R [Can]

Therapeutic Category Acne Products; Antibiotic, Sulfonamide Derivative; Topical Skin Product, Acne

Use Scaling dermatosis (seborrheic); bacterial infections of the skin; acne vulgaris

Dosage Summary

Topical:

Children ≤12 years: Dosage not established
Children >12 years: Apply thin film to affected area 1-4 times/day
Adults: Apply thin film to affected area 1-4 times/day

Dosage Forms

Aerosol, topical:
Ovace®: 10% (70 g)

Cream, topical:
Seb-Prev™: 10% (30 g, 60 g)

Gel, topical:
Seb-Prev™: 10% (30 g, 60 g)

Lotion, topical: 10% (118 mL)
Carmol® Scalp Treatment: 10% (85 g)
Klaron®: 10% (118 mL)
Ovace®: 10% (180 mL, 360 mL)
Ovace® Plus: 10% (480 mL)

Pad, topical: 10% (30s)
Rosula® NS: 10% (30s)

Soap, topical:
Seb-Prev™: 10% (170 mL, 340 mL)

Suspension, topical: 10% (118 mL)

sulfacetamide and prednisolone (sul fa SEE ta mide & pred NIS oh lone)

Sound-Alike/Look-Alike Issues

Blephamide® may be confused with Bleph®-10

Synonyms prednisolone and sulfacetamide

U.S./Canadian Brand Names AK Cide Oph [Can]; Blephamide® [US/Can]; Dioptimyd® [Can]

Therapeutic Category Antibiotic/Corticosteroid, Ophthalmic

Use Steroid-responsive inflammatory ocular conditions in which a corticosteroid is indicated and where infection is present or there is a risk of infection

Dosage Summary

Ophthalmic:

Children <6 years: Dosage not established
Children ≥6 years:
Ointment: Apply ~1/2 inch ribbon 3-4 times/day and 1-2 times at night
Solution, suspension: Instill 2 drops every 4 hours

Adults:
Ointment: Apply ~1/2 inch ribbon 3-4 times/day and 1-2 times at night
Solution, suspension: Instill 2 drops every 4 hours

Dosage Forms

Ointment, ophthalmic:
Blephamide®: Sulfacetamide 10% and prednisolone 0.2% (3.5 g)

Solution, ophthalmic: Sulfacetamide 10% and prednisolone 0.25% (5 mL, 10 mL)

Suspension, ophthalmic:
Blephamide®: Sulfacetamide 10% and prednisolone 0.2% (5 mL, 10 mL)

sulfacetamide and sulfur *see* sulfur and sulfacetamide *on page 903*
sulfacetamide sodium *see* sulfacetamide (topical) *on page 900*
sulfacetamide sodium and fluorometholone *(Discontinued)*
Sulfacet-R [Can] *see* sulfacetamide (topical) *on page 900*
Sulfacet-R® [US/Can] *see* sulfur and sulfacetamide *on page 903*

sulfadiazine (sul fa DYE a zeen)

Sound-Alike/Look-Alike Issues
sulfaDIAZINE may be confused with sulfasalazine, sulfiSOXAZOLE

Tall-Man sulf**ADIAZINE**

Therapeutic Category Sulfonamide

Use Treatment of urinary tract infections and nocardiosis; adjunctive treatment in toxoplasmosis; uncomplicated attack of malaria

Dosage Summary

Oral:
Newborns: 100 mg/kg/day divided every 6 hours
Children 1-2 months: 500 mg once daily **or** 100 mg/kg/day divided every 6 hours
Children 2-12 months: Loading dose: 75 mg/kg **or** 100-200 mg/kg/day divided every 4-6 hours (maximum: 6 g/day) **or** 500 mg once daily
Children 1-12 years: Loading dose: 75 mg/kg **or** 100-200 mg/kg/day divided every 4-6 hours (maximum: 6 g/day) **or** 500 mg twice daily
Children >12 years: Loading dose: 75 mg/kg **or** 100-200 mg/kg/day divided every 4-6 hours (maximum: 6 g/day) **or** 1 g twice daily
Adults: 2-8 g/day divideded every 6 hours **or** 1 g twice daily

Dosage Forms

Tablet, oral: 500 mg

sulfadoxine and pyrimethamine (sul fa DOKS een & peer i METH a meen)

Synonyms pyrimethamine and sulfadoxine

Therapeutic Category Antimalarial Agent

Use Treatment of *Plasmodium falciparum* malaria in patients in whom chloroquine resistance is suspected; malaria prophylaxis for travelers to areas where chloroquine-resistant malaria is endemic

Dosage Summary

Oral:
Children <2 months: Dosage not established
Children 2-11 months: 1/4 tablet as a single dose
Children 1-3 years: 1/2 tablet as a single dose
Children 4-8 years: 1 tablet as a single dose
Children 9-14 years: 2 tablets as a single dose
Children >14 years: 3 tablets as a single dose
Adults: 3 tablets as a single dose

Sulfa-Gyn® *(Discontinued)* *see* sulfabenzamide, sulfacetamide, and sulfathiazole *on page 899*
Sulfamethoprim® *(Discontinued)*

sulfamethoxazole and trimethoprim (sul fa meth OKS a zole & trye METH oh prim)

Sound-Alike/Look-Alike Issues
Bactrim™ may be confused with bacitracin, Bactine®, Bactroban®
co-trimoxazole may be confused with clotrimazole

Septra® may be confused with Ceptaz®, Sectral®
Septra® DS may be confused with Semprex®-D

Synonyms co-trimoxazole; SMZ-TMP; TMP-SMZ; trimethoprim and sulfamethoxazole

U.S./Canadian Brand Names Apo-Sulfatrim® DS [Can]; Apo-Sulfatrim® Pediatric [Can]; Apo-Sulfatrim® [Can]; Bactrim™ DS [US]; Bactrim™ [US]; Novo-Trimel D.S. [Can]; Novo-Trimel [Can]; Nu-Cotrimox [Can]; Septra® DS [US]; Septra® Injection [Can]; Septra® [US]; Sulfatrim® [US]

Therapeutic Category Sulfonamide

Use

Oral treatment of urinary tract infections due to *E. coli*, *Klebsiella* and *Enterobacter* sp, *M. morganii*, *P. mirabilis* and *P. vulgaris*; acute otitis media in children; acute exacerbations of chronic bronchitis in adults due to susceptible strains of *H. influenzae* or *S. pneumoniae*; treatment and prophylaxis of *Pneumocystis jiroveci* pneumonitis (PCP); traveler's diarrhea due to enterotoxigenic *E. coli*; treatment of enteritis caused by *Shigella flexneri* or *Shigella sonnei*

I.V. treatment of severe or complicated infections when oral therapy is not feasible, for documented PCP, empiric treatment of PCP in immune compromised patients; treatment of documented or suspected shigellosis, typhoid fever, *Nocardia asteroides* infection, or other infections caused by susceptible bacteria

Dosage Summary

I.V.:

Children ≤2 months: Dosage not established
Children >2 months: 8-20 mg TMP/kg/day divided every 6-12 hours
Adults: 8-20 mg TMP/kg/day divided every 6-12 hours

Oral:

Children ≤2 months: Dosage not established
Children >2 months: 6-20 mg TMP/kg/day divided every 6-12 hours **or** 150 mg TMP/m^2/day in divided doses every 12-24 hours for 3-7 days/week (maximum: sulfamethoxazole 1600 mg/day; trimethoprim 320 mg/day)
Adults: One or two double strength tablets (sulfamethoxazole 800-1600 mg; trimethoprim 160-320 mg) every 12-24 hours **or** 15-20 mg TMP/kg/day in 3-4 divided doses

Dosage Forms The 5:1 ratio (SMX:TMP) remains constant in all dosage forms.

Injection, solution: Sulfamethoxazole 80 mg and trimethoprim 16 mg per mL (5 mL, 10 mL, 30 mL)
Suspension, oral: Sulfamethoxazole 200 mg and trimethoprim 40 mg per 5 mL
Sulfatrim®: Sulfamethoxazole 200 mg and trimethoprim 40 mg per 5 mL
Tablet: Sulfamethoxazole 400 mg and trimethoprim 80 mg
Bactrim™, Septra®: Sulfamethoxazole 400 mg and trimethoprim 80 mg
Tablet, double strength: Sulfamethoxazole 800 mg and trimethoprim 160 mg
Bactrim™ DS, Septra® DS: Sulfamethoxazole 800 mg and trimethoprim 160 mg

Sulfamide [US] *see* sulfacetamide (ophthalmic) *on page* *899*
Sulfamylon® [US] *see* mafenide *on page* *582*

sulfanilamide (sul fa NIL a mide)

Synonyms p-amino-benzenesulfonamide

U.S./Canadian Brand Names AVC™ [US]

Therapeutic Category Antifungal Agent, Vaginal

Use Treatment of vulvovaginitis caused by *Candida albicans*

Dosage Summary

Intravaginal:

Children: Dosage not established
Adults: 1 applicatorful once or twice daily

Dosage Forms

Cream, vaginal:
AVC™: 15% (120 g)

sulfasalazine (sul fa SAL a zeen)

Sound-Alike/Look-Alike Issues

sulfasalazine may be confused with salsalate, sulfaDIAZINE, sulfiSOXAZOLE
Azulfidine® may be confused with Augmentin®, azaTHIOprine

Synonyms salicylazosulfapyridine

U.S./Canadian Brand Names Alti-Sulfasalazine [Can]; Azulfidine EN-tabs® [US]; Azulfidine® [US]; Salazopyrin En-Tabs® [Can]; Salazopyrin® [Can]

Therapeutic Category 5-Aminosalicylic Acid Derivative

Use Treatment of mild-to-moderate ulcerative colitis or as adjunctive therapy in severe ulcerative colitis; enteric coated tablets are also used for rheumatoid arthritis (including juvenile rheumatoid arthritis) in patients who inadequately respond to analgesics and NSAIDs

Dosage Summary

Oral:

Delayed release:

Children <6 years: Dosage not established

Children ≥6 years: Initial: 1/4 to 1/3 of expected maintenance dose; Maintenance: 30-50 mg/kg/day in 2 divided doses (maximum: 2 g/day); **Note:** Titration is recommended

Adults: Initial: 0.5-1 g/day; Maintenance: 2 g/day in 2 divided doses (maximum: 3 g/day); **Note:** Titration is recommended

Immediate release:

Children <6 years: Dosage not established

Children ≥6 years: Initial: 40-60 mg/kg/day in 3-6 divided doses; Maintenance: 30 mg/kg/day in 4 divided doses

Adults: Initial: 3-4 g/day in evenly divided doses at ≤8-hour intervals; Maintenance: 2 g/day in divided doses at ≤8-hour intervals

Dosage Forms

Tablet, oral: 500 mg

Azulfidine®: 500 mg

Tablet, delayed release, enteric coated, oral: 500 mg

Azulfidine EN-tabs®: 500 mg

Sulfatol® [US] *see* sulfur and sulfacetamide *on page 903*

Sulfatol®-M [US] *see* sulfur and sulfacetamide *on page 903*

Sulfatrim® [US] *see* sulfamethoxazole and trimethoprim *on page 901*

Sulfa-Trip® ***(Discontinued)*** *see* sulfabenzamide, sulfacetamide, and sulfathiazole *on page 899*

sulfinpyrazone ***(Discontinued)***

sulfisoxazole (sul fi SOKS a zole)

Sound-Alike/Look-Alike Issues

sulfiSOXAZOLE may be confused with sulfaDIAZINE, sulfamethoxazole, sulfasalazine

Gantrisin® may be confused with Gastrosed™

Synonyms sulfisoxazole acetyl; sulphafurazole

Tall-Man sulfi**SOXAZOLE**

U.S./Canadian Brand Names Novo-Soxazole [Can]; Sulfizole® [Can]

Therapeutic Category Sulfonamide

Use Treatment of urinary tract infections, otitis media, *Chlamydia*; nocardiosis

Dosage Summary

Oral:

Children ≤2 months: Dosage not established

Children >2 months: Initial: 75 mg/kg as a single dose; Maintenance: 120-150 mg/kg/day divided every 4-6 hours (maximum: 6 g/day)

Adults: Initial: 2-4 g as a single dose; Maintenance: 4-8 g/day divided every 4-6 hours

sulfisoxazole acetyl *see* sulfisoxazole *on page 903*

sulfisoxazole and erythromycin *see* erythromycin and sulfisoxazole *on page 363*

Sulfizole® [Can] *see* sulfisoxazole *on page 903*

sulfur and sulfacetamide (SUL fur & sul fa SEE ta mide)

Synonyms sodium sulfacetamide and sulfur; sulfacetamide and sulfur; sulfur and sulfacetamide sodium

U.S./Canadian Brand Names AVAR™ LS [US]; AVAR™ [US]; AVAR™-e Green [US]; AVAR™-e LS [US]; AVAR™-e [US]; BP Cleansing Wash [US]; BP10-1 [US]; Clarifoam™ EF [US]; Clenia™ [US]; Plexion SCT® [US]; Plexion® [US]; Prascion® FC [US]; Prascion® RA [US]; Prascion® [US]; Rosanil® [US]; Rosula® Clarifying [US]; Rosula® [US]; Sulfacet-R® [US/Can]; Sulfatol® [US]; Sulfatol®-M [US]; Sumaxin™ [US]

Therapeutic Category Antiseborrheic Agent, Topical

Use Aid in the treatment of acne vulgaris, acne rosacea, and seborrheic dermatitis

Dosage Summary

Topical:

Children <12 years: Dosage not established

Children ≥12 years: Apply a thin film 1-3 times/day

Adults: Apply a thin film 1-3 times/day

Dosage Forms

Aerosol, topical [foam]:

Clarifoam™ EF: Sulfur 5% and sulfacetamide 10% (60 g)

Cleanser, topical:

AVAR™: Sulfur 5% and sulfacetamide 10% (228 g)

AVAR™ LS: Sulfur 2% and sulfacetamide 10% (226.8 g)

Plexion®, Prascion®: Sulfur 5% and sulfacetamide 10% (170 g, 340 g)

Rosanil®: Sulfur 5% and sulfacetamide 10% (170 g, 390 g)

Rosula®: Sulfur 5% and sulfacetamide 10% (355 mL)

Cleanser, topical [emulsion-based]:

Sulfatol®: Sulfur 5% and sulfacetamide 10% (355 mL)

Cream, topical:

AVAR™-e, AVAR™-e Green, Prascion® RA, Rosac®: Sulfur 5% and sulfacetamide 10% (45 g)

AVAR™-e LS: Sulfur 2% and sulfacetamide 10% (45 g)

Clenia™: Sulfur 5% and sulfacetamide 10% (28 g)

Plexion SCT®: Sulfur 5% and sulfacetamide 10% (120 g)

Gel, topical:

Rosula®: Sulfur 5% and sulfacetamide 10% (45 g)

Gel, topical [emulsion-based]:

Sulfatol®: Sulfur 5% and sulfacetamide 10% (45 mL)

Lotion, topical: Sulfur 5% and sulfacetamide 10% (25 g, 30 g, 45 g, 60 g)

Sulfacaet-R®, Sulfatol®-M: Sulfur 5% and sulfacetamide 10% (25 g)

Pad, topical [cleansing cloth]: Sulfur 4% and sulfacetamide sodium 10% (60s)

Plexion®, Prascion® FC: Sulfur 5% and sulfacetamide 10% (30s, 60s)

Sumaxin™: Sulfur 4% and sulfacetamide 10% (60s)

Suspension, topical: Sulfur 5% and sulfacetamide 10% (30 g)

Wash, topical: Sulfur 5% and sulfacetamide 10% (170 g, 340 g)

BP10-1: Sulfur 1% and sulfacetamide sodium 10% (170 g)

BP Cleansing Wash, Clenia™: Sulfur 5% and sulfacetamide 10% (170 g, 340 g)

Wash, topical [emulsion-based]:

Rosula® Clarifying: Sulfur 4% and sulfacetamide 10% (473 mL)

sulfur and sulfacetamide sodium *see* sulfur and sulfacetamide *on page 903*

sulindac (SUL in dak)

Sound-Alike/Look-Alike Issues

Clinoril® may be confused with Cleocin®, Clozaril®

U.S./Canadian Brand Names Apo-Sulin® [Can]; Clinoril® [US]; Novo-Sundac [Can]; Nu-Sundac [Can]

Therapeutic Category Analgesic, Nonnarcotic; Nonsteroidal Antiinflammatory Drug (NSAID)

Use Management of inflammatory diseases including osteoarthritis, rheumatoid arthritis, acute gouty arthritis, ankylosing spondylitis, acute painful shoulder (bursitis/tendonitis)

Dosage Summary

Oral:

Children: Dosage not established

Adults: 150-200 mg twice daily (maximum: 400 mg/day)

Dosage Forms

Tablet, oral: 150 mg, 200 mg

Clinoril®: 200 mg

sulphafurazole *see* sulfisoxazole *on page 903*

Sultrin™ *(Discontinued)* *see* sulfabenzamide, sulfacetamide, and sulfathiazole *on page 899*

sumatriptan (soo ma TRIP tan)

Sound-Alike/Look-Alike Issues

SUMAtriptan may be confused with saxagliptin, sitaGLIPtin, somatropin, zolmitriptan

Synonyms sumatriptan succinate

Tall-Man **SUMA**triptan

U.S./Canadian Brand Names Apo-Sumatriptan® [Can]; CO Sumatriptan [Can]; Dom-Sumatriptan [Can]; Gen-Sumatriptan [Can]; Imitrex® DF [Can]; Imitrex® Nasal Spray [Can]; Imitrex® [US/Can]; Mylan-Sumatriptan [Can]; Novo-Sumatriptan [Can]; PHL-Sumatriptan [Can]; PMS-Sumatriptan [Can]; ratio-Sumatriptan [Can]; Rhoxal-sumatriptan [Can]; Riva-Sumatriptan [Can]; Sandoz-Sumatriptan [Can]; Sumatryx [Can]; Sumavel™ DosePro™ [US]

Therapeutic Category Antimigraine Agent

Use

Intranasal, Oral, SubQ: Acute treatment of migraine with or without aura

SubQ: Acute treatment of cluster headache episodes

Dosage Summary

Intranasal:

Children: Dosage not established

Adults: 5-20 mg in one nostril as a single dose (may divide dose into both nostrils); may repeat after 2 hours (maximum: 40 mg/day)

Oral:

Children: Dosage not established

Adults: 25-100 mg as a single dose; may repeat after 2 hours (maximum: 200 mg/day)

SubQ:

Children: Dosage not established

Adults: Initial: Up to 6 mg; may repeat if needed ≥1 hour after initial dose (maximum: Two 6 mg injections per 24-hour period)

Dosage Forms

Injection, solution: 4 mg/0.5 mL (0.5 mL); 6 mg/0.5 mL (0.5 mL)

Imitrex®: 4 mg/0.5 mL (0.5 mL); 6 mg/0.5 mL (0.5 mL)

Sumavel™ DosePro™: 6 mg/0.5 mL (0.5 mL)

Solution, intranasal: 5 mg/0.1 mL (6s); 20 mg/0.1 mL (6s)

Imitrex®: 5 mg/0.1 mL (6s); 20 mg/0.1 mL (6s)

Tablet, oral: 25 mg, 50 mg, 100 mg

Imitrex®: 25 mg, 50 mg, 100 mg

sumatriptan and naproxen (soo ma TRIP tan & na PROKS en)

Sound-Alike/Look-Alike Issues

naproxen may be confused with Natacyn®, Nebcin®, neomycin, niacin

SUMAtriptan may be confused with somatropin, zolmitriptan

Treximet™ may be confused with Trexall™

Synonyms naproxen and sumatriptan; naproxen sodium and sumatriptan; naproxen sodium and sumatriptan succinate; sumatriptan succinate and naproxen; sumatriptan succinate and naproxen sodium

U.S./Canadian Brand Names Treximet™ [US]

Therapeutic Category Antimigraine Agent; Nonsteroidal Antiinflammatory Drug (NSAID); Serotonin 5-$HT_{1B,\ 1D}$ Receptor Agonist

Use Acute treatment of migraine with or without aura

Dosage Summary

Oral:

Children: Dosage not established

Adults: 1 tablet (sumatriptan 85 mg and naproxen 500 mg). If a satisfactory response has not been obtained at 2 hours, a second dose may be administered (maximum: 2 tablets/24 hours)

Dosage Forms

Tablet:

Treximet™ 85/500: Sumatriptan 85 mg and naproxen sodium 500 mg

sumatriptan succinate *see* sumatriptan *on page 904*

sumatriptan succinate and naproxen *see* sumatriptan and naproxen *on page 905*

sumatriptan succinate and naproxen sodium *see* sumatriptan and naproxen *on page 905*

Sumatryx [Can] *see* sumatriptan *on page 904*

Sumavel™ DosePro™ [US] *see* sumatriptan *on page 904*

Sumaxin™ [US] *see* sulfur and sulfacetamide *on page 903*

Summer's Eve® Anti-Itch Maximum Strength [US-OTC] *see* pramoxine *on page 787*

Summer's Eve® Medicated Douche [US-OTC] *see* povidone-iodine (topical) *on page* 784
Summer's Eve® SpecialCare™ Medicated Anti-Itch Cream *(Discontinued)* *see* hydrocortisone (topical) *on page* 483
Sumycin® *(Discontinued)* *see* tetracycline *on page* 922
Sun-Benz® [Can] *see* benzydamine *(Canada only) on page* 130

sunitinib (su NIT e nib)

Sound-Alike/Look-Alike Issues
sunitinib may be confused with imatinib, sorafenib

Synonyms SU011248; SU11248; sunitinib malate

U.S./Canadian Brand Names Sutent® [US/Can]

Therapeutic Category Antineoplastic Agent, Tyrosine Kinase Inhibitor; Vascular Endothelial Growth Factor (VEGF) Inhibitor

Use Treatment of gastrointestinal stromal tumor (GIST) intolerant to or with disease progression on imatinib; treatment of advanced renal cell cancer (RCC)

Dosage Summary Note: Dosage modifications should be done in increments of 12.5 mg; individualize based on safety and tolerability

Oral:
Children: Dosage not established
Adults: 50 mg once daily for 4 weeks of a 6-week treatment cycle

Dosage Forms
Capsule, oral:
Sutent®: 12.5 mg, 25 mg, 50 mg

sunitinib malate *see* sunitinib *on page* 906
Supartz™ [US] *see* hyaluronate and derivatives *on page* 475
Super Calcium 600 [US-OTC] *see* calcium carbonate *on page* 167
Superdophilus® [US-OTC] *see* Lactobacillus *on page* 543
Supeudol® [Can] *see* oxycodone *on page* 714
Suphera™ *(Discontinued)* *see* sulfur and sulfacetamide *on page* 903
Suplasyn® [Can] *see* hyaluronate and derivatives *on page* 475
Suppress® *(Discontinued)* *see* dextromethorphan *on page* 287
Suprane® [US/Can] *see* desflurane *on page* 276
Suprefact® [Can] *see* buserelin acetate *(Canada only) on page* 157
Suprefact® Depot [Can] *see* buserelin acetate *(Canada only) on page* 157
Surgam® [Can] *see* tiaprofenic acid *(Canada only) on page* 931
Surgicel® [US] *see* cellulose, oxidized regenerated *on page* 195
Surgicel® Fibrillar [US] *see* cellulose, oxidized regenerated *on page* 195
Surgicel® NuKnit [US] *see* cellulose, oxidized regenerated *on page* 195
Surmontil® [US/Can] *see* trimipramine *on page* 960
Survanta® [US/Can] *see* beractant *on page* 131
Sus-Phrine® *(Discontinued)* *see* epinephrine (systemic, oral inhalation) *on page* 352
Sustaire® *(Discontinued)* *see* theophylline *on page* 925
Sustiva® [US/Can] *see* efavirenz *on page* 343
SuTan *(Discontinued)* *see* dexchlorpheniramine and pseudoephedrine *on page* 283
Sutent® [US/Can] *see* sunitinib *on page* 906
Su-Tuss DM *(Discontinued)* *see* guaifenesin and dextromethorphan *on page* 455
Su-Tuss®-HD *(Discontinued)*
suxamethonium chloride *see* succinylcholine *on page* 897
Sween Cream® [US-OTC] *see* vitamin A and vitamin D *on page* 988
Symadine® *(Discontinued)*
Symax® DuoTab [US] *see* hyoscyamine *on page* 491
Symax® FasTab [US] *see* hyoscyamine *on page* 491
Symax® SL [US] *see* hyoscyamine *on page* 491
Symax® SR [US] *see* hyoscyamine *on page* 491
Symbicort® [US/Can] *see* budesonide and formoterol *on page* 152

Symbyax® [US] *see* olanzapine and fluoxetine *on page* *697*
Symlin® [US] *see* pramlintide *on page* *786*
Symmetrel® [US/Can] *see* amantadine *on page* *61*
SymTan™ ***(Discontinued)***
synacthen *see* cosyntropin *on page* *253*
Synagis® [US/Can] *see* palivizumab *on page* *721*
Synalar® [Can] *see* fluocinolone (topical) *on page* *411*
Synalar® ***(Discontinued)*** *see* fluocinolone (topical) *on page* *411*
Synalar-HP® Topical ***(Discontinued)*** *see* fluocinolone (topical) *on page* *411*
Synalgos®-DC [US] *see* dihydrocodeine, aspirin, and caffeine *on page* *303*
Synarel® [US/Can] *see* nafarelin *on page* *655*
Synemol® Topical ***(Discontinued)*** *see* fluocinolone (topical) *on page* *411*
Synera™ [US] *see* lidocaine and tetracaine *on page* *565*
Synercid® [US/Can] *see* quinupristin and dalfopristin *on page* *823*
Synphasic® [Can] *see* ethinyl estradiol and norethindrone *on page* *378*
Syntest D.S. ***(Discontinued)*** *see* estrogens (esterified) and methyltestosterone *on page* *372*
Syntest H.S. ***(Discontinued)*** *see* estrogens (esterified) and methyltestosterone *on page* *372*
Synthroid® [US/Can] *see* levothyroxine *on page* *560*
Syntocinon® [Can] *see* oxytocin *on page* *719*
Synvisc® [US] *see* hyaluronate and derivatives *on page* *475*
Synvisc-One™ [US] *see* hyaluronate and derivatives *on page* *475*
Syprine® [US/Can] *see* trientine *on page* *957*
Syrex [US] *see* sodium chloride *on page* *882*
SyringeAvitene™ [US] *see* collagen hemostat *on page* *248*
syrup of ipecac *see* ipecac syrup *on page* *522*
Systane® [US-OTC] *see* artificial tears *on page* *97*
Systane® Free [US-OTC] *see* artificial tears *on page* *97*
Sytobex® ***(Discontinued)*** *see* cyanocobalamin *on page* *257*
T_3/T_4 liotrix *see* liotrix *on page* *568*
T_4 *see* levothyroxine *on page* *560*
T-20 *see* enfuvirtide *on page* *349*
642® Tablet [Can] *see* propoxyphene *on page* *805*
Tabloid® [US] *see* thioguanine *on page* *927*
Tac™-40 Injection ***(Discontinued)***
TachoSil® *see* fibrin sealant *on page* *401*
Taclonex® [US] *see* calcipotriene and betamethasone *on page* *164*
Taclonex Scalp® [US] *see* calcipotriene and betamethasone *on page* *164*
tacrine ***(Discontinued)***

tacrolimus (systemic) (ta KROE li mus)

Sound-Alike/Look-Alike Issues

tacrolimus may be confused with everolimus, pimecrolimus, sirolimus, temsirolimus
Prograf® may be confused with Gengraf®, Prozac®

Synonyms FK506

U.S./Canadian Brand Names Advagraf™ [Can]; Prograf® [US/Can]

Therapeutic Category Calcineurin Inhibitor; Immunosuppressant Agent

Use Prevention of organ rejection in heart, kidney, or liver transplant recipients

Dosage Summary

I.V.:

Children: 0.03-0.05 mg/kg/day as a continuous infusion
Adults: 0.01-0.05 mg/kg/day as a continuous infusion

Oral:

Children: 0.15-0.2 mg/kg/day in divided doses every 12 hours
Adults: 0.075-0.2 mg/kg/day in divided doses every 12 hours

Dosage Forms

Capsule, oral: 0.5 mg, 1 mg, 5 mg

Prograf®: 0.5 mg, 1 mg, 5 mg

Injection, solution:

Prograf®: 5 mg/mL (1 mL)

tacrolimus (topical) (ta KROE li mus)

Sound-Alike/Look-Alike Issues

tacrolimus may be confused with everolimus, pimecrolimus, sirolimus, temsirolimus

U.S./Canadian Brand Names Protopic® [US/Can]

Therapeutic Category Calcineurin Inhibitor; Topical Skin Product

Use Moderate-to-severe atopic dermatitis in patients not responsive to conventional therapy or when conventional therapy is not appropriate

Dosage Summary

Topical:

Children <2 years: Dosage not established

Children ≥2 years: Apply 0.03% to affected area twice daily

Adults: Apply minimum amount of 0.03% or 0.1% to affected area twice daily

Dosage Forms

Ointment, topical:

Protopic®: 0.03% (30 g, 60 g, 100 g); 0.1% (30 g, 60 g, 100 g)

tadalafil (tah DA la fil)

Sound-Alike/Look-Alike Issues

tadalafil may be confused with sildenafil, vardenafil

Adcirca™ may be confused with Advair® Diskus®, Advair® HFA, Advicor®

Synonyms GF196960

U.S./Canadian Brand Names Adcirca™ [US/Can]; Cialis® [US/Can]

Therapeutic Category Phosphodiesterase (Type 5) Enzyme Inhibitor

Use

Adcirca™: Treatment of pulmonary arterial hypertension (PAH) (WHO Group I) to improve exercise ability

Cialis®: Treatment of erectile dysfunction (ED)

Dosage Summary

Oral:

Children: Dosage not established

Adults:

Erectile dysfunction: As-needed dosing: 5-20 mg prior to anticipated sexual activity as a single dose (maximum: 1 dose/day); Once-daily dosing: 2.5-5 mg once daily

Pulmonary arterial hypertension: 40 mg once daily

Dosage Forms

Tablet, oral:

Adcirca™: 20 mg

Cialis®: 2.5 mg, 5 mg, 10 mg, 20 mg

Tagamet® ***(Discontinued)*** *see* cimetidine *on page* 223

Tagamet® HB [Can] *see* cimetidine *on page* 223

Tagamet HB 200® [US-OTC] *see* cimetidine *on page* 223

TAK-375 *see* ramelteon *on page* 826

TAK-390MR *see* dexlansoprazole *on page* 283

talc *see* talc (sterile) *on page* 908

talc for pleurodesis *see* talc (sterile) *on page* 908

talc (sterile) (talk STARE il)

Synonyms intrapleural talc; sterile talc; talc; talc for pleurodesis

U.S./Canadian Brand Names Sclerosol® [US]; Sterile Talc Powder™ [US]

Therapeutic Category Sclerosing Agent

Use Prevention of recurrence of malignant pleural effusion in symptomatic patients

Dosage Summary

Intrapleural:

Children: Dosage not established

Adults: Aerosol: 4-8 g (1-2) cans as a single dose; Instillation: 5 g

Dosage Forms

Aerosol, intrapleural:

Sclerosol®: 4 g (4 g)

Powder, intrapleural:

Sterile Talc Powder™: USP: 100% (5 g)

Talwin® [US/Can] *see* pentazocine *on page 740*

Talwin® Nx *(Discontinued)* *see* pentazocine and naloxone *on page 740*

Tambocor™ [US/Can] *see* flecainide *on page 405*

Tamiflu® [US/Can] *see* oseltamivir *on page 709*

Tamofen® [Can] *see* tamoxifen *on page 909*

tamoxifen (ta MOKS i fen)

Sound-Alike/Look-Alike Issues

tamoxifen may be confused with pentoxifylline, Tambocor™, tamsulosin, temazepam

Synonyms ICI-46474; tamoxifen citras; tamoxifen citrate

U.S./Canadian Brand Names Apo-Tamox® [Can]; Mylan-Tamoxifen [Can]; Nolvadex®-D [Can]; Novo-Tamoxifen [Can]; PMS-Tamoxifen [Can]; Tamofen® [Can]

Therapeutic Category Antineoplastic Agent

Use Treatment of metastatic (female and male) breast cancer; adjuvant treatment of breast cancer; reduce risk of invasive breast cancer in women with ductal carcinoma *in situ* (DCIS); reduce the incidence of breast cancer in women at high risk

Dosage Summary

Oral:

Children: Dosage not established

Adults: 20-40 mg/day in 1-2 divided doses

Dosage Forms

Tablet, oral: 10 mg, 20 mg

tamoxifen citras *see* tamoxifen *on page 909*

tamoxifen citrate *see* tamoxifen *on page 909*

tamsulosin (tam SOO loe sin)

Sound-Alike/Look-Alike Issues

tamsulosin may be confused with tacrolimus, tamoxifen, terazosin

Flomax® may be confused with Flonase®, Flovent®, Foltx®, Fosamax®

Synonyms tamsulosin hydrochloride

U.S./Canadian Brand Names Flomax® CR [Can]; Flomax® [US]; JAMP-Tamsulosin [Can]; Mylan-Tamsulosin [Can]; Novo-Tamsulosin [Can]; RAN™-Tamsulosin [Can]; ratio-Tamsulosin [Can]; Sandoz-Tamsulosin [Can]

Therapeutic Category Alpha-Adrenergic Blocking Agent

Use Treatment of signs and symptoms of benign prostatic hyperplasia (BPH)

Dosage Summary

Oral:

Children: Dosage not established

Adults: Initial: 0.4 mg once daily; Maintenance: 0.4-0.8 mg once daily

Dosage Forms

Capsule, oral: 0.4 mg

Flomax®: 0.4 mg

tamsulosin and dutasteride *see* dutasteride and tamsulosin *on page 337*

tamsulosin hydrochloride *see* tamsulosin *on page 909*

tamsulosin hydrochloride and dutasteride *see* dutasteride and tamsulosin *on page 337*

Tanac® [US-OTC] *see* benzocaine *on page 124*

TanaCof-XR [US] *see* brompheniramine *on page 147*

Tanafed® *(Discontinued)* *see* chlorpheniramine and pseudoephedrine *on page 209*

Tanafed DMX™ [US] *see* chlorpheniramine, pseudoephedrine, and dextromethorphan *on page 214*
Tandem® DHA [US] *see* vitamins (multiple/prenatal) *on page 991*
Tandem® OB [US] *see* vitamins (multiple/prenatal) *on page 991*
Tannate-V-DM *(Discontinued)* *see* phenylephrine, pyrilamine, and dextromethorphan *on page 755*
Tannate 12 S *(Discontinued)* *see* carbetapentane and chlorpheniramine *on page 179*
Tannate PD-DM [US] *see* chlorpheniramine, pseudoephedrine, and dextromethorphan *on page 214*
Tannate Pediatric [US] *see* chlorpheniramine and phenylephrine *on page 208*
Tannic-12 *(Discontinued)* *see* carbetapentane and chlorpheniramine *on page 179*
Tannic-12 S *(Discontinued)* *see* carbetapentane and chlorpheniramine *on page 179*
Tannihist-12 D *(Discontinued)* *see* carbetapentane, phenylephrine, and pyrilamine *on page 181*
Tannihist-12 RF *(Discontinued)* *see* carbetapentane and chlorpheniramine *on page 179*
Tanta-Orciprenaline® [Can] *see* metaproterenol *on page 609*
Tantum® [Can] *see* benzydamine *(Canada only) on page 130*
TAP-144 *see* leuprolide *on page 554*
Tapazole® [US/Can] *see* methimazole *on page 613*

tapentadol (ta PEN ta dol)

Sound-Alike/Look-Alike Issues
tapentadol may be confused with traMADol
Synonyms CG5503; tapentadol hydrochloride
U.S./Canadian Brand Names Nucynta™ [US]
Therapeutic Category Analgesic, Opioid
Controlled Substance C-II
Use Relief of moderate-to-severe acute pain
Dosage Summary
Oral:
Children: Dosage not established
Adults: Day 1: 50-100 mg every 4-6 hours as needed; may administer a second dose ≥1 hour after the initial dose (maximum dose on first day: 700 mg/day); Day 2 and subsequent dosing: 50-100 mg every 4-6 hours as needed (maximum: 600 mg/day)
Dosage Forms
Tablet, oral:
Nucynta™: 50 mg, 75 mg, 100 mg

tapentadol hydrochloride *see* tapentadol *on page 910*
Tarabine® PFS *(Discontinued)* *see* cytarabine *on page 263*
Tarceva® [US/Can] *see* erlotinib *on page 360*
Targel® [Can] *see* coal tar *on page 242*
Targretin® [US/Can] *see* bexarotene (systemic) *on page 136*
Targretin® [US/Can] *see* bexarotene (topical) *on page 136*
Tarka® [US/Can] *see* trandolapril and verapamil *on page 947*
Taro-Amcinonide [Can] *see* amcinonide *on page 62*
Taro-Carbamazepine Chewable [Can] *see* carbamazepine *on page 177*
Taro-Ciprofloxacin [Can] *see* ciprofloxacin (systemic) *on page 224*
Taro-Clindamycin [Can] *see* clindamycin (topical) *on page 232*
Taro-Clobetasol [Can] *see* clobetasol *on page 235*
Taro-Desoximetasone [Can] *see* desoximetasone *on page 280*
Taro-Enalapril [Can] *see* enalapril *on page 348*
Taro-Fluconazole [Can] *see* fluconazole *on page 407*
Taro-Mometasone [Can] *see* mometasone (topical) *on page 641*
Taro-Simvastatin [Can] *see* simvastatin *on page 877*
Taro-Sone [Can] *see* betamethasone *on page 133*
Taro-Warfarin [Can] *see* warfarin *on page 993*
Tarsum® [US-OTC] *see* coal tar and salicylic acid *on page 243*
Tasigna® [US/Can] *see* nilotinib *on page 676*

Tasmar® [US] *see* tolcapone *on page* 940
Tavist® Allergy [US-OTC] *see* clemastine *on page* 231
Tavist® ND Allergy [US-OTC] *see* loratadine *on page* 575
Taxol® [Can] *see* paclitaxel *on page* 719
Taxol® *(Discontinued)* *see* paclitaxel *on page* 719
Taxotere® [US/Can] *see* docetaxel *on page* 321

tazarotene (taz AR oh teen)

U.S./Canadian Brand Names Avage™ [US]; Tazorac® [US/Can]

Therapeutic Category Keratolytic Agent

Use Topical treatment of facial acne vulgaris; topical treatment of stable plaque psoriasis of up to 20% body surface area involvement; mitigation (palliation) of facial skin wrinkling, facial mottled hyper-/ hypopigmentation, and benign facial lentigines

Dosage Summary

Topical:

Children <12 years: Dosage not established

Children ≥12 years: Apply a thin film **or** 2 mg/cm^2 once daily, in the evening

Adults: Apply a thin film **or** 2 mg/cm^2 once daily, in the evening

Dosage Forms

Cream, topical:

Avage™: 0.1% (30 g)

Tazorac®: 0.05% (30 g, 60 g); 0.1% (30 g, 60 g)

Gel, topical:

Tazorac®: 0.05% (30 g, 100 g); 0.1% (30 g, 100 g)

Tazicef® [US] *see* ceftazidime *on page* 192
tazobactam and piperacillin *see* piperacillin and tazobactam sodium *on page* 763
Tazocin® [Can] *see* piperacillin and tazobactam sodium *on page* 763
Tazorac® [US/Can] *see* tazarotene *on page* 911
Taztia XT® [US] *see* diltiazem *on page* 306
TB skin test *see* tuberculin tests *on page* 965
3TC® [Can] *see* lamivudine *on page* 545
3TC, abacavir, and zidovudine *see* abacavir, lamivudine, and zidovudine *on page* 18
T-cell growth factor *see* aldesleukin *on page* 46
TCGF *see* aldesleukin *on page* 46
TCN *see* tetracycline *on page* 922
Td *see* diphtheria and tetanus toxoid *on page* 313
TD-6424 *see* telavancin *on page* 912
Td Adsorbed [Can] *see* diphtheria and tetanus toxoid *on page* 313
Tdap *see* diphtheria, tetanus toxoids, and acellular pertussis vaccine *on page* 316
TDF *see* tenofovir *on page* 916
Teardrops® [Can] *see* artificial tears *on page* 97
Tear Drop® Solution *(Discontinued)* *see* artificial tears *on page* 97
TearGard® Ophthalmic Solution *(Discontinued)* *see* artificial tears *on page* 97
Teargen® [US-OTC] *see* artificial tears *on page* 97
Teargen® II [US-OTC] *see* artificial tears *on page* 97
Tearisol® [US-OTC] *see* artificial tears *on page* 97
Tears Again® [US-OTC] *see* artificial tears *on page* 97
Tears Again® MC Gel Drops™ [US-OTC] *see* hydroxypropyl methylcellulose *on page* 489
Tears Again® Gel Drops™ [US-OTC] *see* carboxymethylcellulose *on page* 184
Tears Again® Night and Day™ [US-OTC] *see* carboxymethylcellulose *on page* 184
Tears Naturale® [US-OTC] *see* artificial tears *on page* 97
Tears Naturale® II [US-OTC] *see* artificial tears *on page* 97
Tears Naturale® Free [US-OTC] *see* artificial tears *on page* 97
Tears Plus® [US-OTC] *see* artificial tears *on page* 97
Tears Renewed® [US-OTC] *see* artificial tears *on page* 97

TEAS *see* trolamine *on page 963*
Tebrazid™ [Can] *see* pyrazinamide *on page 816*
Tecnal C 1/2 [Can] *see* butalbital, aspirin, caffeine, and codeine *on page 160*
Tecnal C 1/4 [Can] *see* butalbital, aspirin, caffeine, and codeine *on page 160*
Tecta™ [Can] *see* pantoprazole *on page 725*

tegaserod (teg a SER od)

Synonyms HTF919; tegaserod maleate

U.S./Canadian Brand Names Zelnorm® [US]

Therapeutic Category Serotonin 5-HT_4 Receptor Agonist

Use Emergency treatment of irritable bowel syndrome with constipation (IBS-C) and chronic idiopathic constipation (CIC) in women (<55 years of age) in which no alternative therapy exists

Dosage Summary

Oral:

Children: Dosage not established

Adults:

Females <55 years of age: 6 mg twice daily, before meals

Females ≥55 years of age: Use is contraindicated.

Dosage Forms

Tablet, oral:

Zelnorm®: 2 mg, 6 mg

tegaserod maleate *see* tegaserod *on page 912*
Tega-Vert® Oral *(Discontinued)* *see* dimenhydrinate *on page 307*
Tegretol® [US/Can] *see* carbamazepine *on page 177*
Tegretol®-XR [US] *see* carbamazepine *on page 177*
TEI-6720 *see* febuxostat *on page 392*
Tekturna® [US] *see* aliskiren *on page 50*
Tekturna HCT® [US] *see* aliskiren and hydrochlorothiazide *on page 50*
Telachlor® Oral *(Discontinued)* *see* chlorpheniramine *on page 207*
Teladar® Topical *(Discontinued)*

telavancin (tel a VAN sin)

Sound-Alike/Look-Alike Issues

telavancin may be confused with telithromycin

Vibativ™ may be confused with Viactiv®, Vibramycin®, vigabatrin

Synonyms TD-6424; telavancin hydrochloride

U.S./Canadian Brand Names Vibativ™ [US]

Therapeutic Category Antibiotic, Miscellaneous

Use Treatment of complicated skin and skin structure infections caused by susceptible gram-positive organisms including methicillin-susceptible or -resistant *Staphylococcus aureus*, vancomycin-susceptible *Enterococcus faecalis*, and *Streptococcus pyogenes*, *Streptococcus agalactiae*, or *Streptococcus anginosus* group

Dosage Summary

I.V.:

Children: Dosage not established

Adults: 10 mg/kg every 24 hours for 1-2 weeks

Dosage Forms

Injection, powder for reconstitution:

Vibativ™: 250 mg, 750 mg

telavancin hydrochloride *see* telavancin *on page 912*

telbivudine (tel BI vyoo deen)

Synonyms L-deoxythymidine; LdT

U.S./Canadian Brand Names Sebivo® [Can]; Tyzeka® [US]

Therapeutic Category Antiretroviral Agent, Reverse Transcriptase Inhibitor (Nucleoside)

Use Treatment of chronic hepatitis B with evidence of viral replication and either persistent transaminase elevations or histologically-active disease

Dosage Summary

Oral:

Children <16 years: Dosage not established.

Children ≥16 years: 600 mg once daily

Adults: 600 mg once daily

Product Availability Tyzeka® oral solution: FDA approved April 2009; anticipated availability is currently undetermined

Dosage Forms

Tablet, oral:

Tyzeka®: 600 mg

Teldrin® HBP [US-OTC] *see* chlorpheniramine *on page* 207

Teldrin® Oral *(Discontinued)* *see* chlorpheniramine *on page* 207

telithromycin (tel ith roe MYE sin)

Sound-Alike/Look-Alike Issues

telithromycin may be confused with telavancin

Synonyms HMR 3647

U.S./Canadian Brand Names Ketek® [US/Can]

Therapeutic Category Antibiotic, Ketolide

Use Treatment of community-acquired pneumonia (mild-to-moderate) caused by susceptible strains of *Streptococcus pneumoniae* (including multidrug-resistant isolates), *Haemophilus influenzae*, *Chlamydophila pneumoniae*, *Moraxella catarrhalis*, and *Mycoplasma pneumoniae*

Dosage Summary

Oral:

Children <13 years: Dosage not established

Adults: 800 mg once daily

Dosage Forms

Tablet, oral:

Ketek®: 300 mg, 400 mg

Dosage Forms - Canada

Tablet:

Ketek®: 400 mg

telmisartan (tel mi SAR tan)

U.S./Canadian Brand Names Micardis® [US/Can]

Therapeutic Category Angiotensin II Receptor Antagonist

Use Treatment of hypertension (may be used alone or in combination with other antihypertensive agents); cardiovascular risk reduction in patients ≥55 years of age unable to take ACE inhibitors and who are at high risk of major cardiovascular events (eg, MI, stroke, death)

Dosage Summary

Oral:

Children: Dosage not established

Adults: Initial: 40-80 mg once daily; Maintenance: 20-80 mg/day once daily

Elderly: Initial: 20-80 mg once daily; Maintenance: 20-80 mg/day once daily

Dosage Forms

Tablet, oral:

Micardis®: 20 mg, 40 mg, 80 mg

telmisartan and amlodipine (tel mi SAR tan & am LOE di peen)

Synonyms amlodipine and telmisartan; amlodipine besylate and telmisartan

U.S./Canadian Brand Names Twynsta® [US]

Therapeutic Category Angiotensin II Receptor Blocker; Calcium Channel Blocker; Calcium Channel Blocker, Dihydropyridine

Use Treatment of hypertension, including initial treatment in patients who will require multiple antihypertensives for adequate control

Dosage Summary

Oral:

Children: Dosage not established.

Adults: Amlodipine 5-10 mg and telmisartan 40-80 mg once daily (maximum: 10 mg/day [amlodipine]; 80 mg/day [telmisartan]); **Note:** Titration is recommended

Dosage Forms

Tablet, oral:

Twynsta® 40/5: Telmisartan 40 mg and amlodipine 5 mg; Twynsta® 40/10: telmisartan 40 mg and amlodipine 10 mg; Twynsta® 80/5: telmisartan 80 mg and amlodipine 5 mg; Twynsta® 80/10: telmisartan 80 mg and amlodipine10 mg

telmisartan and hydrochlorothiazide (tel mi SAR tan & hye droe klor oh THYE a zide)

Synonyms hydrochlorothiazide and telmisartan

U.S./Canadian Brand Names Micardis® HCT [US]; Micardis® Plus [Can]

Therapeutic Category Antihypertensive Agent, Combination

Use Treatment of hypertension; combination product should not be used for initial therapy

Dosage Summary

Oral:

Children: Dosage not established

Adults: Initial: Telmisartan 80 mg and hydrochlorothiazide 12.5-25 mg once daily; Maintenance: Telmisartan 80-160 mg and hydrochlorothiazide 12.5-25 mg once daily

Dosage Forms

Tablet, oral:

Micardis® HCT: 40/12.5: Telmisartan 40 mg and hydrochlorothiazide 12.5 mg; 80/12.5: Telmisartan 80 mg and hydrochlorothiazide 12.5 mg; 80/25: Telmisartan 80 mg and hydrochlorothiazide 25 mg

Dosage Forms - Canada

Tablet, oral:

Micardis® Plus: 80/25: Telmisartan 80 mg and hydrochlorothiazide 25 mg

Telzir® [Can] *see* fosamprenavir *on page 426*

temazepam (te MAZ e pam)

Sound-Alike/Look-Alike Issues

temazepam may be confused with flurazepam, LORazepam, tamoxifen

Restoril™ may be confused with, Risperdal®, Vistaril®, Zestril®

U.S./Canadian Brand Names Apo-Temazepam® [Can]; CO Temazepam [Can]; Dom-Temazepam [Can]; Gen-Temazepam [Can]; Novo-Temazepam [Can]; Nu-Temazepam [Can]; PHL-Temazepam [Can]; PMS-Temazepam [Can]; ratio-Temazepam [Can]; Restoril™ [US/Can]

Therapeutic Category Benzodiazepine

Controlled Substance C-IV

Use Short-term treatment of insomnia

Dosage Summary

Oral:

Children: Dosage not established

Adults: 15-30 mg at bedtime

Elderly: 15 mg at bedtime

Dosage Forms

Capsule, oral: 7.5 mg, 15 mg, 22.5 mg, 30 mg

Restoril™: 7.5 mg, 15 mg, 22.5 mg, 30 mg

Temodal® [Can] *see* temozolomide *on page 914*
Temodar® [US] *see* temozolomide *on page 914*
Temovate® [US] *see* clobetasol *on page 235*
Temovate E® [US] *see* clobetasol *on page 235*

temozolomide (te moe ZOE loe mide)

Sound-Alike/Look-Alike Issues

Temodar® may be confused with Tambocor®

Synonyms TMZ

U.S./Canadian Brand Names Temodal® [Can]; Temodar® [US]

Therapeutic Category Antineoplastic Agent, Alkylating Agent

Use Treatment of newly-diagnosed glioblastoma multiforme (initially in combination with radiotherapy, then as maintenance treatment); treatment of refractory anaplastic astrocytoma

Note: The following use is approved in Canada (not an approved indication in the U.S.): Treatment of recurrent glioblastoma multiforme

Dosage Summary

Oral:

Children: Dosage not established

Adults: Initial: 150 mg/m^2/day for 5 days; Subsequent doses: 100-200 mg/m^2/day for 5 days every 28 days, based upon hematologic tolerance **or** Concomitant phase: 75 mg/m^2/day for 42 days with radiotherapy (60Gy administered in 30 fractions); Maintenance phase: 100-200 mg/m^2/day for 5 days every 28 days, based upon hematologic tolerance (maximum: 6 cycles)

I.V.:

Children: Dosage not established

Adults: Initial: 150 mg/m^2/day for 5 days; Subsequent doses: 100-200 mg/m^2/day for 5 days every 28 days, based upon hematologic tolerance or Concomitant phase: 75 mg/m^2/day for 42 days with radiotherapy (60Gy administered in 30 fractions); Maintenance phase: 100-200 mg/m^2/day for 5 days every 28 days, based upon hematologic tolerance (maximum: 6 cycles)

Dosage Forms

Capsule, oral:

Temodar®: 5 mg, 20 mg, 100 mg, 140 mg, 180 mg, 250 mg

Injection, powder for reconstitution:

Temodar®: 100 mg

Tempra® [Can] *see* acetaminophen *on page 21*

Tempra® *(Discontinued)* *see* acetaminophen *on page 21*

temsirolimus (tem sir OH li mus)

Sound-Alike/Look-Alike Issues

temsirolimus may be confused with everolimus, sirolimus, tacrolimus, temozolomide

Synonyms CCI-779

U.S./Canadian Brand Names Torisel® [US/Can]

Therapeutic Category Antineoplastic Agent, mTOR Kinase Inhibitor

Use Treatment of advanced renal cell cancer (RCC)

Dosage Summary

I.V.:

Children: Dosage not established

Adults: 25 mg once weekly

Dosage Forms

Injection, solution:

Torisel®: 25 mg/mL (1s)

Tenar™ DM [US] *see* guaifenesin, pseudoephedrine, and dextromethorphan *on page 460*

Tenar™ PSE [US] *see* guaifenesin and pseudoephedrine *on page 457*

tenecteplase (ten EK te plase)

Sound-Alike/Look-Alike Issues

TNKase® may be confused with Activase®, t-PA

TNK (occasional abbreviation for TNKase®) is an error-prone abbreviation (mistaken as TPA)

U.S./Canadian Brand Names TNKase® [US/Can]

Therapeutic Category Thrombolytic Agent

Use Thrombolytic agent used in the management of ST-elevation myocardial infarction (STEMI) for the lysis of thrombi in the coronary vasculature to restore perfusion and reduce mortality.

Recommended criteria for treatment: STEMI: Chest pain ≥20 minutes duration, onset of chest pain within 12 hours of treatment (or within prior 12-24 hours in patients with continuing ischemic symptoms), and S-T segment elevation >0.1 mV in at least two contiguous precordial leads or two adjacent limb leads on ECG or new or presumably new left bundle branch block (LBBB)

Dosage Summary

I.V.:

Children: Dosage not established
Adults <60 kg: 30 mg single dose over 5 seconds
Adults ≥60 to <70 kg: 35 mg single dose over 5 seconds
Adults ≥70 to <80 kg: 40 mg single dose over 5 seconds
Adults ≥80 to <90 kg: 45 mg single dose over 5 seconds
Adults ≥90 kg: 50 mg single dose over 5 seconds

Dosage Forms

Injection, powder for reconstitution:
TNKase®: 50 mg

Tenex® [US/Can] *see* guanfacine *on page 461*

teniposide (ten i POE side)

Sound-Alike/Look-Alike Issues
teniposide may be confused with etoposide

Synonyms EPT; PTG; VM-26

U.S./Canadian Brand Names Vumon® [US/Can]

Therapeutic Category Antineoplastic Agent

Use Treatment of refractory childhood acute lymphoblastic leukemia (ALL)

Dosage Summary

I.V.:

Children: 165 mg/m^2 twice weekly for 8-9 doses **or** 250 mg/m^2 weekly for 4-8 weeks

Dosage Forms

Injection, solution:
Vumon®: 10 mg/mL (5 mL)

Ten-K® ***(Discontinued)*** *see* potassium chloride *on page 781*

tenofovir (te NOE fo veer)

Synonyms PMPA; TDF; tenofovir disoproxil fumarate

U.S./Canadian Brand Names Viread® [US/Can]

Therapeutic Category Antiretroviral Agent, Reverse Transcriptase Inhibitor (Nucleotide)

Use Management of HIV infections in combination with at least two other antiretroviral agents; treatment of chronic hepatitis B virus (HBV)

Dosage Summary

Oral:

Children <12 years: Dosage not established
Children ≥12 years and <35 kg: Dosage not established
Children ≥12 years and ≥35 kg: 300 mg once daily
Adults: 300 mg once daily

Dosage Forms

Tablet, oral:
Viread®: 300 mg

tenofovir and emtricitabine *see* emtricitabine and tenofovir *on page 347*

tenofovir disoproxil fumarate *see* tenofovir *on page 916*

tenofovir disoproxil fumarate, efavirenz, and emtricitabine *see* efavirenz, emtricitabine, and tenofovir *on page 343*

Tenoretic® [US/Can] *see* atenolol and chlorthalidone *on page 103*

Tenormin® [US/Can] *see* atenolol *on page 102*

Tensilon® [Can] *see* edrophonium *on page 342*

Tenuate® [Can] *see* diethylpropion *on page 300*

Tenuate® ***(Discontinued)*** *see* diethylpropion *on page 300*

Tenuate® Dospan® [Can] *see* diethylpropion *on page 300*

Tenuate® Dospan® ***(Discontinued)*** *see* diethylpropion *on page 300*

Tequin® ***(Discontinued)*** *see* gatifloxacin *on page 438*

Tera-Gel™ [US-OTC] *see* coal tar *on page 242*

Terazol® [Can] *see* terconazole *on page* 918
Terazol® 3 [US] *see* terconazole *on page* 918
Terazol® 7 [US] *see* terconazole *on page* 918

terazosin (ter AY zoe sin)

U.S./Canadian Brand Names Apo-Terazosin® [Can]; Dom-Terazosin [Can]; Hytrin® [Can]; Nu-Terazosin [Can]; PHL-Terazosin [Can]; PMS-Terazosin [Can]; ratio-Terazosin [Can]; Teva-Terazosin [Can]

Therapeutic Category Alpha-Adrenergic Blocking Agent

Use Management of mild-to-moderate hypertension; alone or in combination with other agents such as diuretics or beta-blockers; benign prostate hyperplasia (BPH)

Dosage Summary

Oral:

Adults: Initial: 1 mg at bedtime; Maintenance: 1-20 mg once daily (maximum: 20 mg/day)

Dosage Forms

Capsule, oral: 1 mg, 2 mg, 5 mg, 10 mg

terbinafine (systemic) (TER bin a feen)

Sound-Alike/Look-Alike Issues

terbinafine may be confused with terbutaline
Lamisil® may be confused with Lamictal®, Lomotil®

Synonyms terbinafine hydrochloride

U.S./Canadian Brand Names Apo-Terbinafine® [Can]; CO Terbinafine [Can]; Lamisil® [US/Can]; Novo-Terbinafine [Can]; PHL-Terbinafine [Can]; PMS-Terbinafine [Can]; Riva-Terbinafine [Can]; Sandoz-Terbinafine [Can]

Therapeutic Category Antifungal Agent, Oral

Use Active against most strains of *Trichophyton mentagrophytes*, *Trichophyton rubrum*; may be effective for infections of *Microsporum gypseum* and *M. nanum*, *Trichophyton verrucosum*, *Epidermophyton floccosum*, *Candida albicans*, and *Scopulariopsis brevicaulis*

Onychomycosis of the toenail or fingernail due to susceptible dermatophytes; treatment of tinea capitis

Dosage Summary

Oral granules:

Children <4 years: Dosage not established
Children ≥4 years:
<25 kg: 125 mg once daily for 6 weeks
25-35 kg: 187.5 mg once daily for 6 weeks
>35 kg: 250 mg once daily for 6 weeks

Oral tablet:

Children: Dosage not established
Adults: 250-500 mg daily in 1-2 divided doses

Dosage Forms

Granules, oral:
Lamisil®: 125 mg/packet (14s, 42s); 187.5 mg/packet (14s, 42s)

Tablet, oral: 250 mg
Lamisil®: 250 mg

terbinafine (topical) (TER bin a feen)

Sound-Alike/Look-Alike Issues

terbinafine may be confused with terbutaline

Synonyms terbinafine hydrochloride

U.S./Canadian Brand Names Lamisil AT® [US-OTC]; Lamisil® [Can]

Therapeutic Category Antifungal Agent, Topical

Use Antifungal for the treatment of tinea pedis (athlete's foot), tinea cruris (jock itch), and tinea corporis (ringworm) [OTC/prescription formulations]; tinea versicolor [prescription formulations]

Dosage Summary

Topical:

Children <12 years: Dosage not established
Children ≥12 years: Apply to affected area once or twice daily
Adults: Apply to affected area once or twice daily

Dosage Forms

Cream, topical: 1% (12 g, 15 g, 24 g, 30 g)
Lamisil AT® [OTC]: 1% (12 g, 15 g, 24 g, 30 g, 36 g)

Gel, topical:
Lamisil AT® [OTC]: 1% (6 g, 12 g)

Solution, topical:
Lamisil AT® [OTC]: 1% (30 mL)

Dosage Forms - Canada

Cream, topical:
Lamisil®: 1% (15 g, 30 g)

Solution, topical [spray]:
Lamisil®: 1% (30 mL)

terbinafine hydrochloride *see* terbinafine (systemic) *on page* *917*
terbinafine hydrochloride *see* terbinafine (topical) *on page* *917*

terbutaline (ter BYOO ta leen)

Sound-Alike/Look-Alike Issues
terbutaline may be confused with terbinafine, TOLBUTamide
brethine may be confused with Methergine®

Synonyms brethine

U.S./Canadian Brand Names Bricanyl® [Can]

Therapeutic Category Adrenergic Agonist Agent

Use Bronchodilator in reversible airway obstruction and bronchial asthma

Dosage Summary

Oral:
Children 12-15 years: 2.5 mg every 6 hours 3 times/day (maximum: 7.5 mg/day)
Children >15 years: 2.5-5 mg every 6 hours 3 times/day (maximum: 15 mg/day)
Adults: 2.5-5 mg every 6 hours 3 times/day (maximum: 15 mg/day)

SubQ:
Children ≥12 years: 0.25 mg/dose; may repeat in 15-30 minutes (maximum: 0.5 mg/4-hour period)
Adults: 0.25 mg/dose; may repeat in 15-30 minutes (maximum: 0.5 mg/4 hour period)

Dosage Forms

Injection, solution: 1 mg/mL (1 mL)
Tablet, oral: 2.5 mg, 5 mg

Dosage Forms - Canada

Powder for oral inhalation:
Bricanyl® Turbuhaler: 500 mcg/actuation [50 or 200 metered actuations]

terconazole (ter KONE a zole)

Sound-Alike/Look-Alike Issues
terconazole may be confused with tioconazole

Synonyms triaconazole

U.S./Canadian Brand Names Terazol® 3 [US]; Terazol® 7 [US]; Terazol® [Can]; Zazole™ [US]

Therapeutic Category Antifungal Agent

Use Local treatment of vulvovaginal candidiasis

Dosage Summary

Intravaginal:
Children: Dosage not established
Adults: Insert 1 applicatorful or suppository at bedtime

Dosage Forms

Cream, vaginal: 0.4% (45 g); 0.8% (20 g)
Terazol® 7: 0.4% (45 g)
Terazol® 3: 0.8% (20 g)
Zazole™: 0.4% (45 g); 0.8% (20 g)

Suppository, vaginal: 80 mg (3s)
Terazol® 3: 80 mg (3s)

Terfluzine [Can] *see* trifluoperazine *on page* *957*

teriparatide (ter i PAR a tide)

Synonyms parathyroid hormone (1-34); recombinant human parathyroid hormone (1-34); rhPTH(1-34)

U.S./Canadian Brand Names Forteo® [US/Can]

Therapeutic Category Diagnostic Agent

Use Treatment of osteoporosis in postmenopausal women at high risk of fracture; treatment of primary or hypogonadal osteoporosis in men at high risk of fracture; treatment of glucocorticoid-induced osteoporosis in men and women at high risk for fracture

Dosage Summary

SubQ:

Children: Dosage not established

Adults: 20 mcg once daily

Dosage Forms

Injection, solution:

Forteo®: 250 mcg/mL (2.4 mL)

terpin hydrate *(Discontinued)*

Terra-Cortril® Ophthalmic Suspension *(Discontinued)*

Terramycin® I.M. *(Discontinued)*

Terramycin® Oral *(Discontinued)*

Terrell™ [US] *see* isoflurane *on page 527*

Tersi [US] *see* selenium sulfide *on page 869*

Tesamone® Injection *(Discontinued)* *see* testosterone *on page 919*

Teslac® *(Discontinued)*

TESPA *see* thiotepa *on page 928*

Tessalon® [US/Can] *see* benzonatate *on page 128*

tessalon perles *see* benzonatate *on page 128*

Testim® [US/Can] *see* testosterone *on page 919*

Testoderm® *(Discontinued)* *see* testosterone *on page 919*

Testoderm® TTS *(Discontinued)* *see* testosterone *on page 919*

Testoderm® With Adhesive *(Discontinued)* *see* testosterone *on page 919*

testolactone *(Discontinued)*

Testomar® *(Discontinued)* *see* yohimbine *on page 996*

Testopel® [US] *see* testosterone *on page 919*

Testopel® Pellet *(Discontinued)* *see* testosterone *on page 919*

testosterone (tes TOS ter one)

Sound-Alike/Look-Alike Issues

testosterone may be confused with testolactone

Testoderm® may be confused with Estraderm®

Synonyms testosterone cypionate; testosterone enanthate

U.S./Canadian Brand Names Andriol® [Can]; Androderm® [US/Can]; AndroGel® [US/Can]; Andropository [Can]; Delatestryl® [US/Can]; Depotest® 100 [Can]; Depo®-Testosterone [US]; Everone® 200 [Can]; First®-Testosterone MC [US]; First®-Testosterone [US]; PMS-Testosterone [Can]; Striant® [US]; Testim® [US/Can]; Testopel® [US]

Therapeutic Category Androgen

Controlled Substance C-III

Use

Injection: Androgen replacement therapy in the treatment of delayed male puberty; male hypogonadism (primary or hypogonadotropic); inoperable metastatic female breast cancer (enanthate only)

Pellet: Androgen replacement therapy in the treatment of delayed male puberty; male hypogonadism (primary or hypogonadotropic)

Buccal system, topical gel, transdermal system: Male hypogonadism (primary or hypogonadotropic)

Capsule (not available in U.S.): Androgen replacement therapy in the treatment of delayed male puberty; male hypogonadism (primary or hypogonadotropic); replacement therapy in impotence or for male climacteric symptoms due to androgen deficiency

Dosage Summary

Buccal:

Children: Dosage not established

Adults (males): 30 mg every 12 hours

I.M.:

Children: Dosage not established

Adolescents (males): 50-400 mg every 2-4 weeks

Adults: 50-400 mg every 2-4 weeks

SubQ:

Children: Dosage not established

Adolescents (males): 150-450 mg every 3-6 months

Adults (males): 150-450 mg every 3-6 months

Transdermal:

Androderm®:

Children: Dosage not established

Adults (males): Apply 2.5-7.5 mg/day at night time

AndroGel®, Testim®:

Children: Dosage not established

Adults (males): 5-10 g (50-100 mg testosterone) applied once daily in the morning (maximum: 10 g/day)

Dosage Forms

Cream, topical:

First®-Testosterone MC: 2% (60 g)

Gel, topical:

AndroGel®: 1% [5 g gel/packet] (30s); 1% [2.5 g gel/packet] (30s); 1% [1.25 g gel/actuation] (75 g)

Testim®: 1% [5 g gel/tube] (30s)

Implant, subcutaneous:

Testopel®: 75 mg (10s, 100s)

Injection, oil: 100 mg/mL (10 mL); 200 mg/mL (1 mL, 5 mL, 10 mL)

Delatestryl®: 200 mg/mL (1 mL, 5 mL)

Depo®-Testosterone: 100 mg/mL (10 mL); 200 mg/mL (1 mL, 10 mL)

Mucoadhesive, for buccal application:

Striant®: 30 mg (60s)

Ointment, topical:

First®-Testosterone: 2% (60 g)

Patch, transdermal:

Androderm®: 2.5 mg/24 hours (60s); 5 mg/24 hours (30s)

Dosage Forms - Canada

Capsule, gelatin:

Andriol™: 40 mg (10s)

testosterone cypionate *see* testosterone *on page 919*

testosterone enanthate *see* testosterone *on page 919*

Testred® [US] *see* methyltestosterone *on page 624*

tetanus and diphtheria toxoid *see* diphtheria and tetanus toxoid *on page 313*

tetanus immune globulin (human) (TET a nus i MYUN GLOB yoo lin HYU man)

Synonyms TIG

U.S./Canadian Brand Names HyperTET™ S/D [US/Can]

Therapeutic Category Immune Globulin

Use Prophylaxis against tetanus following injury in patients where immunization status is not known or uncertain

The Advisory Committee on Immunization Practices (ACIP) recommends passive immunization with TIG for the following:

- Persons with a wound that is not clean or minor and in whom contraindications to a tetanus-toxoid containing vaccine exist and they have not completed a primary series of tetanus toxoid immunization.
- Persons who are wounded in bombings or similar mass casualty events who have penetrating injuries or nonintact skin exposure and who cannot confirm receipt of a tetanus booster within the previous 5 years. In case of shortage, use should be reserved for persons ≥60 years of age.

Dosage Summary

I.M.:

Children <7 years: Prophylaxis: 4 units/kg

Children ≥7 years: Prophylaxis: 250 units

Children: Treatment: 500-6000 units

Adults: Prophylaxis: 250 units; Treatment: 500-6000 units

Dosage Forms

Injection, solution [preservative free]:

HyperTET™ S/D: 250 units/mL (~1 mL)

tetanus toxoid *see* diphtheria and tetanus toxoids, acellular pertussis, poliovirus and *Haemophilus* b conjugate vaccine *on page 314*

tetanus toxoid (adsorbed) (TET a nus TOKS oyd, ad SORBED)

Sound-Alike/Look-Alike Issues

Tetanus toxoid products may be confused with influenza virus vaccine and tuberculin products. Medication errors have occurred when tetanus toxoid products have been inadvertently administered instead of tuberculin skin tests (PPD) and influenza virus vaccine. These products are refrigerated and often stored in close proximity to each other.

Synonyms TT

Therapeutic Category Toxoid

Use Active immunization against tetanus when combination antigen preparations are not indicated. **Note:** Tetanus and diphtheria toxoids for adult use (Td) is the preferred immunizing agent for most adults and for children after their seventh birthday. Young children should receive trivalent DTaP (diphtheria/tetanus/acellular pertussis) as part of their childhood immunization program, unless pertussis is contraindicated, then DT is warranted.

Dosage Summary

I.M.:

Children <7 years: Dosage not established

Children ≥7 years: Initial: 0.5 mL; repeat at 4-8 weeks after first dose and 6-12 months after second dose; Booster: 0.5 mL every 10 years

Adults: Initial: 0.5 mL; repeat at 4-8 weeks after first dose and 6-12 months after second dose; Booster: 0.5 mL every 10 years

Dosage Forms

Injection, suspension: 5 Lf units/0.5 mL (0.5 mL, 5 mL)

tetanus toxoid (fluid) ***(Discontinued)***

tetanus toxoid, reduced diphtheria toxoid, and acellular pertussis, adsorbed *see* diphtheria, tetanus toxoids, and acellular pertussis vaccine *on page 316*

tetrabenazine (tet ra BEN a zeen)

U.S./Canadian Brand Names Nitoman™ [Can]; Xenazine® [US]

Therapeutic Category Monoamine Depleting Agent

Use Treatment of chorea associated with Huntington disease

Canadian labeling: Treatment of hyperkinetic movement disorders, including Huntington chorea, hemiballismus, senile chorea, Tourette syndrome, and tardive dyskinesia

Dosage Summary

Oral:

Children: Dosage not established.

Adults: 12.5 mg once daily; Maintenance: 25-100 mg/day in 2-3 divided doses; **Note:** Titration is recommended

Dosage Forms

Tablet, oral:

Xenazine®: 12.5 mg, 25 mg

Dosage Forms - Canada

Tablet:

Nitoman™: 25 mg

tetracaine (systemic) (TET ra kane)

Synonyms amethocaine hydrochloride; tetracaine hydrochloride

U.S./Canadian Brand Names Pontocaine® [Can]

Therapeutic Category Local Anesthetic

Use Spinal anesthesia

Dosage Summary

Subarachnoid injection:

Children: Dosage not established

Adults: 2-15 mg (maximum: 20 mg)

Dosage Forms

Injection, solution [preservative free]: 1% [10 mg/mL] (2 mL)

tetracaine (ophthalmic) (TET ra kane)

Synonyms amethocaine hydrochloride; tetracaine hydrochloride

U.S./Canadian Brand Names Pontocaine® [Can]

Therapeutic Category Local Anesthetic

Use Local anesthesia in the eye for various diagnostic and examination purposes

Dosage Summary

Ophthalmic:

Children: Dosage not established

Adults: Instill 1-2 drops into eye(s)

Dosage Forms

Solution, ophthalmic: 0.5% [5 mg/mL] (2 mL, 15 mL)

tetracaine (topical) (TET ra kane)

Synonyms amethocaine hydrochloride; tetracaine hydrochloride

U.S./Canadian Brand Names Ametop™ [Can]; Pontocaine® [US/Can]

Therapeutic Category Local Anesthetic

Use Applied to nose and throat for diagnostic procedures

Dosage Summary

Topical:

Children: Dosage not established

Adults: 0.25 % or 0.5% by direct application or nebulization (maximum: 20 mg total)

Dosage Forms

Solution, topical:

Pontocaine®: 2% [20 mg/mL] (30 mL, 118 mL)

tetracaine and lidocaine *see* lidocaine and tetracaine *on page 565*
tetracaine, benzocaine, and butamben *see* benzocaine, butamben, and tetracaine *on page 127*
tetracaine hydrochloride *see* tetracaine (ophthalmic) *on page 922*
tetracaine hydrochloride *see* tetracaine (systemic) *on page 921*
tetracaine hydrochloride *see* tetracaine (topical) *on page 922*
Tetracap® ***(Discontinued)*** *see* tetracycline *on page 922*
tetracosactide *see* cosyntropin *on page 253*

tetracycline (tet ra SYE kleen)

Sound-Alike/Look-Alike Issues

tetracycline may be confused with tetradecyl sulfate

achromycin may be confused with actinomycin, Adriamycin PFS®

Synonyms achromycin; TCN; tetracycline hydrochloride

U.S./Canadian Brand Names Apo-Tetra® [Can]; Nu-Tetra [Can]

Therapeutic Category Tetracycline Derivative

Use Treatment of susceptible bacterial infections of both gram-positive and gram-negative organisms; also infections due to *Mycoplasma*, *Chlamydia*, and *Rickettsia*; indicated for acne, exacerbations of chronic bronchitis, and treatment of gonorrhea and syphilis in patients who are allergic to penicillin; as part of a multidrug regimen for *H. pylori* eradication to reduce the risk of duodenal ulcer recurrence

Dosage Summary

Oral:

Children ≤8 years: Dosage not established

Children >8 years: 25-50 mg/kg/day divided every 6 hours

Adults: 250-500 mg 2-4 times/day

Dosage Forms

Capsule, oral: 250 mg, 500 mg

tetracycline hydrochloride *see* tetracycline *on page 922*

tetracycline, metronidazole, and bismuth subcitrate potassium *see* bismuth, metronidazole, and tetracycline *on page 140*

tetracycline, metronidazole, and bismuth subsalicylate *see* bismuth, metronidazole, and tetracycline *on page 140*

tetrahydrocannabinol *see* dronabinol *on page 333*

tetrahydrocannabinol and cannabidiol *(Canada only)*

(TET ra hye droe can NAB e nol & can nab e DYE ol)

Synonyms cannabidiol and tetrahydrocannabinol; delta-9-tetrahydrocannabinol and cannabinol; GW-1000-02; THC and CBD

U.S./Canadian Brand Names Sativex® [Can]

Therapeutic Category Analgesic, Miscellaneous

Controlled Substance CDSA-II

Use Adjunctive treatment of neuropathic pain or spasticity in multiple sclerosis; adjunctive treatment of moderate-to-severe pain in advanced cancer

Dosage Summary

Buccal:

Children: Dosage not established

Adults: Initial: One spray twice daily; Maintenance: Titration recommended; Usual maximum: 12 sprays/day

Dosage Forms - Canada

Solution, buccal [spray]:

Sativex®: Delta-9 tetrahydrocannabinol 27 mg/mL and cannabidiol 25 mg/mL (5.5 mL)

tetrahydrozoline (nasal) (tet ra hye DROZ a leen)

Synonyms tetrahydrozoline hydrochloride; tetryzoline

U.S./Canadian Brand Names Tyzine® Pediatric [US]; Tyzine® [US]

Therapeutic Category Adrenergic Agonist Agent; Imidazoline Derivative

Use Symptomatic relief of nasal congestion

Dosage Summary

Intranasal:

Children <2 years: Dosage not established

Children 2-6 years: Instill 2-3 drops (0.05%) into each nostril every 4-6 hours as needed (maximum: Every 3 hours)

Children >6 years: Instill 2-4 drops (0.1%) **or** 3-4 sprays (0.1%) into each nostril every 3-4 hours as needed (maximum: Every 3 hours)

Adults: Instill 2-4 drops (0.1%) **or** 3-4 sprays (0.1%) into each nostril every 3-4 hours as needed (maximum: Every 3 hours)

Dosage Forms

Solution, intranasal:

Tyzine®: 0.1% (15 mL, 30 mL)

Tyzine® Pediatric: 0.05% (15 mL)

tetrahydrozoline (ophthalmic) (tet ra hye DROZ a leen)

Sound-Alike/Look-Alike Issues

Visine® may be confused with Visken®

Synonyms tetrahydrozoline hydrochloride; tetryzoline

U.S./Canadian Brand Names Murine® Tears Plus [US-OTC]; Opti-Clear [US-OTC]; Visine® Advanced Relief [US-OTC]; Visine® Original [US-OTC]

Therapeutic Category Adrenergic Agonist Agent; Imidazoline Derivative; Ophthalmic Agent, Vasoconstrictor

Use Symptomatic relief of conjunctival congestion

Dosage Summary

Ophthalmic:

Children: Dosage not established

Adults: Instill 1-2 drops in each eye 2-4 times/day

Dosage Forms

Solution, ophthalmic: 0.05% (15 mL)
Murine® Tears Plus [OTC]: 0.05% (15 mL)
Opti-Clear [OTC]: 0.05% (15 mL)
Visine® Advanced Relief [OTC]: 0.05% (15 mL, 30 mL)
Visine® Original [OTC]: 0.05% (15 mL, 30 mL)

tetrahydrozoline hydrochloride *see* tetrahydrozoline (nasal) *on page 923*
tetrahydrozoline hydrochloride *see* tetrahydrozoline (ophthalmic) *on page 923*
2,2,2-tetramine *see* trientine *on page 957*
Tetramune® ***(Discontinued)***
Tetrasine® Extra Ophthalmic ***(Discontinued)*** *see* tetrahydrozoline (ophthalmic) *on page 923*
Tetrasine® Ophthalmic ***(Discontinued)*** *see* tetrahydrozoline (ophthalmic) *on page 923*

tetrastarch (TET ra starch)

Synonyms HES; HES 130/0.4; hydroxyethyl starch

U.S./Canadian Brand Names Voluven® [US/Can]

Therapeutic Category Plasma Volume Expander, Colloid

Use Blood volume expander used in treatment and prevention of hypovolemia

Dosage Summary

I.V. infusion:
Children <2 years: Average dose: 7-25 mL/kg
Children 2-12 years: Not studied
Children >12 years: Maximum dose: 50 mL/kg/day
Adults: Maximum dose: 50 mL/kg/day

Dosage Forms

Infusion, premixed in NS:
Voluven®: 6% (500 mL)

Tetra Tannate Pediatric [US] *see* chlorpheniramine, ephedrine, phenylephrine, and carbetapentane *on page 210*
tetryzoline *see* tetrahydrozoline (nasal) *on page 923*
tetryzoline *see* tetrahydrozoline (ophthalmic) *on page 923*
Teva-Alendronate [Can] *see* alendronate *on page 47*
Teva-Amiodarone [Can] *see* amiodarone *on page 67*
Teva-Amlodipine [Can] *see* amlodipine *on page 68*
Teva-Atenolol [Can] *see* atenolol *on page 102*
Teva-Azathioprine [Can] *see* azathioprine *on page 109*
Teva-Fosinopril [Can] *see* fosinopril *on page 428*
Teva-Gabapentin [Can] *see* gabapentin *on page 433*
Teva-Meloxicam [Can] *see* meloxicam *on page 598*
Teva-Naproxen Sodium [Can] *see* naproxen *on page 659*
Teva-Naproxen Sodium DS [Can] *see* naproxen *on page 659*
Teva-Olanzapine [Can] *see* olanzapine *on page 696*
Teva-Olanzapine OD [Can] *see* olanzapine *on page 696*
Teva-Paroxetine [Can] *see* paroxetine *on page 729*
Teva-Ramipril [Can] *see* ramipril *on page 826*
Teva-Simvastatin [Can] *see* simvastatin *on page 877*
Teva-Terazosin [Can] *see* terazosin *on page 917*
Teva-Venlafaxine XR [Can] *see* venlafaxine *on page 981*
Teveten® [US/Can] *see* eprosartan *on page 357*
Teveten® HCT [US/Can] *see* eprosartan and hydrochlorothiazide *on page 357*
Teveten® Plus [Can] *see* eprosartan and hydrochlorothiazide *on page 357*
Tev-Tropin® [US] *see* somatropin *on page 889*
Texacort® [US] *see* hydrocortisone (topical) *on page 483*
TG *see* thioguanine *on page 927*

T/Gel® Daily Control 2 in 1 Dandruff Shampoo Plus Conditioner [US-OTC] *see* pyrithione zinc *on page 819*

T/Gel® Daily Control Dandruff Shampoo [US-OTC] *see* pyrithione zinc *on page 819*

T-Gen® *(Discontinued)* *see* trimethobenzamide *on page 959*

thalidomide (tha LI doe mide)

Sound-Alike/Look-Alike Issues

thalidomide may be confused with flutamide, lenalidomide

Thalomid® may be confused with thiamine

U.S./Canadian Brand Names Thalomid® [US/Can]

Therapeutic Category Immunosuppressant Agent

Use Treatment of multiple myeloma; treatment and maintenance of cutaneous manifestations of erythema nodosum leprosum (ENL)

Dosage Summary

Oral:

Children: Dosage not established

Adults:

Cutaneous ENL: Initial: 100-300 mg once daily at bedtime (400 mg/day in severe cases); Maintenance: Continue initial dose until active reaction subsides then taper in 50 mg decrements every 2-4 weeks

Multiple myeloma: 200 mg once daily

Dosage Forms

Capsule, oral:

Thalomid®: 50 mg, 100 mg, 150 mg, 200 mg

Thalitone® [US] *see* chlorthalidone *on page 217*

Thalomid® [US/Can] *see* thalidomide *on page 925*

THAM® [US] *see* tromethamine *on page 963*

THC *see* dronabinol *on page 333*

THC and CBD *see* tetrahydrocannabinol and cannabidiol *(Canada only) on page 923*

Thelin™ [Can] *see* sitaxsentan *(Canada only) on page 880*

Theo-X® *(Discontinued)* *see* theophylline *on page 925*

Theo-24® [US] *see* theophylline *on page 925*

Theobid® *(Discontinued)* *see* theophylline *on page 925*

Theochron™ [US] *see* theophylline *on page 925*

Theochron® SR [Can] *see* theophylline *on page 925*

Theoclear-80® *(Discontinued)* *see* theophylline *on page 925*

Theoclear®-L.A. *(Discontinued)* *see* theophylline *on page 925*

Theo-Dur® (all products) *(Discontinued)* *see* theophylline *on page 925*

Theolair-SR® *(Discontinued)* *see* theophylline *on page 925*

Theolate *(Discontinued)*

theophylline (thee OFF i lin)

Synonyms theophylline anhydrous

U.S./Canadian Brand Names Apo-Theo LA® [Can]; Elixophyllin® [US]; Novo-Theophyl SR [Can]; PMS-Theophylline [Can]; Pulmophylline [Can]; ratio-Theo-Bronc [Can]; Theo-24® [US]; Theochron® SR [Can]; Theochron™ [US]; Uniphyl® SRT [Can]

Therapeutic Category Theophylline Derivative

Use Treatment of symptoms and reversible airway obstruction due to chronic asthma, or other chronic lung diseases; apnea of prematurity

Note: The National Heart, Lung, and Blood Institute Guidelines (2007) do not recommend oral theophylline as a long-term control medication for asthma in children ≤4 years of age; use may be considered as an alternative (but not preferred) agent in older children and adults. The guidelines do not recommend theophylline I.V. for the treatment of exacerbations of asthma.

Dosage Summary

I.V.:

Neonates ≤24 days: 1 mg/kg every 12 hours

Neonates >24 days: 1.5 mg/kg every 12 hours

Infants 6-52 weeks: mg/kg/hour = (0.008) (age in weeks) + 0.21
Children 1-9 years: 0.8 mg/kg/hour
Children 9-12 years: 0.7 mg/kg/hour
Adolescents 12-16 years (cigarette or marijuana smokers): 0.7 mg/kg/hour
Adolescents 12-16 years (nonsmokers): 0.5 mg/kg/hour; maximum 900 mg/day unless serum levels indicate need for larger dose
Adults 16-60 years (otherwise healthy, nonsmokers): 0.4 mg/kg/hour; maximum 900 mg/day unless serum levels indicate need for larger dose
Adults >60 years: 0.3 mg/kg/hour; maximum 400 mg/day unless serum levels indicate need for larger dose
Cardiac decompensation, cor pulmonale, hepatic dysfunction, sepsis with multiorgan failure, shock: 0.2 mg/kg/hour; maximum 400 mg/day unless serum levels indicate need for larger dose

Oral:
Premature Neonates <24 days postnatal age: 1 mg/kg/dose every 12 hours
Premature Neonates ≥24 days postnatal age: 1.5 mg/kg/dose every 12 hours
Full-term Infants and Infants <26 weeks: Total daily dose (mg) = [(0.2 x age in weeks) +5] x (weight in kg); divide dose into 3 equal amounts and administer at 8-hour intervals
Full-term Infants and Infants ≥26 weeks and <52 weeks: Total daily dose (mg) = [(0.2 x age in weeks) +5] x (weight in kg); divide dose into 4 equal amounts and administer at 6-hour intervals
Children 1-15 years and <45 kg ***without*** *risk factors for impaired theophylline clearance:* Initial: 12-14 mg/kg/day in divided doses (maximum dose: 300 mg/day), titrate to maintenance dose: 20 mg/kg/day in divided doses every 4-6 hours (maximum dose: 600 mg/day)
Adults 16-60 years ***without*** *risk factors for impaired theophylline clearance:* Initial: 300 mg/day in divided doses, titrate to maintenance dose: 600 mg/day in divided doses every 6-8 hours
Adults >60 years: Do not exceed a dose of 400 mg/day

Dosage Forms

Capsule, extended release, oral:
Theo-24®: 100 mg, 200 mg, 300 mg, 400 mg

Elixir, oral:
Elixophyllin®: 80 mg/15 mL (473 mL)

Infusion, premixed in D_5W: 400 mg (100 mL, 250 mL, 500 mL, 1000 mL); 800 mg (250 mL, 500 mL, 1000 mL)

Solution, oral: 80 mg/15 mL (15 mL)

Tablet, extended release, oral: 100 mg, 200 mg, 300 mg, 400 mg, 450 mg, 600 mg
Theochron™: 100 mg, 200 mg, 300 mg, 450 mg

theophylline and guaifenesin *(Discontinued)*

theophylline anhydrous *see* theophylline *on page 925*

theophylline ethylenediamine *see* aminophylline *on page 66*

Theo-Sav® *(Discontinued)* *see* theophylline *on page 925*

Theospan®-SR *(Discontinued)* *see* theophylline *on page 925*

Theostat-80® *(Discontinued)* *see* theophylline *on page 925*

Theovent® *(Discontinued)* *see* theophylline *on page 925*

Therabid® *(Discontinued)*

TheraCys® [US] *see* BCG *on page 118*

Theraflu® Daytime Severe Cold & Cough [US-OTC] *see* acetaminophen, dextromethorphan, and phenylephrine *on page 29*

Theraflu® Nighttime Severe Cold & Cough [US-OTC] *see* acetaminophen, diphenhydramine, and phenylephrine *on page 30*

Thera-Flur® *(Discontinued)* *see* fluoride *on page 413*

Thera-Flur-N® *(Discontinued)* *see* fluoride *on page 413*

Thera-Flu® Severe Cold Non-Drowsy *(Discontinued)*

Theraflu® Sugar-Free Nighttime Severe Cold & Cough [US-OTC] *see* acetaminophen, diphenhydramine, and phenylephrine *on page 30*

Theraflu® Thin Strips® Multi Symptom [US-OTC] *see* diphenhydramine (systemic) *on page 310*

Theraflu® Warming Relief Daytime Severe Cold & Cough [US-OTC] *see* acetaminophen, dextromethorphan, and phenylephrine *on page 29*

Theraflu® Warming Relief ™ Flu & Sore Throat [US-OTC] *see* acetaminophen, diphenhydramine, and phenylephrine *on page 30*

Theraflu® Warming Relief™ Nighttime Severe Cold & Cough [US-OTC] *see* acetaminophen, diphenhydramine, and phenylephrine *on page* *30*

Thera-Gel [US-OTC] *see* coal tar *on page* *242*

Thera-Gesic® [US-OTC] *see* methyl salicylate and menthol *on page* *623*

Thera-Gesic® Plus [US-OTC] *see* methyl salicylate and menthol *on page* *623*

Theragran-M® Advanced Formula *(Discontinued)* *see* vitamins (multiple/oral) *on page* *990*

Theragran® Heart Right™ *(Discontinued)* *see* vitamins (multiple/oral) *on page* *990*

TheraPatch® Warm *(Discontinued)* *see* capsaicin *on page* *175*

therapeutic multivitamins *see* vitamins (multiple/oral) *on page* *990*

Thera-Sal [US-OTC] *see* salicylic acid *on page* *858*

Theratears® [US] *see* carboxymethylcellulose *on page* *184*

Thermazene® [US] *see* silver sulfadiazine *on page* *875*

thiabendazole *(Discontinued)*

thiamazole *see* methimazole *on page* *613*

thiamin *see* thiamine *on page* *927*

thiamine (THYE a min)

Sound-Alike/Look-Alike Issues

thiamine may be confused with Tenormin®, Thalomid®, Thorazine®

Synonyms aneurine hydrochloride; thiamin; thiamine hydrochloride; thiaminium chloride hydrochloride; vitamin B_1

U.S./Canadian Brand Names Betaxin® [Can]

Therapeutic Category Vitamin, Water Soluble

Use Treatment of thiamine deficiency including beriberi, Wernicke encephalopathy, Korsakoff syndrome, neuritis associated with pregnancy, or in alcoholic patients; dietary supplement

Dosage Summary

I.M.:

Children: 10-25 mg/dose daily (thiamine deficiency)

Adults: 5-30 mg/dose 3 times/day (thiamine deficiency) **or** 50-250 mg/day (Wernicke encephalopathy)

I.V.:

Children: 10-25 mg/dose daily (thiamine deficiency)

Adults: 5-30 mg/dose 3 times/day (thiamine deficiency) **or** 50-1500 mg/day (Wernicke encephalopathy)

Oral:

Infants: 0.2-0.3 mg/day (adequate intake)

Children: 0.5-1.4 mg/day (recommended daily intake) **or** 5-50 mg/day (thiamine deficiency)

Adults: 1.1-1.4 mg/day (recommended daily intake) **or** 5-30 mg/day in 1-3 divided doses (thiamine deficiency)

Dosage Forms

Injection, solution: 100 mg/mL (2 mL)

Tablet, oral: 50 mg, 100 mg, 250 mg, 500 mg

thiamine hydrochloride *see* thiamine *on page* *927*

thiaminium chloride hydrochloride *see* thiamine *on page* *927*

thioguanine (thye oh GWAH neen)

Sound-Alike/Look-Alike Issues

thioguanine may be confused with thiotepa

6-TG (error-prone abbreviation)

6-thioguanine and 6-TG are error-prone abbreviations (associated with sixfold overdoses of thioguanine)

Synonyms 2-amino-6-mercaptopurine; TG; tioguanine

U.S./Canadian Brand Names Lanvis® [Can]; Tabloid® [US]

Therapeutic Category Antineoplastic Agent

Use Treatment of acute myelogenous (nonlymphocytic) leukemia (AML)

Dosage Summary

Oral:

Children <1 year: Dosage not established.

Adults: Dosage not established.

Dosage Forms
Tablet, oral:
Tabloid®: 40 mg

Thiola® [US/Can] *see* tiopronin *on page 935*

thiopental (thye oh PEN tal)

Synonyms thiopental sodium
U.S./Canadian Brand Names Pentothal® [US/Can]
Therapeutic Category Barbiturate
Controlled Substance C-III
Use Induction of anesthesia; control of convulsive states; treatment of elevated intracranial pressure
Dosage Summary
I.V.:
Infants <1 year: Anesthesia induction: 5-8 mg/kg
Children 1-12 years: Anesthesia induction: 5-6 mg/kg; Maintenance: 1 mg/kg as needed **or** 1.5-5 mg/kg/dose, repeat as needed
Children >12 years: Maintenance: 1 mg/kg as needed **or** 1.5-5 mg/kg/dose, repeat as needed
Adults: Anesthesia induction: 3-5 mg/kg; Maintenance: 25-100 mg as needed **or** 1.5-5 mg/kg/dose, repeat as needed **or** 75-250 mg/dose, repeat as needed
Dosage Forms
Injection, powder for reconstitution:
Pentothal®: 400 mg, 500 mg, 1 g

thiopental sodium *see* thiopental *on page 928*
thiophosphoramide *see* thiotepa *on page 928*
Thioplex® *(Discontinued)* *see* thiotepa *on page 928*

thioridazine (thye oh RID a zeen)

Sound-Alike/Look-Alike Issues
thioridazine may be confused with thiothixene, Thorazine®
Mellaril® may be confused with Elavil®, Mebaral®
Synonyms thioridazine hydrochloride
Therapeutic Category Phenothiazine Derivative
Use Management of schizophrenic patients who fail to respond adequately to treatment with other antipsychotic drugs, either because of insufficient effectiveness or the inability to achieve an effective dose due to intolerable adverse effects from those medications
Dosage Summary
Oral:
Children ≤2 years: Dosage not established
Children >2-12 years: 0.5-3 mg/kg/day in 2-3 divided doses **or** 10-25 mg 2-3 times/day (maximum: 3 mg/kg/day); **Note:** Titration is recommended
Children >12 years: Initial: 50-100 mg 3 times/day, maintenance: 150-800 mg/day in 2-4 divided doses (maximum: 800 mg/day) **or** 25 mg 3 times/day; maintenance: 20-200 mg day; **Note:** Titration is recommended
Adults: Initial: 50-100 mg 3 times/day, maintenance: 150-800 mg/day in 2-4 divided doses (maximum: 800 mg/day) **or** 25 mg 3 times/day; maintenance: 20-200 mg day; **Note:** Titration is recommended
Elderly: Initial: 10-25 mg 1-2 times/day; maintenance: 10-400 mg/day in 1-2 divided doses (maximum: 400 mg/day); **Note:** Titration is recommended
Dosage Forms
Tablet, oral: 10 mg, 25 mg, 50 mg, 100 mg

thioridazine hydrochloride *see* thioridazine *on page 928*
thiosulfuric acid disodium salt *see* sodium thiosulfate *on page 888*

thiotepa (thye oh TEP a)

Sound-Alike/Look-Alike Issues
thiotepa may be confused with thioguanine
Synonyms TESPA; thiophosphoramide; triethylenethiophosphoramide; TSPA
Therapeutic Category Antineoplastic Agent

Use Treatment of superficial papillary bladder cancer; palliative treatment of adenocarcinoma of breast or ovary; controlling intracavitary effusions caused by metastatic tumors

Dosage Summary

I.V.:

Adults: 0.3-0.4 mg/kg every 1-4 weeks

Intracavitary:

Children: Dosage not established

Adults: 0.6-0.8 mg/kg

Intravesical:

Children: Dosage not established

Adults: 60 mg in 30-60 mL NS retained for 2 hours once weekly for 4 weeks

Dosage Forms

Injection, powder for reconstitution: 15 mg

thiothixene (thye oh THIKS een)

Sound-Alike/Look-Alike Issues

thiothixene may be confused with FLUoxetine, thioridazine

Navane® may be confused with Norvasc®, Nubain®

Synonyms tiotixene

U.S./Canadian Brand Names Navane® [US/Can]

Therapeutic Category Thioxanthene Derivative

Use Management of schizophrenia

Dosage Summary

Oral:

Adults: Initial: 6-10 mg/day in 2-3 divided doses; Maintenance: 20-60 mg/day in 2-3 divided doses (maximum: 60 mg/day)

Dosage Forms

Capsule, oral: 1 mg, 2 mg, 5 mg, 10 mg

Navane®: 2 mg, 5 mg, 10 mg, 20 mg

thonzonium, neomycin, colistin, and hydrocortisone *see* neomycin, colistin, hydrocortisone, and thonzonium *on page 666*

Thorazine® ***(Discontinued)*** *see* chlorpromazine *on page 216*

Thorets [US-OTC] *see* benzocaine *on page 124*

Thrive™ [US-OTC] *see* nicotine *on page 674*

Thrombate III® [US/Can] *see* antithrombin III *on page 83*

Thrombi-Gel® [US] *see* thrombin (topical) *on page 929*

Thrombinar® ***(Discontinued)*** *see* thrombin (topical) *on page 929*

Thrombin-JMI® [US] *see* thrombin (topical) *on page 929*

Thrombin-JMI® Epistaxis Kit [US] *see* thrombin (topical) *on page 929*

Thrombin-JMI® Spray Kit [US] *see* thrombin (topical) *on page 929*

Thrombin-JMI® Syringe Spray Kit [US] *see* thrombin (topical) *on page 929*

thrombin (topical) (THROM bin, TOP i kal)

U.S./Canadian Brand Names Evithrom™ [US]; Recothrom™ [US]; Thrombi-Gel® [US]; Thrombi-Pad® [US]; Thrombin-JMI® Epistaxis Kit [US]; Thrombin-JMI® Spray Kit [US]; Thrombin-JMI® Syringe Spray Kit [US]; Thrombin-JMI® [US]

Therapeutic Category Hemostatic Agent

Use Hemostasis whenever minor bleeding from capillaries and small venules is accessible

Thrombi-Gel®; Thrombi-Pad®: Temporary control as trauma dressing for moderate-to-severe bleeding wounds; control of surface bleeding from vascular access sites and percutaneous catheter/tubes

Dosage Summary

Topical:

Children: Dose based on severity of bleeding

Adults: Dose based on severity of bleeding

Dosage Forms

Pad, topical [preservative free]:

Thrombi-Pad® 3x3: ≥200 units

Powder for reconstitution, topical:
Thrombin-JMI®: 5000 int. units, 20,000 int. units
Thrombin-JMI® Epistaxis kit: 5000 int. units
Thrombin-JMI® Spray Kit, Thrombin-JMI® Syringe Spray Kit: 20,000 int. units
Powder for reconstitution, topical [preservative free]:
Recothrom™: 5000 int. units; 20,000 int. units
Solution, topical:
Evithrom™: 800-1200 int. units/mL (2 mL, 5 mL, 20 mL)
Sponge, topical [preservative free]:
Thrombi-Gel® 10: ≥1000 units (10s)
Thrombi-Gel® 40: ≥1000 units (5s)
Thrombi-Gel® 100: ≥2000 units (5s)

Thrombi-Pad® [US] *see* thrombin (topical) *on page 929*
Thrombostat® ***(Discontinued)*** *see* thrombin (topical) *on page 929*
thymocyte stimulating factor *see* aldesleukin *on page 46*
Thymoglobulin® [US] *see* antithymocyte globulin (rabbit) *on page 84*
Thyrar® ***(Discontinued)*** *see* thyroid, desiccated *on page 930*
Thyrel® TRH ***(Discontinued)***
Thyro-Block® ***(Discontinued)*** *see* potassium iodide *on page 782*
Thyrogen® [US/Can] *see* thyrotropin alpha *on page 930*

thyroid, desiccated (THYE roid DES i kay tid)

Synonyms desiccated thyroid; thyroid extract; thyroid USP
U.S./Canadian Brand Names Armour® Thyroid [US]; Nature-Throid™ [US]; Westhroid™ [US]
Therapeutic Category Thyroid Product
Use Replacement or supplemental therapy in hypothyroidism; pituitary TSH suppressants (thyroid nodules, thyroiditis, multinodular goiter, thyroid cancer), thyrotoxicosis, diagnostic suppression tests

Dosage Summary
Oral:
Children 0-6 months: 15-30 mg/day **or** 4.8-6 mg/kg/day
Children 6-12 months: 30-45 mg/day **or** 3.6-4.8 mg/kg/day
Children 1-5 years: 45-60 mg/day **or** 3-3.6 mg/kg/day
Children 6-12 years: 60-90 mg/day **or** 2.4-3 mg/kg/day
Children >12 years: >90 mg/day **or** 1.2-1.8 mg/kg/day
Adults: Initial: 15-30 mg/day; Maintenance: 60-120 mg/day; **Note:** Titration is recommended

Dosage Forms
Tablet, oral:
Armour® Thyroid: 15 mg, 30 mg, 60 mg, 90 mg, 120 mg, 180 mg, 240 mg, 300 mg
Nature-Throid™: 16.25 mg, 32.5 mg, 65 mg, 130 mg, 195 mg
Westhroid™: 32.5 mg, 65 mg, 130 mg

thyroid extract *see* thyroid, desiccated *on page 930*
Thyroid Strong® ***(Discontinued)*** *see* thyroid, desiccated *on page 930*
thyroid USP *see* thyroid, desiccated *on page 930*
Thyrolar® [US/Can] *see* liotrix *on page 568*
ThyroSafe™ [US] *see* potassium iodide *on page 782*
Thyroshield™ [US-OTC] *see* potassium iodide *on page 782*

thyrotropin alpha (thye roe TROH pin AL fa)

Sound-Alike/Look-Alike Issues
Thyrogen® may be confused with Thyrolar®
Synonyms human thyroid stimulating hormone; recombinant human thyrotropin; Rh-TSH; TSH
U.S./Canadian Brand Names Thyrogen® [US/Can]
Therapeutic Category Diagnostic Agent
Use As an adjunctive diagnostic tool for serum thyroglobulin (Tg) testing; adjunctive treatment for radioiodine ablation of thyroid tissue remnants after total or near-total thyroidectomy in patients with well-differentiated thyroid cancer without evidence of metastatic disease

Potential clinical uses include: Patients with an undetectable Tg on thyroid hormone suppressive therapy to exclude the diagnosis of residual or recurrent thyroid cancer, patients requiring serum Tg testing and radioiodine imaging who are unwilling to undergo thyroid hormone withdrawal testing and whose treating physician believes that use of a less sensitive test is justified, patients who are either unable to mount an adequate endogenous TSH response to thyroid hormone withdrawal or in whom withdrawal is medically contraindicated, and patients without evidence of metastatic disease to ablate thyroid remnants (in combination with radioiodine [I^{131}]) following near-total thyroidectomy.

Dosage Summary

I.M.:

Children ≤16 years: Dosage not established

Children >16 years: 0.9 mg, followed 24 hours later by a second 0.9 mg dose

Adults: 0.9 mg, followed 24 hours later by a second 0.9 mg dose

Dosage Forms

Injection, powder for reconstitution:

Thyrogen®: 1.1 mg

tiagabine (tye AG a been)

Sound-Alike/Look-Alike Issues

tiaGABine may be confused with tiZANidine

Synonyms tiagabine hydrochloride

Tall-Man tia**GAB**ine

U.S./Canadian Brand Names Gabitril® [US/Can]

Therapeutic Category Anticonvulsant

Use Adjunctive therapy in adults and children ≥12 years of age in the treatment of partial seizures

Dosage Summary **Note:** The estimated plasma concentrations of tiagabine in patients **not** taking enzyme-inducing medications is twice that of patients receiving enzyme-inducing AEDs. Lower doses are required; slower titration may be necessary.

Oral:

Children <12 years: Dosage not established

Children 12-18 years: Patients receiving enzyme-inducing AED regimens: Initial: 4 mg once daily; Maintenance: 8-32 mg/day in 2-4 divided doses; **Note:** Titration is recommended

Adults: Patients receiving enzyme-inducing AED regimens: Initial: 4 mg once daily; Maintenance: 8-56 mg/day in 2-4 divided doses; **Note:** Titration is recommended

Dosage Forms

Tablet, oral:

Gabitril®: 2 mg, 4 mg, 12 mg, 16 mg

tiagabine hydrochloride *see* tiagabine *on page* 931

Tiamate® *(Discontinued)* *see* diltiazem *on page* 306

Tiamol® [Can] *see* fluocinonide *on page* 411

Tiaprofenic-200 [Can] *see* tiaprofenic acid *(Canada only) on page* 931

Tiaprofenic-300 [Can] *see* tiaprofenic acid *(Canada only) on page* 931

tiaprofenic acid *(Canada only)* (tye ah PRO fen ik AS id)

U.S./Canadian Brand Names Apo-Tiaprofenic® [Can]; Dom-Tiaprofenic [Can]; Novo-Tiaprofenic [Can]; Nu-Tiaprofenic [Can]; PMS-Tiaprofenic [Can]; Surgam® [Can]; Tiaprofenic-200 [Can]; Tiaprofenic-300 [Can]

Therapeutic Category Nonsteroidal Antiinflammatory Drug (NSAID)

Use Relief of signs and symptoms of rheumatoid arthritis and osteoarthritis (degenerative joint disease)

Dosage Summary

Oral:

Regular release:

Children: Dosage not established

Adults: 600 mg/day in 2-3 divided doses (maximum: 600 mg/day)

Sustained release:

Children: Dosage not established

Adults: 600 mg once daily

Dosage Forms - Canada

Capsule, sustained release: 300 mg

Tablet: 200 mg, 300 mg

Tiazac® [US/Can] *see* diltiazem *on page* 306

Tiazac® XC [Can] *see* diltiazem *on page 306*

ticarcillin and clavulanate potassium (tye kar SIL in & klav yoo LAN ate poe TASS ee um)

Synonyms ticarcillin and clavulanic acid

U.S./Canadian Brand Names Timentin® [US/Can]

Therapeutic Category Penicillin

Use Treatment of lower respiratory tract, urinary tract, skin and skin structures, bone and joint, gynecologic (endometritis) and intraabdominal (peritonitis) infections, and septicemia caused by susceptible organisms. Clavulanate expands activity of ticarcillin to include beta-lactamase producing strains of *S. aureus*, *H. influenzae*, *Bacteroides* species, and some other gram-negative bacilli

Dosage Summary

I.V.:

Children <60 kg: 200-300 mg of ticarcillin component/kg/day in divided doses every 4-6 hours

Children ≥60 kg: 3.1 g (ticarcillin 3 g plus clavulanic acid 0.1 g) every 4-6 hours (maximum: 24 g of ticarcillin component/day)

Adults <60 kg: 200-300 mg of ticarcillin component/kg/day in divided doses every 4-6 hours

Adults ≥60 kg: 3.1 g (ticarcillin 3 g plus clavulanic acid 0.1 g) every 4-6 hours (maximum: 24 g of ticarcillin component/day)

Dosage Forms

Infusion [premixed, frozen]:

Timentin®: Ticarcillin 3 g and clavulanic acid 0.1 g (100 mL)

Injection, powder for reconstitution:

Timentin®: Ticarcillin 3 g and clavulanic acid 0.1 g (3.1 g, 31 g)

ticarcillin and clavulanic acid *see* ticarcillin and clavulanate potassium *on page 932*

ticarcillin *(Discontinued)*

Ticar® *(Discontinued)*

TICE® BCG [US] *see* BCG *on page 118*

Ticlid® [Can] *see* ticlopidine *on page 932*

Ticlid® *(Discontinued)* *see* ticlopidine *on page 932*

ticlopidine (tye KLOE pi deen)

Synonyms ticlopidine hydrochloride

U.S./Canadian Brand Names Alti-Ticlopidine [Can]; Apo-Ticlopidine® [Can]; Gen-Ticlopidine [Can]; Mylan-Ticlopidine [Can]; Novo-Ticlopidine [Can]; Nu-Ticlopidine [Can]; Rhoxal-ticlopidine [Can]; Sandoz-Ticlopidine [Can]; Ticlid® [Can]

Therapeutic Category Antiplatelet Agent

Use Platelet aggregation inhibitor that reduces the risk of thrombotic stroke in patients who have had a stroke or stroke precursors. **Note:** Due to its association with life-threatening hematologic disorders, ticlopidine should be reserved for patients who are intolerant to aspirin, or who have failed aspirin therapy. Adjunctive therapy (with aspirin) following successful coronary stent implantation to reduce the incidence of subacute stent thrombosis.

Dosage Summary

Oral:

Children: Dosage not established

Adults: 250 mg twice daily with food

Dosage Forms

Tablet, oral: 250 mg

ticlopidine hydrochloride *see* ticlopidine *on page 932*

Ticon® *(Discontinued)* *see* trimethobenzamide *on page 959*

TIG *see* tetanus immune globulin (human) *on page 920*

Tigan® [US/Can] *see* trimethobenzamide *on page 959*

tigecycline (tye ge SYE kleen)

Synonyms GAR-936

U.S./Canadian Brand Names Tygacil® [US/Can]

Therapeutic Category Antibiotic, Glycylcycline

Use Treatment of complicated skin and skin structure infections caused by susceptible organisms, including methicillin-resistant *Staphylococcus aureus* and vancomycin-sensitive *Enterococcus faecalis*; complicated intraabdominal infections; community-acquired pneumonia

Dosage Summary

I.V.:

Children: Dosage not established

Adults: Initial: 100 mg as a single dose; Maintenance: 50 mg every 12 hours

Dosage Forms

Injection, powder for reconstitution:

Tygacil®: 50 mg

Tikosyn® [US/Can] *see* dofetilide *on page 323*

Tilade® [Can] *see* nedocromil *on page 664*

Tilia™ Fe [US] *see* ethinyl estradiol and norethindrone *on page 378*

tiludronate (tye LOO droe nate)

Synonyms tiludronate disodium

U.S./Canadian Brand Names Skelid® [US]

Therapeutic Category Bisphosphonate Derivative

Use Treatment of Paget disease of the bone (osteitis deformans) in patients who have a level of serum alkaline phosphatase (SAP) at least twice the upper limit of normal, or who are symptomatic, or who are at risk for future complications of their disease

Dosage Summary

Oral:

Children: Dosage not established

Adults: 400 mg once daily for 3 months

Dosage Forms

Tablet, oral:

Skelid®: 200 mg

tiludronate disodium *see* tiludronate *on page 933*

Tim-AK [Can] *see* timolol (ophthalmic) *on page 933*

Time-C [US-OTC] *see* ascorbic acid *on page 98*

Timecelles® ***(Discontinued)*** *see* ascorbic acid *on page 98*

Timentin® [US/Can] *see* ticarcillin and clavulanate potassium *on page 932*

timolol (systemic) (TIM oh lol)

Sound-Alike/Look-Alike Issues

timolol may be confused with atenolol, Tylenol®

Synonyms timolol maleate

U.S./Canadian Brand Names Apo-Timol® [Can]; Nu-Timolol [Can]

Therapeutic Category Beta-Adrenergic Blocker, Nonselective

Use Treatment of hypertension and angina; to reduce mortality following myocardial infarction; prophylaxis of migraine

Dosage Summary

Oral:

Children: Dosage not established

Adults: Initial: 10 mg twice daily; Maintenance: 20-60 mg/day in 2 divided doses (maximum: 60 mg/day)

Dosage Forms

Tablet, oral: 5 mg, 10 mg, 20 mg

timolol (ophthalmic) (TIM oh lol)

Sound-Alike/Look-Alike Issues

timolol may be confused with atenolol, Tylenol®

Timoptic® may be confused with Betoptic® S, Talacen®, Viroptic®

Synonyms timolol hemihydrate; timolol maleate

U.S./Canadian Brand Names Apo-Timop® [Can]; Betimol® [US]; Dom-Timolol [Can]; Istalol® [US]; Med-Timolol [Can]; Mylan-Timolol [Can]; PMS-Timolol [Can]; Rhoxal-Timolol [Can]; Sandoz-Timolol [Can]; Tim-AK [Can]; Timolol GFS [US]; Timoptic-XE® [US/Can]; Timoptic® in OcuDose® [US]; Timoptic® [US/Can]

Therapeutic Category Beta-Adrenergic Blocker, Nonselective; Ophthalmic Agent, Antiglaucoma

Use Treatment of elevated intraocular pressure such as glaucoma or ocular hypertension

Dosage Summary

Ophthalmic:

Gel-forming solution:

Children: Instill 1 drop (0.25% or 0.5%) once daily

Adults: Instill 1 drop (0.25% or 0.5%) once daily

Solution:

Children: Initial: Instill 1 drop (0.25%) twice daily; Maintenance: Instill 1 drop (0.25% or 0.5%) 1-2 times daily (maximum: 2 drops/day [0.5%])

Adults: Initial: Instill 1 drop (0.25%) twice daily; Maintenance: Instill 1 drop (0.25% or 0.5%) 1-2 times daily (maximum: 2 drops/day [0.5%])

Dosage Forms

Gel forming solution, ophthalmic:

Timolol GFS: 0.25% (5 mL); 0.5% (5 mL)

Timoptic-XE®: 0.25% (5 mL); 0.5% (5 mL)

Solution, ophthalmic: 0.25% (5 mL, 10 mL, 15 mL); 0.5% (5 mL, 10 mL, 15 mL)

Betimol®: 0.25% (5 mL); 0.5% (5 mL, 10 mL, 15 mL)

Istalol®: 0.5% (2.5 mL, 5 mL)

Timoptic®: 0.25% (5 mL); 0.5% (5 mL, 10 mL)

Solution, ophthalmic [preservative free]:

Timoptic® in OcuDose®: 0.25% (0.2 mL); 0.5% (0.2 mL)

timolol and brimonidine *see* brimonidine and timolol *on page 145*

timolol and dorzolamide *see* dorzolamide and timolol *on page 327*

Timolol GFS [US] *see* timolol (ophthalmic) *on page 933*

timolol hemihydrate *see* timolol (ophthalmic) *on page 933*

timolol maleate *see* timolol (ophthalmic) *on page 933*

timolol maleate *see* timolol (systemic) *on page 933*

timolol maleate and brinzolamide *see* brinzolamide and timolol *(Canada only) on page 145*

timolol maleate and latanoprost *see* latanoprost and timolol *(Canada only) on page 551*

timolol maleate and travoprost *see* travoprost and timolol *(Canada only) on page 950*

Timoptic® [US/Can] *see* timolol (ophthalmic) *on page 933*

Timoptic® in OcuDose® [US] *see* timolol (ophthalmic) *on page 933*

Timoptic-XE® [US/Can] *see* timolol (ophthalmic) *on page 933*

Tinactin® Antifungal [US-OTC] *see* tolnaftate *on page 940*

Tinactin® Antifungal Deodorant [US-OTC] *see* tolnaftate *on page 940*

Tinactin® Antifungal Jock Itch [US-OTC] *see* tolnaftate *on page 940*

Tinaderm [US-OTC] *see* tolnaftate *on page 940*

Tinamed® Corn and Callus Remover [US-OTC] *see* salicylic acid *on page 858*

Tinamed® Wart Remover [US-OTC] *see* salicylic acid *on page 858*

TinBen® ***(Discontinued)*** *see* benzoin *on page 127*

tincture of opium *see* opium tincture *on page 705*

Tindamax® [US] *see* tinidazole *on page 934*

Ting® Cream [US-OTC] *see* tolnaftate *on page 940*

Ting® Spray Liquid [US-OTC] *see* tolnaftate *on page 940*

Ting® Spray Powder [US-OTC] *see* miconazole (topical) *on page 630*

tinidazole (tye NI da zole)

U.S./Canadian Brand Names Tindamax® [US]

Therapeutic Category Amebicide; Antibiotic, Miscellaneous; Antiprotozoal, Nitroimidazole

Use Treatment of trichomoniasis caused by *T. vaginalis*; treatment of giardiasis caused by *G. duodenalis* (*G. lamblia*); treatment of intestinal amebiasis and amebic liver abscess caused by *E. histolytica*; treatment of bacterial vaginosis caused by *Bacteroides* spp, *Gardnerella vaginalis*, and *Prevotella* spp in nonpregnant females

Dosage Summary

Oral:

Children ≤3 years: Dosage not established
Children >3 years: 50 mg/kg/day (maximum: 2 g/day)
Adults: 1-2 g/day

Dosage Forms

Tablet, oral:

Tindamax®: 250 mg, 500 mg

Tinver® ***(Discontinued)*** *see* sodium thiosulfate *on page* *888*

tinzaparin (tin ZA pa rin)

Synonyms tinzaparin sodium

U.S./Canadian Brand Names Innohep® [US/Can]

Therapeutic Category Anticoagulant (Other)

Use Treatment of acute symptomatic deep vein thrombosis, with or without pulmonary embolism, in conjunction with warfarin sodium

Dosage Summary

SubQ:

Children: Dosage not established
Adults: 175 anti-Xa int. units/kg of body weight once daily

Dosage Forms

Injection, solution:

Innohep®: 20,000 anti-Xa int. units/mL (2 mL)

tinzaparin sodium *see* tinzaparin *on page* *935*

tioconazole (tye oh KONE a zole)

Sound-Alike/Look-Alike Issues

tioconazole may be confused with terconazole

U.S./Canadian Brand Names 1-Day™ [US-OTC]; Vagistat®-1 [US-OTC]

Therapeutic Category Antifungal Agent

Use Local treatment of vulvovaginal candidiasis

Dosage Summary

Intravaginal:

Children: Dosage not established
Adults: Insert 1 applicatorful prior to bedtime, as a single dose

Dosage Forms

Ointment, vaginal:

1-Day™ [OTC]: 6.5% (4.6 g)
Vagistat®-1 [OTC]: 6.5% (4.6 g)

tioguanine *see* thioguanine *on page* *927*

tiopronin (tye oh PROE nin)

U.S./Canadian Brand Names Thiola® [US/Can]

Therapeutic Category Urinary Tract Product

Use Prevention of kidney stone (cystine) formation in patients with severe homozygous cystinuric who have urinary cystine >500 mg/day who are resistant to treatment with high fluid intake, alkali, and diet modification, or who have had adverse reactions to penicillamine

Dosage Summary

Oral:

Children: Dosage not established
Adults: Initial: 800 mg/day; Average dose: 1000 mg/day

Dosage Forms

Tablet, oral:

Thiola®: 100 mg

tiotixene *see* thiothixene *on page* *929*

tiotropium (ty oh TRO pee um)

Sound-Alike/Look-Alike Issues

tiotropium may be confused with ipratropium

Spiriva® may be confused with Inspra™, Serevent®

Synonyms tiotropium bromide monohydrate

U.S./Canadian Brand Names Spiriva® HandiHaler® [US]; Spiriva® [Can]

Therapeutic Category Anticholinergic Agent

Use Maintenance treatment of bronchospasm associated with COPD (including bronchitis and emphysema); reduction of COPD exacerbations

Dosage Summary

Inhalation:

Children: Dosage not established

Adults: Contents of 1 capsule (18 mcg) once daily. **Note:** To ensure drug delivery the contents of each capsule should be inhaled twice.

Dosage Forms

Powder, for oral inhalation:

Spiriva® HandiHaler®: 18 mcg/capsule (5s, 30s, 90s)

tiotropium bromide monohydrate *see* tiotropium *on page 936*

tipranavir (tip RA na veer)

Synonyms PNU-140690E; TPV

U.S./Canadian Brand Names Aptivus® [US/Can]

Therapeutic Category Antiretroviral Agent, Protease Inhibitor

Use Treatment of HIV-1 infections in combination with ritonavir and other antiretroviral agents; limited to highly treatment-experienced or multiprotease inhibitor-resistant patients.

Dosage Summary

Oral:

Children <2 years: Dosage not established

Children ≥2 years: 12-14 mg/kg or 290-375 mg/m^2 (maximum: 500 mg/dose) twice daily

Adults: 500 mg twice daily

Dosage Forms

Capsule, soft gelatin, oral:

Aptivus®: 250 mg

Solution, oral:

Aptivus®: 100 mg/mL (95 mL)

TipTapToe *(Discontinued)* *see* tolnaftate *on page 940*

tirofiban (tye roe FYE ban)

Sound-Alike/Look-Alike Issues

Aggrastat® may be confused with Aggrenox®, argatroban

Synonyms MK383; tirofiban hydrochloride

U.S./Canadian Brand Names Aggrastat® [US/Can]

Therapeutic Category Antiplatelet Agent

Use Treatment of acute coronary syndrome (ie, unstable angina/non-ST-elevation myocardial infarction [UA/NSTEMI]) in combination with heparin

Dosage Summary

I.V.:

Children: Dosage not established

Adults: Initial: 0.4 mcg/kg/minute for 30 minutes; Maintenance infusion: 0.1 mcg/kg/minute

Dosage Forms

Infusion, premixed in NS [preservative free]:

Aggrastat®: 50 mcg/mL (100 mL, 250 mL)

tirofiban hydrochloride *see* tirofiban *on page 936*

Tisseel® VH [Can] *see* fibrin sealant *on page 401*

Tisseel® VH S/D [US] *see* fibrin sealant *on page 401*

Titralac™ [US-OTC] *see* calcium carbonate *on page 167*

Titralac® Plus [US-OTC] *see* calcium carbonate and simethicone *on page 168*

Ti-U-Lac® H [Can] *see* urea and hydrocortisone *on page 971*

tizanidine (tye ZAN i deen)

Sound-Alike/Look-Alike Issues

tiZANidine may be confused with tiaGABine

Zanaflex® may be confused with Xiaflex™

Tall-Man ti**ZAN**idine

U.S./Canadian Brand Names Apo-Tizanidine® [Can]; Gen-Tizanidine [Can]; Mylan-Tizanidine [Can]; Zanaflex Capsules® [US]; Zanaflex® [US/Can]

Therapeutic Category Alpha$_2$-Adrenergic Agonist Agent

Use Skeletal muscle relaxant used for treatment of muscle spasticity

Dosage Summary

Oral:

Children: Dosage not established

Adults: Initial: 2-4 mg 3 times/day; Maintenance: 6-36 mg/day in 3 divided doses (maximum: 36 mg/day)

Dosage Forms

Capsule, oral:

Zanaflex Capsules®: 2 mg, 4 mg, 6 mg

Tablet, oral: 2 mg, 4 mg

Zanaflex®: 4 mg

TMC-114 *see* darunavir *on page 270*

TMC125 *see* etravirine *on page 385*

TMP *see* trimethoprim *on page 959*

TMP-SMZ *see* sulfamethoxazole and trimethoprim *on page 901*

TMX-67 *see* febuxostat *on page 392*

TMZ *see* temozolomide *on page 914*

T.N. Dickinson's® Hazelets [US-OTC] *see* witch hazel *on page 994*

T. N. Dickinson's® Witch Hazel® Astringent [US-OTC] *see* witch hazel *on page 994*

T. N. Dickinson's® Witch Hazel® Hemorrhoidal [US-OTC] *see* witch hazel *on page 994*

TNKase® [US/Can] *see* tenecteplase *on page 915*

TOBI® [US/Can] *see* tobramycin (systemic, oral inhalation) *on page 937*

TobraDex® [US/Can] *see* tobramycin and dexamethasone *on page 938*

tobramycin (systemic, oral inhalation) (toe bra MYE sin)

Sound-Alike/Look-Alike Issues

tobramycin may be confused with Trobicin®, vancomycin

Nebcin® may be confused with Inapsine®, Naprosyn®, Nubain®

Synonyms tobramycin sulfate

U.S./Canadian Brand Names TOBI® [US/Can]; Tobramycin Injection, USP [Can]

Therapeutic Category Antibiotic, Aminoglycoside

Use Treatment of documented or suspected infections caused by susceptible gram-negative bacilli, including *Pseudomonas aeruginosa*. Tobramycin solution for inhalation is indicated for the management of cystic fibrosis patients (>6 years of age) with *Pseudomonas aeruginosa*.

Dosage Summary

I.M.:

Infants: 2.5 mg/kg every 8 hours

Children <5 years: 2.5 mg/kg every 8 hours

Children ≥5 years: 2-3.3 mg/kg every 6-8 hours

Adults: 1-2.5 mg/kg every 8-12 hours (1 mg/kg used for synergy) **or** 4-7 mg/kg/day as a single daily dose

Elderly: 1.5-5 mg/kg/day in 1-2 divided doses

I.V.:

Infants: 2.5 mg/kg every 8 hours

Children <5 years: 2.5 mg/kg every 8 hours

Children ≥5 years: 2-3.3 mg/kg every 6-8 hours

Adults: 1-2.5 mg/kg every 8-12 hours (1 mg/kg/dose used for synergy) **or** 4-7 mg/kg/day as a single daily dose

Elderly: 1.5-5 mg/kg/day in 1-2 divided doses **or** 5-7 mg/kg given every 24, 36, or 48 hours based on Cl_{cr}

Inhalation:

Children <6 years: Dosage not established

Children ≥6 years: 300 mg every 12 hours [TOBI®]

Adults: 300 mg every 12 hours [TOBI®]

Dosage Forms

Infusion, premixed in NS: 60 mg (50 mL); 80 mg (100 mL)

Injection, powder for reconstitution: 1.2 g

Injection, solution: 10 mg/mL (2 mL, 8 mL); 40 mg/mL (2 mL, 30 mL, 50 mL)

Solution, for nebulization [preservative free]:

TOBI®: 300 mg/5 mL (56s)

tobramycin (ophthalmic) (toe bra MYE sin)

Sound-Alike/Look-Alike Issues

tobramycin may be confused with Trobicin®, vancomycin

AK-Tob™ may be confused with AK-Trol®

Tobrex® may be confused with TobraDex®

Synonyms tobramycin sulfate

U.S./Canadian Brand Names AK-Tob™ [US]; PMS-Tobramycin [Can]; Sandoz-Tobramycin [Can]; Tobrex® [US/Can]

Therapeutic Category Antibiotic, Aminoglycoside; Antibiotic, Ophthalmic

Use Treatment of superficial ophthalmic infections caused by susceptible bacteria

Dosage Summary

Ophthalmic:

Ointment:

Children <2 months: Dosage not established

Children ≥2 months: Apply 2-3 times/day; for severe infections, apply every 3-4 hours

Adults: Apply 2-3 times/day; for severe infections, apply every 3-4 hours

Solution:

Children <2 months: Dosage not established

Children ≥2 months: Instill 1-2 drops every 2-4 hours

Adults: Instill 1-2 drops every 2-4 hours

Dosage Forms

Ointment, ophthalmic:

Tobrex®: 0.3% (3.5 g)

Solution, ophthalmic: 0.3% (5 mL)

AK-Tob™: 0.3% (5 mL)

Tobrex®: 0.3% (5 mL)

tobramycin and dexamethasone (toe bra MYE sin & deks a METH a sone)

Sound-Alike/Look-Alike Issues

TobraDex® may be confused with Tobrex®

Synonyms dexamethasone and tobramycin

U.S./Canadian Brand Names TobraDex® [US/Can]

Therapeutic Category Antibiotic/Corticosteroid, Ophthalmic

Use Treatment of external ocular infection caused by susceptible gram-negative bacteria and steroid responsive inflammatory conditions of the palpebral and bulbar conjunctiva, cornea, and anterior segment of the globe

Dosage Summary

Ophthalmic:

Ointment:

Children <2 years: Dosage not established

Children ≥2 years: Apply ~1/2-inch ribbon up to 3-4 times/day

Adults: Apply ~1/2-inch ribbon up to 3-4 times/day

Suspension:

Children <2 years: Dosage not established

Children ≥2 years: Instill 1-2 drops every every 4-6 hours, may increase to 1-2 drops every 2 hours for 24-48 hours

Adults: Instill 1-2 drops every every 4-6 hours, may increase to 1-2 drops every 2 hours for 24-48 hours

Dosage Forms

Ointment, ophthalmic:

TobraDex®: Tobramycin 0.3% and dexamethasone 0.1% (3.5 g)

Suspension, ophthalmic: Tobramycin 0.3% and dexamethasone 0.1% (2.5 mL, 5 mL, 10 mL)

TobraDex®: Tobramycin 0.3% and dexamethasone 0.1% (2.5 mL, 5 mL, 10 mL)

tobramycin and loteprednol etabonate *see* loteprednol and tobramycin *on page 578*

Tobramycin Injection, USP [Can] *see* tobramycin (systemic, oral inhalation) *on page 937*

tobramycin sulfate *see* tobramycin (ophthalmic) *on page 938*

tobramycin sulfate *see* tobramycin (systemic, oral inhalation) *on page 937*

Tobrex® [US/Can] *see* tobramycin (ophthalmic) *on page 938*

tocilizumab (toe si LIZ oo mab)

Synonyms atlizumab; MRA; R-1569; RoActemra®

U.S./Canadian Brand Names Actemra® [US]

Therapeutic Category Antirheumatic, Disease Modifying; Interleukin-6 Receptor Antagonist

Use Treatment of moderately- to severely-active rheumatoid arthritis in adult patients who have had an inadequate response to one or more TNF antagonists (as monotherapy or in combination with nonbiological disease-modifying antirheumatic drugs [DMARDs])

Dosage Summary

I.V.:

Children: Dosage not established

Adults: 4-8 mg/kg every 4 weeks (maximum: 800 mg per infusion)

Dosage Forms

Injection, solution [preservative free]:

Actemra®: 20 mg/mL (4 mL, 10 mL, 20 mL)

tocophersolan *(Discontinued)*

Today® [US-OTC] *see* nonoxynol 9 *on page 681*

Tofranil® [US/Can] *see* imipramine *on page 500*

Tofranil-PM® [US] *see* imipramine *on page 500*

tolazamide (tole AZ a mide)

Sound-Alike/Look-Alike Issues

TOLAZamide may be confused with tolazoline, TOLBUTamide

Tolinase® may be confused with Orinase®

Tall-Man TOLAZamide

U.S./Canadian Brand Names Tolinase® [Can]

Therapeutic Category Antidiabetic Agent, Oral

Use Adjunct to diet for the management of mild-to-moderately severe, stable, type 2 diabetes mellitus (noninsulin-dependent, NIDDM)

Dosage Summary

Oral:

Children: Dosage not established

Adults: Initial: 100-250 mg/day with first main meal of day; Maintenance: 100-1000 mg/day in 1-2 (doses >500 mg) divided doses (maximum: 1 g/day); **Note:** Titration is recommended

Dosage Forms

Tablet, oral: 250 mg, 500 mg

tolazoline *(Discontinued)*

tolbutamide (tole BYOO ta mide)

Sound-Alike/Look-Alike Issues

TOLBUTamide may be confused with terbutaline, TOLAZamide

Orinase® may be confused with Orabase®, Ornex®, Tolinase®

Synonyms tolbutamide sodium
Tall-Man **TOLBUT**amide
U.S./Canadian Brand Names Apo-Tolbutamide® [Can]
Therapeutic Category Antidiabetic Agent, Oral
Use Adjunct to diet for the management of type 2 diabetes mellitus (noninsulin-dependent, NIDDM)
Dosage Summary
Oral:
Children: Dosage not established
Adults: Initial: 1-2 g/day as a single dose or divided doses throughout the day; Maintenance: 0.25-3 g/day as a single dose or divided doses throughout the day
Elderly: Initial: 250 mg 1-3 times/day; Maintenance: 500-2000 mg/day in 1-3 divided doses (maximum: 3 g/day)
Dosage Forms
Tablet, oral: 500 mg

tolbutamide sodium *see* tolbutamide *on page 939*

tolcapone (TOLE ka pone)

U.S./Canadian Brand Names Tasmar® [US]
Therapeutic Category Anti-Parkinson Agent
Use Adjunct to levodopa and carbidopa for the treatment of signs and symptoms of idiopathic Parkinson disease in patients with motor fluctuations not responsive to other therapies
Dosage Summary
Oral:
Children: Dosage not established
Adults: Initial: 100 mg 3 times/day; Maintenance: 100-200 mg 3 times/day
Dosage Forms
Tablet, oral:
Tasmar®: 100 mg

Tolectin® DS *(Discontinued)* *see* tolmetin *on page 940*
Tolinase® [Can] *see* tolazamide *on page 939*
Tolinase® *(Discontinued)* *see* tolazamide *on page 939*

tolmetin (TOLE met in)

Synonyms tolmetin sodium
Therapeutic Category Analgesic, Nonnarcotic; Nonsteroidal Antiinflammatory Drug (NSAID)
Use Treatment of rheumatoid arthritis and osteoarthritis, juvenile rheumatoid arthritis
Dosage Summary
Oral:
Children <2 years: Dosage not established
Children ≥2 years: Initial: 20 mg/kg/day in 3-4 divided doses; Maintenance: 15-30 mg/kg/day in 3-4 divided doses (maximum: 30 mg/kg/day)
Adults: Initial: 400 mg 3 times/day; Maintenance: 600-1800 mg/day in 3 divided doses (maximum: 1.8 g/day)
Dosage Forms
Capsule, oral: 400 mg
Tablet, oral: 200 mg, 600 mg

tolmetin sodium *see* tolmetin *on page 940*

tolnaftate (tole NAF tate)

Sound-Alike/Look-Alike Issues
tolnaftate may be confused with Tornalate®
Tinactin® may be confused with Talacen®
U.S./Canadian Brand Names Blis-To-Sol® [US-OTC]; Mycocide® NS [US-OTC]; Pitrex [Can]; Podactin Powder [US-OTC]; Tinactin® Antifungal Deodorant [US-OTC]; Tinactin® Antifungal Jock Itch [US-OTC]; Tinactin® Antifungal [US-OTC]; Tinaderm [US-OTC]; Ting® Cream [US-OTC]; Ting® Spray Liquid [US-OTC]
Therapeutic Category Antifungal Agent

Use Treatment of tinea pedis, tinea cruris, tinea corporis

Dosage Summary

Topical:

Children <2 years: Dosage not established
Children ≥2 years: Apply to affected areas 2 times/day
Adults: Apply to affected areas 2 times/day

Dosage Forms

Aerosol, topical:
Tinactin® Antifungal [OTC]: 1% (133 g, 150 g)
Tinactin® Antifungal Deodorant [OTC]: 1% (133 g)
Tinactin® Antifungal Jock Itch [OTC]: 1% (133 g)
Ting® Spray Liquid [OTC]: 1% (128 g)

Cream, topical: 1% (15 g, 30 g, 114 g)
Tinactin® Antifungal [OTC]: 1% (15 g, 30 g)
Tinactin® Antifungal Jock Itch [OTC]: 1% (15 g)
Ting® Cream [OTC]: 1% (15 g)

Liquid, topical:
Blis-To-Sol® [OTC]: 1% (30 mL, 55 mL)
Tinactin® Antifungal [OTC]: 1% (59 mL)

Powder, topical: 1% (45 g); 1% (45 g)
Podactin Powder [OTC]: 1% (60 g)
Tinactin® Antifungal [OTC]: 1% (108 g)

Solution, topical:
Mycocide® NS [OTC]: 1% (30 mL)
Tinaderm [OTC]: 1% (10 mL)

Toloxin® [Can] *see* digoxin *on page* 302

tolterodine (tole TER oh deen)

Sound-Alike/Look-Alike Issues

tolterodine may be confused with fesoterodine
Detrol® may be confused with Ditropan®

Synonyms tolterodine tartrate

U.S./Canadian Brand Names Detrol® LA [US/Can]; Detrol® [US/Can]; Unidet® [Can]

Therapeutic Category Anticholinergic Agent

Use Treatment of patients with an overactive bladder with symptoms of urinary frequency, urgency, or urge incontinence

Dosage Summary

Oral:

Extended release:
Children: Dosage not established
Adults: 2-4 mg once daily

Immediate release:
Children: Dosage not established
Adults: 1-2 mg twice daily

Dosage Forms

Capsule, extended release, oral:
Detrol® LA: 2 mg, 4 mg

Tablet, oral:
Detrol®: 1 mg, 2 mg

tolterodine tartrate *see* tolterodine *on page* 941

tolvaptan (tol VAP tan)

Synonyms OPC-41061

U.S./Canadian Brand Names Samsca™ [US]

Therapeutic Category Vasopressin Antagonist

Use Treatment of clinically significant hypervolemic or euvolemic hyponatremia (associated with heart failure, cirrhosis or SIADH) with either a serum sodium <125 mEq/L or less marked hyponatremia that is symptomatic and resistant to fluid restriction

Dosage Summary

Oral:

Children: Dosage not established

Adults: 15-60 mg once daily

Dosage Forms

Tablet, oral:

Samsca™: 15 mg, 30 mg

Tomocat® 1000 ***(Discontinued)*** *see* barium *on page 117*

Tomocat® ***(Discontinued)*** *see* barium *on page 117*

tomoxetine *see* atomoxetine *on page 103*

Tomudex® [Can] *see* raltitrexed *(Canada only) on page 826*

Tomycine® ***(Discontinued)*** *see* tobramycin (ophthalmic) *on page 938*

Tonocard® ***(Discontinued)***

Tonojug ***(Discontinued)*** *see* barium *on page 117*

Tonopaque ***(Discontinued)*** *see* barium *on page 117*

Topactin [Can] *see* fluocinonide *on page 411*

Topamax® [US/Can] *see* topiramate *on page 942*

Topamax® 200 mg Tablet ***(Discontinued)*** *see* topiramate *on page 942*

Topicaine® [US-OTC] *see* lidocaine (topical) *on page 562*

Topicort® [US/Can] *see* desoximetasone *on page 280*

Topicort®-LP [US] *see* desoximetasone *on page 280*

Topicycline® Topical ***(Discontinued)*** *see* tetracycline *on page 922*

Topilene® [Can] *see* betamethasone *on page 133*

topiramate (toe PYRE a mate)

Sound-Alike/Look-Alike Issues

Topamax® may be confused with Sporanox®, Tegretol®, Tegretol®-XR, Toprol-XL®

U.S./Canadian Brand Names Apo-Topiramate® [Can]; CO Topiramate [Can]; Dom-Topiramate [Can]; Mint-Topiramate [Can]; Mylan-Topiramate [Can]; Novo-Topiramate [Can]; PHL-Topiramate [Can]; PMS-Topiramate [Can]; PRO-Topiramate [Can]; ratio-Topiramate [Can]; Sandoz-Topiramate [Can]; Topamax® [US/Can]; ZYM-Topiramate [Can]

Therapeutic Category Anticonvulsant

Use Monotherapy or adjunctive therapy for partial onset seizures and primary generalized tonic-clonic seizures; adjunctive treatment of seizures associated with Lennox-Gastaut syndrome; prophylaxis of migraine headache

Dosage Summary

Oral:

Children <2 years: Dosage not established

Children 2-9 years: Initial: 1-3 mg/kg/day (maximum: 25 mg) given once nightly; Maintenance: 5-9 mg/kg/day given once nightly; **Note:** Titration is recommended

Children 10-16 years: Initial: 1-3 mg/kg/day (maximum: 25 mg) given once nightly; Maintenance: 5-9 mg/kg/day given once nightly **or** 25-200 mg twice daily (maximum: 400 mg/day); **Note:** Titration is recommended

Children ≥17 years: Initial: 25 mg once or twice daily; Maintenance: 100-200 mg twice daily; **Note:** Titration is recommended

Adults: Initial: 25-50 mg/day in 1-2 divided doses; Maintenance: 50-200 mg twice daily; **Note:** Titration is recommended

Dosage Forms

Capsule, sprinkle, oral: 15 mg, 25 mg

Topamax®: 15 mg, 25 mg

Tablet, oral: 25 mg, 50 mg, 100 mg, 200 mg

Topamax®: 25 mg, 50 mg, 100 mg, 200 mg

Topisone® [Can] *see* betamethasone *on page 133*

Toposar® [US] *see* etoposide *on page 384*

topotecan (toe poe TEE kan)

Sound-Alike/Look-Alike Issues

Hycamtin® may be confused with Hycomine®, Mycamine®

Synonyms hycamptamine; SKF 104864; SKF 104864-A; topotecan hydrochloride

U.S./Canadian Brand Names Hycamtin® [US/Can]; Topotecan For Injection [Can]

Therapeutic Category Antineoplastic Agent

Use Treatment of ovarian cancer and small cell lung cancer; cervical cancer (in combination with cisplatin)

Dosage Summary

Oral:

Children: Dosage not established

Adults: 2.3 mg/m^2/day for 5 days; repeated every 21 days

I.V.:

Children: Dosage not established

Adults: IVPB: 1.5 mg/m^2/day for 5 days; repeated every 21 days **or** 0.75 mg/m^2/day for 3 days every 21 days

Dosage Forms

Capsule, oral:

Hycamtin®: 0.25 mg, 1 mg

Injection, powder for reconstitution:

Hycamtin®: 4 mg

Topotecan For Injection [Can] *see* topotecan *on page 943*
topotecan hydrochloride *see* topotecan *on page 943*
Toprol-XL® [US] *see* metoprolol *on page 625*
Topsyn® [Can] *see* fluocinonide *on page 411*
Toradol® [Can] *see* ketorolac (systemic) *on page 537*
Toradol® IM [Can] *see* ketorolac (systemic) *on page 537*

toremifene (tore EM i feen)

Synonyms FC1157a; toremifene citrate

U.S./Canadian Brand Names Fareston® [US/Can]

Therapeutic Category Antineoplastic Agent

Use Treatment of postmenopausal metastatic breast cancer (estrogen receptor positive or estrogen receptor status unknown)

Dosage Summary

Oral:

Children: Dosage not established

Adults: 60 mg once daily

Dosage Forms

Tablet, oral:

Fareston®: 60 mg

toremifene citrate *see* toremifene *on page 943*
Torisel® [US/Can] *see* temsirolimus *on page 915*

torsemide (TORE se mide)

Sound-Alike/Look-Alike Issues

torsemide may be confused with furosemide

Demadex® may be confused with Denorex®

U.S./Canadian Brand Names Demadex® [US]

Therapeutic Category Diuretic, Loop

Use Management of edema associated with heart failure and hepatic or renal disease (including chronic renal failure); treatment of hypertension

Dosage Summary

I.V.:

Children: Dosage not established

Oral:

Children: Dosage not established

Adults: 5-200 mg once daily (maximum: 200 mg/day)

Dosage Forms

Injection, solution: 10 mg/mL (2 mL, 5 mL)

Tablet, oral: 5 mg, 10 mg, 20 mg, 100 mg

Demadex®: 5 mg, 10 mg, 20 mg, 100 mg

tositumomab I-131 *see* tositumomab and iodine I 131 tositumomab *on page 944*

tositumomab and iodine I 131 tositumomab

(toe si TYOO mo mab & EYE oh dyne eye one THUR tee one toe si TYOO mo mab)

Synonyms 131 I anti-B1 antibody; 131 I-anti-B1 monoclonal antibody; anti-CD20-murine monoclonal antibody I-131; iodine I 131 tositumomab and tositumomab; tositumomab I-131

U.S./Canadian Brand Names Bexxar® [US]

Therapeutic Category Antineoplastic Agent, Monoclonal Antibody; Radiopharmaceutical

Use Treatment of relapsed or refractory CD20 positive, low-grade, follicular, or transformed non-Hodgkin lymphoma (NHL)

Dosage Summary

I.V.:

Tositumomab:

Children: Dosage not established

Adults: Step 1: 450 mg in NS 50 mL over 60 minutes; Step 2: 450 mg in NS 50 mL over 60 minutes

Iodine I-131 tositumomab (Given after tositumomab):

Children: Dosage not established

Adults: Step 1: I-131 5 mCi and tositumomab 35 mg in NS 30 mL over 20 minutes; Step 2: I-131 (calculated to deliver 65-75 cGy total body irradiation) and tositumomab 35 mg over 20 minutes

Dosage Forms

Kit [dosimetric package]:

Bexxar®: Tositumomab 225 mg/16.1 mL [2 vials], tositumomab 35 mg/2.5 mL [1 vial], and iodine I 131 tositumomab 0.1 mg/mL and 0.61mCi/mL (20 mL) [1 vial]

Kit [therapeutic package]:

Bexxar®: Tositumomab 225 mg/16.1 mL [2 vials], tositumomab 35 mg/2.5 mL [1 vial], and iodine I 131 tositumomab 1.1 mg/mL and 5.6 mCi/mL (20 mL) [1 or 2 vials]

Totacillin® ***(Discontinued)*** *see* ampicillin *on page 75*

total parenteral nutrition (TOE tal par EN ter al noo TRISH un)

Synonyms hyperal; hyperalimentation; parenteral nutrition; PN; TPN

Therapeutic Category Caloric Agent; Intravenous Nutritional Therapy

Use Infusion of nutrient solutions into the bloodstream to support nutritional needs during a time when patient is unable to absorb nutrients via the gastrointestinal tract, cannot take adequate nutrition orally or enterally, or have had (or are expected to have) inadequate oral intake for 7-14 days.

Dosage Summary

I.V.:

Calories:

Neonates (preterm): 90-120 kcal/kg/day

Neonates (term): 85-105 kcal/kg/day

Children <6 months: 85-105 kcal/kg/day

Children 6-12 months: 80-100 kcal/kg/day

Children 1-7 years: 75-90 kcal/kg/day

Children: 7-12 years: 50-75 kcal/kg/day

Children 12-18 years: 30-50 kcal/kg/day

Adults: 20-40 kcal/kg/day

Carbohydrates:

Neonates (premature): Initial: 6 mg/kg/minute; Goal: 10-13 mg/kg/minute

Neonates (term): Initial: 6-8 mg/kg/minute; Goal: 10-14 mg/kg/minute

Children <1 year: Initial: 6-8 mg/kg/minute; Goal: 10-14 mg/kg/minute

Children 1-10 years: Initial: 10% to 12.5% of total caloric intake (maximum: 15 mg/kg/minute)

Children >10 years: 10% to 15% of total caloric intake (maximum: 8.5 mg/kg/minute)

Adults: 5 g/kg/day **or** 3.5 mg/kg/minute (maximum: 4-7 mg/kg/minute)

Fat:

Neonates (preterm): Initial: 0.25-0.5 g/kg/day (maximum: 3 g/kg/day)

Neonates (term): Initial: 0.5-1 g/kg/day (maximum: 3 g/kg/day)

Children: Initial: 1 g/kg/day (maximum: 3 g/kg/day)

Adults: 20-40 % of total caloric intake (maximum: 60% of total calories **or** 2.5 g/kg/day)
Fluid:
Neonates <1.5 kg: 130-150 mL/kg/day
Neonates 1.5-2 kg: 110-130 mL/kg/day
Neonates and Children 2-10 kg: 100 mL /kg/day
Children >10-20 kg: 1000 mL for 10 kg plus 50 mL/kg for each kg >10
Children >20 kg: 1500 mL for 10 kg plus 20 mL/kg for each kg >20
Adults: 30-40 mL/kg
Protein:
Neonates (premature): Initial: 1-1.5 g/kg/day; Goal: 3.5-3.85 g/kg/day
Neonates (term): Initial: 2.5 g/kg/day; Goal: 3 g/kg/day
Children 1-12 months: Initial: 2-3 g/kg/day (maximum: 3 g/kg/day)
Children 1-10 years: Initial: 1-2 g/kg/day (maximum: 2.5 g/kg/day)
Children >10 years: Initial: 0.8-1.5 g/kg/day (maximum: 2 g/kg/day)
Adults: 0.6-2 g/kg/day

Dosage Forms TPN is usually compounded from optimal combinations of macronutrients (water, protein, dextrose, and lipids) and micronutrients (electrolytes, trace elements, and vitamins) to meet the specific nutritional requirements of a patient. Individual hospitals may have designated standard TPN formulas. There are a few commercially-available amino acids with electrolytes solutions; however, these products may not meet an individual's specific nutrition requirements.

Totect® [US] *see* dexrazoxane *on page* *284*

Touro Ex® ***(Discontinued)*** *see* guaifenesin *on page* *454*

Touro® HC ***(Discontinued)***

Toviaz™ [US] *see* fesoterodine *on page* *399*

tPA *see* alteplase *on page* *56*

TPN *see* total parenteral nutrition *on page* *944*

TPV *see* tipranavir *on page* *936*

tRA *see* tretinoin (systemic) *on page* *951*

4 Trace Elements [US] *see* trace metals *on page* *945*

Trace Elements 4 Pediatric [US] *see* trace metals *on page* *945*

trace metals (trase MET als)

Synonyms chromium; copper; iodine; manganese; molybdenum; neonatal trace metals; selenium; zinc

U.S./Canadian Brand Names 4 Trace Elements [US]; Multitrace®-4 Concentrate [US]; Multitrace®-4 Neonatal [US]; Multitrace®-4 Pediatric [US]; Multitrace®-4 [US]; Multitrace®-5 Concentrate [US]; Multitrace®-5 [US]; Trace Elements 4 Pediatric [US]

Therapeutic Category Trace Element

Use Prevention and correction of trace metal deficiencies

Dosage Summary

I.V.:
Chromium:
Infants: 0.2 mcg/kg/day
Children: 0.2 mcg/kg/day (maximum: 5 mcg/day)
Adults: 10-15 mcg/day
Copper:
Infants: 20 mcg/kg/day
Children: 20 mcg/kg/day (maximum: 300 mcg/day)
Adults: 0.5-1.5 mg/day
Manganese:
Infants: 1 mcg/kg/day
Children: 1 mcg/kg/day (maximum: 50 mcg/day)
Adults: 150-800 mcg/day
Molybdenum:
Infants: 0.25 mcg/kg/day
Children: 0.25 mcg/kg/day (maximum: 5 mcg/day)
Adults: 20-120 mcg/day
Selenium:
Infants: 2 mcg/kg/day
Children: 2 mcg/kg/day (maximum: 30 mcg/day)
Adults: 20-40 mcg/day

Zinc:

Infants, preterm: 400 mcg/kg/day

Infants, term <3 months: 250 mcg/kg/day

Infants, term ≥3 months: 100 mcg/kg/day

Children: 50 mcg/kg/day (maximum: 5 mg/day)

Adults: 2.5-4 mg/day

Dosage Forms

Injection, solution [combination products]:

Multitrace®-4: Chromium 4 mcg, copper 0.4 mg, manganese 0.1 mg, and zinc 1 mg per 1 mL (10 mL)

Multitrace®-4 Concentrate: Chromium 10 mcg, copper 1 mg, manganese 0.5 mg, and zinc 5 mg per 1 mL (1 mL, 10 mL)

Multitrace®-4 Neonatal: Chromium 0.85 mcg, copper 0.1 mg, manganese 0.025 mg, and zinc 1.5 mg per 1 mL (2 mL)

Multitrace®-5: Chromium 4 mcg, copper 0.4 mg, manganese 0.1 mg, selenium 20 mcg, and zinc 1 mg per 1 mL (10 mL)

Multitrace®-5 Concentrate: Chromium 10 mcg, copper 1 mg, manganese 0.5 mg, selenium 60 mcg, and zinc 5 mg per 1 mL (1 mL, 10 mL)

Trace Elements 4 Pediatric: Chromium 1 mcg, copper 0.1 mg, manganese 0.03 mg, and zinc 0.5 mg per 1 mL (10 mL)

Injection, solution [combination products, preservative free]:

4 Trace Elements: Chromium 2 mcg, copper 0.2 mg, manganese 0.16 mg, and zinc 0.8 mg per 1 mL (5 mL, 50 mL)

Multitrace®-4 Pediatric: Chromium 1 mcg, copper 0.1 mg, manganese 0.025 mg, and zinc 1 mg per 1 mL (3 mL)

Tracleer® [US/Can] *see* bosentan *on page 143*

Tramacet [Can] *see* acetaminophen and tramadol *on page 27*

tramadol (TRA ma dole)

Sound-Alike/Look-Alike Issues

traMADol may be confused with tapentadol, Toradol®, Trandate®, traZODone, Voltaren®

Ultram® may be confused with Ultane®, Ultracet®, Voltaren®

Synonyms tramadol hydrochloride

Tall-Man tra**MAD**ol

U.S./Canadian Brand Names Ralivia™ ER [Can]; Rybix™ ODT [US]; Ryzolt™ [US]; Tridural™ [Can]; Ultram® ER [US]; Ultram® [US]; Zytram® XL [Can]

Therapeutic Category Analgesic, Nonnarcotic

Use Relief of moderate to moderately-severe pain

Extended release formulations are indicated for patients requiring around-the-clock management of moderate to moderately-severe pain for an extended period of time

Dosage Summary

Oral:

Immediate release:

Children <17 years: Dosage not established.

Children ≥17 years: 50-100 mg every 4-6 hours (maximum: 400 mg/day)

Adults: 50-100 mg every 4-6 hours (maximum: 400 mg/day)

Elderly >75 years: 50-100 mg every 4-6 hours (maximum: 300 mg/day)

Extended release:

Children: Dosage not established.

Adults: 100-300 once daily (maximum: 300 mg/day); **Note:** Maximum dose of Zytram® XL [CAN] is 400 mg/day per product labeling.

Dosage Forms

Tablet, oral: 50 mg

Ultram®: 50 mg

Tablet, extended release, oral: 100 mg, 200 mg

Ryzolt™: 100 mg, 200 mg, 300 mg

Ultram® ER: 100 mg, 200 mg, 300 mg

Tablet, orally disintegrating, oral:

Rybix™ ODT: 50 mg

Dosage Forms - Canada

Tablet, extended release:

Ralivia™ ER, Tridural™: 100 mg, 200 mg, 300 mg
Zytram® XL: 150 mg, 200 mg, 300 mg, 400 mg

tramadol hydrochloride *see* tramadol *on page* 946

tramadol hydrochloride and acetaminophen *see* acetaminophen and tramadol *on page* 27

Trandate® [US/Can] *see* labetalol *on page* 541

trandolapril (tran DOE la pril)

U.S./Canadian Brand Names Mavik® [US/Can]

Therapeutic Category Angiotensin-Converting Enzyme (ACE) Inhibitor

Use Treatment of hypertension alone or in combination with other antihypertensive agents; treatment of heart failure (HF) or left ventricular (LV) dysfunction after myocardial infarction (MI)

Dosage Summary

Oral:

Children: Dosage not established
Adults: Initial: 1-2 mg once daily; Maintenance: 1-4 mg once daily

Dosage Forms

Tablet, oral: 1 mg, 2 mg, 4 mg
Mavik®: 1 mg, 2 mg, 4 mg

trandolapril and verapamil (tran DOE la pril & ver AP a mil)

Synonyms verapamil and trandolapril

U.S./Canadian Brand Names Tarka® [US/Can]

Therapeutic Category Antihypertensive Agent, Combination

Use Treatment of hypertension; however, not indicated for initial treatment of hypertension

Dosage Summary

Oral:

Children: Dosage not established
Adults: Trandolapril 1-4 mg and verapamil 180-240 mg once daily

Dosage Forms

Tablet, variable release: Trandolapril 2 mg [immediate release] and verapamil 180 mg [sustained release]; Trandolapril 2 mg [immediate release] and verapamil 240 mg [sustained release]; Trandolapril 4 mg [immediate release] and verapamil 240 mg [sustained release]

Tarka®:
1/240: Trandolapril 1 mg [immediate release] and verapamil 240 mg [sustained release]
2/180: Trandolapril 2 mg [immediate release] and verapamil 180 mg [sustained release]
2/240: Trandolapril 2 mg [immediate release] and verapamil 240 mg [sustained release]
4/240: Trandolapril 4 mg [immediate release] and verapamil 240 mg [sustained release]

tranexamic acid (tran eks AM ik AS id)

Sound-Alike/Look-Alike Issues

Cyklokapron® may be confused with cycloSPORINE

U.S./Canadian Brand Names Cyklokapron® [US/Can]; Lysteda™ [US]; Tranexamic Acid Injection BP [Can]

Therapeutic Category Antihemophilic Agent

Use

Solution for injection: Short-term use (2-8 days) in hemophilia patients to reduce or prevent hemorrhage and reduce need for replacement therapy during and following tooth extraction
Tablet: Treatment of cyclic heavy menstrual bleeding

Dosage Summary

I.V.:

Children: Initial: 10 mg/kg before surgery; Maintenance: 10 mg/kg/dose 3-4 times/day
Adults: Initial: 10 mg/kg before surgery; Maintenance: 10 mg/kg/dose 3-4 times/day

Oral:

Children: Dosage not established
Adults: 1300 mg 3 times daily (3900 mg/day) for up to 5 days

Dosage Forms

Injection, solution:
Cyklokapron®: 100 mg/mL (10 mL)

Tablet, oral:
Lysteda™: 650 mg

Tranexamic Acid Injection BP [Can] *see* tranexamic acid *on page 947*
transamine sulphate *see* tranylcypromine *on page 948*
Transderm-V® [Can] *see* scopolamine derivatives (systemic) *on page 866*
Transdermal-NTG® Patch *(Discontinued)* *see* nitroglycerin *on page 679*
Transderm-Nitro® [Can] *see* nitroglycerin *on page 679*
Transderm Scōp® [US] *see* scopolamine derivatives (systemic) *on page 866*
Trans-Plantar® [Can] *see* salicylic acid *on page 858*
Trans-Plantar® Transdermal Patch *(Discontinued)* *see* salicylic acid *on page 858*
***trans*-retinoic acid** *see* tretinoin (systemic) *on page 951*
***trans*-retinoic acid** *see* tretinoin (topical) *on page 951*
Trans-Ver-Sal® [US-OTC/Can] *see* salicylic acid *on page 858*
***trans* vitamin A acid** *see* tretinoin (systemic) *on page 951*
Tranxene®-SD *(Discontinued)* *see* clorazepate *on page 239*
Tranxene®-SD Half Strength *(Discontinued)* *see* clorazepate *on page 239*
Tranxene® T-Tab® [US] *see* clorazepate *on page 239*

tranylcypromine (tran il SIP roe meen)

Synonyms transamine sulphate; tranylcypromine sulfate

U.S./Canadian Brand Names Parnate® [US/Can]

Therapeutic Category Antidepressant, Monoamine Oxidase Inhibitor

Use Treatment of major depressive episode without melancholia

Dosage Summary

Oral:
Children: Dosage not established
Adults: 10-30 mg twice daily (maximum: 60 mg/day)

Dosage Forms

Tablet, oral: 10 mg
Parnate®: 10 mg

tranylcypromine sulfate *see* tranylcypromine *on page 948*

trastuzumab (tras TU zoo mab)

Synonyms anti-c-erB-2; anti-ERB-2; MOAB HER2; rhuMAb HER2

U.S./Canadian Brand Names Herceptin® [US/Can]

Therapeutic Category Antineoplastic Agent

Use Adjuvant treatment of HER-2 overexpressing breast cancer; treatment of HER-2 overexpressing metastatic breast cancer

Canadian labeling: Additional approved use (unlabeled use in the U.S.): Treatment of HER-2 overexpressing, advanced adenocarcinoma of the stomach or gastroesophageal junction

Dosage Summary

I.V.:
Children: Dosage not established
Adults: Loading dose: 4 mg/kg; Maintenance: 2 mg/kg once weekly **or** Loading dose: 8 mg/kg; Maintenance: 6 mg/kg every 3 weeks

Dosage Forms

Injection, powder for reconstitution:
Herceptin®: 440 mg

Trasylol® [Can] *see* aprotinin *on page 92*
Trav-L-Tabs® [US-OTC] *see* meclizine *on page 595*
Travasol® [US] *see* amino acid injection *on page 64*
Travatan® [US/Can] *see* travoprost *on page 949*
Travatan® Z [US/Can] *see* travoprost *on page 949*

traveler's diarrhea and cholera vaccine *(Canada only)*

(TRAV uh lerz dahy uh REE uh & KOL er uh vak SEEN)

Synonyms *Vibrio cholera* and enterotoxigenic *Escherichia coli vaccine*; cholera and traveler's diarrhea vaccine; cholera vaccine; enterotoxigenic *Escherichia coli* and *Vibrio cholera* vaccine; oral cholera vaccine; traveller's diarrhea vaccine and cholera

U.S./Canadian Brand Names Dukoral® [Can]

Therapeutic Category Vaccine

Use Protection against traveler's diarrhea and/or cholera in adults and children ≥2 years of age who will be visiting areas where there is a risk of contracting traveler's diarrhea caused by enterotoxigenic *E. coli* (ETEC) or cholera caused by *V. cholerae* O1 (classical and El Tor biotypes; Inaba and Ogawa serotypes)

Dosage Summary

Oral:

Children <2 years: Dosage not established

Children 2-6 years:

Cholera:

Primary immunization: 3 doses given at intervals of ≥1 week

Booster:

6 months to 5 years **since last dose**: 1 booster dose

>5 years **since last dose**: Repeat primary immunization schedule

Children ≥2 years:

ETEC:

Primary immunization: 2 doses given at intervals of ≥1 week

Booster:

3 months to 5 years **since last dose**: 1 booster dose

>5 years **since last dose**: Repeat primary immunization schedule

Children >6 years:

Cholera:

Primary immunization: 2 doses given at intervals of ≥1 week

Booster:

2-5 years **since last dose**: 1 booster dose

>5 years **since last dose**: Repeat primary immunization schedule

Adults:

Cholera:

Primary immunization: 2 doses given at intervals of ≥1 week

Booster:

2-5 years **since last dose**: 1 booster dose

>5 years **since last dose**: Repeat primary immunization schedule

ETEC:

Primary immunization: 2 doses given at intervals of ≥1 week

Booster:

3 months to 5 years **since last dose**: 1 booster dose

>5 years **since last dose**: Repeat primary immunization schedule

Dosage Forms - Canada

Suspension [vial]:

Dukoral®: 2.5×10^{10} of each of the following *Vibrio cholerae* O1 strains: Inaba classic (heat inactivated), Inaba El Tor (formalin inactivated), Ogawa classic (heat inactivated), Ogawa classic (formalin inactivated), and 1 mg recombinant cholera toxin B subunit (rCTB) (3 mL)

traveller's diarrhea vaccine and cholera *see* traveler's diarrhea and cholera vaccine *(Canada only) on page 949*

travoprost (TRA voe prost)

Sound-Alike/Look-Alike Issues

Travatan® may be confused with Xalatan®

U.S./Canadian Brand Names Travatan® Z [US/Can]; Travatan® [US/Can]

Therapeutic Category Prostaglandin, Ophthalmic

Use Reduction of elevated intraocular pressure in patients with open-angle glaucoma or ocular hypertension who are intolerant of the other IOP-lowering medications or insufficiently responsive (failed to achieve target IOP determined after multiple measurements over time) to another IOP-lowering medication

Dosage Summary

Ophthalmic:

Children: Dosage not established

Adults: Instill 1 drop into affected eye(s) once daily in the evening

Dosage Forms

Solution, ophthalmic:

Travatan®: 0.004% (2.5 mL, 5 mL)

Travatan® Z: 0.004% (2.5 mL, 5 mL)

travoprost and timolol *(Canada only)* (TRA voe prost & TIM oh lol)

Sound-Alike/Look-Alike Issues

DuoTrav™ may be confused with DuoNeb®

Synonyms timolol maleate and travoprost

U.S./Canadian Brand Names DuoTrav™ [Can]

Therapeutic Category Beta Blocker, Nonselective; Ophthalmic Agent, Antiglaucoma; Prostaglandin, Ophthalmic

Use Reduction of intraocular pressure (IOP) in patients with open-angle glaucoma or ocular hypertension who are insufficiently responsive to topical beta-blockers, prostaglandin analogues, or other IOP-reducing agents and in whom combination therapy is appropriate

Dosage Summary

Ophthalmic:

Children: Dosage not established

Adults: Instill 1 drop into affected eye(s) once daily in morning.

Dosage Forms - Canada

Solution, ophthalmic:

DuoTrav™: Travoprost 0.004% and timolol 0.5%: (2.5 mL, 5 mL)

trazodone (TRAZ oh done)

Sound-Alike/Look-Alike Issues

traZODone may be confused with traMADol

Desyrel® may be confused with Demerol®, Delsym®, Zestril®

Synonyms Oleptro™; trazodone hydrochloride

Tall-Man tra**ZOD**one

U.S./Canadian Brand Names Apo-Trazodone D® [Can]; Apo-Trazodone® [Can]; Dom-Trazodone [Can]; Mylan-Trazodone [Can]; Novo-Trazodone [Can]; Nu-Trazodone [Can]; Oleptro™ [US]; PHL-Trazodone [Can]; PMS-Trazodone [Can]; ratio-Trazodone [Can]; Trazorel® [Can]; ZYM-Trazodone [Can]

Therapeutic Category Antidepressant, Triazolopyridine

Use Treatment of major depressive disorder

Dosage Summary

Oral:

Children <6 years: Dosage not established

Adults: Immediate release: Initial: 150 mg/day in 3 divided doses; Maintenance: 150-600 mg/day in 3 divided doses; Extended-release: Initial: 150 mg once daily at bedtime; maximum dose: 375 mg/day. **Note:** Titration is recommended

Elderly: Immediate release: Initial: 25-50 mg at bedtime; Maintenance: 25-150 mg/day at bedtime; Extended-release: Initial: 150 mg once daily at bedtime; maximum dose: 375 mg/day; **Note:** Titration is recommended

Dosage Forms

Tablet, oral: 50 mg, 100 mg, 150 mg, 300 mg

Tablet, extended release, oral:

Oleptro™: 150 mg, 300 mg

trazodone hydrochloride *see* trazodone *on page 950*

Trazorel® [Can] *see* trazodone *on page 950*

Treanda® [US] *see* bendamustine *on page 122*

Trecator® [US/Can] *see* ethionamide *on page 381*

Trelstar® [US/Can] *see* triptorelin *on page 962*

Trendar® ***(Discontinued)*** *see* ibuprofen *on page 494*

Trental® [US/Can] *see* pentoxifylline *on page 742*

treprostinil (tre PROST in il)

Synonyms treprostinil sodium

U.S./Canadian Brand Names Remodulin® [US/Can]; Tyvaso™ [US]

Therapeutic Category Vasodilator

Use

Injection: Treatment of pulmonary arterial hypertension (PAH) in patients with NYHA Class II-IV symptoms to decrease exercise-associated symptoms; to diminish clinical deterioration when transitioning from epoprostenol (I.V.)

Inhalation: Treatment of pulmonary arterial hypertension (PAH) in patients with NYHA Class III symptoms to increase walk distance. **Note:** Nearly all controlled clinical trial experience has been with concomitant bosentan or sildenafil.

Dosage Summary

Inhalation:

Children: Dosage not established.

Adults: Initial: 18 mcg (or 3 inhalations) every 4 hours 4 times/day; maintenance: If tolerated, increase dose by an additional 3 inhalations at approximately 1- to 2-weeks intervals; maximum dose: 54 mcg (or 9 inhalations) 4 times/day.

I.V. Infusion:

Children: Dosage not established

Adults: Initial: 0.625-1.25 ng/kg/minute; Maintenance: 1.25-40 ng/kg/minute; **Note:** Titration is recommended; **Note:** This dosing is for patients new to prostacyclin therapy.

SubQ:

Children: Dosage not established

Adults: Initial: 0.625-1.25 ng/kg/minute; Maintenance: 1.25-40 ng/kg/minute; **Note:** Titration is recommended

Dosage Forms

Injection, solution:

Remodulin®: 1 mg/mL (20 mL); 2.5 mg/mL (20 mL); 5 mg/mL (20 mL); 10 mg/mL (20 mL)

Solution, for oral inhalation:

Tyvaso™: 0.6 mg/mL (2.9 mL)

treprostinil sodium *see* treprostinil *on page 951*

Tretin-X™ [US] *see* tretinoin (topical) *on page 951*

tretinoin and clindamycin *see* clindamycin and tretinoin *on page 233*

tretinoin and mequinol *see* mequinol and tretinoin *on page 606*

tretinoin, fluocinolone acetonide, and hydroquinone *see* fluocinolone, hydroquinone, and tretinoin *on page 411*

tretinoin (systemic) (TRET i noyn, sis TEM ik)

Sound-Alike/Look-Alike Issues

tretinoin may be confused with isotretinoin, Tenormin®, triamcinolone, trientine

Synonyms *trans* vitamin A acid; *trans*-retinoic acid; all-*trans* retinoic acid; all-*trans* vitamin A acid; ATRA; Ro 5488; tRA; tretinoinum

U.S./Canadian Brand Names Vesanoid® [Can]

Therapeutic Category Antineoplastic Agent

Use Induction of remission in patients with acute promyelocytic leukemia (APL), French American British (FAB) classification M3 (including the M3 variant) characterized by t(15;17) translocation and/or PML/RARα gene presence

Dosage Summary

Oral:

Children: Induction: 45 mg/m^2/day in 2 divided doses (maximum duration of treatment: 90 days)

Adults: Induction: 45 mg/m^2/day in 2 divided doses (maximum duration of treatment: 90 days)

Dosage Forms

Capsule, oral: 10 mg

tretinoin (topical) (TRET i noyn TOP i kal)

Sound-Alike/Look-Alike Issues

tretinoin may be confused with isotretinoin, Tenormin®, triamcinolone, trientine

Synonyms *trans*-retinoic acid; retinoic acid; vitamin A acid

U.S./Canadian Brand Names Atralin™ [US]; Avita® [US]; Refissa™ [US]; Rejuva-A® [Can]; Renova® [US/Can]; Retin-A Micro® [US/Can]; Retin-A® [US/Can]; Retinova® [Can]; Stieva-A [Can]; Tretin-X™ [US]

Therapeutic Category Retinoic Acid Derivative

Use Treatment of acne vulgaris; photodamaged skin; palliation of fine wrinkles, mottled hyperpigmentation, and tactile roughness of facial skin as part of a comprehensive skin care and sun avoidance program

Dosage Summary

Topical:

Children ≤12 years: Dosage not established

Children >12 years: Apply once daily **or** every other day in evening to acne lesions

Adults: Apply once daily or every other day in evening to face

Dosage Forms

Cream, topical: 0.025% (20 g, 45 g); 0.05% (20 g, 45 g); 0.1% (20 g, 45 g)

Avita®: 0.025% (20 g, 45 g)

Refissa™: 0.05% (40 g)

Renova®: 0.02% (40 g, 44 g, 60 g)

Retin-A®: 0.025% (20 g, 45 g); 0.05% (20 g, 45 g); 0.1% (20 g, 45 g)

Tretin-X™: 0.025% (35 g); 0.05% (35 g); 0.1% (35 g)

Gel, topical: 0.01% (15 g, 45 g); 0.025% (15 g, 45 g)

Atralin™: 0.05% (45 g)

Avita®: 0.025% (20 g, 45 g)

Retin-A Micro®: 0.04% (20 g, 45 g, 50 g); 0.1% (20 g, 45 g, 50 g)

Retin-A®: 0.01% (15 g, 45 g); 0.025% (15 g, 45 g)

Tretin-X™: 0.01% (35 g); 0.025% (35 g)

tretinoinum *see* tretinoin (systemic) *on page 951*

Trexall™ [US] *see* methotrexate *on page 614*

Treximet™ [US] *see* sumatriptan and naproxen *on page 905*

Trezix® [US] *see* acetaminophen, caffeine, and dihydrocodeine *on page 28*

triacetin (trye a SEE tin)

Sound-Alike/Look-Alike Issues

triacetin may be confused with Triacin®

Synonyms glycerol triacetate

U.S./Canadian Brand Names Myco-Nail [US-OTC]

Therapeutic Category Antifungal Agent

Use Fungistat for athlete's foot and other superficial fungal infections

Dosage Summary

Topical:

Children: Dosage not established

Adults: Apply twice daily to affected areas

Dosage Forms

Liquid, topical:

Myco-Nail [OTC]: 25% (30 mL)

Triacin-C® ***(Discontinued)*** *see* triprolidine, pseudoephedrine, and codeine *(Canada only) on page 961*

triaconazole *see* terconazole *on page 918*

Triaderm [Can] *see* triamcinolone (topical) *on page 954*

Triafed® ***(Discontinued)*** *see* triprolidine and pseudoephedrine *on page 961*

Triall™ [US] *see* chlorpheniramine, phenylephrine, and methscopolamine *on page 212*

triamcinolone (systemic, oral inhalation) (trye am SIN oh lone)

Sound-Alike/Look-Alike Issues

Kenalog® may be confused with Ketalar®

TAC (occasional abbreviation for triamcinolone) is an error-prone abbreviation (mistaken as tetracaine-adrenaline-cocaine)

Synonyms triamcinolone acetonide, aerosol; triamcinolone acetonide, parenteral; triamcinolone hexacetonide

U.S./Canadian Brand Names Aristospan® [US/Can]; Kenalog®-10 [Can]; Kenalog®-40 [Can]

Therapeutic Category Corticosteroid, Inhalant (Oral); Corticosteroid, Systemic

Use

Intraarticular (soft tissue): Acute gouty arthritis, acute/subacute bursitis, acute tenosynovitis, epicondylitis, rheumatoid arthritis, synovitis of osteoarthritis

Intralesional: Alopecia areata, discoid lupus erythematosus, keloids, granuloma annulare lesions (localized hypertrophic, infiltrated, or inflammatory), lichen planus plaques, lichen simplex chronicus plaques, psoriatic plaques, necrobiosis lipoidica diabeticorum, cystic tumors of aponeurosis or tendon (ganglia)

Oral inhalation: Control of bronchial asthma and related bronchospastic conditions

Systemic: Adrenocortical insufficiency, dermatologic diseases, endocrine disorders, gastrointestinal diseases, hematologic and neoplastic disorders, nervous system disorders, nephrotic syndrome, rheumatic disorders, allergic states, respiratory diseases, systemic lupus erythematosus (SLE), and other diseases requiring antiinflammatory or immunosuppressive effects

Dosage Summary

Inhalation: Oral:

Children <6 years: Dosage not established

Children 6-12 years: 75-150 mcg 3-4 times/day **or** 150-300 mcg twice daily (maximum dose: 900 mcg/day)

Children >12 years: 150 mcg 3-4 times/day **or** 300 mcg twice daily (maximum dose: 1200 mcg/day)

Adults: 150 mcg 3-4 times/day **or** 300 mcg twice daily (maximum dose: 1200 mcg/day)

I.M.:

Children: Initial: 0.11-1.6 mg/kg/day in 3-4 divided doses

Children 6-12 years: Acetonide: Initial: 40 mg; Range: 2.5-100 mg/day

Children >12 years: Acetonide: Initial: 60 mg; Range: 2.5-100 mg/day

Adults: Acetonide: Initial: 60 mg; Range: 2.5-100 mg/day, may repeat with 20-100 mg when symptoms recur; Multiple sclerosis: 160 mg/day for 1 week, then 64 mg every other day

Intraarticular:

Children: Dosage not established

Adults: Acetonide: 2.5-80 mg; Hexacetonide: 2-20 mg

Intradermal:

Children: Dosage not established

Adults: Acetonide: 1 mg/site

Intralesional:

Children: Dosage not established

Adults: Acetonide: 1-30 mg (usually 1 mg/injection site); Hexacetonide: Up to 0.5 mg/sq inch

Intrasynovial:

Children: Dosage not established

Adults: Acetonide: 5-40 mg

Tendon Sheath:

Children: Dosage not established

Adults: Acetonide: 2.5-10 mg

Dosage Forms

Injection, suspension:

Aristospan®: 5 mg/mL (5 mL); 20 mg/mL (1 mL, 5 mL)

Kenalog®-10: 10 mg/mL (5 mL)

Kenalog®-40: 40 mg/mL (1 mL, 5 mL, 10 mL)

triamcinolone (nasal) (trye am SIN oh lone)

Sound-Alike/Look-Alike Issues

Nasacort® may be confused with NasalCrom®

TAC (occasional abbreviation for triamcinolone) is an error-prone abbreviation (mistaken as tetracaine-adrenaline-cocaine)

Synonyms triamcinolone acetonide

U.S./Canadian Brand Names Nasacort® AQ [US/Can]; Trinasal® [Can]

Therapeutic Category Corticosteroid, Nasal

Use Management of seasonal and perennial allergic rhinitis

Dosage Summary

Inhalation:

Nasal inhaler:

Children <6 years: Dosage not established

Children 6-11 years: 220 mcg/day as 2 sprays in each nostril once daily

Children ≥12 years: 220-440 mcg/day as 2-4 sprays in each nostril 1-4 times/day

Adults: 220-440 mcg/day as 2-4 sprays in each nostril 1-4 times/day

Nasal spray:

Children <2 years: Dosage not established

Children 2-5 years: 110 mcg/day as 1 spray in each nostril once daily (maximum: 110 mcg/day)

Children 6-11 years: Initial: 110 mcg/day as 1 spray in each nostril once daily; may increase to 220 mcg/day as 2 sprays in each nostril

Children ≥12 years: 110-220 mcg/day as 1-2 sprays in each nostril once daily

Adults: 110-220 mcg/day as 1-2 sprays in each nostril once daily

Dosage Forms

Suspension, intranasal:

Nasacort® AQ: 55 mcg/inhalation (16.5 g)

triamcinolone (ophthalmic) (trye am SIN oh lone)

Sound-Alike/Look-Alike Issues

TAC (occasional abbreviation for triamcinolone) is an error-prone abbreviation (mistaken as tetracaine-adrenaline-cocaine)

Synonyms triamcinolone acetonide

U.S./Canadian Brand Names Triesence™ [US]

Therapeutic Category Corticosteroid, Ophthalmic

Use

Intavitreal: Treatment of sympathetic ophthalmia, temporal arteritis, uveitis, ocular inflammatory conditions unresponsive to topical corticosteroids

Triesence™: Visualization during vitrectomy

Dosage Summary

Intravitreal:

Children: Ocular disease: 4 mg as needed; visualization during vitrectomy: 1-4 mg

Adults: Ocular disease: 4 mg as needed; visualization during vitrectomy: 1-4 mg

Dosage Forms

Injection, suspension, ophthalmic:

Triesence™: 40 mg/mL (1 mL)

triamcinolone (topical) (trye am SIN oh lone)

Sound-Alike/Look-Alike Issues

Kenalog® may be confused with Ketalar®

TAC (occasional abbreviation for triamcinolone) is an error-prone abbreviation (mistaken as tetracaine-adrenaline-cocaine)

U.S./Canadian Brand Names Kenalog® [US/Can]; Oracort [Can]; Oralone® [US]; Triaderm [Can]; Triderm® [US]

Therapeutic Category Corticosteroid, Topical

Use

Oral topical: Adjunctive treatment and temporary relief of symptoms associated with oral inflammatory lesions and ulcerative lesions resulting from trauma

Topical: Inflammatory dermatoses responsive to steroids

Dosage Summary Topical:

Children: Dosage not established

Adults: Cream, ointment: Apply thin film to affected areas 2-4 times/day; Oral: Press a small dab (about 1/4 inch) to the lesion until a thin film develops; Spray: Apply to affected area 3-4 times/day

Dosage Forms

Aerosol, topical:

Kenalog®: 0.2 mg/2-second spray (63 g)

Cream, topical: 0.025% (15 g, 80 g, 454 g); 0.1% (15 g, 30 g, 80 g, 454 g, 2240 g, 2270 g); 0.5% (15 g)

Triderm®: 0.1% (30 g, 85 g)

Lotion, topical: 0.025% (60 mL); 0.1% (60 mL)

Ointment, topical: 0.025% (15 g, 80 g, 454 g); 0.05% (430 g); 0.1% (15 g, 80 g, 454 g); 0.5% (15 g)
Paste, oral, topical: 0.1% (5 g)
Oralone®: 0.1% (5 g)
Powder, topical: USP: 100% (5 g)

triamcinolone acetonide *see* triamcinolone (nasal) *on page 953*

triamcinolone acetonide *see* triamcinolone (ophthalmic) *on page 954*

triamcinolone acetonide, aerosol *see* triamcinolone (systemic, oral inhalation) *on page 952*

triamcinolone acetonide, parenteral *see* triamcinolone (systemic, oral inhalation) *on page 952*

triamcinolone and nystatin *see* nystatin and triamcinolone *on page 693*

triamcinolone hexacetonide *see* triamcinolone (systemic, oral inhalation) *on page 952*

Triaminic® Children's Cough Long Acting [US-OTC] *see* dextromethorphan *on page 287*

Triaminic® Children's Night Time Cold & Cough [US-OTC] *see* diphenhydramine and phenylephrine *on page 312*

Triaminic® Children's Softchews® Cough & Runny Nose [US-OTC] *see* dextromethorphan and chlorpheniramine *on page 288*

Triaminic® Children's Thin Strips® Night Time Cold & Cough [US-OTC] *see* diphenhydramine and phenylephrine *on page 312*

Triaminic® Cold & Allergy [Can] *see* chlorpheniramine and pseudoephedrine *on page 209*

Triaminic® Cold and Allergy [US-OTC] *see* chlorpheniramine and phenylephrine *on page 208*

Triaminic® Cold and Cough *(Discontinued)* *see* chlorpheniramine, pseudoephedrine, and dextromethorphan *on page 214*

Triaminic® Cough and Sore Throat Formula *(Discontinued)*

Triaminic® Cough *(Discontinued)* *see* pseudoephedrine and dextromethorphan *on page 812*

Triaminic® Cough & Nasal Congestion *(Discontinued)* *see* pseudoephedrine and dextromethorphan *on page 812*

Triaminic® Day Time Cold & Cough [US-OTC] *see* dextromethorphan and phenylephrine *on page 289*

Triaminic® Expectorant *(Discontinued)*

Triaminic® Infant Thin Strips® Decongestant *(Discontinued)* *see* phenylephrine (systemic) *on page 751*

Triaminic® Night Time Cough and Cold *(Discontinued)* *see* chlorpheniramine, pseudoephedrine, and dextromethorphan *on page 214*

Triaminic Thin Strips® Children's Cough & Runny Nose [US-OTC] *see* diphenhydramine (systemic) *on page 310*

Triaminic® Thin Strips® Children's Long Acting Cough [US-OTC] *see* dextromethorphan *on page 287*

Triaminic Thin Strips® Children's Cold with Stuffy Nose [US-OTC] *see* phenylephrine (systemic) *on page 751*

Triaminic Thin Strips® Children's Day Time Cold & Cough [US-OTC] *see* dextromethorphan and phenylephrine *on page 289*

Triaminic Thin Strips® Cold *(Discontinued)* *see* phenylephrine (systemic) *on page 751*

Triamonide® Injection *(Discontinued)*

triamterene (trye AM ter een)

Sound-Alike/Look-Alike Issues
triamterene may be confused with trimipramine
Dyrenium® may be confused with Pyridium®

U.S./Canadian Brand Names Dyrenium® [US]

Therapeutic Category Diuretic, Potassium Sparing

Use Alone or in combination with other diuretics in treatment of edema and hypertension; decreases potassium excretion caused by kaliuretic diuretics

Dosage Summary
Oral:
Adults: 50-300 mg/day in 1-2 divided doses (maximum: 300 mg/day)

Dosage Forms
Capsule, oral:
Dyrenium®: 50 mg, 100 mg

triamterene and hydrochlorothiazide *see* hydrochlorothiazide and triamterene *on page 479*
Triant-HC™ [US] *see* phenylephrine, hydrocodone, and chlorpheniramine *on page 754*
Triapin® ***(Discontinued)***
Triatec-8 [Can] *see* acetaminophen and codeine *on page 23*
Triatec-8 Strong [Can] *see* acetaminophen and codeine *on page 23*
Triatec-30 [Can] *see* acetaminophen and codeine *on page 23*
Triavil® ***(Discontinued)*** *see* amitriptyline and perphenazine *on page 68*
Triaz® [US] *see* benzoyl peroxide *on page 128*

triazolam (trye AY zoe lam)

Sound-Alike/Look-Alike Issues
triazolam may be confused with alPRAZolam
Halcion® may be confused with halcinonide, Haldol®

U.S./Canadian Brand Names Apo-Triazo® [Can]; Gen-Triazolam [Can]; Halcion® [US/Can]; Mylan-Triazolam [Can]

Therapeutic Category Benzodiazepine

Controlled Substance C-IV

Use Short-term treatment of insomnia

Dosage Summary
Oral:
Children: Dosage not established
Adults: 0.125-0.25 mg at bedtime (maximum: 0.5 mg/day)
Elderly: Initial: 0.125 mg at bedtime (maximum: 0.25 mg/day)

Dosage Forms
Tablet, oral: 0.125 mg, 0.25 mg
Halcion®: 0.25 mg

tribavirin *see* ribavirin *on page 839*
Tribenzor™ [US] *see* olmesartan, amlodipine, and hydrochlorothiazide *on page 698*
Tri Biozene [US-OTC] *see* bacitracin, neomycin, polymyxin B, and pramoxine *on page 115*
Tri-Buffered Aspirin [US-OTC] *see* aspirin *on page 100*
tricalcium phosphate *see* calcium phosphate (tribasic) *on page 171*
Tricardio B [US] *see* folic acid, cyanocobalamin, and pyridoxine *on page 423*
Tri-Chlor® [US] *see* trichloroacetic acid *on page 956*
Trichlor Fresh Pac™ [US] *see* trichloroacetic acid *on page 956*
trichloroacetaldehyde monohydrate *see* chloral hydrate *on page 202*

trichloroacetic acid (trye klor oh a SEE tik AS id)

U.S./Canadian Brand Names Tri-Chlor® [US]; Trichlor Fresh Pac™ [US]

Therapeutic Category Keratolytic Agent

Use Chemical used in compounding agents for the treatment of warts, skin resurfacing (chemical peels)

Dosage Forms
Liquid, topical:
Tri-Chlor®: 80% (15 mL)
Powder for reconstitution, topical:
Trichlor Fresh Pac™: 10% (28 mL); 15% (28 mL); 20% (28 mL); 25% (28 mL); 30% (28 mL); 35% (28 mL); 40% (28 mL); 50% (28 mL)

trichloromonofluoromethane and dichlorodifluoromethane *see* dichlorodifluoromethane and trichloromonofluoromethane *on page 296*

Trichophyton skin test (trye koe FYE ton skin test)

Therapeutic Category Diagnostic Agent

Use Assess cell-mediated immunity

Dosage Summary
Intradermal:
Children: Dosage not established
Adults: 0.1 mL, examine reaction site in 24-48 hours

Dosage Forms

Injection, solution: 1:200 (2 mL)

Tricitrates [US] *see* citric acid, sodium citrate, and potassium citrate *on page* *228*

Tri-Clear® Expectorant *(Discontinued)*

TriCor® [US] *see* fenofibrate *on page* *393*

tricosal *see* choline magnesium trisalicylate *on page* *219*

Tri-Cyclen® [Can] *see* ethinyl estradiol and norgestimate *on page* *380*

Tri-Cyclen® Lo [Can] *see* ethinyl estradiol and norgestimate *on page* *380*

Triderm® [US] *see* triamcinolone (topical) *on page* *954*

Tridil® Injection *(Discontinued)* *see* nitroglycerin *on page* *679*

Tridione® *(Discontinued)*

Tridural™ [Can] *see* tramadol *on page* *946*

trien *see* trientine *on page* *957*

trientine (TRYE en teen)

Sound-Alike/Look-Alike Issues

trientine may be confused with Trental®, tretinoin

Synonyms 2,2,2-tetramine; trien; trientine hydrochloride; triethylene tetramine dihydrochloride

U.S./Canadian Brand Names Syprine® [US/Can]

Therapeutic Category Chelating Agent

Use Treatment of Wilson disease in patients intolerant to penicillamine

Dosage Summary

Oral:

Children <12 years: 20 mg/kg or 500-750 mg/day in 2-4 divided doses (maximum: 1.5 g/day)

Children ≥12 years: 750-1500 mg/day in 2-4 divided doses (maximum: 2 g/day)

Adults: 750-1500 mg/day in 2-4 divided doses (maximum: 2 g/day)

Dosage Forms

Capsule, oral:

Syprine®: 250 mg

trientine hydrochloride *see* trientine *on page* *957*

Triesence™ [US] *see* triamcinolone (ophthalmic) *on page* *954*

triethanolamine salicylate *see* trolamine *on page* *963*

triethylene tetramine dihydrochloride *see* trientine *on page* *957*

triethylenethiophosphoramide *see* thiotepa *on page* *928*

Trifed-C® *(Discontinued)* *see* triprolidine, pseudoephedrine, and codeine *(Canada only) on page* *961*

trifluoperazine (trye floo oh PER a zeen)

Sound-Alike/Look-Alike Issues

trifluoperazine may be confused with triflupromazine, trihexyphenidyl

Stelazine® may be confused with selegiline

Synonyms trifluoperazine hydrochloride

U.S./Canadian Brand Names Apo-Trifluoperazine® [Can]; Novo-Trifluzine [Can]; PMS-Trifluoperazine [Can]; Terfluzine [Can]

Therapeutic Category Phenothiazine Derivative

Use Treatment of schizophrenia; short-term treatment of generalized nonpsychotic anxiety

Dosage Summary

Oral:

Children <6 years: Dosage not established

Children 6-12 years: Initial: 1 mg 1-2 times/day; Maintenance: 1-15 mg/day in 1-2 divided doses (maximum: 15 mg/day)

Children >12 years: Inpatient: Initial: 2-5 mg twice daily; Maintenance: 15-40 mg/day in 2 divided doses (maximum: 40 mg/day); Outpatient: 1-3 mg twice daily (maximum: 6 mg/day)

Adults: Inpatient: Initial: 2-5 mg twice daily; Maintenance: 15-40 mg/day in 2 divided doses (maximum: 40 mg/day); Outpatient: Initial: 1-3 mg twice daily (maximum: 40 mg/day; exceptions occur [indication specific])

Dosage Forms
Tablet, oral: 1 mg, 2 mg, 5 mg, 10 mg

trifluoperazine hydrochloride *see* trifluoperazine *on page 957*
trifluorothymidine *see* trifluridine *on page 958*

trifluridine (trye FLURE i deen)

Sound-Alike/Look-Alike Issues
Viroptic® may be confused with Timoptic®
Synonyms F_3T; trifluorothymidine
U.S./Canadian Brand Names Sandoz-Trifluridine [Can]; Viroptic® [US/Can]
Therapeutic Category Antiviral Agent
Use Treatment of primary keratoconjunctivitis and recurrent epithelial keratitis caused by herpes simplex virus types I and II
Dosage Summary
Ophthalmic:
Children: Dosage not established
Adults: Initial: Instill 1 drop into affected eye(s) every 2 hours while awake (maximum: 9 drops/day); After re-epithelialization of corneal ulcer: 1 drop every 4 hours (maximum: 21 days of treatment)
Dosage Forms
Solution, ophthalmic: 1% (7.5 mL)
Viroptic®: 1% (7.5 mL)

Triglide® [US] *see* fenofibrate *on page 393*
triglycerides, medium chain *see* medium chain triglycerides *on page 596*
Trihexyphen [Can] *see* trihexyphenidyl *on page 958*

trihexyphenidyl (trye heks ee FEN i dil)

Sound-Alike/Look-Alike Issues
trihexyphenidyl may be confused with trifluoperazine
Synonyms benzhexol hydrochloride; trihexyphenidyl hydrochloride
U.S./Canadian Brand Names PMS-Trihexyphenidyl [Can]; Trihexyphen [Can]; Trihexyphenidyl [Can]
Therapeutic Category Anti-Parkinson Agent; Anticholinergic Agent
Use Adjunctive treatment of Parkinson disease; treatment of drug-induced extrapyramidal symptoms
Dosage Summary
Oral:
Children: Dosage not established
Adults: Initial: 1 mg/day; Maintenance: 3-15 mg/day in 3-4 divided doses; **Note:** Titration is recommended
Dosage Forms
Elixir, oral: 2 mg/5 mL (473 mL)
Tablet, oral: 2 mg, 5 mg

Trihexyphenidyl [Can] *see* trihexyphenidyl *on page 958*
trihexyphenidyl hydrochloride *see* trihexyphenidyl *on page 958*
TriHIBit® [US] *see* diphtheria, tetanus toxoids, and acellular pertussis vaccine and *Haemophilus influenzae* b conjugate vaccine *on page 317*
Tri-Hist *(Discontinued)* *see* chlorpheniramine, pyrilamine, and phenylephrine *on page 215*
Trikof-D® *(Discontinued)* *see* guaifenesin, pseudoephedrine, and dextromethorphan *on page 460*
Tri-Kort® Injection *(Discontinued)*
Trilafon® *(Discontinued)* *see* perphenazine *on page 745*
Tri-Legest™ Fe [US] *see* ethinyl estradiol and norethindrone *on page 378*
Trileptal® [US/Can] *see* oxcarbazepine *on page 712*
Tri-Levlen® *(Discontinued)* *see* ethinyl estradiol and levonorgestrel *on page 376*
TriLipix® [US] *see* fenofibric acid *on page 394*
Trilisate® *(Discontinued)* *see* choline magnesium trisalicylate *on page 219*
Trilog® Injection *(Discontinued)*
Trilone® Injection *(Discontinued)*
Tri-Luma™ [US] *see* fluocinolone, hydroquinone, and tretinoin *on page 411*

TriLyte® [US] *see* polyethylene glycol-electrolyte solution *on page 775*
Trimazide® ***(Discontinued)*** *see* trimethobenzamide *on page 959*

trimebutine *(Canada only)* (trye me BYOO teen)

Synonyms trimebutine maleate

U.S./Canadian Brand Names Apo-Trimebutine® [Can]; Modulon® [Can]

Therapeutic Category Antispasmodic Agent, Gastrointestinal

Use Treatment and relief of symptoms associated with irritable bowel syndrome (IBS) (spastic colon). In postoperative paralytic ileus in order to accelerate the resumption of the intestinal transit following abdominal surgery.

Dosage Summary

Oral:

Children <12 years: Dosage not established
Children ≥12 years: 200 mg 3 times/day before meals
Adults: 200 mg 3 times/day before meals

Dosage Forms - Canada Tablet: 100 mg, 200 mg

trimebutine maleate *see* trimebutine *(Canada only) on page 959*
trimethadione ***(Discontinued)***

trimethobenzamide (trye meth oh BEN za mide)

Sound-Alike/Look-Alike Issues

trimethobenzamide may be confused with metoclopramide, trimethoprim
Tigan® may be confused with Tiazac®, Ticar®, Ticlid®

Synonyms trimethobenzamide hydrochloride

U.S./Canadian Brand Names Tigan® [US/Can]

Therapeutic Category Anticholinergic Agent; Antiemetic

Use Treatment of postoperative nausea and vomiting; treatment of nausea associated with gastroenteritis

Dosage Summary

I.M.:

Children: Dosage not established
Adults: 200 mg 3-4 times/day **or** 200 mg as a single dose, repeat 1 hour later

Oral:

Children ≤40 kg: Unable to administer recommended dose with available product
Children >40 kg: 300 mg 3-4 times/day
Adults: 300 mg 3-4 times/day

Dosage Forms

Capsule, oral: 300 mg
Tigan®: 300 mg
Injection, solution: 100 mg/mL (2 mL)
Tigan®: 100 mg/mL (20 mL)
Injection, solution [preservative free]:
Tigan®: 100 mg/mL (2 mL)

trimethobenzamide hydrochloride *see* trimethobenzamide *on page 959*

trimethoprim (trye METH oh prim)

Sound-Alike/Look-Alike Issues

trimethoprim may be confused with trimethaphan

Synonyms TMP

U.S./Canadian Brand Names Apo-Trimethoprim® [Can]; Primsol® [US]

Therapeutic Category Antibiotic, Miscellaneous

Use Treatment of urinary tract infections due to susceptible strains of *E. coli*, *P. mirabilis*, *K. pneumoniae*, *Enterobacter* sp and coagulase-negative *Staphylococcus* including *S. saprophyticus*; acute otitis media in children; acute exacerbations of chronic bronchitis in adults; in combination with other agents for treatment of toxoplasmosis, *Pneumocystis jiroveci*; treatment of superficial ocular infections involving the conjunctiva and cornea

Dosage Summary

Oral:

Children ≤2 months: Dosage not established

Children >2 months: 4 mg/kg/day in divided doses every 12 hours
Adults: 100 mg every 12 hours **or** 200 mg every 24 hours; up to 15-20 mg/kg/day may be necessary [indication specific]

Dosage Forms

Solution, oral:
Primsol®: 50 mg (base)/5 mL (473 mL)
Tablet, oral: 100 mg

trimethoprim and polymyxin B (trye METH oh prim & pol i MIKS in bee)

Synonyms polymyxin B and trimethoprim

U.S./Canadian Brand Names PMS-Polytrimethoprim [Can]; Polytrim® [US/Can]

Therapeutic Category Antibiotic, Ophthalmic

Use Treatment of surface ocular bacterial conjunctivitis and blepharoconjunctivitis

Dosage Summary

Ophthalmic:
Children: Dosage not established
Adults: Instill 1-2 drops in eye(s) every 4-6 hours

Dosage Forms

Solution, ophthalmic: Trimethoprim 1 mg and polymyxin B 10,000 units per mL (10 mL)
Polytrim®: Trimethoprim 1 mg and polymyxin B 10,000 units per mL (10 mL)

trimethoprim and sulfamethoxazole *see* sulfamethoxazole and trimethoprim *on page 901*

trimetrexate *(Discontinued)*

trimipramine (trye MI pra meen)

Sound-Alike/Look-Alike Issues
trimipramine may be confused with triamterene, trimeprazine

Synonyms trimipramine maleate

U.S./Canadian Brand Names Apo-Trimip® [Can]; Nu-Trimipramine [Can]; Rhotrimine® [Can]; Surmontil® [US/Can]

Therapeutic Category Antidepressant, Tricyclic (Tertiary Amine)

Use Treatment of depression

Dosage Summary

Oral:
Children: Dosage not established
Adults: 50-200 mg at bedtime (maximum: 200 mg/day [outpatient] or 300 mg/day [inpatient])
Elderly: 25-100 mg at bedtime (maximum: 100 mg/day)

Dosage Forms

Capsule, oral:
Surmontil®: 25 mg, 50 mg, 100 mg

trimipramine maleate *see* trimipramine *on page 960*
Trimox® *(Discontinued)* *see* amoxicillin *on page 72*
Trimpex® *(Discontinued)* *see* trimethoprim *on page 959*
Trinasal® [Can] *see* triamcinolone (nasal) *on page 953*
Tri-Nasal® *(Discontinued)* *see* triamcinolone (nasal) *on page 953*
Trinate [US-OTC] *see* vitamins (multiple/prenatal) *on page 991*
TriNessa® [US] *see* ethinyl estradiol and norgestimate *on page 380*
Trinipatch® 0.2 [Can] *see* nitroglycerin *on page 679*
Trinipatch® 0.4 [Can] *see* nitroglycerin *on page 679*
Trinipatch® 0.6 [Can] *see* nitroglycerin *on page 679*
Tri-Norinyl® [US] *see* ethinyl estradiol and norethindrone *on page 378*
Trinsicon® *(Discontinued)* *see* vitamin B complex combinations *on page 988*
Triofed® Syrup *(Discontinued)* *see* triprolidine and pseudoephedrine *on page 961*
Trionate® *(Discontinued)* *see* carbetapentane and chlorpheniramine *on page 179*
Triostat® [US] *see* liothyronine *on page 568*
Tripedia® [US] *see* diphtheria, tetanus toxoids, and acellular pertussis vaccine *on page 316*
Triphasil® [US/Can] *see* ethinyl estradiol and levonorgestrel *on page 376*

Triphenyl® Expectorant ***(Discontinued)***

triple antibiotic *see* bacitracin, neomycin, and polymyxin B *on page 114*

triple sulfa *see* sulfabenzamide, sulfacetamide, and sulfathiazole *on page 899*

Triplex™ AD [US] *see* chlorpheniramine, pyrilamine, and phenylephrine *on page 215*

Tripohist™ D [US] *see* triprolidine and pseudoephedrine *on page 961*

Triposed® Syrup ***(Discontinued)*** *see* triprolidine and pseudoephedrine *on page 961*

Tri-Previfem® ***(Discontinued)*** *see* ethinyl estradiol and norgestimate *on page 380*

triprolidine and pseudoephedrine (trye PROE li deen & soo doe e FED rin)

Sound-Alike/Look-Alike Issues

Aprodine may be confused with Aphrodyne®

Synonyms pseudoephedrine and triprolidine

U.S./Canadian Brand Names Actifed® [Can]; Allerfrim [US-OTC]; Aprodine [US-OTC]; Genac™ [US-OTC]; Pediatex® TD [US]; Silafed [US-OTC]; Tripohist™ D [US]

Therapeutic Category Antihistamine/Decongestant Combination

Use Temporary relief of nasal congestion, decongest sinus openings, running nose, sneezing, itching of nose or throat and itchy, watery eyes due to common cold, hay fever, or other upper respiratory allergies

Dosage Summary

Oral:

Children <6 years: Dosage not established

Children 6-12 years:

Allerfrim, Aprodine: 5 mL every 4-6 hours (maximum 4 doses/24 hours)

Aprodine tablet: 1/2 tablet every 4-6 hours (maximum 4 doses/24 hours)

Pediatex® TD: 1.33 mL every 6 hours (maximum: 4 doses/24 hours)

Tripohist™ D: 2.5-5 mL every 4-6 hours (maximum pseudoephedrine: 120 mg/24 hours)

Children >12 years:

Allerfrim, Aprodine: 10 mL every 4-6 hours (maximum 4 doses/24 hours)

Aprodine tablet: One tablet every 4-6 hours (maximum 4 doses/24 hours)

Pediatex® TD: 2.67 mL every 6 hours (maximum: 4 doses/24 hours)

Tripohist™ D: 5-10 mL every 4-6 hours (maximum pseudoephedrine: 240 mg/24 hours)

Adults:

Allerfrim, Aprodine: 10 mL every 4-6 hours (maximum 4 doses/24 hours)

Aprodine tablet: One tablet every 4-6 hours (maximum 4 doses/24 hours)

Pediatex® TD: 2.67 mL every 6 hours (maximum: 4 doses/24 hours)

Tripohist™ D: 5-10 mL every 4-6 hours (maximum pseudoephedrine: 240 mg/24 hours)

Dosage Forms

Liquid, oral:

Pediatex® TD: Triprolidine 0.938 mg and pseudoephedrine 10 mg per 1 mL

Tripohist™ D: Triprolidine 1.25 mg and pseudoephedrine 45 mg per 5 mL

Syrup, oral:

Allerfrim [OTC], Aprodine [OTC], Silafed [OTC]: Triprolidine 1.25 mg and pseudoephedrine 30 mg per 5 mL

Tablet, oral:

Allerfrim [OTC], Aprodine [OTC], Genac™ [OTC]: Triprolidine 2.5 mg and pseudoephedrine 60 mg

triprolidine, codeine, and pseudoephedrine *see* triprolidine, pseudoephedrine, and codeine *(Canada only) on page 961*

triprolidine, pseudoephedrine, and codeine *(Canada only)*

(trye PROE li deen, soo doe e FED rin, & KOE deen)

Sound-Alike/Look-Alike Issues

Triacin-C® may be confused with triacetin

Synonyms codeine, pseudoephedrine, and triprolidine; codeine, triprolidine, and pseudoephedrine; pseudoephedrine, codeine, and triprolidine; pseudoephedrine, triprolidine, and codeine; triprolidine, codeine, and pseudoephedrine

U.S./Canadian Brand Names CoActifed® [Can]; CoVan® [Can]; ratio-Cotridin [Can]

Therapeutic Category Antihistamine/Decongestant/Antitussive

Controlled Substance C-V (CDSA-I)

Use Symptomatic relief of upper respiratory symptoms and cough

Dosage Summary

Oral:

Children <2 years: Dosage not established
Children 2-6 years: 2.5 mL 4 times/day
Children 7-12 years: 5 mL 4 times/day **or** 1/2 tablet 4 times/day
Children >12 years: 10 mL 4 times/day **or** 1 tablet 4 times/day
Adults: 10 mL 4 times/day **or** 1 tablet 4 times/day

Dosage Forms - Canada

Syrup:

CoActifed®, ratio-Cotridin: Triprolidine 2 mg, pseudoephedrine 30 mg, and codeine 10 mg per 5 mL
CoVan®: Triprolidine 2 mg, pseudoephedrine 30 mg, and codeine 10 mg per 5 mL (500 mL)

Tablet:

CoActifed®: Triprolidine 4 mg, pseudoephedrine 60 mg, and codeine 20 mg (50s)

Tri-Pseudo® *(Discontinued)* *see* triprolidine and pseudoephedrine *on page 961*
TripTone® [US-OTC] *see* dimenhydrinate *on page 307*

triptorelin (trip toe REL in)

Synonyms AY-25650; CL-118,532; D-Trp(6)-LHRH; detryptoreline; triptorelin pamoate; tryptoreline

U.S./Canadian Brand Names Trelstar® [US/Can]

Therapeutic Category Luteinizing Hormone-Releasing Hormone Analog

Use Palliative treatment of advanced prostate cancer

Dosage Summary

I.M.:

Children: Dosage not established
Adults: 3.75 mg once every 4 weeks **or** 11.25 mg once every 12 weeks **or** 22.5 mg once every 24 weeks

Dosage Forms

Injection, powder for reconstitution:

Trelstar®: 3.75 mg, 11.25 mg, 22.5 mg

triptorelin pamoate *see* triptorelin *on page 962*
Triquilar® [Can] *see* ethinyl estradiol and levonorgestrel *on page 376*
tris buffer *see* tromethamine *on page 963*
Trisenox® [US] *see* arsenic trioxide *on page 95*
tris(hydroxymethyl)aminomethane *see* tromethamine *on page 963*
trisodium calcium diethylenetriaminepentaacetate (Ca-DTPA) *see* diethylene triamine pentaacetic acid *on page 300*
Tri-Sprintec® [US] *see* ethinyl estradiol and norgestimate *on page 380*
Tri-Statin® II Topical *(Discontinued)* *see* nystatin and triamcinolone *on page 693*
Tristoject® Injection *(Discontinued)*
Trisudex® *(Discontinued)* *see* triprolidine and pseudoephedrine *on page 961*
Tri-Sudo® *(Discontinued)* *see* triprolidine and pseudoephedrine *on page 961*
Trital DM [US] *see* chlorpheniramine, phenylephrine, and dextromethorphan *on page 211*
Tri-Tannate Plus® *(Discontinued)* *see* chlorpheniramine, ephedrine, phenylephrine, and carbetapentane *on page 210*
TriTuss® [US] *see* guaifenesin, dextromethorphan, and phenylephrine *on page 458*
TriTuss® ER [US] *see* guaifenesin, dextromethorphan, and phenylephrine *on page 458*
Trivagizole-3® [Can] *see* clotrimazole (topical) *on page 240*
Trivagizole-3® *(Discontinued)* *see* clotrimazole (topical) *on page 240*
trivalent inactivated influenza vaccine (TIV) *see* influenza virus vaccine (inactivated) *on page 507*
Tri-Vent™ DM *(Discontinued)* *see* guaifenesin, pseudoephedrine, and dextromethorphan *on page 460*
Tri-Vent™ DPC *(Discontinued)* *see* chlorpheniramine, phenylephrine, and dextromethorphan *on page 211*
Tri-Vent™ HC *(Discontinued)*
Tri-Vi-Sol® [US-OTC] *see* vitamins (multiple/pediatric) *on page 990*
Tri-Vi-Sol® With Iron [US-OTC] *see* vitamins (multiple/pediatric) *on page 990*

Trivora® [US] *see* ethinyl estradiol and levonorgestrel *on page* 376
Trizivir® [US/Can] *see* abacavir, lamivudine, and zidovudine *on page* 18
Trobicin® ***(Discontinued)***
Trocaine® [US-OTC] *see* benzocaine *on page* 124
Trocal® [US-OTC] *see* dextromethorphan *on page* 287

trolamine (TROLE a meen)

Sound-Alike/Look-Alike Issues
Myoflex® may be confused with Mycelex®

Synonyms TEAS; triethanolamine salicylate; trolamine salicylate

U.S./Canadian Brand Names Antiphlogistine Rub A-535 No Odour [Can]; Aspercreme® [US-OTC]; Flex-Power [US-OTC]; Mobisyl® [US-OTC]; Myoflex® [US-OTC/Can]; Sportscreme® [US-OTC]

Therapeutic Category Analgesic, Topical

Use Relief of pain of muscular aches, rheumatism, neuralgia, sprains, arthritis on intact skin

Dosage Summary

Topical:
Children: Dosage not established
Adults: Apply to area as needed

Dosage Forms

Cream, topical:
Aspercreme® [OTC]: 10% (35 g, 85 g, 142 g)
Flex-Power [OTC]: 10% (57 g, 113 g)
Mobisyl® [OTC]: 10% (100 g, 227 g)
Myoflex® [OTC]: 10% (57 g, 113 g)
Sportscreme® [OTC]: 10% (35 g, 85 g)

Lotion, topical:
Aspercreme® [OTC]: 10% (180 mL)

trolamine salicylate *see* trolamine *on page* 963
Trombovar® [Can] *see* sodium tetradecyl *on page* 888

tromethamine (troe METH a meen)

Sound-Alike/Look-Alike Issues
tromethamine may be confused with TrophAmine®

Synonyms tris buffer; tris(hydroxymethyl)aminomethane

U.S./Canadian Brand Names THAM® [US]

Therapeutic Category Alkalinizing Agent

Use Correction of metabolic acidosis associated with cardiac bypass surgery or cardiac arrest; to correct excess acidity of stored blood that is preserved with acid citrate dextrose (ACD); indicated in infants needing alkalinization after receiving maximum sodium bicarbonate (8-10 mEq/kg/24 hours)

Dosage Summary

I.V.:
Neonates: Initial: Approximately 1 mL/kg for each pH unit below 7.4; additional doses determined by changes in PaO_2, pH, and pCO_2
Infants: Initial: Approximately 1 mL/kg for each pH unit below 7.4; additional doses determined by changes in PaO_2, pH, and pCO_2
Adults: 3.6-10.8 g (111-333 mL) **or** 9 mL/kg (maximum: 500 mg/kg) **or** 15-77 mL added to each 500 mL of blood

Intravenrticular:
Adults: 3.6-10.8 g (111-333 mL) **or** 9 mL/kg (maximum: 500 mg/kg) **or** 15-77 mL added to each 500 mL of blood

Dosage Forms

Injection, solution:
THAM®: 18 g (500 mL)

Tronolane® Cream [US-OTC] *see* pramoxine *on page* 787
Tronolane® Suppository [US-OTC] *see* phenylephrine (topical) *on page* 752
TrophAmine® [US] *see* amino acid injection *on page* 64
Tropicacyl® [US] *see* tropicamide *on page* 964

tropicamide (troe PIK a mide)

Synonyms bistropamide

U.S./Canadian Brand Names Diotrope® [Can]; Mydral™ [US]; Mydriacyl® [US/Can]; Tropicacyl® [US]

Therapeutic Category Anticholinergic Agent

Use Short-acting mydriatic used in diagnostic procedures; as well as preoperatively and postoperatively; treatment of some cases of acute iritis, iridocyclitis, and keratitis

Dosage Summary

Ophthalmic:

Children: 0.5%: Instill 1-2 drops 15-20 minutes before exam, may repeat; 1%: Instill 1-2 drops, may repeat in 5 minutes

Adults: 0.5%: Instill 1-2 drops 15-20 minutes before exam, may repeat; 1%: Instill 1-2 drops, may repeat in 5 minutes

Dosage Forms

Solution, ophthalmic: 0.5% (15 mL); 1% (2 mL, 3 mL, 15 mL)

Mydral™: 0.5% (15 mL); 1% (15 mL)

Mydriacyl®: 1% (3 mL, 15 mL)

Tropicacyl®: 0.5% (15 mL); 1% (15 mL)

tropicamide and hydroxyamphetamine *see* hydroxyamphetamine and tropicamide *on page 488*

Trosec [Can] *see* trospium *on page 964*

trospium (TROSE pee um)

Synonyms trospium chloride

U.S./Canadian Brand Names Sanctura® XR [US/Can]; Sanctura® [US]; Trosec [Can]

Therapeutic Category Anticholinergic Agent

Use Treatment of overactive bladder with symptoms of urgency, incontinence, and urinary frequency

Dosage Summary

Oral:

Children: Dosage not established

Adults: Immediate release formulation: 20 mg twice daily; Extended release formulation: 60 mg once daily

Elderly ≥75 years: Immediate release formulation: Initial: 20 mg at bedtime; Maintenance: 20 mg once or twice daily

Dosage Forms

Capsule, extended release, oral:

Sanctura® XR: 60 mg

Tablet, oral: 20 mg

Sanctura®: 20 mg

trospium chloride *see* trospium *on page 964*

Trovan® ***(Discontinued)***

Truphylline® ***(Discontinued)*** *see* aminophylline *on page 66*

Trusopt® [US/Can] *see* dorzolamide *on page 327*

Truvada® [US/Can] *see* emtricitabine and tenofovir *on page 347*

trypsin, balsam Peru, and castor oil (TRIP sin, BAL sam pe RUE, & KAS tor oyl)

Sound-Alike/Look-Alike Issues

Granulex® may be confused with Regranex®

Synonyms balsam Peru, castor oil, and trypsin; castor oil, trypsin, and balsam Peru

U.S./Canadian Brand Names Granulex® [US]; Optase™ [US]; Xenaderm™ [US]

Therapeutic Category Protectant, Topical

Use Treatment of decubitus ulcers, varicose ulcers, debridement of eschar, dehiscent wounds and sunburn; promote wound healing; reduce odor from necrotic wounds

Dosage Summary

Topical:

Children: Dosage not established

Adults: Apply a minimum of twice daily or as often as necessary

Dosage Forms

Aerosol, topical: Trypsin 0.12 mg, balsam Peru 87 mg, and castor oil 788 mg per gram (120 g)

Granulex®: Trypsin 0.12 mg, balsam Peru 87 mg, and castor oil 788 mg per gram (60 g, 120 g)

Gel, topical:

Optase™: Trypsin 0.12 mg, balsam Peru 87 mg, and castor oil 788 mg per gram (95 g)

Ointment, topical:

Xenaderm™: Trypsin 90 USP units, balsam Peru 87 mg, and castor oil 788 mg per gram (30 g, 60 g)

tryptoreline *see* triptorelin *on page 962*

Trysul® *(Discontinued)* *see* sulfabenzamide, sulfacetamide, and sulfathiazole *on page 899*

TSH *see* thyrotropin alpha *on page 930*

TSPA *see* thiotepa *on page 928*

TST *see* tuberculin tests *on page 965*

T-Stat® *(Discontinued)* *see* erythromycin (topical) *on page 362*

TT *see* tetanus toxoid (adsorbed) *on page 921*

tuberculin purified protein derivative *see* tuberculin tests *on page 965*

tuberculin skin test *see* tuberculin tests *on page 965*

tuberculin tests (too BER kyoo lin tests)

Sound-Alike/Look-Alike Issues

Aplisol® may be confused with Anusol®, A.P.L.®, Aplitest®, Atropisol®

Tuberculin products may be confused with tetanus toxoid products and influenza virus vaccine. Medication errors have occurred when tuberculin skin tests (PPD) have been inadvertently administered instead of tetanus toxoid products and influenza virus vaccine. These products are refrigerated and often stored in close proximity to each other.

Synonyms mantoux; PPD; TB skin test; TST; tuberculin purified protein derivative; tuberculin skin test

U.S./Canadian Brand Names Aplisol® [US]; Tubersol® [US]

Therapeutic Category Diagnostic Agent

Use Skin test in diagnosis of tuberculosis

Dosage Summary

Intradermal:

Children: 0.1 mL

Adults: 0.1 mL

Dosage Forms

Injection, solution:

Aplisol®: 5 TU/0.1 mL (1 mL, 5 mL)

Tubersol®: 5 TU/0.1 mL (1 mL, 5 mL)

Tubersol® [US] *see* tuberculin tests *on page 965*

Tucks® Anti-Itch [US-OTC] *see* hydrocortisone (topical) *on page 483*

Tucks® Hemorrhoidal [US-OTC] *see* pramoxine *on page 787*

Tucks® Take Alongs® [US-OTC] *see* witch hazel *on page 994*

Tuinal® *(Discontinued)*

Tums® [US-OTC] *see* calcium carbonate *on page 167*

Tums® Dual Action [US-OTC] *see* famotidine, calcium carbonate, and magnesium hydroxide *on page 391*

Tums® E-X [US-OTC] *see* calcium carbonate *on page 167*

Tums® Extra Strength Sugar Free [US-OTC] *see* calcium carbonate *on page 167*

Tums® Quickpak [US-OTC] *see* calcium carbonate *on page 167*

Tums® Smoothies™ [US-OTC] *see* calcium carbonate *on page 167*

Tums® Ultra [US-OTC] *see* calcium carbonate *on page 167*

Tusal® *(Discontinued)*

Tusibron® *(Discontinued)* *see* guaifenesin *on page 454*

Tusibron-DM® *(Discontinued)* *see* guaifenesin and dextromethorphan *on page 455*

Tusnel® [US] *see* guaifenesin, pseudoephedrine, and dextromethorphan *on page 460*

Tusnel-DM Pediatric® [US] *see* guaifenesin, pseudoephedrine, and dextromethorphan *on page 460*

Tusnel Pediatric® [US] *see* guaifenesin, pseudoephedrine, and dextromethorphan *on page 460*

Tussafed® *(Discontinued)*

Tylenol® Cold Head Congestion Daytime [US-OTC] *see* acetaminophen, dextromethorphan, and phenylephrine *on page* 29
Tylenol® Cold, Infants *(Discontinued)* *see* acetaminophen and pseudoephedrine *on page* 26
Tylenol® Cold Multi-Symptom Daytime [US-OTC] *see* acetaminophen, dextromethorphan, and phenylephrine *on page* 29
Tylenol® Cough & Sore Throat Nighttime [US-OTC] *see* acetaminophen, dextromethorphan, and doxylamine *on page* 29
Tylenol® Decongestant [Can] *see* acetaminophen and pseudoephedrine *on page* 26
Tylenol® Elixir with Codeine [Can] *see* acetaminophen and codeine *on page* 23
Tylenol® Extra Strength [US-OTC] *see* acetaminophen *on page* 21
Tylenol® Flu Non-Drowsy Maximum Strength *(Discontinued)*
Tylenol® Infant's Concentrated [US-OTC] *see* acetaminophen *on page* 21
Tylenol® Jr. Meltaways [US-OTC] *see* acetaminophen *on page* 21
Tylenol® No. 1 [Can] *see* acetaminophen and codeine *on page* 23
Tylenol® No. 1 Forte [Can] *see* acetaminophen and codeine *on page* 23
Tylenol® No. 2 with Codeine [Can] *see* acetaminophen and codeine *on page* 23
Tylenol® No. 3 with Codeine [Can] *see* acetaminophen and codeine *on page* 23
Tylenol® No. 4 with Codeine [Can] *see* acetaminophen and codeine *on page* 23
Tylenol® Plus Infants Cold & Cough *(Discontinued)* *see* acetaminophen, dextromethorphan, and phenylephrine *on page* 29
Tylenol® PM [US-OTC] *see* acetaminophen and diphenhydramine *on page* 24
Tylenol® Severe Allergy [US-OTC] *see* acetaminophen and diphenhydramine *on page* 24
Tylenol® Sinus [Can] *see* acetaminophen and pseudoephedrine *on page* 26
Tylenol® Sinus Congestion & Pain Daytime [US-OTC] *see* acetaminophen and phenylephrine *on page* 25
Tylenol® with Codeine (Elixir) *(Discontinued)* *see* acetaminophen and codeine *on page* 23
Tylenol® with Codeine No. 3 [US] *see* acetaminophen and codeine *on page* 23
Tylenol® with Codeine No. 4 [US] *see* acetaminophen and codeine *on page* 23
Tylenol® Women's Menstrual Relief [US-OTC] *see* acetaminophen and pamabrom *on page* 25
Tylox® [US] *see* oxycodone and acetaminophen *on page* 715
Typherix® [Can] *see* typhoid vaccine *on page* 967
Typhim Vi® [US/Can] *see* typhoid vaccine *on page* 967

typhoid vaccine (TYE foid vak SEEN)

Synonyms Ty21a vaccine; typhoid vaccine live oral Ty21a; Vi vaccine

U.S./Canadian Brand Names Typherix® [Can]; Typhim Vi® [US/Can]; Vivotif® [US/Can]

Therapeutic Category Vaccine, Inactivated Bacteria

Use Active immunization against typhoid fever caused by *Salmonella typhi*

Not for routine vaccination. In the United States and Canada, use should be limited to:

- Travelers to areas with a prolonged risk of exposure to *S. typhi*
- Persons with intimate exposure to a *S. typhi* carrier
- Laboratory technicians with exposure to *S. typhi*
- Travelers with achlorhydria or hypochlorhydria (Canadian recommendation)

Dosage Summary

I.M.:

Children <2 years: Dosage not established

Children ≥2 years: 0.5 mL given at least 2 weeks prior to expected exposure; may repeat every 2 years

Adults: 0.5 mL given at least 2 weeks prior to expected exposure; may repeat every 2 years

Oral:

Children <6 years: Dosage not established

Children ≥6 years: One capsule on alternate days for a total of 4 doses; may repeat full course every 5 years

Adults: One capsule on alternate days for a total of 4 doses; may repeat full course every 5 years

Dosage Forms

Capsule, enteric coated:

Vivotif®: Viable *S. typhi* Ty21a 2-6.8 x 10^9 colony-forming units and nonviable *S. typhi* Ty21a 5-50 x 10^9 bacterial cells [contains lactose 100-180 mg/capsule and sucrose 26-130 mg/capsule]

Injection, solution:

Typhim Vi®: Purified Vi capsular polysaccharide 25 mcg/0.5 mL (0.5 mL, 10 mL) [derived from *S. typhi* Ty2 strain]

Dosage Forms - Canada

Injection, solution:

Typherix®: Vi capsular polysaccharide 25 mcg/0.5 mL (0.5 mL) [derived from *S. typhi* Ty2 strain]

typhoid vaccine live oral Ty21a *see* typhoid vaccine *on page 967*

Tyrodone® Liquid *(Discontinued)*

Tysabri® [US/Can] *see* natalizumab *on page 662*

Tyvaso™ [US] *see* treprostinil *on page 951*

Tyzeka® [US] *see* telbivudine *on page 912*

Tyzine® [US] *see* tetrahydrozoline (nasal) *on page 923*

Tyzine® Pediatric [US] *see* tetrahydrozoline (nasal) *on page 923*

506U78 *see* nelarabine *on page 664*

U-90152S *see* delavirdine *on page 274*

UAD Otic® *(Discontinued)* *see* neomycin, polymyxin B, and hydrocortisone *on page 667*

UCB-P071 *see* cetirizine *on page 198*

U-Cort™ [US] *see* hydrocortisone (topical) *on page 483*

UK-88,525 *see* darifenacin *on page 270*

UK-427,857 *see* maraviroc *on page 591*

UK92480 *see* sildenafil *on page 874*

UK109496 *see* voriconazole *on page 992*

U-Kera E™ [US] *see* urea *on page 970*

Ulcerease® [US-OTC] *see* phenol *on page 748*

Ulcidine [Can] *see* famotidine *on page 390*

Ulesfia™ [US] *see* benzyl alcohol *on page 131*

ulipristal (ue li PRIS tal)

Sound-Alike/Look-Alike Issues

Sound-alike/look-alike issues:

Ulipristal may be confused with ursodiol

Synonyms ulipristal acetate

U.S./Canadian Brand Names ella® [US]

Therapeutic Category Contraceptive; Progestin

Use Emergency contraception following unprotected intercourse or possible contraceptive failure

Product Availability Ulipristal (ella®): FDA approved in August 2010; expected to be available fourth quarter 2010. Consult prescribing information for additional information

ulipristal acetate *see* ulipristal *on page 968*

Uloric® [US] *see* febuxostat *on page 392*

ULR-LA® *(Discontinued)*

Ultane® [US] *see* sevoflurane *on page 873*

Ultiva® [US/Can] *see* remifentanil *on page 834*

Ultracaine® DS [Can] *see* articaine and epinephrine *on page 96*

Ultracaine® DS Forte [Can] *see* articaine and epinephrine *on page 96*

Ultracaps MT *(Discontinued)* *see* pancrelipase *on page 723*

Ultracet® [US] *see* acetaminophen and tramadol *on page 27*

Ultra Freeda A-Free [US-OTC] *see* vitamins (multiple/oral) *on page 990*

Ultra Freeda Iron-Free [US-OTC] *see* vitamins (multiple/oral) *on page 990*

Ultra Freeda With Iron [US-OTC] *see* vitamins (multiple/oral) *on page 990*

Ultram® [US] *see* tramadol *on page 946*

Ultram® ER [US] *see* tramadol *on page 946*

Ultra Mide 25® [US-OTC/Can] *see* urea *on page 970*

Ultramop™ [Can] *see* methoxsalen (systemic) *on page 616*

Ultra NatalCare® [US] *see* vitamins (multiple/prenatal) *on page 991*

Ultraprin [US-OTC] *see* ibuprofen *on page 494*
Ultraquin™ [Can] *see* hydroquinone *on page 487*
Ultrase® [Can] *see* pancrelipase *on page 723*
Ultrase® *(Discontinued)* *see* pancrelipase *on page 723*
Ultrase® MT [Can] *see* pancrelipase *on page 723*
Ultrase® MT *(Discontinued)* *see* pancrelipase *on page 723*
Ultra Tears® [US-OTC] *see* artificial tears *on page 97*
Ultravate® [US/Can] *see* halobetasol *on page 464*
Ultravist® [US] *see* iopromide *on page 520*
Umecta® [US] *see* urea *on page 970*
Umecta® Nail Film [US] *see* urea *on page 970*
Umecta PD™ [US] *see* urea *on page 970*
Unasyn® [US/Can] *see* ampicillin and sulbactam *on page 76*
Unburn® [US-OTC] *see* lidocaine (topical) *on page 562*

undecylenic acid and derivatives (un de sil EN ik AS id & dah RIV ah tivs)

Synonyms zinc undecylenate
U.S./Canadian Brand Names Fungi-Nail® [US-OTC]
Therapeutic Category Antifungal Agent
Use Treatment of athlete's foot (tinea pedis); ringworm (except nails and scalp)
Dosage Summary
Topical:
Children <2 years: Dosage not established
Children ≥2 years: Apply twice daily to affected area
Adults: Apply twice daily to affected area
Dosage Forms
Solution, topical:
Fungi-Nail® [OTC]: Undecylenic acid 25% (29.57 mL)

Unguentine® *(Discontinued)* *see* benzocaine *on page 124*
Uni-Bent® Cough Syrup *(Discontinued)* *see* diphenhydramine (systemic) *on page 310*
Uni-Cenna *(Discontinued)* *see* senna *on page 870*
Uni-Cof *(Discontinued)* *see* pseudoephedrine, dihydrocodeine, and chlorpheniramine *on page 813*
Unidet® [Can] *see* tolterodine *on page 941*
Uni-Dur® *(Discontinued)* *see* theophylline *on page 925*
Unipen® [Can] *see* nafcillin *on page 655*
Uniphyl® *(Discontinued)* *see* theophylline *on page 925*
Uniphyl® SRT [Can] *see* theophylline *on page 925*
Uni-Pro® *(Discontinued)* *see* ibuprofen *on page 494*
Uniretic® [US/Can] *see* moexipril and hydrochlorothiazide *on page 640*
Unisom®-2 [Can] *see* doxylamine *on page 332*
Unisom® SleepGels® Maximum Strength [US-OTC] *see* diphenhydramine (systemic) *on page 310*
Unisom® SleepMelts™ [US-OTC] *see* diphenhydramine (systemic) *on page 310*
Unithroid® [US] *see* levothyroxine *on page 560*
Unitrol® *(Discontinued)*
Uni-tussin® *(Discontinued)* *see* guaifenesin *on page 454*
Uni-tussin® DM *(Discontinued)* *see* guaifenesin and dextromethorphan *on page 455*
Univasc® [US] *see* moexipril *on page 640*
Unna boot *see* zinc gelatin *on page 1001*
Unna paste *see* zinc gelatin *on page 1001*
Urabeth® *(Discontinued)* *see* bethanechol *on page 135*
Uramaxin™ [US] *see* urea *on page 970*
Urasal® [Can] *see* methenamine *on page 612*
urate oxidase *see* rasburicase *on page 830*

urea (yoor EE a)

Synonyms carbamide

U.S./Canadian Brand Names Aqua Care® [US-OTC]; Aquaphilic® with Carbamide [US-OTC]; BP 50% [US]; Carmol® 10 [US-OTC]; Carmol® 20 [US-OTC]; Carmol® 40 [US]; Carmol® Deep Cleansing [US-OTC]; DPM™ [US-OTC]; Gordon's® Urea [US-OTC]; Gormel® Ten [US-OTC]; Gormel® [US-OTC]; Hydro 40™ [US]; Kerafoam® [US]; Keralac™ Nailstik [US]; Keralac™ [US]; Keratol 40™ [US]; Kerol™ Redi-Cloths [US]; Kerol™ ZX [US]; Kerol™ [US]; Lanaphilic® with Urea [US-OTC]; Nutraplus® [US-OTC]; Rea-Lo® [US-OTC]; U-Kera E™ [US]; Ultra Mide 25® [US-OTC/Can]; Umecta PD™ [US]; Umecta® Nail Film [US]; Umecta® [US]; Uramaxin™ [US]; Ureacin-10® [US-OTC]; Ureacin-20® [US-OTC]; Uremol® [Can]; Urisec® [Can]; X-Viate™ [US]

Therapeutic Category Diuretic, Osmotic; Topical Skin Product

Use Keratolytic agent to soften nails or skin; OTC: Moisturizer for dry, rough skin

Dosage Summary

Topical:

Children: Dosage not established
Adults: Apply 1-3 times/day

Dosage Forms

Aerosol, topical:
Hydro 40™: 40% (150 g)
Kerafoam®: 30% (60 g)
Umecta®: 40% (113.4 g)

Cloth, topical:
Kerol™ Redi-Cloths: 42% (30s)

Cream, topical: 40% (30 g, 85 g, 210 g); 40% (28 g, 85 g, 199 g)
Aqua Care® [OTC]: 10% (75 g)
Carmol® 20 [OTC]: 20% (90 g)
Carmol® 40: 40% (28 g, 85 g, 199 g)
DPM™ [OTC]: 20% (118 g)
Gordon's® Urea [OTC]: 40% (30 g)
Gormel® [OTC]: 20% (75 g, 120 g, 454 g, 2270 g)
Keralac™: 50% (142 g, 255 g)
Keratol 40™: 40% (30 g, 90 g, 210 g)
Nutraplus® [OTC]: 10% (90 g, 454 g)
Rea-Lo® [OTC]: 30% (60 g, 240 g)
U-Kera E™: 40% (28 g)
Uramaxin™: 45% (255 g)
Ureacin-20® [OTC]: 20% (114 g)
X-Viate™: 40% (85 g, 199 g)

Emulsion, topical: 50% (300 g)
BP 50%: 50% (300 g)
Kerol™: 50% (284 g)
Umecta PD™: 40% (198.5 g)
Umecta®: 40% (114 g, 227 g)

Gel, topical: 40% (15 mL); 50% (18 mL)
Carmol® 40: 40% (15 mL)
Keralac™: 50% (18 mL)
Keratol 40™: 40% (15 mL)
Uramaxin™: 45% (28 mL)
X-Viate™: 40% (15 mL)

Lotion, topical: 35% (207 mL, 325 mL); 40% (237 mL, 240 mL)
Aqua Care® [OTC]: 10% (240 mL)
Carmol® 10 [OTC]: 10% (180 mL)
Carmol® 40: 40% (237 mL)
Gormel® Ten [OTC]: 20% (240 mL)
Keralac™: 35% (207 mL, 325 mL)
Keratol 40™: 40% (240 mL)
Nutraplus® [OTC]: 10% (240 mL, 480 mL)
Ultra Mide 25® [OTC]: 25% (120 mL, 240 mL)
Ureacin-10® [OTC]: 10% (237 mL)
X-Viate™: 40% (237 mL)

Ointment, topical: 50% (45 g)
Aquaphilic® with Carbamide [OTC]: 10% (180 g, 454 g); 20% (454 g)
Keralac™: 50% (45 g)
Lanaphilic® with Urea [OTC]: 10% (454 g); 20% (454 g)
Shampoo, topical:
Carmol® Deep Cleansing [OTC]: 10% (240 mL)
Solution, topical: 50% (2.4 mL, 12 mL)
Keralac™ Nailstik: 50% (2.4 mL)
Kerol™ ZX: 50% (12 mL)
Suspension, topical: 40% (18 mL); 50% (284 g)
Kerol™: 50% (284 g)
Umecta PD™: 40% (255.1 g)
Umecta®: 40% (283 g)
Umecta® Nail Film: 40% (18 mL)

urea and hydrocortisone (yoor EE a & hye droe KOR ti sone)

Synonyms hydrocortisone and urea

U.S./Canadian Brand Names Carmol-HC® [US]; Ti-U-Lac® H [Can]; Uremol® HC [Can]

Therapeutic Category Corticosteroid, Topical

Use Inflammation of corticosteroid-responsive dermatoses

Dosage Summary

Topical:
Children: Apply thin film and rub in well 1-4 times/day
Adults: Apply thin film and rub in well 1-4 times/day

Dosage Forms

Cream:
Carmol-HC®: Urea 10% and hydrocortisone 1% (30 g)

Ureacin-10® [US-OTC] *see* urea *on page* *970*
Ureacin-20® [US-OTC] *see* urea *on page* *970*
urea peroxide *see* carbamide peroxide *on page* *178*
Urecholine® [US] *see* bethanechol *on page* *135*
Uremol® [Can] *see* urea *on page* *970*
Uremol® HC [Can] *see* urea and hydrocortisone *on page* *971*
Urex™ [Can] *see* methenamine *on page* *612*
Urex® *(Discontinued)* *see* methenamine *on page* *612*
Urisec® [Can] *see* urea *on page* *970*
Urispas® [US/Can] *see* flavoxate *on page* *405*
Uristat® *(Discontinued)* *see* phenazopyridine *on page* *746*
Urocit®-K [US] *see* potassium citrate *on page* *782*
Urodine® *(Discontinued)* *see* phenazopyridine *on page* *746*

urofollitropin (yoor oh fol li TROE pin)

Synonyms follicle-stimulating hormone, human; FSH; hFSH

U.S./Canadian Brand Names Bravelle® [US/Can]; Fertinorm® H.P. [Can]

Therapeutic Category Gonadotropin; Ovulation Stimulator

Use Ovulation induction in patients who previously received pituitary suppression; development of multiple follicles with Assisted Reproductive Technologies (ART)

Dosage Summary

I.M.:
Children: Dosage not established
Adults (females): Initial: 150 int. units once daily for 5 days; Maintenance: Dose adjustments ≤75-150 int. units can be made every ≥2 days up to 450 int. units/day (maximum: 12 days therapy) [ovulation induction]
Adults (males): Dosage not established

SubQ:
Children: Dosage not established
Adults (females):
ART: Initial: 225 int. units once daily for 5 days; Maintenance: Dose adjustments of 75-150 int. units can be made every ≥2 days up to 450 int. units/day (maximum: 12 days therapy)
Ovulation induction: Initial: 150 int. units once daily for 5 days; Maintenance: Dose adjustments of ≤75-150 int. units can be made every ≥2 days up to 450 int. units/day (maximum: 12 days therapy)
Adults (males): Dosage not established

Dosage Forms
Injection, powder for reconstitution:
Bravelle®: 75 int. units

urokinase *(Discontinued)*

Uro-KP-Neutral® [US] *see* potassium phosphate and sodium phosphate *on page 783*

Urolene Blue® *(Discontinued)* *see* methylene blue *on page 619*

Uro-Mag® [US-OTC] *see* magnesium oxide *on page 587*

Uromax® [Can] *see* oxybutynin *on page 713*

Uromitexan [Can] *see* mesna *on page 608*

Uroplus® DS *(Discontinued)*

Uroplus® SS *(Discontinued)*

Uroxatral® [US] *see* alfuzosin *on page 49*

Urso® [Can] *see* ursodiol *on page 972*

Urso 250® [US] *see* ursodiol *on page 972*

ursodeoxycholic acid *see* ursodiol *on page 972*

ursodiol (ur soe DYE ol)

Sound-Alike/Look-Alike Issues
Sound-alike/look-alike issues:
Ursodiol may be confused with ulipristal

Synonyms ursodeoxycholic acid

U.S./Canadian Brand Names Actigall® [US]; Dom-Ursodiol C [Can]; PHL-Ursodiol C [Can]; PMS-Ursodiol C [Can]; Urso 250® [US]; Urso Forte® [US]; Urso® DS [Can]; Urso® [Can]

Therapeutic Category Gallstone Dissolution Agent

Use
Actigall®: Gallbladder stone dissolution; prevention of gallstones in obese patients experiencing rapid weight loss
Urso®, Urso Forte®: Primary biliary cirrhosis

Dosage Summary
Oral:
Children: Dosage not established
Adults: 8-15 mg/kg/day in 2-4 divided doses **or** 300 mg twice daily

Dosage Forms
Capsule, oral: 300 mg
Actigall®: 300 mg
Tablet, oral: 250 mg, 500 mg
Urso 250®: 250 mg
Urso Forte®: 500 mg

Urso® DS [Can] *see* ursodiol *on page 972*

Urso Forte® [US] *see* ursodiol *on page 972*

ustekinumab (yoo stek in YOO mab)

Sound-Alike/Look-Alike Issues
ustekinumab may be confused with infliximab, rituximab
Stelara™ may be confused with Aldara®

Synonyms CNTO 1275

U.S./Canadian Brand Names Stelara™ [US/Can]

Therapeutic Category Antipsoriatic Agent; Interleukin-12 Inhibitor; Interleukin-23 Inhibitor; Monoclonal Antibody

Use Treatment of moderate-to-severe plaque psoriasis

Dosage Summary

Oral:

Children <18 yrs: Dosage not established

Adults:

≤100 kg: 45 mg at 0- and 4 weeks, and then every 12 weeks thereafter

>100 kg: 45 mg or 90 mg at 0- and 4 weeks, and then every 12 weeks thereafter

Dosage Forms

Injection, solution [preservative free]:

Stelara™: 45 mg/0.5 mL (0.5 mL); 90 mg/mL (1 mL)

UTI Relief® [US-OTC] *see* phenazopyridine *on page 746*

Utradol™ [Can] *see* etodolac *on page 383*

Uvadex® [US] *see* methoxsalen (systemic) *on page 616*

vaccinia immune globulin (intravenous)

(vax IN ee a i MYUN GLOB yoo lin IN tra VEE nus)

Synonyms VIGIV

U.S./Canadian Brand Names CNJ-016® [US]

Therapeutic Category Immune Globulin

Use Treatment of infectious complications of smallpox (vaccinia virus) vaccination, such as eczema vaccinatum, progressive vaccinia, and severe generalized vaccinia; treatment of vaccinia infections in individuals with concurrent skin conditions or accidental virus exposure to eyes (except vaccinia keratitis), mouth, or other areas where viral infection would pose significant risk

CDC guidelines for use:

Use is recommended for:

- Inadvertent inoculation (considering severity, toxicity of affected person, and pain)
- Eczema vaccinatum
- Generalized vaccinia (severe form or if underlying illness is present)
- Progressive vaccinia

Use may be considered for:

- Severe ocular complications except isolated keratitis

Use is not recommended for:

- Inadvertent inoculation that is not severe
- Mild or limited generalized vaccinia
- Nonspecific rashes, erythema multiforme, or Stevens-Johnson syndrome
- Postvaccinial encephalitis or encephalomyelitis

Dosage Summary

I.V.:

Children: Dosage not established

Adults: 6000 units/kg; 9000 units/kg may be considered if no response to initial dose

Elderly: Dosage not established

Dosage Forms

Injection, solution [preservative free; solvent-detergent treated]:

CNJ-016®: ≥50,000 units/15 mL (15 mL)

vaccinia vaccine *see* smallpox vaccine *on page 880*

Vagifem® [US/Can] *see* estradiol (topical) *on page 367*

Vagi-Gard® [US-OTC] *see* povidone-iodine (topical) *on page 784*

Vagistat®-1 [US-OTC] *see* tioconazole *on page 935*

Vagitrol® ***(Discontinued)***

valacyclovir (val ay SYE kloe veer)

Sound-Alike/Look-Alike Issues

valACYclovir may be confused with acyclovir, valGANCIclovir, vancomycin

Valtrex® may be confused with Keflex®, Valcyte®, Zovirax®

Synonyms valacyclovir hydrochloride

Tall-Man val**ACY**clovir

U.S./Canadian Brand Names Apo-Valacyclovir® [Can]; Mylan-Valacyclovir [Can]; PHL-Valacyclovir [Can]; PMS-Valacyclovir [Can]; PRO-Valacyclovir [Can]; Riva-Valacyclovir [Can]; Valtrex® [US/Can]

Therapeutic Category Antiviral Agent

Use Treatment of herpes zoster (shingles) in immunocompetent patients; treatment of first-episode and recurrent genital herpes; suppression of recurrent genital herpes and reduction of heterosexual transmission of genital herpes in immunocompetent patients; suppression of genital herpes in HIV-infected individuals; treatment of herpes labialis (cold sores); chickenpox in immunocompetent children

Dosage Summary

Oral:

Children <2 years: Dosage not established

Children 2 to <12 years: 20 mg/kg/dose 3 times/day (maximum: 1 g 3 times/day)

Children ≥12 to <18 years: 2 g every 12 hours for 1 day **or** 20 mg/kg/dose 3 times/day (maximum: 1 g 3 times/day)

Adults: 500 mg to 1 g 1-3 times/day **or** 2 g every 12 hours for 1 day

Dosage Forms

Caplet, oral: 500 mg, 1 g

Valtrex®: 500 mg, 1 g

Tablet, oral: 500 mg, 1 g

valacyclovir hydrochloride *see* valacyclovir *on page 973*

Valcyte® [US/Can] *see* valganciclovir *on page 974*

23-valent pneumococcal polysaccharide vaccine *see* pneumococcal polysaccharide vaccine (polyvalent) *on page 772*

valganciclovir (val gan SYE kloh veer)

Sound-Alike/Look-Alike Issues

valGANCIclovir may be confused with valACYclovir

Valcyte® may be confused with Valium®, Valtrex®

Synonyms valganciclovir hydrochloride

Tall-Man val**GANCI**clovir

U.S./Canadian Brand Names Valcyte® [US/Can]

Therapeutic Category Antiviral Agent

Use Treatment of cytomegalovirus (CMV) retinitis in patients with acquired immunodeficiency syndrome (AIDS); prevention of CMV disease in high-risk patients (donor CMV positive/recipient CMV negative) undergoing kidney, heart, or kidney/pancreas transplantation

Dosage Summary

Oral:

Children 4 months to 16 years: Dose (mg) = 7 x body surface area x creatinine clearance once daily

Children >16 years: 900 mg 1-2 times/day

Adults: 900 mg 1-2 times/day

Dosage Forms

Powder for solution, oral:

Valcyte®: 50 mg/mL (100 mL)

Tablet, oral:

Valcyte®: 450 mg

valganciclovir hydrochloride *see* valganciclovir *on page 974*

Valisone® Scalp Lotion [Can] *see* betamethasone *on page 133*

Valisone® Topical *(Discontinued)*

Valium® [US/Can] *see* diazepam *on page 294*

Valorin [US-OTC] *see* acetaminophen *on page 21*

Valorin Extra [US-OTC] *see* acetaminophen *on page 21*

valproate semisodium *see* valproic acid *on page 974*

valproate sodium *see* valproic acid *on page 974*

valproic acid (val PROE ik AS id)

Sound-Alike/Look-Alike Issues

valproate sodium may be confused with vecuronium

Depakene® may be confused with Depakote®

Synonyms 2-propylpentanoic acid; 2-propylvaleric acid; dipropylacetic acid; DPA; valproate semisodium; valproate sodium

U.S./Canadian Brand Names Apo-Valproic® [Can]; Depacon® [US]; Depakene® [US/Can]; Epival® I.V. [Can]; Mylan-Valproic [Can]; PHL-Valproic Acid E.C. [Can]; PHL-Valproic Acid [Can]; PMS-Valproic Acid E.C. [Can]; PMS-Valproic Acid [Can]; ratio-Valproic ECC [Can]; ratio-Valproic [Can]; Rhoxal-valproic [Can]; Sandoz-Valproic [Can]; Stavzor™ [US]

Therapeutic Category Anticonvulsant, Miscellaneous; Antimanic Agent; Histone Deacetylase Inhibitor

Use Monotherapy and adjunctive therapy in the treatment of patients with complex partial seizures; monotherapy and adjunctive therapy of simple and complex absence seizures; adjunctive therapy in patients with multiple seizure types that include absence seizures

Stavzor™: Mania associated with bipolar disorder; migraine prophylaxis

Dosage Summary

I.V.:

Children: Simple and complex absence seizures: Initial: 15 mg/kg/day over 60 minutes (≤20 mg/minute); maximum: 60 mg/kg/day. **Note:** Titration may be recommended. Administer doses >250 mg/day in divided doses.

Children ≥10 years: Complex partial seizures: Initial: 10-15 mg/kg/day over 60 minutes (≤20 mg/minute). Administer doses >250 mg/day in divided doses.

Adults: Seizure disorders: Initial: 10-15 mg/kg/day over 60 minutes (≤20 mg/minute); maximum: 60 mg/kg/day. **Note:** Titration may be recommended. Administer doses >250 mg/day in divided doses.

Oral:

Children: Simple and complex absence seizures: Initial: 15 mg/kg/day; increase by 5-10 mg/kg/day at weekly intervals until therapeutic levels are achieved; maximum: 60 mg/kg/day. **Note:** Titration recommended. Administer doses >250 mg/day in divided doses.

Children ≥10 years: Complex partial seizures: Initial: 10-15 mg/kg/day; increase by 5-10 mg/kg/day at weekly intervals until therapeutic levels are achieved; maximum: 60 mg/kg/day. **Note:** Titration recommended. Administer doses >250 mg/day in divided doses.

Children ≥12 years: Migraine prophylaxis: Stavzor™ 250 mg twice daily; adjust dose based on patient response, up to 1000 mg/day

Adults:

Seizure disorders: Initial: 10-15 mg/kg/day in 1-3 divided doses; increase by 5-10 mg/kg/day at weekly intervals until therapeutic levels are achieved; maximum: 60 mg/kg/day. **Note:** Titration recommended. Administer doses >250 mg/day in divided doses.

Mania (Stavzor™): Initial: 750 mg/day in divided doses; dose should be adjusted as rapidly as possible to desired clinical effect; maximum recommended dose: 60 mg/kg/day

Migraine prophylaxis (Stavzor™): 250 mg twice daily; adjust dose based on patient response, up to 1000 mg/day

Dosage Forms

Capsule, softgel, oral: 250 mg

Depakene®: 250 mg

Capsule, softgel, delayed release, oral:

Stavzor™: 125 mg, 250 mg, 500 mg

Injection, solution [preservative free]: 100 mg/mL (5 mL)

Depacon®: 100 mg/mL (5 mL)

Solution, oral: 250 mg/5 mL (473 mL, 480 mL)

Syrup, oral: 250 mg/5 mL (5 mL, 10 mL, 473 mL, 480 mL)

Depakene®: 250 mg/5 mL (473 mL)

valproic acid derivative *see* divalproex *on page* 319

valrubicin (val ROO bi sin)

Sound-Alike/Look-Alike Issues

valrubicin may be confused with DAUNOrubicin, DOXOrubicin, epirubicin, IDArubicin

Valstar® may be confused with valsartan

Synonyms *N*-trifluoroacetyladriamycin-14-valerate; AD32

U.S./Canadian Brand Names Valstar® [US]; Valtaxin® [Can]

Therapeutic Category Antineoplastic Agent, Anthracycline

Use Intravesical therapy of BCG-refractory bladder carcinoma *in situ*

Dosage Summary

Intravesical:

Children: Dosage not established

Adults: 800 mg once weekly for 6 weeks

Dosage Forms

Injection, solution [preservative free]:

Valstar®: 40 mg/mL (5 mL)

valsartan (val SAR tan)

Sound-Alike/Look-Alike Issues

valsartan may be confused with losartan, Valstar™, Valturna®

Diovan® may be confused with Darvon®, Dioval®, Zyban®

U.S./Canadian Brand Names Diovan® [US/Can]

Therapeutic Category Angiotensin II Receptor Antagonist

Use Alone or in combination with other antihypertensive agents in the treatment of essential hypertension; reduction of cardiovascular mortality in patients with left ventricular dysfunction postmyocardial infarction; treatment of heart failure (NYHA Class II-IV)

Dosage Summary

Oral:

Children <6 years: Dosage not established.

Children 6-16 years: Initial: 1.3 mg/kg once daily (maximum: 40 mg/day); Maintenance: Adjust dose based on response (maximum: ≤2.7 mg/kg; 160 mg)

Adults: Initial: 20-40 mg twice daily **or** 80-160 mg once daily; Maintenance: 80-160 mg twice daily (maximum: 320 mg/day); **Note:** Titration is recommended

Dosage Forms

Tablet, oral:

Diovan®: 40 mg, 80 mg, 160 mg, 320 mg

valsartan and aliskiren *see* aliskiren and valsartan *on page 51*

valsartan and amlodipine *see* amlodipine and valsartan *on page 70*

valsartan and hydrochlorothiazide (val SAR tan & hye droe klor oh THYE a zide)

Sound-Alike/Look-Alike Issues

Diovan® may be confused with Darvon®, Dioval®, Zyban®

Synonyms hydrochlorothiazide and valsartan

U.S./Canadian Brand Names Diovan HCT® [US/Can]

Therapeutic Category Antihypertensive Agent, Combination

Use Treatment of hypertension

Dosage Summary

Oral:

Children: Dosage not established

Adults: Valsartan 80-160 mg and hydrochlorothiazide 12.5-25 mg once daily (maximum: 25 mg/day [hydrochlorothiazide]; 320 mg/day [valsartan]); **Note:** Titration is recommended

Dosage Forms

Tablet:

Diovan HCT®: 80 mg/12.5 mg: Valsartan 80 mg and hydrochlorothiazide 12.5 mg; 160 mg/12.5 mg: Valsartan 160 mg and hydrochlorothiazide 12.5 mg; 160 mg/25 mg: Valsartan 160 mg and hydrochlorothiazide 25 mg; 320 mg/12.5 mg: Valsartan 320 mg and hydrochlorothiazide 12.5 mg; 320 mg/25 mg: Valsartan 320 mg and hydrochlorothiazide 25 mg

valsartan, hydrochlorothiazide, and amlodipine *see* amlodipine, valsartan, and hydrochlorothiazide *on page 71*

Valstar® [US] *see* valrubicin *on page 975*

Valtaxin® [Can] *see* valrubicin *on page 975*

Valtrex® [US/Can] *see* valacyclovir *on page 973*

Valturna® [US] *see* aliskiren and valsartan *on page 51*

Vamate® Oral *(Discontinued)* *see* hydroxyzine *on page 490*

Vanatrip® *(Discontinued)* *see* amitriptyline *on page 67*

Vancenase *see* beclomethasone (oral inhalation) *on page 120*

Vancenase® AQ 84 mcg *(Discontinued)* *see* beclomethasone (nasal) *on page 120*

Vancenase® Pockethaler® *(Discontinued)* *see* beclomethasone (nasal) *on page 120*

Vanceril® AEM [Can] *see* beclomethasone (oral inhalation) *on page 120*

Vanceril® *(Discontinued)* *see* beclomethasone (oral inhalation) *on page 120*

Vancocin® [US/Can] *see* vancomycin *on page* 977

vancomycin (van koe MYE sin)

Sound-Alike/Look-Alike Issues

vancomycin may be confused with clindamycin, gentamicin, tobramycin, valACYclovir, vecuronium, Vibramycin®

I.V. vancomycin may be confused with Invanz®

Synonyms vancomycin hydrochloride

U.S./Canadian Brand Names Vancocin® [US/Can]

Therapeutic Category Antibiotic, Miscellaneous

Use Treatment of patients with infections caused by staphylococcal species and streptococcal species; used orally for staphylococcal enterocolitis or for antibiotic-associated pseudomembranous colitis produced by *C. difficile*

Dosage Summary

I.V.:

Infants >1 month: 40-60 mg/kg/day in divided doses every 6 hours

Children: 40-60 mg/kg/day in divided doses every 6 hours **or** 20 mg/kg 1 hour prior to surgery

Adults: 15-20 mg/kg every 6-12 hours **or** 30-60 mg/kg/day in divided doses every 8-12 hours **or** 500-750 mg every 6 hours **or** 1 g 1 hour prior to surgery

Intracatheter:

Children: 2 mg/mL ± 10 units heparin/mL **or** 2.5 mg/mL ± 2500 **or** 5000 units heparin/mL **or** 5 mg/mL ± 5000 units heparin/mL (preferred regimen); instill into catheter port with a volume sufficient to fill the catheter (2-5 mL). **Note:** May use SWFI/NS or D_5W as diluents. Do not mix with any other solutions. Dwell times generally should not exceed 48 hours before renewal of lock solution. Remove lock solution prior to catheter use then replace.

Adults: 2 mg/mL ± 10 units heparin/mL **or** 2.5 mg/mL ± 2500 **or** 5000 units heparin/mL **or** 5 mg/mL ± 5000 units heparin/mL (preferred regimen); instill into catheter port with a volume sufficient to fill the catheter (2-5 mL). **Note:** May use SWFI/NS or D_5W as diluents. Do not mix with any other solutions. Dwell times generally should not exceed 48 hours before renewal of lock solution. Remove lock solution prior to catheter use then replace.

Intrathecal:

Children: 5-20 mg/day

Adults: 5-20 mg/day

Oral:

Children: 40 mg/kg/day in 3-4 divided doses (maximum: 2000 mg/day)

Adults: 500-2000 mg/day in 3-4 divided doses (maximum: 2000 mg/day)

Dosage Forms

Capsule, oral:

Vancocin®: 125 mg, 250 mg

Infusion, premixed iso-osmotic dextrose solution: 500 mg (100 mL); 1 g (200 mL)

Injection, powder for reconstitution: 500 mg, 750 mg, 1 g, 5 g, 10 g

vancomycin hydrochloride *see* vancomycin *on page* 977

Vandazole® [US] *see* metronidazole (topical) *on page* 627

Vanex Forte™-D *(Discontinued)* *see* chlorpheniramine, phenylephrine, and methscopolamine *on page* 212

Vanex-HD® *(Discontinued)* *see* phenylephrine, hydrocodone, and chlorpheniramine *on page* 754

Vaniqa® [US/Can] *see* eflornithine *on page* 344

Vanos™ [US] *see* fluocinonide *on page* 411

Vanoxide® *(Discontinued)* *see* benzoyl peroxide *on page* 128

Vanoxide-HC® [US/Can] *see* benzoyl peroxide and hydrocortisone *on page* 129

Vanquish® Extra Strength Pain Reliever [US-OTC] *see* acetaminophen, aspirin, and caffeine *on page* 27

Vansil™ *(Discontinued)*

Vaponefrin® *(Discontinued)* *see* epinephrine (systemic, oral inhalation) *on page* 352

Vaprisol® [US] *see* conivaptan *on page* 249

VAQTA® [US/Can] *see* hepatitis A vaccine *on page* 468

VAR *see* varicella virus vaccine *on page* 978

vardenafil (var DEN a fil)

Sound-Alike/Look-Alike Issues

vardenafil may be confused with sildenafil, tadalafil

Levitra® may be confused with Kaletra®, Lexiva®

Synonyms Staxyn™; vardenafil hydrochloride

U.S./Canadian Brand Names Levitra® [US/Can]

Therapeutic Category Phosphodiesterase (Type 5) Enzyme Inhibitor

Use Treatment of erectile dysfunction (ED)

Dosage Summary

Oral:

Children: Dosage not established

Adults: Film-coated tablet (Levitra®): 2.5-20 mg 60 minutes prior to sexual activity (maximum: 1 dose/day); Oral disintegrating tablet (Staxyn™): 10 mg 60 minutes prior to sexual activity (maximum: 10 mg/day)

Elderly ≥65 years: 2.5-5 mg 60 minutes prior to sexual activity (maximum: 1 dose/day)

Product Availability

Staxyn™: FDA approved June 2010; availability expected near the end of 2010

Staxyn™ orally disintegrating tablets are indicated for the treatment of erectile dysfunction.

Dosage Forms

Tablet, oral:

Levitra®: 2.5 mg, 5 mg, 10 mg, 20 mg

vardenafil hydrochloride *see* vardenafil *on page 978*

varenicline (var e NI kleen)

Synonyms varenicline tartrate

U.S./Canadian Brand Names Champix® [Can]; Chantix® [US]

Therapeutic Category Partial Nicotine Agonist

Use Treatment to aid in smoking cessation

Dosage Summary

Oral:

Children: Dosage not established

Adults: Days 1-3: 0.5 mg once daily; Days 4-7: 0.5 mg twice daily; Maintenance (≥ Day 8): 1 mg twice daily

Dosage Forms

Combination package, oral:

Chantix®: Tablet: 0.5 mg (11s) [white tablets] and Tablet: 1 mg (42s) [light blue tablets]

Tablet, oral:

Chantix®: 0.5 mg, 1 mg

varenicline tartrate *see* varenicline *on page 978*

Varibar® Honey [US] *see* barium *on page 117*

Varibar® Nectar [US] *see* barium *on page 117*

Varibar® Pudding [US] *see* barium *on page 117*

Varibar® Thin Honey [US] *see* barium *on page 117*

varicella, measles, mumps, and rubella vaccine *see* measles, mumps, rubella, and varicella virus vaccine *on page 593*

varicella virus vaccine (var i SEL a VYE rus vak SEEN)

Sound-Alike/Look-Alike Issues

varicella virus vaccine has been given in error (instead of the indicated varicella immune globulin) to pregnant women exposed to varicella

Synonyms chickenpox vaccine; VAR; varicella-zoster virus (VZV) vaccine (varicella); VZV vaccine (varicella)

U.S./Canadian Brand Names Varilrix® [Can]; Varivax® III [Can]; Varivax® [US]

Therapeutic Category Vaccine, Live Virus

Use Immunization against varicella in children ≥12 months of age and adults

The ACIP recommends vaccination for all children, adolescents, and adults who do not have evidence of immunity. Vaccination is especially important for:

- Persons with close contact to those at high risk for severe disease
- Persons living or working in environments where transmission is likely (teachers, child-care workers, residents and staff of institutional settings)
- Persons in environments where transmission has been reported
- Nonpregnant women of childbearing age
- Adolescents and adults in households with children
- International travelers

Postexposure prophylaxis: Vaccination within 3 days (possibly 5 days) after exposure to rash is effective in preventing illness or modifying severity of disease

Dosage Summary

SubQ:

Children <12 months: Dosage not established
Children 12 months to 12 years: 0.5 mL as a single dose; may repeat in ≥3 months
Children ≥13 years: 2 doses of 0.5 mL separated by 4-8 weeks
Adults: 2 doses of 0.5 mL separated by 4-8 weeks

Dosage Forms

Injection, powder for reconstitution [preservative free]:
Varivax®: 1350 PFU

Dosage Forms - Canada

Injection, powder for reconstitution [preservative free]:
Varivax® III: 1350 plaque-forming units (PFU)

Injection, powder for reconstitution:
Valrilix®: $10^{3.3}$ plaque-forming units (PFU)

varicella-zoster immune globulin (human)

(var i SEL a- ZOS ter i MYUN GLOB yoo lin HYU man)

Sound-Alike/Look-Alike Issues

varicella virus vaccine has been given in error (instead of the indicated varicella immune globulin) to pregnant women exposed to varicella.

Synonyms VZIG

U.S./Canadian Brand Names VariZIG™ [Can]

Therapeutic Category Immune Globulin

Use In pregnant women, for the prevention or reduction in severity of maternal infection within 4 days of exposure to the varicella zoster virus.

Dosage Summary

I.M.:

Children: Dosage not established
Adults: 125 int. units/10 kg (minimum dose: 125 int. units; maximum dose: 625 int. units)

I.V.:

Children: Dosage not established
Adults: 125 int. units/10 kg (minimum dose: 125 int. units; maximum dose: 625 int. units)

Dosage Forms - Canada

Injection, powder for reconstitution [preservative free]:
VariZIG™: 125 int. units [package with diluent] [

varicella-zoster virus (VZV) vaccine (varicella) *see* varicella virus vaccine *on page* 978
varicella-zoster (VZV) vaccine (zoster) *see* zoster vaccine *on page* 1006
Varilrix® [Can] *see* varicella virus vaccine *on page* 978
Varivax® [US] *see* varicella virus vaccine *on page* 978
Varivax® III [Can] *see* varicella virus vaccine *on page* 978
VariZIG™ [Can] *see* varicella-zoster immune globulin (human) *on page* 979
Vaseretic® [US/Can] *see* enalapril and hydrochlorothiazide *on page* 348
VasoClear® *(Discontinued)* *see* naphazoline (ophthalmic) *on page* 658
Vasocon® [Can] *see* naphazoline (ophthalmic) *on page* 658
Vasocon®-A *(Discontinued)*
Vasocon Regular® Ophthalmic *(Discontinued)* *see* naphazoline (ophthalmic) *on page* 658
Vasodilan® *(Discontinued)* *see* isoxsuprine *on page* 530

vasopressin (vay soe PRES in)

Synonyms 8-arginine vasopressin; ADH; antidiuretic hormone; AVP

U.S./Canadian Brand Names Pitressin® [US]; Pressyn® AR [Can]; Pressyn® [Can]

Therapeutic Category Hormone, Posterior Pituitary

Use Treatment of central diabetes insipidus; differential diagnosis of diabetes insipidus

Dosage Summary Note: Administration and dosage varies by indication.

I.M.:

Children: 2.5-10 units 2-4 times/day as needed
Adults: 5-10 units 2-4 times/day as needed

SubQ:

Children: 2.5-10 units 2-4 times/day as needed
Adults: 5-10 units every 2-4 hours as needed

Dosage Forms

Injection, solution: 20 units/mL (0.5 mL, 1 mL, 10 mL)
Pitressin®: 20 units/mL (1 mL)

Vasotec® [US/Can] *see* enalapril *on page* 348
Vasotec® I.V. [Can] *see* enalapril *on page* 348
Vasovist® [Can] *see* gadofosveset *on page* 434
Vaxigrip® [Can] *see* influenza virus vaccine (inactivated) *on page* 507
VCF® [US-OTC] *see* nonoxynol 9 *on page* 681
Vectibix® [US/Can] *see* panitumumab *on page* 724
Vectical™ [US] *see* calcitriol *on page* 165
Vectrin® ***(Discontinued)*** *see* minocycline *on page* 635

vecuronium (vek ue ROE nee um)

Sound-Alike/Look-Alike Issues

vecuronium may be confused with valproate sodium, vancomycin
Norcuron® may be confused with Narcan®

Synonyms ORG NC 45

U.S./Canadian Brand Names Norcuron® [Can]

Therapeutic Category Skeletal Muscle Relaxant

Use To facilitate endotracheal intubation and to relax skeletal muscles during surgery; to facilitate mechanical ventilation in ICU patients; does not relieve pain or produce sedation

Dosage Summary

I.V.:

Children >7 weeks to 1 year: Dosage not established

Children ≥1 year: Initial: 0.08-0.1 mg/kg **or** 0.04-0.06 mg/kg after initial dose of succinylcholine; Maintenance: 0.01-0.015 mg/kg every 12-15 minutes **or** 0.8-1.2 mcg/kg/minute as a continuous infusion

Adults: Initial: 0.08-0.1 mg/kg **or** 0.04-0.06 mg/kg after initial dose of succinylcholine **or** 0.05-0.2 mg/kg bolus; Maintenance: 0.01-0.015 mg/kg every 12-15 minutes **or** 0.8-1.2 mcg/kg/minute as a continuous infusion

Dosage Forms

Injection, powder for reconstitution: 10 mg, 20 mg

velaglucerase alfa (vel a GLOO ser ase AL fa)

Synonyms gene-activated human acid-beta-glucosidase; glcCerase

U.S./Canadian Brand Names VPRIV™ [US]

Therapeutic Category Enzyme

Use Long-term enzyme replacement therapy for patients with type 1 Gaucher disease

Dosage Summary

I.V.:

Children <4 years: Dosage not established
Children ≥4 years 15-60 units/kg every other week
Adults: 15-60 units/kg every other week

Dosage Forms

Injection, powder for reconstitution:
VPRIV™: 400 units

Velban® *(Discontinued)* *see* vinblastine *on page* *985*
Velcade® [US/Can] *see* bortezomib *on page* *143*
Velivet™ [US] *see* ethinyl estradiol and desogestrel *on page* *374*
Velosulin® BR (Buffered) *(Discontinued)*
Veltin™ *see* clindamycin and tretinoin *on page* *233*

venlafaxine (ven la FAX een)

Sound-Alike/Look-Alike Issues
Effexor® may be confused with Effexor XR®

U.S./Canadian Brand Names CO Venlafaxine XR [Can]; Effexor XR® [US/Can]; Effexor® [US]; Mylan-Venlafaxine XR [Can]; PMS-Venlafaxine XR [Can]; ratio-Venlafaxine XR [Can]; Riva-Venlafaxine XR [Can]; Sandoz-Venlafaxine XR [Can]; Teva-Venlafaxine XR [Can]; Venlafaxine XR [Can]

Therapeutic Category Antidepressant, Phenethylamine

Use Treatment of major depressive disorder, generalized anxiety disorder (GAD), social anxiety disorder (social phobia), panic disorder

Dosage Summary

Oral:

Extended release:
Children: Dosage not established
Adults: Initial: 37.5-75 mg/day once daily; Maintenance: 75-225 mg/day once daily (recommended maximum: 225 mg/day); **Note:** Titration is recommended

Immediate release:
Adults: Initial: 75 mg/day in 2-3 divided doses; Maintenance: 75-375 mg/day in 2-3 divided doses (recommended maximum: 375 mg/day); **Note:** Titration is recommended

Dosage Forms

Capsule, extended release, oral: 37.5 mg, 75 mg, 150 mg
Effexor XR®: 37.5 mg, 75 mg, 150 mg
Tablet, oral: 25 mg, 37.5 mg, 50 mg, 75 mg, 100 mg
Effexor®: 50 mg
Tablet, extended release, oral: 37.5 mg, 75 mg, 150 mg, 225 mg

Venlafaxine XR [Can] *see* venlafaxine *on page* *981*
Venofer® [US/Can] *see* iron sucrose *on page* *526*
Venoglobulin®-I *(Discontinued)* *see* immune globulin (intravenous) *on page* *502*
Venoglobulin®-S *(Discontinued)* *see* immune globulin (intravenous) *on page* *502*
Ventavis® [US] *see* iloprost *on page* *499*
Ventolin® [Can] *see* albuterol *on page* *43*
Ventolin® *(Discontinued)* *see* albuterol *on page* *43*
Ventolin® Diskus [Can] *see* albuterol *on page* *43*
Ventolin® HFA [US/Can] *see* albuterol *on page* *43*
Ventolin® Inhaler Aerosol *(Discontinued)* *see* albuterol *on page* *43*
Ventolin® I.V. Infusion [Can] *see* albuterol *on page* *43*
Ventolin® Nebules P.F. [Can] *see* albuterol *on page* *43*
VePesid® *(Discontinued)* *see* etoposide *on page* *384*
Veracolate® [US-OTC] *see* bisacodyl *on page* *138*
Veramyst® [US] *see* fluticasone (nasal) *on page* *419*

verapamil (ver AP a mil)

Sound-Alike/Look-Alike Issues
Calan® may be confused with Colace®, diltiazem
Covera-HS® may be confused with Provera®
Isoptin® may be confused with Isopto® Tears
Verelan® may be confused with Virilon®, Voltaren®

Synonyms iproveratril hydrochloride; verapamil hydrochloride

U.S./Canadian Brand Names Apo-Verap® SR [Can]; Apo-Verap® [Can]; Calan® SR [US]; Calan® [US/Can]; Chronovera® [Can]; Covera-HS® [US/Can]; Covera® [Can]; Dom-Verapamil SR [Can]; Gen-Verapamil SR [Can]; Gen-Verapamil [Can]; Isoptin® SR [US/Can]; Med-Verapamil [Can]; Mylan-Verapamil SR [Can]; Mylan-Verapamil [Can]; Novo-Veramil SR [Can]; Novo-Veramil [Can]; Nu-Verap SR [Can]; Nu-Verap [Can]; PHL-Verapamil SR [Can]; PMS-Verapamil SR [Can]; PRO-Verapamil SR [Can]; Riva-Verapamil SR [Can]; Verapamil Hydrochloride Injection, USP [Can]; Verapamil SR [Can]; Verelan SRC [Can]; Verelan® PM [US]; Verelan® [US]

Therapeutic Category Antiarrhythmic Agent, Class IV; Calcium Channel Blocker

Use

Oral: Treatment of hypertension; angina pectoris (vasospastic, chronic stable, unstable) (Calan®, Covera-HS®); supraventricular tachyarrhythmia (PSVT, atrial fibrillation/flutter [rate control])

I.V.: Supraventricular tachyarrhythmia (PSVT, atrial fibrillation/flutter [rate control])

Dosage Summary

I.V.:

Children <1 year: Dosage not established

Children 1-15 years: 0.1-0.3 mg/kg/dose over 2 minutes; maximum: 5 mg/dose, may repeat dose in 15 minutes if adequate response not achieved; maximum for second dose: 10 mg

Adults: Initial dose: 2.5-5 mg over 2 minutes; Second 5-10 mg after 15-30 minutes if no response (maximum: 20 mg total dose)

Oral:

Extended release:

Children: Dosage not established

Adults: 180-480 mg once daily at bedtime

Elderly: Initial: 100-180 mg once daily at bedtime; Maintenance: 100-480 mg once daily at bedtime

Immediate release:

Children: Dosage not established

Adults: Initial: 80-120 mg 3 times/day; Maintenance: 80-480 mg/day in 2-4 divided doses (maximum: 480 mg/day)

Elderly: 120-480 mg/day in 2-4 divided doses

Sustained release:

Children: Dosage not established

Adults: 120-480 mg/day in 1-2 divided doses (maximum: 480 mg/day)

Elderly: Initial: 120 mg/day once daily; Maintenance: 120-360 mg/day in 1-2 divided doses

Dosage Forms

Caplet, sustained release, oral:

Calan® SR: 120 mg, 180 mg, 240 mg

Capsule, extended release, oral: 120 mg, 180 mg, 240 mg

Capsule, extended release, controlled onset, oral: 100 mg, 200 mg, 300 mg

Verelan® PM: 100 mg, 200 mg, 300 mg

Capsule, sustained release, oral: 120 mg, 180 mg, 240 mg, 360 mg

Verelan®: 120 mg, 180 mg, 240 mg, 360 mg

Injection, solution: 2.5 mg/mL (2 mL, 4 mL)

Tablet, oral: 40 mg, 80 mg, 120 mg

Calan®: 80 mg, 120 mg

Tablet, extended release, oral: 120 mg, 180 mg, 240 mg

Tablet, extended release, controlled onset, oral:

Covera-HS®: 180 mg, 240 mg

Tablet, sustained release, oral: 120 mg, 180 mg, 240 mg

Isoptin® SR: 120 mg, 180 mg, 240 mg

verapamil and trandolapril *see* trandolapril and verapamil *on page* 947

verapamil hydrochloride *see* verapamil *on page* 981

Verapamil Hydrochloride Injection, USP [Can] *see* verapamil *on page* 981

Verapamil SR [Can] *see* verapamil *on page* 981

Verazinc® Oral ***(Discontinued)*** *see* zinc sulfate *on page* 1002

Verdeso™ [US] *see* desonide *on page* 279

Veregen™ [US] *see* sinecatechins *on page* 878

Verelan® [US] *see* verapamil *on page* 981

Verelan® PM [US] *see* verapamil *on page* 981

Verelan SRC [Can] *see* verapamil *on page* 981

Vergogel® Gel *(Discontinued)* *see* salicylic acid *on page 858*
Vergon® *(Discontinued)* *see* meclizine *on page 595*
Veripred™ 20 [US] *see* prednisolone (systemic) *on page 790*
Vermox® [Can] *see* mebendazole *on page 594*
Vermox® *(Discontinued)* *see* mebendazole *on page 594*
Versed® *(Discontinued)* *see* midazolam *on page 632*
Versel® [Can] *see* selenium sulfide *on page 869*
Versiclear™ [US] *see* sodium thiosulfate *on page 888*

verteporfin (ver te POR fin)

U.S./Canadian Brand Names Visudyne® [US/Can]

Therapeutic Category Ophthalmic Agent

Use Treatment of predominantly classic subfoveal choroidal neovascularization due to macular degeneration, presumed ocular histoplasmosis, or pathologic myopia

Dosage Summary

I.V.:

Children: Dosage not established
Adults: 6 mg/m^2 body surface area
Elderly ≥75 years: Were less likely to benefit from therapy in clinical trials

Dosage Forms

Injection, powder for reconstitution:
Visudyne®: 15 mg

Verukan® Solution *(Discontinued)* *see* salicylic acid *on page 858*
Vesanoid® [Can] *see* tretinoin (systemic) *on page 951*
Vesanoid® *(Discontinued)* *see* tretinoin (systemic) *on page 951*
VESIcare® [US] *see* solifenacin *on page 889*
Vexol® [US/Can] *see* rimexolone *on page 844*
VFEND® [US/Can] *see* voriconazole *on page 992*
Viactiv® [US-OTC] *see* vitamins (multiple/oral) *on page 990*
Viactiv® Calcium Flavor Glides™ [US-OTC] *see* vitamins (multiple/oral) *on page 990*
Viactiv® Flavor Glides [US-OTC] *see* vitamins (multiple/oral) *on page 990*
Viactiv® for Teens [US-OTC] *see* vitamins (multiple/oral) *on page 990*
Viactiv® With Calcium [US-OTC] *see* vitamins (multiple/oral) *on page 990*
Viadur® *(Discontinued)* *see* leuprolide *on page 554*
Viagra® [US/Can] *see* sildenafil *on page 874*
Vibativ™ [US] *see* telavancin *on page 912*
Vibramycin® [US/Can] *see* doxycycline *on page 331*
Vibramycin® I.V. *(Discontinued)* *see* doxycycline *on page 331*
Vibra-Tabs® [Can] *see* doxycycline *on page 331*
***Vibrio cholera* and enterotoxigenic *Escherichia coli* vaccine** *see* traveler's diarrhea and cholera vaccine *(Canada only) on page 949*
Vicks® 44® Cough Relief [US-OTC] *see* dextromethorphan *on page 287*
Vicks® 44D Cough & Head Congestion *(Discontinued)* *see* pseudoephedrine and dextromethorphan *on page 812*
Vicks® 44E [US-OTC] *see* guaifenesin and dextromethorphan *on page 455*
Vicks® 44® Non-Drowsy Cold & Cough Liqui-Caps *(Discontinued)* *see* pseudoephedrine and dextromethorphan *on page 812*
Vicks® Casero™ Chest Congestion Relief [US-OTC] *see* guaifenesin *on page 454*
Vicks® Children's Chloraseptic® *(Discontinued)* *see* benzocaine *on page 124*
Vicks® Children's NyQuil® *(Discontinued)* *see* chlorpheniramine, pseudoephedrine, and dextromethorphan *on page 214*
Vicks® Chloraseptic® Sore Throat *(Discontinued)* *see* benzocaine *on page 124*
Vicks® DayQuil® Cold/Flu Multi-Symptom Relief [US-OTC] *see* acetaminophen, dextromethorphan, and phenylephrine *on page 29*
Vicks® DayQuil® Cough [US-OTC] *see* dextromethorphan *on page 287*

Vicks® DayQuil® Mucus Control [US-OTC] *see* guaifenesin *on page 454*
Vicks® DayQuil® Mucus Control DM [US-OTC] *see* guaifenesin and dextromethorphan *on page 455*
Vicks® DayQuil® Multi-Symptom Cold and Flu *(Discontinued)*
Vicks® DayQuil® Sinus [US-OTC] *see* acetaminophen and phenylephrine *on page 25*
Vicks® DayQuil® Sinus Pressure & Congestion Relief *(Discontinued)*
Vicks® Early Defense™ [US-OTC] *see* oxymetazoline (nasal) *on page 716*
Vicks® Formula 44® *(Discontinued)* *see* dextromethorphan *on page 287*
Vicks® Formula 44® Pediatric Formula *(Discontinued)* *see* dextromethorphan *on page 287*
Vicks® Formula 44® Sore Throat [US-OTC] *see* phenol *on page 748*
Vicks® NyQuil® D Cold & Flu Multi-Symptom [US-OTC] *see* acetaminophen, dextromethorphan, doxylamine, and pseudoephedrine *on page 30*
Vicks® NyQuil® Cold & Flu Multi-Symptom [US-OTC] *see* acetaminophen, dextromethorphan, and doxylamine *on page 29*
Vicks® Pediatric 44®m *(Discontinued)* *see* chlorpheniramine, pseudoephedrine, and dextromethorphan *on page 214*
Vicks® Pediatric Formula 44E [US-OTC] *see* guaifenesin and dextromethorphan *on page 455*
Vicks Sinex® 12 Hour *(Discontinued)* *see* oxymetazoline (nasal) *on page 716*
Vicks® Sinex® Nasal Spray *(Discontinued)* *see* phenylephrine (nasal) *on page 751*
Vicks® Sinex® Ultra Fine Mist *(Discontinued)* *see* phenylephrine (nasal) *on page 751*
Vicks® Sinex® VapoSpray™ 4 Hour Decongestant [US-OTC] *see* phenylephrine (nasal) *on page 751*
Vicks® Sinex® VapoSpray 12-Hour [US] *see* oxymetazoline (nasal) *on page 716*
Vicks® Sinex® VapoSpray 12-Hour UltraFine Mist [US-OTC] *see* oxymetazoline (nasal) *on page 716*
Vicks® Sinex® VapoSpray Moisturizing 12-Hour UltraFine Mist [US-OTC] *see* oxymetazoline (nasal) *on page 716*
Vicks® Vitamin C [US-OTC] *see* ascorbic acid *on page 98*
Vicodin® [US] *see* hydrocodone and acetaminophen *on page 479*
Vicodin® ES [US] *see* hydrocodone and acetaminophen *on page 479*
Vicodin® HP [US] *see* hydrocodone and acetaminophen *on page 479*
Vicoprofen® [US/Can] *see* hydrocodone and ibuprofen *on page 481*
Victoza® [US/Can] *see* liraglutide *on page 569*
Vi-Daylin® ADC *(Discontinued)* *see* vitamins (multiple/pediatric) *on page 990*
Vi-Daylin® ADC + Iron *(Discontinued)* *see* vitamins (multiple/pediatric) *on page 990*
Vi-Daylin® Drops *(Discontinued)* *see* vitamins (multiple/pediatric) *on page 990*
Vi-Daylin®/F ADC *(Discontinued)* *see* vitamins (multiple/pediatric) *on page 990*
Vi-Daylin®/F ADC + Iron *(Discontinued)* *see* vitamins (multiple/pediatric) *on page 990*
Vi-Daylin®/F *(Discontinued)* *see* vitamins (multiple/pediatric) *on page 990*
Vi-Daylin®/F + Iron *(Discontinued)* *see* vitamins (multiple/pediatric) *on page 990*
Vi-Daylin® + Iron Drops *(Discontinued)* *see* vitamins (multiple/pediatric) *on page 990*
Vi-Daylin® + Iron Liquid *(Discontinued)* *see* vitamins (multiple/oral) *on page 990*
Vi-Daylin® Liquid *(Discontinued)* *see* vitamins (multiple/oral) *on page 990*
Vidaza® [US] *see* azacitidine *on page 109*
Videx® [US/Can] *see* didanosine *on page 299*
Videx® EC [US/Can] *see* didanosine *on page 299*

vigabatrin (vye GA ba trin)

Sound-Alike/Look-Alike Issues
vigabatrin may be confused with Vibativ™

U.S./Canadian Brand Names Sabril® [US/Can]

Therapeutic Category Anticonvulsant

Use Treatment of infantile spasms; refractory complex partial seizures not controlled by usual treatments

Additional uses in Canadian labeling (not in U.S. labeling): Active management of partial or secondary generalized seizures not controlled by usual treatments

Dosage Summary

Oral:

Infants: 50-150 mg/kg/day in 2 divided doses

Children: Dosage not established

Adults: 1-3 g/day in 2 divided doses

Dosage Forms

Powder for solution, oral:

Sabril®: 500 mg/packet (50s)

Tablet, oral:

Sabril®: 500 mg

Dosage Forms - Canada

Powder for suspension, oral [sachets]:

Sabril®: 0.5 g

Vigamox® [US/Can] *see* moxifloxacin (ophthalmic) *on page 647*

VIGIV *see* vaccinia immune globulin (intravenous) *on page 973*

Vimovo™ [US] *see* naproxen and esomeprazole *on page 660*

Vimpat® [US] *see* lacosamide *on page 541*

vinblastine (vin BLAS teen)

Sound-Alike/Look-Alike Issues

vinBLAStine may be confused with vinCRIStine, vinorelbine

Synonyms vinblastine sulfate; vincaleukoblastine; VLB

Tall-Man vin**BLAS**tine

Therapeutic Category Antineoplastic Agent

Use Treatment of Hodgkin and non-Hodgkin lymphoma; testicular cancer; breast cancer; mycosis fungoides; Kaposi sarcoma; histiocytosis (Letterer-Siwe disease); choriocarcinoma

Dosage Summary Details concerning dosing in combination regimens should also be consulted.

I.V.:

Children: Initial dose: 3-6.5 mg/m^2; do not administer more frequently than every 7 days

Adults: Initial: 3.7 mg/m^2; adjust dose every 7 days (based on white blood cell response) up to 5.5 mg/m^2 (second dose); 7.4 mg/m^2 (third dose); 9.25 mg/m^2 (fourth dose); and 11.1 mg/m^2 (fifth dose); Usual range: 5.5-7.4 mg/m^2 every 7 days; Maximum dose: 18.5 mg/m^2

Dosage Forms

Injection, powder for reconstitution: 10 mg

Injection, solution: 1 mg/mL (10 mL)

vinblastine sulfate *see* vinblastine *on page 985*

vincaleukoblastine *see* vinblastine *on page 985*

Vincasar PFS® [US] *see* vincristine *on page 985*

vincristine (vin KRIS teen)

Sound-Alike/Look-Alike Issues

vinCRIStine may be confused with vinBLAStine

Oncovin® may be confused with Ancobon®

Synonyms leurocristine sulfate; vincristine sulfate

Tall-Man vin**CRIS**tine

U.S./Canadian Brand Names Vincasar PFS® [US]; Vincristine Sulfate Injection [Can]

Therapeutic Category Antineoplastic Agent

Use Treatment of acute lymphocytic leukemia (ALL), Hodgkin lymphoma, non-Hodgkin lymphomas, Wilms tumor, neuroblastoma, rhabdomyosarcoma

Dosage Summary Note: Doses may be capped at a maximum of 2 mg/dose; refer to individual protocol.

I.V.:

Children ≤10 kg: 0.05 mg/kg once weekly (maximum: 2 mg/dose)

Children >10 kg: 1.5-2 mg/m^2/dose (maximum: 2 mg/dose); frequency varies based on protocol

Adults: 1.4 mg/m^2/dose (maximum: 2 mg/dose); frequency varies based on protocol

Dosage Forms

Injection, solution [preservative free]: 1 mg/mL (1 mL, 2 mL)

Vincasar PFS®: 1 mg/mL (1 mL, 2 mL)

vincristine sulfate *see* vincristine *on page 985*
Vincristine Sulfate Injection [Can] *see* vincristine *on page 985*

vinorelbine (vi NOR el been)

Sound-Alike/Look-Alike Issues
vinorelbine may be confused with vinBLAStine

Synonyms dihydroxydeoxynorvinkaleukoblastine; vinorelbine tartrate

U.S./Canadian Brand Names Navelbine® [US/Can]; Vinorelbine Injection, USP [Can]; Vinorelbine Tartrate for Injection [Can]

Therapeutic Category Antineoplastic Agent

Use Treatment of nonsmall cell lung cancer (NSCLC)

Dosage Summary Note: Details concerning dosing in combination regimens should also be consulted.

I.V.:

Children: Dosage not established

Adults: 30 mg/m^2/dose every 7 days **or** 25-30 mg/m^2/dose every 7 days (in combination with cisplatin)

Dosage Forms

Injection, solution [preservative free]: 10 mg/mL (1 mL, 5 mL)

Navelbine®: 10 mg/mL (1 mL, 5 mL)

Vinorelbine Injection, USP [Can] *see* vinorelbine *on page 986*
vinorelbine tartrate *see* vinorelbine *on page 986*
Vinorelbine Tartrate for Injection [Can] *see* vinorelbine *on page 986*
Viokase® [Can] *see* pancrelipase *on page 723*
Viokase® *(Discontinued)* *see* pancrelipase *on page 723*
viosterol *see* ergocalciferol *on page 358*
Vioxx® *(Discontinued)*
Viracept® [US/Can] *see* nelfinavir *on page 665*
Viramune® [US/Can] *see* nevirapine *on page 671*
ViraTan™-DM [US] *see* phenylephrine, pyrilamine, and dextromethorphan *on page 755*
Viravan® *(Discontinued)* *see* phenylephrine and pyrilamine *on page 753*
Virazole® [US/Can] *see* ribavirin *on page 839*
Viread® [US/Can] *see* tenofovir *on page 916*
Viroptic® [US/Can] *see* trifluridine *on page 958*
Viscoat® [US] *see* sodium chondroitin sulfate and sodium hyaluronate *on page 884*
viscous lidocaine *see* lidocaine (topical) *on page 562*
Visicol® [US] *see* sodium phosphates *on page 887*
Visine-A® [US-OTC] *see* naphazoline and pheniramine *on page 659*
Visine® Advanced Allergy [Can] *see* naphazoline and pheniramine *on page 659*
Visine® Advanced Relief [US-OTC] *see* tetrahydrozoline (ophthalmic) *on page 923*
Visine L.R.® [US-OTC] *see* oxymetazoline (ophthalmic) *on page 717*
Visine® Original [US-OTC] *see* tetrahydrozoline (ophthalmic) *on page 923*
Visipaque™ [US/Can] *see* iodixanol *on page 518*
Viskazide® [Can] *see* pindolol and hydrochlorothiazide *(Canada only) on page 762*
Visken® [Can] *see* pindolol *on page 761*
Visken® *(Discontinued)* *see* pindolol *on page 761*
Vistacon-50® Injection *(Discontinued)* *see* hydroxyzine *on page 490*
Vistaquel® Injection *(Discontinued)* *see* hydroxyzine *on page 490*
Vistaril® [US/Can] *see* hydroxyzine *on page 490*
Vistazine® Injection *(Discontinued)* *see* hydroxyzine *on page 490*
Vistide® [US] *see* cidofovir *on page 222*
Vistra 650 *(Discontinued)* *see* acetaminophen and phenyltoloxamine *on page 26*
Visudyne® [US/Can] *see* verteporfin *on page 983*
Vita-C® [US-OTC] *see* ascorbic acid *on page 98*
Vitaball® [US-OTC] *see* vitamins (multiple/pediatric) *on page 990*
Vitaball® Minis [US-OTC] *see* vitamins (multiple/pediatric) *on page 990*

Vitaball® Wild 'N Fruity [US-OTC] *see* vitamins (multiple/pediatric) *on page 990*
VitaCarn® Oral *(Discontinued)* *see* levocarnitine *on page 556*
Vitafol® [US] *see* vitamins (multiple/oral) *on page 990*
Vitafol®-OB [US-OTC] *see* vitamins (multiple/prenatal) *on page 991*
Vitafol®-OB+DHA [US-OTC] *see* vitamins (multiple/prenatal) *on page 991*
Vitafol®-PN [US] *see* vitamins (multiple/prenatal) *on page 991*
Vitalets [US-OTC] *see* vitamins (multiple/pediatric) *on page 990*
Vital HN® [US-OTC] *see* nutritional formula, enteral/oral *on page 692*
vitamin C *see* ascorbic acid *on page 98*
vitamin D_3 and alendronate *see* alendronate and cholecalciferol *on page 47*
vitamin D and calcium carbonate *see* calcium and vitamin D *on page 166*

vitamin A (VYE ta min aye)

Sound-Alike/Look-Alike Issues
Aquasol® may be confused with Anusol®

Synonyms oleovitamin A

U.S./Canadian Brand Names A-25 [US-OTC]; A-Natural [US-OTC]; A-Natural-25 [US-OTC]; Aquasol A® [US]

Therapeutic Category Vitamin, Fat Soluble

Use Treatment and prevention of vitamin A deficiency; parenteral (I.M.) route is indicated when oral administration is not feasible or when absorption is insufficient (malabsorption syndrome)

Dosage Summary

I.M.:

Infants: 7500-15,000 units/day for 10 days
Children 1-8 years: 17,500-35,000 units/day for 10 days
Children >8 years: 100,000 units for 3 days, followed by 50,000 units/day for 2 weeks
Adults: 100,000 units for 3 days, followed by 50,000 units/day for 2 weeks

Oral:

Infants up to 6 months: 1500 units/day **or** 100,000 units every 4-6 months
Infants 6 months to 1 year: 1500-2000 units/day **or** 100,000 units every 4-6 months **or** 100,000 units as a single dose, repeat next day and at 4 weeks
Children 1-3 years: 1500-2000 units/day **or** 200,000 units every 4-6 months **or** 5000-10000 units/kg/day for 5 days **or** 200,000 units as a single dose, repeat next day and at 4 weeks
Children 4-6 years: 2500 units/day **or** 200,000 units every 4-6 months **or** 5000-10,000 units/kg/day for 5 days **or** 200,000 units as a single dose, repeat next day and at 4 weeks
Children 7-8 years: 3300-3500 units/day **or** 200,000 units every 4-6 months **or** 5000-10,000 units/kg/day for 5 days **or** 200,000 units as a single dose, repeat next day and at 4 weeks
Children 9-10 years: 3300-3500 units/day **or** 100,000 units/day for 3 days, then 50,000 units/day for 14 days **or** 500,000 units/day for 3 days, then 50,000 units/day for 14 days, then 10,000-20,000 units/day for 2 months **or** 200,000 units as a single dose, then repeat next day and at 4 weeks **or** 10,000-50,000 units/day of water miscible product (prophylaxis)
Children >10 years: 4000-5000 units/day **or** 100,000 units/day for 3 days, then 50,000 units/day for 14 days **or** 500,000 units/day for 3 days, then 50,000 units/day for 14 days, then 10,000-20,000 units/day for 2 months **or** 200,000 units as a single dose, then repeat next day and at 4 weeks **or** 10,000-50,000 units/day of water miscible product (prophylaxis)
Adults: 4000-5000 units/day **or** 100,000 units/day for 3 days, then 50,000 units/day for 14 days **or** 500,000 units/day for 3 days, then 50,000 units for 14 days, then 10,000-20,000 units/day for 2 months **or** 10,000-50,000 units/day of water miscible product (prophylaxis)

Dosage Forms

Capsule, oral:
A-25 [OTC]: 25,000 units
Capsule, softgel, oral: 10,000 units
A-Natural [OTC]: 10,000 units
A-Natural-25 [OTC]: 25,000 units
Injection, solution:
Aquasol A®: 50,000 units/mL (2 mL)
Tablet, oral: 10,000 units, 15,000 units

vitamin A acid *see* tretinoin (topical) *on page 951*

vitamin A and vitamin D (VYE ta min aye & VYE ta min dee)

Synonyms cod liver oil

U.S./Canadian Brand Names A and D® Original [US-OTC]; Baza® Clear [US-OTC]; Sween Cream® [US-OTC]

Therapeutic Category Protectant, Topical

Use Temporary relief of discomfort due to chapped skin, diaper rash, minor burns, abrasions, as well as irritations associated with ostomy skin care

Dosage Summary

Topical:

Children: Apply locally as needed

Adults: Apply locally as needed

Dosage Forms

Capsule, softgel: Vitamin A 1250 int. units and vitamin D 135 int. units; vitamin A 1250 int. units and vitamin D 130 int. units; vitamin A 5,000 int. units and vitamin D 400 int. units; vitamin A 10,000 int. units and vitamin D 400 int. units; vitamin A 10,000 int. units and vitamin D 5000 int. units; vitamin A 25,000 int. units and vitamin D 1000 int. units

Cream:

Sween Cream® [OTC]: 2 g, 57 g, 85 g, 142 g, 184 g, 339 g

Ointment: 0.9 g, 5 g, 60 g, 120 g, 454 g

A and D® Original [OTC]: 45 g, 120 g, 454 g

Baza® Clear [OTC]: 50 g, 150 g, 240 g

Tablet: Vitamin A 10,000 int. units and vitamin D 400 int. units

vitamin B_1 *see* thiamine *on page 927*

vitamin B_2 *see* riboflavin *on page 840*

vitamin B_3 *see* niacin *on page 671*

vitamin B_3 *see* niacinamide *on page 672*

vitamin B_5 *see* pantothenic acid *on page 726*

vitamin B_6 *see* pyridoxine *on page 818*

vitamin B_{12} *see* cyanocobalamin *on page 257*

vitamin B complex combinations (VYE ta min bee KOM pleks kom bi NAY shuns)

Synonyms B complex combinations; B vitamin combinations

Therapeutic Category Vitamin, Water Soluble

Use Supplement for use in the wasting syndrome in chronic renal failure, uremia, impaired metabolic functions of the kidney, dialysis; labeled for OTC use as a dietary supplement

Dosage Summary

Oral:

Children: Dosage not established

Adults: 1-2 tablets/capsules once daily between meals **or** one teasponful daily **or** two tablespoonsful daily

Dosage Forms Content varies depending on product used. For more detailed information on ingredients in these and other multivitamins, please refer to package labeling.

vitamin D2 *see* ergocalciferol *on page 358*

Vitamin D3 [US-OTC] *see* cholecalciferol *on page 218*

vitamin E (VYE ta min ee)

Sound-Alike/Look-Alike Issues

Aquasol E® may be confused with Anusol®

Synonyms *d*-alpha tocopherol; *dl*-alpha tocopherol

U.S./Canadian Brand Names Alph-E [US-OTC]; Alph-E-Mixed [US-OTC]; Aqua Gem-E™ [US-OTC]; Aquasol E® [US-OTC]; d-Alpha-Gems™ [US-OTC]; E-Gems® Elite [US-OTC]; E-Gems® Plus [US-OTC]; E-Gems® [US-OTC]; E-Gem® Lip Care [US-OTC]; E-Gem® [US-OTC]; Ester-E™ [US-OTC]; Gamma E-Gems® [US-OTC]; Gamma-E PLUS [US-OTC]; High Gamma Vitamin E Complete™ [US-OTC]; Key-E® Kaps [US-OTC]; Key-E® Powder [US-OTC]; Key-E® [US-OTC]

Therapeutic Category Vitamin, Fat Soluble; Vitamin, Topical

Use Dietary supplement

Dosage Summary

Oral:

Children: 1 unit/kg/day **or** 100-400 units/day **or** 750 units/day (beta-thalassemia)

Adults: 30-1600 units/day **or** 1000 units twice daily

Topical:

Children: Dosage varies by product; consult package insert for specific product labeling

Adults: Apply a thin layer over affected area

Dosage Forms

Capsule, oral: 400 int. units, 1000 int. units

Key-E® Kaps [OTC]: 200 int. units, 400 int. units

Capsule, liquid, oral: 400 int. units

Capsule, softgel, oral: 100 int. units, 200 int. units, 400 int. units, 600 int. units, 1000 int. units, 200 units, 1000 units

Alph-E [OTC]: 200 int. units, 400 int. units, 1000 int. units

Alph-E-Mixed [OTC]: 200 int. units, 400 int. units, 1000 int. units

Aqua Gem-E™ [OTC]: 200 int. units, 400 int. units

d-Alpha Gems™ [OTC]: 400 int. units

E-Gems® [OTC]: 30 int. units, 100 int. units, 200 int. units, 400 int. units, 600 int. units, 800 int. units, 1000 int. units, 1200 int. units

E-Gems® Elite [OTC]: 400 int. units

E-Gems® Plus [OTC]: 200 int. units, 400 int. units, 800 int. units

Ester-E™ [OTC]: 400 int. units

Gamma E-Gems® [OTC]: 90 int. units

Gamma-E PLUS [OTC]: 200 int. units

High Gamma Vitamin E Complete™ [OTC]: 200 int. units

Cream, topical: 1000 int. units/120 g (120 g); 100 int. units/g (57 g, 60 g); 30,000 int. units/57 g (57 g)

Key-E® [OTC]: 30 int. units/g (57 g, 120 g, 600 g)

Lip balm, topical:

E-Gem® Lip Care [OTC]: 1000 int. units/tube

Liquid, oral/topical: 1150 int. units/1.25 mL (30 mL, 60 mL, 120 mL)

Oil, oral/topical: 100 int. units/0.25 mL (74 mL)

E-Gem® [OTC]: 10 int. units/drop (15 mL, 60 mL)

Oil, topical:

Alph-E [OTC]: 28,000 int. units/30 mL (30 mL)

Ointment, topical:

Key-E® [OTC]: 30 int. units/g (57 g, 113 g, 500 g)

Powder, oral:

Key-E® Powder [OTC]: 700 int. units per 1/4 teaspoon (15 g, 75 g, 1000 g)

Solution, oral: 15 int. units/0.3 mL (30 mL)

Aquasol E® [OTC]: 15 int. units/0.3 mL (12 mL, 30 mL)

Suppository, rectal/vaginal:

Key-E® [OTC]: 30 int. units (12s, 24s)

Tablet, oral: 100 int. units, 200 int. units, 400 int. units, 500 int. units

Key-E® [OTC]: 200 int. units, 400 int. units

vitamin G *see* riboflavin *on page* 840

vitamin K_1 *see* phytonadione *on page* 759

vitamins (multiple/injectable) (VYE ta mins, MUL ti pul/in JEK ti bal)

U.S./Canadian Brand Names Infuvite® Adult [US]; Infuvite® Pediatric [US]; M.V.I. Adult™ [US]; M.V.I.®-12 [US]; M.V.I.® Pediatric [US]

Therapeutic Category Vitamin

Use Nutritional supplement in patients receiving parenteral nutrition or requiring intravenous administration

Dosage Summary

I.V.:

Children <3 kg: Dosage not established

Children ≥3 kg to 11 years: 5 mL/day (pediatric formulation) added to TPN or ≥100 mL of appropriate solution

Children >11 years: 10 mL/day (adult formulation) added to TPN or ≥500 mL or appropriate solution

Adults: 10 mL/day (adult formulation) added to TPN or ≥500 mL or appropriate solution

Dosage Forms Content varies depending on product used. For more detailed information on ingredients in these and other multivitamins, please refer to package labeling.

vitamins (multiple/oral) (VYE ta mins, MUL ti pul/OR al)

Sound-Alike/Look-Alike Issues

Theragran® may be confused with Phenergan®

Synonyms multiple vitamins; therapeutic multivitamins; vitamins, multiple (oral); vitamins, multiple (therapeutic); vitamins, multiple with iron

U.S./Canadian Brand Names Androvite® [US-OTC]; CalciFolic-D™ [US]; Centamin [US-OTC]; Centrum Cardio® [US-OTC]; Centrum Performance® [US-OTC]; Centrum® Silver® Ultra Men's [US-OTC]; Centrum® Silver® Ultra Women's [US-OTC]; Centrum® Silver® [US-OTC]; Centrum® Ultra Men's [US-OTC]; Centrum® Ultra Women's [US-OTC]; Centrum® [US-OTC]; Diatx®Zn [US]; Drinkables® Fruits and Vegetables [US-OTC]; Drinkables® MultiVitamins [US-OTC]; Encora® [US]; Foltrin® [US]; Freedavite [US-OTC]; Geri-Freeda [US-OTC]; Geriation [US-OTC]; Geritol Complete® [US-OTC]; Geritol Extend® [US-OTC]; Geritol® Tonic [US-OTC]; Glutofac®-MX [US]; Glutofac®-ZX [US]; Gynovite® Plus [US-OTC]; Hemocyte Plus® [US]; Hi-Kovite [US-OTC]; Monocaps [US-OTC]; Myadec® [US-OTC]; Nutrimin-Plus [US-OTC]; Ocuvite® Adult 50+ [US-OTC]; Ocuvite® Extra® [US-OTC]; Ocuvite® Lutein [US-OTC]; Ocuvite® [US-OTC]; One A Day® Cholesterol Plus [US-OTC]; One A Day® Energy [US-OTC]; One A Day® Essential [US-OTC]; One A Day® Maximum [US-OTC]; One A Day® Men's 50+ Advantage [US-OTC]; One A Day® Men's Health Formula [US-OTC]; One A Day® Teen Advantage for Her [US-OTC]; One A Day® Teen Advantage for Him [US-OTC]; One A Day® Weight Smart® Advanced [US-OTC]; One A Day® Women's 50+ Advantage [US-OTC]; One A Day® Women's Active Mind & Body [US-OTC]; One A Day® Women's [US-OTC]; Optivite® P.M.T. [US-OTC]; PreserVision® AREDS [US-OTC]; PreserVision® Lutein [US-OTC]; Quintabs [US-OTC]; Quintabs-M Iron-Free [US-OTC]; Quintabs-M [US-OTC]; Renax® 5.5 [US]; Renax® [US]; Replace Without Iron [US-OTC]; Replace [US-OTC]; Repliva 21/7® [US]; SourceCF® [US]; Strovite® Advance [US]; Strovite® Forte [US]; Strovite® Plus [US]; Strovite® [US]; T-Vites [US-OTC]; Ultra Freeda A-Free [US-OTC]; Ultra Freeda Iron-Free [US-OTC]; Ultra Freeda With Iron [US-OTC]; Viactiv® Calcium Flavor Glides™ [US-OTC]; Viactiv® Flavor Glides [US-OTC]; Viactiv® for Teens [US-OTC]; Viactiv® With Calcium [US-OTC]; Viactiv® [US-OTC]; Vitafol® [US]; Xtramins [US-OTC]; Yelets [US-OTC]

Therapeutic Category Vitamin

Use Prevention/treatment of vitamin and mineral deficiencies; labeled for OTC use as a dietary supplement

Dosage Summary

Oral:

Children: Dosage not established

Adults: One tablet/capsule **or** 5-15 mL once daily

Dosage Forms Content varies depending on product used. For more detailed information on ingredients in these and other multivitamins, please refer to package labeling.

vitamins, multiple (oral) *see* vitamins (multiple/oral) *on page 990*

vitamins (multiple/pediatric) (VYE ta mins, MUL ti pul/pe de AT rik)

Synonyms children's vitamins; multivitamins/fluoride

U.S./Canadian Brand Names ADEKs® [US-OTC]; AquADEKs™ [US-OTC]; Centrum Kids® Complete Dora the Explorer™ [US-OTC]; Centrum Kids® Complete Rugrats™ [US-OTC]; Centrum Kids® Complete SpongeBob SquarePants™ [US-OTC]; Flintstones™ Complete [US-OTC]; Flintstones™ Gummies Vita-Packs [US-OTC]; Flintstones™ Gummies [US-OTC]; Flintstones™ Plus Bone Building Support [US-OTC]; Flintstones™ Plus Immunity Support [US-OTC]; Flintstones™ Plus Iron [US-OTC]; Flintstones™ Sour Gummies [US-OTC]; My First Flintstones™ [US-OTC]; MyKidz Iron FL™ [US]; MyKidz Iron™ [US-OTC]; One A Day® Kids Bugs Bunny and Friends Complete [US-OTC]; One A Day® Kids Scooby-Doo!™ Gummies [US-OTC]; One-A-Day® Kids Scooby-Doo!™ Complete [US-OTC]; One-A-Day® Kids Scooby-Doo!™ Plus Calcium [US-OTC]; Poly-Vi-Sol® with Iron [US-OTC]; Poly-Vi-Sol® [US-OTC]; SourceCF® [US-OTC]; Tri-Vi-Sol® With Iron [US-OTC]; Tri-Vi-Sol® [US-OTC]; Vitaball® Minis [US-OTC]; Vitaball® Wild 'N Fruity [US-OTC]; Vitaball® [US-OTC]; Vitalets [US-OTC]

Therapeutic Category Vitamin

Use Prevention/treatment of vitamin deficiency; products containing fluoride are used to prevent dental caries; labeled for OTC use as a dietary supplement

Dosage Summary

Oral:

Children: Daily dose varies by product; consult package insert for specific product labeling

Adults: Dosage not established

Dosage Forms Content varies depending on product used. For more detailed information on ingredients in these and other multivitamins, please refer to package labeling.

vitamins (multiple/prenatal) (VYE ta mins, MUL ti pul/pree NAY tal)

Sound-Alike/Look-Alike Issues

PreCare® may be confused with Precose®

Synonyms prenatal vitamins

U.S./Canadian Brand Names A-Free Prenatal [US]; Calna [US-OTC]; CitraNatal™ 90 DHA [US]; CitraNatal™ DHA [US]; CitraNatal™ Rx [US]; Duet® DHA [US]; Duet® DHA[ec] [US]; Duet® [US]; KPN Prenatal [US-OTC]; Mini-Prenatal [US-OTC]; NataCaps™ [US]; NataChew® [US-OTC]; NataFort® [US-OTC]; NatalCare® GlossTabs™ [US]; NatalCare® PIC Forte [US]; NatalCare® PIC [US]; NatalCare® Plus [US]; NatalCare® Rx [US]; NatalCare® Three [US]; NataTab™ CFe [US]; NataTab™ FA [US]; NataTab™ Rx [US]; NutriNate® [US]; NutriSpire™ [US]; Néevo® DHA [US]; Néevo® [US]; One A Day® Women's Prenatal [US-OTC]; OptiNate® [US]; PreCare Conceive® [US]; PreCare Premier® [US]; PreCare® [US]; PremesisRx® [US]; Prenatal 19 [US-OTC]; Prenatal AD [US-OTC]; Prenatal One Daily [US-OTC]; Prenatal Rx 1 [US]; Prenatal U [US-OTC]; Prenate DHA™ [US]; Prenate Elite® [US]; PrimaCare® One [US]; PrimaCare® [US]; Select-OB™ [US-OTC]; Stuart Prenatal® [US-OTC]; Tandem® DHA [US]; Tandem® OB [US]; Trinate [US-OTC]; Ultra NatalCare® [US]; Vitafol®-OB [US-OTC]; Vitafol®-OB+DHA [US-OTC]; Vitafol®-PN [US]

Therapeutic Category Vitamin

Use Nutritional supplement for use prior to conception, during pregnancy, and postnatal (in lactating and nonlactating women)

Dosage Summary

Oral:

Children: Dosage not established

Adults: One tablet/capsule once daily **or** 4 teaspoonfuls/day once daily or in divided doses

Dosage Forms Content varies depending on product used. For more detailed information on ingredients in these and other multivitamins, please refer to package labeling.

vitamins, multiple (therapeutic) *see* vitamins (multiple/oral) *on page 990*

vitamins, multiple with iron *see* vitamins (multiple/oral) *on page 990*

Vitaneed™ [US-OTC] *see* nutritional formula, enteral/oral *on page 692*

Vitelle™ Irospan® *(Discontinued)* *see* ferrous sulfate and ascorbic acid *on page 399*

Vitrase® [US] *see* hyaluronidase *on page 476*

Vitrasert™ [US/Can] *see* ganciclovir (ophthalmic) *on page 437*

Vitrax® [US] *see* hyaluronate and derivatives *on page 475*

Vitussin *(Discontinued)*

Vivacaine™ [US] *see* bupivacaine and epinephrine *on page 154*

Vi vaccine *see* typhoid vaccine *on page 967*

Vivactil® [US] *see* protriptyline *on page 810*

Viva-Drops® [US-OTC] *see* artificial tears *on page 97*

Vivaglobin® [US] *see* immune globulin (subcutaneous) *on page 503*

Vivarin® [US-OTC] *see* caffeine *on page 163*

Vivelle® *(Discontinued)* *see* estradiol (topical) *on page 367*

Vivelle-Dot® [US] *see* estradiol (systemic) *on page 366*

Vivitrol™ [US] *see* naltrexone *on page 657*

Vivonex® [US-OTC] *see* nutritional formula, enteral/oral *on page 692*

Vivonex® T.E.N. [US-OTC] *see* nutritional formula, enteral/oral *on page 692*

Vivotif® [US/Can] *see* typhoid vaccine *on page 967*

VLB *see* vinblastine *on page 985*

VM-26 *see* teniposide *on page 916*

Volibris® [Can] *see* ambrisentan *on page 62*

Volmax® *(Discontinued)* *see* albuterol *on page 43*

Voltaren® [Can] *see* diclofenac (systemic) *on page* *296*
Voltaren® *(Discontinued)* *see* diclofenac (systemic) *on page* *296*
Voltaren® Emulgel™ [Can] *see* diclofenac (topical) *on page* *297*
Voltaren® Gel [US] *see* diclofenac (topical) *on page* *297*
Voltaren Ophtha® [Can] *see* diclofenac (ophthalmic) *on page* *297*
Voltaren Ophthalmic® [US] *see* diclofenac (ophthalmic) *on page* *297*
Voltaren Rapide® [Can] *see* diclofenac (systemic) *on page* *296*
Voltaren SR® [Can] *see* diclofenac (systemic) *on page* *296*
Voltaren®-XR [US] *see* diclofenac (systemic) *on page* *296*
VoLumen® [US] *see* barium *on page* *117*
Voluven® [US/Can] *see* tetrastarch *on page* *924*

voriconazole (vor i KOE na zole)

Synonyms UK109496

U.S./Canadian Brand Names VFEND® [US/Can]

Therapeutic Category Antifungal Agent

Use Treatment of invasive aspergillosis; treatment of esophageal candidiasis; treatment of candidemia (in nonneutropenic patients); treatment of disseminated *Candida* infections of the skin and viscera; treatment of serious fungal infections caused by *Scedosporium apiospermum* and *Fusarium* spp (including *Fusarium solani*) in patients intolerant of, or refractory to, other therapy

Dosage Summary

I.V.:

Children <12 years: Dosage not established
Children ≥12 years: Initial: 6 mg/kg every 12 hours for 2 doses; Maintenance: 3-4 mg/kg every 12 hours
Adults: Initial: 6 mg/kg every 12 hours for 2 doses; Maintenance: 3-4 mg/kg every 12 hours

Oral:

Children <12 years: Dosage not established
Children ≥12 years: 100-300 mg every 12 hours
Adults: 100-300 mg every 12 hours

Dosage Forms

Injection, powder for reconstitution:
VFEND®: 200 mg

Powder for suspension, oral:
VFEND®: 40 mg/mL (70 mL)

Tablet, oral:
VFEND®: 50 mg, 200 mg

vorinostat (vor IN oh stat)

Sound-Alike/Look-Alike Issues
vorinostat may be confused with Votrient™

Synonyms SAHA; suberoylanilide hydroxamic acid

U.S./Canadian Brand Names Zolinza™ [US/Can]

Therapeutic Category Antineoplastic Agent, Histone Deacetylase Inhibitor

Use Treatment of progressive, persistent, or recurrent cutaneous T-cell lymphoma (CTCL)

Dosage Summary

Oral:

Children: Dosage not established
Adults: 400 mg once daily

Dosage Forms

Capsule, oral:
Zolinza™: 100 mg

VoSoL® [US] *see* acetic acid *on page* *32*
VoSol® HC [US] *see* acetic acid, propylene glycol diacetate, and hydrocortisone *on page* *33*
VoSpire ER® [US] *see* albuterol *on page* *43*
Votrient™ [US] *see* pazopanib *on page* *730*
VP-16 *see* etoposide *on page* *384*
VP-16-213 *see* etoposide *on page* *384*

VPRIV™ [US] *see* velaglucerase alfa *on page 980*
VSL #3® [US-OTC] *see* Lactobacillus *on page 543*
VSL #3®-DS [US] *see* Lactobacillus *on page 543*
V-Tann™ *(Discontinued)* *see* phenylephrine and pyrilamine *on page 753*
Vumon® [US/Can] *see* teniposide *on page 916*
Vusion® [US] *see* miconazole and zinc oxide *on page 631*
V.V.S.® [US] *see* sulfabenzamide, sulfacetamide, and sulfathiazole *on page 899*
vWF:RCof *see* antihemophilic factor/von Willebrand factor complex (human) *on page 82*
Vytone® [US] *see* iodoquinol and hydrocortisone *on page 519*
Vytorin® [US] *see* ezetimibe and simvastatin *on page 388*
Vyvanse® [US/Can] *see* lisdexamfetamine *on page 569*
VZIG *see* varicella-zoster immune globulin (human) *on page 979*
VZV vaccine (varicella) *see* varicella virus vaccine *on page 978*
VZV vaccine (zoster) *see* zoster vaccine *on page 1006*

warfarin (WAR far in)

Sound-Alike/Look-Alike Issues
Coumadin® may be confused with Avandia®, Cardura®, Compazine®, Kemadrin®
Jantoven® may be confused with Janumet®, Januvia®

Synonyms warfarin sodium

U.S./Canadian Brand Names Apo-Warfarin® [Can]; Coumadin® [US/Can]; Jantoven® [US]; Mylan-Warfarin [Can]; Novo-Warfarin [Can]; Taro-Warfarin [Can]

Therapeutic Category Anticoagulant (Other)

Use Prophylaxis and treatment of thromboembolic disorders (eg, venous, pulmonary) and embolic complications arising from atrial fibrillation or cardiac valve replacement; adjunct to reduce risk of systemic embolism (eg, recurrent MI, stroke) after myocardial infarction

Dosage Summary

I.V.:
Children: Dosage not established
Adults: 2-5 mg/day once daily

Oral:
Children: Dosage not established.
Adults: Initial: 2-5 mg daily for 2 days; Maintenance: 2-10 mg daily adjusted according to INR results
Elderly: Initial: ≤5 mg/day; Maintenance: 2-5 mg/day

Dosage Forms

Injection, powder for reconstitution:
Coumadin®: 5 mg

Tablet, oral: 1 mg, 2 mg, 2.5 mg, 3 mg, 4 mg, 5 mg, 6 mg, 7.5 mg, 10 mg
Coumadin®: 1 mg, 2 mg, 2.5 mg, 3 mg, 4 mg, 5 mg, 6 mg, 7.5 mg, 10 mg
Jantoven®: 1 mg, 2 mg, 2.5 mg, 3 mg, 4 mg, 5 mg, 6 mg, 7.5 mg, 10 mg

warfarin sodium *see* warfarin *on page 993*
Wartec® [Can] *see* podofilox *on page 773*
Wart-Off® Maximum Strength [US-OTC] *see* salicylic acid *on page 858*
4-Way® 12 Hour [US-OTC] *see* oxymetazoline (nasal) *on page 716*
4 Way® Fast Acting [US-OTC] *see* phenylephrine (nasal) *on page 751*
4 Way® Menthol [US-OTC] *see* phenylephrine (nasal) *on page 751*
4-Way® Saline Moisturizing Mist [US-OTC] *see* sodium chloride *on page 882*
Welchol® [US/Can] *see* colesevelam *on page 246*
Wellbutrin® [US] *see* bupropion *on page 156*
Wellbutrin XL® [US/Can] *see* bupropion *on page 156*
Wellbutrin SR® [US/Can] *see* bupropion *on page 156*
Wellcovorin® *(Discontinued)* *see* leucovorin calcium *on page 553*
Westcort® [US/Can] *see* hydrocortisone (topical) *on page 483*
Westhroid™ [US] *see* thyroid, desiccated *on page 930*
40 Winks® *(Discontinued)* *see* diphenhydramine (systemic) *on page 310*
Winpred™ [Can] *see* prednisone *on page 792*

WinRho SD® ***(Discontinued)***
WinRho® SDF [US/Can] *see* Rh_o(D) immune globulin *on page 838*
Winstrol® ***(Discontinued)***

witch hazel (witch HAY zel)

Synonyms hamamelis water

U.S./Canadian Brand Names Dickinson's® Witch Hazel Astringent Cleanser [US-OTC]; Dickinson's® Witch Hazel Cleansing Astringent [US-OTC]; Dickinson's® Witch Hazel [US-OTC]; Medi Pads [US-OTC]; Preparation H® Cleansing Pads [Can]; Preparation H® Medicated Wipes [US-OTC]; T. N. Dickinson's® Witch Hazel® Astringent [US-OTC]; T. N. Dickinson's® Witch Hazel® Hemorrhoidal [US-OTC]; T.N. Dickinson's® Hazelets [US-OTC]; Tucks® Take Alongs® [US-OTC]

Therapeutic Category Astringent

Use After-stool wipe to remove most causes of local irritation; temporary management of vulvitis, pruritus ani and vulva; help relieve the discomfort of simple hemorrhoids, anorectal surgical wounds, and episiotomies

Dosage Summary

Topical:

Children: Dosage not established
Adults: Apply to anorectal area as needed

Dosage Forms

Liquid, topical:

Dickinson's® Witch Hazel Astringent Cleanser [OTC]: 99.5% (3785 mL)
Dickinson's® Witch Hazel Cleansing Astringent [OTC]: 99.5% (59 mL, 237 mL, 473 mL)
T. N. Dickinson's® Witch Hazel® Astringent [OTC]: 100% (59 mL, 237 mL, 473 mL)

Pad, topical:

Dickinson's® Witch Hazel [OTC]: 99% (60s)
Dickinson's® Witch Hazel Cleansing Astringent [OTC]: 99% (20s)
Medi Pads [OTC]: 50% (100s)
Preparation H® Medicated Wipes [OTC]: 50% (8s, 48s, 96s)
T. N. Dickinson's® Hazelets® [OTC]: 100% (50s, 60s)
T. N. Dickinson's® Witch Hazel® Hemorrhoidal [OTC]: 50% (100s)
Tucks® Anti-Itch [OTC]: 50% (40s, 100s)

Towelette, topical:

Tucks® Take Alongs® [OTC]: 50% (12s)

Wolfina® ***(Discontinued)***
Wound Wash Saline™ [US-OTC] *see* sodium chloride *on page 882*
WR-2721 *see* amifostine *on page 63*
WR-139007 *see* dacarbazine *on page 265*
WR-139013 *see* chlorambucil *on page 202*
WR-139021 *see* carmustine *on page 186*
Wycillin® [Can] *see* penicillin G procaine *on page 738*
Wycillin® ***(Discontinued)*** *see* penicillin G procaine *on page 738*
Wydase® ***(Discontinued)*** *see* hyaluronidase *on page 476*
Wygesic® ***(Discontinued)*** *see* propoxyphene and acetaminophen *on page 805*
Wymox® ***(Discontinued)*** *see* amoxicillin *on page 72*
Wytensin® [Can] *see* guanabenz *on page 461*
Wytensin® ***(Discontinued)*** *see* guanabenz *on page 461*
Xalacom™ [Can] *see* latanoprost and timolol *(Canada only) on page 551*
Xalatan® [US/Can] *see* latanoprost *on page 551*
Xamiol® [Can] *see* calcipotriene and betamethasone *on page 164*
Xanax® [US/Can] *see* alprazolam *on page 55*
Xanax TS™ [Can] *see* alprazolam *on page 55*
Xanax XR® [US] *see* alprazolam *on page 55*
Xarelto® [Can] *see* rivaroxaban *(Canada only) on page 848*
Xatral [Can] *see* alfuzosin *on page 49*
Xeloda® [US/Can] *see* capecitabine *on page 174*
Xenaderm™ [US] *see* trypsin, balsam Peru, and castor oil *on page 964*

Xenazine® [US] *see* tetrabenazine *on page 921*
Xenical® [US/Can] *see* orlistat *on page 707*
Xeomin® [US] *see* incobotulinumtoxinA *on page 504*
Xerac AC™ [US] *see* aluminum chloride hexahydrate *on page 58*
Xiaflex™ [US] *see* collagenase (systemic) *on page 247*
Xibrom™ [US] *see* bromfenac *on page 146*
Xifaxan® [US] *see* rifaximin *on page 842*
Xigris® [US/Can] *see* drotrecogin alfa *on page 334*
xilep *see* rufinamide *on page 856*
XiraTuss™ *(Discontinued)* *see* carbetapentane, phenylephrine, and chlorpheniramine *on page 180*
Xodol® 5/300 [US] *see* hydrocodone and acetaminophen *on page 479*
Xodol® 7.5/300 [US] *see* hydrocodone and acetaminophen *on page 479*
Xodol® 10/300 [US] *see* hydrocodone and acetaminophen *on page 479*
Xolair® [US/Can] *see* omalizumab *on page 700*
Xolegel® [US/Can] *see* ketoconazole (topical) *on page 536*
Xopenex® [US/Can] *see* levalbuterol *on page 554*
Xopenex HFA™ [US] *see* levalbuterol *on page 554*
Xpect™ [US-OTC] *see* guaifenesin *on page 454*
Xpect-HC™ *(Discontinued)*
XPECT-PE™ *(Discontinued)* *see* guaifenesin and phenylephrine *on page 456*
X-Prep® *(Discontinued)* *see* senna *on page 870*
XRP6258 *see* cabazitaxel *on page 162*
X-Seb T® Pearl [US-OTC] *see* coal tar and salicylic acid *on page 243*
X-Seb T® Plus [US-OTC] *see* coal tar and salicylic acid *on page 243*
Xtramins [US-OTC] *see* vitamins (multiple/oral) *on page 990*
X-Viate™ [US] *see* urea *on page 970*
Xylocaine® [US] *see* lidocaine (systemic) *on page 561*
Xylocaine® [US/Can] *see* lidocaine (topical) *on page 562*
Xylocaine® Dental [US] *see* lidocaine (systemic) *on page 561*
Xylocaine® MPF [US] *see* lidocaine (systemic) *on page 561*
Xylocaine® MPF With Epinephrine [US] *see* lidocaine and epinephrine *on page 563*
Xylocaine® Viscous *(Discontinued)* *see* lidocaine (topical) *on page 562*
Xylocaine® With Epinephrine [US/Can] *see* lidocaine and epinephrine *on page 563*
Xylocard® [Can] *see* lidocaine (systemic) *on page 561*
Xyntha™ [US] *see* antihemophilic factor (recombinant) *on page 81*
Xyralid™ *(Discontinued)* *see* lidocaine and hydrocortisone *on page 564*
Xyralid™ LP *(Discontinued)* *see* lidocaine and hydrocortisone *on page 564*
Xyralid™ RC *(Discontinued)* *see* lidocaine and hydrocortisone *on page 564*
Xyrem® [US/Can] *see* sodium oxybate *on page 885*
Xyzal® [US] *see* levocetirizine *on page 557*
Y-90 ibritumomab *see* ibritumomab *on page 494*
Y-90 zevalin *see* ibritumomab *on page 494*
Yasmin® [US/Can] *see* ethinyl estradiol and drospirenone *on page 375*
Yaz® [US/Can] *see* ethinyl estradiol and drospirenone *on page 375*
Yelets [US-OTC] *see* vitamins (multiple/oral) *on page 990*

yellow fever vaccine (YEL oh FEE ver vak SEEN)

U.S./Canadian Brand Names YF-VAX® [US/Can]

Therapeutic Category Vaccine, Live Virus

Use Induction of active immunity against yellow fever virus, primarily among persons traveling or living in areas where yellow fever infection exists and laboratory workers who may be exposed to the virus; vaccination may also be required for some international travelers

The Advisory Committee on Immunization Practices (ACIP) recommends vaccination for:

- Persons traveling to or living in areas at risk for yellow fever transmission
- Persons traveling to countries which require vaccination for international travel
- Laboratory personnel who may be exposed to the yellow fever virus or concentrated preparations of the vaccine

Although the vaccine is approved for use in children ≥9 months of age, the CDC recommends use in children as young as 6 months under unusual circumstances (eg, travel to an area where exposure is unavoidable). Children <6 months of age should **never** receive the vaccine.

Dosage Summary

SubQ:

Children <9 months: Dosage not established
Children ≥9 months: Initial: 0.5 mL ≥10 days before travel; Booster: Every 10 years
Adults: Initial: 0.5 mL ≥10 days before travel; Booster: Every 10 years

Dosage Forms

Injection, powder for reconstitution [17D-204 strain]:
YF-VAX®: ≥4.74 Log_{10} plaque-forming units (PFU) per 0.5 mL dose

YF-VAX® [US/Can] *see* yellow fever vaccine *on page* *995*
YM087 *see* conivaptan *on page* *249*
YM905 *see* solifenacin *on page* *889*
YM-08310 *see* amifostine *on page* *63*
Yocon® [US/Can] *see* yohimbine *on page* *996*
Yodoxin® [US] *see* iodoquinol *on page* *519*

yohimbine (yo HIM bine)

Sound-Alike/Look-Alike Issues
Aphrodyne® may be confused with Aprodine®
Yocon® may be confused with Zocor®

Synonyms yohimbine hydrochloride

U.S./Canadian Brand Names PMS-Yohimbine [Can]; Yocon® [US/Can]

Therapeutic Category Miscellaneous Product

Dosage Summary

Oral:

Children: Not indicated

Dosage Forms

Tablet, oral:
Yocon®: 5.4 mg

yohimbine hydrochloride *see* yohimbine *on page* *996*
Yohimex™ *(Discontinued)* *see* yohimbine *on page* *996*
Yutopar® Injection *(Discontinued)*
Z4942 *see* ifosfamide *on page* *498*
Zaditen® [Can] *see* ketotifen *on page* *538*
Zaditor® [US-OTC/Can] *see* ketotifen *on page* *538*

zafirlukast (za FIR loo kast)

Sound-Alike/Look-Alike Issues
Accolate® may be confused with Accupril®, Accutane®, Aclovate®

Synonyms ICI-204,219

U.S./Canadian Brand Names Accolate® [US/Can]

Therapeutic Category Leukotriene Receptor Antagonist

Use Prophylaxis and chronic treatment of asthma in adults and children ≥5 years of age

Dosage Summary

Oral:

Children <5 years: Dosage not established
Children 5-11 years: 10 mg twice daily
Children ≥12 years: 20 mg twice daily
Adults: 20 mg twice daily

Dosage Forms

Tablet, oral:

Accolate®: 10 mg, 20 mg

Zagam® ***(Discontinued)***

zalcitabine ***(Discontinued)***

zaleplon (ZAL e plon)

Sound-Alike/Look-Alike Issues

zaleplon may be confused with zolpidem

Sonata® may be confused with Soriatane®

U.S./Canadian Brand Names Sonata® [US]

Therapeutic Category Hypnotic, Nonbenzodiazepine (Pyrazolopyrimidine)

Controlled Substance C-IV

Use Short-term (7-10 days) treatment of insomnia (has been demonstrated to be effective for up to 5 weeks in controlled trial)

Dosage Summary

Oral:

Children: Dosage not established

Adults: 5-20 mg at bedtime

Elderly: 5 mg at bedtime (maximum: 10 mg/day)

Dosage Forms

Capsule, oral: 5 mg, 10 mg

Sonata®: 5 mg, 10 mg

Zamicet™ [US] *see* hydrocodone and acetaminophen *on page 479*

Zanaflex® [US/Can] *see* tizanidine *on page 937*

Zanaflex Capsules® [US] *see* tizanidine *on page 937*

zanamivir (za NA mi veer)

Sound-Alike/Look-Alike Issues

Relenza® may be confused with Albenza®, Aplenzin™

U.S./Canadian Brand Names Relenza® [US/Can]

Therapeutic Category Antiviral Agent, Inhalation Therapy

Use Treatment of uncomplicated acute illness due to influenza virus A and B in patients who have been symptomatic for no more than 2 days; prophylaxis against influenza virus A and B

The Advisory Committee on Immunization Practices (ACIP) recommends that **treatment** be considered for the following:

- Persons hospitalized with laboratory confirmed influenza (may also have benefit if started >48 hours after onset of illness).
- Persons with laboratory confirmed influenza pneumonia.
- Persons with laboratory confirmed influenza and bacterial infections.
- Persons with laboratory confirmed influenza and who are at higher risk for influenza complications.
- Persons presenting for care within 48 hours of laboratory confirmed influenza onset and who want to decrease duration and/or severity of their symptoms or decrease the risk of transmission to those at high risk for complications.

The ACIP recommends that **prophylaxis** be considered for the following:

- Persons at high risk for influenza infection during the first 2 weeks following vaccination (eg, children <9 years and not previously vaccinated) if the virus is circulating in the community.
- Persons at high risk for influenza infection, but the vaccination is contraindicated.
- Unvaccinated family members or healthcare providers with prolonged exposure to or close contact with high-risk persons, unvaccinated persons, or infants <6 months of age.
- Persons at high risk for influenza infection, their family members and close contacts, and healthcare workers when the circulating strain of influenza is not matched with the vaccine.
- Persons with immune deficiency or those who may not respond to vaccination.
- Unvaccinated staff and persons during response to an outbreak in a closed institutional setting that has patients at high risk for infection (eg, extended care facilities).

Dosage Summary

Oral inhalation:

Children ≥5 years: Prophylaxis: 10 mg once daily

Children ≥7 years: Treatment: 10 mg twice daily
Adolescents: Prophylaxis: 10 mg once daily
Adults:
Prophylaxis: 10 mg once daily
Treatment: 10 mg twice daily

Dosage Forms

Powder, for oral inhalation:
Relenza®: 5 mg/blister (20s)

Zanosar® [US/Can] *see* streptozocin *on page 896*
Zantac® [US/Can] *see* ranitidine *on page 828*
Zantac 75® [US-OTC/Can] *see* ranitidine *on page 828*
Zantac 150® [US-OTC] *see* ranitidine *on page 828*
Zantac® EFFERdose® [US] *see* ranitidine *on page 828*
Zantac Maximum Strength Non-Prescription [Can] *see* ranitidine *on page 828*
Zantryl® *(Discontinued)* *see* phentermine *on page 750*
Zapzyt® [US-OTC] *see* benzoyl peroxide *on page 128*
Zapzyt® Acne Wash [US-OTC] *see* salicylic acid *on page 858*
Zapzyt® Pore Treatment [US-OTC] *see* salicylic acid *on page 858*
Zarontin® [US/Can] *see* ethosuximide *on page 381*
Zaroxolyn® [US/Can] *see* metolazone *on page 625*
Zartan® *(Discontinued)* *see* cephalexin *on page 197*
Zavesca® [US/Can] *see* miglustat *on page 634*
Zazole™ [US] *see* terconazole *on page 918*
Z-chlopenthixol *see* zuclopenthixol *(Canada only) on page 1006*
Z-Cof HC *(Discontinued)* *see* phenylephrine, hydrocodone, and chlorpheniramine *on page 754*
Z-Cof LA™ [US] *see* guaifenesin and dextromethorphan *on page 455*
ZD1033 *see* anastrozole *on page 78*
ZD1694 *see* raltitrexed *(Canada only) on page 826*
ZD1839 *see* gefitinib *on page 439*
ZDV *see* zidovudine *on page 999*
ZDV, abacavir, and lamivudine *see* abacavir, lamivudine, and zidovudine *on page 18*
Zeasorb®-AF [US-OTC] *see* miconazole (topical) *on page 630*
Zebeta® [US] *see* bisoprolol *on page 141*
Zebutal® [US] *see* butalbital, acetaminophen, and caffeine *on page 159*
Zefazone® *(Discontinued)*
Zeftera™ [Can] *see* ceftobiprole *(Canada only) on page 193*
Zegerid® [US] *see* omeprazole and sodium bicarbonate *on page 702*
Zegerid OTC™ [US-OTC] *see* omeprazole and sodium bicarbonate *on page 702*
Zelapar™ [US] *see* selegiline *on page 869*
Zeldox® [Can] *see* ziprasidone *on page 1002*
Zelnorm® [US] *see* tegaserod *on page 912*
Zemaira® [US] *see* alpha$_1$-proteinase inhibitor *on page 54*
Zemplar® [US/Can] *see* paricalcitol *on page 728*
Zemuron® [US/Can] *see* rocuronium *on page 850*
Zenapax® [Can] *see* daclizumab *on page 265*
Zenapax® *(Discontinued)* *see* daclizumab *on page 265*
Zenchent™ [US] *see* ethinyl estradiol and norethindrone *on page 378*
zeneca 182,780 *see* fulvestrant *on page 431*
Zenpep™ [US] *see* pancrelipase *on page 723*
Zephiran® *(Discontinued)* *see* benzalkonium chloride *on page 124*
Zephrex LA® *(Discontinued)* *see* guaifenesin and pseudoephedrine *on page 457*
Zerit® [US/Can] *see* stavudine *on page 894*
ZerLor™ [US] *see* acetaminophen, caffeine, and dihydrocodeine *on page 28*
Zestoretic® [US/Can] *see* lisinopril and hydrochlorothiazide *on page 570*

Zestril® [US/Can] *see* lisinopril *on page* 570
Zetar® [US-OTC] *see* coal tar *on page* 242
Zetia® [US] *see* ezetimibe *on page* 387
Zevalin® [US/Can] *see* ibritumomab *on page* 494
Zgesic [US] *see* acetaminophen and phenyltoloxamine *on page* 26
Ziac® [US/Can] *see* bisoprolol and hydrochlorothiazide *on page* 141
Ziagen® [US/Can] *see* abacavir *on page* 18
Ziana™ [US] *see* clindamycin and tretinoin *on page* 233

ziconotide (zi KOE no tide)

U.S./Canadian Brand Names Prialt® [US]

Therapeutic Category Analgesic, Nonnarcotic; Calcium Channel Blocker, N-Type

Use Management of severe chronic pain in patients requiring intrathecal (I.T.) therapy and who are intolerant or refractory to other therapies

Dosage Summary

I.T.:

Children: Dosage not established

Adults: Initial dose: ≤2.4 mcg/day (0.1 mcg/hour); Maintenance range: 2.4-19.2 mcg/day (0.1-0.8 mcg/hour) (maximum: 19.2 mcg/day [0.8 mcg/hour]); **Note:** Titration is recommended

Dosage Forms

Injection, solution [preservative free]:

Prialt®: 25 mcg/mL (20 mL); 100 mcg/mL (1 mL, 5 mL)

zidovudine (zye DOE vyoo deen)

Sound-Alike/Look-Alike Issues

azidothymidine may be confused with azaTHIOprine, aztreonam
Retrovir® may be confused with acyclovir, ritonavir
AZT is an error-prone abbreviation (mistaken as azathioprine, aztreonam)

Synonyms azidothymidine; compound S; ZDV

U.S./Canadian Brand Names Apo-Zidovudine® [Can]; AZT™ [Can]; Novo-AZT [Can]; Retrovir® (AZT™) [Can]; Retrovir® [US/Can]

Therapeutic Category Antiviral Agent

Use Treatment of HIV infection in combination with at least two other antiretroviral agents; prevention of maternal/fetal HIV transmission as monotherapy

Dosage Summary

I.V.:

Infants <30 weeks gestation at birth: 1.5 mg/kg/dose every 12 hours; at 4 weeks of age advance to 1.5 mg/kg/dose every 8 hours

Infants ≥30 weeks and <35 weeks gestation at birth: 2 mg/kg/dose every 12 hours; at 2 weeks of age, advance to 1.5 mg/kg/dose every 8 hours

Infants (full term): 1.5 mg/kg/dose every 6 hours

Children 6 weeks to <12 years: 120 mg/m^2/dose every 6 hours **or** 20 mg/m^2/hour as a continuous infusion

Children ≥12 years: 1 mg/kg/dose every 4 hours around-the-clock **or** 2 mg/kg bolus followed by 1 mg/kg/hour continuous infusion

Adults: 1 mg/kg/dose every 4 hours around-the-clock **or** 2 mg/kg bolus followed by 1 mg/kg/hour continuous infusion

Oral:

Infants <30 weeks gestation at birth: 2 mg/kg/dose every 12 hours; at 4 weeks of age advance to 2 mg/kg/dose every 8 hours

Infants ≥30 weeks and <35 weeks gestation at birth: 2 mg/kg/dose every 12 hours; at 2 weeks of age, advance to 2 mg/kg/dose every 8 hours

Infants (full term): 2 mg/kg/dose every 6 hours

Children 4 weeks to <18 years: 240 mg/m^2 every 12 hours (maximum 300 mg every 12 hours) **or** 160 mg/m^2/dose every 8 hours (maximum: 200 mg every 8 hours)

4 to <9 kg: 12 mg/kg/dose twice daily **or** 8 mg/kg/dose 3 times/day
≥9 to <30 kg: 9 mg/kg/dose twice daily **or** 6 mg/kg/dose 3 times/day
≥30 kg: 300 mg twice daily **or** 200 mg 3 times/day

Adults: 200 mg 3 times/day **or** 300 mg twice daily

Dosage Forms
Capsule, oral: 100 mg
Retrovir®: 100 mg
Injection, solution [preservative free]:
Retrovir®: 10 mg/mL (20 mL)
Syrup, oral: 50 mg/5 mL (240 mL)
Retrovir®: 50 mg/5 mL (240 mL)
Tablet, oral: 300 mg
Retrovir®: 300 mg

zidovudine, abacavir, and lamivudine *see* abacavir, lamivudine, and zidovudine *on page* 18

zidovudine and lamivudine (zye DOE vyoo deen & la MI vyoo deen)

Sound-Alike/Look-Alike Issues
Combivir® may be confused with Combivent®, Epivir®
AZT is an error-prone abbreviation (mistaken as azaTHIOprine, aztreonam)
AZT + 3TC (error-prone abbreviation)

Synonyms lamivudine and zidovudine

U.S./Canadian Brand Names Combivir® [US/Can]

Therapeutic Category Antiviral Agent

Use Treatment of HIV infection when therapy is warranted based on clinical and/or immunological evidence of disease progression

Dosage Summary
Oral:
Children <30 kg: Dosage not established
Adolescents ≥30 kg: One tablet twice daily
Adults: One tablet twice daily

Dosage Forms
Tablet:
Combivir®: Zidovudine 300 mg and lamivudine 150 mg

Zilactin®-L [US-OTC] *see* benzyl alcohol *on page* 131
Zilactin®-B [US-OTC/Can] *see* benzocaine *on page* 124
Zilactin Baby® [Can] *see* benzocaine *on page* 124
Zilactin® Tooth & Gum Pain [US-OTC] *see* benzocaine *on page* 124

zileuton (zye LOO ton)

U.S./Canadian Brand Names Zyflo CR® [US]

Therapeutic Category 5-Lipoxygenase Inhibitor

Use Prophylaxis and chronic treatment of asthma

Dosage Summary
Oral:
Extended release:
Children <12 years: Dosage not established
Children ≥12 years: 1200 mg twice daily
Adults: 1200 mg twice daily
Immediate release:
Children <12 years: Dosage not established
Children ≥12 years: 600 mg 4 times/day
Adults: 600 mg 4 times/day

Dosage Forms
Tablet, oral:
Zyflo®: 600 mg [scored]
Tablet, extended release, oral:
Zyflo CR®: 600 mg

Zinacef® [US] *see* cefuroxime *on page* 194
zinc *see* trace metals *on page* 945
Zinc 15 [US-OTC] *see* zinc sulfate *on page* 1002

zinc acetate (zink AS e tate)

U.S./Canadian Brand Names Galzin® [US]

Therapeutic Category Trace Element

Use Maintenance treatment of Wilson disease following initial chelation therapy

Dosage Summary

Oral: Dose expressed in mg elemental zinc:

Children <50 kg and >5 years: 75 mg/day in 3 divided doses
Children >50 kg: 150 mg/day in 3 divided doses
Children ≥10 years (manufacturer labeling): 75-150 mg/day in 3 divided doses
Adults:
Pregnant females: 75-150 mg/day in 3 divided doses
Males and nonpregnant females: 150 mg/day in 3 divided doses

Dosage Forms

Capsule, oral:
Galzin®: Elemental zinc 25 mg, Elemental zinc 50 mg

Zincate® [US] *see* zinc sulfate *on page 1002*

zinc chloride (zink KLOR ide)

Therapeutic Category Trace Element

Use Cofactor for replacement therapy to different enzymes; helps maintain normal growth rates, normal skin hydration, and senses of taste and smell

Dosage Summary

I.V.:

Premature infants <1500 g up to 3 kg: 300 mcg/kg/day to I.V. fluid
Infants (full term): 100 mcg/kg/day ot I.V. fluid
Children ≤5 years: 100 mcg/kg/day to I.V. fluid
Adults: 2-6 mg/day (for small bowel fluid loss: up to 12.2 mg/L TPN **or** 17.1 mg/kg of stool or ileostomy output, added to 1000 mL of I.V. fluids)

Dosage Forms

Injection, solution [preservative free]: 1 mg/mL (10 mL)

zinc diethylenetriaminepentaacetate (Zn-DTPA) *see* diethylene triamine penta-acetic acid *on page 300*

Zincfrin® [Can] *see* phenylephrine and zinc sulfate *(Canada only) on page 753*

zinc gelatin (zink JEL ah tin)

Synonyms dome paste bandage; Unna boot; Unna paste; zinc gelatin boot

U.S./Canadian Brand Names Gelucast® [US]

Therapeutic Category Protectant, Topical

Use As a protectant and to support varicosities and similar lesions of the lower limbs

Dosage Summary

Topical:

Children: Dosage not established
Adults: Apply externally as an occlusive boot

Dosage Forms

Bandage: 3" x 10 yards; 4" x 10 yards
Gelucast®: 3" x 10 yards; 4" x 10 yards

zinc gelatin boot *see* zinc gelatin *on page 1001*

Zincofax® [Can] *see* zinc oxide *on page 1001*

Zincon® [US-OTC] *see* pyrithione zinc *on page 819*

zinc oxide (zink OKS ide)

Synonyms base ointment; lassar's zinc paste

U.S./Canadian Brand Names Ammens® Original Medicated [US-OTC]; Ammens® Shower Fresh [US-OTC]; Balmex® [US-OTC]; Boudreaux's® Butt Paste [US-OTC]; Critic-Aid Skin Care® [US-OTC]; Desitin® Creamy [US-OTC]; Desitin® [US-OTC]; Zincofax® [Can]

Therapeutic Category Topical Skin Product

Use Protective coating for mild skin irritations and abrasions; soothing and protective ointment to promote healing of chapped skin, diaper rash

Dosage Summary

Topical:

Children: Apply as required to affected areas several times daily
Adults: Apply as required to affected areas several times daily

Dosage Forms

Cream, topical:
Balmex® [OTC]: 11.3% (60 g, 120 g, 480 g)
Cream, topical [stick]:
Balmex® [OTC]: 11.3% (56 g)
Ointment, topical: 20% (30 g, 60 g, 454 g); 40% (120 g)
Desitin® [OTC]: 40% (30 g, 60 g, 90 g, 120 g, 270 g, 480 g)
Desitin® Creamy [OTC]: 10% (60 g, 120 g)
Paste, topical:
Boudreaux's® Butt Paste [OTC]: 16% (30 g, 60 g, 120 g, 480 g)
Critic-Aid Skin Care® [OTC]: 20% (71 g, 170 g)
Powder, topical:
Ammens® Original Medicated [OTC], Ammens® Shower Fresh [OTC]: 9.1% (312 g)

zinc oxide and miconazole nitrate *see* miconazole and zinc oxide *on page 631*

zinc sulfate (zink SUL fate)

Sound-Alike/Look-Alike Issues

$ZnSO_4$ is an error-prone abbreviation (mistaken as morphine sulfate)

U.S./Canadian Brand Names Anuzinc [Can]; Orazinc® 110 [US-OTC]; Orazinc® 220 [US-OTC]; Rivasol [Can]; Zinc 15 [US-OTC]; Zincate® [US]

Therapeutic Category Electrolyte Supplement, Oral

Use Zinc supplement (oral and parenteral); may improve wound healing in those who are deficient

Dosage Summary

I.V.:

Premature infants (<1500 g up to 3 kg): 300 mcg/kg/day to I.V. fluid or TPN
Infants (full term): 100 mcg/kg/day to I.V. fluid or TPN
Children ≤5 years: 100 mcg/kg/day to I.V. fluid or TPN
Adults: 2.5-6 mg/day **or** 12.2 mg/L of TPN **or** 17.1 mg/kg of stool or ileostomy output added to 1000 mL I.V. fluid

Oral:

Children: 0.5-1 mg elemental zinc/kg/day divided in 1-3 doses
Adults: 110-220 mg (25-50 mg elemental zinc) 3 times/day

Dosage Forms

Capsule, oral: 220 mg
Orazinc® 220 [OTC]: 220 mg
Zincate®: 220 mg
Injection, solution [preservative free]: Elemental zinc 1 mg/mL (10 mL); Elemental zinc 5 mg/mL (5 mL)
Tablet, oral: 220 mg
Orazinc® 110 [OTC]: 110 mg
Zinc 15 [OTC]: 66 mg

zinc sulfate and phenylephrine *see* phenylephrine and zinc sulfate *(Canada only) on page 753*
zinc undecylenate *see* undecylenic acid and derivatives *on page 969*
Zinecard® [US/Can] *see* dexrazoxane *on page 284*
Zingo™ *(Discontinued)* *see* lidocaine (topical) *on page 562*
Ziox 405™ *(Discontinued)*
Ziox™ *(Discontinued)*

ziprasidone (zi PRAS i done)

Sound-Alike/Look-Alike Issues

Sound-alike/look-alike issues:
Ziprasidone may be confused with TraZODone

Synonyms ziprasidone hydrochloride; ziprasidone mesylate

U.S./Canadian Brand Names Geodon® [US]; Zeldox® [Can]

Therapeutic Category Antipsychotic Agent

Use Treatment of schizophrenia; treatment of acute manic or mixed episodes associated with bipolar disorder with or without psychosis; maintenance treatment of bipolar disorder as an adjunct to lithium or valproate; acute agitation in patients with schizophrenia

Dosage Summary

I.M.:

Children: Dosage not established

Adults: 10 mg every 2 hours **or** 20 mg every 4 hours (maximum: 40 mg/day)

Oral:

Children: Dosage not established

Adults: Initial: 20-40 mg twice daily; Maintenance: 20-80 mg twice daily (maximum: 200 mg/day); **Note:** Titration is recommended

Dosage Forms

Capsule, oral:

Geodon®: 20 mg, 40 mg, 60 mg, 80 mg

Injection, powder for reconstitution:

Geodon®: 20 mg

ziprasidone hydrochloride *see* ziprasidone *on page* *1002*

ziprasidone mesylate *see* ziprasidone *on page* *1002*

Zipsor™ [US] *see* diclofenac (systemic) *on page* *296*

Zirgan™ [US] *see* ganciclovir (ophthalmic) *on page* *437*

Zithromax® [US/Can] *see* azithromycin (systemic) *on page* *111*

Zithromax TRI-PAK™ *see* azithromycin (systemic) *on page* *111*

Zithromax Z-PAK® *see* azithromycin (systemic) *on page* *111*

ZM-182,780 *see* fulvestrant *on page* *431*

Zmax® [US] *see* azithromycin (systemic) *on page* *111*

Zn-DTPA [US] *see* diethylene triamine penta-acetic acid *on page* *300*

ZNP® [US-OTC] *see* pyrithione zinc *on page* *819*

Zocor® [US/Can] *see* simvastatin *on page* *877*

Zoderm® [US] *see* benzoyl peroxide *on page* *128*

Zoderm® Hydrating Wash™ [US] *see* benzoyl peroxide *on page* *128*

Zoderm® Redi-Pads™ [US] *see* benzoyl peroxide *on page* *128*

Zofran® [US/Can] *see* ondansetron *on page* *704*

Zofran® ODT [US/Can] *see* ondansetron *on page* *704*

zol 446 *see* zoledronic acid *on page* *1003*

Zoladex® [US/Can] *see* goserelin *on page* *452*

Zoladex® LA [Can] *see* goserelin *on page* *452*

zoledronate *see* zoledronic acid *on page* *1003*

zoledronic acid (zoe le DRON ik AS id)

Sound-Alike/Look-Alike Issues

Zometa® may be confused with Zofran®, Zoladex®

Synonyms CGP-42446; zol 446; zoledronate

U.S./Canadian Brand Names Aclasta® [Can]; Reclast® [US]; Zometa® [US/Can]

Therapeutic Category Bisphosphonate Derivative

Use

Oncology-related uses: Treatment of hypercalcemia of malignancy (albumin-corrected serum calcium >12 mg/dL); treatment of multiple myeloma; treatment of bone metastases of solid tumors

Nononcology uses: Treatment of Paget disease of bone; treatment of osteoporosis in postmenopausal women (to reduce the incidence of fractures or to reduce the incidence of new clinical fractures in patients with low-trauma hip fracture); prevention of osteoporosis in postmenopausal women, treatment of osteoporosis in men (to increase bone mass); treatment and prevention of glucocorticoid-induced osteoporosis (in patients initiating or continuing prednisone ≥7.5 mg/day [or equivalent] and expected to remain on glucocorticoids for at least 12 months)

Dosage Summary

I.V.:

Children: Dosage not established

Adults:

Zometa®: 4 mg as a single dose [hypercalcemia of malignancy] or 4 mg every 3-4 weeks [multiple myeloma or metastatic bone lesions]

Reclast®: 5 mg [Paget disease] or 5 mg once a year or every 2 years [osteoporosis]

Dosage Forms

Infusion, solution, premixed:

Reclast®: 5 mg (100 mL)

Injection, solution:

Zometa®: 4 mg/5 mL (5 mL)

Dosage Forms - Canada

Infusion, solution [premixed]:

Aclasta®: 5 mg (100 mL)

Zolicef® *(Discontinued)* *see* cefazolin *on page* 189

Zolinza™ [US/Can] *see* vorinostat *on page* 992

zolmitriptan (zohl mi TRIP tan)

Sound-Alike/Look-Alike Issues

zolmitriptan may be confused with SUMAtriptan

Synonyms 311C90

U.S./Canadian Brand Names Zomig-ZMT® [US]; Zomig® Nasal Spray [Can]; Zomig® Rapimelt [Can]; Zomig® [US/Can]

Therapeutic Category Antimigraine Agent; Serotonin Agonist

Use Acute treatment of migraine with or without aura

Dosage Summary

Nasal Inhalation:

Children: Dosage not established

Adults: 1 spray (5 mg) at the onset of migraine headache; may repeat in 2 hours if no relief (maximum: 10 mg/24 hours)

Oral:

Children: Dosage not established

Adults: 1.25-2.5 mg at the onset of migraine headache; may repeat in 2 hours if no relief (maximum: 10 mg/24 hours)

Dosage Forms

Solution, intranasal:

Zomig®: 5 mg/0.1 mL (0.1 mL)

Tablet, oral:

Zomig®: 2.5 mg, 5 mg

Tablet, orally disintegrating, oral:

Zomig-ZMT®: 2.5 mg, 5 mg

Zoloft® [US/Can] *see* sertraline *on page* 872

zolpidem (zole PI dem)

Sound-Alike/Look-Alike Issues

zolpidem may be confused with lorazepam, zaleplon

Ambien® may be confused with Abilify®, Ativan®, Ambi 10®

Synonyms zolpidem tartrate; Zolpimist®

U.S./Canadian Brand Names Ambien CR® [US]; Ambien® [US]; Edluar™ [US]

Therapeutic Category Hypnotic, Nonbarbiturate

Controlled Substance C-IV

Use

Ambien®, Edluar™: Short-term treatment of insomnia (with difficulty of sleep onset)

Ambien CR®: Treatment of insomnia (with difficulty of sleep onset and/or sleep maintenance)

Dosage Summary

Oral:

Children: Dosage not established

Adults: 10-12.5 mg immediately before bedtime

Elderly: 5-6.25 mg immediately before bedtime

Product Availability Zolpimist® oral spray: FDA approved December, 2008; availability currently undetermined

Zolpimist® is an oral spray of zolpidem indicated for the short-term treatment of insomnia characterized by difficulties with sleep initiation.

Dosage Forms

Tablet, oral: 5 mg, 10 mg

Ambien®: 5 mg, 10 mg

Tablet, sublingual:

Edluar™: 5 mg, 10 mg

Tablet, extended release, oral:

Ambien CR®: 6.25 mg, 12.5 mg

zolpidem tartrate *see* zolpidem *on page 1004*

Zolpimist® *see* zolpidem *on page 1004*

Zometa® [US/Can] *see* zoledronic acid *on page 1003*

Zomig® [US/Can] *see* zolmitriptan *on page 1004*

Zomig® Nasal Spray [Can] *see* zolmitriptan *on page 1004*

Zomig® Rapimelt [Can] *see* zolmitriptan *on page 1004*

Zomig-ZMT® [US] *see* zolmitriptan *on page 1004*

Zonalon® [US/Can] *see* doxepin (topical) *on page 329*

Zonatuss™ [US] *see* benzonatate *on page 128*

Zonegran® [US] *see* zonisamide *on page 1005*

zonisamide (zoe NIS a mide)

Sound-Alike/Look-Alike Issues

zonisamide may be confused with lacosamide

Zonegran® may be confused with Sinequan®

U.S./Canadian Brand Names Zonegran® [US]

Therapeutic Category Anticonvulsant, Sulfonamide

Use Adjunct treatment of partial seizures in children >16 years of age and adults with epilepsy

Dosage Summary

Oral:

Children ≤16 years: Dosage not established

Children >16 years: Initial: 100 mg/day; Maintenance: 100-600 mg/day (maximum: 600 mg/day); **Note:** Titration is recommended (increase dose by 100 mg/day every 2 weeks)

Adults: Initial: 100 mg/day; Maintenance: 100-600 mg/day (maximum: 600 mg/day); **Note:** Titration is recommended (increase dose by 100 mg/day every 2 weeks)

Dosage Forms

Capsule, oral: 25 mg, 50 mg, 100 mg

Zonegran®: 25 mg, 100 mg

zopiclone *(Canada only)* (ZOE pi clone)

U.S./Canadian Brand Names Apo-Zopiclone® [Can]; CO Zopiclone [Can]; Dom-Zopiclone [Can]; Imovane® [Can]; Mylan-Zopiclone [Can]; Novo-Zopiclone [Can]; Nu-Zopiclone [Can]; PHL-Zopiclone [Can]; PMS-Zopiclone [Can]; PRO-Zopiclone [Can]; RAN™-Zopiclone [Can]; ratio-Zopiclone [Can]; Rhovane® [Can]; Riva-Zopiclone [Can]; Sandoz-Zopiclone [Can]

Therapeutic Category Hypnotic

Use Symptomatic relief of transient and short-term insomnia

Dosage Summary

Oral:

Children: Dosage not established

Adults: 3.75-7.5 mg just before retiring for the night

Elderly: Initial: 3.75 mg just before retiring for the night; may increase to 5-7.5 mg

Dosage Forms - Canada

Tablet:

Apo-Zopiclone®, Gen-Zopiclone, Imovane®, Novo-Zopiclone, Nu-Zopiclone, PMS-Zopiclone, Rhovane®, Rhoxal-zopiclone: 5 mg, 7.5 mg

Zorbtive® [US] *see* somatropin *on page 889*

Zorcaine™ [US/Can] *see* articaine and epinephrine *on page 96*

ZORprin® ***(Discontinued)*** *see* aspirin *on page 100*
Zortress® [US] *see* everolimus *on page 385*
ZOS *see* zoster vaccine *on page 1006*
Zostavax® [US] *see* zoster vaccine *on page 1006*

zoster vaccine (ZOS ter vak SEEN)

Synonyms shingles vaccine; varicella-zoster (VZV) vaccine (zoster); VZV vaccine (zoster); ZOS

U.S./Canadian Brand Names Zostavax® [US]

Therapeutic Category Vaccine

Use Prevention of herpes zoster (shingles) in patients ≥60 years of age

The Advisory Committee on Immunization Practices (ACIP) recommends routine vaccination of all patients ≥60 years of age, including:

- Patients who report a previous episode of zoster.
- Patients with chronic medical conditions (eg, chronic renal failure, diabetes mellitus, rheumatoid arthritis, chronic pulmonary disease) unless those conditions are contraindications.
- Residents of nursing homes and other long-term care facilities ≥60 years of age, without contraindications.

Dosage Summary

SubQ:

Children: Dosage not established
Adults <60 years: Dosage not established
Adults ≥60 years: 0.65 mL administered as a single dose

Dosage Forms

Injection, powder for reconstitution [preservative free]:
Zostavax®: 19,400 PFU

Zostrix® [US-OTC/Can] *see* capsaicin *on page 175*
Zostrix® Diabetic Foot Pain [US-OTC] *see* capsaicin *on page 175*
Zostrix®-HP [US-OTC/Can] *see* capsaicin *on page 175*
Zostrix® Neuropathy ***(Discontinued)*** *see* capsaicin *on page 175*
Zosyn® [US] *see* piperacillin and tazobactam sodium *on page 763*
Zovia® [US] *see* ethinyl estradiol and ethynodiol diacetate *on page 376*
Zovirax® [US/Can] *see* acyclovir (systemic) *on page 36*
Zovirax® [US/Can] *see* acyclovir (topical) *on page 37*
Z-Pak *see* azithromycin (systemic) *on page 111*
Ztuss™ Tablet ***(Discontinued)***
Ztuss™ ZT ***(Discontinued)***
zuclopenthixol acetate *see* zuclopenthixol *(Canada only) on page 1006*

zuclopenthixol *(Canada only)* (zoo kloe pen THIX ol)

Synonyms Z-chlopenthixol; zuclopenthixol acetate; zuclopenthixol decanoate; zuclopenthixol dihydrochloride

U.S./Canadian Brand Names Clopixol-Acuphase® [Can]; Clopixol® Depot [Can]; Clopixol® [Can]

Therapeutic Category Antipsychotic Agent

Use Management of schizophrenia; acetate injection is intended for short-term acute treatment; decanoate injection is for long-term management; dihydrochloride tablets may be used in either phase

Dosage Summary

I.M.:

Children: Dosage not established
Adults: Acetate: Initial: 50-150 mg, may repeat in 2-3 days (maximum: 4 doses or 400 mg/2 week treatment course); Decanoate: Initial: 100 mg as single dose; Maintenance: 100-600 mg every 1-4 weeks (maximum: 600 mg/week)

Oral:

Children: Dosage not established
Adults: Initial: 10-50 mg/day in 2-3 divided doses; Maintenance: 20-100 mg/day in 2-3 divided doses (maximum: 100 mg/day)

Dosage Forms - Canada

Injection:

Clopixol Acuphase®: 50 mg/mL [zuclopenthixol 42.5 mg/mL] (1 mL, 2 mL)

Clopixol® Depot: 200 mg/mL [zuclopenthixol 144.4 mg/mL] (10 mL)

Tablet:

Clopixol®: 10 mg, 25 mg, 40 mg

CHEMOTHERAPY REGIMENS

5 + 2

Use Leukemia, acute myeloid (induction)

Regimen

Cytarabine: I.V.: 100-200 mg/m^2/day continuous infusion days 1 to 5
[total dose/cycle = 500-1000 mg/m^2]

with

Daunorubicin: I.V.: 45 mg/m^2/day days 1 and 2
[total dose/cycle = 90 mg/m^2]

7 + 3 + 7

Use Leukemia, acute myeloid

Regimen

Cytarabine: I.V.: 100 mg/m^2/day continuous infusion days 1 to 7
[total dose/cycle = 700 mg/m^2]
Daunorubicin: I.V.: 50 mg/m^2/day days 1, 2, and 3
[total dose/cycle = 150 mg/m^2]
Etoposide: I.V.: 75 mg/m^2/day days 1 to 7
[total dose/cycle = 525 mg/m^2]
Repeat cycle every 21 days; up to 3 cycles may be given based on individual response

7 + 3 (Daunorubicin)

Use Leukemia, acute myeloid (induction)

Regimen

Cytarabine: I.V.: 100 mg/m^2/day continuous infusion days 1 to 7
[total dose/cycle = 700 mg/m^2]
Daunorubicin: I.V.: 45 mg/m^2/day days 1, 2, and 3
[total dose/cycle = 135 mg/m^2]
Administer one cycle only

7 + 3 (Idarubicin)

Use Leukemia, acute myeloid (induction)

Regimen

Cytarabine: I.V.: 100-200 mg/m^2/day continuous infusion days 1 to 7
[total dose/cycle = 700-1400 mg/m^2]
Idarubicin: I.V.: 12 mg/m^2/day days 1, 2, and 3
[total dose/cycle = 36 mg/m^2]
Administer one cycle only

7 + 3 (Mitoxantrone)

Use Leukemia, acute myeloid (induction)

Regimen

Cytarabine: I.V.: 100-200 mg/m^2/day continuous infusion days 1 to 7
[total dose/cycle = 700-1400 mg/m^2]
Mitoxantrone: I.V.: 12 mg/m^2/day days 1, 2, and 3
[total dose/cycle = 36 mg/m^2]
Administer one cycle only

8 in 1 (Brain Tumors)

Use Brain tumors

Regimen NOTE: Multiple variations are listed below.

Variation 1:

Methylprednisolone: I.V.: 300 mg/m^2 every 6 hours day 1 (3 doses)
[total dose/cycle = 900 mg/m^2]
Vincristine: I.V.: 1.5 mg/m^2 (maximum dose: 2 mg) day 1
Lomustine: Oral: 75 mg/m^2 day 1
Procarbazine: Oral: 75 mg/m^2 day 1; 1 hour after methylprednisolone and vincristine
Hydroxyurea: Oral: 3000 mg/m^2 day 1; 2 hours after methylprednisolone and vincristine
Cisplatin: I.V.: 90 mg/m^2 day 1; 3 hours after methylprednisolone and vincristine
Cytarabine: I.V.: 300 mg/m^2 day 1; 9 hours after methylprednisolone and vincristine
Dacarbazine: I.V.: 150 mg/m^2 day 1; 12 hours after methylprednisolone and vincristine
Repeat cycle every 14 days

Variation 2:
Methylprednisolone: I.V.: 300 mg/m^2 every 6 hours day 1 (3 doses)
[total dose/cycle = 900 mg/m^2]
Vincristine: I.V.: 1.5 mg/m^2 (maximum dose: 2 mg) day 1
Lomustine: Oral: 75 mg/m^2 day 1
Procarbazine: Oral: 75 mg/m^2 day 1; 1 hour after methylprednisolone and vincristine
Hydroxyurea: Oral: 3000 mg/m^2 day 1; 2 hours after methylprednisolone and vincristine
Cisplatin: I.V.: 60 mg/m^2 day 1; 3 hours after methylprednisolone and vincristine
Cytarabine: I.V.: 300 mg/m^2 day 1; 9 hours after methylprednisolone and vincristine
Cyclophosphamide: I.V.: 300 mg/m^2 day 1; 12 hours after methylprednisolone and vincristine
Repeat cycle every 14 days

8 in 1 (Retinoblastoma)

Use Retinoblastoma

Regimen
Vincristine: I.V.: 1.5 mg/m^2 day 1
Methylprednisolone: I.V.: 300 mg/m^2 day 1
Lomustine: Oral: 75 mg/m^2 day 1
Procarbazine: Oral: 75 mg/m^2 day 1
Hydroxyurea: Oral: 1500 mg/m^2 day 1
Cisplatin: I.V.: 60 mg/m^2 day 1
Cytarabine: I.V.: 300 mg/m^2 day 1
Repeat cycle every 28 days

AAV (DD)

Use Wilms tumor

Regimen
Dactinomycin: I.V.: 15 mcg/kg/day days 1 to 5 of weeks 0, 13, 26, 39, 52, and 65
[total dose/cycle = 450 mcg/kg]
Doxorubicin: I.V.: 20 mg/m^2/day days 1, 2, and 3 of weeks 6, 19, 32, 45, and 58
[total dose/cycle = 300 mg/m^2]
Vincristine: I.V.: 1.5 mg/m^2 day 1 of weeks 0-10, 13, 14, 26, 27, 39, 40, 52, 53, 65, and 66
[total dose/cycle = 31.5 mg/m^2]

ABVD

Use Lymphoma, Hodgkin disease

Regimen
Doxorubicin: I.V.: 25 mg/m^2/day days 1 and 15
[total dose/cycle = 50 mg/m^2]
Bleomycin: I.V.: 10 units/m^2/day days 1 and 15
[total dose/cycle = 20 units/m^2]
Vinblastine: I.V.: 6 mg/m^2/day days 1 and 15
[total dose/cycle = 12 mg/m^2]
Dacarbazine: I.V.: 375 mg/m^2/day days 1 and 15
[total dose/cycle = 750 mg/m^2]
Repeat cycle every 28 days

AC

Use Breast cancer

Regimen NOTE: Multiple variations are listed below.
Variation 1: AC (conventional):
Doxorubicin: I.V.: 60 mg/m^2 day 1
[total dose/cycle = 60 mg/m^2]
Cyclophosphamide: I.V.: 600 mg/m^2 day 1
[total dose/cycle = 600 mg/m^2]
Repeat cycle every 21 days

Variation 2:
Cyclophosphamide: Oral: 200 mg/m^2/day days 3 to 6
[total dose/cycle = 800 mg/m^2]
Doxorubicin: I.V.: 40 mg/m^2 day 1
[total dose/cycle = 40 mg/m^2]
Repeat cycle every 3 weeks for 3 cycles, then every 4 weeks

AC/Paclitaxel (Sequential)

Use Breast cancer

Regimen

Variation 1: AC + Paclitaxel (conventional):
Doxorubicin: I.V.: 60 mg/m^2 day 1
[total dose/cycle = 60 mg/m^2]
Cyclophosphamide: I.V.: 600 mg/m^2 day 1
[total dose/cycle = 600 mg/m^2]
Repeat cycle every 21 days for 4 cycles
followed by
Paclitaxel: I.V.: 175 mg/m^2 day 1
[total dose/cycle = 175 mg/m^2]
Repeat cycle every 21 days for 4 cycles

Variation 2: AC + Paclitaxel (dose dense):
Doxorubicin: I.V.: 60 mg/m^2 day 1
[total dose/cycle = 60 mg/m^2]
Cyclophosphamide: I.V.: 600 mg/m^2 day 1
[total dose/cycle = 600 mg/m^2]
Filgrastim: SubQ: 5 mcg/kg/day days 3 to 10
[total dose/cycle = 40 mcg/kg]
Repeat cycle every 14 days for 4 cycles
followed by
Paclitaxel: I.V.: 175 mg/m^2 day 1
[total dose/cycle = 175 mg/m^2]
Filgrastim: SubQ: 5 mcg/kg/day days 3 to 10
[total dose/cycle = 40 mcg/kg]
Repeat cycle every 14 days for 4 cycles

AC-Paclitaxel-Trastuzumab

Use Breast cancer

Regimen NOTE: Multiple variations are listed below.

Variation 1:
Doxorubicin: I.V.: 60 mg/m^2 day 1
[total dose/cycle = 60 mg/m^2]
Cyclophosphamide: I.V.: 600 mg/m^2 day 1
[total dose/cycle = 600 mg/m^2]
Repeat cycle every 21 days for 4 cycles
followed by
Paclitaxel: I.V.: 175 mg/m^2 day 1
[total dose/cycle = 175 mg/m^2]
Trastuzumab: I.V.: 4 mg/kg (loading dose) day 1 (cycle 1 only)
[total dose/cycle = 4 mg/kg]
followed by I.V.: 2 mg/kg/day days 8 and 15 (cycle 1)
[total dose/cycle = 4 mg/kg]
then I.V.: 2 mg/kg/day days 1, 8, and 15 (cycles 2, 3, and 4)
[total dose/cycle = 6 mg/kg]
Repeat cycle every 21 days for 4 cycles
followed by
Trastuzumab: I.V.: 2 mg/kg weekly for 40 weeks

Variation 2:
Doxorubicin: I.V.: 60 mg/m^2 day 1
[total dose/cycle = 60 mg/m^2]
Cyclophosphamide: I.V.: 600 mg/m^2 day 1
[total dose/cycle = 600 mg/m^2]
Repeat cycle every 21 days for 4 cycles
followed by
Paclitaxel: I.V.: 80 mg/m^{2}day 1 week 13
[total dose/cycle = 80 mg/m^2]
Trastuzumab: I.V.: 4 mg/kg (loading dose) day 1 week 13 only
[total dose/cycle = 4 mg/kg]
followed by
Paclitaxel: I.V.: 80 mg/m^2 weekly
[total dose/cycle = 80 mg/m^2]
Trastuzumab: I.V.: 2 mg/kg /weekly
[total dose/cycle = 2 mg/kg]
Repeat cycle every week for 11 cycles
followed by
Trastuzumab: I.V.: 2 mg/kg/weekly for 40 weeks

AD

Use Soft tissue sarcoma
Regimen
Doxorubicin: I.V.: 60 mg/m^2 day 1
[total dose/cycle = 60 mg/m^2]
Dacarbazine: I.V.: 250 mg/m^2/day days 1 to 5
[total dose/cycle = 1250 mg/m^2]
Repeat cycle every 21 days

AI

Use Soft tissue sarcoma
Regimen NOTE: Multiple variations are listed below.
Variation 1:
Doxorubicin: I.V.: 25 mg/m^2/day continuous infusion days 1, 2, and 3
[total dose/cycle = 75 mg/m^2]
Ifosfamide: I.V.: 2 g/m^2/day days 1 to 5
[total dose/cycle = 10 g/m^2]
Mesna: I.V.: 400 mg/m^2 day 1
followed by I.V.: 1200 mg/m^2/day continuous infusion days 1 to 5
[total dose/cycle = 6400 mg/m^2]
Repeat cycle every 3 weeks
Variation 2:
Doxorubicin: I.V.: 30 mg/m^2/day continuous infusion days 1, 2, and 3
[total dose/cycle = 90 mg/m^2]
Ifosfamide: I.V.: 2.5 g/m^2/day days 1 to 4
[total dose/cycle = 10 g/m^2]
Mesna: I.V.: 500 mg/m^2 day 1
followed by I.V.: 1500 mg/m^2/day continuous infusion days 1 to 4
[total dose/cycle = 6500 mg/m^2]
Filgrastim: SubQ: 5 mcg/kg/day days 5 through ANC recovery
Repeat cycle every 3 weeks

AP

Use Endometrial cancer
Regimen
Doxorubicin: I.V.: 60 mg/m^2 day 1
[total dose/cycle = 60 mg/m^2]
Cisplatin: I.V.: 60 mg/m^2 day 1
[total dose/cycle = 60 mg/m^2]
Repeat cycle every 21-28 days

AT

Use Breast cancer

Regimen NOTE: Multiple variations are listed below.

Variation 1:
- Doxorubicin: I.V.: 50 mg/m^2 day 1
  [total dose/cycle = 50 mg/m^2]
- Docetaxel: I.V.: 75 mg/m^2 day 1
  [total dose/cycle = 75 mg/m^2]
- Repeat cycle every 3 weeks

Variation 2:
- Doxorubicin: I.V.: 60 mg/m^2 day 1
  [total dose/cycle = 60 mg/m^2]
- Docetaxel: I.V.: 60 mg/m^2 day 1
  [total dose/cycle = 60 mg/m^2]
- Repeat cycle every 3 weeks

Variation 3:
- Doxorubicin: I.V.: 50 mg/m^2 day 1
  [total dose/cycle = 50 mg/m^2]
- Docetaxel: I.V.: 75 mg/m^2 day 1
  [total dose/cycle = 75 mg/m^2]
- Repeat cycle every 14 days

Variation 4:
- Doxorubicin: I.V.: 50 mg/m^2 day 1
  [total dose/cycle = 50 mg/m^2]
- Docetaxel: I.V.: 60 mg/m^2 day 1
  [total dose/cycle = 60 mg/m^2]
- Repeat cycle every 3 weeks

Variation 5:
- Doxorubicin: I.V.: 50 mg/m^2 day 1
  [total dose/cycle = 50 mg/m^2]
- Docetaxel: I.V.: 60 mg/m^2 day 1
  [total dose/cycle = 60 mg/m^2]
- Repeat cycle every 3-4 weeks

Variation 6:
- Doxorubicin: I.V.: 56 mg/m^2 day 1
  [total dose/cycle = 56 mg/m^2]
- Docetaxel: I.V.: 75 mg/m^2 day 1
  [total dose/cycle = 75 mg/m^2]
- Repeat cycle every 3 weeks

Variation 7:
- Doxorubicin: I.V.: 50 mg/m^2 day 1
  [total dose/cycle = 50 mg/m^2]
- Docetaxel: I.V.: 75 mg/m^2 day 2
  [total dose/cycle = 75 mg/m^2]
- Repeat cycle every 4 weeks

AVD

Use Wilms tumor

Regimen

- Dactinomycin: I.V.: 15 mcg/kg/day days 1 to 5 of weeks 0, 13, 26, 39, 52, and 65
  [total dose/cycle = 450 mcg/kg]
- Doxorubicin: I.V.: 60 mg/m^2 day 1 of weeks 6, 19, 32, 45, and 58
  [total dose/cycle = 300 mg/m^2]
- Vincristine: I.V.: 1.5 mg/m^2 day 1 of weeks 1 to 8, 13, 14, 26, 27, 39, 40, 52, 53, 65, and 66
  [total dose/cycle = 27 mg/m^2]

AV (EE)

Use Wilms tumor

Regimen

Dactinomycin: I.V.: 15 mcg/kg/day days 1 to 5 of weeks 0, 5, 13, and 26
[total dose/cycle = 300 mcg/kg]
Vincristine: I.V.: 1.5 mg/m^2/dose day 1 of weeks 1 to 10, and days 1 and 5 of weeks 13 and 26
[total dose/cycle = 21 mg/m^2]

AV (K)

Use Wilms tumor

Regimen

Dactinomycin: I.V.: 15 mcg/kg/day days 1 to 5 of weeks 0, 5, 13, 22, 31, 40, 49, and 58
[total dose/cycle = 600 mcg/kg]
Vincristine: I.V.: 1.5 mg/m^2/dose day 1 of weeks 0-10, 15-20, 24-29, 33-38, 42-47, 51-56, and 60-65
[total dose/cycle = 70.5 mg/m^2]

AV (L)

Use Wilms tumor

Regimen

Dactinomycin: I.V.: 15 mcg/kg/day days 1 to 5 of weeks 0 and 5
[total dose/cycle = 150 mcg/kg]
Vincristine: I.V.: 1.5 mg/m^2 day 1 of weeks 0-10
[total dose/cycle = 16.5 mg/m^2]

AV (Wilms Tumor)

Use Wilms tumor

Regimen

Dactinomycin: I.V.: 15 mcg/kg/day days 1 to 5 of weeks 0, 13, 26, 39, 52, and 65
[total dose/cycle = 450 mcg/kg]
Vincristine: I.V.: 1.5 mg/m^2/dose day 1 of weeks 1 to 8, 13, 14, 26, 27, 39, 40, 52, 53, 65, and 66
[total dose/cycle = 27 mg/m^2]

BEACOPP-14 (Hodgkin Lymphoma)

Use Lymphoma, Hodgkin disease

Regimen

Bleomycin: I.V.: 10 units/m^2 day 8
[total dose/cycle = 10 units/m^2]
Etoposide: I.V.: 100 mg/m^2/day days 1, 2, and 3
[total dose/cycle = 300 mg/m^2]
Doxorubicin: I.V.: 25 mg/m^2 day 1
[total dose/cycle = 25 mg/m^2]
Cyclophosphamide: I.V.: 650 mg/m^2 day 1
[total dose/cycle = 650 mg/m^2]
Vincristine: I.V.: 1.4 mg/m^2 (maximum dose: 2 mg) day 8
[total dose/cycle = 1.4 mg/m^2; maximum: 2 mg]
Procarbazine: Oral: 100 mg/m^2/day days 1 to 7
[total dose/cycle = 700 mg/m^2]
Prednisone: Oral: 80 mg/m^2/day days 1 to 7
[total dose/cycle = 560 mg/m^2]
Filgrastim: SubQ: 300 or 480 mcg/day days 8 to13
Repeat cycle every 14 days for a total of 8 cycles

BEACOPP Escalated (Hodgkin Lymphoma)

Use Lymphoma, Hodgkin disease

Regimen NOTE: Multiple variations are listed below.

Variation 1:
Bleomycin: I.V.: 10 units/m^2 day 8
[total dose/cycle = 10 units/m^2]

Etoposide: I.V.: 200 mg/m^2/day days 1, 2, and 3
[total dose/cycle = 600 mg/m^2]
Doxorubicin: I.V.: 35 mg/m^2 day 1
[total dose/cycle = 35 mg/m^2]
Cyclophosphamide: I.V.: 1200 mg/m^2 day 1
[total dose/cycle = 1200 mg/m^2]
Vincristine: I.V.: 1.4 mg/m^2 (maximum dose: 2 mg) day 8
[total dose/cycle = 1.4 mg/m^2: maximum: 2 mg]
Procarbazine: Oral: 100 mg/m^2/day days 1 to 7
[total dose/cycle = 700 mg/m^2]
Prednisone: Oral: 40 mg/m^2/day days 1 to 14
[total dose/cycle = 560 mg/m^2]
Filgrastim: SubQ: 300 or 480 mcg/day day 8 until leukocyte recovery (3 days at >1000/mm^3)
Repeat cycle every 21 days for a total of 8 cycles

Variation 2:
Bleomycin: I.V.: 10 units/m^2 day 8
[total dose/cycle = 10 units/m^2]
Etoposide: I.V.: 200 mg/m^2/day days 1, 2, and 3
[total dose/cycle = 600 mg/m^2]
Doxorubicin: I.V.: 35 mg/m^2 day 1
[total dose/cycle = 35 mg/m^2]
Cyclophosphamide: I.V.: 1250 mg/m^2 day 1
[total dose/cycle = 1250 mg/m^2]
Vincristine: I.V.: 1.4 mg/m^2 (maximum dose: 2 mg) day 8
[total dose/cycle = 1.4 mg/m^2; maximum: 2 mg]
Procarbazine: Oral: 100 mg/m^2/day days 1 to 7
total dose/cycle = 700 mg/m^2]
Prednisone: Oral: 40 mg/m^2/day days 1 to 14
[total dose/cycle = 560 mg/m^2]
Filgrastim: SubQ: Daily (dose not specified) beginning day 8 until leukocyte recovery
Repeat cycle every 21 days for a total of 8 cycles

Variation 3:
Bleomycin: I.V.: 10 units/m^2 day 8
[total dose/cycle = 10 units/m^2]
Etoposide: I.V.: 200 mg/m^2/day days 1, 2, and 3
[total dose/cycle = 600 mg/m^2]
Doxorubicin: I.V.: 35 mg/m^2 day 1
[total dose/cycle = 35 mg/m^2]
Cyclophosphamide: I.V.: 1250 mg/m^2 day 1
[total dose/cycle = 1250 mg/m^2]
Mesna: I.V.: 250 mg/m^2 day 1
[total dose/cycle = 250 mg/m^2]
Mesna: Oral: 500 mg/m^2/dose at hour 2 and hour 5 day 1
[total dose/cycle = 1000 mg/m^2]
Vincristine: I.V.: 1.4 mg/m^2 (maximum dose: 2 mg) day 8
[total dose/cycle = 1.4 mg/m^2; maximum: 2 mg]
Procarbazine: Oral: 100 mg/m^2/day days 1 to 7
[total dose/cycle = 700 mg/m^2]
Prednisone: Oral: 40 mg/m^2/day days 1 to 7
[total dose/cycle = 280 mg/m^2]
Filgrastim: SubQ: (dose not specified)
Repeat cycle every 21 days for a total of 6 cycles

Variation 4:
Bleomycin: I.V.: 10 units/m^2 day 8
[total dose/cycle = 10 units/m^2]
Etoposide: I.V.: 200 mg/m^2/day days 1, 2, and 3
[total dose/cycle = 600 mg/m^2]
Doxorubicin: I.V.: 35 mg/m^2 day 1
[total dose/cycle = 35 mg/m^2]
Cyclophosphamide: I.V.: 1250 mg/m^2 day 1
[total dose/cycle = 1250 mg/m^2]
Mesna: I.V.: 250 mg/m^2/dose at hours 0, 4, and 8 day 1
[total dose/cycle = 750 mg/m^2]

Vincristine: I.V.: 1.4 mg/m^2 (maximum dose: 2 mg) day 8
[total dose/cycle = 1.4 mg/m^2; maximum: 2 mg]
Procarbazine: Oral: 100 mg/m^2/day days 1 to 7
[total dose/cycle = 700 mg/m^2]
Prednisone: Oral: 40 mg/m^2/day days 1 to 14
[total dose/cycle = 560 mg/m^2]
Filgrastim: SubQ: 300 or 480 mcg/day day 8 until leukocyte recovery (3 days at >1000/mm^3)
Repeat cycle every 21 days for a total of 8 cycles
Variation 5 (studied in children):
Bleomycin: I.V.: 10 units/m^2 day 8
[total dose/cycle = 10 units/m^2]
Etoposide: I.V.: 200 mg/m^2/day days 1, 2, and 3
[total dose/cycle = 600 mg/m^2]
Doxorubicin: I.V.: 35 mg/m^2 day 1
[total dose/cycle = 35 mg/m^2]
Cyclophosphamide: I.V.: 1200 mg/m^2 day 1
[total dose/cycle = 1200 mg/m^2]
Vincristine: I.V.: 2 mg/m^2 (maximum dose: 2 mg) day 8
[total dose/cycle = 2 mg/m^2; maximum: 2 mg]
Procarbazine: Oral: 100 mg/m^2/day days 1 to 7
[total dose/cycle = 700 mg/m^2]
Prednisone: Oral: 40 mg/m^2/day days 1 to 14
[total dose/cycle = 560 mg/m^2]
Repeat cycle every 21 days for 4 cycles (may repeat with 4 more cycles if "slow early responder")

BEACOPP Standard (Hodgkin Lymphoma)

Use Lymphoma, Hodgkin disease

Regimen NOTE: Multiple variations are listed below.
Variation 1:
Bleomycin: I.V.: 10 units/m^2 day 8
[total dose/cycle = 10 units/m^2]
Etoposide: I.V.: 100 mg/m^2/day days 1, 2, and 3
[total dose/cycle = 300 mg/m^2]
Doxorubicin: I.V.: 25 mg/m^2 day 1
[total dose/cycle = 25 mg/m^2]
Cyclophosphamide: I.V.: 650 mg/m^2 day 1
[total dose/cycle = 650 mg/m^2]
Vincristine: I.V.: 1.4 mg/m^2 (maximum dose: 2 mg) day 8
[total dose/cycle = 1.4 mg/m^2; maximum: 2 mg]
Procarbazine: Oral: 100 mg/m^2/day days 1 to 7
[total dose/cycle = 700 mg/m^2]
Prednisone: Oral: 40 mg/m^2/day days 1 to 14
[total dose/cycle = 560 mg/m^2]
Repeat cycle every 21 days for a total of 8 cycles
Variation 2:
Bleomycin: I.V.: 10 units/m^2 day 8
[total dose/cycle = 10 units/m^2]
Etoposide: I.V.: 100 mg/m^2/day days 1, 2, and 3
[total dose/cycle = 300 mg/m^2]
Doxorubicin: I.V.: 25 mg/m^2 day 1
[total dose/cycle = 25 mg/m^2]
Cyclophosphamide: I.V.: 650 mg/m^2 day 1
[total dose/cycle = 650 mg/m^2]
Vincristine: I.V.: 1.4 mg/m^2 (maximum dose: 2 mg) day 8
[total dose/cycle = 1.4 mg/m^2; maximum: 2 mg]
Procarbazine: Oral: 100 mg/m^2/day days 1 to 7
[total dose/cycle = 700 mg/m^2]
Prednisone: Oral: 40 mg/m^2/day days 1 to 7
[total dose/cycle = 280 mg/m^2]
Repeat cycle every 21 days for a total of 6 cycles

Variation 3:
Bleomycin: I.V.: 10 units/m^2 day 8
[total dose/cycle = 10 units/m^2]
Etoposide: Oral: 50 mg/m^2/day days 3 to 12
[total dose/cycle = 500 mg/m^2]
Doxorubicin: I.V.: 40 mg/m^2 day 1
[total dose/cycle = 40 mg/m^2]
Cyclophosphamide: I.V.: 650 mg/m^2 day 1
[total dose/cycle = 650 mg/m^2]
Vincristine: I.V.: 1.4 mg/m^2 (maximum dose: 2 mg) day 8
[total dose/cycle = 1.4 mg/m^2; maximum: 2 mg]
Procarbazine: Oral: 100 mg/m^2/day days 1 to 7
[total dose/cycle = 700 mg/m^2]
Prednisone: Oral: 40 mg/m^2/day days 1 to 14
[total dose/cycle = 560 mg/m^2]
Repeat cycle every 21 days for a total of 8 cycles
Variation 4:
Bleomycin: I.V.: 10 units/m^2 day 8
[total dose/cycle = 10 units/m^2]
Etoposide: I.V.: 100 mg/m^2/day days 1, 2, and 3
[total dose/cycle = 300 mg/m^2]
Doxorubicin: I.V.: 25 mg/m^2 day 1
[total dose/cycle = 25 mg/m^2]
Cyclophosphamide: I.V.: 650 mg/m^2 day 1
[total dose/cycle = 650 mg/m^2]
Vincristine: I.V.: 2 mg day 8
[total dose/cycle = 2 mg]
Procarbazine: Oral: 100 mg/m^2/day days 1 to 7
[total dose/cycle = 700 mg/m^2]
Prednisone: Oral: 40 mg/m^2/day days 1 to 7
[total dose/cycle = 280 mg/m^2]
Repeat cycle every 21 days for a total of 8 cycles

Bendamustine-Rituximab

Use Lymphoma, non-Hodgkin (mantle cell or low-grade NHL)
Regimen NOTE: Multiple variations are listed below.
Variation 1:
Pretreatment:
Rituximab: I.V.: 375 mg/m^2 1 week before the start of cycle 1
[total dose/pretreatment = 375 mg/m^2]
Cycles:
Rituximab: I.V.: 375 mg/m^2 day 1
[total dose/cycle = 375 mg/m^2]
Bendamustine: I.V.: 90 mg/m^2 days 2 and 3
[total dose/cycle = 180 mg/m^2]
Repeat cycle every 4 weeks for up to 4 cycles
Post-Treatment:
Rituximab: I.V.: 375 mg/m^2 4 weeks after the last cycle
[total dose/post-treatment = 375 mg/m^2]
Variation 2:
Pretreatment:
Rituximab: I.V.: 375 mg/m^2 1 week before the start of cycle 1
[total dose/pretreatment = 375 mg/m^2]
Cycles:
Rituximab: I.V.: 375 mg/m^2 day 1
[total dose/cycle = 375 mg/m^2]
Bendamustine: I.V.: 90 mg/m^2 days 2 and 3
[total dose/cycle = 180 mg/m^2]
Repeat cycle every 4 weeks for 4-6 cycles
Post-Treatment:
Rituximab: I.V.: 375 mg/m^2 4 weeks after the last cycle
[total dose/post-treatment = 375 mg/m^2]

BEP (Ovarian Cancer)

Use Ovarian cancer

Regimen

Bleomycin: I.V.: 20 units/m^2 (maximum dose: 30 units) day 1
[total dose/cycle = 20 units/m^2]
Etoposide: I.V.: 75 mg/m^2/day days 1 to 5
[total dose/cycle = 375 mg/m^2]
or I.V.: 75 mg/m^2/day days 1 to 4 (if received prior radiation therapy)
[total dose/cycle = 300 mg/m^2]
Cisplatin: I.V.: 20 mg/m^2/day days 1 to 5
[total dose/cycle = 100 mg/m^2]
Repeat cycle every 3 weeks for 4 cycles

BEP (Ovarian Cancer, Testicular Cancer)

Use Ovarian cancer; Testicular cancer

Regimen

Bleomycin: I.V.: 30 units/day days 2, 9, and 16
[total dose/cycle = 90 units]
Etoposide: I.V.: 100 mg/m^2/day days 1 to 5
[total dose/cycle = 500 mg/m^2]
or I.V.: 120 mg/m^2/day days 1, 2, and 3
[total dose/cycle = 360 mg/m^2]
Cisplatin: I.V.: 20 mg/m^2/day days 1 to 5
[total dose/cycle = 100 mg/m^2]
Repeat cycle every 21 days

BEP (Testicular Cancer)

Use Testicular cancer

Regimen NOTE: Multiple variations are listed below.

Variation 1:
Bleomycin: I.V.: 30 units/day days 1, 8, and 15
[total dose/cycle = 90 units]
Etoposide: I.V.: 100 mg/m^2/day days 1 to 5
[total dose/cycle = 500 mg/m^2]
Cisplatin: I.V.: 20 mg/m^2/day days 1 to 5
[total dose/cycle = 100 mg/m^2]
Repeat cycle every 21 days for 3-4 cycles

Variation 2:
Bleomycin: I.V.: 30 units/day days 2, 9, and 16
[total dose/cycle = 90 units]
Etoposide: I.V.: 100 mg/m^2/day days 1 to 5
[total dose/cycle = 500 mg/m^2]
Cisplatin: I.V.: 20 mg/m^2/day days 1 to 5
[total dose/cycle = 100 mg/m^2]
Repeat cycle every 21 days

Variation 3:
Bleomycin: I.V.: 30 units once weekly
[total dose/cycle = 90 units]
Etoposide: I.V.: 120 mg/m^2/day days 1, 3, and 5
[total dose/cycle = 360 mg/m^2]
Cisplatin: I.V.: 20 mg/m^2/day days 1 to 5
[total dose/cycle = 100 mg/m^2]
Repeat cycle every 21 days

Variation 4:
Bleomycin: I.V.: 30 units/day days 1, 8, and 15
[total dose/cycle = 90 units]
Etoposide: I.V.: 165 mg/m^2/day days 1, 2, and 3
[total dose/cycle = 495 mg/m^2]
Cisplatin: I.V.: 50 mg/m^2/day days 1 and 2
[total dose/cycle = 100 mg/m^2]
Repeat cycle every 21 days

Bevacizumab-Capecitabine (Breast Cancer)

Use Breast cancer

Regimen NOTE: Multiple variations are listed.

Variation 1:

Capecitabine: Oral: 1250 mg/m^2 twice daily days 1 to 14
[total dose/cycle = 35,000 mg/m^2]

Bevacizumab: I.V.: 15 mg/kg day 1
[total dose/cycle = 15 mg/kg]

Repeat cycle every 21 days for up to 35 cycles

Variation 2:

Capecitabine: Oral: 2000 mg/m^2/day days 1 to 14
[total dose/cycle = 28,000 mg/m^2]

Bevacizumab: I.V.: 15 mg/kg day 1
[total dose/cycle = 15 mg/kg]

Repeat cycle every 21 days

Bevacizumab-Cisplatin-Gemcitabine (NSCLC)

Use Lung cancer, nonsmall cell

Regimen

Bevacizumab: I.V.: 7.5 or 15 mg/kg/dose day 1
[total dose/cycle = 7.5 or 15 mg/kg]

Cisplatin: I.V.: 80 mg/m^2/dose day 1
[total dose/cycle = 80 mg/m^2]

Gemcitabine: I.V.: 1250 mg/m^2/dose days 1 and 8
[total dose/cycle = 2500 mg/m^2]

Repeat cycle every 21 days for up to 6 cycles (bevacizumab monotherapy may be continued thereafter until disease progression)

Bevacizumab-Fluorouracil-Leucovorin

Use Colorectal cancer

Regimen

Bevacizumab: I.V.: 5 mg/kg/day days 1, 15, 29, and 43
[total dose/cycle = 20 mg/kg]

Leucovorin: I.V.: 500 mg/m^2/day days 1, 8, 15, 22, 29, and 36
[total dose/cycle = 3000 mg/m^2]

Fluorouracil: I.V.: 500 mg/m^2/day days 1, 8, 15, 22, 29, and 36
[total dose/cycle = 3000 mg/m^2]

Repeat cycle every 56 days

Bevacizumab-Interferon Alfa (RCC)

Use Renal cell cancer

Regimen NOTE: Multiple variations are listed below

Variation 1:

Interferon Alfa-2a: SubQ: 9 million units 3 times/week
[total dose/cycle = 54 million units]

Bevacizumab: I.V.: 10 mg/kg day 1
[total dose/cycle = 10 mg/kg]

Repeat cycle every 14 days for up to 1 year or until disease progression

Variation 2:

Interferon Alfa-2b: SubQ: 9 million units 3 times/week
[total dose/cycle = 108 million units]

Bevacizumab: I.V.: 10 mg/kg day 1 and 15
[total dose/cycle = 20 mg/kg]

Repeat cycle every 28 days until disease progression or unacceptable toxicity

Bevacizumab-Irinotecan-Fluorouracil-Leucovorin

Use Colorectal cancer

Regimen

Bevacizumab: I.V.: 5 mg/kg/day days 1, 15, and 29
[total dose/cycle = 15 mg/kg]

Irinotecan: I.V.: 125 $mg/m^2/day$ days 1, 8, 15, and 22
[total dose/cycle = 500 mg/m^2]
Fluorouracil: I.V.: 500 $mg/m^2/day$ days 1, 8, 15, and 22
[total dose/cycle = 2000 mg/m^2]
Leucovorin: I.V.: 20 $mg/m^2/day$ days 1, 8, 15, and 22
[total dose/cycle = 80 mg/m^2]
Repeat cycle every 42 days

Bevacizumab-Irinotecan (Glioblastoma)

Use Brain tumors

Regimen Note: Patients receiving concurrent antiepileptic enzyme-inducing drugs received an increased dose of irinotecan (340 $mg/m^2/dose$).
Bevacizumab: I.V.: 10 mg/kg day 1
[total dose/cycle = 10 mg/kg]
Irinotecan: I.V.: 125 mg/m^2 day 1
[total dose/cycle = 125 mg/m^2]
Repeat cycle every 14 days

Bevacizumab-Oxaliplatin-Fluorouracil-Leucovorin

Use Colorectal cancer

Regimen
Bevacizumab: I.V.: 10 mg/kg day 1
[total dose/cycle = 10 mg/kg]
Oxaliplatin: I.V.: 85 mg/m^2 day 1
[total dose/cycle = 85 mg/m^2]
Leucovorin: I.V.: 200 $mg/m^2/day$ days 1 and 2
[total dose/cycle = 400 mg/m^2]
Fluorouracil: I.V. bolus: 400 $mg/m^2/day$ days 1 and 2
followed by I.V.: 600 mg/m^2 continuous infusion over 22 hours days 1 and 2
[total dose/cycle = 2000 mg/m^2]
Repeat cycle every 14 days

Bicalutamide-Goserelin

Use Prostate cancer

Regimen
Bicalutamide: Oral: 50 mg/day
[total dose/cycle = 1400 mg]
Goserelin acetate: SubQ: 3.6 mg day 1
[total dose/cycle = 3.6 mg]
Repeat cycle every 28 days

Bicalutamide-Leuprolide

Use Prostate cancer

Regimen
Bicalutamide: Oral: 50 mg/day
[total dose/cycle = 1400 mg]
Leuprolide depot: I.M.: 7.5 mg day 1
[total dose/cycle = 7.5 mg]
Repeat cycle every 28 days

BOLD

Use Melanoma

Regimen
Dacarbazine: I.V.: 200 $mg/m^2/day$ days 1 to 5
[total dose/cycle = 1000 mg/m^2]
Vincristine: I.V.: 1 $mg/m^2/day$ days 1 and 4
[total dose/cycle = 2 mg/m^2]
Bleomycin: I.V.: 15 units/day days 2 and 5
[total dose/cycle = 30 units]
Lomustine: Oral: 80 mg day 1
[total dose/cycle = 80 mg]
Repeat cycle every 4 weeks

BOLD + Interferon

Use Melanoma

Regimen NOTE: Multiple variations are listed below.

Variation 1:

Bleomycin: I.V.: 15 units/day days 2 and 5
[total dose/cycle = 30 units]

Vincristine: I.V.: 1 mg/m^2/day days 1 and 4
[total dose/cycle = 2 mg/m^2]

Lomustine: Oral: 80 mg day 1
[total dose/cycle = 80 mg]

Dacarbazine: I.V.: 200 mg/m^2/day days 1 to 5
[total dose/cycle = 1000 mg/m^2]

Interferon Alfa-2b: SubQ: 3 million units/day days 8 to 49 (cycles 1 and 2)
[total dose through day 49 = 126 million units]
followed by SubQ: 6 million units 3 times/week (beginning day 50 and subsequent cycles)
[total dose/cycle = 72 million units]

Repeat cycle every 4 weeks

Variation 2:

Bleomycin: I.V.: 30 units day 1
[total dose/cycle = 30 units]

Vincristine: I.V.: 2 mg day 1
[total dose/cycle = 2 mg]

Lomustine: Oral: 80 mg day 1
[total dose/cycle = 80 mg]

Dacarbazine: I.V.: 700 mg/m^2 day 1
[total dose/cycle = 700 mg/m^2]

Interferon Alfa-2b: SubQ: 3 million units 3 times/week
[total dose/cycle = 36 million units]

Repeat cycle every 4 weeks

Variation 3:

Bleomycin: I.V.: 15 units/day days 2 and 5
[total dose/cycle = 30 units]

Vincristine: I.V.: 1-2 mg/day days 1 and 4
[total dose/cycle = 2-4 mg]

Lomustine: Oral: 80 mg day 1
[total dose/cycle = 80 mg]

Dacarbazine: I.V.: 200 mg/m^2/day days 1 to 5
[total dose/cycle = 1000 mg/m^2]

Interferon Alfa-2b: SubQ: 6 million units 3 times/week, for 6 doses, starting day 8
[total dose/cycle = 36 million units]

Repeat cycle every 4 weeks

Variation 4:

Bleomycin: I.V.: 15 units/day days 2 and 5
[total dose/cycle = 30 units]

Vincristine: I.V.: 1 mg/m^2/day (maximum dose: 2 mg) days 1 and 4
[total dose/cycle = 2 mg/m^2]

Lomustine: Oral: 80 mg day 1
[total dose/cycle = 80 mg]

Dacarbazine: I.V.: 200 mg/m^2/day days 1 to 5
[total dose/cycle = 1000 mg/m^2]

Interferon Alfa-2b: SubQ: 3 million units/day days 8, 10, 12, 15, 17, and 19
[total dose/cycle = 18 million units]

Repeat cycle every 4 weeks

BOLD (Melanoma)

Use Melanoma

Regimen NOTE: Multiple variations are listed below.

Variation 1:

Bleomycin: SubQ: 7.5 units/day days 1 and 4 (cycle 1 only)
followed by SubQ: 15 units/day days 1 and 4 (subsequent cycles)
[total dose/cycle = 45 units; maximum total dose (all cycles): 400 units]

Vincristine: I.V.: 1 mg/m^2/day days 1 and 5
[total dose/cycle = 2 mg/m^2]
Lomustine: Oral: 80 mg/m^2 (maximum dose: 150 mg) day 1
[total dose/cycle = 80 mg/m^2]
Dacarbazine: I.V.: 200 mg/m^2/day (maximum dose: 400 mg) days 1 to 5
[total dose/cycle = 1000 mg/m^2; maximum: 2000 mg]
Repeat cycle every 4-6 weeks

Variation 2:
Bleomycin: I.V.: 15 units/day days 1 and 4
[total dose/cycle = 30 units]
Vincristine: I.V.: 1 mg/m^2/day days 1 and 5
[total dose/cycle = 2 mg/m^2]
Lomustine: Oral: 80 mg/m^2 (maximum dose: 150 mg) day 1
[total dose/cycle = 80 mg/m^2]
Dacarbazine: I.V.: 200 mg/m^2/day days 1 to 5
[total dose/cycle = 1000 mg/m^2]
Repeat cycle every 4 weeks

Variation 3:
Bleomycin: I.V.: 15 units/day days 1 and 4
[total dose/cycle = 30 units]
Vincristine: I.V.: 1 mg/m^2 day 1
[total dose/cycle = 1 mg/m^2]
Lomustine: Oral: 80 mg/m^2 day 3 (odd numbered cycles)
[total dose/cycle = 80 mg/m^2; every other cycle]
Dacarbazine: I.V.: 200 mg/m^2/day days 1 to 5
[total dose/cycle = 1000 mg/m^2]
Repeat cycle every 4 weeks

Bortezomib-Dexamethasone

Use Multiple myeloma

Regimen NOTE: Multiple variations are listed below.

Variation 1:
Cycles 1 and 2:
Bortezomib: I.V.: 1.3 mg/m^2/day days 1, 4, 8, and 11
[total dose/cycle = 5.2 mg/m^2]
Dexamethasone: Oral: 40 mg/day days 1 to 4 and days 9 to 12
[total dose/cycle = 320 mg]
Treatment cycle is 21 days
Cycles 3 and 4:
Bortezomib: I.V.: 1.3 mg/m^2/day days 1, 4, 8, and 11
[total dose/cycle = 5.2 mg/m^2]
Dexamethasone: Oral: 40 mg/day days 1 to 4
[total dose/cycle = 160 mg]
Treatment cycle is 21 days

Variation 2:
Cycles 1 and 2:
Bortezomib: I.V.: 1.3 mg/m^2/day days 1, 4, 8, and 11
[total dose/cycle = 5.2 mg/m^2]
Treatment cycle is 21 days
Cycles 3 through 6 (begin dexamethasone after cycle 2 if partial response not achieved or after cycle 4 if complete response not achieved):
Bortezomib: I.V.: 1.3 mg/m^2/day days 1, 4, 8, and 11
[total dose/cycle = 5.2 mg/m^2]
Dexamethasone: Oral: 40 mg/day days 1 and 2
[total dose/cycle = 80 mg]
Treatment cycle is 21 days (for up to a total of 6 cycles)

Bortezomib-Doxorubicin-Dexamethasone

Use Multiple myeloma

Regimen NOTE: Multiple variations are listed below.

Variation 1:

Cycle 1:

Bortezomib: I.V.: 1.3 mg/m^2/day days 1, 4, 8, and 11 [total dose/cycle = 5.2 mg/m^2]

Dexamethasone: Oral: 40 mg/day days 1 to 4, 8 to 11, and 15 to 18 [total dose/cycle = 480 mg]

Doxorubicin: I.V.: 4.5 or 9 mg/m^2/day days 1 to 4 [total dose/cycle = 18 or 36 mg/m^2]

Treatment cycle is 21 days

Cycles 2-4:

Bortezomib: I.V.: 1.3 mg/m^2/day days 1, 4, 8, and 11 [total dose/cycle = 5.2 mg/m^2]

Dexamethasone: Oral: 40 mg/day days 1 to 4 [total dose/cycle = 160 mg]

Doxorubicin: I.V.: 4.5 or 9 mg/m^2/day days 1 to 4 [total dose/cycle = 18 or 36 mg/m^2]

Treatment cycle is 21 days

Variation 2:

Cycle 1:

Bortezomib: I.V.: 1 mg/m^2/day days 1, 4, 8, and 11 [total dose/cycle = 4 mg/m^2]

Dexamethasone: Oral: 40 mg/day days 1 to 4, 8 to 11, and 15 to 18 [total dose/cycle = 480 mg]

Doxorubicin: I.V.: 9 mg/m^2/day days 1 to 4 [total dose/cycle = 36 mg/m^2]

Treatment cycle is 21 days

Cycles 2-4:

Bortezomib: I.V.: 1 mg/m^2/day days 1, 4, 8, and 11 [total dose/cycle = 4 mg/m^2]

Dexamethasone: Oral: 40 mg/day days 1 to 4 [total dose/cycle = 160 mg]

Doxorubicin: I.V.: 9 mg/m^2/day days 1 to 4 [total dose/cycle = 36 mg/m^2]

Treatment cycle is 21 days

Variation 3:

Bortezomib: I.V.: 1.3 mg/m^2/day days 1, 4, 8, and 11 [total dose/cycle = 5.2 mg/m^2]

Dexamethasone: Oral: 40 mg/day days 1 to 4 [total dose/cycle = 160 mg]

Doxorubicin: I.V.: 20 mg/m^2/day days 1 and 4 [total dose/cycle = 40 mg/m^2]

Repeat cycle every 28 days for up to 6 cycles

Bortezomib-Doxorubicin (Liposomal)

Use Multiple myeloma

Regimen

Bortezomib: I.V.: 1.3 mg/m^2/day days 1, 4, 8, and 11 [total dose/cycle = 5.2 mg/m^2]

Doxorubicin (liposomal): I.V.: 30 mg/m^2 day 4 [total dose/cycle = 30 mg/m^2]

Repeat cycle every 21 days for up to 8 cycles

Bortezomib-Doxorubicin (Liposomal)-Dexamethasone

Use Multiple myeloma

Regimen

Bortezomib: I.V.: 1.3 mg/m^2/day days 1, 4, 8, and 11 [total dose/cycle = 5.2 mg/m^2]

Doxorubicin (Liposomal): I.V.: 30 mg/m^2 day 1
[total dose/cycle = 30 mg/m^2]
Dexamethasone: Oral: 40 mg/day days 1 to 4
[total dose/cycle = 160 mg]
Repeat cycle every 28 days for up to 6 cycles

Bortezomib-Melphalan-Prednisone-Thalidomide

Use Multiple myeloma

Regimen

Bortezomib: I.V.: 1-1.3 mg/m^2/day days 1, 4, 15, and 22
[total dose/cycle = 4-5.2 mg/m^2]
Melphalan: Oral: 6 mg/m^2/day days 1 to 5
[total dose/cycle = 30 mg/m^2]
Prednisone: Oral: 60 mg/m^2/day days 1 to 5
[total dose/cycle = 300 mg/m^2]
Thalidomide: Oral: 50 mg/day days 1 to 35
[total dose/cycle = 1750 mg]
Repeat cycle every 35 days for 6 cycles

CA

Use Leukemia, acute myeloid

Regimen

Cytarabine: I.V.: 3000 mg/m^2 every 12 hours days 1 and 2 (4 doses)
[total dose/cycle = 12,000 mg/m^2]
Asparaginase: I.M.: 6000 units/m^2 at hour 42
[total dose/cycle = 6000 units/m^2]
Repeat cycle every 7 days for 2 or 3 cycles

Cabazitaxel-Prednisone (Prostate Cancer)

Use Prostate cancer

Regimen

Cabazitaxel: I.V.: 25 mg/m^2/dose day 1
[total dose/cycle = 25 mg/m^2]
Prednisone: Oral: 10 mg once daily
[total dose/cycle = 210 mg]
Repeat cycle every 21 days

CAD/MOPP/ABV

Use Lymphoma, Hodgkin disease

Regimen

CAD:
Lomustine: Oral: 100 mg/m^2 day 1
[total dose/cycle = 100 mg/m^2]
Melphalan: Oral: 6 mg/m^2/day days 1 to 4
[total dose/cycle = 24 mg/m^2]
Vindesine: I.V.: 3 mg/m^2/day days 1 and 8
[total dose/cycle = 6 mg/m^2]
MOPP:
Mechlorethamine: I.V.: 6 mg/m^2/day days 1 and 8
[total dose/cycle = 12 mg/m^2]
Vincristine: I.V.: 1.4 mg/m^2/day days 1 and 8
[total dose/cycle = 2.8 mg/m^2]
Procarbazine: Oral: 100 mg/m^2/day days 1 to 14
[total dose/cycle = 1400 mg/m^2]
Prednisone: Oral: 40 mg/m^2/day days 1 to 14
[total dose/cycle = 560 mg/m^2]

ABV:

Doxorubicin: I.V.: 25 mg/m^2/day days 1 and 14
[total dose/cycle = 50 mg/m^2]
Bleomycin: SubQ: 6 units/m^2/day days 1 and 14
[total dose/cycle = 12 units/m^2]
Vinblastine: I.V.: 2 mg/m^2 continuous infusion days 4 to 12 and 18 to 26
[total dose/cycle = 36 mg/m^2]

CAD is administered first, then MOPP begins on day 29 or day 37 following CAD. ABV is administered on day 29 following MOPP; CAD recycles on day 29 following ABV.

CAF

Use Breast cancer

Regimen NOTE: Multiple variations are listed below.

Variation 1:
Cyclophosphamide: Oral: 100 mg/m^2/day days 1 to 14
[total dose/cycle = 1400 mg/m^2]
Doxorubicin: I.V.: 30 mg/m^2/day days 1 and 8
[total dose/cycle = 60 mg/m^2]
Fluorouracil: I.V.: 500 mg/m^2/day days 1 and 8
[total dose/cycle = 1000 mg/m^2]
Repeat cycle every 28 days

Variation 2:
Cyclophosphamide: Oral: 100 mg/m^2/day days 1 to 14
[total dose/cycle = 1400 mg/m^2]
Doxorubicin: I.V.: 25 mg/m^2/day days 1 and 8
[total dose/cycle = 50 mg/m^2]
Fluorouracil: I.V.: 500 mg/m^2/day days 1 and 8
[total dose/cycle = 1000 mg/m^2]
Repeat cycle every 28 days

CAP

Use Bladder cancer

Regimen

Cyclophosphamide: I.V.: 400 mg/m^2 day 1
[total dose = 400 mg/m^2]
Doxorubicin: I.V.: 40 mg/m^2 day 1
[total dose = 40 mg/m^2]
Cisplatin: I.V.: 60 mg/m^2 day 1
[total dose = 60 mg/m^2]
Repeat cycle every 21 days

Capecitabine + Docetaxel (Breast Cancer)

Use Breast cancer

Regimen NOTE: Multiple variations are listed below.

Variation 1:
Capecitabine: Oral: 1250 mg/m^2 twice daily days 1 to 14
[total dose/cycle = 35,000 mg/m^2]
Docetaxel: I.V.: 75 mg/m^2 day 1
[total dose/cycle = 75 mg/m^2]
Repeat cycle every 3 weeks

Variation 2:
Capecitabine: Oral: 1000 mg/m^2 twice daily days 2 to 15
[total dose/cycle = 28,000 mg/m^2]
Docetaxel: I.V.: 75 mg/m^2 day 1
[total dose/cycle = 75 mg/m^2]
Repeat cycle every 3 weeks

Variation 3:
Capecitabine: Oral: 937.5 mg/m^2 twice daily days 2 to 15
[total dose/cycle = 26,250 mg/m^2]
Docetaxel: I.V.: 60 mg/m^2 day 1
[total dose/cycle = 60 mg/m^2]
Repeat cycle every 3 weeks

Capecitabine-Docetaxel (Gastric Cancer)

Use Gastric cancer

Regimen NOTE: Multiple variations are listed below

Variation 1:

Capecitabine: Oral: 1000 mg/m^2 twice daily days 1 to 14
[total dose/cycle = 28,000 mg/m^2]

Docetaxel: I.V.: 75 mg/m^2 day 1
[total dose/cycle = 75 mg/m^2]

Repeat cycle every 3 weeks for up to 9 cycles or until disease progression or unacceptable toxicity

Variation 2:

Capecitabine: Oral: 1000 mg/m^2 twice daily days 1 to 14
[total dose/cycle = 28,000 mg/m^2]

Docetaxel: I.V.: 36 mg/m^2 days 1 and 8
[total dose/cycle = 72 mg/m^2]

Repeat cycle every 3 weeks until disease progression or unacceptable toxicity

Variation 3:

Capecitabine: Oral: 825 mg/m^2 twice daily days 1 to 14
[total dose/cycle = 23,100 mg/m^2]

Docetaxel: I.V.: 75 mg/m^2 day 1
[total dose/cycle = 75 mg/m^2]

Repeat cycle every 3 weeks until disease progression

Variation 4:

Capecitabine: Oral: 1250 mg/m^2 twice daily days 1 to 14
[total dose/cycle = 35,000 mg/m^2]

Docetaxel: I.V.: 75 mg/m^2 day 1
[total dose/cycle = 75 mg/m^2]

Repeat cycle every 3 weeks until disease progression for up to a maximum of 6 cycles

Capecitabine-Docetaxel (NSCLC)

Use Lung cancer, nonsmall cell

Regimen NOTE: Multiple variations are listed below

Variation 1:

Capecitabine: Oral: 1000 mg/m^2 twice daily days 1 to 14
[total dose/cycle = 28,000 mg/m^2]

Docetaxel: I.V.: 36 mg/m^2 days 1 and 8
[total dose/cycle = 72 mg/m^2]

Repeat cycle every 3 weeks

Variation 2:

Capecitabine: Oral: 625 mg/m^2 twice daily days 5 to 18
[total dose/cycle = 17,500 mg/m^2]

Docetaxel: I.V.: 36 mg/m^2 days 1, 8, and 15
[total dose/cycle = 108 mg/m^2]

Repeat cycle every 4 weeks

Capecitabine + Lapatinib (Breast Cancer)

Use Breast cancer

Regimen

Capecitabine: Oral: 1000 mg/m^2 twice daily days 1 to 14
[total dose/cycle = 28,000 mg/m^2]

Lapatinib: Oral: 1250 mg/day days 1 to 21
[total dose/cycle = 26,250 mg]

Repeat cycle every 3 weeks

Capecitabine-Trastuzumab

Use Breast cancer

Regimen NOTE: Multiple variations are listed below.

Variation 1:

Cycle 1:

Capecitabine: Oral: 1250 mg/m^2 twice daily days 1 to 14
[total dose/cycle 1 = 35,000 mg/m^2]

Trastuzumab: I.V.: 4 mg/kg (loading dose) day 1 cycle 1
followed by I.V.: 2 mg/kg/day days 8 and 15 cycle 1
[total dose/cycle 1 = 8 mg/kg]
Treatment cycle is 21 days
Subsequent cycles:
Capecitabine: Oral: 1250 mg/m^2 twice daily days 1 to 14
[total dose/cycle = 35,000 mg/m^2]
Trastuzumab: I.V.: 2 mg/kg/day days 1, 8, and 15
[total dose/cycle = 6 mg/kg]
Repeat cycle every 21 days
Variation 2:
Cycle 1:
Capecitabine: Oral: 1250 mg/m^2 twice daily days 1 to 14
[total dose/cycle 1 = 35,000 mg/m^2]
Trastuzumab: I.V.: 8 mg/kg (loading dose) day 1 cycle 1
[total dose/cycle 1 = 8 mg/kg]
Treatment cycle is 21 days
Subsequent cycles:
Capecitabine: Oral: 1250 mg/m^2 twice daily days 1 to 14
[total dose/cycle = 35,000 mg/m^2]
Trastuzumab: I.V.: 6 mg/kg day 1
[total dose/cycle = 6 mg/kg]
Repeat cycle every 21 days

CAPOX (Biliary Cancer)

Use Biliary adenocarcinoma

Regimen

Capecitabine: Oral: 1000 mg/m^2/dose twice daily days 1 to 14
[total dose/cycle = 28,000 mg/m^2]
Oxaliplatin: I.V.: 130 mg/m^2 over 2 hours day 1
[total dose/cycle = 130 mg/m^2]
Repeat cycle every 3 weeks

CAPOX (Colorectal Cancer)

Use Colorectal cancer

Regimen Note: Multiple variations are listed below.

Variation 1:
Oxaliplatin: I.V.: 130 mg/m^2 day 1
[total dose/cycle = 130 mg/m^2]
Capecitabine: Oral: 2500 mg/m^2/day days 1 to 14
[total dose/cycle = 35,000 mg/m^2]
Repeat cycle every 21 days
Variation 2:
Oxaliplatin: I.V.: 85 mg/m^2 day 1
[total dose/cycle = 85 mg/m^2]
Capecitabine: Oral: 3500 mg/m^2/day days 1 to 7
[total dose/cycle = 24,500 mg/m^2]
Repeat cycle every 14 days
Variation 3:
Oxaliplatin: I.V.: 50-80 mg/m^2/day days 1, 8, 22, and 29
[total dose/cycle = 200-320 mg/m^2]
Capecitabine: Oral: 1650 mg/m^2/day days 1 to 14 and 22 to 35
[total dose/cycle = 46,200 mg/m^2]
Variation 4:
Oxaliplatin: I.V.: 70 mg/m^2/day days 1 and 8
[total dose/cycle = 140 mg/m^2]
Capecitabine: Oral: 2000 mg/m^2/day days 1 to 14
[total dose/cycle = 28,000 mg/m^2]
Repeat cycle every 21 days

Variation 5:
Oxaliplatin: I.V.: 120 mg/m^2 day 1
[total dose/cycle = 120 mg/m^2]
Capecitabine: Oral: 2500 mg/m^2/day days 1 to 14
[total dose/cycle = 35,000 mg/m^2]
Repeat cycle every 21 days
Variation 6:
Oxaliplatin: I.V.: 85 mg/m^2 day 1
[total dose/cycle = 85 mg/m^2]
Capecitabine: Oral: 2500 mg/m^2/day days 1 to 7
[total dose/cycle = 17,500 mg/m^2]
or Capecitabine: Oral: 3000 mg/m^2/day days 1 to 7
[total dose/cycle = 21,000 mg/m^2]
or Capecitabine: Oral: 3500 mg/m^2/day days 1 to 7
[total dose/cycle = 24,500 mg/m^2]
or Capecitabine: Oral: 4000 mg/m^2/day days 1 to 7
[total dose/cycle = 28,000 mg/m^2]
Repeat cycle every 14 days
Variation 7:
Oxaliplatin: I.V.: 130 mg/m^2 day 1
[total dose/cycle = 130 mg/m^2]
Capecitabine: Oral: 1000 mg/m^2 twice daily days 1 (beginning with evening dose) to 15 (ending with morning dose)
[total dose/cycle = 28,000 mg/m^2]
Repeat cycle every 21 days

CAPOX (Pancreatic Cancer)

Use Pancreatic cancer

Regimen NOTE: Multiple variations are listed below.
Variation 1 (patients ≤65 years of age or ECOG PS <2):
Capecitabine: Oral: 1000 mg/m^2/dose twice daily days 1 to 14
[total dose/cycle = 28,000 mg/m^2]
Oxaliplatin: I.V.: 130 mg/m^2/dose over 2 hours day 1
[total dose/cycle = 130 mg/m^2]
Repeat cycle every 21 days until disease progression or unacceptable toxicity
Variation 2 (patients >65 years of age or ECOG PS of 2):
Capecitabine: Oral: 750 mg/m^2/dose twice daily days 1 to 14
[total dose/cycle = 21,000 mg/m^2]
Oxaliplatin: I.V.: 110 mg/m^2/dose over 2 hours day 1
[total dose/cycle = 110 mg/m^2]
Repeat cycle every 21 days until disease progression or unacceptable toxicity

Carboplatin-Cetuximab (Head and Neck Cancer)

Use Head and neck cancer

Regimen
Cycle 1:
Cetuximab: I.V.: 400 mg/m^2 (loading dose) day 1 (week 1, cycle 1 only)
[total loading dose = 400 mg/m^2]
followed by I.V.: 250 mg/m^2/day days 8 and 15
[total dose/cycle 1 = 900 mg/m^2]
Carboplatin: I.V.: AUC 5 day 1
[total dose/cycle = AUC = 5]
Treatment cycle is 3 weeks
Subsequent cycles:
Cetuximab: I.V.: 250 mg/m^2/day days 1, 8, and 15
[total dose/cycle = 750 mg/m^2]
Carboplatin: I.V.: AUC 5 day 1
[total dose/cycle = AUC = 5]
Repeat cycle every 3 weeks until disease progression or unacceptable toxicity for up to a maximum of 8 cycles

Carboplatin-Paclitaxel (Cervical Cancer)

Use Cervical cancer

Regimen NOTE: Multiple variations are listed below.

Variation 1:

Paclitaxel: I.V.: 175 mg/m^2 over 3 hours day 1 (reduce to 155 mg/m^2 over 3 hours day 1 if prior pelvic irradiation)
[total dose/cycle = 175 (or 155) mg/m^2]

Carboplatin: I.V.: AUC 5 or 6 day 1
[total dose/cycle = AUC = 5 or 6]

Repeat cycle every 28 days for up to a total of 6-9 cycles

Variation 2:

Paclitaxel: I.V.: 175 mg/m^2 over 3 hours day 1
[total dose/cycle = 175 mg/m^2]

Carboplatin: I.V.: AUC 5 day 1
[total dose/cycle = AUC = 5]

Repeat cycle every 21 days for 6-9 cycles

Carboplatin-Paclitaxel (Ovarian Cancer)

Use Ovarian cancer

Regimen NOTE: Multiple variations are listed below.

Variation 1:

Carboplatin: I.V.: AUC 7.5 day 1
[total dose/cycle = AUC = 7.5]

Paclitaxel: I.V.: 175 mg/m^2 over 3 hours day 1
[total dose/cycle = 175 mg/m^2]

Repeat cycle every 3 weeks for a total for 6 cycles

Variation 2:

Carboplatin: I.V.: AUC 5-6 day 1
[total dose/cycle = AUC = 5-6]

Paclitaxel: I.V.: 175 mg/m^2 over 3 hours day 1
[total dose/cycle = 175 mg/m^2]

Repeat cycle every 3 weeks for a total of 6-8 cycles

Variation 3:

Carboplatin: I.V.: AUC 5 day 1
[total dose/cycle = AUC = 5]

Paclitaxel: I.V.: 175 mg/m^2 over 3 hours day 1
[total dose/cycle = 175 mg/m^2]

Repeat cycle every 3 weeks for 6 cycles

Variation 4:

Carboplatin: I.V.: AUC 6 (maximum dose: 880 mg) day 1
[total dose/cycle = AUC = 6; maximum dose: 880 mg]

Paclitaxel: I.V.: 185 mg/m^2 (maximum dose: 400 mg) over 3 hours day 1
[total dose/cycle = 185 mg/m^2; maximum dose: 400 mg]

Repeat cycle every 3 weeks

Variation 5:

Carboplatin: I.V.: AUC 7.5 day 1
[total dose/cycle = AUC = 7.5]

Paclitaxel: I.V.: 175 mg/m^2 over 3 hours day 1
[total dose/cycle = 175 mg/m^2]

Repeat cycle every 3 weeks for 3-6 cycles

Carboplatin-Paclitaxel (Unknown Primary)

Use Unknown primary (adenocarcinoma)

Regimen

Carboplatin: I.V.: Target AUC 6 day 1
[total dose/cycle = AUC = 6]

followed by

Paclitaxel: I.V.: 200 mg/m^2 infused over 3 hours day 1
[total dose/cycle = 200 mg/m^2]

Filgrastim: SubQ: 300 mcg/day days 5 to 12
[total dose/cycle = 2400 mcg]

Repeat cycle every 21 days for a total of 6 or 8 cycles

Carbo-Tax (NSCLC)

Use Lung cancer, nonsmall cell

Regimen

Paclitaxel: I.V.: 135-215 mg/m^2 infused over 24 hours day 1
[total dose/cycle = 135-215 mg/m^2]
or I.V.: 175 mg/m^2 infused over 3 hours day 1
[total dose/cycle = 175 mg/m^2]
followed by
Carboplatin: I.V.: Target AUC 7.5
[total dose/cycle = AUC = 7.5]
Repeat cycle every 21 days

CaT (NSCLC)

Use Lung cancer, nonsmall cell

Regimen NOTE: Multiple variations are listed below.

Variation 1:
Paclitaxel: I.V.: 175 mg/m^2 day 1
[total dose/cycle = 175 mg/m^2]
or I.V.: 135 mg/m^2 continuous infusion day 1
[total dose/cycle = 135 mg/m^2]
Carboplatin: I.V.: AUC 7.5 day 1 or 2
[total dose/cycle = AUC = 7.5]
Repeat cycle every 21 days

Variation 2:
Paclitaxel: I.V.: 225 mg/m^2 day 1
[total dose/cycle = 225 mg/m^2]
Carboplatin: I.V.: AUC 6 day 1
[total dose/cycle = AUC = 6]
Repeat cycle every 21 days

CAVE

Use Lung cancer, small cell

Regimen

Cyclophosphamide: I.V.: 750 mg/m^2 day 1
[total dose/cycle = 750 mg/m^2]
Doxorubicin: I.V.: 50 mg/m^2 day 1
[total dose/cycle = 50 mg/m^2]
Vincristine: I.V.: 1.4 mg/m^2 (maximum dose: 2 mg) day 1
[total dose/cycle = 1.4 mg/m^2]
Etoposide: I.V.: 60-100 mg/m^2/day days 1, 2, and 3
[total dose/cycle = 180-300 mg/m^2]
Repeat cycle every 21 days

CAV-P/VP

Use Neuroblastoma

Regimen

Course 1, 2, 4, and 6:
Cyclophosphamide: I.V.: 70 mg/kg/day days 1 and 2
[total dose/cycle = 140 mg/kg]
Doxorubicin: I.V.: 25 mg/m^2/day continuous infusion days 1, 2, and 3
[total dose/cycle = 75 mg/m^2]
Vincristine: I.V.: 0.033 mg/kg/day continuous infusion days 1, 2, and 3
[total dose/cycle = 0.099 mg/kg]
Vincristine: I.V.: 1.5 mg/m^2 day 9
[total dose/cycle = 1.5 mg/m^2]

Course 3, 5, and 7:
Etoposide: I.V.: 200 mg/m^2/day days 1, 2, and 3
[total dose/cycle = 600 mg/m^2]
Cisplatin: I.V.: 50 mg/m^2/day days 1 to 4
[total dose/cycle = 200 mg/m^2]

CC

Use Ovarian cancer

Regimen

Carboplatin: I.V.: Target AUC 5-7.5 day 1
[total dose/cycle = AUC = 5-7.5]
Cyclophosphamide: I.V.: 600 mg/m^2 day 1
[total dose/cycle = 600 mg/m^2]
Repeat cycle every 28 days

CCCDE (Retinoblastoma)

Use Retinoblastoma

Regimen

Cyclophosphamide: I.V.: 150 mg/m^2/day days 1 to 7
[total dose/cycle = 1050 mg/m^2]
Cyclophosphamide: Oral: 150 mg/m^2/day days 22 to 28 and 43 to 49
[total dose/cycle = 2100 mg/m^2]
Doxorubicin: I.V.: 35 mg/m^2/day days 10 and 52
[total dose/cycle = 70 mg/m^2]
Cisplatin: I.V.: 90 mg/m^2/day days 8, 50, and 71
[total dose/cycle = 270 mg/m^2]
Etoposide: I.V.: 150 mg/m^2/day continuous infusion days 29, 30, and 31 and 73, 74, and 75
[total dose/cycle = 900 mg/m^2]

CCDT (Melanoma)

Use Melanoma

Regimen

Dacarbazine: I.V.: 220 mg/m^2/day days 1, 2, and 3, every 21 to 28 days
[total dose/cycle = 660 mg/m^2]
Carmustine: I.V.: 150 mg/m^2 day 1, every 42 to 56 days
[total dose/cycle = 150 mg/m^2]
Cisplatin: I.V.: 25 mg/m^2/day days 1, 2, and 3, every 21 to 28 days
[total dose/cycle = 75 mg/m^2]
Tamoxifen: Oral: 20 mg/day (use of tamoxifen is optional)

CDDP/VP-16

Use Brain tumors

Regimen

Cisplatin: I.V.: 90 mg/m^2 day 1
[total dose/cycle = 90 mg/m^2]
Etoposide: I.V.: 150 mg/m^2/day days 3 and 4
[total dose/cycle = 300 mg/m^2]
Repeat cycle every 21 days

CE-CAdO

Use Neuroblastoma

Regimen

Carboplatin: I.V.: 160 mg/m^2/day days 1 to 5
[total dose/cycle = 800 mg/m^2]
Etoposide: I.V.: 100 mg/m^2/day days 1 to 5
[total dose/cycle = 500 mg/m^2]
or
Carboplatin: I.V.: 200 mg/m^2/day days 1, 2, and 3
[total dose/cycle = 600 mg/m^2]
Etoposide: I.V.: 150 mg/m^2/day days 1, 2, and 3
[total dose/cycle = 450 mg/m^2]
and
Cyclophosphamide: I.V.: 300 mg/m^2/day days 1 to 5
[total dose/cycle = 1500 mg/m^2]

Doxorubicin: I.V.: 60 mg/m^2 day 5
[total dose/cycle = 60 mg/m^2]
Vincristine: I.V.: 1.5 mg/m^2/day days 1 and 5
[total dose/cycle = 3 mg/m^2]
Repeat cycle every 21 days

CEF

Use Breast cancer

Regimen

Cyclophosphamide: Oral: 75 mg/m^2/day days 1 to 14
[total dose/cycle = 1050 mg/m^2]
Epirubicin: I.V.: 60 mg/m^2/day days 1 and 8
[total dose/cycle = 120 mg/m^2]
Fluorouracil: I.V.: 500 mg/m^2/day days 1 and 8
[total dose/cycle = 1000 mg/m^2]
Repeat cycle every 28 days

CE (Neuroblastoma)

Use Neuroblastoma

Regimen

Carboplatin: I.V.: 500 mg/m^2/day days 1 and 2
[total dose/cycle = 1000 mg/m^2]
Etoposide: I.V.: 100 mg/m^2/day days 1, 2, and 3
[total dose/cycle = 300 mg/m^2]
Repeat cycle every 21-28 days

CEPP(B)

Use Lymphoma, non-Hodgkin

Regimen

Cyclophosphamide: I.V.: 600-650 mg/m^2/day days 1 and 8
[total dose/cycle = 1200-1300 mg/m^2]
Etoposide: I.V.: 70-85 mg/m^2/day days 1, 2, and 3
[total dose/cycle = 210-255 mg/m^2]
Procarbazine: Oral: 60 mg/m^2/day days 1 to 10
[total dose/cycle = 600 mg/m^2]
Prednisone: Oral: 60 mg/m^2/day days 1 to 10
[total dose/cycle = 600 mg/m^2]
Bleomycin: I.V.: 15 units/m^2/day days 1 and 15 (Bleomycin is sometimes omitted)
[total dose/cycle = 30 units/m^2]
Repeat cycle every 28 days

CE (Retinoblastoma)

Use Retinoblastoma

Regimen

Etoposide: I.V.: 100 mg/m^2/day days 1 to 5
[total dose/cycle = 500 mg/m^2]
Carboplatin: I.V.: 160 mg/m^2/day days 1 to 5
[total dose/cycle = 800 mg/m^2]
Repeat cycle every 21 days

Cetuximab (Biweekly)-Irinotecan

Use Colorectal cancer

Regimen

Cycle 1:
Cetuximab: I.V.: 500 mg/m^2 over 120 minutes day 1 (cycle 1 only)
[total dose/cycle = 500 mg/m^2]
Irinotecan: I.V.: 180 mg/m^2 day 1
[total dose/cycle = 180 mg/m^2]

Subsequent cycles:
Cetuximab: I.V.: 500 mg/m^{2}over 60 minutes day 1
[total dose/cycle = 500 mg/m^2]
Irinotecan: I.V.: 180 mg/m^2 day 1
[total dose/cycle = 180 mg/m^2]
Repeat cycle every 14 days

Cetuximab-Carboplatin-Fluorouracil (Head and Neck Cancer)

Use Head and neck cancer

Regimen

Cycle 1:
Cetuximab: I.V.: 400 mg/m^2 (loading dose) day 1 (week 1, cycle 1 only)
[total loading dose = 400 mg/m^2]
followed by I.V.: 250 mg/m^2/day days 8 and 15
[total dose/cycle 1 = 900 mg/m^2]
Carboplatin: I.V.: AUC 5 day 1
[total dose/cycle = AUC = 5]
Fluorouracil: I.V.: 1000 mg/m^2/day continuous infusion days 1 to 4
[total dose/cycle = 4000 mg/m^2]
Treatment cycle is 3 weeks
Subsequent cycles:
Cetuximab: I.V.: 250 mg/m^2/day days 1, 8, and 15
[total dose/cycle = 750 mg/m^2]
Carboplatin: I.V.: AUC 5 day 1
[total dose/cycle = AUC = 5]
Fluorouracil: I.V.: 1000 mg/m^2/day continuous infusion days 1 to 4
[total dose/cycle = 4000 mg/m^2]
Repeat cycle every 3 weeks for a total of up to 6 cycles (cetuximab monotherapy may be continued thereafter until disease progression or unacceptable toxicity)

Cetuximab-Cisplatin-Fluorouracil (Head and Neck Cancer)

Use Head and neck cancer

Regimen

Cycle 1:
Cetuximab: I.V.: 400 mg/m^2 (loading dose) day 1 (week 1, cycle 1 only)
[total loading dose = 400 mg/m^2]
followed by I.V.: 250 mg/m^2/day days 8 and 15
[total dose/cycle 1 = 900 mg/m^2]
Cisplatin: I.V.: 100 mg/m^2 day 1
[total dose/cycle = 100 mg/m^2]
Fluorouracil: I.V.: 1000 mg/m^2/day continuous infusion days 1 to 4
[total dose/cycle = 4000 mg/m^2]
Treatment cycle is 3 weeks
Subsequent cycles:
Cetuximab: I.V.: 250 mg/m^2/day days 1, 8, and 15
[total dose/cycle = 750 mg/m^2]
Cisplatin: I.V.: 100 mg/m^2 day 1
[total dose/cycle = 100 mg/m^2]
Fluorouracil: I.V.: 1000 mg/m^2/day continuous infusion days 1 to 4
[total dose/cycle = 4000 mg/m^2]
Repeat cycle every 3 weeks for a total of up to 6 cycles (cetuximab monotherapy may be continued thereafter until disease progression or unacceptable toxicity)

Cetuximab-Cisplatin-Vinorelbine

Use Lung cancer, nonsmall cell

Regimen

Cycle 1:
Cetuximab: I.V.: 400 mg/m^2 (loading dose) day 1 (week 1, cycle 1 only)
[total loading dose = 400 mg/m^2]
followed by I.V.: 250 mg/m^2/dose days 8 and 15
[total dose/cycle 1 = 900 mg/m^2]

Cisplatin: I.V.: 80 mg/m^2/dose day 1
[total dose/cycle = 80 mg/m^2]
Vinorelbine: I.V.: 25 mg/m^2/dose days 1 and 8
[total dose/cycle = 50 mg/m^2]
Treatment cycle is 3 weeks
Subsequent cycles:
Cetuximab: I.V.: 250 mg/m^2/day days 1, 8, and 15
[total dose/cycle = 750 mg/m^2]
Cisplatin: I.V.: 80 mg/m^2 day 1
[total dose/cycle = 80 mg/m^2]
Vinorelbine: I.V.: 25 mg/m^2/dose days 1 and 8
[total dose/cycle = 50 mg/m^2]
Repeat cycle every 3 weeks

Cetuximab-FOLFOX4

Use Colorectal cancer

Regimen

Cycle 1:
Cetuximab: I.V.: 400 mg/m^2 (loading dose) day 1 (week 1, cycle 1 only)
followed by I.V.: 250 mg/m^2/day day 8
[total dose/cycle 1 = 650 mg/m^2]
Oxaliplatin: I.V.: 85 mg/m^2 (over 2 hours) day 1
[total dose/cycle = 85 mg/m^2]
Leucovorin: I.V.: 200 mg/m^2/day (over 2 hours) days 1 and 2
[total dose/cycle = 400 mg/m^2]
Fluorouracil: I.V. bolus: 400 mg/m^2/day days 1 and 2
followed by I.V.: 600 mg/m^2 continuous infusion (over 22 hours) days 1 and 2
[total dose/cycle = 2000 mg/m^2]
Note: Bolus fluorouracil and continuous infusion are both given on each day.
Treatment cycle is 14 days
Subsequent cycles:
Cetuximab: I.V.: 250 mg/m^2/day days 1 and 8
[total dose/cycle = 500 mg/m^2]
Oxaliplatin: I.V.: 85 mg/m^2 day 1
[total dose/cycle = 85 mg/m^2]
Leucovorin: I.V.: 200 mg/m^2/day (over 2 hours) days 1 and 2
[total dose/cycle = 400 mg/m^2]
Fluorouracil: I.V. bolus: 400 mg/m^2/day days 1 and 2
followed by I.V.: 600 mg/m^2 continuous infusion (over 22 hours) days 1 and 2
[total dose/cycle = 2000 mg/m^2]
Note: Bolus fluorouracil and continuous infusion are both given on each day.
Repeat cycle every 14 days

Cetuximab-Irinotecan

Use Colorectal cancer

Regimen NOTE: Multiple variations are listed below.

Variation 1:
Cycle 1:
Cetuximab: I.V.: 400 mg/m^2 (loading dose) day 1 (week 1, cycle 1 only)
[total loading dose = 400 mg/m^2]
followed by I.V.: 250 mg/m^2/day days 8, 15, 22, 29, and 36
[total dose/cycle 1 = 1650 mg/m^2]
Irinotecan: I.V.: 125 mg/m^2/day days 1, 8, 15, and 22
[total dose/cycle = 500 mg/m^2]
Subsequent cycles:
Cetuximab: I.V.: 250 mg/m^2/day days 1, 8, 15, 22, 29, and 36
[total dose/cycle = 1500 mg/m^2]
Irinotecan: I.V.: 125 mg/m^2/day days 1, 8, 15, and 22
[total dose/cycle = 500 mg/m^2]
Repeat cycle every 42 days

Variation 2:
Cycle 1:
Cetuximab: I.V.: 400 mg/m^2 (loading dose) day 1 (week 1, cycle 1 only)
[total loading dose = 400 mg/m^2]
followed by I.V.: 250 mg/m^2 day 8
[total dose/cycle 1 = 650 mg/m^2]
Irinotecan: I.V.: 180 mg/m^2 day 1
[total dose/cycle = 180 mg/m^2]
Subsequent cycles:
Cetuximab: I.V.: 250 mg/m^2/day days 1 and 8
[total dose/cycle = 500 mg/m^2]
Irinotecan: I.V.: 180 mg/m^2 day 1
[total dose/cycle = 180 mg/m^2]
Repeat cycle every 14 days
Variation 3:
Cycle 1:
Cetuximab: I.V.: 400 mg/m^2 (loading dose) day 1 (week 1, cycle 1 only)
[total loading dose = 400 mg/m^2]
followed by I.V.: 250 mg/m^2/day days 8 and 15 (cycle 1)
[total dose/cycle 1 = 900 mg/m^2]
Irinotecan: I.V.: 350 mg/m^2 day 1
[total dose/cycle = 350 mg/m^2]
Subsequent cycles:
Cetuximab: I.V.: 250 mg/m^2/day days 1, 8, and 15
[total dose/cycle = 750 mg/m^2]
Irinotecan: I.V.: 350 mg/m^2 day 1
[total dose/cycle = 350 mg/m^2]
Repeat cycle every 21 days

CEV

Use Rhabdomyosarcoma

Regimen

Carboplatin: I.V.: 500 mg/m^2 day 1
[total dose/cycle = 500 mg/m^2]
Epirubicin: I.V.: 150 mg/m^2 day 1
[total dose/cycle = 150 mg/m^2]
Vincristine: I.V.: 1.5 mg/m^2/day days 1 and 7
[total dose/cycle = 3 mg/m^2]
Repeat cycle every 21 days

CFP

Use Breast cancer

Regimen

Cyclophosphamide: I.V.: 150 mg/m^2/day days 1 to 5
[total dose/cycle = 750 mg/m^2]
Fluorouracil: I.V.: 300 mg/m^2/day days 1 to 5
[total dose/cycle = 1500 mg/m^2]
Prednisone: Oral: 30 mg/day days 1 to 14 (cycle 1 only)
followed by Oral: 20 mg/day days 15 to 21 (cycle 1 only)
followed by Oral: 10 mg daily thereafter as maintenance
[total dose/cycle = 700 mg in cycle 1; 350 mg in subsequent cycles]
Repeat cycle every 35 days

CHAMOCA (Modified Bagshawe Regimen)

Use Gestational trophoblastic tumor

Regimen NOTE: Multiple variations are listed below.

Variation 1:
Hydroxyurea: Oral: 500 mg every 6 hours, for 4 doses, day 1 (start at 6 AM)
[total dose/cycle = 2000 mg]
Dactinomycin: I.V.: 0.2 mg/day days 1, 2, and 3 (give at 7 PM)
followed by I.V.: 0.5 mg/day days 4 and 5 (give at 7 PM)
[total dose/cycle = 1.6 mg]

Cyclophosphamide: I.V.: 500 mg/m^2/day days 3 and 8 (give at 7 PM)
[total dose/cycle = 1000 mg/m^2]
Vincristine: I.V.: 1 mg/m^2 (maximum dose: 2 mg) day 2 (give at 7 AM)
[total dose/cycle = 1 mg/m^2; maximum: 2 mg]
Methotrexate: I.V. bolus: 100 mg/m^2 day 2 (give at 7 PM)
followed by I.V.: 200 mg/m^2 continuous infusion over 12 hours day 2
[total dose/cycle = 300 mg/m^2]
Leucovorin: I.M.: 14 mg every 6 hours, for 6 doses, days 3, 4, and 5 (begin at 7 PM on day 3; start 24 hours after the start of methotrexate)
[total dose/cycle = 84 mg]
Doxorubicin: I.V.: 30 mg/m^2 day 8 (give at 7 PM)
[total dose/cycle = 30 mg/m^2]
Repeat cycle every 18 days or as toxicity permits (cycle may be repeated 10 days after last treatment)

Variation 2:
Hydroxyurea: Oral: 500 mg every 12 hours, for 4 doses, days 1 and 2 (usually started in early morning)
[total dose/cycle = 2000 mg]
Dactinomycin: I.V.: 10 mcg/kg/day days 5, 6, and 7
[total dose/cycle = 30 mcg/kg]
Vincristine: I.V.: 1 mg/m^2 day 3
[total dose/cycle = 1 mg/m^2]
Methotrexate: I.V. bolus: 100 mg/m^2 day 3
followed by I.V.: 200 mg/m^2 continuous infusion over 12 hours day 3
[total dose/cycle = 300 mg/m^2]
Leucovorin: I.M.: 10 mg/m^2 every 12 hours, for 4 doses, days 4 and 5 (start 24 hours after the start of methotrexate)
[total dose/cycle = 40 mg/m^2]
Cyclophosphamide: I.V.: 600 mg/m^2 day 5
[total dose/cycle = 600 mg/m^2]
Doxorubicin: I.V.: 30 mg/m^2 day 10
[total dose/cycle = 30 mg/m^2]
Repeat cycle every 3 weeks

Variation 3:
Hydroxyurea: Oral: 500 mg every 12 hours, for 4 doses, days 1 and 2 (usually started in early morning)
[total dose/cycle = 2000 mg/m^2]
Vincristine: I.V.: 1 mg/m^2 day 3
[total dose/cycle = 1 mg/m^2]
Methotrexate: I.V. bolus: 100 mg/m^2 day 3
followed by I.V.: 200 mg/m^{2}continuous infusion over 12 hours day 3
[total dose/cycle = 300 mg/m^2]
Leucovorin: I.M.: 14 mg every 6 hours, for 6 doses, days 4, 5, and 6 (start 24 hours after start of methotrexate)
[total dose/cycle = 84 mg]
Dactinomycin: I.V.: 0.2 mg/day days 2, 3, and 4
followed by I.V.: 0.5 mg/day days 5 and 6
[total dose/cycle = 1.6 mg]
Cyclophosphamide: I.V.: 500 mg/m^2 day 4
[total dose/cycle = 500 mg/m^2]
Doxorubicin: I.V.: 30 mg/m^2 day 9
[total dose/cycle = 30 mg/m^2]
Melphalan: I.V.: 6 mg/m^2 day 9
[total dose/cycle = 6 mg/m^2]
Repeat cycle approximately every 3 weeks

Variation 4:
Hydroxyurea: Oral: 500 mg 4 times/day, for 4 doses, day 1
[total dose/cycle = 2000 mg/m^2]
Vincristine: I.V.: 1 mg/m^2 day 2
[total dose/cycle = 1 mg/m^2]
Methotrexate: I.V. bolus: 100 mg/m^2 day 2
followed by I.V.: 200 mg/m^2 continuous infusion over 12 hours day 2
[total dose/cycle = 300 mg/m^2]

Leucovorin: I.M.: 14 mg every 6 hours, for 6 doses, days 3, 4, and 5 (start 24 hours after the start of methotrexate)
[total dose/cycle = 84 mg]
Dactinomycin: I.V.: 0.2 mg days 1, 2, and 3
followed by I.V.: 0.5 mg days 4 and 5
[total dose/cycle = 1.6 mg]
Cyclophosphamide: I.V.: 500 mg/m^2 day 3
[total dose/cycle = 500 mg/m^2]
Cyclophosphamide: I.V.: 300 mg/m^2 on day 8
[total dose/cycle = 300 mg/m^2]
Doxorubicin: I.V.: 30 mg/m^2 day 8
[total dose/cycle = 30 mg/m^2]
Repeat cycle approximately every 3 weeks

CHAMOMA (Bagshawe Regimen)

Use Gestational trophoblastic tumor

Regimen

Hydroxyurea: Oral: 500 mg every 12 hours, for 4 doses, days 1 and 2
[total dose/cycle = 2000 mg]
Vincristine: I.V.: 1 mg/m^2 day 3
[total dose/cycle = 1 mg/m^2]
Methotrexate: I.V. bolus: 100 mg/m^2 day 3
followed by I.V.: 200 mg/m^2 continuous infusion over 12 hours day 3
[total dose/cycle = 300 mg/m^2]
Leucovorin: I.M.: 12 mg/m^2 every 12 hours, for 4 doses, days 4 and 5 (start 12 hours after the end of methotrexate infusion)
[total dose/cycle = 48 mg/m^2]
Dactinomycin: I.V.: 10 mcg/kg/day days 5, 6, and 7
[total dose/cycle = 30 mcg/kg]
Cyclophosphamide: I.V.: 600 mg/m^2 day 5
[total dose/cycle = 600 mg/m^2]
Doxorubicin: I.V.: 30 mg/m^2 day 10
[total dose/cycle = 30 mg/m^2]
Melphalan: I.V.: 6 mg/m^2 day 10
[total dose/cycle = 6 mg/m^2]
Repeat cycle approximately every 3 weeks

Chlorambucil-VPP (Hodgkin Lymphoma)

Use Lymphoma, Hodgkin disease

Regimen

Chlorambucil: Oral: 6 mg/m^2/day (maximum dose: 10 mg) days 1 to 14
[total dose/cycle = 84 mg/m^2]
Vinblastine: I.V.: 6 mg/m^2/day (maximum dose: 10 mg) days 1 and 8
[total dose/cycle = 12 mg/m^2]
Procarbazine: Oral: 100 mg/m^2/day (maximum dose: 150 mg) days 1 to 14
[total dose/cycle = 1400 mg/m^2]
Prednisone: Oral: 40-50 mg/day days 1 to 14
[total dose/cycle = 560-700 mg]
Repeat cycle every 28 days

CHL + PRED

Use Leukemia, chronic lymphocytic

Regimen

Chlorambucil: Oral: 0.4 mg/kg/day for 1 day every other week; increase initial dose of 0.4 mg/kg by 0.1 mg/kg every 2 weeks until toxicity or disease control is achieved
Prednisone: Oral: 100 mg/day for 2 days every other week

CHOP

Use Lymphoma, non-Hodgkin

Regimen NOTE: Multiple variations are listed below.

Variation 1:

Cyclophosphamide: I.V.: 750 mg/m^2 day 1
[total dose/cycle = 750 mg/m^2]
Doxorubicin: I.V.: 50 mg/m^2 day 1
[total dose/cycle = 50 mg/m^2]
Vincristine: I.V.: 1.4 mg/m^2 (maximum dose: 2 mg) day 1
[total dose/cycle = 1.4 mg/m^2]
Prednisone: Oral: 100 mg/day days 1 to 5
[total dose/cycle = 500 mg]
or Oral: 50 mg/m^2/day days 1 to 5
[total dose/cycle = 250 mg/m^2]
or Oral: 100 mg/m^2/day days 1 to 5
[total dose/cycle = 500 mg/m^2]
Repeat cycle every 21 days

Variation 2:

Cyclophosphamide: I.V.: 750 mg/m^2 day 1
[total dose/cycle = 750 mg/m^2]
Doxorubicin: I.V.: 50 mg/m^2 day 1
[total dose/cycle = 50 mg/m^2]
Vincristine: I.V.: 2 mg day 1
[total dose/cycle = 2 mg]
Prednisone: Oral: 75 mg/day days 1 to 5
[total dose/cycle = 375 mg]
Repeat cycle every 21 days

Variation 3:

Cyclophosphamide: I.V.: 750 mg/m^2/day days 1 and 8
[total dose/cycle = 1500 mg/m^2]
Doxorubicin: I.V.: 25 mg/m^2/day days 1 and 8
[total dose/cycle = 50 mg/m^2]
Vincristine: I.V.: 1.4 mg/m^2/day (maximum dose: 2 mg) days 1 and 8
[total dose/cycle = 2.8 mg/m^2]
Prednisone: Oral: 50 mg/m^2/day days 1 to 8
[total dose/cycle = 400 mg/m^2]
Repeat cycle every 28 days

Variation 4 - "mini-CHOP":

Cyclophosphamide: I.V.: 250 mg/m^2/day days 1, 8, and 15
[total dose/cycle = 750 mg/m^2]
Doxorubicin: I.V.: 16.7 mg/m^2/day days 1, 8, and 15
[total dose/cycle = 50.1 mg/m^2]
Vincristine: I.V.: 0.67 mg/day days 1, 8, and 15
[total dose/cycle = 2.01 mg]
Prednisone: Oral: 75 mg/day days 1 to 5
[total dose/cycle = 375 mg]
Repeat cycle every 21 days

CI (Neuroblastoma)

Use Neuroblastoma

Regimen

Ifosfamide: I.V.: 1500 mg/m^2/day days 1, 2, and 3
[total dose/cycle = 4500 mg/m^2]
Mesna: I.V.: 500 mg/m^2 every 3 hours, for 3 doses each day, days 1, 2, and 3
[total dose/cycle = 4500 mg/m^2]
Carboplatin: I.V.: 400 mg/m^2 day 4
[total dose/cycle = 400 mg/m^2]
Repeat cycle every 21-28 days

CISCA

Use Bladder cancer

Regimen

Cyclophosphamide: I.V.: 650 mg/m^2 day 1
[total dose = 650 mg/m^2]
Doxorubicin: I.V.: 50 mg/m^2 day 1
[total dose = 50 mg/m^2]
Cisplatin: I.V.: 100 mg/m^2 day 2
[total dose = 100 mg/m^2]
Repeat cycle every 21-28 days

Cisplatin-Capecitabine (Esophageal Cancer)

Use Esophageal cancer

Regimen

Cisplatin: I.V.: 80 mg/m^2 over 2 hours day 1
[total dose/cycle = 80 mg/m^2]
Capecitabine: Oral: 1000 mg/m^2/dose twice daily, days 1 to 14
[total dose/cycle = 28,000 mg/m^2]
Repeat cycle every 3 weeks until disease progression or unacceptable toxicity

Cisplatin-Capecitabine (Gastric Cancer)

Use Gastric cancer

Regimen

Cisplatin: I.V.: 80 mg/m^2 over 2 hours day 1
[total dose/cycle = 80 mg/m^2]
Capecitabine: Oral: 1000 mg/m^2/dose twice daily, days 1 to 14
[total dose/cycle = 28,000 mg/m^2]
Repeat cycle every 3 weeks until disease progression or unacceptable toxicity

Cisplatin-Cetuximab (Head and Neck Cancer)

Use Head and neck cancer

Regimen NOTE: Multiple variations are listed below.

Variation 1:
Cycle 1:
Cetuximab: I.V.: 400 mg/m^2 (loading dose) day 1 (week 1, cycle 1 only)
[total loading dose = 400 mg/m^2]
followed by I.V.: 250 mg/m^2/day days 8, 15, and 22
[total dose/cycle 1 = 1150 mg/m^2]
Cisplatin: I.V.: 100 mg/m^2 day 1
[total dose/cycle = 100 mg/m^2]
Treatment cycle is 4 weeks
Subsequent cycles:
Cetuximab: I.V.: 250 mg/m^2/day days 1, 8, 15, and 22
[total dose/cycle = 1000 mg/m^2]
Cisplatin: I.V.: 100 mg/m^2 day 1
[total dose/cycle = 100 mg/m^2]
Repeat cycle every 4 weeks
Variation 2:
Cycle 1:
Cetuximab: I.V.: 400 mg/m^2 (loading dose) day 1 (week 1, cycle 1 only)
[total loading dose = 400 mg/m^2]
followed by I.V.: 250 mg/m^2/day days 8 and 15
[total dose/cycle 1 = 900 mg/m^2]
Cisplatin: I.V.: 75-100 mg/m^2 day 1
[total dose/cycle = 75-100 mg/m^2]
Treatment cycle is 3 weeks

Subsequent cycles:
Cetuximab: I.V.: 250 mg/m^2/day days 1, 8, and 15
[total dose/cycle = 750 mg/m^2]
Cisplatin: I.V.: 75-100 mg/m^2 day 1
[total dose/cycle = 75-100 mg/m^2]
Repeat cycle every 3 weeks

Cisplatin-Cytarabine-Dexamethasone (NHL Regimen)

Use Lymphoma, non-Hodgkin

Regimen NOTE: Multiple variations are listed below.

Variation 1:
Dexamethasone: I.V. or Oral: 40 mg/day days 1 to 4
[total dose/cycle = 160 mg]
Cisplatin: I.V.: 100 mg/m^2 over 24 hours day 1
[total dose/cycle = 100 mg/m^2]
Cytarabine: I.V.: 2000 mg/m^2 every 12 hours for 2 doses day 2 (begins at the end of the cisplatin infusion)
[total dose/cycle = 4000 mg/m^2]
Repeat cycle every 3-4 weeks for 6-10 cycles

Variation 2 (patients >70 years of age):
Dexamethasone: I.V. or Oral: 40 mg/day days 1 to 4
[total dose/cycle = 160 mg]
Cisplatin: I.V.: 100 mg/m^2 over 24 hours day 1
[total dose/cycle = 100 mg/m^2]
Cytarabine: I.V.: 1000 mg/m^2 every 12 hours for 2 doses day 2 (begins at the end of the cisplatin infusion)
[total dose/cycle = 2000 mg/m^2]
Repeat cycle every 3-4 weeks for 6-10 cycles

Cisplatin-Dacarbazine-Carmustine (Melanoma)

Use Melanoma

Regimen NOTE: Multiple variations are listed below.

Variation 1:
Cisplatin: I.V.: 25 mg/m^2/day days 1, 2, and 3
[total dose/cycle = 75 mg/m^2]
Dacarbazine: I.V.: 220 mg/m^2/day days 1, 2, and 3
[total dose/cycle = 660 mg/m^2]
Carmustine: I.V.: 150 mg/m^2 day 1 (every other cycle **[odd cycles]**)
[total dose/**odd** cycles = 150 mg/m^2]
Repeat cycle every 21 days

Variation 2:
Carmustine: I.V.: 150 mg/m^2 day 1
[total dose/cycle = 150 mg/m^2]
Cisplatin: I.V.: 25 mg/m^2/day days 1, 2, 3, 22, 23, and 24
[total dose/cycle = 150 mg/m^2]
Dacarbazine: I.V.: 220 mg/m^2/day days 1, 2, 3, 22, 23, and 24
[total dose/cycle = 1320 mg/m^2]
Repeat cycle every 42 days

Cisplatin-Dacarbazine-Interferon Alfa-2b-Aldesleukin

Use Melanoma

Regimen

Cisplatin: I.V.: 25 mg/m^2/day days 1, 2, and 3
[total dose/cycle = 75 mg/m^2]
Dacarbazine: 250 mg/m^2/day days 1, 2, and 3
[total dose/cycle = 750 mg/m^2]
Interferon Alfa-2b: SubQ: 5 million units/m^2/day days 6, 8, 10, 13, and 15
[total dose/cycle = 25 million units/m^2]
Aldesleukin: I.V.: 18 million units/m^2/day days 6 to 10, 13, 14, and 15
[total dose/cycle = 144 million units/m^2]
Repeat cycle every 28 days

Cisplatin-Etoposide (NSCLC)

Use Lung cancer, nonsmall cell

Regimen NOTE: Multiple variations are listed below.

Variation 1:

Cisplatin: I.V.: 80 mg/m^2 day 1
[total dose/cycle = 80 mg/m^2]

Etoposide: I.V.: 100 mg/m^2/day days 1, 2, and 3
[total dose/cycle = 300 mg/m^2]

Repeat cycle every 21 days for a total of 4 cycles

Variation 2:

Cisplatin: I.V.: 100 mg/m^2 day 1
[total dose/cycle = 100 mg/m^2]

Etoposide: I.V.: 100 mg/m^2/day days 1, 2, and 3
[total dose/cycle = 300 mg/m^2]

Repeat cycle every 28 days for a total of 3 cycles

Variation 3:

Cisplatin: I.V.: 100 mg/m^2 day 1
[total dose/cycle = 100 mg/m^2]

Etoposide: I.V.: 100 mg/m^2/day days 1, 2, and 3
[total dose/cycle = 300 mg/m^2]

Repeat cycle every 28 days for a total of 4 cycles

Variation 4:

Cisplatin: I.V.: 120 mg/m^2/day days 1, 29, and 71
[total dose/treatment = 360 mg/m^2]

Etoposide: I.V.: 100 mg/m^2/day days 1, 2, 3, 29, 30, 31, 71, 72, and 73
[total dose/treatment = 900 mg/m^2]

Variation 5:

Cisplatin: I.V.: 75 mg/m^2 day 1
[total dose/cycle = 75 mg/m^2]

Etoposide: I.V.: 100 mg/m^2/day days 1, 2, and 3
[total dose/cycle = 300 mg/m^2]

Repeat cycle every 21 days for up to 10 cycles

Cisplatin-Fluorouracil (Bladder Cancer)

Use Bladder cancer

Regimen In combination with radiation therapy

Note: Begin infusion(s) 2 hours before radiation therapy on days 1, 3, 15, and 17:

Cisplatin: I.V.: 15 mg/m^2/day over 2 hours days 1, 2, 3, 15, 16, and 17
[total dose/cycle = 90 mg/m^2]

Fluorouracil: I.V.: 400 mg/m^2/day over 2 hours days 1, 2, 3, 15, 16, and 17
[total dose/cycle = 2400 mg/m^2]

Cisplatin-Fluorouracil (Cervical Cancer)

Use Cervical cancer

Regimen NOTE: Multiple variations are listed below.

Variation 1 (with concurrent radiation therapy):

Cisplatin: I.V.: 75 mg/m^2 day 1
[total dose/cycle = 75 mg/m^2]

Fluorouracil: I.V.: 1000 mg/m^2/day continuous infusion days 1 to 4 (96 hours)
[total dose/cycle = 4000 mg/m^2]

Repeat cycle every 21 days for a total 3 cycles

Variation 2 (with concurrent radiation therapy):

Cisplatin: I.V.: 50 mg/m^2 day 1 starting 4 hours before radiotherapy
[total dose/cycle = 50 mg/m^2]

Fluorouracil: I.V.: 1000 mg/m^2/day continuous infusion days 2 to 5 (96 hours)
[total dose/cycle = 4000 mg/m^2]

Repeat cycle every 28 days for a total of 2 cycles

Variation 3 (cycles 1 and 2 are with concurrent radiation therapy):
Cisplatin: I.V.: 70 mg/m^2 day 1
[total dose/cycle = 70 mg/m^2]
Fluorouracil: I.V.: 1000 mg/m^2/day continuous infusion days 1 to 4 (96 hours)
[total dose/cycle = 4000 mg/m^2]
Repeat cycle every 21 days for a total of 4 cycles

Cisplatin-Fluorouracil (Esophageal Cancer)

Use Esophageal cancer

Regimen NOTE: Multiple variations are listed below.

Variation 1:
Cisplatin: I.V.: 100 mg/m^2/dose day 1
[total dose/cycle = 100 mg/m^2]
Fluorouracil: I.V.: 1000 mg/m^2/day continuous infusion days 1 to 5
[total dose/cycle = 5000 mg/m^2]
Repeat cycle every 28 days

Variation 2:
Cycles 1 to 3 (prior to surgery):
Cisplatin: I.V.: 100 mg/m^2/dose day 1
[total dose/cycle = 100 mg/m^2]
Fluorouracil: I.V.: 1000 mg/m^2/day continuous infusion days 1 to 5
[total dose/cycle = 5000 mg/m^2]
Treatment cycles 1-3 are 28 days each
Cycles 4 and 5 (postoperative):
Cisplatin: I.V.: 75 mg/m^2/dose day 1
[total dose/cycle = 75 mg/m^2]
Fluorouracil: I.V.: 1000 mg/m^2/day continuous infusion days 1 to 5
[total dose/cycle = 5000 mg/m^2]
Treatment cycles 4 and 5 are 28 days each

Variation 3 (in combination with radiation therapy):
Cycle 1:
Cisplatin: I.V.: 75 mg/m^2/dose day 1
[total dose/cycle = 75 mg/m^2]
Fluorouracil: I.V.: 1000 mg/m^2/day continuous infusion days 1 to 4
[total dose/cycle = 4000 mg/m^2]
Treatment cycle is 28 days
Cycles 2 to 4:
Cisplatin: I.V.: 75 mg/m^2/dose day 1
[total dose/cycle = 75 mg/m^2]
Fluorouracil: I.V.: 1000 mg/m^2/day continuous infusion days 1 to 4
[total dose/cycle = 4000 mg/m^2]
Repeat cycle every 21 days for 3 more cycles (total of 4 cycles)

Variation 4 (in combination with radiation therapy):
Cisplatin: I.V.: 100 mg/m^2/dose day 1
[total dose/cycle = 100 mg/m^2]
Fluorouracil: I.V.: 1000 mg/m^2/day continuous infusion days 1 to 4
[total dose/cycle = 4000 mg/m^2]
Repeat cycle every 28 days for total of 2 cycles

Variation 5 (in combination with radiation therapy):
Cisplatin: I.V.: 75 mg/m^2/dose day 1
[total dose/cycle = 75 mg/m^2]
Fluorouracil: I.V.: 1000 mg/m^2/day continuous infusion days 1 to 4
[total dose/cycle = 4000 mg/m^2]
Repeat cycle every 28 days for 4 cycles

Variation 6 (in combination with radiation therapy):
Cycles 1 and 2:
Cisplatin: I.V.: 75 mg/m^2/dose day 1
[total dose/cycle = 75 mg/m^2]
Fluorouracil: I.V.: 1000 mg/m^2/day continuous infusion days 1 to 4
[total dose/cycle = 4000 mg/m^2]
Treatment cycles 1 and 2 are 28 days each; cycle 2 is followed by a 2-week rest

Cycles 3 and 4 (begin cycle 3 at week 11):
Cisplatin: I.V.: 75 mg/m^2/dose day 1
[total dose/cycle = 75 mg/m^2]
Fluorouracil: I.V.: 1000 mg/m^2/day continuous infusion days 1 to 4
[total dose/cycle = 4000 mg/m^2]
Treatment cycles 3 and 4 are 28 days each
Variation 7 (in combination with radiation therapy):
Cycles 1 to 4:
Cisplatin: I.V.: 15 mg/m^2/day days 1 to 5
[total dose/cycle = 75 mg/m^2]
Fluorouracil: I.V.: 800 mg/m^2/day continuous infusion days 1 to 5
[total dose/cycle = 4000 mg/m^2]
Repeat cycles 1-4 every 21 days; cycle 4 is followed by a 1-week rest
Cycles 5 (begin cycle 5 at week 14):
Cisplatin: I.V.: 15 mg/m^2/day days 1 to 5
[total dose/cycle = 75 mg/m^2]
Fluorouracil: I.V.: 800 mg/m^2/day continuous infusion days 1 to 5
[total dose/cycle = 4000 mg/m^2]

Cisplatin-Fluorouracil (Gastric Cancer)

Use Gastric cancer

Regimen NOTE: Multiple variations are listed below.
Variation 1:
Cisplatin: I.V.: 100 mg/m^2 day 1
[total dose/cycle = 100 mg/m^2]
Fluorouracil: I.V.: 1000 mg/m^2/day continuous infusion days 1 to 5
[total dose/cycle = 5000 mg/m^2]
Repeat cycle every 4 weeks until disease progression or unacceptable toxicity
Variation 2:
Cisplatin: I.V.: 80 mg/m^2 over 2 hours day 1
[total dose/cycle = 80 mg/m^2]
Fluorouracil: I.V.: 800 mg/m^2/day continuous infusion days 1 to 5
[total dose/cycle = 4000 mg/m^2]
Repeat cycle every 21 days until disease progression or unacceptable toxicity
Variation 3:
Fluorouracil: I.V.: 1000 mg/m^2/day continuous infusion days 1 to 5
[total dose/cycle = 5000 mg/m^2]
Cisplatin: I.V.: 100 mg/m^2 day 2
[total dose/cycle = 100 mg/m^2]
Repeat cycle every 4 weeks

Cisplatin-Fluorouracil (Head and Neck Cancer)

Use Head and neck cancer

Regimen NOTE: Multiple variations are listed below.
Variation 1:
Cisplatin: I.V.: 100 mg/m^2 day 1
[total dose/cycle = 100 mg/m^2]
Fluorouracil: I.V.: 1000 mg/m^2/day continuous infusion days 1 to 4
[total dose/cycle = 4000 mg/m^2]
Repeat cycle every 3 weeks
Variation 2:
Cisplatin: I.V.: 100 mg/m^2 day 1
[total dose/cycle = 100 mg/m^2]
Fluorouracil: I.V.: 1000 mg/m^2/day continuous infusion days 1 to 4
[total dose/cycle = 4000 mg/m^2]
Repeat cycle every 3 or 4 weeks
Variation 3:
Cisplatin: I.V.: 100 mg/m^2 day 1
[total dose/cycle = 100 mg/m^2]
Fluorouracil: I.V.: 1000 mg/m^2/day continuous infusion days 1 to 5
[total dose/cycle = 5000 mg/m^2]
Repeat cycle every 3 or 4 weeks

Variation 4:
- Cisplatin: I.V.: 60 mg/m^2 day 1
  - [total dose/cycle = 60 mg/m^2]
- Fluorouracil: I.V.: 800 mg/m^2/day continuous infusion days 1 to 5
  - [total dose/cycle = 4000 mg/m^2]
- Repeat cycle every 14 days

Variation 5:
- Cisplatin: I.V.: 20 mg/m^2/day days 1 to 5
  - [total dose/cycle = 100 mg/m^2]
- Fluorouracil: I.V.: 200 mg/m^2/day days 1 to 5
  - [total dose/cycle = 1000 mg/m^2]
- Repeat cycle every 3 weeks

Variation 6:
- Cisplatin: I.V.: 80 mg/m^2 continuous infusion day 1
  - [total dose/cycle = 80 mg/m^2]
- Fluorouracil: I.V.: 800 mg/m^2/day continuous infusion days 2 to 6
  - [total dose/cycle = 4000 mg/m^2]
- Repeat cycle every 3 weeks

Variation 7:
- Cisplatin: I.V.: 75 mg/m^2 day 1
  - [total dose/cycle = 75 mg/m^2]
- Fluorouracil: I.V.: 1000 mg/m^2/day continuous infusion days 1 to 4
  - [total dose/cycle = 4000 mg/m^2]
- Repeat cycle every 4 weeks

Variation 8:
- Cisplatin: I.V.: 120 mg/m^2 day 1
  - [total dose/cycle = 120 mg/m^2]
- Fluorouracil: I.V.: 1000 mg/m^2/day continuous infusion days 1 to 5
  - [total dose/cycle = 5000 mg/m^2]
- Repeat cycle every 3 weeks

Variation 9:
- Cisplatin: I.V.: 25 mg/m^2/day continuous infusion days 1 to 4
  - [total dose/cycle = 100 mg/m^2]
- Fluorouracil: I.V.: 1000 mg/m^2/day days 1 to 4
  - [total dose/cycle = 4000 mg/m^2]
- Repeat cycle every 3 weeks

Variation 10:
- Fluorouracil: I.V.: 350 mg/m^2/day continuous infusion days 1 to 5
  - [total dose/cycle = 1750 mg/m^2]
- Cisplatin: I.V.: 50 mg/m^2 day 6
  - [total dose/cycle = 50 mg/m^2]
- Repeat cycle every 3 weeks

Variation 11:
- Cisplatin: I.V.: 5 mg/m^2/day continuous infusion days 1 to 14
  - [total dose/cycle = 70 mg/m^2]
- Fluorouracil: I.V.: 200 mg/m^2/day continuous infusion days 1 to 14
  - [total dose/cycle = 2800 mg/m^2]
- With concurrent radiation therapy, cycle does not repeat

Variation 12 (administer during the final 2 weeks of radiation therapy; weeks 6 and 7):
- Cisplatin: I.V.: 10 mg/m^2/day days 1 to 5 beginning week 6
  - [total dose/week = 50 mg/m^2]
- Fluorouracil: I.V.: 400 mg/m^2/day continuous infusion days 1 to 5 beginning week 6
  - [total dose/week = 2000 mg/m^2]
- Repeat cycle one time in week 7

Variation 13:
Cisplatin: I.V.: 100 mg/m²/day day 1 (concurrent with radiation therapy)
[total dose/cycle = 100 mg/m²]
Repeat cycle every 3 weeks for a total of 3 cycles
Followed by (postradiation chemotherapy; begin 4 weeks after radiotherapy or the last cisplatin dose):
Cisplatin: I.V.: 80 mg/m² day 1
[total dose/cycle = 80 mg/m²]
Fluorouracil: I.V.: 1000 mg/m²/day continuous infusion days 1 to 4
[total dose/cycle = 4000 mg/m²]
Repeat cycle every 4 weeks for a total of 3 cycles

Cisplatin-Gemcitabine (Cervical Cancer)

Use Cervical cancer

Regimen NOTE: Multiple variations are listed below.

Variation 1:
Gemcitabine: I.V.: 1250 mg/m²/day days 1 and 8
[total dose/cycle = 2500 mg/m²]
Cisplatin: I.V.: 50 mg/m² day 1
[total dose/cycle = 50 mg/m²]
Repeat cycle every 21 days for up to a total of 6 cycles

Variation 2:
Gemcitabine: I.V.: 1000 mg/m²/day days 1 and 8
[total dose/cycle = 2000 mg/m²]
Cisplatin: I.V.: 50 mg/m² day 1
[total dose/cycle = 50 mg/m²]
Repeat cycle every 21 days for up to a total of 6 cycles; responders may continue beyond 6 cycles

Cisplatin-Irinotecan (Small Cell Lung Cancer)

Use Lung cancer, small cell

Regimen NOTE: Multiple variations are listed.

Variation 1:
Cisplatin: I.V.: 60 mg/m² day 1
[total dose/cycle = 60 mg/m²]
Irinotecan: I.V.: 60 mg/m²/dose days 1, 8, and 15
[total dose/cycle = 180 mg/m²]
Repeat cycle every 28 days for 4 cycles

Variation 2:
Cisplatin: I.V.: 30 mg/m² days 1 and 8
[total dose/cycle = 60 mg/m²]
Irinotecan: I.V.: 65 mg/m²/dose days 1 and 8
[total dose/cycle = 130 mg/m²]
Repeat cycle every 21 days for at least 4 cycles

Cisplatin-Paclitaxel (Cervical Cancer)

Use Cervical cancer

Regimen

Paclitaxel: I.V.: 135 mg/m² continuous infusion over 24 hours day 1
[total dose/cycle = 135 mg/m²]
Cisplatin: I.V.: 50 mg/m² day 2
[total dose/cycle = 50 mg/m²]
Repeat cycle every 21 days for up to a total of 6 cycles; responders may continue beyond 6 cycles

Cisplatin-Paclitaxel (Head and Neck Cancer)

Use Head and neck cancer

Regimen NOTE: Multiple variations are listed.

Variation 1 (with concurrent radiation therapy):
Paclitaxel: I.V.: 30 mg/m² day 1
[total dose/week = 30 mg/m²]
Cisplatin: I.V.: 20 mg/m² day 2
[total dose/week = 20 mg/m²]
Repeat every week for a total of 7 weeks

Variation 2:
Paclitaxel: I.V.: 175 mg/m^2 dose over 3 hours day 1
[total dose/cycle = 175 mg/m^2]
Cisplatin: I.V.: 75 mg/m^2/dose day 1
[total dose/cycle = 75 mg/m^2]
Repeat cycle every 3 weeks

Cisplatin-Paclitaxel (Intraperitoneal Regimen)

Use Ovarian cancer

Regimen Note: I.P. therapies administered in 2 liters warmed saline
Paclitaxel: I.V.: 135 mg/m^2 continuous infusion (over 24 hours) day 1
[total dose/cycle = 135 mg/m^2]
Cisplatin: I.P.: 100 mg/m^2 day 2
[total dose/cycle = 100 mg/m^2]
Paclitaxel: I.P.: 60 mg/m^2 day 8
[total dose/cycle = 60 mg/m^2]
Repeat cycle every 21 days for 6 cycles

Cisplatin-Paclitaxel (Ovarian Cancer)

Use Ovarian cancer

Regimen NOTE: Multiple variations are listed below.
Variation 1:
Paclitaxel: I.V.: 135 mg/m^2 continuous infusion over 24 hours day 1
[total dose/cycle = 135 mg/m^2]
Cisplatin: I.V.: 75 mg/m^2 day 2
[total dose/cycle = 75 mg/m^2]
Repeat cycle every 21 days for a total of 6 cycles
Variation 2:
Paclitaxel: I.V.: 175 mg/m^2 over 3 hours day 1
[total dose/cycle = 175 mg/m^2]
Cisplatin: I.V.: 75 mg/m^2 day 1
[total dose/cycle = 75 mg/m^2]
Repeat cycle every 21 days for a total of at least 6 cycles
Variation 3:
Paclitaxel: I.V.: 185 mg/m^2 (maximum dose: 400 mg) over 3 hours day 1
[total dose/cycle = 185 mg/m^2; maximum: 400 mg]
Cisplatin: I.V.: 75 mg/m^2 (maximum dose: 165 mg) day 1
[total dose/cycle = 75 mg/m^2; maximum: 165 mg]
Repeat cycle every 21 days

Cisplatin-Pemetrexed (Mesothelioma)

Use Malignant pleural mesothelioma

Regimen
Pemetrexed: I.V.: 500 mg/m^2 infused over 10 minutes day 1
[total dose/cycle = 500 mg/m^2]
Cisplatin: I.V.: 75 mg/m^2 infused over 2 hours day 1 (start 30 minutes after pemetrexed)
[total dose/cycle = 75 mg/m^2]
Repeat cycle every 21 days

Cisplatin-Topotecan (Cervical Cancer)

Use Cervical cancer

Regimen NOTE: Multiple variations are listed below.
Variation 1 (Body surface area capped at 2 m^2 maximum):
Topotecan: I.V.: 0.75 mg/m^2/day days 1, 2, and 3
[total dose/cycle = 2.25 mg/m^2]
Cisplatin: I.V.: 50 mg/m^2 day 1 only
[total dose/cycle = 50 mg/m^2]
Repeat cycle every 21 days for up to a total of 6 cycles; responders may continue beyond 6 cycles

Variation 2:
Topotecan: I.V.: 0.75 mg/m^2/day days 1, 2, and 3
[total dose/cycle = 2.25 mg/m^2]
Cisplatin: I.V.: 50 mg/m^2 day 1 only
[total dose/cycle = 50 mg/m^2]
Repeat cycle every 21 days for up to a total of 6 cycles; responders may continue beyond 6 cycles

Cisplatin-Vinblastine-Dacarbazine (Melanoma)

Use Melanoma

Regimen NOTE: Multiple variations are listed below.

Variation 1:
Cisplatin: I.V.: 20 mg/m^2/day days 2 to 5
[total dose/cycle = 80 mg/m^2]
Vinblastine: I.V.: 1.6 mg/m^2/day days 1 to 5
[total dose/cycle = 8 mg/m^2]
Dacarbazine: I.V.: 800 mg/m^2 day 1
[total dose/cycle = 800 mg/m^2]
Repeat cycle every 21 days

Variation 2:
Cisplatin: I.V.: 20 mg/m^2/day days 1 to 4
[total dose/cycle = 80 mg/m^2]
Vinblastine: I.V.: 2 mg/m^2/day days 1 to 4
[total dose/cycle = 8 mg/m^2]
Dacarbazine: I.V.: 800 mg/m^2 day 1
[total dose/cycle = 800 mg/m^2]
Repeat cycle every 21 days

Cisplatin-Vinblastine (NSCLC)

Use Lung cancer, nonsmall cell

Regimen NOTE: Multiple variations are listed below.

Variation 1:
Cisplatin: I.V.: 80 mg/m^2/day days 1, 22, 43, and 64
[total dose/treatment = 320 mg/m^2]
Vinblastine: I.V.: 4 mg/m^2/day days 1, 8, 15, 22, 29, 43, and 57
[total dose/treatment = 28 mg/m^2]

Variation 2:
Cisplatin: I.V.: 100 mg/m^2/day days 1, 29, and 57
[total dose/treatment = 300 mg/m^2]
Vinblastine: I.V.: 4 mg/m^2/day days 1, 8, 15, 22, 29, 43, and 57
[total dose/treatment = 28 mg/m^2]

Variation 3:
Cisplatin: I.V.: 100 mg/m^2/day days 1, 29, 57, and 85
[total dose/treatment = 400 mg/m^2]
Vinblastine: I.V.: 4 mg/m^2/day days 1, 8, 15, 22, 29, 43, 57, 71, and 85
[total dose/treatment = 36 mg/m^2]

Variation 4:
Cisplatin: I.V.: 120 mg/m^2/day days 1, 29, and 71
[total dose/treatment = 360 mg/m^2]
Vinblastine: I.V.: 4 mg/m^2/day days 1, 8, 15, 22, 29, 43, 57, and 71
[total dose/treatment = 32 mg/m^2]

Cisplatin-Vinorelbine (Cervical Cancer)

Use Cervical cancer

Regimen NOTE: Multiple variations are listed below.

Variation 1:
Cisplatin: I.V.: 50 mg/m^2 day 1
[total dose/cycle = 50 mg/m^2]
Vinorelbine: I.V.: 30 mg/m^2/day days 1 and 8
[total dose/cycle = 60 mg/m^2]
Repeat cycle every 21 days for up to a total of 6 cycles; responders may continue beyond 6 cycles

Variation 2:
Cisplatin: I.V.: 80 mg/m^2 day 1
[total dose/cycle = 80 mg/m^2]
Vinorelbine: I.V.: 25 mg/m^2/day days 1 and 8
[total dose/cycle = 50 mg/m^2]
Repeat cycle every 21 days for a total of 3-6 cycles

CMF

Use Breast cancer

Regimen NOTE: Multiple variations are listed below.
Variation 1:
Methotrexate: I.V.: 40 mg/m^2/day days 1 and 8
[total dose/cycle = 80 mg/m^2]
Fluorouracil: I.V.: 600 mg/m^2/day days 1 and 8
[total dose/cycle = 1200 mg/m^2]
Cyclophosphamide: Oral: 100 mg/m^2/day days 1 to 14
[total dose/cycle = 1400 mg/m^2]
Repeat cycle every 28 days
Variation 2 (>60 years of age):
Methotrexate: I.V.: 30 mg/m^2/day days 1 and 8
[total dose/cycle = 60 mg/m^2]
Fluorouracil: I.V.: 400 mg/m^2/day days 1 and 8
[total dose/cycle = 800 mg/m^2]
Cyclophosphamide: Oral: 100 mg/m^2/day days 1 to 14
[total dose/cycle = 1400 mg/m^2]
Repeat cycle every 28 days

CMF-IV

Use Breast cancer

Regimen
Cyclophosphamide: I.V.: 600 mg/m^2 day 1
[total dose/cycle = 600 mg/m^2]
Methotrexate: I.V.: 40 mg/m^2 day 1
[total dose/cycle = 40 mg/m^2]
Fluorouracil: I.V.: 600 mg/m^2 day 1
[total dose/cycle = 600 mg/m^2]
Repeat cycle every 21 or 28 days

CMFP

Use Breast cancer

Regimen
Cyclophosphamide: Oral: 100 mg/m^2/day days 1 to 14
[total dose = 1400 mg/m^2]
Methotrexate: I.V.: 30 or 40 mg/m^2/day days 1 and 8
[total dose = 60 or 80 mg/m^2]
Fluorouracil: I.V.: 400 or 600 mg/m^2/day days 1 and 8
[total dose = 800 or 1200 mg/m^2]
Prednisone: Oral: 40 mg/m^2/day days 1 to 14
[total dose = 560 mg/m^2]
Repeat cycle every 28 days

CMFVP (Cooper Regimen, VPCMF)

Use Breast cancer

Regimen
Cyclophosphamide: Oral: 2 mg/kg/day days 1 to 252
[total dose/cycle = 504 mg/kg]
Methotrexate: I.V.: 0.7 mg/kg day 1, weeks 1 to 8, 10, 12, 14, 16, 18, 20, 22, 24, 26, 28, 30, 32, 34, and 36
[total dose/cycle = 15.4 mg/kg]
Fluorouracil: I.V.: 12 mg/kg day 1, weeks 1 to 8, 10, 12, 14, 16, 18, 20, 22, 24, 26, 28, 30, 32, 34, and 36
[total dose/cycle = 264 mg/kg]

Vincristine: I.V.: 0.035 mg/kg (maximum dose: 2 mg) day 1, weeks 1 to 5, 8, 12, 16, 20, 24, 28, 32, and 36
[total dose/cycle = 0.455 mg/kg]
Prednisone: Oral: 0.75 mg/kg/day days 1 to 10, taper off over next 40 days
Administer one cycle only

CMV

Use Bladder cancer

Regimen

Cisplatin: I.V.: 100 mg/m^2 infused over 4 hours (start at least 12 hours after methotrexate) day 2
[total dose = 100 mg/m^2]
Methotrexate: I.V.: 30 mg/m^2/day days 1 and 8
[total dose = 60 mg/m^2]
Vinblastine: I.V.: 4 mg/m^2/day days 1 and 8
[total dose = 8 mg/m^2]
Repeat cycle every 21 days

CNOP

Use Lymphoma, non-Hodgkin

Regimen

Cyclophosphamide: I.V.: 750 mg/m^2 day 1
[total dose/cycle = 750 mg/m^2]
Mitoxantrone: I.V.: 10 mg/m^2 day 1
[total dose/cycle = 10 mg/m^2]
Vincristine: I.V.: 1.4 mg/m^2 day 1
[total dose/cycle = 1.4 mg/m^2]
Prednisone: Oral: 50 mg/m^2/day days 1 to 5
[total dose/cycle = 250 mg/m^2]
Repeat cycle every 21 days

CO

Use Retinoblastoma

Regimen

Cyclophosphamide: I.V.: 10 mg/kg/day days 1, 2, and 3
[total dose/cycle = 30 mg/kg]
Vincristine: I.V.: 1.5 mg/m^2 day 1
[total dose/cycle = 1.5 mg/m^2]
Repeat cycle every 21 days

CODOX-M

Use Lymphoma, non-Hodgkin

Regimen

Cytarabine: I.T.: 70 mg/day days 1 and 3
[total dose/cycle = 140 mg]
Cyclophosphamide: I.V.: 800 mg/m^2 day 1
followed by I.V.: 200 mg/m^2/day days 2 to 5
[total dose/cycle = 1600 mg/m^2]
Vincristine: I.V.: 1.5 mg/m^2/day days 1 and 8 (cycle 1); days 1, 8, and 15 (cycle 3)
[total dose/cycle = 3-4.5 mg/m^2]
Doxorubicin: I.V.: 40 mg/m^2 day 1
[total dose/cycle = 40 mg/m^2]
Methotrexate:
I.T.: 12 mg day 15
[total dose/cycle = 12 mg]
I.V.: 1200 mg/m^2 loading dose
followed by I.V.: 240 mg/m^2/hour for 23 hours day 10
[total dose/cycle = 6720 mg/m^2]
Leucovorin: I.V.: 192 mg/m^2 day 11
followed by I.V.: 12 mg/m^2 every 6 hours until methotrexate level <5 X 10^{-8}M (begin 36 hours after the start of methotrexate infusion)
Sargramostim: SubQ: 7.5 mcg/kg/day day 13 until ANC >1000 cells/mm^3
Repeat cycle when ANC >1000 cells/mm^3

CODOX-M/IVAC

Use Lymphoma, non-Hodgkin (Burkitt)

Regimen

CODOX-M

Cyclophosphamide: I.V.: 800 mg/m^2/day days 1 and 2
[total dose/cycle = 1600 mg/m^2]
Vincristine: I.V.: 1.4 mg/m^2/day (maximum dose: 2 mg) days 1 and 10
[total dose/cycle = 2.8 mg/m^2; maximum: 4 mg/cycle]
Doxorubicin: I.V.: 50 mg/m^2 day 1
[total dose/cycle = 50 mg/m^2]
Methotrexate: I.V.: 3 g/m^2 day 10
[total dose/cycle = 3 g/m^2]
Leucovorin: I.V.: 200 mg/m^2 day 11
followed by Oral, I.V.: 15 mg/m^2 every 6 hours until methotrexate level <0.1 Mmol/L
Cytarabine: I.T.: 50 mg/day days 1 and 3
[total dose/cycle = 100 mg]
Methotrexate: I.T.: 12 mg day 1
[total dose/cycle = 12 mg]
Filgrastim: SubQ: Dose not specified, days 3 to 8 and day 12 until ANC >1000 cells/mm^3
Cycle alternates with IVAC (cycles begin when ANC >1000 cells/mm^3)

Note: Hydrocortisone 50 mg may be added to intrathecal therapy to reduce the incidence of side effects/ chemical arachnoiditis.

IVAC

Ifosfamide: I.V.: 1500 mg/m^2/day days 1 to 5
[total dose/cycle = 7500 mg/m^2]
Mesna: I.V.: 1500 mg/m^2/day (in divided doses) days 1 to 5
[total dose/cycle = 7500 mg/m^2]
Etoposide: I.V.: 60 mg/m^2/day days 1 to 5
[total dose/cycle = 300 mg/m^2]
Cytarabine: I.V.: 2 g/m^2 every 12 hours, for 4 doses, days 1 and 2
[total dose/cycle = 8 g/m^2]
Methotrexate: I.T.: 12 mg day 5
[total dose/cycle = 12 mg]
Filgrastim: SubQ: Dose not specified, day 6 until ANC >1000 cells/mm^3
Cycle alternates with CODOX-M (cycles begin when ANC >1000 cells/mm^3)

Note: Hydrocortisone 50 mg may be added to intrathecal therapy to reduce the incidence of side effects/ chemical arachnoiditis.

COMLA

Use Lymphoma, non-Hodgkin

Regimen

Cyclophosphamide: I.V.: 1500 mg/m^2 day 1
[total dose/cycle = 1500 mg/m^2]
Vincristine: I.V.: 1.4 mg/m^2/day (maximum dose: 2 mg) days 1, 8, and 15
[total dose/cycle = 4.2 mg/m^2]
Methotrexate: I.V.: 120 mg/m^2/day days 22, 29, 36, 43, 50, 57, 64, and 71
[total dose/cycle = 960 mg/m^2]
Leucovorin: Oral: 25 mg/m^2 every 6 hours for 4 doses (beginning 24 hours after each methotrexate dose)
[total dose/cycle = 800 mg/m^2]
Cytarabine: I.V.: 300 mg/m^2/day days 22, 29, 36, 43, 50, 57, 64, and 71
[total dose/cycle = 2400 mg/m^2]
Repeat cycle every 85 days

COMP

Use Lymphoma, Hodgkin disease; Lymphoma, non-Hodgkin disease

Regimen

Cyclophosphamide: I.V.: 1200 mg/m^2 day 1, cycle 1
[total dose/cycle = 1200 mg/m^2]
followed by I.V.: 1000 mg/m^2 day 1 on subsequent cycles
[total dose/cycle = 1000 mg/m^2]

Vincristine: I.V.: 2 mg/m^2/day (maximum dose: 2 mg) days 3, 10, 17, 24, cycle 1
[total dose/cycle = 8 mg/m^2]
followed by I.V.: 1.5 mg/m^2/day days 1 and 4, on subsequent cycles
[total dose/cycle = 3 mg/m^2]
Methotrexate: I.V.: 300 mg/m^2 day 12
[total dose/cycle = 300 mg/m^2]
Prednisone: Oral: 60 mg/m^2/day (maximum dose: 60 mg) days 3 to 30 then taper over next 7 days, cycle 1
[total dose/cycle = 1680 mg/m^2 then taper over next 7 days]
followed by Oral: 60 mg/m^2 (maximum dose: 60 mg) days 1 to 5, on subsequent cycles
[total dose/cycle = 300 mg/m^2]
Maintenance cycles repeat every 28 days

COP-BLAM

Use Lymphoma, non-Hodgkin

Regimen

Cyclophosphamide: I.V.: 400 mg/m^2 day 1
[total dose/cycle = 400 mg/m^2]
Vincristine: I.V.: 1 mg/m^2 day 1
[total dose/cycle = 1 mg/m^2]
Prednisone: Oral: 40 mg/m^2/day days 1 to 10
[total dose/cycle = 400 mg/m^2]
Bleomycin: I.V.: 15 mg day 14
[total dose/cycle = 15 mg]
Doxorubicin: I.V.: 40 mg/m^2 day 1
[total dose/cycle = 40 mg/m^2]
Procarbazine: Oral: 100 mg/m^2/day days 1 to 10
[total dose/cycle = 1000 mg/m^2]

COPE

Use Brain tumors

Regimen

Cycle A:
Vincristine: I.V.: 0.065 mg/kg/day (maximum dose: 1.5 mg) days 1 and 8
[total dose/cycle = 0.13 mg/kg]
Cyclophosphamide: I.V.: 65 mg/kg day 1
[total dose/cycle = 65 mg/kg]
Cycle B:
Cisplatin: I.V.: 4 mg/kg day 1
[total dose/cycle = 4 mg/kg]
Etoposide: I.V.: 6.5 mg/kg/day days 3 and 4
[total dose/cycle = 13 mg/kg]
Repeat cycle every 28 days in the following sequence: AABAAB

COPP

Use Lymphoma, non-Hodgkin

Regimen

Cyclophosphamide: I.V.: 450-650 mg/m^2/day days 1 and 8
[total dose/cycle = 900-1300 mg/m^2]
Vincristine: I.V.: 1.4-2 mg/m^2/day (maximum dose: 2 mg) days 1 and 8
[total dose/cycle = 2.8-4 mg/m^2]
Procarbazine: Oral: 100 mg/m^2/day days 1 to 14
[total dose/cycle = 1400 mg/m^2]
Prednisone: Oral: 40 mg/m^2/day days 1 to 14
[total dose/cycle = 560 mg/m^2]
Repeat cycle every 3-4 weeks

CP (Leukemia)

Use Leukemia, chronic lymphocytic

Regimen

Chlorambucil: Oral: 30 mg/m^2 day 1
[total dose/cycle = 30 mg/m^2]
Prednisone: Oral: 80 mg/day days 1 to 5
[total dose/cycle = 400 mg]
Repeat cycle every 14 days

CP (Ovarian Cancer)

Use Ovarian cancer

Regimen

Cyclophosphamide: I.V.: 750 mg/m^2 day 1
[total dose/cycle = 750 mg/m^2]
Cisplatin: I.V.: 75 mg/m^2 day 1
[total dose/cycle = 75 mg/m^2]
Repeat cycle every 21 days

CV

Use Retinoblastoma

Regimen

Cyclophosphamide: I.V.: 300 mg/m^2
[total dose/cycle = 300 mg/m^2]
Vincristine: I.V.: 1.5 mg/m^2
[total dose/cycle = 1.5 mg/m^2]
Repeat weekly for 6 weeks
followed by
Cyclophosphamide: I.V.: 200 mg/m^2
[total dose/cycle = 200 mg/m^2]
Vincristine: I.V.: 1.5 mg/m^2
[total dose/cycle = 1.5 mg/m^2]
Repeat weekly for 42 weeks

CVD-Interleukin-Interferon (Melanoma)

Use Melanoma

Regimen NOTE: Multiple variations are listed below.

Variation 1:
Cisplatin: I.V.: 20 mg/m^2/day days 1 to 4 and 22 to 25
[total dose/cycle = 160 mg/m^2]
Vinblastine: I.V.: 1.5 mg/m^2/day days 1 to 4 and 22 to 25
[total dose/cycle = 12 mg/m^2]
Dacarbazine: I.V.: 800 mg/m^2/day days 1 and 22
[total dose/cycle = 1600 mg/m^2]
Aldesleukin: I.V.: 9 million units/m^2/day continuous infusion days 5 to 8, 17 to 20, and 26 to 29
[total dose/cycle = 108 million units/m^2]
Interferon alfa-2b: SubQ: 5 million units/m^2/day days 5 to 9, 17 to 21, and 26 to 30
[total dose/cycle = 75 million units/m^2]
Repeat every 42 days (maximum of five 21-day cycles for cytokine [interleukin and interferon] component)

Variation 2:
Cisplatin: I.V.: 20 mg/m^2/day days 1 to 4
[total dose/cycle = 80 mg/m^2]
Vinblastine: I.V.: 1.6 mg/m^2/day days 1 to 4
[total dose/cycle = 6.4 mg/m^2]
Dacarbazine: I.V.: 800 mg/m^2 day 1
[total dose/cycle = 800 mg/m^2]
Aldesleukin: I.V.: 9 million units/m^2/day continuous infusion days 1 to 4
[total dose/cycle = 36 million units/m^2]

Interferon alfa-2a: SubQ: 5 million units/m^2/day days 1 to 5, 7, 9, 11, and 13
[total dose/cycle = 45 million units/m^2]
Repeat cycle every 21 days for a total of 6 cycles

Variation 3:
Cisplatin: I.V.: 20 mg/m^2/day days 1 to 4
[total dose/cycle = 80 mg/m^2]
Vinblastine: I.V.: 1.2 mg/m^2/day days 1 to 4
[total dose/cycle = 4.8 mg/m^2]
Dacarbazine: I.V.: 800 mg/m^2 day 1
[total dose/cycle = 800 mg/m^2]
Aldesleukin: I.V.: 9 million units/m^2/day continuous infusion days 1 to 4
[total dose/cycle = 36 million units/m^2]
Interferon alfa-2b: SubQ: 5 million units/m^2/day days 1 to 5, 8, 10, and 12
[total dose/cycle = 40 million units/m^2]
Repeat cycle every 21 days (maximum: 4 cycles)

CVP (Leukemia)

Use Leukemia, chronic lymphocytic

Regimen NOTE: Multiple variations are listed below.

Variation 1:
Cyclophosphamide: Oral: 300 or 400 mg/m^2/day days 1 to 5
[total dose/cycle = 1500 or 2000 mg/m^2]
Vincristine: I.V.: 1.4 mg/m^2 (maximum dose: 2 mg) day 1
[total dose/cycle = 1.4 mg/m^2]
Prednisone: Oral: 100 mg/m^2/day days 1 to 5
[total dose/cycle = 500 mg/m^2]
Repeat cycle every 21 days

Variation 2:
Cyclophosphamide: I.V.: 800 mg/m^2 day 1
[total dose/cycle = 800 mg/m^2]
Vincristine: I.V.: 1.4 mg/m^2 (maximum dose: 2 mg) day 1
[total dose/cycle = 1.4 mg/m^2]
Prednisone: Oral: 100 mg/m^2/day days 1 to 5
[total dose/cycle = 500 mg/m^2]
Repeat cycle every 21 days

CVP (Lymphoma, non-Hodgkin)

Use Lymphoma, non-Hodgkin

Regimen NOTE: Multiple variations are listed below.

Variation 1:
Cyclophosphamide: I.V.: 750 mg/m^2 day 1
[total dose/cycle = 750 mg/m^2]
Vincristine: I.V.: 1.2 mg/m^2 day 1
[total dose/cycle = 1.2 mg/m^2]
Prednisone: Oral: 40 mg/m^2/day days 1 to 5
[total dose/cycle = 200 mg/m^2]
Repeat cycle every 21 days for up to 10 cycles

Variation 2:
Cyclophosphamide: I.V.: 750 mg/m^2 day 1
[total dose/cycle = 750 mg/m^2]
Vincristine: I.V.: 1.2 mg/m^2 day 1 (maximum dose: 2 mg)
[total dose/cycle = 1.2 mg/m^2 (maximum: 2 mg)]
Prednisone: Oral: 40 mg/m^2/day days 1 to 5
[total dose/cycle = 200 mg/m^2]
Repeat cycle every 28 days for up to 8 cycles

Variation 3:
Cyclophosphamide: I.V.: 750 mg/m^2 day 1
[total dose/cycle = 750 mg/m^2]
Vincristine: I.V.: 1.4 mg/m^2 day 1 (maximum dose: 2 mg)
[total dose/cycle = 1.4 mg/m^2 (maximum: 2 mg)]
Prednisone: Oral: 40 mg/m^2/day days 1 to 5
[total dose/cycle = 200 mg/m^2]
Repeat cycle every 21 days for up to 8 cycles

Variation 4:
Cyclophosphamide: Oral: 400 mg/m^2/day days 1 to 5
[total dose/cycle = 2000 mg/m^2]
Vincristine: I.V.: 1.4 mg/m^2 day 1 (maximum dose: 2 mg)
[total dose/cycle = 1.4 mg/m^2 (maximum: 2 mg)]
Prednisone: Oral: 100 mg/m^2/day days 1 to 5
[total dose/cycle = 500 mg/m^2]
Repeat cycle every 21 days

Cyclophosphamide-Fludarabine-Alemtuzumab-Rituximab (CLL)

Use Leukemia, chronic lymphocytic

Regimen

Variation 1:
Cyclophosphamide: I.V.: 200 mg/m^2/day days 3, 4, and 5
[total dose/cycle = 600 mg/m^2]
Fludarabine: I.V.: 20 mg/m^2/day days 3, 4, and 5
[total dose/cycle = 60 mg/m^2]
Rituximab: I.V.: 375-500 mg/m^2/dose day 2
[total dose/cycle = 375-500 mg/m^2]
Alemtuzumab: I.V.: 30 mg/dose days 1, 3, and 5
[total dose/cycle = 90 mg]
Repeat cycle every 28 days for up to a total of 6 cycles
Variation 2:
Cyclophosphamide: I.V.: 200 mg/m^2/day days 3, 4, and 5
[total dose/cycle = 600 mg/m^2]
Fludarabine: I.V.: 20 mg/m^2/day days 3, 4, and 5
[total dose/cycle = 60 mg/m^2]
Rituximab: I.V.: 375-500 mg/m^2/dose day 2
[total dose/cycle = 375-500 mg/m^2]
Alemtuzumab: I.V.: 30 mg/dose days 1, 3, and 5
[total dose/cycle = 90 mg]
Pegfilgrastim: SubQ: 6 mg with each cycle
Repeat cycle every 28 days for a total of 6 cycles
Variation 3:
Cyclophosphamide: I.V.: 250 mg/m^2/day days 3, 4, and 5
[total dose/cycle = 750 mg/m^2]
Fludarabine: I.V.: 25 mg/m^2/day days 3, 4, and 5
[total dose/cycle = 75 mg/m^2]
Rituximab: I.V.: 375-500 mg/m^2/dose day 2
[total dose/cycle = 375-500 mg/m^2]
Alemtuzumab: I.V.: 30 mg/dose days 1, 3, and 5
[total dose/cycle = 90 mg]
Repeat cycle every 28 days for a total of 6 cycles

CYVADIC

Use Sarcoma

Regimen

Cyclophosphamide: I.V.: 500 mg/m^2 day 1
[total dose/cycle = 500 mg/m^2]
Vincristine: I.V.: 1.4 mg/m^2/day days 1 and 5
[total dose/cycle = 2.8 mg/m^2]
Doxorubicin: I.V.: 50 mg/m^2 day 1
[total dose/cycle = 50 mg/m^2]
Dacarbazine: I.V.: 250 mg/m^2/day days 1 to 5
[total dose/cycle = 1250 mg/m^2]
Repeat cycle every 21 days

DA

Use Leukemia, acute myeloid (induction)

Regimen Induction:

Daunorubicin: I.V.: 45 mg/m^2/day days 1, 2, and 3
[total dose/cycle = 135 mg/m^2]
Cytarabine: I.V.: 100 mg/m^2/day continuous infusion days 1 to 7
[total dose/cycle = 700 mg/m^2]

Dacarbazine-Carboplatin-Aldesleukin-Interferon

Use Melanoma

Regimen

Dacarbazine: I.V.: 750 mg/m^2/day days 1 and 22
[total dose/cycle = 1500 mg/m^2]
Carboplatin: I.V.: 400 mg/m^2/day days 1 and 22
[total dose/cycle = 800 mg/m^2]
Aldesleukin: SubQ: 4,800,000 units every 8 hours days 36 and 57
[total dose/cycle = 28,800,000 units]
then 4,800,000 units every 12 hours days 37 and 58
[total dose/cycle = 19,200,000 units]
then 4,800,000 units/day days 38 to 40, 43 to 47, 50 to 54, 59 to 61, 65 to 68, 71 to 75
[total dose/cycle = 120,000,000 units]
Interferon alpha-2a: SubQ: 6,000,000 units days 38, 40, 43, 45, 47, 50, 52, 54, 59, 61, 64, 66, 68, 71, 73, and 75
[total dose/cycle = 96,000,000 units]
Repeat cycle every 78 days for 3 cycles

Dartmouth Regimen

Use Melanoma

Regimen NOTE: Multiple variations are listed below.

Variation 1:
Cisplatin: I.V.: 25 mg/m^2/day days 1, 2, and 3
[total dose/cycle = 75 mg/m^2]
Dacarbazine: I.V.: 220 mg/m^2/day days 1, 2, and 3
[total dose/cycle = 660 mg/m^2]
Carmustine: I.V.: 150 mg/m^2 day 1 (every other cycle)
[total dose/cycle = 150 mg/m^2; every other cycle]
Tamoxifen: Oral: 10 mg twice daily (begin 1 week before chemotherapy)
[total dose/cycle = 420 mg]
Repeat cycle every 21 days

Variation 2:
Carmustine: I.V.: 150 mg/m^2 day 1
[total dose/cycle = 150 mg/m^2]
Cisplatin: I.V.: 25 mg/m^2/day days 1, 2, 3, 22, 23, and 24
[total dose/cycle = 150 mg/m^2]
Dacarbazine: I.V.: 220 mg/m^2/day days 1, 2, 3, 22, 23, and 24
[total dose/cycle = 1320 mg/m^2]
Tamoxifen: Oral: 10 mg twice daily days 1 to 42
[total dose/cycle = 840 mg]
Repeat cycle every 42 days

Variation 3:
Carmustine: I.V.: 150 mg/m^2 day 1
[total dose/cycle = 150 mg/m^2]
Cisplatin: I.V.: 25 mg/m^2/day days 1, 2, 3, 22, 23, and 24
[total dose/cycle = 150 mg/m^2]
Dacarbazine: I.V.: 220 mg/m^2/day days 1, 2, 3, 22, 23, and 24
[total dose/cycle = 1320 mg/m^2]

Tamoxifen: Oral: 160 mg/day days -6 to 0 (cycle 1 only)
[total dose/cycle = 1120 mg]
followed by Oral: 40 mg/day days 1 to 42
[total dose/cycle = 1680 mg]
Repeat cycle every 42 days

Variation 4:
Carmustine: I.V.: 150 mg/m^2 day 1
[total dose/cycle = 150 mg/m^2]
Cisplatin: I.V.: 25 mg/m^2/day days 1, 2, 3, 29, 30, and 31
[total dose/cycle = 150 mg/m^2]
Dacarbazine: I.V.: 220 mg/m^2/day days 1, 2, 3, 29, 30, and 31
[total dose/cycle = 1320 mg/m^2]
Tamoxifen: Oral: 10-20 mg twice daily days 1 to 56
[total dose/cycle = 1120-2240 mg]
Repeat cycle every 56 days

Variation 5:
Cisplatin: I.V.: 25 mg/m^2/day days 1, 2, and 3
[total dose/cycle = 75 mg/m^2]
Dacarbazine: I.V.: 220 mg/m^2/day days 1, 2, and 3
[total dose/cycle = 660 mg/m^2]
Carmustine: I.V.: 100 mg/m^2 day 1 (give in cycles 1, 3, and 6 **only**)
[total dose/cycles 1, 3, and 6 = 100 mg/m^2]
Tamoxifen: Oral: 160 mg loading dose immediately before cycle 1
[total dose/loading dose + cycle 1 = 580 mg]
followed by Oral: 20 mg daily days 1 to 21
[total dose/subsequent cycles = 420 mg]
Repeat cycle every 21 days
Note: Tamoxifen is continued until 3 weeks after last cycle.

DAV

Use Leukemia, acute myeloid

Regimen

Daunorubicin: I.V.: 60 mg/m^2/day days 3, 4, and 5
[total dose/cycle = 180 mg/m^2]
Cytarabine I.V.: 100 mg/m^2/day continuous infusion days 1 and 2
[total dose/cycle = 200 mg/m^2]
followed by I.V.: 100 mg/m^2 over 30 minutes every 12 hours days 3 to 8 (12 doses)
[total dose/cycle = 1200 mg/m^2]
Etoposide: I.V.: 150 mg/m^2/day days 6, 7, and 8
[total dose/cycle = 450 mg/m^2]
Administer one cycle only

Decitabine (Low Dose Regimen)

Use Leukemia, chronic myelogenous; Myelodysplastic syndrome

Regimen

Decitabine: I.V.: 20 mg/m^2/day days 1 to 5
[total dose/cycle = 100 mg/m^2]
Repeat cycle every 28 days for at least 3 cycles

Docetaxel-Bevacizumab

Use Breast cancer

Regimen NOTE: Multiple variations are listed below.

Variation 1:
Docetaxel: I.V.: 100 mg/m^2 day 1
[total dose/cycle = 100 mg/m^2]
Bevacizumab: I.V.: 7.5 mg/kg day 1
[total dose/cycle = 7.5 mg/kg]
Repeat cycle every 21 days (administer docetaxel for up to 9 cycles, bevacizumab until disease progression or unacceptable toxicity)

Variation 2:

Docetaxel: I.V.: 100 mg/m^2 day 1
[total dose/cycle = 100 mg/m^2]

Bevacizumab: I.V.: 15 mg/kg day 1
[total dose/cycle = 15 mg/kg]

Repeat cycle every 21 days (administer docetaxel for up to 9 cycles, bevacizumab until disease progression or unacceptable toxicity)

Docetaxel-Carboplatin (Ovarian Cancer)

Use Ovarian cancer

Regimen NOTE: Multiple variations are listed below.

Variation 1:

Docetaxel: I.V.: 60 mg/m^2 day 1
[total dose/cycle = 60 mg/m^2]

Carboplatin: I.V.: Target AUC 6
[total dose/cycle = AUC = 6]

Repeat cycle every 21 days for 6 cycles

Variation 2:

Docetaxel: I.V.: 75 mg/m^2 day 1
[total dose/cycle = 75 mg/m^2]

Carboplatin: I.V.: AUC 5 day 1
[total dose/cycle = AUC = 5]

Repeat cycle every 21 days for 6 cycles

Docetaxel-Carboplatin (Unknown Primary)

Use Unknown primary (adenocarcinoma)

Regimen

Docetaxel: I.V.: 65 mg/m^2 infused over 1 hour day 1
[total dose/cycle = 65 mg/m^2]

followed by

Carboplatin: I.V.: Target AUC 6 day 1
[total dose/cycle = AUC = 6]

Repeat cycle every 21 days for up to a total of 8 cycles

Docetaxel-Cisplatin

Use Lung cancer, nonsmall cell

Regimen

Docetaxel: I.V.: 75 mg/m^2 day 1
[total dose/cycle = 75 mg/m^2]

Cisplatin: I.V.: 75 mg/m^2 day 1
[total dose/cycle = 75 mg/m^2]

Repeat cycle every 21 days

Docetaxel-Cisplatin-Fluorouracil (Gastric/Esophageal Cancer)

Use Esophageal cancer; Gastric cancer

Regimen NOTE: Multiple variations are listed below.

Variation 1:

Docetaxel: I.V.: 75 mg/m^2 day 1
[total dose/cycle = 75 mg/m^2]

Cisplatin: I.V.: 75 mg/m^2 day 1
[total dose/cycle = 75 mg/m^2]

Fluorouracil: I.V.: 750 mg/m^2/day continuous infusion days 1 to 5
[total dose/cycle = 3750 mg/m^2]

Repeat cycle every 21 days until disease progression or unacceptable toxicity

Variation 2:

Docetaxel: I.V.: 75 mg/m^2 day 1
[total dose/cycle = 75 mg/m^2]

Cisplatin: I.V.: 75 mg/m^2 over 4 hours day 1
[total dose/cycle = 75 mg/m^2]

Fluorouracil: I.V.: 300 mg/m^2/day continuous infusion days 1 to 14
[total dose/cycle = 4200 mg/m^2]

Repeat cycle every 21 days until disease progression or unacceptable toxicity for up to a maximum of 8 cycles

Docetaxel-Cisplatin-Fluorouracil (Head and Neck Cancer)

Use Head and neck cancer

Regimen NOTE: Multiple variations are listed below.

Variation 1:

Docetaxel: I.V.: 75 mg/m^2 day 1
[total dose/cycle = 75 mg/m^2]

Cisplatin: I.V.: 75 mg/m^2 day 1
[total dose/cycle = 75 mg/m^2]

Fluorouracil: I.V.: 750 mg/m^2/day continuous infusion days 1 to 5
[total dose/cycle = 3750 mg/m^2]

Repeat cycle every 21 days for 4 cycles

Variation 2:

Docetaxel: I.V.: 75 mg/m^2 day 1
[total dose/cycle = 75 mg/m^2]

Cisplatin: I.V.: 75-100 mg/m^2 day 1
[total dose/cycle = 75-100 mg/m^2]

Fluorouracil: I.V.: 1000 mg/m^2/day continuous infusion days 1 to 4
[total dose/cycle = 4000 mg/m^2]

Repeat cycle every 21 days for total of 3 cycles

Docetaxel-Cisplatin (Unknown Primary)

Use Unknown primary (adenocarcinoma)

Regimen

Docetaxel: I.V.: 75 mg/m^2 infused over 1 hour day 1
[total dose/cycle = 75 mg/m^2]

followed by

Cisplatin: I.V.: 75 mg/m^2 infused over 1 hour day 1
[total dose/cycle = 75 mg/m^2]

Repeat cycle every 21 days for up to a total of 8 cycles

Docetaxel-Cyclophosphamide (TC)

Use Breast cancer

Regimen

Docetaxel: I.V.: 75 mg/m^2 day 1
[total dose/cycle = 75 mg/m^2]

Cyclophosphamide: I.V.: 600 mg/m^2 day 1
[total dose/cycle = 600 mg/m^2]

Repeat cycle every 21 days for 4 cycles

Docetaxel-FEC

Use Breast cancer

Regimen

Cycles 1, 2, and 3:

Docetaxel: I.V.: 80-100 mg/m^2 day 1
[total dose/cycle = 80-100 mg/m^2]

Repeat cycle every 21 days for 3 cycles

Cycles 4, 5, and 6 (FEC):

Fluorouracil: I.V.: 600 mg/m^2 day 1
[total dose/cycle = 600 mg/m^2]

Epirubicin: I.V.: 60 mg/m^2 day 1
[total dose/cycle = 60 mg/m^2]

Cyclophosphamide: I.V.: 600 mg/m^2 day 1
[total dose/cycle = 600 mg/m^2]

Repeat FEC cycle every 21 days for total of 3 cycles

Docetaxel-Oxaliplatin (Ovarian Cancer)

Use Ovarian cancer

Regimen

Docetaxel: I.V.: 75 mg/m^2/dose over 60 minutes day 1
[total dose/cycle = 75 mg/m^2]
Oxaliplatin: I.V.: 100 mg/m^2/dose over 2 hours day 1
[total dose/cycle = 100 mg/m^2]
Repeat cycle every 21 days

Docetaxel-Prednisone

Use Prostate cancer

Regimen

Docetaxel: I.V.: 75 mg/m^2 day 1
[total dose/cycle = 75 mg/m^2]
Prednisone: Oral: 5 mg twice daily
[total dose/cycle = 210 mg]
Repeat cycle every 21 days for up to 10 cycles

Docetaxel-Thalidomide

Use Prostate cancer

Regimen

Docetaxel: I.V.: 30 mg/m^2/day days 1, 8, and 15
[total dose/cycle = 90 mg/m^2]
Thalidomide: Oral: 200 mg daily (at bedtime)
[total dose/cycle = 5600 mg]
Repeat cycle every 28 days

Docetaxel-Trastuzumab

Use Breast cancer

Regimen

Cycle 1:
Docetaxel: I.V.: 100 mg/m^2 day 1
[total dose/cycle 1 = 100 mg/m^2]
Trastuzumab: I.V.: 4 mg/kg (loading dose) day 1 cycle 1
followed by I.V.: 2 mg/kg/day days 8 and 15 cycle 1
[total dose/cycle 1 = 8 mg/kg]
Treatment cycle is 21 days
Subsequent cycles:
Docetaxel: I.V.: 100 mg/m^2 day 1
[total dose/cycle = 100 mg/m^2]
Trastuzumab: I.V.: 2 mg/kg/day days 1, 8, and 15
[total dose/cycle = 6 mg/kg]
Repeat cycle every 21 days for a total of at least 6 cycles (continue weekly trastuzumab until disease progression)

Docetaxel-Trastuzumab-Carboplatin

Use Breast cancer

Regimen

Cycle 1:
Trastuzumab: I.V.: 4 mg/kg (loading dose) day 1 cycle 1
followed by I.V.: 2 mg/kg/day days 8 and 15 cycle 1
[total dose/cycle 1 = 8 mg/kg]
Docetaxel: I.V.: 75 mg/m^2 day 2
[total dose/cycle 1 = 75 mg/m^2]
Carboplatin: I.V.: AUC 6 day 2
[total dose/cycle 1 = AUC = 6]
Treatment cycle is 21 days

Subsequent cycles:

Trastuzumab: I.V.: 2 mg/kg/day days 1, 8, and 15
[total dose/cycle = 6 mg/kg]

Docetaxel: I.V.: 75 mg/m^2 day 1
[total dose/cycle = 75 mg/m^2]

Carboplatin: I.V.: AUC 6 day 1
[total dose/cycle = AUC = 6]

Repeat cycle every 21 days for a total of ~6 cycles (continue weekly trastuzumab for 1 year after chemotherapy, or until disease progression or unacceptable toxicity)

Docetaxel-Trastuzumab-Cisplatin

Use Breast cancer

Regimen

Cycle 1:

Trastuzumab: I.V.: 4 mg/kg (loading dose) day 1 cycle 1
followed by I.V.: 2 mg/kg/day days 8 and 15 cycle 1
[total dose/cycle 1 = 8 mg/kg]

Docetaxel: I.V.: 75 mg/m^2 day 2
[total dose/cycle 1 = 75 mg/m^2]

Cisplatin: I.V.: 75 mg/m^2 day 2
[total dose/cycle 1 = 75 mg/m^2]

Treatment cycle is 21 days

Subsequent cycles:

Trastuzumab: I.V.: 2 mg/kg/day days 1, 8, and 15
[total dose/cycle = 6 mg/kg]

Docetaxel: I.V.: 75 mg/m^2 day 1
[total dose/cycle = 75 mg/m^2]

Cisplatin: I.V.: 75 mg/m^2 day 1
[total dose/cycle = 75 mg/m^2]

Repeat cycle every 21 days for a total of ~6 cycles (continue weekly trastuzumab for 1 year after chemotherapy, or until disease progression or unacceptable toxicity)

Docetaxel-Trastuzumab-FEC

Use Breast cancer

Regimen

Cycle 1:

Trastuzumab: I.V.: 4 mg/kg (loading dose) day 1 cycle 1
followed by I.V.: 2 mg/kg/day days 8 and 15 cycle 1
[total dose/cycle 1 = 8 mg/kg]

Docetaxel: I.V.: 80-100 mg/m^2 day 1
[total dose/cycle 1 = 80-100 mg/m^2]

Treatment cycle is 21 days

Cycles 2 and 3:

Trastuzumab: I.V.: 2 mg/kg/day days 1, 8, and 15
[total dose/cycle = 6 mg/kg]

Docetaxel: I.V.: 80-100 mg/m^2 day 1
[total dose/cycle = 80-100 mg/m^2]

Treatment cycle is 21 days

Cycles 4, 5, and 6 (FEC):

Fluorouracil: I.V.: 600 mg/m^2 day 1
[total dose/cycle = 600 mg/m^2]

Epirubicin: I.V.: 60 mg/m^2 day 1
[total dose/cycle = 60 mg/m^2]

Cyclophosphamide: I.V.: 600 mg/m^2 day 1
[total dose/cycle = 600 mg/m^2]

Repeat FEC cycle every 21 days for total of 3 cycles

Docetaxel (Weekly Regimen)

Use Prostate cancer

Regimen

Docetaxel: I.V.: 40 mg/m^2 days 1, 8, and 15
[total dose/cycle = 120 mg/m^2]
Repeat cycle every 4 weeks

Docetaxel (Weekly)-Trastuzumab

Use Breast cancer

Regimen

Cycle 1:
Docetaxel: I.V.: 35 mg/m^2/day days 1, 8, and 15
[total dose/cycle 1 = 105 mg/m^2]
Trastuzumab: I.V.: 4 mg/kg (loading dose) day 0 cycle 1
followed by I.V.: 2 mg/kg/day days 8 and 15 cycle 1
[total dose/cycle 1 = 8 mg/kg]
Treatment cycle is 28 days
Subsequent cycles:
Docetaxel: I.V.: 35 mg/m^2/day days 1, 8, and 15
[total dose/cycle = 105 mg/m^2]
Trastuzumab: I.V.: 2 mg/kg/day days 1, 8, and 15
[total dose/cycle = 6 mg/kg]
Repeat cycle every 28 days

Dox-CMF (Sequential)

Use Breast cancer

Regimen

Doxorubicin: I.V.: 75 mg/m^2 day 1
[total dose/cycle = 75 mg/m^2]
Repeat cycle every 21 days for 4 cycles
followed by (after completing Cycle 4)
Cyclophosphamide: I.V.: 600 mg/m^2 day 1
[total dose/cycle = 600 mg/m^2]
Methotrexate: I.V.: 40 mg/m^2 day 1
[total dose/cycle = 40 mg/m^2]
Fluorouracil: I.V.: 600 mg/m^2 day 1
[total dose/cycle = 600 mg/m^2]
Repeat cycle every 21 days for 8 cycles

Doxorubicin + Ketoconazole

Use Prostate cancer

Regimen

Doxorubicin: I.V.: 20 mg/m^2 continuous infusion day 1
[total dose/cycle = 20 mg/m^2]
Ketoconazole: Oral: 400 mg 3 times/day days 1 to 7
[total dose/cycle = 8400 mg]
Repeat cycle every 7 days

Doxorubicin + Ketoconazole/Estramustine + Vinblastine

Use Prostate cancer

Regimen

Doxorubicin: I.V.: 20 mg/m^2/day days 1, 15, and 29
[total dose/cycle = 60 mg/m^2]
Ketoconazole: Oral: 400 mg 3 times/day days 1 to 7, 15 to 21, and 29 to 35
[total dose/cycle = 25,200 mg]
Estramustine: Oral: 140 mg 3 times/day days 8 to 14, 22 to 28, and 36 to 42
[total dose/cycle = 8820 mg]
Vinblastine: I.V.: 5 mg/m^2/day days 8, 22, and 36
[total dose/cycle = 15 mg/m^2]
Repeat cycle every 8 weeks

Doxorubicin (Liposomal)-Docetaxel (Breast Cancer)

Use Breast cancer

Regimen

Doxorubicin (liposomal): I.V.: 30 mg/m^2 over 1 hour day 1
[total dose/cycle = 30 mg/m^2]
Docetaxel: I.V.: 60 mg/m^2 over 1 hour day 1
[total dose/cycle = 60 mg/m^2]
Repeat cycle every 3 weeks until disease progression or unacceptable toxicity

Doxorubicin (Liposomal)-Vincristine-Dexamethasone

Use Multiple myeloma

Regimen NOTE: Multiple variations are listed below.

Variation 1:
Doxorubicin, liposomal: I.V.: 40 mg/m^2 day 1
[total dose/cycle = 40 mg/m^2]
Vincristine: I.V.: 2 mg day 1
[total dose/cycle = 2 mg]
Dexamethasone: Oral or I.V.: 40 mg/day days 1 to 4
[total dose/cycle = 160 mg]
Repeat cycle every 4 weeks

Variation 2:
Doxorubicin, liposomal: I.V.: 40 mg/m^2 day 1
[total dose/cycle = 40 mg/m^2]
Vincristine: I.V.: 1.4 mg/m^2 (maximum dose: 2 mg) day 1
[total dose/cycle = 1.4 mg/m^2; maximum: 2 mg]
Dexamethasone: Oral: 40 mg/day days 1 to 4
[total dose/cycle = 160 mg]
Repeat cycle every 4 weeks

DTPACE

Use Multiple myeloma

Regimen

Dexamethasone: Oral: 40 mg/day days 1 to 4
[total dose/cycle = 160 mg]
Thalidomide: Oral: 400 mg/day
[total dose/cycle = 11,200 - 16,800 mg]
Cisplatin: I.V.: 10 mg/m^2/day continuous infusion days 1 to 4
[total dose/cycle = 40 mg/m^2]
Doxorubicin: I.V.: 10 mg/m^2/day continuous infusion days 1 to 4
[total dose/cycle = 40 mg/m^2]
Cyclophosphamide: I.V.: 400 mg/m^2 continuous infusion days 1 to 4
[total dose/cycle = 1600 mg/m^2]
Etoposide: I.V.: 40 mg/m^2 continuous infusion days 1 to 4
[total dose/cycle = 160 mg/m^2]
Repeat cycle every 4-6 weeks

DVP

Use Leukemia, acute lymphocytic

Regimen Induction:

Daunorubicin: I.V.: 25 mg/m^2/day days 1, 8, and 15
[total dose/cycle = 75 mg/m^2]
Vincristine: I.V.: 1.5 mg/m^2/day (maximum dose: 2 mg) days 1, 8, 15, and 22
[total dose/cycle = 6 mg/m^2]
Prednisone: Oral: 60 mg/m^2/day days 1 to 28 then taper over next 14 days
[total dose/cycle = 1680 mg/m^2 + taper over next 14 days]
Administer single cycle; used in conjunction with intrathecal chemotherapy

EC (NSCLC)

Use Lung cancer, nonsmall cell

Regimen

Etoposide: I.V.: 120 mg/m^2/day days 1, 2, and 3
[total dose/cycle = 360 mg/m^2]
Carboplatin: I.V.: AUC 6 day 1
[total dose/cycle = AUC = 6]
Repeat cycle every 21-28 days

EC (Small Cell Lung Cancer)

Use Lung cancer, small cell

Regimen NOTE: Multiple variations are listed below.

Variation 1:
Etoposide: I.V.: 100-120 mg/m^2/day days 1, 2, and 3
[total dose/cycle = 300-360 mg/m^2]
Carboplatin: I.V.: 325-400 mg/m^2 day 1
[total dose/cycle = 325-400 mg/m^2]
Repeat cycle every 28 days

Variation 2:
Etoposide: I.V.: 120 mg/m^2/day days 1, 2, and 3
[total dose/cycle = 360 mg/m^2]
Carboplatin: I.V.: AUC 6 day 1
[total dose/cycle = AUC = 6]
Repeat cycle every 21-28 days

EE

Use Wilms tumor

Regimen

Dactinomycin: I.V.: 15 mcg/kg/day days 1 to 5 of weeks 0, 5, 13, and 24
[total dose/cycle = 300 mcg/kg]
Vincristine: I.V.: 1.5 mg/m^2 day 1 of weeks 1-10, 13, 14, 24, and 25
[total dose/cycle = 21 mg/m^2]

EE-4A

Use Wilms tumor

Regimen

Dactinomycin: I.V.: 45 mcg/kg day 1 of weeks 0, 3, 6, 9, 12, 15, and 18
[total dose/cycle = 315 mcg/kg]
Vincristine: I.V.: 2 mg/m^2 day 1 of weeks 1-10, 12, 15, and 18
[total dose/cycle = 26 mg/m^2]

EMA 86

Use Leukemia, acute myeloid

Regimen

Mitoxantrone: I.V.: 12 mg/m^2/day days 1, 2, and 3
[total dose/cycle = 36 mg/m^2]
Etoposide: I.V.: 200 mg/m^2/day continuous infusion days 8, 9, and 10
[total dose/cycle = 600 mg/m^2]
Cytarabine: I.V.: 500 mg/m^2/day continuous infusion days 1, 2, and 3 and days 8, 9, and 10
[total dose/cycle = 3000 mg/m^2]
Administer one cycle only

EMA/CO

Use Gestational trophoblastic tumor

Regimen NOTE: Multiple variations are listed below.

Variation 1:
Etoposide: I.V.: 100 mg/m^2/day days 1 and 2
[total dose/cycle = 200 mg/m^2]

Methotrexate: I.V.: 300 mg/m^2 continuous infusion over 12 hours day 1
[total dose/cycle = 300 mg/m^2]
Dactinomycin: I.V. push: 0.5 mg/day days 1 and 2
[total dose/cycle = 1 mg]
Leucovorin: Oral, I.M.: 15 mg twice daily for 2 days (start 24 hours after the start of methotrexate) days 2 and 3
[total dose/cycle = 60 mg]
Alternate weekly with:
Cyclophosphamide: I.V.: 600 mg/m^2 day 1
[total dose/cycle = 600 mg/m^2]
Vincristine: I.V. push: 0.8 mg/m^2 (maximum dose: 2 mg) day 1
[total dose/cycle = 0.8 mg/m^2]
Repeat cycle every 2 weeks

Variation 2:
Dactinomycin: I.V.: 0.5 mg/day days 1 and 2
[total dose/cycle = 1 mg]
Etoposide: I.V.: 100 mg/m^2/day days 1 and 2
[total dose/cycle = 200 mg/m^2]
Methotrexate: I.V. bolus: 100 mg/m^2 then 200 mg/m^2 continuous infusion over 12 hours day 1
[total dose/cycle = 300 mg/m^2]
Leucovorin: Oral, I.M.: 15 mg every 12 hours for 4 doses (start 24 hours after methotrexate) days 2 and 3
[total dose/cycle = 60 mg]
Vincristine: I.V.: 1 mg/m^2 day 8
[total dose/cycle = 1 mg/m^2]
Cyclophosphamide: I.V.: 600 mg/m^2 day 8
[total dose/cycle = 600 mg/m^2]
Repeat cycle every 2 weeks

Variation 3:
Dactinomycin: I.V.: 0.5 mg/day days 1 and 2
[total dose/cycle = 1 mg]
Etoposide: I.V.: 100 mg/m^2/day days 1 and 2
[total dose/cycle = 200 mg/m^2]
Methotrexate: I.V.: 300 mg/m^2 continuous infusion over 12 hours day 1
[total dose/cycle = 300 mg/m^2]
Leucovorin: Oral, I.M.: 15 mg every 12 hours for 4 doses (start 24 hours after start of methotrexate) days 2 and 3
[total dose/cycle = 60 mg]
Vincristine: I.V.: 1 mg/m^2 day 8
[total dose/cycle = 1 mg/m^2]
Cyclophosphamide: I.V.: 600 mg/m^2 day 8
[total dose/cycle = 600 mg/m^2]
Repeat cycle every 2 weeks

Variation 4:
Dactinomycin: I.V.: 0.35 mg/m^2/day days 1 and 2
[total dose/cycle = 0.7 mg/m^2]
Etoposide: I.V.: 100 mg/m^2/day days 1 and 2
[total dose/cycle = 200 mg/m^2]
Methotrexate: I.V. bolus: 100 mg/m^2 then 200 mg/m^2 continuous infusion over 12 hours day 1
[total dose/cycle = 300 mg/m^2]
Leucovorin: Oral, I.M.: 15 mg every 12 hours for 4 doses (start 24 hours after start of methotrexate) days 2 and 3
[total dose/cycle = 60 mg]
Vincristine: I.V.: 1 mg/m^2 day 8
[total dose/cycle = 1 mg/m^2]
Cyclophosphamide: I.V.: 600 mg/m^2 day 8
[total dose/cycle = 600 mg/m^2]
Repeat cycle every 2 weeks

Variation 5 (patients with brain metastases):
Dactinomycin: I.V.: 0.5 mg/day days 1 and 2
[total dose/cycle = 1 mg]

Etoposide:I.V.: 100 mg/m^2/day days 1 and 2
[total dose/cycle = 200 mg/m^2]
Methotrexate: I.V.: 1 g/m^2 continuous infusion over 12 hours day 1
[total dose/cycle = 1 g/m^2]
Leucovorin: I.M.: 20 mg/m^2 every 6 hours for 12 doses (start 24 hours after start of methotrexate) days 2, 3, and 4
[total dose/cycle = 240 mg/m^2]
Vincristine: I.V.: 1 mg/m^2 day 8
[total dose/cycle = 1 mg/m^2]
Cyclophosphamide: I.V.: 600 mg/m^2 day 8
[total dose/cycle = 600 mg/m^2]
Repeat cycle every 2 weeks

Variation 6 (patients with brain metastases):
Dactinomycin: I.V.: 0.5 mg/day days 1 and 2
[total dose/cycle = 1 mg]
Etoposide: I.V.: 100 mg/m^2/day days 1 and 2
[total dose/cycle = 200 mg/m^2]
Methotrexate: I.V.: 1 g/m^2 continuous infusion over 12 hours day 1
[total dose/cycle = 1 g/m^2]
Leucovorin: Oral, I.M.: 30 mg/m^2 every 12 hours for 6 doses (start 32 hours after start of methotrexate) days 2, 3, and 4
[total dose/cycle = 180 mg/m^2]
Vincristine: I.V.: 1 mg/m^2 day 8
[total dose/cycle = 1 mg/m^2]
Cyclophosphamide: I.V.: 600 mg/m^2 day 8
[total dose/cycle = 600 mg/m^2]
Repeat cycle every 2 weeks

Variation 7:
Dactinomycin: I.V.: 0.5 mg/day days 1 and 2
[total dose/cycle = 1 mg]
Etoposide: I.V.: 100 mg/m^2/day days 1 and 2
[total dose/cycle = 200 mg/m^2]
Methotrexate: I.V.: 1 g/m^2 continuous infusion over 24 hours day 1
[total dose/cycle = 1 g/m^2]
Leucovorin: Oral, I.M.: 15 mg every 8 hours for 9 doses (start 32 hours after start of methotrexate) days 2, 3, and 4
[total dose/cycle = 135 mg/m^2]
Vincristine: I.V.: 1 mg/m^2 day 8
[total dose/cycle = 1 mg/m^2]
Cyclophosphamide: I.V.: 600 mg/m^2 day 8
[total dose/cycle = 600 mg/m^2]
Repeat cycle every 2 weeks

Variation 8 (patients with lung metastases):
Dactinomycin: I.V.: 0.5 mg/day days 1 and 2
[total dose/cycle = 1 mg]
Etoposide: I.V.: 100 mg/m^2/day days 1 and 2
[total dose/cycle = 200 mg/m^2]
Methotrexate: I.V. bolus: 100 mg/m^2 then 200 mg/m^2 continuous infusion over 12 hours day 1
[total dose/cycle = 300 mg/m^2]
Leucovorin: Oral, I.M.: 15 mg every 12 hours for 4 doses (start 24 hours after start of methotrexate) days 2 and 3
[total dose/cycle = 60 mg]
Vincristine: I.V.: 1 mg/m^2 day 8
[total dose/cycle = 1 mg/m^2]
Cyclophosphamide: I.V.: 600 mg/m^2 day 8
[total dose/cycle = 600 mg/m^2]
Methotrexate: I.T.: 10 mg day 1 (every other cycle)
[total dose/cycle = 10 mg, every other cycle]
Repeat cycle every 2 weeks

Variation 9 (patients with lung metastases):
Dactinomycin: I.V.: 0.5 mg/day days 1 and 2
[total dose/cycle = 1 mg]

Etoposide: I.V.: 100 mg/m^2/day days 1 and 2
[total dose/cycle = 200 mg/m^2]
Methotrexate: I.V. bolus: 100 mg/m^2 then 200 mg/m^2 continuous infusion over 12 hours day 1
[total dose/cycle = 300 mg/m^2]
Leucovorin: Oral, I.M.: 15 mg every 12 hours for 4 doses (start 24 hours after start of methotrexate) days 2 and 3
[total dose/cycle = 60 mg]
Vincristine: I.V.: 1 mg/m^2 day 8
[total dose/cycle = 1 mg/m^2]
Cyclophosphamide: I.V.: 600 mg/m^2 day 8
[total dose/cycle = 600 mg/m^2]
Methotrexate: I.T.: 12.5 mg day 8
[total dose/cycle = 12.5 mg]
Repeat cycle every 2 weeks

EP (Small Cell Lung Cancer)

Use Lung cancer, small cell

Regimen NOTE: Multiple variations are listed below.

Variation 1:
Etoposide: I.V.: 100 mg/m^2/day days 1, 2, and 3
[total dose/cycle = 300 mg/m^2]
Cisplatin: I.V.: 100 mg/m^2 day 1
[total dose/cycle = 100 mg/m^2]
Repeat cycle every 21 days

Variation 2:
Etoposide: I.V.: 80 mg/m^2/day days 1, 2, and 3
[total dose/cycle = 240 mg/m^2]
Cisplatin: I.V.: 80 mg/m^2 day 1
[total dose/cycle = 80 mg/m^2]
Repeat cycle every 21-28 days

EP/EMA

Use Gestational trophoblastic tumor

Regimen NOTE: Multiple variations are listed below.

Variation 1:
Etoposide: I.V.: 150 mg/m^2 day 1
[total dose/cycle = 150 mg/m^2]
Cisplatin: I.V.: 25 mg/m^2 infused over 4 hours for 3 consecutive doses, day 1
[total dose/cycle = 75 mg/m^2]
Alternate weekly with:
Etoposide: I.V.: 100 mg/m^2 day 1
[total dose/cycle = 100 mg/m^2]
Methotrexate: I.V.: 300 mg/m^2 infused over 12 hours day 1
[total dose/cycle = 300 mg/m^2]
Dactinomycin: I.V. push: 0.5 mg day 1
[total dose/cycle = 0.5 mg]
Leucovorin: Oral, I.M.: 15 mg twice daily for 2 days (start 24 hours after the start of methotrexate) days 2 and 3
[total dose/cycle = 60 mg]

Variation 2:
Dactinomycin: I.V.: 0.5 mg/day days 1 and 2
[total dose/cycle = 1 mg]
Etoposide: I.V.: 100 mg/m^2/day days 1 and 2
[total dose/cycle = 200 mg/m^2]
Methotrexate: I.V.: 300 mg/m^2 continuous infusion over 12 hours day 1
[total dose/cycle = 300 mg/m^2]
Leucovorin: Oral, I.M.: 15 mg every 12 hours for 4 doses (start 24 hours after start of methotrexate) days 2 and 3
[total dose/cycle = 60 mg]
Etoposide: I.V.: 150 mg/m^2 day 8
[total dose/cycle = 150 mg/m^2]

Cisplatin: I.V.: 75 mg/m^2 day 8
[total dose/cycle = 75 mg/m^2]
Repeat cycle every 2 weeks

Epirubicin-Cisplatin-Capecitabine (Esophageal Cancer)

Use Esophageal cancer

Regimen

Epirubicin: I.V.: 50 mg/m^2 day 1
[total dose/cycle = 50 mg/m^2]
Cisplatin: I.V.: 60 mg/m^2 day 1
[total dose/cycle = 60 mg/m^2]
Capecitabine: Oral: 625 mg/m^2 twice daily days 1 to 21
[total dose/cycle = 26,250 mg/m^2]
Repeat cycle every 21 days for up to 8 cycles

Epirubicin-Cisplatin-Fluorouracil (Gastric/Esophageal Cancer)

Use Esophageal cancer; Gastric cancer

Regimen NOTE: Multiple variations are listed below.

Variation 1:
Epirubicin: I.V.: 50 mg/m^2 day 1
[total dose/cycle = 50 mg/m^2]
Cisplatin: I.V.: 60 mg/m^2 day 1
[total dose/cycle = 60 mg/m^2]
Fluorouracil: I.V.: 200 mg/m^2/day continuous infusion days 1 to 21
[total dose/cycle = 4200 mg/m^2]
Repeat cycle every 3 weeks for up to a maximum of 8 cycles

Variation 2:
Epirubicin: I.V.: 50 mg/m^2 day 1
[total dose/cycle = 50 mg/m^2]
Cisplatin: I.V.: 60 mg/m^2 day 1
[total dose/cycle = 60 mg/m^2]
Fluorouracil: I.V.: 200 mg/m^2/day continuous infusion days 1 to 21
[total dose/cycle = 4200 mg/m^2]
Repeat cycle every 3 weeks for up to 6 cycles (3 cycles before surgery and 3 cycles postoperatively)

Epirubicin-Oxaliplatin-Capecitabine

Use Esophageal cancer; Gastric cancer

Regimen

Epirubicin: I.V.: 50 mg/m^2 day 1
[total dose/cycle = 50 mg/m^2]
Oxaliplatin: I.V.: 130 mg/m^2 day 1
[total dose/cycle = 130 mg/m^2]
Capecitabine: Oral: 625 mg/m^2 twice daily days 1 to 21
[total dose/cycle = 26,250 mg/m^2]
Repeat cycle every 21 days for up to 8 cycles

Epirubicin-Oxaliplatin-Fluorouracil (Esophageal Cancer)

Use Esophageal cancer

Regimen

Epirubicin: I.V.: 50 mg/m^2 day 1
[total dose/cycle = 50 mg/m^2]
Oxaliplatin: I.V.: 130 mg/m^2 day 1
[total dose/cycle = 130 mg/m^2]
Fluorouracil: I.V.: 200 mg/m^2/day continuous infusion days 1 to 21
[total dose/cycle = 4200 mg/m^2]
Repeat cycle every 21 days for up to 8 cycles

EP (NSCLC)

Use Lung cancer, nonsmall cell

Regimen

Etoposide: I.V.: 80-120 mg/m^2/day days 1, 2, and 3
[total dose/cycle = 240-360 mg/m^2]
Cisplatin: I.V.: 80-100 mg/m^2 day 1
[total dose/cycle = 80-100 mg/m^2]
Repeat cycle every 21-28 days

EPOCH Dose-Adjusted (AIDS-Related Lymphoma)

Use Lymphoma, AIDS-related

Regimen

Etoposide: I.V.: 50 mg/m^2/day continuous infusion days 1 to 4
[total dose/cycle = 200 mg/m^2]
Vincristine: I.V.: 0.4 mg/m^2/day continuous infusion days 1 to 4
[total dose/cycle = 1.6 mg/m^2]
Doxorubicin: I.V.: 10 mg/m^2/day continuous infusion days 1 to 4
[total dose/cycle = 40 mg/m^2]
Cyclophosphamide: I.V.: 375 mg/m^2 day 5 for CD4+ cells ≥100/mm^3 **or** 187 mg/m^2 day 5 for CD4+ cells <100/mm^3
[total dose/cycle = 187-375 mg/m^2]
Prednisone: Oral: 60 mg/m^2/day days 1 to 5
[total dose/cycle = 300 mg/m^2]
Filgrastim: SubQ: 5 mcg/kg/day beginning day 6; continue until ANC >5000/mm^3 (past nadir)
Repeat cycle every 21 days for 6 cycles with cyclophosphamide dose adjusted based on previous cycle nadir according to the following schedule:
Nadir ANC >500/mm^3: Increase cyclophosphamide dose by 187 mg/m^2 above previous cycle dose (maximum dose: 750 mg/m^2)
Nadir ANC <500/mm^3 or platelet <25,000/mm^3: Decrease cyclophosphamide dose by 187 mg/m^2 below previous cycle dose

EPOCH Dose-Adjusted (NHL)

Use Lymphoma, non-Hodgkin

Regimen

Etoposide: I.V.: 50 mg/m^2/day continuous infusion days 1 to 4
[total dose/cycle = 200 mg/m^2]
Vincristine: I.V.: 0.4 mg/m^2/day continuous infusion days 1 to 4
[total dose/cycle = 1.6 mg/m^2]
Doxorubicin: I.V.: 10 mg/m^2/day continuous infusion days 1 to 4
[total dose/cycle = 40 mg/m^2]
Cyclophosphamide: I.V.: 750 mg/m^2 day 5
[total dose/cycle = 750 mg/m^2]
Prednisone: Oral: 60 mg/m^2 twice daily days 1 to 5
total dose/cycle = 600 mg/m^2]
Filgrastim: SubQ: 5 mcg/kg/day beginning day 6; continue until ANC >5000/mm^3
Repeat cycle every 21 days with etoposide, doxorubicin, and cyclophosphamide dose adjustments (based on CBC 2 times/week) according to the following schedule:
Nadir ANC ≥500/mm^3: 20% increase (above previous cycle) for etoposide, doxorubicin, and cyclophosphamide
Nadir ANC <500/mm^3 (on 1 or 2 measurements): Same doses as previous cycle
Nadir ANC <500/mm^3 (on ≥3 measurements) or nadir platelet <25,000/mm^3 (on 1 measurement): 20% decrease below previous cycle for etoposide, doxorubicin, and cyclophosphamide (dosing adjustments below starting dose levels only apply to cyclophosphamide)

EPOCH (Dose-Adjusted)-Rituximab (NHL)

Use Lymphoma, non-Hodgkin

Regimen NOTE: Multiple variations are listed below.

Variation 1:
Rituximab: I.V.: 375 mg/m^2 day 1
[total dose/cycle = 375 mg/m^2]

Etoposide: I.V.: 50 mg/m^2/day continuous infusion days 1 to 4
[total dose/cycle = 200 mg/m^2]
Vincristine: I.V.: 0.4 mg/m^2/day continuous infusion days 1 to 4
[total dose/cycle = 1.6 mg/m^2]
Doxorubicin: I.V.: 10 mg/m^2/day continuous infusion days 1 to 4
[total dose/cycle = 40 mg/m^2]
Cyclophosphamide: I.V.: 750 mg/m^2 day 5
[total dose/cycle = 750 mg/m^2]
Prednisone: Oral: 60 mg/m^2 twice daily days 1 to 5
[total dose/cycle = 600 mg/m^2]
Filgrastim: SubQ: 5 mcg/kg/day beginning day 6; continue until ANC >5000/mm^3
Repeat cycle every 21 days (for at least 2 cycles beyond best response; minimum of 6 cycles) with etoposide, doxorubicin, and cyclophosphamide dose adjustments (based on CBC 2 times/week) according to the following schedule:
Nadir ANC ≥500/mm^3: 20% increase (above previous cycle) for etoposide, doxorubicin, and cyclophosphamide
Nadir ANC <500/mm^3 (on 1 or 2 measurements): Same doses as previous cycle
Nadir ANC <500/mm^3 (on ≥3 measurements): 20% decrease below previous cycle for etoposide, doxorubicin, and cyclophosphamide (dosing adjustments below starting dose levels only apply to cyclophosphamide)

Variation 2:
Rituximab: I.V.: 375 mg/m^2 day 1
[total dose/cycle = 375 mg/m^2]
Etoposide: I.V.: 50 mg/m^2/day continuous infusion days 1 to 4
[total dose/cycle = 200 mg/m^2]
Vincristine: I.V.: 0.4 mg/m^2/day continuous infusion days 1 to 4
[total dose/cycle = 1.6 mg/m^2]
Doxorubicin: I.V.: 10 mg/m^2/day continuous infusion days 1 to 4
[total dose/cycle = 40 mg/m^2]
Cyclophosphamide: I.V.: 750 mg/m^2 day 5
[total dose/cycle = 750 mg/m^2]
Prednisone: Oral: 60 mg/m^2/day days 1 to 5
[total dose/cycle = 300 mg/m^2]
Filgrastim: SubQ: 5 mcg/kg/day beginning day 6; continue until ANC >500/mm^3
Repeat cycle every 21 days (for 6-8 cycles); refer to variation 1 for dose adjustments

EPOCH (NHL)

Use Lymphoma, non-Hodgkin

Regimen NOTE: Multiple variations are listed below.

Variation 1:
Etoposide: I.V.: 50 mg/m^2/day continuous infusion days 1 to 4
[total dose/cycle = 200 mg/m^2]
Vincristine: I.V.: 0.4 mg/m^2/day continuous infusion days 1 to 4
[total dose/cycle = 1.6 mg/m^2]
Doxorubicin: I.V.: 10 mg/m^2/day continuous infusion days 1 to 4
[total dose/cycle = 40 mg/m^2]
Cyclophosphamide: I.V.: 750 mg/m^2 day 5
[total dose/cycle = 750 mg/m^2]
Prednisone: Oral: 60 mg/m^2/day days 1 to 5
[total dose/cycle = 300 mg/m^2]
Repeat cycle (with cyclophosphamide dose adjustments if needed based on ANC) every 21 days (best response seen in a median of 4 cycles)

Variation 2:
Etoposide: I.V.: 50 mg/m^2/day continuous infusion days 1 to 4
[total dose/cycle = 200 mg/m^2]
Vincristine: I.V.: 0.4 mg/m^2/day continuous infusion days 1 to 4
[total dose/cycle = 1.6 mg/m^2]
Doxorubicin: I.V.: 10 mg/m^2/day continuous infusion days 1 to 4
[total dose/cycle = 40 mg/m^2]
Cyclophosphamide: I.V.: 750 mg/m^2 day 6
[total dose/cycle = 750 mg/m^2]

Prednisone: Oral: 60 mg/m^2/day days 1 to 6
[total dose/cycle = 360 mg/m^2]
Repeat cycle (with cyclophosphamide dose adjustments if needed based on ANC) every 21 days (best response seen in a median of 4 cycles)

EPOCH-Rituximab (NHL)

Use Lymphoma, non-Hodgkin

Regimen

Rituximab: I.V.: 375 mg/m^2 day 1
[total dose/cycle = 375 mg/m^2]
Etoposide: I.V.: 65 mg/m^2/day continuous infusion days 2, 3, and 4
[total dose/cycle = 195 mg/m^2]
Vincristine: I.V.: 0.5 mg/m^2/day continuous infusion days 2, 3, and 4
[total dose/cycle = 1.5 mg/m^2]
Doxorubicin: I.V.: 15 mg/m^2/day continuous infusion days 2, 3, and 4
[total dose/cycle = 45 mg/m^2]
Cyclophosphamide: I.V.: 750 mg/m^2 day 5
[total dose/cycle = 750 mg/m^2]
Prednisone: Oral: 60 mg/m^2/day days 1 to 14
[total dose/cycle = 840 mg/m^2]
Repeat cycle every 21 days for 4-6 cycles

EP/PE

Use Lung cancer, nonsmall cell

Regimen

Etoposide: I.V.: 120 mg/m^2/day days 1, 2, and 3
[total dose/cycle = 360 mg/m^2]
Cisplatin: I.V.: 60-120 mg/m^2 day 1
[total dose/cycle = 60-120 mg/m^2]
Repeat cycle every 21-28 days

EP (Testicular Cancer)

Use Testicular cancer

Regimen NOTE: Multiple variations are listed below.

Variation 1:
Etoposide: I.V.: 100 mg/m^2/day days 1 to 5
[total dose/cycle = 500 mg/m^2]
Cisplatin: I.V.: 20 mg/m^2/day days 1 to 5
[total dose/cycle = 100 mg/m^2]
Repeat cycle every 21 days

Variation 2:
Etoposide: I.V.: 120 mg/m^2/day days 1, 2, and 3
[total dose/cycle = 360 mg/m^2]
Cisplatin: I.V.: 20 mg/m^2/day days 1 to 5
[total dose/cycle = 100 mg/m^2]
Repeat cycle every 3 or 4 weeks

Variation 3:
Etoposide: I.V.: 120 mg/m^2/day days 1, 3, and 5
[total dose/cycle = 360 mg/m^2]
Cisplatin: I.V.: 20 mg/m^2/day days 1 to 5
[total dose/cycle = 100 mg/m^2]
Repeat cycle every 3 weeks

ESHAP

Use Lymphoma, non-Hodgkin

Regimen NOTE: Multiple variations are listed below.

Variation 1:
Etoposide: I.V.: 40 mg/m^2/day days 1 to 4
[total dose/cycle = 160 mg/m^2]
Methylprednisolone: I.V.: 250-500 mg/day days 1 to 5
[total dose/cycle = 1250-2500 mg]

Cytarabine: I.V.: 2000 mg/m^2 day 5
[total dose/cycle = 2000 mg/m^2]
Cisplatin: I.V.: 25 mg/m^2/day continuous infusion days 1 to 4
[total dose/cycle = 100 mg/m^2]
Repeat cycle every 21-28 days

Variation 2:
Etoposide: I.V.: 40 mg/m^2/day days 1 to 4
[total dose/cycle = 160 mg/m^2]
Methylprednisolone: I.V.: 500 mg/day days 1 to 5
[total dose/cycle = 2500 mg]
Cytarabine: I.V.: 2000 mg/m^2 day 5
[total dose/cycle = 2000 mg/m^2]
Cisplatin: I.V.: 25 mg/m^2/day continuous infusion days 1 to 4
[total dose/cycle = 100 mg/m^2]
Repeat cycle every 21-28 days

Variation 3:
Etoposide: I.V.: 60 mg/m^2/day days 1 to 4
[total dose/cycle = 240 mg/m^2]
Methylprednisolone: I.V.: 500 mg/day days 1 to 4
[total dose/cycle = 2000 mg]
Cytarabine: I.V.: 2000 mg/m^2 day 5
[total dose/cycle = 2000 mg/m^2]
Cisplatin: I.V.: 25 mg/m^2/day continuous infusion days 1 to 4
[total dose/cycle = 100 mg/m^2]
Repeat cycle every 21 days

Estramustine + Docetaxel

Use Prostate cancer

Regimen NOTE: Multiple variations are listed below.

Variation 1:
Docetaxel: I.V.: 20-80 mg/m^2 day 2
[total dose/cycle = 20-80 mg/m^2]
Estramustine: Oral: 280 mg 3 times/day days 1 to 5
[total dose/cycle = 4200 mg]
Repeat cycle every 21 days

Variation 2:
Docetaxel: I.V.: 20-80 mg/m^2 day 2
[total dose/cycle = 20-80 mg/m^2]
Estramustine: Oral: 14 mg/kg/day days 1 to 21
[total dose/cycle = 294 mg/kg]
Repeat cycle every 21 days

Variation 3:
Docetaxel: I.V.: 35 mg/m^2/day days 2 and 9
[total dose/cycle = 70 mg/m^2]
Estramustine: Oral: 420 mg 3 times/day for 4 doses, then 280 mg 3 times/day for 5 doses days 1, 2, 3, 8, 9, and 10
[total dose/cycle = 6160 mg]
Repeat cycle every 21 days

Variation 4:
Docetaxel: I.V.: 60 mg/m^2 day 2 cycle 1
[total dose/cycle = 60 mg/m^2]
followed by I.V.: 60-70 mg/m^2 day 2 (subsequent cycles)
[total dose/cycle = 60-70 mg/m^2]
Estramustine: Oral: 280 mg 3 times/day days 1 to 5
[total dose/cycle = 4200 mg]
Repeat cycle every 21 days for up to 12 cycles

Estramustine + Docetaxel + Calcitriol

Use Prostate cancer

Regimen

Cycle 1:
Calcitriol: Oral: 60 mcg (in divided doses) day 1
[total dose/cycle = 60 mcg]

Estramustine: Oral: 280 mg 3 times/day days 1 to 5
[total dose/cycle = 4200 mg]
Docetaxel: I.V.: 60 mg/m^2 day 2
[total dose/cycle = 60 mg/m^2]
Treatment cycle is 21 days
Subsequent cycles:
Calcitriol: Oral: 60 mcg (in divided doses) day 1
[total dose/cycle = 60 mcg]
Estramustine: Oral: 280 mg 3 times/day days 1 to 5
[total dose/cycle = 4200 mg]
Docetaxel: I.V.: 70 mg/m^2 day 2
[total dose/cycle = 70 mg/m^2]
Repeat cycle every 21 days for up to 12 cycles

Estramustine + Docetaxel + Carboplatin

Use Prostate cancer

Regimen

Docetaxel: I.V.: 70 mg/m^2 day 2
[total dose/cycle = 70 mg/m^2]
Estramustine: Oral: 280 mg 3 times/day days 1 to 5
[total dose/cycle = 4200 mg]
Carboplatin: I.V.: Target AUC 5 day 2
[total dose/cycle = AUC = 5]
Repeat cycle every 3 weeks

Estramustine + Docetaxel + Hydrocortisone

Use Prostate cancer

Regimen

Docetaxel: I.V.: 70 mg/m^2 day 2
[total dose/cycle = 70 mg/m^2]
Estramustine: Oral: 10 mg/kg/day days 1 to 5
[total dose/cycle = 50 mg/kg]
Hydrocortisone: Oral: 40 mg daily
[total dose/cycle = 840 mg]
Repeat cycle every 3 weeks

Estramustine + Docetaxel + Prednisone

Use Prostate cancer

Regimen

Estramustine: Oral: 280 mg 3 times/day days 1 to 5 and days 7 to 11
[total dose/cycle = 8400 mg]
Docetaxel: I.V.: 70 mg/m^2 day 2
[total dose/cycle = 70 mg/m^2]
Prednisone: Oral: 10 mg daily
[total dose/cycle = 210 mg]
Repeat cycle every 21 days for up to 6 cycles

Estramustine + Etoposide

Use Prostate cancer

Regimen NOTE: Multiple variations are listed below.

Variation 1:
Estramustine: Oral: 15 mg/kg/day days 1 to 21
[total dose/cycle = 315 mg/kg]
Etoposide: Oral: 50 mg/m^2/day days 1 to 21
[total dose/cycle = 1050 mg/m^2]
Repeat cycle every 4 weeks

Variation 2:
Estramustine: Oral: 10 mg/kg/day days 1 to 21
[total dose/cycle = 210 mg/kg]
Etoposide: Oral: 50 mg/m^2/day days 1 to 21
[total dose/cycle = 1050 mg/m^2]
Repeat cycle every 4 weeks
Variation 3:
Estramustine: Oral: 140 mg 3 times/day days 1 to 21
[total dose/cycle = 8820 mg]
Etoposide: Oral: 50 mg/m^2/day days 1 to 21
[total dose/cycle = 1050 mg/m^2]
Repeat cycle every 4 weeks

Estramustine-Paclitaxel

Use Prostate cancer

Regimen NOTE: Multiple variations are listed below.
Variation 1:
Paclitaxel: I.V.: 30-35 mg/m^2/day continuous infusion (given in 2-3 divided doses daily) either days 1 to 4 or days 2 to 5
[total dose/cycle = 120-140 mg/m^2]
Estramustine: Oral: 600 mg/m^2/day days 1 to 21
[total dose/cycle = 12,600 mg/m^2]
Repeat cycle every 21 days
Variation 2:
Paclitaxel: I.V. 60-107 mg/m^2 infused over 3 hours weekly for 6 weeks
[total dose/cycle = 360-642 mg/m^2]
Estramustine: Oral: 280 mg twice daily 3 days/week for 6 weeks
[total dose/cycle = 3360 mg]
Repeat cycle every 8 weeks
Variation 3:
Paclitaxel: I.V. 150 mg/m^2/day days 2, 9, and 16
[total dose/cycle = 450 mg/m^2]
Estramustine: Oral: 280 mg 3 times/day days 1, 2, 3, 8, 9, 10, 15, 16, and 17
[total dose/week = 7560 mg/m^2]
Repeat cycle every 4 weeks
Variation 4:
Paclitaxel: I.V.: 100 mg/m^2/day days 2, 9, and 16
[total dose/cycle = 300 mg/m^2]
Estramustine: Oral: 280 mg 3 times/day days 1, 2, 3, 8, 9, 10, 15, 16, and 17
[total dose/cycle = 7560 mg]
Repeat cycle every 4 weeks

Estramustine-Vinblastine

Use Prostate cancer

Regimen NOTE: Multiple variations are listed below.
Variation 1:
Estramustine: Oral: 10 mg/kg/day days 1 to 42
[total dose/cycle = 420 mg/kg]
Vinblastine: I.V.: 4 mg/m^2/day days 1, 8, 15, 22, 29, and 36
[total dose/cycle = 24 mg/m^2]
Repeat cycle every 8 weeks
Variation 2:
Estramustine: Oral: 600 mg/m^2/day days 1 to 42
[total dose/cycle = 25,200 mg/m^2]
Vinblastine: I.V.: 4 mg/m^2/day days 1, 8, 15, 22, 29, and 36
[total dose/cycle = 24 mg/m^2]
Repeat cycle every 8 weeks

Estramustine + Vinorelbine

Use Prostate cancer

Regimen NOTE: Multiple variations are listed below.

Variation 1:

Estramustine: Oral: 140 mg 3 times/day days 1 to 14
[total dose/cycle = 5880 mg]

Vinorelbine: I.V.: 25 mg/m^2/day days 1 and 8
[total dose/cycle = 50 mg/m^2]

Repeat cycle every 21 days

Variation 2:

Estramustine: Oral: 280 mg 3 times/day days 1, 2, and 3
[total dose/cycle = 2520 mg/m^2]

Vinorelbine: I.V.: 15 or 20 mg/m^2 day 2
[total dose/cycle = 15 or 20 mg/m^2]

Repeat cycle weekly for 8 weeks, then every other week

Etoposide-Carboplatin (Ovarian Cancer)

Use Ovarian cancer

Regimen

Etoposide: I.V.: 120 mg/m^2/day days 1, 2, and 3
[total dose/cycle = 360 mg/m^2]

Carboplatin: I.V.: 400 mg/m^2 day 1
[total dose/cycle = 400 mg/m^2]

Repeat cycle every 28 days for a total of 3 cycles

Etoposide-Vinblastine-Doxorubicin (Hodgkin)

Use Lymphoma, Hodgkin disease

Regimen

Etoposide: I.V.: 100 mg/m^2/day days 1, 2, and 3
[total dose/cycle = 300 mg/m^2]

Vinblastine: I.V.: 6 mg/m^2 day 1
[total dose/cycle = 6 mg/m^2]

Doxorubicin: I.V.: 50 mg/m^2 day 1
[total dose/cycle = 50 mg/m^2]

Repeat cycle every 28 days

FAC

Use Breast cancer

Regimen NOTE: Multiple variations are listed below.

Variation 1:

Fluorouracil: I.V.: 500 mg/m^2/day days 1 and 8
[total dose/cycle = 1000 mg/m^2]
or 500 mg/m^2 day 1
[total dose/cycle = 500 mg/m^2]

Doxorubicin: I.V.: 50 mg/m^2 day 1
[total dose/cycle = 50 mg/m^2]

Cyclophosphamide: I.V.: 500 mg/m^2 day 1
[total dose/cycle = 500 mg/m^2]

Repeat cycle every 21-28 days

Variation 2:

Fluorouracil: I.V.: 200 mg/m^2/day days 1, 2, and 3
[total dose/cycle = 600 mg/m^2]

Doxorubicin: I.V.: 40 mg/m^2 day 1
[total dose/cycle = 40 mg/m^2]

Cyclophosphamide: I.V.: 400 mg/m^2 day 1
[total dose/cycle = 400 mg/m^2]

Repeat cycle every 28 days

Variation 3:
Fluorouracil: I.V.: 400 mg/m^2/day days 1 and 8
[total dose/cycle = 800 mg/m^2]
Doxorubicin: I.V.: 40 mg/m^2 day 1
[total dose/cycle = 40 mg/m^2]
Cyclophosphamide: I.V.: 400 mg/m^2 day 1
[total dose/cycle = 400 mg/m^2]
Repeat cycle every 28 days
Variation 4:
Fluorouracil: I.V.: 600 mg/m^2/day days 1 and 8
[total dose/cycle = 1200 mg/m^2]
Doxorubicin: I.V.: 60 mg/m^2 day 1
[total dose/cycle = 60 mg/m^2]
Cyclophosphamide: I.V.: 600 mg/m^2 day 1
[total dose/cycle = 600 mg/m^2]
Repeat cycle every 28 days
Variation 5:
Fluorouracil: I.V.: 300 mg/m^2/day days 1 and 8
[total dose/cycle = 600 mg/m^2]
Doxorubicin: I.V.: 30 mg/m^2 day 1
[total dose/cycle = 30 mg/m^2]
Cyclophosphamide: I.V.: 300 mg/m^2 day 1
[total dose/cycle = 300 mg/m^2]
Repeat cycle every 28 days

FEC

Use Breast cancer

Regimen
Fluorouracil: I.V.: 500 mg/m^2 day 1
[total dose/cycle = 500 mg/m^2]
Cyclophosphamide: I.V.: 500 mg/m^2 day 1
[total dose/cycle = 500 mg/m^2]
Epirubicin: I.V.: 100 mg/m^2 day 1
[total dose/cycle = 100 mg/m^2]
Repeat cycle every 21 days

FL

Use Prostate cancer

Regimen NOTE: Multiple variations are listed below.
Variation 1:
Flutamide: Oral: 250 mg every 8 hours
[total dose/cycle = 21,000 mg]
Leuprolide acetate: SubQ: 1 mg/day
[total dose/cycle = 28 mg]
Repeat cycle every 28 days
Variation 2:
Flutamide: Oral: 250 mg every 8 hours
[total dose/cycle = 67,500 mg]
Leuprolide acetate depot: I.M.: 22.5 mg day 1
[total dose/cycle = 22.5 mg]
Repeat cycle every 3 months

FLAG (AML)

Use Leukemia, acute myeloid

Regimen NOTE: Multiple variations are listed below.
Variation 1:
Fludarabine: I.V.: 30 mg/m^2/day over 30 minutes days 1 to 5
[total dose/cycle = 150 mg/m^2]
Cytarabine: I.V.: 2 g/m^2/day over 4 hours days 1 to 5 (begin 4 hours after fludarabine infusion)
[total dose/cycle = 10 g/m^2]

Filgrastim: SubQ: 300 mcg 12 hours prior to start of fludarabine then 300 mcg/day days 2 through 5
[total dose/cycle = 1500 mcg]
followed by Filgrastim: SubQ: 300 mcg/day beginning one week after the end of treatment and continuing until complete neutrophil recovery

Variation 2:
Fludarabine: I.V.: 30 mg/m^2/day over 30 minutes days 1 to 5
[total dose/cycle = 150 mg/m^2]
Cytarabine: I.V.: 2 g/m^2/day over 4 hours days 1 to 5 (begin 3.5 hours after end of fludarabine infusion)
[total dose/cycle = 10 g/m^2]
Filgrastim: SubQ: 5 mcg/kg/day beginning 24 hours prior to start of fludarabine and continuing until ANC >500 cells/mm^3
May repeat cycle one time for partial remission

Variation 3:
Fludarabine: I.V.: 30 mg/m^2/day over 30 minutes days 1 to 5
[total dose/cycle = 150 mg/m^2]
Cytarabine: I.V.: 2 g/m^2/day over 2 hours days 1 to 5 (begin 4 hours after the start of fludarabine infusion)
[total dose/cycle = 10 g/m^2]
Filgrastim: SubQ or I.V.: 300 mcg/day beginning the day prior to start of chemotherapy and continuing during chemotherapy and until ANC >1000 cells/mm^3
May receive a second cycle

Variation 4:
Fludarabine: I.V.: 25 mg/m^2/day over 30 minutes days 1 to 5
[total dose/cycle = 125 mg/m^2]
Cytarabine: I.V.: 2 g/m^2/day over 4 hours days 1 to 5 (begin 4 hours after start of fludarabine infusion)
[total dose/cycle = 10 g/m^2]
Filgrastim: SubQ: 5 mcg/kg/day beginning 24 hours prior to start of cytarabine and continuing until ANC >500 cells/mm^3

FLAG-IDA

Use Leukemia, acute myeloid

Regimen

Fludarabine: I.V.: 30 mg/m^2/day days 1 to 5
[total dose/cycle = 150 mg/m^2]
Cytarabine: I.V.: 2 g/m^2/day days 1 to 5
[total dose/cycle = 10 g/m^2]
Idarubicin: I.V.: 10 mg/m^2/day days 1, 2, and 3
[total dose/cycle = 30 mg/m^2]
Filgrastim: 5 mcg/kg from day 6 until neutrophil recovery
Administer one cycle only

FLOX (Nordic FLOX)

Use Colorectal cancer

Regimen

Oxaliplatin: I.V.: 85 mg/m^2 day 1
[total dose/cycle = 85 mg/m^2]
Fluorouracil: I.V.: 500 mg/m^2/day days 1 and 2
[total dose/cycle = 1000 mg/m^2]
Leucovorin: I.V.: 60 mg/m^2/day days 1 and 2
[total dose/cycle = 120 mg/m^2]
Repeat cycle every 2 weeks

Fludarabine-Alemtuzumab (CLL)

Use Leukemia, chronic lymphocytic

Regimen

Prior to Cycle 1 (days -14 to -1):
Alemtuzumab dose escalation (on consecutive days): I.V.: 3 mg/dose/day (repeat until tolerated); when tolerated, increase to 10 mg/dose/day (repeat until tolerated); when tolerated, increase to 30 mg/dose
Cycle 1 (begin when alemtuzumab successfully escalated to 30 mg, but no more than 14 days from dose escalation protocol):
Alemtuzumab: I.V.: 30 mg/dose over 2 hours days 1, 2, and 3
[total dose/cycle = 90 mg]

Fludarabine: I.V.: 30 mg/m^2/day over 15-30 minutes days 1, 2, and 3 (begin with alemtuzumab at full dose)
[total dose/cycle = 90 mg/m^2]
Repeat cycle in 28 days
Cycles 2-4:
Alemtuzumab: I.V.: 30 mg/dose (over 4 hours day 1; over 2 hours days 2 and 3) days 1, 2, and 3
[total dose/cycle = 90 mg]
Fludarabine: I.V.: 30 mg/m^2/day over 15-30 minutes days 1, 2, and 3
[total dose/cycle = 90 mg/m^2]
Repeat cycle every 28 days; may administer an additional 2 cycles (cycles 5 and 6) if respond (and tolerate)

Fludarabine-Cyclophosphamide (CLL)

Use Leukemia, chronic lymphocytic

Regimen NOTE: Multiple variations are listed below.

Variation 1:
Fludarabine: I.V.: 25 mg/m^2/day days 1, 2, and 3
[total dose/cycle = 75 mg/m^2]
Cyclophosphamide: I.V.: 250 mg/m^2/day days 1, 2, and 3
[total dose/cycle = 750 mg/m^2]
Repeat cycle every 4 weeks for up to 6 cycles

Variation 2:
Fludarabine: I.V.: 30 mg/m^2/day days 1, 2, and 3
[total dose/cycle = 90 mg/m^2]
Cyclophosphamide: I.V.: 250 mg/m^2/day days 1, 2, and 3
[total dose/cycle = 750 mg/m^2]
Repeat cycle every 4 weeks for up to 6 cycles

Variation 3:
Cyclophosphamide: I.V.: 600 mg/m^2 day 1
[total dose/cycle = 600 mg/m^2]
Fludarabine: I.V.: 20 mg/m^2/day days 1 to 5
[total dose/cycle = 100 mg/m^2]
Repeat cycle every 4 weeks for up to 6 cycles

Variation 4:
Fludarabine: I.V.: 30 mg/m^2/day days 1, 2, and 3
[total dose/cycle = 90 mg/m^2]
Cyclophosphamide: I.V.: 300 mg/m^2/day days 1, 2, and 3
[total dose/cycle = 900 mg/m^2]
Repeat cycle every 4 weeks for up to 6 cycles

Variation 5:
Fludarabine: I.V.: 30 mg/m^2/day days 1, 2, and 3
[total dose/cycle = 90 mg/m^2]
Cyclophosphamide: I.V.: 300 mg/m^2/day days 1, 2, and 3
[total dose/cycle = 900 mg/m^2]
Repeat cycle every 4-6 weeks for up to 6 cycles

Fludarabine-Cyclophosphamide-Mitoxantrone-Rituximab

Use Lymphoma, non-Hodgkin

Regimen NOTE: Multiple variations are listed below.

Consider pretherapy cytoreduction with cyclophosphamide 200 mg/m^2/day for 3-5 days for patients with high tumor burden and/or lymphocytes >20,000/mm^3

Variation 1:
Rituximab: I.V.: 375 mg/m^2/dose day 1
[total dose/cycle = 375 mg/m^2]
Fludarabine: I.V.: 25 mg/m^2/day days 2, 3, and 4
[total dose/cycle = 75 mg/m^2]
Cyclophosphamide: I.V.: 200 mg/m^2/day days 2, 3, and 4
[total dose/cycle = 600 mg/m^2]
Mitoxantrone: I.V.: 8 mg/m^2/dose day 2
[total dose/cycle = 8 mg/m^2]
Repeat cycle every 28 days for total of 4 cycles

Variation 2 (with maintenance rituximab):
Rituximab: I.V.: 375 mg/m^2/dose day 1
[total dose/cycle = 375 mg/m^2]
Fludarabine: I.V.: 25 mg/m^2/day days 2, 3, and 4
[total dose/cycle = 75 mg/m^2]
Cyclophosphamide: I.V.: 200 mg/m^2/day days 2, 3, and 4
[total dose/cycle = 600 mg/m^2]
Mitoxantrone: I.V.: 8 mg/m^2/dose day 2
[total dose/cycle = 8 mg/m^2]
Repeat cycle every 28 days for total of 4 cycles
followed by:
Maintenance rituximab (begin 3 months after completion of cycle 4):
Rituximab: I.V.: 375 mg/m^2/dose day 1, 8, 15, and 22
[total dose/cycle = 1500 mg/m^2]
Repeat maintenance cycle (once) in 6 months

Fludarabine-Cyclophosphamide (NHL-Mantle Cell)

Use Lymphoma, non-Hodgkin (mantle cell)

Regimen NOTE: Multiple variations are listed below.
Variation 1:
Fludarabine: I.V.: 20 mg/m^2/day days 1 to 5
[total dose/cycle = 100 mg/m^2]
Cyclophosphamide: I.V.: 800 mg/m^2/dose day 1
[total dose/cycle = 800 mg/m^2]
Repeat cycle every 3-4 weeks for up to a total of 5 cycles
Variation 2:
Fludarabine: I.V.: 20 mg/m^2/day days 1 to 5
[total dose/cycle = 100 mg/m^2]
Cyclophosphamide: I.V.: 1000 mg/m^2/dose day 1
[total dose/cycle = 1000 mg/m^2]
Repeat cycle every 3-4 weeks for up to a total of 5 cycles
Variation 3:
Fludarabine: I.V.: 25 mg/m^2/day days 1 to 4
[total dose/cycle = 100 mg/m^2]
Cyclophosphamide: I.V.: 1000 mg/m^2/dose day 1
[total dose/cycle = 1000 mg/m^2]
Repeat cycle every 3-4 weeks for up to a total of 5 cycles

Fludarabine-Cyclophosphamide-Rituximab (CLL)

Use Leukemia, chronic lymphocytic

Regimen
Cycle 1:
Rituximab: I.V.: 375 mg/m^2 day 1
[total dose/cycle = 375 mg/m^2]
Fludarabine: I.V.: 25 mg/m^2/day days 2, 3, and 4
[total dose/cycle = 75 mg/m^2]
Cyclophosphamide: I.V.: 250 mg/m^2/day days 2, 3, and 4
[total dose/cycle = 750 mg/m^2]
Treatment cycle is 4 weeks
Cycles 2-6:
Rituximab: I.V.: 500 mg/m^2 day 1
[total dose/cycle = 500 mg/m^2]
Fludarabine: I.V.: 25 mg/m^2/day days 1, 2, and 3
[total dose/cycle = 75 mg/m^2]
Cyclophosphamide: I.V.: 250 mg/m^2/day days 1, 2, and 3
[total dose/cycle = 750 mg/m^2]
Repeat cycle every 4 weeks

Fludarabine-Cyclophosphamide-Rituximab (NHL-Follicular)

Use Lymphoma, non-Hodgkin (Follicular lymphoma)

Regimen

Cycle 1:

Rituximab: I.V.: 375 mg/m^2 day 15
[total dose/cycle = 375 mg/m^2]

Fludarabine: I.V.: 25 mg/m^2/day days 1, 2, and 3
[total dose/cycle = 75 mg/m^2]

Cyclophosphamide: I.V.: 300 mg/m^2/day days 1, 2, and 3
[total dose/cycle = 900 mg/m^2]

Treatment cycle is 3 weeks

Cycles 2-4:

Rituximab: I.V.: 375 mg/m^2 day 1
[total dose/cycle = 375 mg/m^2]

Fludarabine: I.V.: 25 mg/m^2/day days 1, 2, and 3
[total dose/cycle = 75 mg/m^2]

Cyclophosphamide: I.V.: 300 mg/m^2/day days 1, 2, and 3
[total dose/cycle = 900 mg/m^2]

Each treatment cycle is 3 weeks

Fludarabine-Mitoxantrone

Use Lymphoma, non-Hodgkin

Regimen

Fludarabine: I.V.: 25 mg/m^2/day days 1, 2, and 3
[total dose/cycle = 75 mg/m^2]

Mitoxantrone: I.V.: 10 mg/m^2/dose day 1
[total dose/cycle = 10 mg/m^2]

Repeat cycle every 21 days for total of 6 cycles

Fludarabine-Mitoxantrone-Dexamethasone (NHL)

Use Lymphoma, non-Hodgkin

Regimen

Fludarabine: I.V.: 25 mg/m^2/day days 1, 2, and 3
[total dose/cycle = 75 mg/m^2]

Mitoxantrone: I.V.: 10 mg/m^2/dose day 1
[total dose/cycle = 10 mg/m^2]

Dexamethasone: I.V. or Oral: 20 mg/day days 1 to 5
[total dose/cycle = 100 mg]

Repeat cycle every 28 days for up to a total of 8 cycles

Fludarabine-Mitoxantrone-Dexamethasone-Rituximab

Use Lymphoma, non-Hodgkin

Regimen

Cycle 1:

Rituximab: I.V.: 375 mg/m^2/day days 1 and 8
[total dose/cycle = 750 mg/m^2]

Fludarabine: I.V.: 25 mg/m^2/day days 1, 2, and 3
[total dose/cycle = 75 mg/m^2]

Mitoxantrone: I.V.: 10 mg/m^2/dose day 1
[total dose/cycle = 10 mg/m^2]

Dexamethasone: I.V. or Oral: 20 mg/m^2/day days 1 to 5
[total dose/cycle = 100 mg/m^2]

Treatment cycle is 28 days

Cycles 2-5:

Rituximab: I.V.: 375 mg/m^2 day 1
[total dose/cycle = 375 mg/m^2]

Fludarabine: I.V.: 25 mg/m^2/day days 2, 3, and 4
[total dose/cycle = 75 mg/m^2]

Mitoxantrone: I.V.: 10 mg/m^2/dose day 2
[total dose/cycle = 10 mg/m^2]
Dexamethasone: I.V. or Oral: 20 mg/m^2/day days 1 to 5
[total dose/cycle = 100 mg/m^2]
Repeat cycle every 28 days
Cycles 6-8:
Fludarabine: I.V.: 25 mg/m^2/day days 1, 2, and 3
[total dose/cycle = 75 mg/m^2]
Mitoxantrone: I.V.: 10 mg/m^2/dose day 1
[total dose/cycle = 10 mg/m^2]
Dexamethasone: I.V. or Oral: 20 mg/m^2/day days 1 to 5
[total dose/cycle = 100 mg/m^2]
Repeat cycle every 28 days
followed by:
Interferon maintenance:
Interferon alfa-2b: SubQ: 3 million units/m^2 days 1 to 14
[total dose/cycle = 42 million units/m^2]
Dexamethasone: Oral: 8 mg/day days 1, 2, and 3
[total dose/cycle = 24 mg]
Repeat cycle every month for 1 year

Fludarabine-Mitoxantrone-Rituximab

Use Lymphoma, non-Hodgkin

Regimen

Fludarabine: I.V.: 25 mg/m^2/day days 1, 2, and 3
[total dose/cycle = 75 mg/m^2]
Mitoxantrone: I.V.: 10 mg/m^2/dose day 1
[total dose/cycle = 10 mg/m^2]
Repeat cycle every 21 days for total of 6 cycles
followed by:
Sequential rituximab (after completion of cycle 6):
Rituximab: I.V.: 375 mg/m^2/dose weekly for 4 doses
[total dose/4 weeks = 1500 mg/m^2]

Fludarabine-Rituximab (CLL)

Use Leukemia, chronic lymphocytic

Regimen

Rituximab: I.V.: 375 mg/m^2/day days 1 and 4 (cycle 1); day 1 (cycles 2 to 6)
Fludarabine: I.V.: 25 mg/m^2/day days 1 to 5
Repeat cycle every 4 weeks

Fludarabine-Rituximab (NHL-Follicular)

Use Lymphoma, non-Hodgkin (follicular lymphoma)

Regimen

Week 1:
Rituximab: I.V.: 375 mg/m^2/dose for 2 doses 4 days apart
[total dose/week = 750 mg/m^2]
Week 2:
Fludarabine: I.V.: 25 mg/m^2/day days 1 to 5
[total dose/week = 125 mg/m^2]
Week 5:
Rituximab: I.V.: 375 mg/m^2/dose day 5
[total dose/week = 375 mg/m^2]
Week 6:
Fludarabine: I.V.: 25 mg/m^2/day days 1 to 5
[total dose/week = 125 mg/m^2]
Week 10:
Fludarabine: I.V.: 25 mg/m^2/day days 1 to 5
[total dose/week = 125 mg/m^2]

Week 13:
Rituximab: I.V.: 375 mg/m^2/dose day 5
[total dose/week = 375 mg/m^2]
Week 14:
Fludarabine: I.V.: 25 mg/m^2/day days 1 to 5
[total dose/week = 125 mg/m^2]
Week 18:
Fludarabine: I.V.: 25 mg/m^2/day days 1 to 5
[total dose/week = 125 mg/m^2]
Week 21:
Rituximab: I.V.: 375 mg/m^2/dose day 5
[total dose/week = 375 mg/m^2]
Week 22:
Fludarabine: I.V.: 25 mg/m^2/day days 1 to 5
[total dose/week = 125 mg/m^2]
Week 26:
Rituximab: I.V.: 375 mg/m^2/dose for 2 doses 4 days apart
[total dose/week = 750 mg/m^2]

Fluorouracil-Carboplatin (Head and Neck Cancer)

Use Head and neck cancer

Regimen NOTE: Multiple variations are listed below.

Variation 1:
Fluorouracil: I.V.: 600 mg/m^2/day continuous infusion days 1 to 4
[total dose/cycle = 2400 mg/m^2]
Carboplatin: I.V.: 70 mg/m^2/day days 1 to 4
[total dose/cycle = 280 mg/m^2]
Repeat cycle every 3 weeks for 3 cycles
Variation 2:
Fluorouracil: I.V.: 1000 mg/m^2/day continuous infusion days 1 to 4
[total dose/cycle = 4000 mg/m^2]
Carboplatin: I.V.: 300 mg/m^2/dose day 1 (may escalate to 360 mg/m^2/dose in future cycles for grade 0 or 1 hematologic toxicity)
[total dose/cycle = 300-360 mg/m^2]
Repeat cycle every 28 weeks
Variation 3:
Carboplatin: I.V.: 400 mg/m^2 day 1
[total dose/cycle = 400 mg/m^2]
Fluorouracil: I.V.: 1000 mg/m^2/day continuous infusion days 1 to 4
[total dose/cycle = 4000 mg/m^2]
Repeat cycle every 28 days for a total of 2 or 3 cycles

Fluorouracil-Hydroxyurea (Head and Neck Cancer)

Use Head and neck cancer

Regimen NOTE: Administered with concurrent radiation therapy
Fluorouracil: I.V.: 800 mg/m^2/day continuous infusion days 1 to 5
[total dose/cycle = 4000 mg/m^2]
Hydroxyurea: Oral: 1000 mg/dose every 12 hours for 11 doses beginning day 1
[total dose/cycle = 11,000 mg]
Repeat cycle every other week for a total therapy duration of 13 weeks

Fluorouracil-Leucovorin

Use Colorectal cancer

Regimen NOTE: Multiple variations are listed below.

Variation 1 (Mayo Regimen):
Fluorouracil: I.V.: 370-425 mg/m^2/day days 1 to 5
[total dose/cycle = 1850-2125 mg/m^2]
Leucovorin: I.V.: 20 mg/m^2/day days 1 to 5
[total dose/cycle = 100 mg/m^2]
Repeat cycle at 4 weeks, 8 weeks, and every 5 weeks thereafter

Variation 2:
Fluorouracil: I.V.: 400 mg/m^2/day days 1 to 5
[total dose/cycle = 2000 mg/m^2]
Leucovorin: I.V.: 20 mg/m^2/day days 1 to 5
[total dose/cycle = 100 mg/m^2]
Repeat cycle every 28 days
Variation 3:
Fluorouracil: I.V.: 500 mg/m^2 day 1
[total dose/cycle = 500 mg/m^2]
Leucovorin: I.V.: 20 mg/m^2 (2-hour infusion) day 1
[total dose/cycle = 20 mg/m^2]
Repeat cycle weekly
Variation 4:
Fluorouracil: I.V.: 600 mg/m^2 weekly for 6 weeks
[total dose/cycle = 3600 mg/m^2]
Leucovorin: I.V.: 500 mg/m^2 (3-hour infusion) weekly for 6 weeks
[total dose/cycle = 3000 mg/m^2]
Repeat cycle every 8 weeks
Variation 5:
Fluorouracil: I.V.: 600 mg/m^2 weekly for 6 weeks
[total dose/cycle = 3600 mg/m^2]
Leucovorin: I.V.: 500 mg/m^2 (2-hour infusion) weekly for 6 weeks
[total dose/cycle = 3000 mg/m^2]
Repeat cycle every 8 weeks
Variation 6:
Fluorouracil: I.V.: 600 mg/m^2 weekly
[total dose/cycle = 600 mg/m^2]
Leucovorin: I.V.: 500 mg/m^2 (2-hour infusion) weekly
[total dose/cycle = 500 mg/m^2]
Repeat cycle weekly
Variation 7:
Fluorouracil: I.V.: 2600 mg/m^2 continuous infusion over 24 hours day 1
[total dose/cycle = 2600 mg/m^2]
Leucovorin: I.V.: 500 mg/m^2 continuous infusion over 24 hours day 1
[total dose/cycle = 500 mg/m^2]
Repeat cycle weekly
Variation 8:
Fluorouracil: I.V.: 2600 mg/m^2 continuous infusion over 24 hours day 1
[total dose/cycle = 2600 mg/m^2]
Leucovorin: I.V.: 300 mg/m^2 (maximum dose: 500 mg) continuous infusion over 24 hours day 1
[total dose/cycle = 300 mg/m^2; maximum: 500 mg]
Repeat cycle weekly
Variation 9:
Fluorouracil: I.V.: 2600 mg/m^2 continuous infusion over 24 hours once weekly for 6 weeks
[total dose/cycle = 15,600 mg/m^2]
Leucovorin: I.V.: 500 mg/m^2 over 2 hours once weekly for 6 weeks
[total dose/cycle = 3000 mg/m^2]
Repeat cycle every 8 weeks
Variation 10:
Fluorouracil: I.V.: 2300 mg/m^2 continuous infusion over 24 hours day 1
[total dose/cycle = 2300 mg/m^2]
Leucovorin: I.V.: 50 mg/m^2 continuous infusion over 24 hours day 1
[total dose/cycle = 50 mg/m^2]
Repeat cycle weekly
Variation 11:
Fluorouracil: I.V.: 200 mg/m^2/day continuous infusion days 1 to 14
[total dose/cycle = 2800 mg/m^2]
Leucovorin: I.V.: 5 mg/m^2/day continuous infusion days 1 to 14
[total dose/cycle = 70 mg/m^2]
Repeat cycle every 28 days

Variation 12:
Cycle 1:
Fluorouracil: I.V.: 200 mg/m^2/day continuous infusion for 4 weeks
[total dose/cycle = 5600 mg/m^2]
Leucovorin: I.V.: 20 mg/m^2/day days 1, 8, 15, 22
[total dose/cycle = 80 mg/m^2]
Treatment cycle is 6 weeks
Subsequent cycles (starting week 7):
Fluorouracil: 200 mg/m^2 continuous infusion days 1 to 21
[total dose/cycle = 4200 mg/m^2]
Leucovorin: I.V.: 20 mg/m^2/day days 1, 8, and 15
[total dose/cycle = 60 mg/m^2]
Repeat cycle every 4 weeks

Fluorouracil-Leucovorin-Irinotecan (Saltz Regimen)

Use Colorectal cancer

Regimen
Fluorouracil: I.V.: 500 mg/m^2/day days 1, 8, 15, and 22
[total dose/cycle = 2000 mg/m^2]
Leucovorin: I.V.: 20 mg/m^2/day days 1, 8, 15, and 22
[total dose/cycle = 80 mg/m^2]
Irinotecan: I.V.: 125 mg/m^2/day days 1, 8, 15, and 22
[total dose/cycle = 500 mg/m^2]
Repeat cycle every 42 days

Fluorouracil-Leucovorin-Oxaliplatin (Esophageal Cancer)

Use Esophageal Cancer

Regimen NOTE: Multiple variations are listed below.
Variation 1:
Oxaliplatin: I.V.: 85 mg/m^2/dose over 2 hours day 1
[total dose/cycle = 85 mg/m^2]
Leucovorin: I.V.: 200 mg/m^2/dose over 2 hours day 1
[total dose/cycle = 200 mg/m^2]
Fluorouracil: I.V.: 2600 mg/m^2/dose continuous infusion over 24 hours day 1
[total dose/cycle = 2600 mg/m^2]
Repeat cycle every 2 weeks
Variation 2:
Oxaliplatin: I.V.: 85 mg/m^2/dose over 2 hours day 1
[total dose/cycle = 85 mg/m^2]
Leucovorin: I.V.: 500 mg/m^2/day over 2 hours days 1 and 2
[total dose/cycle = 1000 mg/m^2]
Fluorouracil: I.V. bolus: 400 mg/m^2/day days 1 and 2
followed by I.V.: 600 mg/m^2/day continuous infusion over 22 hours days 1 and 2
[total dose/cycle = 2000 mg/m^2]
Note: Bolus fluorouracil and continuous infusion are both given on days 1 and 2.
Repeat cycle every 2 weeks

Fluorouracil-Leucovorin-Oxaliplatin (Gastric Cancer)

Use Gastric cancer

Regimen NOTE: Multiple variations are listed below.
Variation 1:
Oxaliplatin: I.V.: 85 mg/m^2/dose over 2 hours day 1
[total dose/cycle = 85 mg/m^2]
Leucovorin: I.V.: 200 mg/m^2/dose over 2 hours day 1
[total dose/cycle = 200 mg/m^2]
Fluorouracil: I.V.: 2600 mg/m^2/dose continuous infusion over 24 hours day 1
[total dose/cycle = 2600 mg/m^2]
Repeat cycle every 2 weeks until disease progression or unacceptable toxicity
Variation 2:
Oxaliplatin: I.V.: 100 mg/m^2/dose over 2 hours day 1
[total dose/cycle = 100 mg/m^2]

Leucovorin: I.V.: 400 mg/m^2/dose over 2 hours day 1
[total dose/cycle = 400 mg/m^2]
Fluorouracil: I.V. bolus: 400 mg/m^2/dose over 10 minutes day 1
followed by I.V.: 3000 mg/m^2 continuous infusion over 46 hours beginning day 1
[total dose/cycle = 3400 mg/m^2]
Repeat cycle every 2 weeks until disease progression or unacceptable toxicity for at least 6 cycles
Variation 3:
Oxaliplatin: I.V.: 85 mg/m^2/dose over 2 hours day 1
[total dose/cycle = 85 mg/m^2]
Leucovorin: I.V.: 500 mg/m^2/dose over 2 hours day 1
[total dose/cycle = 500 mg/m^2]
Fluorouracil: I.V.: 2600 mg/m^2/dose continuous infusion over 24 hours day 1
[total dose/cycle = 2600 mg/m^2]
Repeat cycle every 2 weeks until disease progression or unacceptable toxicity

Fluorouracil-Mitomycin (Anal Cancer)

Use Anal cancer

Regimen NOTE: Multiple variations are listed below.
Variation 1 (in combination with radiotherapy):
Fluorouracil: I.V.: 1000 mg/m^2/day continuous infusion days 1 to 4 and days 29 to 32
[total dose/cycle = 8000 mg/m^2]
Mitomycin: I.V.: 10 mg/m^2/day (maximum dose: 20 mg) days 1 and 29
[total dose/cycle = 20 mg/m^2; maximum: 40 mg]
Variation 2 (in combination with radiotherapy):
Fluorouracil: I.V.: 1000 mg/m^2/day continuous infusion days 1 to 4
[total dose/cycle = 4000 mg/m^2]
Mitomycin: I.V.: 10 mg/m^2/dose (maximum dose: 20 mg) day 1
[total dose/cycle = 10 mg/m^2; maximum: 20 mg]
Repeat cycle in 28 days (total of 2 cycles)

FOIL (Colorectal Cancer)

Use Colorectal cancer

Regimen
Irinotecan: I.V.: 175 mg/m^2 day 1
[total dose/cycle = 175 mg/m^2]
Oxaliplatin: I.V.: 100 mg/m^2 day 1
[total dose/cycle = 100 mg/m^2]
Leucovorin: I.V.: 200 mg/m^2 day 1
[total dose/cycle = 200 mg/m^2]
Fluorouracil: I.V.: 3800 mg/m^2/day continuous infusion days 1 and 2
[total dose/cycle = 7600 mg/m^2]
Repeat cycle every 14 days

FOLFIRI (Colorectal Cancer)

Use Colorectal cancer

Regimen NOTE: Multiple variations are listed below.
Variation 1:
Cycles 1 and 2:
Irinotecan: I.V.: 180 mg/m^2 over 90 minutes day 1
[total dose/cycle = 180 mg/m^2]
Leucovorin: I.V.: 400 mg/m^2 over 2 hours day 1
[total dose/cycle = 400 mg/m^2]
Fluorouracil: I.V. bolus: 400 mg/m^2 day 1
followed by I.V.: 2400 mg/m^2 continuous infusion (over 46 hours) beginning day 1
[total fluorouracil dose/cycle = 2800 mg/m^2]
Repeat cycle in 14 days
Subsequent cycles:
Irinotecan: I.V.: 180 mg/m^2 over 90 minutes day 1
[total dose/cycle = 180 mg/m^2]
Leucovorin: I.V.: 400 mg/m^2 over 2 hours day 1
[total dose/cycle = 400 mg/m^2]

Fluorouracil: I.V. bolus: 400 mg/m^2 day 1
followed by I.V.: 3000 mg/m^2 continuous infusion (over 46 hours) beginning day 1
[total fluorouracil dose/cycle = 3400 mg/m^2]
Repeat cycle every 14 days until disease progression or unacceptable toxicity

Variation 2:
Irinotecan: I.V.: 180 mg/m^2 over 90 minutes day 1
[total dose/cycle = 180 mg/m^2]
Leucovorin: I.V.: 200 mg/m^2/day over 2 hours days 1 and 2
[total dose/cycle = 400 mg/m^2]
Fluorouracil: I.V. bolus: 400 mg/m^2/day days 1 and 2
followed by I.V.: 600 mg/m^2/day continuous infusion (over 22 hours each day) on days 1 and 2
[total fluorouracil dose/cycle = 2000 mg/m^2]
Repeat cycle every 14 days until disease progression or unacceptable toxicity

Variation 3:
Irinotecan: I.V.: 180 mg/m^2 over 1 hour day 1
[total dose/cycle = 180 mg/m^2]
Leucovorin: I.V.: 100 mg/m^2/day over 2 hours days 1 and 2
[total dose/cycle = 200 mg/m^2]
Fluorouracil: I.V. bolus: 400 mg/m^2/day days 1 and 2
followed by I.V.: 600 mg/m^2/day continuous infusion (over 22 hours each day) on days 1 and 2
[total fluorouracil dose/cycle = 2000 mg/m^2]
Repeat cycle every 14 days for up to 12 cycles or until disease progression or unacceptable toxicity

Variation 4:
Irinotecan: I.V.: 180 mg/m^2 over 90 minutes day 1
[total dose/cycle = 180 mg/m^2]
Leucovorin: I.V.: 400 mg/m^2 over 2 hours day 1
[total dose/cycle = 400 mg/m^2]
Fluorouracil: I.V. bolus: 400 mg/m^2 day 1
followed by I.V.: 2400 mg/m^2 continuous infusion (over 46 hours) beginning day 1
[total fluorouracil dose/cycle = 2800 mg/m^2]
Repeat cycle every 14 days until disease progression or unacceptable toxicity

FOLFIRINOX (Pancreatic Cancer)

Use Pancreatic cancer

Regimen

Oxaliplatin: I.V.: 85 mg/m^2/dose over 2 hours day 1
[total dose/cycle = 85 mg/m^2]
Irinotecan: I.V.: 180 mg/m^2/dose over 90 minutes day 1
[total dose/cycle = 180 mg/m^2]
Leucovorin: I.V.: 400 mg/m^2/dose over 2 hours day 1
[total dose/cycle = 400 mg/m^2]
Fluorouracil: I.V. bolus: 400 mg/m^2/dose day 1
followed by I.V.: 2400 mg/m^2 continuous infusion over 46 hours beginning day 1
[total dose/cycle = 2800 mg/m^2]
Note: Bolus fluorouracil and continuous infusion are both given on day 1.
Repeat cycle every 14 days for 12 cycles or until disease progression or unacceptable toxicity

FOLFOX 1

Use Colorectal cancer

Regimen

Oxaliplatin: I.V.: 130 mg/m^2 day 1 (every other cycle)
[total dose/cycle = 130 mg/m^2]
Leucovorin: I.V.: 500 mg/m^2/day days 1 and 2
[total dose/cycle = 1000 mg/m^2]
Fluorouracil: I.V.: 1.5-2 g/m^2/day continuous infusion days 1 and 2
[total dose/cycle = 3-4 g/m^2]
Repeat cycle every 14 days

FOLFOX 2

Use Colorectal cancer

Regimen

Oxaliplatin: I.V.: 100 mg/m^2 day 1
[total dose/cycle = 100 mg/m^2]
Leucovorin: I.V.: 500 mg/m^2/day days 1 and 2
[total dose/cycle = 1000 mg/m^2]
Fluorouracil: I.V.: 1.5-2 g/m^2/day continuous infusion days 1 and 2
[total dose/cycle = 3-4 g/m^2]
Repeat cycle every 14 days

FOLFOX 3

Use Colorectal cancer

Regimen

Oxaliplatin: I.V.: 85 mg/m^2 day 1
[total dose/cycle = 85 mg/m^2]
Leucovorin: I.V.: 500 mg/m^2/day days 1 and 2
[total dose/cycle = 1000 mg/m^2]
Fluorouracil: I.V.: 1.5-2 g/m^2/day continuous infusion days 1 and 2
[total dose/cycle = 3-4 g/m^2]
Repeat cycle every 14 days

FOLFOX 4

Use Colorectal cancer

Regimen

Oxaliplatin: I.V.: 85 mg/m^2 day 1
[total dose/cycle = 85 mg/m^2]
Leucovorin: I.V.: 200 mg/m^2/day days 1 and 2
[total dose/cycle = 400 mg/m^2]
Fluorouracil: I.V. bolus: 400 mg/m^2/day days 1 and 2
[total dose/cycle = 800 mg/m^2]
followed by I.V.: 600 mg/m^2 continuous infusion (over 22 hours) days 1 and 2
[total dose/cycle = 1200 mg/m^2]
Note: Bolus fluorouracil and continuous infusion are both given on each day.
Repeat cycle every 14 days

FOLFOX 6

Use Colorectal cancer

Regimen

Oxaliplatin: I.V.: 100 mg/m^2 day 1
[total dose/cycle = 100 mg/m^2]
Leucovorin: I.V.: 400 mg/m^2 day 1
[total dose/cycle = 400 mg/m^2]
Fluorouracil: I.V. bolus: 400 mg/m^2 day 1
[total dose/cycle = 400 mg/m^2]
followed by I.V.: 2.4-3 g/m^2 continuous infusion (46 hours) extending over days 1 and 2
[total dose/cycle = 2.4-3 g/m^2]
Repeat cycle every 14 days

FOLFOX 7

Use Colorectal cancer

Regimen

Oxaliplatin: I.V.: 130 mg/m^2 day 1
[total dose/cycle = 130 mg/m^2]
Leucovorin: I.V.: 400 mg/m^2 day 1
[total dose/cycle = 400 mg/m^2]

Fluorouracil: I.V. bolus: 400 mg/m^2 day 1
[total dose/cycle = 400 mg/m^2]
followed by I.V.: 2.4 g/m^2 continuous infusion (46 hours) extending over days 1 and 2
[total dose/cycle = 2.4 g/m^2]
Repeat cycle every 14 days

FOLFOXIRI (Colorectal Cancer)

Use Colorectal cancer

Regimen

Irinotecan: I.V.: 165 mg/m^2 over 1 hour day 1
[total dose/cycle = 165 mg/m^2]
Oxaliplatin: I.V.: 85 mg/m^2 over 2 hours day 1
[total dose/cycle = 85 mg/m^2]
Leucovorin: I.V.: 200 mg/m^2 over 2 hours day 1
[total dose/cycle = 200 mg/m^2]
Fluorouracil: I.V.: 3200 mg/m^2/day continuous infusion over 48 hours beginning day 1
[total dose/cycle = 6400 mg/m^2]
Repeat cycle every 14 days (maximum: 12 cycles)

FU-LV-CPT-11

Use Colorectal cancer

Regimen NOTE: Multiple variations are listed below.

Variation 1:
Irinotecan: I.V.: 350 mg/m^2 day 1
[total dose/cycle = 350 mg/m^2]
Leucovorin: I.V.: 20 mg/m^2/day days 22 to 26
[total dose/cycle = 100 mg/m^2]
Fluorouracil: I.V.: 425 mg/m^2/day days 22 to 26
[total dose/cycle = 2125 mg/m^2]
Repeat cycle every 6 weeks

Variation 2:
Irinotecan: I.V.: 80 mg/m^2 day 1
[total dose/cycle = 80 mg/m^2]
Fluorouracil: I.V.: 2300 mg/m^2 continuous infusion day 1
[total dose/cycle = 2300 mg/m^2]
Leucovorin: I.V.: 500 mg/m^2 day 1
[total dose/cycle = 500 mg/m^2]
Repeat cycle weekly
or
Irinotecan: I.V.: 180 mg/m^2 day 1
[total dose/cycle = 180 mg/m^2]
Leucovorin: I.V.: 200 mg/m^2/day days 1 and 2
[total dose/cycle = 400 mg/m^2]
Fluorouracil: I.V.: 400 mg/m^2/day days 1 and 2
[total dose/cycle = 800 mg/m^2]
followed by I.V.: 600 mg/m^2/day continuous infusion days 1 and 2
[total dose/cycle = 1200 mg/m^2]
Repeat cycle every 2 weeks

Variation 3:
Irinotecan: I.V.: 175 mg/m^2 day 1
[total dose/cycle = 175 mg/m^2]
Leucovorin: I.V.: 250 mg/m^2 day 2
[total dose/cycle = 250 mg/m^2]
Fluorouracil: I.V.: 950 mg/m^2 day 2
[total dose/cycle = 950 mg/m^2]
or
Irinotecan: I.V.: 200 mg/m^2 day 1
[total dose/cycle = 200 mg/m^2]
Leucovorin: I.V.: 250 mg/m^2 day 2
[total dose/cycle = 250 mg/m^2]
Fluorouracil: I.V.: 850 mg/m^2 day 2
[total dose/cycle = 850 mg/m^2]
Repeat cycle every other week

FZ

Use Prostate cancer

Regimen NOTE: Multiple variations are listed below.

Variation 1:

Flutamide: Oral: 250 mg every 8 hours
[total dose/cycle = 21,000 mg]

Goserelin acetate: SubQ: 3.6 mg day 1
[total dose/cycle = 3.6 mg]

Repeat cycle every 28 days

Variation 2:

Flutamide: Oral: 250 mg every 8 hours
[total dose/cycle = 67,500 mg]

Goserelin acetate: SubQ: 10.8 mg day 1
[total dose/cycle = 10.8 mg]

Repeat cycle every 3 months

Gemcitabine-Capecitabine (Biliary Cancer)

Use Biliary adenocarcinoma

Regimen

Gemcitabine: I.V.: 1000 mg/m^2/day over 30 minutes days 1 and 8
[total dose/cycle = 2000 mg/m^2]

Capecitabine: Oral: 650 mg/m^2 twice daily days 1 to 14
[total dose/cycle = 18,200 mg/m^2]

Repeat cycle every 21 days until disease progression or unacceptable toxicity

Gemcitabine-Capecitabine (Pancreatic Cancer)

Use Pancreatic cancer

Regimen NOTE: Multiple variations are listed below.

Variation 1:

Gemcitabine: I.V.: 1000 mg/m^2/day over 30 minutes days 1 and 8
[total dose/cycle = 2000 mg/m^2]

Capecitabine: Oral: 650 mg/m^2/dose twice daily days 1 to 14
[total dose/cycle = 18,200 mg/m^2]

Repeat cycle every 21 days until disease progression (maximum duration: 24 weeks)

Variation 2:

Gemcitabine: I.V.: 1000 mg/m^2/day over 30 minutes days 1, 8, and 15
[total dose/cycle = 3000 mg/m^2]

Capecitabine: Oral: 830 mg/m^2/dose twice daily days 1 to 21
[total dose/cycle = 34,860 mg/m^2]

Repeat cycle every 28 days until disease progression or unacceptable toxicity

Gemcitabine-Capecitabine (RCC)

Use Renal cell cancer

Regimen NOTE: Multiple variations are listed below.

Variation 1:

Gemcitabine: I.V.: 1000 mg/m^2/day days 1, 8, and 15
[total dose/cycle = 3000 mg/m^2]

Capecitabine: Oral: 830 mg/m^2/dose twice daily on days 1 to 21
[total dose/cycle = 34,860 mg/m^2]

Repeat cycle every 28 days

Variation 2 (for patients with Cl_{cr} 30-50 mL/minute):

Gemcitabine: I.V.: 1000 mg/m^2/day days 1, 8, and 15
[total dose/cycle = 3000 mg/m^2]

Capecitabine: Oral: 622 mg/m^2/dose twice daily on days 1 to 21
[total dose/cycle = 26,124 mg/m^2]

Repeat cycle every 28 days

Variation 3:

Gemcitabine: I.V.: 1200 mg/m^2/day days 1 and 8
[total dose/cycle = 2400 mg/m^2]

Capecitabine: Oral: 1300 mg/m^2/dose twice daily on days 1 to 14
[total dose/cycle = 36,400 mg/m^2]
Repeat cycle every 21 days for up to 6 cycles

Gemcitabine-Carboplatin (Bladder Cancer)

Use Bladder cancer

Regimen

Gemcitabine: I.V.: 1000 mg/m^2/day days 1 and 8
[total dose/cycle = 2000 mg/m^2]
Carboplatin: I.V.: AUC 5 day 1
[total dose/cycle = AUC = 5]
Repeat cycle every 21 days for up to 6 cycles

Gemcitabine-Carboplatin (NSCLC)

Use Lung cancer, nonsmall cell

Regimen NOTE: Multiple variations are listed below.

Variation 1:
Gemcitabine: I.V.: 1000 mg/m^2/dose days 1, 8, and 15
[total dose/cycle = 3000 mg/m^2]
Carboplatin: I.V.: AUC 5 day 1
[total dose/cycle = AUC = 5]
Repeat cycle every 28 days for up to 4 cycles

Variation 2:
Gemcitabine: I.V.: 1000 or 1100 mg/m^2/day days 1 and 8
[total dose/cycle = 2000 or 2200 mg/m^2]
Carboplatin: I.V.: AUC 5 day 8
[total dose/cycle = AUC = 5]
Repeat cycle every 28 days

Gemcitabine-Carboplatin (Ovarian Cancer)

Use Ovarian cancer

Regimen

Gemcitabine: I.V.: 1000 mg/m^2/day days 1 and 8
[total dose/cycle = 2000 mg/m^2]
Carboplatin: I.V.: AUC 4 day 1
[total dose/cycle = AUC = 4]
Repeat cycle every 21 days for 6-10 cycles

Gemcitabine-Cisplatin (Biliary Cancer)

Use Biliary adenocarcinoma

Regimen NOTE: Multiple variations are listed below.

Variation 1:
Gemcitabine: I.V.: 1250 mg/m^2/dose days 1 and 8
[total dose/cycle = 2500 mg/m^2]
Cisplatin: I.V.: 75 mg/m^2/dose day 1
[total dose/cycle = 75 mg/m^2]
Repeat cycle every 3 weeks

Variation 2:
Gemcitabine: I.V.: 1000 mg/m^2/dose days 1 and 8
[total dose/cycle = 2000 mg/m^2]
Cisplatin: I.V.: 70 mg/m^2/dose day 1
[total dose/cycle = 70 mg/m^2]
Repeat cycle every 3 weeks (maximum: 6 cycles)

Gemcitabine-Cisplatin (Bladder Cancer)

Use Bladder cancer

Regimen

Gemcitabine: I.V.: 1000 mg/m^2/day days 1, 8, and 15
[total dose/cycle = 3000 mg/m^2]
Cisplatin: I.V.: 70 mg/m^2 day 2
[total dose/cycle = 70 mg/m^2]
Repeat cycle every 28 days for 6 cycles

Gemcitabine-Cisplatin (Mesothelioma)

Use Malignant pleural mesothelioma

Regimen NOTE: Multiple variations are listed below.

Variation 1:

Cisplatin: I.V.: 100 mg/m^2 infused over 1 hour day 1
[total dose/cycle = 100 mg/m^2]

Gemcitabine: I.V.: 1000 mg/m^2/dose over 30 minutes days 1, 8, and 15
[total dose/cycle = 3000 mg/m^2]

Repeat cycle every 28 days for up to a total of 6 cycles

Variation 2:

Gemcitabine: I.V.: 1250 mg/m^2/dose over 30 minutes days 1 and 8
[total dose/cycle = 2500 mg/m^2]

Cisplatin: I.V.: 80 mg/m^2 infused over 3 hours day 1
[total dose/cycle = 80 mg/m^2]

Repeat cycle every 21 days for up to a total of 6 cycles

Gemcitabine-Cisplatin (NSCLC)

Use Lung cancer, nonsmall cell

Regimen NOTE: Multiple variations are listed below.

Variation 1:

Gemcitabine: I.V.: 1000 mg/m^2/day days 1, 8, and 15
[total dose/cycle = 3000 mg/m^2]

Cisplatin: I.V.: 100 mg/m^2 day 1
[total dose/cycle = 100 mg/m^2]

Repeat cycle every 28 days

Variation 2:

Gemcitabine: I.V.: 1250 mg/m^2/day days 1 and 8
[total dose/cycle = 2500 mg/m^2]

Cisplatin: I.V.: 100 mg/m^2 day 1
[total dose/cycle = 100 mg/m^2]

Repeat cycle every 21 days

Variation 3:

Gemcitabine: I.V.: 1000 mg/m^2/day days 1 and 8
[total dose/cycle = 2000 mg/m^2]

Cisplatin: I.V.: 80 mg/m^2 day 1
[total dose/cycle = 80 mg/m^2]

Repeat cycle every 21 days

Variation 4:

Gemcitabine: I.V.: 1250 mg/m^2/day days 1 and 8
[total dose/cycle = 2500 mg/m^2]

Cisplatin: I.V.: 75 mg/m^2 day 1
[total dose/cycle = 75 mg/m^2]

Repeat cycle every 21 days for up to 6 cycles

Variation 5:

Gemcitabine: I.V.: 1000 mg/m^2/day days 1, 8, and 15
[total dose/cycle = 3000 mg/m^2]

Cisplatin: I.V.: 100 mg/m^2 day 15
[total dose/cycle = 100 mg/m^2]

Repeat cycle every 28 days

Variation 6:

Gemcitabine: I.V.: 1000 mg/m^2/day days 1, 8, and 15
[total dose/cycle = 3000 mg/m^2]

Cisplatin: I.V.: 100 mg/m^2 day 2
[total dose/cycle = 100 mg/m^2]

Repeat cycle every 28 days for 5 cycles

Variation 7:

Gemcitabine: I.V.: 1200 mg/m^2/day days 1, 8, and 15
[total dose/cycle = 3600 mg/m^2]

Cisplatin: I.V.: 100 mg/m^2 day 15
[total dose/cycle = 100 mg/m^2]

Repeat cycle every 28 days for up to 6 cycles

Variation 8 (patients ≥70 years of age):
Gemcitabine: I.V.: 1000 mg/m^2/day days 1 and 8
[total dose/cycle = 2000 mg/m^2]
Cisplatin: I.V.: 60 mg/m^2 day 1
[total dose/cycle = 60 mg/m^2]
Repeat cycle every 21 days for up to 6 cycles

Gemcitabine-Cisplatin (Pancreatic Cancer)

Use Pancreatic cancer

Regimen

Cisplatin: I.V.: 50 mg/m^2 infused over 1 hour days 1 and 15
[total dose/cycle = 100 mg/m^2]
Gemcitabine: I.V.: 1000 mg/m^2/dose over 30 minutes days 1 and 15
[total dose/cycle = 2000 mg/m^2]
Repeat cycle every 28 days

Gemcitabine-Cisplatin (Unknown Primary)

Use Unknown primary (adenocarcinoma)

Regimen

Gemcitabine: I.V.: 1250 mg/m^2/day days 1 and 8
[total dose/cycle = 2500 mg/m^2]
Cisplatin: I.V.: 100 mg/m^2 infused over 1 hour day 1
[total dose/cycle = 100 mg/m^2]
Repeat cycle every 21 days

Gemcitabine-Docetaxel (Sarcoma)

Use Osteosarcoma; Soft tissue sarcoma

Regimen

Gemcitabine: I.V.: 675 mg/m^2/day days 1 and 8
[total dose/cycle = 1350 mg/m^2]
Docetaxel: I.V.: 100 mg/m^2 day 8
[total dose/cycle = 100 mg/m^2]
Repeat cycle every 21 days

Gemcitabine-Docetaxel (Unknown Primary)

Use Unknown primary (adenocarcinoma)

Regimen

Gemcitabine: I.V.: 1000 mg/m^2/day days 1 and 8
[total dose/cycle = 2000 mg/m^2]
Docetaxel: I.V.: 75 mg/m^2 infused over 1 hour day 8
[total dose/cycle = 75 mg/m^2]
Repeat cycle every 21 days for up to a total of 6 cycles

Gemcitabine-Erlotinib (Pancreatic Cancer)

Use Pancreatic cancer

Regimen

Cycle 1:
Gemcitabine: I.V.: 1000 mg/m^2/day days 1, 8, 15, 22, 29, 36, and 43 (cycle 1 only)
[total dose/cycle 1 = 7000 mg/m^2]
Erlotinib: Oral: 100 mg once daily days 1 to 56
[total dose/cycle 1 = 5600 mg]
Treatment cycle is 56 days
Subsequent cycles:
Gemcitabine: I.V.: 1000 mg/m^2/day days 1, 8, and 15
[total dose/cycle = 3000 mg/m^2]
Erlotinib: Oral: 100 mg once daily days 1 to 28
[total dose/cycle = 2800 mg]
Repeat cycle every 28 days

Gemcitabine-Fluorouracil (RCC)

Use Renal cell cancer

Regimen

Gemcitabine: I.V.: 600 mg/m^2/day days 1, 8, and 15
[total dose/cycle = 1800 mg/m^2]
Fluorouracil: I.V.: 150 mg/m^2/day continuous infusion days 1 to 21
[total dose/cycle = 3150 mg/m^2]
Repeat cycle every 28 days for at least 2 cycles

Gemcitabine-Oxaliplatin (Pancreatic Cancer)

Use Pancreatic cancer

Regimen

Gemcitabine: I.V.: 1000 mg/m^2/day (infused at 10 mg/m^2/minute) day 1
[total dose/cycle = 1000 mg/m^2]
Oxaliplatin: I.V.: 100 mg/m^2/day (over 2 hours) day 2
[total dose/cycle = 100 mg/m^2]
Repeat cycle every 14 days

Gemcitabine-Oxaliplatin-Rituximab (NHL)

Use Lymphoma, non-Hodgkin

Regimen

Oxaliplatin: I.V.: 100 mg/m^2/dose day 1
[total dose/cycle = 100 mg/m^2]
Gemcitabine: I.V.: 1000 mg/m^2/dose day 1
[total dose/cycle = 1000 mg/m^2]
Rituximab: I.V.: 375 mg/m^2/dose day 1
[total dose/cycle = 375 mg/m^2]
Repeat cycle every 3 weeks (for a total of 6-8 cycles)

Gemcitabine-Paclitaxel

Use Ovarian cancer

Regimen

Paclitaxel: I.V.: 80 mg/m^2 (infused over 60 minutes) days 1, 8, and 15
[total dose/cycle = 240 mg/m^2]
Gemcitabine: I.V.: 1000 mg/m^2/day (start at end of paclitaxel infusion) days 1, 8, and 15
[total dose/cycle = 3000 mg/m^2]
Repeat cycle every 4 weeks

Gemcitabine-Paclitaxel (Breast Cancer)

Use Breast cancer

Regimen

Paclitaxel: I.V.: 175 mg/m^2 (infused over 3 hours) day 1
[total dose/cycle = 175 mg/m^2]
Gemcitabine: I.V.: 1250 mg/m^2/day days 1 and 8
[total dose/cycle = 2500 mg/m^2]
Repeat cycle every 21 days until disease progression or unacceptable toxicity

Gemcitabine-Vinorelbine

Use Lung cancer, nonsmall cell

Regimen NOTE: Multiple variations are listed below.

Variation 1:
Gemcitabine: I.V.: 1200 mg/m^2/day days 1 and 8
[total dose/cycle = 2400 mg/m^2]
Vinorelbine: I.V.: 30 mg/m^2/day days 1 and 8
[total dose/cycle = 60 mg/m^2]
Repeat cycle every 21 days for 6 cycles

Variation 2:
Gemcitabine: I.V.: 1000 mg/m^2/day days 1, 8, and 15
[total dose/cycle = 3000 mg/m^2]
Vinorelbine: I.V.: 20 mg/m^2/day days 1, 8, and 15
[total dose/cycle = 60 mg/m^2]
Repeat cycle every 28 days for 6 cycles

Gemcitabine-Vinorelbine-Doxorubicin (Liposomal)

Use Lymphoma, Hodgkin disease

Regimen NOTE: Multiple variations are listed below.
Variation 1 (for transplant-naive patients):
Vinorelbine: I.V.: 20 mg/m^2/day days 1 and 8
[total dose/cycle = 40 mg/m^2]
Gemcitabine: I.V.: 1000 mg/m^2/day days 1 and 8
[total dose/cycle = 2000 mg/m^2]
Doxorubicin liposomal: I.V.: 15 mg/m^2/day days 1 and 8
[total dose/cycle = 30 mg/m^2]
Repeat cycle every 21 days for 2-6 cycles
Variation 2 (for patients with prior transplant):
Vinorelbine: I.V.: 15 mg/m^2/day days 1 and 8
[total dose/cycle = 30 mg/m^2]
Gemcitabine: I.V.: 800 mg/m^2/day days 1 and 8
[total dose/cycle = 1600 mg/m^2]
Doxorubicin liposomal: I.V.: 10 mg/m^2/day days 1 and 8
[total dose/cycle = 20 mg/m^2]
Repeat cycle every 21 days for 2-6 cycles

Gemcitabine-Vinorelbine (Sarcoma)

Use Soft tissue sarcoma

Regimen NOTE: Multiple variations are listed.
Variation 1:
Vinorelbine: I.V.: 25 mg/m^2/dose over 10 minutes days 1 and 8
[total dose/cycle = 50 mg/m^2]
Gemcitabine: I.V.: 800 mg/m^2/dose over 90 minutes days 1 and 8
[total dose/cycle = 1600 mg/m^2]
Repeat cycle every 21 days until disease progression or unacceptable toxicity
Variation 2 (modification for toxicity):
Vinorelbine: I.V.: 25 mg/m^2/dose over 10 minutes days 1 and 15
[total dose/cycle = 50 mg/m^2]
Gemcitabine: I.V.: 800 mg/m^2/dose over 90 minutes days 1 and 15
[total dose/cycle = 1600 mg/m^2]
Repeat cycle every 28 days until disease progression or unacceptable toxicity

GEMOX (Biliary Cancer)

Use Biliary adenocarcinoma

Regimen
Gemcitabine: I.V.: 1000 mg/m^2 day 1
[total dose/cycle = 1000 mg/m^2]
Oxaliplatin: I.V.: 100 mg/m^2 day 2
[total dose/cycle = 100 mg/m^2]
Repeat cycle every 2 weeks

GEMOX (Testicular Cancer)

Use Testicular cancer

Regimen NOTE: Multiple variations are listed below.
Variation 1:
Gemcitabine: I.V.: 1000 mg/m^2/dose over 30 minutes days 1 and 8
[total dose/cycle = 2000 mg/m^2]
Oxaliplatin: I.V.: 130 mg/m^2/dose over 2 hours day 1
[total dose/cycle = 130 mg/m^2]
Repeat cycle every 21 days for a total of at least 2 cycles (maximum: 6 cycles)

Variation 2:
Gemcitabine: I.V.: 1250 mg/m^2/dose over 30 minutes days 1 and 8
[total dose/cycle = 2500 mg/m^2]
Oxaliplatin: I.V.: 130 mg/m^2/dose over 2 hours day 1
[total dose/cycle = 130 mg/m^2]
Repeat cycle every 21 days

HDMTX

Use Osteosarcoma

Regimen

Methotrexate: I.V.: 12 g/m^2/week for 2-12 weeks
[total dose/cycle = 24-144 g/m^2]
Leucovorin calcium rescue: Oral, I.V.: 15 mg/m^2 every 6 hours (beginning 30 hours after the beginning of the 4-hour methotrexate infusion) for 10 doses; **serum methotrexate levels must be monitored**
[total dose/cycle = 150 mg/m^2]

HIPE-IVAD

Use Neuroblastoma

Regimen

Cisplatin: I.V.: 40 mg/m^2/day days 1 to 5
[total dose/cycle = 200 mg/m^2]
Etoposide: I.V.: 100 mg/m^2/day days 1 to 5
[total dose/cycle = 500 mg/m^2]
Ifosfamide: I.V.: 3 g/m^2/day days 21 to 23
[total dose/cycle = 9 g/m^2]
Mesna: I.V.: 3 g/m^2/day continuous infusion days 21, 22, and 23
[total dose/cycle = 9 g/m^2]
Vincristine: I.V.: 1.5 mg/m^2 day 21
[total dose/cycle = 1.5 mg/m^2]
Doxorubicin: I.V.: 60 mg/m^2 day 23
[total dose/cycle = 60 mg/m^2]
Repeat cycle every 28 days

Hyper-CVAD + Imatinib

Use Leukemia, acute lymphocytic

Regimen

Cycle A: (Cycles 1, 3, 5, and 7)
Imatinib: Oral: 400 mg/day days 1 to 14
[total dose/cycle = 5600 mg]
Cyclophosphamide: I.V.: 300 mg/m^2 every 12 hours, for 6 doses, days 1, 2, and 3
[total dose/cycle = 1800 mg/m^2]
Mesna: I.V. 600 mg/m^2/day continuous infusion days 1, 2, and 3
[total dose/cycle = 1800 mg/m^2]
Vincristine: I.V.: 2 mg/day days 4 and 11
[total dose/cycle = 4 mg]
Doxorubicin: I.V.: 50 mg/m^2/day continuous infusion day 4
[total dose/cycle = 50 mg/m^2]
Dexamethasone: Oral, I.V.: 40 mg/day days 1 to 4 and 11 to 14
[total dose/cycle = 320 mg]
Cycle B: (Cycles 2, 4, 6, and 8)
Imatinib: Oral: 400 mg/day days 1 to 14
[total dose/cycle = 5600 mg]
Methotrexate: I.V.: 1 g/m^2/day continuous infusion day 1
[total dose/cycle = 1 g/m^2]
Leucovorin: I.V.: 50 mg then 15 mg every 6 hours, for 8 doses (start 12 hours after the end of the methotrexate infusion)
[total dose/cycle = 170 mg]
Cytarabine: I.V.: 3 g/m^2 every 12 hours for 4 doses, days 2 and 3
[total dose/cycle = 12 g/m^2]
Repeat every 6 weeks in the following sequence: ABABABAB

CNS Prophylaxis
Methotrexate: I.T.: 12 mg/day day 2
[total dose/cycle = 12 mg/day]
or 6 mg into Ommaya day 2
[total dose/cycle = 6 mg/day]
Cytarabine: I.T.: 100 mg/day day 7 or 8
[total dose/cycle = 100 mg/day]
Repeat cycle every 3 weeks for 3 or 4 cycles

Maintenance (POMP)
Imatinib: Oral: 600 mg/day
[total dose/cycle = 18,000 mg]
Vincristine: I.V.: 2 mg/day day 1
[total dose/cycle = 2 mg]
Prednisone: Oral: 200 mg/day days 1 to 5
[total dose/cycle = 1000 mg/m^2]
Repeat cycle every month (except months 6 and 13) for 13 months

Intensification
Imatinib: Oral: 400 mg/day days 1 to 14
[total dose/cycle = 5600 mg]
Cyclophosphamide: I.V.: 300 mg/m^2 every 12 hours, for 6 doses, days 1, 2, and 3
[total dose/cycle = 1800 mg/m^2]
Mesna: I.V.: 600 mg/m^2/day continuous infusion days 1, 2, and 3
[total dose/cycle = 1800 mg/m^2]
Vincristine: I.V.: 2 mg/day days 4 and 11
[total dose/cycle = 4 mg]
Doxorubicin: 50 mg/m^2/day continuous infusion day 4
[total dose/cycle = 50 mg/m^2]
Dexamethasone: I.V. or Oral: 40 mg/day days 1 to 4 and 11 to 14
[total dose/cycle = 320 mg]
Cycle is given in months 6 and 13 during maintenance

Hyper-CVAD (Leukemia, Acute Lymphocytic)

Use Leukemia, acute lymphocytic

Regimen NOTE: Multiple variations are listed below.

Variation 1:

Cycle A: (Cycles 1, 3, 5, and 7)
Cyclophosphamide: I.V.: 300 mg/m^2 every 12 hours, for 6 doses, days 1, 2, and 3
[total dose/cycle = 1800 mg/m^2]
Mesna: I.V.: 1200 mg/m^2/day continuous infusion days 1, 2, and 3
[total dose/cycle = 3600 mg/m^2]
Vincristine: I.V.: 2 mg/day days 4 and 11
[total dose/cycle = 4 mg]
Doxorubicin: I.V.: 50 mg/m^2 day 4
[total dose/cycle = 50 mg/m^2]
Dexamethasone: (route not specified): 40 mg/day days 1 to 4 and 11 to 14
[total dose/cycle = 320 mg]

Cycle B: (Cycles 2, 4, 6, and 8)
Methotrexate: I.V.: 1 g/m^2 continuous infusion day 1
[total dose/cycle = 1g/m^2]
Leucovorin: (route not specified): 15 mg every 6 hours, for 8 doses (start 12 hours after end of methotrexate infusion)
[total dose/cycle = 120 mg]
Cytarabine: I.V.: 3 g/m^2 every 12 hours, for 4 doses, days 2 and 3
[total dose/cycle = 12 g/m^2]
Methylprednisolone: I.V.: 50 mg twice daily, for 6 doses, days 1, 2, and 3
[total dose/cycle = 300 mg/m^2]
Repeat every 6 weeks in the following sequence: ABABABAB

CNS Prophylaxis
Methotrexate: I.T.: 12 mg/day day 2
[total dose/cycle = 12 mg]
or 6 mg/day into Ommaya day 2
[total dose/cycle = 6 mg]

Cytarabine: I.T: 100 mg day 8
[total dose/cycle = 100 mg]
Repeat cycle every 3 weeks

Maintenance (POMP)

Mercaptopurine: Oral: 50 mg 3 times/day
[total dose/cycle = 4200-4650 mg]
Vincristine: I.V.: 2 mg day 1
[total dose/cycle = 2 mg]
Methotrexate: Oral: 20 mg/m^2/day days 1, 8, 15, and 22
[total dose/cycle = 80 mg/m^2]
Prednisone: Oral: 200 mg/day days 1 to 5
[total dose/cycle = 1000 mg/m^2]

or

Mercaptopurine: I.V.: 1 g/m^2/day days 1 to 5
[total dose/cycle = 5 g/m^2]
Vincristine: I.V.: 2 mg day 1
[total dose/cycle = 2 mg]
Methotrexate: I.V.: 10 mg/m^2/day days 1 to 5
[total dose/cycle = 50 mg/m^2]
Prednisone: Oral: 200 mg/day days 1 to 5
[total dose/cycle = 1000 mg/m^2]
Repeat cycles every month for 2 years

Variation 2:

Cycle A: (Cycles 1, 3, 5, and 7)

Cyclophosphamide: I.V.: 300 mg/m^2 every 12 hours, for 6 doses, days 1, 2, and 3
[total dose/cycle = 1800 mg/m^2]
Mesna: I.V.: 600 mg/m^2/day continuous infusion days 1, 2, and 3
[total dose/cycle = 1800 mg/m^2]
Vincristine: I.V.: 2 mg/day days 4 and 11
[total dose/cycle = 4 mg]
Doxorubicin: I.V.: 50 mg/m^2 day 4
[total dose/cycle = 50 mg/m^2]
Dexamethasone: Oral, I.V.: 40 mg/day days 1 to 4 and 11 to 14
[total dose/cycle = 320 mg]

Cycle B: (Cycles 2, 4, 6, and 8)

Methotrexate: I.V.: 1 g/m^2 continuous infusion day 1
[total dose/cycle = 1 g/m^2]
Leucovorin: I.V.: 50 mg (start 12 hours after end of methotrexate infusion)
followed by I.V.: 15 mg every 6 hours, for 8 doses
[total dose/cycle = 170 mg]
Cytarabine: I.V.: 3 g/m^2 every 12 hours, for 4 doses, days 2 and 3
[total dose/cycle = 12 g/m^2]
Repeat every 6 weeks in the following sequence: ABABABAB

CNS Prophylaxis

Methotrexate: I.T.: 12 mg day 2
[total dose/cycle = 12 mg]
or 6 mg into Ommaya day 2
[total dose/cycle = 6 mg]
Cytarabine: I.T.: 100 mg day 7
[total dose/cycle = 100 mg]
Repeat cycle every 3 weeks

Variation 3:

Cycle A: (Cycles 1, 3, 5, and 7)

Cyclophosphamide: I.V.: 300 mg/m^2 every 12 hours, for 6 doses, days 1, 2, and 3
[total dose/cycle = 1800 mg/m^2]
Mesna: I.V.: 600 mg/m^2/day continuous infusion days 1, 2, and 3
[total dose/cycle = 1800 mg/m^2]
Vincristine: I.V.: 2 mg/day days 4 and 11
[total dose/cycle = 4 mg]
Doxorubicin: I.V.: 50 mg/m^2 continuous infusion day 4
[total dose/cycle = 50 mg/m^2]

Dexamethasone: Oral, I.V.: 40 mg/day days 1 to 4 and 11 to 14
[total dose/cycle = 320 mg]
Cycle B: (Cycles 2, 4, 6, and 8)
Methotrexate: I.V.: 200 mg/m^2 day 1
followed by I.V.: 800 mg/m^2 continuous infusion day 1
[total dose/cycle = 1 g/m^2]
Leucovorin: I.V.: 50 mg (start 12 hours after end of methotrexate infusion)
followed by I.V.: 15 mg every 6 hours, for 8 doses
[total dose/cycle = 170 mg/m^2]
Cytarabine: I.V.: 3 g/m^2 every 12 hours, for 4 doses, days 2 and 3
[total dose/cycle = 12 g/m^2]
Repeat every 6 weeks in the following sequence: ABABABAB
CNS Prophylaxis
Methotrexate: I.T.: 12 mg day 2
[total dose/cycle = 12 mg]
or 6 mg into Ommaya day 2
[total dose/cycle = 6 mg]
Cytarabine: I.T.: 100 mg day 7 **or** 8
[total dose/cycle = 100 mg]
Repeat cycles every 3 weeks for 6 or 8 cycles
Maintenance (POMP)
Mercaptopurine: Oral: 50 mg 3 times/day
[total dose/cycle = 4200-4650 mg]
Vincristine: I.V.: 2 mg day 1
[total dose/cycle = 2 mg]
Methotrexate: Oral, I V: 20 mg/m^2/ day days 1, 8, 15, and 22
[total dose/cycle = 80 mg/m^2]
Prednisone: Oral: 200 mg/day days 1 to 5
[total dose/cycle = 1000 mg/m^2]
or
Mercaptopurine: I.V.: 1 g/m^2/day days 1 to 5
[total dose/cycle = 5 g/m^2]
Vincristine: I.V.: 2 mg day 1
[total dose/cycle = 2 mg]
Methotrexate: I.V.: 10 mg/m^2/day days 1 to 5
[total dose/cycle = 50 mg/m^2]
Prednisone: Oral: 200 mg/day days 1 to 5
[total dose/cycle = 1000 mg]
Repeat cycles every month (except months 7 and 11 or 9 and 12) for 2 years
Intensification
Etoposide: I.V.: 100 mg/m^2/day days 1 to 5
[total dose/cycle = 500 mg/m^2]
Pegaspargase: I.V.: 2500 units/m^2 day 1
[total dose/cycle = 2500 units/m^2]
Given during months 9 and 12 of maintenance
or
Methotrexate: I.V.: 100 mg/m^2/day days 1, 8, 15, and 22
[total dose/cycle = 400 mg/m^2]
Asparaginase: I.V.: 20,000 units/day days 2, 9, 16, and 23
[total dose/cycle = 80,000 units]
Given during months 7 and 11 of maintenance
Variation 4:
Cycle A: (Cycles 1, 3, 5, and 7)
Cyclophosphamide: I.V.: 300 mg/m^2 every 12 hours, for 6 doses, days 1, 2, and 3
[total dose/cycle = 1800 mg/m^2]
Mesna: I.V.: 600 mg/m^2/day continuous infusion days 1, 2, and 3
[total dose/cycle = 1800 mg/m^2]
Vincristine: I.V.: 2 mg/day days 4 and 11
[total dose/cycle = 4 mg]
Doxorubicin: I.V.: 50 mg/m^2day 4
[total dose/cycle = 50 mg/m^2]

Dexamethasone: (route not specified): 40 mg/day days 1 to 4 and 11 to 14
[total dose/cycle = 320 mg]
Cycle B: (Cycles 2, 4, 6, and 8)
Methotrexate: I.V.: 200 mg/m^2 day 1
followed by I.V.: 800 mg/m^2 continuous infusion day 1
[total dose/cycle = 1 g/m^2]
Leucovorin: (route not specified): 15 mg every 6 hours, for 8 doses (start 24 hours after end of methotrexate infusion)
[total dose/cycle = 120 mg]
Cytarabine: I.V.: 3 g/m^2 every 12 hours, for 4 doses, days 2 and 3
[total dose/cycle = 12 g/m^2]
Repeat every 6 weeks in the following sequence: ABABABAB
CNS Prophylaxis
Methotrexate: I.T.: 12 mg day 2
[total dose/cycle = 12 mg]
Cytarabine: I.T.: 100 mg day 8
[total dose/cycle = 100 mg]
Repeat cycle every 3 weeks for 4 or 8 cycles
Maintenance (POMP)
Mercaptopurine: Oral: 50 mg 3 times/day
[total dose/cycle = 4200-4650 mg]
Vincristine: I.V.: 2 mg day 1
[total dose/cycle = 2 mg]
Methotrexate: Oral: 20 mg/m^2/day days 1, 8, 15, and 22
[total dose/cycle = 80 mg/m^2]
Prednisone: Oral: 200 mg/day days 1 to 5
[total dose/cycle = 1000 mg/m^2]
or
Mercaptopurine: I.V.: 1 g/m^2/day days 1 to 5
[total dose/cycle = 5 g/m^2]
Vincristine: I.V.: 2 mg day 1
[total dose/cycle = 2 mg]
Methotrexate: I.V.: 10 mg/m^2/day days 1 to 5
[total dose/cycle = 50 mg/m^2]
Prednisone: Oral: 200 mg/day days 1 to 5
[total dose/cycle = 1000 mg/m^2]
or
Interferon alfa: SubQ: 5 million units/m^2 daily
[total dose/cycle = 140-155 million units/m^2]
Cytarabine: SubQ: 10 mg daily
[total dose/cycle = 280-310 mg]
Repeat cycles every month for 2 years
Variation 5:
Cycle A: (Cycles 1, 4, 6, and 8)
Cyclophosphamide: I.V.: 300 mg/m^2 every 12 hours, for 6 doses, days 1, 2, and 3
[total dose/cycle = 1800 mg/m^2]
Mesna: I.V.: 600 mg/m^2/day continuous infusion days 1, 2, and 3
[total dose/cycle = 1800 mg/m^2]
Vincristine: I.V.: 2 mg/day days 4 and 11
[total dose/cycle = 4 mg]
Doxorubicin: I.V.: 50 mg/m^2 continuous infusion day 4
[total dose/cycle = 50 mg/m^2]
Dexamethasone: Oral, I.V.: 40 mg/day days 1 to 4 and 11 to 14
[total dose/cycle = 320 mg]
Cycle B: (Cycles 3, 5, 7, and 9)
Methotrexate: I.V.: 200 mg/m^2 day 1
followed by I.V.: 800 mg/m^2 continuous infusion day 1
[total dose/cycle = 1 g/m^2]
Leucovorin: I.V.: 50 mg (start 12 hours after end of methotrexate infusion)
followed by I.V.: 15 mg every 6 hours, for 8 doses
[total dose/cycle = 170 mg]

Cytarabine: I.V.: 3 g/m^2 every 12 hours, for 4 doses, days 2 and 3
[total dose/cycle = 12 g/m^2]
Cycle C: Liposomal Daunorubicin/Cytarabine (Cycle 2):
Daunorubicin, liposomal: I.V.: 150 mg/m^2/day days 1 and 2
[total dose/cycle = 300 mg/m^2]
Cytarabine: I.V.: 1.5 g/m^2/day continuous infusion days 1 and 2
[total dose/cycle = 3 g/m^2]
Prednisone: Oral: 200 mg/day days 1 to 5
[total dose/cycle = 1000 mg]
Administer in the following sequence: ACBABABA (Cycle C does not repeat)

CNS Prophylaxis

Methotrexate: I.T.: 12 mg day 2
[total dose/cycle = 12 mg]
or 6 mg into Ommaya day 2
[total dose/cycle = 6 mg]
Cytarabine: I.T.: 100 mg day 7 **or** 8
[total dose/cycle = 100 mg]
Repeat cycle every 3 weeks for 6 or 8 cycles

Maintenance (POMP)

Mercaptopurine: I.V.: 1 g/m^2/day days 1 to 5
[total dose/cycle = 5 g/m^2]
Vincristine: I.V.: 2 mg day 1
[total dose/cycle = 2 mg]
Methotrexate: I.V.: 10 mg/m^2/day days 1 to 5
[total dose/cycle = 50 mg/m^2]
Prednisone: Oral: 200 mg/day days 1 to 5
[total dose/cycle = 1000 mg]
Repeat cycles monthly, except months 6, 7, 18, and 19 for 3 years

Intensification

Methotrexate: I.V.: 100 mg/m^2/day days 1, 8, 15, and 22
[total dose/cycle = 400 mg/m^2]
Asparaginase: I.V.: 20,000 units/day days 2, 9, 16, and 23
[total dose/cycle = 80,000 units]
Given during months 6 and 18 of maintenance
Cyclophosphamide: I.V.: 300 mg/m^2 every 12 hours, for 6 doses, days 1, 2, and 3
[total dose/cycle = 1800 mg/m^2]
Mesna: I.V.: 600 mg/m^2/day continuous infusion days 1, 2, and 3
[total dose/cycle = 1800 mg/m^2]
Vincristine: I.V.: 2 mg/day days 4 and 11
[total dose/cycle = 4 mg]
Doxorubicin: I.V.: 50 mg/m^2/day continuous infusion day 4
[total dose/cycle = 50 mg/m^2]
Dexamethasone: Oral, I.V.: 40 mg/day days 1 to 4 and 11 to 14
[total dose/cycle = 320 mg]
Given during months 7 and 19 of maintenance

Hyper-CVAD (Lymphoma, non-Hodgkin)

Use Lymphoma, non-Hodgkin

Regimen

Cycle A: (Cycles 1, 3, 5, and 7)
Cyclophosphamide: I.V.: 300 mg/m^2 every 12 hours, for 6 doses, days 1, 2, and 3
[total dose/cycle = 1800 mg/m^2]
Vincristine: I.V.: 2 mg/day days 4 and 11
[total dose/cycle = 4 mg]
Doxorubicin: I.V.: 25 mg/m^2/day continuous infusion days 4 and 5
[total dose/cycle = 50 mg/m^2]
Dexamethasone: Oral, I.V.: 40 mg/day days 1 to 4 and 11 to 14
[total dose/cycle = 320 mg]
Cycle B: (Cycles 2, 4, 6, and 8)
Methotrexate: I.V.: 200 mg/m^2 day 1
followed by I.V.: 800 mg/m^2 continuous infusion day 1
[total dose/cycle = 1 g/m^2]

Leucovorin: Oral: 50 mg
followed by Oral: 15 mg every 6 hours, for 8 doses (start 24 hours after end of methotrexate infusion)
[total dose/cycle = 170 mg]
Cytarabine: I.V.: 3 g/m^2 every 12 hours, for 4 doses, days 2 and 3
[total dose/cycle = 12 g/m^2]
Repeat every 6 weeks in the following sequence: ABABABAB

Hyper-CVAD (Multiple Myeloma)

Use Multiple myeloma

Regimen

Cyclophosphamide: I.V.: 300 mg/m^2 every 12 hours, for 6 doses, days 1, 2, and 3
[total dose/cycle = 1800 mg/m^2]
Mesna: I.V.: 600 mg/m^2/day continuous infusion days 1, 2, and 3
[total dose/cycle = 1800 mg/m^2]
Doxorubicin: I.V.: 25 mg/m^2/day continuous infusion days 4 and 5
[total dose/cycle = 50 mg/m^2]
Vincristine: I.V.: 1 mg/day continuous infusion days 4 and 5
followed by I.V.: 2 mg day 11
[total dose/cycle = 4 mg]
Dexamethasone: Oral, I.V.: 20 mg/m^2/day days 1 to 5 and 11 to 14
[total dose/cycle = 180 mg/m^2]
Repeat cycle once if ≥50% reduction in myeloma protein

Maintenance

Cyclophosphamide: Oral: 125 mg/m^2 every 12 hours, for 10 doses, days 1 to 5
[total dose/cycle = 1250 mg/m^2]
Dexamethasone: Oral: 20 mg/m^2/day days 1 to 5
[total dose/cycle = 100 mg/m^2]
Repeat maintenance cycle every 5 weeks

Hyper-CVAD + Rituximab

Use Lymphona, non-Hodgkin (mantle cell)

Regimen

Cycle A: (Cycles 1, 3, 5 [and 7, if needed])
Rituximab: I.V.: 375 mg/m^2 day 1
[total dose/cycle = 375 mg/m^2]
Cyclophosphamide: I.V.: 300 mg/m^2 every 12 hours, for 6 doses, days 2, 3, and 4
[total dose/cycle = 1800 mg/m^2]
Mesna: I.V.: 600 mg/m^2 continuous infusion days 2, 3, and 4
[total dose/cycle = 1800 mg/m^2]
Vincristine: I.V.: 1.4 mg/m^2 (maximum dose: 2 mg) days 5 and 12
[total dose/cycle = 2.8 mg/m^2; maximum: 4 mg]
Doxorubicin: I.V.: 16.7 mg/m^2 continuous infusion days 5, 6, and 7
[total dose/cycle = 50.1 mg/m^2]
Dexamethasone: Oral, I.V.: 40 mg/day days 2 to 5 and 12 to 15
[total dose/cycle = 320 mg]
Cycle B: (Cycles 2, 4, 6 [and 8, if needed])
Rituximab: I.V.: 375 mg/m^2 day 1
[total dose/cycle = 375 mg/m^2]
Methotrexate: I.V.: 200 mg/m^2 day 2
followed by I.V.: 800 mg/m^2 continuous infusion day 2
[total dose/cycle = 1000 mg/m^2]
Leucovorin: Oral: 50 mg (start 12 hours after the end of the methotrexate infusion)
followed by Oral: 15 mg every 6 hours, for 8 doses
[total dose/cycle = 170 mg]
Cytarabine: I.V.: 3 g/m^2 every 12 hours, for 4 doses, day 3 and 4
[total dose/cycle = 12 g/m^2]
Repeat every 6 weeks in the following sequence: ABABABAB

ICE (Lymphoma, non-Hodgkin)

Use Lymphoma, non-Hodgkin

Regimen

Etoposide: I.V.: 100 mg/m^2/day days 1, 2, and 3
[total dose/cycle = 300 mg/m^2]
Carboplatin: I.V.: AUC 5 (maximum dose: 800 mg) day 2
[total dose/cycle = AUC = 5]
Ifosfamide: I.V.: 5000 mg/m^2 continuous infusion day 2
[total dose/cycle = 5000 mg/m^2]
Mesna: I.V.: 5000 mg/m^2 continuous infusion day 2
[total dose/cycle = 5000 mg/m^2]
Filgrastim: SubQ: 5 mcg/kg/day days 5-12 (cycles 1 and 2 only)
[total dose/cycle = 40 mcg/kg]
followed by SubQ: 10 mcg/kg/day day 5 through completion of leukaphoresis (cycle 3 only)
Repeat cycle every 2 weeks for 3 cycles

ICE (Sarcoma)

Use Osteosarcoma; Soft tissue sarcoma

Regimen

Ifosfamide: I.V.: 1500 mg/m^2/day days 1, 2, and 3
[total dose/cycle = 4500 mg/m^2]
Carboplatin: I.V.: 300-635 mg/m^2 day 3
[total dose/cycle = 300-635 mg/m^2]
Etoposide: I.V.: 100 mg/m^2/day days 1, 2, and 3
[total dose/cycle = 300 mg/m^2]
Mesna: I.V.: 500 mg/m^2 prior to each ifosfamide, and every 3 hours for 2 more doses/day days 1, 2, and 3
[total dose/cycle = 4500 mg/m^2]
Repeat cycle every 21-28 days

ICE-T

Use Breast cancer; Soft tissue sarcoma

Regimen

Ifosfamide: I.V.: 1250 mg/m^2/day days 1, 2, and 3
[total dose/cycle = 3750 mg/m^2]
Carboplatin: I.V.: 300 mg/m^2 day 1
[total dose/cycle = 300 mg/m^2]
Etoposide: I.V.: 80 mg/m^2/day days 1, 2, and 3
[total dose/cycle = 240 mg/m^2]
Paclitaxel: I.V.: 175 mg/m^2 day 4
[total dose/cycle = 175 mg/m^2]
Mesna: I.V.: 250 mg prior to ifosfamide days 1, 2, and 3
followed by: Oral: 500 mg at 4 and 8 hours after ifosfamide days 1, 2, and 3
[total dose/cycle = I.V. 750 mg; Oral: 3000 mg]
or
Mesna: I.V.: 1250 mg/m^2/day over 6 hours, days 1, 2, and 3
[total dose/cycle = 3750 mg/m^2]
Repeat cycle every 28 days

Idarubicin, Cytarabine, Etoposide (ICE Protocol)

Use Leukemia, acute myeloid

Regimen

Idarubicin: I.V.: 6 mg/m^2/day days 1 to 5
[total dose/cycle = 30 mg/m^2]
Cytarabine: I.V.: 600 mg/m^2/day days 1 to 5
[total dose/cycle = 3000 mg/m^2]
Etoposide: I.V.: 150 mg/m^2/day days 1, 2, and 3
[total dose/cycle = 450 mg/m^2]
Administer one cycle only

Idarubicin-Cytarabine (High Dose)-Etoposide (AML)

Use Leukemia, acute myeloid

Regimen Induction:

Idarubicin: I.V.: 5 mg/m^2/day days 1 to 5
[total dose/cycle = 25 mg/m^2]
Cytarabine: I.V.: 2000 mg/m^2 every 12 hours for 10 doses days 1 to 5
[total dose/cycle = 20,000 mg/m^2]
Etoposide: I.V.: 100 mg/m^2/day days 1 to 5
[total dose/cycle = 500 mg/m^2]

IE

Use Soft tissue sarcoma

Regimen

Etoposide: I.V.: 100 mg/m^2/day days 1, 2, and 3
[total dose/cycle = 300 mg/m^2]
Ifosfamide: I.V.: 2500 mg/m^2/day days 1, 2, and 3
[total dose/cycle = 7500 mg/m^2]
Mesna: I.V.: 500 mg/m^2 prior to ifosfamide, after ifosfamide, and every 4 hours for 3 more doses (total of 5 doses/day) days 1, 2, and 3
[total dose/cycle = 7500 mg/m^2]
Repeat cycle every 28 days

IMVP-16

Use Lymphoma, non-Hodgkin

Regimen

Ifosfamide: I.V.: 4 g/m^2 continuous infusion over 24 hours day 1
[total dose/cycle = 4 g/m^2]
Mesna: I.V.: 800 mg/m^2 bolus prior to ifosfamide, then 4 g/m^2 continuous infusion over 12 hours concurrent with ifosfamide, then 2.4 g/m^2 continuous infusion over 12 hours after ifosfamide infusion day 1
[total dose/cycle = 7.2 g/m^2]
Methotrexate: I.V.: 30 mg/m^2/day days 3 and 10
[total dose/cycle = 60 mg/m^2]
Etoposide: I.V.: 100 mg/m^2/day days 1, 2, and 3
[total dose/cycle = 300 mg/m^2]
Repeat cycle every 21-28 days

Interleukin 2-Interferon Alfa-2 (RCC)

Use Renal cell cancer

Regimen

Induction (2 cycles):
Aldesleukin: I.V.: 18 million units/m^2/day continuous infusion days 1 to 5 and days 12 to 16
[total dose/cycle = 180 million units/m^2]
Repeat aldesleukin induction cycle one time (total of 2 cycles) after a 3-week rest between cycles
Interferon Alfa-2: SubQ: 6 million units/dose 3 times weekly continuously (no rest break) during induction cycles
[total dose/week = 18 million units/week]
Maintenance (begin after a 3-week aldesleukin rest):
Aldesleukin: I.V.: 18 million units/m^2/day continuous infusion days 1 to 5
[total dose/cycle = 90 million units/m^2]
Repeat aldesleukin maintenance cycle 3 times (total of 4 maintenance cycles) after 3-week rest between cycles
Interferon Alfa-2: SubQ: 6 million units/dose 3 times weekly continuously (no rest break) during maintenance cycles
[total dose/week = 18 million units/week]

IPA

Use Hepatoblastoma

Regimen

Ifosfamide: I.V.: 500 mg/m^2 day 1
[total dose/cycle = 500 mg/m^2]
followed by I.V.: 1000 mg/m^2/day continuous infusion days 1 to 3
[total dose/cycle = 3000 mg/m^2]
Cisplatin: I.V.: 20 mg/m^2/day days 4 to 8
[total dose/cycle = 100 mg/m^2]
Doxorubicin: I.V.: 30 mg/m^2/day continuous infusion days 9 and 10
[total dose/cycle = 60 mg/m^2]
Repeat cycle every 21 days

Irinotecan-Cisplatin (Esophageal Cancer)

Use Esophageal cancer

Regimen

Cisplatin: I.V.: 30 mg/m^2/day days 1, 8, 15, and 22
[total dose/cycle = 120 mg/m^2]
Irinotecan: I.V.: 65 mg/m^2/day days 1, 8, 15, and 22
[total dose/cycle = 260 mg/m^2]
Repeat cycle every 6 weeks

Irinotecan-Cisplatin (Gastric Cancer)

Use Gastric cancer

Regimen

Irinotecan: I.V.: 65 mg/m^2/dose over 90 minutes days 1, 8, 15, and 22
[total dose/cycle = 260 mg/m^2]
Cisplatin: I.V.: 30 mg/m^2/dose over 1 hour days 1, 8, 15, and 22
[total dose/cycle = 120 mg/m^2]
Repeat cycle every 6 weeks until disease progression or unacceptable toxicity

Irinotecan-Leucovorin-Fluorouracil (Gastric Cancer)

Use Gastric cancer

Regimen NOTE: Multiple variations are listed below.

Variation 1:
Irinotecan: I.V.: 80 mg/m^2/dose day 1
[total dose/week = 80 mg/m^2]
Leucovorin: I.V.: 500 mg/m^2/dose over 2 hours day 1
[total dose/week = 500 mg/m^2]
Fluorouracil: I.V.: 2000 mg/m^2/dose continuous infusion over 22 hours day 1
[total dose/week = 2000 mg/m^2]
Repeat cycle weekly for 6 weeks followed by a 1-week rest; repeat until disease progression or unacceptable toxicity

Variation 2:
Irinotecan: I.V.: 180 mg/m^2/dose day 1
[total dose/cycle = 180 mg/m^2]
Leucovorin: I.V.: 200 mg/m^2/dose over 2 hours days 1 and 2
[total dose/cycle = 400 mg/m^2]
Fluorouracil: I.V. bolus: 400 mg/m^2 days 1 and 2
followed by I.V.: 600 mg/m^2/dose continuous infusion over 22 hours days 1 and 2
[total dose/cycle = 2000 mg/m^2]
Repeat cycle every 14 days for at least 4 cycles or until disease progression or unacceptable toxicity

IVAC

Use Lymphoma, non-Hodgkin

Regimen

Ifosfamide: I.V.: 1500 mg/m^2/day days 1 to 5
[total dose/cycle = 7500 mg/m^2]

Etoposide: I.V.: 60 mg/m^2/day days 1 to 5
[total dose/cycle = 300 mg/m^2]
Cytarabine: I.V.: 2 g/m^2 every 12 hours days 1 and 2
[total dose/cycle = 8 g/m^2]
Mesna: I.V.: 360 mg/m^2 every 3 hours days 1 to 5
[total dose/cycle = 14,400 mg/m^2]
Methotrexate: I.T.: 12 mg day 5
Sargramostim: SubQ: 7.5 mcg/kg day 7 until ANC >1000 cells/mm^3
Repeat when ANC >1000 cells/mm^3

Ixabepilone-Capecitabine

Use Breast cancer

Regimen

Capecitabine: Oral: 1000 mg/m^2 twice daily days 1 to 14
[total dose/cycle = 28,000 mg/m^2]
Ixabepilone: I.V.: 40 mg/m^2 day 1
[total dose/cycle = 40 mg/m^2]
Repeat cycle every 3 weeks

Lapatinib-Letrozole (Breast Cancer)

Use Breast cancer

Regimen

Lapatinib: Oral: 1500 mg/day days 1 to 28
[total dose/cycle = 42,000 mg]
Letrozole: Oral: 2.5 mg/day days 1 to 28
[total dose/cycle = 70 mg]
Repeat cycle every 28 days until disease progression

Lapatinib-Trastuzumab (Breast Cancer)

Use Breast cancer

Regimen

Week 1:
Trastuzumab: I.V.: 4 mg/kg (loading dose) day 1
[total dose/week 1 = 4 mg/kg]
Lapatinib: Oral: 1000 mg/day days 1 to 7
[total dose/week = 7000 mg]
Subsequent weeks:
Trastuzumab: I.V.: 2 mg/kg day 1
[total dose/week = 2 mg/kg]
Lapatinib: Oral: 1000 mg/day days 1 to 7
[total dose/week = 7000 mg]
Repeat weekly

Larson Regimen

Use Leukemia, acute lymphocytic

Regimen

Cyclophosphamide: I.V.: 1200 mg/m^2 day 1
[total dose/cycle = 1200 mg/m^2]
Daunorubicin: I.V.: 45 mg/m^2/day days 1, 2, and 3
[total dose/cycle = 135 mg/m^2]
Vincristine: I.V.: 2 mg/day days 1, 8, 15, and 22
[total dose/cycle = 8 mg]
Prednisone: Oral or I.V.: 60 mg/m^2/day days 1 to 21
[total dose/cycle = 1260 mg/m^2]
Asparaginase: SubQ: 6000 units/m^2/day days 5, 8, 11, 15, 18, and 22
[total dose/cycle = 36,000 units/m^2]
Administer one cycle only

Lenalidomide-Dexamethasone

Use Multiple myeloma

Regimen

Lenalidomide: Oral: 25 mg/day days 1 to 21
[total dose/cycle = 525 mg]
Dexamethasone: Oral: 40 mg/day days 1 to 4, 9 to 12, and 17 to 20 (cycles 1 to 4)
[total dose/cycle = 480 mg]
Dexamethasone: Oral 40 mg/day days 1 to 4 (cycle 5 and beyond)
[total dose/cycle = 160 mg]
Repeat cycle every 28 days

Lenalidomide-Dexamethasone (Low Dose)

Use Multiple myeloma

Regimen

Lenalidomide: Oral: 25 mg/day days 1 to 21
[total dose/cycle = 525 mg]
Dexamethasone: Oral: 40 mg/day days 1, 8, 15, and 22
[total dose/cycle = 160 mg]
Repeat cycle every 28 days

Linker Protocol (ALL)

Use Leukemia, acute lymphocytic

Regimen

Remission induction:

Daunorubicin: I.V.: 50 mg/m^2/day days 1, 2, and 3
[total dose/cycle = 150 mg/m^2]
Vincristine: I.V.: 2 mg/day days 1, 8, 15, and 22
[total dose/cycle = 8 mg]
Prednisone: Oral: 60 mg/m^2/day days 1 to 28
[total dose/cycle = 1680 mg/m^2]
Asparaginase: I.M.: 6000 units/m^2/day days 17 to 28
[total dose/cycle = 72,000 units/m^2]

If residual leukemia in bone marrow on day 14:

Daunorubicin: I.V.: 50 mg/m^2 day 15
[total dose/cycle = 50 mg/m^2]

If residual leukemia in bone marrow on day 28:

Daunorubicin: I.V.: 50 mg/m^2/day days 29 and 30
[total dose/cycle = 100 mg/m^2]
Vincristine: I.V.: 2 mg/day days 29 and 36
[total dose/cycle = 4 mg]
Prednisone: Oral: 60 mg/m^2/day days 29 to 42
[total dose/cycle = 840 mg/m^2]
Asparaginase: I.M.: 6000 units/m^2/day days 29 to 35
[total dose/cycle = 42,000 units/m^2]

Consolidation therapy:

Treatment A (cycles 1, 3, 5, and 7)
Daunorubicin: I.V.: 50 mg/m^2/day days 1 and 2
[total dose/cycle = 100 mg/m^2]
Vincristine: I.V.: 2 mg/day days 1 and 8
[total dose/cycle = 4 mg]
Prednisone: Oral: 60 mg/m^2/day days 1 to 14
[total dose/cycle = 840 mg/m^2]
Asparaginase: I.M.: 12,000 units/m^2/day days 2, 4, 7, 9, 11, and 14
[total dose/cycle = 72,000 units/m^2]

Treatment B (cycles 2, 4, 6, and 8)
Teniposide: I.V.: 165 mg/m^2/day days 1, 4, 8, and 11
[total dose/cycle = 660 mg/m^2]
Cytarabine: I.V.: 300 mg/m^2/day days 1, 4, 8, and 11
[total dose/cycle = 1200 mg/m^2]

Treatment C (cycle 9)
Methotrexate: I.V.: 690 mg/m^2 continuous infusion over 42 hours day 1
[total dose/cycle = 690 mg/m^2]
Leucovorin: I.V.: 15 mg/m^2 every 6 hours for 12 doses (start at end of methotrexate infusion)
[total dose/cycle = 180 mg/m^2]
Administer remission induction regimen for one cycle only. Repeat consolidation cycle every 28 days.

LOPP

Use Lymphoma, Hodgkin disease

Regimen

Chlorambucil: Oral: 10 mg/day days 1 to 10
[total dose/cycle = 100 mg/m^2]
Vincristine: I.V.: 1.4 mg/m^2/day (maximum dose: 2 mg) days 1 and 8
[total dose/cycle = 2.8 mg/m^2]
Procarbazine: Oral: 100 mg/m^2/day days 1 to 10
[total dose/cycle = 1000 mg/m^2]
Prednisone: Oral: 25 mg/m^2/day (maximum dose: 60 mg) days 1 to 14
[total dose/cycle = 350 mg/m^2]
or
Prednisolone: Oral: 25 mg/m^2/day (maximum dose: 60 mg) days 1 to 14
[total dose/cycle = 350 mg/m^2]
Repeat cycle every 28 days

M-2

Use Multiple myeloma

Regimen

Vincristine: I.V.: 0.03 mg/kg (maximum dose: 2 mg) day 1
[total dose/cycle = 0.03 mg/kg]
Carmustine: I.V.: 0.5-1 mg/kg day 1
[total dose/cycle = 0.5-1 mg/kg]
Cyclophosphamide: I.V.: 10 mg/kg day 1
[total dose/cycle = 10 mg/kg]
Melphalan: Oral: 0.25 mg/kg/day days 1 to 4
[total dose/cycle = 1 mg/kg]
or 0.1 mg/kg/day days 1 to 7 or 1 to 10
[total dose/cycle = 0.7 or 1 mg/kg]
Prednisone: Oral: 1 mg/kg/day days 1 to 7
[total dose/cycle = 7 mg/kg]
Repeat cycle every 35-42 days

MACOP-B

Use Lymphoma, non-Hodgkin

Regimen

Methotrexate: I.V. bolus: 100 mg/m^2 weeks 2, 6, 10
followed by I.V.: 300 mg/m^2 over 4 hours weeks 2, 6, and 10
[total dose/cycle = 1200 mg/m^2]
Doxorubicin: I.V.: 50 mg/m^2 weeks 1, 3, 5, 7, 9, and 11
[total dose/cycle = 300 mg/m^2]
Cyclophosphamide: I.V.: 350 mg/m^2 weeks 1, 3, 5, 7, 9, and 11
[total dose/cycle = 2100 mg/m^2]
Vincristine: I.V.: 1.4 mg/m^2 (maximum dose: 2 mg) weeks 2, 4, 6, 8, 10, and 12
[total dose/cycle = 8.4 mg/m^2; maximum: 12 mg]
Bleomycin: I.V.: 10 units/m^2 weeks 4, 8, and 12
[total dose/cycle = 30 units/m^2]
Prednisone: Oral: 75 mg/day for 12 weeks, then taper over 2 weeks
Leucovorin calcium: Oral: 15 mg/m^2 every 6 hours, for 6 doses (beginning 24 hours after methotrexate) weeks 2, 6, and 10
[total dose/cycle = 270 mg/m^2]
Administer one cycle

MAID (Sarcoma)

Use Soft tissue sarcoma

Regimen NOTE: Multiple variations are listed.

Variation 1:

Mesna: I.V.: 2000 mg/m^2/day continuous infusion days 1 to 4 [total dose/cycle = 8000 mg/m^2]

Doxorubicin: I.V.: 15 mg/m^2/day continuous infusion days 1 to 4 [total dose/cycle = 60 mg/m^2]

Ifosfamide: I.V.: 2000 mg/m^2/day continuous infusion days 1, 2, and 3 [total dose/cycle = 6000 mg/m^2]

Dacarbazine: I.V.: 250 mg/m^2/day continuous infusion days 1 to 4 [total dose/cycle = 1000 mg/m^2]

Repeat cycle every 21days until disease progression or until maximum cumulative doxorubicin dose of 450 mg/m^2

Variation 2 (with concurrent radiotherapy):

Mesna: I.V.: 2500 mg/m^2/day continuous infusion days 1 to 4 [total dose/cycle = 10,000 mg/m^2]

Doxorubicin: I.V.: 20 mg/m^2/day continuous infusion days 1, 2, and 3 [total dose/cycle = 60 mg/m^2]

Ifosfamide: I.V.: 2000 mg/m^2/day continuous infusion days 1, 2, and 3 [total dose/cycle = 6000 mg/m^2]

Dacarbazine: I.V.: 250 mg/m^2/day continuous infusion days 1 to 4 [total dose/cycle = 1000 mg/m^2]

Filgrastim (optional): SubQ: 5 mcg/kg/day beginning day 5

Repeat cycle every 21days pre-op, followed 3 weeks later by surgery, followed by post-op chemotherapy 3-5 weeks after surgery (if not receiving post-op radiotherapy) or after post-op radiotherapy

Variation 3:

Mesna: I.V.: 2500 mg/m^2/day continuous infusion days 1 to 4 [total dose/cycle = 10,000 mg/m^2]

Doxorubicin: I.V.: 20 mg/m^2/day continuous infusion days 1, 2, and 3 [total dose/cycle = 60 mg/m^2]

Ifosfamide: I.V.: 2500 mg/m^2/day continuous infusion days 1, 2, and 3 [total dose/cycle = 7500 mg/m^2]

Dacarbazine: I.V.: 300 mg/m^2/day continuous infusion days 1, 2, and 3 [total dose/cycle = 900 mg/m^2]

Repeat cycle every 21 days (delay 1 week for leukopenia or thrombocytopenia)

m-BACOD

Use Lymphoma, non-Hodgkin

Regimen

Methotrexate: I.V.: 200 mg/m^2/day days 8 and 15 [total dose/cycle = 400 mg/m^2]

Leucovorin calcium: Oral: 10 mg/m^2 every 6 hours for 8 doses (beginning 24 hours after each methotrexate dose) days 9 and 16 [total dose/cycle = 160 mg/m^2]

Bleomycin: I.V.: 4 units/m^2 day 1 [total dose/cycle = 4 units/m^2]

Doxorubicin: I.V.: 45 mg/m^2 day 1 [total dose/cycle = 45 mg/m^2]

Cyclophosphamide: I.V.: 600 mg/m^2 day 1 [total dose/cycle = 600 mg/m^2]

Vincristine: I.V.: 1 mg/m^2 day 1 [total dose/cycle = 1 mg/m^2]

Dexamethasone: Oral: 6 mg/m^2/day days 1 to 5 [total dose/cycle = 30 mg/m^2]

Repeat cycle every 21 days

Melphalan-Prednisone-Bortezomib (Multiple Myeloma)

Use Multiple myeloma

Regimen NOTE: Multiple variations are listed below.

Variation 1:

Bortezomib: I.V.: 1.3 mg/m^2/day days 1, 4, 8, 11, 22, 25, 29, and 32
[total dose/cycle = 10.4 mg/m^2]

Melphalan: Oral: 9 mg/m^2/day days 1 to 4
[total dose/cycle = 36 mg/m^2]

Prednisone: Oral: 60 mg/m^2/day days 1 to 4
[total dose/cycle = 240 mg/m^2]

Repeat cycle every 42 days for 4 cycles

followed by

Bortezomib: I.V.: 1.3 mg/m^2/day days 1, 8, 22, and 29
[total dose/cycle = 5.2 mg/m^2]

Melphalan: Oral: 9 mg/m^2/day days 1 to 4
[total dose/cycle = 36 mg/m^2]

Prednisone: Oral: 60 mg/m^2/day days 1 to 4
[total dose/cycle = 240 mg/m^2]

Repeat cycle every 42 days for 5 cycles

Variation 2:

Bortezomib: I.V.: 1-1.3 mg/m^2/day days 1, 4, 8, 11, 22, 25, 29, and 32
[total dose/cycle = 8-10.4 mg/m^2]

Melphalan: Oral: 9 mg/m^2/day days 1 to 4
[total dose/cycle = 36 mg/m^2]

Prednisone: Oral: 60 mg/m^2/day days 1 to 4
[total dose/cycle = 240 mg/m^2]

Repeat cycle every 42 days for 4 cycles

followed by

Bortezomib: I.V.: 1-1.3 mg/m^2/day days 1, 8, 15, and 22
[total dose/cycle = 4-5.2 mg/m^2]

Melphalan: Oral: 9 mg/m^2/day days 1 to 4
[total dose/cycle = 36 mg/m^2]

Prednisone: Oral: 60 mg/m^2/day days 1 to 4
[total dose/cycle = 240 mg/m^2]

Repeat cycle every 35 days for 5 cycles

Melphalan-Prednisone (Multiple Myeloma)

Use Multiple myeloma

Regimen NOTE: Multiple variations are listed below.

Variation 1:

Melphalan: Oral: 0.25 mg/kg/dose days 1 to 4
[total dose/cycle = 1 mg/kg]

Prednisone: Oral: 2 mg/kg/dose days 1 to 4
[total dose/cycle = 8 mg/kg]

Repeat cycle every 6 weeks for a total of 12 cycles

Variation 2:

Melphalan: Oral: 4 mg/m^2/dose days 1 to 7
[total dose/cycle = 28 mg/m^2]

Prednisone: Oral: 40 mg/m^2/dose days 1 to 7
[total dose/cycle = 280 mg/m^2]

Repeat cycle every 4 weeks for a total of 6 cycles

Variation 3:

Melphalan: Oral: 9 mg/m^2/dose days 1 to 4
[total dose/cycle = 36 mg/m^2]

Prednisone: Oral: 60 mg/m^2/dose days 1 to 4
[total dose/cycle = 240 mg/m^2]

Repeat cycle every 6 weeks for a total of 9 cycles

Variation 4:
Melphalan: Oral: 6 mg/m^2/dose days 1 to 7
[total dose/cycle = 42 mg/m^2]
Prednisone: Oral: 60 mg/m^2/dose days 1 to 7
[total dose/cycle = 420 mg/m^2]
Repeat cycle every 4 weeks for a total of 6 cycles
Followed by (in responders):
Interferon alfa: SubQ: 3 million units/dose 3 times/week until relapse
Dexamethasone: Oral: 40 mg/dose days 1 to 4 every 2 months until relapse

Melphalan-Prednisone-Thalidomide (Multiple Myeloma)

Use Multiple myeloma

Regimen NOTE: Multiple variations are listed below.

Variation 1:
Melphalan: Oral: 4 mg/m^2/day days 1 to 7
[total dose/cycle = 28 mg/m^2]
Prednisone: Oral: 40 mg/m^2/day days 1 to 7
[total dose/cycle = 280 mg/m^2]
Thalidomide: Oral: 100 mg/day days 1 to 28
[total dose/cycle = 2800 mg]
Repeat cycle every 28 days for 6 cycles
followed by
Thalidomide: Oral: 100 mg daily (as maintenance)

Variation 2:
Melphalan: Oral: 0.25 mg/kg/dose days 1 to 4
[total dose/cycle = 1 mg/kg]
Prednisone: Oral: 2 mg/kg/dose days 1 to 4
[total dose/cycle = 8 mg/kg]
Thalidomide: Oral: 100-400 mg/day days 1 to 42
[total dose/cycle = 4200-16,800 mg]
Repeat cycle every 6 weeks for a total of 12 cycles (discontinue thalidomide on day 4 of the last cycle)

Methotrexate-Vinblastine (Desmoid Tumor)

Use Soft tissue sarcoma (desmoid tumor)

Regimen

Methotrexate: I.V.: 30 mg/m^2 every 7-10 days
[total dose/treatment = 30 mg/m^2]
Vinblastine: I.V.: 6 mg/m^2 every 7-10 days
[total dose/treatment = 6 mg/m^2]
Continue treatment for 1 year (52 treatments)

MF

Use Breast cancer

Regimen

Methotrexate: I.V. 100 mg/m^2/day days 1 and 8
[total dose/cycle = 200 mg/m^2]
Fluorouracil: I.V.: 600 mg/m^2/day (start 1 hour after methotrexate) days 1 and 8
[total dose/cycle = 1200 mg/m^2]
Leucovorin: Oral, I.V.: 10 mg/m^2 every 6 hours for 6 doses (start 24 hours after methotrexate)
[total dose/cycle = 60 mg/m^2]
Repeat cycle every 28 days for 12 cycles

MINE

Use Lymphoma, non-Hodgkin

Regimen

Mesna: I.V.: 1.33 g/m^2/day concurrent with ifosfamide dose, then 500 mg orally (4 hours after each ifosfamide infusion) days 1, 2, and 3
[total dose/cycle = 3.99 g/m^2/1500 mg]
Ifosfamide: I.V.: 1.33 g/m^2/day days 1, 2, and 3
[total dose/cycle = 3.99 g/m^2]

Mitoxantrone: I.V.: 8 mg/m^2 day 1
[total dose/cycle = 8 mg/m^2]
Etoposide: I.V.: 65 mg/m^2/day days 1, 2, and 3
[total dose/cycle = 195 mg/m^2]
Repeat cycle every 28 days

MINE-ESHAP

Use Lymphoma, non-Hodgkin

Regimen

Mesna: I.V.: 1.33 g/m^2 concurrent with ifosfamide dose, then 500 mg orally (4 hours after ifosfamide) days 1, 2, and 3
[total dose/cycle = 4 g/m^2/1500 mg]
Ifosfamide: I.V.: 1.33 g/m^2/day days 1, 2, and 3
[total dose/cycle = 4 g/m^2]
Mitoxantrone: I.V.: 8 mg/m^2 day 1
[total dose/cycle = 8 mg/m^2]
Etoposide: I.V.: 65 mg/m^2/day days 1, 2, and 3
[total dose/cycle = 195 mg/m^2]
Repeat cycle every 21 days for 6 cycles, followed by 3-6 cycles of ESHAP

mini-BEAM

Use Lymphoma, Hodgkin disease

Regimen

Carmustine: I.V.: 60 mg/m^2 day 1
[total dose/cycle = 60 mg/m^2]
Etoposide: I.V.: 75 mg/m^2/day days 2 to 5
[total dose/cycle = 300 mg/m^2]
Cytarabine: I.V.: 100 mg/m^2 every 12 hours for 8 doses days 2 to 5
[total dose/cycle = 800 mg/m^2]
Melphalan: I.V.: 30 mg/m^2 day 6
[total dose/cycle = 30 mg/m^2]
Repeat cycle every 4-6 weeks

Mitomycin-Vinblastine

Use Breast cancer

Regimen

Mitomycin: I.V.: 20 mg/m^2 day 1
[total dose/cycle = 20 mg/m^2]
Vinblastine: I.V.: 0.15 mg/kg/day days 1 and 21
[total dose/cycle = 0.3 mg/kg]
Repeat cycle every 6-8 weeks

Mitoxantrone + Hydrocortisone

Use Prostate cancer

Regimen

Mitoxantrone: I.V.: 14 mg/m^2 day 1
[total dose/cycle = 14 mg/m^2]
Hydrocortisone: Oral: 40 mg daily
[total dose/cycle = 840 mg]
Repeat cycle every 3 weeks

Mitoxantrone-Prednisone (Prostate Cancer)

Use Prostate cancer

Regimen NOTE: Multiple variations are listed below.

Variation 1:
Mitoxantrone: I.V.: 12 mg/m^2 day 1
[total dose/cycle = 12 mg/m^2]
Prednisone: Oral: 5 mg twice daily
[total dose/cycle = 210 mg]
Repeat cycle every 21 days for up to a total of 10 cycles

Variation 2:
Cycle 1:
Mitoxantrone: I.V.: 12 mg/m^2 day 1
[total dose/cycle = 12 mg/m^2]
Prednisone: Oral: 5 mg twice daily
[total dose/cycle = 210 mg]
Treatment cycle is 21 days
Cycle 2 and beyond:
Mitoxantrone: I.V.: 12-14 mg/m^2 day 1 (increase to 14 mg/m^2 if no grade 3/4 adverse events)
[total dose/cycle = 12-14 mg/m^2]
Prednisone: Oral: 5 mg twice daily
[total dose/cycle = 210 mg]
Repeat cycle every 21 days for up to a maximum cumulative mitoxantrone dose of 144 mg/m^2
Variation 3:
Cycle 1:
Mitoxantrone: I.V.: 12 mg/m^2 day 1
[total dose/cycle = 12 mg/m^2]
Prednisone: Oral: 5 mg twice daily
[total dose/cycle = 210 mg]
Treatment cycle is 21 days
Cycles 2-8:
Mitoxantrone: I.V.: 12-14 mg/m^2 day 1 (increase to 14 mg/m^2 if granulocyte nadir is >1000/mm^3 and platelet nadir >50,000/ mm^3)
[total dose/cycle = 12-14 mg/m^2]
Prednisone: Oral: 5 mg twice daily
[total dose/cycle = 210 mg]
Treatment cycle is 21 days for up to a total of 8 cycles

MOP

Use Brain tumors

Regimen

Mechlorethamine: I.V.: 6 mg/m^2/day days 1 and 8
[total dose/cycle = 12 mg/m^2]
Vincristine: I.V.: 1.5 mg/m^2/day (maximum dose: 2 mg) days 1 and 8
[total dose/cycle = 3 mg/m^2]
Procarbazine: Oral: 100 mg/m^2/day days 1 to 14
[total dose/cycle = 1400 mg/m^2]
Repeat cycle every 28 days

MOPP/ABVD

Use Lymphoma, Hodgkin disease

Regimen NOTE: Multiple variations are listed below.

Variation 1:
Mechlorethamine: I.V.: 6 mg/m^2/day days 1 and 8
[total dose/cycle = 12 mg/m^2]
Vincristine: I.V.: 1.4 mg/m^2/day (maximum dose: 2 mg) days 1 and 8
[total dose/cycle = 2.8 mg/m^2]
Procarbazine: I.V.: 100 mg/m^2/day days 1 to 14
[total dose/cycle = 1400 mg/m^2]
Prednisone: Oral: 40 mg/m^2/day days 1 to 14 (during cycles 1, 4, 7, and 10 only)
[total dose/cycle = 560 mg/m^2]
Doxorubicin: I.V.: 25 mg/m^2/day days 29 and 43
[total dose/cycle = 50 mg/m^2]
Bleomycin: I.V.: 10 units/m^2/day days 29 and 43
[total dose/cycle = 20 units/m^2]
Vinblastine: I.V.: 6 mg/m^2/day days 29 and 43
[total dose/cycle = 12 mg/m^2]
Dacarbazine: I.V.: 375 mg/m^2/day days 29 and 43
[total dose/cycle = 750 mg/m^2]
Repeat cycle every 56 days

Variation 2:
Mechlorethamine: I.V.: 6 mg/m^2/day days 1 and 8
[total dose/cycle = 12 mg/m^2]
Vincristine: I.V.: 1.4 mg/m^2/day (maximum dose: 2 mg) days 1 and 8
[total dose/cycle = 2.8 mg/m^2]
Procarbazine: I.V.: 100 mg/m^2/day days 1 to 14
[total dose/cycle = 1400 mg/m^2]
Prednisone: Oral: 40 mg/m^2/day days 1 to 14 (during cycles 1 and 7 only)
[total dose/cycle = 560 mg/m^2]
Doxorubicin: I.V.: 25 mg/m^2/day days 29 and 43
[total dose/cycle = 50 mg/m^2]
Bleomycin: I.V.: 10 units/m^2/day days 29 and 43
[total dose/cycle = 20 units/m^2]
Vinblastine: I.V.: 6 mg/m^2/day days 29 and 43
[total dose/cycle = 12 mg/m^2]
Dacarbazine: I.V.: 375 mg/m^2/day days 29 and 43
[total dose/cycle = 750 mg/m^2]
Repeat cycle every 56 days
Variation 3:
Mechlorethamine: I.V.: 6 mg/m^2/day days 1 and 8
[total dose/cycle = 12 mg/m^2]
Vincristine: I.V.: 1.4 mg/m^2/day (maximum dose: 2 mg) days 1 and 8
[total dose/cycle = 2.8 mg/m^2]
Procarbazine: I.V.: 100 mg/m^2/day days 1 to 14
[total dose/cycle = 1400 mg/m^2]
Prednisone: Oral: 40 mg/m^2/day days 1 to 14 (every cycle)
[total dose/cycle = 560 mg/m^2]
Doxorubicin: I.V.: 25 mg/m^2/day days 29 and 43
[total dose/cycle = 50 mg/m^2]
Bleomycin: I.V.: 10 units/m^2/day days 29 and 43
[total dose/cycle = 20 units/m^2]
Vinblastine: I.V.: 6 mg/m^2/day days 29 and 43
[total dose/cycle = 12 mg/m^2]
Dacarbazine: I.V.: 375 mg/m^2/day days 29 and 43
[total dose/cycle = 750 mg/m^2]
Repeat cycle every 56 days
Variation 4:
MOPP Regimen:
Mechlorethamine: I.V.: 6 mg/m^2/day days 1 and 8
[total dose/cycle = 12 mg/m^2]
Vincristine: I.V.: 1.4 mg/m^2/day (maximum dose: 2 mg) days 1 and 8
[total dose/cycle = 2.8 mg/m^2]
Procarbazine: I.V.: 100 mg/m^2/day days 1 to 14
[total dose/cycle = 1400 mg/m^2]
Prednisone: Oral: 25 mg/m^2/day days 1 to 14
[total dose/cycle = 350 mg/m^2]
ABVD Regimen:
Doxorubicin: I.V.: 25 mg/m^2/day days 1 and 15
[total dose/cycle = 50 mg/m^2]
Bleomycin: I.V.: 6 units/m^2/day days 1 and 15
[total dose/cycle = 12 units/m^2]
Vinblastine: I.V.: 6 mg/m^2/day days 1 and 15
[total dose/cycle = 12 mg/m^2]
Dacarbazine: I.V.: 250 mg/m^2/day days 1 and 15
[total dose/cycle = 500 mg/m^2]
Each regimen cycle is 28 days. Administer regimens in alternating fashion as follows: 2 cycles of MOPP alternating with 2 cycles of ABVD for a total of 8 cycles
Variation 5 (pediatrics):
Mechlorethamine: I.V.: 6 mg/m^2/day days 1 and 8
[total dose/cycle = 12 mg/m^2]
Vincristine: I.V.: 1.4 mg/m^2/day days 1 and 8
[total dose/cycle = 2.8 mg/m^2]

Procarbazine: Oral: 100 mg/m^2/day days 1 to 14 [total dose/cycle = 1400 mg/m^2]
Prednisone: Oral: 40 mg/m^2/day days 1 to 14 [total dose/cycle = 560 mg/m^2]
Doxorubicin: I.V.: 25 mg/m^2/day days 29 and 42 [total dose/cycle = 50 mg/m^2]
Bleomycin: I.V.: 10 units/m^2/day days 29 and 42 [total dose/cycle = 20 units/m^2]
Vinblastine: I.V.: 6 mg/m^2/day days 29 and 42 [total dose/cycle = 12 mg/m^2]
Dacarbazine: I.V.: 150 mg/m^2/day days 29 to 33 [total dose/cycle = 750 mg/m^2]
Repeat cycle every 56 days for 4 cycles

Variation 6 (pediatrics):
Mechlorethamine: I.V.: 6 mg/m^2/day days 1 and 8 [total dose/cycle = 12 mg/m^2]
Vincristine: I.V.: 1.4 mg/m^2/day days 1 and 8 [total dose/cycle = 2.8 mg/m^2]
Procarbazine: Oral: 100 mg/m^2/day days 1 to 14 [total dose/cycle = 1400 mg/m^2]
Prednisone: Oral: 40 mg/m^2/day days 1 to 14 [total dose/cycle = 560 mg/m^2]
Doxorubicin: I.V.: 25 mg/m^2/day days 29 and 42 [total dose/cycle = 50 mg/m^2]
Bleomycin: I.V.: 10 units/m^2/day days 29 and 42 [total dose/cycle = 20 units/m^2]
Vinblastine: I.V.: 6 mg/m^2/day days 29 and 42 [total dose/cycle = 12 mg/m^2]
Dacarbazine: I.V.: 375 mg/m^2/day days 29 and 43 [total dose/cycle = 750 mg/m^2]
Repeat cycle every 56 days for 4 cycles

MOPP/ABV Hybrid

Use Lymphoma, Hodgkin disease

Regimen

Mechlorethamine: I.V.: 6 mg/m^2 day 1 [total dose/cycle = 6 mg/m^2]
Vincristine: I.V.: 1.4 mg/m^2 (maximum dose: 2 mg) day 1 [total dose/cycle = 1.4 mg/m^2]
Procarbazine: Oral: 100 mg/m^2/day days 1 to 7 [total dose/cycle = 700 mg/m^2]
Prednisone: Oral: 40 mg/m^2/day days 1 to 14 [total dose/cycle = 560 mg/m^2]
Doxorubicin: I.V.: 35 mg/m^2 day 8 [total dose/cycle = 35 mg/m^2]
Bleomycin: I.V.: 10 units/m^2 day 8 [total dose/cycle = 10 units/m^2]
Vinblastine: I.V.: 6 mg/m^2 day 8 [total dose/cycle = 6 mg/m^2]
Repeat cycle every 28 days

MOPP (Lymphoma, Hodgkin Disease)

Use Lymphoma, Hodgkin disease

Regimen NOTE: Multiple variations are listed below.

Variation 1:
Mechlorethamine: I.V.: 6 mg/m^2/day days 1 and 8 [total dose/cycle = 12 mg/m^2]
Vincristine: I.V.: 1.4 mg/m^2/day days 1 and 8 [total dose/cycle = 2.8 mg/m^2]
Procarbazine: Oral: 100 mg/m^2/day days 1 to 14 [total dose/cycle = 1400 mg/m^2]

Prednisone: Oral: 40 mg/m^2/day days 1 to 14 (cycles 1 and 4)
[total dose/cycle = 560 mg/m^2]
Repeat cycle every 28 days for 6-8 cycles
Variation 2:
Mechlorethamine: I.V.: 6 mg/m^2/day (maximum dose: 15 mg) days 1 and 8
[total dose/cycle = 12 mg/m^2]
Vincristine: I.V.: 1.4 mg/m^2/day (maximum dose: 2 mg) days 1 and 8
[total dose/cycle = 2.8 mg/m^2]
Procarbazine: Oral: 100 mg/m^2/day days 1 to 10
[total dose/cycle = 1000 mg/m^2]
Prednisone: Oral: 25 mg/m^2/day (maximum dose: 60 mg) days 1 to 14
[total dose/cycle = 350 mg/m^2]
or
Prednisolone: Oral: 25 mg/m^2/day (maximum dose: 60 mg) days 1 to 14
[total dose/cycle = 350 mg/m^2]
Repeat cycle every 28 days
Variation 3:
Mechlorethamine: I.V.: 6 mg/m^2/day days 1 and 8
[total dose/cycle = 12 mg/m^2]
Vincristine: I.V.: 1.4 mg/m^2/day days 1 and 8
[total dose/cycle = 2.8 mg/m^2]
Procarbazine: Oral: 50 mg day 1, 100 mg day 2, 100 mg/m^2/day days 3 to 14
[total dose/cycle = 150 mg / 1200 mg/m^2]
Prednisone: Oral: 40 mg/m^2/day days 1 to 14
[total dose/cycle = 560 mg/m^2]
Repeat cycle every 28 days
Variation 4:
Mechlorethamine: I.V.: 6 mg/m^2/day days 1 and 8
[total dose/cycle = 12 mg/m^2]
Vincristine: I.V.: 1.4 mg/m^2/day days 1 and 8
[total dose/cycle = 2.8 mg/m^2]
Procarbazine: Oral: 50 mg day 1, 100 mg day 2, 100 mg/m^2/day days 3 to 10
[total dose/cycle = 150 mg / 800 mg/m^2]
Prednisone: Oral: 40 mg/m^2/day days 1 to 14
[total dose/cycle = 560 mg/m^2]
Repeat cycle every 28 days
Variation 5:
Mechlorethamine: I.V.: 6 mg/m^2/day days 1 and 8
[total dose/cycle = 12 mg/m^2]
Vincristine: I.V.: 1.4 mg/m^2/day days 1 and 8
[total dose/cycle = 2.8 mg/m^2]
Procarbazine: Oral: 50 mg/m^2 day 1, then 100 mg/m^2/day days 2 to 14
[total dose/cycle = 1350 mg/m^2]
Prednisone: Oral: 40 mg/m^2/day days 1 to 14
[total dose/cycle = 560 mg/m^2]
Repeat cycle every 28 days

MOPP (Medulloblastoma)

Use Brain tumors

Regimen

Mechlorethamine: I.V.: 3 mg/m^2/day days 1 and 8
[total dose/cycle = 6 mg/m^2]
Vincristine: I.V.: 1.4 mg/m^2/day (maximum dose: 2 mg) days 1 and 8
[total dose/cycle = 2.8 mg/m^2]
Prednisone: Oral: 40 mg/m^2/day days 1 to 10
[total dose/cycle = 400 mg/m^2]
Procarbazine: Oral: 50 mg day 1
[total dose/cycle = 50 mg]
followed by Oral: 100 mg day 2
[total dose/cycle = 100 mg]
followed by Oral: 100 mg/m^2/day days 3 to 10
[total dose/cycle = 800 mg/m^2]
Repeat cycle every 28 days

MTX/6-MP/VP (Maintenance)

Use Leukemia, acute lymphocytic

Regimen

Methotrexate: Oral: 20 mg/m^2 weekly
[total dose/cycle = 80 mg/m^2]
Mercaptopurine: Oral: 75 mg/m^2/day
[total dose/cycle = 2250 mg/m^2]
Vincristine: I.V.: 1.5 mg/m^2 day 1
[total dose/cycle = 1.5 mg/m^2]
Prednisone: Oral: 40 mg/m^2/day days 1 to 5
[total dose/cycle = 200 mg/m^2]
Repeat monthly for 2-3 years

MTX-CDDPAdr

Use Osteosarcoma

Regimen

Cisplatin: I.V.: 75 mg/m^2 day 1 of cycles 1-7, then 120 mg/m^2 for cycles 8, 9, and 10
Doxorubicin: I.V.: 25 mg/m^2/day days 1, 2, and 3 of cycles 1 to 7
Methotrexate: I.V.: 12 g/m^2/day days 21 and 28
Leucovorin calcium rescue: I.V.: 20 mg/m^2 every 3 hours (beginning 16 hours after completion of methotrexate) for 8 doses, then orally every 6 hours for 8 doses

MV

Use Leukemia, acute myeloid

Regimen Induction:

Mitoxantrone: I.V.: 10 mg/m^2/day days 1 to 5
[total dose/cycle = 50 mg/m^2]
Etoposide: I.V.: 100 mg/m^2/day days 1 to 5
[total dose/cycle = 500 mg/m^2]
Second cycle may be given based on individual response; time between cycles not specified

M-VAC (Bladder Cancer)

Use Bladder cancer

Regimen NOTE: Multiple variations are listed below.

Variation 1:
Methotrexate: I.V.: 30 mg/m^2/day days 1, 15, and 22
[total dose/cycle = 90 mg/m^2]
Vinblastine: I.V.: 3 mg/m^2/day days 2, 15, and 22
[total dose/cycle = 9 mg/m^2]
Doxorubicin: I.V.: 30 mg/m^2 day 2
[total dose/cycle = 30 mg/m^2]
Cisplatin: I.V.: 70 mg/m^2 day 2
[total dose/cycle = 70 mg/m^2]
Repeat cycle every 4 weeks

Variation 2:
Methotrexate: I.V.: 40 or 50 mg/m^2/day days 1, 15, and 22
[total dose/cycle = 120 or 150 mg/m^2]
Vinblastine: I.V.: 4 or 5 mg/m^2/day days 2, 15, and 22
[total dose/cycle = 12 or 15 mg/m^2]
Doxorubicin: I.V.: 40 or 50 mg/m^2 day 2
[total dose/cycle = 40 or 50 mg/m^2]
Cisplatin: I.V.: 100 mg/m^2 day 2
[total dose/cycle = 100 mg/m^2]
Repeat cycle every 4 weeks

Variation 3:
Methotrexate: I.V.: 30 mg/m^2/day days 1, 15, and 22
[total dose/cycle = 90 mg/m^2]
Vinblastine: I.V.: 3 mg/m^2 day 2
[total dose/cycle = 3 mg/m^2]

Doxorubicin: I.V.: 30 mg/m^2 day 2
[total dose/cycle = 30 mg/m^2]
Cisplatin: I.V.: 70 mg/m^2 day 2
[total dose/cycle = 70 mg/m^2]
Repeat cycle every 4 weeks
Variation 4:
Methotrexate: I.V.: 60 mg/m^2 day 1
[total dose/cycle = 60 mg/m^2]
followed by I.V.: 30 mg/m^2 day 16
[total dose/cycle = 30 mg/m^2]
Vinblastine: I.V.: 4 mg/m^2/day days 2 and 16
[total dose/cycle = 8 mg/m^2]
Doxorubicin: I.V.: 60 mg/m^2 day 2
[total dose/cycle = 60 mg/m^2]
Cisplatin: I.V.: 100 mg/m^2 day 2
[total dose/cycle = 100 mg/m^2]
Repeat cycle every 23 days
Variation 5:
Methotrexate: I.V.: 30 mg/m^2/day days 1, 16, and 23
[total dose/cycle = 90 mg/m^2]
Vinblastine: I.V.: 4 mg/m^2/day days 1, 16, and 23
[total dose/cycle = 12 mg/m^2]
Doxorubicin: I.V.: 60 mg/m^2 day 2
[total dose/cycle = 60 mg/m^2]
Cisplatin: I.V.: 100 mg/m^2 day 2
[total dose/cycle = 100 mg/m^2]
Repeat cycle every 23 days
Variation 6:
Methotrexate: I.V.: 30 or 35 mg/m^2 day 1
[total dose/cycle = 30 or 35 mg/m^2]
Vinblastine: I.V.: 3 or 3.5 mg/m^2 day 2
[total dose/cycle = 3 or 3.5 mg/m^2]
Doxorubicin: I.V.: 30 or 35 mg/m^2 day 2
[total dose/cycle = 30 or 35 mg/m^2]
Cisplatin: I.V.: 70 or 80 mg/m^2 day 2
[total dose/cycle = 70 or 80 mg/m^2]
Repeat cycle every 2 weeks
Variation 7:
Methotrexate: I.V.: 30 mg/m^2 day 1
[total dose/cycle = 30 mg/m^2]
Vinblastine: I.V.: 3 mg/m^2 day 2
[total dose/cycle = 3 mg/m^2]
Doxorubicin: I.V.: 30 mg/m^2 day 2
[total dose/cycle = 30 mg/m^2]
Cisplatin: I.V.: 70 mg/m^2 day 2
[total dose/cycle = 70 mg/m^2]
Repeat cycle every 14 days
Variation 8:
Methotrexate: I.V.: 30 mg/m^2/day days 1, 15, and 22
[total dose/cycle = 90 mg/m^2]
Vinblastine: I.V.: 3 mg/m^2/day days 1, 15, and 22
[total dose/cycle = 9 mg/m^2]
Doxorubicin: I.V.: 45 mg/m^2 day 2
[total dose/cycle = 45 mg/m^2]
Cisplatin: I.V.: 70 mg/m^2 day 2
[total dose/cycle = 70 mg/m^2]
Repeat cycle every 4 weeks
Variation 9:
Methotrexate: I.V.: 40 mg/m^2/day days 1 and 15
[total dose/cycle = 80 mg/m^2]
Vinblastine: I.V.: 4 mg/m^2/day days 1, 16, and 23
[total dose/cycle = 12 mg/m^2]

Doxorubicin: I.V.: 60 mg/m^2 day 2
[total dose/cycle = 60 mg/m^2]
Cisplatin: I.V.: 100 mg/m^2 day 2
[total dose/cycle = 100 mg/m^2]
Repeat cycle every 23 days

Variation 10:
Methotrexate: I.V.: 30 mg/m^2/day days 1, 15, and 22
[total dose/cycle = 90 mg/m^2]
Vinblastine: I.V.: 3 mg/m^2/day days 1, 16, and 22
[total dose/cycle = 9 mg/m^2]
Doxorubicin: I.V.: 30 mg/m^2 day 1
[total dose/cycle = 30 mg/m^2]
Cisplatin: I.V.: 70 mg/m^2 day 1
[total dose/cycle = 70 mg/m^2]
Repeat cycle every 4 weeks

Variation 11:
Methotrexate: I.V.: 30 mg/m^2/day days 1, 15, and 22
[total dose/cycle = 90 mg/m^2]
Vinblastine: I.V.: 3 mg/m^2/day days 2, 15, and 22
[total dose/cycle = 9 mg/m^2]
Doxorubicin: I.V.: 30 mg/m^2 day 2
[total dose/cycle = 30 mg/m^2]
Cisplatin: I.V.: 70 mg/m^2 day 2
[total dose/cycle = 70 mg/m^2]
Leucovorin: Oral: 15 mg every 6 hours for 4 doses days 2, 16, and 23
[total dose/cycle = 180 mg]
Repeat cycle every 4 weeks

Variation 12:
Methotrexate: I.V.: 30 mg/m^2/day days 1 and 15
[total dose/cycle = 60 mg/m^2]
Vinblastine: I.V.: 3 mg/m^2/day days 2 and 15
[total dose/cycle = 6 mg/m^2]
Doxorubicin: I.V.: 30 or 40 mg/m^2 day 3
[total dose/cycle = 30 or 40 mg/m^2]
Cisplatin: I.V.: 70 mg/m^2 day 2
[total dose/cycle = 70 mg/m^2]
Repeat cycle every 4 weeks

Variation 13:
Methotrexate: I.V.: 30 mg/m^2/day days 1 and 15
[total dose/cycle = 60 mg/m^2]
Vinblastine: I.V.: 3 mg/m^2/day days 2 and 15
[total dose/cycle = 6 mg/m^2]
Doxorubicin: I.V.: 30 or 40 mg/m^2 day 2
[total dose/cycle = 30 or 40 mg/m^2]
Cisplatin: I.V.: 70 mg/m^2 day 2
[total dose/cycle = 70 mg/m^2]
Repeat cycle every 4 weeks

M-VAC (Breast Cancer)

Use Breast cancer

Regimen

Methotrexate: I.V.: 30 mg/m^2/day days 1, 15, and 22
[total dose/cycle = 90 mg/m^2]
Vinblastine: I.V.: 3 mg/m^2/day days 2, 15, and 22
[total dose/cycle = 9 mg/m^2]
Doxorubicin: I.V.: 30 mg/m^2 day 2
[total dose/cycle = 30 mg/m^2]
Cisplatin: I.V.: 70 mg/m^2 day 2
[total dose/cycle = 70 mg/m^2]
Leucovorin: Oral: 10 mg every 6 hours for 6 doses days 2, 16, and 23
[total dose/cycle = 180 mg]
Repeat cycle every 4 weeks

M-VAC (Endometrial Cancer)

Use Endometrial cancer

Regimen

Methotrexate: I.V.: 30 mg/m^2/day days 1, 15, and 22
[total dose/cycle = 90 mg/m^2]
Vinblastine: I.V.: 3 mg/m^2/day days 2, 15, and 22
[total dose/cycle = 9 mg/m^2]
Doxorubicin: I.V.: 30 mg/m^2/day day 2
[total dose/cycle = 30 mg/m^2]
Cisplatin: I.V.: 70 mg/m^2/day day 2
[total dose/cycle = 70 mg/m^2]
Repeat cycle every 4 weeks

MVPP

Use Lymphoma, Hodgkin disease

Regimen

Mechlorethamine: I.V.: 6 mg/m^2/day days 1 and 8
[total dose/cycle = 12 mg/m^2]
Vinblastine: I.V.: 4 mg/m^2/day days 1 and 8
[total dose/cycle = 8 mg/m^2]
Procarbazine: Oral: 100 mg/m^2/day days 1 to 14
[total dose/cycle = 1400 mg/m^2]
Prednisone: Oral: 40 mg/m^2/day days 1 to 14
[total dose/cycle = 560 mg/m^2]
Repeat cycle every 4-6 weeks

N4SE Protocol

Use Neuroblastoma

Regimen

Vincristine: I.V.: 0.05 mg/kg/day days 1 and 2
[total dose/cycle = 0.1 mg/kg]
Doxorubicin: I.V.: 15 mg/m^2/day days 1 and 2
[total dose/cycle = 30 mg/m^2]
Cyclophosphamide: I.V.: 30 mg/kg/day days 1 and 2
[total dose/cycle = 60 mg/kg]
Fluorouracil: I.V.: 1 mg/kg/day days 3, 8, and 9
[total dose/cycle = 3 mg/kg]
Cytarabine: I.V.: 3 mg/kg/day days 3, 8, and 9
[total dose/cycle = 9 mg/kg]
Hydroxyurea: Oral: 40 mg/kg/day days 3, 8, and 9
[total dose/cycle = 120 mg/kg]
Repeat cycle every 21-28 days

N6 Protocol

Use Neuroblastoma

Regimen

Course 1, 2, 4, and 6:
Cyclophosphamide: I.V.: 70 mg/kg/day days 1 and 2
[total dose/cycle = 140 mg/kg]
Doxorubicin: I.V.: 25 mg/m^2/day continuous infusion days 1, 2, and 3
[total dose/cycle = 75 mg/m^2]
Vincristine: I.V.: 0.033 mg/kg/day continuous infusion days 1, 2, and 3
[total dose/cycle = 0.099 mg/kg]
Vincristine: I.V.: 1.5 mg/m^2 day 9
[total dose/cycle = 1.5 mg/m^2]
Course 3, 5, and 7:
Etoposide: I.V.: 200 mg/m^2/day days 1, 2, and 3
[total dose/cycle = 600 mg/m^2]
Cisplatin: I.V.: 50 mg/m^2/day days 1 to 4
[total dose/cycle = 200 mg/m^2]

OFAR (CLL)

Use Leukemia, chronic lymphocytic

Regimen

Cycle 1:

Oxaliplatin: I.V.: 25 mg/m^2/dose day 1 to 4
[total dose/cycle = 100 mg/m^2]

Fludarabine: I.V.: 30 mg/m^2/dose days 2 and 3
[total dose/cycle = 60 mg/m^2]

Cytarabine: I.V.: 1000 mg/m^2/dose over 2 hours days 2 and 3
[total dose/cycle = 2000 mg/m^2]

Rituximab: I.V.: 375 mg/m^2 day 3
[total dose/cycle = 375 mg/m^2]

Treatment cycle is 4 weeks

Cycles 2-6:

Oxaliplatin: I.V.: 25 mg/m^2/dose day 1 to 4
[total dose/cycle = 100 mg/m^2]

Fludarabine: I.V.: 30 mg/m^2/dose days 2 and 3
[total dose/cycle = 60 mg/m^2]

Cytarabine: I.V.: 1000 mg/m^2/dose over 2 hours days 2 and 3
[total dose/cycle = 2000 mg/m^2]

Rituximab: I.V.: 375 mg/m^2 day 1
[total dose/cycle = 375 mg/m^2]

Repeat cycle every 4 weeks (maximum: 6 cycles)

OPA

Use Lymphoma, Hodgkin disease

Regimen

Vincristine: I.V.: 1.5 mg/m^2/day (maximum dose: 2 mg) days 1, 8, and 15
[total dose/cycle = 4.5 mg/m^2]

Prednisone: Oral: 60 mg/m^2/day in 3 divided doses days 1 to 15
[total dose/cycle = 900 mg/m^2]

Doxorubicin: I.V.: 40 mg/m^2/day days 1 and 15
[total dose/cycle = 80 mg/m^2]

Second cycle may be given based on individual response; time between cycles not specified

OPPA

Use Lymphoma, Hodgkin disease

Regimen

Vincristine: I.V.: 1.5 mg/m^2/day (maximum dose: 2 mg) days 1, 8, and 15
[total dose/cycle = 4.5 mg/m^2]

Prednisone: Oral: 60 mg/m^2/day in 3 divided doses days 1 to 15
[total dose/cycle = 900 mg/m^2]

Doxorubicin: I.V.: 40 mg/m^2/day days 1 and 15
[total dose/cycle = 80 mg/m^2]

Procarbazine: Oral: 100 mg/m^2/day in 2 or 3 divided doses days 1 to 15
[total dose/cycle = 1500 mg/m^2]

Second cycle may be given based on individual response; time between cycles not specified

Oxaliplatin-Cytarabine-Dexamethasone (NHL Regimen)

Use Lymphoma, non-Hodgkin

Regimen

Dexamethasone: I.V. or Oral: 40 mg/day days 1 to 4
[total dose/cycle = 160 mg]

Oxaliplatin: I.V.: 130 mg/m^2 over 2 hours day 1
[total dose/cycle = 130 mg/m^2]

Cytarabine: I.V.: 2000 mg/m^2 over 3 hours every 12 hours for 2 doses day 2
[total dose/cycle = 4000 mg/m^2]

Repeat cycle every 3 weeks

Oxaliplatin-Fluorouracil (Esophageal Cancer)

Use Esophageal cancer

Regimen In combination with radiation therapy:

Oxaliplatin: I.V.: 85 mg/m^2/day over 2 hours days 1, 15, and 29
[total dose/cycle = 255 mg/m^2]

Fluorouracil: I.V.: 180 mg/m^2/day continuous infusion days 8 to 42
[total dose/cycle = 6300 mg/m^2]

PAC (CAP)

Use Ovarian cancer

Regimen

Cisplatin: I.V.: 50 mg/m^2 day 1
[total dose/cycle = 50 mg/m^2]

Doxorubicin: I.V.: 50 mg/m^2 day 1
[total dose/cycle = 50 mg/m^2]

Cyclophosphamide: I.V.: 1000 mg/m^2 day 1
[total dose/cycle = 1000 mg/m^2]

Repeat cycle every 21 days for 8 cycles

PA-CI

Use Hepatoblastoma

Regimen NOTE: Multiple variations are listed below.

Variation 1:

Cisplatin: I.V.: 90 mg/m^2 day 1
[total dose/cycle = 90 mg/m^2]

Doxorubicin: I.V.: 20 mg/m^2/day continuous infusion days 2 to 5
[total dose/cycle = 80 mg/m^2]

Repeat cycle every 21 days

Variation 2:

Cisplatin: I.V.: 20 mg/m^2/day days 1 to 4
[total dose/cycle = 80 mg/m^2]

Doxorubicin: I.V.: 100 mg/m^2 continuous infusion day 1
[total dose/cycle = 100 mg/m^2]

Repeat cycle every 21-28 days

Paclitaxel-Bevacizumab

Use Breast cancer

Regimen

Paclitaxel: I.V.: 90 mg/m^2/day days 1, 8, and 15
[total dose/cycle = 270 mg/m^2]

Bevacizumab: I.V.: 10 mg/kg/day days 1 and 15
[total dose/cycle = 20 mg/kg]

Repeat cycle every 28 days

Paclitaxel-Carboplatin-Bevacizumab

Use Lung cancer, nonsquamous, nonsmall cell

Regimen

Paclitaxel: I.V.: 200 mg/m^2 infused over 3 hours day 1
[total dose/cycle = 200 mg/m^2]

followed by

Carboplatin: I.V.: Target AUC 6 day 1
[total dose/cycle = AUC = 6]

followed by

Bevacizumab: I.V.: 15 mg/kg day 1
[total dose/cycle = 15 mg/kg]

Repeat cycle every 21 days for 6 cycles

Paclitaxel-Carboplatin (Bladder Cancer)

Use Bladder cancer

Regimen

Paclitaxel: I.V.: 200 mg/m^2 or 225 mg/m^2 day 1
[total dose/cycle = 200 or 225 mg/m^2]
Carboplatin: I.V.: AUC 5-6 day 1
[total dose/cycle = AUC = 5-6]
Repeat cycle every 21 days

Paclitaxel-Carboplatin-Etoposide (Unknown Primary)

Use Unknown primary, adenocarcinoma

Regimen

Paclitaxel: I.V.: 200 mg/m^2 infused over 1 hour day 1
[total dose/cycle = 200 mg/m^2]
followed by
Carboplatin: I.V.: Target AUC 6 day 1
[total dose/cycle = AUC = 6]
Etoposide: Oral: 50 mg/day days 1, 3, 5, 7, and 9
and Oral: 100 mg/day days 2, 4, 6, 8, and 10
[total dose/cycle = 750 mg]
Repeat cycle every 21 days for a total of 4-8 cycles

Paclitaxel-Carboplatin-Gemcitabine

Use Bladder cancer

Regimen

Paclitaxel: I.V.: 200 mg/m^2 day 1
[total dose/cycle = 200 mg/m^2]
Gemcitabine: I.V.: 1000 mg/m^2/day days 1 and 8
[total dose/cycle = 2000 mg/m^2]
Carboplatin: I.V.: AUC 5 day 1
[total dose/cycle = AUC = 5]
Repeat cycle every 21 days

Paclitaxel-Carboplatin-Gemcitabine (Unknown Primary)

Use Unknown primary (adenocarcinoma)

Regimen

Paclitaxel: I.V.: 200 mg/m^2 infused over 1 hour day 1
[total dose/cycle = 200 mg/m^2]
Carboplatin: I.V.: Target AUC 5 day 1
[total dose/cycle = AUC = 5]
Gemcitabine: I.V.: 1000 mg/m^2/dose days 1 and 8
[total dose/cycle = 2000 mg/m^2]
Repeat cycle every 21 days for a total of 4 cycles

Paclitaxel-Cetuximab

Use Head and neck cancer

Regimen

Week 1:
Paclitaxel: I.V.: 80 mg/m^2 day 1
[total dose/week 1 = 80 mg/m^2]
Cetuximab: I.V.: 400 mg/m^2 (loading dose) day 1 (week 1 only)
[total loading dose (week 1) = 400 mg/m^2]
Subsequent weeks:
Paclitaxel: I.V.: 80 mg/m^2 day 1
[total dose/week = 80 mg/m^2]
Cetuximab: I.V.: 250 mg/m^2 day 1
[total dose/week = 250 mg/m^2]

Paclitaxel-Cisplatin-Fluorouracil (Esophageal Cancer)

Use Esophageal cancer

Regimen

Paclitaxel: I.V.: 175 mg/m^2 over 3 hours day 1
[total dose/cycle = 175 mg/m^2]
Cisplatin: I.V.: 20 mg/m^2/day days 1 to 5 for cycles 1, 2, and 3
[total dose/cycle = 100 mg/m^2]
then 15 mg/m^2/day days 1 to 5
[total dose/cycle = 75 mg/m^2]
Fluorouracil: I.V.: 750 mg/m^2/day continuous infusion days 1 to 5
[total dose/cycle = 3750 mg/m^2]
Repeat cycle every 28 days

Paclitaxel-Cisplatin-Fluorouracil (Unknown Primary)

Use Unknown primary (squamous cell)

Regimen

Paclitaxel: I.V.: 175 mg/m^2 over 3 hours day 1
[total dose/cycle = 175 mg/m^2]
Cisplatin: I.V.: 100 mg/m^2 day 2
[total dose/cycle = 100 mg/m^2]
Fluorouracil: I.V.: 500 mg/m^2/day continuous infusion days 2 to 6
[total dose/cycle = 2500 mg/m^2]
Repeat cycle every 21 days for a total of 3 cycles

Paclitaxel + Estramustine + Carboplatin

Use Prostate cancer

Regimen

Paclitaxel: I.V.: 100 mg/m^2 day 3 each week
[total dose/cycle = 400 mg/m^2]
Estramustine: Oral: 10 mg/kg/day days 1 to 5 each week
[total dose/cycle = 200 mg/kg]
Carboplatin: I.V.: Target AUC 6 day 3
[total dose/cycle = AUC = 6]
Repeat cycle every 28 days

Paclitaxel + Estramustine + Etoposide

Use Prostate cancer

Regimen

Paclitaxel: I.V.: 135 mg/m^2 day 2
[total dose/cycle = 135 mg/m^2]
Estramustine: Oral: 280 mg 3 times/day days 1 to 14
[total dose/cycle = 11,760 mg]
Etoposide: Oral: 100 mg/day days 1 to 14
[total dose/cycle = 1400 mg]
Repeat cycle every 21 days

Paclitaxel-Gemcitabine

Use Bladder cancer

Regimen

Paclitaxel: I.V.: 200 mg/m^2 day 1
[total dose/cycle = 200 mg/m^2]
Gemcitabine: I.V.: 1000 mg/m^2/day days 1, 8, and 15
[total dose/cycle = 3000 mg/m^2]
Repeat cycle every 21 days for a maximum of 6 cycles

Paclitaxel-Ifosfamide-Cisplatin

Use Testicular cancer

Regimen

Paclitaxel: I.V.: 250 mg/m^2 continuous infusion day 1
[total dose/cycle = 250 mg/m^2]

Ifosfamide: I.V.: 1500 mg/m^2/day days 2 to 5
[total dose/cycle = 6000 mg/m^2]
Cisplatin: I.V.: 25 mg/m^2/day days 2 to 5
[total dose/cycle = 100 mg/m^2]
Mesna: I.V.: 500 mg/m^2 prior to ifosfamide and every 4 hours for 2 doses, days 2 to 5
[total dose/cycle = 6000 mg/m^2]
Repeat cycle every 21 days for 4 cycles

Paclitaxel-Vinorelbine

Use Breast cancer

Regimen NOTE: Multiple variations are listed below.

Variation 1:
Paclitaxel: I.V.: 135 mg/m^2 day 1
[total dose/cycle = 135 mg/m^2]
Vinorelbine: I.V.: 30 mg/m^2 day 1
[total dose/cycle = 30 mg/m^2]
Repeat cycle every 21 days

Variation 2:
Paclitaxel: I.V.: 150 mg/m^2 day 1
[total dose/cycle = 150 mg/m^2]
Vinorelbine: I.V.: 25 mg/m^2 day 1
[total dose/cycle = 25 mg/m^2]
Repeat cycle every 21 days

Variation 3:
Paclitaxel: I.V.: 135 mg/m^2 day 1
[total dose/cycle = 135 mg/m^2]
Vinorelbine: I.V.: 30 mg/m^2/day days 1 and 8
[total dose/cycle = 60 mg/m^2]
Repeat cycle every 28 days

PC (NSCLC)

Use Lung cancer, nonsmall cell

Regimen NOTE: Multiple variations are listed below.

Variation 1:
Paclitaxel: I.V.: 175-225 mg/m^2 day 1
[total dose/cycle = 175-225 mg/m^2]
Carboplatin: I.V.: Target AUC 5-7 day 1
[total dose/cycle = AUC = 5-7]
Repeat cycle every 21 days for 2-8 cycles

Variation 2:
Paclitaxel: I.V.: 175 mg/m^2 day 1
[total dose/cycle = 175 mg/m^2]
Cisplatin: I.V.: 80 mg/m^2 day 1
[total dose/cycle = 80 mg/m^2]
Repeat cycle every 21 days

Variation 3:
Paclitaxel: I.V.: 135 mg/m^2 continuous infusion day 1
[total dose/cycle = 135 mg/m^2]
Carboplatin: I.V.: AUC 7.5 day 2
[total dose/cycle = AUC = 7.5]
Repeat cycle every 21 days

Variation 4:
Paclitaxel: I.V.: 135 mg/m^2 continuous infusion day 1
[total dose/cycle = 135 mg/m^2]
Cisplatin: I.V.: 75 mg/m^2 day 2
[total dose/cycle = 75 mg/m^2]
Repeat cycle every 21 days

PCR

Use Leukemia, chronic lymphocytic

Regimen NOTE: Multiple variations are listed below.

Variation 1:

Cycle 1:

Cyclophosphamide: I.V.: 600 mg/m^2 day 1
[total dose/cycle = 600 mg/m^2]

Pentostatin: I.V.: 4 mg/m^2 day 1
[total dose/cycle = 4 mg/m^2]

Treatment cycle is 3 weeks

Cycles 2-6:

Cyclophosphamide: I.V.: 600 mg/m^2 day 1
[total dose/cycle = 600 mg/m^2]

Pentostatin: I.V.: 4 mg/m^2 day 1
[total dose/cycle = 4 mg/m^2]

Rituximab: I.V.: 375 mg/m^2 day 1
[total dose/cycle = 375 mg/m^2]

Repeat cycle every 3 weeks

Variation 2:

Cycle 1:

Pentostatin: I.V.: 2 mg/m^2 day 1
[total dose/cycle = 2 mg/m^2]

Cyclophosphamide: I.V.: 600 mg/m^2 day 1
[total dose/cycle = 600 mg/m^2]

Rituximab: I.V.: 100 mg/m^2 day 1 only
followed by I.V.: 375 mg/m^2/day days 3 and 5 only
[total dose/cycle 1 = 850 mg/m^2]

Treatment cycle is 3 weeks

Cycles 2-6:

Pentostatin: I.V.: 2 mg/m^2 day 1
[total dose/cycle = 2 mg/m^2]

Cyclophosphamide: I.V.: 600 mg/m^2 day 1
[total dose/cycle = 600 mg/m^2]

Rituximab: I.V.: 375 mg/m^2 day 1
[total dose/cycle = 375 mg/m^2]

Repeat cycle every 3 weeks

PCV (Brain Tumor Regimen)

Use Brain tumors

Regimen NOTE: Multiple variations are listed below.

Variation 1:

Lomustine: Oral: 110 mg/m^2 day 1
[total dose/cycle = 110 mg/m^2]

Procarbazine: Oral: 60 mg/m^2/day days 8 to 21
[total dose/cycle = 840 mg/m^2]

Vincristine: I.V.: 1.4 mg/m^2/day (maximum dose: 2 mg) days 8 and 29
[total dose/cycle = 2.8 mg/m^2; maximum: 4 mg]

Repeat cycle every 6 weeks for a total of 6 cycles

Variation 2:

Lomustine: Oral: 110 mg/m^2 day 1
[total dose/cycle = 110 mg/m^2]

Procarbazine: Oral: 60 mg/m^2/day days 8 to 21
[total dose/cycle = 840 mg/m^2]

Vincristine: I.V.: 1.4 mg/m^2/day (maximum dose: 2 mg) days 8 and 29
[total dose/cycle = 2.8 mg/m^2; maximum: 4 mg]

Repeat cycle every 6 weeks for a total of 7 cycles

Variation 3:
Procarbazine: Oral: 75 mg/m^2/day days 8 to 21
[total dose/cycle = 1050 mg/m^2]
Lomustine: Oral: 130 mg/m^2 day 1
[total dose/cycle = 130 mg/m^2]
Vincristine: I.V.: 1.4 mg/m^2/day (no maximum) days 8 and 29
[total dose/cycle = 2.8 mg/m^2; no maximum]
Repeat cycle every 6 weeks for a total of 6 cycles

Variation 4:
Procarbazine: Oral: 75 mg/m^2/day days 8 to 21
[total dose/cycle = 1050 mg/m^2]
Lomustine: Oral: 130 mg/m^2 day 1
[total dose/cycle = 130 mg/m^2]
Vincristine: I.V.: 1.4 mg/m^2/day (no maximum) days 8 and 29
[total dose/cycle = 2.8 mg/m^2; no maximum]
Repeat cycle every 6 weeks for up to a total of 4 cycles

Variation 5:
Lomustine: Oral: 110 mg/m^2 day 1
[total dose/cycle = 110 mg/m^2]
Procarbazine: Oral: 60 mg/m^2/day days 8 to 21
[total dose/cycle = 840 mg/m^2]
Vincristine: I.V.: 1.4 mg/m^2/day days 8 and 29
[total dose/cycle = 2.8 mg/m^2]
Repeat cycle every 6-8 weeks for 1 year

Pemetrexed (Bladder Cancer Regimen)

Use Bladder cancer

Regimen

Pemetrexed: I.V.: 500 mg/m^2 infused over 10 minutes day 1
[total dose/cycle = 500 mg/m^2]
Repeat cycle every 21 days

Pemetrexed-Carboplatin (Mesothelioma)

Use Malignant pleural mesothelioma

Regimen

Pemetrexed: I.V.: 500 mg/m^2 infused over 10 minutes day 1
[total dose/cycle = 500 mg/m^2]
Carboplatin: I.V.: AUC 5 infused over 30 minutes day 1 (start 30 minutes after pemetrexed)
[total dose/cycle = AUC = 5]
Repeat cycle every 21 days

Pemetrexed-Cisplatin (NSCLC)

Use Lung cancer, nonsmall cell

Regimen

Pemetrexed: I.V.: 500 mg/m^2/dose day 1
[total dose/cycle = 500 mg/m^2]
Cisplatin: I.V.: 75 mg/m^2/dose day 1
[total dose/cycle = 75 mg/m^2]
Repeat cycle every 21 days for up to 6 cycles

Pentostatin-Cyclophosphamide

Use Leukemia, chronic lymphocytic

Regimen

Cyclophosphamide: I.V.: 600 mg/m^2 day 1
[total dose/cycle = 600 mg/m^2]
Pentostatin: I.V.: 4 mg/m^2 day 1
[total dose/cycle = 4 mg/m^2]
Repeat cycle every 3 weeks for up to 6 cycles

PFL (Colorectal Cancer)

Use Colorectal cancer

Regimen

Cisplatin: I.V.: 25 mg/m^2/day continuous infusion days 1 to 5
[total dose/cycle = 125 mg/m^2]
Fluorouracil: I.V.: 800 mg/m^2/day continuous infusion days 2 to 5
[total dose/cycle = 3200 mg/m^2]
Leucovorin calcium: I.V.: 500 mg/m^2/day continuous infusion days 1 to 5
[total dose/cycle = 2500 mg/m^2]
Repeat cycle every 28 days

POC

Use Brain tumors

Regimen

Prednisone: Oral: 40 mg/m^2/day days 1 to 14
[total dose/cycle = 560 mg/m^2]
Vincristine: I.V.: 1.5 mg/m^2/day (maximum dose: 2 mg) days 1, 8, and 15
[total dose/cycle = 4.5 mg/m^2]
Lomustine: Oral: 100 mg/m^2 day 1
[total dose/cycle = 100 mg/m^2]
Repeat cycle every 6 weeks

POG-8651

Use Osteosarcoma

Regimen

(Surgery at week 10)
Methotrexate: I.V.: 12 g/m^2 weeks 0, 1, 5, 6, 13, 14, 18, 19, 23, 24, 37, and 38
[total dose/cycle = 144 g/m^2]
Leucovorin: (route not specified): 15 mg every 6 hours for 10 doses, weeks 0, 1, 5, 6, 13, 14, 18, 19, 23, 24, 37, and 38
[total dose/cycle = 1800 mg]
Doxorubicin: I.V.: 37.5 mg/m^2/dose days 1 and 2 of weeks 2, 7, 25, and 28
followed by I.V.: 30 mg/m^2/dose days 1, 2, and 3 of week 20
[total dose/cycle = 390 mg/m^2]
Cisplatin: I.V.: 60 mg/m^2/day days 1 and 2, weeks 2, 7, 25, and 28
[total dose/cycle = 480 mg/m^2]
Cyclophosphamide: I.V.: 600 mg/m^2/day days 1, 2, and 3, weeks 15, 31, 34, 39, and 42
[total dose/cycle = 9000 mg/m^2]
Bleomycin: I.V.: 15 units/m^2/day days 1, 2, and 3, weeks 15, 31, 34, 39, and 42
[total dose/cycle = 225 units/m^2]
Dactinomycin: I.V.: 0.6 mg/m^2/day days 1, 2, and 3, weeks 15, 31, 34, 39, and 42
[total dose/cycle = 9 mg/m^2]
or
(Surgery at week 0)
Methotrexate: 12 g/m^2 weeks 3, 4, 8, 9, 13, 14, 18, 19, 23, 24, 37, and 38
[total dose/cycle = 144 g/m^2]
Leucovorin: (route not specified): 15 mg every 6 hours for 10 doses, weeks 3, 4, 8, 9, 13, 14, 18, 19, 23, 24, 37, and 38
[total dose/cycle = 1800 mg]
Doxorubicin: I.V.: 37.5 mg/m^2/day days 1 and 2, weeks 5, 10, 25, and 28 and 30 mg/m^2 days 1, 2, and 3, week 20
[total dose/cycle = 390 mg/m^2]
Cisplatin: I.V.: 60 mg/m^2/day days 1 and 2, weeks 5, 10, 25, and 28
[total dose/cycle = 480 mg/m^2]
Cyclophosphamide: I.V.: 600 mg/m^2/day days 1, 2, and 3, weeks 15, 31, 34, 39, and 42
[total dose/cycle = 9000 mg/m^2]
Bleomycin: I.V.: 15 units/m^2/day days 1, 2, and 3, weeks 15, 31, 34, 39, and 42
[total dose/cycle = 225 units/m^2]

Dactinomycin: I.V.: 0.6 mg/m^2/day days 1, 2, and 3, weeks 15, 31, 34, 39, and 42
[total dose/cycle = 9 mg/m^2]

POMP

Use Leukemia, acute lymphocytic

Regimen Maintenance:

Mercaptopurine: Oral: 50 mg 3 times/day
[total dose/cycle = 4200-4650 mg]
Methotrexate: Oral: 20 mg/m^2 once weekly
[total dose/cycle = 80 mg/m^2]
Vincristine: I.V.: 2 mg day 1
[total dose/cycle = 2 mg]
Prednisone: Oral: 200 mg/day days 1 to 5
[total dose/cycle = 1000 mg]
Repeat cycle monthly for 2 years

Pro-MACE-CytaBOM

Use Lymphoma, non-Hodgkin

Regimen

Prednisone: Oral: 60 mg/m^2/day days 1 to 14
[total dose/cycle = 840 mg/m^2]
Doxorubicin: I.V.: 25 mg/m^2 day 1
[total dose/cycle = 25 mg/m^2]
Cyclophosphamide: I.V.: 650 mg/m^2 day 1
[total dose/cycle = 650 mg/m^2]
Etoposide: I.V.: 120 mg/m^2 day 1
[total dose/cycle = 120 mg/m^2]
Cytarabine: I.V.: 300 mg/m^2 day 8
[total dose/cycle = 300 mg/m^2]
Bleomycin: I.V.: 5 units/m^2 day 8
[total dose/cycle = 5 units/m^2]
Vincristine: I.V.: 1.4 mg/m^2 (maximum dose: 2 mg) day 8
[total dose/cycle = 1.4 mg/m^2]
Methotrexate: I.V.: 120 mg/m^2 day 8
[total dose/cycle = 120 mg/m^2]
Leucovorin: Oral: 25 mg/m^2 every 6 hours for 4 doses (start 24 hours after methotrexate dose) day 9
[total dose/cycle = 100 mg/m^2]
Repeat cycle every 21 days

PVA (POG 8602)

Use Leukemia, acute lymphocytic

Regimen

Induction:

Prednisone: Oral: 40 mg/m^2/day (maximum dose: 60 mg) given in 3 divided doses days 0 to 28
[total dose/cycle = 1160 mg/m^2]
Vincristine: I.V.: 1.5 mg/m^2/day (maximum dose: 2 mg) days 0, 7, 14, and 21
[total dose/cycle = 6 mg/m^2; maximum: 8 mg]
Asparaginase: I.M.: 6000 units/m^2 3 times per week for 2 weeks
[total dose/cycle = 36,000 units/m^2]
Intrathecal therapy (triple): Days 0 and 22
Leucovorin: Route and dose not specified: Single dose 24 hours after every intrathecal treatment days 1 and 23
Administer one cycle only

CNS consolidation:

Mercaptopurine: Oral: 75 mg/m^2/day days 29 to 43
[total dose/cycle = 1125 mg/m^2]
Intrathecal therapy (triple): Days 29 and 36
Leucovorin: Route and dose not specified: Single dose 24 hours after every intrathecal treatment days 30 and 37
Administer one cycle only

Intensification:

Regimen A:

Methotrexate: I.V.: 1000 mg/m^2 continuous infusion over 24 hours day 1
[total dose/cycle = 1000 mg/m^2]

Cytarabine: I.V.: 1000 mg/m^2 continuous infusion over 24 hours day 1 (start 12 hours after start of methotrexate)
[total dose/cycle = 1000 mg/m^2]

Leucovorin: I.M., I.V., or Oral: 30 mg/m^2 at 24 and 36 hours after the start of methotrexate
[total dose/cycle = 60 mg/m^2]

followed by I.M., I.V., or Oral: 3 mg/m^2 at 48, 60, and 72 hours after the start of methotrexate
[total dose/cycle = 9 mg/m^2]

Repeat cycle every 3 weeks for 6 cycles (administered weeks 7, 10, 13, 16, 19, and 22)

Intrathecal therapy (triple): Weeks 9, 12, 15, and 18

Leucovorin: Route and dose not specified: Single dose 24 hours after every intrathecal treatment weeks 9, 12, 15, and 18

or

Regimen B:

Methotrexate: I.V.: 1000 mg/m^2 continuous infusion over 24 hours day 1
[total dose/cycle = 1000 mg/m^2]

Cytarabine: I.V.: 1000 mg/m^2 continuous infusion over 24 hours day 1 (start 12 hours after methotrexate)
[total dose/cycle = 1000 mg/m^2]

Leucovorin: I.M., I.V., or Oral: 30 mg/m^2 at 24 and 36 hours after the start of methotrexate
[total dose/cycle = 60 mg/m^2]

followed by I.M., I.V., or Oral: 3 mg/m^2 at 48, 60, and 72 hours after the start of methotrexate
[total dose/cycle = 9 mg/m^2]

Repeat cycle every 12 weeks for 6 cycles (administer weeks 7, 19, 31, 43, 55, and 67)

Intrathecal therapy (triple): Weeks 9, 12, 15, and 18

Leucovorin: Route and dose not specified: Single dose 24 hours after every intrathecal treatment weeks 9, 12, 15, and 18

Maintenance:

Regimen A:

Methotrexate: I.M.: 20 mg/m^2 weekly, weeks 25 to 156
[total dose/cycle = 2640 mg/m^2]

Mercaptopurine: Oral: 75 mg/m^2 daily, weeks 25 to 156
[total dose/cycle = 69,300 mg/m^2]

Intrathecal therapy (triple): Every 8 weeks, weeks 26 through 105

Leucovorin: Route and dose not specified: Single dose 24 hours after every intrathecal treatment weeks 26 through 105

Prednisone: Oral: 40 mg/m^2/day (maximum dose: 60 mg) days 1 to 7 (given in 3 divided doses), weeks 8, 17, 25, 41, 57, 73, 89, and 105
[total dose/cycle = 2240 mg/m^2; maximum: 3360 mg]

Vincristine: I.V.: 1.5 mg/m^2/day (maximum dose: 2 mg) day 1, weeks 8, 9, 17, 18, 25, 26, 41, 42, 57, 58, 73, 74, 89, 90, 105, and 106
[total dose/cycle = 24 mg/m^2; maximum: 32 mg]

or

Regimen B:

Methotrexate: I.M.: 20 mg/m^2 weekly, weeks 22-28, 34-40, 46-52, and 58-64
[total dose/cycle = 560 mg/m^2]

Mercaptopurine: Oral: 75 mg/m^2 daily for 7 weeks, weeks 22-28, 34-40, 46-52, and 58-64
[total dose/cycle = 14700 mg/m^2]

followed by

Methotrexate: I.M.: 20 mg/m^2 weekly, weeks 70 to 156
[total dose/cycle = 1720 mg/m^2]

Mercaptopurine: Oral: 75 mg/m^2 daily, weeks 70 to 156
[total dose/cycle = 45,150 mg/m^2]

Intrathecal therapy (triple): Every 8 weeks, weeks 26 through 105

Leucovorin: Route and dose not specified: Single dose 24 hours after every intrathecal treatment weeks 26 through 105

Prednisone: Oral: 40 mg/m^2/day (maximum dose: 60 mg) days 1 to 7 (given in 3 divided doses), weeks 8, 17, 25, 41, 57, 73, 89, and 105
[total dose/cycle = 2240 mg/m^2]

Vincristine: I.V.: 1.5 mg/m^2/day (maximum dose: 2 mg) day 1, weeks 8, 9, 17, 18, 25, 26, 41, 42, 57, 58, 73, 74, 89, 90, 105, and 106
[total dose/cycle = 24 mg/m^2; maximum dose: 32 mg]

PVB

Use Testicular cancer

Regimen NOTE: Multiple variations are listed below.

Variation 1:
Cisplatin: I.V.: 20 mg/m^2/day days 1 to 5
[total dose/cycle = 100 mg/m^2]
Vinblastine: I.V.: 0.2 mg/kg/day days 1 and 2
[total dose/cycle = 0.4 mg/kg]
Bleomycin: I.V.: 30 units/day days 2, 9, and 16
[total dose/cycle = 90 units]
Repeat cycle every 3 weeks

Variation 2:
Cisplatin: I.V.: 20 mg/m^2/day days 1 to 5
[total dose/cycle = 100 mg/m^2]
Vinblastine: I.V.: 0.15 mg/kg/day days 1 and 2
[total dose/cycle = 0.3 mg/kg]
Bleomycin: I.V.: 30 units/day days 2, 9, and 16
[total dose/cycle = 90 units]
Repeat cycle every 3 weeks

Variation 3:
Cisplatin: I.V.: 20 mg/m^2/day days 1 to 5
[total dose/cycle = 100 mg/m^2]
Vinblastine: I.V.: 6 mg/m^2/day days 1 and 2
[total dose/cycle = 12 mg/m^2]
Bleomycin: I.M.: 30 units/day days 2, 9, and 16
[total dose/cycle = 90 units]
Repeat cycle every 3 weeks

PVDA

Use Leukemia, acute lymphocytic

Regimen Induction:
Prednisone: Oral: 60 mg/m^2/day days 1 to 28
[total dose/cycle = 1680 mg/m^2]
Vincristine: I.V.: 1.5 mg/m^2/day days 1, 8, 15, and 22
[total dose/cycle = 6 mg/m^2]
Daunorubicin: I.V.: 25 mg/m^2/day days 1, 8, 15, and 22
[total dose/cycle = 100 mg/m^2]
Asparaginase: I.M., SubQ, or I.V.: 5000 units/m^2/day days 1 to 14
[total dose/cycle = 70,000 units/m^2]
Administer one cycle only; used in conjunction with intrathecal chemotherapy

R-CVP

Use Lymphoma, non-Hodgkin

Regimen
Rituximab: I.V.: 375 mg/m^2 day 1
[total dose/cycle = 375 mg/m^2]
Cyclophosphamide: I.V.: 750 mg/m^2 day 1
[total dose/cycle = 750 mg/m^2]
Vincristine: I.V.: 1.4 mg/m^2 day 1
[total dose/cycle = 1.4 mg/m^2]
Prednisone: Oral: 40 mg/m^2/day days 1 to 5
[total dose/cycle = 200 mg/m^2]
Repeat cycle every 21 days

Regimen A1

Use Neuroblastoma

Regimen

Cyclophosphamide: I.V.: 1.2 g/m^2 day 1
[total dose/cycle = 1.2 g/m^2]
Vincristine: I.V.: 1.5 mg/m^2 day 1
[total dose/cycle = 1.5 mg/m^2]
Doxorubicin: I.V.: 40 mg/m^2 day 3
[total dose/cycle = 40 mg/m^2]
Cisplatin: I.V.: 90 mg/m^2 day 5
[total dose/cycle = 90 mg/m^2]
Repeat cycle every 28 days

Regimen A2

Use Neuroblastoma

Regimen

Cyclophosphamide: I.V.: 1.2 g/m^2 day 1
[total dose/cycle = 1.2 g/m^2]
Etoposide: I.V.: 100 mg/m^2/day days 1 to 5
[total dose/cycle = 500 mg/m^2]
Doxorubicin: I.V.: 40 mg/m^2 day 3
[total dose/cycle = 40 mg/m^2]
Cisplatin: I.V.: 90 mg/m^2 day 5
[total dose/cycle = 90 mg/m^2]
Repeat cycle every 28 days

RICE

Use Lymphoma, non-Hodgkin

Regimen

Rituximab: I.V.: 375 mg/m^2/day days -2 and 1 (cycle 1)
[total dose/cycle = 750 mg/m^2]
Rituximab: I.V.: 375 mg/m^2 day 1 (cycles 2 and 3)
[total dose/cycle = 375 mg/m^2]
Etoposide: I.V.: 100 mg/m^2/day days 3, 4, and 5
[total dose/cycle = 300 mg/m^2]
Carboplatin: I.V.: AUC = 5 (maximum dose: 800 mg) day 4
[total dose/cycle = AUC = 5]
Ifosfamide: I.V.: 5000 mg/m^2 continuous infusion day 4
[total dose/cycle = 5000 mg/m^2]
Mesna: I.V.: 5000 mg/m^2 continuous infusion day 4
[total dose/cycle = 5000 mg/m^2]
Filgrastim: SubQ: 5 mcg/kg/day days 7 to 14 (cycles 1 and 2)
[total dose/cycle = 40 mcg/kg]
Filgrastim: SubQ: 10 mcg/kg/day days 7 to 14 (cycle 3)
[total dose/cycle = 80 mcg/kg]
Repeat cycle every 2 weeks

Rituximab-CHOP

Use Lymphoma, non-Hodgkin

Regimen

Rituximab: I.V.: 375 mg/m^2 day 1
[total dose/cycle = 375 mg/m^2]
Cyclophosphamide: I.V.: 750 mg/m^2 day 1
[total dose/cycle = 750 mg/m^2]
Doxorubicin: I.V.: 50 mg/m^2 day 1
[total dose/cycle = 50 mg/m^2]
Vincristine: I.V.: 1.4 mg/m^2 (maximum dose: 2 mg) day 1
[total dose/cycle = 1.4 mg/m^2; maximum: 2 mg]

Prednisone: Oral: 40 mg/m^2/day days 1 to 5
[total dose/cycle = 200 mg/m^2]
Repeat cycle every 21 days

Stanford V Regimen

Use Lymphoma, Hodgkin disease

Regimen NOTE: Multiple variations are listed below.

Variation 1:
Mechlorethamine: I.V.: 6 mg/m^2 day 1
[total dose/cycle = 6 mg/m^2]
Doxorubicin: I.V.: 25 mg/m^2/day days 1 and 15
[total dose/cycle = 50 mg/m^2]
Vinblastine: I.V.: 6 mg/m^2/day days 1 and 15
[total dose/cycle = 12 mg/m^2]
Vincristine: I.V.: 1.4 mg/m^2/day (maximum dose: 2 mg) days 8 and 22
[total dose/cycle = 2.8 mg/m^2; maximum: 4 mg]
Bleomycin: I.V.: 5 units/m^2/day days 8 and 22
[total dose/cycle = 10 units/m^2]
Etoposide: I.V.: 60 mg/m^2/day days 15 and 16
[total dose/cycle = 120 mg/m^2]
Prednisone: Oral: 40 mg/m^2 every other day for 9 weeks
followed by tapering of dose by 10 mg every other day, beginning at week 10
Repeat cycle every 28 days for 3 cycles; **Note:** In cycle 3, for patients ≥50 years of age, decrease vinblastine dose to 4 mg/m^2/dose and decrease vincristine dose to 1 mg/m^2/dose

Variation 2:
Mechlorethamine: I.V.: 6 mg/m^2/dose weeks 1, 5, and 9
[total dose/cycle = 18 mg/m^2]
Doxorubicin: I.V.: 25 mg/m^2/dose weeks 1, 3, 5, 7, 9, and 11
[total dose/cycle = 150 mg/m^2]
Vinblastine: I.V.: 6 mg/m^2/dose weeks 1, 3, 5, 7, 9, and 11
[total dose/cycle = 36 mg/m^2]
Vincristine: I.V.: 1.4 mg/m^2/dose (maximum dose: 2 mg) weeks 2, 4, 6, 8, 10, and 12
[total dose/cycle = 8.4 mg/m^2; maximum: 12 mg]
Bleomycin: I.V.: 5 units/m^2/dose weeks 2, 4, 6, 8, 10, and 12
[total dose/cycle = 30 units/m^2]
Etoposide: I.V.: 60 mg/m^2/day for 2 consecutive days, weeks 3, 7, and 11
[total dose/cycle = 360 mg/m^2]
Prednisone: Oral: 40 mg/m^2 every other day for 10 weeks
[total dose prior to taper = 1400 mg/m^2]
followed by tapering of prednisone dose during weeks 11 and 12
Treatment cycle is 12 weeks

TAC

Use Breast cancer

Regimen NOTE: Multiple variations are listed below.

Variation 1:
Docetaxel: I.V.: 75 mg/m^2 day 1
[total dose/cycle = 75 mg/m^2]
Doxorubicin: I.V.: 50 mg/m^2 day 1
[total dose/cycle = 50 mg/m^2]
Cyclophosphamide: I.V.: 500 mg/m^2 day 1
[total dose/cycle = 500 mg/m^2]
Repeat cycle every 3 weeks

Variation 2:
Docetaxel: I.V.: 60 mg/m^2 day 1
[total dose/cycle = 60 mg/m^2]
Doxorubicin: I.V.: 60 mg/m^2 day 1
[total dose/cycle = 60 mg/m^2]
Cyclophosphamide: I.V.: 600 mg/m^2 day 1
[total dose/cycle = 600 mg/m^2]
Repeat cycle every 3 weeks

Tamoxifen-Epirubicin

Use Breast cancer

Regimen

Tamoxifen: Oral: 20 mg daily
[total dose/cycle = 560 mg]
Epirubicin: I.V.: 50 mg/m^2/day days 1 and 8
[total dose/cycle = 100 mg/m^2]
Repeat epirubicin cycle every 28 days for 6 cycles; continue tamoxifen for 4 years

Temozolomide-Rituximab (CNS Lymphoma)

Use Primary CNS lymphoma

Regimen NOTE: Multiple variations are listed.

Variation 1:
Combination therapy (cycles 1-4):
Rituximab: I.V.: 375 mg/m^2/dose day 1
[total dose/cycle = 375 mg/m^2]
Temozolomide: Oral: 150 mg/m^2/day days 1 to 5
[total dose/cycle = 750 mg/m^2]
Repeat cycle every 28 days for a total of 4 cycles
followed by
Maintenance therapy:
Temozolomide: Oral: 150 mg/m^2/day days 1 to 5
[total dose/cycle = 750 mg/m^2]
Repeat cycle every 28 days for a total of 8 cycles
Variation 2:
Combination therapy (cycles 1 and 2):
Rituximab: I.V.: 750 mg/m^2/dose days 1, 8, 15, and 22
[total dose/cycle = 3000 mg/m^2]
Temozolomide: Oral: 150 mg/m^2/day days 1 to 7
[total dose/cycle = 1050 mg/m^2]
Repeat cycle every 28 days for a total of 2 cycles
followed by
Maintenance therapy:
Temozolomide: Oral: 150 mg/m^2/day days 1 to 5
[total dose/cycle = 750 mg/m^2]
Repeat cycle every 28 days

TEX (Capecitabine + Docetaxel + Epirubicin)

Use Breast cancer

Regimen

Capecitabine: Oral: 1000 mg/m^2 twice daily days 1 to 14
[total dose/cycle = 28,000 mg/m^2]
Docetaxel: I.V.: 75 mg/m^2 day 1
[total dose/cycle = 75 mg/m^2]
Epirubicin: I.V.: 75 mg/m^2 day 1
[total dose/cycle = 75 mg/m^2]
Repeat cycle every 3 weeks

Thalidomide-Dexamethasone

Use Multiple myeloma

Regimen Note: Multiple variations are listed below.

Variation 1:
Thalidomide: Oral: 100 mg/day days 1 to 28
[total dose/cycle = 2800 mg]
Dexamethasone: Oral: 40 mg/day days 1 to 4
[total dose/cycle = 160 mg]
Repeat cycle every 28 days
Variation 2:
Thalidomide: Oral: 200 mg/day days 1 to 14 cycle 1
followed by Oral: 400 mg/day days 15 to 28 cycle 1
[total dose/cycle = 8400 mg]

Thalidomide: Oral: 400 mg/day days 1 to 28 (subsequent cycles)
[total dose/cycle = 11,200 mg]
Dexamethasone: Oral: 20 mg/m^2/day days 1 to 4, 9 to 12, and 17 to 20 cycle 1 (subsequent cycles)
[total dose/cycle = 240 mg/m^2]
followed by Oral: 20 mg/m^2/day days 1 to 4 (subsequent cycles)
[total dose/cycle = 80 mg/m^2]
Repeat cycle every 28 days

Variation 3:
Thalidomide: Oral: 100 mg/day days 1 to 7, 150 mg/day days 8 to 14, 200 mg/day days 15 to 21, 250 mg/day days 22 to 28, and 300 mg/day days 29 to 35 (cycle 1)
[total dose/cycle = 7000 mg]
Thalidomide: Oral: 300 mg/day days 1 to 35 (subsequent cycles)
[total dose/cycle = 10,500 mg]
Dexamethasone: Oral: 20 mg/m^2/day days 1 to 4, 9 to 12, and 17 to 20
[total dose/cycle = 240 mg/m^2]
Repeat cycle every 35 days

Variation 4:
Thalidomide: Oral: 200 mg/day days 1 to 28
[total dose/cycle = 5600 mg]
Dexamethasone: Oral: 40 mg/day days 1 to 4, 9 to 12, and 17 to 20 (odd cycles)
[total dose/cycle = 480 mg]
Dexamethasone: Oral: 40 mg/day days 1 to 4 (even cycles)
[total dose/cycle = 160 mg]
Repeat cycle every 28 days

Topotecan (Oral Regimen)

Use Lung cancer, nonsmall cell; Lung cancer, small cell; Ovarian cancer

Regimen

Topotecan: Oral: 2.3 mg/m^2/day days 1 to 5
[total dose/cycle = 11.5 mg/m^2]
Repeat cycle every 21 days

Topotecan (Oral)-Cisplatin

Use Lung cancer, small cell

Regimen

Topotecan: Oral: 1.7 mg/m^2/day days 1 to 5
[total dose/cycle = 8.5 mg/m^2]
Cisplatin: I.V.: 60 mg/m^2 day 5 only
[total dose/cycle = 60 mg/m^2]
Repeat cycle every 21 days for 4 cycles (or for 2 cycles beyond best response)

Topotecan (Weekly)

Use Lung cancer, small cell; Ovarian cancer

Regimen

Topotecan: I.V.: 4 mg/m^2/day days 1, 8, and 15
[total dose/cycle = 12 mg/m^2]
Repeat cycle every 28 days

Trastuzumab-Paclitaxel

Use Breast cancer

Regimen NOTE: Multiple variations are listed below.

Variation 1:
Cycle 1:
Paclitaxel: I.V.: 175 mg/m^2 day 1
[total dose/cycle = 175 mg/m^2]
Trastuzumab: I.V.: 4 mg/kg (loading dose) day 1
followed by I.V.: 2 mg/kg/day days 8 and 15
[total dose/cycle 1 = 8 mg/kg]
Treatment cycle is 21 days

Subsequent cycles:
Paclitaxel: I.V.: 175 mg/m^2 day 1
[total dose/cycle = 175 mg/m^2]
Trastuzumab: I.V.: 2 mg/kg/day days 1, 8, and 15
[total dose/cycle = 6 mg/kg]
Repeat cycle every 21 days for a total of at least 6 cycles

Variation 2:
Cycle 1:
Trastuzumab: I.V.: 4 mg/kg (loading dose) day 1
followed by I.V.: 2 mg/kg/day days 8 and 15
[total dose/cycle 1 = 8 mg/kg]
Paclitaxel: I.V.: 175 mg/m^2 day 2
[total dose/cycle = 175 mg/m^2]
Treatment cycle is 21 days
Subsequent cycles:
Trastuzumab: I.V.: 2 mg/kg/day days 1, 8, and 15
[total dose/cycle = 6 mg/kg]
Paclitaxel: I.V.: 175 mg/m^2 day 2
[total dose/cycle = 175 mg/m^2]
Repeat cycle every 21 days for a total of at least 6 cycles (continue weekly trastuzumab after chemotherapy until disease progression or unacceptable toxicity)

Trastuzumab-Paclitaxel-Carboplatin

Use Breast cancer

Regimen

Cycle 1:
Trastuzumab: I.V.: 4 mg/kg (loading dose) day 1
followed by I.V.: 2 mg/kg/day days 8 and 15
[total dose/cycle 1 = 8 mg/kg]
Paclitaxel: I.V.: 175 mg/m^2 day 2
[total dose/cycle = 175 mg/m^2]
Carboplatin: I.V.: AUC 6 day 2
[total dose/cycle = AUC = 6]
Treatment cycle is 21 days
Subsequent cycles:
Trastuzumab: I.V.: 2 mg/kg/day days 1, 8, and 15
[total dose/cycle = 6 mg/kg]
Paclitaxel: I.V.: 175 mg/m^2 day 2
[total dose/cycle = 175 mg/m^2]
Carboplatin: I.V.: AUC 6 day 2
[total dose/cycle = AUC = 6]
Repeat cycle every 21 days for a total of at least 6 cycles (continue weekly trastuzumab after chemotherapy until disease progression or unacceptable toxicity)

Trastuzumab-Paclitaxel (Weekly)

Use Breast cancer

Regimen NOTE: Multiple variations are listed below.

Variation 1:
Week 1:
Trastuzumab: I.V.: 4 mg/kg (loading dose) day 1
[total dose/week 1 = 4 mg/kg]
Paclitaxel: I.V.: 90 mg/m^2 day 2
[total dose/week 1 = 90 mg/m^2]
Subsequent weeks:
Paclitaxel: I.V.: 90 mg/m^2 day 1
[total dose/week = 90 mg/m^2]
Trastuzumab: I.V.: 2 mg/kg day 1
[total dose/week = 2 mg/kg]
Repeat weekly

Variation 2:
Week 1:
Trastuzumab: I.V.: 4 mg/kg (loading dose) day 1
[total dose/week 1 = 4 mg/kg]
Paclitaxel: I.V.: 80 mg/m^2 day 1
[total dose/week 1 = 80 mg/m^2]
Subsequent weeks:
Trastuzumab: I.V.: 2 mg/kg day 1
[total dose/week = 2 mg/kg]
Paclitaxel: I.V.: 80 mg/m^2 day 1
[total dose/week = 80 mg/m^2]
Repeat weekly

Tretinoin-Arsenic Trioxide (APL)

Use Leukemia, acute promyelocytic

Regimen

Induction (continue until <5% blasts in marrow and no abnormal promyelocytes):
Tretinoin: Oral: 45 mg/m^2/day (in 2 divided doses) day 1 up to day 85
[total induction dose = up to 3825 mg/m^2]
Arsenic Trioxide: I.V.: 0.15 mg/kg/day over 1 hour beginning day 10 up to day 85
[total induction dose = up to 11.25 mg/kg]
Postremission therapy (beginning with complete remission):
Tretinoin: Oral: 45 mg/m^2/day weeks 1, 2, 5, 6, 9, 10, 13, 14, 17, 18, 21, 22, 25, 26
[total postremission dose = 4410 mg/m^2]
Arsenic Trioxide: I.V.: 0.15 mg/kg/day Monday through Friday weeks 1 to 4, 9 to 12, 17 to 20, and 25 to 28
[total postremission dose = 12 mg/kg]

Tretinoin-Daunorubicin (APL)

Use Leukemia, acute promyelocytic

Regimen

Induction:
Tretinoin: Oral: 45 mg/m^2/day (in 2 divided doses) day 1 until hematologic complete remission
Daunorubicin: I.V.: 60 mg/m^2/day days 1, 2, and 3
[total dose/cycle = 180 mg/m^2]

Consolidation:
Course 1:
Daunorubicin: I.V.: 60 mg/m^2/day days 1, 2, and 3
[total dose/cycle = 180 mg/m^2]
Course 2:
Daunorubicin: I.V.: 45 mg/m^2/day days 1, 2, and 3
[total dose/cycle = 135 mg/m^2]

Maintenance:
Mercaptopurine: Oral: 90 mg/m^2 daily
[total dose/cycle = 8100 mg/m^2 (90 days)]
Methotrexate: Oral: 15 mg/m^2 weekly
[total dose/cycle = 180 mg/m^2]
Tretinoin: Oral: 45 mg/m^2/day (in 2 divided doses) days 1 to 15
[total dose/cycle = 675 mg/m^2]
Repeat cycle every 3 months for 2 years

Tretinoin-Daunorubicin-Cytarabine (APL)

Use Leukemia, acute promyelocytic

Regimen NOTE: Multiple variations are listed below.

Variation 1 (patients ≤60 years of age and WBC <10,000/mm^3):
Induction:
Tretinoin: Oral: 45 mg/m^2/day (in 2 divided doses) day 1 until hematologic complete remission
Daunorubicin: I.V.: 60 mg/m^2/day days 1, 2, and 3
[total dose/cycle = 180 mg/m^2]
Cytarabine: I.V.: 200 mg/m^2/day days 3 to 10
[total dose/cycle = 1400 mg/m^2]

Consolidation:
Course 1:
Daunorubicin: I.V.: 60 mg/m^2/day days 1, 2, and 3
[total dose/cycle = 180 mg/m^2]
Cytarabine: I.V.: 200 mg/m^2/day days 1 to 7
[total dose/cycle = 1400 mg/m^2]
Course 2:
Daunorubicin: I.V.: 45 mg/m^2/day days 1, 2, and 3
[total dose/cycle = 135 mg/m^2]
Cytarabine: I.V.: 1000 mg/m^2/dose every 12 hours for 8 doses
[total dose/cycle = 8000 mg/m^2]
Maintenance:
Mercaptopurine: Oral: 90 mg/m^2 daily
[total dose/cycle = 8100 mg/m^2 (90 days)]
Methotrexate: Oral: 15 mg/m^2 weekly
[total dose/cycle = 180 mg/m^2]
Tretinoin: Oral: 45 mg/m^2/day (in 2 divided doses) days 1 to 15
[total dose/cycle = 675 mg/m^2]
Repeat cycle every 3 months for 2 years
Variation 2 (patients ≤60 years of age and WBC ≥10,000/mm^3):
Induction:
Tretinoin: Oral: 45 mg/m^2/day (in 2 divided doses) day 1 until hematologic complete remission
Daunorubicin: I.V.: 60 mg/m^2/day days 1, 2, and 3
[total dose/cycle = 180 mg/m^2]
Cytarabine: I.V.: 200 mg/m^2/day days 3 to 10
[total dose/cycle = 1400 mg/m^2]
Consolidation:
Course 1:
Daunorubicin: I.V.: 60 mg/m^2/day days 1, 2, and 3
[total dose/cycle = 180 mg/m^2]
Cytarabine: I.V.: 200 mg/m^2/day days 1 to 7
[total dose/cycle = 1400 mg/m^2]
Course 2:
Daunorubicin: I.V.: 45 mg/m^2/day days 1, 2, and 3
[total dose/cycle = 135 mg/m^2]
Cytarabine: I.V.: 2000 mg/m^2/dose every 12 hours for 10 doses
[total dose/cycle = 20,000 mg/m^2]
Intrathecal prophylaxis: Five intrathecal injections: First dose in between induction and consolidation and 2 doses during each consolidation phase:
Methotrexate (preservative free): I.T.: 15 mg
Cytarabine (preservative free): I.T.: 50 mg
Corticosteroids (preservative free): I.T.: Dose unspecified
Maintenance:
Mercaptopurine: Oral: 90 mg/m^2 daily
[total dose/cycle = 8100 mg/m^2 (90 days)]
Methotrexate: Oral: 15 mg/m^2 weekly
[total dose/cycle = 180 mg/m^2]
Tretinoin: Oral: 45 mg/m^2/day (in 2 divided doses) days 1 to 15
[total dose/cycle = 675 mg/m^2]
Repeat cycle every 3 months for 2 years
Variation 3 (patients >60 years of age and WBC >10,000/mm^3):
Induction:
Tretinoin: Oral: 45 mg/m^2/day (in 2 divided doses) day 1 until hematologic complete remission
Daunorubicin: I.V.: 60 mg/m^2/day days 1, 2, and 3
[total dose/cycle = 180 mg/m^2]
Cytarabine: I.V.: 200 mg/m^2/day days 3 to 10
[total dose/cycle = 1400 mg/m^2]
Consolidation:
Course 1:
Daunorubicin: I.V.: 60 mg/m^2/day days 1, 2, and 3
[total dose/cycle = 180 mg/m^2]

Cytarabine: I.V.: 200 mg/m^2/day days 1 to 7
[total dose/cycle = 1400 mg/m^2]
Course 2:
Daunorubicin: I.V.: 45 mg/m^2/day days 1, 2, and 3
[total dose/cycle = 135 mg/m^2]
Cytarabine: I.V.: 1000 mg/m^2/dose every 12 hours for 8 doses
[total dose/cycle = 8,000 mg/m^2]

Intrathecal prophylaxis: Five intrathecal injections: First dose in between induction and consolidation and 2 doses during each consolidation phase:
Methotrexate (preservative free): I.T.: 15 mg
Cytarabine (preservative free): I.T.: 50 mg
Corticosteroids (preservative free): I.T.: Dose unspecified

Maintenance:
Mercaptopurine: Oral: 90 mg/m^2 daily
[total dose/cycle = 8100 mg/m^2 (90 days)]
Methotrexate: Oral: 15 mg/m^2 weekly
[total dose/cycle = 180 mg/m^2]
Tretinoin: Oral: 45 mg/m^2/day (in 2 divided doses) days 1 to 15
[total dose/cycle = 675 mg/m^2]
Repeat cycle every 3 months for 2 years

Tretinoin-Idarubicin (APL)

Use Leukemia, acute promyelocytic

Regimen NOTE: Multiple variations are listed below.

Variation 1:

Induction:
Tretinoin: Oral: 45 mg/m^2/day (in 2 divided doses) day 1 up to 90 days
[total dose/cycle = up to 4050 mg/m^2]
≤20 years: Oral: 25 mg/m^2/day (in 2 divided doses) day 1 up to 90 days
[total dose/cycle = up to 2250 mg/m^2]
Idarubicin: I.V.: 12 mg/m^2/day days 2, 4, 6, and 8 (omit day 8 for patients >70 years of age)
[total dose/cycle = 36-48 mg/m^2]

Consolidation (administer courses sequentially at 1-month intervals for 3 months):
Course 1:
Idarubicin: I.V.: 5 mg/m^2/day days 1 to 4
[total dose/cycle = 20 mg/m^2]
or
Idarubicin: I.V.: 7 mg/m^2/day days 1 to 4
[total dose/cycle = 28 mg/m^2]
Tretinoin: Oral: 45 mg/m^2/day (in 2 divided doses) days 1 to 15
[total dose/cycle = 675 mg/m^2]
Course 2:
Mitoxantrone: I.V.: 10 mg/m^2/day days 1 to 5
[total dose/cycle = 50 mg/m^2]
or
Mitoxantrone: I.V.: 10 mg/m^2/day days 1 to 5
[total dose/cycle = 50 mg/m^2]
Tretinoin: Oral: 45 mg/m^2/day (in 2 divided doses) days 1 to 15
[total dose/cycle = 675 mg/m^2]
Course 3:
Idarubicin: I.V.: 12 mg/m^2 day 1
[total dose/cycle = 12 mg/m^2]
or
Idarubicin: I.V.: 12 mg/m^2/day days 1 and 2
[total dose/cycle = 24 mg/m^2]
Tretinoin: Oral: 45 mg/m^2/day (in 2 divided doses) days 1 to 15
[total dose/cycle = 675 mg/m^2]

Maintenance:
Mercaptopurine: Oral: 50 mg/m^2 daily
[total dose/cycle = 4500 mg/m^2 (90 days)]
Methotrexate: I.M.: 15 mg/m^2 weekly
[total dose/cycle = 180 mg/m^2]

Tretinoin: Oral: 45 mg/m^2/day (in 2 divided doses) days 1 to 15
[total dose/cycle = 675 mg/m^2]
Repeat cycle every 3 months for 2 years

Variation 2:

Induction:

Tretinoin: Oral: 45 mg/m^2/day (in 2 divided doses) day 1 up to 90 days
[total dose/cycle = up to 4050 mg/m^2]
<15 years: Oral: 25 mg/m^2/day (in 2 divided doses) day 1 up to 90 days
[total dose/cycle = up to 2250 mg/m^2]
Idarubicin: I.V.: 12 mg/m^2/day days 2, 4, 6, and 8
[total dose/cycle = 48 mg/m^2]

Consolidation (administer courses sequentially at 1-month intervals for 3 months):

Course 1:
Idarubicin: I.V.: 5 mg/m^2/day days 1 to 4
[total dose/cycle = 20 mg/m^2]

Course 2:
Mitoxantrone: I.V.: 10 mg/m^2/day days 1 to 5
[total dose/cycle = 50 mg/m^2]

Course 3:
Idarubicin: I.V.: 12 mg/m^2 day 1
[total dose/cycle = 12 mg/m^2]

Maintenance:

Mercaptopurine: Oral: 90 mg/m^2 daily
[total dose/cycle = 8100 mg/m^2(90 days)]
Methotrexate: I.M.: 15 mg/m^2 weekly
[total dose/cycle = 180 mg/m^2]
Tretinoin: Oral: 45 mg/m^2/day (in 2 divided doses) days 1 to 15
[total dose/cycle = 675 mg/m^2]
Repeat cycle every 3 months for 2 years

Variation 3 (patients ≥60 years of age):

Induction:

Tretinoin: Oral: 45 mg/m^2/day (in 2 divided doses) day 1 up to 90 days
[total dose/cycle = up to 4050 mg/m^2]
Idarubicin: I.V.: 12 mg/m^2/day days 2, 4, 6, and 8 (omit day 8 for patients ≥70 years of age)
[total dose/cycle = 36-48 mg/m^2]

Consolidation (administer courses sequentially at 1-month intervals for 3 months):

Course 1:
Idarubicin: I.V.: 5 mg/m^2/day days 1 to 4
[total dose/cycle = 20 mg/m^2]
Tretinoin: Oral: 45 mg/m^2/day (in 2 divided doses) days 1 to 15 (if intermediate or high risk)
[total dose/cycle = 675 mg/m^2]

Course 2:
Mitoxantrone: I.V.: 10 mg/m^2/day days 1 to 5
[total dose/cycle = 50 mg/m^2]
Tretinoin: Oral: 45 mg/m^2/day (in 2 divided doses) days 1 to 15 (if intermediate or high risk)
[total dose/cycle = 675 mg/m^2]

Course 3:
Idarubicin: I.V.: 12 mg/m^2 day 1
[total dose/cycle = 12 mg/m^2]
Tretinoin: Oral: 45 mg/m^2/day (in 2 divided doses) days 1 to 15 (if intermediate or high risk)
[total dose/cycle = 675 mg/m^2]

Maintenance:

Mercaptopurine: Oral: 50 mg/m^2 daily
[total dose/cycle = 4500 mg/m^2 (90 days)]
Methotrexate: I.M.: 15 mg/m^2 weekly
[total dose/cycle = 180 mg/m^2]
Tretinoin: Oral: 45 mg/m^2/day (in 2 divided doses) days 1 to 15
[total dose/cycle = 675 mg/m^2]
Repeat cycle every 3 months for 2 years

TVTG

Use Leukemia, acute lymphocytic; Leukemia, acute myeloid

Regimen

Topotecan: I.V.: 1 mg/m^2/day continuous infusion days 1 to 5
[total dose/cycle = 5 mg/m^2]
Vinorelbine: I.V.: 20 mg/m^2/day days 0, 7, 14, and 21
[total dose/cycle = 80 mg/m^2]
Thiotepa: I.V.: 15 mg/m^2 day 2
Gemcitabine: I.V.: 3600 mg/m^2 day 7
Dexamethasone: Oral or I.V.: 45 mg/m^2/day days 7 to 14 (given in 3 divided doses)
[total dose/cycle = 315 mg/m^2]
Repeat cycle when ANC >500 cells/mm^3 and platelet count >75,000 cells/mm^3

VAC Alternating With IE (Ewing Sarcoma)

Use Ewing sarcoma

Regimen

Cycle A: (Odd numbered cycles)
Cyclophosphamide: I.V.: 1200 mg/m^2 day 1 (followed by mesna; dose not specified)
[total dose/cycle = 1200 mg/m^2]
Vincristine: I.V.: 2 mg/m^2 (maximum dose: 2 mg) day 1
[total dose/cycle = 2 mg/m^2; maximum: 2 mg]
Doxorubicin: I.V.: 75 mg/m^2 day 1, for 5 cycles (maximum cumulative dose: 375 mg/m^2)
[total dose/cycle = 75 mg/m^2; maximum cumulative dose: 375 mg/m^2]
Dactinomycin: I.V.: 1.25 mg/m^2 day 1, begin cycle 11 (after reaching maximum cumulative doxorubicin dose)
[total dose/cycle = 1.25 mg/m^2]
Cycle B: (Even numbered cycles)
Ifosfamide: I.V.: 1800 mg/m^2/day days 1 to 5 (given with mesna)
[total dose/cycle = 9000 mg/m^2]
Etoposide: I.V.: 100 mg/m^2/day days 1 to 5
[total dose/cycle = 500 mg/m^2]
Alternate Cycles A and B, administering a cycle every 3 weeks (alternating in the following sequence: ABABAB) for 17 cycles

VAC Pulse

Use Rhabdomyosarcoma

Regimen

Vincristine: I.V.: 2 mg/m^2/dose (maximum dose: 2 mg/dose) every 7 days, for 12 weeks
Dactinomycin: I.V.: 0.015 mg/kg/day (maximum dose: 0.5 mg/day) days 1 to 5, every 3 months for 5 courses
Cyclophosphamide: Oral, I.V.: 10 mg/kg/day for 7 days, repeat every 6 weeks

VAC (Rhabdomyosarcoma)

Use Rhabdomyosarcoma

Regimen

Induction (weeks 1 to 17):
Vincristine: I.V. push: 1.5 mg/m^2 (maximum dose: 2 mg) day 1 of weeks 1 to 13, then one dose at week 17
Dactinomycin: I.V. push: 0.015 mg/kg/day (maximum dose: 0.5 mg) days 1 to 5 of weeks 1, 4, 7, and 17
Cyclophosphamide: I.V.: 2.2 g/m^2 day 1 of weeks 1, 4, 7, 10, 13, and 17
Continuation (weeks 21 to 44):
Vincristine: I.V. push: 1.5 mg/m^2 (maximum dose: 2 mg) day 1 of weeks 21 to 26, 30 to 35, and 39 to 44
Dactinomycin: I.V. push: 0.015 mg/kg/day (maximum dose: 0.5 mg) days 1 to 5 of weeks 21, 24, 30, 33, 39, and 42
Cyclophosphamide: I.V.: 2.2 g/m^2 day 1 of weeks 21, 24, 30, 33, 39, and 42

VAD

Use Multiple myeloma

Regimen

Vincristine: I.V.: 0.4 mg/day continuous infusion days 1 to 4
[total dose/cycle = 1.6 mg]
Doxorubicin: I.V.: 9 mg/m^2/day continuous infusion days 1 to 4
[total dose/cycle = 36 mg/m^2]
Dexamethasone: Oral: 40 mg/day days 1 to 4, 9 to 12, and 17 to 20
[total dose/cycle = 480 mg]
Repeat cycle every 28-35 days

VAD/CVAD

Use Leukemia, acute lymphocytic

Regimen Induction cycle:

Vincristine: I.V.: 0.4 mg/day continuous infusion days 1 to 4 and 24 to 27
[total dose/cycle = 3.2 mg]
Doxorubicin: I.V.: 12 mg/m^2/day continuous infusion days 1 to 4 and 24 to 27
[total dose/cycle = 96 mg/m^2]
Dexamethasone: Oral: 40 mg/day days 1 to 4, 9 to 12, 17 to 20, 24 to 27, 32 to 35, and 40 to 43
[total dose/cycle = 960 mg]
Cyclophosphamide: I.V.: 1 g/m^2 day 24
[total dose/cycle = 1 g/m^2]
Administer one cycle only

VBAP

Use Multiple myeloma

Regimen

Vincristine: I.V.: 1 mg day 1
[total dose/cycle = 1 mg]
Carmustine: I.V.: 30 mg/m^2 day 1
[total dose/cycle = 30 mg/m^2]
Doxorubicin: I.V.: 30 mg/m^2 day 1
[total dose/cycle = 30 mg/m^2]
Prednisone: Oral: 100 mg/day days 1 to 4
[total dose/cycle = 400 mg]
Repeat cycle every 21 days

VBMCP

Use Multiple myeloma

Regimen

Vincristine: I.V.: 1.2 mg/m^2 (maximum dose: 2 mg) day 1
[total dose/cycle = 1.2 mg/m^2; maximum: 2 mg]
Carmustine: I.V.: 20 mg/m^2 day 1
[total dose/cycle = 20 mg/m^2]
Melphalan: Oral: 8 mg/m^2/day days 1 to 4
[total dose/cycle = 32 mg/m^2]
Cyclophosphamide: I.V.: 400 mg/m^2 day 1
[total dose/cycle = 400 mg/m^2]
Prednisone: Oral: 40 mg/m^2/day days 1 to 7 (all cycles)
[total dose/cycle = 280 mg/m^2]
followed by Oral: 20 mg/m^2/day days 8 to 14 (first 3 cycles only)
[total dose/cycle = 140 mg/m^2]
Repeat cycle every 35 days

VBP

Use Testicular cancer

Regimen

Vinblastine: I.V.: 0.15 mg/kg/day days 1 and 2
[total dose/cycle = 0.3 mg/kg]

Bleomycin: I.V.: 30 units/day days 2, 9, and 16
[total dose/cycle = 90 units]
Cisplatin: I.V.: 20 mg/m^2/day days 1 to 5
[total dose/cycle = 100 mg/m^2]
Repeat cycle every 21 days for 4 cycles

VCAP

Use Multiple myeloma

Regimen

Vincristine: I.V.: 1 mg/m^2 (maximum dose: 1.5 mg) day 1
[total dose/cycle = 1 mg/m^2]
Cyclophosphamide: Oral: 125 mg/m^2/day days 1 to 4
[total dose/cycle = 500 mg/m^2]
Doxorubicin: I.V.: 30 mg/m^2 day 1
[total dose/cycle = 30 mg/m^2]
Prednisone: Oral: 60 mg/m^2/day days 1 to 4
[total dose/cycle = 240 mg/m^2]
Repeat cycle every 21 days for 6-12 months

VDA-C (Wilms Tumor)

Use Wilms tumor

Regimen

Dactinomycin: I.V.: 15 mcg/kg/day days 1 to 5 of weeks 0, 13, 26, 39, 52, and 65
[total dose/cycle = 450 mcg/kg]
Cyclophosphamide: I.V.: 10 mg/kg/day days 1, 2, and 3 of weeks 6, 13, 19, 26, 32, 39, 45, 52, 58, and 65
[total dose/cycle = 300 mg/kg]
Doxorubicin: I.V.: 20 mg/m^2/day days 1, 2, and 3 of weeks 6, 19, 32, 45, and 58
[total dose/cycle = 300 mg/m^2]
Vincristine: I.V.: 1.5 mg/m^2 day 1 of weeks 1-10, 13, 14, 19, 20, 26, 27, 32, 33, 39, 40, 45, 46, 52, 53, 58, 59, 65, and 66
[total dose/cycle = 42 mg/m^2]

VIM-D (Hodgkin Lymphoma)

Use Lymphoma, Hodgkin disease

Regimen

Cycle 1:
Etoposide: I.V.: 100 mg/m^2 day 1
[total dose/cycle = 100 mg/m^2]
Ifosfamide: I.V.: 4 g/m^2 continuous infusion over 24 hours day 1
[total dose/cycle = 4 g/m^2]
Mesna: I.V.: 1 g/m^2 bolus day 1, followed by 6 g/m^2 continuous infusion over 36 hours
[total dose/cycle = 7 g/m^2]
Mitoxantrone: I.V.: 10 mg/m^2 day 1
[total dose/cycle = 10 mg/m^2]
Dexamethasone: Oral: 40 mg/day days 1 to 5
[total dose/cycle = 200 mg]
Treatment cycle is 28 days

Cycle 2 and subsequent cycles (if mid-cycle neutrophil count >1500/mm^3; if not, continue with cycle 1 regimen):
Etoposide: I.V.: 100 mg/m^2/day days 1 and 2
[total dose/cycle = 200 mg/m^2]
Ifosfamide: I.V.: 4 g/m^2 continuous infusion over 24 hours day 1
[total dose/cycle = 4 g/m^2]
Mesna: I.V.: 1 g/m^2 bolus day 1, followed by 6 g/m^2 continuous infusion over 36 hours
[total dose/cycle = 7 g/m^2]
Mitoxantrone: I.V.: 10 mg/m^2 day 1
[total dose/cycle = 10 mg/m^2]
Dexamethasone: Oral: 40 mg/day days 1 to 5
[total dose/cycle = 200 mg]
Repeat cycle every 28 days for up to 6 cycles

Vincristine-Dactinomycin-Cyclophosphamide (Ovarian Cancer)

Use Ovarian cancer (germ cell tumor)

Regimen NOTE: Multiple variations are listed below.

Variation 1:
- Vincristine: I.V.: 1.5 mg/m^2 (maximum dose: 2 mg) days 1, 8, 15, and 22 for 2-3 cycles
  [total dose/cycle = 6 mg/m^2 (maximum: 8 mg)] for 2-3 cycles
- Dactinomycin: I.V.: 300 mcg/m^2/day days 1 to 5
  [total dose/cycle = 1500 mcg/m^2]
- Cyclophosphamide: I.V.: 150 mg/m^2/day days 1 to 5
  [total dose/cycle = 750 mg/m^2]
- Repeat cycle every 4 weeks for at least 10 cycles; vincristine is only administered for 8-12 weeks

Variation 2:
- Vincristine: I.V.: 1-1.5 mg/m^2 day 1
  [total dose/cycle = 1-1.5 mg/m^2]
- Dactinomycin: I.V.: 500 mcg/day days 1 to 5
  [total dose/cycle = 2500 mcg]
- Cyclophosphamide: I.V.: 5-7 mg/kg/day days 1 to 5
  [total dose/cycle = 25-35 mg/kg]
- Repeat cycle every 4 weeks for up to 12 cycles

Vinorelbine-Cisplatin

Use Lung cancer, nonsmall cell

Regimen NOTE: Multiple variations are listed below.

Variation 1:
- Cisplatin: I.V.: 50 mg/m^2/day days 1 and 8
  [total dose/cycle = 100 mg/m^2]
- Vinorelbine: I.V.: 25 mg/m^2/day days 1, 8, 15, and 22
  [total dose/cycle = 100 mg/m^2]
- Repeat cycle every 28 days for total of 4 cycles

Variation 2:
- Vinorelbine: I.V.: 25 mg/m^2/day days 1, 8, 15, and 22
  [total dose/cycle = 100 mg/m^2]
- Cisplatin: I.V.: 100 mg/m^2 day 1
  [total dose/cycle = 100 mg/m^2]
- Repeat cycle every 28 days

Variation 3:
- Vinorelbine: I.V.: 30 mg/m^2 weekly
- Cisplatin: I.V.: 120 mg/m^2/day days 1 and 29, then once every 6 weeks

Variation 4:
- Vinorelbine: I.V.: 30 mg/m^2/day days 1, 8, and 15
  [total dose/cycle = 90 mg/m^2]
- Cisplatin: I.V.: 80 mg/m^2 day 1
  [total dose/cycle = 80 mg/m^2]
- Repeat cycle every 21 days for total of 4 cycles
- **Note:** Vinorelbine treatment is discontinued after day 1 of cycle 4

Variation 5:
- Vinorelbine: I.V.: 30 mg/m^2/day days 1, 8, 15, and 22
  [total dose/cycle = 120 mg/m^2]
- Cisplatin: I.V.: 100 mg/m^2 day 1
  [total dose/cycle = 100 mg/m^2]
- Repeat cycle every 28 days for total of 3 or 4 cycles
- **Note:** Vinorelbine treatment is discontinued after day 1 of last treatment cycle

Vinorelbine-FEC

Use Breast cancer

Regimen

Cycles 1 and 2:
- Vinorelbine: I.V.: 25 mg/m^2/day days 1, 8, and 15
  [total dose/cycle = 75 mg/m^2]
- Treatment cycle is 21 days

Cycle 3:
Vinorelbine: I.V.: 25 mg/m^2/day days 1 and 8
[total dose/cycle 3 = 50 mg/m^2]
Treatment cycle is 21 days
Cycles 4, 5, and 6 (FEC):
Fluorouracil: I.V.: 600 mg/m^2 day 1
[total dose/cycle = 600 mg/m^2]
Epirubicin: I.V.: 60 mg/m^2 day 1
[total dose/cycle = 60 mg/m^2]
Cyclophosphamide: I.V.: 600 mg/m^2 day 1
[total dose/cycle = 600 mg/m^2]
Repeat FEC cycle every 21 days for total of 3 cycles

Vinorelbine-Gemcitabine

Use Lung cancer, nonsmall cell

Regimen

Vinorelbine: I.V.: 20 mg/m^2/day days 1, 8, and 15
[total dose/cycle = 60 mg/m^2]
Gemcitabine: I.V.: 800 mg/m^2/day days 1, 8, and 15
[total dose/cycle = 2400 mg/m^2]
Repeat cycle every 28 days

Vinorelbine-Trastuzumab

Use Breast cancer

Regimen

Week 1:
Trastuzumab: I.V.: 4 mg/kg (loading dose) day 1 week 1
[total dose/week 1 = 4 mg/kg]
Vinorelbine: I.V.: 25 mg/m^2 day 1
[total dose/week 1 = 25 mg/m^2]
Subsequent weeks:
Trastuzumab: I.V.: 2 mg/kg (loading dose) day 1
[total dose/week = 2 mg/kg]
Vinorelbine: I.V.: 25 mg/m^2 day 1
[total dose/week = 25 mg/m^2]
Repeat weekly

Vinorelbine-Trastuzumab-FEC

Use Breast cancer

Regimen

Cycle 1:
Trastuzumab: I.V.: 4 mg/kg (loading dose) day 1 cycle 1
followed by I.V.: 2 mg/kg/day days 8 and 15 cycle 1
[total dose/cycle 1 = 8 mg/kg]
Vinorelbine: I.V.: 25 mg/m^2/day days 1, 8, and 15
[total dose/cycle 1 = 75 mg/m^2]
Treatment cycle is 21 days
Cycle 2:
Trastuzumab: I.V.: 2 mg/kg/day days 1, 8, and 15
[total dose/cycle = 6 mg/kg]
Vinorelbine: I.V.: 25 mg/m^2/day days 1, 8, and 15
[total dose/cycle 2 = 75 mg/m^2]
Treatment cycle is 21 days
Cycle 3:
Trastuzumab: I.V.: 2 mg/kg/day days 1, 8, and 15
[total dose/cycle = 6 mg/kg]
Vinorelbine: I.V.: 25 mg/m^2/day days 1 and 8
[total dose/cycle 3 = 50 mg/m^2]
Treatment cycle is 21 days

Cycles 4, 5, and 6 (FEC):
Fluorouracil: I.V.: 600 mg/m^2 day 1
[total dose/cycle = 600 mg/m^2]
Epirubicin: I.V.: 60 mg/m^2 day 1
[total dose/cycle = 60 mg/m^2]
Cyclophosphamide: I.V.: 600 mg/m^2 day 1
[total dose/cycle = 600 mg/m^2]
Repeat FEC cycle every 21 days for total of 3 cycles

VIP (Etoposide) (Testicular Cancer)

Use Testicular cancer

Regimen NOTE: Multiple variations are listed below.

Variation 1:
Etoposide: I.V.: 75 mg/m^2/day days 1 to 5
[total dose/cycle = 375 mg/m^2]
Ifosfamide: I.V.: 1200 mg/m^2/day days 1 to 5
[total dose/cycle = 6000 mg/m^2]
Cisplatin: I.V.: 20 mg/m^2/day days 1 to 5
[total dose/cycle = 100 mg/m^2]
Mesna: I.V.: 400 mg day 1 only
followed by I.V.: 1200 mg/day continuous infusion days 1 to 5
[total dose/cycle = 6400 mg]
Repeat cycle every 21 days for 4 cycles

Variation 2:
Etoposide: I.V.: 100 mg/m^2/day days 1 to 5
[total dose/cycle = 500 mg/m^2]
Ifosfamide: I.V.: 1200 mg/m^2/day days 1 to 5
[total dose/cycle = 6000 mg/m^2]
Cisplatin: I.V.: 20 mg/m^2/day days 1 to 5
[total dose/cycle = 100 mg/m^2]
Mesna: I.V.: 200 mg/m^2 every 4 hours, for 3 doses each day, days 1, 2, and 3
[total dose/cycle = 1800 mg/m^2]
Repeat cycle every 21 days

Variation 3:
Ifosfamide: I.V.: 2500 mg/m^2/day days 1 and 2
[total dose/cycle = 5000 mg/m^2]
Mesna: I.V.: 2400 mg/m^2/day days 1 and 2
[total dose/cycle = 4800 mg/m^2]
Etoposide: I.V.: 100 mg/m^2/day days 3, 4, and 5
[total dose/cycle = 300 mg/m^2]
Cisplatin: I.V.: 40 mg/m^2/day days 3, 4, and 5
[total dose/cycle = 120 mg/m^2]
Repeat cycle every 21 days

Variation 4:
Etoposide: I.V.: 75 mg/m^2/day days 1 to 5
[total dose/cycle = 375 mg/m^2]
Ifosfamide: I.V.: 1200 mg/m^2/day days 1 to 5
[total dose/cycle = 6000 mg/m^2]
Cisplatin: I.V.: 20 mg/m^2/day days 1 to 5
[total dose/cycle = 100 mg/m^2]
Mesna: I.V.: 120 mg/m^2 day 1 only
followed by I.V.: 1200 mg/m^2/day continuous infusion days 1 to 5
[total dose/cycle = 6120 mg/m^2]
Repeat cycle every 21 days for 4 cycles

VIP (Small Cell Lung Cancer)

Use Lung cancer, small cell

Regimen

Etoposide: I.V.: 75 mg/m^2/day days 1 to 4
[total dose/cycle = 300 mg/m^2]
Ifosfamide: I.V.: 1200 mg/m^2/day days 1 to 4
[total dose/cycle = 4800 mg/m^2]
Cisplatin: I.V.: 20 mg/m^2/day days 1 to 4
[total dose/cycle = 80 mg/m^2]
Mesna: I.V.: 300 mg/m^2 day 1 only
followed by I.V.: 1200 mg/m^2/day continuous infusion days 1 to 4
[total dose/cycle = 5100 mg/m^2]
Repeat cycle every 21 days

VIP (Vinblastine) (Testicular Cancer)

Use Testicular cancer

Regimen NOTE: Multiple variations are listed below.

Variation 1:
Vinblastine: I.V.: 0.11 mg/kg/day days 1 and 2
[total dose/cycle = 0.22 mg/kg]
Ifosfamide: I.V.: 1200 mg/m^2/day days 1 to 5
[total dose/cycle = 6000 mg/m^2]
Cisplatin: I.V.: 20 mg/m^2/day days 1 to 5
[total dose/cycle = 100 mg/m^2]
Mesna: I.V.: 400 mg day 1
followed by I.V.: 1200 mg/day continuous infusion days 1 to 5
[total dose/cycle = 6400 mg]
Repeat cycle every 21 days for 4 cycles

Variation 2:
Vinblastine: I.V.: 6 mg/m^2/day days 1 and 2
[total dose/cycle = 12 mg/m^2]
Ifosfamide: I.V.: 1500 mg/m^2/day days 1 to 5
[total dose/cycle = 7500 mg/m^2]
Cisplatin: I.V.: 20 mg/m^2/day days 1 to 5
[total dose/cycle = 100 mg/m^2]
Mesna: I.V.: 300 mg/m^2 3 times/day days 1 to 5
[total dose/cycle = 4500 mg/m^2]
Repeat cycle every 21 days for 4 cycles

VM

Use Breast cancer

Regimen

Variation 1:
Mitomycin: I.V.: 10 mg/m^2 days 1 and 28 for 2 cycles
[total dose/cycle = 20 mg/m^2]
followed by I.V.: 10 mg/m^2 day 1 only for subsequent cycles
[total dose/cycle = 10 mg/m^2]
Vinblastine: I.V.: 5 mg/m^2/day days 1, 14, 28, and 42 for 2 cycles
[total dose/cycle = 20 mg/m^2]
followed by I.V.: 5 mg/m^2/day days 1 and 21
[total dose/cycle = 10 mg/m^2]
Repeat cycle every 6-8 weeks

Variation 2:

Mitomycin: I.V.: 10 mg/m^2/day days 1 and 28 for 2 cycles
[total dose/cycle = 20 mg/m^2]
followed by I.V.: 10 mg/m^2 day 1 only for subsequent cycles
[total dose/cycle = 10 mg/m^2]

Vindesine: I.V.: 2 mg/m^2/day days 1, 14, 28, and 42 for 2 cycles
[total dose/cycle = 8 mg/m^2]
followed by I.V.: 2 mg/m^2/ day days 1 and 21 for subsequent cycles
[total dose/cycle = 4 mg/m^2]

Repeat cycle every 6-8 weeks

VP (Small Cell Lung Cancer)

Use Lung cancer, small cell

Regimen

Etoposide: I.V.: 100 mg/m^2/day days 1 to 4
[total dose/cycle = 400 mg/m^2]

Cisplatin: I.V.: 20 mg/m^2/day days 1 to 4
[total dose/cycle = 80 mg/m^2]

Repeat cycle every 21 days

CHEMOTHERAPY REGIMEN INDEX

BRAIN TUMORS

Neuroblastoma

Primary CNS Lymphoma

BREAST CANCER

GASTROINTESTINAL

Anal Cancer

Biliary Adenocarcinoma

Colorectal Cancer

Esophageal Cancer

Gastric Cancer

Hepatoblastoma

Pancreatic Cancer

GENITOURINARY

Bladder Cancer

Prostate Cancer

Renal Cell Cancer

Testicular Cancer

Wilms Tumor

GYNECOLOGIC

Cervical Cancer

Endometrial Cancer

Gestational Trophoblastic Tumor

Ovarian Cancer

HEAD AND NECK CANCER

HEMATOLOGIC/LEUKEMIA

Leukemia, Acute Lymphocytic

Leukemia, Acute Myeloid

Leukemia, Acute Promyelocytic

Leukemia, Chronic Lymphocytic

Leukemia, Chronic Myelogenous

LUNG CANCER

Nonsmall Cell Cancer

MYELODYSPLASTIC SYNDROME

RETINOBLASTOMA

SARCOMA

Osteosarcoma

Rhabdomyosarcoma

Soft Tissue Sarcoma

UNKNOWN PRIMARY (ADENOCARCINOMA)

UNKNOWN PRIMARY (SQUAMOUS CELL)

APPENDIX TABLE OF CONTENTS

Visit thePoint http://thepoint.lww.com/QL2011 for exclusive access to:

- Apothecary/Metric Conversions
- Pounds/Kilograms Conversion
- Temperature Conversion
- Pharmaceutical Manufacturers and Distributors
- Multivitamin Products

Refer to the inside front cover of this book for your online access code.

ABBREVIATIONS & SYMBOLS COMMONLY USED IN MEDICAL ORDERS

Abbreviations Which May Be Used in This Reference

Abbreviation	Meaning
5-HT	5-hydroxytryptamine
AAP	American Academy of Pediatrics
ABG	arterial blood gases
ABW	adjusted body weight
AACT	American Academy of Clinical Toxicology
ACC	American College of Cardiology
ACE	angiotensin converting enzyme
ACLS	advanced cardiac life support
ACOG	American College of Obstetricians and Gynecologists
ACTH	adrenocorticotrophic hormone
ADH	alcohol dehydrogenase
ADHD	attention-deficit/hyperactivity disorder
ADLs	activities of daily living
AED	antiepileptic drug
AHA	American Heart Association
AIDS	acquired immune deficiency syndrome
AIMS	Abnormal Involuntary Movement Scale
ALS	amyotrophic lateral sclerosis
ALT	alanine aminotransferase
AMA	American Medical Association
ANC	absolute neutrophil count
aPTT	activated partial thromboplastin
ARB	angiotensin receptor blocker
ARDS	acute respiratory distress syndrome
AST	aspartate aminotransferase
AUC	area under the curve
BDI	Beck Depression Inventory
BEC	blood ethanol concentration
BLS	basic life support
BMI	body mass index
BMT	bone marrow transplant
BP	blood pressure
BPH	benign prostatic hyperplasia
BPRS	Brief Psychiatric Rating Scale
BSA	body surface area
BUN	blood urea nitrogen
CABG	coronary artery bypass graft
CAD	coronary artery disease
CAN	Canadian

Abbreviations Which May Be Used in This Reference *(continued)*

Abbreviation	Meaning
CAPD	continuous ambulatory peritoneal dialysis
CAS	chemical abstract service
CBC	complete blood count
CBT	cognitive behavioral therapy
Cl_{cr}	creatinine clearance
CDC	Centers for Disease Control and Prevention
CF	cystic fibrosis
CGI	Clinical Global Impression
CHD	coronary heart disease
CHF	congestive heart failure; chronic heart failure
CIE	chemotherapy-induced emesis
C-II	schedule two controlled substance
C-III	schedule three controlled substance
C-IV	schedule four controlled substance
C-V	schedule five controlled substance
CIV	continuous I.V. infusion
C_{max}	maximum plasma concentration
C_{min}	minimum plasma concentration
CMV	cytomegalovirus
CNS	central nervous system or coagulase negative staphylococcus
COLD	chronic obstructive lung disease
COPD	chronic obstructive pulmonary disease
COX	cyclooxygenase
CPK	creatine phosphokinase
CRF	chronic renal failure
CRP	C-reactive protein
CRRT	continuous renal replacement therapy
CSF	cerebrospinal fluid
CSII	continuous subcutaneous insulin infusion
CT	computed tomography
CVA	cerebrovascular accident
CVVH	continuous venovenous hemofiltration
CVVHD	continuous venovenous hemodialysis
CVVHDF	continuous venovenous hemodiafiltration
CYP	cytochrome
D_5W	dextrose 5% in water
DBP	diastolic blood pressure
DEHP	di(3-ethylhexyl)phthalate
DIC	disseminated intravascular coagulation
DM	diabetes mellitus
DMARD	disease modifying antirheumatic drug
DSC	discontinued
DSM-IV	Diagnostic and Statistical Manual
DVT	deep vein thrombosis

Abbreviations Which May Be Used in This Reference *(continued)*

Abbreviation	Meaning
EBV	Epstein-Barr virus
ECG	electrocardiogram
ECMO	extracorporeal membrane oxygenation
ECT	electroconvulsive therapy
ED	emergency department
EEG	electroencephalogram
EF	ejection fraction
EG	ethylene glycol
EGA	estimated gestational age
EIA	enzyme immunoassay
ELISA	enzyme-linked immunosorbent assay
EPS	extrapyramidal side effects
ESR	erythrocyte sedimentation rate
ESRD	end stage renal disease
EtOH	alcohol
FDA	Food and Drug Administration
FTT	failure to thrive
GABA	gamma-aminobutyric acid
GAD	generalized anxiety disorder
GERD	gastroesophageal reflux disease
GFR	glomerular filtration rate
GGT	gamma-glutamyltransferase
GI	gastrointestinal
GU	genitourinary
GVHD	graft versus host disease
HAM-A	Hamilton Anxiety Scale
HAM-D	Hamilton Depression Scale
HDL	high density lipoprotein
HF	heart failure
HFSA	Heart Failure Society of America
HIV	human immunodeficiency virus
HMG-CoA	3-hydroxy-3-methylglutaryl-coenzyme A
HOCM	hypertrophic obstructive cardiomyopathy
HPA	hypothalamic-pituitary-adrenal
HSV	herpes simplex virus
HTN	hypertension
HUS	hemolytic uremic syndrome
IBD	inflammatory bowel disease
IBS	irritable bowel syndrome
IBW	ideal body weight
ICD	implantable cardioverter defibrillator
ICH	intracranial hemorrhage
ICP	intracranial pressure
IDDM	insulin dependent diabetes mellitus

Abbreviations Which May Be Used in This Reference *(continued)*

Abbreviation	Meaning
IDSA	Infectious Diseases Society of America
IHSS	idiopathic hypertrophic subaortic stenosis
I.M.	intramuscular
INR	international normalized ration
Int. unit	international unit
IOP	intraocular pressure
IUGR	intrauterine growth retardation
I.V.	intravenous
JIA	juvenile idiopathic arthritis
JNC	Joint National Committee
KIU	kallikrein inhibitor unit
LAMM	L-α-acetyl methadol
LDH	lactate dehydrogenase
LDL	low density lipoprotein
LFT	liver function test
LGA	large for gestational age
LR	lactated ringers
LVEF	left ventricular ejection fraction
LVH	left ventricular hypertrophy
MADRS	Montgomery Asbery Depression Rating Scale
MAOIs	monamine oxidase inhibitors
MDD	major depressive disorder
MDRD	modification of diet in renal disease
MDRSP	multidrug resistant *streptococcus pneumoniae*
mEq	milliequivalent
mg	milligram
MI	myocardial infarction
mL	milliliter
mm	millimeter
mM	millimolar
mm Hg	millimeters of mercury
MMSE	mini mental status examination
M/P	milk to plasma ratio
MPS I	mucopolysaccharidosis I
MRHD	maximum recommended human dose
MRI	magnetic resonance imaging
MUGA	multiple gated acquisition scan
NAS	neonatal abstinence syndrome
NF	National Formulary
NFD	Nephrogenic fibrosing dermopathy
ng	nanogram
NIDDM	Noninsulin dependent diabetes mellitus
NKA	no known allergies
NKDA	No known drug allergies

Abbreviations Which May Be Used in This Reference *(continued)*

Abbreviation	Meaning
NMDA	n-methyl-d-aspartic acid
NMS	neuroleptic malignant syndrome
NNRTI	nonnucleoside reverse transcriptase inhibitor
NRTI	nucleoside reverse transcriptase inhibitor
NS	normal saline
NSAID	nonsteroidal antiinflammatory drug
NSF	nephrogenic systemic fibrosis
NSTEMI	Non-ST-elevation myocardial infarction
OA	osteoarthritis
OCD	obsessive-compulsive disorder
OHSS	ovarian hyperstimulation syndrome
OTC	over-the-counter
PAT	paroxysmal atrial tachycardia
PD	Parkinson disease; peritoneal dialysis
PDA	patent ductus arteriosus
PDE-5	phosphodiesterase-5
PE	pulmonary embolus
PEG tube	percutaneous endoscopic gastrostomy tube
PHN	post-herpetic neuralgia
PID	pelvic inflammatory disease
PMDD	premenstrual dysphoric disorder
PONV	postoperative nausea and vomiting
PPN	peripheral parenteral nutrition
PROM	premature rupture of membranes
PSVT	paroxysmal supraventricular tachycardia
PT	prothrombin time
PTSD	post-traumatic stress disorder
PTT	partial thromboplastin time
PUD	peptic ulcer disease
PVD	peripheral vascular disease
QT_c	corrected QT interval
QT_c-F	corrected QT interval by Fredricia formula
RA	rheumatoid arthritis
REM	rapid eye movement
RPLS	reversible posterior leukoencephalopathy syndrome
SA	sinoatrial
SAD	seasonal affective disorder
SAH	subarachnoid hemorrhage
SBE	subacute bacterial endocarditis
SBP	systolic blood pressure
S_{Cr}	serum creatinine
SERM	selective estrogen receptor modulator
SGA	small for gestational age
SGOT	serum glutamic oxaloacetic aminotransferase

Abbreviations Which May Be Used in This Reference *(continued)*

Abbreviation	Meaning
SGPT	serum glutamic pyruvate transaminase
SI	International System of Units or Systeme international d'Unites
SIADH	syndrome of inappropriate antidiuretic hormone secretion
SLE	systemic lupus erythematosus
SNRI	serotonin norepinephrine reuptake inhibitor
SSKI	saturated solution of potassium iodide
SSRIs	selective serotonin reuptake inhibitors
STD	sexually transmitted disease
STEM I	ST-elevation myocardial infarction
SubQ	subcutaneous
supp	suppository
SVT	supraventricular tachycardia
SWFI	sterile water for injection
syr	syrup
$T_{1/2}$	half-life
tab	tablet
TB	tuberculosis
TC	total cholesterol
TCA	tricyclic antidepressant
TD	tardive dyskinesia
TG	triglyceride
TIA	transient ischemic attack
TMA	thrombotic microangiopathy
T_{max}	time to maximum observed concentration, plasma
TNF	Tumor necrosis factor
TPN	total parenteral nutrition
tr, tinct	tincture
tsp	teaspoonful
UC	ulcerative colitis
ULN	upper limits of normal
URI	upper respiratory infection
USAN	United States Adopted Names
USP	United States Pharmacopeia
UTI	urinary tract infection
UV	ultraviolet
V_d	volume of distribution
VEGF	vascular endothelial growth factor
VF	ventricular fibrillation
VT	ventricular tachycardia
VTE	venous thromboembolism
vWD	von Willebrand disease
VZV	varicella zoster virus
YBOC	Yale Brown Obsessive-Compulsive Scale
YMRS	Young Mania Rating Scale

ABBREVIATIONS & SYMBOLS COMMONLY USED IN MEDICAL ORDERS

Common Weights, Measures, or Apothecary Abbreviations

Abbreviation	Meaning
<[1]	less than
>[1]	greater than
≤	less than or equal to
≥	greater than or equal to
ac	before meals or food
ad	to, up to
ad lib	at pleasure
AM	morning
AMA	against medical advice
amp	ampul
amt	amount
aq	water
aq. dest.	distilled water
ASAP	as soon as possible
a.u.[1]	each ear
bid	twice daily
bm	bowel movement
C	Celsius, centigrade
cal	calorie
cap	capsule
cc[1]	cubic centimeter
cm	centimeter
comp	compound
cont	continue
d	day
d/c[1]	discharge
dil	dilute
disp	dispense
div	divide
dtd	give of such a dose
Dx	diagnosis
elix, el	elixir
emp	as directed
et	and
ex aq	in water
F	Fahrenheit
f, ft	make, let be made
g	gram
gr	grain
gtt	a drop
h	hour

Common Weights, Measures, or Apothecary Abbreviations *(continued)*

Abbreviation	Meaning
hs[1]	at bedtime
kcal	kilocalorie
kg	kilogram
L	liter
liq	a liquor, solution
M	molar
mcg	microgram
m. dict	as directed
mEq	milliequivalent
mg	milligram
microL	microliter
mL	milliliter
mm	millimeter
mM	millimolar
mm Hg	millimeters of mercury
ng	nanogram
no.	number
noc	in the night
non rep	do not repeat, no refills
NPO	nothing by mouth
NV	nausea and vomiting
O, Oct	a pint
o.d.[1]	right eye
o.l.	left eye
o.s.[1]	left eye
o.u.[1]	each eye, both eyes together
pc, post cib	after meals
PM	afternoon or evening
P.O.	by mouth
P.R.	rectally
prn	as needed
pulv	a powder
q	every
qad	every other day
qd[1,2]	every day, daily
qh	every hour
qid	four times a day
qod[1,2]	every other day
qs	a sufficient quantity
qs ad	a sufficient quantity to make
Rx	take, a recipe
SL	sublingual
stat	at once, immediately
SubQ	subcutaneous

Common Weights, Measures, or Apothecary Abbreviations *(continued)*

Abbreviation	Meaning
supp	suppository
syr	syrup
tab	tablet
tal	such
tid	three times a day
tr, tinct	tincture
trit	triturate
tsp	teaspoon
u.d.	as directed
ung	ointment
v.o.	verbal order
w.a.	while awake
x3	3 times
x4	4 times

[1]ISMP error-prone abbreviation.

[2]JCAHO Do Not Use list.

Additional abbreviations used and defined within a specific monograph or text piece may only apply to that text.

References

The Institute for Safe Medication Practices (ISMP) list of Error-Prone Abbreviations, Symbols, and Dose Designations. Available at: http://www.ismp.org/Tools/errorproneabbreviations.pdf.

The Joint Commission Official "Do Not Use" list. Available at: http://www.jointcommission.org/PatientSafety/DoNotUseList/.

NORMAL LABORATORY VALUES FOR ADULTS

CHEMISTRY

Test	Values	Remarks
Serum / Plasma		
Acetone	Negative	
Albumin	3.2-5 g/dL	
Alcohol, ethyl	Negative	
Aldolase	1.2-7.6 IU/L	
Ammonia	20-70 mcg/dL	Specimen to be placed on ice as soon as collected.
Amylase	30-110 units/L	
Bilirubin, direct	0-0.3 mg/dL	
Bilirubin, total	0.1-1.2 mg/dL	
Calcium	8.6-10.3 mg/dL	
Calcium, ionized	2.24-2.46 mEq/L	
Chloride	95-108 mEq/L	
Cholesterol, total	≤200 mg/dL	Fasted blood required – normal value affected by dietary habits. This reference range is for a general adult population.
HDL cholesterol	40-60 mg/dL	Fasted blood required – normal value affected by dietary habits.
LDL cholesterol	<160 mg/dL	If triglyceride is >400 mg/dL, LDL cannot be calculated accurately (Friedewald equation). Target LDL-C depends on patient's risk factors.
CO_2	23-30 mEq/L	
Creatine kinase (CK) isoenzymes		
CK-BB	0%	
CK-MB (cardiac)	0%-3.9%	
CK-MM (muscle)	96%-100%	
CK-MB levels must be both ≥4% and 10 IU/L to meet diagnostic criteria for CK-MB positive result consistent with myocardial injury.		
Creatine phosphokinase (CPK)	8-150 IU/L	
Creatinine	0.5-1.4 mg/dL	
Ferritin	13-300 ng/mL	
Folate	3.6-20 ng/dL	
GGT (gamma-glutamyltranspeptidase)		
male	11-63 IU/L	
female	8-35 IU/L	
GLDH	To be determined	
Glucose (preprandial)	<115 mg/dL	Goals different for diabetics.
Glucose, fasting	60-110 mg/dL	Goals different for diabetics.
Glucose, nonfasting (2-h postprandial)	<120 mg/dL	Goals different for diabetics.
Hemoglobin A_{1c}	<8	
Hemoglobin, plasma free	<2.5 mg/100 mL	
Hemoglobin, total glycosolated (Hb A_1)	4%-8%	
Iron	65-150 mcg/dL	
Iron binding capacity, total (TIBC)	250-420 mcg/dL	
Lactic acid	0.7-2.1 mEq/L	Specimen to be kept on ice and sent to lab as soon as possible.
Lactate dehydrogenase (LDH)	56-194 IU/L	

CHEMISTRY *(continued)*

Test	Values	Remarks
Lactate dehydrogenase (LDH) isoenzymes		
LD_1	20%-34%	
LD_2	29%-41%	
LD_3	15%-25%	
LD_4	1%-12%	
LD_5	1%-15%	
Flipped LD_1/LD_2 ratios (>1 may be consistent with myocardial injury) particularly when considered in combination with a recent CK-MB positive result.		
Lipase	23-208 units/L	
Magnesium	1.6-2.5 mg/dL	Increased by slight hemolysis.
Osmolality	289-308 mOsm/kg	
Phosphatase, alkaline		
adults 25-60 y	33-131 IU/L	
adults ≥61 y	51-153 IU/L	
infancy-adolescence	Values range up to 3-5 times higher than adults	
Phosphate, inorganic	2.8-4.2 mg/dL	
Potassium	3.5-5.2 mEq/L	Increased by slight hemolysis.
Prealbumin	>15 mg/dL	
Protein, total	6.5-7.9 g/dL	
AST	<35 IU/L (20-48)	
ALT (10-35)	<35 IU/L	
Sodium	134-149 mEq/L	
Thyroid stimulating hormone (TSH)		
adults ≤20 y	0.7-6.4 mIU/L	
21-54 y	0.4-4.2 mIU/L	
55-87 y	0.5-8.9 mIU/L	
Transferrin	>200 mg/dL	
Triglycerides	45-155 mg/dL	Fasted blood required.
Troponin I	<1.5 ng/mL	
Urea nitrogen (BUN)	7-20 mg/dL	
Uric acid		
male	2-8 mg/dL	
female	2-7.5 mg/dL	
Cerebrospinal Fluid		
Glucose	50-70 mg/dL	
Protein	15-45 mg/dL	CSF obtained by lumbar puncture.
Note: Bloody specimen gives erroneously high value due to contamination with blood proteins		
Urine (24-hour specimen is required for all these tests unless specified)		
Amylase	32-641 units/L	The value is in units/L and **not** calculated for total volume.
Amylase, fluid (random samples)		Interpretation of value left for physician, depends on the nature of fluid.
Calcium	Depends upon dietary intake	
Creatine		
male	150 mg/24 h	Higher value on children and during pregnancy.
female	250 mg/24 h	
Creatinine	1000-2000 mg/24 h	
Creatinine clearance (endogenous)		
male	85-125 mL/min	
female	75-115 mL/min	A blood sample must accompany urine specimen.

CHEMISTRY *(continued)*

Test	Values	Remarks
Glucose	1 g/24 h	
5-hydroxyindoleacetic acid	2-8 mg/24 h	
Iron	0.15 mg/24 h	Acid washed container required.
Magnesium	146-209 mg/24 h	
Osmolality	500-800 mOsm/kg	With normal fluid intake.
Oxalate	10-40 mg/24 h	
Phosphate	400-1300 mg/24 h	
Potassium	25-120 mEq/24 h	Varies with diet; the interpretation of urine electrolytes and osmolality should be left for the physician.
Sodium	40-220 mEq/24 h	
Porphobilinogen, qualitative	Negative	
Porphyrins, qualitative	Negative	
Proteins	0.05-0.1 g/24 h	
Salicylate	Negative	
Urea clearance	60-95 mL/min	A blood sample must accompany specimen.
Urea N	10-40 g/24 h	Dependent on protein intake.
Uric acid	250-750 mg/24 h	Dependent on diet and therapy.
Urobilinogen	0.5-3.5 mg/24 h	For qualitative determination on random urine, send sample to urinalysis section in Hematology Lab.
Xylose absorption test		
children	16%-33% of ingested xylose	
Feces		
Fat, 3-day collection	<5 g/d	Value depends on fat intake of 100 g/d for 3 days preceding and during collection.
Gastric Acidity		
Acidity, total, 12 h	10-60 mEq/L	Titrated at pH 7.

Blood Gases

	Arterial	Capillary	Venous
pH	7.35-7.45	7.35-7.45	7.32-7.42
pCO_2 (mm Hg)	35-45	35-45	38-52
pO_2 (mm Hg)	70-100	60-80	24-48
HCO_3 (mEq/L)	19-25	19-25	19-25
TCO_2 (mEq/L)	19-29	19-29	23-33
O_2 saturation (%)	90-95	90-95	40-70
Base excess (mEq/L)	-5 to +5	-5 to +5	-5 to +5

HEMATOLOGY

Complete Blood Count

Age	Hgb (g/dL)	Hct (%)	RBC (mill/mm^3)	RDW
0-3 d	15.0-20.0	45-61	4.0-5.9	<18
1-2 wk	12.5-18.5	39-57	3.6-5.5	<17
1-6 mo	10.0-13.0	29-42	3.1-4.3	<16.5
7 mo to 2 y	10.5-13.0	33-38	3.7-4.9	<16
2-5 y	11.5-13.0	34-39	3.9-5.0	<15
5-8 y	11.5-14.5	35-42	4.0-4.9	<15
13-18 y	12.0-15.2	36-47	4.5-5.1	<14.5
Adult male	13.5-16.5	41-50	4.5-5.5	<14.5
Adult female	12.0-15.0	36-44	4.0-4.9	<14.5

Age	MCV (fL)	MCH (pg)	MCHC (%)	Plts (x 10^3/mm^3)
0-3 d	95-115	31-37	29-37	250-450
1-2 wk	86-110	28-36	28-38	250-450
1-6 mo	74-96	25-35	30-36	300-700
7 mo to 2 y	70-84	23-30	31-37	250-600
2-5 y	75-87	24-30	31-37	250-550
5-8 y	77-95	25-33	31-37	250-550
13-18 y	78-96	25-35	31-37	150-450
Adult male	80-100	26-34	31-37	150-450
Adult female	80-100	26-34	31-37	150-450

WBC and Differential

Age	WBC (x 10^3/mm^3)	Segs	Bands	Lymphs	Monos
0-3 d	9.0-35.0	32-62	10-18	19-29	5-7
1-2 wk	5.0-20.0	14-34	6-14	36-45	6-10
1-6 mo	6.0-17.5	13-33	4-12	41-71	4-7
7 mo to 2 y	6.0-17.0	15-35	5-11	45-76	3-6
2-5 y	5.5-15.5	23-45	5-11	35-65	3-6
5-8 y	5.0-14.5	32-54	5-11	28-48	3-6
13-18 y	4.5-13.0	34-64	5-11	25-45	3-6
Adults	4.5-11.0	35-66	5-11	24-44	3-6

Age	Eosinophils	Basophils	Atypical Lymphs	No. of NRBCs
0-3 d	0-2	0-1	0-8	0-2
1-2 wk	0-2	0-1	0-8	0
1-6 mo	0-3	0-1	0-8	0
7 mo to 2 y	0-3	0-1	0-8	0
2-5 y	0-3	0-1	0-8	0
5-8 y	0-3	0-1	0-8	0
13-18 y	0-3	0-1	0-8	0
Adults	0-3	0-1	0-8	0

Segs = segmented neutrophils.

Bands = band neutrophils.

Lymphs = lymphocytes.

Monos = monocytes.

Erythrocyte Sedimentation Rates and Reticulocyte Counts

Sedimentation rate, Westergren	Children	0-20 mm/h
	Adult male	0-15 mm/h
	Adult female	0-20 mm/h
Sedimentation rate, Wintrobe	Children	0-13 mm/h
	Adult male	0-10 mm/h
	Adult female	0-15 mm/h
Reticulocyte count	Newborns	2%-6%
	1-6 mo	0%-2.8%
	Adults	0.5%-1.5%

NORMAL LABORATORY VALUES FOR CHILDREN

		Normal Values
CHEMISTRY		
Albumin	0-1 y	2-4 g/dL
	1 y to adult	3.5-5.5 g/dL
Ammonia	Newborns	90-150 mcg/dL
	Children	40-120 mcg/dL
	Adults	18-54 mcg/dL
Amylase	Newborns	0-60 units/L
	Adults	30-110 units/L
Bilirubin, conjugated, direct	Newborns	<1.5 mg/dL
	1 mo to adult	0-0.5 mg/dL
Bilirubin, total	0-3 d	2-10 mg/dL
	1 mo to adult	0-1.5 mg/dL
Bilirubin, unconjugated, indirect		0.6-10.5 mg/dL
Calcium	Newborns	7-12 mg/dL
	0-2 y	8.8-11.2 mg/dL
	2 y to adult	9-11 mg/dL
Calcium, ionized, whole blood		4.4-5.4 mg/dL
Carbon dioxide, total		23-33 mEq/L
Chloride		95-105 mEq/L
Cholesterol	Newborns	45-170 mg/dL
	0-1 y	65-175 mg/dL
	1-20 y	120-230 mg/dL
Creatinine	0-1 y	≤0.6 mg/dL
	1 y to adult	0.5-1.5 mg/dL
Glucose	Newborns	30-90 mg/dL
	0-2 y	60-105 mg/dL
	Children to Adults	70-110 mg/dL
Iron		
	Newborns	110-270 mcg/dL
	Infants	30-70 mcg/dL
	Children	55-120 mcg/dL
	Adults	70-180 mcg/dL
Iron binding	Newborns	59-175 mcg/dL
	Infants	100-400 mcg/dL
	Adults	250-400 mcg/dL
Lactic acid, lactate		2-20 mg/dL
Lead, whole blood		<10 mcg/dL
Lipase		
	Children	20-140 units/L
	Adults	0-190 units/L
Magnesium		1.5-2.5 mEq/L
Osmolality, serum		275-296 mOsm/kg
Osmolality, urine		50-1400 mOsm/kg

		Normal Values
Phosphorus	Newborns	4.2-9 mg/dL
	6 wk to 19 mo	3.8-6.7 mg/dL
	19 mo to 3 y	2.9-5.9 mg/dL
	3-15 y	3.6-5.6 mg/dL
	>15 y	2.5-5 mg/dL
Potassium, plasma	Newborns	4.5-7.2 mEq/L
	2 d to 3 mo	4-6.2 mEq/L
	3 mo to 1 y	3.7-5.6 mEq/L
	1-16 y	3.5-5 mEq/L
Protein, total	0-2 y	4.2-7.4 g/dL
	>2 y	6-8 g/dL
Sodium		136-145 mEq/L
Triglycerides	Infants	0-171 mg/dL
	Children	20-130 mg/dL
	Adults	30-200 mg/dL
Urea nitrogen, blood	0-2 y	4-15 mg/dL
	2 y to Adult	5-20 mg/dL
Uric acid	Male	3-7 mg/dL
	Female	2-6 mg/dL
ENZYMES		
Alanine aminotransferase (ALT)	0-2 mo	8-78 units/L
	>2 mo	8-36 units/L
Alkaline phosphatase (ALKP)	Newborns	60-130 units/L
	0-16 y	85-400 units/L
	>16 y	30-115 units/L
Aspartate aminotransferase (AST)	Infants	18-74 units/L
	Children	15-46 units/L
	Adults	5-35 units/L
Creatine kinase (CK)	Infants	20-200 units/L
	Children	10-90 units/L
	Adult male	0-206 units/L
	Adult female	0-175 units/L
Lactate dehydrogenase (LDH)	Newborns	290-501 units/L
	1 mo to 2 y	110-144 units/L
	>16 y	60-170 units/L

Blood Gases

	Arterial	Capillary	Venous
pH	7.35-7.45	7.35-7.45	7.32-7.42
pCO_2 (mm Hg)	35-45	35-45	38-52
pO_2 (mm Hg)	70-100	60-80	24-48
HCO_3 (mEq/L)	19-25	19-25	19-25
TCO_2 (mEq/L)	19-29	19-29	23-33
O_2 saturation (%)	90-95	90-95	40-70
Base excess (mEq/L)	-5 to +5	-5 to +5	-5 to +5

Thyroid Function Tests

T_4 (thyroxine)	1-7 d	10.1-20.9 mcg/dL
	8-14 d	9.8-16.6 mcg/dL
	1 mo to 1 y	5.5-16 mcg/dL
	>1 y	4-12 mcg/dL
FTI	1-3 d	9.3-26.6
	1-4 wk	7.6-20.8
	1-4 mo	7.4-17.9
	4-12 mo	5.1-14.5
	1-6 y	5.7-13.3
	>6 y	4.8-14
T_3 by RIA	Newborns	100-470 ng/dL
	1-5 y	100-260 ng/dL
	5-10 y	90-240 ng/dL
	10 y to Adult	70-210 ng/dL
T_3 uptake		35%-45%
TSH	Cord	3-22 μIU/mL
	1-3 d	<40 μIU/mL
	3-7 d	<25 μIU/mL
	>7 d	0-10 μIU/mL

ACQUIRED IMMUNODEFICIENCY SYNDROME (AIDS) - LAB TESTS AND APPROVED DRUGS FOR HIV INFECTION AND AIDS-RELATED CONDITIONS

This list of tests is not intended in any way to suggest patterns of physician's orders, nor is it complete. These tests may support possible clinical diagnoses or rule out other diagnostic possibilities. Each laboratory test relevant to AIDS is listed and weighted. Two symbols (**) indicate that the test is diagnostic, that is, documents the diagnosis if the expected is found. A single symbol (*) indicates a test frequently used in the diagnosis or management of the disease. The other listed tests are useful on a selective basis with consideration of clinical factors and specific aspects of the case.

Acid-Fast Stain
Acid-Fast Stain, Modified, *Nocardia* Species
Antimicrobial Susceptibility Testing, Fungi
Antimicrobial Susceptibility Testing, Mycobacteria
Arthropod Identification
Babesiosis Serological Test
Bacteremia Detection, Buffy Coat Micromethod
Bacterial Culture, Blood
Bacterial Culture, Bronchoscopy Specimen
Bacterial Culture, Sputum
Bacterial Culture, Stool
Bacterial Culture, Throat
Bacterial Culture, Urine, Clean Catch
Beta$_2$-Microglobulin
Blood and Fluid Precautions, Specimen Collection
Bronchial Washings Cytology
Bronchoalveolar Lavage Cytology
Brushings Cytology
Candida Antigen
Candidiasis Serologic Test
Cat Scratch Disease Serology
CD4/CD8 Enumeration
Cerebrospinal Fluid Cytology
Cryptococcal Antigen Titer
Cryptosporidium Diagnostic Procedures
Cytomegalic Inclusion Disease Cytology
Cytomegalovirus Antibody
Cytomegalovirus Antigen Detection
Cytomegalovirus Culture
Cytomegalovirus DNA Detection
Darkfield Examination, Syphilis
Electron Microscopy
Folic Acid, Serum
Fungal Culture, Biopsy or Body Fluid
Fungal Culture, Blood
Fungal Culture, Cerebrospinal Fluid
Fungal Culture, Sputum
Fungal Culture, Stool
Fungal Culture, Urine
Hemoglobin A_2
Hepatitis B Surface Antigen
Herpes Cytology
Herpes Simplex Virus Antigen Detection
Herpes Simplex Virus Culture
Histopathology
Histoplasmosis Antibody
Histoplasmosis Antigen
**HIV-1/HIV-2 Serology
HTLV-I/II Antibody
*Human Immunodeficiency Virus Culture
*Human Immunodeficiency Virus DNA Amplification

India Ink Preparation
Inhibitor, Lupus, Phospholipid Type
KOH Preparation
Leishmaniasis Serological Test
Leukocyte Immunophenotyping
Lymphocyte Enumeration Test
Lymphocyte Transformation Test
Microsporidia Diagnostic Procedures
Mycobacteria by DNA Probe
Mycobacterial Culture, Biopsy or Body Fluid
Mycobacterial Culture, Cerebrospinal Fluid
Mycobacterial Culture, Cutaneous and Subcutaneous Tissue
Mycobacterial Culture, Sputum
Mycobacterial Culture, Stool
Neisseria gonorrhoeae Culture and Smear
Nocardia Culture
Ova and Parasites, Stool
*p24 Antigen
Platelet Count
Pneumocystis carinii Preparation
Pneumocystis Immunofluorescence
Polymerase Chain Reaction
Red Blood Cell Indices
Risks of Transfusion
Skin Biopsy
Sputum Cytology
Toxoplasmosis Serology
VDRL, Serum
Viral Culture
Viral Culture, Blood
Viral Culture, Body Fluid
Viral Culture, Central Nervous System Symptoms
Viral Culture, Dermatological Symptoms
Viral Culture, Tissue
Virus, Direct Detection by Fluorescent Antibody
White Blood Count

FDA-APPROVED AND INVESTIGATIONAL ANTIRETROVIRAL DRUGS

Antiretroviral Drugs

Generic Name	Also Known As	Brand Name	FDA Status
NUCLEOSIDE/NUCLEOTIDE ANALOG REVERSE TRANSCRIPTASE INHIBITORS (NRTIs)			
abacavir	ABC	Ziagen®	Approved
apricitabine	AVX754	—	Investigational
didanosine	ddl	Videx®; Videx® EC	Approved
elvucitabine	ACH-126,443; Beta-L-Fd4C	—	Investigational
emtricitabine	FTC	Emtriva®	Approved
lamivudine	3TC	Epivir®	Approved
stavudine	d4T	Zerit®	Approved
tenofovir	TDF	Viread®	Approved
zidovudine	ZDV	Retrovir®	Approved
—	RCV	Racivir	Investigational
NONNUCLEOSIDE REVERSE TRANSCRIPTASE INHIBITORS (NNRTIs)			
delavirdine	DLV	Rescriptor®	Approved
efavirenz	EFV	Sustiva®	Approved
etravirine	TMC 125	Intelence™	Approved
nevirapine	NVP	Viramune®	Approved
rilpivirine	TMC 278	—	Investigational
PROTEASE INHIBITORS (PIs)			
atazanavir	ATV	Reyataz®	Approved
darunavir	DRV	Prezista™	Approved
fosamprenavir	FPV	Lexiva®	Approved
indinavir	IDV	Crixivan®	Approved
lopinavir and ritonavir	LPV/RTV	Kaletra®	Approved
nelfinavir	NFV	Viracept®	Approved
ritonavir	RTV	Norvir®	Approved
saquinavir	SQV	Invirase®	Approved
tipranavir	TPV	Aptivus®	Approved
FIXED-DOSE COMBINATION PRODUCTS			
abacavir and lamivudine	ABC/3TC	Epzicom®, Kivexa™	Approved
abacavir, lamivudine, and zidovudine	ABC/3TC/ZDV	Trizivir®	Approved
efavirenz, emtricitabine and tenofovir	EFV/FTC/TDF	Atripla™	Approved
emtricitabine and tenofovir	FTC/TDF	Truvada®	Approved
zidovudine and lamivudine	ZDV/3TC	Combivir®	Approved
FUSION INHIBITORS			
enfuvirtide	ENF	Fuzeon®	Approved
—	TNX-355	—	Investigational

Antiretroviral Drugs *(continued)*

Generic Name	Also Known As	Brand Name	FDA Status
CHEMOKINE CORECEPTOR ANTAGONIST			
maraviroc	MVC	Selzentry™	Approved
vicriviroc	SCH-417690; SCH-D	—	Investigational
—	PRO 140	—	Investigational
—	INCB9741	—	Investigational
INTEGRASE INHIBITORS			
elvitegravir	GS-9137	—	Investigational
raltegravir	RAL	Isentress™	Approved
—	GSK364735	—	Investigational
MATURATION INHIBITORS			
bevirimat	PA-457	—	Investigational

DRUGS USED TO TREAT COMPLICATIONS OF HIV / AIDS

Brand Name	Generic Name (Synonym)	Use
Abelcet®, AmBisome®	amphotericin B, ABLC	Antifungal for aspergillosis
Bactrim™, Septra®	sulfamethoxazole and trimethoprim, SMZ/TMP	Antiprotozoal antibiotic used to treat and prevent *Pneumocystis carinii* pneumonia
Biaxin®	clarithromycin	Antibiotic used to treat and prevent *Mycobacterium avium*
Cytovene®	ganciclovir, DHPG	Antiviral used to treat CMV retinitis
DaunoXome®	daunorubicin citrate (liposomal)	Chemotherapy for Kaposi sarcoma
Diflucan®	fluconazole	Antifungal for candidiasis, cryptococcal meningitis
Doxil®	doxorubicin (liposomal)	Chemotherapy for Kaposi sarcoma
Eraxis™	anidulafungin	Antifungal (intravenous), used to treat *Candida* infections in the esophagus (candidiasis), blood stream (candidemia), and other forms of *Candida* infections, including abdominal abscesses and peritonitis (inflammation of the lining of the abdominal cavity)
Famvir®	famciclovir	Antiviral used to treat herpes
Foscavir®	foscarnet	Antiviral used to treat herpes and CMV retinitis
Gamimune® N	immune globulin, gamma globulin, IGIV	Immune booster used to prevent bacterial infections in children
Intron® A	interferon alfa-2b	Treat Kaposi sarcoma and hepatitis C
Marinol®	dronabinol	Treat loss of appetite
Megace®	megestrol acetate	Treat loss of appetite and weight
Mepron®	atovaquone	Antiprotozoal antibiotic used to treat and prevent *Pneumocystis carinii* pneumonia
Mycobutin®	rifabutin	Antimycobacterial used to prevent *Mycobacterium avium*
NebuPent®	pentamidine	Antiprotozoal antibiotic used to prevent *Pneumocystis carinii* pneumonia
Neutrexin®	trimetrexate glucuronate and leucovorin	Antiprotozoal antibiotic used to treat *Pneumocystis carinii* pneumonia
Panretin® Gel	alitretinoin gel 0.1%	AIDS-related Kaposi sarcoma
Procrit®, Epogen®	erythropoietin, EPO	Treat anemia related to AZT therapy
Roferon-A®	interferon alfa-2a	Treat Kaposi sarcoma and hepatitis C

DRUGS USED TO TREAT COMPLICATIONS OF HIV / AIDS *(continued)*

Brand Name	Generic Name (Synonym)	Use
Serostim®	somatropin rDNA	Treat weight loss
Sporanox®	itraconazole	Antifungal used to treat blastomycosis, histoplasmosis, aspergillosis, and candidiasis
Taxol®	paclitaxel	Kaposi sarcoma
Valcyte™	valganciclovir	Antiviral used to treat CMV retinitis
VFEND®	voriconazole	Antifungal for invasive aspergillosis and serious fungal infections due to *Fusarium sporotrichoides* and *Scedosporium apiospermum*, and Esophageal Candidiasis
Vistide®	cidofovir, HPMPC	Antiviral used to treat cytomegalovirus (CMV)
Vitrasert® Implant	ganciclovir insert	Antiviral used to treat CMV retinitis
Vitravene™ intravitreal injection	fomivirsen sodium injection	Antiviral used to treat CMV retinitis
Zithromax®	azithromycin	Antibiotic used to treat *Mycobacterium avium*

HERBS AND COMMON NATURAL AGENTS

The authors have chosen to include this list of natural products and their reported uses. Due to limited scientific evidence to support these uses, the information provided here is not intended as a cure for any disease, and should not be construed as curative or healing. In addition, the reader is strongly encouraged to seek other references that discuss this information in more detail, and that discuss important issues such as contraindications, warnings, precautions, adverse reactions, and interactions.

PROPOSED MEDICINAL CLAIMS

Herb	Reported Uses
Acetyl-L-carnitine (ALC)	AIDS; alcoholism; Alzheimer disease; angina; cerebral ischemia; congestive heart failure; coronary artery disease; dementia; depression; diabetes mellitus; diabetic peripheral neuropathy; erectile dysfunction; fatigue; fibromyalgia; fragile X syndrome; Huntington disease; hyperlipoproteinemia; infertility; liver disease; mood disorder; myocardial infarction; neurologic function; neuropathy; nutritional deficiency; Parkinson disease; peripheral vascular disease; Peyronie disease; sickle cell disease; surgical uses; sperm motility; tuberculosis
Adrenal extract	Depression; fatigue; fibromyalgia; stress
Aloe (*Aloe* spp)	Aphthous stomatitis; cancer (prevention); constipation; diabetes; dry skin; genital herpes; gingivitis; healing agent for wounds, minor burns, and other minor skin irritations; human immunodeficiency virus (HIV); irritable bowel syndrome; lichen planus; mucositis; pressure ulcers; psoriasis vulgaris; radiation dermatitis; seborrheic dermatitis; skin burns; ulcerative colitis
Alpha-Lipoic acid	Alcohol-induced liver damage; Alzheimer disease; antioxidant; burning mouth syndrome; cancer; cardiovascular outcomes (in end-state renal disease); carpal tunnel syndrome; cataract prevention; chemotherapy and radiation (adjunct); circulation; cognitive function; coronary artery disease; diabetes, diabetic peripheral neuropathy; drug-induced cardiotoxicity; glaucoma; hypertension; insulin resistance; liver protective effects; multiple sclerosis; neuralgias; neurologic disorders, including stroke (preventive); peripheral artery disease; radiation injuries; skin aging; weight gain; wound healing
Andrographis (*Andrographis paniculata*)	Familial Mediterranean Fever (FMF); influenza; upper respiratory tract infection (treatment and prevention)
Aortic extract	Circulation structure, function, and integrity (arteries and veins); prevention of vascular disease including atherosclerosis, cerebral and peripheral arterial insufficiency, varicose veins, hemorrhoids, and vascular retinopathies such as macular degeneration
Arabinoxylan	Cancer; diabetes, type 2; HIV; immune support (antiviral and anticancer activity); leukopenia (chemotherapy-induced)
Arginine	Adrenoleukodystrophy (ALD); anal fissures; angina; burns; cancer; cardiovascular disease; chronic heart failure; circulation; critical illness; dental pain; diabetes (diabetic complications); erectile dysfunction; gastrointestinal cancer surgery; growth hormone reserve test/pituitary disorder diagnosis; heart protection during CABG; hypercholesterolemia; hypertension; immune support; inborn errors of urea synthesis; inflammatory bowel disease; increases lean body mass; kidney disease; male infertility; MELAS syndrome; migraine headache; myocardial infarction; neonatal outcomes; obesity (in type 2 diabetic patients); peripheral vascular disease/claudication; preeclampsia; pressure ulcers; recovery after surgery; sexual vitality and enhancement; transplants; wound healing
Arnica (*Arnica montana*)	Bruising; coagulation; diabetic retinopathy; osteoarthritis; pain; swelling (postoperative); trauma
Artichoke (*Cynara scolymus*)	Bile flow; dyspepsia (nonulcer); eczema and other dermatologic problems; hepatic protection/stimulation; hypercholesterolemia; indigestion; irritable bowel syndrome (IBS)
Ashwagandha (*Withania somnifera*)	Adaptogen/tonic (promote wellness); chemotherapy and radiation (adjunct); diabetes (type 2); diuresis; hypercholesterolemia; longevity/anti-aging; osteoarthritis; Parkinson disease; stress, fatigue, nervous exhaustion

PROPOSED MEDICINAL CLAIMS *(continued)*

Herb	Reported Uses
Astragalus (*Astragalus membranaceus*) [Milk Vetch]	Adaptogen/tonic (promote wellness); antiviral activity; athletic performance (enhancement); burns; chemotherapy and radiation (adjunct); coronary artery disease; diabetes; heart failure; immune support; liver protection; mental performance; multiple sclerosis; otitis media; renal failure; smoking cessation; tissue oxygenation; tuberculosis
Bacopa (*Bacopa monniera*)	Alzheimer disease/senility; anxiety; epilepsy; irritable bowel syndrome (IBS); memory enhancement and improvement of cognitive function
Barberry (*Berberis vulgaris*)	Bladder infection; bronchitis; sore throat; yeast infection
Beta-Carotene	Age-related maculopathy; AIDS; asthma; breast cancer; carotenoid deficiency; cataract prevention; cervical dysplasia; chromosome damage (reduction); chronic obstructive pulmonary disease (COPD); coronary heart disease (risk reduction; in combination); cystic fibrosis; diabetes; diabetes, type 2; esophageal cancer; gastric cancer; immune support; laryngeal cancer; LDL oxidation (decrease in males); lung cancer (preventive); lung function; macular degeneration; memory and cognition; night blindness; oral leukoplakia; osteoarthritis; photoprotection (erythropoietic protoporphyria); pregnancy-related complications
Betaine hydrochloride	Cardiovascular disease (in homocystinuric patients); cholesterol levels; digestive aid (hypochlorhydria and achlorhydria); hyperhomocysteinemia; hyperhomocysteinemia (in chronic renal failure patients); rosacea; steatohepatitis (nonalcoholic); weight loss
Bifidobacterium bifidum (*bifidus*)	Atopic dermatitis; constipation; Crohn disease; diarrhea; gastrointestinal microflora recolonization (anaerobic); *Helicobacter pylori* infection; immune function; irritable bowel syndrome (IBS); pouchitis; ulcerative colitis
Bilberry (*Vaccinium myrtillus*)	Circulation, peripheral; diabetes; diarrhea; dysmenorrhea; fibrocystic breast disease (FBD); hemorrhoids; ophthalmologic disorders (antioxidant) including myopia, diminished acuity, glaucoma; dark adaptation, macular degeneration, night blindness, diabetic retinopathy, cataracts; peptic ulcer disease; scleroderma; vascular disorders including varicose veins, capillary permeability/stability, phlebitis
Biotin (Vitamin H)	Cardiovascular disease (risk reduction; in combination); diabetes; diabetic peripheral neuropathy; hypertriglyceridemia; nails, brittle; pregnancy supplementation; seborrheic dermatitis; total parenteral nutrition (TPN); uncombable hair syndrome
Bismuth	Diarrhea; ulcers
Bitter melon (*Momordica charantia*)	Antiviral; cancer; diabetes, including impaired glucose tolerance; human immunodeficiency virus (HIV)
Black cohosh (*Cimicifuga racemosa*)	Arthritis; depression (mild); hot flashes (related to breast cancer treatment); menopause symptoms (including vasomotor); migraine; premenstrual syndrome (PMS)
Bladderwrack (*Fucus vesiculosus*)	Anticoagulant; antioxidant; bacterial and fungal infections; cancer; diabetes; fibrocystic breast disease (FBD); hypothyroidism; nutrient (rich source of iodine, potassium, magnesium, calcium, and iron); weight loss
Borage (*Borago officinalis*)	Acute respiratory distress syndrome; alcohol hangover; asthma; atopic dermatitis (treatment and prophylaxis); atopic eczema; cystic fibrosis; diabetic neuropathy; fatty acids (preterm infants); growth and development (infants); hyperlipidemia; infantile seborrheic dermatitis; malnutrition-inflammation complex syndrome; periodontitis; rheumatoid arthritis; stress; weight regain
Boron	Cognitive function improvement; osteoarthritis; osteoporosis; rheumatoid arthritis; vaginitis
Boswellia (*Boswellia serrata*)	Antiinflammatory; arthritis; asthma; brain tumors; Crohn disease; ulcerative colitis
Branched-chain amino acids (BCAAs)	Amyotrophic lateral sclerosis; anorexia; cardiac atrophy; cirrhosis; diabetes; energy metabolism improvement (in cirrhosis patients); exercise performance; hepatic encephalopathy; muscle development and lean body mass (increase); muscle fatigue and soreness; protein metabolism (in COPD patients); tardive dyskinesia
Bromelain (*Anas comosus*)	Arthritis (antiinflammatory; proteolytic); burn debridement; cancer; cervical dysplasia; chronic obstructive pulmonary disease (COPD); digestive enzyme; inflammation/pain; muscle soreness; osteoarthritis of the knee; rash; rheumatoid arthritis; sinusitis; steatorrhea; urinary tract infection (UTI)

PROPOSED MEDICINAL CLAIMS *(continued)*

Herb	Reported Uses
Bupleurum (*Bupleurum falcatum*)	Brain damage (minimal, children); chronic inflammatory disease; fatigue; hepatic protection; hepatitis; systemic lupus erythematosus (SLE); thrombocytopenic purpura
Calcium	Antacid; black widow spider bite; blood pressure regulation; bone loss; bone stress injury prevention; cancer (prevention); colon cancer (distal); colorectal adenomas (recurrence); growth; hypercholesterolemia; hyperkalemia; hypermagnesemia; hyperparathyroidism; hyperphosphatemia; hypertension; kidney stones; lead toxicity; osteomalacia/rickets; osteoporosis (preventive); poison ivy (topical; lactate form); preeclampsia; pregnancy; premenstrual syndrome (PMS); weight loss in type 2 diabetic patients, fat metabolism, and weight gain prevention (in postmenopausal women); vaginal atrophy
Calendula (*Calendula officinalis*)	Antibacterial, antifungal, antiviral, antiprotozoal; otitis media; radiation dermatitis; skin inflammation; venous leg ulcers; wound healing
Caprylic acid	Antifungal/antiyeast; candidiasis; Crohn disease; dysbiosis; epilepsy (children)
Caprylidene	Alzheimer disease
Carnitine	Acute myocardial infarction (mortality); angina; arrhythmia; athletic performance (enhancement); attention-deficit hyperactivity disorder (ADHD); chronic obstructive pulmonary disease (COPD); congestive heart failure (CHF); diabetes; dialysis; diphtheria; erectile dysfunction; exercise performance; fatigue; hepatic encephalopathy; HIV/AIDS; Huntington disease; hypercholesterolemia; hyperlipoproteinemia; hyperthyroidism; male infertility; myocardial infarction; neonatal growth and breathing; obesity; peripheral vascular disease; postexercise metabolic stress and muscle damage; quality of life (maintenance hemodialysis patients); renal failure/dialysis; respiratory distress; sperm motility; surgical uses; weight loss
Cascara (*Rhamnus purshiana*)	Laxative
Cat's claw (*Uncaria tomentosa*)	Allergies; antiinflammatory; antimicrobial (antibacterial, antifungal, antiviral); antioxidant; arthritis; cancer; cervical dysplasia; Crohn disease; diverticulitis; endometriosis; fibromyalgia; immune support; multiple sclerosis; rosacea; systemic lupus erythematosus (SLE)
Cayenne (*Capsicum annuum, Capsicum frutescens*)	Antiinflammatory and analgesic (topical); cardiovascular circulatory support; cluster headache; concentration/stimulant; digestive stimulant; duodenal ulcer; dyspepsia; fibromyalgia; *H. pylori*; low back pain; nausea/vomiting (postoperative); pain (postoperative); postherpetic neuralgia; pruritus; rhinitis
Chamomile, German (*Matricaria chamomilla, Matricaria recutita*)	Acute radiation skin reaction; anxiolytic; cardiovascular conditions; carminative, antispasmodic; colic; common cold; diaper rash; diarrhea (children); eczema; hemorrhagic cystitis; hemorrhoids; indigestion; insomnia (mild sedative); minor injury (topical antiinflammatory); mucositis (from chemotherapy); nausea/vomiting; oral health (as mouth rinse/gargle); stress/anxiety; teething; uterine tonic; vaginitis
Chasteberry (*Vitex agnus-castus*)	Acne vulgaris; cervical dysplasia; corpus luteum insufficiency; hyperprolactinemia and insufficient lactation; cyclic mastalgia; menopause; menorrhagia; menstrual disorders including amenorrhea, endometriosis, premenstrual syndrome (PMS); rosacea
Chitosan	Antibacterial; dental plaque; hyperlipidemia; periodontitis; renal failure; weight loss; wound healing
Chlorophyll	Antiinflammatory, antioxidant, and wound healing properties; bacteriostatic; cancer; chemoprevention; fibrocystic breast disease; herpes simplex, herpes zoster; leukopenia; odor absorbent/suppressant (breath freshener, toothpaste, mouthwash, and deodorant); pancreatitis; pneumonia; poisoning; protectant; rheumatoid arthritis; tuberculosis
Chondroitin sulfate	Coronary artery disease; interstitial cystitis; iron absorption enhancement; muscle soreness, delayed onset; ophthalmologic uses; osteoarthritis; overactive bladder; psoriasis

PROPOSED MEDICINAL CLAIMS *(continued)*

Herb	Reported Uses
Chromium	Atherosclerosis; bipolar disorder; bone loss (postmenopausal women); cardiovascular disease (risk reduction; in combination); depression; diabetes; diabetes, type 1; diabetes, type 2; glaucoma; hypercholesterolemia; hypertriglyceridemia; hypothyroidism; immunosuppression; insulin sensitivity (obese women with polycystic ovarian syndrome); premenstrual syndrome (PMS); weight loss
Clove (*Syzygium aromaticum*)	Anal fissures (topical); analgesic (toothache and teething); anesthetic; antiseptic; fever; mosquito repellent; premature ejaculation (combination preparation)
Coenzyme Q_{10}	Acute myocardial infarction; AIDS; Alzheimer disease; amyotrophic lateral sclerosis (ALS); angina; antioxidant; asthenozoospermia (idiopathic); cancer (preventive); cardiomyopathy; cardioprotection during surgery; chemotherapy (adjunct); chronic fatigue syndrome; congestive heart failure (CHF); Down syndrome; exercise performance; fibromyalgia; Friedreich ataxia; gingivitis; hypercholesterolemia; hypertension; migraine; mitochondrial disease and Kearns-Sayre syndrome; multiple sclerosis; muscle pain (associated with HMG-CoA reductase inhibitors); muscular dystrophy; myelodysplastic syndromes; Parkinson disease; periodontal disease; renal failure; tinnitus; weight loss
Coleus (*Coleus forskohlii*)	Antiinflammatory action after cardiopulmonary bypass; asthma and allergies; eczema; erectile dysfunction; glaucoma; hypertension and congestive heart failure; lactagogue; psoriasis
Collagen (Type II)	Arthritis (osteo and rheumatoid); burns (first- and second-degree); soft tissue correction; surgical and traumatic wounds; ulcers (pressure, venous stasis, diabetic); wound healing (topical)
Colostrum	Antiviral (mild); athletic performance (enhancement); body composition; colitis; cryptosporidiosis; diarrhea; flu prevention; HIV-associated diarrhea; *H. Pylori*; immune support; multiple sclerosis; oral hygiene; prevention of NSAID-induced GI injury; rotavirus-associated diarrhea; shigellosis; sore throat; surgery recovery; upper respiratory tract infection
Conjugated linoleic acid (CLA)	Cancer; diabetes; hypercholesterolemia; immune support; muscle development and lean body mass (increase); obesity; oxidative stress and inflammatory disease in obese men; preeclampsia (in combination with calcium)
Copper	Age-related macular degeneration; anemia; arthritis; atherosclerosis; copper deficiency; dental enamel demineralization (in combination with fluoride); growth promotion (children); marasmus; osteoporosis; plaque prevention; rheumatoid arthritis; systemic lupus erythematosus
Cordyceps (*Cordyceps sinensis*)	Adaptogen/tonic (promote wellness); antioxidant; asthma; chemotherapy and radiation (adjunct); endurance and stamina; fatigue; fibromyalgia; hepatitis B; hepatoprotection; hyperlipidemia; immunomodulator; lung, liver, and kidney function (general support); organ transplant; sexual vitality (males and females); tissue oxygenation
Cranberry (*Vaccinium macrocarpon*)	Achlorhydria and B_{12} absorption; antioxidant; bacterial and fungal infections; cancer (prevention); *H. pylori* infection; plaque; reduction of urinary odors; urinary tract infection, including prevention
Creatine	Athletic performance (enhancement) as energy production and protein synthesis for muscle building; bone density; chronic obstructive pulmonary disease; congestive heart failure (CHF); dermatomyositis/polymyositis; GAMT deficiency; hemodialysis-associated muscle cramps; Huntington disease; hyperlipidemia; ischemic heart disease; McArdle disease; mitochondrial diseases; muscle function and strength; mood; muscular dystrophy; Parkinson disease; resistance training in patients with Parkinson disease; schizophrenia; spinal cord injury; surgery (adjunct); traumatic brain injury, prevention of complications (children)
Cyclo-hispro	Diabetes, type 2; hypoglycemia
Damiana (*Turnera diffusa*)	Female sexual dysfunction; weight loss/obesity
Dandelion (*Taraxacum officinale*)	Leaf used as a diuretic; root used to increase bile secretion (choleretic), appetite stimulation, and dyspepsia

PROPOSED MEDICINAL CLAIMS *(continued)*

Herb	Reported Uses
Dehydroepiandrosterone (DHEA)	Adrenal insufficiency; AIDS/HIV; antiaging; cardiovascular disease; cervical cancer; chronic fatigue syndrome; cocaine withdrawal; cognitive function; Crohn disease; dementia; depression; diabetes, type 2; erectile dysfunction; extrapyramidal symptoms; fatigue; fibromyalgia; induction of labor; infertility; libido (premenopausal women); lupus; muscle mass and strength; obesity; perimenopausal symptoms; psoriasis; rheumatoid arthritis; schizophrenia; Sjögren syndrome
Devil's claw (*Harpagophytum procumbens*)	Antiinflammatory; back pain; osteoarthritis, gout, and other inflammatory conditions
Docosahexaenoic acid (DHA)	Alzheimer disease; angina pectoris; appetite; arrhythmias; asthma; attention-deficit disorder and attention-deficit hyperactivity disorder (ADD/ADHD); bipolar disorder; cancer (prevention); cardiovascular disease; colon cancer; coronary heart disease (risk reduction); Crohn disease; cystic fibrosis; depression; diabetes; diabetes, type 2; dysmenorrhea; eczema; hypercholesterolemia; hypertension; hypertriglyceridemia; IgA nephropathy; immune support; infant eye/brain development; infection; lupus; nephrotic syndrome; postpartum depression; preeclampsia; prevention of graft failure after heart bypass surgery; protection from cyclosporine toxicity in organ transplant patients; psoriasis; rheumatoid arthritis; schizophrenia; stroke (risk reduction); ulcerative colitis
Dong quai (*Angelica sinensis*)	Anemia; energy enhancement (particularly in females); hypertension; menopause, dysmenorrhea, premenstrual syndrome (PMS), and amenorrhea; menorrhagia; phytoestrogen; pulmonary hypertension
Echinacea (*Echinacea purpurea, Echinacea angustifolia*)	Antibacterial (topical; boils, abscesses, tonsillitis, poison ivy); antiviral; arthritis (*E. augustifolia*); genital herpes; immune support (cold and other upper respiratory infections); otitis media; radiation-associated leucopenia; upper respiratory infection; uveitis
Elder (*Sambucus nigra, Sambucus canadensis*)	Berry used as an antiviral, antioxidant, and for influenza; flower used as an antiinflammatory, for colds and influenza, diaphoretic, diuretic, fever, sinusitis, and sore throat
Ephedra (*Ephedra sinica*)	Allergies, sinusitis, hay fever; asthma; hypotension; sexual arousal; weight loss (monotherapy); weight loss (combination therapy)
Evening primrose (*Oenothera biennis*)	Amenorrhea; atopic dermatitis; attention-deficit disorder; bronchitis; depression; diabetes; diabetic peripheral neuropathy; eczema, dermatitis, and psoriasis; endometriosis; fatigue; fibrocystic breast disease (FBD); hypercholesterolemia; ichthyosis vulgaris; irritable bowel syndrome (IBS); mastalgia; menorrhagia; multiple sclerosis; obesity; omega-6 fatty acid supplementation; preeclampsia; premenstrual syndrome (PMS) and menopause; Raynaud phenomenon; rheumatoid arthritis; rosacea; scleroderma
Eyebright (*Euphrasia officinalis*)	Conjunctivitis; eye fatigue; catarrh of the eyes; hepatoprotection
Fennel (*Foeniculum vulgare* Mill.)	ACE inhibitor-associated cough; colic, infantile; dysmenorrhea; ultraviolet skin protection
Fenugreek (*Trigonella foenum-graecum*)	Diabetes; galactagogue; hypercholesterolemia
Feverfew (*Tanacetum parthenium*)	Antiinflammatory, rheumatoid arthritis; migraine headache (preventive); muscle soreness
Fish oils	Acne vulgaris; angina pectoris; arrhythmias; asthma; bipolar disorder; body weight improvement; cancer (prevention); cardiac death (sudden; preventive); cardiac support (general; proposed benefits); cardiovascular disease; circulation; cognitive performance; colon cancer; coronary heart disease (preventive); Crohn disease; cystic fibrosis; depression; diabetes, type 2; dysmenorrhea; eczema, psoriasis; fatigue; headache; heart disease and heart attack (risk reduction), including women and antiinflammatory effects in heart failure patients; herpes simplex 2; hypercholesterolemia; hypertension; hypertriglyceridemia; IgA nephropathy; immune support; infant eye/brain development; lupus; memory enhancement; multiple sclerosis; nephrotic syndrome; preeclampsia; premenstrual syndrome (PMS); prevention of graft failure after heart bypass surgery; protection from cyclosporine toxicity in organ transplant patients; psoriasis; Raynaud phenomenon; rheumatoid arthritis; rosacea; schizophrenia; scleroderma; stroke (risk reduction); ulcerative colitis

PROPOSED MEDICINAL CLAIMS *(continued)*

Herb	Reported Uses
Flaxseed oil	Acne vulgaris; arthritis (rheumatoid); asthma; attention deficit hyperactivity disorder (ADHD); constipation; coronary heart disease (risk reduction); diabetes; dry eyes (Sjögren syndrome); hemorrhoids; hyperlipidemia; hypertension; menopausal symptoms; multiple sclerosis; omega-3 essential fatty acid source (cell wall and cellular membrane structure; cholesterol transport and oxidation); premenstrual syndrome (PMS); prostaglandins production; psoriasis; stroke (risk reduction); systemic lupus erythematosus (SLE)
Folic acid	Alcoholism; Alzheimer disease; anemia; atherosclerosis; beta-thalassemia; cancer (preventive; colon and breast); cardiovascular morbidity or mortality in patients with chronic renal failure; cervical dysplasia; chronic fatigue syndrome; cognitive function; coronary heart disease (risk reduction); coronary restenosis (rate reduction by decreasing plasma homocysteine levels); Crohn disease; dementia and Alzheimer disease (risk reduction); depression; endothelial dysfunction (in type 2 diabetes); fragile X syndrome; gingivitis; hearing loss (slows progression); homocysteine (reduction); methotrexate toxicity; nitrate tolerance; osteoporosis; phenytoin-induced gingival hyperplasia; pregnancy (prevention of birth defects) and lactation; schizophrenia (risk reduction, by decreasing homocysteine levels); stroke; ulcer, aphthous; vitiligo
Gamma Linolenic Acid (GLA)	Acute respiratory distress syndrome; atopic dermatitis; attention-deficit hyperactivity disorder (ADHD); blood pressure control; cancer treatment (adjunct); diabetic neuropathy; immune enhancement; mastalgia; menopausal hot flashes; migraine; osteoporosis; preeclampsia; premenstrual syndrome (PMS); pruritus; rheumatoid arthritis; Sjögren syndrome; ulcerative colitis
Garcinia (*Garcinia cambogia*)	Exercise performance; halitosis; pancreatic function (supportive) and glucose regulation; weight loss
Garlic (*Allium sativum*)	Alopecia; antimicrobial (bacterial and fungal) including *Helicobacter pylori* infection and tinea pedis; antioxidant (practitioners should be aware that aged garlic extracts have been reported to improve this benefit); atherosclerosis; cancer (prevention); coagulation (mild inhibitor of platelet-activating factor); cryptococcal meningitis; cutaneous microcirculation; diabetes; hyperlipidemia; hypertension; immune support; peripheral vascular disease; tick repellant; upper respiratory tract infection
Ginger (*Zingiber officinale*)	Antiemetic (for nausea and vomiting in pregnancy, motion sickness, and chemotherapy); antiinflammatory (musculoskeletal); diverticulitis; gonarthritis; indigestion/heartburn; labor (shortening duration); osteoarthritis; rheumatoid arthritis
Ginkgo (*Ginkgo biloba*)	Acute ischemic stroke; Alzheimer disease, dementia, age-related memory impairment; anxiety; asthma; cerebral insufficiency; chemotherapy (adjunct); chronic cochleovestibular disorders; cocaine dependence; cognitive function; depression; diabetic neuropathy; dyslexia; epilepsy; functional measures (in patients with multiple sclerosis); gastric cancer; glaucoma; headache; intermittent claudication; macular degeneration; memory enhancement; mountain sickness; multiple sclerosis; ocular blood flow; Parkinson disease; peripheral blood flow (cerebral vascular disease, peripheral vascular insufficiency, impotence, tinnitus, and depression); premenstrual syndrome (PMS); quality of life; Raynaud phenomenon; retinopathy; seasonal affective disorder (SAD); schizophrenia; seizures; sexual dysfunction (antidepressant-induced); tinnitus; vertigo; vitiligo
Ginseng, Panax (*Panax ginseng*)	Adrenal tonic; brain injury; bronchitis; cancer; congestive heart failure; COPD; dementia; diabetes; diabetic nephropathy; energy enhancement; erectile dysfunction; hepatoprotection; hyperlipidemia; hypertension; immune support; mental health; physical and mental performance; radiation therapy side effects
Ginseng, Siberian (*Eleutherococcus senticosus*)	Adaptogen/tonic (promote wellness); athletic performance (enhancement); stress (decreased fatigue); herpes simplex, type 2; immune support; neurocirculatory hypotension
Glucosamine	Chronic venous insufficiency; inflammatory bowel disease; knee injury recovery; osteoarthritis and joint structure support; rheumatoid arthritis and other inflammatory conditions; temporomandibular joint (TMJ)
Glutamine	Alcoholism; athletic performance (enhancement); cancer (adjunct); catabolic wasting; chemotherapy (prevention of adverse effects); critical illness; fibromyalgia; HIV (adjunct); HIV wasting; immune support; muscular dystrophy; peptic ulcer disease; postsurgical healing; ulcerative colitis and other inflammatory bowel diseases

PROPOSED MEDICINAL CLAIMS *(continued)*

Herb	Reported Uses
Glutathione	Antioxidant, chemoprotection; hepatoprotection (alcohol-induced liver damage); immune support; male infertility; peptic ulcer disease; peripheral artery disease
Golden seal (*Hydrastis canadensis*)	Antimicrobial (antibacterial/antifungal); bronchitis, cystitis, and infectious diarrhea; fever; gallbladder; gastritis; heart failure; hypercholesterolemia; immune stimulation; infectious diarrhea; malaria (chloroquine resistant); mucous membrane tonifying (used in inflammation of mucosal membranes); narcotic concealment (urine analysis); sinusitis; sore throat; trachoma; urinary tract infection (UTI)
Gotu kola (*Centella asiatica*)	Anxiety; cirrhosis; connective tissue (support); diabetic microangiopathy; hemorrhoids (topical); macular degeneration; memory enhancement; psoriasis; venous insufficiency; wound healing (topical)
Grapefruit seed (*Citrus paradisi*)	Antifungal, antibacterial, and antiparasitic agent; diarrhea; diverticulitis; eczema; endometriosis; heart disease; irritable bowel syndrome (IBS); kidney stones; metabolic syndrome; rosacea; sinusitis; sore throat; ulcerative colitis; urinary tract infection (UTI)
Grapeseed (*Vitis vinifera*)	Agitation (aromatherapy); allergies, antiinflammatory, asthma; antioxidant; cardiovascular health; chloasma; circulation, platelet aggregation inhibitor, capillary fragility, arterial/venous insufficiency (intermittent claudification, varicose veins); diabetic retinopathy; edema; gingivitis; glaucoma; hyperlipidemia; macular degeneration; multiple sclerosis; pancreatitis; Parkinson disease; premenstrual syndrome; scleroderma; sun protection; vision problems
Green tea (*Camellia sinensis*)	Antioxidant; cancer (prevention); cardiovascular disease (preventive); cardiovascular disease (reduction of risks); chemotherapy and radiation (adjunct); common cold (prevention); diabetes; diarrhea; genital warts; gingivitis (prevention); human T-cell lymphocytic virus; hypercholesterolemia; hypertension; hypertriglyceridemia; macular degeneration; photoprotection; platelet aggregation inhibition; weight loss
Ground Ivy (*Glechoma hederacea*)	No reported therapeutic uses
Guggul (*Commiphora mukul*)	Acne vulgaris; hypercholesterolemia; hypothyroidism; obesity; osteoarthritis; rheumatoid arthritis; weight loss
Gymnema (*Gymnema sylvestre*)	Diabetes, blood sugar regulation; hyperlipidemia; weight loss
Hawthorn (*Crataegus oxyacantha*)	Angina, hypotension, hypertension, peripheral vascular disease, and tachycardia; cardiotonic; congestive heart failure; heart failure
Hops (*Humulus lupulus*)	Menopausal symptoms; sedative/hypnotic (mild); rheumatic disease
Horse chestnut (*Aesculus hippocastanum*)	Scleroderma; venous insufficiency (varicose veins, hemorrhoids, deep venous thrombosis, lower extremity edema [oral and topical])
Horseradish (*Armoracia rusticana, Cochlearia armoracia*)	No reported therapeutic uses
Horsetail (*Equisetum arvense*)	Bone and connective tissue strengthening (including osteoporosis); diuretic; high mineral content (including silicic acid)
HuperzineA (*Huperzia serrata*)	Myasthenia gravis; senile dementia and Alzheimer disease
Hyaluronic acid	Aging; antioxidant; arthritis; immune system stimulant; osteoarthritis; skin conditions; urinary tract infections
Hydroxymethyl butyrate (HMB)	AIDS wasting; athletic performance (enhancement); muscle damage
5-Hydroxytryptophan (5-HTP)	Anxiety; cerebellar ataxia; depression; fibromyalgia; headache; migraine; schizophrenia; sleep disorders, insomnia (stimulates the production of melatonin); weight loss/obesity
Hyssop (*Hyssopus officinalis*)	Kidney inflammation
Inositol hexaphosphate (IP-6)	Cancer (preventive); intermittent claudication

PROPOSED MEDICINAL CLAIMS *(continued)*

Herb	Reported Uses
Iodine	Bacterial conjunctivitis; bladder irrigation; bowel irrigation; cancer; cognitive function; corpus vitreous degeneration; fibrocystic breast disease (FBD); filarial lymphoedema; goiter (preventive); Graves disease; hypothyroidism; molluscum; mucolytic; ophthalmia neonatorum (preventive); oral intubation; periodontitis/gingivitis; pneumonia; postcesarean endometriosis; renal pelvic instillation sclerotherapy; skin disinfectant (wound cleansing); thyrotoxicosis; water purification
Ipriflavone	Menopausal symptoms; prevention of osteoporosis (men and women)
Iron	ACE inhibitor-associated cough; anemia (infants); athletic performance; attention-deficit hyperactivity disorder (ADHD); blood transfusions (reduction); cognitive performance; hyposalivation; menorrhagia; nutritional status (infants/children); pregnancy; restless legs syndrome
Isoflavones (soy)	Antioxidant; athletic performance; benign prostatic hyperplasia (BPH); bone mineral density (increase); cancer (preventive); cardiovascular effects; cervical dysplasia; chemotherapy (adjunct); cognitive function; Crohn disease; cyclical breast pain; diabetes; diarrhea; endometriosis; food allergies; hypercholesterolemia; hypertension; immune function; kidney disease; menopausal symptoms; menstrual migraine; osteoarthritis; osteoporosis; platelet function; premenstrual syndrome (PMS); skin aging; weight loss
Kava kava (*Piper methysticum*)	Fibromyalgia; insomnia (anxiety/stress, skeletal muscle relaxation, postischemic episodes); muscle soreness
Kudzu (*Pueraria lobata*)	Alcoholism; cardiovascular disease/angina; deafness; diabetes; diabetic retinopathy; glaucoma; ischemic stroke; menopausal symptoms
Lactobacillus acidophilus	Allergies; bacterial vaginosis; colitis (collagenous); constipation; diarrhea (infantile, prevention, and chronic); eczema (preventive); gastrointestinal microflora recolonization; hepatic encephalopathy; hypercholesterolemia; immune support; irritable bowel syndrome (IBS); lactose intolerance; necrotizing enterocolitis; vaginal candidiasis
Lavender (*Lavendula officinalis*)	Anxiety; attention; cancer; dementia (behavior disturbances); depression; hypnotic/sleep (aromatherapy); pain; perineal discomfort following childbirth; spasmolytic (oral); wound healing including minor burns (topical)
Lecithin	Acne vulgaris; dementia; dry skin; extrapyramidal disorders; gallstones; hepatic steatosis; hypercholesterolemia; mania; tardive dyskinesia
Lemon balm/Melissa (*Melissa officinalis*)	Agitation in dementia; antiviral (oral herpes virus); anxiety; attention-deficit hyperactivity disorder (ADHD); cognitive performance; colitis; dyspepsia; sedation (pediatrics); sleep quality; teething (topical)
Licorice (*Glycyrrhiza glabra*)	Adrenal insufficiency (licorice); aphthous ulcers/canker sores; atopic dermatitis; body fat mass reduction; Crohn disease; croup; expectorant and antitussive (licorice); familial Mediterranean fever (FMF); gastric mucosal damage by aspirin; gastrointestinal ulceration (DGL chewable products); herpes simplex; HIV/AIDS; hyperkalemia; peptic ulcer disease; sore throat (postoperative); viral hepatitis
Liver extract	Chronic fatigue syndrome; hepatitis; liver tonic; pernicious anemia
Lutein	Antioxidant; breast cancer; cardiovascular disease; cataracts; colon cancer; diabetes; macular degeneration; preeclampsia; visual acuity and function
Lycopene	Asthma (exercise induced); atherosclerosis; benign prostate hypertrophy; cancer (preventive; especially colon, lung, prostate and kidney); diabetes; gingivitis; hypertension; immune enhancement; infertility; macular degeneration; oral submucous fibrosis; preeclampsia
Lysine	Angina pectoris; growth and development (children); herpes simplex; osteoporosis; ulcer, aphthous

PROPOSED MEDICINAL CLAIMS *(continued)*

Herb	Reported Uses
Magnesium	Acute tocolysis of preterm labor; arrhythmias/torsade de pointes; asthma; athletic performance; attention-deficit hyperactivity disorder (ADHD); cardiovascular disease; chronic obstructive pulmonary disease; circulation; colic (magnesium salt); congestive heart failure (CHF); constipation; coronary artery disease; diabetes; dysmenorrhea; epilepsy; fatigue; fibromyalgia (magnesium salt); gallbladder (magnesium salt); hearing loss; heart disease; heart failure (endothelial function); hypertension; hypoglycemia; insomnia; kidney stones; leg cramps (during pregnancy); migraine headache; mitral valve prolapse (MVP); multiple sclerosis; muscle cramps; myocardial infarction; nervousness; neuropathic pain; osteoporosis; pain; preeclampsia/eclampsia; premenstrual syndrome (PMS); stress/anxiety; tension headache (prevention)
Maitake (*Grifola frondosa*)	Cancer; diabetes; immune stimulation
Malic acid	Aluminum toxicity; fibromyalgia
Manganese	Diabetes; epilepsy; menstrual symptoms; osteoporosis
Marshmallow (*Althaea officinalis*)	Cough; croup; mucilaginous, demulcent; peptic ulcer disease; skin inflammatory conditions; sore throat
Mastic (*Pistacia lentiscus*)	Dental plaque; *H. pylori* inhibitor; peptic ulcer disease
Melatonin	Age-related macular degeneration; Alzheimer disease (sleep disorders); anxiety (preoperative); athletic performance; autism (sleep disorders); benzodiazepine tapering; bipolar disorder; cancer; cardioprotection; chemotherapy adverse effects; chronic fatigue syndrome; cognitive impairment; delayed sleep phase syndrome; depression (sleep disturbances); duodenal ulcer; dyspepsia; glaucoma; glycemic control; headache prevention; HIV/AIDS; hypertension; insomnia including elderly, children, and individuals with intellectual disabilities; irritable bowel syndrome; jet lag; menopause; nocturia; nocturnal hypertension; oxidative stress in dialysis patients (preventive); Parkinson disease; periodic limb movement disorder; preoperative sedation/anxiolysis; Rett syndrome; sarcoidosis, chronic; schizophrenia (sleep disorders); seasonal affective disorder (SAD); sedation (children); seizure disorders; skin damage; sleep disturbances (in blind people and children with developmental disabilities); stroke; tardive dyskinesia; thermoregulation; thrombocytopenia; tinnitus (sleep disorders); tuberous sclerosis; work-shift sleep disorder
Methionine	Acetaminophen toxicity; cobalamin deficiency; liver detoxification
Methyl sulfonyl methane (MSM)	Allergies; analgesic; arthritis (osteo and rheumatoid); interstitial cystitis; lupus; seasonal allergic rhinitis
Milk thistle (*Silybum marianum*)	*Amanita phalloides* mushroom toxicity; antidote for poisoning by Death Cup mushroom; antioxidant (specifically hepatic cells), acute/chronic hepatitis, jaundice, and stimulation of bile secretion/cholagogue; chemotherapy and radiation (adjunct); cirrhosis; constipation; diabetes; eczema; gallbladder; halitosis; hepatoprotective, including drug toxicities (ie, phenothiazines, butyrophenones, ethanol, and acetaminophen); hyperlipidemia; hyperthyroidism; liver disease (chronic, alcoholic, viral); psoriasis; rosacea
Modified citrus pectin (MCP)	Anticarcinogenic; detoxification (toxic elements); diarrhea; hypercholesterolemia; prostate cancer
Muira puama (*Ptychopetalum olacoides*)	Athletic performance (enhancement); erectile dysfunction; sexual vitality (males)
N-Acetyl cysteine (NAC)	Acetaminophen toxicity; acute respiratory distress syndrome (ARDS); acute respiratory infection; AIDS; angina; asthma (mucolytic, antioxidant); atelectasis; bronchitis; cancer; cardioprotection (during chemotherapy); cerebral adrenoleukodystrophy; chemotherapy adverse effects; chronic obstructive pulmonary disease (COPD); cystic fibrosis; fatigue; glutathione production; heavy metal detoxification; HIV/AIDS; hyperthyroidism; hypothyroidism; influenza prevention; macular degeneration; multiple sclerosis; myocardial infarction; nephropathy (preventive); ovulation (induction in polycystic ovary syndrome); Parkinson disease; polycystic ovarian syndrome; renal impairment; scleroderma; sepsis; Sjögren syndrome; systemic lupus erythematosus (SLE); trichotillomania
Nicotinamide adenine dinucleotide (NADH)	Chronic fatigue syndrome; dementia; diabetes, type 1; hepatitis; Parkinson disease; stamina and energy

PROPOSED MEDICINAL CLAIMS *(continued)*

Herb	Reported Uses
Octacosanol	Amyotrophic lateral sclerosis (ALS); hypercholesterolemia; Parkinson disease
Olive leaf (*Olea europaea*)	Acne vulgaris; antibacterial; antifungal, antiviral; Crohn disease; diabetes; diarrhea; diverticulitis; eczema; endometriosis; hypertension; multiple sclerosis; scleroderma; ulcerative colitis; urinary tract infection (UTI)
Pancreatic extract	Antiinflammatory; cancer (adjunct); celiac disease; digestive disturbances; food allergies; immune complex diseases; malabsorption
Para-Aminobenzoic acid (PABA)	Asthma; autoimmune disorders (pemphigus vulgaris adjuvant); cancer pain; dermatomyositis; hair loss; herpes labialis infection (prevention); herpetic keratitis; lichen sclerosus; morphea; pemphigus; Peyronie disease; scleroderma; sunburn; vitiligo
Parsley (*Petroselinum crispum*)	Antibacterial; antifungal; halitosis
Passion flower (*Passiflora spp*)	Anxiety; congestive heart failure (CHF); hyperthyroidism; insomnia (sedative); opiate withdrawal
Peppermint (*Mentha piperita*)	Brain injury (aromatherapy); carminative, spasmolytic; colic; cough; cracked nipples (prevention); dyspepsia; gastrointestinal disorders, antispasmodic; indigestion; irritable bowel syndrome (IBS); motion sickness; nasal congestion; postherpetic neuralgia; postoperative nausea (inhalation); tension headache (topical)
Periwinkle (*Vinca minor*)	No reported therapeutic uses
Phenylalanine	Addiction (reward deficiency syndrome); analgesic; attention-deficit/ hyperactivity disorder; depression; pain; Parkinson disease; vitiligo
Phosphatidyl choline (PC)	Alcohol-induced liver damage; Alzheimer disease; fat deposits; gallstones; hepatitis; hypercholesterolemia; lipoma; memory; peritoneal dialysis; periorbital fat pad herniation; tardive dyskinesia
Phosphatidyl serine (PS)	Alzheimer disease; depression; memory and cognitive enhancement; physical stress
Phosphorus	Bowel cleansing; burns; diabetic ketoacidosis; exercise performance; hypercalcemia; hypercalciuria; hyperparathyroidism; hypophosphatemia; kidney stones; refeeding syndrome prevention; total parenteral nutrition (TPN); vitamin D resistant rickets
Policosanol	Coronary heart disease; hypercholesterolemia; intermittent claudication; platelet aggregation inhibition; reactivity/brain activity
Potassium	Bone loss; cardiac arrhythmias; congestive heart failure (CHF); hypercalciuria; hypertension; kidney stones; molluscum contagiosum (topical); QT prolongation; stroke
Pregnenolone	Arthritis; hormone precursor (DHEA, cortisol, progesterone, estrogens, and testosterone); mental performance
Progesterone	Brain injury; breast cancer (preventive); dysmenorrhea; endometriosis; infertility; menopause; osteoporosis; premenstrual syndromes (PMS); preterm birth
Psyllium (*Plantago ovata, Plantago isphagula*)	Anal fissures; bulk-forming laxative (containing 10% to 30% mucilage); colon cancer; colonoscopy preparation; constipation; diarrhea; flatulence; halitosis; hemorrhoids; hypercholesterolemia; hyperglycemia; induction of labor; inflammatory bowel disease; irritable bowel syndrome (IBS); obesity
Pycnogenol (*Pinus pinaster*)	Aging; asthma; attention-deficit hyperactivity disorder (ADHD); chronic venous insufficiency; climacteric syndrome; diabetes, type 2; diabetic microangiopathy; erectile dysfunction; gingival bleeding/plaque; hypertension; osteoarthritis; platelet aggregation (smokers); prevention of blood clots during long airplane flights; retinopathy; systemic lupus erythematosus (SLE); venous leg ulcers
Pygeum (*Pygeum africanum, Prunus africana*)	Benign prostatic hyperplasia (BPH)
Pyruvate	Athletic performance (enhancement); hyperlipidemia; photoaging; weight loss
Quercetin	Allergies; asthma; atherosclerosis; cancer prevention (lung, ovarian, pancreatic); cardiovascular disease; cataracts; hypertension; immune function; kidney transplant; peptic ulcer disease; prostatitis; sinusitis

PROPOSED MEDICINAL CLAIMS *(continued)*

Herb	Reported Uses
Red clover (*Trifolium pratense*)	Benign prostatic hyperplasia (BPH); cognitive function; endometriosis; hypercholesterolemia; hypertension; liver and kidney detoxification (liquid extract); menopause; menorrhagia; osteoporosis; prostate cancer
Red yeast rice (*Monascus purpureus*)	Coronary heart disease; diabetes; hypercholesterolemia
Rehmannia (*Rehmannia glutinosa*)	Aplastic anemia (adjuvant); rheumatoid arthritis; Sheehan syndrome; systemic lupus erythematosus (SLE)
Reishi (*Ganoderma lucidum*)	Chemotherapy and radiation (adjunct); chronic hepatitis B; coronary heart disease; diabetes, type 2; fatigue; hypertension; immune support; poisoning (*Russula subnigricans*); postherpetic neuralgia; proteinuria; seizure disorder
Rose Hips (*Rosa canina*, *Various Rosa* spp)	Antioxidant; osteoarthritis
SAMe (S-adenosyl methionine)	AIDS-related myelopathy; attention-deficit/hyperactivity disorder (ADHD); cardiovascular disease; cholestasis (pregnancy); depression; fibromyalgia; headache; insomnia; liver disease; osteoarthritis; rheumatoid arthritis
Saw palmetto (*Serenoa repens*)	Androgenetic alopecia (topical); benign prostatic hyperplasia (BPH); prostatitis
Schisandra (*Schizandra chinensis*)	Adaptogen/tonic (to promote wellness); hepatic protection and detoxification; chemotherapy and radiation (adjunct); endurance, stamina, and work performance (enhancement); decreases fatigue
Selenium	Acne vulgaris (with vitamin E); AIDS/HIV; asthma; atherosclerosis; bronchial asthma; burns; cancer (preventive); cardiomyopathy; cardiovascular disease; cataracts; chemotherapy and radiation (adjunct); chromosome damage (reduction); circulation; cystic fibrosis; dandruff; diabetes; dialysis; eczema; epilepsy; esophageal cancer; gastric cancer; hemorrhoids; herpes simplex 1 and 2; hypothyroidism; infection; infertility; intracranial pressure symptoms; low birth weight; lymphedema; macular degeneration; myotonic dystrophy; osteoarthritis; pancreatitis; preeclampsia; prostate cancer (preventive); psoriasis; rheumatoid arthritis; sepsis; thyroid conditions; tinea capitis; tinea versicolor; ulcerative colitis; uveitis
Senna (*Cassia senna*)	Bowel preparation for colonoscopy; laxative
Shark cartilage	Analgesia; cancer therapy; Kaposi sarcoma; macular degeneration; osteoarthritis, rheumatoid arthritis; psoriasis
Silibinin	Cancer; hepatoprotection (acute/chronic hepatitis, jaundice, and stimulation of bile secretion/cholagogue)
Skullcap (*Scutellaria lateriflora*)	Anxiety; cancer (*in vitro*); inflammation (*in vitro*)
Slippery Elm (*Ulmus fulva, Ulmus rubra*)	Cancer; diarrhea; gastrointestinal disorders; sore throat
Sodium	No reported therapeutic uses
Spirulina	Allergic rhinitis; arsenic poisoning; blepharospasm; chronic viral hepatitis; diabetes, type 2; fatigue; hypercholesterolemia; malnutrition; oral leukoplakia/cancer; skeletal muscle damage; weight loss
Spleen extract	Chemotherapy and radiation (adjunct); cold/influenza; fatigue; spleen function (supportive)
Stinging nettle (*Urtica dioica*)	Leaf used for allergic rhinitis, allergy and hay fever symptoms, arthritis, joint pain, sinusitis, uric acid excretion; root used for benign prostatic hyperplasia (BPH)
St John's wort (*Hypericum perforatum*)	ADHD; antibacterial, antiinflammatory (topical: minor wounds, infections, bruises, muscle soreness, and sprains); antiviral; anxiety; atopic dermatitis; autism; burning mouth syndrome; climacteric symptoms (combination therapy); mild to moderate depression, depression (children), seasonal affective disorder (SAD), melancholia, stress and anxiety, major depression; HIV; irritable bowel syndrome (IBS); obsessive compulsive disorder (OCD); perimenopausal symptoms; premenstrual syndrome (PMS); smoking cessation; social phobia; somatoform disorders
Taurine	Congestive heart failure (CHF); cystic fibrosis; diabetes; energy; gallbladder; hypercholesterolemia; hypertension; iron deficiency anemia; liver disease; myotonic dystrophy; nutritional supplement (infant formula); nutritional support (TPN); obesity; seizure disorders; surgery; vaccine adjunct; vision problems

PROPOSED MEDICINAL CLAIMS *(continued)*

Herb	Reported Uses
Tea tree (*Melaleuca alternifolia*)	**Not for ingestion**; acne vulgaris; antifungal, antibacterial; mouthwash for dental and oral health; burns, cuts, scrapes, insect bites, dandruff, lice, MRSA, onychomycosis, or thrush
Thyme (*Thymus vulgaris*)	Alopecia areata; antifungal; bronchitis with cough; cough (upper respiratory origin); croup; dental plaque; inflammatory skin disorders
Thymus extract	Alopecia; arthritis; asthma; burns; cancer; cardiomyopathy; chemotherapy (adjunct); chronic obstructive pulmonary disease; diabetes; eczema; fatigue; food allergies; glaucoma; herpetic keratitis; HIV/AIDS; human papilloma virus; immune support; liver disease; otitis media; respiratory tract infection; sinusitis; systemic lupus erythematosus (SLE)
Thyroid extract	Fatigue; immune support; fibromyalgia; hypothyroidism
Tocotrienols	Atherosclerosis; cancer (preventive); heart disease; hypercholesterolemia; skin (supportive, protective)
Tribulus (*Tribulus terrestris*)	Athletic performance (enhancement); coronary artery disease; infertility; muscle strength; sexual vitality
Turmeric (*Curcuma longa*)	Antioxidant; antiinflammatory; antirheumatic; cancer; cholelithiasis prevention, gallbladder disease; hypercholesterolemia; dysmenorrhea; dyspepsia; HIV; muscle soreness; osteoarthritis; peptic ulcer disease; rheumatoid arthritis; scabies; uveitis
Tylophora (*Tylophora asthmatica*)	Allergies; asthma
Tyrosine	Alzheimer disease; attention-deficit disorder and attention-deficit hyperactivity disorder (ADD/ADHD); cocaine cravings; cognitive performance; depression; hypertension; hypothyroidism; narcolepsy; phenylketonuria (PKU); Rett syndrome; schizophrenia; stress; substance abuse
Uva Ursi (*Arctostaphylos uva-ursi*)	Hyperpigmentation; urinary tract infections and kidney stone prevention
Valerian (*Valeriana officinalis*)	Anxiety; depression; hyperthyroidism; insomnia (sedative/hypnotic); premenstrual syndrome (PMS), menopause; restless motor syndromes and muscle spasms
Vanadium	Allergic rhinitis; diabetes, type 1; diabetes, type 2; hypercholesterolemia; hypoglycemia; pneumonia
Vinpocetine	Acute ischemic stroke; Alzheimer disease and senility; cerebrovascular disease; cognitive function; hearing impairment; joint disorders; urinary incontinence
Vitamin A (Retinol)	Acne vulgaris; acute promyelocytic leukemia; AIDS; breast cancer; cancer (preventive); cataract preventive; cervical dysplasia; chemotherapy adverse effects; circulation; cold/influenza; Crohn disease; diarrhea; diverticulitis; eczema; esophageal cancer; fibrocystic breast disease (FBD); gastric cancer; glaucoma; goiter; hemorrhoids; HIV transmission; immune function; infant mortality; iron deficiency anemia; lung cancer; malaria; measles; menorrhagia; night blindness; norovirus; otitis media; pancreatic cancer; parasitic infections; photorefractive keratectomy; pneumonia; polyp prevention; pregnancy related complications; premenstrual syndrome (PMS); psoriasis; respiratory infection; retinitis pigmentosa; rosacea; skin aging, wrinkles; skin cancer preventive; sore throat; ulcerative colitis; urinary tract infection (UTI); weight loss; wound healing; xerophthalmia
Vitamin B_1 (Thiamine)	Alcoholism; Alzheimer disease; anemia (megaloblastic); cancer; cataract prevention; congestive heart failure (CHF); Crohn disease; diabetes; endothelial function; fibromyalgia; heart failure (cardiomyopathy); insomnia; metabolic disorders; neurological conditions (Bell palsy, trigeminal neuralgia, sciatica, sensory neuropathies); psychiatric illness; pyruvate dehydrogenase deficiency (PDH); total parenteral nutrition (TPN); Wernicke-Korsakoff syndrome (WKS); Wolfram syndrome (DIDMOAD)
Vitamin B_2	Anemia; anorexia/bulimia; cataracts; depression; esophageal cancer; ethylmalonic encephalopathy; malaria; migraine; neonatal jaundice; preeclampsia

PROPOSED MEDICINAL CLAIMS *(continued)*

Herb	Reported Uses
Vitamin B_3	Acne vulgaris (4% niacinamide topical gel); age-related macular degeneration; atherosclerosis; cataracts; coronary disease (preventive), antioxidant; diabetes, type 1; diabetes, type 2; headache; hypercholesterolemia; hyperlipidemia; hypertriglyceridemia; impaired glucose tolerance; intermittent claudication; myocardial infarction (risk reduction); osteoarthritis; pellagra; phosphate control; Raynaud phenomenon; rheumatoid arthritis; schizophrenia; skin conditions
Vitamin B_5 (Pantothenic acid)	Adrenal support; allergies; arthritis; athletic performance (enhancement); attention-deficit hyperactivity disorder (ADHD); constipation; hyperlipidemia (pantethine, but not pantothenic acid, lowers cholesterol and triglycerides); osteoarthritis; radiation skin irritation; rheumatoid arthritis; wound healing
Vitamin B_6 (Pyridoxine)	Adverse effects of cycloserine (prevention); akathisia; Alzheimer disease; angioplasty; arthritis; asthma; attention-deficit hyperactivity disorder (ADHD); autism; birth outcomes; cardiovascular disease; carpal tunnel syndrome; coronary heart disease (risk reduction); coronary restenosis (rate reduction by lowering plasma homocysteine levels); dementia (risk reduction); depression (associated with oral contraceptives); diabetic peripheral neuropathy; epilepsy, B_6-dependant; headache; hereditary sideroblastic anemia; homocysteine (reduction); hyperkinetic syndrome; immune function; insomnia; kidney stones; lactation suppression; monosodium glutamate (MSG) sensitivity; nausea and vomiting (in pregnancy); peptic ulcer disease; premenstrual syndrome (PMS); pyridoxine-dependent seizures in newborns; tardive dyskinesia
Vitamin B_{12} (Cobalamin)	AIDS; angioplasty; asthma; atherosclerosis (due to homocysteine elevation); atopic dermatitis; breast cancer; coronary heart disease; coronary restenosis (rate reduction by lowering plasma homocysteine levels); Crohn disease; dementia and Alzheimer disease (risk reduction); depression; diabetic peripheral neuropathy; fatigue; homocysteine (reduction); Imerslund-Grasbeck disease; male infertility; megaloblastic anemia; memory loss; multiple sclerosis; pernicious anemia; radiation-induced mucosal injury; shaky leg syndrome; sickle cell disease; stroke; sulfite sensitivity
Vitamin B complex-25	See individual B vitamins
Vitamin C	AIDS; alkaptonuria; allergies; Alzheimer disease; antioxidant; asthma; atherosclerosis; bronchitis; cancer; cardiovascular disease; cataracts; cervical dysplasia; chromosome damage (reduction); circulation; cold; constipation; contrast-mediated nephropathy; coronary heart disease (preventive, in patients taking lipid-lowering agents); Crohn disease; diabetes; diverticulitis; eczema; endometriosis; erythema; fatigue; fever; fibrocystic breast disease (FBD); fibromyalgia; gallbladder disease (risk reduction); gastroprotection; gingivitis; glaucoma; gout; *helicobacter pylori*; herpes simplex virus 1 and 2; hypertension; immune support; interferon-related retinopathy; iron absorption enhancement; irritable bowel syndrome (IBS); ischemic heart disease; LDL oxidation (decrease in males); lead toxicity; leukemia; macular degeneration; mortality; multiple sclerosis; myocardial infarction (risk reduction); nitrate tolerance (preventive); osteoporosis; otitis media; pain (complex regional pain syndrome with wrist fracture); Parkinson disease; peptic ulcer disease; plaque; pregnancy; psoriasis; radiation dermatitis; reflex sympathetic dystrophy (preventive); sinusitis; sore throat; stress/anxiety; stroke (preventive); sunburn; ulcerative colitis; urinary tract infection (UTI); vaginitis; wound healing; wrinkled skin
Vitamin D	Cancer; cardiovascular disease; congestive heart failure; Crohn disease; diabetes; epilepsy (during anticonvulsant therapy); fall prevention; familial hypophosphatemia; Fanconi syndrome; hearing loss; hepatic osteodystrophy; hyperparathyroidism; hypertension; hypocalcemia; immune response (prevents reactivation of latent tuberculosis infection); immune response to hepatitis B vaccine; multiple sclerosis (protective effect); muscle weakness; Myelodysplastic syndrome; nutritional status (breast-feeding women and infants); osteogenesis imperfecta; osteomalacia; osteoporosis including increase bone mineral density; physical performance; pigmented lesions; premenstrual syndrome; prostate cancer; proximal myopathy; psoriasis; renal osteodystrophy; rheumatoid arthritis; rickets; scleroderma; seasonal affective disorder (SAD); senile warts; statin-induced myalgia; tooth retention; weight loss (combination therapy)

PROPOSED MEDICINAL CLAIMS *(continued)*

Herb	Reported Uses
Vitamin E	Acne vulgaris (with selenium); allergic rhinitis; Alzheimer disease; anemia; angina; arterial elasticity; asthma; ataxia with vitamin E deficiency (AVED); atherosclerosis; benign prostatic hyperplasia (BPH); beta-thalassemia; bladder cancer; breast cancer; bronchopulmonary dysplasia; cancer (preventive); cardiovascular disease; cataracts; cervical dysplasia; chromosome damage (reduction); circulation; colon cancer (preventive); congestive heart failure; diabetes; diabetes, type 2; dyslipidemias; dysmenorrhea; eczema; endometriosis; epilepsy; esophageal cancer; fibrocystic breast disease (FBD); G6PD deficiency; gallbladder; gastric cancer; glomerulosclerosis (kidney disease); hemorrhoids; Huntington disease; hyperlipidemia; immune support; infertility; intermittent claudication; ischemic reperfusion injury; LDL oxidation (decrease in males); macular degeneration; mucositis (chemotherapy-induced); multiple sclerosis; myocardial infarction (risk reduction); neurotoxicity; osteoarthritis; Parkinson disease; peptic ulcer disease; peripheral circulation; photorefractive keratectomy; platelet aggregation; premenstrual syndrome (PMS); prostate cancer; psoriasis; respiratory infection (preventive); rheumatoid arthritis; scar prevention; scleroderma; steatohepatitis; sunburn; systemic lupus erythematosus (SLE); tardive dyskinesia; ulcerative colitis; uveitis; venous thromboembolism
Vitamin K	Bone strength; coronary heart disease; hemorrhagic disease (in newborns); hepatitis C (preventive effects); hepatocellular carcinoma; hypercholesterolemia; osteoporosis; synthesis of blood clotting factors; warfarin toxicity
White oak (*Quercus alba*)	Antiinflammatory (mild: throat and mouth as a soothing agent)
White willow (*Salix alba*)	Antiinflammatory; antipyretic; headache; low back pain; osteoarthritis; rheumatoid arthritis
Wild yam (*Dioscorea villosa*)	Female vitality (conversion to progesterone in the body is poor); hyperlipidemia; menopause
Yohimbe (*Pausinystalia yohimbe*)	Athletic performance; autonomic failure; male erectile dysfunction; platelet aggregation inhibition; sexual side effects of SSRIs; sexual vitality (men and women); xerostomia (psychotropic drug induced)
Zinc	Acne vulgaris; acrodermatitis enteropathica; AIDS-related opportunistic infections; alopecia areata; anorexia nervosa; aphthous ulcers; attention-deficit hyperactivity disorder (ADHD); benign prostatic hyperplasia (BPH); beta-thalassemia; boils; burns; cirrhosis; closed head injuries; cognitive deficits (children); common cold; Crohn disease; cystic fibrosis; dandruff; diabetes; diabetic neuropathy; diaper rash; diarrhea; diverticulitis; Down syndrome; exercise performance; fungal infections; gastric ulcer healing; Gilbert syndrome; halitosis; hepatic encephalopathy; hepatitis C; herpes simplex; HIV/AIDS; hyperlipidemia; immune support; infection; infertility; kwashiorkor; leg ulcers; leprosy; lower respiratory tract infection (children); macular degeneration; malaria; mucositis; muscle cramps; osteoporosis; otitis media; parasite infection; plaque/gingivitis; pneumonia; poisoning (arsenic); pregnancy; pregnancy-related iron deficiency; prostatitis (chronic); respiratory papillomatosis; rheumatoid arthritis; rosacea; sexual vitality (men); sickle cell anemia; skin conditions, eczema, psoriasis; sore throat; stomatitis; taste perception; tinnitus; trichomoniasis; ulcerative colitis; urecemic hypogeusia; viral warts; Wilson disease; wound healing

NEW DRUGS ADDED SINCE LAST EDITION

Brand Name	Generic Name	Use
Actemra®	tocilizumab	Rheumatoid arthritis
Ampyra™	dalfampridine	Multiple sclerosis (MS)
Arzerra™	ofatumumab	Leukemia
Asclera™	polidocanol	Varicose veins
Bepreve™	bepotastine	Allergic conjunctivitis
Carbaglu®	carglumic acid	Chronic hyperammonemia
Cervarix®	papillomavirus (types 16, 18) vaccine (human, recombinant)	Prevention of cervical cancer
Chenodal™	chenodiol	Cholesterol gallstones
Dulera®	mometasone and formoterol	Asthma
ella®	ulipristal	Emergency contraception
Embeda™	morphine and naltrexone	Pain
Folotyn™	pralatrexate	Lymphoma
Galzin®	zinc acetate	Wilson disease
Iprivask®	desirudin	Deep vein thrombosis (DVT)
Istodax®	romidepsin	Lymphoma
Jalyn™	dutasteride and tamsulosin	Benign prostatic hyperplasia (BPH)
Jevtana®	cabazitaxel	Carcinoma
Kalbitor®	ecallantide	Hereditary angioedema (HAE)
Lastacaft™	alcaftadine	Allergic conjunctivitis
Livalo®	pitavastatin	Primary hyperlipidemia and mixed dyslipidemia
MagneBind® 400 Rx	magnesium carbonate, calcium carbonate, and folic acid	Nutritional deficiencies
Natazia™	estradiol and dienogest	Hypermenorrhea
Prevnar 13™	pneumococcal conjugate vaccine (13-valent)	Pneumonia
Prolia™	denosumab	Osteoporosis
Provenge®	sipuleucel-T	Carcinoma
Sabril®	vigabatrin	Infantile spasms
Tribenzor™	olmesartan, amlodipine, and hydrochlorothiazide	Hypertension
Twynsta®	telmisartan and amlodipine	Hypertension
Valturna®	aliskiren and valsartan	Hypertension
Vibativ™	telavancin	Complicated skin and skin structure infections
Victoza®	liraglutide	Type II diabetes
Vimovo™	naproxen and esomeprazole	Rheumatoid arthritis, osteoarthritis, and ankylosing spondylitis
Voluven®	tetrastarch	Blood volume expander
Votrient™	pazopanib	Carcinoma
VPRIV™	velaglucerase alfa	Gaucher disease

PENDING DRUGS OR DRUGS IN CLINICAL TRIALS

Proposed Brand Name or Synonym	Generic Name	Use
Abstral™	fentanyl	Pain
Afrezza™	insulin human [rDNA origin]	Oral inhalation insulin
AR-100	iclaprim	Diaminopyrimidine antibiotic (MRSA)
Benlysta™	belimumab	Systemic lupus erythematosus
Brilinta™	ticagrelor	Acute coronary syndrome (ACS)
Ceftera™	ceftobiprole	Cephalosporin (MRSA)
Ceplene™	histamine dihydrochloride	Leukemia
Civanex™	zucapsaicin	Osteoarthritis
Contrave™	naltrexone and bupropion	Obesity
Cystoran™	cysteamine hydrochloride	Cystinosis
Daxas™	roflumilast	Chronic obstructive pulmonary disease (COPD)
Duexa™	famotidine and ibuprofen	Pain
Fortesta™	testosterone	Male hypogonadism
Gilenia™	fingolimod	Multiple sclerosis (MS)
Iluvien™	flucocinolone acetonide	Diabetic macular edema
JZP-6	sodium oxybate	Fibromyalgia
LibiGel™	testosterone	Hypoactive sexual desire disorder
Luveniq™	voclosporin	Noninfectious uveitis
Naproxcinod	nitronaproxen	Osteoarthritis
Neotrofin T	leteprinim potassium	Alzheimer disease
Omapro™	omacetaxine mepesuccinate	Leukemia
Qnexa™	phentermine and topiramate	Obesity
Solzira™	gabapentin enacarbil	Restless legs syndrome
Surfaxin™	lucinactant	Respiratory distress syndrome
TMC278	rilpivirine	HIV
TR-701	torezolide	Oxazolidone antibiotic (MRSA)
TSX TH	tesamorelin	HIV
Uplyso™	taliglucerase alfa	Gaucher disease
Zalbin™	albinterferon alfa-2b	Hepatitis C
Zenvia™	dextromethrophan and quinidine	Diabetic peripheral neuropathic (DPN) pain
Zeven™	dalbavancin	Glycopeptide antibiotic (MRSA)

INDICATION / THERAPEUTIC CATEGORY INDEX

ANESTHESIA (LOCAL)

Analgesic, Topical

Local Anesthetic

Local Anesthetic, Ophthalmic

ANESTHESIA (OPHTHALMIC)

Diagnostic Agent

Local Anesthetic

ANGINA PECTORIS

Beta-Adrenergic Blocker

ARTHRITIS (RHEUMATOID)

ATTENTION DEFICIT/HYPERACTIVITY DISORDER (ADHD)

Antimanic Agent

Antipsychotic Agent

Antipsychotic Agent, Atypical

Antipsychotic Agent, Benzisoxazole

Antipsychotic Agent, Quinolone

Antipsychotic Agent, Thienobenzodiaepine

Histone Deacetylase Inhibitor

Sulfonamide

Sympathomimetic

Tetracycline Derivative

Theophylline Derivative

BRONCHOCONSTRICTION

$Beta_2$-Adrenergic Agonist

BRONCHOSPASM

Adrenergic Agonist Agent

$Beta_2$-Adrenergic Agonist Agent

Bronchodilator

BRUCELLOSIS

Antibiotic, Aminoglycoside

Tetracycline Derivative

BULLOUS SKIN DISEASE

Antibacterial, Topical

Immunosuppressant Agent

BURNS

Analgesic, Topical

CACHEXIA

Antineoplastic Agent

Growth Hormone

Progestin

CALCIUM CHANNEL BLOCKER TOXICITY

Electrolyte Supplement, Oral

CANDIDIASIS

Antifungal Agent

CANKER SORE

CARCINOMA

Antineoplastic Agent, Alkylating Agent

Antineoplastic Agent, Anthracycline

Antineoplastic Agent, Antibiotic

Antineoplastic Agent, Antimetabolite

Antineoplastic Agent, Antimetabolite (Pyrimidine Analog)

Antineoplastic Agent, Antimicrotubular

Antineoplastic Agent, Epothilone B Analog

Antineoplastic Agent, Estrogen Receptor Antagonist

Corticosteroid, Topical

Monoclonal Antibody

COLLAGEN DISORDERS

Adrenal Corticosteroid

Antiinflammatory Agent

Corticosteroid, Inhalant (Oral)

Corticosteroid, Systemic

Decongestant

Decongestant/Analgesic

Expectorant/Decongestant

Histamine H_1 Antagonist

Histamine H_1 Antagonist, First Generation

Imidazoline Derivative

Sympathomimetic

CONJUNCTIVITIS

CONJUNCTIVITIS (ALLERGIC)

CONSTIPATION

Ammonium Detoxicant

Anticonvulsant

Gastrointestinal Agent, Miscellaneous

Gastrointestinal Agent, Prokinetic

Genitourinary Irrigant

Laxative

Laxative, Osmotic

Laxative, Stimulant

Opioid Antagonist, Peripherally-Acting

Serotonin 5-HT_4 Receptor Agonist

Radiological/Contrast Media, Nonionic (Iso-Osmolality)

Radiological/Contrast Media, Paramagnetic Agent

CORNEAL EDEMA

Ophthalmic Agent, Miscellaneous

COUGH

Alpha/Beta Agonist

Analgesic, Miscellaneous

Analgesic, Narcotic

Antihistamine

Antihistamine/Antitussive

Antihistamine/Decongestant/Antitussive

Antihistamine/Decongestant/Antitussive/Expectorant

Antihistamine/Decongestant Combination

Antitussive

Antitussive/Decongestant

Antitussive/Decongestant/Expectorant

Antitussive/Expectorant

Cold Preparation

Cough Preparation

Decongestant

Expectorant

Expectorant/Decongestant

Expectorant/Decongestant/Antitussive

Histamine H_1 Antagonist

DEPRESSION

Antidepressant

Antidepressant, Alpha-2 Antagonist

Antidepressant, Aminoketone

Antidepressant, Miscellaneous

Antidepressant, Monoamine Oxidase Inhibitor

Antidepressant, Phenethylamine

Antidepressant/Phenothiazine

Antidepressant, Selective Serotonin Reuptake Inhibitor

Corticosteroid, Topical

DIARRHEA (TRAVELER'S)

Antibiotic, Miscellaneous

Antidiarrheal

Vaccine

DIETARY SUPPLEMENT

Dietary Supplement

DIGITALIS GLYCOSIDE POISONING

Antidote

DIPHTHERIA

Antitoxin

DISCOID LUPUS ERYTHEMATOSUS (DLE)

Corticosteroid, Topical

Immune Response Modifier

Immunosuppressant Agent

Topical Skin Product

Nonsteroidal Antiinflammatory Drug (NSAID), COX-2 Selective

DYSURIA

Analgesic, Urinary

Antispasmodic Agent, Urinary

Estrogen Derivative

EAR WAX

Otic Agent, Analgesic

Otic Agent, Ceruminolytic

EATON-LAMBERT SYNDROME

Cholinergic Agent

ECHOCARDIOGRAM AID

Diagnostic Agent

ECLAMPSIA

Anticonvulsant

Barbiturate

FAMILIAL MEDITERRANEAN FEVER (FMF)

Antigout Agent

FATTY ACID DEFICIENCY

Intravenous Nutritional Therapy

Nutritional Supplement

FEBRILE NEUTROPENIA

Antibiotic, Quinolone

Antifungal Agent, Systemic

Cephalosporin (Fourth Generation)

Colony-Stimulating Factor

Penicillin

FEVER

Antipyretic

Antitussive/Decongestant

Cold Preparation

Decongestant

Histamine H_1 Antagonist

HIV INFECTIONS

HODGKIN DISEASE

HOMOCYSTINURIA

HOOKWORMS

HORMONAL IMBALANCE (FEMALE)

HMG-CoA Reductase Inhibitor

Vitamin, Water Soluble

HYPERHIDROSIS

Topical Skin Product

HYPERHOMOCYSTEINEMIA

Dietary Supplement

HYPERKALEMIA

Alkalinizing Agent

Antacid

Antidote

Electrolyte Supplement, Oral

HYPERPARATHYROIDISM

Calcimimetic

Vitamin D Analog

HYPERPHOSPHATEMIA

Electrolyte Supplement, Oral

Phosphate Binder

HYPERPIGMENTATION

Topical Skin Product

HYPERPROLACTINEMIA

Ergot Alkaloid and Derivative

Ergot-like Derivative

HYPERTENSION

Adrenergic Agonist Agent

Alpha-Adrenergic Agonist

Alpha-Adrenergic Blocking Agent

Antihypertensive Agent, Combination

Beta-Adrenergic Blocker

Beta-Adrenergic Blocker, Nonselective

Beta Blocker, Beta-1 Selective

Beta Blocker With Intrinsic Sympathomimetic Activity

Calcium Channel Blocker

Calcium Channel Blocker, Dihydropyridine

Diagnostic Agent

Diuretic, Combination

MIGRAINE

Analgesic, Narcotic

Analgesic, Nonnarcotic

Antimigraine Agent

Beta-Adrenergic Blocker

Beta-Adrenergic Blocker, Nonselective

Calcium-Entry Blocker (Selective)

Ergot Alkaloid and Derivative

Ergot Derivative

Histone Deacetylase Inhibitor

OSTEOPOROSIS

Calcium Salt

Contraceptive, Oral

Diagnostic Agent

Electrolyte Supplement, Oral

OVULATION INDUCTION

Gonadotropin

PAGET DISEASE OF BONE

Bisphosphonate Derivative

Polypeptide Hormone

PAIN

Analgesic Combination (Opioid)

Analgesic, Miscellaneous

Analgesic, Narcotic

Analgesic, Nonnarcotic

Analgesic, Opioid

Androgen

Antihistamine

Nonsteroidal Antiinflammatory Drug (NSAID)

PARACOCCIDIOIDOMYCOSIS

Antifungal Agent, Oral

PARALYTIC ILEUS (PROPHYLAXIS)

Gastrointestinal Agent, Stimulant

PARKINSONISM

Anti-Parkinson Agent

Anti-Parkinson Agent, COMT Inhibitor

Anti-Parkinson Agent (Dopamine Agonist)

Anti-Parkinson Agent, MAO Type B Inhibitor

Antiviral Agent

Dopaminergic Agent (Anti-Parkinson)

Ergot Alkaloid and Derivative

Histamine H_1 Antagonist

Bile Acid Sequestrant

Corticosteroid, Topical

Histamine H_1 Antagonist

Histamine H_1 Antagonist, First Generation

Local Anesthetic

Corticosteroid, Topical

Immunosuppressant Agent

Interleukin-12 Inhibitor

Interleukin-23 Inhibitor

Keratolytic Agent

REPLACEMENT SOLUTION

Alkalinizing Agent

Electrolyte Supplement

RESPIRATORY DISTRESS SYNDROME (RDS)

Lung Surfactant

RESPIRATORY SYNCYTIAL VIRUS (RSV)

Antiviral Agent

Monoclonal Antibody

RESPIRATORY TRACT INFECTION

Amebicide

Aminoglycoside (Antibiotic)

Antibiotic, Aminoglycoside

Antibiotic, Lincosamide

Antibiotic, Macrolide

Antibiotic, Miscellaneous

Antibiotic, Quinolone

Antiprotozoal, Nitroimidazole

Carbapenem (Antibiotic)

Cephalosporin (First Generation)

Cephalosporin (Second Generation)

Cephalosporin (Third Generation)

Cephalosporin (Fourth Generation)

Macrolide (Antibiotic)

Penicillin

Respiratory Fluoroquinolone

Sulfonamide

Tetracycline Derivative

Antihistamine

Antihistamine/Decongestant/Anticholinergic

Antihistamine/Decongestant/Antitussive

Antihistamine/Decongestant Combination

Antihistamine/Decongestant Combination, Nonsedating

Antihistamine, Nonsedating

Antitussive

Corticosteroid, Inhalant (Oral)

Corticosteroid, Nasal

Corticosteroid, Systemic

Decongestant

Decongestant/Analgesic

Decongestant/Anticholingeric Combination

Expectorant

Histamine H_1 Antagonist

Histamine H_1 Antagonist, First Generation

Histamine H_1 Antagonist, Second Generation

Imidazoline Derivative

SCLERODERMA

Aminoquinoline (Antimalarial)

SCURVY

Vitamin, Water Soluble

SEBORRHEIC DERMATITIS

Antiseborrheic Agent, Topical

SEDATION

Alpha-Adrenergic Agonist - Central-Acting (Alpha$_2$-Agonists)

SEDATION

SORE THROAT

Local Anesthetic

SPASTICITY

Alpha$_2$-Adrenergic Agonist Agent

Benzodiazepine

Skeletal Muscle Relaxant

SPINAL CORD INJURY

Bisphosphonate Derivative

Skeletal Muscle Relaxant

STATUS EPILEPTICUS

Anticonvulsant

Benzodiazepine

Hydantoin

STOMATITIS

Gastrointestinal Agent, Miscellaneous

Local Anesthetic

TOTAL PARENTERAL NUTRITION

Intravenous Nutritional Therapy

TOURETTE DISEASE

Antipsychotic Agent, Butyrophenone

Monoamine Depleting Agent

Neuroleptic Agent

Phenothiazine Derivative

TOXICITY, NONSPECIFIC (TREATMENT)

Antacid

Antidote

ULCER (PEPTIC)

Antineoplastic Agent

Electrolyte Supplement, Oral

Gastric Acid Secretion Inhibitor

Histamine H_2 Antagonist

Prostaglandin

Proton Pump Inhibitor

Substituted Benzimidazole

ZOLLINGER-ELLISON SYNDROME (DIAGNOSTIC)

Diagnostic Agent

2010

QUICK LOOK DRUG BOOK

Top 200 Prescribed Tablets and Capsules with Images

The Quick Look Drug Book 2010 Top 200 Prescribed Drugs insert displays actual colór photographs of the most commonly prescribed tablets and capsules.

Drugs are listed alphabetically by generic name, and, where applicable, the trade name is listed. Dosages appear under each individual image.

Use the white scale at the bottom of each image to determine the actual size. The distance between each division on the scale is equivalent to 1/8 inch or 3.175 mm.

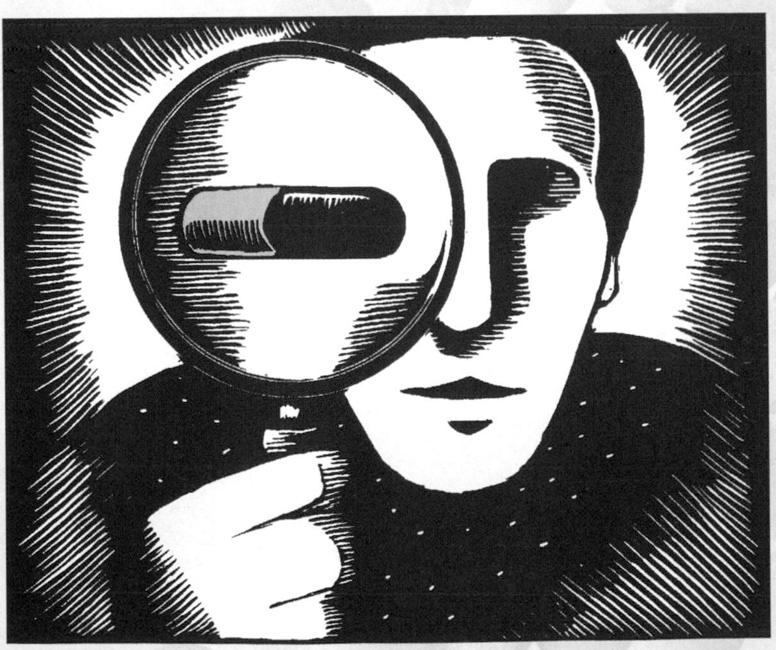

Acetaminophen

(generic)

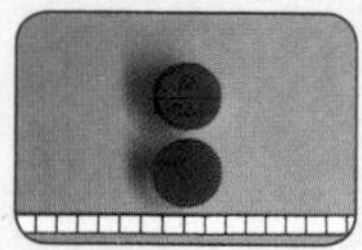

80 mg

325 mg

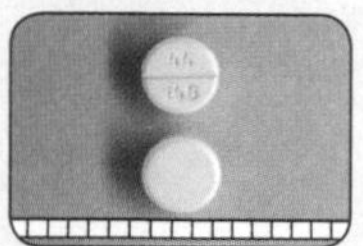

500 mg

Acyclovir

(generic)

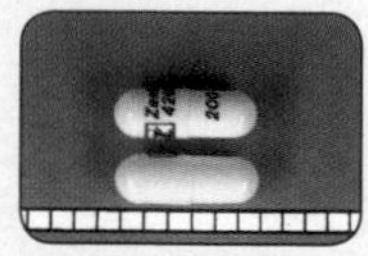

200 mg

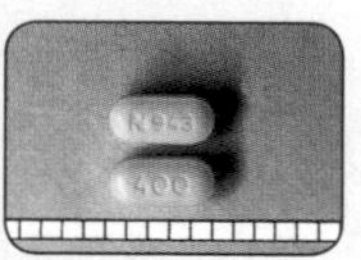

400 mg

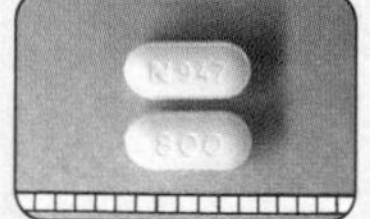

800 mg

Albuterol

(generic)

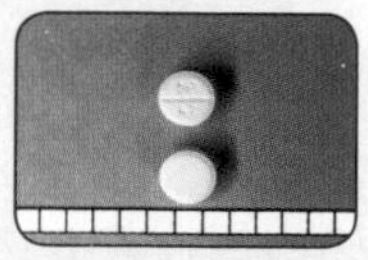

2 mg

Alendronate

(generic)

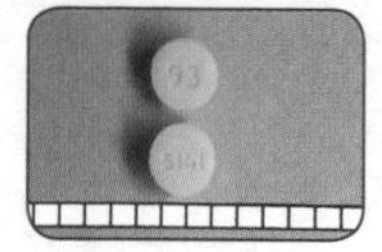

10 mg

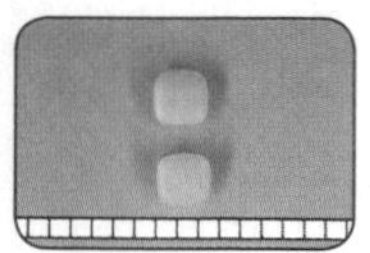

70 mg

Allopurinol

(generic)

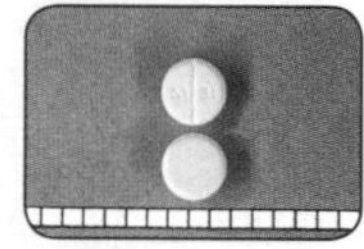

100 mg

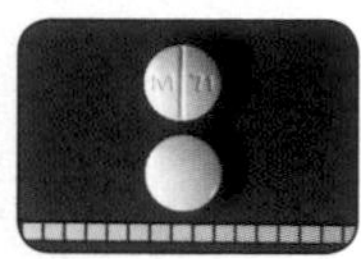

300 mg

Alprazolam

(generic)

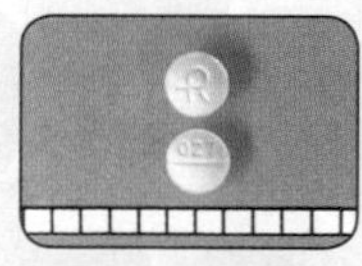

0.25 mg

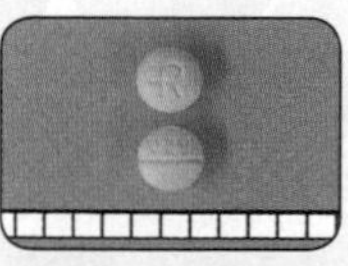

0.5 mg

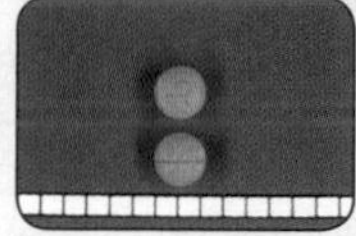

1 mg

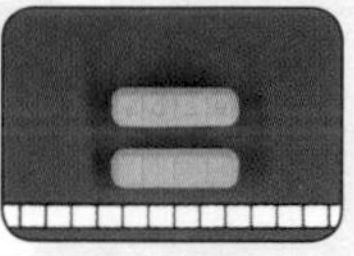

2 mg

Amitriptyline

(generic)

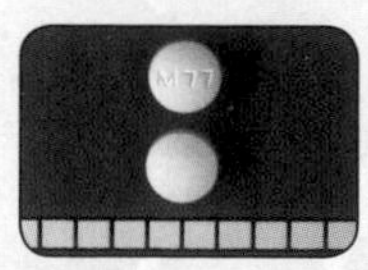

10 mg

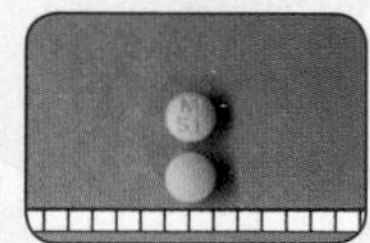

25 mg

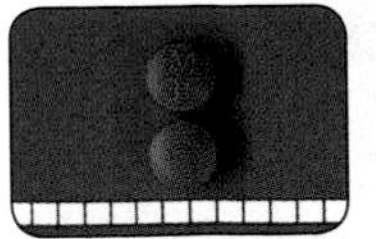
50 mg

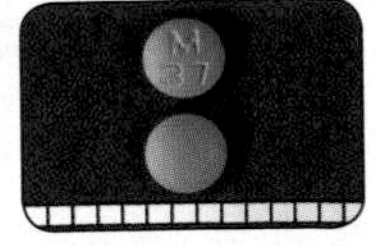
75 mg

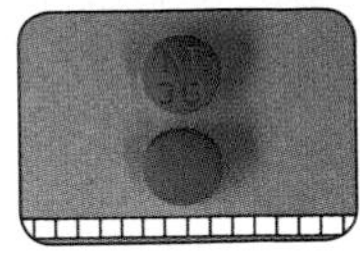
100 mg

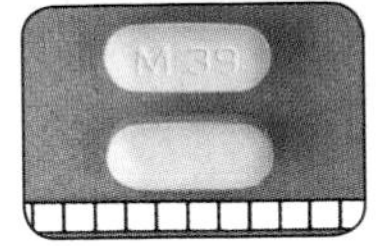
150 mg

Amlodipine

(generic)

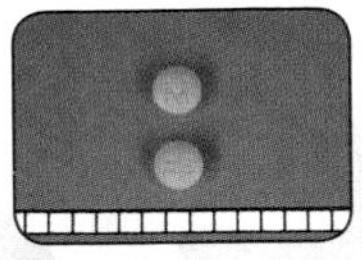
2.5 mg

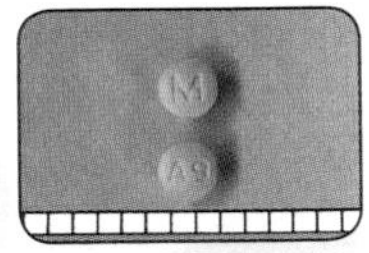
5 mg

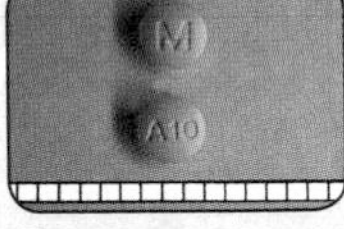
10 mg

Amlodipine and Benazepril

(generic)

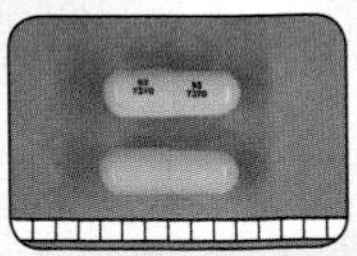
2.5/10 mg

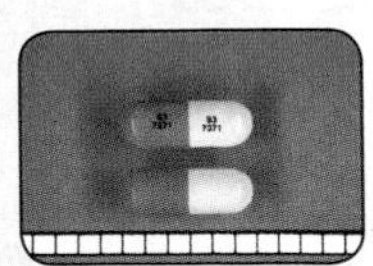
5/10 mg

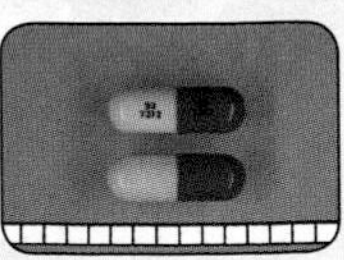
5/20 mg

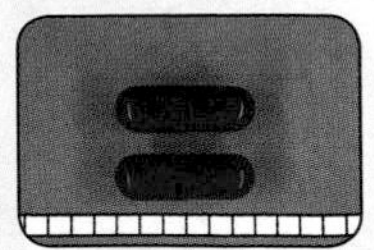
10/20 mg

Amoxicillin

(generic)

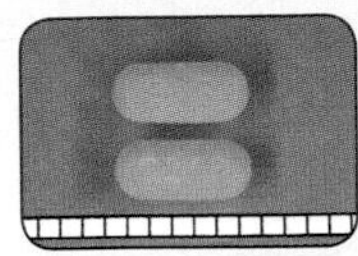
250 mg

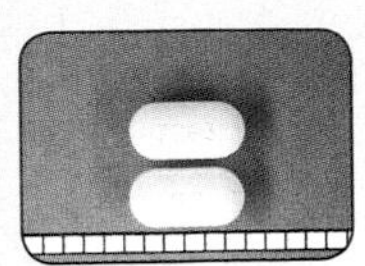
500 mg

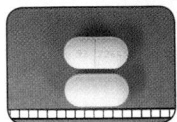

875 mg

Amoxicillin and Clavulanate Potassium

(generic)

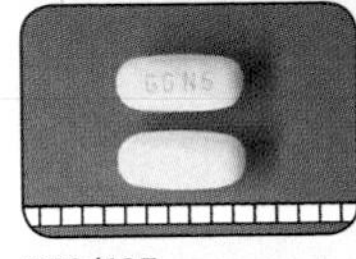
250/125 mg

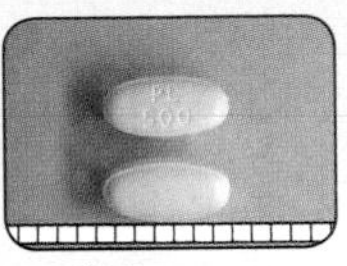
500/125 mg

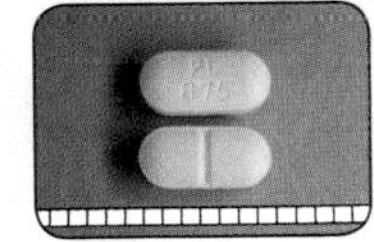
875/125 mg

Aripiprazole

Abilify®

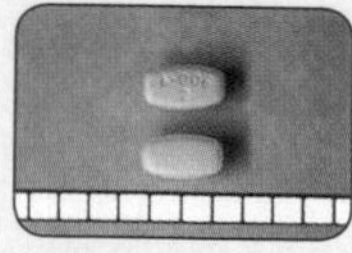
2 mg

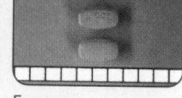

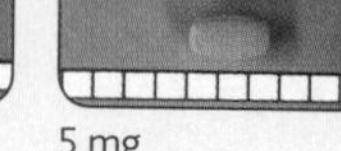
5 mg

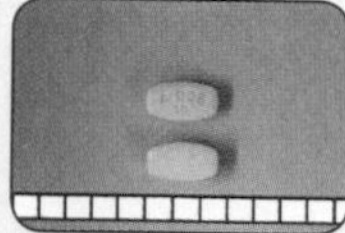
10 mg

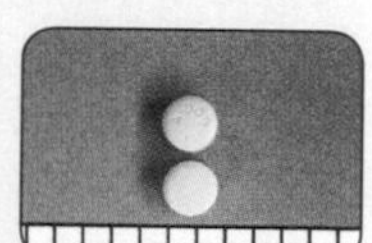
15 mg

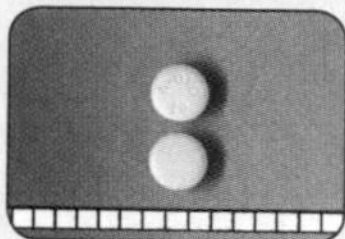
20 mg

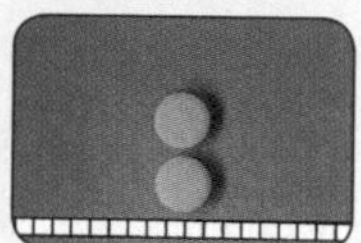
30 mg

Atenolol

(generic)

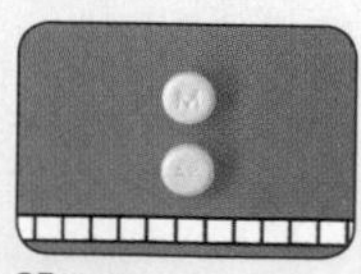
25 mg

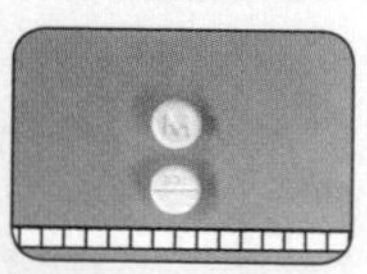
50 mg

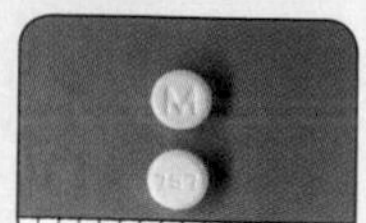
100 mg

Azithromycin

(generic)

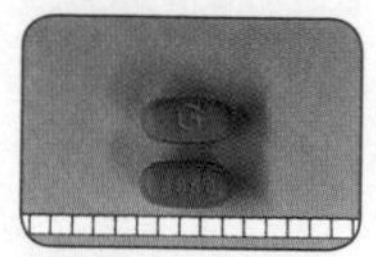
250 mg

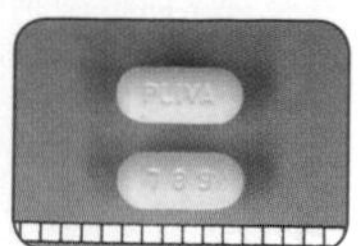
600 mg

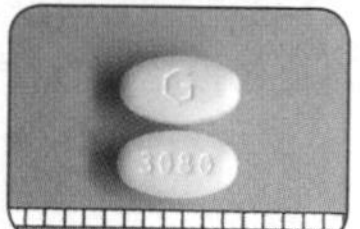

600 mg

Benazepril

(generic)

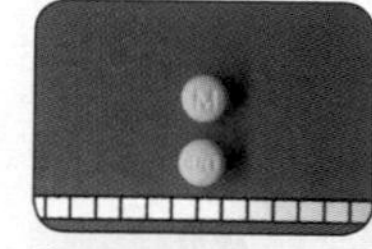
5 mg

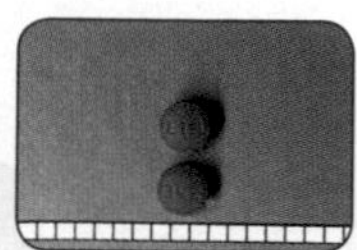
10 mg

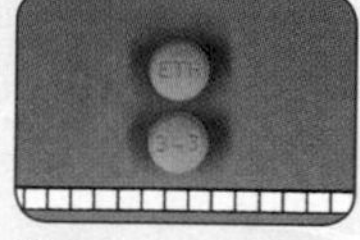
20 mg

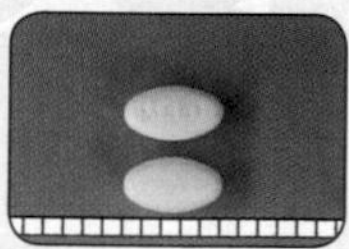
40 mg

Benzonatate

(generic)

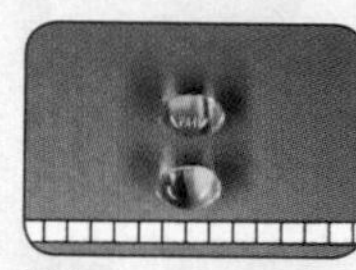
100 mg

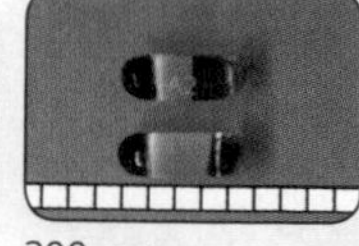
200 mg

Bisoprolol and Hydrochlorothiazide

(generic)

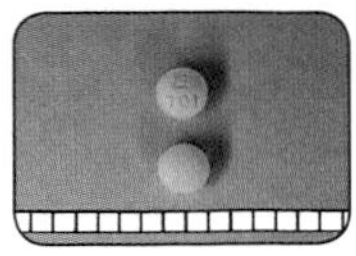

2.5/6.25 mg

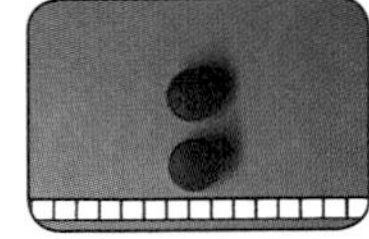

5/6.25 mg

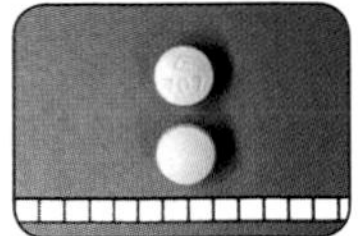

10/6.25 mg

Buprenorphine and Naloxone

Suboxone®

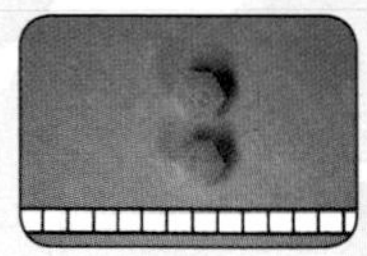

2/0.5 mg

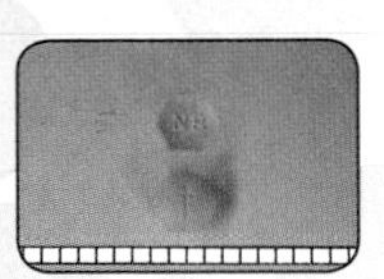

8/2 mg

Bupropion

(generic)

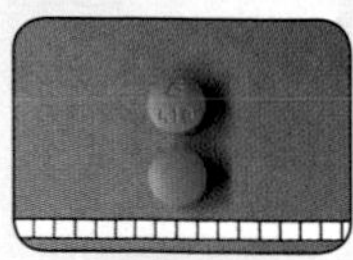

100 mg

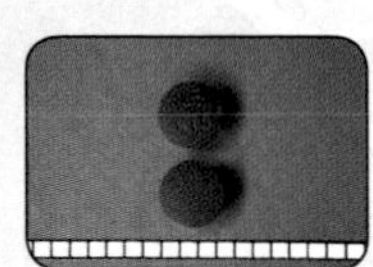

150 mg

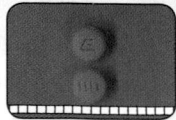

200 mg

Budeprion XL®

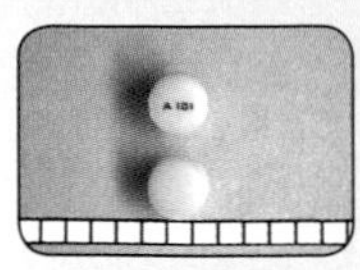

150 mg

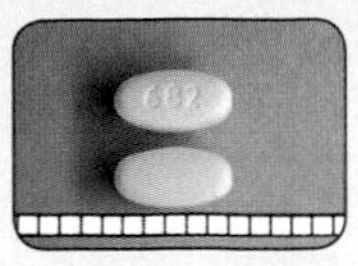

300 mg

Buspirone

(generic)

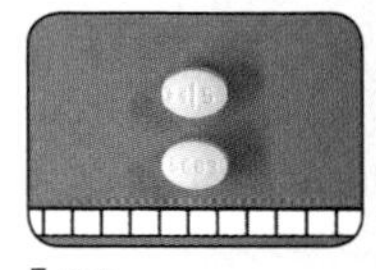

5 mg

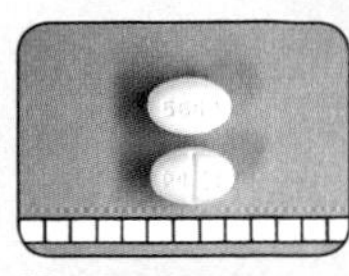

10 mg

Butalbital, Acetaminophen, and Caffeine

(generic)

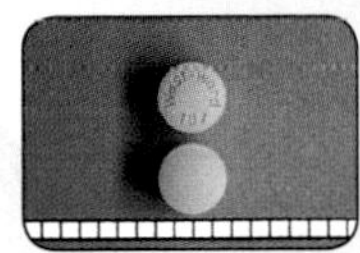

50/325/40 mg

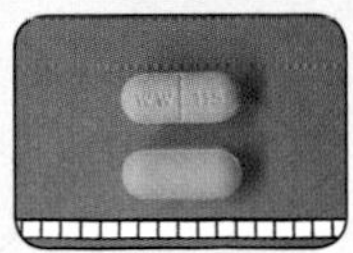

50/500/40 mg

Carisoprodol

Soma®

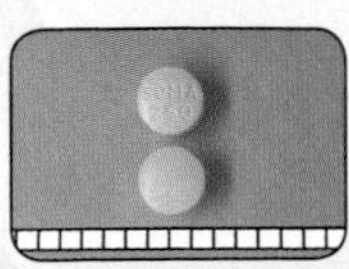

250 mg

Carvedilol

(generic)

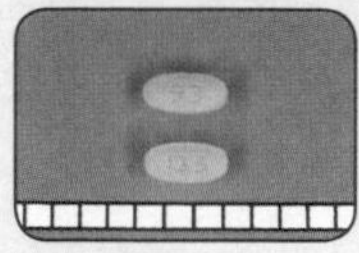
6.25 mg

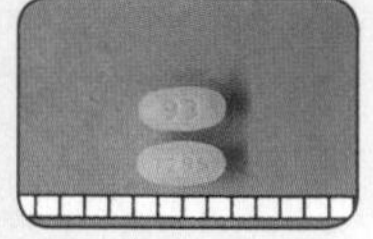
12.5 mg

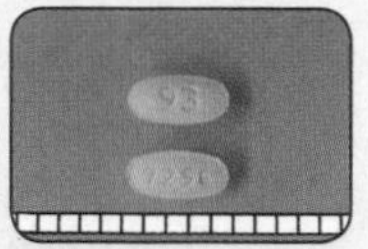
25 mg

Cefdinir

(generic)

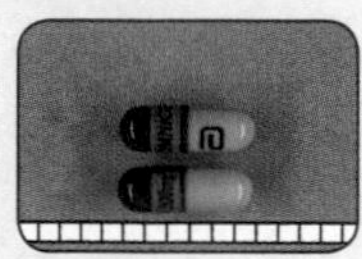
300 mg

Celecoxib

Celebrex®

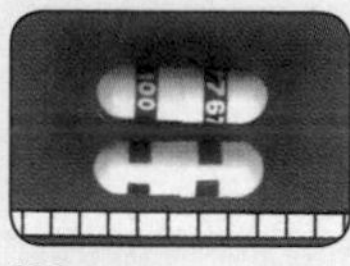
100 mg

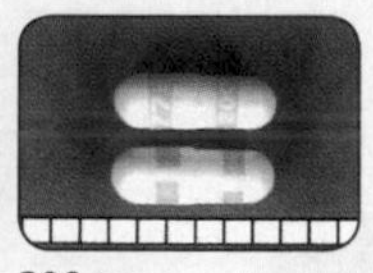
200 mg

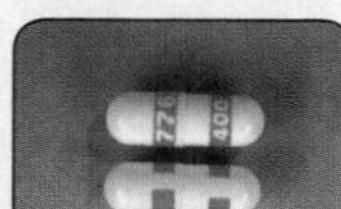
400 mg

Cephalexin

(generic)

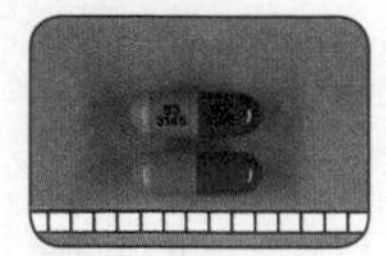
250 mg

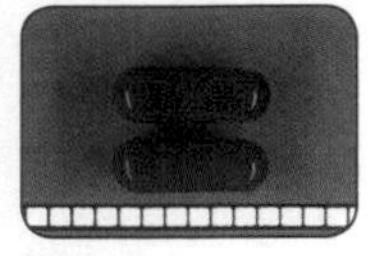
500 mg

Ciprofloxacin

(generic)

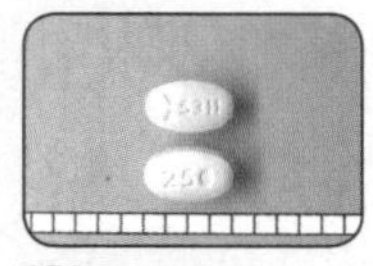
250 mg

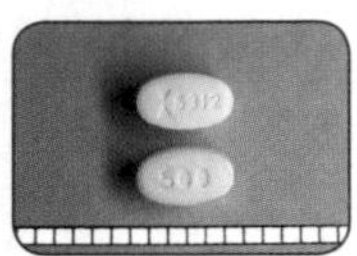
500 mg

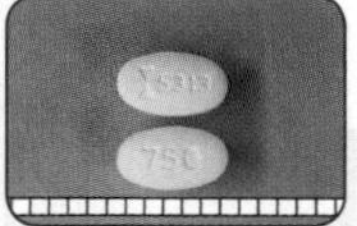
750 mg

Citalopram

(generic)

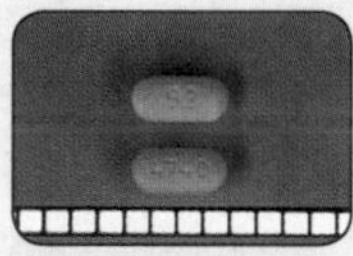
10 mg

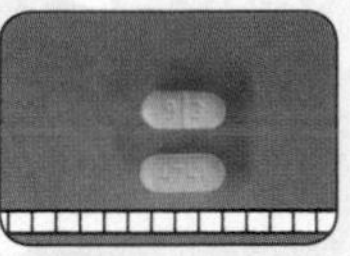
20 mg

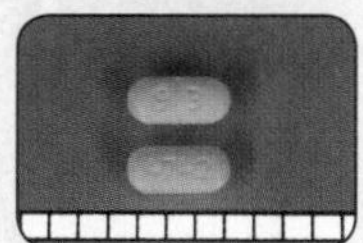
40 mg

Clindamycin

(generic)

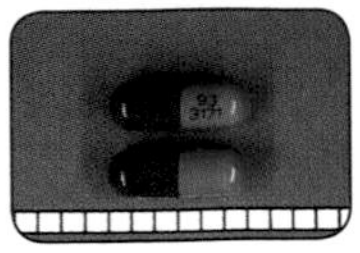
150 mg

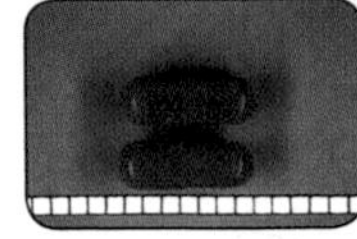
300 mg

Clonazepam

(generic)

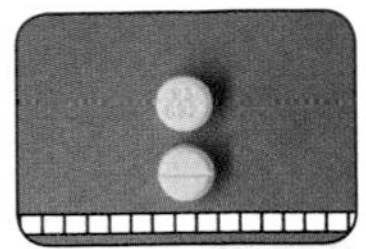
0.5 mg

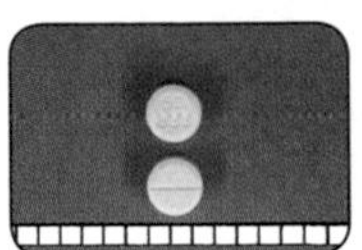
1 mg

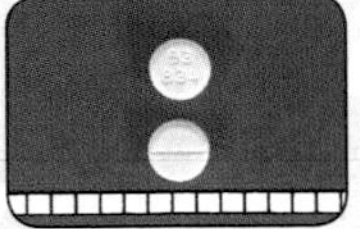
2 mg

Clonidine

(generic)

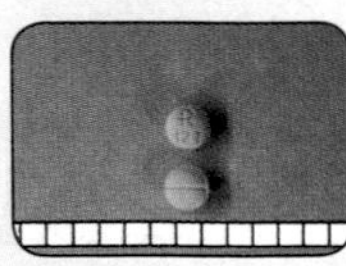
0.1 mg

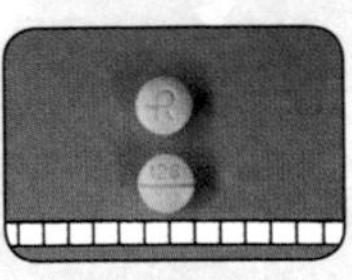
0.2 mg

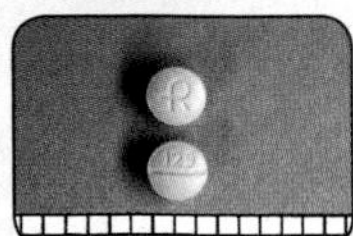
0.3 mg

Clopidogrel

Plavix®

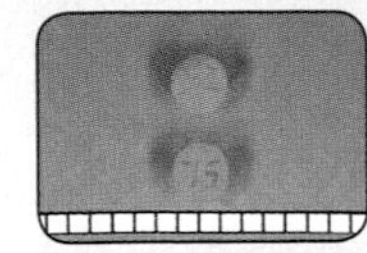
75 mg

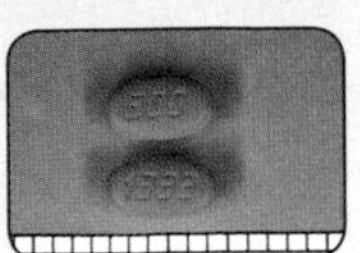
300 mg

Cyclobenzaprine

(generic)

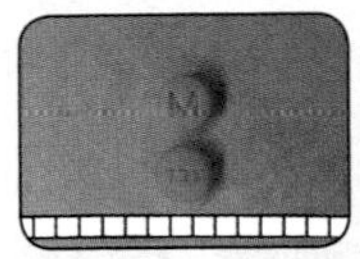
5 mg

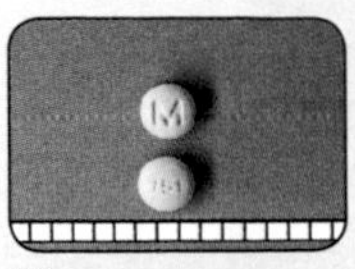
10 mg

Dextroamphetamine and Amphetamine

(generic)

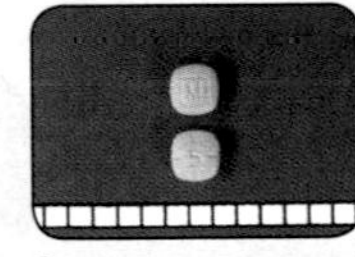
5 mg

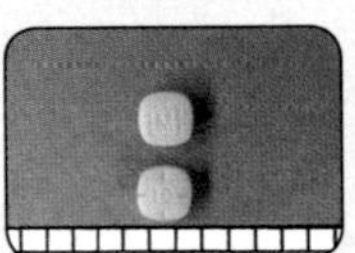
10 mg

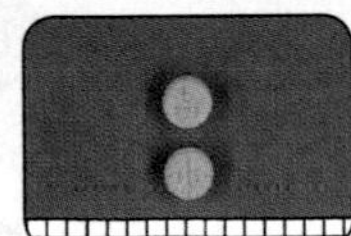
15 mg

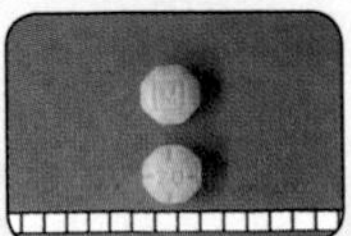
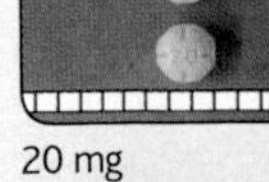
20 mg

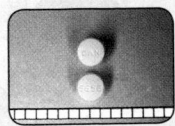

30 mg

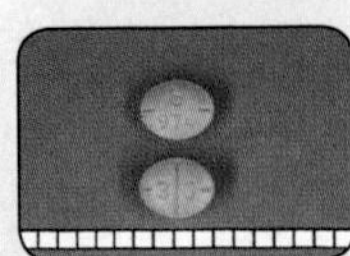
30 mg

Adderall®

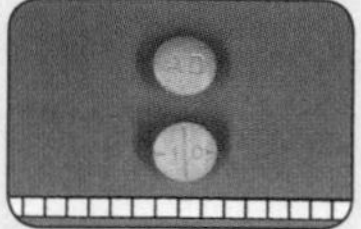
10 mg

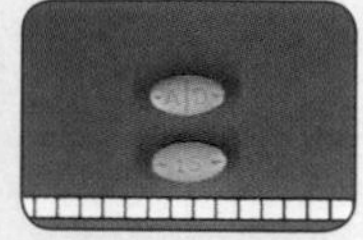
15 mg

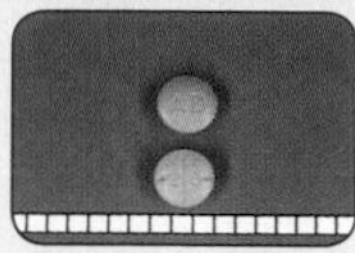
20 mg

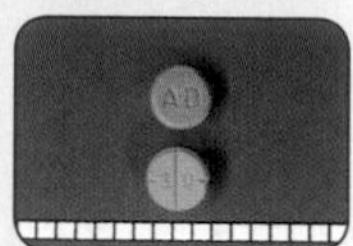
30 mg

Diazepam

(generic)

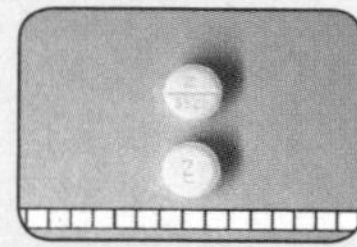
2 mg

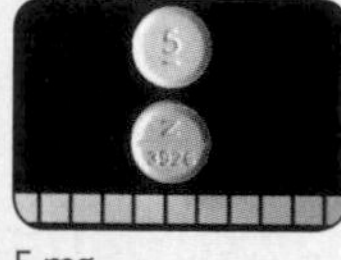
5 mg

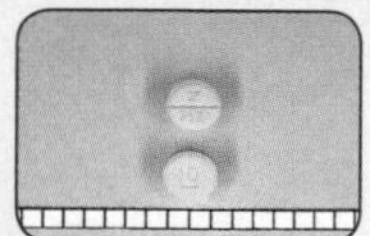
10 mg

Diclofenac

(generic)

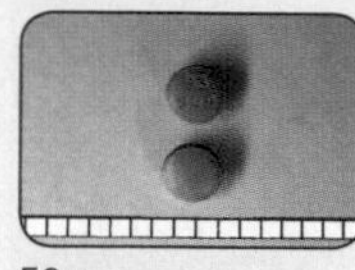
50 mg

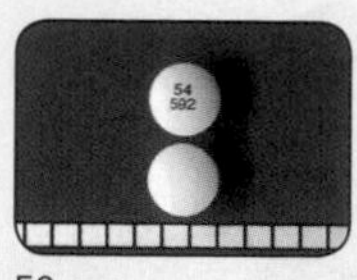

50 mg

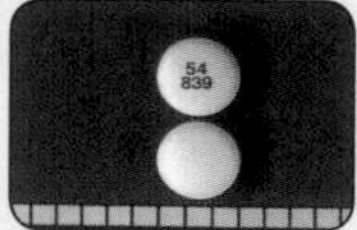

75 mg

Digoxin

(generic)

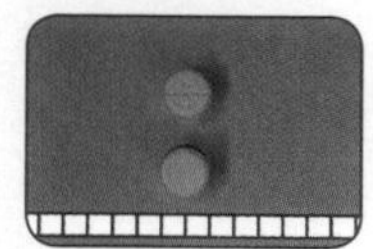
125 mcg

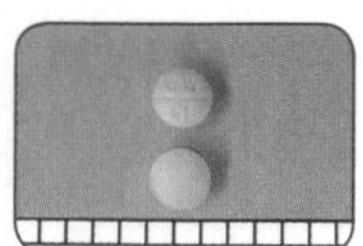
250 mcg

Diltiazem

(generic)

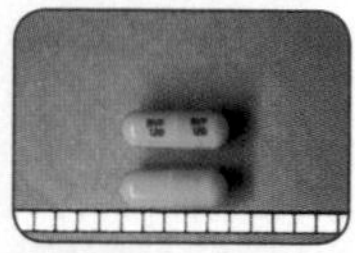
120 mg

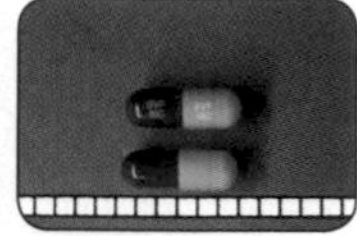
180 mg

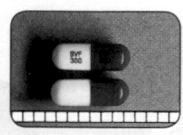

240 mg

300 mg

Divalproex

(generic)

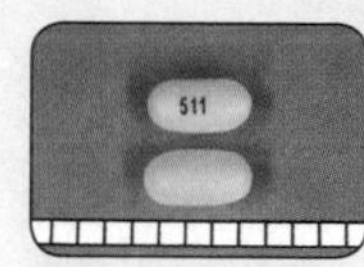

125 mg

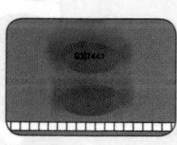

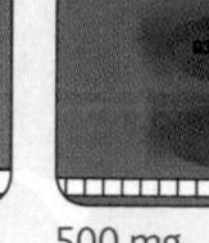
500 mg

Donepezil

Aricept®

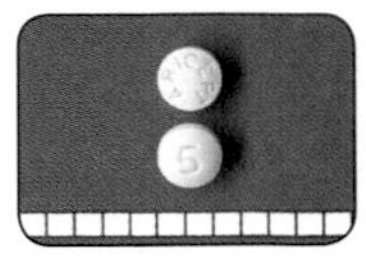

5 mg

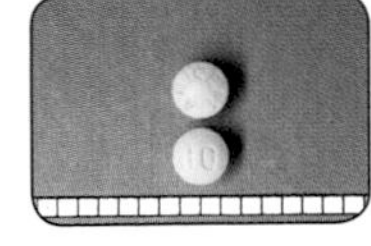

10 mg

Doxazosin

(generic)

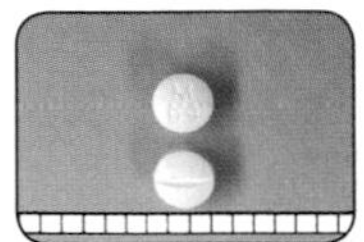

1 mg

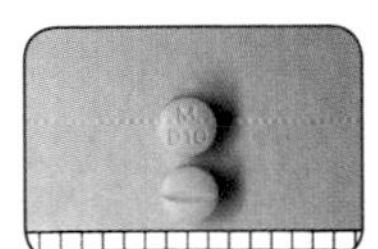

2 mg

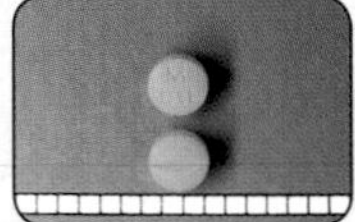

4 mg

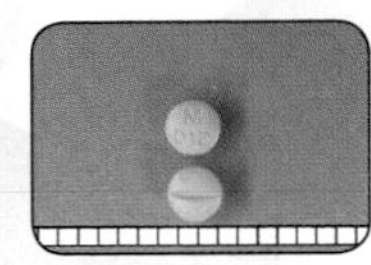

8 mg

Doxycycline

(generic)

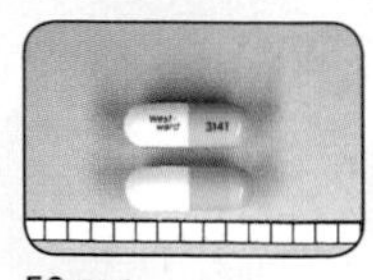

50 mg

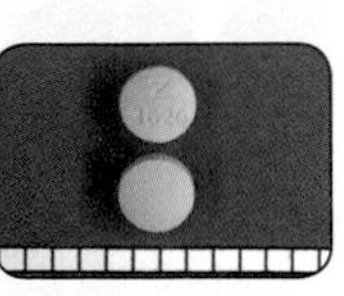

100 mg

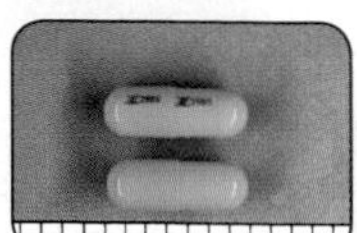

100 mg

Duloxetine

Cymbalta®

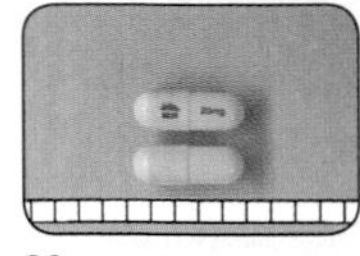

20 mg

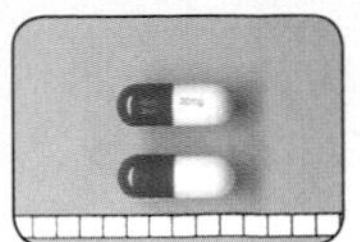

30 mg

60 mg

Enalapril

(generic)

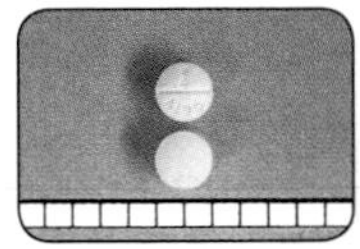

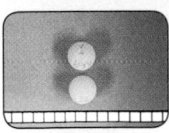

2.5 mg

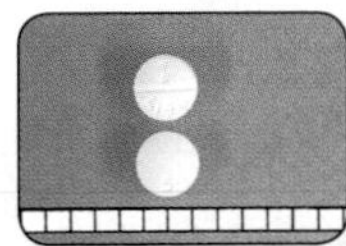

5 mg

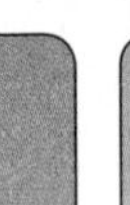

10 mg

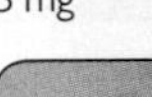

20 mg

Esomeprazole

Nexium®

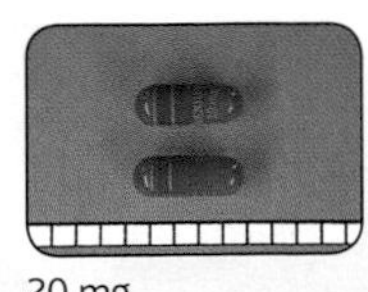

20 mg

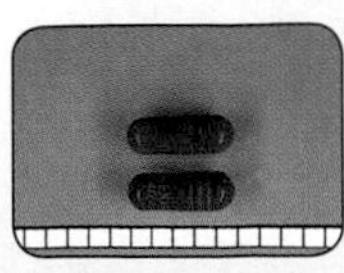

40 mg

Estradiol

(generic)

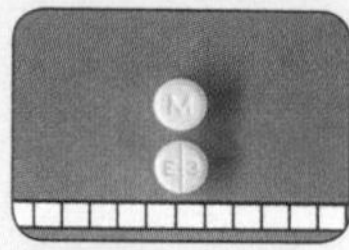

0.5 mg

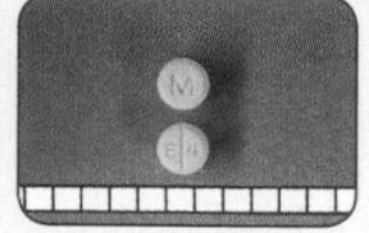

1 mg

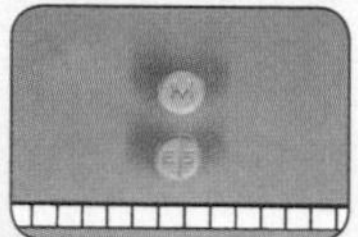

2 mg

Estrogens (Conjugated/Equine)

Premarin®

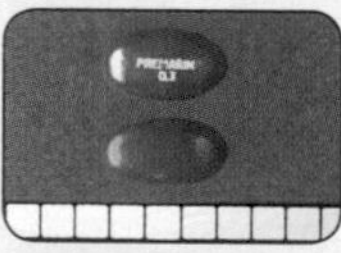

0.3 mg

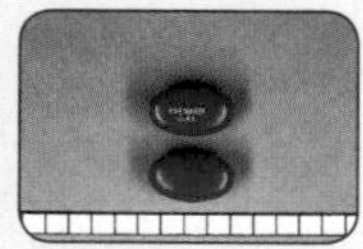

0.45 mg

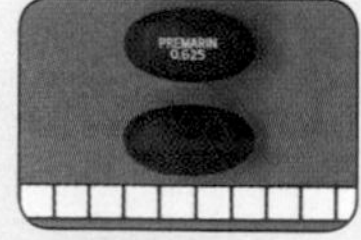

0.625 mg

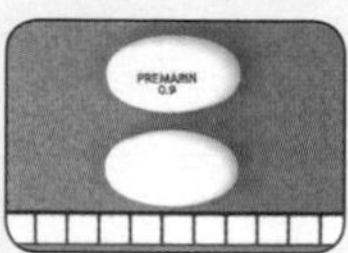

0.9 mg

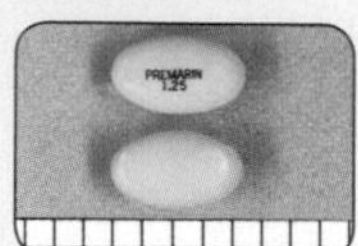

1.25 mg

Eszopiclone

Lunesta®

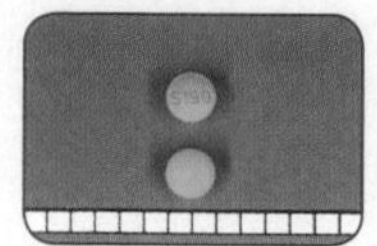

1 mg

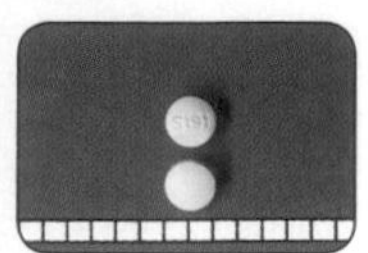

2 mg

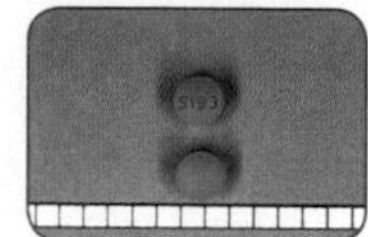

3 mg

Ethinyl Estradiol and Drospirenone

Ocella®

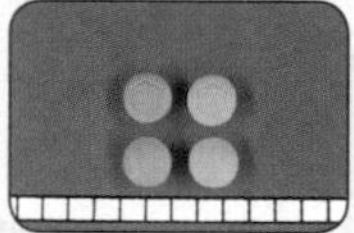

0.03/3 mg

Yaz®

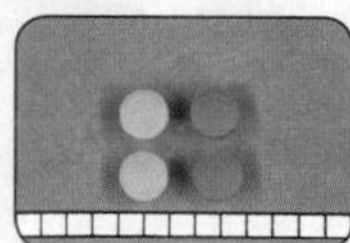

0.02/3 mg

Ethinyl Estradiol and Norgestimate

Sprintec®

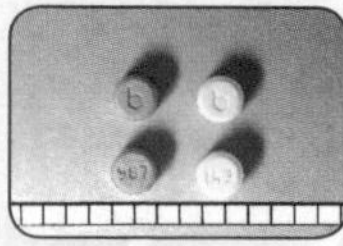

0.035/0.25 mg

TriNessa®

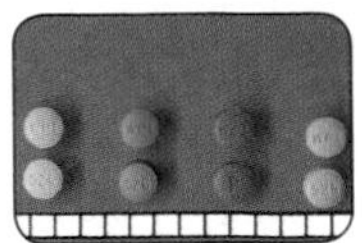

multiple # dosages

Ezetimibe

Zetia®

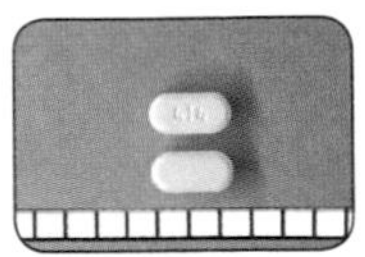

10 mg

Ezetimibe and Simvastatin

Vytorin®

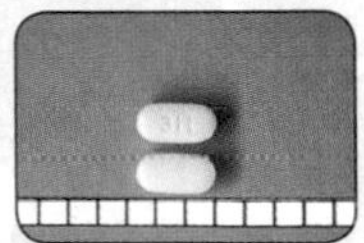

10/10 mg

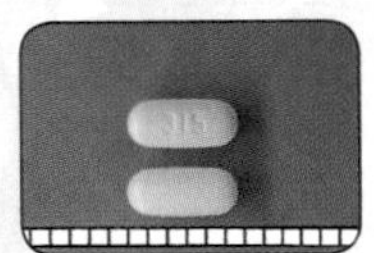

10/20 mg

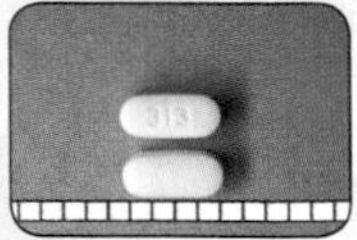

10/40 mg

10/80 mg

Famotidine

(generic)

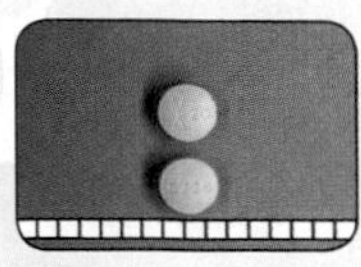

20 mg

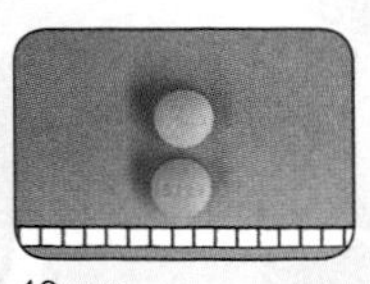

40 mg

Fenofibrate

TriCor®

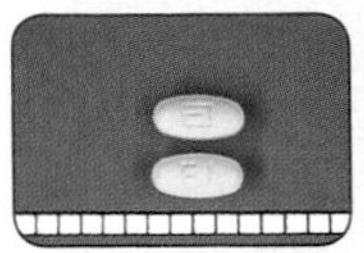

48 mg

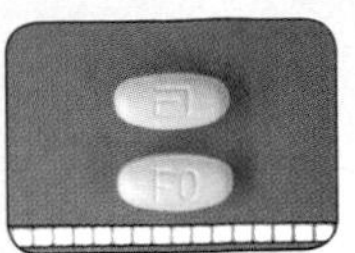

145 mg

Fexofenadine

(generic)

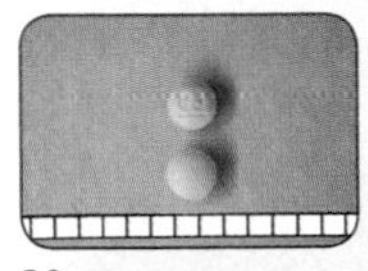

30 mg

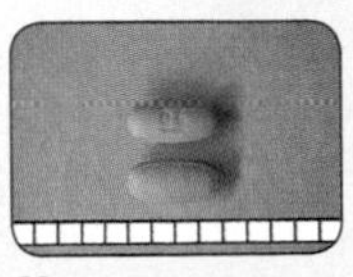

60 mg

180 mg

Finasteride

(generic)

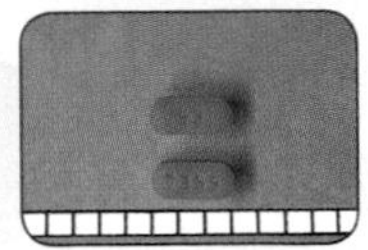

5 mg

Fluoxetine

(generic)

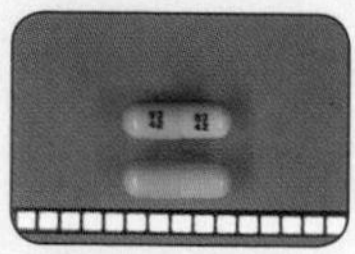
10 mg

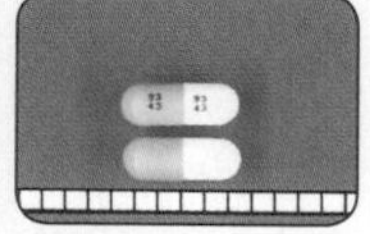
20 mg

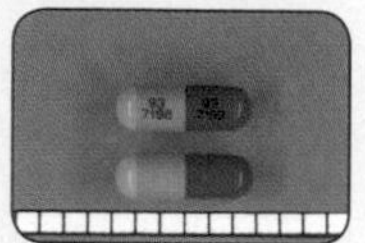
40 mg

Fluconazole

(generic)

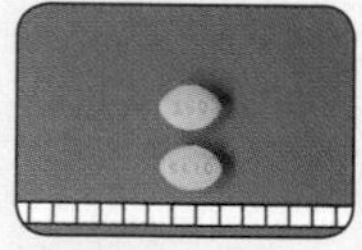
50 mg

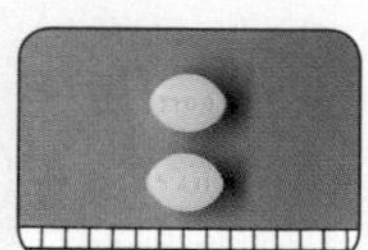
100 mg

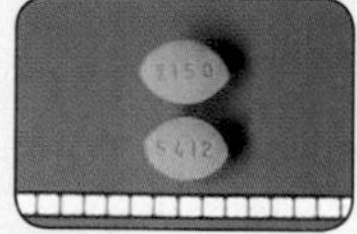
150 mg

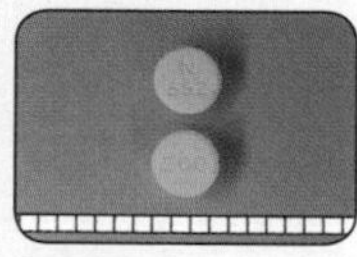
200 mg

Folic Acid

(generic)

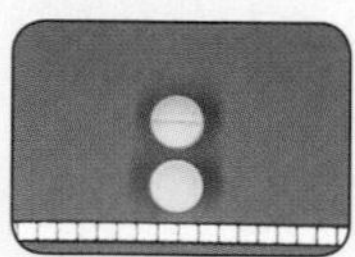
0.8 mg

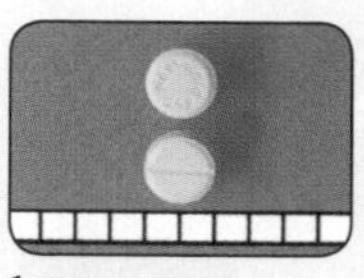
1 mg

Furosemide

(generic)

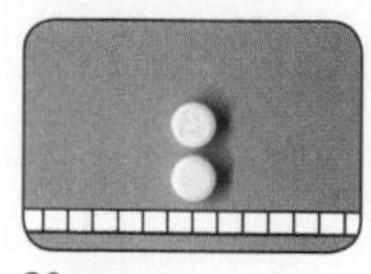
20 mg

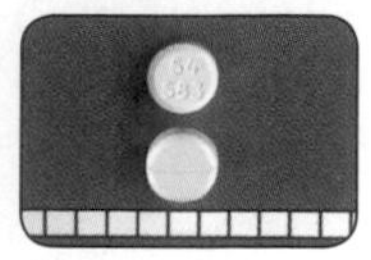
40 mg

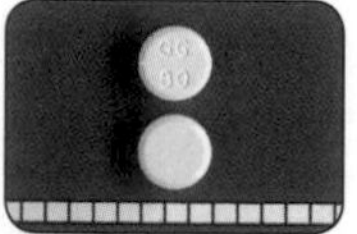
80 mg

Gabapentin

(generic)

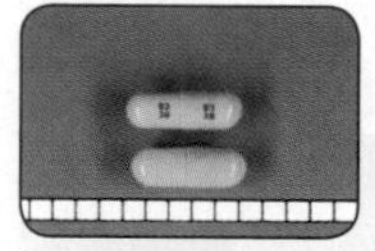
100 mg

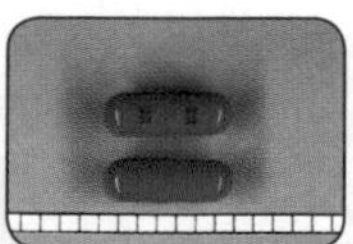
300 mg

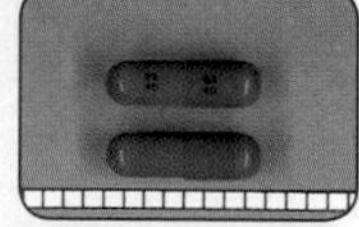
400 mg

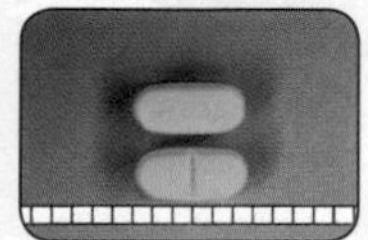
600 mg

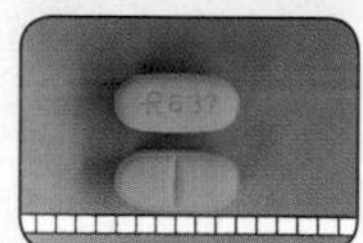
800 mg

Gemfibrozil

(generic)

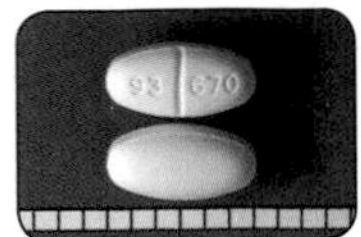

600 mg

Glimepiride

(generic)

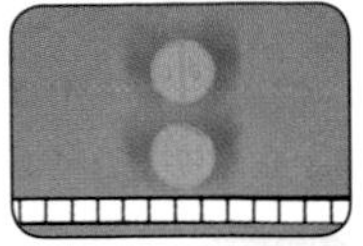

1 mg

2 mg

4 mg

Glipizide

(generic)

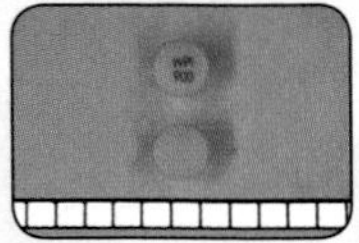

2.5 mg

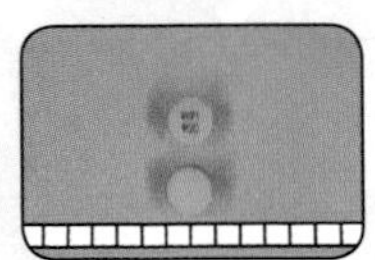

2.5 mg

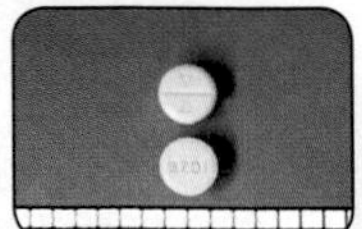

5 mg

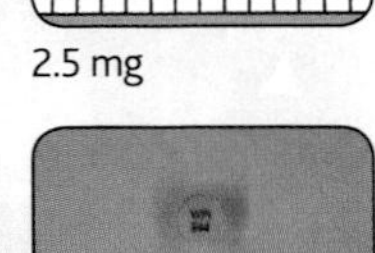

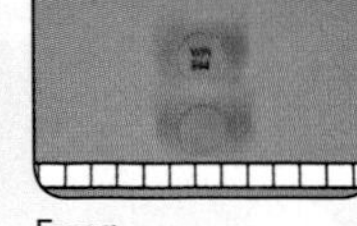

5 mg

10 mg

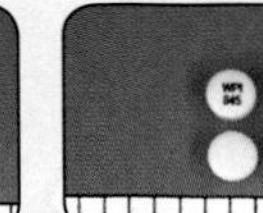

10 mg

Glyburide

(generic)

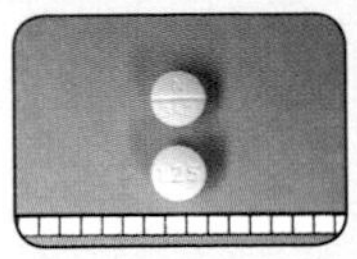

1.25 mg

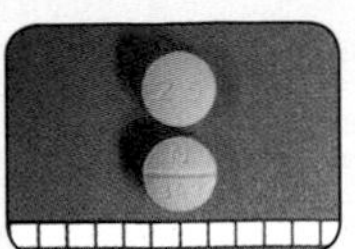

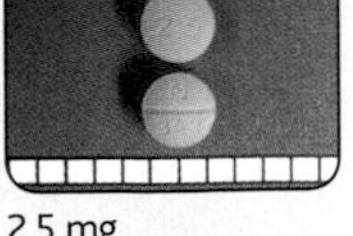

2.5 mg

3 mg

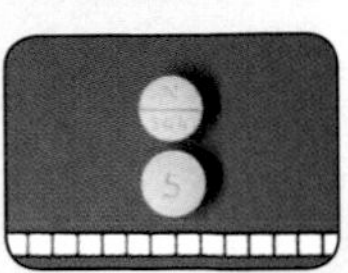

5 mg

6 mg

Glyburide Metformin

(generic)

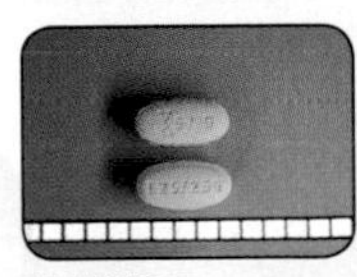

1.25/250 mg

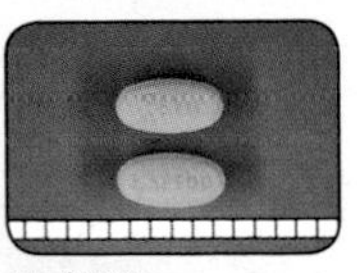

2.5/500 mg

5/500 mg

Hydrochlorothiazide

(generic)

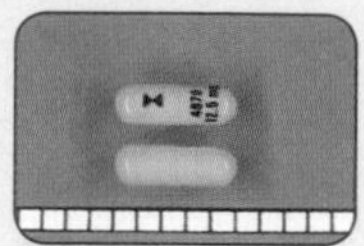

12.5 mg

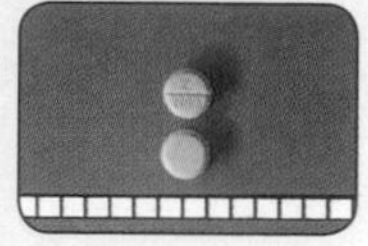

25 mg

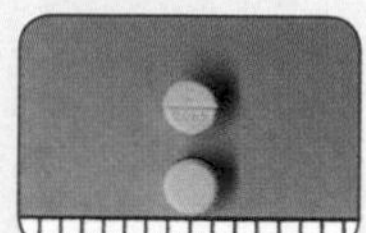

50 mg

Hydrocodone and Acetaminophen

(generic)

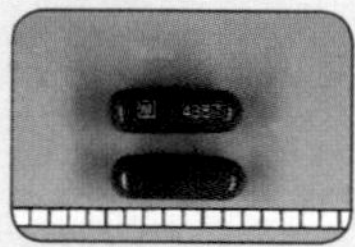

5/500 mg

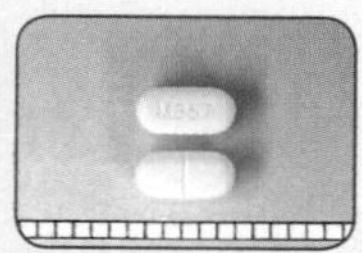

5/500 mg

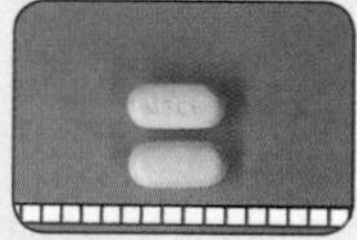

7.5/325 mg mg

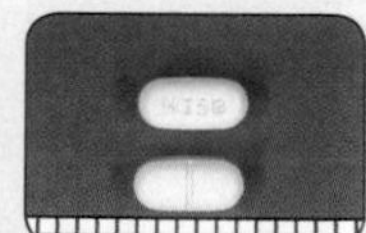

7.5/500 mg mg

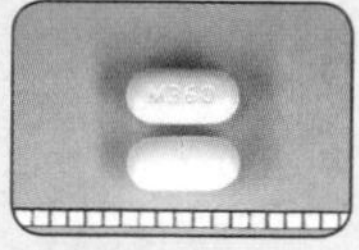

7.5/750 mg mg

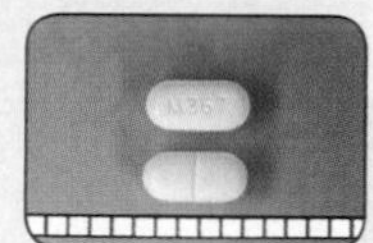

10/325 mg

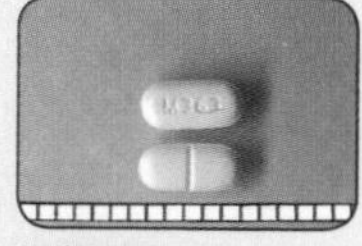

10/500 mg

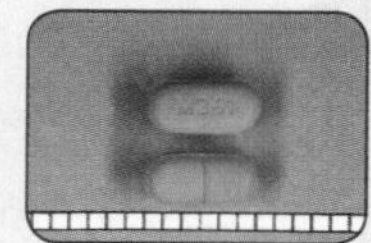

10/650 mg

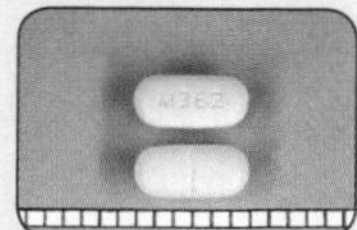

10/660 mg

Hydroxyzine

(generic)

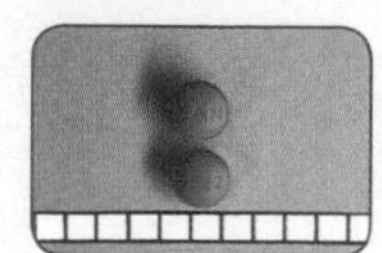

10 mg

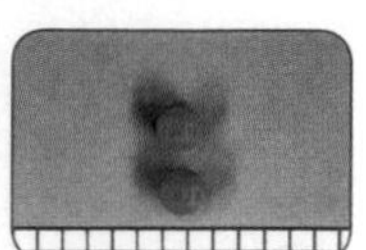

25 mg

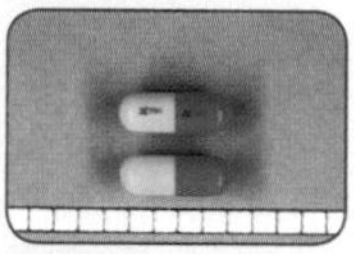

25 mg

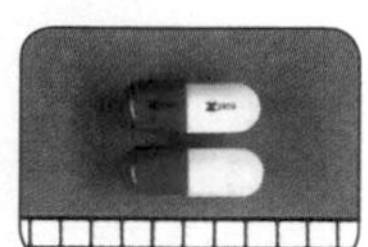

50 mg

Ibandronate

Boniva®

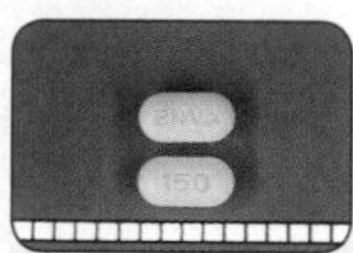

150 mg

Irbesartan

Avapro®

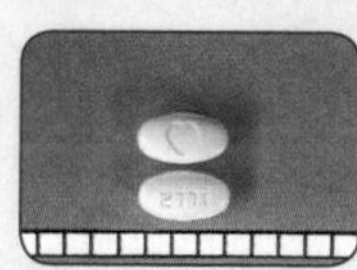

75 mg

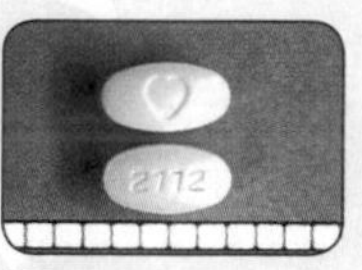

150 mg

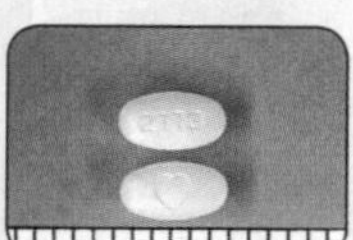

300 mg

Lansoprazole

Prevacid®

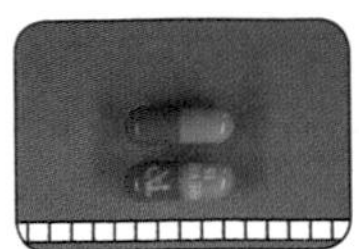
15 mg

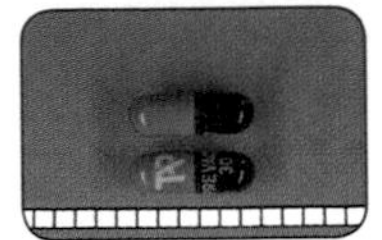
30 mg

Prevacid® SoluTab™

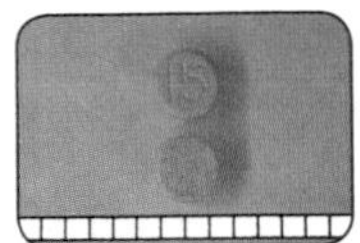
15 mg

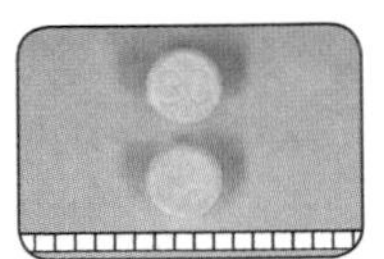
30 mg

Levothyroxine

(generic)

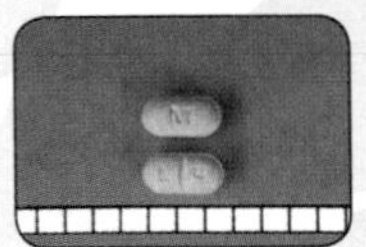
25 mcg

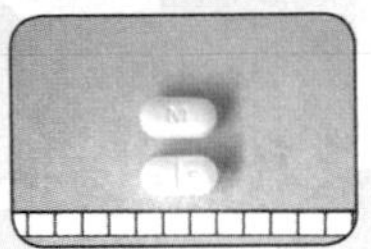
50 mcg

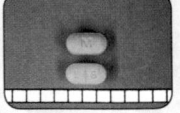

75 mcg

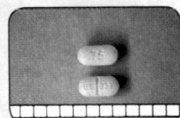

75 mcg

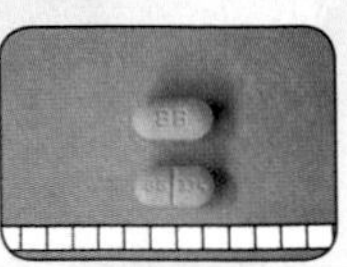
88 mcg

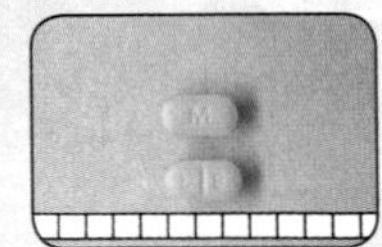
100 mcg

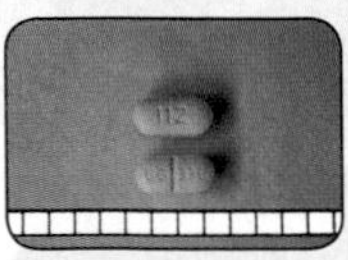
112 mcg

125 mcg

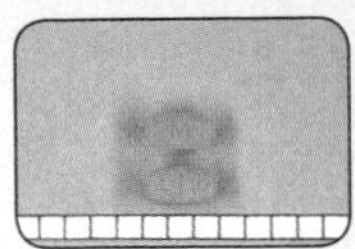
125 mcg

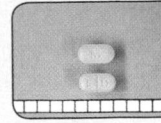

137 mcg

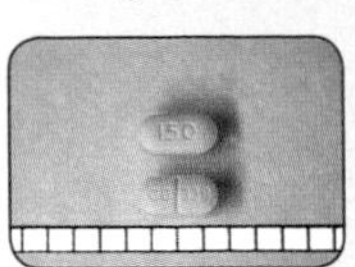
150 mcg

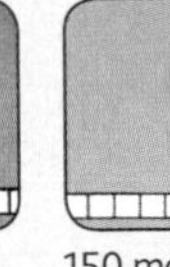

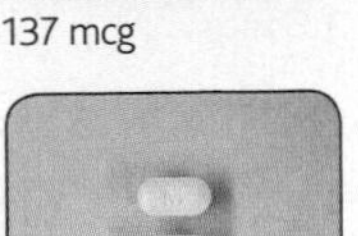
150 mcg

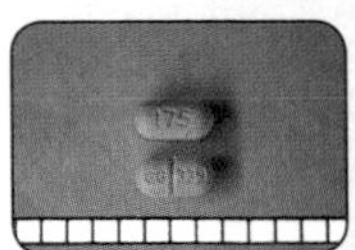
175 mcg

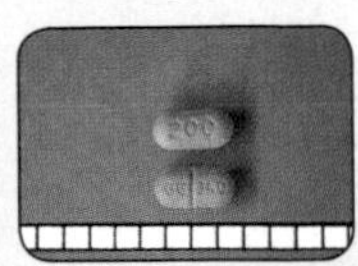
200 mcg

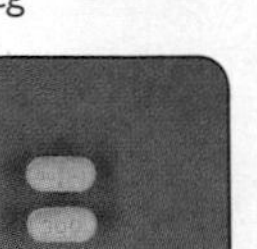
300 mcg

Synthroid®

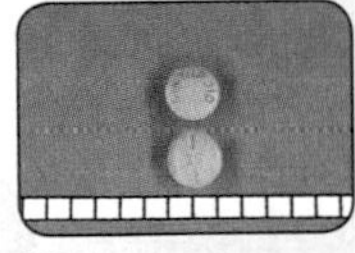
25 mcg

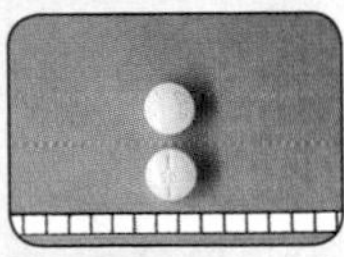
50 mcg

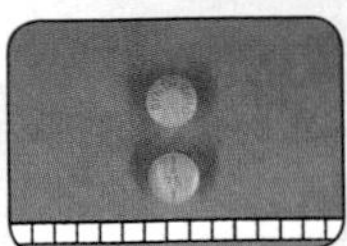
75 mcg

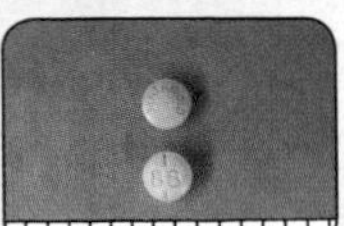
88 mcg

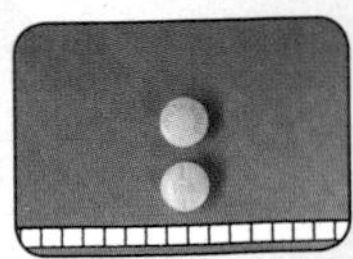
100 mcg

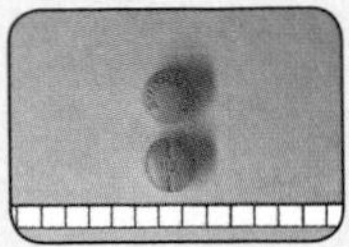
112 mcg

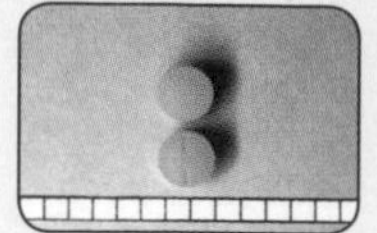
125 mcg

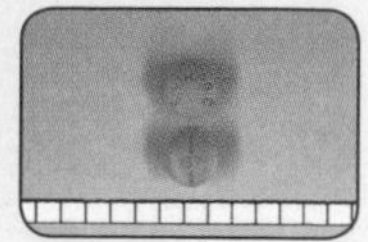
137 mcg

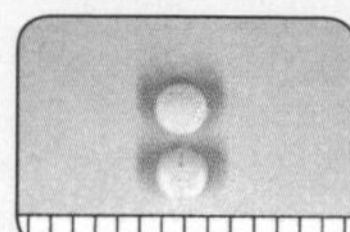
150 mcg

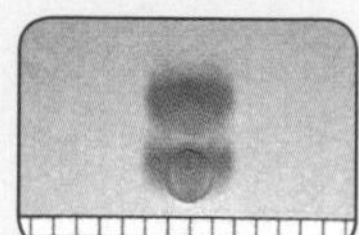
175 mcg

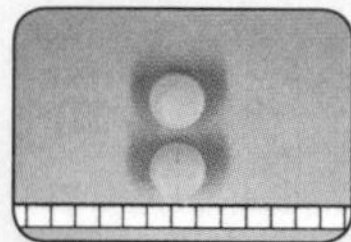
200 mcg

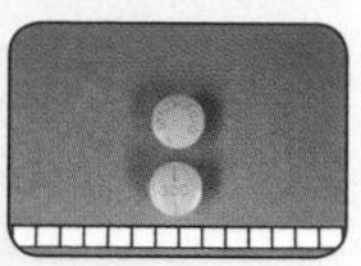
300 mcg

Lisdexamfetamine

Vyvanse®

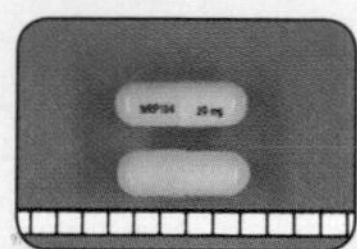
20 mg

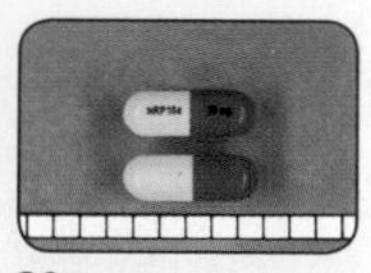
30 mg

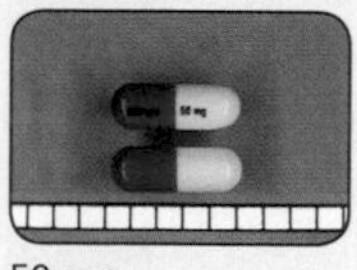
50 mg

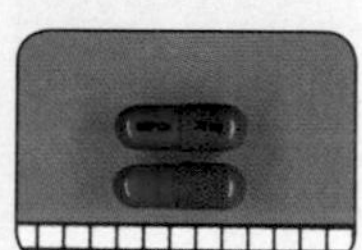
70 mg

Lisinopril

(generic)

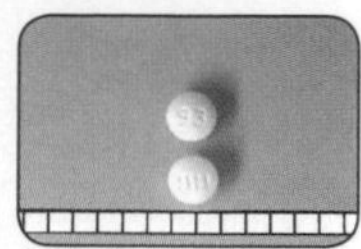
2.5 mg

Losartan

Cozaar®

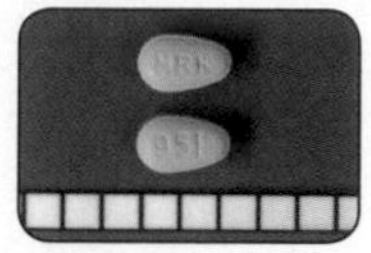

25 mg

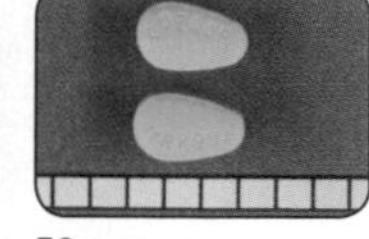
50 mg

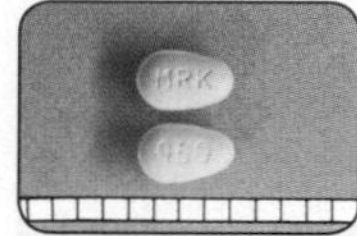

100 mg

Losartan and Hydrochlorothiazide

Hyzaar®

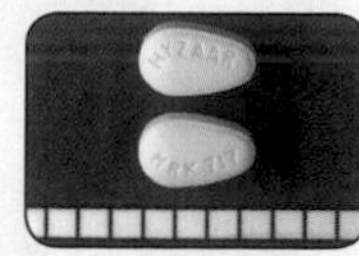
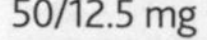
50/12.5 mg

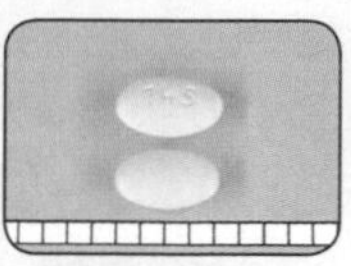
100/12.5 mg

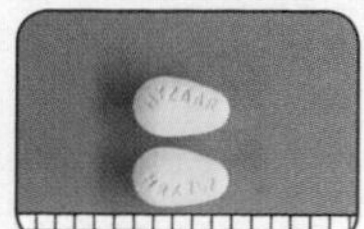
100/25 mg

Meclizine

(generic)

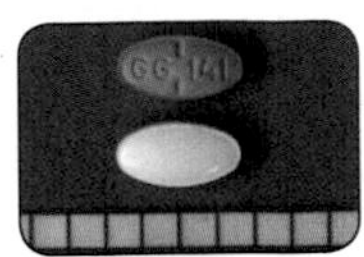
12.5 mg

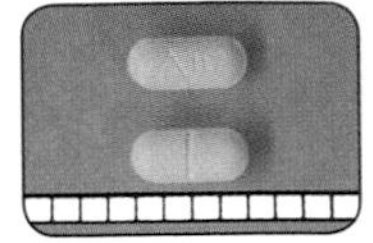
12.5 mg

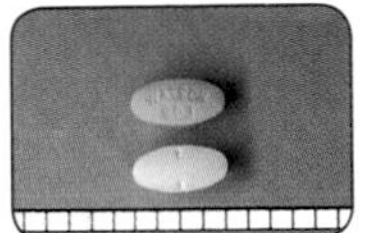
25 mg

Meloxicam

(generic)

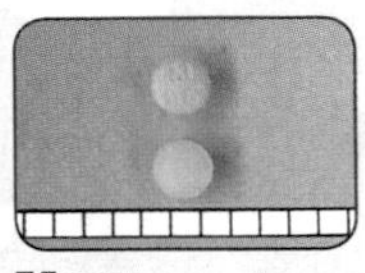
7.5 mg

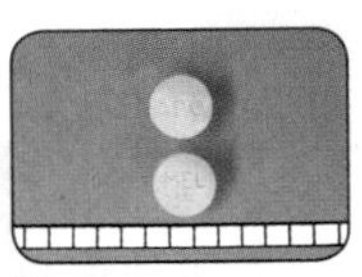
15 mg

Memantine

Namenda®

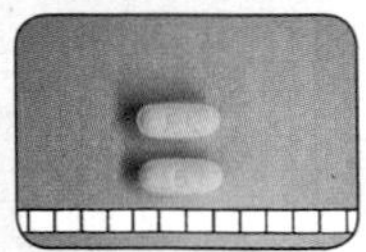
5 mg

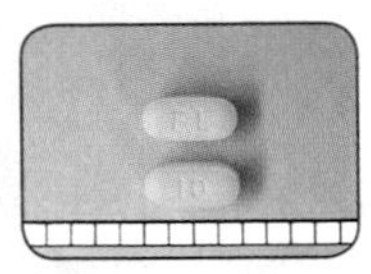
10 mg

Metformin

(generic)

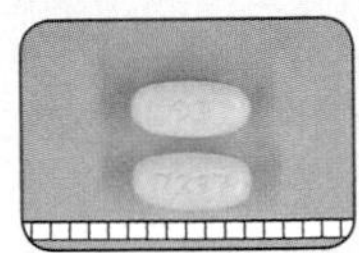
500 mg

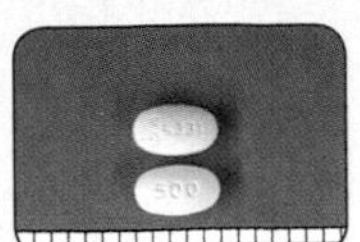
500 mg

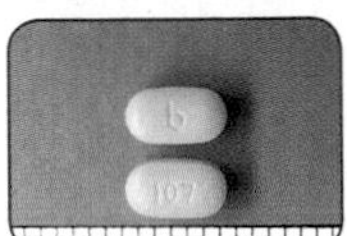
750 mg

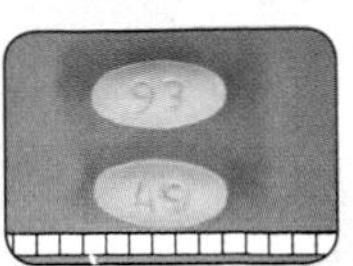
850 mg

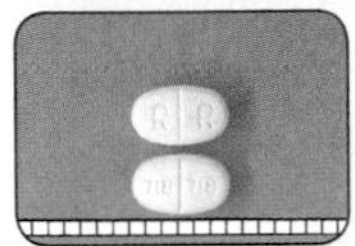
1000 mg

Methadone

(generic)

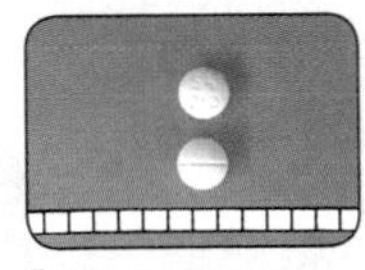
5 mg

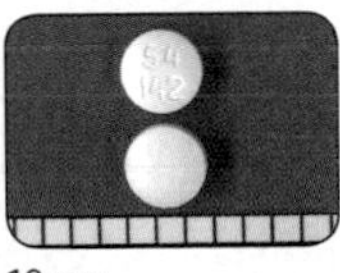
10 mg

Methocarbamol

(generic)

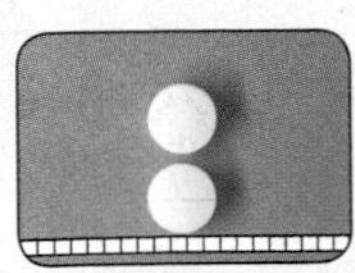
500 mg

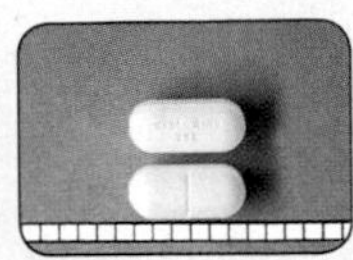
750 mg

Methotrexate

(generic)

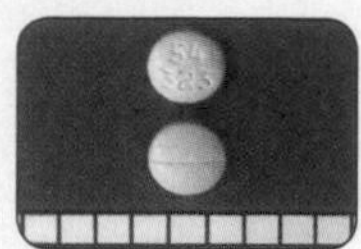

2.5 mg

Methylphenidate

Concerta®

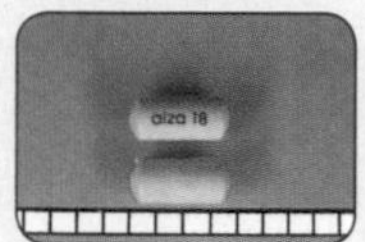

18 mg

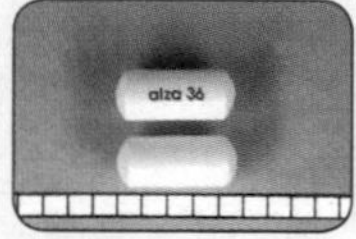

27 mg

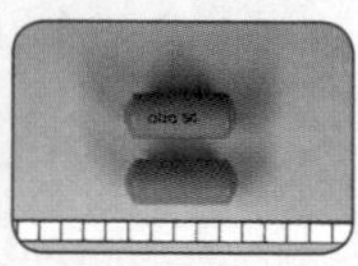

36 mg

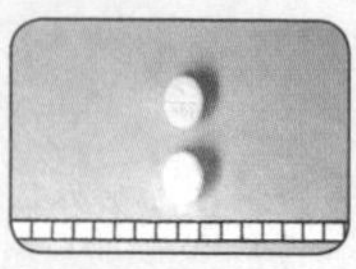

54 mg

Methylprednisolone

(generic)

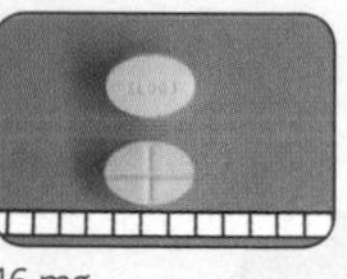

4 mg

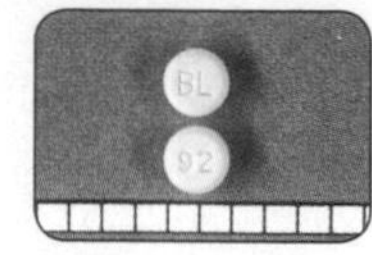

16 mg

Metoclopramide

(generic)

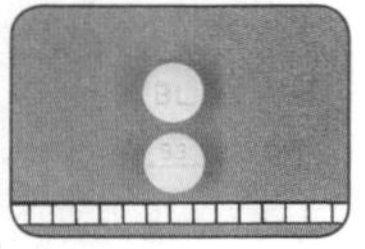

5 mg

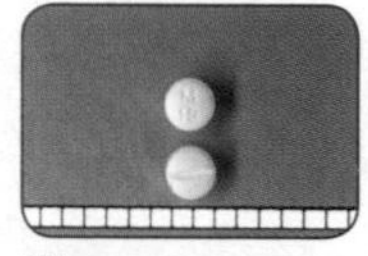

10 mg

Metoprolol

(generic)

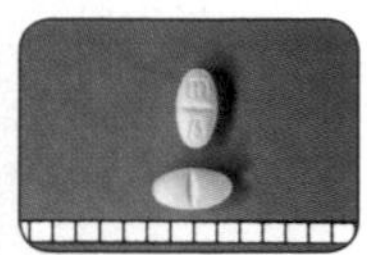

25 mg

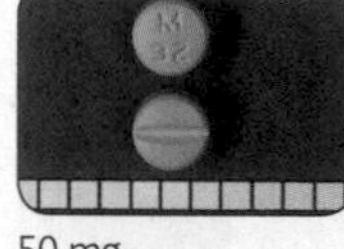

25 mg

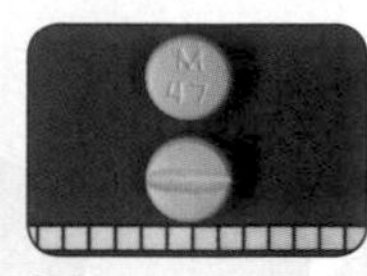

50 mg

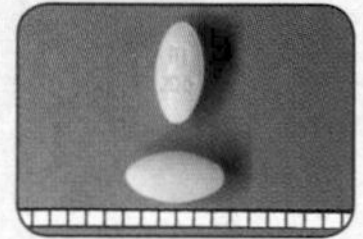

100 mg

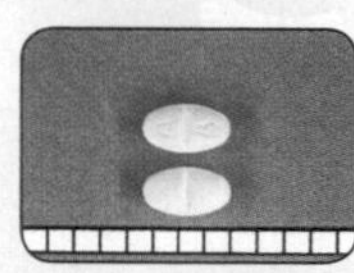

200 mg

Toprol-XL®

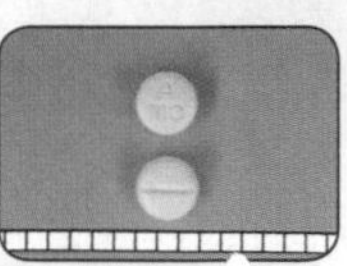

25 mg

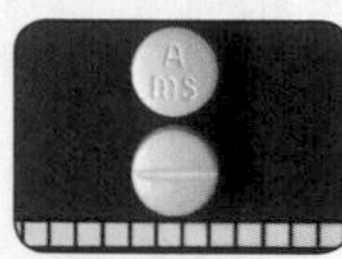

50 mg

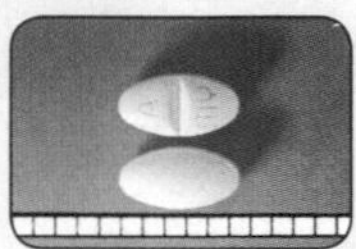

100 mg

200 mg

Metronidazole

(generic)

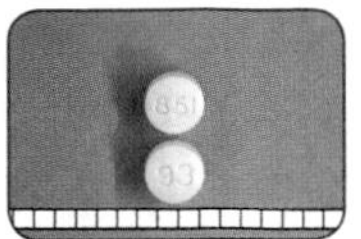
250 mg

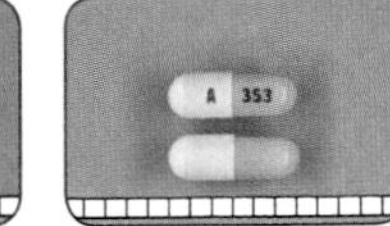

375 mg

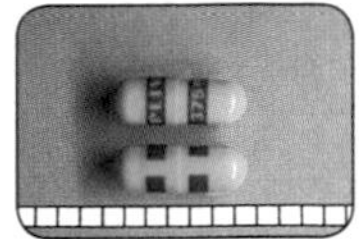
375 mg

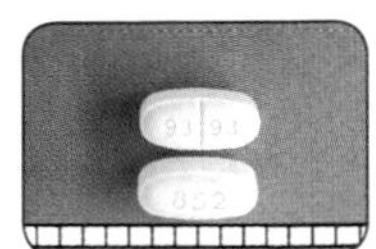
500 mg

Mirtazapine

(generic)

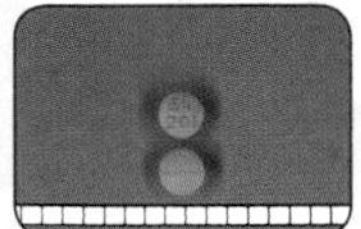
15 mg

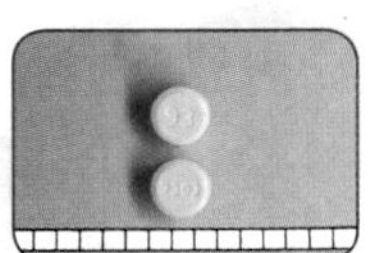
15 mg

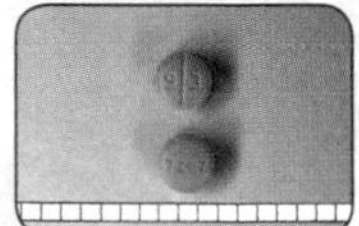
30 mg

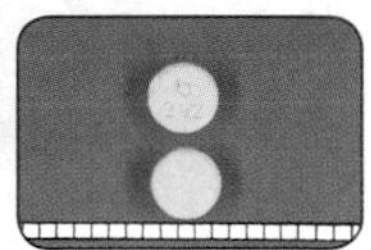
30 mg

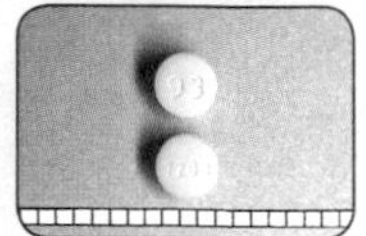
45 mg

Montelukast

Singulair®

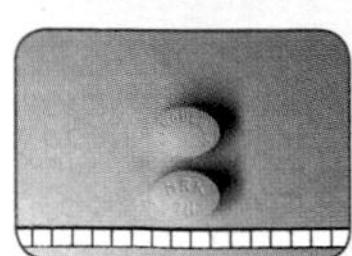
4 mg

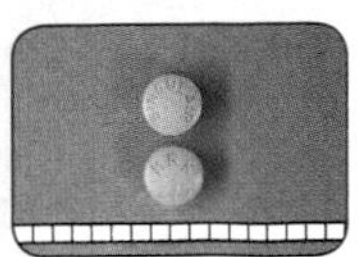
5 mg

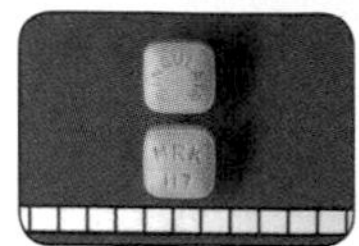
10 mg

Naproxen

(generic)

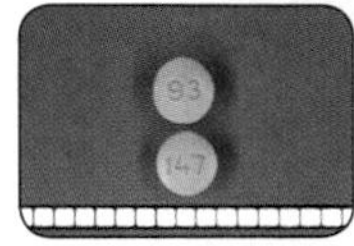
250 mg

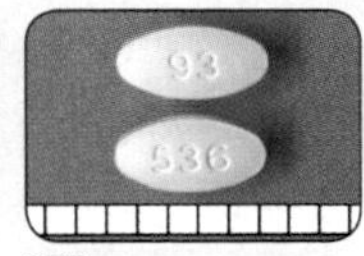

275 mg

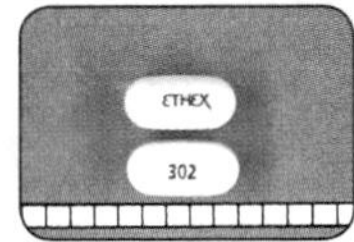

375 mg

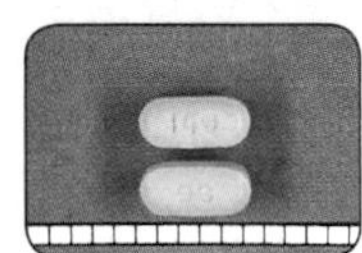
500 mg

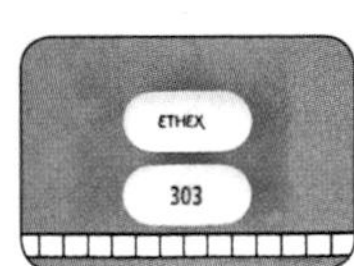

500 mg

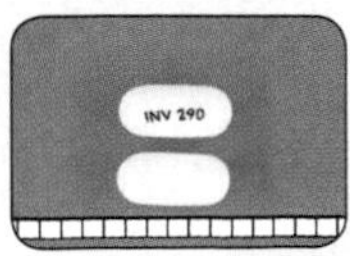

500 mg

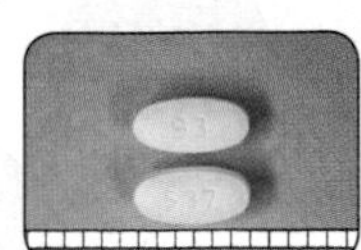
550 mg

Niacin

Niaspan®

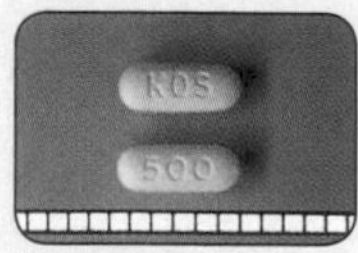

500 mg

750 mg

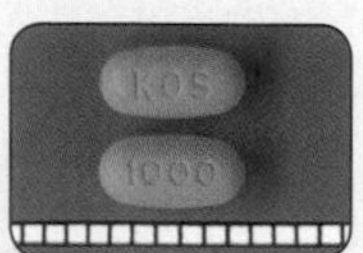

1000 mg

Nifedipine

(generic)

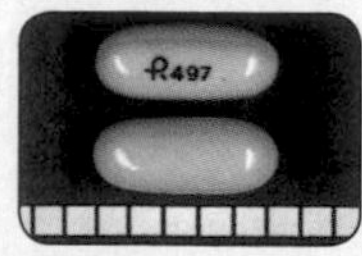

10 mg

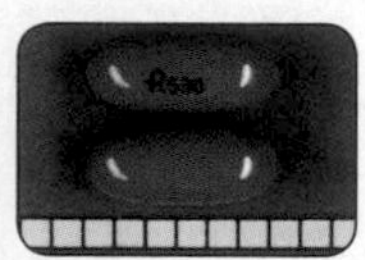
20 mg

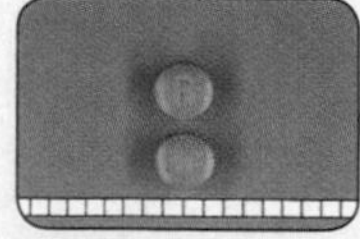
30 mg

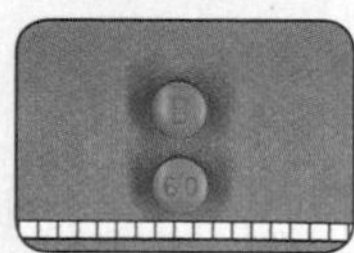
60 mg

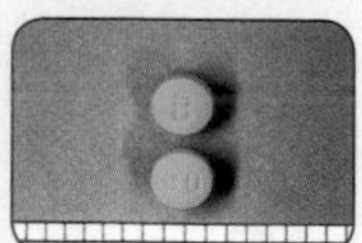
90 mg

Nitrofurantoin

(generic)

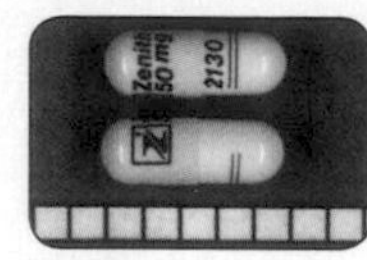

50 mg

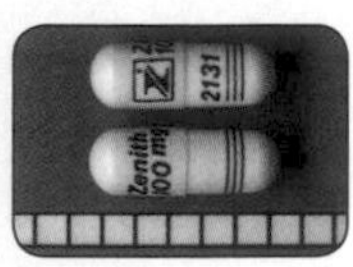

100 mg

Nitroglycerin

(generic)

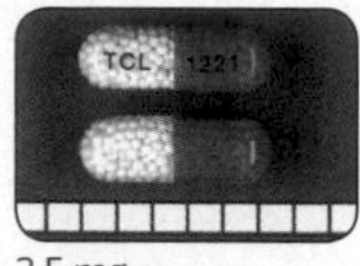

2.5 mg

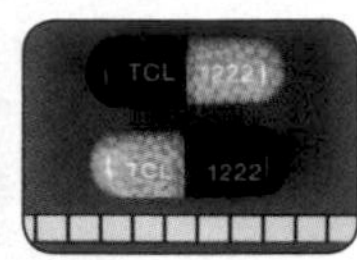

6.5 mg

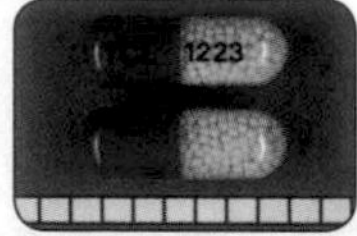

9 mg

Olmesartan

Benicar®

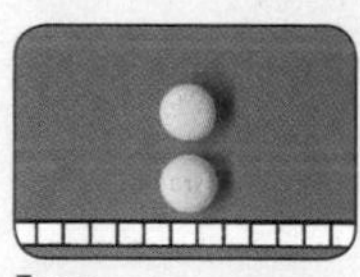
5 mg

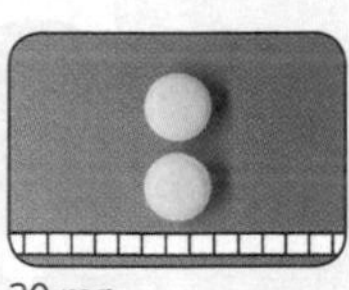
20 mg

40 mg

Olmesartan and Hydrochlorothiazide

Benicar HCT®

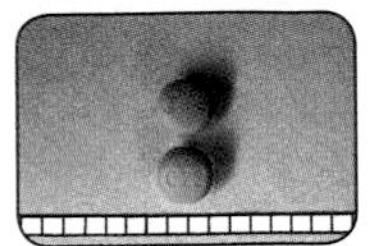
20/12.5 mg

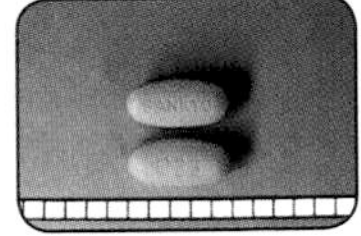
40/12.5 mg

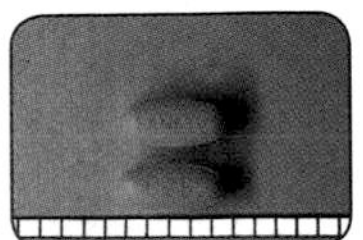
40/25 mg

Omega-3-Acid Ethyl Esters

Lovaza®

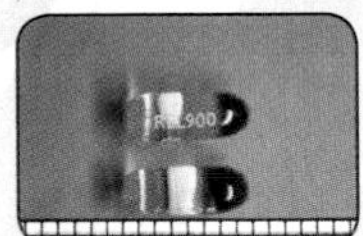
1 g

Omeprazole

(generic)

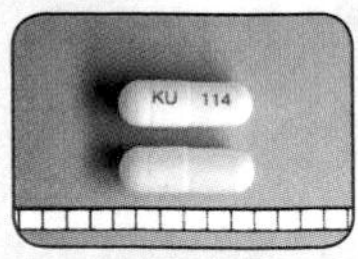

10 mg

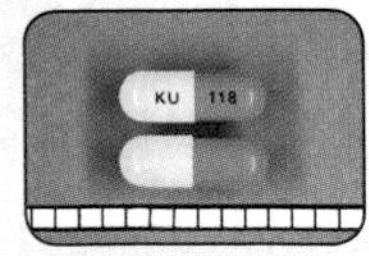

20 mg

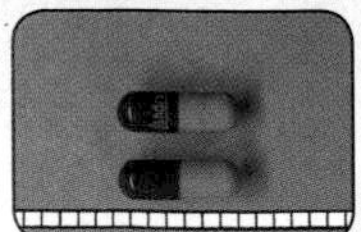
40 mg

Ondansetron

(generic)

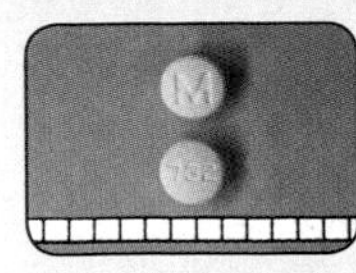
4 mg

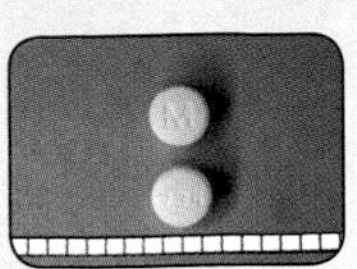
8 mg

8 mg

Oseltamivir

Tamiflu®

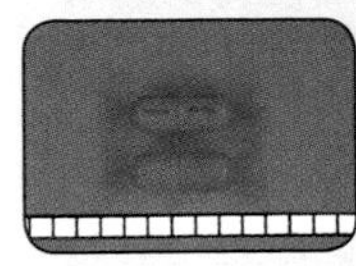
45 mg

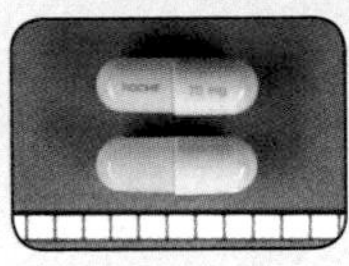
75 mg

Oxycodone

(generic)

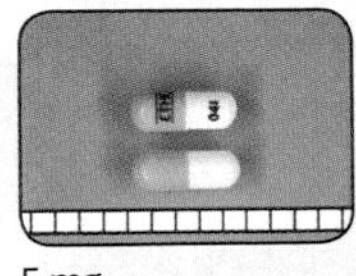
5 mg

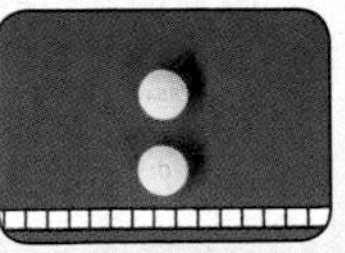
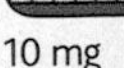
10 mg

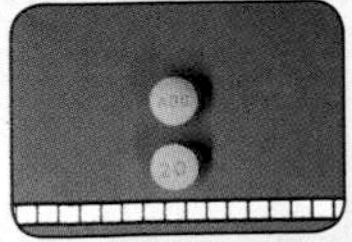
20 mg

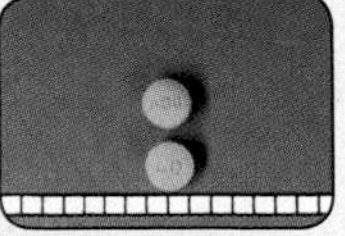
40 mg

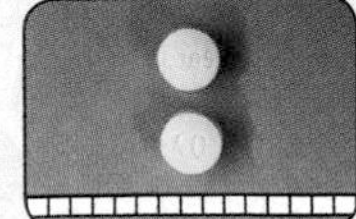
80 mg

OxyContin®

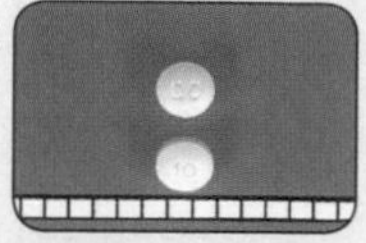
10 mg

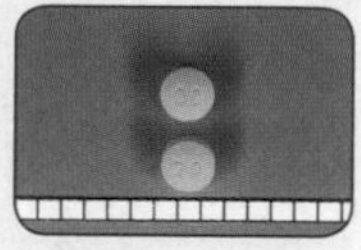
20 mg

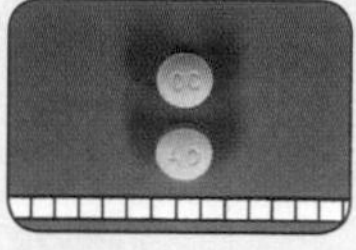
40 mg

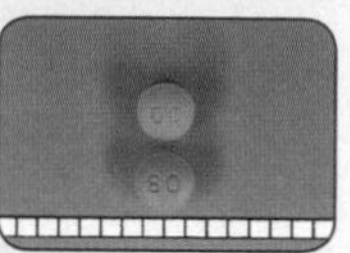
80 mg

Oxycodone and Acetaminophen

(generic)

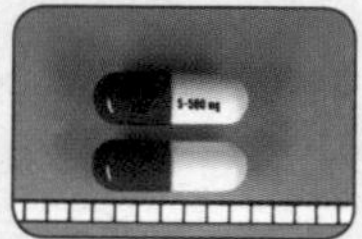
5/500 mg

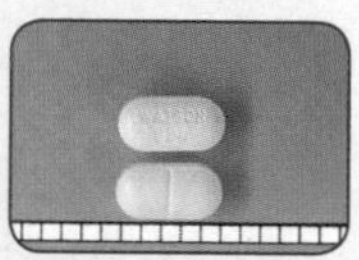
7.5/500 mg

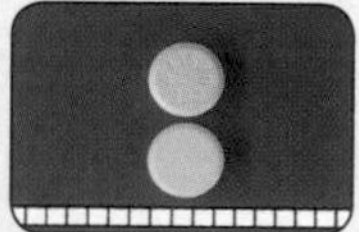
10/325 mg

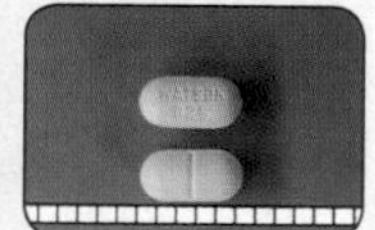
10/650 mg

Endocet®

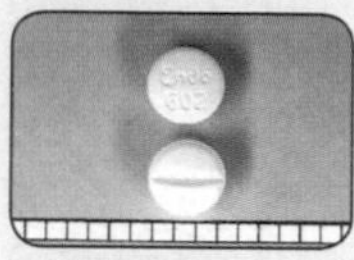
5/325 mg

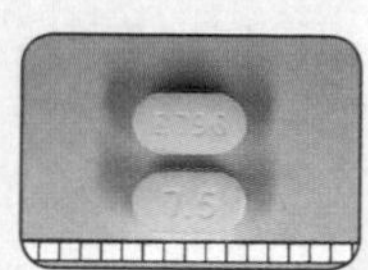
7.5/500 mg

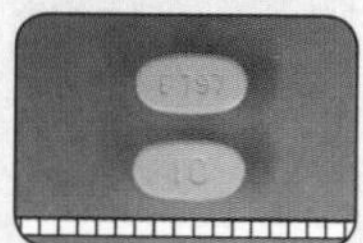
10/650 mg

Pantoprazole

(generic)

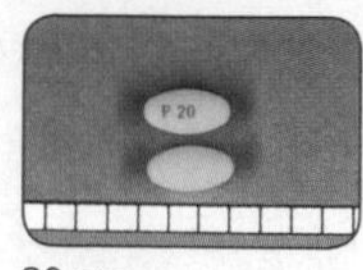
20 mg

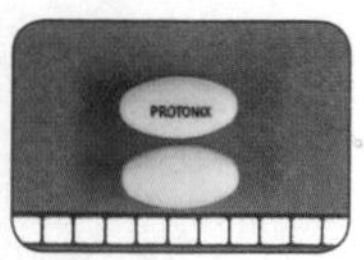
40 mg

Paroxetine

(generic)

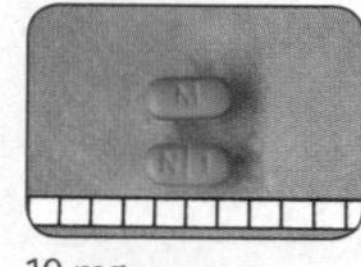
10 mg

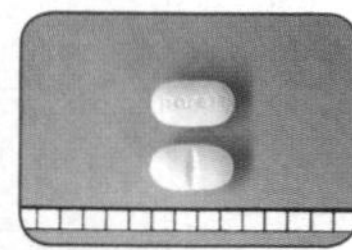
20 mg

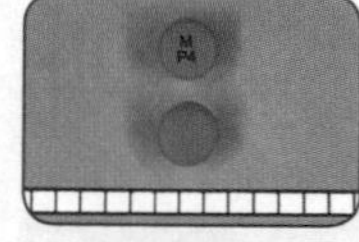
25 mg

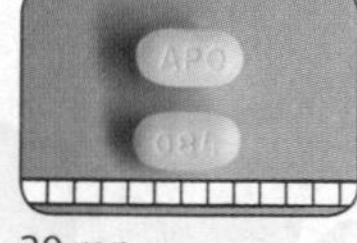
30 mg

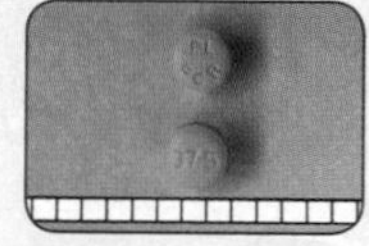
37.5 mg

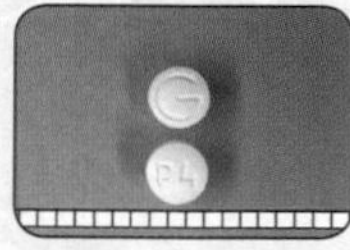
40 mg

Penicillin V Potassium

(generic)

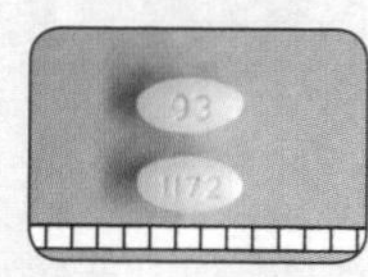
250 mg

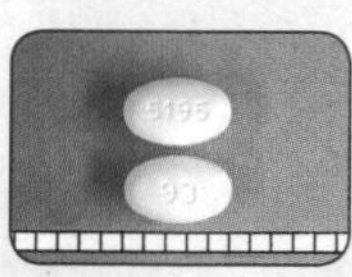
500 mg

Phentermin

(generic)

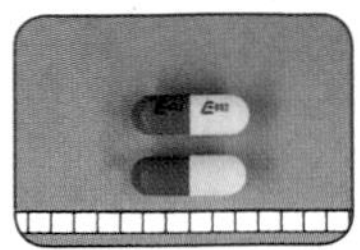
15 mg

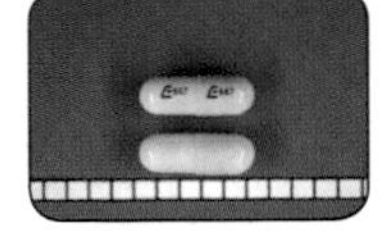
30 mg

Pioglitazone

Actos®

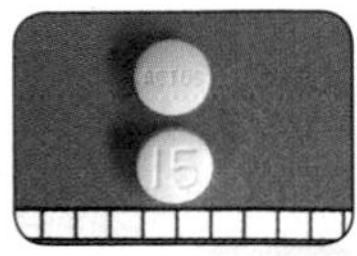

15 mg

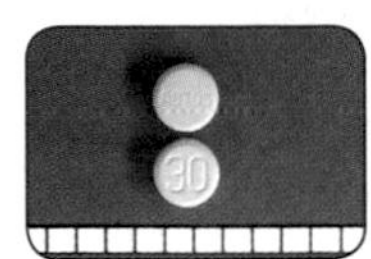

30 mg

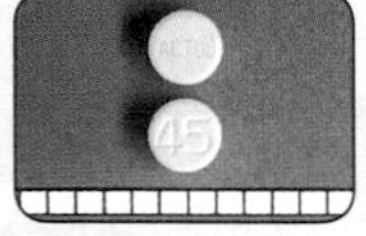

45 mg

Pravastatin

(generic)

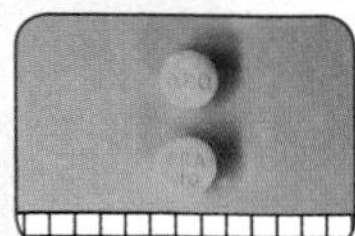
10 mg

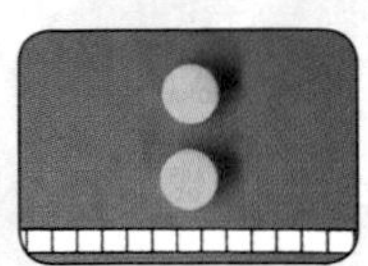
20 mg

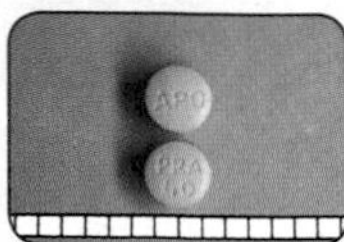
40 mg

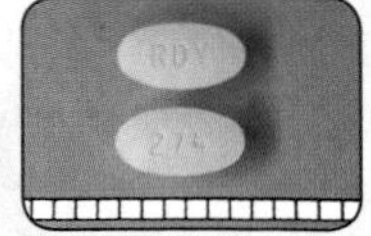

80 mg

Prednisone

(generic)

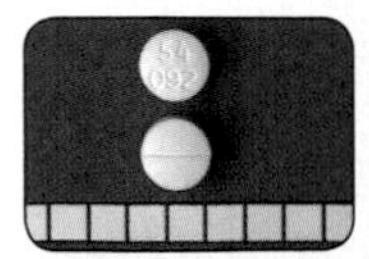
1 mg

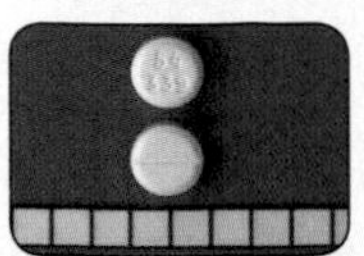
2.5 mg

5 mg

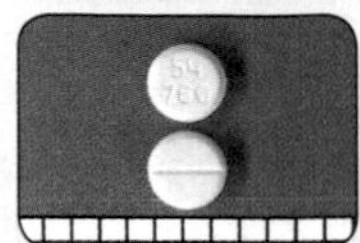
20 mg

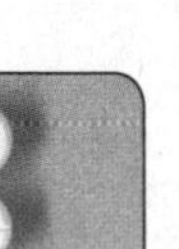
50 mg

Pregabalin

Lyrica®

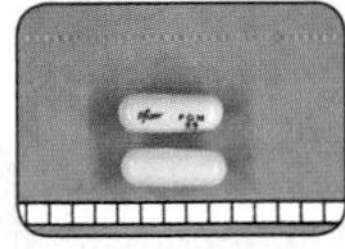
25 mg

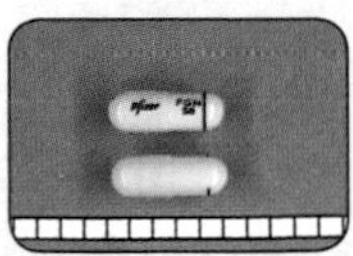
50 mg

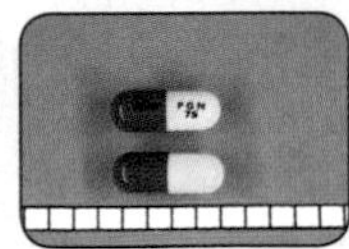
75 mg

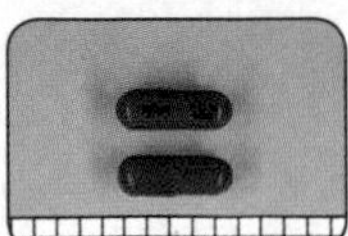
100 mg

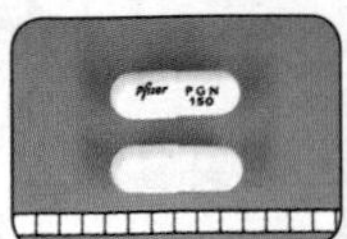

150 mg

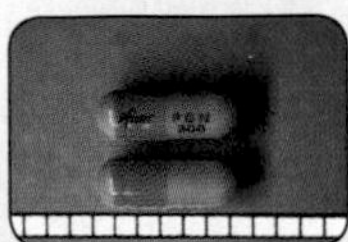
200 mg

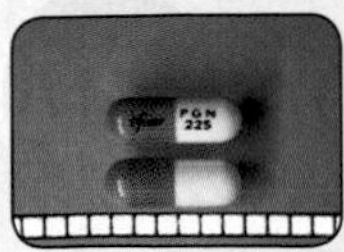

225 mg

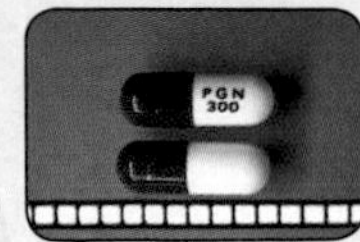

300 mg

Propoxyphene and Acetaminophen

(generic)

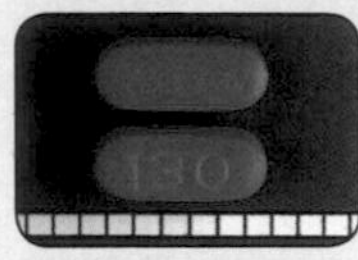

65/650 mg

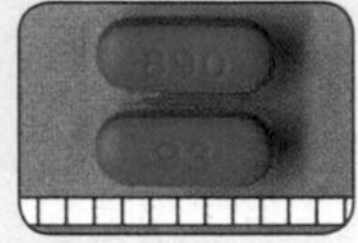

100/650 mg

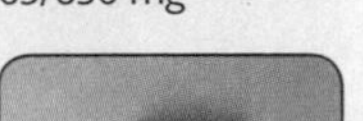
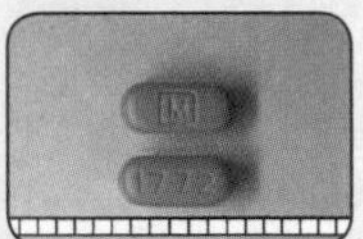

100/650 mg

Propranolol

(generic)

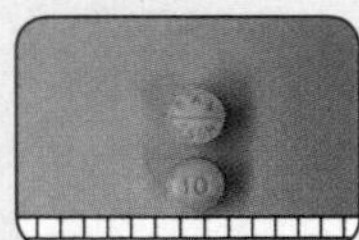

10 mg

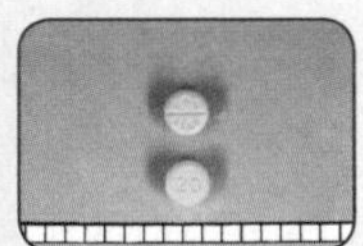

20 mg

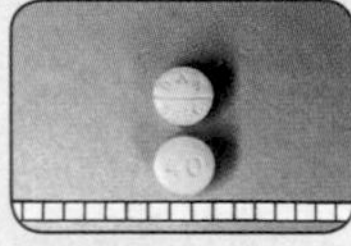

40 mg

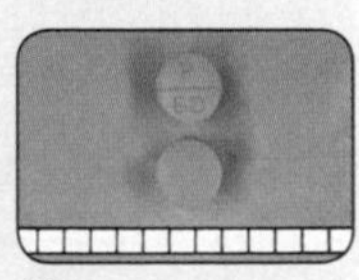

60 mg

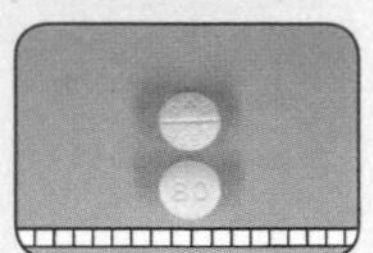

80 mg

Quetiapine

Seroquel®

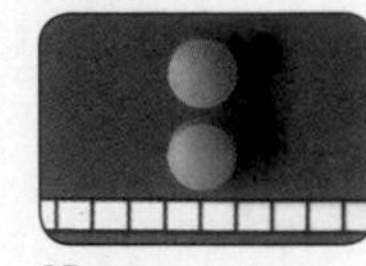

25 mg

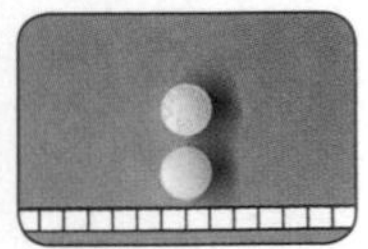

50 mg

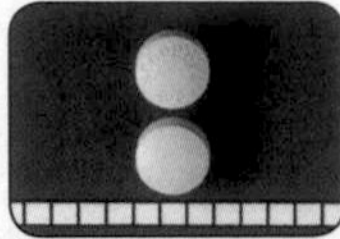

100 mg

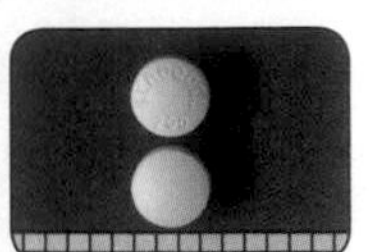

200 mg

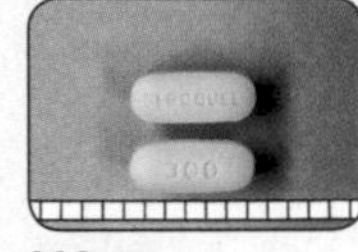

300 mg

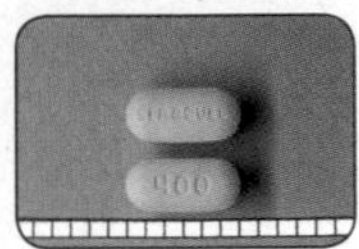

400 mg

Quinapril

(generic)

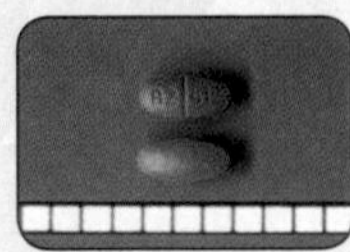

5 mg

Rabeprazole

AcipHex®

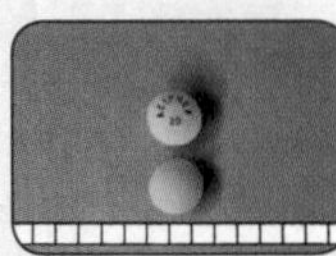

20 mg

Raloxifene

Evista®

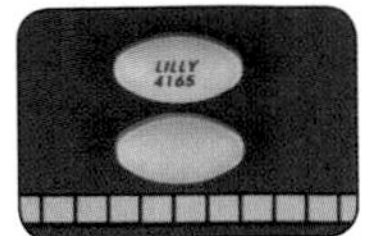

60 mg

Ramipril

(generic)

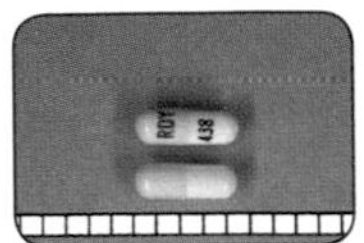

1.25 mg

2.5 mg

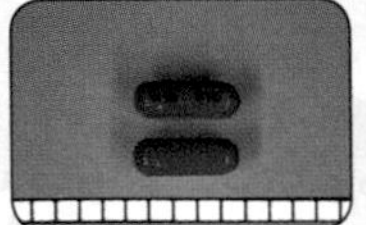

5 mg

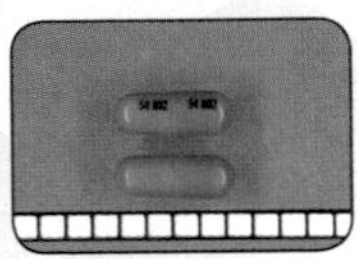

10 mg

Ranitidine

(generic)

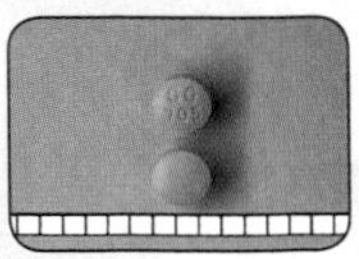

150 mg

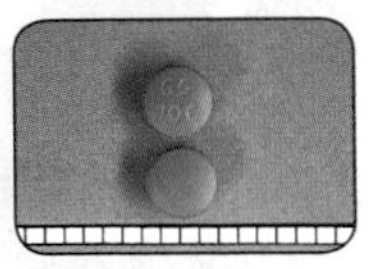

300 mg

Risedronate

Actonel®

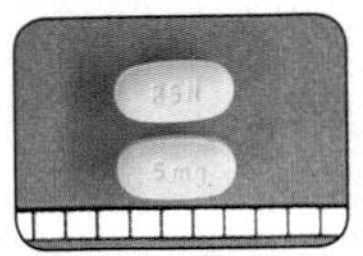

5 mg

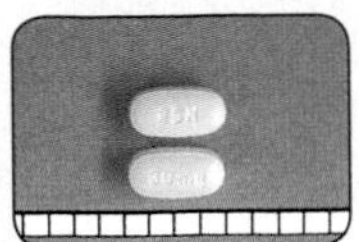

30 mg

35 mg

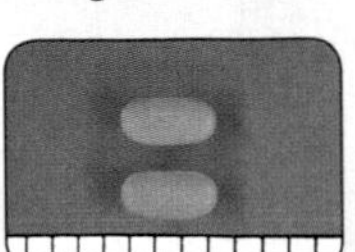

150 mg

Risperidone

(generic)

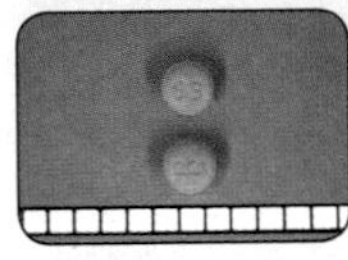

0.25 mg

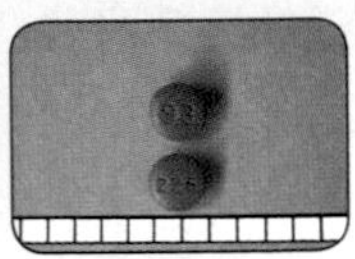

0.5 mg

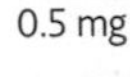

1 mg

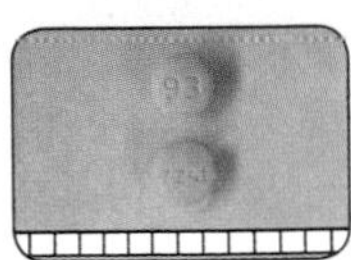

2 mg

4 mg

Rosuvastatin

Crestor®

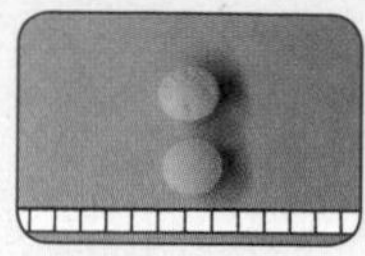

5 mg

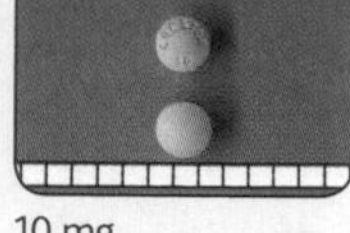

10 mg

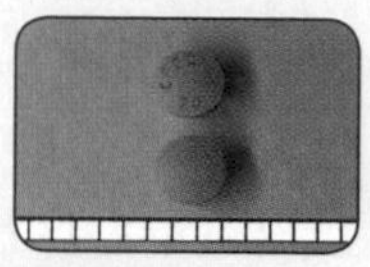

20 mg

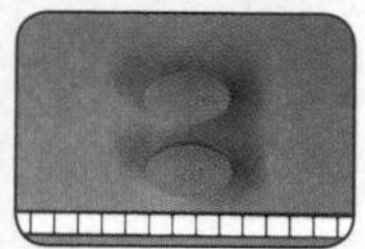

40 mg

Sertraline

(generic)

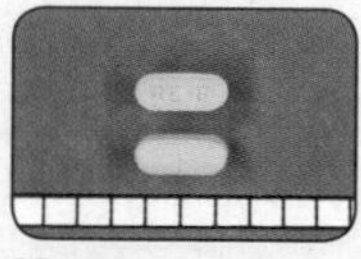

25 mg

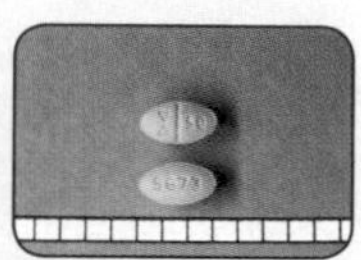

50 mg

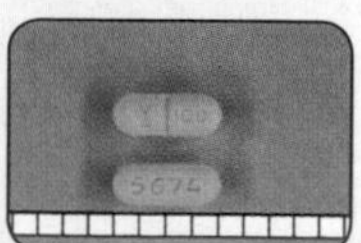

100 mg

Sildenafil

Viagra®

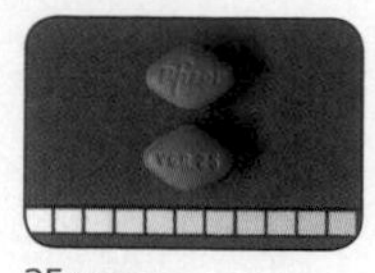

25 mg

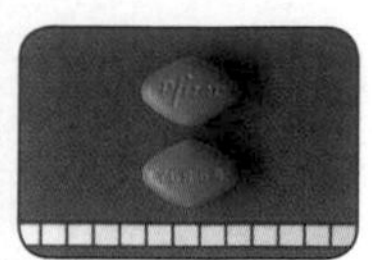

50 mg

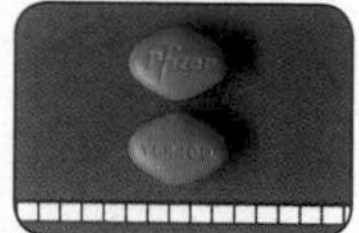

100 mg

Simvastin

(generic)

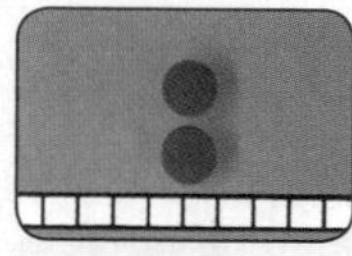

5 mg

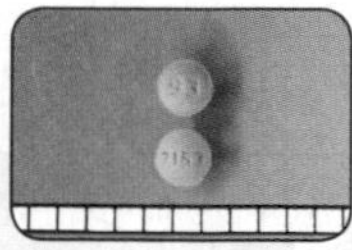

10 mg

40 mg

Spironolactone

(generic)

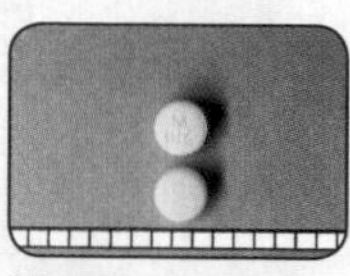

25 mg

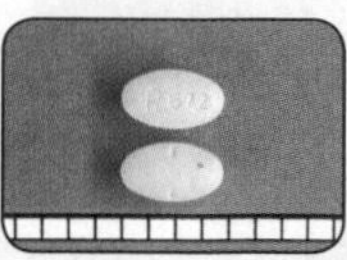

50 mg

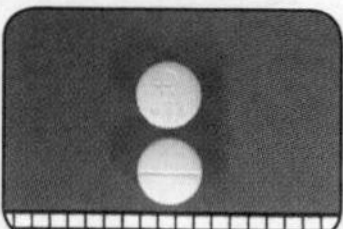

100 mg